Tumors of the Lymph Nodes and Spleen

AFIP Atlas
of
Tumor Pathology

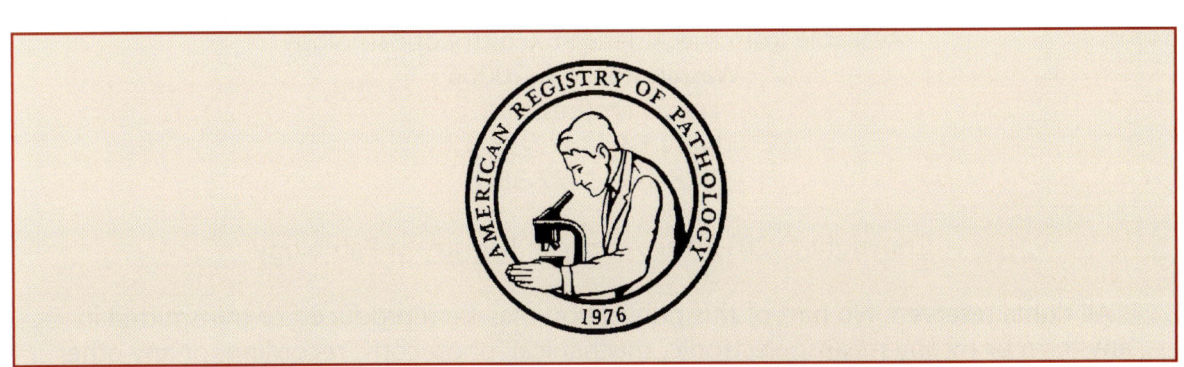

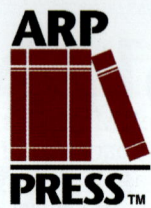

ARP PRESS

Washington, DC

Editorial Director: Mirlinda Q. Caton
Production Editor: Dian S. Thomas
Editorial Assistant: Magdalena C. Silva
Editorial Assistant: Alana N. Black
Copyeditor: Audrey Kahn

Available from the American Registry of Pathology
Washington, DC 20006
www.arppress.org
ISBN 1-933477-38-5
978-1-933477-38-1

AFIP ATLAS OF TUMOR PATHOLOGY

Fourth Series
Fascicle 25

TUMORS OF THE
LYMPH NODES AND SPLEEN

by

L. Jeffrey Medeiros, MD
Professor and Chair, Department of Hematopathology
The University of Texas MD Anderson Cancer Center
Houston, Texas

Dennis P. O'Malley, MD
Pathologist, Neogenomics, Aliso Viejo, California
Adjunct Associate Professor, Department of Hematopathology
The University of Texas MD Anderson Cancer Center
Houston, Texas

Nancy P. Caraway, MD
Professor, Department of Anatomic Pathology
The University of Texas MD Anderson Cancer Center
Houston, Texas

Francisco Vega, MD, PhD
Professor of Pathology, Department of Pathology and Laboratory Medicine
University of Miami/Sylvester Comprehensive Cancer Center
Miami, Florida

Kojo S. J. Elenitoba-Johnson, MD
Peter C. Nowell, MD, Endowed Chair
Professor, Department of Pathology and Laboratory Medicine
Perelman School of Medicine, University of Pennsylvania
Founding Director, PENN Center for Personalized Diagnostics
Founding Director, Division of Precision and Computational Diagnostics
Philadelphia, Pennsylvania

Megan S. Lim, MD, PhD
Professor and Director, Division of Hematopathology
Department of Pathology and Laboratory Medicine
Perelman School of Medicine, University of Pennsylvania
Philadelphia, Pennsylvania

Published by the
American Registry of Pathology
Washington, DC
2017

AFIP ATLAS OF TUMOR PATHOLOGY

EDITORS' NOTE

The Atlas of Tumor Pathology has a long and distinguished history. It was first conceived at a cancer research meeting held in St. Louis in September 1947, as an attempt to standardize the nomenclature of neoplastic diseases. The first series was sponsored by the National Academy of Sciences-National Research Council. The organization of this formidable effort was entrusted to the Subcommittee on Oncology of the Committee on Pathology, and Dr. Arthur Purdy Stout was the first editor-in-chief. Many of the illustrations were provided by the Medical Illustration Service of the Armed Forces Institute of Pathology (AFIP), the type was set by the Government Printing Office, and the final printing was done at the Armed Forces Institute of Pathology. The American Registry of Pathology (ARP) purchased the Fascicles from the Government Printing Office and sold them virtually at cost. Over a period of 20 years, approximately 15,000 copies each of nearly 40 Fascicles were produced. The worldwide impact of these publications over the years has largely surpassed the original goal. They quickly became among the most influential publications on tumor pathology, primarily because of their overall high quality, but also because their low cost made them easily accessible the world over to pathologists and other students of oncology.

Upon completion of the first series, the National Academy of Sciences-National Research Council handed further pursuit of the project over to the newly created Universities Associated for Research and Education in Pathology (UAREP). A second series was started, generously supported by grants from the AFIP, the National Cancer Institute, and the American Cancer Society. Dr. Harlan I. Firminger became the editor-in-chief and was succeeded by Dr. William H. Hartmann. The second series' Fascicles were produced as bound volumes instead of loose leaflets. They featured a more comprehensive coverage of the subjects, to the extent that the Fascicles could no longer be regarded as "atlases" but rather as monographs describing and illustrating in detail the tumors and tumor-like conditions of the various organs and systems.

Once the second series was completed, with a success that matched that of the first, ARP, UAREP, and AFIP decided to embark on a third series. Dr. Juan Rosai was appointed as editor-in-chief, and Dr. Leslie Sobin became associate editor. A distinguished Editorial Advisory Board was also convened, and these outstanding pathologists and educators played a major role in the success of this series, the first publication of which appeared in 1991 and the last (number 32) in 2003.

The same organizational framework applies to the current fourth series, but with UAREP and AFIP no longer functioning, ARP is now the responsible organization. New features include a hardbound cover and illustrations almost exclusively in color. There is also an increased emphasis on the cytopathologic (intraoperative, exfoliative, or fine needle aspiration) and molecular features that are important in diagnosis and prognosis. What does not change from the three previous series, however, is the goal of providing the practicing pathologist with thorough, concise, and up-to-date information on the nomenclature and classification; epidemiologic, clinical, and pathogenetic features; and, most importantly, guidance in the diagnosis of the tumors and tumorlike lesions of all major organ systems and body sites.

As in the third series, a continuous attempt is made to correlate, whenever possible, the nomenclature used in the Fascicles with that proposed by the World Health Organization's Classification of Tumors, as well as to ensure a consistency of style. Close cooperation between the various authors and their respective liaisons from the Editorial Board will continue to be emphasized in order to minimize unnecessary repetition and discrepancies in the text and illustrations.

Particular thanks are due to the members of the Editorial Advisory Board, the reviewers, the editorial and production staff, and the individual Fascicle authors for their ongoing efforts to ensure that this series is a worthy successor to the previous three.

Steven G. Silverberg, MD

Ronald A. DeLellis, MD

Leslie H. Sobin, MD

ACKNOWLEDGMENTS

I am very grateful to the coauthors of this Fascicle. Their knowledge, effort, patience, and good humor were essential to the completion of this work.

I thank my colleagues at MD Anderson Cancer Center in Houston and at other hospitals, who generously contributed schematic and microscopic images. I particularly thank Drs. Sanam Loghavi, Chi Young Ok, Mariko Yabe, and H. Deniz Gur, who as fellows at MD Anderson Cancer Center, critically read chapters and made helpful suggestions.

My coauthors and I thank Dr. Steven Silverberg for asking us to take on this project and Drs. Nadine Aguilera, Addam Bagg, William Frable, and Ronald DeLellis for reviewing the volume. Their comments were invaluable. We also thank Mirlinda Caton and her colleagues, Dian Thomas and Magdalena Silva, at the American Registry of Pathology for their efforts to bring this book to fruition.

All pathologists have training experiences that were instrumental in helping them become successful pathologists. My lucky break came when I was accepted into the surgical pathology fellowship program at Stanford University Medical Center, co-directed by Drs. Ronald F. Dorfman and Richard L. Kempson. I was also fortunate that Dr. Roger A. Warnke gave me the opportunity to stay at Stanford a second year working in his laboratory. I am very grateful. My two years at Stanford gave me the privilege to watch outstanding academic surgical pathologists do the job, and they opened my eyes to what was possible in my own future.

Lastly, I dedicate this fascicle to my wife Carrie and our two daughters Christina and Caroline, who were very supportive of this effort.

L. Jeffrey Medeiros, MD

Permission to use copyrighted illustrations has been granted by:

College of American Pathologists
Arch Pathol Lab Med 2014;138:1211-1212. For figures 49-14 and 49-15.

Elsevier
Cancer Epidemiol 2009;33:345. For figure 8-5.
Human Pathol 2010;41:461-476. For figures 50-8 and 50-9.
J Invest Dermatol 1961;37:51-64. For figure 55-8.
Lancet 1964;283:702. For figure 9-2, top.

IARC Press
GLOBOCAN 2008 Cancer Incidence and Mortality Worldwide: IARC CancerBase No. 10.
  Lyon: IARC. For figure 8-6.

LWW/Wolters Kluwer
Am J Surg Pathol 2003;27:1351. For figure 42-8.

Medicina Oral
Med Oral Patol Cir Bucal 201;19:e32. For figure 25-1.

Nature
Mod Pathol 2013;26(Suppl 1):S112. For tables 7-1 and 7-2.

Sage
Toxicol Pathol 2006;34:411. For figure 1-2.

CONTENTS

1. Normal Anatomy and Function of Lymph Nodes and Spleen 1
   Lymph Node 1
      Gross Anatomy 1
      Microscopic Anatomy 1
      Lymph Node Cortex 2
      Cellular Elements of Germinal Centers 4
      Germinal Center-Associated Events 7
      Lymph Node Paracortex 8
      Lymph Node Medulla 11
      Lymph Node Sinuses 11
   Spleen 12
      Gross Anatomy 12
      Microscopic Anatomy 12

2. Processing Lymph Node and Spleen Specimens 17
   Excisional Biopsy Versus Needle Biopsy 17
   Gross Evaluation 17
   Fixation and Routine Histologic Stains 18
   Immunophenotypic Analysis 18
      Immunohistochemistry 19
      Flow Cytometry 22
   Cytogenetic and Molecular Analysis 25
   Common Techniques in Diagnostic Cytogenetics 25
      Conventional Karyotyping 26
      Fluorescence in Situ Hybridization 26
   Types of Cytogenetic Abnormalities in Lymphomas 28
      MYC Translocations: t(8;14)(q24;q32), t(2;8)(p11;q24), and t(8;22)q24;q11) . . . 28
      BCL2 Translocation: t(14;18)(132;q21) 29
      BCL6 Translocations: t(3;var)(q27;var) 29
      CCND1 Translocation: t(11;14)(q13;q32) 30
      NPM-ALK: t(2;5)(p23;q35) 30
      API2-MALT1; t(11;18)(q21;q21) and Other MALT Lymphoma Translocations . . . 31
   Common Techniques Used in Molecular Diagnostics 31
      Southern Blot Hybridization 31
      Polymerase Chain Reaction 31
      Quantitative and Real-Time PCR 32
      In Situ Hybridization 32

Common Applications of Molecular Testing in Lymphomas 33
   Detection of Clonality in Lymphoid Lesions 33
   Lineage Infidelity 34
   Detection of Clonality in Nonlymphoid Cells 35
High-Throughput Techniques Used in Molecular Diagnostics 35
   Comparative Genomic Hybridization 35
   Single Nucleotide Polymorphism Arrays 36
   Gene Expression Profiling 36
   MicroRNA Analysis 36
   Proteomics 36
   Mutational Analysis 38
Reporting Pathology Results: the Integrated Report 38

3. Needle Core Biopsy and Fine-Needle Aspiration for the Diagnosis of Lymphopro-
     liferative Disorders 43
Needle Core Biopsy 43
   Diagnostic Approach Emphasizing Limitations 44
Fine-Needle Aspiration Biopsy 47
   Fine-Needle Aspiration Technique 49
   Diagnostic Approach Emphasizing Limitations 52
Role of Immunophenotypic Analysis 58
Role of Cytogenetic and Molecular Analysis 60

4. Classification of Lymphomas 65
Historical Background 65
   Hodgkin Lymphomas 65
   Non-Hodgkin Lymphomas 67
Current Lymphoma Classification Scheme 71
Composite Lymphoma 75
Discordant Histology 76

5. Histologic Transformation 79
Histologic Transformation of Follicular Lymphoma 79
   Frequency 79
   Clinical Features 80
   Pathologic Findings 80
   Molecular Genetic Findings 80
   Prognosis 84
Histologic Transformation of Other Types of Low-Grade Lymphoma 84
   Chronic Lymphocytic Leukemia/Small Lymphocytic Lymphoma 85
   Waldenstrom Macroglobulinemia 89
   Marginal Zone Lymphoma 89
   Mycosis Fungoides 91

Nodular Lymphocyte-Predominant Hodgkin Lymphoma 91

Low-Grade Lymphoma Following High-Grade Lymphoma. 92

6. In Situ Neoplasia/Early Lesions 97

In Situ Follicular Neoplasia 98

In Situ Mantle Cell Neoplasia 101

Nodular Lymphocyte-Predominant Hodgkin Lymphoma in Situ 102

Monoclonal B-Cell Lymphocytosis. 103

CLL-Like MBL 104

MBL with Atypical CLL-Like Immunophenotype 106

MBL with a Mantle Cell Lymphoma-Like Immunophenotype. 106

MBL with a Non-CLL Immunophenotype. 107

7. Clinical Workup, Stage, and Prognostic Factors of Lymphoma 109

Clinical Workup 109

Stage. 110

Hodgkin Lymphomas. 110

Non-Hodgkin Lymphomas 111

Prognostic Factors 112

Prognostic Scoring Systems for Lymphoma Patients. 112

Prognostic Biomarkers 114

Non-Hodgkin Lymphomas Divided into Prognostic Groups 115

Grading 116

8. Epidemiology of Hodgkin and Non-Hodgkin Lymphomas 119

Overall Statistics 119

Relative Frequency of Lymphomas. 119

Age 120

Sex and Race 123

Geographic Variation 123

Risk Factors for Hodgkin Lymphomas 125

Risk Factors for Non-Hodgkin Lymphomas 125

9. Infectious Organisms and Lymphomas. 129

Organisms with Direct Oncogenic Effects 130

Epstein-Barr Virus. 130

EBV-Associated Lymphomas 132

Human Herpesvirus 8. 137

Human Herpesvirus-8-Associated Lymphomas 138

Human T-Cell Lymphotropic Virus Type 1 140

Indirect Oncogenic Effects 141

Bacteria 141

Hepatitis C-Associated Lymphomas. 143

Human Immunodeficiency Virus 145

10. B-Lymphoblastic Leukemia/Lymphoma 149
     General Features 149
     Clinical Features 151
     Histologic Findings 151
     Cytologic Findings 153
     Immunophenotypic Findings. 153
     Molecular Genetic Findings 159
         BCL-ABL1-Like or Philadelphia Chromosome-Like B-ALL 161
         B-ALL with Functional Pre-B-Cell Receptor Signaling. 162
     Differential Diagnosis 162
     Treatment and Prognosis 163
11. Chronic Lymphocytic Leukemia/Small Lymphocytic Lymphoma. 167
     General Features 167
     Clinical Features 167
     Histologic Findings 168
         Lymph Nodes 168
         Peripheral Blood. 169
         Bone Marrow 171
         Other Sites 171
     Cytologic Findings 172
     Immunophenotypic Findings. 172
     Molecular Genetic Findings 174
     Transformation 177
     Differential Diagnosis 178
     Treatment and Prognosis 179
12. Mantle Cell Lymphoma. 183
     General Features 183
     Clinical Features 183
     Histologic Findings 184
         Lymph Nodes 184
         Indolent Variants of MCL 187
         Histologically Aggressive Variants of MCL 188
         MCL Associated with Other Lymphoma Types (Composite Lymphoma) 189
         Gastrointestinal Tract. 191
         Bone Marrow and Peripheral Blood. 191
         Spleen and Liver. 191
     Cytologic Findings 191
     Immunophenotypic Findings. 195
     Molecular Genetic Findings 197
         Cyclin D1-Negative MCL 200

Differential Diagnosis 200

Treatment and Prognosis 201

13. Follicular Lymphoma. 205

    General Features 205

        Role of t(14;18)(q32;q21)/*IGH-BCL2* in Pathogenesis 205

    Clinical Features 206

    Histologic Findings 206

        Lymph Nodes 206

        Grading. 210

        Morphologic Variants of Follicular Lymphoma. 214

        Liver and Spleen 217

        Bone Marrow 217

        Peripheral Blood 217

    Specific Types of Follicular Lymphoma 218

        CD5-Positive Follicular Lymphoma. 218

        Duodenal-Type Follicular Lymphoma 218

        Follicular Lymphoma in Children 221

        Follicular Lymphoma with *IRF4* Rearrangement. 222

        Follicular Lymphoma of the Testis. 225

        Follicular Lymphoma with del1p36/ *TNFRSF14* Abnormalities 225

        Primary Cutaneous Follicular Lymphoma. 225

        Epstein-Barr Virus-Positive Follicular Lymphoma 225

    Cytologic Findings 227

    Immunophenotypic Findings. 227

    Molecular Genetic Findings 230

        Follicular Lymphoma Microenvironment 232

    Differential Diagnosis 233

    Treatment and Prognosis 234

14. Nodal Marginal Zone Lymphoma. 239

    General Features 239

    Clinical Features 239

    Histologic Findings 239

        Lymph Nodes 239

        Bone Marrow 242

    Cytologic Findings 244

    Immunophenotypic Findings. 244

    Molecular Genetic Findings 246

    Differential Diagnosis 246

    Treatment and Prognosis 248

15. Extranodal Marginal Zone Lymphoma of Mucosa-Associated Lymphoid Tissue 251
    General Features 251
    Clinical Features 251
    Histologic Findings 252
        Extranodal Sites 252
        Lymph Nodes 256
        Bone Marrow 256
    Cytologic Findings 256
    Immunophenotypic Findings 256
    Molecular Genetic Findings 257
    Differential Diagnosis 261
    Treatment and Prognosis 263

16. Lymphoplasmacytic Lymphoma and Waldenstrom Macroglobulinemia 267
    General Features 267
    Clinical Features 267
    Histologic Findings 268
        Lymph Nodes and Other Tissues 268
        Peripheral Blood 272
        Bone Marrow 273
    Cytologic Findings 273
    Immunophenotypic Findings 273
    Molecular Genetic Findings 274
    Differential Diagnosis 278
    Treatment and Prognosis 279

17. Diffuse Large B-Cell Lymphoma, Not Otherwise Specified 283
    General Features 283
    Clinical Features 285
    Histologic Findings 285
        Lymph Node 285
        Bone Marrow 290
        Peripheral Blood 293
        Other Extranodal Sites 294
    Other Extranodal Large B-Cell Lymphomas 295
        Primary DLBCL of the Central Nervous System 295
        Intravascular Large B-Cell Lymphoma 296
        Diffuse Large B-Cell Lymphoma Associated with Chronic Inflammation 298
        Primary Cutaneous DLBCL, Leg Type 298
        Lymphomatoid Granulomatosis 298
        Diffuse Large B-Cell Lymphoma Arising at Other Extranodal Sites 302
    Cytologic Findings 303

Immunophenotypic Findings. 303

Molecular Genetic Findings 311

    Chromosomal Abnormalities. 311

    Gene Expression Profiling 312

    Gene Mutations 313

Transformed DLBCL 314

Differential Diagnosis 314

Treatment 315

Prognosis. 316

    Clinical Features. 316

    Morphologic Features. 317

    Gene Expression Profile 317

    Immunophenotypic Findings 317

    Cytogenetic Findings 318

    Gene Mutations 319

18. T-Cell/Histiocyte-Rich Large B-Cell Lymphoma 325

General Features 325

Clinical Features 325

Histologic Findings 325

    Lymph Node. 325

    Spleen and Liver 325

    Bone Marrow 328

Cytologic Findings 328

Immunophenotypic Findings. 330

Molecular Genetic Findings 332

Differential Diagnosis 332

Treatment and Prognosis 333

19. Epstein-Barr Virus-Positive Diffuse Large B-Cell Lymphoma 335

General Features 335

Clinical Features 336

Histologic Findings 336

Cytologic Findings 337

Immunophenotypic Findings. 337

    Epstein-Barr Virus. 337

Molecular Genetic Findings 339

Differential Diagnosis 339

Treatment and Prognosis 340

20. Primary Mediastinal Large B-Cell Lymphoma 343

General Features 343

Clinical Features 343

Histologic Findings 343

    Mediastinum 343

    Lymph Nodes 344

Cytologic Findings 344

Immunophenotypic Findings 348

Molecular Genetic Findings 348

Differential Diagnosis 351

Treatment and Prognosis 351

21. Anaplastic Lymphoma Kinase-Positive Large B-Cell Lymphoma 355

General Features 355

Clinical Features 355

Histologic Findings 355

Cytologic Findings 355

Immunophenotypic Findings 358

Molecular Genetic Findings 358

    ALK Expression Pattern and Molecular Abnormalities 359

Differential Diagnosis 360

Treatment and Prognosis 361

22. Human Herpesvirus 8-Positve Large B-Cell Lymphomas and Associated Diseases 363

HHV-8-Positive Multicentric Castleman Disease 363

Large B-Cell Lymphoma Arising in HHV-8-Positive

    Multicentric Castleman Disease 368

HHV-8-Positive Germinotropic Lymphoproliferative Disorder 370

HHV-8-Positive Diffuse Large B-Cell Lymphoma, Not Otherwise pecified 369

23. Plasmablastic Lymphoma 375

General Features 375

Clinical Features 375

    HIV-Positive PBL 375

    Immunocompetent Patients with PBL 377

    Transplantation-Associated PBL 377

    Autoimmune Diseases Associated with PBL 377

Histologic Findings 377

Cytologic Findings 378

Immunophenotypic Findings 378

Molecular Genetic Findings 384

Differential Diagnosis 385

Treatment and Prognosis 386

24. Plasmacytoma 389

General Features 389

Clinical Features 390

Histologic Findings 391

Cytologic Findings 391

Immunophenotypic Findings. 391

Epstein-Barr Virus in Extramedullary Plasmacytoma 391

Molecular Genetic Findings 394

Differential Diagnosis 396

Treatment and Prognosis 398

Monoclonal Immunoglobulin-Deposition Diseases. 399

Amyloidosis 399

Crystal-Storing Histiocytosis 399

25. Burkitt Lymphoma 403

General Features 403

Pathogenesis 404

Cofactors Thought Likely to Be Involved in BL Pathogenesis. 404

Clinical Features 405

Endermic Variant 405

Sporadic Variant 405

Immunodeficiency-Associated Variant 406

Histologic Findings 406

Lymph Nodes 406

Extranodal Sites 409

Cytologic Findings 410

Immunophenotypic Findings. 412

Molecular Genetic Findings 412

Differential Diagnosis 417

Treatment and Prognosis 418

26. High-Grade B-Cell Lymphoma, Not Otherwise Specified. 421

General Features 421

Clinical Features 421

Histologic Findings 421

Cytologic Findings 423

Immunophenotypic Findings. 423

Molecular Genetic Findings 423

Double-Hit Lymphomas. 426

Differential Diagnosis 426

Treatment and Prognosis 426

27. Double-Hit Lymphomas 429

General Features 429

Clinical Features 429

Histologic Findings 430

MYC/BCL2 Double-Hit Lymphoma 430

MYC/BCL6 Double-Hit Lymphoma 433

MYC/BCL2/BCL6 Triple-Hit Lymphoma 433

Bone Marrow 434

Cytologic Findings 435

Immunophenotypic Findings 435

Double-Positive or Double-Expressor Lymphoma 437

Molecular Genetic Findings 437

Atypical *MYC/BCL2* Double-Hit Lymphoma 437

Lymphomas with *BCL2* and *BCL6* Translocations 438

Differential Diagnosis 438

Treatment and Prognosis 438

28. B-Cell Lymphomas, Unclassifiable, with Features Between Diffuse Large B-Cell
Lymphoma and Classic Hodgkin Lymphoma (Gray Zone Lymphoma) 441

General Features 441

Clinical Features 441

Histologic Findings 442

Cytologic Findings 443

Immunophenotypic Findings 444

Molecular Genetic Findings 445

Differential Diagnosis 446

Treatment and Prognosis 447

29. T-Lymphoblastic Leukemia/Lymphoma 449

General Features 449

Clinical Features 449

Histologic Findings 449

Lymph Nodes 449

Other Tissue Sites 449

Peripheral Blood and Bone Marrow 450

Cytologic Findings 453

Immunophenotypic Findings 453

Molecular Genetic Findings 455

Early T-Cell Acute Precursor Leukemia 458

ETP-ALL Compared to Immature T-ALL 460

Differential Diagnosis 460

Treatment and Prognosis 461

30. Peripheral T-Cell Lymphoma, Not Otherwise Specified 465

General Features 465

Advances in T-Cell and NK-Cell Immunity Contribute to sification 465

Clinical Features 466

Histologic Findings 466

Morphologic Variants 468

    Lymphoepithelioid Variant 468

    T-Zone Variant 468

    Follicular Variant 469

Cytologic Findings 472

Immunophenotypic Findings 472

Molecular Genetic Findings 477

Differential Diagnosis 479

Treatment and Prognosis 480

31. Angioimmunoblastic T-Cell Lymphoma 483

General Features 483

Clinical Features 484

Histologic Findings 484

    Lymph Node 484

    Histologic Variants of Angioimmunoblastic T-Cell Lymphoma 486

    Bone Marrow 488

    Peripheral Blood 488

    Other Sites of Involvement 489

Cytologic Findings 490

Immunohistochemical Findings 490

    Prominent B-Cell or Plasma Cell Population in ATL 495

Molecular Genetic Findings 495

    Is AITL Related to T_{FH} Cell Lymphomas 496

Risk of Other Lymphomas 496

Differential Diagnosis 496

Treatment and Prognosis 498

32. Adult T-Cell Leukemia/Lymphoma 501

General Features 501

    HTLV-1 Virus 501

    Epidemiology of HTLV-1 Infection 501

    HTLV-1-Associated Diseases 503

Clinical Features 503

    Clinical Variants 504

Histologic Findings 505

    Lymph Node 505

    Peripheral Blood and Bone Marrow 507

    Skin 508

    Other Organ Systems 509

Cytologic Findings 509

Immunophenotypic Findings 510

Molecular Genetic Findings 511

Differential Diagnosis 513

Treatment and Prognosis 513

33. ALK-Positive Anaplastic Large Cell Lymphoma 517

General Features 517

Clinical Features 518

Histologic Findings 518

Lymph Node 518

Peripheral Blood and Bone Marrow 522

Cytologic Findings 526

Immunohistophenotypic Findings 528

Molecular Genetic Findings 532

Differential Diagnosis 534

Treatment and Prognosis 536

34. ALK-Negative Anaplastic Large Cell Lymphoma 539

General Features 539

Clinical Features 539

Histologic Findings 539

Cytologic Findings 540

Immunohistophenotypic Findings 540

Molecular Genetic Findings 543

Differential Diagnosis 548

Treatment and Prognosis 552

35. Extranodal NK/T-Cell Lymphoma, Nasal Type 555

General Features 555

Clinical Features 555

Histologic Findings 556

Lymph Node 556

Nasal Region/Upper Aerodigestive Tract 557

Extranasal Sites 557

Cytologic Findings 563

Immunohistochemical Findings 563

Molecular Genetic Findings 566

Differential Diagnosis 568

Treatment and Prognosis 569

36. Mycosis Fungoides 573

General Features 573

Clinical Features 573

Histologic Findings 575

Lymph Node. 575

Skin 578

Peripheral Blood and Bone Marrow. 380

Viscera. 581

Cytologic Findings 581

Immunohistophenotypic Findings. 582

Molecular Genetic Findings 586

Sézary Syndrome. 586

Differential Diagnosis 588

Treatment and Prognosis 590

37.   Overview of Hodgkin Lymphomas 593

General Features 593

Bimodal Incidence of HL 595

Epstein-Barr Virus in HL. 595

Risk Factors for Classic HL 596

Clinical Features 596

Patterns of Spread and Relapse in Patients with Classic HL 597

Histologic Findings 597

Immunophenotypic Findings. 597

Molecular Genetic Findings 601

Differential Diagnosis 602

Treatment and Prognosis 603

Prognostic Factors 603

38.   Nodular Sclerosis Hodgkin Lymphoma. 611

General Features 611

Clinical Features 611

Histologic Findings. 611

Lymph Nodes. 611

Thymus. 616

Spleen and Liver. 616

Bone Marrow 617

Cytologic Findings 617

Immunohistochemical Findings. 620

Does T-Cell Classic HL Exist? 621

Molecular Genetic Findings 621

Differential Diagnosis 623

Treatment and Prognosis 624

39.   Lymphocyte-Rich Classic Hodgkin Lymphoma 627

General Features 627

Clinical Features 627

Histologic Findings 627

  Lymph Nodes 627

  Other Sites 628

  The Relationship of LRCHL to Nodular Sclerosis HL. 630

Cytologic Findings 631

Immunohistochemical Findings. 631

Molecular Genetic Findings 633

Differential Diagnosis 633

Treatment and Prognosis 634

40. Mixed Cellularity Hodgkin Lymphoma 637

General Features 637

Clinical Features 637

Histologic Findings 637

  Lymph Nodes 637

  Spleen, Liver, and Bone Marrow 641

Cytologic Findings 641

Immunophenotypic Findings. 641

Molecular Genetic Findings 641

Differential Diagnosis 643

Treatment and Prognosis 644

41. Lymphocyte-Depleted Hodgkin Lymphoma. 645

General Features 645

Clinical Features 645

Histologic Findings 645

  Lymph Nodes 645

Cytologic Findings 648

Immunophenotypic Findings. 648

Molecular Genetic Findings 648

Differential Diagnosis 648

Treatment and Prognosis 649

42. Nodular Lymphocyte-Predominant Hodgkin Lymphoma 651

General Features 651

Clinical Features 652

Histologic Findings 653

  Lymph Nodes 653

  Spleen, Liver, and Bone Marrow 659

Cytologic Findings 659

Immunophenotypic Findings. 659

Molecular Genetic Findings 667

Diffuse Large B-Cell Lymphoma in Patients with NLPHL 668

Diffuse Lymphocyte-Predominant Hodgkin Lymphoma. 670

Differential Diagnosis 670

Treatment and Prognosis 671

43. Human Immunodeficiency Virus-Associated Lymphoproliferative rders. 675

General Features 675

Viral Structure and Replication 675

Natural History of HIV Infection 676

HIV-Associated Benign Lymphadenopathy 677

Risk of Lymphoma 677

Clinical Features 679

Lymphomas Characteristic of HIV Infection 680

HIV-Positive Multicentric Castleman Disease and Associated Large

B-Cell Lymphoma 680

Primary Effusion Lymphoma 680

AIDS-Related Polymorphic Lymphoproliferative Disorder 684

Lymphomas that also Occur in Immunocompetent Patients 685

Burkitt Lymphoma 685

Diffuse Large B-Cell Lymphoma 686

Primary DLBCL of the Central Nervous System 687

Plasmablastic Lymphoma. 688

Hodgkin Lymphoma 688

Other Lymphomas 688

Treatment and Prognosis 689

44. Iatrogenic Lymphoproliferative Disorders 693

General Features 693

Clinical Features 694

Histologic and Immunophenotypic Findings 695

Diffuse Large B-Cell Lymphoma 695

Classic Hodgkin Lymphoma and Hodgkin-Like Lesions. 695

Polymorphic Lymphoproliferative Disorders 697

EBV-Positive Mucocutaneous Ulcer 699

Other Iatrogenic LPDs 700

Cytologic Findings 703

Molecular Genetic Findings 703

Differential Diagnosis 704

Treatment and Prognosis 704

Diffuse Large B-Cell Lymphoma 705

Classic Hodgkin Lymphoma and Hodgkin-Like Lesion 704

Polymorphic LPD EBV-Positive Mucocutaneous Ulcer 704

45. Cancer Therapy-Associated Lymphoproliferative Disorders 707
    General Features 707
    Clinical Features 708
    Histologic Findings 709
    Cytologic Findings 709
    Immunophenotypic Findings. 709
    Molecular Genetic Findings 709
    Differential Diagnosis 709
    Treatment and Prognosis 712
46. Primary Immunodeficiency-Associated Lymphoproliferative Disorders 715
    General Features 715
    Clinical Features 718
    Types of PID 718
        Common Variable Immunodeficiency Syndrome. 718
        Ataxia-Telangiectasia 720
        Severe Combined Immunodeficiency 721
        Wiskott-Aldrich Syndrome. 721
        Hyper-IgM Syndrome. 721
        Nijmegen Breakage Syndrome 721
        X-Linked Agammaglobulinemia 722
        Cartilage Hair Hypoplasia Syndrome. 722
        X-Linked Lymphoproliferative Syndrome. 722
        Autoimmune Lymphoproliferative Syndrome 723
        Activated Phosphoinositide 3-Kinase Syndrome. 724
        Interleukin-2-Inducible T-Cell Kinase Deficiency 725
        Other Immunodeficiency Disorders Likely Associated with an Increased Risk of
        Lymphoma 725
    Histologic Findings. 725
    Cytologic Findings 727
    Immunophenotypic Findings. 727
    Molecular Genetic Findings 727
    Differential Diagnosis. 727
    Treatment and Prognosis 727
47. Post-Transplant Lymphoproliferative Disorders 731
    General Features 731
    Clinical Features 732
    Histologic and Immunohenotypic Findings 733
        Nondestructive Lesions 733
        Polymorphic Lesions 735
        Monomorphic Lesions: B Cell 738

Classic Hodgkin Lymphoma 741

Monomorphic Lesions: T Cell 743

Cytologic Findings 744

Molecular Genetic Findings 744

Differential Diagnosis 746

Treatment and Prognosis 746

48. Blastic Plasmacytoid Dendritic Cell Neoplasm 751

General Features 751

Clinical Features 751

Histologic Findings 751

Lymph Node 751

Skin 751

Bone Marrow 754

Peripheral Blood 754

Cytologic Findings 754

Cytochemical Findings 755

Immunophenotypic Findings 755

Molecular Genetic Findings 758

Differential Diagnosis 758

Treatment and Prognosis 761

49. Mastocytosis 763

General Features 763

Clinical Features 764

Cutaneous Mastocytosis 764

Systemic Mastocytosis 765

Histologic Findings 767

Cutaneous Mastocytosis 767

Systemic Mastocytosis 768

Cytologic Findings 779

Cytochemical Findings 779

Immunophetypic Findings 779

Molecular Genetic Findings 780

Differential Diagnosis 781

Treatment and Prognosis 782

50. Blastic Hematopoietic Neoplasms Associated with t(8;13)(p11;q12)/ZMYM2-FGFR1   787

General Features 787

Clinical Features 788

Histologic Findings 788

Lymph Nodes 788

Bone Marrow 790

Cytologic Findings 790

Immunophenotypic Findings. 790

Molecular Genetic Findings 791

Differential Diagnosis 794

Treatment and Prognosis 795

51. Myeloid Sarcoma 797

General Features 797

Clinical Features 797

Histologic Findings 799

Lymph Node. 801

Skin 803

Other Sites 803

Cytologic Findings 803

Cytochemical Findings. 807

Immunophenotypic Findings. 807

Molecular Genetic Findings 807

Differential Diagnosis 809

Treatment and Prognosis 810

52. Histiocytic Sarcoma 813

General Features 813

Clinical Features 813

Histologic Findings 816

Cytologic Findings 816

Ultrastructural and Immunophenotypic Findings. 816

Molecular Genetic Findings 818

Differential Diagnosis 821

Treatment and Prognosis 822

53. Follicular Dendritic Cell Sarcoma 825

General Features 825

Clinical Features 825

Histologic Findings 825

Cytologic Findings 830

Ultrastructural and Immunophenotypic Findings. 830

Molecular Genetic Findings 831

Differential Diagnosis 832

Treatment and Prognosis 835

54. Intradigitating Dendritic Cell Sarcoma 837

General Features 837

Clinical Features 837

Histologic Findings 837

Cytologic Findings 839
Immunophenotypic Findings. 839
Ultrastructural Findings 840
Molecular Genetic Findings 840
Differential Diagnosis 840
Treatment and Prognosis 841

55. Langerhans Cell Tumors 843
    Langerhans Cell Histiocytosis. 843
        General Features. 843
        Clinical Features. 844
        Histologic Findings. 844
        Tumor-Associated Langerhans Cell Histiocytosis 847
        Cytologic Findings 847
        Immunophenotypic Findings 847
        Ultrastructural Findings 850
        Molecular Genetic Findings. 850
        Differential Diagnosis. 851
        Treatment and Prognosis 852
    Langerhans Cell Sarcoma 855
        General Features. 855
        Clinical Features. 855
        Histologic Findings. 855
        Cytologic Findings 855
        Immunophenotypic Findings 855
        Molecular Genetic Findings. 855
        Treatment and Prognosis 855

56. Hairy Cell Leukemia 861
    General Features 861
    Clinical Features 861
    Gross Findings. 862
    Histologic Findings 862
        Spleen 862
        Blood and Bone Marrow 862
        Lymph Node and Extranodal Sites. 864
    Cytologic Findings 864
    Immunophenotypic Findings. 867
    Ultrastructural Findings 869
    Molecular Genetic Findings 869
    Differential Diagnosis 870
    Treatment and Prognosis 871

57. Hairy Cell Leukemia-Variant 875

    General Features 875

    Clinical Features 875

    Gross and Histologic Findings 876

        Spleen 876

        Peripheral Blood 876

        Bone Marrow 877

        Other Tissues 877

    Cytologic Findings 879

    Immunophenotypic Findings 879

    Molecular Genetic Findings 879

    Differential Diagnosis 880

    Treatment and Prognosis 881

58. Splenic Marginal Zone Lymphoma 885

    General Features 885

    Clinical Features 885

    Gross and Histologic Findings 886

        Spleen 886

        Lymph Nodes 887

        Bone Marrow 889

        Peripheral Blood 889

        Liver 891

    Cytologic Findings 891

    Immunophenotypic Findings 891

    Molecular Genetic Findings 892

    Differential Diagnosis 894

    Treatment and Prognosis 896

59. Splenic Diffuse Red Pulp Small B-Cell Lymphoma 899

    General Features 899

    Clinical Features 899

    Gross and Histologic Findings 899

        Spleen 899

        Bone Marrow 900

        Blood 900

        Other Sites 900

    Immunophenotypic Findings 900

    Molecular Genetic Findings 903

    Differential Diagnosis 903

    Treatment and Prognosis 903

60. Primary Splenic Large B-Cell Lymphoma 905
       General Features 905
       Clinical Features 905
       Gross Findings 906
       Histologic Findings 906
       Cytologic Findings 907
       Immunophenotypic Findings 907
       Molecular Genetic Findings 908
       Differential Diagnosis 908
       Treatment and Prognosis 912
61. Hepatosplenic T-Cell Lymphoma 915
       General Features 915
       Clinical Features 915
       Gross and Histologic Findings 916
          Spleen 916
          Other Sites 918
          Bone Marrow 920
       Cytologic Findings 923
       Immunophenotypic Findings 923
       Molecular Genetic Findings 924
       Differential Diagnosis 925
       Treatment and Prognosis 926
62. Myeloid Neoplasms Involving the Spleen 929
       Myeloproliferative Neoplasms 929
       Mastocytosis 933
       Myelodysplastic/Myeloproliferative Neoplasms 935
       Myelodysplastic Syndromes 938
       Myeloid Sarcoma 941
63. Vascular Tumors of the Spleen 945
       Hamartoma 945
       Hemangioma 950
       Littoral Cell Angioma 953
       Hemangioendothelioma 954
       Kaposi Sarcoma 958
       Angiosarcoma 959
64. Stromal Tumors and Tumor-Like Lesions of the Spleen 967
       General Features 967
       Clinical Features 967
       Gross and Histologic Findings 967
          Inflammatory Pseudotumor 968

       Inflammatory Pseudotumor-Like Follicular Dendritic Cell Tumor 971

       Inflammatory Myofibroblastic Tumor 971

    Immunophenotypic Findings 972

       Inflammatory Pseudotumor of Spleen 972

       Inflammatory Pseudotumor-Like Follicular Dendritic Cell Tumor 973

       Inflammatory Myofibroblastic Tumor 973

    Molecular Genetic Findings 973

    Differential Diagnosis 974

    Treatment and Prognosis 975

65. Cysts of Spleen 977

    General Features 977

    Clinical Features 977

    Gross and Histologic Findings 977

       Mesothelial Cyst 977

       Epidermoid/Epithelial Cyst 978

       Pseudocyst 978

       Echinococcal Cyst 978

       Other Types of Cysts 980

    Cytologic Findings 980

    Immunophenotypic Findings 981

    Treatment and Prognosis 981

66. Nonhematolymphoid Tumors and Tumor-Like Lesions 983

    Inflammatory Pseudotumor 983

    Palisaded Myofibroblastoma 987

    Angiomyolipoma 989

    Lymphangioleiomyomatosis 990

    Leiomyomatosis 991

    Angiomyomatous Hamartoma 992

    Lymphangioma and Lymphangiomatosis 992

    Limpomatosis and Lipoma 993

    Vascular Transformation of Lymph Node Sinuses 994

    Lymphangiectasia 995

    Peliosis 996

    Hemangioma 997

67. Metastatic Tumors 1001

    General Features 1001

       Lymph Node Versus Spleen 1001

       Biology of Metastases 1001

       Role of Metastases in Staging 1002

    Clinical Features 1002

Gross Findings. 1004

Histologic Findings 1004

Morphologic Differentiation of Metastases 1006

    Small Cell Tumors 1007

    Epithelioid Tumors. 1010

    Anaplastic Tumors 1014

    Spindle Cell Tumors. 1015

    Metastatic Solid Tumors Associated with a Prominent Infiltrate of Benign

        Hematopoietic Cells 1019

Potential Pitfalls Using Immunohistochemistry 1019

    Epithelial- and Mesenchymal-Related Antigens in Hematopoietic Tumors 1021

    Common Hematopoietic Antigens in Epithelial and Mesenchymal Tumors. . . . 1021

    Normal Cells Usually Not Appreciated in Routinely Stained Tissue Sections. . . . 1023

Other Ancillary Methods for Diagnosis of Metastases 1025

Spleen 1025

Index 1029

1 NORMAL ANATOMY AND FUNCTION OF LYMPH NODES AND SPLEEN

The immune system is dedicated to the recognition of foreign antigens and defense from invading microorganisms. It consists of primary (central) and secondary (peripheral) lymphoid tissues. The primary lymphoid tissues are the bone marrow and thymus gland, which contain the precursors of the lymphoid cells and support initial antigen-independent differentiation from the immature to mature stage. The secondary lymphoid tissues include lymph nodes, spleen, and sites of mucosa-associated lymphoid tissue (MALT) including tonsils, appendix, and Peyer patches of the gastrointestinal tract. Secondary lymphoid tissues are the sites of antigen-dependent proliferation and differentiation of lymphoid cells.

LYMPH NODE

Gross Anatomy

The lymph nodes are small, ovoid or bean-shaped encapsulated lymphoid tissues, generally less than 1 cm in greatest dimension. The human body contains about 450 lymph nodes. They are located adjacent to lymphatic vessels, particularly in areas where these vessels converge. Lymph nodes are abundant in neck, axilla, mediastinum, retroperitoneum, and inguinal regions, and generally in those areas draining organs/tissues in contact to the external environment (fig. 1-1). They are connected to the blood circulation via an artery and vein, and to the lymphatic system through afferent and efferent lymphatic vessels. The lymph node is the site where circulating naïve lymphocytes encounter antigens and antigen-presenting cells (APC), which travel from peripheral tissues through the lymph. This system provides effective immune surveillance for the screening of foreign pathogens.

Microscopic Anatomy

Traditionally, lymph node anatomy is organized into discrete compartments: cortex, paracortex, medulla, and sinuses. More recently, an anatomic and functional unit of the lymph node parenchyma, termed the "lymphoid lobule," has been proposed as an addition, although its relevance has not been widely recognized (5,15,26,54). In this model, each lymph node contains one or several functional units, or lobules, dependent on the size of the lymph node. A lobule represents a portion of lymph node parenchyma between two transverse sinuses, centered under one afferent lymphatic vessel and including the superficial cortex with

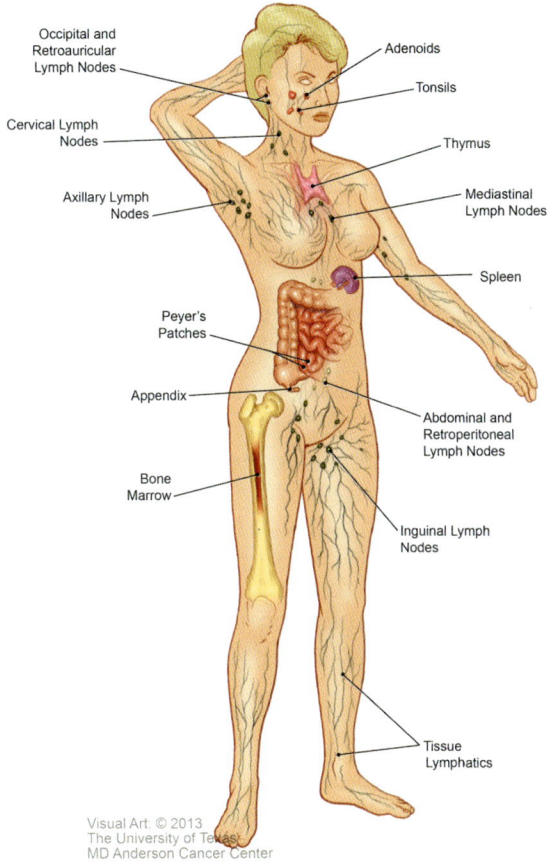

Figure 1-1

LYMPH NODES AND EXTRANODAL LYMPHOID TISSUES

Schematic showing sites of lymph node groups and extranodal sites of lymphoid tissue throughout the body.

1

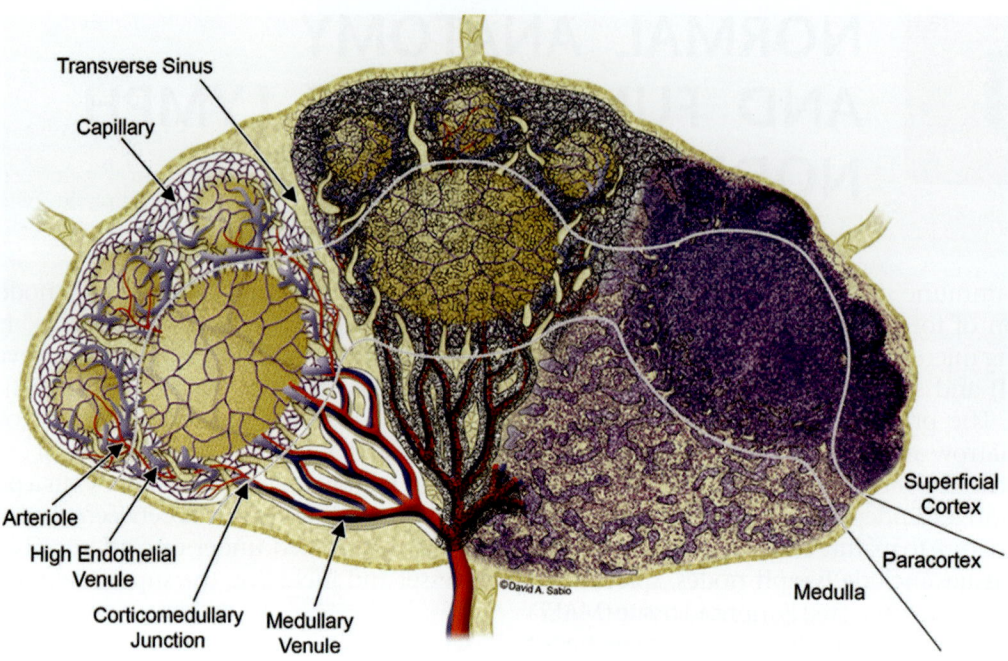

Transverse Sinus

Capillary

Arteriole

High Endothelial
Venule

Corticomedullary Medullary
Junction   Venule

©David A. Sabio

Superficial
Cortex

Paracortex

Medulla

Figure 1-2

LYMPH NODE

Schematic diagram of a mid-sagittal section of a lymph node containing three lymphoid "lobules." Each lobule is centered under its own afferent lymphatic vessel. The follicles and interfollicular cortex of these lobules constitute the superficial cortex, the deep cortex constitutes the paracortex, and the medullary cords and medullary sinuses constitute the medulla.

Left lobule: Arterioles (red) and venules (blue) converge in the medullary cords. Arterioles arborize in the paracortical cords and interfollicular cortex and give rise to capillary beds (purple). Capillaries are present in the follicles but are less dense than in the other areas (omitted from the medullary cords shown here for clarity). Capillaries empty into high endothelial venules.

Center lobule: This lobule is shown with the reticular meshwork superimposed on the vasculature. The center lobule is separated from the left lobule by a transverse sinus.

Right lobule: The lobule is shown as it appears in histologic sections. Densely packed lymphoid cells fill the lobular reticular meshwork. Five cortical follicles are represented. The paracortex and medulla constitute the remainder of the lobule. (Fig. 2 from Willard-Mack C. Normal structure, function and histology of lymph nodes. Toxicol Pathol 2006;34:411.)

lymphoid follicles, paracortex, and medulla (fig. 1-2). As each afferent lymphatic vessel collects from a different drainage field, each lobule is potentially exposed to a different set of antigens, an arrangement that may explain why areas within a lymph node may show different levels of immunologic activity (fig. 1-3).

Lymph Node Cortex

The major component of the lymph node cortex is the B-cell compartment, basically represented by primary and secondary lymphoid follicles.

Primary Follicles. Primary follicles are round aggregates of activated small B cells within a small network of follicular dendritic cells (FDCs). These cells express immunoglobulin (Ig)M, IgD, CD23, and CD38, and are negative for CD10 and CD27.

Circulating naïve B cells enter the lymph node, are activated in the paracortex by CD4-positive T cells and dendritic cells, and move into the primary follicle (34,40). Once in the primary follicle, a subset of these activated B cells begins to rapidly proliferate to form a germinal center (GC). The GCs are surrounded by a darker corona (mantle zone) of displaced IgM- and IgD-positive activated B cells, establishing the structure known as a secondary lymphoid follicle (21).

Secondary Follicles. Secondary follicles are defined by the presence of GCs, the main sites of antibody affinity maturation and where plasma cells and a subset of memory B cells are generated. The GC reaction results in selective survival and expansion of B-cell clones with a high affinity for antigens, resulting in a substantially more effective immune response.

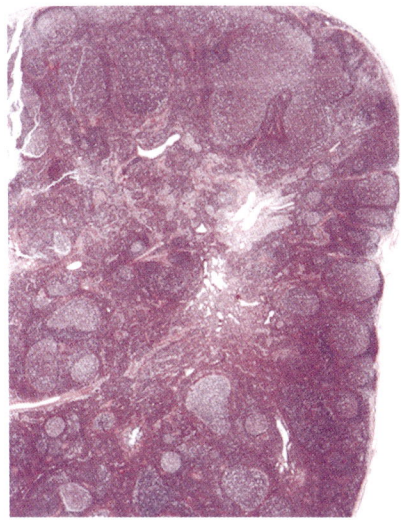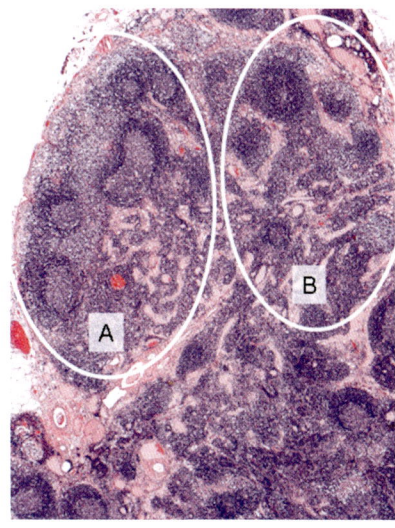

Figure 1-3

LYMPH NODE

Left: A section of a lymph node shows the prominent cortex and medulla. Follicular hyperplasia is seen. The cortex has numerous secondary lymphoid follicles with germinal centers of different sizes, including some forming geographic configurations (top of the lymph node).

Right: Five secondary follicles are present in region A and mainly primary follicles in region B. These different regions of the same lymph node represent two different lobules collecting lymph from different drainage fields, and thus exposed to a different set of antigens.

Germinal Centers. GCs are dynamic structures. A few days after exposure to an antigen, a GC develops in the center of a primary follicle, reaches its maximum size within approximately 2 weeks, and thereafter slowly involutes within several weeks as antigen levels decrease. The kinetics of GC formation and involution are variable and depend on the nature of the antigen and the ability of the immune system to clear the antigen. For some viral or other types of chronic infection, GC reactions may persist longer, up to several months. The GC reaction ends with involution of the GC and dissolution of the follicle. Follicular dissolution can adopt several histologic patterns (23). The histologic pattern of follicular dissolution is, in part, related to the nature and duration of antigenic stimulation.

The most conspicuous morphologic feature of the GC is the presence of two distinct compartments, the dark and light zones (fig. 1-4) (7). The dark zone consists almost entirely of centroblasts (mitotically active B cells) and few FDCs, thus appearing "dark" by light microscopy. By contrast, the light zone is occupied by large and small centrocytes (nondividing B cells) interspersed among a rich network of FDCs, which imparts its "lighter" appearance by light microscopy. The light zone also contains naïve IgD-positive B cells, in transit through the GC, and T cells, most of which are CD4-positive. Tingible body macrophages, which phagocytose apoptotic B cells, are also found throughout the GC (31).

In the dark zone, B-cell proliferation occurs along with somatic hypermutation of the vari-able regions of the Ig heavy and light chain genes, resulting in a diversity of B-cell receptors with varying affinities for antigen. The light zone is where the B cells are selected to generate plasma cells and memory B cells based on the affinity for antigen of their mutated surface Ig (i.e., B-cell receptor).

The dark and light zones have a unique distribution within the GC. The dark zone usually lies nearest the paracortex and the light zone is often polarized toward the site of antigen entry, the subcapsular sinus (which receives the afferent lymphatic drainage) in the case of lymph nodes, or the mucosal surface in the case of tonsils, appendix, or Peyer patches of the ileum (37). The organization of the GC into dark and light zones depends on the differential expression of chemokines and chemokine receptors. Expression of the chemokine receptor CXCR4 by GC B cells is tightly controlled and is a major factor controlling cell position within the dark versus light zone (fig. 1-5). CXCL12 (previously known as SDF1) is the ligand of CXCR4 and is more abundant in the dark zone where CXCL12 is produced locally by stromal cells (1). CXCL13, the ligand for CXCR5, is more abundant in the light zone, where it is produced by FDCs. Alternating upregulation and downregulation of CXCR4 and CXCR5 expression, as well as MYC expression by GC B cells, promotes the cycling of cells back and forth between the dark and light zones (1,10). Recent live-imaging studies have shown that GC B cells move bidirectionally between the two

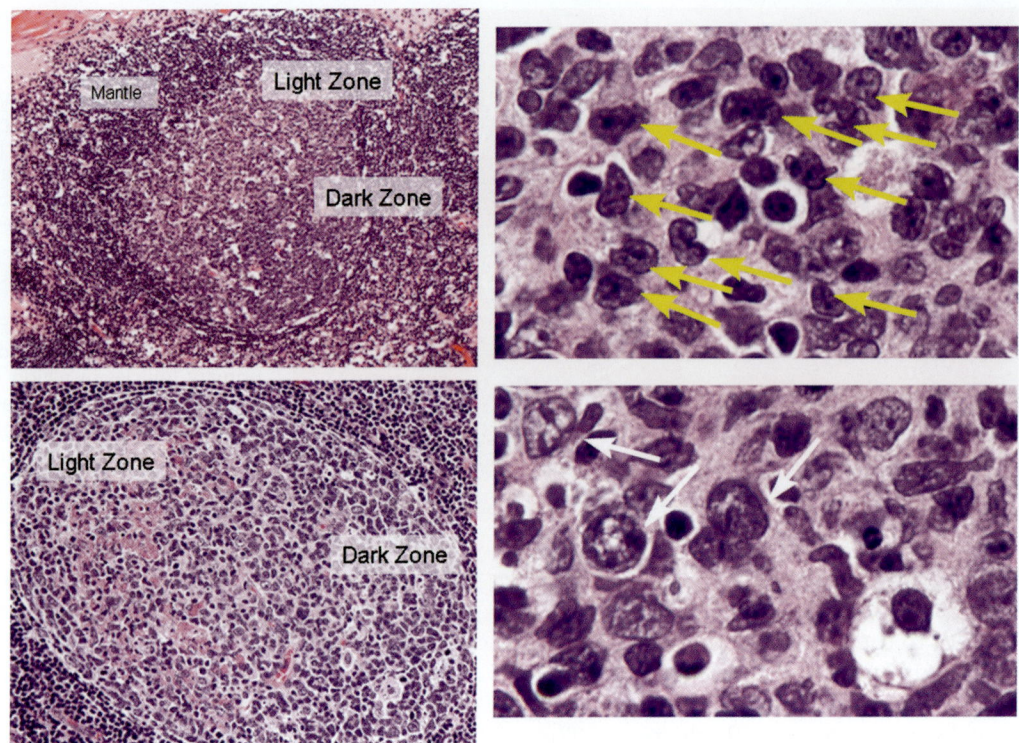

Figure 1-4

SECONDARY LYMPHOID FOLLICLE

Upper left: A secondary lymphoid follicle with a reactive germinal center is surrounded by the mantle zone. The germinal center shows distinct light (top) and dark (bottom) zones. The mantle zone is thicker in the subcapsular aspect (top) of the lymphoid follicle and thinner in the opposite site.

Lower left: Another secondary lymphoid follicle with a reactive germinal center has polarized light and dark zones.

Upper right: the light zone is mainly composed of centrocytes (small cleaved cells) (yellow arrows). Lower right: the dark zone is mainly composed of centroblasts (large noncleaved cells) (white arrows).

GC zones; B cells also reenter the dark zone for additional rounds of proliferation and somatic hypermutation (10,18,45).

Marginal Zone. The lymph nodes occasionally exhibit a well-developed marginal zone. The marginal zone is a distinct pale-appearing corona composed of small cells with slightly irregular nuclei and clear cytoplasm surrounding mantle zones. In particular, lymph nodes located in the mesenteric region often show a marginal zone. The marginal zone is usually more prominent in the spleen (see below) and in MALT (e.g., Peyer patches) than in lymph nodes. In some reactive and neoplastic conditions, marginal zones are expanded. A related finding is monocytoid B-cell hyperplasia, which usually fills and distends nearby sinuses but can spill into marginal zones. Monocytoid B cells are of intermediate to large size, have abundant pale cytoplasm

imparting a monocytoid appearance, and are commonly admixed with neutrophils (fig. 1-6).

Cellular Elements of Germinal Centers

B Cells. Most cells in the GC are activated B cells that consist of small and large centrocytes (cleaved cells) and small and large centroblasts (noncleaved cells). A putative GC B-founder cell (known as a pro-GC cell) has been identified and characterized in human tonsils (29).

Centroblasts are medium to large B cells with an oval nucleus and open chromatin, containing one to three small nucleoli often opposed to the nuclear membrane and a rim of basophilic cytoplasm. *Centrocytes* are small to large B cells with irregular to cleaved nuclei, dense nuclear chromatin, inconspicuous nucleoli, and scant cytoplasm (fig. 1-4). Large centrocytes are generally smaller than centroblasts.

The GC B cells have the following immunophenotype: CD38(+hi), CD20(+hi), CD27(+), and IgD(-). GC B cells also express BCL6, CD10, LIM domain only 2 (LMO2), activation-induced cytidine deaminase (AID), and telomerase (20). CXCR4 expression delineates a homogeneous GC B-cell subpopulation that corresponds to centroblasts (8). GC B cells are characteristically negative for BCL2 and other antiapoptotic family members. The characteristic immunophenotypic profile of reactive GCs as detected by immunohistochemical studies is illustrated in figures 1-7 and 1-8.

Gene expression studies have shown differences between centrocytes and centroblasts (8,52). Centroblasts upregulate genes involved in cell proliferation and mitosis whereas centrocytes upregulate genes related to selection and affinity maturation events including genes related to the NF-κB, B-cell receptor, and CD40 signaling pathways. Centrocytes that fail to be selected are enriched in the GC light zone where they eventually undergo apoptosis, as suggested by enhanced expression of proapoptotic genes in this zone.

Follicular Dendritic Cells. FDCs are stromal cells that form a network of processes in primary follicles and GCs. FDCs have the ability to capture large amounts of antigen in the form of immune complexes in highly ordered units designated as iccosomes (9). In GCs, FDCs are more densely

concentrated in the light zone. The cell of origin of the FDC has not been established definitively, but FDCs are not derived from hematopoietic

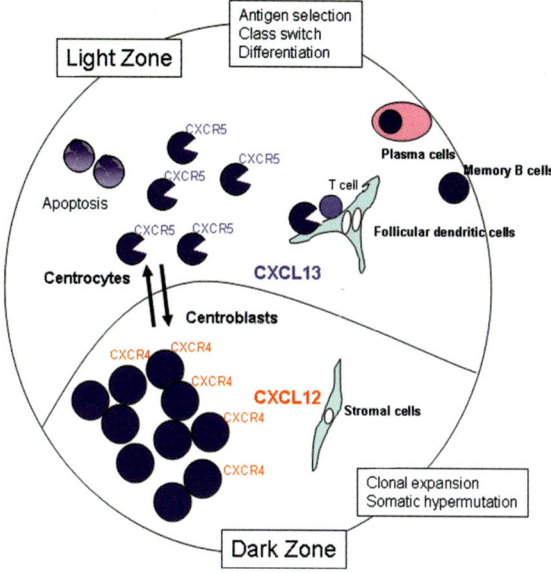

Figure 1-5

GERMINAL CENTER

A simplified schematic diagram shows the cellular composition of the germinal center. The centroblasts (large round blue cells) and centrocytes (small cleaved blue cells) are distributed in the dark and light zones, respectively. The centroblasts express CXCR4, a receptor for CXCL12 that is secreted by the local stromal cells of the dark zone. The centrocytes express CXCR5, a receptor for CXCL13 that is secreted by follicular dendritic cells of the light zone.

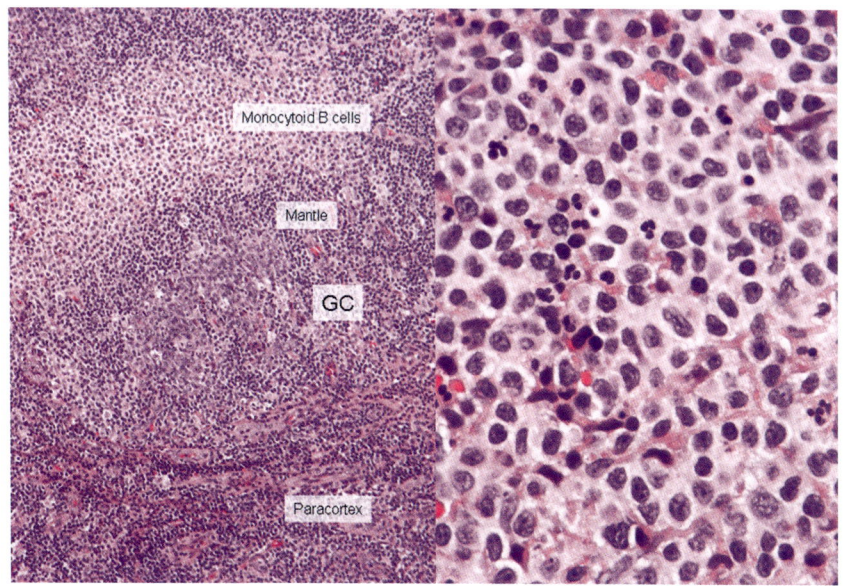

Figure 1-6

SECONDARY LYMPHOID FOLLICLE

Left: Monocytoid B cells are close to a secondary lymphoid follicle. At low-power magnification, the cluster of monocytoid B cells is paler than the reactive germinal center.

Right: High-power magnification of monocytoid B cells. These cells are intermediate to large, with round to slightly irregular nuclei and a moderate amount of clear cytoplasm. Neutrophils are frequently admixed with the monocytoid B cells.

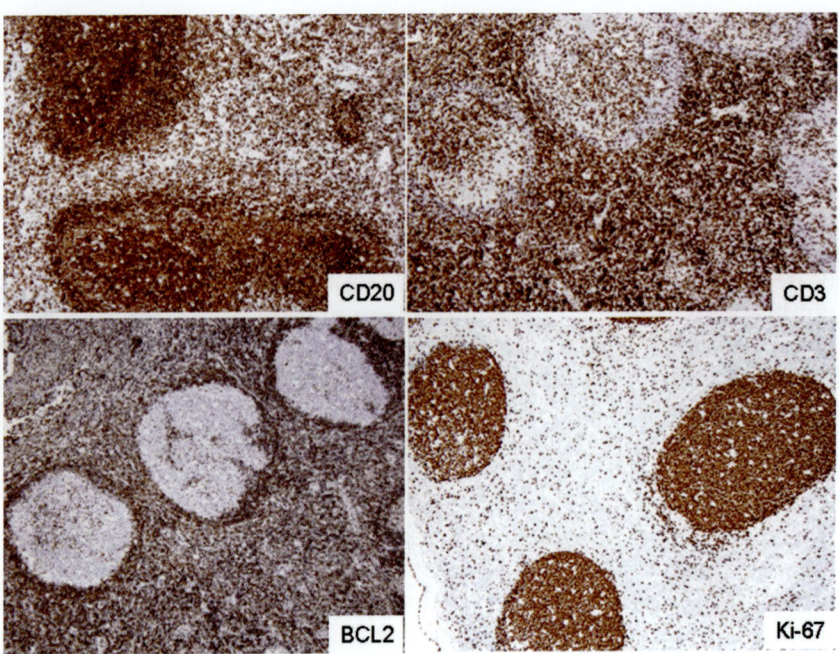

Figure 1-7

TYPICAL IMMUNOPHENOTYPE OF SECONDARY LYMPHOID FOLLICLES

The germinal centers of the B cells are positive for CD20 and negative for BCL2. CD3 highlights scattered germinal center T cells. The characteristic high proliferation rate of the germinal center cells is easily demonstrated using a marker of cell proliferation, such as Ki-67.

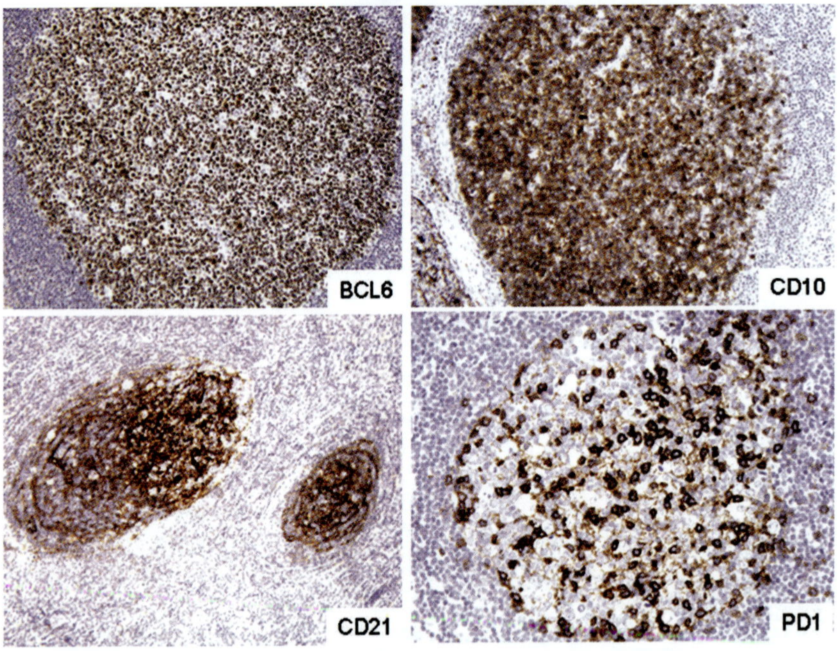

Figure 1-8

TYPICAL IMMUNOPHENOTYPE OF SECONDARY LYMPHOID FOLLICLES

The germinal center B cells are positive for BCL6 and CD10. CD21 is a follicular dendritic cell-associated antigen and immunohistochemistry highlights meshworks of follicular dendritic cells inside the lymphoid follicles. The programmed cell death protein 1 (PD1[CD279]) is expressed by a subset of germinal center T cells (T-follicular helper cells).

precursors and most likely develop from local resident mesenchymal cells in the GC.

FDCs are recognized morphologically by the presence of double oval to rectangular-shaped nuclei with vesicular chromatin and small nucleoli. FDCs express Fc receptors such as FcγRIIb (CD32); they also express FcγRII (CD23) and complement receptors such as CR1 (CD35), CR2 (CD21) (fig. 1-8), CR3 (CD11b/CD18), vascular cell adhesion molecule 1 (VCAM-1), and intercellular adhesion molecule 1 (ICAM-1) (30).

The maintenance of the GC structure and GC B cells is dependent on the presence of FDCs. FDCs support the migration and positioning of GC cells by secreting chemokines and survival factors. CXCL13 is perhaps the most important chemokine as it is the major chemoattractant for B cells and follicular T cells. Survival factors

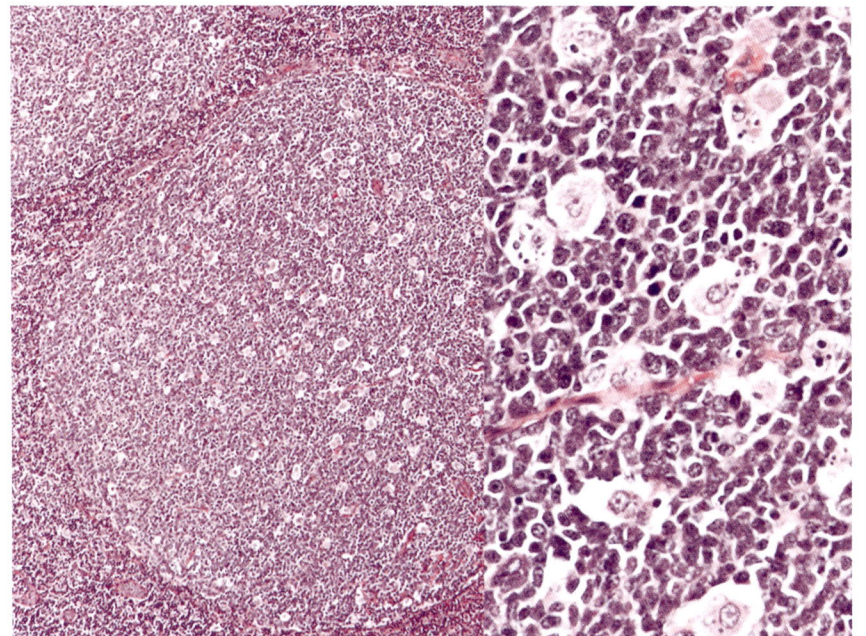

Figure 1-9

TINGIBLE BODY MACROPHAGES

Left: The presence of tingible body macrophages is a char- acteristic feature of reactive germinal centers.

Right: High magnification showing macrophages with phagocytized lymphocytes and cellular debris (tingible bodies) inside their cytoplasm.

for GC cells include IL-6, BAFF (B-cell activating factor), and hedgehog ligands (44).

T Cells. T cells represent a minor (5 to 20 percent) population in GCs but their function is essential for GC maintenance (19). GC T cells are heterogeneous. One population is positive for CD40L (CD154); has a T-helper (Th) immunophenotype; is positive for CD4, CXCR5 (required for follicular homing), ICOS, PD1 (CD279) (fig.1-7), IL-21, and CD57; and is characterized by the secretion of IL-4. These cells are designated as follicular helper T cells (27,46). IL-21 promotes T- and B-cell survival. Other T-cell populations residing in the GC include CD8-positive T cells, Th17 cells, and FOXP3-positive regulatory cells, all of which play functional roles in regulating the GC reaction.

GC T cells express BCL6, which is essential for CXCR5 expression, T-cell follicular homing, and GC formation. The importance of GC T cells is highlighted by the fact that a loss of function mutation in either CD40L (CD154) or CD40 (constitutively expressed by B cells) results in the complete absence of GCs (13). Conversely, defects in T-cell apoptosis can lead to an exaggerated GC reaction.

Tingible Body Macrophages and Bone Marrow-Derived Dendritic Cells. The GC also contains a population of tingible body macrophages (fig. 1-9) and a small population of bone

marrow-derived dendritic cells. Tingible body macrophages eliminate apoptotic B cells inside GCs. Defects in the internalization of apoptotic cells by macrophages have been reported in patients with systemic lupus erythematosus (4). The clearance of apoptotic cells by macrophages may be important to avoid immune responses to nuclear antigens exposed during the process of apoptosis. GC-resident dendritic cells were first identified in human tonsils by immunohisto-chemistry, however, the function of these cells in the GC is not yet elucidated (16).

Germinal Center-Associated Events

The GC is a highly specialized and regulated compartment where many cellular and molecular events occur that result in the production of high-affinity antibody-secreting plasma cells and memory B cells (26). These events include: 1) B-cell clonal expansion, 2) somatic hypermutation, 3) class switch recombination, and 4) affinity-based selection and differentiation of B cells into plasma cells and memory B cells.

B-cell clonal expansion occurs mainly in centroblasts (53). Centroblasts are among the fastest proliferating cells in the human body, with a cell cycle estimated between 6 and 12 hours. Centroblasts express genes involved in cell proliferation and DNA replication, highlighting the fact that these cells are proliferating and undergoing somatic hypermutation of the variable regions of the Ig heavy and light chain genes. Centroblasts activate telomerase to prevent the shortening of telomeres in each cell cycle, downregulate antiapoptotic genes, and upregulate proapoptotic genes. The result of this proapoptotic default program is to facilitate the survival of only those GC cells that receive survival signals.

Somatic hypermutation of the Ig variable region genes occurs in centroblasts and increases the affinity of the Ig variable region (encoded by a VDJ rearrangement) for a particular antigen. This process of mutation, mainly single-nucleotide exchanges or small insertions or deletions of DNA, occurs after exposure to an antigen. Somatic mutations arise via double-stranded DNA breaks prior to the mutational event and depend on the activity of the enzyme activation-induced cytidine deaminase (AID) (32,41). This process results in B-cell clones with increased affinity for antigen. Class switch recombination occurs in centroblasts and is a process by which the heavy chain class of an antibody produced by a GC B-cell clone changes from IgM (usually associated with IgD) to IgG, IgA, or IgE. Since the variable region does not change, class switching does not alter antigen specificity. Instead, the antibody retains affinity for the same antigen, but can interact with different effector molecules. Class switch recommendation is mediated also by AID.

In the light zone, GC B cells with increased affinity for antigen are selected over those with lower affinity; the end result is a substantially more effective immune response. The selection process involves the following steps: interaction between centrocytes with the antigen retained on FDCs, processing of antigen by B cells, and presentation of antigen to follicular T-helper cells. FDC-activated T cells provide survival signals to the selected centrocytes. These selected centrocytes may return to the dark zone for further rounds of proliferation and selection, whereas apoptotic centrocytes are removed from GCs by tingible body macrophages.

All of these GC events are tightly regulated by a complex network of transcription factors. BCL6 is the master regulator of the GC reaction and is required for GC formation. BCL6 is a 95-kD nuclear phosphoprotein that belongs to a large family of nuclear factors that contain zinc-finger motifs to mediate specific DNA binding. BCL6 acts as a transcriptional repressor (28) and is strongly upregulated by GC B cells (centroblasts and most, but not all, centrocytes) and GC T cells (fig. 1-8). It controls several important functions in the biology of GC cells (reviewed in references 28 and 52). BCL6 silences the antiapoptotic molecule BCL2, ensuring that GC B cells are eliminated by apoptosis if they are not selected and rescued by survival signals. BCL6 also silences sensors of DNA damage, such as the *TP53* and ataxia-telangiectasia-mutated (*ATM*) and Rad3-related (*ATR*) genes that help to suppress DNA-damage responses, allowing GC B cells to sustain the genotoxic stress associated with high proliferation. BCL6 also silences Blimp-1, a transcription factor, and thus controls the differentiation of GC B cells into plasma cells. Lastly, BCL6 promotes the expression of T-follicular/helper cell-related genes, such as *CXCR5*, *PD1*, and *ICOS*. T cells lacking BCL6 fail to differentiate into GC Th cells and fail to support GC responses (22).

Lymph Node Paracortex

The paracortex is located between the superficial cortex, the area with the lymphoid follicles, and the medulla. The paracortex is enriched with T cells, but also contains dendritic cells of the interdigitating dendritic subtype, fibroblastic reticular cells (FRC), scattered large B cells, plasmacytoid dendritic cells, and high endothelial venules (HEVs). The paracortex is the region where T cells encounter antigen-presenting cells (APC) such as interdigitating dendritic cells. APC and dendritic cells migrate into the lymph nodes via afferent lymphatics while most circulating naïve T lymphocytes enter the lymph node from the blood via HEVs (fig. 1-10). The homing of naïve T cells and migratory dendritic cells to the nodal paracortex is mediated by CCR7, a chemokine receptor in dendritic cells and naïve T cells, and by the ligands CCL19 and CCL21 expressed by FRCs and HEVs (12). Subsequent downregulation of CCR7 and upregulation of CXCR5 contribute to follicular homing of activated T cells.

Fibroblastic Reticular Cell. The FRC is a distinct type of cell in the paracortex that has hybrid features between epithelial and fibroblastic cells. These cells are difficult to recognize in routine hematoxylin and eosin (H&E)-stained sections,

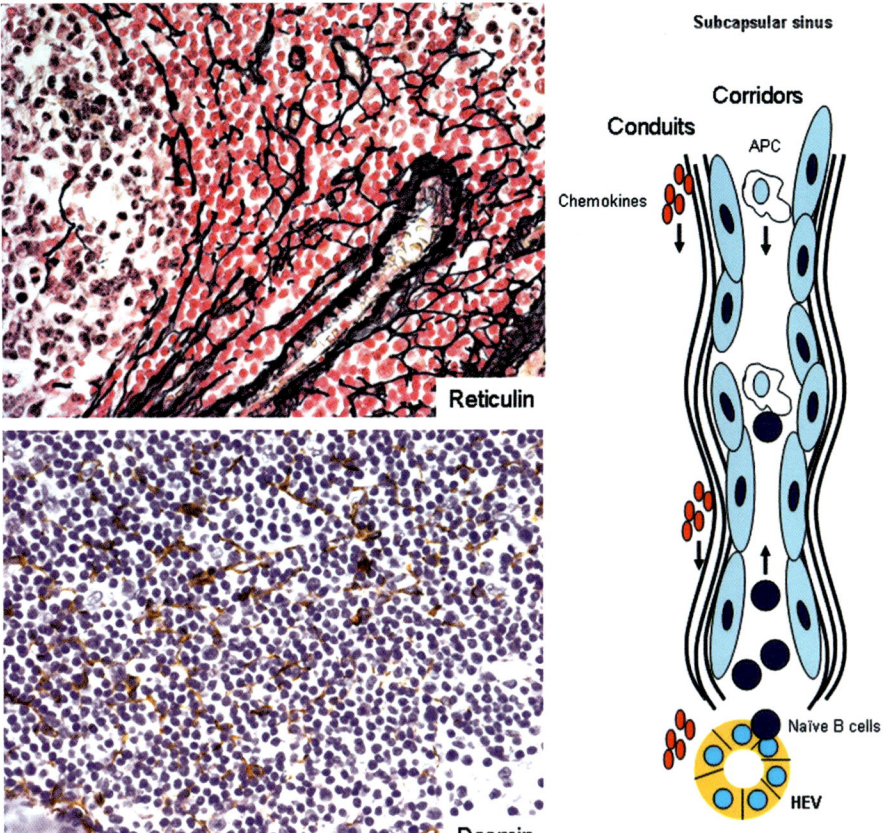

Figure 1-10

T-CELL PARACORTEX

Left: Silver stains (reticulin shown) highlight the reticular fiber network and the "corridors" of the paracortex (upper left). The reticular network is produced and maintained by fibroblastic reticular cells. Fibroblastic reticular cells are variably positive for desmin (lower left) and cytokeratins 8 and 18.

Right: A schematic representation of the "corridors and conduits" of the paracortex.

but can be identified with immunohistochemical studies (fig. 1-10). FRCs have long slender cytoplasmic processes; express cytokeratins 8 and 18, vimentin, smooth muscle actin, and desmin; and form tight junctions with each other.

The connective tissue skeletal network of the lymph node is composed of a thin external fibrous capsule with internal prolongations or trabeculae, and by a complex meshwork of reticular fibers (fig. 1-10). FRCs produce, ensheathe, and maintain this reticular fiber network (15). The network has been conceptualized as a concentric arrangement of nested cylinders or "corridors" lined by FRCs that encircle the HEVs and radiate outwards to the sinuses (15). FRCs form an epithelium-like monolayer separating the corridors from the interstitial reticular matrix (fig. 1-10). The corridors are filled with lymphocytes, and provide spaces for cell trafficking and for antigen-presenting cells and lymphocytes to meet. Another space between FRCs and the basal membrane, termed a "conduit," has been postulated to mediate lymph flow from the sinuses

to the perivascular spaces (24). Cytokines and other soluble substances entering lymph nodes from sites of inflammation through the subcapsular sinuses use these conduits to modulate the adhesive properties of the HEVs and thus allow for entry of lymphocytes into the lymph node.

FRCs participate dynamically in the cytokine microenvironment of the paracortex as well as in the regulation of cell trafficking and access of T cells into the paracortex (2,49,51). FRCs secrete several homeostatic chemokines, such as CCL19, CCL21, and CXCL12, and present on their surface immobilized CCR7 ligands that provide signals to maintain the motility of paracortical naïve T cells.

Plasmacytoid Dendritic Cells. Clusters of plasmacytoid dendritic cells (previously known as plasmacytoid T cells or plasmacytoid monocytes) are occasionally seen in lymph nodes in H&E-stained sections. They are easily identified by immunostains using antibodies against CD68, CD123, CD303, or TCL1 (figs. 1-11, 1-12). The number of plasmacytoid dendritic

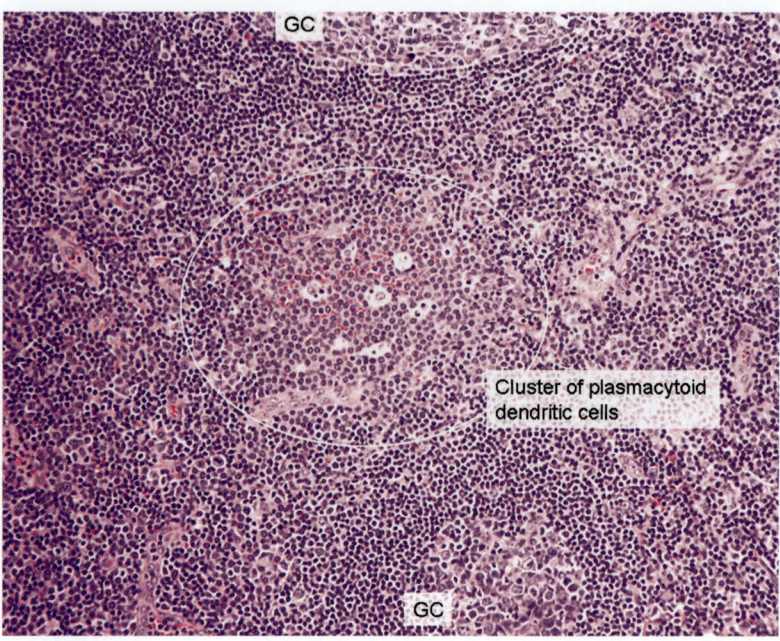

Figure 1-11

**PLASMACYTOID
DENDRITIC CELLS**

Cluster of plasmacytoid dendritic cells between two secondary lymphoid follicles. Scattered tingible body macrophages are admixed with the plasmacytoid dendritic cells.

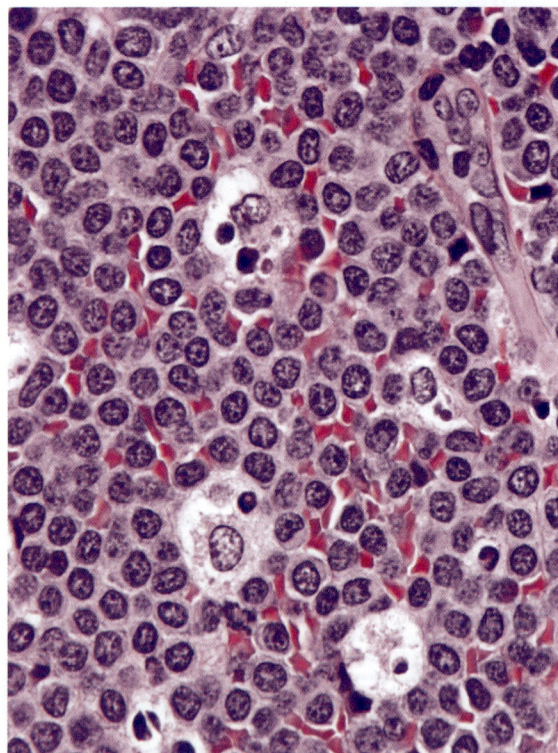

Figure 1-12

PLASMACYTOID DENDRITIC CELLS

High-power magnification of figure 1-10. The plasmacytoid dendritic cells are intermediate to large, with round to oval and slightly eccentrically located nuclei with clumped nuclear chromatin (plasmacytoid appearance). Tingible body macrophages are present.

cells increases in certain inflammatory and neoplastic conditions, for example, hyaline-vascular Castleman disease and Kikuchi-Fujimoto lymphadenopathy (11,17). Plasmacytoid dendritic cells are bone marrow derived, enter lymph nodes through the HEVs, and are a major source of interferon-α.

High Endothelial Venules. HEVs are postcapillary venules located in the paracortex of lymph nodes and other secondary lymphoid organs (except the spleen), specialized for the recruitment of B and T cells into the paracortex. HEVs are lined by unique endothelial cells with distinctive, almost cuboidal morphology, unlike the flat morphology of typical endothelial cells. Experimental data suggest that these morphologic features are a result of continuous but transient accumulation of lymphocytes between the endothelial cells and the underlying basal layer (38). Pockets of four to five lymphocytes are frequently observed underneath endothelial cells of the HEV. The endothelial cells express high levels of sulphated carbohydrate ligands for L-selectin, which can be recognized by the monoclonal antibody MECA-79.

Lymphocyte adhesion to HEV endothelial cells is mediated by vascular addressins expressed by the endothelial cells. These addressins bind to homing receptors, such as L-selectin and α4β2 integrins, expressed on the

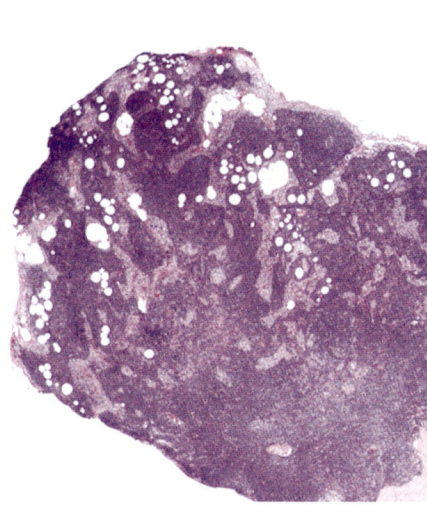

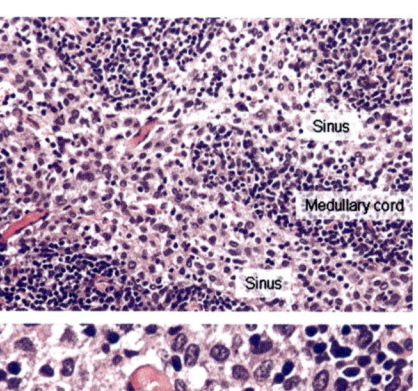

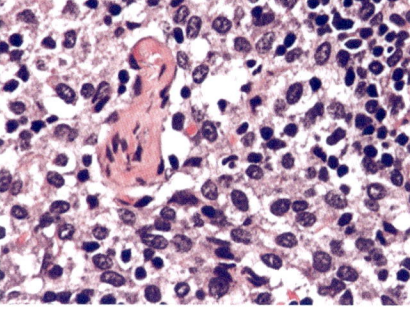

Figure 1-13

MEDULLARY CORDS AND SINUSES

This lymph node biopsy specimen (left) shows predominantly medulla, focal adipose tissue metaplasia, and, in the right lower corner, a small portion of paracortex. The medulla is composed of sinuses and medullary cords (upper and lower right). The sinuses contain macrophages and small lymphocytes.

surface of circulating lymphocytes (6,36). Lymphocyte recruitment by HEVs also is modulated remotely by chemokines produced by FRCs and dendritic cells in the lymph node microenvironment (39,43). Postcapillary venules in other tissues do not express lymphocyte adhesion molecules unless they are stimulated by inflammatory mediators (36). HEVs can develop in nonlymphoid tissues involved by chronic inflammatory diseases or cancer and are associated with high levels of lymphocyte infiltration into these affected tissue sites.

Lymph Node Medulla

The medulla is located in the inner or hilar portion of the lymph node and is composed of cords and sinuses (fig. 1-13). The medullary cords are usually clearly delineated because their dense cellularity contrasts with the sparse cellularity of the surrounding medullary sinuses. The medullary cords contain B cells, T cells, plasma cells, macrophages, mast cells, and dendritic cells. A paired arteriole and venule runs along the central axis of each medullary cord and is surrounded by the FRC network.

Lymph Node Sinuses

The afferent lymphatics contain lymph that drains into the subcapsular sinus. This lymph originates in the interstitial spaces of most of the tissues and contains antigens, APC, chemokines,

and other signaling agents generated by local inflammatory conditions in tissues draining to lymph nodes. The sinuses are the channels that carry lymph from the afferent lymphatics to the efferent lymph vessels at the hilum. There are cortical and medullary sinuses. Most of the cortical sinuses seem to be blunt-ended and are in proximity to HEVs. There are also sinuses, frequently located adjacent to lymphoid follicles, connecting the subcapsular and medullary sinuses.

The sinuses are lined, at least in part, by endothelial cells. There are some differences in the composition and structure of the lining between the subcapsular and medullary sinuses. The floor of the subcapsular sinus is lined by lymphatic endothelial cells interspersed with subcapsular sinus macrophages (CD169 positive). These macrophages have a head that protrudes into the sinus lumens and a long tail of processes that extends into the underlying lymphoid follicles. Sinus macrophages capture large antigens that enter the lymph node through the lymph, and display them to B cells.

In addition to being sites of B-cell encounter with large soluble antigens, the cortical and medullary sinuses are the major gateways for lymphocytes exiting the lymph node. Experimental data show that expansion of cortical and medullary sinuses participates in regulating lymphocyte egress from lymph nodes during prolonged inflammation, providing exit routes

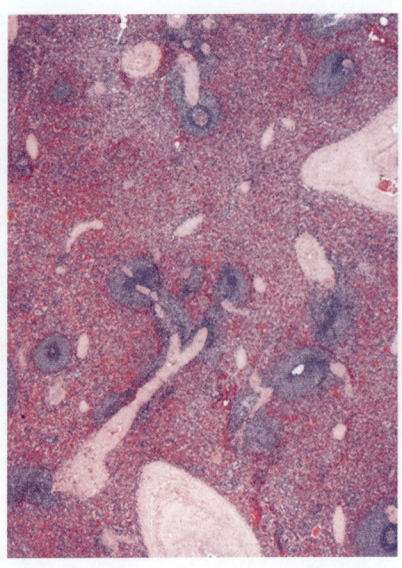 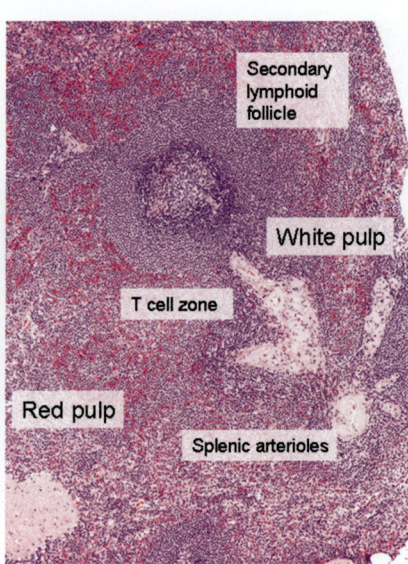

Figure 1-14

SPLEEN SHOWING WHITE AND RED PULP

The white pulp consists of T-cell zones that surround the splenic arterioles (also known as periarteriolar T-cell–rich lymphoid sheets, or PALS) and B-cell follicles (primary or secondary), usually at the periphery of the sheets of T cells.

for lymphocytes (48). Spingosine 1-phosphate (S1P) receptors on endothelial cells lining the sinuses and CD69 on lymphocytes control the passage of lymphocytes into the sinuses to alter exit from the lymph node. The lymphatic system converges onto a single lymphatic vessel, the thoracic duct, which drains the lymph into the bloodstream.

SPLEEN

Gross Anatomy

The spleen is the largest secondary lymphoid organ and is responsible for defense against blood-borne pathogens (the spleen filters the blood as lymph nodes filter lymph). In particular, the spleen has a key role in the removal of encapsulated bacteria. Patients with splenectomy or with splenic dysfunction need routine prophylaxis to prevent *Streptococcus pneumoniae*, *Haemophilus influenzae*, and *Neisseria meningitides* infections. Other relevant functions of the spleen include filtering the blood to remove old or damaged erythrocytes and recycling iron (35). The spleen lacks an afferent lymphatic system, but receives a fair amount of the blood supply, about 5 percent of cardiac output.

The spleen is an elongated, dark red organ, surrounded by a thin capsule of connective tissue. In younger adults, the spleen weights 150 to 250 g, but the size decreases with age. Normally, the spleen is located in the abdomen in the left hypochondrium, attached by the gastrosplenic and

splenorenal ligaments. When these ligaments have not developed properly, the spleen can be aberrantly located in other sites of the abdomen or pelvis (ectopic spleen). Single or multiple accessory spleens are found in about 10 percent of the general population; usually accessory spleens are of small size and located near the hilum of the spleen or the pancreatic tail. Splenosis is the implantation of splenic tissues into the peritoneum (and often throughout the abdomen) following traumatic rupture of the spleen. The spleen has two major distinct compartments, the white pulp and the red pulp (fig. 1-14), with distinctive morphologic features and function.

Microscopic Anatomy

White Pulp. The white pulp is a continuous layer of lymphoid tissue that surrounds the branching splenic arterioles. The white pulp consists of T-cell zones (also known as the periarteriolar lymphoid sheath, or PALS) and B-cell follicles (primary and secondary) (figs. 1-14, 1-15), resembling the organization of the lymph node, except for the apparent absence of HEVs.

The organization of the white pulp is controlled by specific chemokines that attract T and B cells to their specific compartments: B cells are attracted by CXCL13 (produced by FDC and stromal cells) whereas T cells are attracted by CCL19 and CCL21 (mainly produced by stromal cells in the T zone). Lymphoid follicles are frequently observed at the periphery of T-cell aggregates and have histologic and immunophenotypic features identical

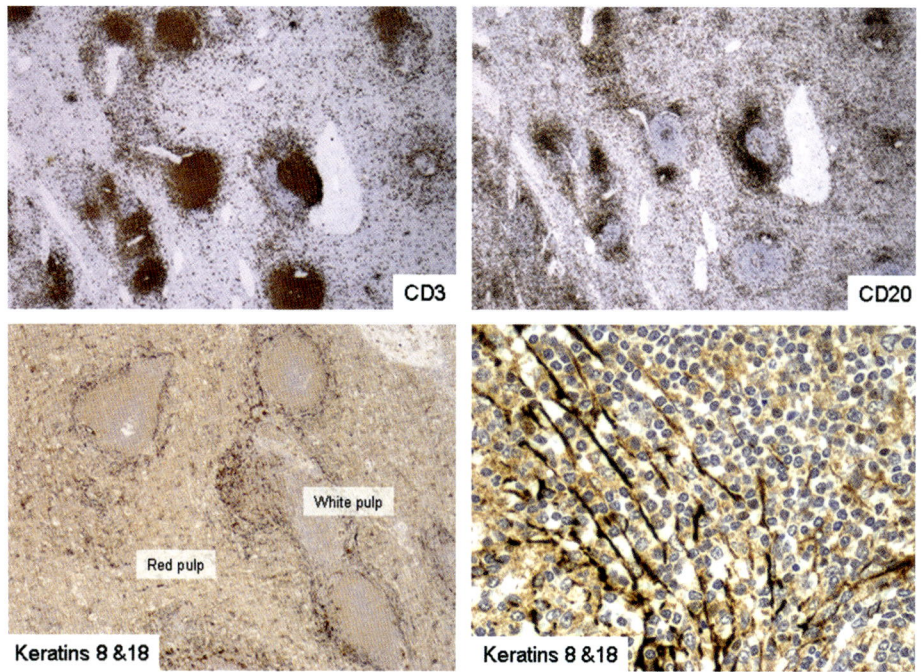

Figure 1-15

SPLEEN: WHITE PULP

CD3 immunostain highlights the T-cell zone that surrounds the splenic arterioles and CD20 immunostain identifies the B-cell compartment, in this case represented mostly by primary follicles. The white pulp contains also a network of fibroblastic reticular cells, highlighted by cytokeratins 8 and 18, which provide the corridors or physical roads for T cells in the white pulp.

Figure 1-16

SPLENIC SECONDARY LYMPHOID FOLLICLE

Splenic secondary lymphoid follicle with a germinal center, mantle zone, and marginal zone. The mantle zone, represented by a thin rim of dark small lymphocytes, surrounds the germinal center. The marginal zone is the corona that surrounds the mantle zone. The marginal zone is composed of medium-sized lymphoid cells with abundant pale cytoplasm and slightly irregular nuclear contours (monocytoid appearance).

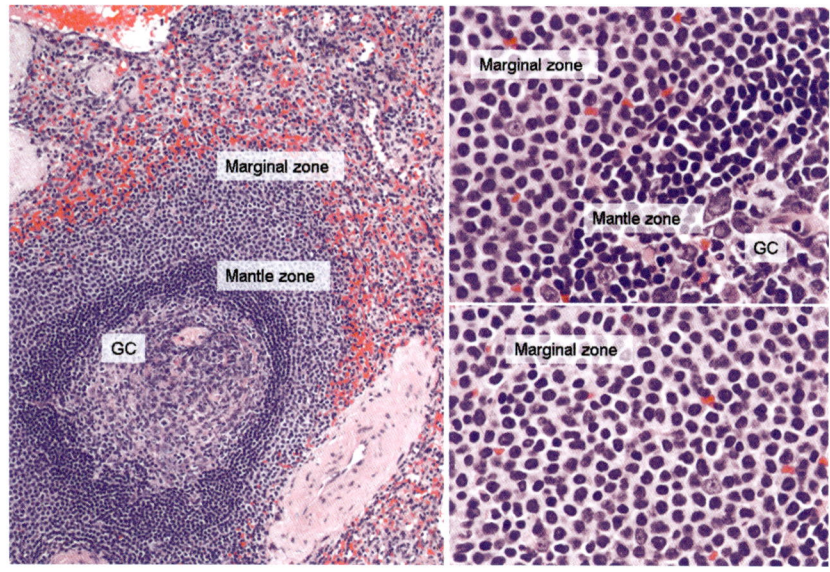

to those of primary and secondary follicles of the lymph node. In splenic lymphoid follicles, the processes described in lymph node secondary follicles also occur, including clonal expansion of activated B cells, somatic hypermutation, and isotype switching. Similar to the lymph node paracortex, the white pulp of the spleen contains a network of FRCs (positive for cytokeratins 8 and 18) that provide physical corridors to the T cells and participate in T-cell distribution within the white pulp (fig. 1-15) (3).

Localized between the white and red pulp is the splenic marginal zone (fig. 1-16) (33). The spleen lacks a marginal zone sinus and the arterioles open in a large perifollicular area, poor in reticulin fibers, located at the outer aspect of the marginal zone. This area is recognized in routine H&E-stained sections by the presence of pools of erythrocytes (fig. 1-17). It has been suggested that blood flow is retarded in this area. In humans, the splenic marginal zone is limited to the follicular compartment and does not extend along the T-cell zone (47).

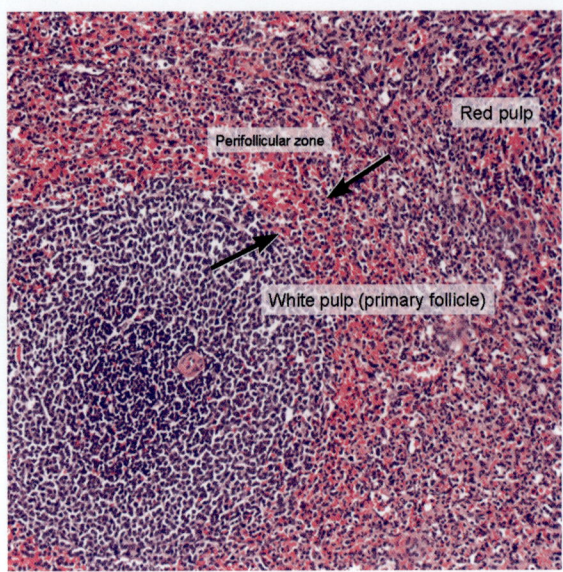

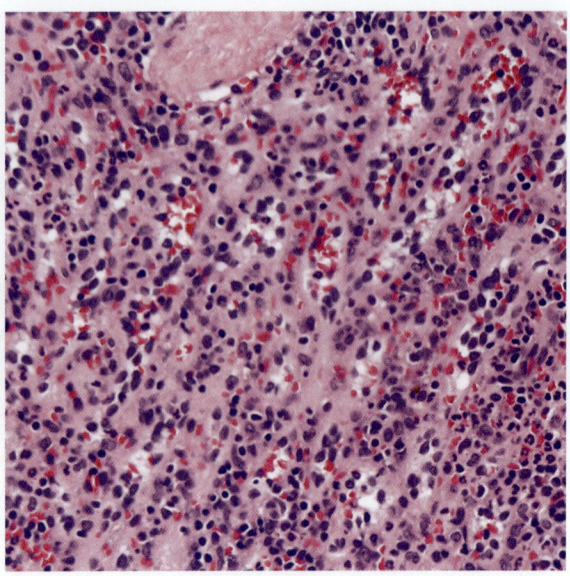

Figure 1-17	**Figure 1-18**
SPLENIC ARTERIOLES	**SPLENIC RED PULP**

In the human spleen, the splenic arterioles open in a perifollicular area, poor in reticulin fibers, located immediately peripheral to the marginal zones where the blood flow seems to be retarded. This area is recognized in routine hematoxylin and eosin (H&E)-stained sections by the presence of a corona of erythrocytes.

The red pulp is composed of a network of cords and venous sinuses. The sinuses are lined by sinusoidal cells that express endothelial markers as well as CD8.

The splenic marginal zone is an important transit area between the bloodstream and white pulp, and is involved in both innate and adaptive immunity. The splenic marginal zone has a specific and distinct cell composition that contains a population of resident macrophages and marginal zone B cells. The macrophages express unique specific receptors, such as the C-type lectin SIGNR1 and the type I scavenger receptor MARCO (macrophage receptor with collagenous structure) (14,25). SIGNR1 binds polysaccharide antigens and participates in the uptake and clearance of *Mycobacterium tuberculosis* and *Streptococcus pneumoniae*. MARCO recognizes many pathogens, including *Escherichia coli* and *Staphylococcus aureus*. In addition to the clearance of encapsulated bacteria, marginal zone macrophages are important for the clearance of viruses. Marginal zone B cells are considered to represent a first line of defense against blood-borne pathogens, particularly encapsulated bacteria. Marginal zone B cells are IgM(+), IgD(+/-), CD21(+), CD23(+/-), CD1c(+), and CD27(+) and seem to represent recirculating IgM-positive memory cells (42).

Red Pulp. The red pulp is the most abundant compartment of the spleen and is composed of a network of cords (about 70 percent) and venous sinuses (about 30 percent) (fig. 1-18) (50). The capillaries open to the splenic cords, which form an open blood system without an endothelial lining and contains reticular fibers, myofibroblasts, plasma cells, plasmablasts, and numerous macrophages that remove old and damaged erythrocytes.

From the cords, blood passes into venous sinuses lined by sinusoidal cells. These sinusoidal cells are positive for endothelial markers such as factor VIII, and are also strongly positive for CD8. A set of stress fibers extending underneath the basal plasma membrane of sinusoidal cells forms slits. These slits are difficult for ageing erythrocytes with stiff membranes to pass through. The blood cells that cannot pass through sinusoidal cells are destroyed by macrophages residing in the cords. As a consequence of cell destruction in the red pulp, pigments such as hemosiderin and lipofuscin (less abundant), accumulate and are frequently observed in the cytoplasm of macrophages.

REFERENCES

1. Allen CD, Ansel KM, Low C, et al. Germinal center dark and light zone organization is mediated by CXCR4 and CXCR5. Nat Immunol 2004;5:943-952.
2. Bajenoff M, Egen JG, Koo LY, et al. Stromal cell networks regulate lymphocyte entry, migration, and territoriality in lymph nodes. Immunity 2006;25:989-1001.
3. Bajenoff M, Glaichenhaus N, Germain RN. Fibroblastic reticular cells guide T lymphocyte entry into and migration within the splenic T cell zone. J Immunol 2008;181:3947-3954.
4. Baumann I, Kolowos W, Voll RE, et al. Impaired uptake of apoptotic cells into tingible body macrophages in germinal centers of patients with systemic lupus erythematosus. Arthritis Rheum 2002;46:191-201.
5. Belisle C, Sainte-Marie G. Blood vascular network of the rat lymph node: tridimensional studies by light and scanning electron microscopy. Am J Anat 1990;189:111-126.
6. Berlin C, Berg EL, Briskin MJ, et al. Alpha 4 beta 7 integrin mediates lymphocyte binding to the mucosal vascular addressin MAdCAM-1. Cell 1993;74:185-195.
7. Camacho SA, Kosco-Vilbois MH, Berek C. The dynamic structure of the germinal center. Immunol Today 1998;19:511-514.
8. Caron G, Le Gallou S, Lamy T, Tarte K, Fest T. CXCR4 expression functionally discriminates centroblasts versus centrocytes within human germinal center B cells. J Immunol 2009;182: 7595-7602.
9. Cyster JG, Ansel KM, Reif K, et al. Follicular stromal cells and lymphocyte homing to follicles. Immunol Rev 2000;176:181-193.
10. Dominguez-Sola D, Victora GD, Ying CY, et al. The proto-oncogene MYC is requried for selection in the germinal center and cyclin reentry. Nat Immunol 2012;13:1083-1091.
11. Facchetti F, de Wolf-Peeters C, van den Oord JJ, de Vos R, Desmet VJ. Plasmacytoid monocytes (so-called plasmacytoid T-cells) in Kikuchi's lymphadenitis. An immunohistologic study. Am J Clin Pathol 1989;92:42-50.
12. Forster R, Davalos-Misslitz AC, Rot A. CCR7 and its ligands: balancing immunity and tolerance. Nat Rev Immunol 2008;8:362-371.
13. Foy TM, Laman JD, Ledbetter JA, Aruffo A, Claassen E, Noelle RJ. gp39-CD40 interactions are essential for germinal center formation and the development of B cell memory. J Exp Med 1994;180:157-163.
14. Geijtenbeek TB, Groot PC, Nolte MA, et al. Marginal zone macrophages express a murine homologue of DC-SIGN that captures blood-borne antigens in vivo. Blood 2002;100:2908-2916.
15. Gretz JE, Anderson AO, Shaw S. Cords, channels, corridors and conduits: critical architectural elements facilitating cell interactions in the lymph node cortex. Immunol Rev 1997;156:11-24.
16. Grouard G, Durand I, Filgueira L, Banchereau J, Liu YJ. Dendritic cells capable of stimulating T cells in germinal centres. Nature 1996;384:364-367.
17. Harris NL, Bhan AK. "Plasmacytoid T cells" in Castleman's disease. Immunohistologic phenotype. Am J Surg Pathol 1987;11:109-113.
18. Hauser AE, Junt T, Mempel TR, et al. Definition of germinal-center B cell migration in vivo reveals predominant intrazonal circulation patterns. Immunity 2007;26:655-667.
19. Haynes NM, Allen CD, Lesley R, Ansel KM, Killeen N, Cyster JG. Role of CXCR5 and CCR7 in follicular Th cell positioning and appearance of a programmed cell death gene-1 high germinal center-associated subpopulation. J Immunol 2007;179:5099-5108.
20. Hu BT, Lee SC, Marin E, Ryan DH, Insel RA. Telomerase is up-regulated in human germinal center B cells in vivo and can be re-expressed in memory B cells activated in vitro. J Immunol 1997;159:1068-1071.
21. Jacob J, Kassir R, Kelsoe G. In situ studies of the primary immune response to (4-hydroxy-3-nitrophenyl)acetyl. I. The architecture and dynamics of responding cell populations. J Exp Med 1991;173:1165-1175.
22. Johnston RJ, Poholek AC, DiToro D, et al. Bcl6 and Blimp-1 are reciprocal and antagonistic regulators of T follicular helper cell differentiation. Science 2009;325:1006-1010.
23. Jones D. Dismantling the germinal center: comparing the processes of transformation, regression, and fragmentation of the lymphoid follicle. Adv Anat Pathol 2002;9:129-138.
24. Kaldjian EP, Gretz JE, Anderson AO, Shi Y, Shaw S. Spatial and molecular organization of lymph node T cell cortex: a labyrinthine cavity bounded by an epithelium-like monolayer of fibroblastic reticular cells anchored to basement membrane-like extracellular matrix. Int Immunol 2001;13:1243-1253.
25. Kang YS, Kim JY, Bruening SA, et al. The C-type lectin SIGN-R1 mediates uptake of the capsular polysaccharide of Streptococcus pneumoniae in the marginal zone of mouse spleen. Proc Natl Acad Sci U S A 2004;101:215-220.
26. Kelly RH. Functional anatomy of lymph nodes. I. The paracortical cords. Int Arch Allergy Appl Immunol 1975;48:836-849.

27. Kim CH, Rott LS, Clark-Lewis I, Campbell DJ, Wu L, Butcher EC. Subspecialization of CXCR5+ T cells: B helper activity is focused in a germinal center-localized subset of CXCR5+ T cells. J Exp Med 2001;193:1373-1381.

28. Klein U, Dalla-Favera R. Germinal centres: role in B-cell physiology and malignancy. Nat Rev Immunol 2008;8:22-33.

29. Kolar GR, Mehta D, Pelayo R, Capra JD. A novel human B cell subpopulation representing the initial germinal center population to express AID. Blood 2007;109:2545-2552.

30. Koopman G, Parmentier HK, Schuurman HJ, Newman W, Meijer CJ, Pals ST. Adhesion of human B cells to follicular dendritic cells involves both the lymphocyte function-associated antigen 1/intercellular adhesion molecule 1 and very late antigen 4/vascular cell adhesion molecule 1 pathways. J Exp Med 1991;173:1297-1304.

31. Kroese FG, Timens W, Nieuwenhuis P. Germinal center reaction and B lymphocytes: morphology and function. Curr Top Pathol 1990;84(Pt 1):103-148.

32. Kuppers R, Zhao M, Hansmann ML, Rajewsky K. Tracing B cell development in human germinal centres by molecular analysis of single cells picked from histological sections. EMBO J 1993;12:4955-4967.

33. Lyons AB, Parish CR. Are murine marginal-zone macrophages the splenic white pulp analog of high endothelial venules? Eur J Immunol 1995;25:3165-3172.

34. MacLennan IC. Germinal centers. Annu Rev Immunol 1994;12:117-139.

35. Mebius RE, Kraal G. Structure and function of the spleen. Nat Rev Immunol 2005;5:606-616.

36. Michie SA, Streeter PR, Bolt PA, Butcher EC, Picker LJ. The human peripheral lymph node vascular addressin. An inducible endothelial antigen involved in lymphocyte homing. Am J Pathol 1993;143:1688-1698.

37. Millikin PD. Anatomy of germinal centers in human lymphoid tissue. Arch Pathol 1966;82:499-505.

38. Mionnet C, Sanos SL, Mondor I, et al. High endothelial venules as traffic control points maintaining lymphocyte population homeostasis in lymph nodes. Blood 2011;118:6115-6122.

39. Moussion C, Girard JP. Dendritic cells control lymphocyte entry to lymph nodes through high endothelial venules. Nature 2011;479:542-546.

40. Okada T, Miller MJ, Parker I, et al. Antigen-engaged B cells undergo chemotaxis toward the T zone and form motile conjugates with helper T cells. PLoS Biol 2005;3:e150.

41. Pasqualucci L, Guglielmino R, Houldsworth J, et al. Expression of the AID protein in normal and neoplastic B cells. Blood 2004;104:3318-3325.

42. Pillai S, Cariappa A, Moran ST. Marginal zone B cells. Annu Rev Immunol 2005;23:161-196.

43. Rot A. In situ binding assay for studying chemokine interactions with endothelial cells. J Immunol Methods 2003;273:63-71.

44. Sacedon R, Diez B, Nunez V, et al. Sonic hedgehog is produced by follicular dendritic cells and protects germinal center B cells from apoptosis. J Immunol 2005;174:1456-1461.

45. Schwickert TA, Lindquist RL, Shakhar G, et al. In vivo imaging of germinal centres reveals a dynamic open structure. Nature 2007;446:83-87.

46. Shulman Z, Gitlin AD, Targ S, et al. T follicular helper cell dynamics in germinal centers. Science 2013;341:673-677.

47. Steiniger B, Timphus EM, Barth PJ. The splenic marginal zone in humans and rodents: an enigmatic compartment and its inhabitants. Histochem Cell Biol 2006;126:641-648.

48. Tan KW, Yeo KP, Wong FH, et al. Expansion of cortical and medullary sinuses restrains lymph node hypertrophy during prolonged inflammation. J Immunol 2012;188:4065-4080.

49. Thomazy VA, Vega F, Medeiros LJ, Davies PJ, Jones D. Phenotypic modulation of the stromal reticular network in normal and neoplastic lymph nodes: tissue transglutaminase reveals coordinate regulation of multiple cell types. Am J Pathol 2003;163:165-174.

50. van Krieken JH, Te Velde J, Hermans J, Welvaart K. The splenic red pulp; a histomorphometrical study in splenectomy specimens embedded in methylmethacrylate. Histopathology 1985;9:401-416.

51. Vega F, Coombes KR, Thomazy VA, Patel K, Lang W, Jones D. Tissue-specific function of lymph node fibroblastic reticulum cells. Pathobiology 2006;73:71-81.

52. Victora GD, Nussenzweig MC. Germinal centers. Annu Rev Immunol 2012;30:429-457.

53. Victora GD, Schwickert TA, Fooksman DR, et al. Germinal center dynamics revealed by multiphoton microscopy with a photoactivatable fluorescent reporter. Cell 2010;143:592-605.

54. Willard-Mack CL. Normal structure, function, and histology of lymph nodes. Toxicol Pathol 2006;34:409-424.

2 PROCESSING LYMPH NODE AND SPLEEN SPECIMENS

EXCISIONAL BIOPSY VERSUS NEEDLE BIOPSY

In recent years, there has been an increasing tendency to avoid excisional lymph node biopsy and, instead, perform core needle biopsy with or without fine-needle aspiration (FNA). Core needle biopsy and FNA are highly useful, complimentary techniques that are indicated when performing an excisional lymph node biopsy would be hazardous, for example, in a patient with difficult to access lymph nodes (see chapter 3). When needle biopsy and cytologic smear morphologic findings are integrated with immunophenotypic features and, in some cases, cytogenetic and/or molecular data, many lymphoma diagnoses can be established. In some circumstances, however, these specimen types are inadequate for diagnosis (42). This is attributable to the small size of specimens, which precludes assessment of the architecture, and sampling error. These limitations make it difficult to establish the diagnosis of some types of lymphoma (e.g., nodular lymphocyte-predominant Hodgkin lymphoma versus T-cell/histiocyte-rich large B-cell lymphoma). Therefore, excisional biopsy of an intact lymph node remains the procedure of choice for evaluating a patient with suspected lymphoma and the pathologist should not hesitate to defer diagnosis and request an excisional biopsy if core needle biopsy or FNA are insufficient to establish a clinically useful diagnosis.

GROSS EVALUATION

Lymph nodes, spleen, and other types of extranodal specimens involved by hematopoietic tumors should be received intact, fresh, and unfixed. The pathologist should be notified at the time of the surgical excision to avoid a delay in the handling of the specimen. In many centers, it is most convenient to do initial specimen assessment in the frozen section room. Lymph nodes should be measured and cut in approximately 2- to 3-mm slices perpendicular to the long axis. This orientation provides the best assessment of the nodal architecture. Large lymph nodes should be bisected and further sectioned into 2- to 3-mm slices. The gross appearance of the cut surface should be recorded including color, nodularity, and the presence of necrosis.

A splenectomy specimen should be measured and weighed, and a search for hilar lymph nodes is mandatory. A spleen should be sectioned in 5-mm intervals, or if very large, 1-cm intervals, searching for grossly identifiable lesions. When a delay in the processing of a specimen cannot be avoided, lymph node and spleen specimens can be maintained at 4°C for a few hours.

Determining the adequacy of a specimen for diagnosis and dividing the specimen to provide tissue for various ancillary studies are essential as part of the initial evaluation. Traditionally, an excisional lymph node biopsy specimen is examined by frozen section and preparation of touch imprints of the cut surface of the specimen are helpful in informing these decisions. A frozen section is most useful for assessing the architecture of the specimen, but cytologic features are somewhat compromised by this technique. Frozen sections are stained with hematoxylin and eosin (H&E), although other stains can be used. Touch imprints greatly facilitate the appreciation of the cytologic features of the cell population(s). It is essential that imprints to be stained with H&E or Papanicolaou be fixed immediately to avoid air-drying artifact. By contrast, imprints for Romanowsky stains, such as Wright-Giemsa or Diff-Quik (fig. 2-1), must be completely air-dried before staining to avoid staining artifacts. Morphologic examination of stained imprints can facilitate the recognition of dysplasia for suspected myeloid neoplasms and Wright-Giemsa or Diff-Quik stains are helpful for highlighting eosinophils, basophils, and mast cells. Imprints also can be used for cytochemistry (e.g., myeloperoxidase) and are suitable for fluorescence in situ hybridization (FISH) analysis since cells with whole nuclei lie on the slide surface. Imprints can be stored at -70 C° for future use.

It must be emphasized, however, that the traditional frozen section approach cannot be used for needle biopsy specimens as the specimen is small and tissue needs to be conserved. In this circumstance, the clinical history and the results of fine-needle aspiration (if performed in the past) can inform the triage process.

If an infectious process is suspected, fresh tissue should be sent for microbiologic studies and special stains for organisms (e.g., acid fast or methenamine silver) ordered. If lymphoma is suspected, a cell suspension can be prepared from a portion of the lymph node and sent for flow cytometry immunophenotypic analysis, with the results often available the same day. Additional portions of the specimen can be sent for conventional cytogenetic analysis and molecular analysis, if indicated. If the specimen is sufficient, saving a portion in a tumor bank is valuable in the event that other testing is needed in the future.

As important as all of these ancillary tests are, it is essential that adequate specimen is submitted for histologic examination. If a surgical specimen is composed of multiple lymph nodes, all lymph nodes should be submitted for histologic examination. For splenectomy specimens, representative sections of the gross lesion as well as sections of uninvolved spleen and hilar lymph nodes should be submitted for histologic examination.

FIXATION AND ROUTINE HISTOLOGIC STAINS

The preparation of high-quality histologic sections is essential for the interpretation of morphologic findings and for reliable immunohistochemical results. Poor fixation is the leading cause of uninterpretable tissue sections of lymph node and spleen specimens. Poor fixation can also compromise molecular results for assays designed to assess fixed, paraffin-embedded tissue.

Lymph nodes and spleen are usually fixed in 10 percent neutral buffered formalin. Neutral buffered formalin is inexpensive, provides good

morphologic preservation, and can be used for immunohistochemical and polymerase chain reaction (PCR)-based molecular studies. Buffered formalin is also adequate for long-term storage of fixed tissue. A variety of other fixatives can be used. Some fixatives (Zenker, B5) provide excellent morphologic preservation and facilitate assessment of nuclear detail, but compromise the efficiency of using some ancillary techniques, for example, PCR.

After fixation, lymph node and spleen sections are embedded in paraffin and cut on a microtome at not more than 4-µm thickness; sections of 5-µm or greater thickness compromise morphologic and immunohistochemical analysis. Lymph node and spleen sections are most often stained with H&E, which is the stain used most often for the morphologic assessment of lymphomas (fig. 2-1). In Europe, the Giemsa stain is commonly used for evaluating the morphologic features of lymph node biopsy specimens. Giemsa is a metachromatic stain which provides good nuclear detail and distinguishes the cytoplasm of centroblasts from immunoblasts. The Giemsa stain also highlights mast cells. The periodic acid–Schiff (PAS) reaction, often combined with diastase digestion, is helpful for assessing the spleen since it highlights the red pulp architecture.

The role of "old fashioned" special stains in the diagnosis of lymphomas has diminished over time and these stains are currently used infrequently because they have been mostly replaced by immunohistochemical methods. Stains that were used frequently to evaluate lymph nodes in the past, and which still can be helpful in certain scenarios, include a reticulin stain to assess overall architecture, the metachromatic stain toluidine blue, napthol-ASD-chloroacetate esterase which highlights myeloid precursors and mast cells, and methyl green-pyronin which highlights plasma cells.

IMMUNOPHENOTYPIC ANALYSIS

Immunophenotypic information is important not only for establishing a diagnosis of lymphoma but for determining cell lineage, which is essential for lymphoma classification. There are two major methods routinely used to immunophenotype lymphomas, immunohistochemistry and flow cytometry.

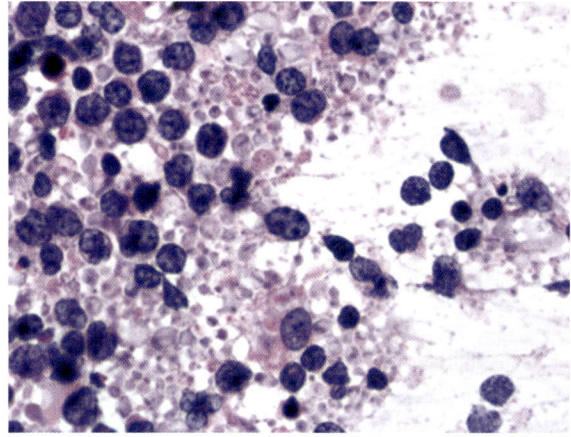

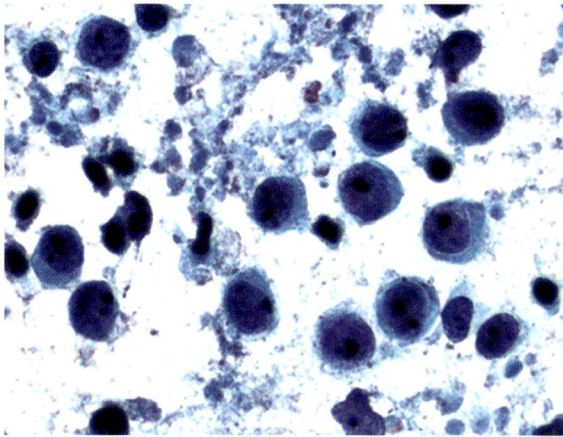

Figure 2-1

DIFFUSE LARGE B-CELL LYMPHOMA (DLBCL)

Top: Hematoxylin and eosin (H&E) stain of touch imprint shows medium to large lymphoid cells, some with small nucleoli close to the nuclear membrane. A few cleaved cells are also seen.

Bottom: Large lymphoid cells with central nucleoli and a plasmacytoid appearance in touch imprint.

Immunohistochemistry

Immunohistochemistry refers to the process of detecting antigens in cells present in a tissue section by exploiting the principle of specific antibody-antigen binding (44). Many of the relevant antigens for the diagnosis of lymphoma are designated by a cluster of differentiation (CD) number. The CD nomenclature was proposed and established at the 1st International Workshop and Conference on Human Leukocyte Differentiation Antigens, which was held in Paris in 1982 (5). This system was intended for the classification of the many monoclonal antibod-

ies (mAbs) generated by different laboratories around the world against epitopes of leukocyte surface molecules. The CD nomenclature since has been expanded to many other cell types, and over 300 unique CDs have been identified. The proposed surface molecule is assigned a CD number once two specific mAbs are shown to bind to the molecule. For an antigen that is not well-characterized, or if there is only one known mAb that reacts with the antigen, a CD number is usually further specified by using the provisional indicator "w" (meaning workshop).

Immunohistochemistry can be performed using frozen or routinely processed tissue sections as well as smears (44). The number of antigens that can be detected by this method is theoretically innumerable, as any substance that is antigenic and whose antigenicity is retained in tissue sections can be demonstrated by immunohistochemical methods. In addition, the number of antibodies reactive in routinely processed tissue sections has progressively increased in the past 20 years. Some of the most relevant antibodies that are used in fixed, paraffin-embedded tissue sections for the diagnosis of lymphomas are discussed here.

CD20. This is a pan-B-cell antigen expressed by most B-cell lymphomas and a small subset of plasma cell neoplasms. CD20 is important for establishing B-cell lineage. Rare T-cell lymphomas express CD20. CD20 is expressed on mature and late pre-B cells (expressed after CD19 and CD10 but before cytoplasmic µ chain) but not in mature plasma cells. CD20 expression can be lost after immunotherapy using anti-CD20 antibodies (rituximab).

Paired Box Protein 5 (PAX5). This is a transcription factor, also known as B-cell-specific activator protein (BSAP), required for the rearrangement of immunoglobulin (Ig)H-variable gene segments and for commitment and maintenance of B-cell differentiation. PAX5 is useful for demonstrating B-cell lineage. The tumor cells of classic Hodgkin lymphoma usually express PAX5 in the nuclei more weakly than the reactive B cells (fig. 2-2). PAX5 expression is not affected by rituximab therapy.

CD3. This is a pan-T-cell marker expressed by most mature T-cell lymphomas and a subset of immature T-cell lymphomas. Surface CD3 expression is the most specific T-cell marker, although

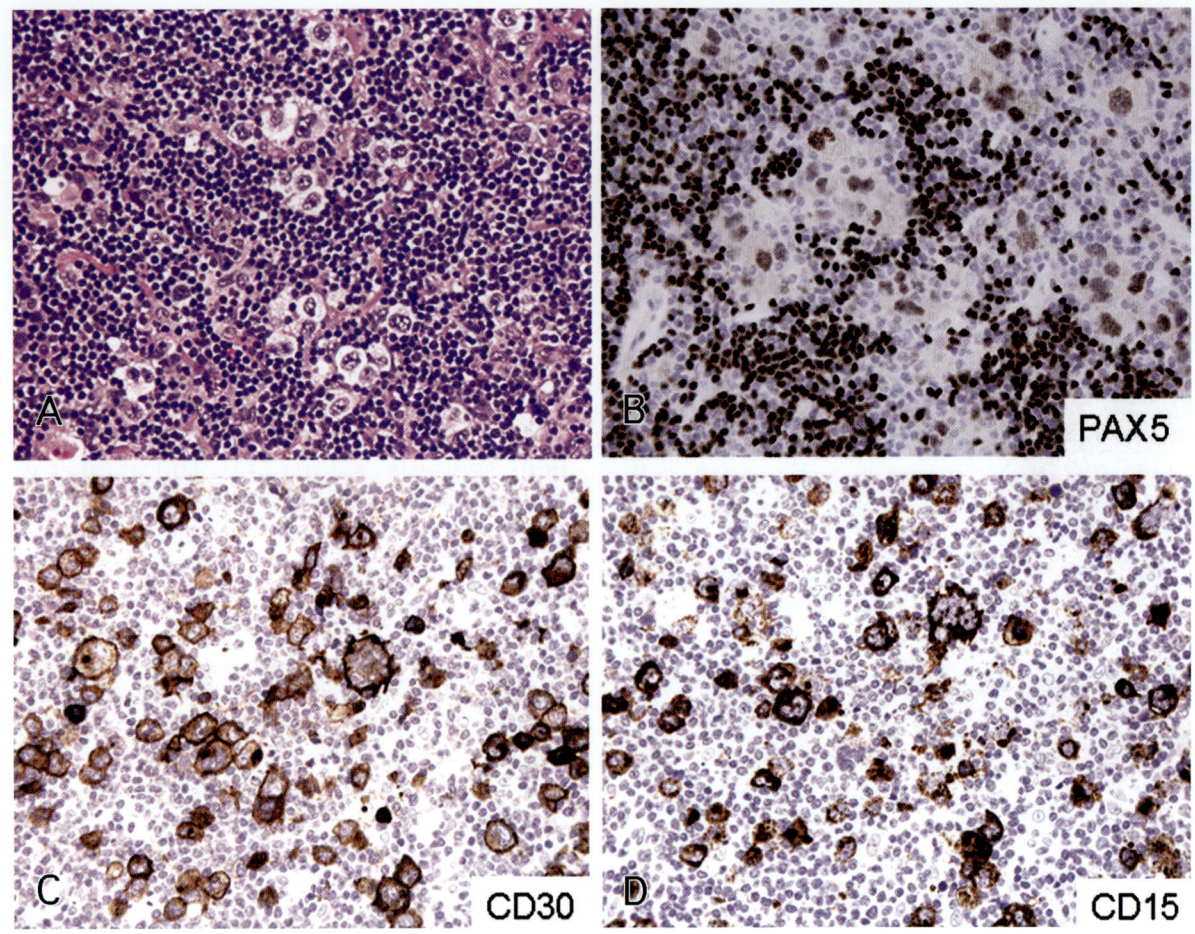

Figure 2-2

HODGKIN LYMPHOMA

A: Excisional biopsy of a lymph node shows scattered, large atypical lymphoid cells consistent with Hodgkin and Reed-Sternberg cells admixed with inflammatory cells.

B–D: Immunohistochemical studies confirmed the diagnosis of classic Hodgkin lymphoma. The tumor cells are weakly positive for PAX5, CD30, and CD15 (hematoxylin and eosin [H&E] stain).

it is expressed very rarely by other hematopoietic neoplasms. Cytoplasmic CD3 is more sensitive than surface expression, but cytoplasmic CD3 is less specific and is expressed by the cells of extranodal natural killer (NK)/T-cell lymphoma and infrequent B-cell lymphomas and plasma cell neoplasms. In addition, aberrant T-cell antigen expression by Reed-Sternberg and Hodgkin cells of classic Hodgkin lymphoma, including CD3, can occur in 10 to 15 percent of cases.

CD5. This T-cell marker is also often expressed dimly by NK cells and by a small subset of normal B cells in the mantle zones of follicles. CD5 is expressed by most mature and immature T-cell lymphomas, but hepatosplenic T-cell lymphoma

and enteropathy-associated T-cell lymphoma are characteristically negative. CD5 is also expressed in a subset of B-cell lymphomas including chronic lymphocytic leukemia/small lymphocytic lymphoma (CLL/SLL), mantle cell lymphoma, and about 5 percent of diffuse large B-cell lymphomas. CD5 is often included in the antibody panel used to classify small B-cell proliferations.

Cyclin D1. Cyclin D1 is a regulator of cell cycle progression from the G1 to S phase. Almost all mantle cell lymphomas are positive for cyclin D1 (fig. 2-3). Other lymphomas also may express cyclin D1, including less than 5 percent of diffuse large B-cell lymphomas (usually variable or focal), approximately half of hairy cell leukemia

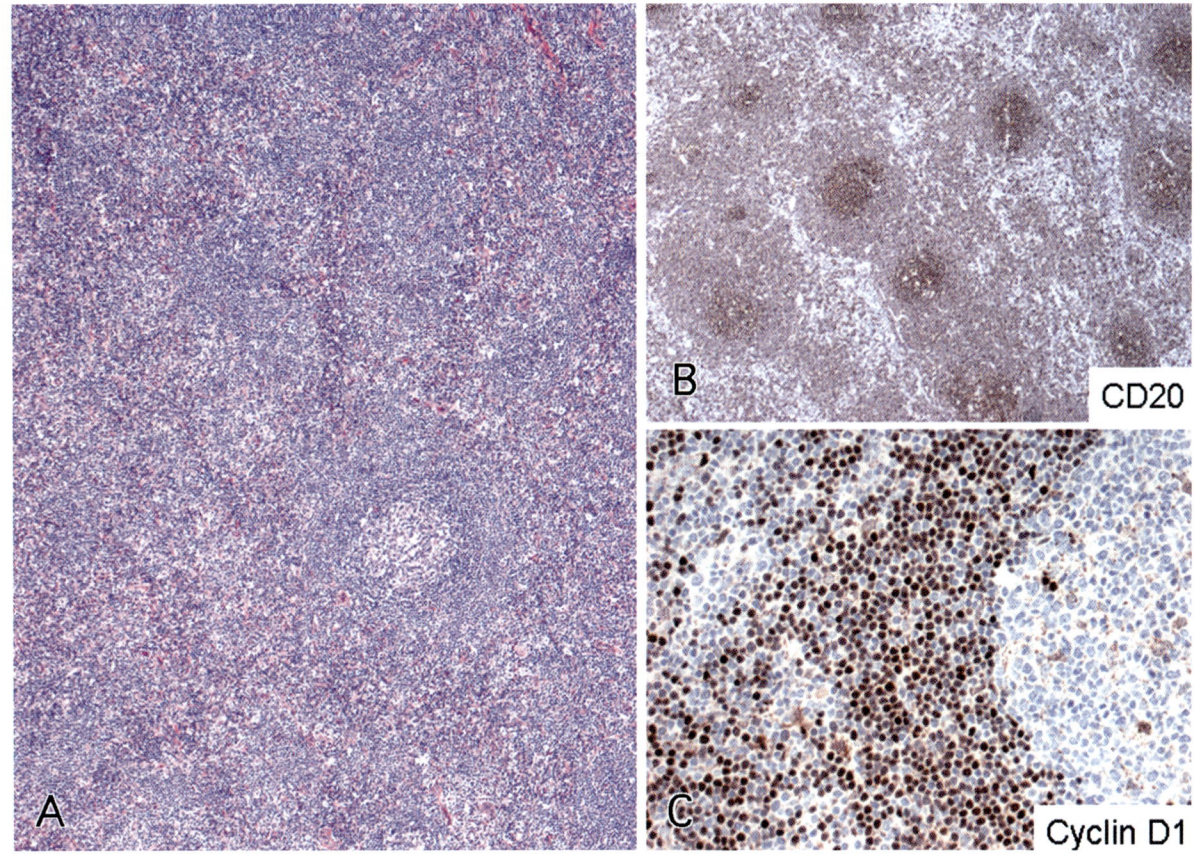

Figure 2-3

MANTLE CELL LYMPHOMA

A: This excisional biopsy lymph node specimen shows lymph nodes with expanded mantle zones.

B,C: Immunohistochemical studies confirmed that the mantle zones are expanded by a population of B cells positive for CD20 and cyclin D1. The germinal center cells express CD20 more strongly than the neoplastic cells. These findings are diagnostic of mantle cell lymphoma.

cases (usually weak), and a third of plasma cell myelomas, most strongly in cases with t(11;14) (q13;q32) or trisomy 11. Cyclin D1 expression has been described in a subset of cells within the proliferation centers of 10 to 20 percent of cases of CLL/SLL (15).

CD30. CD30 is a transmembrane glycoprotein of the tumor necrosis factor (TNF) receptor family. Uniform and bright CD30 expression is characteristic of Reed-Sternberg and Hodgkin cells of classic Hodgkin lymphoma (fig. 2-2) and anaplastic large cell lymphoma, and therefore, is an important marker of these neoplasms. CD30 is also expressed in approximately 10 to 15 percent of diffuse large B-cell lymphoma (with and without anaplastic features), follicular lymphoma (often a small subset of cells), and in a large

number of nonlymphoid malignant neoplasms including carcinomas. CD30 is emerging as an important target for monoclonal antibody therapy in patients with CD30-positive malignancies.

CD10. CD10 is a 100-kDa cell surface metalloendopeptidase, known as common acute lymphoblastic leukemia antigen (CALLA). CD10 is expressed in immature and mature lymphoid neoplasms, including B- and T-lymphoblastic lymphoma, follicular lymphoma, diffuse large B-cell lymphoma with a germinal center immunophenotype, Burkitt lymphoma, angioimmunoblastic T-cell lymphoma (AILT), and rarely, other T-cell lymphomas (38).

BCL2 (B-Cell Lymphoma 2). BCL2 is frequently expressed in malignant lymphomas including approximately half of diffuse large

B-cell lymphomas. About 80 percent of follicular lymphomas express BCL2, whereas reactive germinal center B cells do not, making BCL2 useful for distinguishing follicular lymphoma from reactive follicular hyperplasia. A subset of follicular lymphomas, including pediatric-type nodal follicular lymphoma and some extranodal follicular lymphomas, are BCL2 negative (33). BCL2 is characteristically negative in Burkitt lymphoma.

Ki-67. Ki-67 is a nuclear protein associated with cellular proliferation and expressed in all phases of the cell cycle except G0 (53). In Burkitt lymphoma, virtually all the neoplastic cells are uniformly and strongly positive for Ki-67; this pattern, although uncommon, can occur in diffuse large B-cell lymphoma. Ki-67 may help distinguish follicular hyperplasia from follicular lymphoma, since follicular hyperplasia shows a high proliferation rate and Ki-67 highlights the polarization of light and dark zones. Low-grade follicular lymphomas usually have a low Ki-67 index and follicle polarization is not highlighted.

Flow Cytometry

Flow cytometry immunophenotypic analysis quantifies various cellular parameters as a suspension of cells flows through a laser at an appropriate wavelength (22,70). The sample is incubated with antibodies of interest, followed by washing, fixation, and analysis. The antibodies are conjugated with fluorochromes that are excited by laser(s) in the flow cytometer. Flow cytometry immunophenotyping can detect a vast number of cell surface antigens, including pan-B and pan-T markers, markers of B and T subsets, and markers associated with other leukocytes including granulocytes, monocytes, histiocytes, basophils, and mast cells. For antigens located within the cell cytoplasm (BCL2, cIgM) or nuclear antigens (TdT, Ki-67) cells have to be permeabilized before flow cytometry can be performed.

Flow cytometry immunophenotyping is a useful tool for the diagnosis and classification of nodal and extranodal lymphomas (figs. 2-4, 2-5) and can also assist in supporting the absence of lymphoma (11,13,70). The use of multiple fluorochromes allows the assessment of multiple antigens simultaneously, allowing greater discrimination between various cell populations present simultaneously, and thus flow cytom-

etry can be used for the detection of minimal residual disease, allowing for monitoring the response to therapy and for documenting disease relapse or progression (12). The turnaround time of flow cytometry is much less than that of immunohistochemistry, and flow cytometry can analyze thousands of cells within seconds. Flow cytometry immunophenotyping has higher sensitivity than immunohistochemistry and therefore antigens negative by immunohistochemistry may be detected by flow cytometry (usually dim expression).

A disadvantage of using flow cytometry is the need for a liquid cell suspension and therefore morphologic features cannot be correlated with immunophenotype. Some lymphomas characterized by a low number of tumor cells, i.e., classic Hodgkin lymphoma or T-cell/histiocyte-rich large B-cell lymphoma, are difficult to detect by conventional flow cytometry immunophenotyping. In addition, some antibodies that work well in paraffin tissue sections and are frequently used for the diagnosis of malignant lymphomas, such as cyclin D1, are difficult to detect reliably using flow cytometry.

When a specimen is received for flow cytometry immunophenotyping, a decision must be made regarding the panel of antibodies to be employed, and this decision is based on medical information, suspected diagnosis, clinical history, and the results of other laboratory tests. In low volume laboratories, a single "scout" tube containing B-, T-, and myeloid cell antibodies can be used to direct selection of an optimal antibody panel. Flow cytometry immunophenotypic analysis usually involves a process of cell gating, which selects the cell subsets of interest. For example, if a B-cell lymphoma is suspected, B cells can be gated by focusing on CD19-positive cells (figs. 2-4, 2-5). If a T/NK-cell lymphoma is suspected, cells can be gated for analysis using CD3 expression. Once the gate is established, expression levels of a series of other antigens are evaluated. This approach allows the antigenic signature of the tumor cells to be determined and immunophenotypic aberrancies detected that are helpful for classifying the lymphoma. Examples of immunophenotypic aberrancies include: expression of antigen(s) not usually present in a particular cell lineage (e.g., CD5 or CD43 expression by B-cell lymphomas),

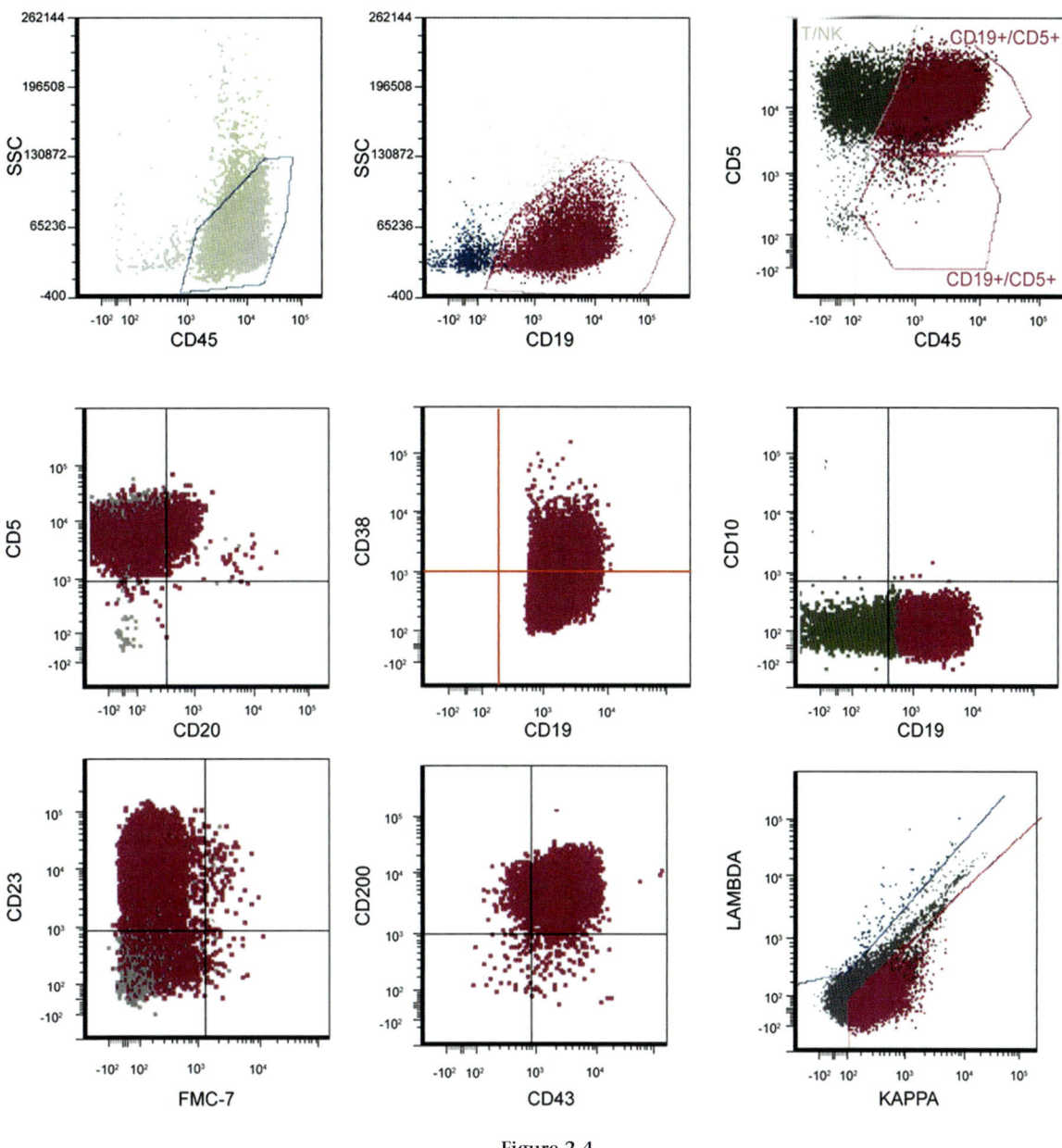

Figure 2-4

CHRONIC LYMPHOCYTIC LEUKEMIA/SMALL LYMPHOCYTIC LYMPHOMA

By flow cytometry, the tumor cells of the lymph node express CD5, CD19, CD23, CD43, and CD200, and weakly express surface immunoglobulin kappa. There is the dim expression of CD20 with partial expression of CD38.

absence (or loss) of antigen(s) usually expressed by a certain cell lineage (e.g., absence of CD3 in T-cell lymphomas), and levels of antigen expression that are lower or higher than normal levels for a cell lineage (e.g., dim CD20 in CLL/SLL or bright CD20 in marginal zone lymphomas).

In addition to pan-B-cell markers and immunoglobulin light chains, expression of other an-

tigens is useful for classifying B-cell lymphomas including: CD5, CD10, CD23, CD25, FMC-7, CD123, and CD200. B-cell lymphomas that are CD5-positive and CD10-negative include CLL/SLL (fig. 2-3), mantle cell lymphoma, a subset of diffuse large B-cell lymphoma, and small subsets of marginal zone lymphoma and lymphoplasmacytic lymphoma. CLL/SLL is a B-cell neoplasm

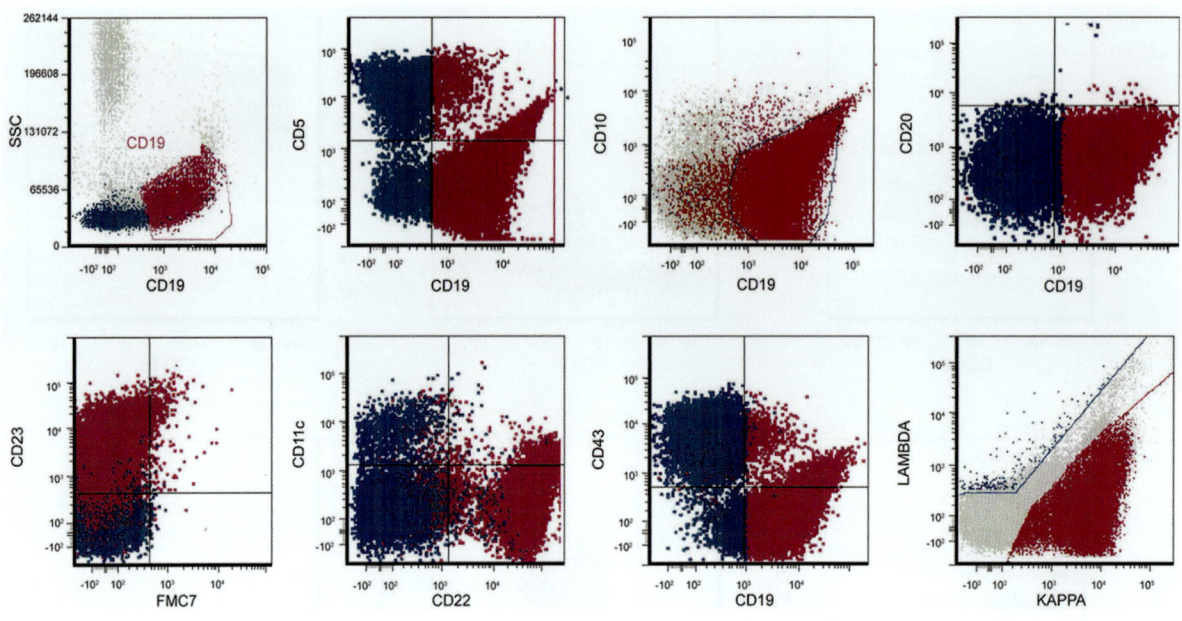

Figure 2-5

SPLENIC MARGINAL ZONE LYMPHOMA

The lymphoma cells express CD19, CD20, CD22, CD23, and surface immunoglobulin kappa light chain. The lymphoma cells are negative for CD5, CD10, CD11c, CD20, CD43, and FMC-7. This patient was previously treated with rituximab.

characterized by the expression of CD23 and CD200 and the absence of FMC-7 (fig. 2-4). Mantle cell lymphoma is also a B-cell neoplasm that is CD5-positive, but usually negative for CD23 and CD200. CD123 and CD25 are useful for the diagnosis of hairy cell leukemia and CD10 expression is frequently present in follicular lymphoma and diffuse large B-cell lymphoma with a germinal center cell immunophenotype. Splenic marginal zone lymphoma is usually positive for pan-B-cell antigens and monotypic surface immunoglobulin light chain, and negative for cyclin D1, CD10, and CD43 (fig. 2-4).

Antibodies frequently used for the diagnosis of T/NK-cell lymphomas include reagents specific for: CD2, CD3, CD4, CD5, CD7, CD8, CD10, CD16, CD25, CD56, CD57, TCRα/β, and TCRγ/δ (6,70). Expression of TdT is useful as it is characteristically expressed by immature tumors such T-lymphoblastic lymphoma. Flow cytometric immunophenotypic analysis helps in establishing the diagnosis of T-cell lymphomas by detecting aberrant expression (complete loss, altered expression levels) of some of the above markers. Approximately one third of T-cell lymphomas aberrantly do not express

(or have "lost" or "deleted") at least one pan-T-cell antigen. Some T-cell lymphomas have a distinctive immunophenotype, for example, the tumor cells of hepatosplenic T-cell lymphoma are usually positive for CD56 and TCRγ/δ and negative for CD4, CD5, and CD57 (61). T-cell large granular lymphocytic leukemia is usually positive for CD8, CD16, and CD57, and is negative for CD56, with dim or absent CD5 expression. Expression of CD10 is a common feature of angioimmunoblastic T-cell lymphoma (38). High expression of CD25 (interleukin-2 receptor) is a characteristic (although not specific) finding in adult T-cell leukemia/lymphoma (66). Similarly, uniform and bright CD30 expression is a characteristic (although not specific) finding in anaplastic large cell lymphoma. Enteropathy-associated T-cell lymphoma usually shows a double negative CD4 and CD8 immunophenotype, with expression of the intestine homing adhesion molecule CD103 (αE integrin).

NK-cell lymphomas express T-cell-associated markers, such as CD2 and CD43, but are negative for surface CD3 and CD5. NK-cell markers should be analyzed, such as CD16, CD56, CD57, and CD94. Immunohistochemistry is more convenient than flow cytometry for the assessment of cytotoxic markers (TIA-1, granzyme B, and perforin). In situ hybridization is the best approach for showing Epstein-Barr virus (EBV)–encoded RNA (EBER) in extranodal NK/T-cell lymphomas of nasal type.

Flow cytometry immunophenotyping also detects clonality in T- and NK-cell proliferations. Assessment of expression of TCR-Vβ family subtypes provides a specific assay for the detection and quantification of monoclonal T cells (14). Reactive T cells include a mixture of cells with variable expression of the Vβ family subtypes. In T-cell lymphoma, there is expansion of a population of T cells expressing the same Vβ family subtype. However, flow cytometric analysis of TCR-Vβ expression is labor intensive and covers only 65 percent of the TCR-Vβ repertoire. Therefore, TCR-Vβ restriction cannot be detected in one third of T-cell lymphomas (54).

NK cells do not rearrange their T-cell receptor genes and do not express T-cell markers associated with clonality. NK cells, however, express a set of killer immunoglobulin-like receptors (KIRs) and also a set of C-type lectins of CD94/NKG2 heterodimers (using NKG2A, -B or -C). Each NK cell selectively expresses one or a few subtypes of KIR (KIR repertoire) and also expresses one of the heterodimers CD94-NKG2A, -B, or -C. Demonstration of a skewed NK-cell repertoire using antibodies against KIRs and CD94/NKG2A supports the presence of a monoclonal NK-cell population (52). Expression of KIRs and CD94, however, is also observed in a subset of cytotoxic T-cell lymphomas (19).

CYTOGENETIC AND MOLECULAR ANALYSIS

Cytogenetic and molecular techniques contribute to the diagnosis and classification of malignant lymphomas in two ways: detection of clonality and detection of specific molecular abnormalities that either define or help to classify specific types of lymphoma. Detection of clonality is achieved by conventional cytogenetics but, in general, this application is not widely used because fresh tissue is required for cell culture and turnaround time is slow. Instead, conventional cytogenetics and fluorescence in situ hybridization (FISH) are more helpful for detecting the chromosomal translocations that are highly characteristic of certain types

of lymphoma. For example, t(14;18)(q32,q21)/*IGH-BCL2* is common in follicular lymphoma; mantle cell lymphoma is essentially defined by t(11;14)(q13;q32)/*CCND1-IGH*.

FISH, which can be applied to routinely processed tissue sections, is valuable for prognostic stratification of patients with certain types of lymphoma. For example, FISH assessment has shown that some patients with diffuse large B-cell lymphoma have concurrent *MYC* and either *BCL2* or *BCL6* gene rearrangements, so called "double hit" or "triple hit" lymphomas (30,45), and these patients have a poor prognosis if treated with standard therapy

A variety of molecular methods have been used to study lymphomas. Assessment for immunoglobulin (IG) or T-cell receptor (TCR) gene rearrangements helps to establish clonality in lymphomas. In general, PCR methods are employed most often for this purpose. The detection of IG or TCR gene rearrangements helps support an initial diagnosis of lymphoma. PCR-based detection of antigen receptor gene rearrangements is not sufficient to follow disease response because of limited sensitivity.

Molecular methods to detect chromosomal translocations are helpful for the classification of lymphomas and to assess minimal residual disease following therapy. With the advent of next-generation sequencing, which has shown recurrent gene mutations in certain types of lymphoma that can be exploited for the rational design of targeted therapies, it is expected that the role of molecular techniques in diagnosis, prognostication, and selection of therapy for patients with malignant lymphoma will continue to expand.

COMMON TECHNIQUES IN DIAGNOSTIC CYTOGENETICS

Hematologic malignancies represent the area in which conventional cytogenetics has had the greatest impact in advancing our understanding of cancer. This is true because lymphomas (and leukemias) often exhibit single, distinctive, nonrandom chromosomal abnormalities that define specific tumor subtypes. In contrast, the most common epithelial cancers exhibit considerable variability in the number and degree of complexity of chromosomal aberrations, with multiple and often random numerical and structural chromosomal abnormalities. The identification of

G-banded metaphases

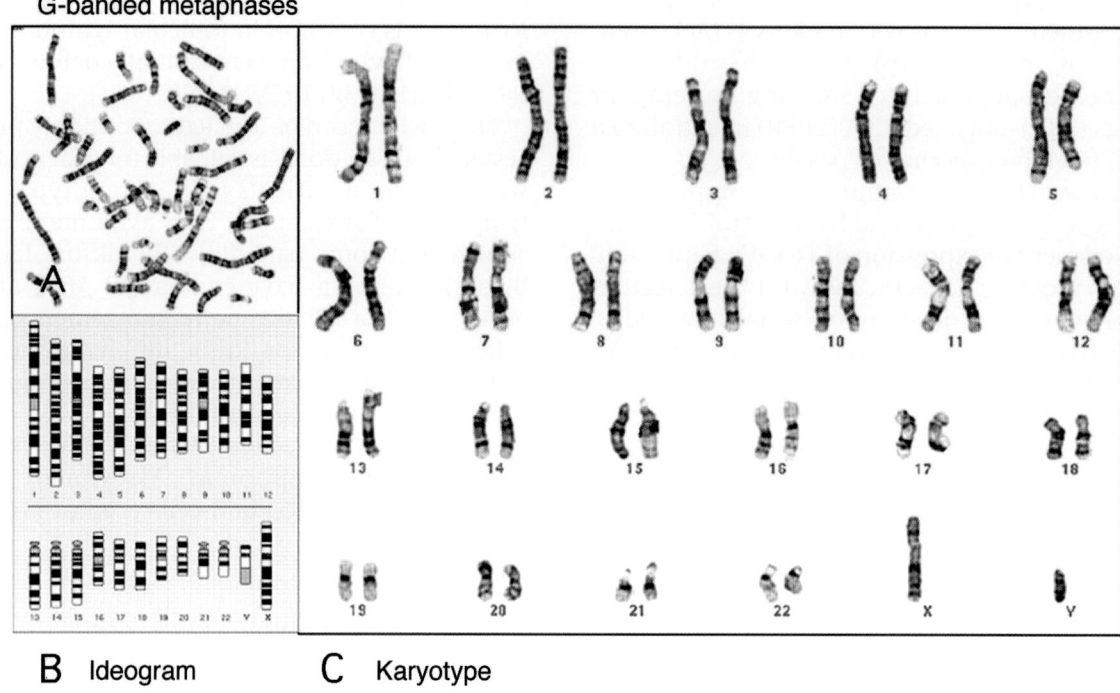

B Ideogram   C Karyotype

Figure 2-6

G-BANDED KARYOTYPING

A: The chromosomes from a single cell are seen in a metaphase chromosome spread.
B: Diploid male karyotype, 46, XY.
C: Normal ideogram representing the 22 human autosomal chromosomes and the sex chromosomes.

nonrandom distinctive abnormalities in these tumors is a difficult task. The most common cytogenetic techniques used for the diagnosis of malignant lymphomas are discussed here.

Conventional Karyotyping

In the 1950s and 1960s, chromosomes were studied using Giemsa and Wright stains. With these techniques, chromosomes could be counted and grouped together on the basis of similar size and shape, but they could not be distinguished within morphologically similar groups. In the 1970s, the development of chromosome banding allowed precise identification of each chromosome and parts of chromosomes. Currently, the most commonly used banding technique is Giemsa banding (G-banding) (73). G-banding requires pretreatment of cells with trypsin, which removes proteins from chromatin and results in a defined pattern of alternating light and dark regions. Each chromosome has a characteristic banding pattern that allows

its recognition and, when altered, allows for identification of structural abnormalities (fig. 2-6). Fresh tumor cells are cultured, and cells in metaphase are obtained for staining and visualization under the microscope. Conventional karyotyping provides a complete overview of all chromosomal changes within a tumor cell and is performed as part of the routine evaluation of hematopoietic and nonhematopoietic malignancies in many institutions.

Fluorescence in Situ Hybridization

This technique involves the hybridization of DNA-specific probes onto interphase and metaphase chromosomal DNA. The ability to localize fluorescent signals to specific interphase nuclei in nondividing cells is a principal advantage of FISH. A schematic representation of the FISH technique (interphase and metaphase analysis) is shown in figure 2-7.

There are three basic types of probes. Unique sequence probes hybridize to a locus-specific site

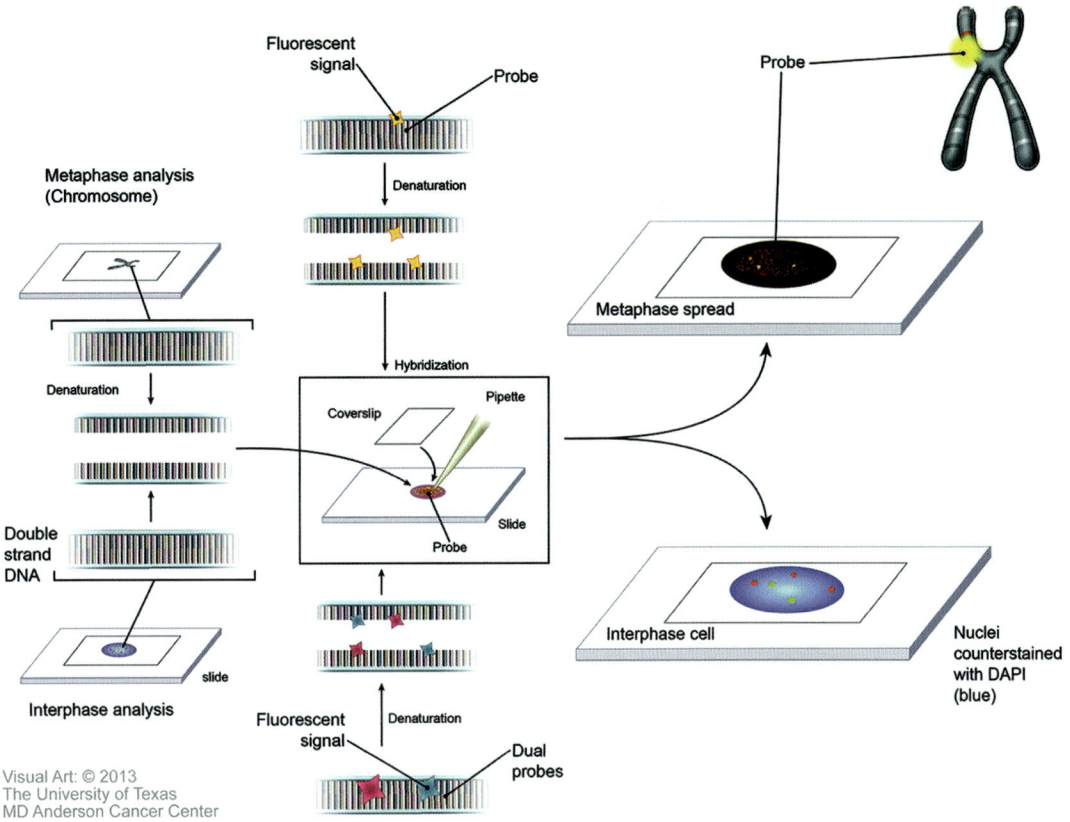

Figure 2-7

FLUORESCENCE IN SITU HYBRIDIZATION (FISH)

Schematic representation of the FISH technique (interphase and metaphase analysis). First, cells are permeabilized and DNA is denatured to allow the probe to hybridize specifically with its target. The probes are tagged directly with fluorochromes. A single "unique sequence" probe or two different probes labeled with two different fluorochromes can be used, as shown in this figure. "Unique sequence" probes hybridize to a locus-specific site. These probes can be used to detect deletions, gene amplifications, and gene rearrangements (split of the signal). Using two different "unique sequence" probes labeled with two different fluorochromes, fusion genes also are detected.

in the human genome. These probes are used to detect fusion genes, deletions, and amplification. Chromosome painting probes represent a cocktail of many unique DNA fragments designed to mark the entire chromosome of interest. These probes are mostly useful in the study of translocations, identifying the origin of marker chromosomes and derivative chromosomes, and clarifying complex rearrangements. Repeat sequence probes are isolated from telomere or centromere regions. Centromeric probes are often used to enumerate specific chromosomal gains or losses. Telomere probes are often used to characterize cryptic rearrangements.

Two strategies are used to detect chromosomal translocations: break-apart and fusion. With the break-apart strategy, probes are labeled with two different fluorescent chromophores (fluorochromes), often orange/red and green, which hybridize to sequences that flank a known chromosomal breakpoint region (fig. 2-8). When these two probes hybridize with an intact gene/locus, they are in close proximity and appear as a combined or single signal (usually yellow) because of the mixture of the dye spectra of these two probes. When a translocation occurs in the gene, the signals from the two probes are split, and separate orange/red and green signals are detected, along with the remaining intact yellow signal representing the nonrearranged locus/chromosome. The break-apart strategy offers the advantage of demonstrating any

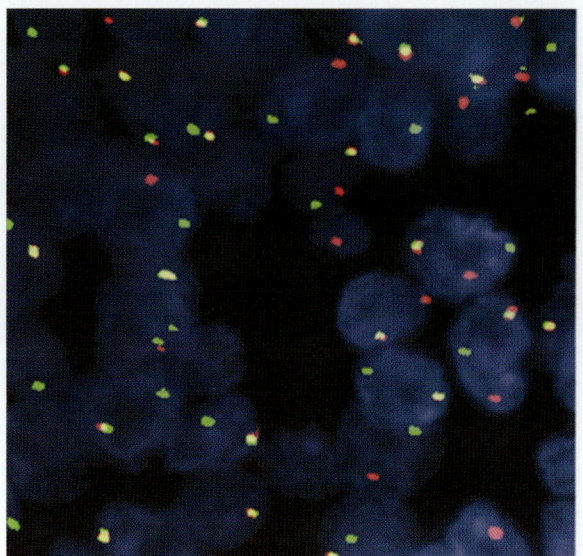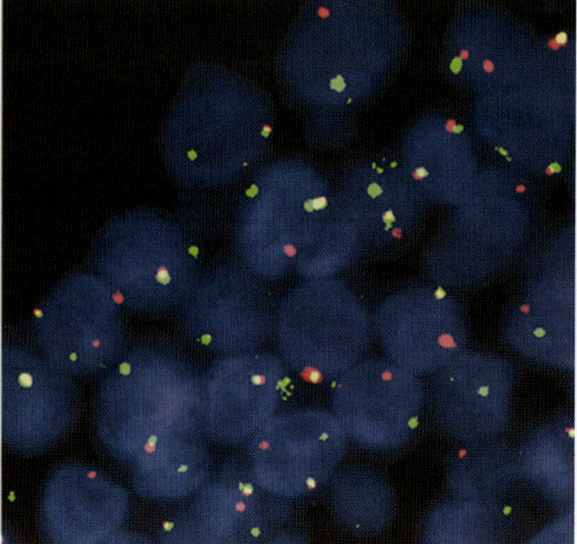

Figure 2-8

BREAK-APART (RED/GREEN) FUSION PROBES

When the probes hybridize with an intact gene/locus, they are in close proximity and appear as a combined or single yellow signal because of the mixture of the dye spectra of these two probes. When a translocation occurs in the gene, the signals from the two probes are split, and separate red and green signals are detected, along with the remaining intact yellow signal representing the nonrearranged locus/chromosome. (FISH methods using a *MALT1* break-apart probe, left; FISH methods using a *MYC* break-apart probe, right.)

rearrangement at the locus probed, but it cannot identify the translocation partner.

In the fusion strategy, two probes are used (labeled with two distinct chromophores) targeted to the two loci that are known to recombine (giving 2 red signals and 2 green signals in cells negative for the fusion event). A translocation involving two probed loci generates nuclei with 3 or 4 signals, 1 or 2 yellow (indicating the recombination product) and 1 red and 1 green signal (corresponding to the other loci not involved in the translocation) (fig. 2-9).

One convenient advantage of FISH is that it can be used to assess touch imprint preparations, fresh tissue, karyotype preparations, frozen specimens, and histologic sections cut from formalin-fixed paraffin-embedded samples.

TYPES OF CYTOGENETIC ABNORMALITIES IN LYMPHOMAS

Chromosomal translocations are of two general types. In the first type, an oncogene is juxtaposed via translocation with a promoter and/or enhancer element of another gene (i.e., antigen receptor gene). As a result of the trans-

location, the oncogene becomes deregulated. This type of rearrangement occurs frequently in lymphomas. In the second type of chromosomal translocation, two coding regions are disrupted and juxtaposed, resulting in a fusion gene, chimeric RNA, and a novel protein with new or altered activity. This type of rearrangement occurs in some types of lymphoma, such as anaplastic large cell lymphoma (ALCL) or extranodal marginal zone lymphoma of mucosa-associated lymphoid tissue (MALT) type, but is more frequent in acute and chronic leukemias and sarcomas. Common or characteristic translocations are discussed below.

MYC Translocations: t(8;14)(q24;q32), t(2;8)(p11;q24), and t(8;22)(q24;q11)

Burkitt lymphoma is characterized by one of three translocations: most cases (80 to 85 percent) carry t(8;14)(q24;q32) (35); two other translocations, t(2;8)(p11;q24) and t(8;22) (q24;q11), also known as the variant translocations, occur in 10 to 15 percent of cases. Because of these rearrangements, the *MYC* gene becomes constitutively expressed owing

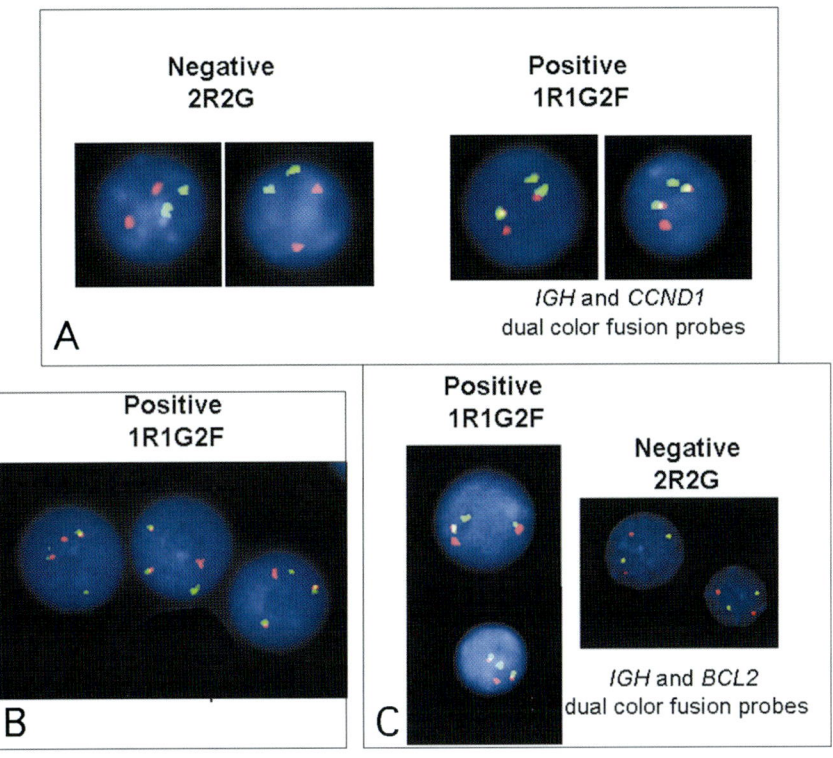

Negative 2R2G

Positive 1R1G2F

IGH and *CCND1* dual color fusion probes

A

Positive 1R1G2F

B

Positive 1R1G2F

Negative 2R2G

IGH and *BCL2* dual color fusion probes

C

Figure 2-9

DUAL COLOR (RED/GREEN) FUSION PROBES

A: FISH using *CCND1/IGH* dual color fusion probes. The two left nuclei show no evidence of rearrangements between *IGH* (at 14q32) and *CCND1* (at 11q13) genes, thus 2 red and 2 green signals are seen per nucleus (normal signal pattern: 2R2G). If the cells are carrying the t(11;14), the abnormal nuclei show the 1R1G2F signal pattern.

B: FISH methods using *MYC/IGH* dual color fusion probes. The presence of dual fusion signals in the three cells indicates the presence of the t(8;14).

C: FISH methods using *BCL2/IGH* dual color fusion probes. The presence of dual fusion signals in the two cells on the left indicates the presence of the t(14;18).

to the influence of regulatory elements of the IG genes. *MYC* alterations are usually detected by conventional cytogenetic methods or FISH. PCR approaches are suboptimal because *MYC* breakpoints are widely scattered and there are three partner chromosomes. FISH methods have the advantage that fresh material is not required, and the large size of the *MYC* probes (break-apart type) allows detection of virtually all 8q24 breakpoints (fig. 2-8). In addition to the IG genes, *MYC* can partner with other chromosomal loci; this occurs in a subset of diffuse large B-cell lymphomas (DLBCL).

BCL2 Translocation: t(14;18)(q32;q21)

The t(14;18) as detected by conventional cytogenetics, is present in 80 to 90 percent of follicular lymphomas (72). It is also found in 20 to 30 percent of cases of DLBCL, presumably of germinal center origin (20). In t(14;18), the *BCL2* gene on 18q21 is juxtaposed with the *IGH* gene on 14q32, resulting in overexpression of structurally intact and functional BCL2 protein (52). The breakpoints on chromosome 14 are tightly clustered, occurring immediately 5' to the IGH joining regions, usually JH5 or JH6. The breakpoints on chromosome 18 occur predom-

inantly in a tight cluster, the major breakpoint cluster region (MBR) (60). The MBR is involved in 50 to 70 percent of cases of follicular lymphoma. Other lower frequency cluster regions also have been characterized (1). For diagnosis, FISH methods using *BCL2* and *IGH* probes to detect fusion signals are the preferred method (fig. 2-10). The tight clustering of the MBR and minor cluster region (MCR) breakpoints is also amenable to standard PCR assays, which are commonly used in the assessment of minimal residual disease. Using two sets of primers specific for the MBR and MCR, PCR can detect the t(14;18) in 60 to 80 percent of cases.

BCL6 Translocations: t(3;var)(q27;var)

Rearrangements of the *BCL6* gene are found in approximately 30 percent of DLBCLs, approximately 20 percent of acquired immunodeficiency syndrome-associated DLBCLs, and 5 to 15 percent of follicular lymphomas (71). Translocations involving *BCL6* do not involve its coding regions and thus result in overexpression of structurally intact BCL6 protein (57). The *BCL6* gene is highly promiscuous, as it can be juxtaposed with a number of partner chromosome loci (more than 20) in addition

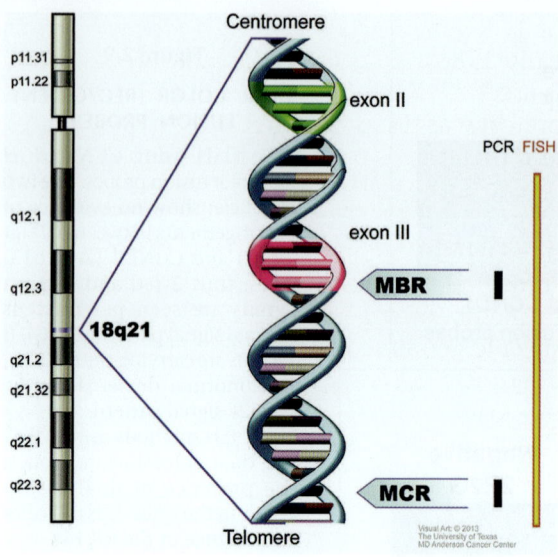

Figure 2-10

FOLLICULAR LYMPHOMA: CHROMOSOME 18q21 REGION INVOLVED IN t(14;18)

Most of the BCL2 breakpoints occur in the major breakpoint region (MBR) with a smaller subset in the minor breakpoint cluster region (MCR) (other cluster regions not shown). The black and red/yellow rectangles (vertical on right) span the breakpoints detected using polymerase chain reaction (PCR) and FISH, respectively. FISH methods have the potential to detect virtually all follicular lymphoma cases with the t(14;18).

to *IGH*, including 4p13, 6p21.3, 9p22, 14q11, and the *IG* loci: 14q32 (*IGH*), 2p12 (*IGκ*), and 22q11 (*IGλ*) (41). The large number of partner chromosomes precludes routine PCR analysis in the clinical laboratory. Conventional cytogenetics is the only approach that can identify all the possible partner loci, of which *IGH* is most common. FISH analysis using a break-apart probe provides a simple and rapid method for detecting chromosomal translocations involving *BCL6*, but does not identify the partner chromosome.

CCND1 Translocation: t(11;14)(q13;q32)

The t(11;14)(q13;q32) is present in virtually all cases of mantle cell lymphoma and is thought to be a primary event in pathogenesis (36,68). As a result of t(11;14), the *CCND1* gene is juxtaposed near an enhancer of the *IGH* gene on the derivative 14q32, resulting in overexpression of cyclin D1. Approximately 30 to 40 percent of these translocations are clustered within an 80-100 base pair region known as the major

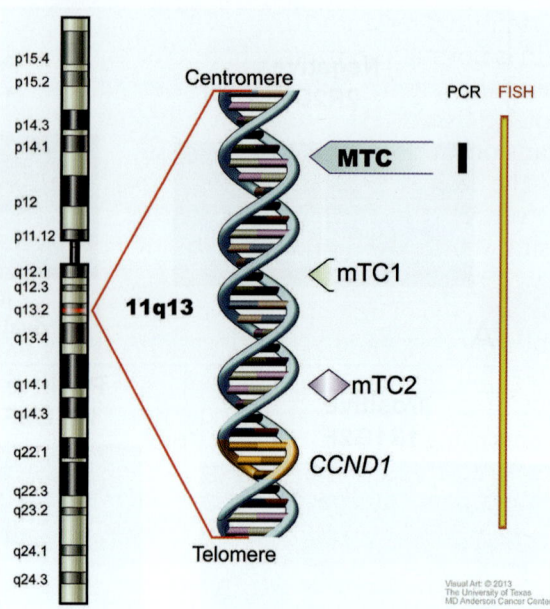

Figure 2-11

MANTLE CELL LYMPHOMA: CHROMOSOME 11q13 REGION INVOLVED IN t(11;14)

The *CCND1* gene is indicated in an orange box. The MTC region accounts for 30 to 40 percent of all translocations. Minor breakpoint clusters are indicated as mTC1 and mTC2. The breakpoints of this translocation detected using PCR and FISH are indicated as black and red/yellow rectangles (vertical on right).

translocation cluster (MTC) region on chromosome 11q13. The remainder of the chromosome 11 breakpoints, however, are widely scattered over approximately 120 kb. The breakpoints on chromosome 14 occur within the 5' region of one of six joining regions of the *IGH* gene. For diagnosis, dual-probe FISH to detect fusion signals is preferred and can detect t(11;14) in up to 95 percent of the cases (fig. 2-11) (47). Translocations involving the MTC are amenable to routine PCR analysis (34).

NPM-ALK: t(2;5)(p23;q35)

The t(2;5)(p23;q35) is the most common translocation in anaplastic lymphoma kinase (ALK)-positive ALCL, a neoplasm that is most common in younger patients (25). The t(2;5) fuses the nucleophosmin (*NPM1*) gene at 5q35 with the *ALK* gene at 2p23, forming a fusion gene that encodes an 80-kD chimeric protein. The 117 aminoterminal residues of NPM are linked to the intracytoplasmic portion of ALK

(C-terminal residues 1058-1620) (39). ALK protein is normally expressed in cells of the central nervous system, but not in normal hematopoietic tissues. As a result of t(2;5) or variant translocations, ALK is overexpressed.

The lack of tight clustering within the involved *NPM* and *ALK* introns precludes analysis using standard PCR methods, but reverse transcriptase (RT)-PCR or long-range PCR methods can be used. These methods detect t(2;5), but not the other variant translocations involving *ALK* that have been reported in ALK-positive ALCL (25). FISH methods detect *ALK* rearrangements using break-apart probes for *ALK*, and can detect all translocations, although the partner is unknown. Immunohistochemistry for ALK overexpression is convenient for detecting all cases of ALK-positive ALCL (25).

API2-MALT1; t(11;18)(q21;q21) and Other MALT Lymphoma Translocations

In MALT lymphomas, four well-established translocations are known, of which t(11;18)(q21;q21) is the most common. This translocation results in a chimeric *API2-MALT1* gene. MALT lymphomas associated with t(11;18) arise most often in the lung (40 percent) and stomach (30 percent) (58). Assays are available that can detect t(11;18) by RT-PCR and FISH (fig. 2-8, right).

Three other translocations have been well characterized in MALT lymphomas: *IGH-MALT1*/t(14;18)(q32;q21), which is more common in MALT lymphomas of the orbit; *FOXP1-IGH*/t(3;14)(p14.1;q32), which is more common in MALT1 lymphomas of the thyroid gland; and *BCL10-IGH*/t(1;14)(p22;q32), a rare translocation most common in the MALT lymphomas of the intestine (58). A MALT1 break-apart probe detects any translocation that involves the *MALT1* gene. There are additional potential or proved chromosomal translocations reported in MALT lymphomas, all at low frequency (63).

COMMON TECHNIQUES USED IN MOLECULAR DIAGNOSTICS

Southern Blot Hybridization

Southern blotting, also known as restriction fragment length analysis, was reported by Edwin Southern in 1975 (56) and was widely used in molecular diagnostic laboratories to detect IG or TCR gene rearrangements beginning in the early 1980s. Currently, Southern blot analysis is used in few clinical molecular diagnostic laboratories as it has been replaced by PCR assays and therefore is mostly of historical interest.

The first step in Southern blot analysis is to use restriction endonucleases to cut germline DNA into fragments. These fragments are subjected to electrophoresis and transferred to membranes; genes are then detected using specific genomic cDNA probes. In lymphoma diagnosis, Southern blot analysis was used most often to detect the physiological variable (V)-diversity (D)-joining (J) segment recombination, which by deleting restriction enzyme sites, changes the size and the banding pattern of the germline fragments. Using J or constant (C) region probes, the Southern blot technique can examine large segments of the IG and TCR genes (up to 25 kb) with a sensitivity of approximately 5 percent. In other words, the neoplastic B or T cells need to represent at least 5 percent of the entire cell population assessed. Southern blotting is a labor-intensive technique with a relatively long turnaround time (at least 1 week for routine testing), and requires appreciable amounts of high-quality (nondegraded) DNA. Therefore, Southern blot analysis cannot be performed on DNA extracted from fixed, paraffin-embedded tissue.

Polymerase Chain Reaction

PCR is a technology that is designed to permit selective amplification of specific DNA sequences. This method was developed by Kary Mullis in 1983 (40), and consists of a series of cycles of three types of reactions: 1) denaturation (separation) of double-stranded DNA at high temperature (93 to 95°C for human genomic DNA); 2) annealing of primers to a DNA template at a lower temperature (50°C to 70°C); and 3) extension of the primer to create a new copy using heat-stable DNA polymerase (the enzyme was originally isolated from the bacterial species *Thermus aquaticus*, but now recombinant enzyme is used) typically at about 70 to 75°C. In standard assays, PCR can amplify up to 1 kb of DNA, but efficiency is best for fragments less than 500 bp (for fresh or frozen tissue) and less than 200 bp (for fixed paraffin-embedded tissue).

Figure 2-12

TaqMan® REAL-TIME PCR

First, the primers and the TaqMan probe hybridize to the target during the annealing step of each PCR cycle. During the extension step, the TaqMan probe is hydrolyzed by the 5′ exonuclease activity of Taq polymerase. When the TaqMan probe is hydrolyzed, the reporter is detached from the adjacent quencher molecule and fluoresces in an amount proportional to the degree of PCR product amplification. Forward (F) and reverse (R) primers are represented with red and green boxes. R, reporter; Q, quencher.

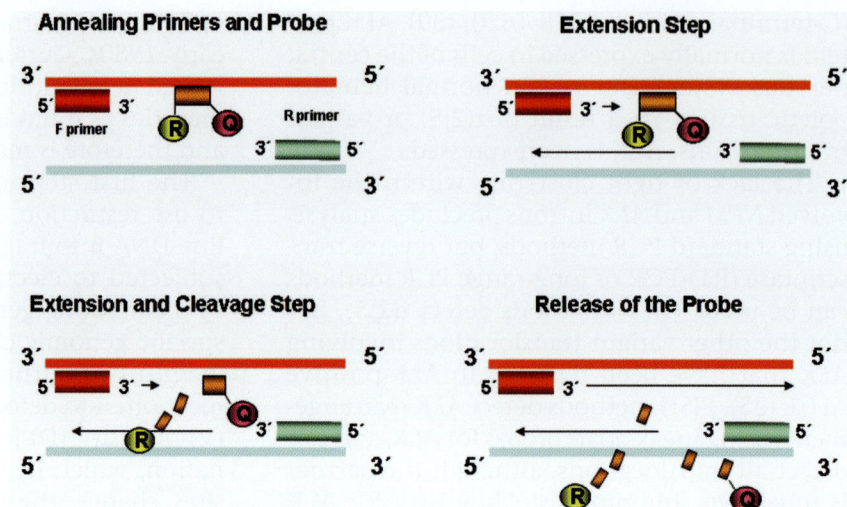

PCR-based assays are now performed in many clinical laboratories using capillary electrophoresis, where one of the primers is labeled with a fluorochrome that is incorporated into the PCR products during amplification. The PCR products separate as they migrate through the capillary due to their electrophoretic mobility. At the outlet of the capillary, a laser excites the fluorochrome and the mobility of the PCR products is compared with that of reference size standards. Capillary electrophoresis can readily separate PCR products that differ from each other by as little as one or two base pairs. The high sensitivity of PCR, depending on the target, allows for detection of minimal residual disease (17).

Quantitative and Real-Time PCR

This PCR method is used to amplify and simultaneously quantify a targeted DNA molecule. In quantitative (q) PCR, amplicons are detected and quantified during the exponential expansion phase in real time, as the reaction progresses. By contrast, in conventional PCR, the product of the reaction is detected at the end of the cycling (plateau) phase when logarithmic doubling has ceased.

Two common methods for detection of products in real-time PCR are: 1) nonspecific fluorescent dyes (e.g., SYBR green dye) that intercalate into any double-stranded DNA; and 2) sequence-specific DNA probes (e.g., TaqMan®). The latter consist of oligonucleotides that are labeled with a fluorescent reporter at their 5′ and a quencher at their 3′ ends. This design permits detection only after hybridization of the probe with its complementary DNA target (fig. 2-12). The probe hybridizes to its target amplicon during the annealing step of each PCR cycle and is then hydrolyzed by the 5′ exonuclease activity of Taq polymerase during DNA extension. When the TaqMan probe is hydrolyzed, the reporter is detached from the adjacent quencher molecule and fluoresces in an amount proportional to the degree of PCR product amplification. *BCL2/IGH* and *CCND1/IGH* real-time PCR assays have been developed (17,49,50).

In Situ Hybridization

In clinical practice, in situ hybridization is most commonly used for three purposes: 1) to detect chromosomal abnormalities, including translocations, isochromosomes, and changes in copy number; 2) to demonstrate clonality by detecting cytoplasmic mRNA expression of kappa and lambda light chains; and 3) to detect evidence of viral infections, especially latent EBV infection. The large number of EBV-encoded RNA (EBER) copies in infected cells makes this assay highly sensitive.

In situ hybridization can be performed on fresh cells in smears or touch imprints or fixed, paraffin-embedded tissue sections. Semi-quantification of cells with a specific abnormality can be achieved by manual or automated counting, usually of up to 200 cell nuclei. Counting is less reliable in fixed, paraffin-embedded tissue sections because not all cells are in the same plane of section (unlike smears or imprints).

COMMON APPLICATIONS OF MOLECULAR TESTING IN LYMPHOMAS

Detection of Clonality in Lymphoid Lesions

Assessment of the configuration of the immunoglobulin and T-cell receptor genes is a highly useful tool for assessing clonality because the antigen-receptor genes typically rearrange physiologically before neoplastic transformation occurs, and therefore, lymphoma cells all have the same gene rearrangements (35). The presence of monoclonal gene rearrangement helps distinguish benign from malignant lymphoid lesions, as most lymphomas are monoclonal and gene rearrangements are uncommon in benign lesions. This general rule is not absolute, however, and clonality is not equivalent to malignancy. Detection of clonality using molecular methods is generally more sensitive than immunophenotypic or conventional cytogenetic analysis.

The surface B-cell receptor (BCR) is an immunoglobulin composed of one Ig light chain (kappa or lambda) and one heavy chain. B cells express only one clonotypic type of Ig (i.e., only one heavy and light chain protein per cell). Similarly, T cells express either TCRα/β or TCRγ/δ receptors. Functional antigen-receptor genes are assembled from separate germline coding sequences by a site-specific V(D)J DNA recombination. The V(D)J recombination is the main mechanism for generating antigen-receptor diversity, with the generation of an almost unlimited repertoire of different antigen receptors with unique specificities.

Immunoglobulin and T-cell receptor gene rearrangements are lineage specific, at least in mature B and T cells (i.e., immunoglobulin gene assembly occurs in B cells but not in T cells and T-cell receptor gene assembly occurs in T cells but in B cells). There is also a developmental hierarchy of gene rearrangements. In B cells, *IGH* rearranges before *IGK*. If *IGK* does not rearrange functionally, then *IGL* rearranges (known as the principle of allelic exclusion). In T cells, *TRD* rearranges (and is often deleted) before *TRG* rearranges, followed by *TRB* and then *TRA*.

The anatomy of the antigen-receptor genes and the mechanism of gene rearrangements are well-described elsewhere (10,35). As *IGH*, *TRG*, and *TRB* are most often used for clonality testing by PCR in routine diagnosis, the unique anatomic structures of these three genes are described briefly. *IGH* (located at chromosome 14q32.3) in its germline configuration has approximately 129 V regions (many nonfunctional), up to 27 D regions, 9 J regions, and 11 C regions. The process of *IGH* gene rearrangement selects one V, D, and J, first DJ and then VDJ, to form a continuous and intact VDJ segment, which is then spliced together with one of the C regions during transcription to create a single transcript encoding IgM/IgD or (after class switch) IgA, IgG, or IgE. The *TRG* gene (at chromosome 7p15-p14) has 15 V regions (4 nonfunctional), 5 J regions, 2 C regions, whereas the *TRB* gene (at chromosome 7q34) has 67 V regions, 2 D regions, 14 J regions, and 2 C regions (28).

In the germline configuration, the discontinuous V and J regions are widely separated, precluding PCR amplification. In contrast, a rearranged gene has V and J regions in close proximity allowing PCR amplification. Monoclonal lymphocytes contain one or two rearranged antigen-receptor alleles; therefore, PCR will amplify one or two predominant bands/peaks per cells, and a cell population will show that these peaks predominate. In contrast, each polyclonal lymphocyte carries a distinctive gene rearrangement of slightly different size due to CDR3 diversity, and a cell population will show a Gaussian/normal distribution (smear pattern) of amplified bands. Using conventional PCR, one monoclonal B or T cell in up to 10^2 to 10^4 B or T cells can be detected, depending on the number of polyclonal lymphocytes present.

IGH **PCR.** PCR assessment of *IGH* is the most frequently used test to assess clonality in B-cell neoplasms (fig. 2-13). Forward PCR primers are derived from conserved sequences in the framework regions of the V segments (framework 1, 2, and 3). Reverse PCR primers are derived from a conserved sequence within the J_H region. One disadvantage of PCR is a high percentage of false negative results in a subset of B-cell lymphomas that arise from B cells that pass through the germinal center and therefore carry a number of somatic mutations. Each mutation can preclude primer annealing to the DNA template and therefore no amplification of PCR products occurs. Examples of tumors with many somatic mutations include follicular lymphoma, marginal zone lymphomas, and plasma cell myeloma. In follicular lymphoma, *IGH* is not amplified in up to 40 percent of tumors. False negative results

33

are therefore not uncommon and occur when a consensus primer does not anneal with all V regions. On the other hand, monoclonal *IGH* rearrangements can occur in clinically benign lesions. From the clinical perspective these results are considered false positive although the result is showing a true, usually small, monoclonal gene rearrangement.

TCR **PCR.** The four *TCR* genes encode, respectively, the four varieties of the *TCR* gene chain: α and β, which form the common αβ heterodimer, plus γ and δ, which form the less frequent γδ heterodimer. Of the four *TCR* genes, *TRA* is too complex, and *TRD* is frequently rearranged and then deleted in mature T cells (24). Thus, PCR assays to detect T-cell clonality have focused on the *TRB* or *TRG* genes. The *TRG* gene is much less complex than *TRB*. *TRG* has only 11 functional V segments that can be grouped into four homologous families and 5 J segments that can be grouped into two highly homologous groups (22,51). Thus, most of the *TRG* gene rearrangements can be detected using a small set of primers (fig. 2-13) (59,62).

Currently, there are multiplex PCR assays that assess the *TRB* gene. Consensus PCR primers, developed by the BIOMED-2 group, are highly sensitive, with false negative rates in T-cell lymphomas of only 5 to 10 percent with either the *TRG* or *TRB* assay. Somatic mutations rarely occur in the *TCR* genes, false negative results are usually attributable to the consensus primers not annealing with all V regions. Similar to *IGH* results, monoclonal *TCR* rearrangements can occur in clinically non-neoplastic lesions. As a result, the diagnosis of lymphoma cannot rely exclusively on clonality studies by PCR.

Although underemphasized in the literature, there was a tradeoff when PCR methods replaced Southern blot analysis for IG and TCR clonality testing. The problem of false negative results attributable to somatic mutations of the V genes or the use of consensus primers did not exist when using Southern blot analysis because large probes were used. The problem of false positive results was also less of an issue because Southern blotting is much less sensitive than PCR and small monoclonal IG or TCR rearrangements were not detected. Southern blot analysis is more reliable than PCR-based methods to assess clonality when DNA is adequate

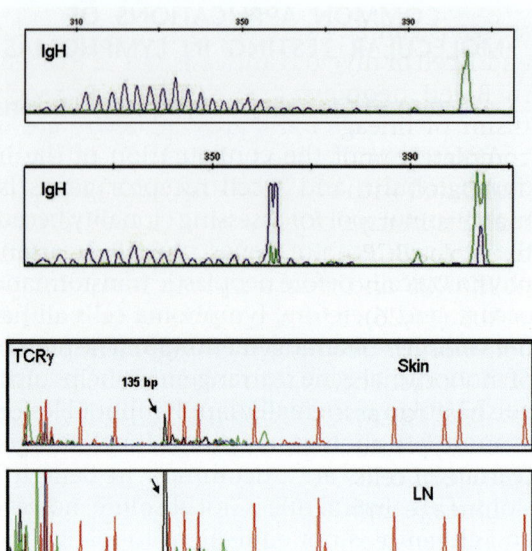

Figure 2-13

PCR IGH AND TCRγ ASSESSMENT

Top: *IGH*-PCR analysis of a reactive lymph node (top) and diffuse large B-cell lymphoma (DLBCL) (bottom). The reactive lymph node shows a polyclonal population of B cells (in blue). The green peak is the internal control to demonstrate DNA integrity. In the DLBCL, a monoclonal *IGH* peak is present in a polyclonal background of B cells. Again, the green peak is the internal control.

Bottom: *TRG*-PCR analysis of a skin biopsy specimen involved by mycosis fungoides and the regional lymph node (LN) showing a common clonal gene rearrangement. Both monoclonal gene rearrangements have the same signature. Both peaks are black, indicating that they are using the same family (VγIII) and they are the same size (135 bp). Red peaks correspond to internal size standards.

and involvement by lymphoma is greater than 5 percent. However, the need for high-quality DNA, the labor intensive nature of Southern blotting, and the long turnaround time are sufficient drawbacks to Southern blot analysis so that most clinical laboratories have replaced this method with PCR.

Lineage Infidelity

Lineage infidelity (or lineage promiscuity) is defined as the occurrence of TCR gene rearrangements in B-cell neoplasms or IG gene rearrangements in T-cell neoplasms (10,35). Lineage infidelity is common in immature lymphoid neoplasms such as acute lymphoblastic leukemia/lymphoma (ALL), and is not restricted to gene rearrangements since B-cell or myeloid antigens can be expressed in T-cell neoplasms and T-cell or myeloid antigens can be expressed in B-cell neoplasms. Although the mechanisms of lineage ambiguity/plasticity are not completely understood, genetic alterations are associated with the upregulation of lymphoid markers in myeloid tumors and vice versa. For example, *BCR-ABL1* induces aberrant splicing of *IKAROS* and results in lineage infidelity in B-ALL (16,26). Lineage infidelity is much less common in neoplasms arising from mature B and T cells. For this reason, molecular studies are best for assessing clonality, but immunophenotypic analysis is better for assessing the lineage of cells.

Lineage infidelity, as shown by detection of antigen-receptor gene rearrangements, also has been shown in nonlymphoid tumors. Rearrangements of the IG or TCR genes are detected in 15 to 20 percent of acute myeloid leukemias, most often in the most immature neoplasms (so-called M0 tumors). Rearrangements of the IG or TCR genes also have been reported in a subset of histiocytic neoplasms (8,64).

Detection of Clonality in Nonlymphoid Cells

Antigen-receptor genes do not rearrange in NK cells or nonlymphoid cells, and as a result, cannot be used to assess clonality in tumors arising from nonlymphoid cells. Another method used to assess clonality in nonlymphoid cells is the human androgen receptor assay (HUMARA) technique, which is useful for showing clonality in Langerhans cell histiocytosis (69) and nonhematopoietic tumors. The androgen receptor locus is highly polymorphic in the human population. As a tumor arises from a single cell, only one form of the polymorphic locus is reproduced in the neoplastic cell population (loss of heterozygosity) compared with a benign lesion in which heterozygosity remains present.

EBV also has been used for the assessment of clonality in tumors infected by EBV (18), such as nasopharyngeal carcinoma and extranodal NK/T-cell lymphoma of nasal type. In this approach, only a single form of viral episome is usually present in a cell before it undergoes neoplastic transformation. As a result, there is only one form of episome in a neoplastic cell population versus a number of different episomal forms in a benign population.

HIGH-THROUGHPUT TECHNIQUES USED IN MOLECULAR DIAGNOSTICS

A number of high-throughput methods to analyze lymphoid neoplasms have been developed in the past decade. Currently, these techniques have been applied sparingly to routine patient care. It seems likely, however, that high-throughput methods will assume greater importance and become a much greater part routine clinical care in the future. A detailed description of the methods involved is beyond the scope of this chapter, but a brief description of methods and their implications are discussed here.

Comparative Genomic Hybridization

Classic comparative genomic hybridization (CGH) was developed in the 1990s. CGH is a double-color hybridization procedure that provides a genome-wide view of DNA copy number changes in a single experiment (23). Total genomic DNA is isolated from a tumor and reference cell populations, labeled with different fluorochromes (e.g., green for normal DNA and red for tumor DNA), and then hybridized with metaphase chromosomes (fig. 2-14). If the tumor sample has a gain in a particular chromosomal region, a predominance of tumor DNA (red signal) is detected, and if there is a loss of a chromosomal region, a predominance of reference DNA (green signal) is detected.

The newer oligonucleotide array-based CGH (aCGH) has much higher resolution and accuracy (4,55). Oligonucleotide-array probes, usually 50 to 75 nucleotides (50 to 75-mer), are designed in silico for any sequenced region of the genome (custom arrays), thus allowing region-specific or whole genome coverage with a high number of probes. Arrays also can be constructed that are disease specific. Another advantage of aCGH is that this method detects genomic imbalances at the level of single genetic loci. A disadvantage is the inability of the method to detect chromosomal inversions or translocations where there is no net loss or gain of chromosomal material. In addition, some small gains or losses of chromosomal material are known to be present in the genome and can resemble copy number variations (46). Array CGH is well integrated into research laboratories, but more recently has been implemented in some diagnostic laboratories; it can be used to study fixed, paraffin-embedded tissue specimens.

Single Nucleotide Polymorphism Arrays

Single nucleotide polymorphism (SNP) arrays are similar to aCGH arrays except that the probes are short oligonucleotides (25-mer) (7). SNP arrays are designed to detect genetic variations (polymorphisms) as well as larger segments of DNA that are present in variable copy number, also known as copy number variants, in constitutional DNA. SNP arrays can show differences between tumor and normal host DNA, and also help to assess associations between specific diseases and genome-wide variations. A major advantage of SNP arrays is that uniparental disomy (UPD) can be detected. In UPD, stretches of DNA are composed of two identical strands and all SNPs are therefore homozygous. One possible explanation for UPD is that one allele is deleted and the other allele is duplicated. The risk of UPD is that a heterozygous state can be converted to a homozygous gene defect. Similar to aCGH, SNP arrays can be used to study fixed, paraffin-embedded tissues.

Gene Expression Profiling

The most common form of gene expression profiling (GEP) that has been applied to the study of lymphomas involves preparation of tumor RNA and hybridization to a solid platform (array) on which DNA probes are immobilized (7). The RNA is labeled with fluorochrome and the signal following hybridization is a measure of overexpression or underexpression of corresponding transcripts. As this approach can yield thousands of data points, bioinformatic analysis is challenging.

Gene expression profiling has allowed the recognition of specific genes or cellular pathways in different types of tumors. The data derived from these studies have contributed to better insights into pathogenesis as well as the recognition of potential targets for therapy. In addition, GEP studies have identified new biomarkers helpful in diagnosis or prognostication that already are being used in clinical practice, for example, ZAP70 in CLL/SLL and SOX11 in mantle cell lymphoma (7).

In some types of lymphomas, GEP also has been used to try and improve lymphoma classification or to tease out new entities. The results are somewhat mixed, and are discussed in subsequent chapters as they pertain to various lymphoma types. Since GEP has had its greatest impact on classification of DLBCL it is briefly discussed here.

In 2000, Alizadeh et al. (3) used GEP data to subdivide cases of DLBCL into two subsets: germinal center B-cell (GCB) cases and activated B-cell (ABC) cases, with the former having a better prognosis independent of the International Prognostic Index. A number of subsequent studies (but not all) have found that the cell-of-origin classification has prognostic importance and that the NF-kappa B pathway is overexpressed and likely involved in the pathogenesis of the ABC type of DLBCL (2,7,29). In general, cell-of-origin classification is most helpful in the assessment of patients with nodal DLBCL and is less helpful for primary extranodal DLBCL cases.

MicroRNA Analysis

MicroRNAs (miRNAs) are a class of small (20 to 22 nucleotides) noncoding RNA molecules that play crucial roles in regulating gene expression, by either inducing mRNA degradation or inhibiting translation (21,27,32). These noncoding RNA molecules can simultaneously target up to one third of all genes, thereby controlling a wide range of biological functions including differentiation, proliferation, and apoptosis. Deregulation of miRNA expression has been shown to play an important role in cancer pathogenesis and has been described in solid cancers, leukemias, and lymphomas.

Arrays have been designed to assess miRNA signatures in various diseases including lymphomas. To date, most miRNA studies have been focused on B-cell lymphomas (21,27). Two miRNAs that appear to be particularly important are MIR-155 and the MIR17-92 cluster. Much less is known about T-cell lymphomas, but a recent study on ALCLs has shown different miRNA signatures for ALK-positive and ALK-negative ALCL (32).

Proteomics

Proteomics is a term that describes the large-scale interrogation of proteins, usually in cells, tissues, or organisms (31). Proteomic analysis allows the development of a highly detailed view of disease biomarkers and protein-protein interactions involved in signaling pathways, and is helpful in characterizing drug targets.

Conventional CGH

aCGH

Tumor

Normal (Ref)

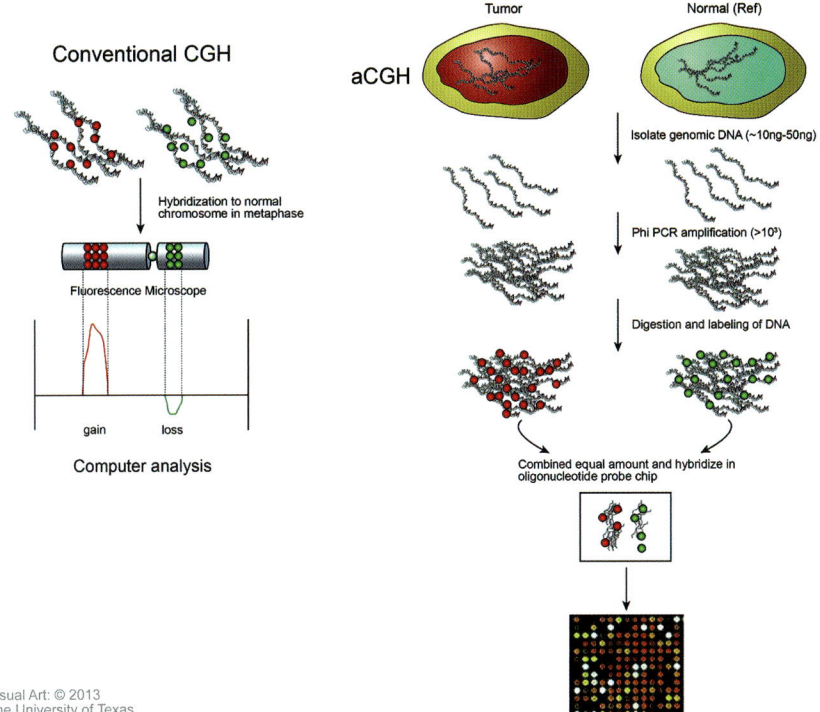

Isolate genomic DNA (~10ng-50ng)

Phi PCR amplification (>10³)

Digestion and labeling of DNA

Hybridization to normal
chromosome in metaphase

Fluorescence Microscope

gain   loss

Computer analysis

Combined equal amount and hybridize in
oligonucleotide probe chip

Figure 2-14

**CONVENTIONAL
COMPARATIVE GENOMIC
HYBRIDIZATION (CGH)
AND ARRAY-CGH METHODS**

DNA from tumor (in red) and from non-neoplastic (ref) tissue (in green) are each labeled with different fluorochromes (tags). After mixing tumor and reference DNA along with unlabeled human cot-1 DNA (placental DNA that is enriched for repetitive DNA sequences such as the Alu and Kpn family) to suppress repetitive DNA sequences, the mix is hybridized to normal metaphase chromosomes, in the case of conventional CGH, or to a slide containing thousands of defined DNA probes, in the case of aCGH. Using fluorescence microscopy and quantitative image analysis, regional differences in the fluorescence ratio of gains/losses compared to control DNA are detected and used for identifying abnormal regions in tumors.

Protein microarrays are one application of proteomics. These assays are designed to allow proteins, usually in a fluid state, to interact with capture-reagents (e.g., antibodies). In forward-phase arrays, proteins are isolated from biological samples by capture reagents immobilized on a solid matrix (array). In reverse-phase arrays, multiple biological samples are immobilized on a solid matrix and the array is incubated with a specific molecule or antibody. In clinical diagnostics, protein microarrays are often used to detect infectious organisms.

Mass spectrometry-based proteomic analysis is another important proteomic approach (31). All mass spectrophotometers have four components: an ionization source, ion optics, a mass analyzer, and a detector. Proteins or peptides are first ionized, usually using a laser, and these ions are then collected and analyzed. A common approach used to ionize proteins is matrix-assisted laser desorption/ionization (MALDI). Ions in the gas phase are then collected into the analyzer by a series of ion optics. The analyzer measures the ions based on their mass-to-charge ratio and directs the ions to an electron multiplier. The ions are then detected, allowing characterization of the protein or peptide being analyzed with great specificity.

A common approach for identifying proteins involves using a proteolytic enzyme, such as trypsin, to digest complex protein mixtures into peptides. The peptides are then separated by liquid chromatography and analyzed by tandem mass spectrophotometry. The results of the analysis are then matched against known databases, allowing protein identification. Peptide fragmentation generally occurs in a highly predictable manner, yielding structural information such as the amino acid sequence.

One common use of mass spectrometry-driven proteomics in clinical diagnostics is the characterization of amyloid (65). Amyloid deposits can be microdissected from tissue biopsy specimens and analyzed by mass spectrophotometry. The amyloids that have been defined using this approach include AL (lambda/kappa), heavy chain amyloidosis, AA, and other more uncommon types. The use of proteomics to identify amyloidosis is an improvement over Congo red staining and polarized light to identify apple-green birefringence. Mass spectrometry proteomics also has been used to identify lymphoma-associated fusion proteins, such as NPM-ALK, as well as proteins that interact with fusion proteins (9,31).

Mutational Analysis

Traditional DNA sequencing for cancer was initially focused on the detection of cancer predisposition in the patient's germline (67). The "gold standard" method used for sequencing has been the method developed by Sanger (51). This method is considered "first-generation" technology, and newer methods that recently have been become available are referred to as "next-generation sequencing" (NGS), or massive parallel sequencing (37,48). Next-generation sequencing is a powerful, high-throughput method that allows the simultaneous detection of base substitutions, deletions, insertions, copy number alterations, and translocations in a single tube. Using NGS methods, the whole exome or genome can be sequenced within hours, although the analysis of the sequence is often far more time consuming.

From a research perspective, the identification of lymphoma driver somatic mutations may help define new subgroups of lymphoma with distinct clinical and biological characteristics. The identification of specific somatic mutations that alter cellular pathways also may reveal possible vulnerabilities of cancer cells to specific drugs. For example, a mutation that results in the activation of an oncoprotein may allow a clinician to choose the appropriate drug that inhibits that protein. It is now widely anticipated that NGS will enable in-depth characterization of the cancer cell genome and further advance the field of personalized medicine for patients with lymphomas and other cancers as well. It also seems likely that knowledge of gene mutations, particularly if specific targeted therapies become available, will lead to modifications of current lymphoma classification schemes.

REPORTING PATHOLOGY RESULTS: THE INTEGRATED REPORT

Election of the best therapy, which is the ultimate goal of the diagnostic process, is based on a multi-dimensional approach that includes the integration of clinical findings with intrinsic tumor qualities. In the "old days," the pathology report included data derived only from gross and microscopic evaluation of a lymphoma. As technology has evolved, the pathology report has expanded to include data from immunophenotypic (always), cytogenetic, and molecular analyses. With the advent of high-throughput molecular methods to the analysis of lymphoid lesions, it is expected that the number of data elements will be greatly increased in the near future. The hematopathologist is perhaps best positioned to integrate and deliver this information to clinicians. It would be highly convenient to have all this relevant information available in a single pathology report.

Relevant tumor qualities that need be reported include essential histologic variables such as the morphologic appearance of the lymphoma, degree of differentiation, growth pattern; the immunophenotype of the lymphoma cells, including cell lineage; proliferation rate (usually quantifying Ki-67 expression); and cytogenetic and molecular data such as gene rearrangements or translocations that help in the diagnosis and classification of the lymphoma (e.g., t(14;18)(q32;q21)/*IGH-BCL2* in follicular lymphoma or t(8;14)(q24;q32) in Burkitt lymphoma).

To date, the predominant role of the pathologist has been to determine the diagnosis and convey that information to the clinician. This role has evolved and now involves providing prognostic data. For example, in patients with DLBCL, knowledge of *MYC* rearrangement is essential for prognosis. In other examples, deletions in chromosomal regions 11q23 and 17p, usually shown by FISH, are associated with aggressive disease in patients with CLL/SLL and gene aberrations in the p53/MDM2 pathway, observed in a subset of mantle cell lymphoma patients, are associated with aggressive clinical behavior.

The pathologist's role also has evolved to include qualitative or quantitative assessment of molecules that can be targeted for therapy that is now required for many lymphoma patients. For example, the anti-CD20 agent, rituximab, has been available for over a decade and CD20 expression needs to be assessed prior to therapy with this agent. Antibody-drug conjugates have been developed as therapies (e.g., brentuximab verdotin) and therefore the expression of targets (e.g., CD30) needs to be assessed. There is also growing evidence to support the value of targeting cell signaling pathways that are activated in lymphomas, and either immunophenotypic assessment to show overexpression or genetic studies to prove the presence of activating mutations will need to be reported.

Parameter	Results
Clinical data	Inguinal and retroperitoneal lymphadenopathy. No history of lymphoma
Tissue site/procedure	Lymph node, right inguinal; excisional biopsy
Diagnosis	Diffuse large B-cell lymphoma with a germinal center cell signature
Immunophenotype	CD20+, CD19(+ decreased), CD38(+ decreased), CD10(+), BCL2(+), BCL6(+), MYC(+) MUM-1(+), CD5(-), FOXP1(-), PTEN(-), CD30(-)
EBER[a] in situ hybridization	Negative
Proliferation index (Ki-67)	50-60%
FISH	*MYC/BCL2/BCL6* are not rearranged
aCGH	Heterozygous deletion of 10q23 (*PTEN*)
Gene expression profile	Germinal center, stromal-1
2-gene score	High *LMO2*, high *TNFRSF9* (CD137) (good prognosis)
Sequencing	No mutation of *PTEN* (phosphatase and C2 domain)

Summary: Germinal center (GCB) DLBCL with stromal-1 signature, deletion of PTEN, and activation of PI3K/AKT. The neoplasm is likely associated with a good prognosis and seems to be dependent of PI3K/AKT activation (as indicated by the heterozygous deletion of *PTEN*). MYC expression is likely a consequence of PI3K/AKT activation and not due to the presence of *MYC* gene amplification/rearrangements.

Suggestions for therapy: The neoplasm may be susceptible to a combination of PI3K inhibitors, MYC and inhibitors of connective tissue growth factors.

Suggested References:
Lenz G, Wright G, Dave SS, et al. Stromal gene signatures in large B cell lymphomas. N Engl J Med 2008;359:2313 (29).
Pfeifer M, Grau M, Lenze D, et al. PTEN loss defines a PI3K/AKT pathway-dependent germinal center subtype of diffuse large B-cell lymphoma. Proc Natl Acad Sci USA 2013;110:12420 (43).
Alizadeh AA, Gentiles AJ, Alencar AJ, et al. Prediction of survival in diffuse large B-cell lymphoma based on the expression of 2 genes reflecting tumor and microenvironment. Blood 2011;118:1350 (2).

[a]EBER = Epstein-Barr virus encoded RNA; FISH = fluorescence in situ hybridization; aCGH = array comparative genomic hybridization.

Figure 2-15

EXAMPLE OF PATHOLOGY REPORT FOR DIFFUSE LARGE B-CELL LYMPHOMA

The diagnosis of DLBCL requires the integration of morphologic findings, immunophenotypic results, and the results of molecular testing. In the future, molecular testing will likely include the results of high-throughput methods such as next-generation sequencing. This approach will provide the prognostic and therapeutic information needed to be included in the pathology report.

The pathology report, like the pathologist, needs to evolve (fig. 2-15). The report should include all relevant pathologic information for a comprehensive diagnosis and must also include those factors that have been validated or considered to contribute to predict prognosis or to choose a particular therapy. The sets of relevant pathologic data differ for various lymphoma types and patient subsets, and thus the pathology report must be customized. Creating such a report will unlikely be a "once and done" effort because the data typically become available at different times. Pathology reports need to be updated (sometimes multiple times) to integrate all findings. A format that is "granular," allowing for the extraction of relevant data points for clinical and translation research efforts in the future, will be ideal. Improved bioinformatic design of the pathology report and ongoing support are important for creating an integrated report.

REFERENCES

1. Albinger-Hegyi A, Hochreutener B, Abdou MT, et al. High frequency of t(14;18)-translocation breakpoints outside of major breakpoint and minor cluster regions in follicular lymphomas: improved polymerase chain reaction protocols for their detection. Am J Pathol 2002;160:823-832.

2. Alizadeh AA, Gentiles AJ, Alencar AJ, et al. Prediction of survival in diffuse large B-cell lymphoma based on the expression of 2 genes reflecting tumor and microenvironment. Blood 2011;118:1350-1358.

3. Alizadeh AA, Eisen MB, Davis RE, et al. Distinct types of diffuse large B-cell lymphoma identified by gene expression profiling. Nature 2000;403:503-511.

4. Barrett MT, Scheffer A, Ben-Dor A, et al. Comparative genomic hybridization using oligonucleotide microarrays and total genomic DNA. Proc Natl Acad Sci USA 2004;101:17765-17770.

5. Bernard A, Boumsell L. [Human leukocyte differentiation antigens.] Presse Med 1984;13:2311-2316. [French]

6. Cady FM, Morice WG. Flow cytometric assessment of T-cell chronic lymphoproliferative disorders. Clin Lab Med 2007;27:513-532, vi.

7. Campo E. Whole genome profiling and other high throughput technologies in lymphoid neoplasms—current contributions and future hopes. Mod Pathol 2013;26:S97-S110.

8. Castro EC, Blazquez C, Boyd J, et al. Clinicopathologic features of histiocytic lesions following ALL, with a review of the literature. Pediatr Dev Pathol 2010;13:225-237.

9. Conlon KP, Basrur V, Rolland D, et al. Fusion peptides from oncogeneic chimeric proetins as specific biomarkers of cancer. Mol Cell Proteomics 2013;12:2714-2723.

10. Cossman J, Uppenkamp M, Andrade R, Medeiros LJ. T-cell receptor gene rearrangements and the diagnosis of human T-cell neoplasms. Crit Rev Oncol Hematol 1990;10:267-281.

11. Craig FE, Foon KA. Flow cytometric immunophenotyping for hematologic neoplasms. Blood 2008;111:3941-3967.

12. Davis BH, Holden JT, Bene MC, et al. 2006 Bethesda International Consensus recommendations on the flow cytometric immunophenotypic analysis of hematolymphoid neoplasia: medical indications. Cytometry B Clin Cytom 2007;72(Suppl 1):S5-13.

13. Demurtas A, Stacchini A, Aliberti S, Chiusa L, Chiarle R, Novero D. Tissue flow cytometry immunophenotyping in the diagnosis and classification of non-Hodgkin's lymphomas: a retrospective evaluation of 1,792 cases. Cytometry B Clin Cytom 2013;84:82-95.

14. Feng B, Jorgensen JL, Jones D, et al. Flow cytometric detection of peripheral blood involvement by mycosis fungoides and Sezary syndrome using T-cell receptor Vbeta chain antibodies and its application in blood staging. Mod Pathol 2010;23:284-295.

15. Gradowski JF, Sargent RL, Craig FE, et al. Chronic lymphocytic leukemia/small lymphocytic lymphoma with cyclin D1 positive proliferation centers do not have CCND1 translocations or gains and lack SOX11 expression. Am J Clin Pathol 2012;138:132-139.

16. Greif PA, Konstandin NP, Metzeler KH, et al. RUNX1 mutations in cytogenetically normal acute myeloid leukemia are associated with a poor prognosis and up-regulation of lymphoid genes. Haematologica 2012;97:1909-1215.

17. Gribben JG. Monitoring disease in lymphoma and CLL patients using molecular techniques. Best Pract Res Clin Haematol 2002;15:179-195.

18. Gulley ML, Raab-Traub N. Detection of Epstein-Barr virus in human tissues by molecular genetic techniques. Arch Pathol Lab Med 1993;117:1115-1120.

19. Haedicke W, Ho FC, Chott A, et al. Expression of CD94/NKG2A and killer immunoglobulin-like receptors in NK cells and a subset of extranodal cytotoxic T-cell lymphomas. Blood 2000;95:3628-3630.

20. Jacobson JO, Wilkes BM, Kwiatkowski DJ, Medeiros LJ, Aisenberg AC, Harris NL. bcl-2 rearrangements in de novo diffuse large cell lymphoma. Association with distinctive clinical features. Cancer 1993;72:231-236.

21. Jardin F, Figeac M. MicroRNAs in lymphoma, from diagnosis to targeted therapy. Curr Opin Oncol 2013;25:480-486.

22. Jorgensen JL. State of the Art Symposium: flow cytometry in the diagnosis of lymphoproliferative disorders by fine-needle aspiration. Cancer 2005;105:443-51.

23. Kallioniemi OP, Kallioniemi A, Sudar D, et al. Comparative genomic hybridization: a rapid new method for detecting and mapping DNA amplification in tumors. Semin Cancer Biol 1993;4:41-46.

24. Kanavaros, P, Farcet JP, Gaulard P, et al. Recombinative events of the T cell antigen receptor delta gene in peripheral T cell lymphomas. J Clin Invest 1991;87:666-672.

25. Kinney MC, Higgins RA, Medina EA. Anaplastic large cell lymphoma: twenty-five years of discovery. Arch Pathol Lab Med 2011;135:19-43.

26. Klein F, Feldhahn N, Herzog S, et al. BCR-ABL1 induces aberrant splicing of IKAROS and lineage infidelity in pre-B lymphoblastic leukemia cells. Oncogene 2006;25:1118-1124.

27. Lawrie CH. MicroRNAs and lymphomagenesis: a functional review. Br J Haematol 2013;160:571-581.

28. Lefranc MP, Rabbitts TH. The human T-cell receptor gamma (TRG) genes. Trends Biochem Sci 1989;14:214-218.

29. Lenz G, Wright G, Dave SS, et al. Stromal gene signatures in large B cell lymphomas. N Engl J Med 2008;359:2313-2323.

30. Li S, Lin P, Fayad LE, et al. B-cell lymphomas with MYC/8q24 rearrangements and IGH@ BCL2/t(14;18)(q32;q21): an aggressive disease with heterogeneous histology, germinal center B-cell immunophenotype and poor outcome. Mod Pathol 2012;25:145-156.

31. Lim MS, Elenitoba-Johnson KS. Proteomics in pathology research. Lab Invest 2004;84:1227-1244.

32. Liu C, Iqbal J, Teruya-Feldstein J, et al. MicroRNA expression profiling identified molecular signatures associated with anaplastic large cell lymphoma. Blood 2013;122:2083-2092.

33. Louissaint A Jr, Ackerman AM, Dias-Santagata D, et al. Pediatric-type nodal follicular lymphoma: an indolent clonal proliferation in children and adults with high proliferation index and no BCL2 rearrangement. Blood 2012;120:2395-2404.

34. Luthra R, Sarris AH, Hai S, et al. Real-time 5′->3′ exonuclease-based PCR assay for detection of the t(11;14)(q13;q32). Am J Clin Pathol 1999;112:524-530.

35. Medeiros LJ, Carr J. Overview of the role of molecular methods in the diagnosis of malignant lymphomas. Arch Pathol Lab Med 1999;123:1189-1207.

36. Medeiros LJ, Van Krieken JH, Jaffe ES, Raffeld M. Association of bcl-1 rearrangements with lymphocytic lymphoma of intermediate differentiation. Blood 1990;76:2086-2090.

37. Metzker ML. Sequencing technologies—the next generation. Nat Rev Genet 2010;11:31-46.

38. Meyerson HJ, Awadallah A, Pavlidakey P, Cooper K, Honda K, Miedler J. Follicular center helper T-cell (TFH) marker positive mycosis fungoides/ Sezary syndrome. Mod Pathol 2013;26:32-43.

39. Morris SW, Kirstein MN, Valentine MB, et al. Fusion of a kinase gene, ALK, to a nucleolar protein gene, NPM, in non-Hodgkin's lymphoma. Science 1994;263:1281-1284.

40. Mullis KB. The unusual origin of the polymerase chain reaction. Sci Am 1990;262:56-61, 64-65.

41. Ohshima A, Miura I, Hashimoto K, et al. Rearrangements of the BCL6 gene and chromosome aberrations affecting 3q27 in 54 patients with non-Hodgkin's lymphoma. Leuk Lymphoma 1997;27:329-334.

42. Orucevic A, Reddy VB, Selvaggi SM, Green L, Spitz DJ, Gattuso P. Fine-needle aspiration of extranodal and extramedullary hematopoietic malignancies. Diagn Cytopathol 2000;23:318-321.

43. Pfeifer M, Grau M, Lenze D, et al. PTEN loss defines a PI3K/AKT pathway-dependent germinal center subtype of diffuse large B-cell lymphoma. Proc Natl Acad Sci USA 2013;110:12420-12425.

44. Picker LJ, Weiss LM, Medeiros LJ, Wood GS, Warnke RA. Immunophenotypic criteria for the diagnosis of non-Hodgkin's lymphoma. Am J Pathol 1987;128:181-201.

45. Pillai RK, Sathanoori M, Van Oss SB, Swerdlow SH. Double-hit B-cell lymphomas with BCL6 and MYC translocations are aggressive, frequently extranodal lymphomas distinct from BCL2 double-hit B-cell lymphomas. Am J Surg Pathol 2013;37:323-332.

46. Redon R, Ishikawa S, Fitch KR, et al. Global variation in copy number in the human genome. Nature 2006;444:444-454.

47. Remstein ED, Kurtin PJ, Buno I, et al. Diagnostic utility of fluorescence in situ hybridization in mantle-cell lymphoma. Br J Haematol 2000;110:856-862.

48. Ross JS, Cronin M. Whole cancer genome sequencing by next-generation methods. Am J Clin Pathol 2011;136:527-539.

49. Sanchez-Vega B, Vega F, Hai S, Medeiros LJ, Luthra R. Real-Time t(14;18)(q32;q21) PCR assay combined with high-resolution capillary electrophoresis: a novel and rapid approach that allows accurate quantitation and size determination of bcl-2/JH fusion sequences. Mod Pathol 2002;15:448-453.

50. Sanchez-Vega B, Vega F, Medeiros LJ, Lee MS, Luthra R. Quantification of bcl-2/JH fusion sequences and a control gene by multiplex real-time PCR coupled with automated amplicon sizing by capillary electrophoresis. J Mol Diagn 2002;4:223-229.

51. Sanger F, Nicklen S, Coulson AR. DNA sequencing with chain-terminating inhibitors. Proc Natl Acad Sci USA 1977;74:5463-5467.

52. Sawada A, Sato E, Koyama M, et al. NK-cell repertoire is feasible for diagnosing Epstein-Barr virus-infected NK-cell lymphoproliferative disease and evaluating the treatment effect. Am J Hematol 2006;81:576-581.

53. Scholzen T, Gerdes J. The Ki-67 protein: from the known and the unknown. J Cell Physiol 2000;182:311-322.

54. Schwab C, Willers J, Niederer E, et al. The use of anti-T-cell receptor-Vbeta antibodies for the estimation of treatment success and phenotypic characterization of clonal T-cell populations in cutaneous T-cell lymphomas. Br J Haematol 2002;118:1019-1026.

55. Schwaenen C, Nessling M, Wessendorf S, et al. Automated array-based genomic profiling in chronic lymphocytic leukemia: development of a clinical tool and discovery of recurrent genomic alterations. Proc Natl Acad Sci U S A 2004;101:1039-1044.

56. Southern EM. Detection of specific sequences among DNA fragments separated by gel electrophoresis. J Mol Biol 1975;98:503-517.

57. Staudt LM, Dent, AL, Shaffer AL, Yu X. Regulation of lymphocyte cell fate decisions and lymphomagenesis by BCL-6. Int Rev Immunol 1999;18:381-403.

58. Streubel B, Simonitsch-Klupp I, Mullauer L, et al. Variable frequencies of MALT lymphoma-associated genetic aberrations in MALT lymphomas of different sites. Leukemia 2004;18:1722-1726.

59. Theodorou I, Raphael M, Bigorgne C, et al. Recombination pattern of the TCR gamma locus in human peripheral T-cell lymphomas. J Pathol 1994;174:233-242.

60. Tsujimoto Y, Cossman J, Jaffe E, Croce CM. Involvement of the bcl-2 gene in human follicular lymphoma. Science 1985;228:1440-1443.

61. Vega F, Medeiros LJ, Bueso-Ramos C, et al. Hepatosplenic gamma/delta T-cell lymphoma in bone marrow. A sinusoidal neoplasm with blastic cytologic features. Am J Clin Pathol 2001;116:410-419.

62. Vega F, Medeiros LJ, Jones D, et al. A novel four-color PCR assay to assess T-cell receptor gamma gene rearrangements in lymphoproliferative lesions. Am J Clin Pathol 2001;116:17-24.

63. Vinatzer U, Gollinger M, Mullauer L, Raderer M, Chott A, Streubel B. Mucosa-associated lymphoid tissue lymphoma: novel translocations including rearrangements of ODZ2, JMJD2C, and CNN3. Clin Cancer Res 2008;6426-6431.

64. Vos JA, Abbondanzo SL, Barekman CL, Andriko JW, Miettinen M, Aguilera NS. Histiocytic sarcoma: a study of five cases including the histiocyte marker CD163. Mod Pathol 2005;18:693-704.

65. Vrana JA, Gamez JD, Madden BJ, Theis JD, Bergen HR 3rd, Dogan A. Classification of amyloidosis by laser microdissection and mass spectrophotometry-based proteomic analysis in clinical biopsy specimens. Blood 2009; 114: 4957-4599.

66. Waldmann TA, White JD, Goldman CK, et al. The interleukin-2 receptor: a target for monoclonal antibody treatment of human T-cell lymphotrophic virus I-induced adult T-cell leukemia. Blood 1993;82:1701-1712.

67. Weinstein JL, Ayyanar K, Watral MA. Cancer predisposition syndromes. Cancer Treat Res 2009;150:223-238.

68. Williams ME, Swerdlow SH, Rosenberg CL, Arnold A. Chromosome 11 translocation breakpoints at the PRAD1/cyclin D1 gene locus in centrocytic lymphoma. Leukemia 1993;7:241-245.

69. Willman CL, Busque L, Griffith BB, et al. Langerhans'-cell histiocytosis (histiocytosis X)—a clonal proliferative disease. N Engl J Med 1994;331:154-160.

70. Wu D, Wood BL, Fromm JR. Flow cytometry for non-Hodgkin and classical Hodgkin lymphoma. Methods Mol Biol 2013;971:27-47.

71. Ye BH, Chaganti S, Chang CC, et al. Chromosomal translocations cause deregulated BCL6 expression by promoter substitution in B cell lymphoma. Embo J 1995;14:6209-6217.

72. Yunis JJ, Frizzera G, Oken MM, McKenna J, Theologides A, Arnesen M. Multiple recurrent genomic defects in follicular lymphoma. A possible model for cancer. N Engl J Med 1987;316:79-84.

73. Yunis JJ, Sanchez O. G-banding and chromosome structure. Chromosoma 1973;44:15-23.

3

NEEDLE CORE BIOPSY AND FINE-NEEDLE ASPIRATION FOR THE DIAGNOSIS OF LYMPHOPROLIFERATIVE DISORDERS

One traditional approach to the evaluation of biopsy specimens is to study the pathologic findings and establish a diagnosis or differential diagnosis before correlating with the history. In this way, the pathologist initially evaluates the morphologic findings without bias. This approach is less helpful in the evaluation of small needle core biopsy and fine-needle aspiration (FNA) specimens. The clinical setting, including the patient age, the distribution of disease, the anatomic site of the biopsy, and the relevant history, are important for diagnosis. If the lesion is nonpalpable, then communication during the procedure between the pathologist and the physician obtaining the specimen is essential.

Needle core biopsy and FNA have advantages and disadvantages, and in many ways, these techniques are complementary. The needle core biopsy, if well done, allows appreciation of the nodal architecture, which is helpful because some lymphoid diseases are difficult to distinguish without such knowledge. FNA smears often allow better assessment of the cytologic features of the lymphoid cells. Although the needle core biopsy often yields a larger specimen for analysis, this is not always the case. In our experience, FNA can yield larger numbers of cells as well as small tissue fragments that, in aggregate, are more abundant than that obtained by needle core biopsy. In part, the different yields obtained by needle core biopsy and FNA depend on the type of lymphoma and presence or absence of sclerosis. Performing needle core biopsy and FNA concurrently enhances the chances of establishing a solid diagnosis.

It is mandatory that immunophenotypic analysis be performed with needle core biopsy and FNA, often further supported by cytogenetic or molecular studies. The diagnosis of lymphoma requires the integration of morphologic findings with cell lineage (B versus T cell) and often specific molecular findings. A review of the English-language literature found that FNA and needle core biopsy (with ancillary studies) establish a diagnosis adequate for treatment decisions in 65 to 75 percent of patients with lymphoma (14).

NEEDLE CORE BIOPSY

In the past decade, many institutions have observed a rapid rise in the frequency of lymph node needle core biopsies. While the material obtained by needle core biopsy is more limited than that obtained by an excisional lymph node biopsy, there are a number of reasons for the increasing popularity of this procedure (Table 3-1). First, needle core biopsy can spare the patient a surgical procedure. The operating room is not needed, recuperation time is minimal, and the

Table 3-1

ADVANTAGES AND DISADVANTAGES OF NEEDLE CORE BIOPSY

Advantages
Less complex than excisional biopsy
Lymph nodes difficult to excise can be sampled using image guidance
The most abnormal lymph node can be sampled, rather than the most accessible
Little morbidity
Patient does not require admission to the hospital
No operating room or surgeon is required
Less expensive
Small specimens can be rapidly processed

Disadvantages
Difficult to establish certain diagnoses, especially if architecture is needed
Small specimen size can lead to sampling error
Artifactual distortion of cytologic features (e.g., fibrotic specimens)
Workup results in paraffin block being exhausted[a]

[a]Exhaustion of the paraffin block can be problematic if material is needed subsequently to assess for therapy targets (e.g., assessment of antigen expression or next-generation sequencing).

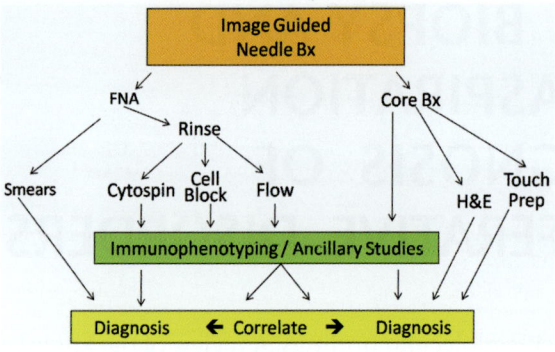

Figure 3-1

TRIAGING IMAGE-GUIDED BIOPSY SPECIMENS

A schematic illustrating the components of fine-needle aspiration (FNA) and needle core biopsy (Bx) specimens and their potential applications to arrive at a diagnosis.

risk of complications such as infection, poor wound healing, or excessive bleeding is minimized. Apart from such benefits to the patient, there are substantial savings of resources. Lachar et al. (17) estimated that a needle core biopsy performed to assess a superficial lymph node suspected of being involved by lymphoma is approximately 75 percent less expensive than an excisional lymph node biopsy. The savings are likely to be greater for patients with deep-seated lymph nodes.

Needle core biopsy is valuable for excluding nonhematopoietic neoplasms, staging patients with known lymphoma, and assessing for relapse in lymphoma patients. In these scenarios, the goal is to document the presence of lymphoma and address a potential change in the histologic findings (i.e., transformation or second tumor). By contrast, using needle core biopsy as an initial diagnostic approach, in other words to establish a de novo diagnosis of lymphoma, is more challenging. Although an adequate diagnosis often can be established, issues of sampling error and adequacy of tissue for ancillary studies arise. These issues can be addressed, at least in part, by optimizing tissue sampling (fig. 3-1). Optimization includes the use of an adequately sized needle to perform the core biopsy and obtaining multiple passes to ensure that adequate material is procured, not only for histologic analysis, but for ancillary studies such as flow cytometric immunophenotyping and immunohistochemical analysis. In some

cases, material should be sent for cytogenetic and molecular studies as well.

Diagnostic Approach Emphasizing Limitations

When evaluating needle core biopsy specimens, sampling is the most important issue. Some samples have features that are recognizable as a distinct type of lymphoma. More often, the features are suggestive of an entity, but the diagnosis can only be established with immunophenotypic data. To optimize evaluation, it is important to have a well-preserved specimen and to sample different areas of the lesion. Several studies have reported higher diagnostic accuracy when tissue cores were obtained using an 18-gauge needle (or larger) and when 4 to 5 cores were obtained (1–3,9,11,19,21). However, tissue retrieval is highly variable in published studies and there are no uniform guidelines.

Since needle core biopsy specimens are small, they can be fixed in formalin and processed, either overnight or on the same day. In our practice, we request hematoxylin and eosin (H&E)-stained slides on the first and last levels of the paraffin block, with at least eight unstained slides in between, up front, for ancillary testing. Usually immunohistochemical studies, but also fluorescence in situ hybridization (FISH) and polymerase chain reaction (PCR)-based tests can be performed on unstained slides.

Touch imprints of the needle core biopsy specimen (fig. 3-2) are helpful for evaluating specimen adequacy and assessing cytomorphologic findings. Touch imprints are air-dried and assessed with Romanowsky stains (Wright-Giemsa, May-Grunwald-Giemsa, or Diff-Quik) or are alcohol-fixed and stained with Papanicolaou (Pap) or H&E. These stains highlight different cellular features and are useful in combination. Touch imprints show morphologic features similar to aspirate smears although the cytologic features are less well preserved, and stripped cytoplasm and distorted nuclear shapes are more common (see Fine-Needle Aspiration Biopsy).

Large B-cell lymphomas are often diagnosed by core needle biopsy. The presence of cytologically atypical, large lymphoid cells with a B-cell immunophenotype is sufficient to render a diagnosis (fig. 3-3). Similarly, small B-cell lymphomas are often diagnosed by needle biopsy although small neoplastic lymphocytes may be mistaken

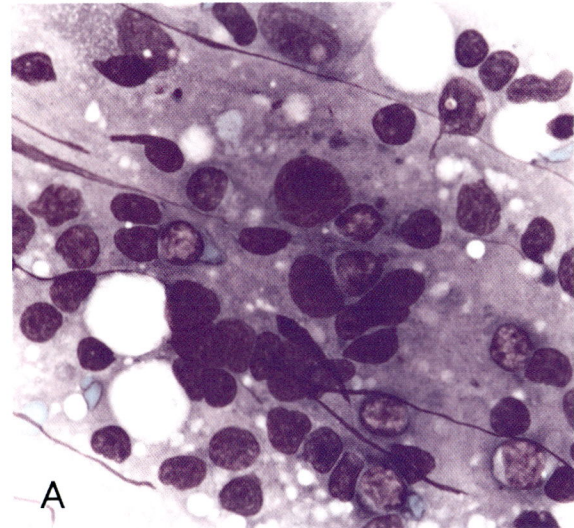

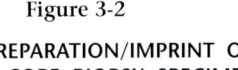

Figure 3-2

TOUCH PREPARATION/IMPRINT OF A NEEDLE CORE BIOPSY SPECIMEN

A: A large atypical cell with a prominent nucleolus suggestive of a Hodgkin cell is seen in a background of small lymphocytes (Wright-Giemsa stain).

B: High-power magnification of a needle core biopsy specimen of Hodgkin lymphoma showing large atypical mononuclear and binucleated cells in a background of small lymphocytes and eosinophils (hematoxylin and eosin [H&E] stain).

C: The large atypical cells are positive for CD30.

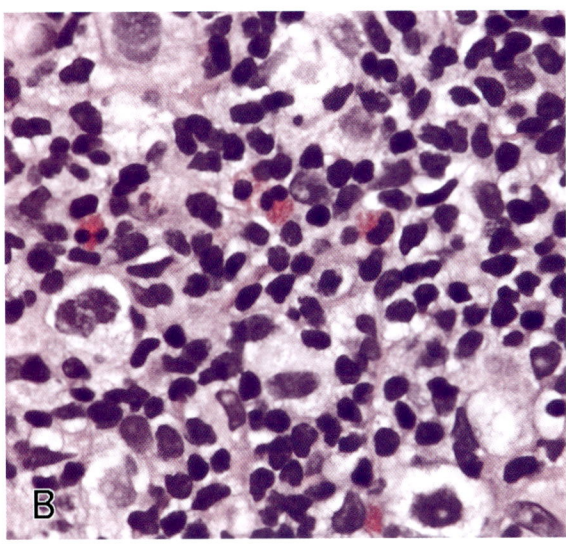

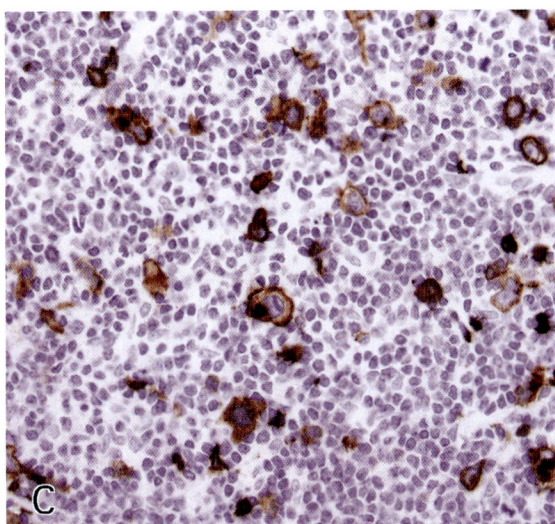

for non-neoplastic elements if large lymphoid cells are also present. The presence of a monotypic B-cell population supports a diagnosis of small B-cell lymphoma, and other markers facilitate more complete classification (16), for example, cyclin D1 expression supports mantle cell lymphoma (fig. 3-4). It can be difficult to subclassify small B-cell lymphomas, however, when the results of flow cytometry immunophenotyping studies are not representative, or immunohistochemical results are equivocal (10).

Small needle core biopsy specimens can preclude assessment of architecture, in part because of their size, but also because the specimen is often fragmented. Any lymphoma diagnosis that depends on or is aided by the architecture

of a neoplasm can be problematic using this technique. A good example is the distinction between nodular lymphocyte-predominant Hodgkin lymphoma and T-cell/histiocyte-rich large B-cell lymphoma. These two entities can be composed of cytologically similar cell populations and the large B cells have a similar B-cell immunophenotype. Therefore, assessment of architecture is very helpful. In an appreciable subset of needle core biopsy specimens, however, the architecture cannot be assessed reliably, particularly if small gauge needles are used (15,24). Another potential source of error is a sample in which a benign structure, incompletely sampled, mimics lymphoma. In particular, large follicles may not be well seen or may be only partially

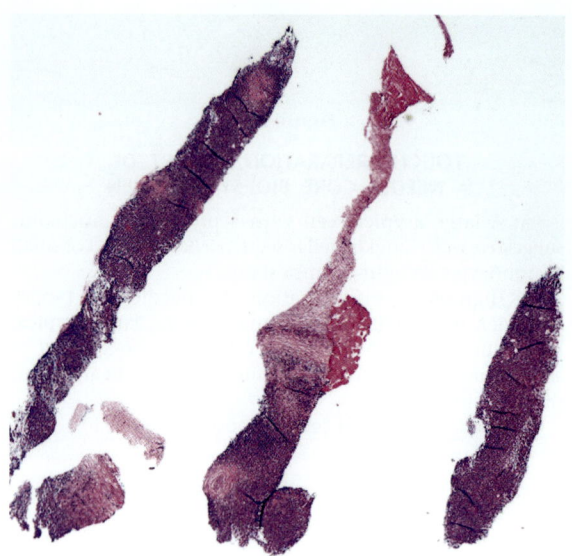
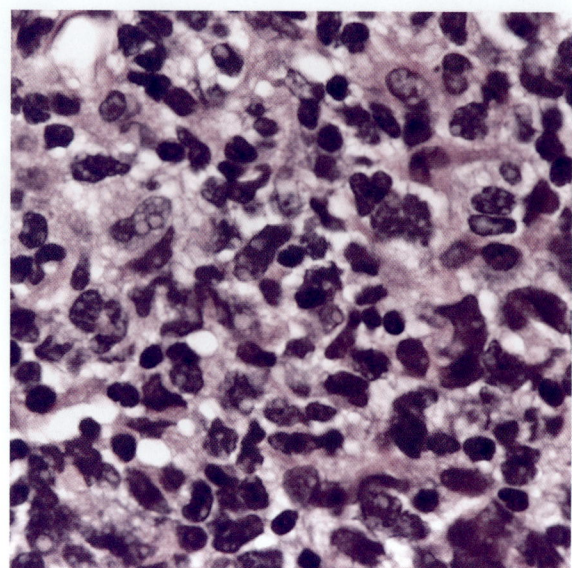

Figure 3-3

NEEDLE CORE BIOPSY SPECIMEN OF LARGE B-CELL LYMPHOMA

Left: 20-gauge needle cores of large B-cell lymphoma are shown (H&E stain).
Right: A diffuse infiltrate of large cells with irregular nuclei and prominent nucleoli is seen (H&E stain).

sampled in needle core biopsy specimens and can mimic large B-cell lymphoma (18).

In follicular lymphoma, architectural pattern is not required for diagnosis but it is recommended that the follicular pattern in a tumor be estimated as a percentage of the entire tumor (26). Although antibodies specific for follicular dendritic cells (e.g., CD21) (fig. 3-5) help to highlight tumor follicles, an estimation of the percentage of the follicular pattern in a follicular lymphoma is likely to be unreliable in small needle biopsy specimens (3).

The grading of follicular lymphomas can be another problem in core needle biopsy specimens. It is well known that the neoplastic follicles exhibit a range of grades from follicle to follicle. A small biopsy specimen, due to sampling error, may not reliably reflect the overall grade. Radiologic studies need to be correlated with the pathologic findings in this circumstance, as discordance between tumor grade and positron emission tomography (PET) activity suggests that the needle biopsy specimen is not representative of the tumor grade.

For lymphomas that exhibit a wide spectrum of morphologic findings, such as anaplastic large cell lymphoma (fig. 3-6), a small needle core biopsy specimen can be misinterpreted as another type of lymphoma or possibly as a nonlymphoid malignancy. In these cases, the diagnosis hinges on the recognition of morphologic clues, such as the presence of cells with horseshoe-shaped nuclei (hallmark cells) particularly around blood vessels, an aberrant T-cell immunophenotype, and positivity for CD30 and anaplastic lymphoma kinase (ALK)-1. The reliability and interpretation of the immunohistochemical markers in these cases are crucial.

For lymphomas that require extensive immunophenotypic or molecular studies for complete classification, such as natural killer (NK)-cell lymphomas, a needle core biopsy specimen may be inadequate for diagnosis. In this case, adequate FNA material for complete flow cytometry immunophenotypic studies is essential (25).

The presence of extensive necrosis or sclerosis is another common problem that can hinder a diagnosis of lymphoma in a needle core biopsy specimen. Necrosis is observed in high-grade lymphomas or in lymph nodes status post-therapy. In some patients, an optimally sized needle core biopsy specimen may consist of only necrotic tissue. In this scenario, the material submitted for flow cytometry may be viable and helpful for diagnosis, or may be necrotic and useless. Immunohistochemical

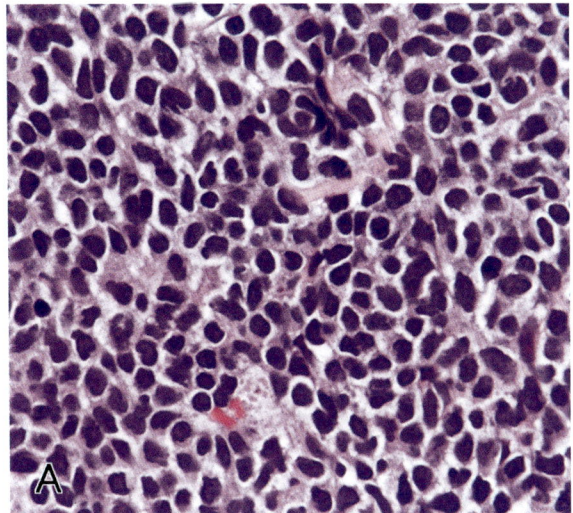

Figure 3-4

NEEDLE CORE BIOPSY SPECIMEN OF MANTLE CELL LYMPHOMA

A: There is a predominantly small lymphoid population (H&E stain).

B,C: Most of the cells are reactive for cyclin D1 (B) and PAX5 (C).

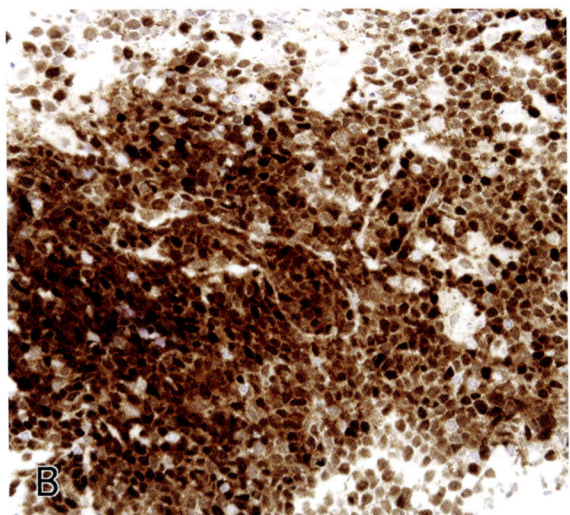

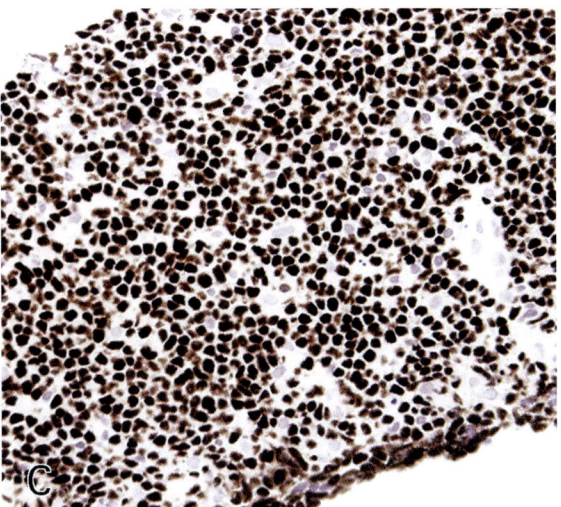

stains of necrotic tissue can suggest lineage, for example, CD20 reactivity, but these results are difficult to interpret and many antibodies are not reliable in the assessment of necrotic tissue. The diagnosis of classic Hodgkin lymphoma may be problematic because these tumors may be necrotic, or more often, fibrotic (fig. 3-7), resulting in limited cellularity. Reed-Sternberg and Hodgkin cells can be sparse in the needle core biopsy specimens, or the sample may not capture the full spectrum of histologic features, thereby compromising diagnostic accuracy.

FINE-NEEDLE ASPIRATION BIOPSY

Traditionally, both architectural and cytologic features have been instrumental in establishing the diagnosis, as well as the classification, of lym-

phoma. The major limitation of cytologic preparations is the lack of architectural clarity (Table 3-2). While architecture is important, the advent of ancillary studies, especially immunophenotypic methods, has made the diagnosis and classification of many lymphoma entities possible using the current World Health Organization (WHO) classification system. The value of cytologic evaluation of lymphoproliferative disorders, combined with the results of appropriate ancillary studies, is currently well established (7,12,27).

The cytologic examination of lymph nodes for suspected lymphoma is not simply the morphologic examination of aspirate smears. A complete FNA workup includes the preparation of a cell block from tiny tissue fragments that often come out of the needle, if possible. It is

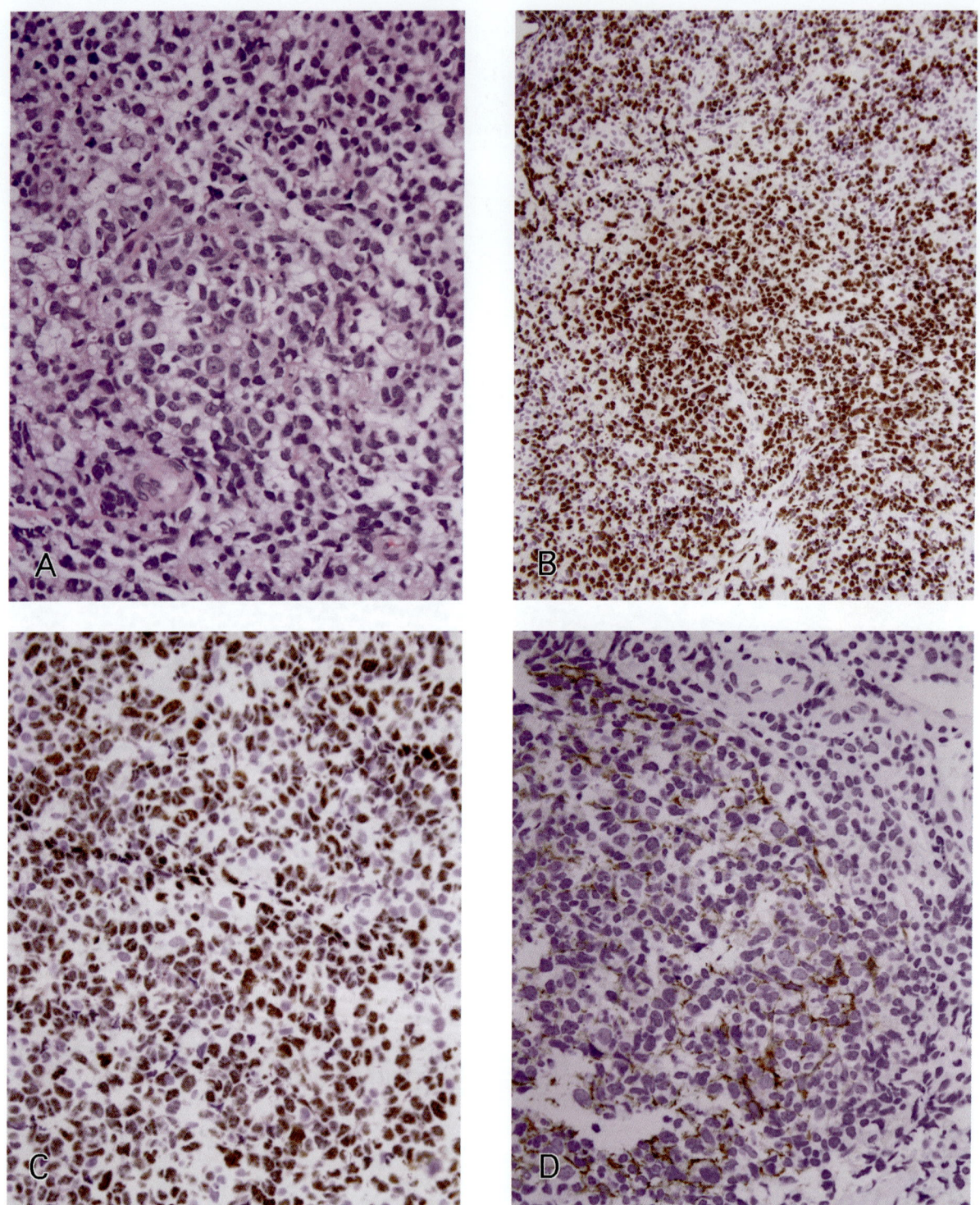

Figure 3-5

NEEDLE CORE BIOPSY SPECIMEN OF FOLLICULAR LYMPHOMA, GRADE 2

A: A mixture of centrocytes and centroblasts is shown (H&E stain).
B,C: The large lymphoid cells are reactive for PAX5 (B) and BCL6.
D: CD21 expression highlights follicular dendritic cells in a follicle.

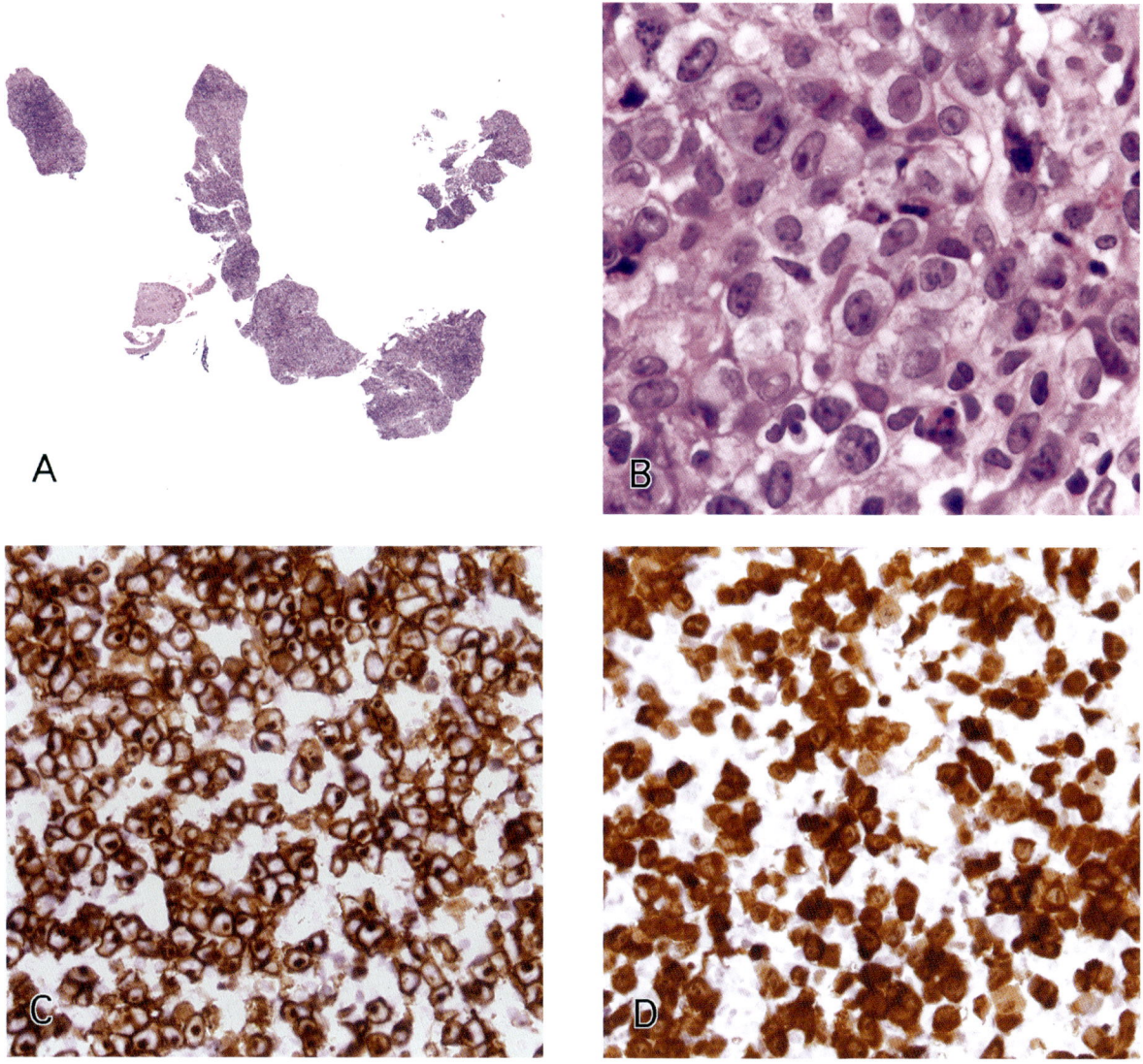

Figure 3-6

NEEDLE CORE BIOPSY SPECIMEN OF ANAPLASTIC LARGE CELL LYMPHOMA

A,B: There is a diffuse infiltrate of large neoplastic cells (H&E stain).
C,D: The tumor cells are positive for CD30 (C) and ALK-1 (D).

also imperative that these cytologic specimens be interpreted using a multiparameter approach. This approach includes analysis of the cytomorphologic features in conjunction with other ancillary studies such as immunophenotyping and molecular studies (4). Not all of these studies are necessary in every case; however, immunophenotypic analysis is imperative for a diagnosis with specific classification. Flow cytometric analysis is an essential component of an FNA workup of lymph nodes or tumors suspected to be lymphoma and several passes may be necessary to obtain sufficient material. Furthermore, experience is required to obtain the specimen and interpret the results.

Fine-Needle Aspiration Technique

For enlarged lymph nodes that are superficial, palpation is used to guide the FNA biopsy, but for deep seated lymph nodes, radiographic guidance is required. For superficial palpable lymph nodes, after cleaning the skin, the selected lymph node

---

Table 3-2

**INDICATIONS FOR FINE-NEEDLE ASPIRATION (FNA)
AND ADVANTAGES OF CONCURRENT NEEDLE CORE BIOPSY AND FNA**

Indications for FNA
　Primary diagnosis in selected cases, especially low-grade lymphomas
　Document relapse and cell type
　Clarify stage
　Rule out transformation of low-grade lymphomas
　Diagnose second primary neoplasms
　Obtain tissue for immunophenotypic, cytogenetic, and FISH[a] analysis

Advantages of Concurrent Needle Core Biopsy and FNA
　Both procedures can be performed in an outpatient setting
　Increased likelihood of definitive diagnosis when cytologic and histologic findings are integrated and correlated with
　　ancillary data
　Optimal for directing the sampling of problematic specimens (e.g., necrotic or fibrotic)
　Can assess specimen adequacy for flow cytometry immunophenotypic analysis[b]

---

[a]FISH = fluorescence in situ hybridization.
[b]Abundant peripheral blood, fat, or necrotic debris may cause erroneously elevated cell counts in FNA specimens.

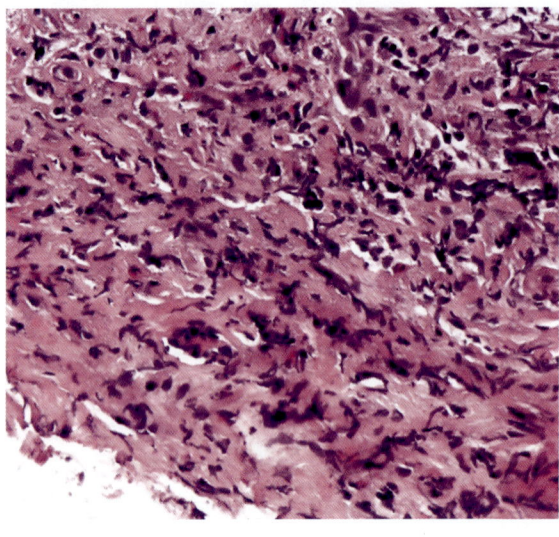

Figure 3-7

**NEEDLE CORE BIOPSY SPECIMEN FROM A PATIENT
WITH A HISTORY OF HODGKIN LYMPHOMA**

Abundant sclerosis is infiltrated by large atypical cells (H & E). The atypical cells were positive for CD30 and CD15 and negative for CD20, consistent with recurrent disease.

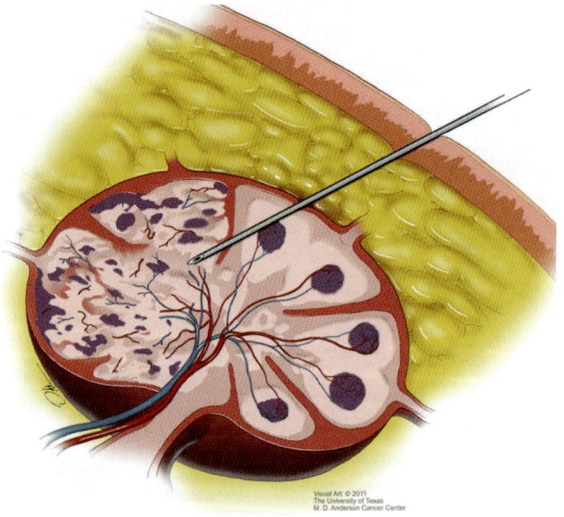

Figure 3-8

FINE-NEEDLE ASPIRATION

Diagram depicting FNA sampling of a lymph node partially involved by lymphoma.

is immobilized between the fingers of one hand and aspirated with the dominant hand. This insures that the needle tip does not displace the target lymph node. In nonpalpable lesions, the needle is guided to the target area using various imaging modalities such as ultrasound or computerized tomography (CT).

The FNA technique is essentially the same for all organ sites, both palpable and nonpalpable

(fig. 3-8). A small drop of the aspirated material is placed on slides and smeared. The smeared slides can be air-dried or immediately fixed in alcohol. The remainder of the material is rinsed into a cell media solution such as RPMI which can be triaged for immunophenotyping and, if needed, molecular studies (fig. 3-9).

It is often necessary to aspirate the lymph node several times to obtain adequate material for cytologic examination and ancillary studies. An automated cell counter helps ensure that

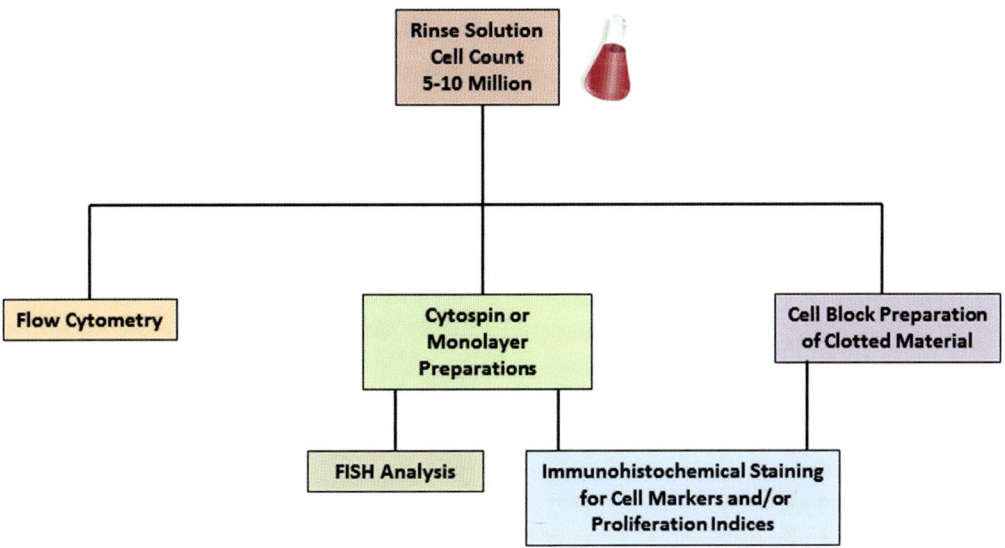

Figure 3-9

FINE-NEEDLE ASPIRATION

Algorithm for triaging FNA rinse solutions for ancillary studies.

adequate numbers of lymphocytes have been collected. An optimal cell count for immunophenotypic analysis is approximately 10 million cells. The cellularity on the slides should be correlated with the cell count. Cell counts may be falsely elevated in cases with extensive necrosis, adipose tissue, or excessive peripheral blood contamination that is not properly lysed. When both FNA and core biopsies are performed, the FNA biopsy should be done prior to the core biopsy so that there is less peripheral blood contamination.

Immediate assessment of the aspirate smears helps to optimize adequate sampling. Adequacy can be assessed using air-dried smears stained with Romanowsky stains or alcohol-fixed smears stained with Pap or H&E (fig. 3-10). As these stains highlight different cellular features, using a combination of stains is helpful. The Romanowsky stain accentuates cytoplasmic features whereas cytoplasmic granules are best seen in preparations stained with Wright-Giemsa. The Diff-Quik method is rapid and easier to perform than Wright-Giemsa, but cytoplasmic granules are not as well visualized. The Pap method is optimal for evaluating cell size and nuclear features. Although performing a Pap stain takes more time compared with the Diff-Quik method, it can

usually be done in less than 5 minutes using a modified staining method. H&E-stained slides, similar to the Pap method, are helpful for assessing cell size and nuclear features. In addition, surgical pathologists with limited experience in the evaluation of cytologic smears may be more comfortable with H&E-stained slides since they are used in surgical pathology.

Cytologic features also can be assessed on slides prepared from the rinse solution, such as cytospin and liquid-based preparations (22). While these methods typically show good cytologic detail, liquid-based preparations should be used with caution since the cells often appear smaller, nucleoli are more prominent, aggregates of cells are fragmented, lymphocytes may aggregate into tight clusters, and background elements are more difficult to recognize (22). Likewise on cytospin preparations, lymphocytes often have artifactually induced irregular nuclear contours.

If the aspirates are paucicellular on immediate assessment, additional material can be obtained with a needle core biopsy. The presence of extensive necrosis may be an indicator to redirect the needle to the outer edge or a less necrotic area, to sample a different lesion, or to send material for

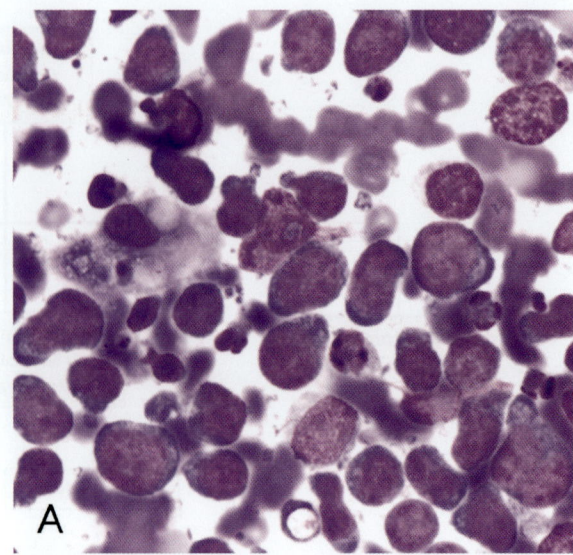

Figure 3-10

CYTOLOGIC PREPARATIONS OF BURKITT LYMPHOMA
A: Aspirate smear (Diff-Quik stain).
B: Cytospin preparation (Diff-Quik stain).
C: Touch imprint (Wright-Giemsa stain).

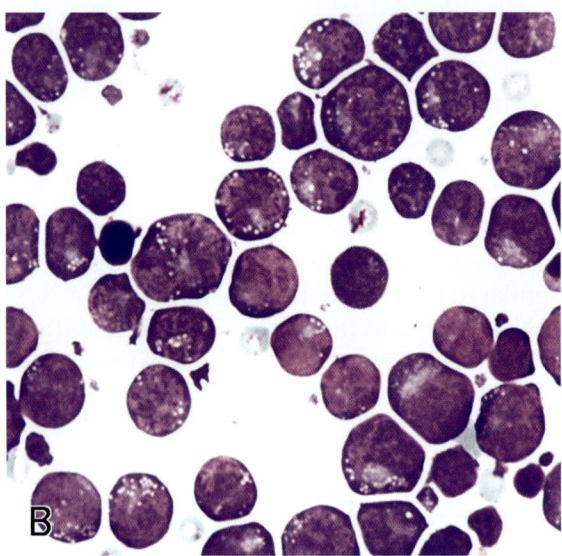

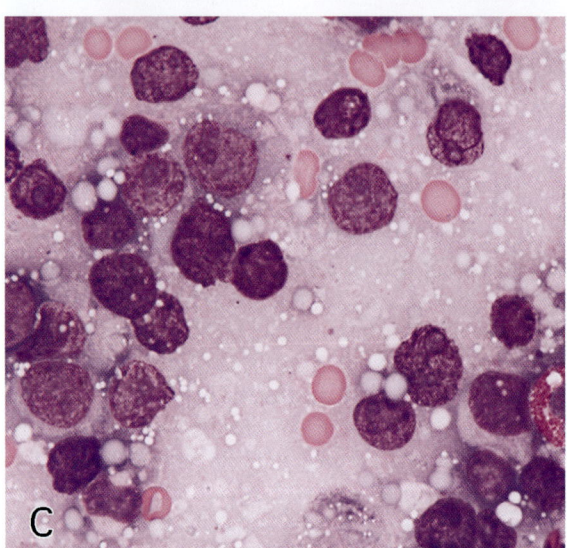

cultures in the appropriate clinical/radiographic setting. In cases suspected to be Hodgkin lymphoma, a core needle biopsy should be considered, especially for the initial diagnosis (23).

Diagnostic Approach Emphasizing Limitations

Evaluation of the cytomorphologic features is essential in developing a differential diagnosis. Most lymphoproliferative processes show a dispersed population of cells with relatively scant cytoplasm compared with epithelioid neoplasms which tend to have larger cells and be more cohesive. The presence of lymphoglandular bodies (also known as Soderstrom bodies), small detached cytoplasmic fragments in the background, is a helpful indicator of a lymphoproliferative process. Lymphoglandular bodies are more common in B-cell neoplasms, but have been described in T-cell, myeloid, and rarely, nonlymphoid neoplasms (13).

One approach to evaluating the cytomorphologic features is to determine whether the lymphoid population is polymorphic or monomorphic (fig. 3-11). In lesions composed of a polymorphic lymphoid population, the differential diagnosis typically includes reactive conditions versus lymphoma/leukemia. Since most lymphomas are of B-cell lineage,

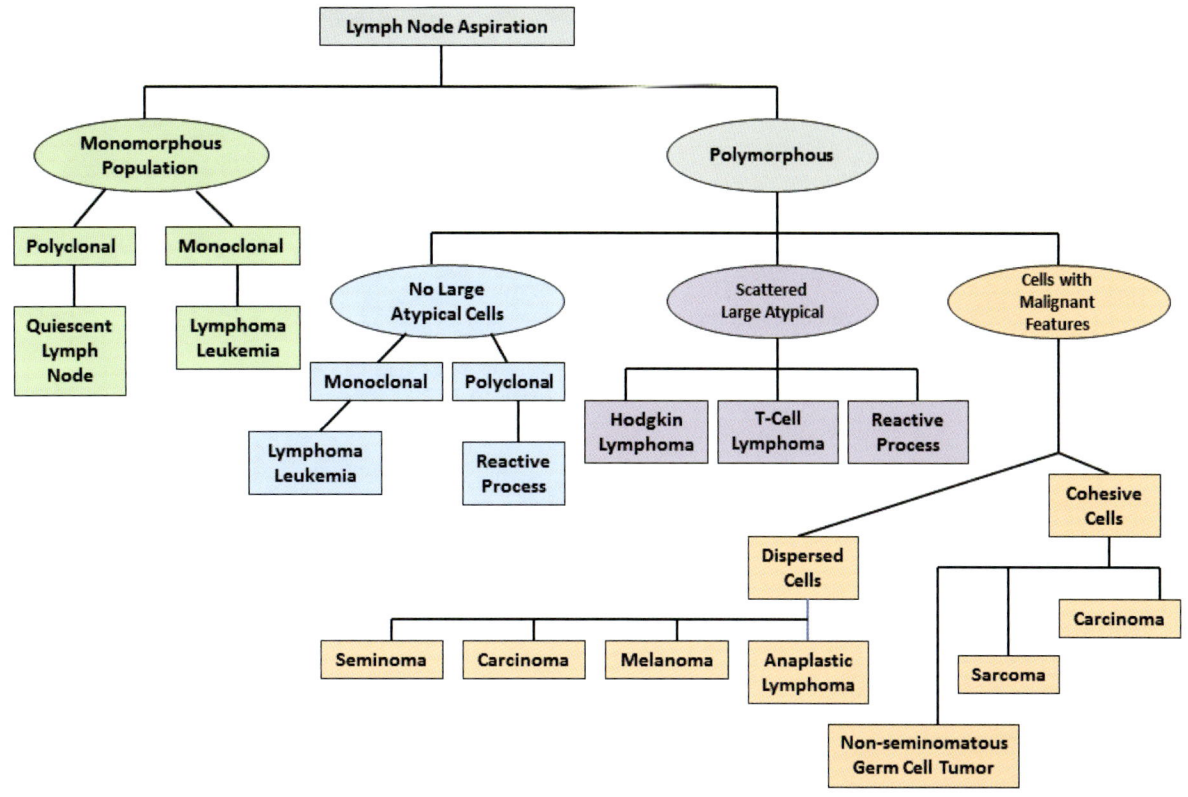

Figure 3-11

FINE-NEEDLE ASPIRATION

Algorithm for interpreting lymph node FNA biopsy specimens.

assessment of immunoglobulin light chain restriction is essential. In lesions composed of a monomorphic lymphoid population, the differential diagnosis is based on cell size: small, intermediate, or large cells (4). Small lymphocytes vary in size, similar to or greater than that of an erythrocyte, but less than the size of a neutrophil. Large lymphocytes are at least three times greater in size than an erythrocyte and larger than a histiocyte nucleus. Intermediate-sized lymphocytes are approximately the size of histiocyte nuclei.

Small B-cell lymphomas composed of a fairly monotonous population of small cells can be challenging to classify if based on cytologic features alone (Table 3-3). Distinguishing cytologic features include prolymphocytes and paraimmunoblasts in chronic lymphocytic leukemia/small lymphocytic lymphoma (CLL/SLL) and centrocytes forming follicular aggregates in follicular lymphoma. Lymphoplasmacytic and

marginal zone lymphomas are often composed of a mixture of lymphocytes and plasma cells. The lymphocytes in marginal zone lymphomas can have abundant pale (monocytoid) cytoplasm. Mantle cell lymphomas may have epithelioid histiocytes and the cell population is particularly monotonous.

Although these cytologic clues are helpful, immunophenotypic studies are essential for the reliable diagnosis of small B-cell lymphomas. CLL/SLL and mantle cell lymphomas (fig. 3-12) typically express CD5, CD19, and CD20; CLL/SLL usually express CD23 and dim CD20. In contrast, CD20 is expressed with greater intensity in mantle cell lymphoma, and CD23 is usually negative (16). Cyclin D1 expression in mantle cell lymphoma (not expressed in CLL/SLL) is also helpful, and usually assessed by immunohistochemical analysis using a cell block. Follicular lymphomas characteristically express CD10 and BCL6.

53

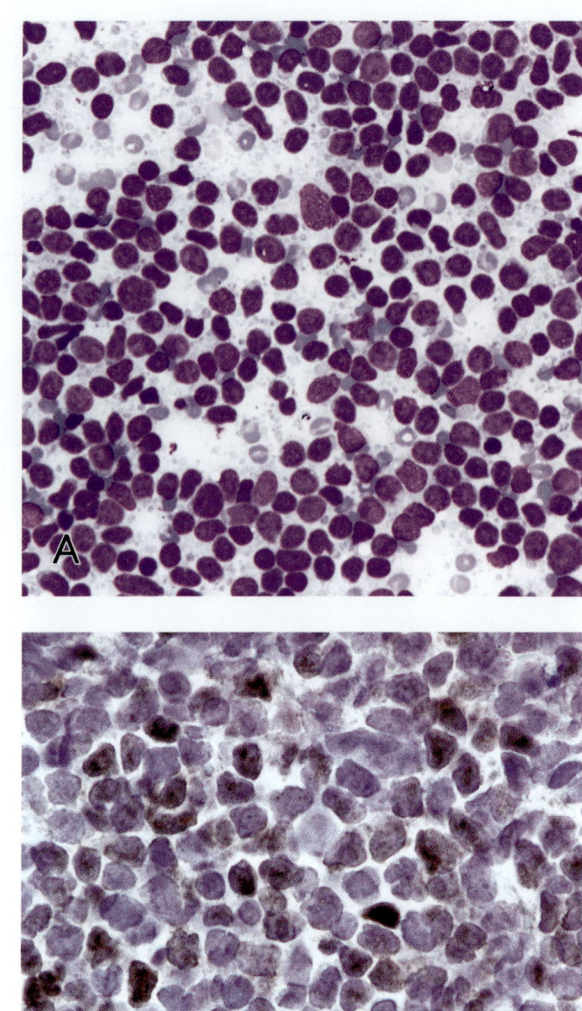

Figure 3-12

**FINE-NEEDLE ASPIRATION
OF MANTLE CELL LYMPHOMA**

A: Primarily small lymphoid cells are present (Diff-Quik stain).

B: The cell block preparation contains well-preserved lymphoid cells (H&E stain).

C: The cells are reactive for cyclin D1, albeit weakly in this case, supporting the diagnosis.

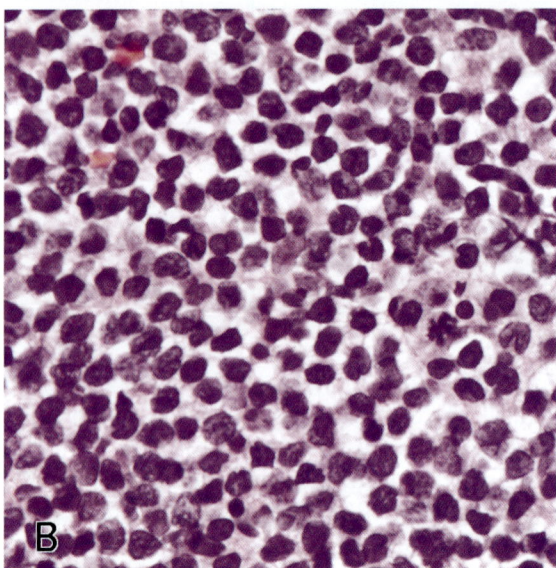

As already stated, architecture cannot be reliably assessed in most FNA specimens and therefore pattern cannot be determined in follicular lymphoma or mantle cell lymphoma. Although the mantle zone pattern is considered more indolent and may be treated differently in some institutions, in general, pattern is not required for diagnosis or therapeutic decisions for patients with small B-cell lymphomas.

The differential diagnosis of a monomorphic population of intermediate-sized cells includes Burkitt lymphoma (fig. 3-10), lymphoblastic lymphoma (LBL), a small subset of cases of dif-

fuse large B-cell lymphoma (DLBCL) (fig. 3-13) composed of intermediately sized cells (so-called small centroblastic), and the blastoid variant of mantle cell lymphoma. Aspirates of Burkitt lymphoma typically show round hyperchromatic cells with scant, vacuolated cytoplasm. Burkitt lymphoma is usually positive for CD10 and BCL6 and negative for BCL2, and has a very high proliferation rate as assessed by Ki-67 (16,26). *MYC* rearrangements are typical of Burkitt lymphoma and are uncommon in other entities in the differential diagnosis and therefore FISH analysis is useful. LBL is composed of convoluted to

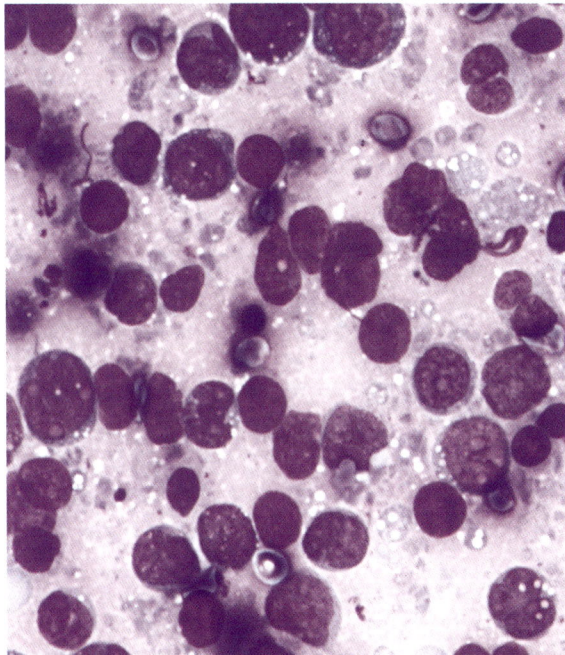
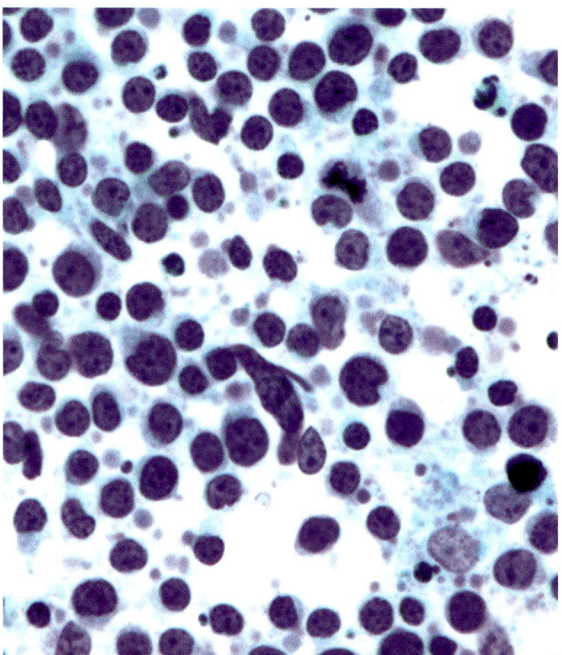

Figure 3-13

FINE-NEEDLE ASPIRATION OF LARGE B-CELL LYMPHOMA

This lymphoma had high-grade features including cytoplasmic vacuoles, apoptotic bodies, and tingible body macrophages mimicking Burkitt lymphoma (Diff-Quik [left] and Pap [right] stains).

round blastic cells. Most cases of LBL are of T-cell lineage, but uncommon cases of B-cell LBL are present in extranodal sites. Both T- and B-cell LBL commonly express CD10 and TdT.

When FNA of the mediastinum is performed, it is important to remember that the lymphocytes of lymphocyte-rich thymoma also have an immature immunophenotype very similar to T-LBL. As T-LBL usually occurs in adolescents and young adults, the differential diagnosis includes other small round blue cell tumors (Table 3-2).

The blastoid variant of mantle cell lymphoma is another entity with intermediate-sized cells, with fine chromatin and small nucleoli. The diagnosis is supported by its characteristic immunophenotypic profile including cyclin D1 expression; FISH is helpful to show t(11;14)(q13;q32)/*IGH-CCND1*.

Most large B-cell lymphomas are diagnosed on cytologic specimens (16). The lymphoma cells can be round, cleaved, or lobulated, and have centroblastic or immunoblastic features; immunoblasts have prominent central nucleoli. A small subset of large B-cell lymphomas may not express immunoglobulin; however, these lymphomas usually express B-cell antigens, and the absence of immunoglobulin is aberrant and supports an abnormal cell population (15).

It is difficult to distinguish grade 3 follicular lymphoma from DLBCL on aspirate smears, since both tumors can be CD10 positive and the architecture cannot be assessed (Table 3-3). Aspirates of T-cell/histiocyte-rich large B-cell lymphoma may be misinterpreted as a reactive process or Hodgkin lymphoma because there are less than 10 percent large cells; these cells can be easily missed on both cytologic preparations and flow cytometric analysis. In some cases of large B-cell lymphoma (fig. 3-13), the differential diagnosis may be expanded to include metastatic carcinoma (fig. 3-14), melanoma (fig. 3-15), seminoma (fig. 3-16), and myeloid sarcoma. Rarely, lymph node aspirates contain concomitant metastatic carcinoma and lymphoma, and the latter, if a small B-cell tumor, can be easily missed (6).

Some types of T-cell lymphoma, histiocytic sarcoma, and Hodgkin lymphoma are difficult to diagnose on FNA specimens. Angioimmunoblastic T-cell lymphoma (fig. 3-17), for example, is composed of a mixture of reactive and neoplastic

Table 3-3

CHALLENGES WHEN USING FNA TO ASSESS LYMPHOMAS

Identifying lymphoma in specimens with partial involvement

CLL/SLL with prominent pseudofollicles versus Richter syndrome

Assessment of pattern in follicular and mantle cell lymphomas

Grading of follicular lymphoma; however, low versus high is often achievable

Diffuse large B-cell lymphoma versus Burkitt lymphoma

Assessment of "gray zone" lymphomas

Angioimmunoblastic T-cell lymphoma versus reactive lymphadenopathy

Angioimmunoblastic T-cell lymphoma versus peripheral T-cell lymphoma

Variants of ALK-positive ALCL[a], especially the lymphohistiocytic and small cell variants

ALK-negative ALCL versus classic Hodgkin lymphoma

ALK-negative ALCL versus CD30-positive peripheral T-cell lymphoma

Classification of natural killer cell lymphomas

Nodular lymphocyte-predominant Hodgkin lymphoma versus progressive transformation of germinal centers

Nodular lymphocyte-predominant Hodgkin lymphoma versus T-cell/histiocyte-rich large B-cell lymphoma

Subclassification of classic Hodgkin lymphoma

Recognition of composite lymphoma

[a]ALK = anaplastic lymphoma kinase; ALCL = anaplastic large cell lymphoma.

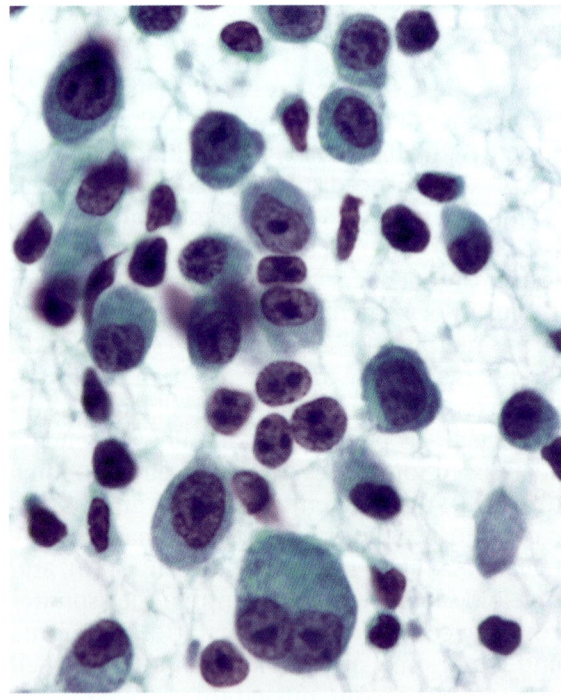

Figure 3-14

FINE-NEEDLE ASPIRATION OF METASTATIC ADENOCARCINOMA FROM ESOPHAGUS

The lesion mimics a lymphoproliferative neoplasm (Pap stain).

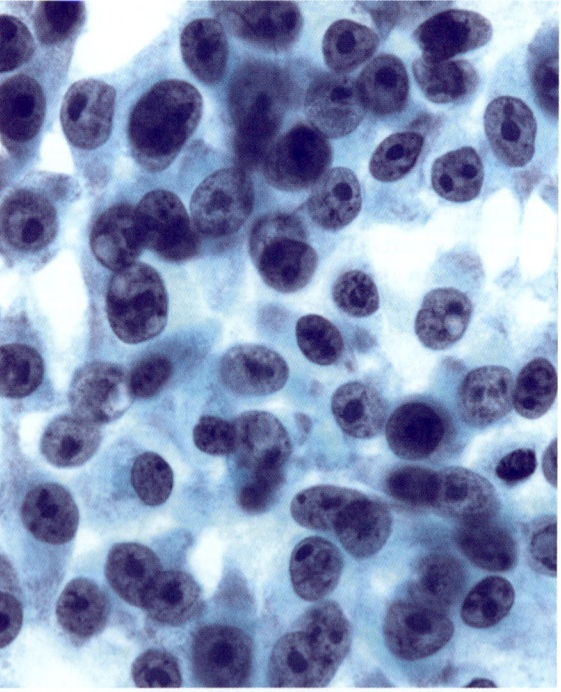

Figure 3-15

FINE-NEEDLE ASPIRATION OF METASTATIC MELANOMA

This may be misinterpreted as large cell lymphoma with immunoblastic features (Pap stain).

cells and can mimic a reactive process in cytology specimens (fig. 3-18). The problem is exacerbated when there are small numbers of neoplastic cells, an aberrant immunophenotype is not detected by flow cytometry immunophenotyping, or a monoclonal T-cell receptor gene rearrangement is not detected using standard PCR methods.

Aspirates of ALK-negative anaplastic large cell lymphoma (ALCL) (fig. 3-19) can be difficult to distinguish from classic Hodgkin lymphoma (fig. 3-20) because the neoplastic cells in both entities may resemble each other and are CD30 positive. Furthermore, variants of ALK-positive ALCL have bizarre cells mimicking carcinoma or sarcoma. CD13, a myeloid-associated antigen, is also commonly expressed by ALK-positive ALCL and can lead to misdiagnosis as myeloid sarcoma. Histiocytic sarcomas, in general, lack characteristic cytologic features and can mimic other entities, and expression of CD45/LCA can lead to an erroneous diagnosis of lymphoma.

Hodgkin lymphomas can be diagnosed on FNA specimens (23); tissue confirmation is recommended, however, when rendering an initial diagnosis because of overlapping cytomorphologic features with other entities. Also, classic Hodgkin lymphoma cannot be reliably subclassified on FNA specimens. A cytologic diagnosis of Hodgkin lymphoma is

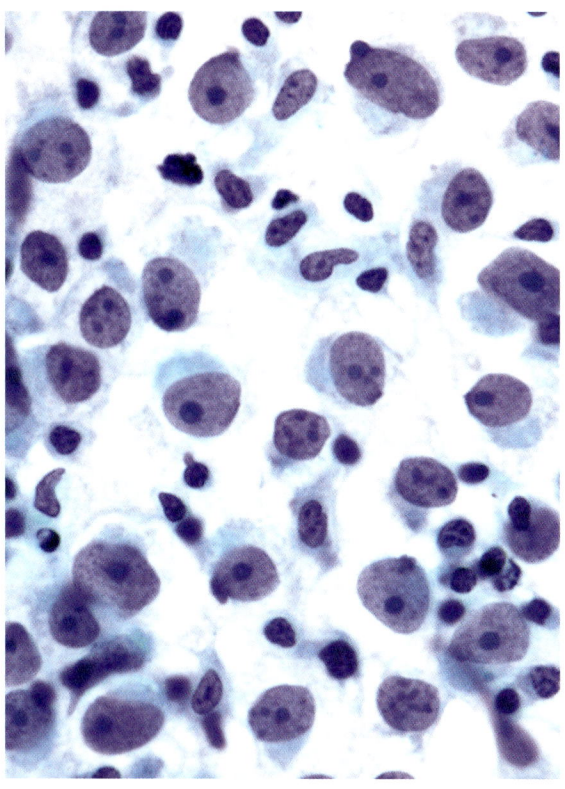

Figure 3-16

FINE-NEEDLE ASPIRATION OF METASTATIC SEMINOMA

The dispersed cell population may be mistaken for a large cell lymphoma (Pap stain).

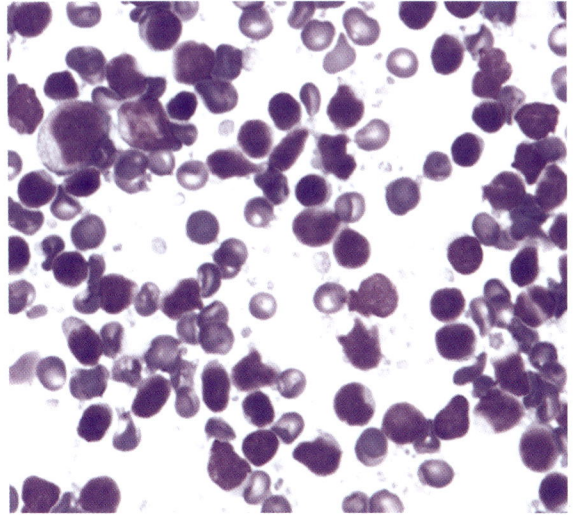 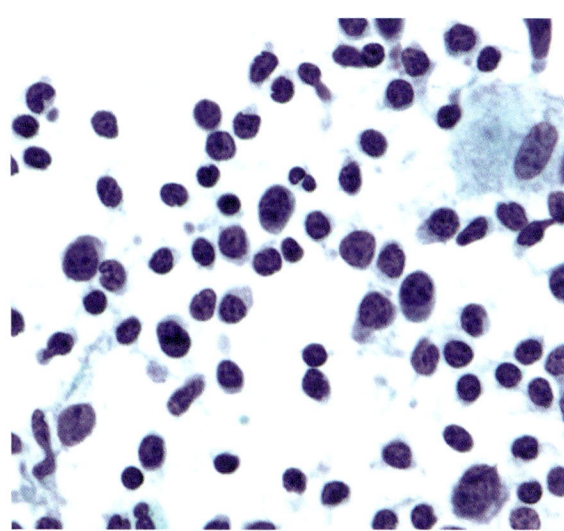

Figure 3-17

FINE-NEEDLE ASPIRATION OF ANGIOIMMUNOBLASTIC T-CELL LYMPHOMA

The polymorphous lymphoid population may be mistaken for a reactive process (Diff-Quik [left] and Pap [right] stains).

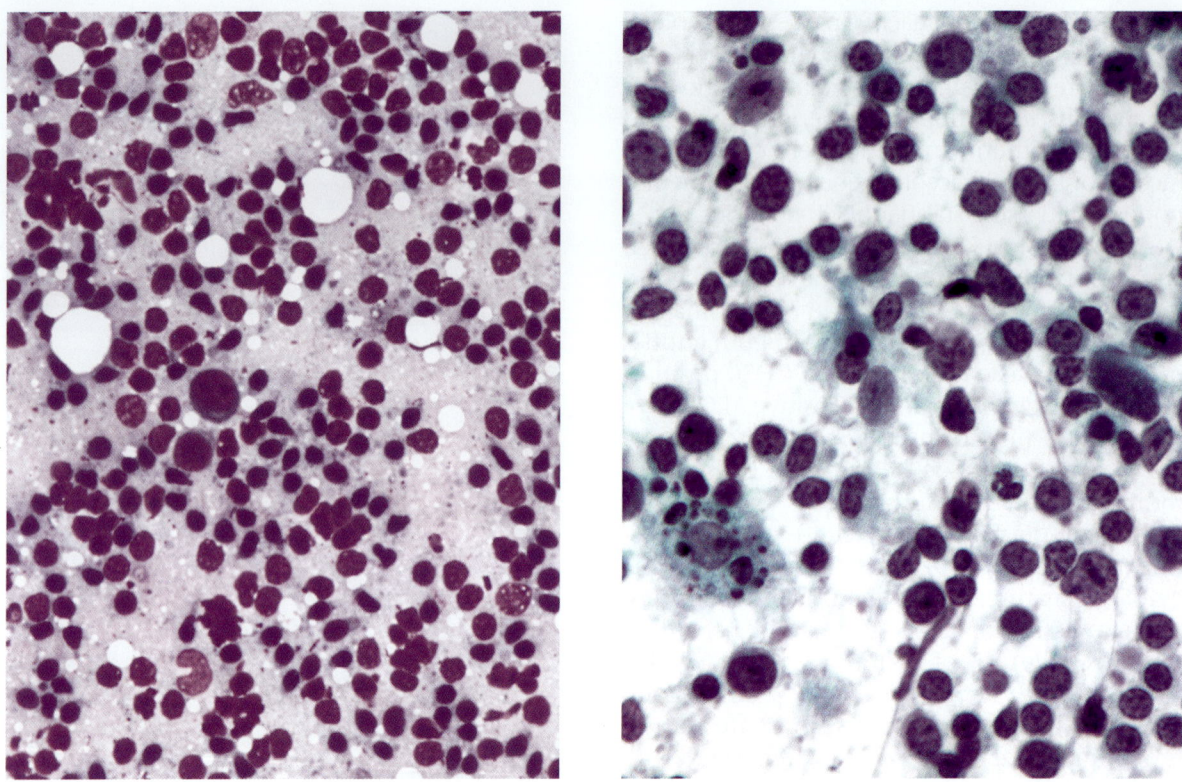

Figure 3-18

FINE-NEEDLE ASPIRATION OF A REACTIVE LYMPH NODE

A polymorphous lymphoid population is seen (Diff-Quik [left] and Pap [right] stains).

primarily based on the presence of Reed-Stern-berg cells and mononuclear Hodgkin cells in a background of lymphocytes, plasma cells, eosinophils, and histiocytes. It is not uncommon for aspirates of Hodgkin lymphoma to be hypocellular and contain primarily inflammatory cells with few or no Reed-Sternberg cells. Reed-Sternberg-like cells and variants also may be observed in non-neoplastic conditions (e.g., infectious mononucleosis and drug reactions), other types of lymphoma, and nonlymphoid tumors. Aspirates of nodular lymphocyte-predominant Hodgkin lymphoma may be difficult to distinguish from reactive processes as well as T-cell/histiocyte-rich B-cell lymphoma.

ROLE OF IMMUNOPHENOTYPIC ANALYSIS

The diagnosis of lymphoma by FNA and needle core biopsy requires immunophenotypic studies. Cell lineage must be assessed for treatment implications. For example, a diagnosis of "large cell lymphoma" is insufficient because the therapies for DLBCL and peripheral T-cell lymphoma composed of large cells are different. Based on the clinical history and initial morphologic review of the specimen, panels of antibodies can be designed to aid in the differential diagnosis as well as in lymphoma subclassification (Table 3-4).

Flow cytometry immunophenotypic and immunohistochemical analyses have distinct advantages. Flow cytometry is more sensitive, can evaluate a large number of cells, offers greater objectivity through automation, has the ability to collect a number of parameters on the cells and assess many antigens at once on a single cell population, and is a rapid procedure with short turnaround time (25). This technique also allows for a more precise gating of the cells, which is particularly useful in those specimens containing small numbers of neoplastic cells. The data derived by flow cytometry immunophenotyping can be helpful in establishing monoclonality in B-cell populations and establishing an

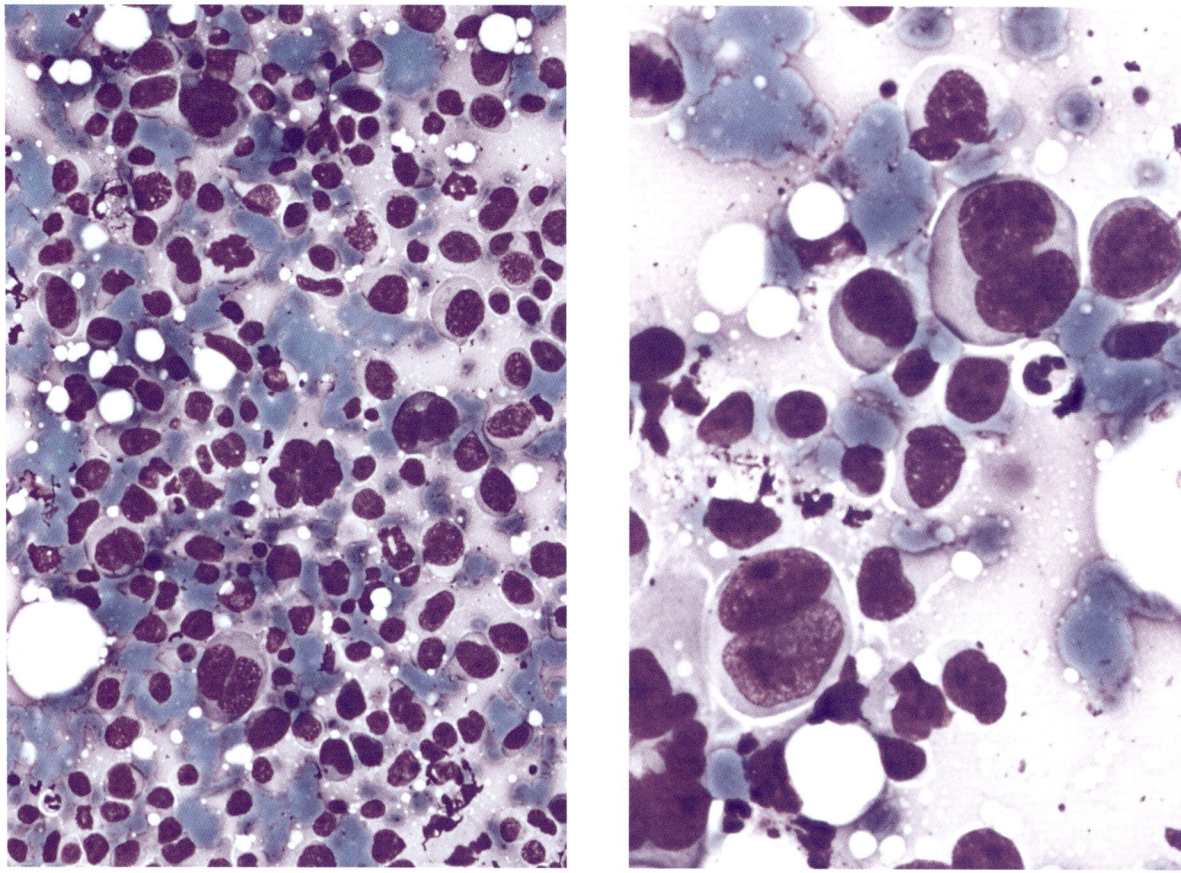

Figure 3-19

FINE-NEEDLE ASPIRATION OF ALK-NEGATIVE ANAPLASTIC LARGE CELL LYMPHOMA

Large mononucleated, binucleated, and multinucleated pleomorphic cells are seen at low (left) and high (right) power magnification (Diff-Quik stain).

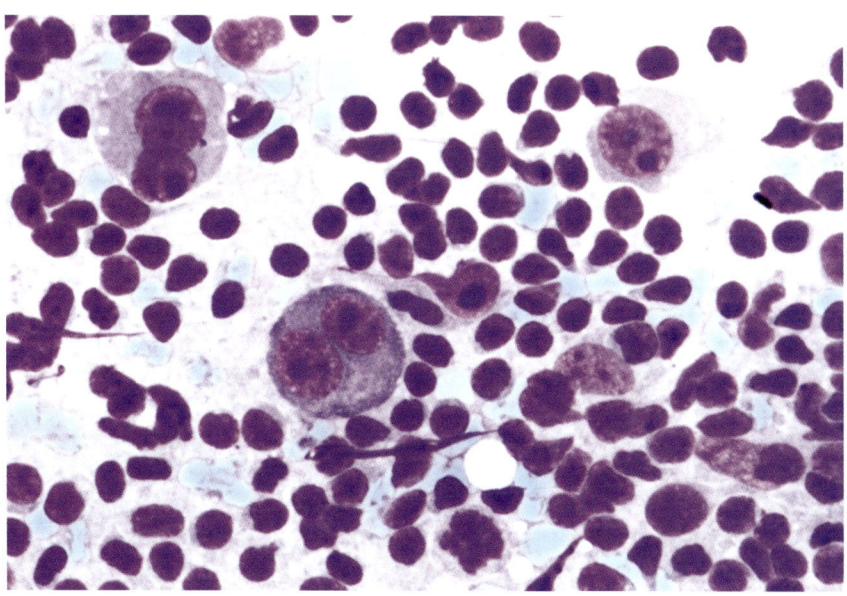

Figure 3-20

FINE-NEEDLE ASPIRATION OF HODGKIN LYMPHOMA

Large mononucleated and binucleated atypical cells in a background of lymphocytes (Diff-Quik stain).

Table 3-4

SELECTED ANTIBODY PANELS HELPFUL TO SUPPORT A LYMPHOMA DIAGNOSIS

Lymphoma Type	Antibody Panel
Nodular lymphocyte-predominant Hodgkin lymphoma	CD3, CD15, CD20, CD21, CD30, CD45/LCA, PAX5, BCL6
Classic Hodgkin lymphoma	CD3, CD15, CD20, CD30, CD45/LCA, PAX5, EBER1[a]
B-lymphoblastic lymphoma	CD1a, CD3, CD5, CD10, CD20, CD34, PAX5, TdT, Ki-67
Small B-cell lymphoma	CD3, CD5, CD10, CD20, CD23, BCL6, cyclin D1
Diffuse large B-cell lymphoma	CD3, CD5, CD10, CD20, CD10, BCL6, MUM1, Ki-67, MYC
Burkitt lymphoma	CD3, CD5, CD10, CD20, BCL2, BCL6, Ki-67
T-lymphoblastic lymphoma	CD1a, CD3, CD5, CD10, CD20, CD34, PAX5, TdT, Ki-67
Peripheral T-cell lymphoma	CD2, CD3, CD5, CD7, CD20, CD30, Ki-67
Angioimmunoblastic T-cell lymphoma	CD3, CD5, CD10, CD20, CD30, BCL6, CD279/PD-1, CXCL13
Anaplastic large cell lymphoma	CD2, CD3, CD4, CD5, CD20, CD30, ALK, cytotoxic markers
Natural killer cell lymphoma	CD2, CD3, CD5, CD20, CD56, CD57, EBER1[a]

[a]EBER1 = Epstein-Barr virus-encoded RNA1 assessed by in situ hybridization.

immunophenotype that is characteristic of a lymphoma. One limitation is that flow cytometry does not allow direct visual evaluation of the gated population being analyzed (16).

Immunohistochemistry, by contrast, offers two great advantages: the studies can be performed on fixed, paraffin-embedded tissue sections and the pathologist can directly observe the patterns of antigen expression. Also, immunohistochemistry often allows the observer to better appreciate the architecture in a needle core biopsy specimen, especially if it is markedly fragmented, or fixed poorly. For example, in some reactive cases, small fragments of lymph node can appear to be replaced when stained with H&E, but immunohistochemical studies highlight the lymph node compartments, supporting a reactive process. The patterns of certain lymphoma types (e.g., follicular lymphoma) also may be better appreciated by immunohistochemistry studies in some cases.

In addition to core needle biopsy specimens, immunohistochemical analysis can be performed on FNA cell block preparations. The clotted material at the bottom of the rinse solution, not utilized for flow cytometric immunophenotyping, often contains tissue fragments that contribute to the diagnosis (fig. 3-21). To expedite diagnosis, it is useful to order H&E-stained slides as well as 6 to 8 unstained slides for potential immunohistochemical studies at the time the cell block is cut initially.

Immunohistochemical studies also can be performed on cytospin slides prepared using the density gradient (ficoll-hypaque) method (i.e., immunocytochemistry). This technique isolates mononuclear cells and decreases blood antigens that can cause high interstitial (background) immunoreactivity. The density gradient method offers advantages: the ability to isolate mononuclear cells in aspirates with low cell counts and immunophenotypic results can be correlated with the cytomorphology findings (fig. 3-22). A limiting factor is that the density gradient procedure is not routinely performed in most laboratories. Other drawbacks include the inability to directly assess coexpression of antigens and limited resources for appropriate controls on cytology specimens.

ROLE OF CYTOGENETIC AND MOLECULAR ANALYSIS

Cytogenetic and molecular studies are not routinely performed on needle core biopsy specimens or FNA aspirates, but these studies are available for selected cases in which the cytomorphologic and immunophenotypic findings are inconclusive (20). Typically, a needle core biopsy specimen is too small to send a portion for conventional cytogenetic analysis. Karyotyping can be performed on FNA specimens submitted in sterile media; turnaround time is a limitation as the results are not available in time for diagnosis.

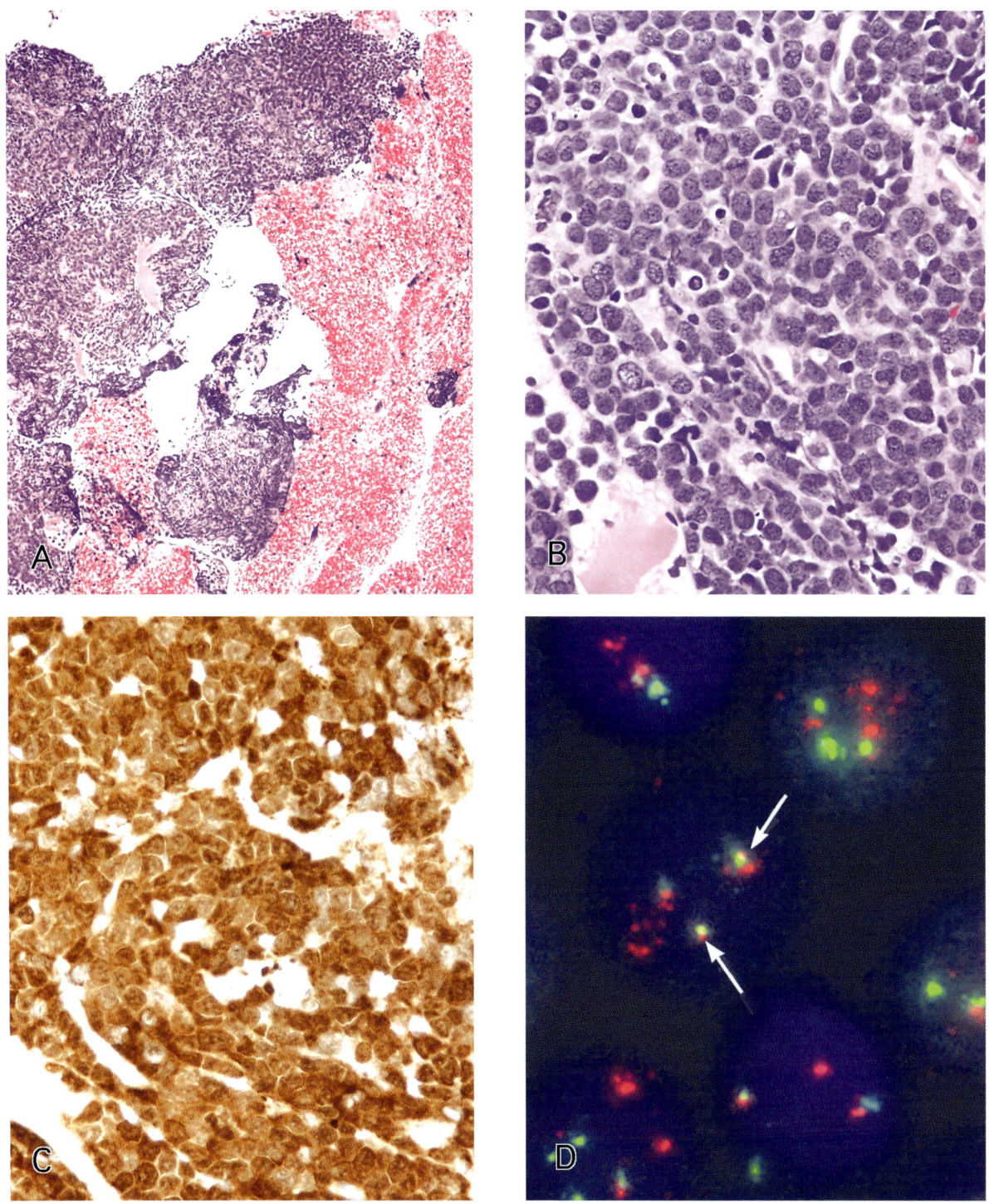

Figure 3-21

CELL BLOCK PREPARATION

A,B: Low (A) and high (B) power magnification of a cell block preparation showing the blastoid variant of mantle cell lymphoma (H&E stain).

C: Cyclin D1 performed on the cell block supports the diagnosis.

D: FISH analysis performed on a cytospin preparation demonstrates the presence of *CCND1-IGH*.

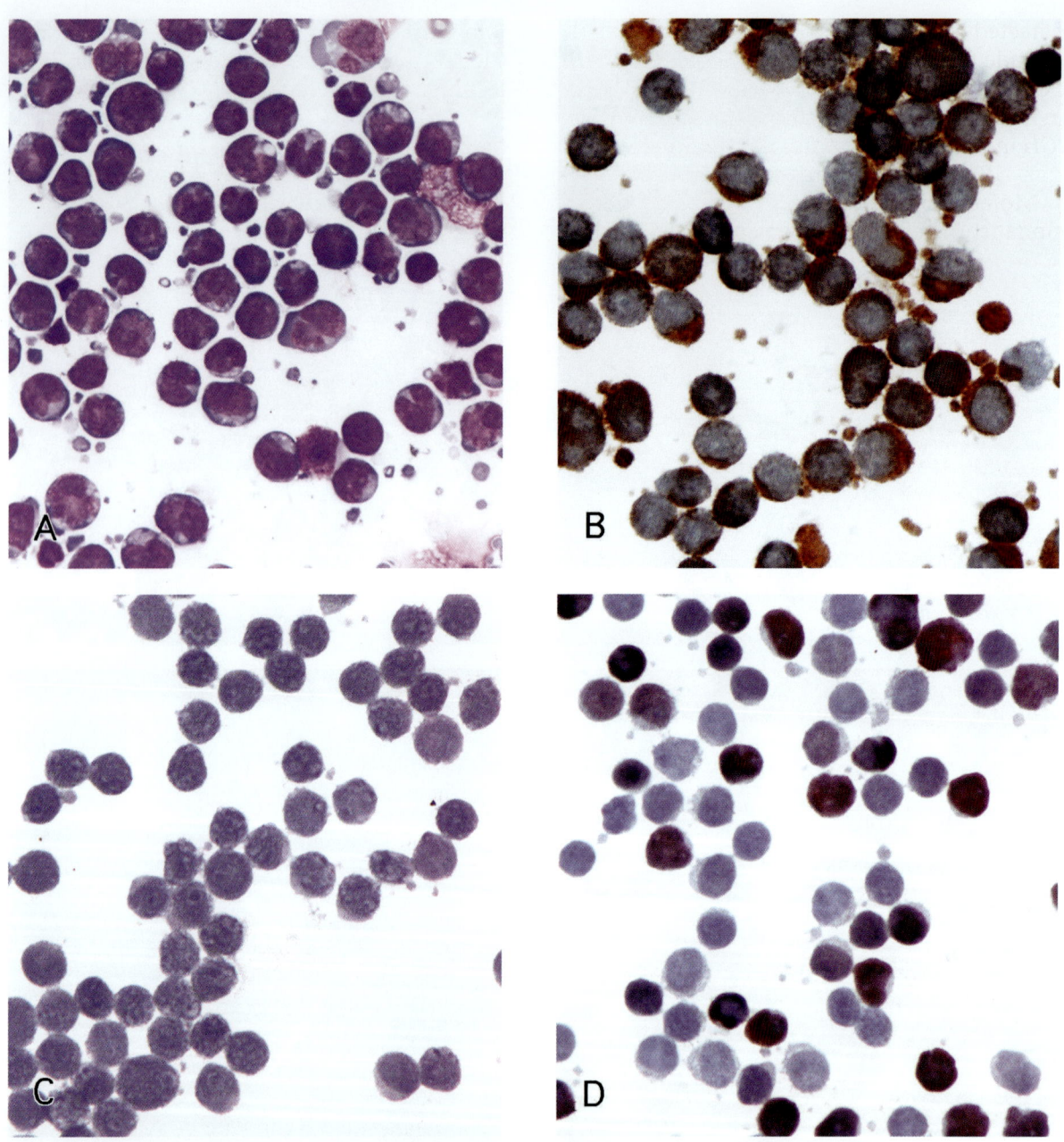

Figure 3-22

CYTOSPIN PREPARATIONS OF LARGE B-CELL LYMPHOMA

A: Cytomorphology of large lymphoma cells (Diff-Quik stain).
B: Kappa reactivity (positive).
C: Lambda reactivity (negative).
D: Ki-67 shows that about 40 percent of cells are positive.

FISH analysis can be performed on touch imprints, FNA aspirate smears, monolayers, cytospin preparations (5,8), nuclei extracted from fixed and paraffin-embedded tissue, or fixed and paraffin-embedded tissue sections. Touch imprints or extracted nuclei are easy to count, and therefore, it is easy to quantify the abnormality. Specific chromosomal translocations detected by FISH that support subclassification include t(1l;14)(q13;q32)/*CCND1-IGH* in mantle cell lymphoma, t(14;18)(q32;q21)/*IGH-BCL2* in follicular lymphoma, t(8:14)(q24;q32)/*MYC-IGH* in Burkitt lymphoma, and t(2;5)(p23;q35)/*ALK-NPM1* in ALK-positive ALCL.

Molecular analysis can be used to detect clonality or gene rearrangements when the histologic findings are suspicious or inconclusive. Clonality is usually determined using PCR. This technique can assess clonality of the IG and TCR genes using either fixed, paraffin-embedded tissue or the rinse of FNA specimens. PCR also can be used to detect specific breakpoint clusters of chromosomal translocations, such as t(14;18)(q32;q21) and t(11;14)(q13;q32).

REFERENCES

1. Agid R, Sklair-Levy M, Bloom AI, et al. CT-guided biopsy with cutting-edge needle for the diagnosis of malignant lymphoma: experience of 267 biopsies. Clin Radiol 2003;58:143-147.

2. Amador-Ortiz C, Chen L, Hassan A, et al. Combined core needle biopsy and fine-needle aspiration with ancillary studies correlate highly with traditional techniques in the diagnosis of nodal-based lymphoma. Am J Clin Pathol 2011; 135:516-524.

3. Ben-Yehuda D, Polliack A, Okon E, et al. Image-guided core-needle biopsy in malignant lymphoma: experience with 100 patients that suggests the technique is reliable. J Clin Oncol 1996;14:2431-2434.

4. Caraway NP. Strategies to diagnose lymphoproliferative disorders by fine-needle aspiration by using ancillary studies. Cancer 2005;105:432-442.

5. Caraway NP, Gu J, Lin P, Romaguera JE, Glassman A, Katz R. The utility of interphase fluorescence in situ hybridization for the detection of the translocation t(11;14)(q13;q32) in the diagnosis of mantle cell lymphoma on fine-needle aspiration specimens. Cancer 2005;105:110-118.

6. Caraway NP, Wojcik EM, Saboorian HM, Katz RL. Concomitant lymphoma and metastatic carcinoma in a lymph node: diagnosis by fine-needle aspiration biopsy in two cases. Diagn Cytopathol 1997;17:287-291.

7. Coe A, Conway J, Evans J, Goebel M, Mishra G. The yield of EUS-FNA in undiagnosed upper abdominal adenopathy is very high. J Clin Ultrasound 2013;41:210-213.

8. da Cunha Santos G, Ko HM, Geddie WR, et al. Targeted use of fluorescence in situ hybridization (FISH) in cytospin preparations: results of 298 fine needle aspirates of B-cell non-Hodgkin lymphoma. Cancer Cytopathol 2010;118:250-258.

9. de Kerviler E, Benet C, Briere J, de Bazelaire C. Image-guided needle biopsy for diagnosis and molecular biology in lymphomas. Best pract Res Clin Haematol 2012;25:29-39.

10. de Larrinoa AF, del Cura J, Zabala R, Fuertes E, Bilbao F, Lopez JI. Value of ultrasound-guided core biopsy in the diagnosis of malignant lymphoma. J Clin Ultrasound 2007;35:295-301.

11. Demharter J, Muller P, Wagner T, Schlimok G, Haude K, Bohndorf K. Percutaneous core-needle biopsy of enlarged lymph nodes in the diagnosis and subclassification of malignant lymphomas. Eur Radiol 2001;11:276-283.

12. Ensani F, Mehravaran S, Irvanlou G, et al. Fine-needle aspiration cytology and flow cytometric immunophenotyping in diagnosis and classification of non-Hodgkin lymphoma in comparison to histopathology. Diagn Cytopathol 2012;40:305-310.

13. Francis IM, Das DK, al-Rubah NA, Gupta SK. Lymphoglandular bodies in lymphoid lesions and non-lymphoid round cell tumours: a quantitative assessment. Diagn Cytopathol 1994;11:23-27.

14. Frederiksen JK, Sharma M, Casulo C, Burack WR. Systematic review of the effectiveness of fine-needle aspiration and/or core needle biopsy for subclassifying lymphoma. Arch Pathol Lab Med 2015;139: 245-251.

15. Hu Q, Naushad H, Xie Q, Al-Howaidi I, Wang M, Fu K. Needle-core biopsy in the pathologic diagnosis of malignant lymphoma showing high reproducibility among pathologists. Am J Clin Pathol 2013;140:238-247.

16. Jorgensen JL. State of the Art Symposium: flow cytometry in the diagnosis of lymphoproliferative disorders by fine-needle aspiration. Cancer 2005;105:443-451.

17. Lachar WA, Shahab I, Saad AJ. Accuracy and cost-effectiveness of core needle biopsy in the evaluation of suspected lymphoma: a study of 101 cases. Arch Pathol Lab Med 2007;131:1033-1039.

18. Li L, Wu QL, Liu LZ, et al. Value of CT-guided core-needle biopsy in diagnosis and classification of malignant lymphomas using automated biopsy gun. World J Gastroenterol 2005;11:4843-4847.

19. Loubeyre P, McKee TA, Copercini M, Rosset A, Dietrich PY. Diagnostic precision of image-guided multisampling core needle biopsy of suspected lymphomas in a primary care hospital. Br J Cancer 2009;100:1771-1776.

20. Medeiros LJ, Carr J. Overview of the role of molecular methods in the diagnosis of malignant lymphomas. Arch Pathol Lab Med 1999;123:1189-1207.

21. Metzgeroth G, Schneider S, Walz C, et al. Fine needle aspiration and core needle biopsy in the diagnosis of lymphadenopathy of unknown aetiology. Ann Hematol 2012;91:1477-1484.

22. Michael CW, Hunter B. Interpretation of fine-needle aspirates processed by the ThinPrep technique: cytologic artifacts and diagnostic pitfalls. Diagn Cytopathol 2000;23:6-13.

23. Moreland WS, Geisinger KR. Utility and outcomes of fine-needle aspiration biopsy in Hodgkin's disease. Diagn Cytopathol 2002;26:278-282.

24. Pedersen OM, Aarstad HJ, Lokeland T, Bostad L. Diagnostic yield of biopsies of cervical lymph nodes using a large (14-gauge) core biopsy needle. APMIS 2013;121:1119-1130.

25. Simsir A, Fetsch P, Stetler-Stevenson M, Abati A. Immunophenotypic analysis of non-Hodgkin's lymphomas in cytologic specimens: a correlative study of immunocytochemical and flow cytometric techniques. Diagn Cytopathol 1999; 20:278-284.

26. Swerdlow SH, Campo E, Harris NL, et al, eds Tumours of haematopoietic and lymphoid tissues. Lyon: IARC Press; 2008. World Health Organization Classification of Tumours.

27. Zeppa P, Marino G, Troncone G, et al. Fine-needle cytology and flow cytometry immunophenotyping and subclassification of non-Hodgkin lymphoma: a critical review of 307 cases with technical suggestions. Cancer 2004;102:55-65.

4 CLASSIFICATION OF LYMPHOMAS

There has been enormous progress in our understanding of lymphomas as can be observed by comparing older systems with the current World Health Organization (WHO) lymphoma classification system (51,51a). Most of this progress has occurred in the past 40 to 50 years. As reviewed by Taylor and Hartsock (53), progress has been driven by advances in technology. Initial efforts to study lymphomas relied only on observations of gross pathology. It was only in the late 19th and early 20th centuries that observations derived from light microscopic examination were used to inform classification systems. In the second half of the 20th century, technological advances accelerated, allowing for the application of multiple ancillary techniques to the study of the normal immune system and lymphomas. Electron microscopy, cytochemistry, histochemistry, and most importantly, monoclonal antibody technology and immunophenotypic analysis (flow cytometry and immunohistochemistry) contributed greatly to the characterization of lymphomas in successive decades beginning in the 1960s.

It became clear that lymphomas are neoplasms of the immune system that correspond to normal B-, T-, or natural killer (NK)-cell counterparts. The application of conventional cytogenetic analysis and molecular techniques has advanced our knowledge of lymphomas. These advances are reflected in successive lymphoma classification systems. Even with this explosion of knowledge, however, our understanding of the normal immune system and lymphomas remains incomplete. High-throughput molecular methods that are currently being applied to the study of lymphomas will likely further contribute to this understanding.

HISTORICAL BACKGROUND

Hodgkin Lymphomas

Most historians begin the history of the classification of lymphomas with Thomas Hodgkin (fig. 4-1) who in 1832, as Inspector of the Dead and Curator of the Museum at Guy's Hospital in London, England, described seven patients with lymphoma (15). Hodgkin made his conclusions

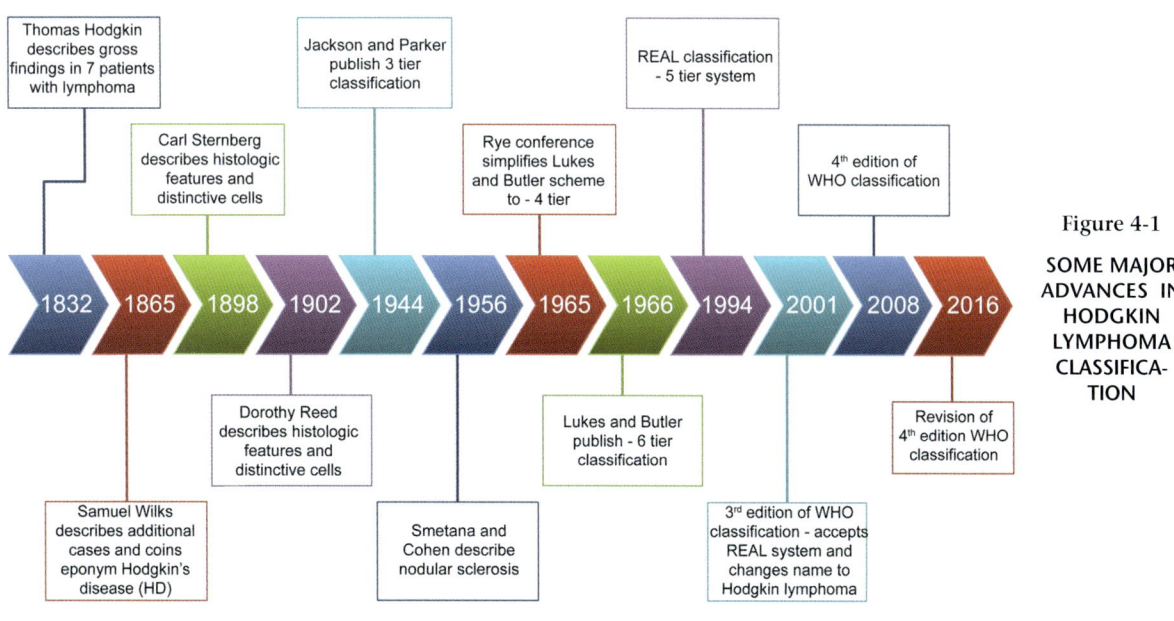

Figure 4-1

SOME MAJOR ADVANCES IN HODGKIN LYMPHOMA CLASSIFICATION

Thomas Hodgkin describes gross findings in 7 patients with lymphoma

Carl Sternberg describes histologic features and distinctive cells

Jackson and Parker publish 3 tier classification

Rye conference simplifies Lukes and Butler scheme to - 4 tier

REAL classification - 5 tier system

4ᵗʰ edition of WHO classification

1832 1865 1898 1902 1944 1956 1965 1966 1994 2001 2008 2016

Samuel Wilks describes additional cases and coins eponym Hodgkin's disease (HD)

Dorothy Reed describes histologic features and distinctive cells

Smetana and Cohen describe nodular sclerosis

Lukes and Butler publish - 6 tier classification

3ʳᵈ edition of WHO classification - accepts REAL system and changes name to Hodgkin lymphoma

Revision of 4ᵗʰ edition WHO classification

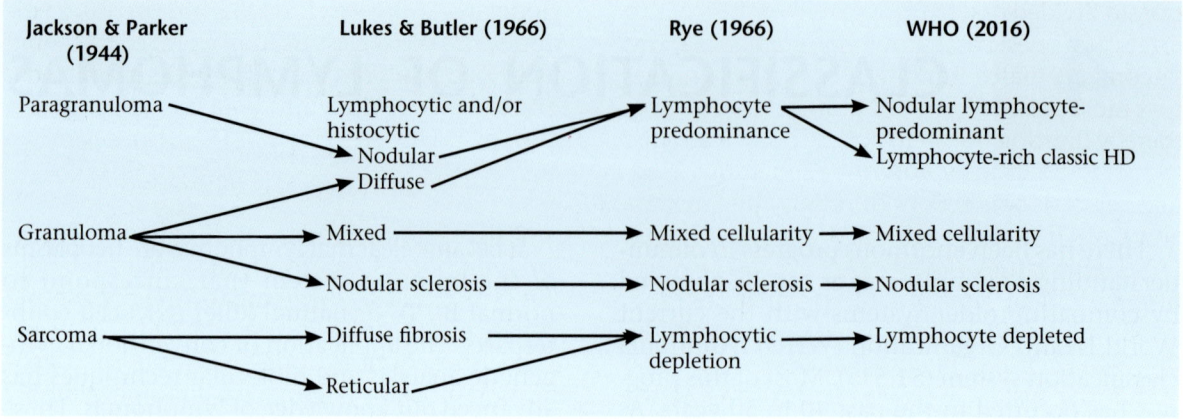

Figue 4-2

HODGKIN LYMPHOMA CLASSIFICATION: PAST AND PRESENT

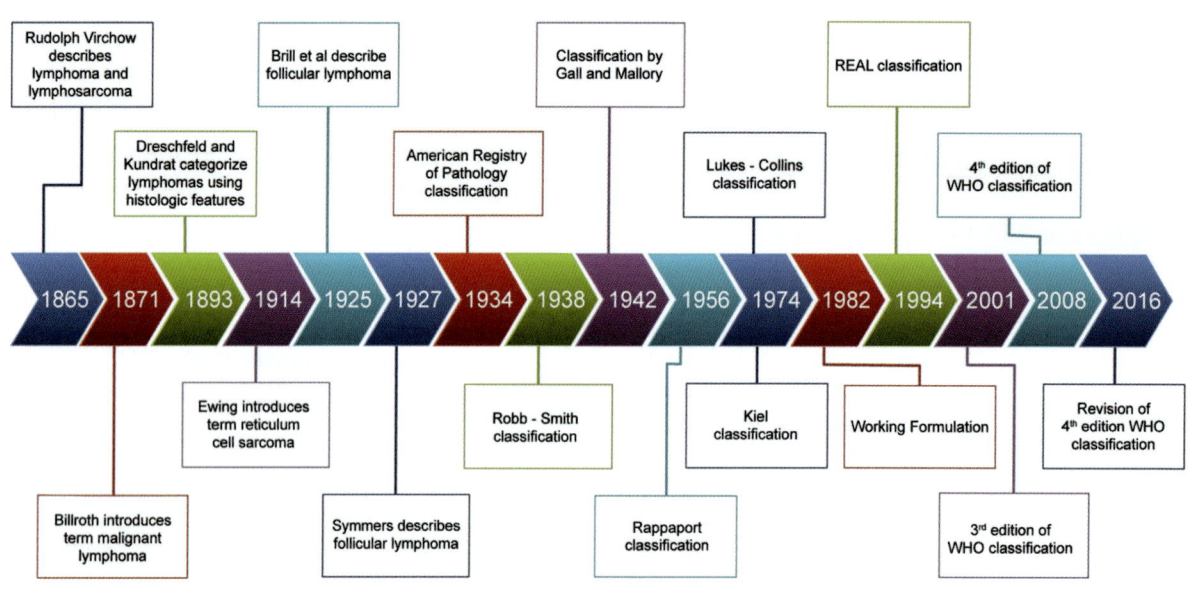

Figure 4-3

SOME MAJOR ADVANCES IN NON-HODGKIN LYMPHOMA CLASSIFCATION

based on observations of the gross pathology of specimens, without benefit of light microscopy and, in retrospect, some of these cases were actually non-Hodgkin lymphomas (41). Hodgkin, therefore, described the gross features of both Hodgkin and non-Hodgkin lymphomas. When Hodgkin presented his paper, it had little impact at the time and his work may have been forgotten if not for Sir Samuel Wilks who described the gross features of Hodgkin lymphoma and acknowledged the earlier work of Hodgkin (56).

Subsequent contributions to the understanding of Hodgkin lymphoma came with the description of the histologic findings, including the distinctive large neoplastic cells by Carl Sternberg in 1898 (50) and Dorothy Reed in 1902 (43). Sternberg was a physician in Austria and Reed was a 28-year-old trainee in pathology at Johns Hopkins at the time they wrote their papers.

The first widely used classification of Hodgkin lymphoma was proposed by Henry Jackson, Jr. and Francis Parker, Jr. in 1944 (fig. 4-2) (16). This system divided cases of Hodgkin lymphoma into three categories: paragranuloma, granuloma, and sarcoma. A major limitation of this system was that most cases fell into the granuloma category, thereby limiting the ability of the classification to stratify patients into prognostic subgroups. Nodular sclerosis was reported initially by Smetana and Cohen in 1956 (48). Subsequently, Robert Lukes and James Butler proposed a classification system of Hodgkin lymphomas in 1965, published in 1966, that included six categories (fig. 4-2) (27). The major advances of the Lukes and Butler system were the recognition of the nodular and diffuse variants of lymphocytic-predominance Hodgkin lymphoma and the emphasis on nodular sclerosis.

In September of 1965, a conference titled "On obstacles to the control of Hodgkin's disease" was held in Rye, New York, sponsored by the American College of Surgeons and the National Cancer Institute, and organized by Henry Kaplan, a leading radiation oncologist of the time. Sidney Farber, one of only 42 attendees, suggested to Lukes that six categories for Hodgkin lymphoma were excessive (17). Lukes then compressed the Lukes-Butler system into four categories: lymphocyte predominance, nodular sclerosis, mixed cellularity, and lymphocyte depletion, which came to be known as the Rye Classification (28). In retrospect, this compression over-simplified the lymphocyte-predominance category and important information was lost. This information was recovered subsequently in the Revised European American Lymphoma (REAL) (14) and WHO classifications (18,51).

The application of monoclonal antibodies and molecular techniques to the study of Hodgkin lymphomas has been essential to the development of current concepts. Results of studies using these methods showed that the Reed-Sternberg and Hodgkin cells of Hodgkin lymphoma are of germinal center B-cell origin. The neoplastic cells express some B-cell antigens and single-cell polymerase chain reaction (PCR) and sequencing studies have shown that the neoplastic cells of nodular lymphocyte-predominant and classic Hodgkin lymphomas virtually always carry immunoglobulin (IG) gene rearrangements and somatic mutations of the variable regions of the IG genes (reviewed in 45,49). As a result of these efforts, the controversy over the cell of origin of

Hodgkin disease was resolved and the third edition of the WHO classification changed the name from Hodgkin's disease to Hodgkin lymphoma. The term Hodgkin lymphoma is retained in the current WHO classification (51,51a).

Non-Hodgkin Lymphomas

Progress in the understanding of non-Hodgkin lymphomas was slower than that for Hodgkin lymphomas, with many of the conceptual advances occurring in the last 30 to 40 years. The history of non-Hodgkin lymphoma classification probably begins with Rudolph Virchow (fig. 4-3) who described lymphoid neoplasms using the terms *lymphoma* in 1858 and *lymphosarcoma* in 1865 (54,55). The use of the term *malignant lymphoma* has been attributed to Bilroth in 1871 (2).

Initial attempts to classify non-Hodgkin lymphomas by using light microscopy began as the 20th century approached. Dreschfeld (7) and Kundrat (22) were two investigators in the 1890s who subdivided lymphomas into different types. Follicular lymphoma was one the first non-Hodgkin lymphomas to be recognized as a distinct entity, by Ghon and Roman (12) in 1916, and subsequently recognized and described in the English literature by Brill et al. (3) and Symmers (52) in 1925 and 1927, respectively, although the malignant nature of follicular lymphomas was considered uncertain at that time. Gall (9) recognized that follicular lymphoma arose in germinal centers of reactive lymphoid tissue and published histologic criteria to distinguish follicular hyperplasia from follicular lymphoma in 1941 (9). The term reticulum cell sarcoma for lymphoid neoplasms composed of large cells was used by Ewing in 1914 and subsequently by Olberding in 1928 (39).

In the first half of the 20th century, three morphologic classifications of non-Hodgkin lymphoma had impact on the field, especially that of Robb-Smith (44) in 1938 in Europe. In the United States, classifications were proposed by Callender for the American Registry of Pathology in 1934 and Gall and Mallory in 1942 (8).

The last (and best received at the time) purely morphologic classification of non-Hodgkin lymphoma was proposed by Henry Rappaport who initially had collaborated with Gall (10). The Rappaport classification, initially proposed in 1956 (42), and subsequently updated (36),

---

Table 4-1

UPDATED RAPPAPORT CLASSIFICATION OF NON-HODGKIN LYMPHOMAS (1976)

Nodular
  Lymphocytic, poorly differentiated
  Mixed lymphocytic-histiocytic
  Histiocytic

Diffuse
  Lymphocytic, well-differentiated
  Lymphocytic, intermediately differentiated
  Lymphocytic, poorly differentiated
  Mixed lymphocytic-histiocytic
  Undifferentiated, Burkitt type
  Undifferentiated, non-Burkitt type
  Histiocytic
  Lymphoblastic

---

was very popular for the next 20 years (Table 4-1). Rappaport proposed dividing lymphomas by pattern, either nodular or diffuse, and then further subdividing tumors on the basis of cytologic features. Rappaport thought the term nodular was preferable to follicular because at that time there was no proof that nodular neoplasms were derived from the germinal center. (In retrospect, this was a step back from Gall's correct position.) Tumors composed of small lymphocytes that closely resembled normal lymphocytes were designated as well differentiated. Poorly differentiated tumors were composed of slightly larger, but still small lymphoid cells with irregular nuclear contours that less closely resembled normal lymphocytes. Non-Hodgkin lymphomas composed of large cells were designated as histiocytic on the basis of their resemblance to normal histiocytes. Undifferentiated lymphomas were composed of cells of intermediate size that failed to demonstrate cytologic features of either lymphoid or histiocytic origin. Mixed non-Hodgkin lymphomas were composed of a mixture of poorly differentiated lymphocytes and histiocytes.

Rappaport's classification was popular because it was clinically useful, recognizing patients with clinically indolent versus aggressive lymphomas that required vastly different therapeutic approaches. Rappaport's classification, however, depended only on morphologic features and was developed when there was little knowledge of the immune system. So why was the Rappaport

classification so useful clinically? The emphasis placed on pattern in the Rappaport system separated, in large part, clinically indolent nodular lymphomas from clinically aggressive diffuse lymphomas, in retrospect, follicular lymphomas and diffuse large B-cell lymphomas, which represent 50 to 60 percent of all non-Hodgkin lymphomas in the United States and Europe.

As knowledge of immunology grew, it was proved that lymphomas are tumors of the immune system. Normal lymphocytes can be divided into B, T, and NK cells, and each group is highly heterogeneous and composed of many lymphocyte subsets. The morphologic categories of lymphoma in the Rappaport system did not recognize the heterogeneity of lymphocytes. In addition, the concept of lymphocytic differentiation was not scientifically accurate. Well or poorly differentiated lymphocytes, as designated in the Rappaport system, did not truly reflect stages of differentiation. Therefore, despite updates to the Rappaport system that incorporated newer disease categories that emerged from advances in our understanding of the immunology of lymphomas (36), some of the basic tenets of the Rappaport classification were flawed.

With the advent of immunologic data, a number of classifications were proposed to replace the Rappaport system in the 1970s, but with the benefit of hindsight, only two of these classifications stand out: the Lukes-Collins and the Kiel classifications. Both of these classifications focused on immunologic (or functional) data and tried to combine morphologic and immunologic data into their classification proposals. It is worth reviewing these classifications briefly because their terminology is still in common use today.

Robert Lukes and Robert Collins initially proposed their classification in 1974 (30) and they provided an update of this classification in their Fasicle submitted for publication in 1988 (Table 4-2) (31). This system divided lymphomas into T-cell, B-cell, phagocytic, and unclassified tumors. The initial version of this classification also included tumors of undefined cell type which, in retrospect, represented acute lymphoblastic leukemia/lymphoma cases (30). The Lukes-Collins classification relied primarily on morphologic observations, but these findings were correlated with immunophenotypic data. In 1977, Lukes

Table 4-2

UPDATED LUKES AND COLLINS CLASSIFICATION OF NON-HODGKIN LYMPHOMAS (1988)

B-Cell Lymphomas
    B-cell acute lymphocytic leukemia (ALL), including
    B-precursor ALL
        Prolymphocytic leukemia
        Small B-cell neoplasms (including chronic lympho-
        cytic leukemia)
    B-cell neoplasms with plasmacytic differentiation
        (including plasmacytoid lymphocytic lymphoma
        and multiple myeloma)
    Hairy cell leukemia
    Mantle zone lymphoma
    Marginal zone lymphoma
    Parafollicular (monocytoid) B-cell lymphoma
    Follicular center cell lymphomas, including Burkitt
        and non-Burkitt types
    Immunoblastic lymphoma of B cells
    Large B-cell lymphomas

T-Cell Lymphomas
    T-cell acute lymphocytic leukemia
    Adult T-cell leukemia
    Small T-cell neoplasms (including T-chronic lympho-
        cytic leukemia)
    Convoluted T-cell lymphoma/lymphoblastic (thymic
        lymphoma)
    Immunoblastic T-cell lymphoma, including periph-
        eral T-cell lymphoma
    Other T-cell neoplasms (lymphoepithelioid/Lennert
        lymphoma, T-zone lymphoma)
    Cerebriform T-cell lymphoma (mycosis fungoides and
        Sézary syndrome)
    Extranodal T-cell lymphomas

Mononuclear Phagocyte System
    Macrophage/histiocytic neoplasms
    Follicular dendritic cell type
    Interdigitating cell type
    Langerhans cell type

Unclassifiable

and Collins used their system to review cases from their home institutions and reported their results. They made the following claims: 1) lymphomas correspond to neoplasms of either B or T cells and the immunophenotype can be predicted, in large part, by the morphologic features; 2) nodular lymphomas are, in fact, B-cell lymphomas that arise from the germinal center and are better designated as follicular lymphomas; and 3) so-called histiocytic neoplasms of the Rappaport classification are rarely derived from histiocytes and instead are derived from transformed B or T lymphocytes. Lukes and Collins

further suggested that additional clinical-morphologic lymphoma variants would be recognized with additional integration of clinical, morphologic, and immunologic findings (29). Lukes and Collins were correct in large part. The only claim never validated (and controversial at the time) is that morphologic/cytologic findings could be used to predict immunophenotype. This claim is true for only a few lymphoma types (e.g., follicular lymphomas).

Karl Lennert et al. proposed a non-Hodgkin lymphoma classification in a letter to the journal Lancet first authored by Gerard-Marchant in 1974 (11). This classification came to be known as the Kiel classification, which was updated subsequently, most recently in 1992 (Table 4-3) (26). Lennert et al. were part of the European Lymphoma Club (the precursor of the European Association for Haematopathology) and the members regularly met to discuss lymphoma cases over decades (24). Like the Lukes-Collins system, the Kiel classification was primarily a morphologic classification, but it sought to integrate immunologic data whenever possible. The Kiel classification initially focused almost exclusively on B-cell lymphomas, with T-cell lymphomas receiving relatively little attention (11). Subsequent updates of the Kiel classification were based on additional immunologic and subsequently molecular data and focused more on T-cell tumors, greatly expanding this aspect of the classification (26). The Kiel classification strived to achieve two goals: 1) track each lymphoma back to its normal B- or T-cell counterpart of the normal immune system; and 2) provide a histologic grade of malignancy, based on the numbers of cytes (small cells), blasts (large cells), and mitotic figures. The Kiel classification achieved widespread popularity in Europe and, in large part, provided a scaffold for the REAL classification in 1994 (14,25).

By the late 1970s, six lymphoma classifications were in use throughout the world: Rappaport, Lukes-Collins, and Kiel, as well as three other classifications proposed by Dorfman (6), the British National Lymphoma Investigation group (1), and initial editions of the WHO classification (33). The latter three classification systems are not reviewed here in detail as they add little to this discussion. In general, these classifications were an attempt to integrate

Table 4-3

UPDATED KIEL CLASSIFICATION OF NON-HODGKIN LYMPHOMAS (1992)

B Cell	T Cell
Low-grade malignant lymphomas	
Lymphocytic	Lymphocytic
Chronic lymphocytic leukemia	Chronic lymphocytic leukemia
Prolymphocytic leukemia	Prolymphocytic leukemia
Hairy cell leukemia	Small cell, cerebriform
Lymphoplasmacytic/cytoid (immunocytoma)	Mycosis fungoides/Sezary syndrome
Plasmacytic	Lymphoepithelioid (Lennert lymphoma)
Centroblastic-centrocytic (follicular ± diffuse; diffuse)	Angioimmunoblastic (AILD)[a]
Centrocytic (mantle cell)	T-zone lymphoma
Monocytoid, including marginal zone cell	Pleomorphic, small cell (HTLV-1±)[a]
High-grade malignant lymphomas	
Centroblastic	Pleomorphic, medium-sized and large cell (HTLV-1±)
Immunoblastic	Immunoblastic (HTLV-1±)
Burkitt's lymphoma	Large cell anaplastic (Ki-1+)
Large cell anaplastic	Lymphoblastic
Lymphoblastic	

[a]AILD = angiommunoblastic lymphadenopathy with dysproteinemia; HTLV = human T-cell leukemia-lymphoma virus.

immunologic advances into the framework of the Rappaport classification. As the many classification systems and terminologies were confusing to pathologists and clinicians alike, and proponents of each classification system had difficultly achieving any sort of consensus, the National Cancer Institute funded an international study to test each of the six classifications on 1,175 non-Hodgkin lymphomas staged and treated in a fairly consistent manner (37). The study was designed by Costan Berard, then Chief of the Hematopathology Section in the Laboratory of Pathology of the National Cancer Institute. On the basis of the results of this study, it was concluded that each of the systems was useful in separating large numbers of patients into subgroups with varying survival rates and clinical features. Consequently, study investigators jointly developed a Working Formulation (Table 4-4). In this formulation, non-Hodgkin lymphomas were divided into three groups based on clinical outcome: low grade, intermediate grade, and high grade. The authors also emphasized that the Working Formulation was not intended as a classification per se, but rather it was to be used as a common language (in association with another classification system) that could translate one classification scheme into another. Despite reservations expressed by Lukes and Lennert, two of the principal participants in the

study (37), the Working Formulation was soon used as a de facto classification for lymphomas in the United States for the next decade. In Europe, the Kiel classification continued to be used as the primary lymphoma classification.

The Working Formulation, by simplifying terminology and reducing confusion, was an immediate boon to clinical research, and thus achieved the most important goal of the study. Nevertheless, the Working Formulation was based purely on histologic data and the participants recognized the limitations of this approach at the time.

About the time the Working Formulation was published, a virtual avalanche of studies applying newly developed immunophenotypic and molecular methods to the study of hematolymphoid neoplasms made it clear that the Working Formulation was inadequate as a stand-alone classification. The categories of the Working Formulation were immunologically and molecularly heterogeneous. Almost immediately, pathologists began to informally modify the Working Formulation by including immunophenotypic and molecular data. By the early 1990s, virtually all hematopathologists who used the Working Formulation were using a more complex version that included histologic, immunophenotypic, molecular, and cytogenetic data, but in a nonstandardized fashion. In the meantime, new research into lymphomas also

Table 4-4

INTERNATIONAL WORKING FORMULATION OF NON-HODGKIN LYMPHOMAS (1982)

Low Grade
A. Malignant lymphoma, small lymphocytic
    Consistent with chronic lymphocytic leukemia
    Plasmacytoid
B. Malignant lymphoma, follicular, predominantly
        small cleaved cell
    Diffuse areas
    Sclerosis
C. Malignant lymphoma, follicular, mixed small
        cleaved and large cell
    Diffuse areas
    Sclerosis

Intermediate Grade
D. Malignant lymphoma, follicular, predominantly
        large cell
    Diffuse areas
    Sclerosis
E. Malignant lymphoma, diffuse, small cleaved cell
    Sclerosis
F. Malignant lymphoma, diffuse, mixed cell
    Sclerosis
    Epithelioid cell component
G. Malignant lymphoma, diffuse, large cell
    Cleaved
    Noncleaved

High Grade
H. Malignant lymphoma, large cell immunoblastic
    Plasmacytoid
    Clear cell
    Polymorphous
    Epithelioid cell
I. Malignant lymphoma, lymphoblastic
    Convoluted cell
    Nonconvoluted cell
J. Malignant lymphoma, small noncleaved
    Burkitt
    Non-Burkitt
K. Miscellaneous
    Composite
    Mycosis fungoides
    Histiocytic
    Extramedullary plasmacytoma
    Unclassifiable

showed that the Kiel classification needed updating and this classification was also modified to incorporate new concepts (26).

The REAL classification (14) was proposed by members of the International Lymphoma Study Group, a group of pathologists interested in lymphomas who initially met ad hoc in 1991 in London. This group took on the challenge of proposing a new lymphoma classification in 1993 and 1994, as reviewed by Pileri et al. (Table 4-5) (40). The International Lymphoma Study Group chose to propose a classification based on all available data to create "real" entities. Therefore, each category in the system incorporated all available clinical, morphologic, immunophenotypic, cytogenetic, and molecular data. Although this approach was novel, the entities included in the classification were not; all entities had been published in the medical literature and therefore, in a sense, the REAL classification was a both a review of the literature and a list of entities. The REAL classification also expanded the number of diseases traditionally included in a lymphoma classification scheme by including plasma cell neoplasms and lymphoid leukemias, as there is substantial overlap between clinical presentations of leukemia versus lymphoma, and this distinction can seem arbitrary (14).

There were criticisms of the REAL system at the time. Perhaps the most important issues were the need for the REAL system to be tested for clinical relevance and the need for input from clinicians. These issues were addressed in an important validation study of the REAL classification organized by Dennis Weisenburger and James Armitage at the University of Nebraska (38). Weisenburger et al. also organized a meeting for pathologists and clinicians to discuss the REAL classification in Omaha, Nebraska. Once the REAL classification was published, and particularly after the Omaha meeting, the REAL classification became widely accepted by clinicians and pathologists worldwide. The REAL classification paper published in the journal Blood has been cited almost 5,000 times (at time of writing). The REAL classification, in spirit and largely in content, became the basis for the third and fourth editions of the WHO classification (18,51). The transition from REAL to WHO has been reviewed by Pileri et al. (40).

CURRENT LYMPHOMA CLASSIFICATION SCHEME

The fourth edition of the WHO classification is shown in Tables 4-6 to 4-8. An update and revision of the 2008 classification also has been published in preliminary form in 2016 (51a). Compared with the lack of consensus regarding lymphoma classification in the 1970s, the worldwide use of the WHO "blue book" is

Table 4-5

REVISED EUROPEAN AMERICAN CLASSIFICATION OF LYMPHOID NEOPLASMS (1994)

B-Cell Neoplasms

  I. Precursor B-cell neoplasm: precursor B-lymphoblastic leukemia/lymphoma
 II. Peripheral B-cell neoplasms
   1. B-cell chronic lymphocytic leukemia/prolymphocytic leukemia/small lymphocytic lymphoma
   2. Lymphoplasmacytoid lymphoma/immunocytoma
   3. Mantle cell lymphoma
   4. Follicle center lymphoma, follicular
      Provisional cytologic grades: I (small cell), II (mixed small and large cell), III (large cell)
   5. Marginal zone B-cell lymphoma
      Extranodal (MALT type[a] ± monocytoid B cells)
   6. Provisional entity: splenic marginal zone lymphoma (± villous lymphocytes)
   7. Hairy cell leukemia
   8. Plasmacytoma/plasma cell myeloma
   9. Diffuse large B-cell lymphoma[b]
  10. Burkitt lymphoma
  11. Provisional entity: high-grade B-cell lymphoma, Burkitt-like[b]

T-Cell and Putative NK-Cell Neoplasms

  I. Precursor T-cell neoplasms: precursor T-lymphoblastic lymphoma/leukemia
 II. Peripheral T-cell and NK-cell neoplasms
   1. T-cell chronic lymphocytic leukemia/prolymphocytic leukemia
   2. Large granular lymphocytic leukemia (LGL) T-cell type
   3. Mycosis fungoides/Sézary syndrome
   4. Peripheral T-cell lymphomas, unspecified[b]
      Provisional cytologic categories: medium-sized cell, mixed medium and large-cell, large-cell, lympho-
         epithelioid cell
      Provisional subtype: hepatosplenic γδ T-cell lymphoma
      Provisional subtype: subcutaneous panniculitic T-cell lymphoma
   5. Angioimmunoblastic T-cell lymphoma (AILD)
   6. Angiocentric lymphoma
   7. Intestinal T-cell lymphoma (± enteropathy-associated)
   8. Adult T-cell lymphoma/leukemia (ATL)
   9. Anaplastic large cell lymphoma (ALCL), CD30-, T-, and null-cell types
  10. Provisional entity: anaplastic large-cell lymphoma, Hodgkin-like

Hodgkin Disease

  I. Lymphocyte predominance
 II. Nodular sclerosis
III. Mixed cellularity
 IV. Lymphocyte depletion
  V. Provisional entity: lymphocyte-rich classical Hodgkin disease

[a]MALT = mucosa-associated lymphoid tissue.
[b]Categories thought likely to include more than one disease.

remarkable. The general principles of the WHO classification are as follows: 1) following the approach of the REAL classification, the WHO system is based on utilization of all clinical, pathologic, and laboratory information that is available. As a corollary to this first tenet, immunophenotype is essential to the classification of any lymphoid neoplasm; 2) the classification emphasizes the value of the clinical features, for more accurate diagnosis and, in some instances, in defining some diseases; 3) the classification recognizes that there is overlap between B-cell non-Hodgkin lymphomas and classic Hodgkin lymphoma that, in some instances, can be marked. This overlap is recognized in two "gray zone" B-cell categories. In addition to these principles, the authors of the WHO book state that reliance on a single feature of a disease may not be reliable. Using the example of immunophenotypic analysis, the authors point out that within a given disease there is variation of the immunophenotype. There is also evidence of lineage plasticity, where tumors can switch lineage, more common in immature tumors (e.g., acute lymphoblastic leukemia) than in lymphomas derived from mature lymphocytes. Therefore, reliance on a single marker can lead to misdiagnosis.

Although the WHO classification and its approach are widely accepted, there are some minor issues with its use. The inclusion of all data in establishing a diagnosis, although clearly valuable, leads to a rather holistic approach to establishing a lymphoma diagnosis. Although usually a good thing, a drawback to this approach is that two pathologists, by emphasizing different aspects of a case, can arrive at a different diagnosis. For example, more emphasis on the clinical location of a neoplasm might support one diagnosis whereas another pathologist might emphasize immunophenotypic or molecular findings to support another diagnosis. With the current state of knowledge, either position may be correct. This type of disagreement seems most likely to occur in the diagnosis of T-cell lymphomas in the WHO system because clinical data assume greater importance. More objective data, likely to come from molecular studies, are needed for entities in which clinical data currently play a major role in establishing a diagnosis in the current WHO system.

A second issue with the WHO classification is that incorporating cytogenetic or molecular data into a lymphoma classification can introduce delays in establishing a diagnosis. Lymphoma diagnosis is now becoming similar to the diagnosis of acute leukemias, where morphology and immunophenotypic data are available quickly, and molecular and then cytogenetic data may not be available for 1 to 2 weeks.

A third issue involves the results of high-throughput genetic and proteomic methods that will likely show a number of important findings in lymphomas targetable for therapy. It is unclear whether the inclusion of specific genetic data (e.g., mutation status) into the definition of a disease, as has been done in the current WHO classification for some diseases, will be ultimately practical. As it is, B-acute lymphoblastic leukemia in the current WHO classification is already divided into eight molecular subsets, and much more mutation data has become available in recent years.

The inclusion of provisional entities into the WHO classification also has drawbacks. As the classification has become the standard in the field of lymphomas, the inclusion of a provisional entity gives the entity a status that may not be supported by the data.

The 2008 WHO system for lymphoid neoplasms included 62 entities, as well as additional provisional entities and morphologic variants. These entities were divided into six subsections: precursor lymphoid neoplasms, mature B-cell neoplasms, mature T-cell and NK-cell neoplasms, Hodgkin lymphomas, immunodeficiency-associated lymphoproliferative disorders, and histiocytic and dendritic cell neoplasms. The 2016 revision (Table 4-9) to the WHO system adds another 17 entities and modifies terminology (51a). Although lymphoma classification is becoming more complex with each new version of the WHO system, lymphoid neoplasms (and all cancers) are complicated, and attempts at designing conceptual classification systems in the past were over-simplifying the complex issues involved.

In the approach to lymphoma diagnosis, morphologic features are important but immunophenotype is equally important and essential for establishing a diagnosis. In general, cytogenetic and molecular data, although important, currently have a lesser role in classification.

The general approach to B- and T/NK-cell lymphomas is somewhat different. By far, knowledge is most advanced for B-cell lymphomas, which represent 85 to 90 percent of all lymphoma cases. Based on the recognition of the structures and cytologic features in the normal lymph node, the cell of origin and its function for many B-cell lymphomas are known. Immunophenotypic markers that correspond to normal structures are also available. As a result, the option of designating a mature B-cell lymphoma as "not otherwise classified" is the last option, used uncommonly. By contrast, T-cell lymphomas represent about 10 to 15 percent of lymphomas and little is known of their normal cell of origin or function. As a result, the designation of a mature T-cell lymphoma as "not otherwise specified" is often a first choice and other data are required to move the tumor into a more specific category. In general, specific types of T-cell lymphoma that are more developed or advanced have characteristic morphologic features whereas earlier lesions are less distinctive and show greater morphologic overlap with peripheral T-cell lymphoma, not otherwise specified.

Table 4-6

WORLD HEALTH ORGANIZATION (WHO) CLASSIFICATION OF B-CELL NEOPLASMS (2008)

Precursor B-Cell Neoplasms
B-lymphoblastic leukemia/lymphoma, not otherwise specified
B-lymphoblastic leukemia/lymphoma, with recurrent genetic abnormalities
    B-lymphoblastic leukemia/lymphoma with t(9;22)(q34;q11,2);*BCR-ABL1*
    B-lymphoblastic leukemia/lymphoma with t(v;11q23);*MLL* rearranged
    B-lymphoblastic leukemia/lymphoma with t(12;21)(p13;q22);*TEL-AML1 (ETV6-RUNX1)*
    B-lymphoblastic leukemia/lymphoma with hyperdiploidy
    B-lymphoblastic leukemia/lymphoma with hypodiploidy (hypodiploid ALL)[a]
    B-lymphoblastic leukemia/lymphoma with t(5;14)(q31;q32);IL3-*IGH*
    B-lymphoblastic leukemia/lymphoma with t(1;19)(q23;p13.3);*E2A-PBX (TCF3-PBX1)*

Mature B-Cell Neoplasms
Chronic lymphocytic leukemia/small lymphocytic lymphoma
B-cell prolymphocytic leukemia
Splenic marginal zone B-cell lymphoma
Hairy cell leukemia
Splenic B-cell lymphoma/leukemia unclassifiable[b]
    Splenic diffuse red pulp small B-cell lymphoma
    Hairy cell leukemia-variant
Lymphoplasmacytic lymphoma
    Waldenstrom macroglobulinemia
Heavy chain diseases
    Alpha heavy chain disease
    Gamma heavy chain disease
    Mu heavy chain disease
Plasma cell myeloma
Solitary plasmacytoma of bone
Extraosseous plasmacytoma
Extranodal marginal zone B-cell lymphoma of mucosa-associated lymphoid tissue (MALT)
Nodal marginal zone B-cell lymphoma
    Pediatric nodal marginal zone lymphoma
Follicular lymphoma
    Pediatric follicular lymphoma
Primary cutaneous follicle center cell lymphoma
Mantle cell lymphoma
Diffuse large B-cell lymphoma (DLBCL), not otherwise specified
    T-cell/histiocyte-rich large B-cell lymphoma
    Primary DLBCL of the central nervous system
    Primary cutaneous DLBCL, leg type
    EBV+ DLBCL of the elderly
    DLBCL associated with chronic inflammation
    Lymphomatoid granulomatosis
    Primary mediastinal (thymic) large B-cell lymphoma
    Intravascular large B-cell lymphoma
    ALK-positive large B-cell lymphoma
    Plasmablastic lymphoma
    Large B-cell lymphoma arising in HHV8-associated multicentric Castleman disease
    Primary effusion lymphoma
    Burkitt lymphoma
B-cell lymphoma, unclassifiable, with features intermediate between DLBCL and Burkitt lymphoma
B-cell lymphoma, unclassifiable, with features intermediate between DLBCL and classic Hodgkin lymphoma

[a]ALL = acute lymphoblastic leukemia; EBV = Epstein-Barr virus; ALK = anaplastic lymphoma kinase; HHV = human herpesvirus.
[b]Italics denotes provisional entities.

Table 4-7

WHO CLASSIFICATION OF T- AND NK-CELL NEOPLASMS (2008)

Precursor T-Cell Neoplasm
T-lymphoblastic lymphoma/leukemia

Mature T-Cell and NK-Cell Neoplasms
T-cell prolymphocytic leukemia
T-cell large granular lymphocytic leukemia
  Chronic lymphoproliferative disorder of NK cells[a]
Aggressive NK-cell leukemia
Systemic EBV+ T-cell lymphoproliferative diseases of
  childhood
Hydroa vacciniforme-like lymphoma
Adult T-cell lymphoma/leukemia
Extranodal NK/T-cell lymphoma, nasal type
Enteropathy-associated T-cell lymphoma
Hepatosplenic T-cell lymphoma
Subcutaneous panniculitis-like T-cell lymphoma
Mycosis fungoides
Sezary syndrome
Primary cutaneous CD30+ T-cell lymphoproliferative
  disorders
Primary cutaneous peripheral T-cell lymphomas, rare
  subtypes
  Primary cutaneous gamma-delta T-cell lymphoma
  Primary cutaneous CD8+ aggressive epidermotropic
    cytotoxic T-cell lymphoma
  Primary cutaneous CD4+ small/medium T-cell
    lymphoma
Peripheral T-cell lymphoma, not otherwise specified
Angioimmunoblastic T-cell lymphoma
Anaplastic large cell lymphoma, ALK+
Anaplastic large cell lymphoma, ALK-

[a]Italics denotes provisional entities.
[b]EBV = Epstein-Barr virus; ALK = anaplastic lymphoma kinase.

Table 4-8

WHO CLASSIFICATION OF HODGKIN LYMPHOMAS (2008)

Nodular lymphocyte-predominant Hodgkin lymphoma

Classical Hodgkin lymphoma
  Nodular sclerosis classical Hodgkin lymphoma
  Lymphocyte-rich classical Hodgkin lymphoma
  Mixed cellularity classical Hodgkin lymphoma
  Lymphocyte-depletion classical Hodgkin lymphoma

Although the complete update of the fourth edition of the WHO classification is not available at the time of this writing, a preliminary version has been published. The upcoming changes include minor alterations of terminology and new provisional entities (Table 4-9).

COMPOSITE LYMPHOMA

The term *composite lymphoma* was coined by Philip Custer (5) for a patient who had two or more types of lymphoma as defined at the light microscopic level. In Custer's definition, the lymphomas could involve the same or different anatomic sites. Kim et al. (20) and subsequently others (13) refined the definition, suggesting that composite lymphoma be defined as two lymphomas involving the same anatomic site. Inherent in this definition was the assumption that the two tumors were not clonally related. Subsequent immunophenotypic studies of presumed composite lymphomas, however, showed in many cases that the two histologic components shared the same immunophenotype and were likely related. In a lymph node specimen involved by both low-grade follicular lymphoma and diffuse large B-cell lymphoma, for example, it was recognized that both components were derived from the same tumor clone, with the higher-grade component representing histologic transformation as a result of clonal evolution. Such cases were then excluded from the designation of composite lymphoma by most pathologists.

The concept of composite lymphoma further evolved with the advent of molecular genetic techniques and particularly single cell PCR studies (45,46). These studies have shown that some cases of composite lymphoma with widely divergent histologic components are in fact clonally related at the molecular level. Furthermore, the two components often share

Regarding Hodgkin lymphomas, other than the change of the name from Hodgkin's disease to Hodgkin lymphoma (Table 4-8), the categories and terminology used in the current WHO classification have changed little from those of the Lukes-Butler classification (fig. 4-2). It is important to recognize, however, that the classification of Hodgkin lymphomas has evolved greatly over the past 50 years, driven by a shift from using purely histologic criteria to using immunophenotypic data for diagnosis, particularly immunohistochemical studies. There is also less emphasis on the identification of classic Reed-Sternberg cells in some types of Hodgkin lymphoma. One can liken the changes in Hodgkin lymphoma classification to that of the make of an automobile in 1966 as compared with today; the name of the vehicle may be the same, but the automobile itself has changed greatly in the past 50 years.

Table 4-9

ADDITIONS AND CHANGES IN 2016 REVISION OF WORLD HEALTH ORGANIZATION CLASSIFICATION[a]

Additions
Monoclonal B-cell lymphocytosis
Monoclonal gammopathy of undetermined significance, IgM or IgG/A
Monoclonal immunoglobulin deposition diseases
In situ follicular neoplasia
Duodenal-type follicular lymphoma
Large B-cell lymphoma with *IRF4* rearrangement
In situ mantle cell neoplasia
Diffuse large B-cell lymphoma (DLBCL): specification as germinal center B-cell vs. activated B-cell type
EBV+ mucocutaneous ulcer
Burkitt-like lymphoma with 11q aberration
Systemic EBV+ T-cell lymphoma of childhood
Hydroa vacciniforme-like lymphoproliferative disorder
Indolent T-cell lymphoproliferative disorder of GI tract
Primary cutaneous acral CD8+ T-cell lymphoma
Follicular T-cell lymphoma
Nodal peripheral T-cell lymphoma with TFH phenotype
Breast implant-associated anaplastic large-cell lymphoma

Changes in Terminology

From	To
EBV+ DLBCL of elderly	EBV+ DLBCL
Large B-cell lymphoma arising in HHV8+ multicentric Castleman disease	HHV8+ DLBCL, not otherwise specified (NOS)
B-cell lymphoma, unclassifiable, with features intermediate between DLBCL and Burkitt lymphoma	High-grade B-cell lymphoma with MYC and BCL2 and/or BCL6 rearrangements
	High-grade B-cell lymphoma, NOS
Enteropathy-associated T-cell lymphoma, type II	Monomorphic epitheliotropic intestinal T-cell lymphoma
Primary cutaneous CD4+ small/medium T-cell lymphoma	Primary cutaneous CD4+ small/medium T-cell lymphoproliferative disorder

[a]Derived from reference 51a. Immunodeficiency-associated lymphoid lesions and histiocytic disorders are not included.

some molecular lesions but do not share other mutations (23,32,46). These findings suggest that the two histologic components may have arisen from a common ancestor cell, with the parallel evolution of each component, rather than transformation from one component to the other. These results also imply, based on the definition of composite lymphoma resting on clonal unrelatedness, that molecular analysis of both histologic components is required to establish the diagnosis of composite lymphoma. As the clonal relationship is often unknown in cases that morphologically appear to represent composite lymphoma, the practicality of establishing the diagnosis of composite lymphoma becomes an issue.

Mueller-Hermelink et al. (35) suggested a compromise for using the designation of composite lymphoma that is workable. They suggested using the term in a descriptive manner for lymphomas that have two or more distinctive morphologic components, irrespective of a clonal relationship. The pathogenesis for clonally related lymphomas with divergent morphologic components is unknown, but origin from a multipotential stem cell is a possible explanation. An underlying genetic predisposition or a coincidental relationship is possible for clonally unrelated tumors.

DISCORDANT HISTOLOGY

The term *discordant histology* is used for a patient who has two (or more) biopsy specimens from different anatomic sites involved by morphologically different lymphomas (34). The two lymphomas may be present simultaneously or detected in a sequential manner, and may be clonally related or unrelated (19). The most common example of discordant histology in daily practice occurs in patients with diffuse large B-cell lymphoma who have a small B-cell lymphoma involving the bone marrow, most often low-grade follicular lymphoma (4,21,47). The implications of a patient having two discordant lymphomas are probably similar to a patient with composite lymphoma. Typically, the treatment plan is aimed at the more aggressive lymphoma component.

REFERENCES

1. Bennett MH, Farrer-Brown G, Henry K, et al. Classification of non-Hodgkin's lymphomas. Lancet 1974;304:405-408.
2. Billroth T. Multiple Lymphome: Erfolgreiche Behandlung mit Arsenik. Wien Med Wochenschr 1871; 21: 1066-1067.
3. Brill NE, Baehr G, Rosenthal N. Generalized giant lymph follicle hyperplasia of the lymph nodes and spleen: a hitherto undescribed type. JAMA 1925;84:668-671.
4. Chung R, Lai R, Weis P, et al. Concordant but not discordant bone marrow involvement in diffuse large B-cell lymphoma predicts a poor clinical outcome independent of the International Prognostic Index. Blood 2007;110:1278-1282.
5. Custer RP. Pitfalls in the diagnosis of lymphoma and leukemia from a pathologist's point of view. Proceedings of the 2nd National Cancer Conference. New York. American Cancer Society, 1954: 554-557.
6. Dorfman RF. Classification of non-Hodgkin's lymphoma. Lancet 1974;303:1295-1296.
7. Dreschfield J. Ein Beitrag zur Lehre von den Lymphosarkomen. Dtsch Med Wochenschr 1893;17: 1175-1177.
8. Gall EA, Mallory TB. Malignant lymphoma: A clinico-pathologic survey of 618 cases. Am J Pathol 1942;18:381-429.
9. Gall EA, Morrison HR, Scott AT. The follicular type of malignant lymphoma: A survey of 63 cases. Ann Intern Med 1941;14:2073-2090.
10. Gall EA, Rappaport H. Seminar on disease of lymph nodes and spleen. In McDonald, JR (Ed.): Proceedings of 23rd Seminar, American Society of Clinical Pathology. Chicago, The American Society of Clinical Pathology, 1957.
11. Garard-Marchant R, Hamlin I, Lennert K, Rilke F, Stansfeld AG, Van Unnik JA. Classification of non-Hodgkin's lymphomas. Lancet 1974; 304:405-408.
12. Ghon A, Roman B. Uber das Lymphosarkom. Frankfurt Z Pathol 1916;19:1-138.
13. Gonzalez CL, Medeiros LJ, Jaffe ES. Composite lymphoma. A clinicopathologic analysis of nine patients with Hodgkin's disease and B-cell non-Hodgkin's lymphoma. Am J Clin Pathol 1991; 96:81-89.
14. Harris NL, Jaffe ES, Stein H, et al. A revised European-American classification of lymphoid neoplasms: a proposal from the International Lymphoma Study Group. Blood 1994;84:1361-1392.
15. Hodgkin T. On some morbid appearances of the absorbent glands and spleen. Med Chir Trans 1832;17:68-114.
16. Jackson HJ, Jr, Parker F, Jr. Hodgkin's Disease and Allied Disorders. Oxford University Press, New York, 1947.
17. Jacobs CD. Henry Kaplan and the story of Hodgkin's disease. Stanford, CA: Stanford General Books; 2012:164.
18. Jaffe ES, Harris NL, Stein H, Vardiman JW (eds.). Pathology and Genetics of Tumours of the Haematopoietic and Lymphoid Tissues. IARC Press, Lyon, 2001
19. Jaffe ES, Zarate-Osorno A, Medeiros LJ. The interrelationship between Hodgkin's disease and non-Hodgkin's lymphomas—lessons learned from composite and sequential malignancies. Semin Diagn Pathol 1992;9:297-303.
20. Kim H, Hendrickson M, Dorfman RF. Composite lymphoma. Cancer 1977;40:959-976.
21. Kremer M, Spitzer M, Mandl-Weber S, et al. Discordant bone marrow involvement in diffuse large B-cell lymphoma: comparative molecular analysis reveals a heterogeneous group of disorders. Lab Invest 2003;83:107-114.
22. Kundrat H. Ueber Lympho-sarkomatosis. Wien Klin Wochenschr 1893;6:211-213, 234-239.
23. Kuppers R, Sousa AB, Baur AS, Strickler JG, Rajewsky K, Hansmann ML. Common germinal-center B-cell origin of the malignant cells in two composite lymphomas, involving classical Hodgkin's disease and either follicular lymphoma or B-CLL. Mol Med 2001;7:285-292.
24. Lennert K (translated by M Siehring). History of the European Association for Haematopathology. Springer-Verlag, Berlin, 2006.
25. Lennert K. The proposal for a Revised European American Lymphoma classification - a new start of a transatlantic discussion. Histopathology 1995;26:481-483.
26. Lennert K, Feller AC. Histopathology of non-Hodgkin's lymphomas. (Based on the updated Kiel classification; translated by M. Soehring). Berlin, Springer-Verlag, 1992:16.
27. Lukes RJ, Butler JJ. The pathology and nomenclature of Hodgkin's disease. Cancer Res 1966;26:1063-1081.

28. Lukes RJ, Craver LF, Hall TC, Rappaport H, Ruben P. Report of the nomenclature committee. Cancer Res 1966;26: 1311.

29. Lukes RJ, Collins RD. Lukes-Collins classification and its significance. Cancer Treat Rep 1977;61:971-979.

30. Lukes RJ, Collins RD. Immunologic characterization of human malignant lymphomas. Cancer 1974;34(suppl):1488-1503.

31. Lukes RJ, Collins RD. Tumors of the Hematopoietic System. Atlas of Tumor Pathology, 2nd Series, Fascicle 28, Washington DC: Armed Forces Institute of Pathology; 1992:29.

32. Marafioti T, Hummel M, Anagnostopoulos I, Foss HD, Huhn D, Stein H. Classical Hodgkin's disease and follicular lymphoma originating from the same germinal center B cell. J Clin Oncol 1999;17:3804-3809.

33. Mathe G, Rappaport H, O'Conor GT, Torloni H. Histological and cytological typing of neoplastic diseases of hematopoietic and lymphoid tissues. WHO International Histological Classification of Tumours, No. 14. Geneva: World Health Organization; 1976.

34. Mead GM, Kushlan P, O'Neil M, Burke JS, Rosenberg SA. Clinical aspects of non-Hodgkin's lymphomas presenting with discordant histologic subtypes. Cancer 1983;52:1496-1501.

35. Mueller-Hermelink HK, Zettl A, Pfeifer W, Ott G. Pathology of lymphoma progression. Histopathology 2001;38:285-306.

36. Nathwani BN. A critical analysis of the classification of non-Hodgkin's lymphoma. Cancer 1979;44:347-384.

37. [No authors listed.] National Cancer Institute sponsored study of classifications of non-Hodgkin's lymphomas: summary and description of a Working Formulation for clinical usage. The Non-Hodgkin's Lymphoma Pathologic Classification Project. Cancer 1982;15:2112-2135.

38. [No authors listed.] A clinical evaluation of the International Lymphoma Study Group. Classification of non-Hodgkin's lymphoma. The Non-Hodgkin's Lymphoma Classification Project. Blood 1997;89:3909-3918.

39. Oberling C. Les reticulosarcomes et les reticulo-en-dotheliosarcomes de la moelle osseuse (sarcomes d'Ewing). Bull Assoc Fr Etud Cancer 1928;17:290-296.

40. Pileri SA, Agostinelli C, Sabattini E, et al. Lymphomas classification: the quiet after the storm. Sem Diagn Pathol 2011;28:113-123.

41. Poston RN. A new look at the original cases of Hodgkin's disease. Cancer Treat Rev 1999;25:151-155.

42. Rappaport H, Winter WJ, Hicks EB. Follicular lymphoma; a re-evaluation of its position in the scheme of malignant lymphoma, based on a survey of 253 cases. Cancer 1956;9:792-821.

43. Reed DM. On the pathological changes in Hodgkin's disease, with especial reference to its relation to tuberculosis. The Johns Hopkins Hospital Reports 1902;10:133-196.

44. Robb-Smith AHT. Reticulosis and reticulosarcoma: a histological classification. J Pathol 1938; XLVII:457-480.

45. Schmitz R. Stanelle J, Hansmann ML, Küppers R. Pathogenesis of classical and lymphocyte-predominant Hodgkin lymphoma. Annu Rev Pathol 2009;4:151-174.

46. Schneider S, Crescenzi B, Schneider M, et al. Subclonal evolution of a classical Hodgkin lymphoma from a germinal center B-cell derived mantle cell lymphoma. Int J Cancer 2014; 134:832-843.

47. Shim H, Oh JI, Park SH, et al. Prognostic impact of concordant and discordant cytomorphology of bone marrow involvement in patients with diffuse large B-cell lymphoma treated with R-CHOP. J Clin Pathol 2013;66:420-425.

48. Smetana HF, Cohen BM. Mortality in relation to histologic type in Hodgkin's disease. Blood 1956;11:211-224.

49. Stein H, Hummel M. Cellular origin and clonality of classic Hodgkin lymphoma: immunophenotypic and molecular studies. Semin Hematol 1999;36:233-241.

50. Sternberg C. Uber eine eigenarige unter dem Bilder der Pseudoleukamie verlaufende Tuberkulose des lymphatischen Apparates. Zeitschrift Heilkunde 1898;19:21-90.

51. Swerdlow SH, Campo E, Harris NL, et al. WHO Classification of Tumours of Haematopoietic and Lymphoid Tissues. IARC; Lyon, 2008.

51a. Swerdlow SH, Campo E, Pileri SA, et al. The 2016 revision of the World Health Organization classification of lymphoid neoplasms. Blood 2016;127:2375-2390.

52. Symmers D. Follicular lymphadenopathy with splenomegaly: A newly recognized disease of the lymphatic system. Arch Pathol 1927;3:816-820.

53. Taylor CR, Hartsock RJ. Classifications of lymphoma; reflections of time and technology. Virchows Arch 2011;458:637-648

54. Virchow R. Die cellularpathologie in ihrer Begruendung auf physiologische und pathologische Gewebelehre. Berlin, Hirschwald, 1859.

55. Virchow RIK. Die Krankhaftern Geschwulste, Berlin, Hirschwald 1865;2:728-738.

56. Wilks S. Cases of enlargement of the lymphatic glands and spleen (or Hodgkin's disease), with remarks. Guys Hosp Rep 1865;11:56-67.

5   HISTOLOGIC TRANSFORMATION

The term *histologic transformation* is commonly used for the clinical circumstance in which a patient with clinically indolent (low-grade) non-Hodgkin lymphoma (NHL), after a variable time interval, suddenly develops an aggressive (high-grade) lymphoma. At the time of histologic transformation, patients usually show the clinical manifestations of a change in the pace of their disease. Histologically, the transformed lymphoma is most often classified as diffuse large B-cell lymphoma (DLBCL), although other morphologic manifestations of transformation occur. Proof of a clonal relationship between the indolent and aggressive lymphoma is required in the ideal definition of histologic transformation.

Biopsy specimens in which low-grade follicular lymphoma and DLBCL coexist at initial diagnosis, although likely clonally related and a manifestation of histologic transformation, are usually not included in the category of histologic transformation per se. These patients are not included because they tend to have a better prognosis than patients who have low-grade follicular lymphoma and subsequently develop DLBCL (34). One possible explanation may be that patients with de novo coexistent follicular lymphoma and DLBCL have not been treated, avoiding the risks of acquiring increased genetic complexity or chemoresistance after therapy.

The term *histologic progression* has been used by some authors as a synonym for histologic transformation. In this chapter, however, we use the term histologic progression to characterize morphologic changes in a neoplasm that often occur over time and that are usually not associated with a sudden change in clinical manifestations. For example, in patients with follicular lymphoma, it is not unusual for the neoplasm in sequential biopsy specimens to acquire, at least in part, a diffuse pattern or an increase of large cells resulting in a change of grade from grade 1 or 2 to 3A. Other types of NHL, for example T-cell lymphomas, also undergo histologic progression. Over time these tumors often accrue larger cells and become more proliferative. Histologic progression also occurs in patients with Hodgkin lymphomas. Progressive depletion of background small reactive lymphocytes and increased numbers of neoplastic cells are observed. Therapy effects and the acquisition of therapy resistance are also likely manifested in the morphologic changes of histologic progression.

HISTOLOGIC TRANSFORMATION OF FOLLICULAR LYMPHOMA

Frequency

Histologic transformation is best understood in patients with follicular lymphoma and this lymphoma is emphasized in this chapter. A "ballpark" frequency for histologic transformation in follicular lymphoma patients is 2 to 3 percent per year (12,14,33,37). The risk is cumulative over time. A few studies have suggested that risk may plateau after a number of years (33), but in other studies, risk rises indefinitely for each year after diagnosis. Historically, the prognosis was poor once histologic transformation arose, but recent studies have shown a better prognosis than historical data suggested (2,33). Possible explanations for the better prognosis of patients at time of histologic transformation include more powerful imaging and pathologic techniques making possible the diagnosis of transformation sooner, improved therapy for the follicular lymphoma at the time of initial diagnosis, and better treatment options at the time of transformation, such as autologous stem cell transplantation. In one study, follicular lymphoma patients who were initially managed by watchful waiting had an almost 4-fold higher risk of histologic transformation compared with patients who received therapy that included rituximab (33).

The incidence of histologic transformation in patients with follicular lymphoma is difficult to derive from the literature. The incidence has ranged from 10 to 60 percent in various studies, explained, in part, by the different methods used to assess for transformation (14,33,37). In general, studies that reported a lower frequency of histologic transformation have tended to require biopsy proof of transformation. Studies with prolonged clinical follow-up or studies that included autopsy data have reported a higher frequency of histologic transformation. More extensive tumor sampling or selection of patients who responded poorly to therapy and died may explain the higher reported frequency of histologic transformation in autopsy studies. In most studies in the literature focused on histologic transformation, the authors did not perform clonality studies to prove a clonal relationship between the low-grade follicular lymphoma and the transformed tumor, a potential drawback of the data reported.

Clinical Features

At the time of transformation, patients commonly develop B-type symptoms, rapidly progressive lymphadenopathy (localized or disseminated), or new extranodal sites of involvement with or without an extranodal mass (14,33,37). Laboratory studies may show a rapid rise in serum lactate dehydrogenase (LDH) or β-2-microglubulin levels. Imaging studies may show new-onset masses and sudden enlargement of lymph nodes, or a fluorodeoxyglucose-positron emission tomography (FDG-PET) scan may show a sudden change in uptake, indicating the presence of a more proliferative tumor. In rare patients, histologic transformation is an incidental finding.

Pathologic Findings

Tumors that arise by histologic transformation from a low-grade lymphoma share many morphologic features with de novo lymphomas, but they are not identical. Often, histologically transformed tumors have some evidence of persistent low-grade lymphoma in the background. In addition, the cell size is often not the same as the cells in de novo NHLs. In particular, the neoplastic cells in the transformed lymphoma are intermediate in size or there may be a spectrum of sizes from intermediate to large.

In patients with follicular lymphoma, the most common morphologic manifestation of histologic transformation is a lymphoma that is best classified as DLBCL (fig. 5-1) (14,37). In these tumors, the follicular pattern is lost and numerous large cells are present, often in sheets. The large cells most often resemble centroblasts, but may be immunoblasts, or uncommonly, the cells are pleomorphic or anaplastic (fig. 5-2) (1,14). Mitotic figures are usually numerous. In some cases, some small centrocytes are observed in the background, often in association with small residual follicles. Immunophenotypic studies show that these neoplasms usually have a germinal center B-cell immunophenotype (positivity for pan-B, CD10, LMO2, and BCL6) and have a high proliferation rate shown by assessment of Ki-67. BCL2 is commonly positive. Reactive T cells in the background are decreased, and few (if any) follicular dendritic cells are present.

There are other unusual morphologic manifestations of histologic transformation (Table 5-1). In a subset of cases, the transformed neoplasm retains its follicular architecture but is composed almost entirely of large cells, supporting follicular lymphoma, grade 3B. The transformed neoplasm can have a high-grade (Burkitt-like) appearance, with a prominent starry sky pattern and some cells of intermediate size. These tumors are usually strongly BCL2 positive and have a very high proliferation rate, and were classified previously as B-cell lymphoma, unclassifiable, with features intermediate between DLBCL and Burkitt lymphoma (2008 WHO). Currently these tumors are classified as high-grade B-cell lymphoma (WHO update) (56a).

Follicular lymphoma can transform to a neoplasm composed of small blastoid cells that are TdT positive (fig. 5-3) or negative (20,40). The TdT-positive tumors are often classified as B-lymphoblastic lymphomas, but this terminology seems to be problematic since patients with these transformed tumors usually have a poorer prognosis than patients with de novo B-acute lymphoblastic leukemia/lymphoblastic lymphoma (20). Rare cases of follicular lymphoma transform to a lymphoma with a CD138 positive/CD20 negative immunophenotype and plasmablastic cytologic features (36) or acquire large CD30-positive cells and have a Hodgkin lymphoma-like appearance (3).

Molecular Genetic Findings

In many studies, proof is lacking that the initial low-grade follicular lymphoma and the histologically transformed tumor are clonally

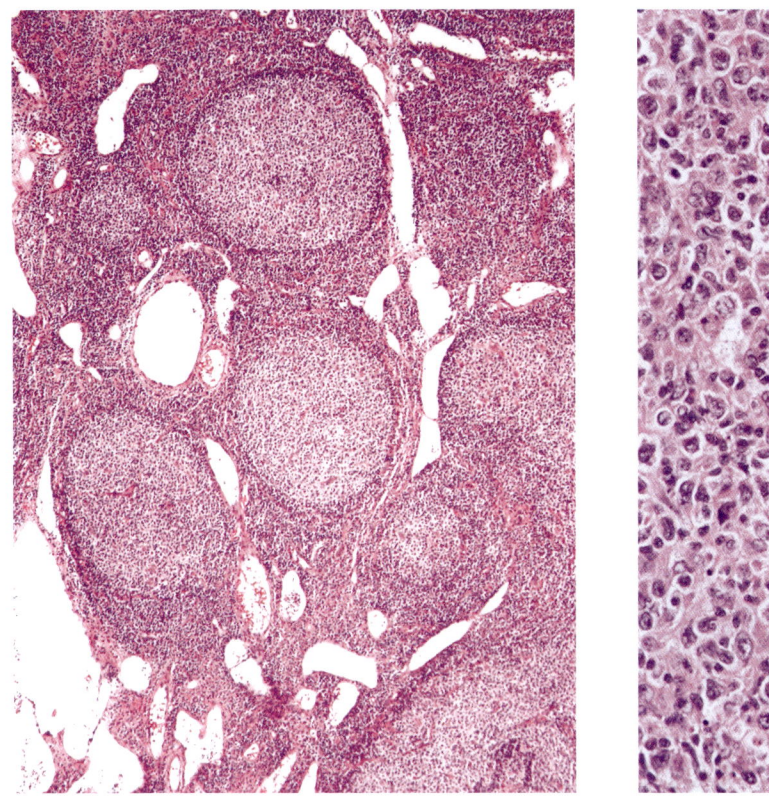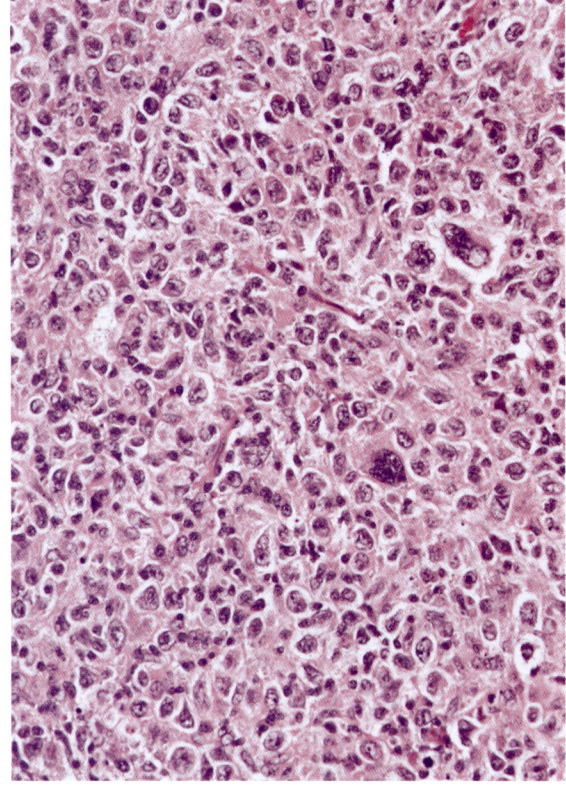

Figure 5-1

HISTOLOGIC TRANSFORMATION

A patient with grade 1 follicular lymphoma (left) subsequently transformed to diffuse large B-cell lymphoma (DLBCL) (right) 2 years later (hematoxylin and eosin [H&E] stain).

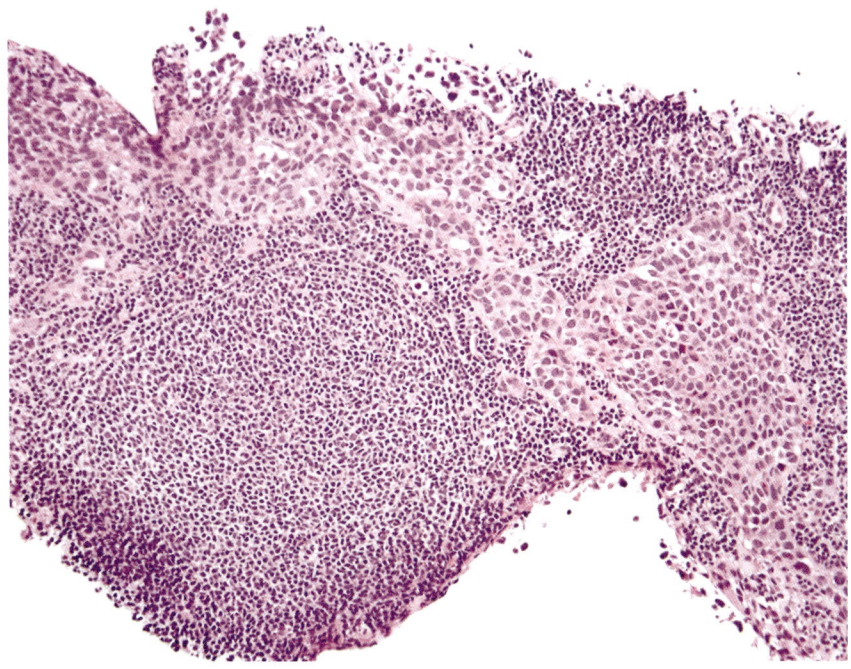

Figure 5-2

HISTOLOGIC TRANSFORMATION

A patient with a history of low-grade lymphoma (not shown) showed transformation 8 months later. The subsequent needle biopsy specimen shows both grade 1 follicular lymphoma and sinusoidal involvement by DLBCL. The sinusoidal large cell lymphoma was CD30 positive (not shown) (H&E stain).

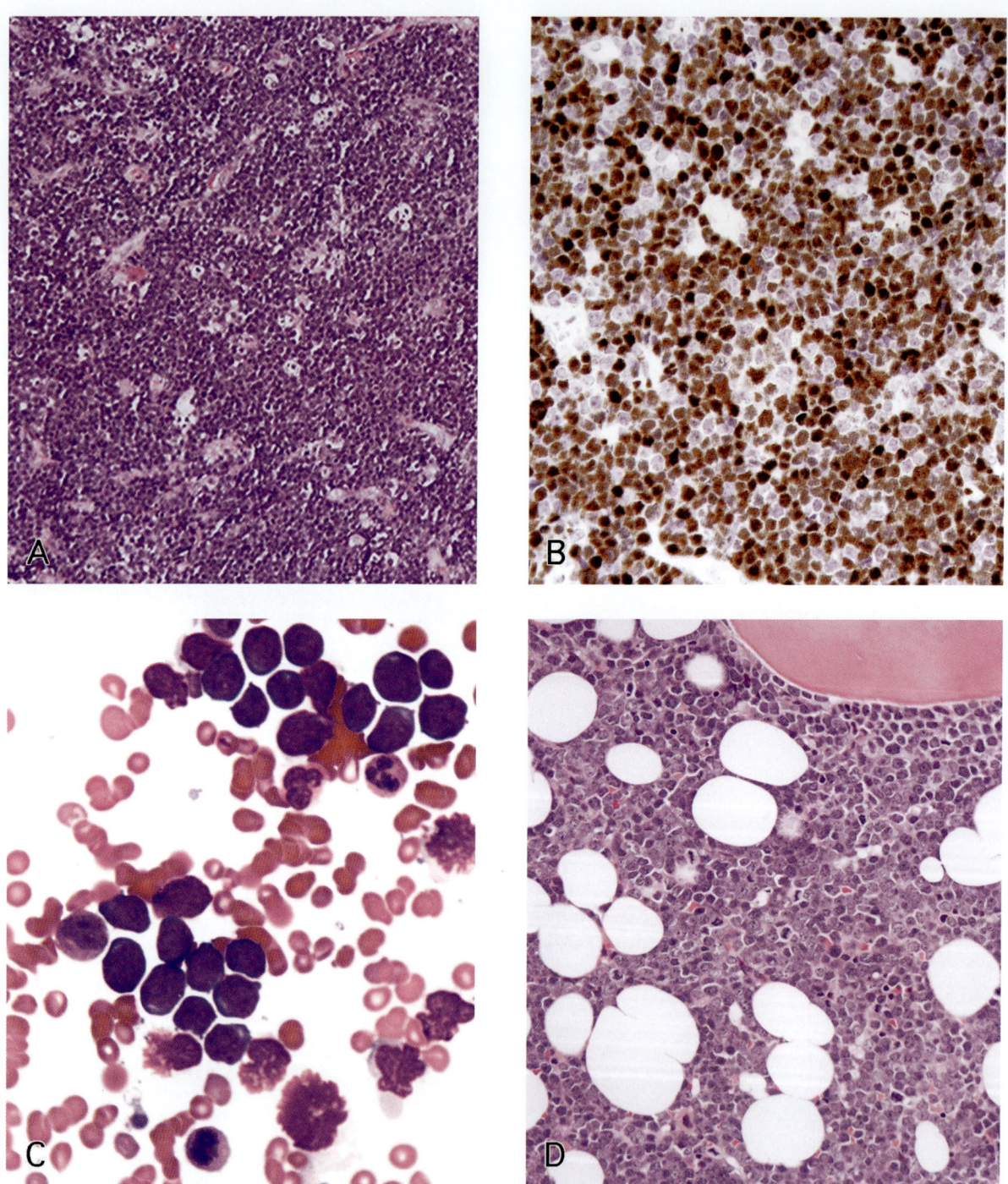

Figure 5-3

HISTOLOGIC TRANSFORMATION

A patient with grade 2 follicular lymphoma (not shown) subsequently developed extensive lymphadenopathy and bone marrow disease involved by a TdT-positive B-cell lymphoma resembling acute lymphoblastic leukemia.

A,B: A lymph node biopsy specimen was totally effaced by the neoplasm that was positive for TdT (B), PAX5 (not shown), and CD10 (not shown).

C,D: The bone marrow aspirate smear (C) shows many small blasts and the biopsy specimen (D) shows total effacement of the medullary space (A,D: H&E stain; B: immunohistochemistry with hematoxylin counterstain; C: Wright-Giemsa stain).

related. Nevertheless, the studies that have performed this comparison have shown that a clonal relationship is usually the case (14,37). Risk of histologic transformation does not seem to differ in patients treated with chemotherapy versus patients treated conservatively (watchful waiting), suggesting that histologic transformation is an inherent feature of follicular lymphoma; in other words, probably related to secondary genetic events in the neoplastic cells (14,37).

Cytogenetic or molecular studies usually identify t(14;18)(q32;q21)/*IGH-BCL2* in transformed cases of follicular lymphoma. One likely (but overly simplistic) hypothesis is that the neoplastic cells, by overexpressing BCL2 as a result of t(14;18), have a prolonged lifespan. In addition, t(14;18)-positive B-cell clones are genetically unstable and the combination of longer lifespan and genetic instability maximizes the chances of additional genetic events, which can lead eventually to histologic transformation.

Cytogenetic findings at the time of histologic transformation are usually complex and suggest that histologic transformation of low-grade follicular lymphoma can follow different pathways (14,59). Coexistent *MYC* and *BCL2* rearrangements, or less often, coexistent *MYC* and *BCL6* rearrangements occur in follicular lymphomas that undergo histologic transformation. These tumors, also known as double-hit lymphomas (or triple-hit when all three genes are rearranged), are often associated with high-grade morphologic features (26,31). A number of chromosomal abnormalities or specific gene abnormalities occur more commonly in follicular lymphomas that have undergone histologic transformation including: *CDKN2a/p16* deletion; *TP53* deletion/mutation; chromosomal deletions of 1p36.3, 6q, 10q (*FAS*), and 16p; and gains in chromosome 7 and 12q13-14/*MDM2* (7,16,49). *TNFRSF14* (located at 1p36.3), *EZH2*, and *KMT2D* (*MLL2*) are commonly mutated during the course of disease evolution or at transformation (18). Chromosome 8q24 abnormalities, *MYC* amplification, or overexpression of *MYC* via other mechanisms are involved in some types of histologic transformation (12,14,30). *BCL2* mutations and *BCL6* mutations and translocations also have been reported more frequently in histologically transformed follicular lymphomas (7,14). In recent studies using next-generation sequencing and other

Table 5-1
VARIANTS OF HISTOLOGIC TRANSFORMATION IN FOLLICULAR LYMPHOMA
Diffuse large B-cell lymphoma (centroblastic, immunoblastic, and rarely, anaplastic)
High-grade B-cell (Burkitt-like) lymphoma
Small blastoid with mature B-cell immunophenotype (TdT negative)
Lymphoblastic with immature B-cell immunophenotype (TdT positive)
Plasmablastic lymphoma
Hodgkin lymphoma-like (CD30-positive large cells)

high-throughput methods, mutations of genes in the JAK-STAT and NF-κB pathways and B-cell development genes or corresponding gene expression signatures have been associated with histologic transformation (7,8,44).

Some studies have suggested that transformation of follicular lymphoma is commonly a reflection of branched (or divergent) evolution (fig. 5-4) (49). In other words, the low-grade follicular lymphoma and the transformed tumor, usually DLBCL, share some genetic abnormalities, but other mutations are unique to either the follicular lymphoma or the DLBCL. A possible explanation is that the DLBCL arises from a progenitor (or stem) cell common to the follicular lymphoma and the DLBCL (15,37,49). Another possible explanation is that the cells of follicular lymphoma are clonally related but not genetically identical. The daughter cells in a transformed tumor, theoretically derived from a single follicular lymphoma cell, therefore show genetic differences from many of the cells in the initial follicular lymphoma. This second explanation is somewhat similar to linear evolution (discussed below).

The tumor microenvironment has a role in follicular lymphoma pathogenesis and also may be involved in histologic transformation. One study has shown that follicular lymphoma cells can develop impaired B-cell receptor signaling, perhaps related to defects in the interactions between lymphoma cells and reactive T cells, and this finding correlates with poorer patient survival (24). The ability of reactive T cells infiltrating follicular lymphoma to respond to cytokines is also suppressed, perhaps compromising

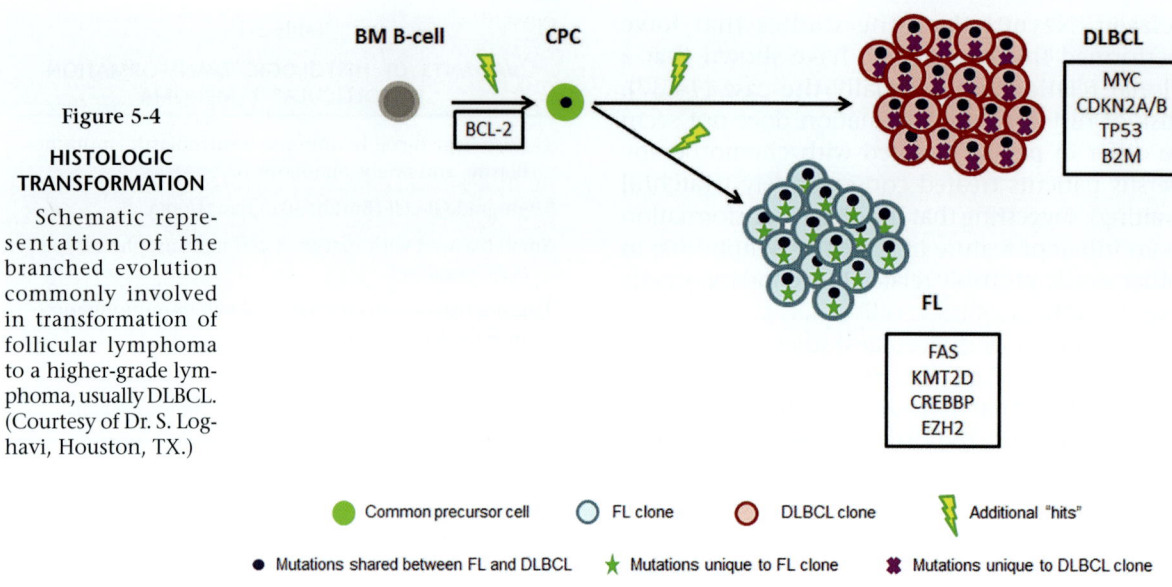

Figure 5-4

HISTOLOGIC TRANSFORMATION

Schematic representation of the branched evolution commonly involved in transformation of follicular lymphoma to a higher-grade lymphoma, usually DLBCL. (Courtesy of Dr. S. Loghavi, Houston, TX.)

the ability of these T cells to inhibit lymphoma cells (39). This is a highly active area of research and the mechanisms for the possible role of the tumor microenvironment in histologic transformation of follicular lymphoma will likely be more fully elucidated.

Prognosis

The prognosis and therapeutic options for patients with transformed follicular lymphomas have been reviewed by Casulo et al. (10). The median survival rate of follicular lymphoma patients who undergo histologic transformation is significantly decreased compared with patients with de novo DLBCL, and traditionally the prognosis of the former patients was poor (14,37). More recent studies, however, have shown that complete remission and prolonged survival may be attained in patients with histologically transformed follicular lymphoma with current therapeutic approaches (2,10,33,60). Link et al. (33) reported a median overall survival rate of 50 percent at 50 months (33). These authors also suggested that patients with early histologic transformation, defined as less than 18 months, had a worse prognosis than patients who develop histologic transformation later.

Despite these data, it remains that patients with follicular lymphoma who develop histologic transformation, most often DLBCL, have a worse prognosis than patients with de novo DLBCL. This prognostic difference is likely attributable

to the genetic complexity of the histologically transformed lymphoma. In addition, patients with transformed lymphomas often have been treated previously, acquiring chemoresistance or compromising the patient's ability to receive certain therapeutic agents or optimal doses of therapy at the time of histologic transformation.

HISTOLOGIC TRANSFORMATION OF OTHER TYPES OF LOW-GRADE LYMPHOMA

Virtually all types of clinically indolent (low-grade) lymphoma can potentially undergo histologic transformation. Discussed here are low-grade lymphomas other than follicular lymphoma that may undergo transformation to a clinically aggressive (high-grade) lymphoma.

The clinical features of patients with nodal low-grade lymphomas at the time of histologic transformation are similar to those of follicular lymphoma patients who undergo histologic transformation. There is a clear change in the pace of the patient's disease, with variable degrees of progressive lymphadenopathy, B-type symptoms, elevated serum LDH and β-2-microglobulin levels, and radiologic findings that show evidence of rapid tumor growth. When patients with nodular lymphocyte-predominant Hodgkin lymphoma transform to DLBCL they also commonly develop extranodal sites of involvement, including liver, spleen, bones, and bone marrow (28). Patients with extranodal marginal zone lymphoma may develop a change in the size of an extranodal mass. Skin manifestations dominate in patients with mycosis fungoides who undergo histologic transformation. These patients may develop new skin nodules or tumors or a sudden change in growth of preexisting skin lesions. In mycosis fungoides, patients may develop widespread lymphadenopathy or extracutaneous sites of disease at the time of histologic transformation.

Chronic Lymphocytic Leukemia/ Small Lymphocytic Lymphoma

The eponym *Richter syndrome*, named for Maurice Richter who described a single case in 1928 (52), is used to describe a patient with chronic lymphocytic leukemia/small lymphocytic lymphoma (CLL/SLL) who subsequently develops an aggressive B-cell lymphoma that most often resembles DLBCL. The frequency of Richter syndrome in CLL/SLL patients ranges from 2 to 10 percent in various studies (1a,38). In a recent Mayo Clinic report, the risk of developing an aggressive lymphoma was approximately 2 to 3 percent overall and about 0.5 percent per year after the diagnosis of CLL/SLL (48).

Clonality studies of paired CLL/SLL and high-grade B-cell lymphoma (mostly DLBCL) samples have shown that 70 to 80 percent of CLL/SLL patients who develop Richter syndrome have a clonally related high-grade B-cell lymphoma (35,38,48). The term *Richter transformation* is a more specific designation for this event, although Richter syndrome and transformation are often used interchangeably in the literature. Richter syndrome is more likely to arise in CLL/SLL patients with advanced tumor stage, high-risk genetic abnormalities such as del(11q22) and del(17p13), unmutated immunoglobulin-variable region (*IGV*) genes, and expression of ZAP70 and CD38 (35,55). The risk of Richter syndrome is also increased in patients who have been treated with nucleoside analogs and alkylating agents (48). Patients with a clonally related high-grade B-cell lymphoma have a poorer prognosis than patients with a clonally unrelated tumor (55).

Histologically, the most common morphologic manifestation of histologic transformation in CLL/SLL is DLBCL (figs. 5-5, 5-6). Approximately 80 percent of all cases of Richter syndrome in tissue biopsy specimens are histologically best classified as DLBCL (38). The neoplastic cells resemble centroblasts or immunoblasts, or a mixture of the two. Terminally, the large tumor cells can become leukemic. Other morphologic manifestations of Richter syndrome also can occur. Some cases of CLL/SLL transform to high-grade (Burkitt-like) B-cell lymphoma (38) or plasmablastic lymphoma (36,46).

At time of Richter syndrome, the mitotic and apoptotic rates are higher than would be expected in CLL/SLL and the tumor may have a starry sky pattern, coagulative necrosis, or both. In some cases, evidence of residual CLL/SLL is observed at the margins of the biopsy specimen or small CD5 positive B cells are intermixed within the DLBCL. At time of Richter transformation, CD5 and CD23 expression by the large cells is often retained, but one or both of these antigens can be absent in the DLBCL (38).

In lymph node biopsy specimens, distinguishing between CLL/SLL and "early" histologic transformation to a higher grade B-cell lymphoma can be problematic. These cases have been referred to as *accelerated phase CLL/SLL*. The percentage of prolymphocytes, the size of the proliferation centers, and the proliferation rate as assessed by mitotic count or Ki-67 percentage have been suggested as indicators of histologic transformation, but these findings need to be validated. It is helpful to compare the initial CLL/SLL specimen to a follow-up specimen in which histologic transformation is suspected. If the follow-up specimen shows obvious changes in the number of larger cells or the mitotic rate, then the diagnosis of Richter transformation (at an early stage) is likely, even if sheets of large cells are absent.

In blood smears, a prolymphocyte count of greater than 10 percent has been reported to indicate a poorer prognosis, but for an individual patient the prognostic significance of a prolymphocyte count in the range of 10 to 20 percent is uncertain. The higher the prolymphocyte percentage, the more likely that transformation to a more aggressive tumor has occurred. When patients have a high percentage of prolymphocytes (40 percent or higher), they often also have rapidly increasing leukocytosis and absolute lymphocytosis, and B-type symptoms. The term *prolymphocytoid transformation of CLL/SLL* is used to describe this occurrence (fig. 5-7),

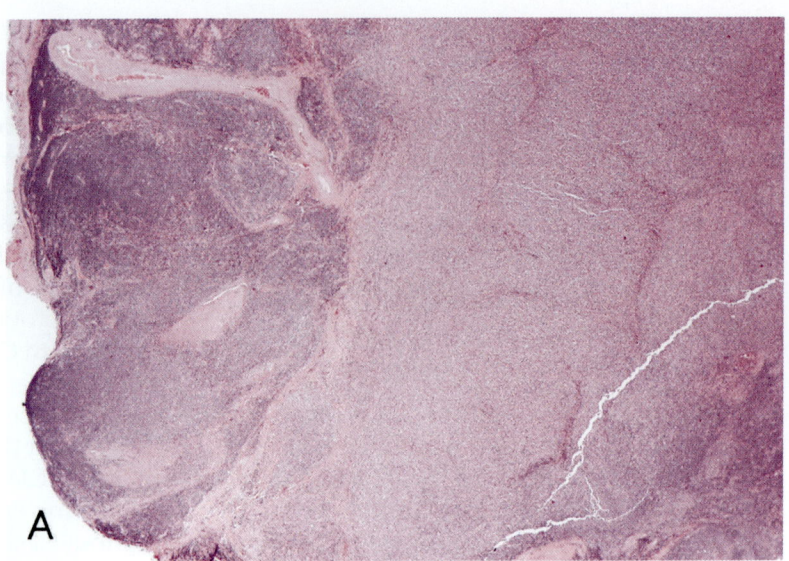

Figure 5-5

**RICHTER SYNDROME
INVOLVING TONSIL**

A: Low-magnification view shows chronic lymphocytic leukemia/small lymphocytic lymphoma (CLL/SLL) on the left and DLBCL on the right.

B: High-power magnification of CLL/SLL.

C: High-power magnification of DLBCL (A–C: H&E stain).

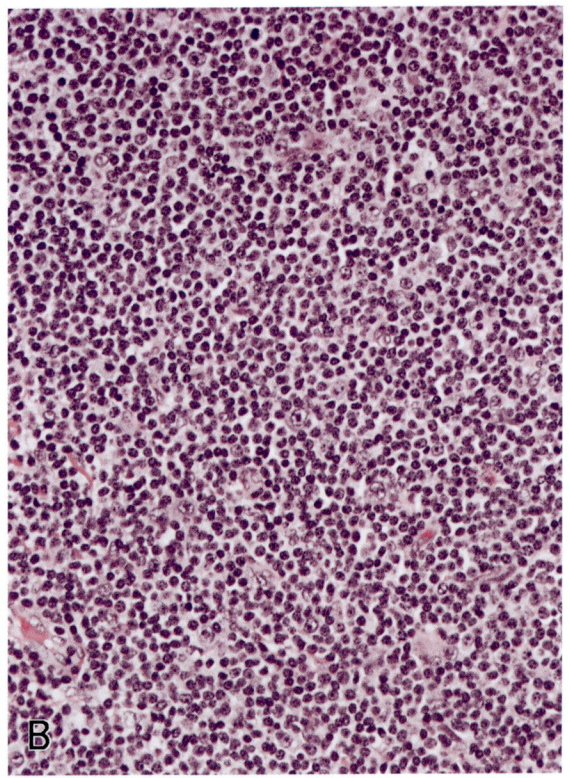

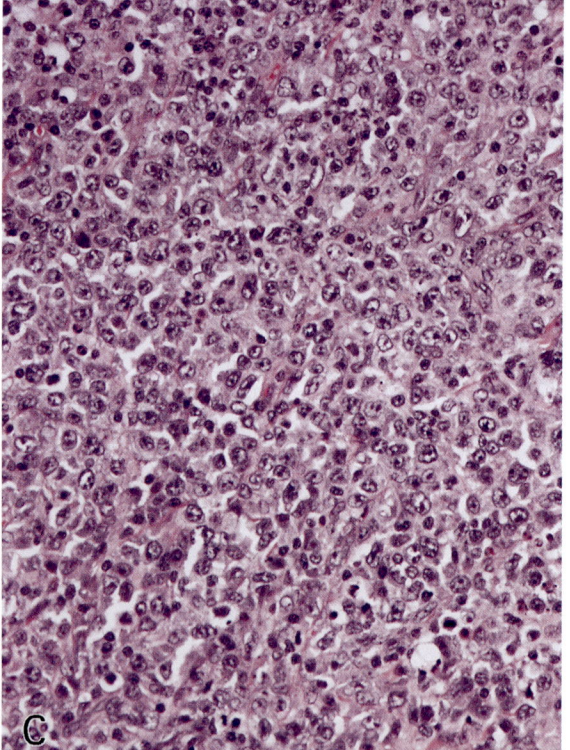

which is likely another manifestation of histologic transformation (38).

There are other uncommon histologic manifestations of Richter syndrome. Patients with CLL/SLL can develop classic Hodgkin lymphoma (6,47). In a large study of 3,887 CLL patients at the Mayo Clinic, 26 (0.7 percent) developed Hodgkin lymphoma (47). Classic Hodgkin lymphoma is characterized by Reed-Sternberg and Hodgkin cells in an appropriate inflammatory cellular background. The neoplastic cells express CD15 and CD30 and are commonly positive for Epstein-Barr virus (EBV) (figs. 5-8, 5-9) (6,38). Clonality has been assessed in very few paired CLL/SLL and classic Hodgkin lymphoma samples: Ohno et al. (43) showed shared clonality in 2 of 3 pairs

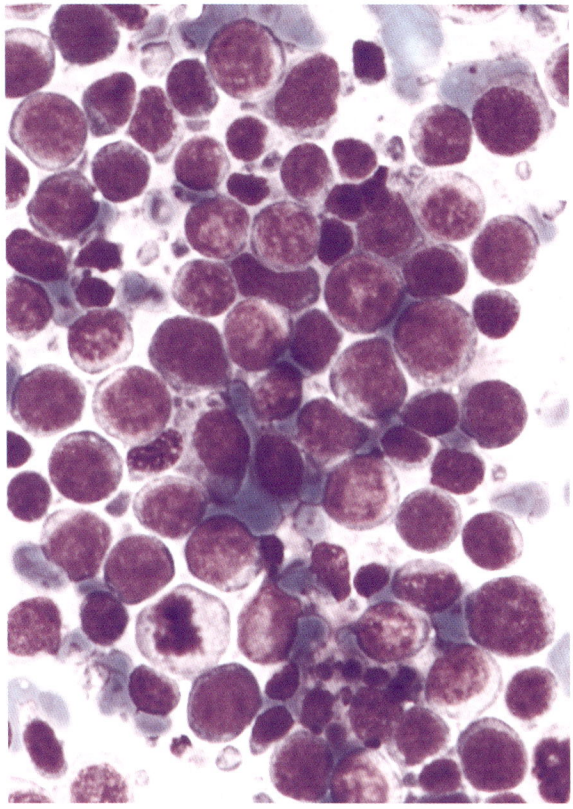

Figure 5-6

RICHTER SYNDROME

A patient with CLL who developed rapidly increasing lymphadenopathy underwent fine-needle aspiration for suspected Richter syndrome. The smear shows numerous large cells consistent with large B-cell lymphoma, supporting the clinical suspicion (Diff-Quik stain).

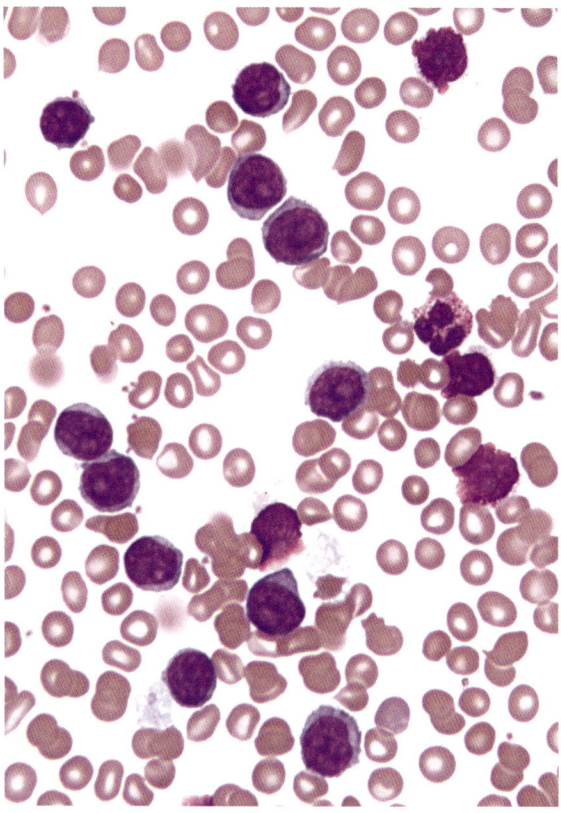

Figure 5-7

PROLYMPHOCYTOID TRANSFORMATION OF CLL

This field shows leukocytosis with many prolymphocytes charactererized by medium cell size, a moderate amount cytoplasm, and prominent central nucleoli accentuated by a prominent rim of chromatin (Wright-Giemsa stain).

assessed and Mao et al. (35) studied two pairs that were clonally unrelated.

The development of classic Hodgkin lymphoma is more likely in CLL/SLL patients with mutated *IGV* (35). Patients who develop Hodgkin lymphoma in the setting of CLL/SLL have a poorer prognosis than patients with de novo classic Hodgkin lymphoma (47). Rarely, CLL/SLL patients develop isolated Reed-Sternberg or Hodgkin cells, often EBV positive, in a background of CLL/SLL. A mixed inflammatory background (i.e., eosinophils or plasma cells) is absent. The classification of these tumors is controversial. In our opinion, these cases do not qualify as Hodgkin lymphoma, although some patients go on to develop true classic Hodgkin lymphoma.

Rare CLL/SLL patients develop peripheral T-cell lymphoma. This phenomenon also has

been included under the Richter syndrome umbrella, is not clonally related, and the prognosis is thought to be predicted by the nature of the T-cell neoplasm. The occurrence of T-cell lymphoma in this context may be related to the inherent host genetic predisposition, compromised immunosurveillance as is known to occur CLL/SLL patients, or a coincidental occurrence.

Molecular studies of cases of Richter syndrome have shown that pathogenesis is diverse. Unlike the situation in follicular lymphoma, transformation of CLL/SLL to DLBCL is thought to result from linear evolution (fig. 5-10) (17). In other words, the CLL/SLL and DLBCL share a common mutational profile, but the DLBCL cells have additional mutations thought to lead to transformation. In clonally related CLL/SLL and DLBCL, the DLBCL component has an

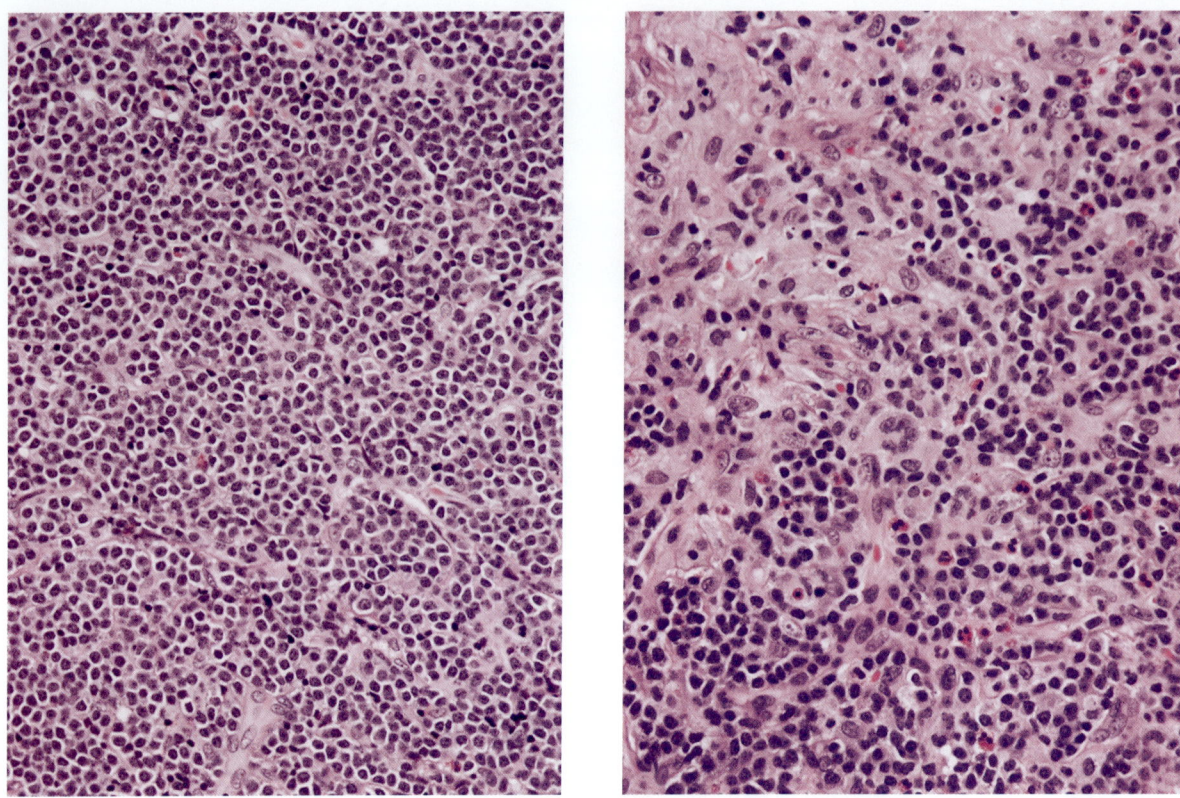

Figure 5-8

HODGKIN VARIANT OF RICHTER SYNDROME

Left: Representative field shows CLL/SLL.

Right: One year later the patient developed B symptoms and increasing lymphadenopathy. The biopsy showed features of classic Hodgkin lymphoma (left, right: H&E stain).

Figure 5-9

HODGKIN VARIANT OF RICHTER SYNDROME

A fine-needle aspirate smear shows a large Hodgkin cell in a background of reactive cells consistent with classic Hodgkin lymphoma in a patient with a history of CLL (Diff-Quik stain).

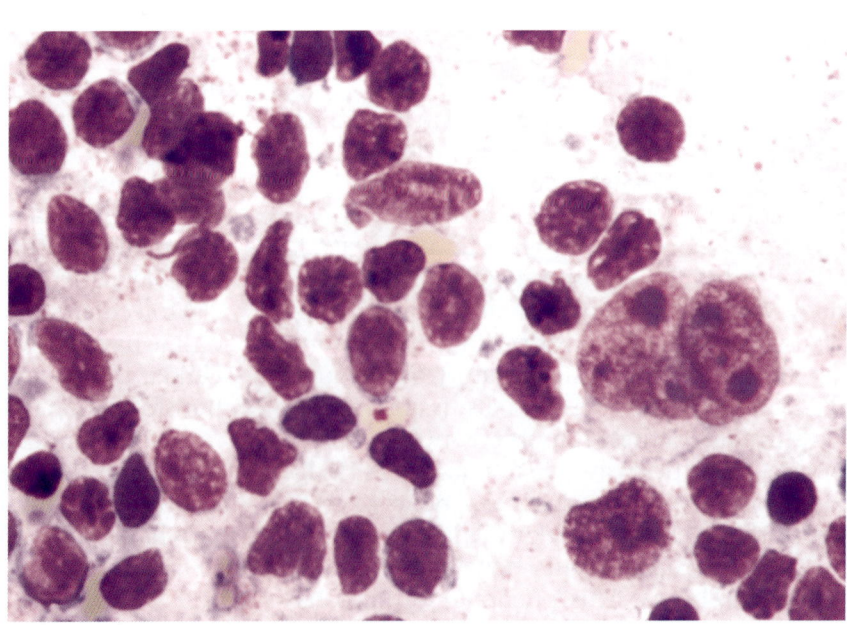

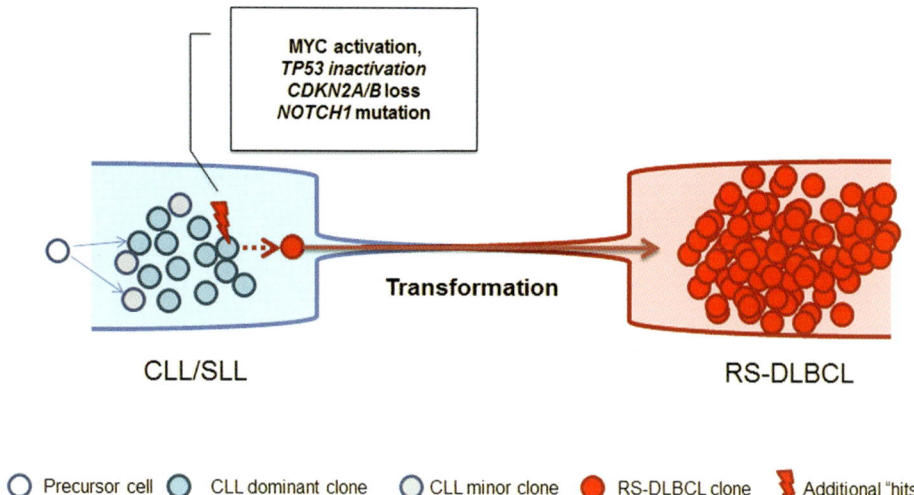

Figure 5-10

TRANSFORMATION OF CLL/SLL TO HIGHER-GRADE LYMPHOMA

Schematic representation of the linear evolution that is commonly involved in the transformation of CLL/SLL to higher-grade lymphoma, usually DLBCL (Richter syndrome). (Courtesy of Dr. S. Loghavi, Houston, TX.)

average of 22 mutations not identified in the CLL/SLL component (17). Common abnormalities include *TP53* disruption in about 60 percent of cases, *CDKN2A/p16* deletion in about 30 percent, *MYC* translocations/activation in about 30 percent, and *NOTCH1* mutations. Richter syndrome cases can be divided into three overall pathways: 1) *TP53-MYC-CDKN2a*; 2) *NOTCH1* and trisomy 12; and 3) a less distinctive pathway in about 20 percent of cases (11,17). Many cell pathways are dysregulated in Richter syndrome, especially apoptosis, proliferation, and the cell cycle. In one study that assessed methylation of various gene promoters, the transformed lymphoma cells acquired features of a stem cell phenotype (53). The overall genetic findings in cases of Richter syndrome/DLBCL differ greatly from cases of de novo DLBCL (11,17,53).

Waldenstrom Macroglobulinemia

Patients with Waldenstrom macroglobulinemia (WM) have a risk of developing high-grade lymphoma that ranges from 3.8 to 13.0 percent in different studies (9a,29,32). The risk of developing another lymphoma is higher in patients who have been treated with nucleoside analogue therapy (29). Histologically, most cases of high-grade lymphoma are classified as DLBCL (fig. 5-11). Little molecular data are available comparing the initial WM with the subsequent DLBCL, but the rare cases studied have been clonally related (56). Other rare second lymphomas in WM patients, usually clonally unrelated, include classic Hodgkin lymphoma, plasma cell-rich lesions that can resemble plasmacytoma, and peripheral T-cell lymphoma (45,54). EBV is uncommonly involved in transformation (45).

Marginal Zone Lymphoma

Patients with all types of *marginal zone lymphoma* (MZL) undergo histologic transformation to a higher-grade B-cell lymphoma; 6 to 11 percent of patients with splenic MZL undergo transformation to DLBCL (9,10a,30,63). The frequency of transformation is lower in patients with extranodal or nodal MZL, 4 and 3 percent respectively, in one study (19). The percentage of sheets of large cells with high mitotic and apoptotic rates supports the diagnosis of DLBCL in this context. As this criterion is somewhat stringent, and MZLs can have a fair number of large cells, although not in sheets, the estimates of transformation may be conservative. A small subset of patients with MZL develops classic Hodgkin lymphoma. Patients with splenic MZL can, rarely, undergo prolymphocytoid transformation resembling B-prolymphocytic leukemia (22).

Clonality studies have shown identical clones in some paired samples of MZL and DLBCL, but otherwise little molecular data are available to explain pathogenesis. Huang et al. (23) have suggested that MYC expression by 20 percent or more of extranodal MZL cells correlates with an increased frequency of transformation to DLBCL. In one study of gastric MZLs that used single nucleotide polymorphism arrays, genomic

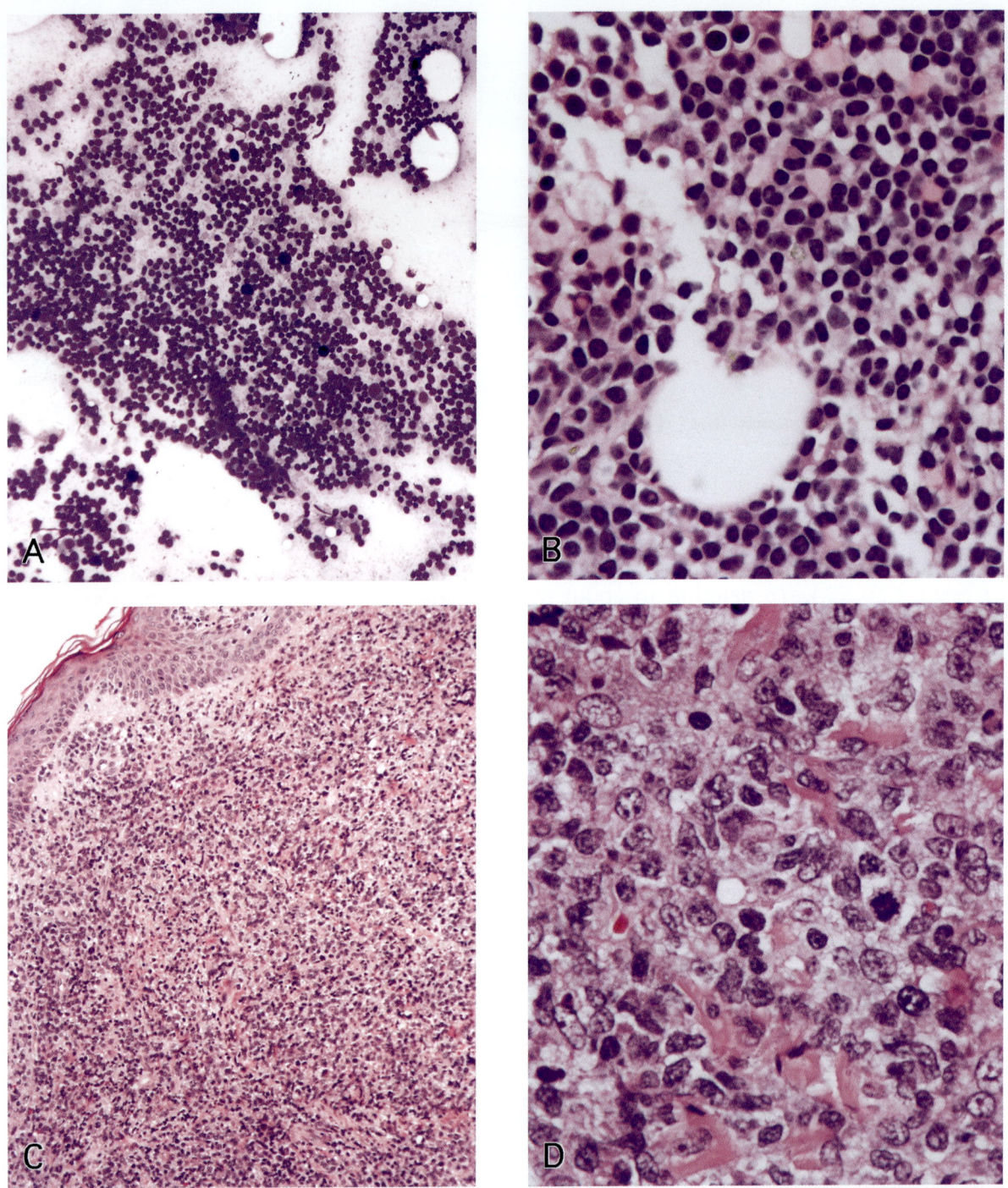

Figure 5-11

TRANSFORMATION OF WALDENSTROM MACROGLOBULINEMIA

A patient with Waldenstrom macroglobulinemia/lymphoplasmacytic lymphoma subsequently developed DLBCL involving skin.
A: The bone marrow aspirate smear shows many small lymphocytes, plasmacytoid lymphocytes, and scattered mast cells.
B: The aspirate clot specimen shows small lymphocytes and plasmacytoid lymphocytes.
C: Dermis of the skin is replaced by DLBCL.
D: High-magnification view of DLBCL. Most of the neoplastic cells have centroblastic features (A: Wright-Giemsa stain; B–D: H&E stain).

complexity was shown to be much greater in gastric DLBCL than in low-grade gastric MZL (18). This was also true in composite lymphomas composed of low-grade MZL and DLBCL in the stomach. Gains of a number of genes were identified only in the DLBCL component, including *REL, BCL11A, KRAS,* and *PTEN*, among others. The authors further suggested that multiple subclones are present in low-grade gastric MZL that compete with each other during progression to DLBCL (18). Gene mutations likely involved in histologic transformation of MZLs include *NOTCH2* and *TNFAIP3* (in spleen) and *TP16/ CDKN2A* (extranodal) (10a). EBV infection is rarely detected in cases of MZL that have undergone histologic transformation.

Mycosis Fungoides

Patients with *mycosis fungoides* (MF) have skin lesions that are characterized as patches, plaques, or tumor nodules. It is the natural history of MF for the initial manifestation of the disease to be patches, which can be followed subsequently by the onset of plaques and tumor nodules, and then spread to lymph nodes or viscera. Typically, the patch stage is prolonged, often for many years, but plaque and tumor stages persist for a shorter interval (4,25,58). Presumably, progression from patch to tumor stage is accompanied by genetic evolution to a more aggressive and unstable clone. Decreased host immunosurveillance also may play a role in MF progression.

The histologic transformation of MF to a morphologically higher-grade T-cell lymphoma occurs in a subset of patients, most often when the patient has tumor phase disease, and less often at the plaque stage. In skin, a cutoff of 25 percent large cells or micronodules of large cells is used as the criterion for histologic transformation (fig. 5-12) (13,58). Usually, histologic transformation is accompanied by increased mitotic figures; in a subset of cases, the large cells express CD30.

In lymph nodes, transformed MF can resemble peripheral T-cell lymphoma composed of a mixture of small and large cells or mostly large cells. In addition, some cases of transformed MF are characterized by Reed-Sternberg-like or Hodgkin-like cells that express CD15 and CD30, resembling classic Hodgkin lymphoma (51). There is a good correlation between histologic transformation of MF and the on-set of lymphadenopathy or involvement of other noncutaneous extranodal sites. In some patients, however, histologic transformation occurs after the patient develops lymphadenopathy. Histologic transformation often heralds a poorer prognosis, but some patients maintain a clinically indolent course, especially if they have low-stage disease (4).

Clonality studies have shown that patch stage MF lesions are usually monoclonal or oligoclonal, but about 10 percent are polyclonal (57). Large cell transformation of MF usually shares the same clone as the preceding low-grade lesion. Comparative genomic hybridization analysis of MF at the time of histologic transformation has shown a high frequency of chromosomal imbalances, with gains of chromosome regions 1p36, 7, 9q34, 17, 19, and losses of 2q36-ter, 9p21, and 17p the most common (50).

Nodular Lymphocyte-Predominant Hodgkin Lymphoma

In one large study, the cumulative risk at 10 years of patients with nodular lymphocyte-predominant Hodgkin lymphoma (NLPHL) undergoing histologic transformation to DLBCL was 12 percent (5). Patients with advanced stage disease, and particularly those with splenic involvement, have a higher risk of subsequent transformation (62). Histologically, the high-grade lymphoma resembles typical DLBCL (centroblastic or immunoblastic variant) or T-cell/histiocyte-rich large B-cell lymphoma (fig. 5-13) (28). Molecular analyses of paired samples have shown a clonal relationship in many cases (21,41,56).

Little is known about the sequence of molecular events involved in the transformation of NLPHL to DLBCL. In one gene expression profiling study that compared NLPHL with T-cell/histiocyte-rich large B-cell lymphoma, no unique gene expression patterns were identified (21). The authors suggested that the differences in the lymphoma microenvironment or patient immune status at time of diagnosis may explain the differences in the clinical behavior of the two lymphomas (21). Complicating the analysis of patients with T-cell/histiocyte-rich large B-cell lymphoma, it can be difficult to distinguish cases of true transformation from the so-called variant E pattern that closely resembles T-cell/histiocyte-rich large B-cell lymphoma (see chapter 42).

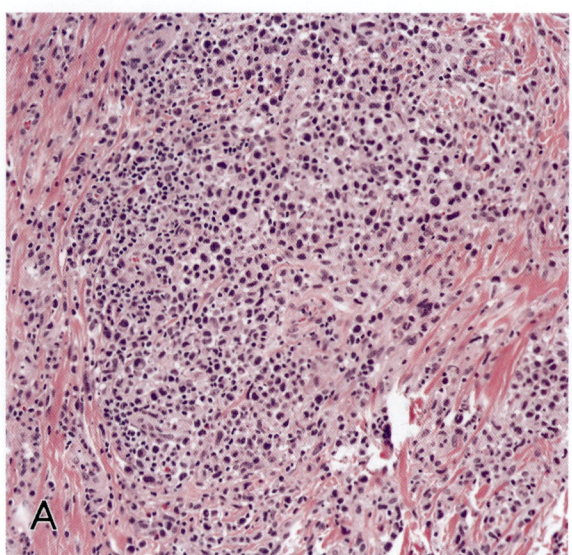

Figure 5-12

TRANSFORMATION OF MYCOSIS FUNGOIDES

A patient with longstanding mycosis fungoides developed more rapidly growing skin nodules. A skin biopsy showed an increased number of large cells that were CD30 positive, supporting large cell transformation.

A,B: Numerous large cells are in a background of small cerebriform lymphocytes within the dermis.

C: CD30 is expressed by many cells in this field. (A,B: H&E stain; C: immunohistochemistry with hematoxylin counterstain).

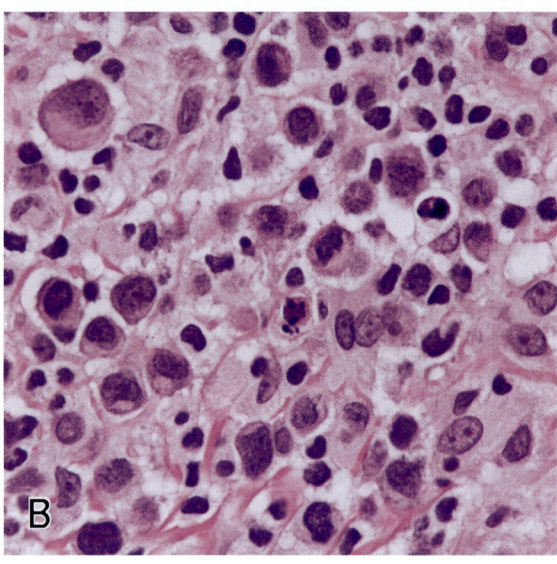

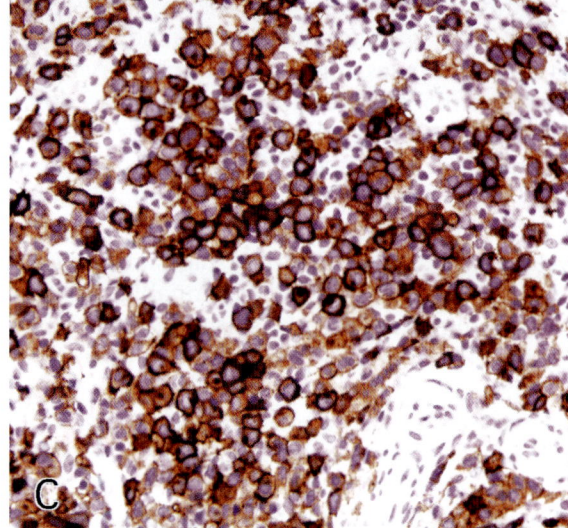

LOW-GRADE LYMPHOMA FOLLOWING HIGH-GRADE LYMPHOMA

Some patients with DLBCL, after treatment with combination chemotherapy with resultant complete remission, subsequently relapse with low-grade B-cell lymphoma. This clinical phenomenon is most common in patients with follicular lymphoma, but is also observed in patients with other types of small B-cell NHL. The term *histologic downgrading of lymphoma* has been used by some (27) for this occurrence, although the term is not in widespread use.

One hypothesis to explain histologic downgrading is that the initial DLBCL may represent histologic transformation of an underlying and undetected low-grade B-cell lymphoma. Combination chemotherapy is effective against the DLBCL component, whereas the low-grade B-cell lymphoma is often less responsive and may either persist or respond and then relapse. This explanation, however, is likely simplistic and other possible explanations need to be excluded, such as an independent, second low-grade B-cell lymphoma. Few studies have compared paired samples in patients who undergo histologic downgrading. Ogata et al. (41) reported one case in which the DLBCL and subsequent follicular lymphoma were not clonally related.

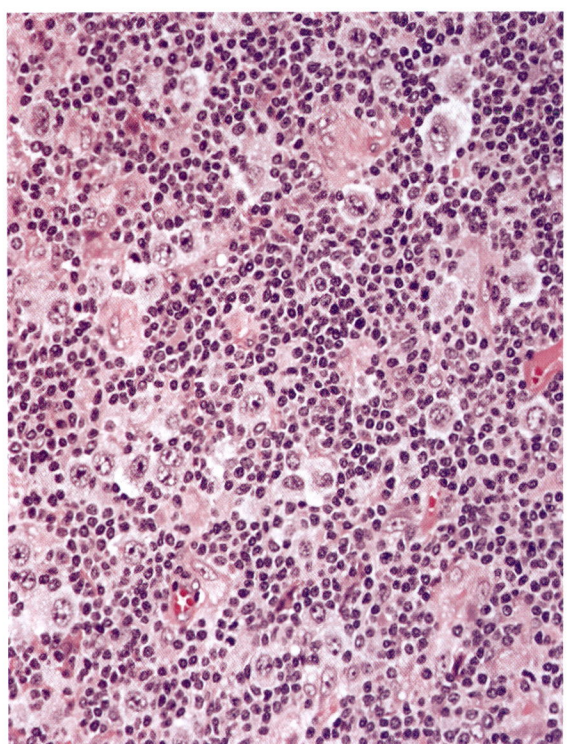 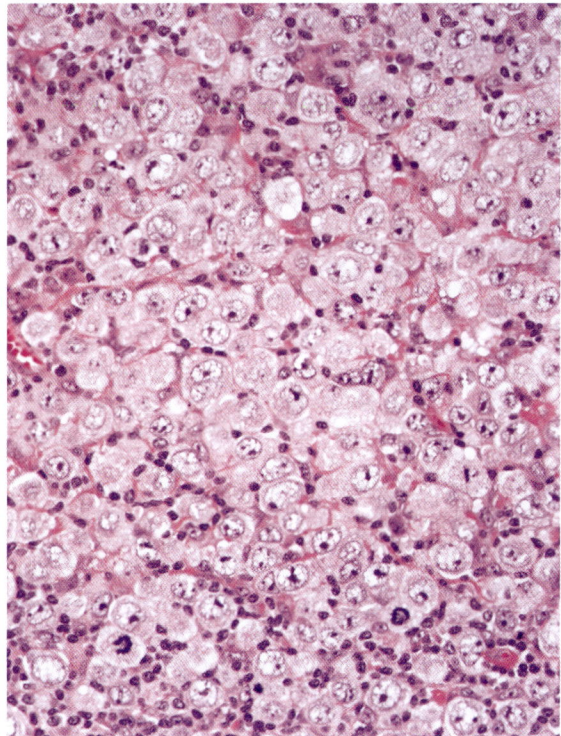

Figure 5-13

TRANSFORMATION OF LYMPHOCYTE-PREDOMINANT HODGKIN LYMPHOMA

A patient with nodular lymphocyte-predominant Hodgkin lymphoma (NLPHL) developed DLBCL 1 year later.

Left: This field shows scattered large lymphocyte-predominant cells of NLPHL in a background of small lymphocytes and fewer histiocytes.

Right: The subsequent biopsy specimen shows sheets of large cells that were CD20 positive (not shown), supporting the diagnosis of DLBCL (left, right: H&E stain).

REFERENCES

1. Alsabeh R, Medeiros LJ, Glackin C, Weiss LM. Transformation of follicular lymphoma into CD30-large cell lymphoma with anaplastic cytologic features. Am J Surg Pathol 1997;21:528-536.

1a. Agbay RL, Jain N, Loghavi S, Medeiros LJ, Khoury JD. Histologic transformation of chronic lymphocytic leukemia/small lymphocytic lymphoma. Am J Hematol 2016;91:1036-1043.

2. Ban-Hoefen M, Vanderplas A, Crosby-Thompson AL, et al. Transformed non-Hodgkin lymphoma in the rituximab era: analysis of the NCCN outcomes database. Br J Haematol 2013;163:487-495.

3. Bayerl MG, Bentley G, Bellan C, Leoncini L, Ehmann WC, Palutke M. Lacunar and Reed-Sternberg-like cells in follicular lymphomas are clonally related to the centrocytic and centroblastic cells as demonstrated by laser capture microdissection. Am J Clin Pathol 2004;122:858-864.

4. Benner MF, Jansen PM, Vermeer MH, Willemze R. Prognostic factors in transformed mycosis fungoides: a retrospective analysis of 100 cases. Blood 2012;119:1643-1649.

5. Biasoli I, Stamatoullas A, Meignin V, et al. Nodular, lymphocyte-predominant Hodgkin lymphoma: a long-term study and analysis of transformation to diffuse large B-cell lymphoma in a cohort of 164 patients from the Adult Lymphoma Study Group. Cancer 2010;116:631-639.

6. Bockorny B, Codreanu I, Dasanu CA. Hodgkin lymphoma as Richter transformation in chronic lymphocytic leukaemia: a retrospective analysis of world literature. Br J Haematol 2012;156:50-66.

7. Bouska A, McKeithan TW, Deffenbacher KE, et al. Genome-wide copy number analyses reveal genomic abnormalities involved in transformation of follicular lymphoma. Blood 2014;123:1681-1690.

8. Brodtkorb M, Lingjaered OC, Huse K, et al. Whole-genome integrative analysis reveals expression signatures predicting transformation in follicular lymphoma. Blood 2014;123:1051-1054.

9. Camacho FI, Mollejo M, Mateo MS, et al. Progression to large B-cell lymphoma in splenic marginal zone lymphoma: a description of a series of 12 cases. Am J Surg Pathol 2001;25:1268-1276.

9a. Castillo JJ, Gustine J, Meid K, Dubeau T, Hunter ZR, Treon SP. Histological transformation to diffuse large B-cell lymphoma in patients with Waldenström macroglobulinemia. Am J Hematol 2016;91:1032-1035.

10. Casulo C, Burack WR, Friedberg JW. Transformed follicular non-Hodgkin lymphoma. Blood 2015;125:40-47.

10a. Casulo C, Friedberg J. Transformation of marginal zone lymphoma (and association with other lymphomas). Best Pract Res Clin Haematol 2017;30:131-138.

11. Chigrinova E, Rinaldi A, Kwee I, et al. Two main genetic pathways lead to the transformation of chronic lymphocytic leukemia to Richter syndrome. Blood 2013;122:2673-2682.

12. Conconi A, Ponzio C, Lobetti-Bodoni C, et al. Incidence, risk factors and outcome of histological transformation in follicular lymphoma. Br J Haematol 2012;157:188-196.

13. Diamandidou E, Colome-Grimmer M, Fayad L, Duvic M, Kurzrock R. Transformation of mycosis fungoides/Sezary syndrome: clinical characteristics and prognosis. Blood 1998;92:1150-1159.

14. De Jong D, De Boer JP. Predicting transformation in follicular lymphoma. Leuk Lymphoma 2009;50:1406-1411.

15. Eide MB, Liestol K, Lingiaerde OC, et al. Genomic alterations reveal potential for potential for higher grade transformation in follicular lymphoma and confirm parallel evolution of tumor cell clones. Blood 2010;116:1489-1497.

16. Elenitoba-Johnson KSJ, Gascoyne RD, Lim MS, Chhanabai M, Jaffe ES, Raffeld M. Homozygous deletions at chromosome 9p21 involving p16 and p15 are associated with histological progression in follicle center cell lymphoma. Blood 1998;91:4677-4685.

17. Fabbri G, Khiabanian H, Holmes AB, et al. Genetic lesions associated with chronic lymphocytic leukemia transformation to Richter syndrome. J Exp Med 2013;210:2273-2288.

18. Flossbach L, Holzmann K, Mattfeldt T, et al. High-resolution genomic profiling reveals clonal evolution and compatetition in gastrointestinal marginal zone B-cell lymphoma and its large cell variant. Int J Cancer 2013;132;E116-E127.

19. Franceschetti F, Conconi A, Von Hohenstaufen KA, et al. Histological transformation in marginal zone lymphomas. Abstract # 1571. 54th American Society of Hematology Annual Meeting. Atlanta, GA; December 8-11, 2012.

20. Geyer JT, Subramaniyam S, Jiang Y, et al. Lymphoblastic transformation of follicular lymphoma: a clinicopathologic and molecular analysis of 7 patients. Hum Pathol 2015;46:260-271.

21. Hartmann S, Doring C, Jakobus C, et al. Nodular lymphocyte predominant Hodgkin lymphoma and T cell histiocyte rich large B cell lymphoma—endpoints of a spectrum of one disease? PLoS One 2013;8:e78812.

22. Hoehn D, Miranda RN, Kanagal-Shamana R, Lin P, Medeiros LJ. Splenic B-cell lymphomas with more than 55% prolymphocytes in blood: evidence for prolymphocytoid transformation. Hum Pathol 2012;43:1828-1838.

23. Huang W, Guo L, Liu H, Zheng B, Ying J, Lv N. C-MYC overexpression predicts aggressive transformation and a poor outcome in mucosa-associated lymphoid tissue lymphomas. Int J Clin Exp Pathol 2014;7:5634-5644.

24. Irish JM, Myklebust JH, Alizadeh AA, et al. B-cell signaling networks reveal a negative prognostic human lymphoma cell subset that emerges during tumor progression. Blood 2010;107:12747-12754.

25. Kamarashev J, Theler B, Dummer R, Burg G. Mycosis fungoides—analysis of the duration of disease stages in patients who progress and the time point of high-grade transformation. Int J Dermatol 2007;46:930-935.

26. Kanagal-Shamanna R, Medeiros LJ, Lu G, et al. High-grade B cell lymphoma, unclassifiable, with blastoid features: an unusual morphological subgroup associated frequently with BCL2 and/or MYC gene rearrangements and a poor prognosis. Histopathology 2012;61:945-954.

27. Kerrigan DP, Foucar K, Dressler L. High-grade non-Hodgkin lymphoma relapsing as low-grade follicular lymphoma: so-called downgraded lymphoma. Am J Hematol 1989;30:36-41.

28. Khoury JD, Jones D, Yared MA, et al. Bone marrow involvement in patients with nodular lymphocyte predominant Hodgkin lymphoma. Am J Surg Pathol 2004;28:489-495.

29. Leleu X, Soumerai J, Roccaro A, et al. Increased incidence of transformation and myelodysplasia/acute leukemia in patients with Waldenström macroglobulinemia treated with nucleoside analogs. J Clin Oncol 2009;27:250-255.

30. Lenglet J, Traullé C, Mounier N, et al. Long-term follow-up analysis of 100 patients with splenic marginal zone lymphoma treated with splenectomy as first-line treatment. Leuk Lymphoma 2014;55:1854-1860.

31. Li S, Lin P, Fayad LE, et al. B-cell lymphomas with MYC/8q24 rearrangements and IGH@ BCL2/t(14;18)(q232;q21): an aggressive disease with heterogeneous histology, germinal center B-cell immunophenotype and poor outcome. Mod Pathol 2012;25:145-156.

32. Lin P, Mansoor A, Bueso-Ramos C, Hao S, Lai R, Medeiros LJ. Diffuse large B-cell lymphoma occurring in patients with lymphoplasmacytic lymphoma/Waldenström macroglobulinemia. Clinicopathologic features of 12 cases. Am J Clin Pathol 2003;120:246-253.

33. Link BK, Maurer MJ, Nowakowski GS, et al. Rates and outcomes of follicular lymphoma transformation in the immunochemotherapy era: a report from the University of Iowa/Mayo Clinic Specialized Program of Research Excellence Molecular Epidemiology Resource. J Clin Oncol 2013;31:3272-3278.

34. Maeshima AM, Taniguchi H, Fukuhara S, et al. Clinicopathological prognostic indicators in 107 patients with diffuse large B-cell lymphoma transformed from follicular lymphoma. Cancer Sci 2013;104:952-957.

35. Mao Z, Quintanilla-Martinez L, Raffeld M, et al. IgVH mutational status and clonality analysis of Richter's transformation: diffuse large B-cell lymphoma and Hodgkin lymphoma in association with B-cell chronic lymphocytic leukemia (B-CLL) represent 2 different pathways of disease evolution. Am J Surg Pathol 2007;31:1605-1614.

36. Martinez D, Valera A, Perez NS, et al. Plasmablastic transformation of low-grade B-cell lymphomas: report of 6 cases. Am J Surg Pathol 2013;37:272-281.

37. Montoto S, Fitzgibbons J. Transformation of indolent B-cell lymphomas. J Clin Oncol 2011;29:1627-1634.

38. Muller-Hermelink HK, Montserrat E, Catovsky D, et al. Chronic lymphocytic leukemia/small lymphocytic lymphoma. In: Swerdlow SH, Campo E, Harris NL, et al., eds. WHO classification of tumours of haematopoietic and lymphoid tissues, Lyon: IARC Press; 2008:180-182.

39. Myklebust JH, Irish JM, Brody J, et al. High PD-1 expression and suppressed cytokine signaling distinguish T cells infiltrating follicular lymphoma tumors from peripheral T cells. Blood 2013;121:1367-1376.

40. Natkunam Y, Warnke RA, Zehnder JL, Jones CD, Milatovich-Cherry A, Cornbleet PJ. Blastic/blastoid transformation of follicular lymphoma: immunohistologic and molecular analyses of five cases. Am J Surg Pathol 2000;24:525-534.

41. Ogata Y, Setoguchi M, Tahara T, Takahashi M. Downgraded non-Hodgkin's lymphoma in the neck occurring as a secondary malignancy. ORL J Otorhinolaryngol Relat Spec 1998;60:295-300.

42. Ohno T, Huang JZ, Wu G, Park KH, Weisenburger DD, Chan WC. The tumor cells in nodular lymphocyte-predominant Hodgkin disease are clonally related to the large cell lymphoma occurring in the same individual. Direct demonstration by single cell analysis. Am J Clin Pathol 2001;116:506-511.

43. Ohno T, Smir BN, Weisenburger DD, Gascoyne RD, Hinrichs SD, Chan WC. Origin of the Hodgkin/Reed-Sternberg cells in chronic lymphocytic leukemia with "Hodgkin's transformation." Blood 1998;91:1757-1761.

44. Okosun J, Bödör C, Wang J, et al. Integrated genomic analysis identifies recurrent mutations and evolution patterns driving the initiation and progression of follicular lymphoma. Nat Genet 2014;46:176-181.

45. Owen RG, Bynoe AG, Varghese A, de Tute RM, Rawstron AC. Heterogeneity of histological transformation events in Waldenström's macroglobulinemia (WM) and related disorders. Clin Lymphoma Myeloma Leuk 2011;11:176-179.

46. Pan Z, Xie Q, Repertinger S, Richendollar BG, Chan WC, Huang Q. Plasmablastic transformation of low-grade CD5+ B-cell lymphoproliferative disorder with MYC gene rearrangements. Hum Pathol 2013;44:2139-2148.

47. Parikh SA, Habermann TM, Chaffee KG, et al. Hodgkin transformation of chronic lymphocytic leukemia: incidence, outcomes and comparison to de novo Hodgkin lymphoma. Am J Hematol 2015;90:334-338.

48. Parikh SA, Rabe KG, Call TG, et al. Diffuse large B-cell lymphoma (Richter syndrome) in patients with chronic lymphocytic leukaemia (CLL): a cohort study of newly diagnosed patients. Br J Haematol 2013;162:774-782.

49. Pasqualicci L, Khiabanian H, Fangazio M, et al. Genetics of follicular lymphoma transformation. Cell Rep 2014;6:130-140.

50. Prochazkova M, Chevret E, Mainhaguiet G, et al. Common chromosomal abnormalities in mycosis fungoides transformation. Genes Chromosomes Cancer 2007;46:828-838.

51. Reddi DM, Sebastian S, Wang E. Acquisition of CD30 and CD15 accompanied with simultaneous loss of all pan-T-cell antigens in a case of histological transformation of mycosis fungoides with involvement of regional lymph node: an immunophenotypic alteration resembling classical Hodgkin lymphoma. Am J Dermatopathol 2015;37:249-253.

52. Richter MN. Generalized reticular cell sarcoma of lymph nodes associated with lymphatic leukemia. Am J Pathol 1928;4:285-292.

53. Rinaldi A, Mensah AA, Kwee I, et al. Promoter methylation patterns in Richter syndrome affect stem-cell maintenance and cell cycle regulation and differ from de novo diffuse large B-cell lymphoma. Br J Haematol 2013;163:194-204.

54. Rosales CM, Lin P, Mansoor A, Bueso-Ramos C, Medeiros LJ. Lymphoplasmacytic lymphoma/ Waldenstrom macroglobulinemia. Am J Clin Pathol 2001;116:34-40.

55. Rossi D, Spina V, Deambrogi C, et al. The genetics of Richter syndrome reveals disease heterogeneity and predicts survival after transformation. Blood 2011;117:3391-3401.

56. Shiseki M, Masuda A, Watanabe N, et al. Development of diffuse large B-cell lymphoma in a patient with Waldenström's macroglobulinemia/ lymphoplasmacytic lymphoma: clonal identity between two B-cell neoplasms. Hematol Rep 2011;3:e10.

56a. Swerdlow SH, Campo E, Pileri SA, et al. The 2016 revision of the World Health Organization classification of lymphoid neoplasms. Blood 2016;127:2375-2390.

57. Vega F, Luthra R, Medeiros LJ, et al. Clonal heterogeneity in mycosis fungoides and its relationship to clinical course. Blood 2002;100:3369-3373.

58. Vergier B, de Muret A, Beylot-Barry M, et al. Transformation of mycosis fungoides: clinicopathological and prognostic features of 45 cases. French Study Group of Cutaneous Lymphomas. Blood 2000; 95:2212-2218.

59. Viardot A, Barth TF, Moller P, Döhner H, Bentz M. Cytogenetic evolution of follicular lymphoma. Semin Cancer Biol 2003;13:183-190.

60. Wagner-Johnston ND, Link BK, Byrtek M, et al. Outcomes of transformed follicular lymphoma in the modern era: a report from the National LymphoCare Study (NLCS). Blood 2015;126:851-857.

61. Wickert RS. Weisenburger DD, Tierens A, Greiner TC, Chan WC. Clonal relationship between lymphocytic predominance Hodgkin's disease and concurrent or subsequent large-cell lymphoma of B lineage. Blood 1995;86:2312-2320.

62. Xing KH, Connors JM, Lai A, et al. Advanced-stage nodular lymphocyte predominant Hodgkin lymphoma compared with classical Hodgkin lymphoma: a matched pair outcome analysis. Blood 2014;123:3567-3573.

63. Xing KH, Kahlon A, Skinnider BF, et al. Outcomes in splenic marginal zone lymphoma: analysis of 107 patients treated in British Columbia. Br J Haematol 2015;169:520-527.

6 IN SITU NEOPLASIA/ EARLY LESIONS

The term in situ in the context of neoplasia is most often used to describe a lesion that has neoplastic cytologic features, but is confined to the tissue compartment where the lesion has arisen. This concept was initially designed for the study of uterine cervical carcinoma in which in situ carcinoma is confined to the epithelium and does not invade the underlying basal membrane. Unlike epithelial cells, lymphocytes typically do not invade through a basement membrane, but rather disseminate via lymphatic and vascular channels. Use of the term in situ neoplasia is therefore scientifically problematic because many of these early lesions are likely systemic at their onset. In this chapter, *in situ neoplasia* is defined as a lesion in which the neoplastic cells occupy the tissue compartment where the normal cell equivalent resides, without any evidence of invasion into other tissue compartments (5).

It is difficult (and in some cases impossible) to recognize in situ neoplasia by routine histologic examination. Using immunohistochemistry and antibodies such as BCL2 or cyclin D1, however, such lesions are recognizable. In situ neoplasia is most often detected incidentally in patients with no other sites of lymphoma. Some patients with an in situ lesion, however, have had overt (symptomatic) lymphoma in the past, may have overt lymphoma at another anatomic site at the time the in situ lesion is diagnosed (5,20), or may develop overt lymphoma in the future (15,20).

For patients who have an isolated in situ lymphoid neoplasm the rate of progression to overt lymphoma is low, less than 10 percent (15). Therefore, an important consideration for these patients is the risk of overtreatment. As many patients with in situ neoplasia do not progress clinically, it seems unnecessary to treat a patient who has an isolated in situ lesion because the potential harm from therapy outweighs the potential benefits (5).

The pathogenesis of in situ lymphoid neoplasia is currently poorly understood. For in situ follicular neoplasia (ISFN), which is the best studied, it seems unlikely that the lesion arises at the anatomic site biopsied. Instead, t(14;18) (q32;q21)/*IGH-BCL2*-positive naïve B cells arise in the bone marrow and are thought to migrate via the bloodstream to germinal centers of reactive lymphoid tissues (fig. 6-1) (24). Typically, these t(14;18)-positive B cells are present at low levels in the blood, from 0.001 to 1 x 10^9/L, and their detection correlates with age, being absent in children and present in 50 to 60 percent of adults (17). It is hypothesized that BCL2 overexpression, by prolonging B-cell survival, predisposes B cells to additional genetic "hits," which are required for overt lymphoma to develop. These additional "hits" are thought to occur in the germinal center, making this microenvironment essential in follicular lymphoma pathogenesis. The circulating t(14;18)/*IGH-BCL2*-positive B cells enter germinal centers of reactive lymphoid tissues where they undergo somatic mutation of their immunoglobulin variable region genes as well as isotype switching (5,8). Mistakes in these processes result in mutations that contribute to the neoplastic phenotype, if they confer a selective growth advantage. At this point, these B cells express CD27, a marker of memory B cells, and can emerge from germinal centers, disseminate via the peripheral blood, and seed germinal centers at other anatomic sites (8,28). Overall, the iterative process of t(14;18)-positive B cells entering and exiting germinal centers increases the likelihood that the cells will undergo additional mutations, thereby maximizing the chances of the developing follicular lymphoma (8,24).

Some experts have suggested that ISFN is a benign or preneoplastic lesion. Others, based on genetic data, have suggested that ISFN is clearly neoplastic, but these lesions represent an early stage of disease evolution. In part, these differences are

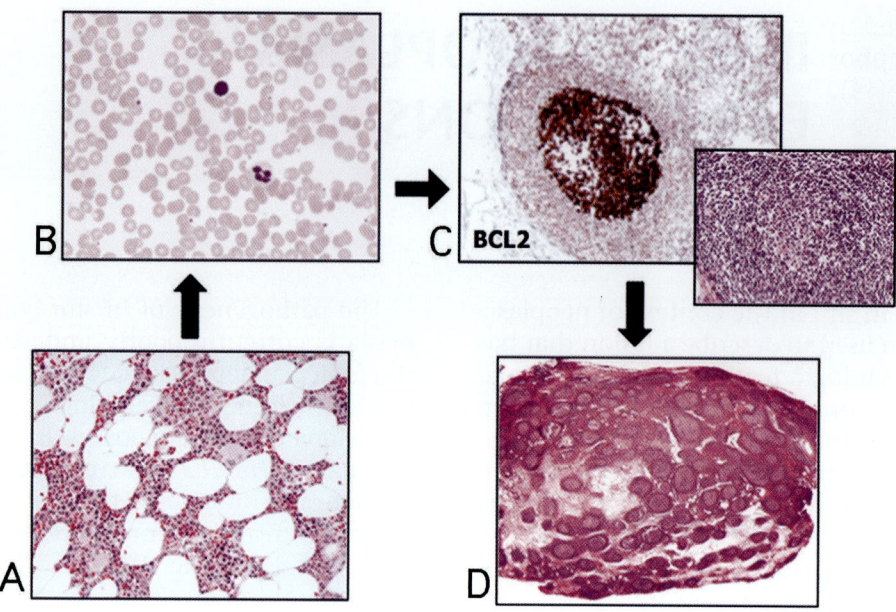

Figure 6-1

PATHOGENESIS OF FOLLICULAR LYMPHOMA

The potential sequence of events is as follows:

A: t(14;18)(q32;q21) arises as a mistake during physiologic immunoglobulin gene rearrangement in B cells in the bone marrow. The translocation, by itself, is insufficient to cause follicular lymphoma.

B: B cells with t(14;18)(q32;q21) enter and circulate in the peripheral blood. These cells are rare, representing 1×10^6/L to 1×10^9/L B cells, and resemble memory B cells (CD27 positive) suggesting that they have traversed germinal centers of reactive lymphoid tissue.

C: In a germinal center of a lymph node, additional genetic mutations occur, resulting in the development of in situ follicular neoplasia. The neoplasm overexpresses BCL2 and is confined to the germinal center at this stage. Mutations acquired at this stage may be the result of the somatic mutations that usually occur in the germinal center and therefore the microenvironment is essential to pathogenesis.

D: Additional genetic events result in fully developed follicular lymphoma.

semantic in nature. Regardless of whether ISFN is benign/preneoplastic or neoplastic, the data suggest that these lesions are less genetically complex than their fully developed lymphoma counterparts (18,26). Therefore, additional genetic "hits" are required for ISFN to progress to a clinically significant neoplasm that requires therapy, and progression is a low frequency event. Nevertheless, some patients with ISFN also have coexistent systemic lymphoma elsewhere. This occurrence suggests another possibility: that a fully developed lymphoma can disseminate and resemble an in situ lesion in a biopsy specimen, especially in a small needle biopsy specimen (16). These two possible explanations for an in situ lesion are probably not mutually exclusive.

As stated, the concept of in situ neoplasia is best developed for follicular lymphoma, but has been described as well for mantle cell lymphoma (MCL) and recently for nodular lymphocyte-predominant Hodgkin lymphoma. Although monoclonal B-cell lymphocytosis (MBL) is not an in situ neoplasm per se, the issues for patients with MBL are somewhat similar to those for patients with in situ neoplasia. Furthermore, a tissue equivalent of MBL has been proposed.

IN SITU FOLLICULAR NEOPLASIA

General Features. *In situ follicular neoplasia* is the currently preferred term in the World Health Organization (WHO) classification (27a). Others have used the terms *follicular lymphoma in situ, intrafollicular neoplasia, follicular lymphoma-like B cells of uncertain significance,* and *incipient follicular lymphoma* for these lesions (5,15). The frequency of ISFN in lymph nodes is low. In a study of 1,294 lymph nodes in patients who underwent excision for a variety of cancers and did not have evidence of systemic follicular lymphoma, ISFN was detected in 29 (2.3 percent) (14). As this frequency is higher than the frequency of follicular lymphoma in the general population, it is inferred that ISFN is a preneoplastic or early lesion in the pathogenesis of follicular lymphoma.

Microscopic Findings. Morphologically, ISFN is difficult to recognize in routine hematoxylin and eosin (H&E)-stained tissue sections. Jegalian et al. (15) proposed rigorous criteria for ISFN (Table 6-1). The lymph node architecture is normal, with widely scattered follicles that are of normal size and inconspicuous (fig. 6-2). Typically, more than one germinal center is involved by ISFN in a biopsy specimen (5,15,20). These germinal centers have a sharp peripheral margin and are composed almost exclusively of centrocytes. The presence of highly monotonous germinal centers composed of centrocytes with few tingible body macrophages is a morphologic clue to the diagnosis of ISFN, but these changes are often subtle. In some patients, ISFN is associated with systemic follicular lymphoma in the same biopsy specimen (fig. 6-3), or in biopsy specimens derived from other anatomic sites.

Immunohistochemical Findings. Immunohistochemical analysis shows that the germinal center cells in affected follicles are strongly positive for BCL2 and CD10 (fig. 6-2). Typically, the BCL2 expression level by the cells of ISFN is brighter than the expression level by mantle zone cells surrounding the germinal center. The cells of ISFN also express pan-B-cell antigens (e.g., CD19, CD20, CD22, PAX5) and other germinal center B-cell markers such as BCL6 and LMO2, and are negative for IgD and T-cell markers (5,15).

Molecular Genetic Findings. Cytogenetic and molecular studies have shown that the cells of ISFN carry t(14;18)(q32;q21) and monoclonal immunoglobulin gene rearrangements (5,15,16). Array comparative genomic hybridization and other methods performed on ISFN lesions have confirmed that the cells carry the t(14;18), but have relatively few secondary genetic abnormalities in contrast with fully developed follicular lymphoma (3,18,26). *EZH2* mutations have been detected in ISFN, suggesting that this is another early lesion in follicular lymphoma pathogenesis.

Table 6-1

FEATURES OF IN SITU FOLLICULAR NEOPLASIA

Intact architecture

Normal follicle size

Involved follicles are widely scattered

Normal mantle zones with sharp edge to germinal centers

Strong expression of BCL2 and CD10

Almost pure centrocytes

Atypical cells confined to germinal center

In patients with both ISFN and systemic (fully developed) follicular lymphoma, the ISFN cells have been shown to be clonally related to the systemic follicular lymphoma cells. In most cases tested, the overt follicular lymphoma is characterized by a greater number of genomic lesions including del(1p36) and gains of chromosomes 7p and 12q (18,26), supporting the concept that in most cases ISFN is an early step in follicular lymphoma pathogenesis. Some ISFN lesions have been more genetically complex, however, similar to the systemic lymphoma, suggesting seeding of the germinal center by systemic lymphoma (16,26).

ISFN in Patients with, or Who Subsequently Develop, Overt Lymphoma. Some patients with ISFN also have evidence of overt lymphoma. In the study by Jegalian et al. (15), 6 of 34 (17.6 percent) patients with ISFN had overt lymphoma previously or concurrently and 1 of 21 (4.8 percent) patients with negative staging at diagnosis of ISFN subsequently developed lymphoma. In addition, some patients with ISFN subsequently develop a histologically discordant type of lymphoma. These cases suggest that ISFN may be a marker of genetic instability or a marker of genetic predisposition to lymphoma. Lymphomas reported in association with ISFN include classic Hodgkin lymphoma, splenic marginal zone lymphoma, chronic lymphocytic leukemia/small lymphocytic lymphoma (CLL/SLL) (fig. 6-4), lymphoplasmacytic lymphoma, and rarely, T-cell lymphomas (5,6,20).

Treatment and Prognosis. The data suggest that ISFN is a neoplastic process representing an early step in follicular lymphoma pathogenesis that is unlikely to affect patient survival if it is an isolated finding. Nevertheless, some

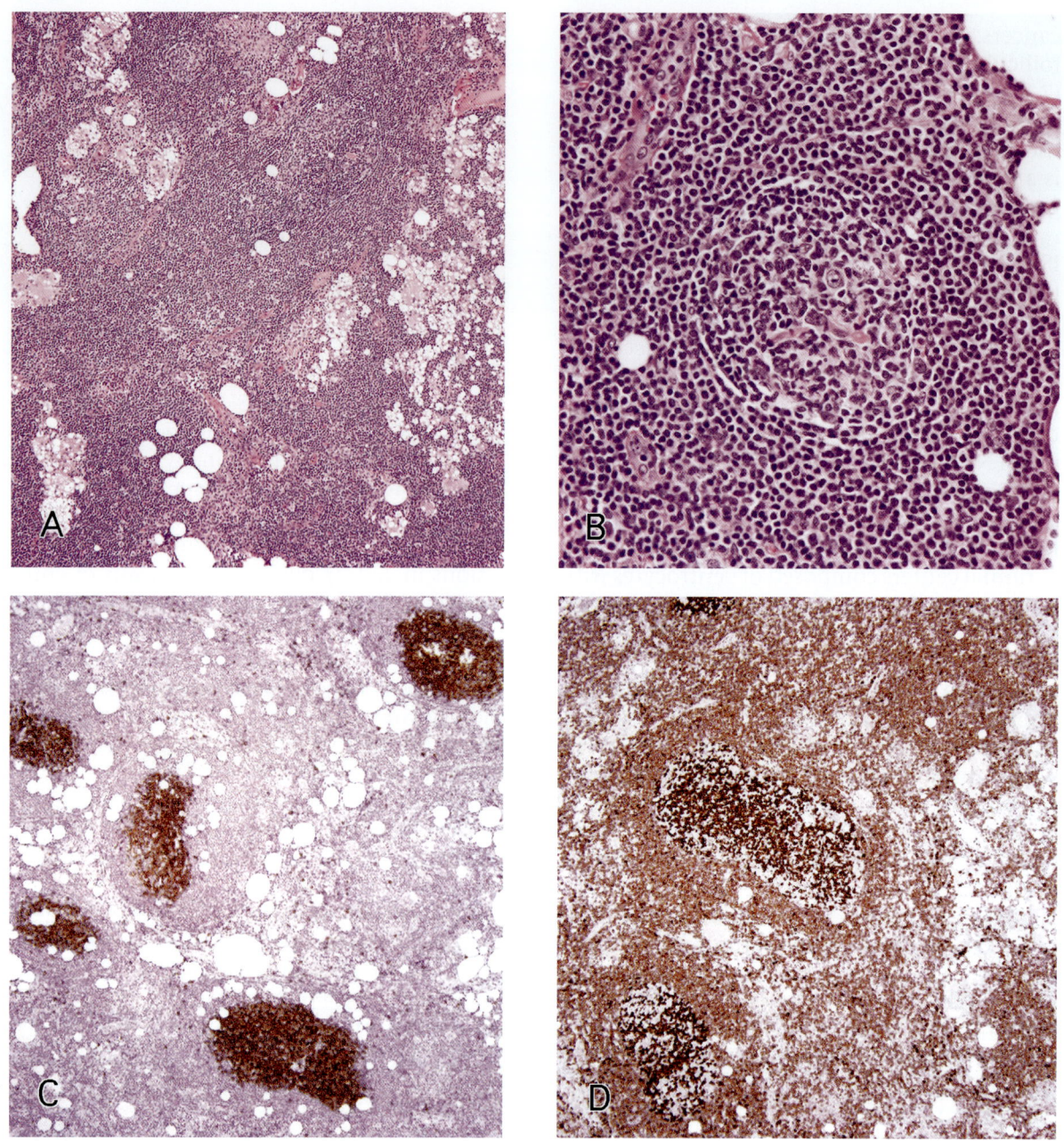

Figure 6-2

IN SITU FOLLICULAR NEOPLASIA (ISFN) INVOLVING ABDOMINAL LYMPH NODE

A: At low magnification, scattered, inconspicuous lymphoid follicles are present.

B: One follicle in which the germinal center is composed mostly of centrocytes.

C,D: Scattered germinal centers are brightly positive for CD10 (C) and BCL2 (D). Many lipogranulomas are also present in this biopsy specimen (A,B: hematoxylin and eosin [H&E] stain; C,D: immunohistochemistry with hematoxylin counterstain).

patients with ISFN have overt lymphoma at other anatomic sites and a few will develop overt follicular lymphoma subsequently. Therefore, the management of a patient with ISFN requires clinical judgment. Staging studies seem to be indicated, but if ISFN is the only disease discovered, overtreatment is to be avoided and watchful waiting is adequate.

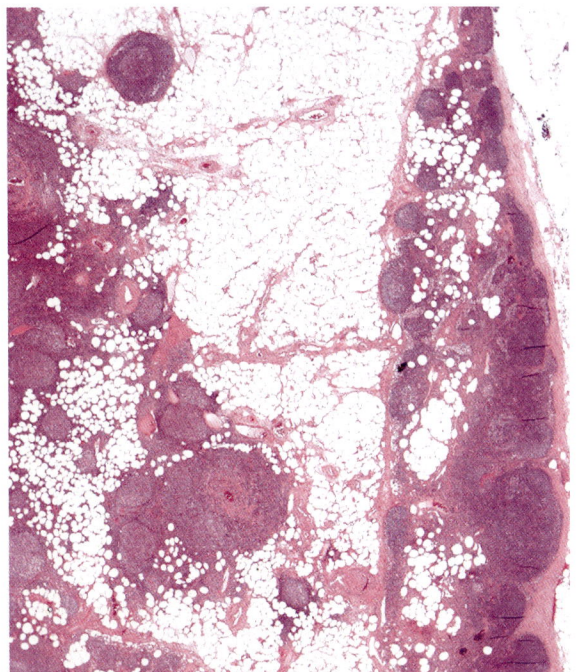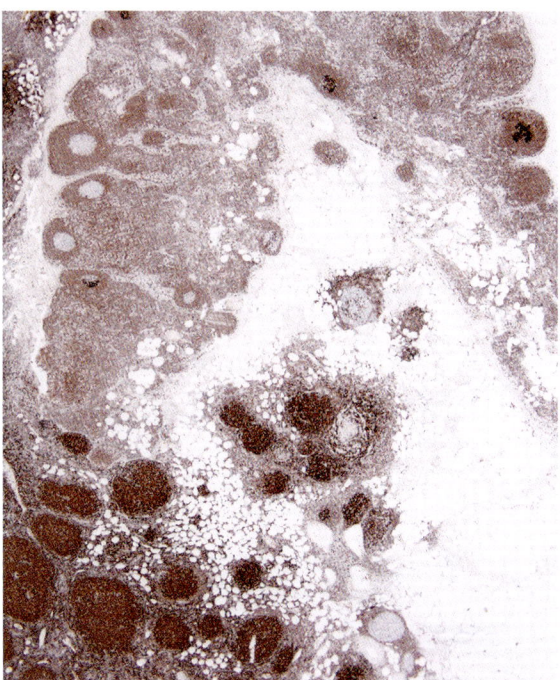

Figure 6-3

ISFN ASSOCIATED WITH FULLY DEVELOPED FOLLICULAR LYMPHOMA

Left: Large follicles of fully developed follicular lymphoma (left of field) are present. ISFN is also present in lymph node parenchyma but cannot be appreciated in this field (H&E stain).

Right: BCL2 highlights fully developed follicular lymphoma and ISFN (top of field) in lymph node parenchyma. Cases such as this raise the possibility that the fully developed lymphoma can seed germinal centers of preexistent follicles and mimic ISFN. Alternatively, the ISFN and fully developed lymphoma are at different stages of evolution (immunohistochemistry with hematoxylin counterstain).

IN SITU MANTLE CELL NEOPLASIA

General Features. The current WHO classification prefers the term *in situ mantle cell neoplasia* (ISMCN). The terms *mantle cell lymphoma in situ* and *mantle cell lymphoma-like cells of uncertain significance* also have been suggested for these lesions (7). In one large study of reactive lymph nodes by Adam et al. (1), not a single case of ISMCN was detected. In patients who developed overt MCL, however, up to one third had evidence of ISMCN in biopsy specimens obtained prior to the development of overt disease (1). Similar to the scenarios described above for patients with ISFN, patients can have a history of overt MCL, or can have histologically discordant types of lymphoma at the time of ISMCN diagnosis. Other lymphoma types reported in patients with ISMCN include follicular lymphoma, CLL/SLL, marginal zone lymphoma, and classic Hodgkin lymphoma (7,29).

Microscopic Findings. Morphologically, ISMCN is defined as a lymph node or other lymphoid organ with normal architecture and reactive follicles surrounded by inconspicuous mantle zones that often appear reactive or normal in routine H&E-stained tissue sections (fig. 6-5).

Immunohistochemical Findings. Immunohistochemical analysis is required for the recognition of ISMCN (figs. 6-5, 6-6). The cells of ISMCN overexpress cyclin D1 and are confined to the mantle zones of follicles. Although difficult to assess when minimal, the cells are usually positive for CD5 and approximately half of cases are positive for SOX11.

Molecular Genetic Findings. Cytogenetic and molecular studies have shown the presence of t(11;14)(q13;q32) and monoclonal immunoglobulin gene rearrangements in patients with ISMCN. Few other molecular analyses have been performed at this time.

Figure 6-4

ISFN ASSOCIATED WITH CHRONIC LYMPHOCYTIC LEUKEMIA/SMALL LYMPHOCYTIC LYMPHOMA (CLL/SLL)

A: Low-magnification view of a lymph node replaced by CLL/SLL. Many proliferation centers are seen in the field. Scattered small germinal centers are also present but are difficult to appreciate at this magnification (A,B: H&E stain).

B: High-power magnification of ISFN surrounded by CLL/SLL.

C: BCL2 is expressed by both the CLL/SLL and the ISFN (bright) (immunohistochemistry with hematoxylin counterstain).

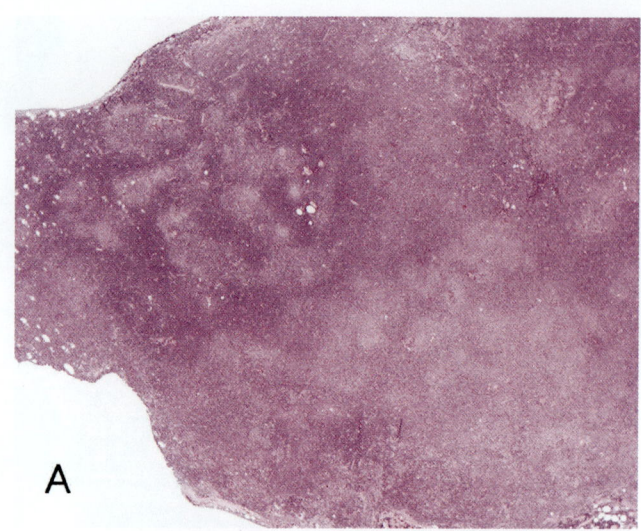

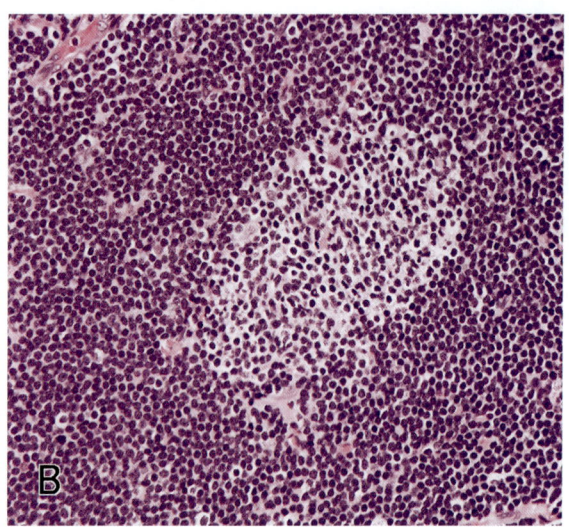

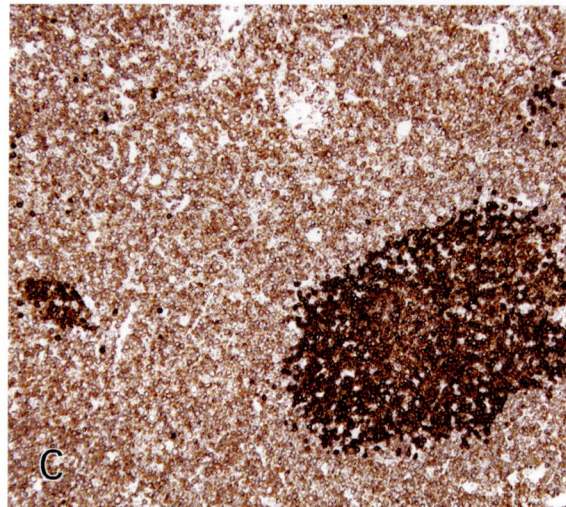

Treatment and Prognosis. Currently, there are no consensus recommendations for managing patients with ISMCN. The issue of avoiding overtreatment is even more important for patients with ISMCN than those with ISFN because aggressive chemotherapy regimens are commonly used to treat patients with overt MCL. In one study (7), only 1 of 12 (8.3 percent) patients with ISMCN and no other sites of disease subsequently developed overt MCL. This study suggested conservative management, although the follow-up time of this study was short. SOX11 expression was suggested to correlate with risk of progression in one study (7). Clinical judgment is essential in patient management to avoid overtreatment of patients with ISMCN. A diagnosis of ISMCN is an indication for rigorous clinical staging and careful follow-up.

NODULAR LYMPHOCYTE-PREDOMINANT HODGKIN LYMPHOMA IN SITU

Recently, Carbone et al. (4) proposed the concept of *nodular lymphocyte-predominant Hodgkin lymphoma (NLPHL) in situ*. This concept has yet to be fully vetted and is not included in the most recent version of the WHO classification of lymphomas.

Morphologically, NLPHL in situ is a nodule composed of one or more reactive germinal centers and scattered neoplastic lymphocyte-predominant (LP) cells in a background of small, reactive mantle zone lymphocytes (fig. 6-7). The LP cells are confined within the nodule and do

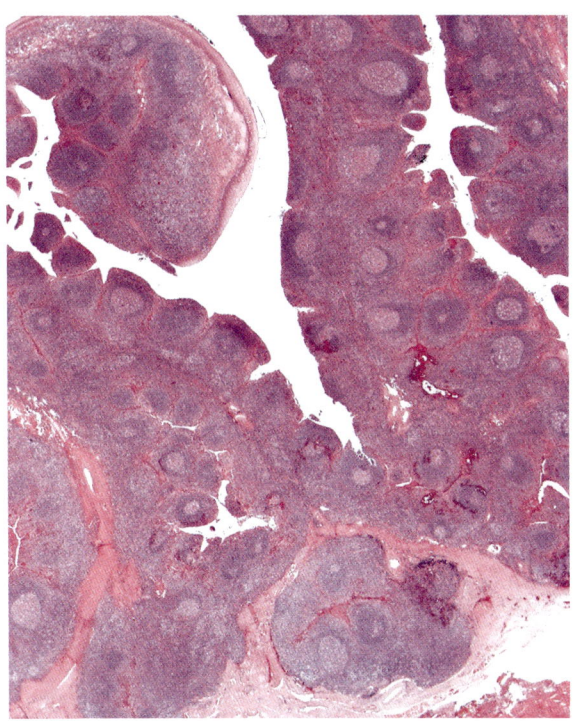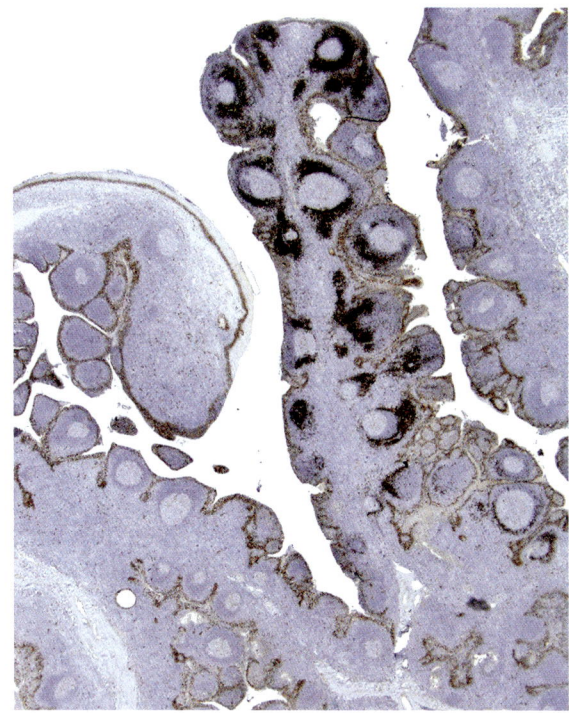

Figure 6-5

IN SITU MANTLE CELL NEOPLASIA INVOLVING A TONSIL

This previously healthy woman underwent bilateral tonsillectomy. Both tonsils were involved and staging studies performed subsequently showed no evidence of systemic lymphoma.

Left: At low magnification, the tonsil shows only reactive follicular hyperplasia (H&E stain).

Right: The anti-cyclin D1 antibody highlights many brightly positive cells in the mantle zones, supporting a diagnosis of ISMCN. These cells were also positive for SOX11 (not shown) (immunohistochemistry with hematoxylin counterstain).

not extend (or invade) into the perinodular tissue. Immunohistochemical analysis shows that the LP cells are B cells with a germinal center immunophenotype positive for CD20 and BCL6. The LP cells are surrounded by rosettes of T cells (CD3 positive) that are positive for PD1 (CD279). The LP cells appear to be entrapped by follicular dendritic cells (CD21 positive, CD23 positive, or both). The mantle zone small B cells are positive for IgD and a swath of IgD-positive cells is present at the periphery of the nodules between more central LP cells and the perinodular tissue.

There is little information regarding clinical outcome for patients who have NLPHL in situ. This pattern is commonly associated with fully developed NLPHL, complicating assessment of the clinical impact of the in situ lesion. Carbone (4) followed four patients with NLPHL in situ treated by surgical excision who had long-term, benign clinical follow-up.

MONOCLONAL B-CELL LYMPHOCYTOSIS

Monoclonal B-cell lymphocytosis (MBL) is defined as a monotypic B-cell expansion in peripheral blood that is less than $5 \times 10^9/L$ in a patient with no evidence of other signs or symptoms of a lymphoproliferative disorder (e.g., lymphadenopathy or related autoimmune disease) (13,19,23). An older name of MBL was *monoclonal B-cell lymphocytosis of uncertain significance*. This term is rarely used currently, in part to reduce patient anxiety, nevertheless, this term highlights that the model for MBL is a monoclonal gammopathy of undetermined significance, an early precursor of plasma cell myeloma that is detected in the bone marrow.

Cases of MBL have been subclassified into three categories: CLL-like immunophenotype [CD5(+), CD20(dim+)], atypical CLL immunophenotype [CD5(+), CD20(bright+)], and non-CLL immunophenotype [CD5(-),

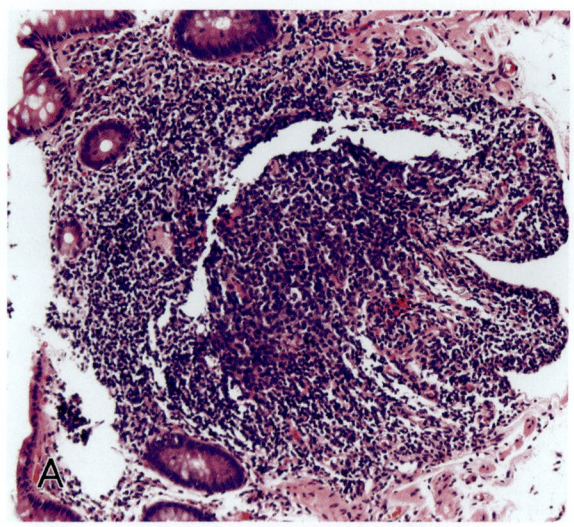

Figure 6-6

IN SITU MANTLE CELL NEOPLASIA INVOLVING THE GASTROINTESTINAL TRACT

This woman had a 10-year history of systemic mantle cell lymphoma, treated with aggressive chemotherapy at time of initial diagnosis.

A: A small lymphoid follicle is present. The mantle zone does not appear to be expanded (H&E stain).

B,C: The neoplastic cells are positive for cyclin D1 (B) and SOX11 (C) (immunohistochemistry with hematoxylin counterstain).

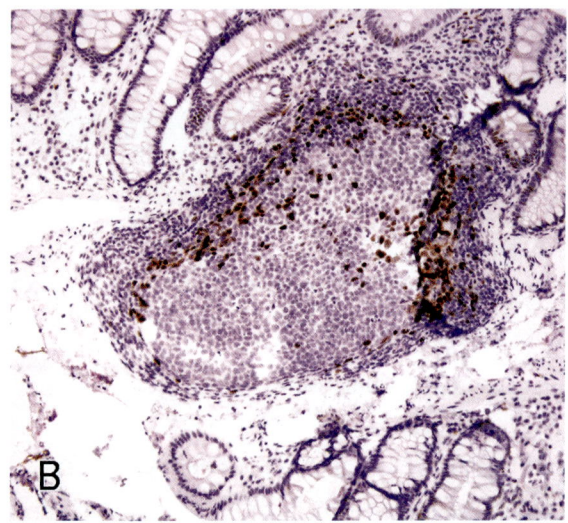

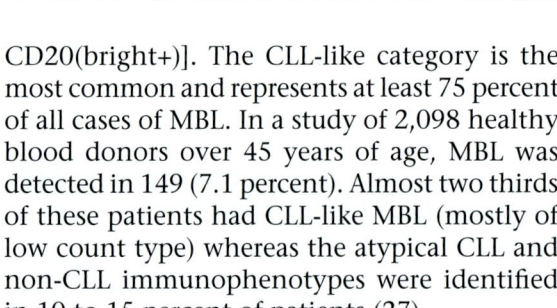

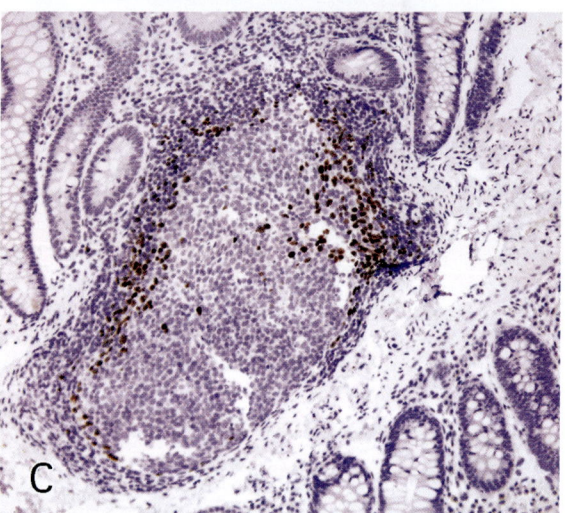

CD20(bright+)]. The CLL-like category is the most common and represents at least 75 percent of all cases of MBL. In a study of 2,098 healthy blood donors over 45 years of age, MBL was detected in 149 (7.1 percent). Almost two thirds of these patients had CLL-like MBL (mostly of low count type) whereas the atypical CLL and non-CLL immunophenotypes were identified in 10 to 15 percent of patients (27).

CLL-Like MBL

The overall frequency of *CLL-like MBL* in the general population has ranged in various studies from 3.5 to 12 percent. The frequency of CLL-like MBL is higher when sensitive (multi-color) flow cytometry techniques are used for detection, explaining, in part, the range reported in

the literature. The frequency of CLL-like MBL increases with age, and over half of all patients are over 90 years of age.

The distribution of absolute lymphocyte counts in patients with CLL-like MBL is not a bell-shaped curve. Instead, most patients have a very low CD5(+) CD20(dim+) B-cell count, less than 0.5×10^9/L. A second, smaller subset of patients has a CD5(+) CD20(dim+) B-cell count at least 1.5×10^9/L or higher. These data support two subsets, or variants, of CLL-like MBL: low-count CLL-like MBL and clinical (high count) CLL-like MBL.

Low-Count CLL-Like MBL. *Low-count CLL-like MBL*, defined as less than 0.05×10^9/L monotypic CD5(+), CD20(dim+) B cells in the peripheral blood of a healthy patient who does not have lymphocytosis, accounts for a large

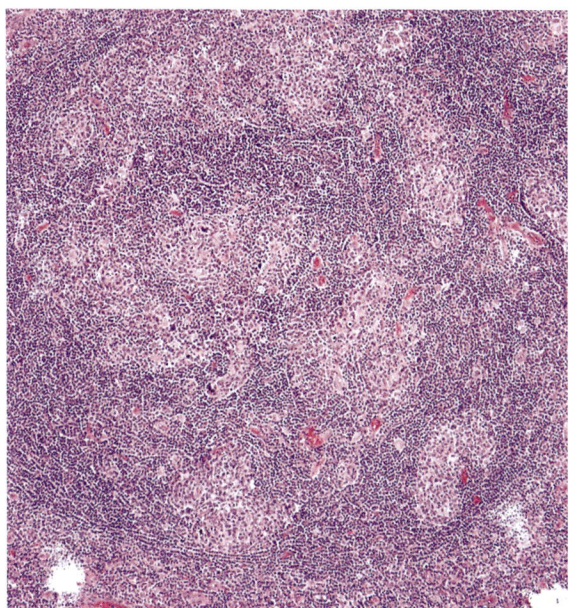
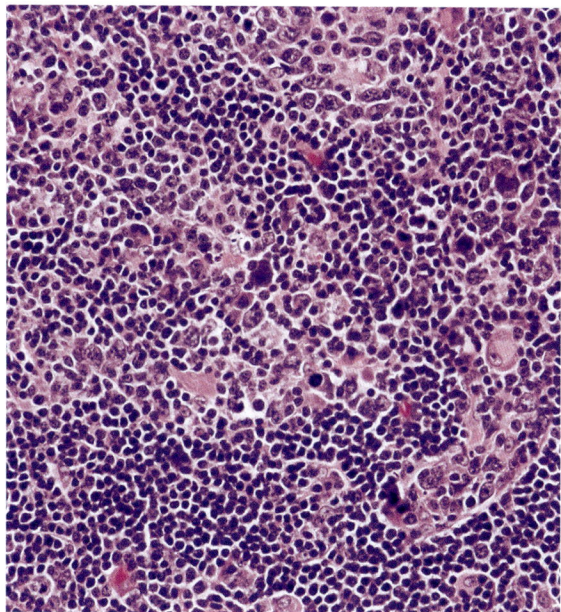

Figure 6-7

NODULAR LYMPHOCYTE-PREDOMINANT HODGKIN LYMPHOMA (NLPHL) IN SITU

This patient had fully developed NLPHL elsewhere in this lymph node biopsy specimen (not shown).

Left: A large nodule shows features of progressive transformation of germinal centers. A few large and apoptotic cells are observed.

Right: High-power magnification shows large apoptotic cells and occasional large, multilobated cells intermixed with germinal center cells (H&E stain).

proportion of cases of CLL-like MBL detected in the general population. The frequency of low-count CLL-like MBL is substantially higher than true CLL, up to 100-fold higher, suggesting that low-count CLL-like MBL is an early or precursor lesion (rather than an early phase of true CLL).

At the molecular level, low-count CLL-like MBL is usually monoclonal, but some cases reported are oligoclonal or polyclonal. The cells of CLL-like MBL do not show preferential use of immunoglobulin heavy chain variable regions or stereotypy, both common findings in true CLL, but deletions of 13q14 are seen in up to half of low-count CLL-like MBL cases, similar to true CLL. Small T-cell clones also have been identified in some patients with low-count CLL-like MBL (10).

Long-term follow-up studies have shown that patients with low count CLL-like MBL tend to have stable monotypic B-cell populations and they do not progress to true CLL (10). Nor do patients with low-count CLL-like MBL have a higher risk of infections or other manifestations seen in patients with true CLL. Therefore, low-count CLL-like MBL is not clinically important and patients do not need to be closely followed.

The etiology of low-count CLL-like MBL is unknown but it is thought to develop as a result of immunosenescence. It is unclear, however, whether the small T-cell clones in some patients can be attributed to immunosenescence. There is also some evidence that low count CLL-like MBL is more common in patients with viral infections, such as hepatitis C (25).

Clinical CLL-like MBL. *Clinical CLL-like MBL*, also known as high-count MBL, is defined as a monotypic CD5(+) CD20(dim+) B-cell population that is at least 1.5×10^9/L. The overall frequency of clinical CLL-like MBL in the general population is much lower than low-count CLL-like MBL, but slightly higher than the frequency of true, early stage (Rai 0) CLL. Almost all patients who develop CLL have an antecedent clinical CLL-like MBL phase.

The data suggest that clinical CLL-like MBL and Rai stage 0 CLL are overlapping groups at the clinical, cytogenetic, and molecular levels. Many patients with clinical CLL-like MBL have bone marrow involvement similar to that observed in patients with Rai stage 0 CLL. The bone marrow is usually involved in a nodular or focally interstitial pattern by monotypic B cells (21). At the molecular level, clinical CLL-like MBL cells often show del(13q14) and similar immunoglobulin variable gene usage and stereotypy as occurs in Rai stage 0 CLL.

As many patients with clinical CLL-like MBL have a clinically indolent course after detection, observation is usually the recommended therapeutic approach (22,23). However, 1 to 2 percent of patients progress to true CLL and some progress quickly. Currently, it is not possible to reliably predict which patients with CLL-like MBL will progress to true CLL. The absolute lymphocyte count is the most predictive factor. Most patients with a CD5(+) CD20(dim+) B-cell count over 3.5×10^9/L will eventually progress to CLL and in a study from the United Kingdom (23), a CD5(+) CD20(dim+) cell count of 3.2×10^9/L was the threshold value that best correlated with patient survival.

Scarfo et al. (25) suggested that rather than struggle with the labels of CLL-like MBL and Rai stage 0 CLL, it may be better to group these patients with the goal of subdividing patients into those who will develop progressive CLL requiring therapy versus those who will never require therapy. Although the absolute count of monotypic B cells has predictive value, it is clearly an imperfect predictor, and increased knowledge of the biology of clinical CLL-like MBL is needed to assign patients to the likely to progress versus clinically indolent groups (23,25). Ferrajoli et al. (11) have shown that CLL-like MBL patients have lower levels of microRNA-155 (miR-155) than patients with CLL, suggesting that miR-155 may be involved in progression. Next-generation sequencing studies have shown mutations in a number of genes in CLL-like MBL with a profile similar to CLL. In both patient groups, the presence of mutations in *SF3B1* (about 8 percent), *NOTCH1* (about 5 percent), and genes mutated at lower (about 1 percent) frequency predict a shorter time to when patients need therapy (2a,30). *TP53* and *XPO1* mutations are rare in CLL-like MBL (2a).

The concept of clinical CLL-like MBL is relevant to lymph node diagnosis because a small percentage of patients who undergo surgery for carcinoma (or other nonlymphoid tumors) can have an incidentally detected CD5-positive B-cell lymphoproliferative disorder in a lymph node(s) usually removed for staging purposes. Typically,

the lesions only partially replace the architecture of the lymph node biopsy specimen and there is no evidence of other sites of lymphadenopathy, hepatosplenomegaly, or absolute lymphocytosis. In one study, approximately 10 percent of patients with these findings progressed to overt CLL/SLL (12). Gibson et al. (12) proposed that the concept of clinical CLL-like MBL can be extended to lymph node biopsy specimens. They suggested that a lymph node biopsy specimen involved (usually partially) by a B-cell infiltrate with a CLL immunophenotype, but without proliferation centers, is the tissue equivalent of clinical CLL-like MBL if the patient has a peripheral blood monoclonal B-cell count of less than 5×10^9/L and the lymph nodes were smaller than 1.5 cm as shown by imaging studies. Gibson et al. used the term *CLL/SLL-like cells of uncertain significance* for this scenario.

MBL with an Atypical CLL-Like Immunophenotype

Monoclonal B-cell lymphocytosis with an atypical CLL immunophenotype is defined as the presence of a monotypic CD5-positive B-cell population in the peripheral blood of a patient with an absolute lymphocyte count of less than 5×10^9/L. In these cases, the atypical features are bright CD20 expression and CD23 is often negative or dim. The overall prevalence of MBL with an atypical CLL-like immunophenotype in the general population is about 1 to 2 percent. Little is known about this entity. The overall survival rate of these patients is lower than those with clinical CLL-like MBL and this is attributed to more extensive bone marrow involvement or lymphadenopathy (22). A subset of these patients has so-called atypical CLL; another subset likely has MBL with a MCL-like immunophenotype.

MBL with a Mantle Cell Lymphoma-Like Immunophenotype

Monoclonal B-cell lymphocytosis with a mantle cell lymphoma (MCL)-like immunophenotype is defined here as the presence of a monotypic CD5(+) cyclin D1(+) B-cell population in the peripheral blood of a patient with an absolute lymphocyte count less than 5×10^9/L. The lymphocytes also carry t(11;14)(q13;q32)/*IGH-CCND1*. This is an uncommon form of MBL. Espinet et al. (9) have used the term *monoclonal asymptomatic lymphocytosis, cyclin D1-positive* for this type of MBL.

In general, MBL with a MCL-like immunophenotype cannot be recognized in tissue biopsy specimens without immunohistochemical analysis for cyclin D1. Flow cytometry immunophenotypic analysis helps distinguish this entity from clinically important MCL (i.e., patients who require therapy). Lymphocytes of MBL with a MCL-like immunophenotype are usually CD38 negative (or low) and CD200 positive; the converse is true for typical cases of MCL (9). SOX11 expression was negative in one study (9). When compared with typical MCL, gene expression profiling showed enrichment of the proliferation signature in MCL and evidence for immune activation, likely related to inflammation, in MBL with a MCL-like immunophenotype (9).

The therapeutic implications for patients with MBL with a MCL-like immunophenotype are likely to be greater than for patients with other types of MBL. These patients should undergo rigorous clinical evaluation and be followed closely.

MBL with a Non-CLL Immunophenotype

Monoclonal B-cell lymphocytosis with a non-CLL immunophenotype is defined as the presence of a monotypic CD5(-), often CD20(bright+) B-cell population in the peripheral blood of a patient with an absolute lymphocyte count less than 5 x 10^9/L. The overall prevalence of non-CLL MBL is approximately 2 to 3 percent (22). Most patients with non-CLL MBL have an immunophenotype similar to that of marginal zone lymphoma or Waldenstrom macroglobulinemia. Clonal cytogenetic abnormalities are common in these B-cell populations, including del(7q), as is common in splenic marginal zone lymphoma (2).

In one clinical follow-up study of 102 patients, approximately 15 percent developed splenomegaly, suggesting that they had progressed to splenic marginal zone lymphoma (31). A few other patients in this study developed lymphadenopathy and the bone marrow was involved in approximately 70 percent. The patterns of involvement in bone marrow have been variable; a mixed pattern of paratrabecular and nonparatrabecular involvement as is seen in patients with marginal zone lymphomas is common.

It is rare for CD10 to be expressed in cases of MBL (22). This is true despite the fact that healthy adults commonly carry t(14;18)(q32;q21)/*IGH-BCL2* in the peripheral blood. Therefore, patients who present with an absolute CD10-positive monotypic B-cell population of less than 5 x 10^9/L need to undergo a complete clinical workup to exclude follicular lymphoma. Patients with CD10-positive low-level B-cell populations have a high frequency of systemic diseases and overall poorer survival rates than patients with clinical CLL-like MBL (22).

REFERENCES

1. Adam P, Schiefer AI, Prill S, et al. Incidence of preclinical manifestations of mantle cell lymphoma and mantle cell lymphoma in situ in reactive lymphoid tissues. Mod Pathol 2012;25:1629-1636.
2. Amato D, Oscier DG, Davis Z, et al. Cytotgenetic aberrations and immunoglobulin VH gene mutations in clinically benign CD5-monoclonal B-cell lymphocytosis. Am J Clin Pathol 2007;128:333-338.
2a. Barrio S, Shanafelt TD, Ojha J, et al. Genomic characterization of high-count MBL cases indicates that early detection of driver mutations and subclonal expansion are predictors of adverse clinical outcome. Leukemia 2017; 31:170-176.
2b. Bermudez G, González de Villambrosía S, Martínez-López A, et al. Incidental and isolated follicular lymphoma in situ and mantle cell lymphoma in situ lack clinical significance. Am J Surg Pathol 2016;40:943-949.
3. Bonzheim I, Salaverria I, Haake A, et al. A unique case of follicular lymphoma provides insights to the clonal evolution from follicular lymphoma in situ to manifest follicular lymphoma. Blood 2011;118:3442-3444.
4. Carbone A, Gloghini A. "Intrafollicular neoplasia" of nodular lymphocyte predominant Hodgkin lymphoma: description of a hypothetic early step of the disease. Hum Pathol 2012;43:619-628.
5. Carbone A, Gloghini A. Emerging issues after the recognition of in situ follicular lymphoma. Leuk Lymphoma 2014;55:482-490.
6. Carbone A, Tibiletti MG, Zannier L, Selva A, Sulfaro S, Gloghini A. A unique case of extranodal DLBCL sharing genetic abnormalities with a synchronous ileal lymphoma exhibiting immunoarchitectural features of in situ follicular lymphoma. Am J Hematol 2012;87:E134-E135.

7. Carvajal-Cuenca A, Sua LF, Silva NM, et al. In situ mantle cell lymphoma: clinical implications of an incidental finding with indolent clinical behavior. Haematologica 2012;97:270-278.

8. Cheung MC, Bailey D, Pennell N, et al. In situ localization of follicular lymphoma: evidence for a subclinical systemic disease with detection of an identical BCL-2/IGH fusion gene in blood and lymph node. Leukemia 2009;23:1176-1179.

9. Espinet B, Ferrer A, Bellosillo B, et al. Distinction between asymptomatic monoclonal B-cell lymphocytosis with cyclin D1 expression and mantle cell lymphoma: from molecular profiling to flow cytometry. Clin Cancer Res 2013;20:1007-1019.

10. Fazi C, Scarfo L, Pecciarini L, et al. General population low-count CLL-like MBL persists over time without clinical progression, though carrying the same cytogenetic abnormalities of CLL. Blood 2011;118:6618-6625.

11. Ferrajoli A, Shanafelt TD, Ivan C, et al. Prognostic value of miR-155 in individuals with monoclonal B-cell lymphocytosis and patients with chronic lymphocytic leukemia. Blood 2013;122:1891-1899.

12. Gibson SE, Swerdlow SH, Ferry JA, et al. Reassessment of small lymphocytic lymphoma in the era of monoclonal B-cell lymphocytosis. Haematologica 2011;96:1144-1152.

13. Hallek M, Cheson BD, Catovsky D, et al. Guidelines for the diagnosis and treatment of chronic lymphocytic leukemia: a report from the International Workshop on Chronic Lymphocytic Leukemia updating the National Cancer Institute-Working Group 1996 guidelines. Blood 2008;111:5446-5456.

14. Henopp T, Quintanilla-Martinez L, Fend F, Adam P. Prevalence of follicular lymphoma in situ in consecutively analyzed reactive lymph nodes. Histopathology 2011;59:139-142.

15. Jegalian AC, Eberle FC, Pack SD, et al. Follicular lymphoma in situ: clinical implications and comparisons with partial involvement by follicular lymphoma. Blood 2011;118:2976-2984.

16. Lee JC, Hoehn D, Schecter J, et al. Lymphoid follicle colonization by Bcl-2(bright+)CD10(+) B-cells ("follicular lymphoma in situ") at nodal and extranodal sites can be a manifestation of follicular homing of lymphoma. Hum Pathol 2013;44:1328-1340.

17. Liu Y, Hernandez AM, Shibata D, Cortopassi GA. BCL2 translocation frequency rises with age in humans. Proc Natl Acad Sci U S A 1994;91:8910-8914.

18. Mamessier E, Song JY, Eberle FC, et al. Early lesions of follicular lymphoma: a genetic perspective. Haematologica 2014;99:481-488.

19. Marti GE, Rawstrom AC, Ghia P, et al. Diagnostic criteria for monoclonal B-cell lymphocytosis. Br J Haematol 2005;130:325-332.

20. Montes-Moreno S, Castro Y, Rodriguez-Pinilla SM, et al. Intra-follicular neoplasia/in situ follicular lymphoma: review of a series of 13 cases. Histopathology 2010;56:658-662.

21. Randen U, Tierens AM, Tjonnfiord GE, Delabie J. Bone marrow histology in monoclonal B-cell lymphocytosis shows various B-cell infiltration patterns. Am J Clin Pathol 2013;139:390-395.

22. Rawstrom AC. Occult B-cell lymphoproliferative disorders. Histopathology 2011;58:81-89.

23. Rawstrom AC, Bennett FL, O'Connor SJ, et al. Monoclonal B-cell lymphocytosis and chronic lymphocytic leukemia. N Engl J Med 2008;359:575-583.

24. Roulland S, Navarro JM, Grenot P, et al. Follicular lymphoma-like B cells in healthy individuals: a novel intermediate step in early lymphomagenesis. J Exp Med 2006;203:2425-31. Erratum in: J Exp Med 2006;203:2563.

25. Scarfo L, Fazi C, Ghia P. MBL versus CLL. How important is the distinction? Hematol Oncol Clin N Am 2013;27:251-265.

26. Schmidt J, Salaverria I, Haake A, et al. Increasing genomic and epigenomic complexity in the clonal evolution from in situ to manifest t(14;18) positive follicular lymphoma. Leukemia 2014;28:1103-1112.

27. Shim YK, Rachel JM, Ghia P, et al. Monoclonal B-cell lymphocytosis in healthy blood donors: an unexpectedly common finding. Blood 2014;123:1319-1326.

27a. Swerdlow SH, Campo E, Pileri SA, et al. The 2016 revision of the World Health Organization classification of lymphoid neoplasms. Blood 2016;127:2375-2390.

28. Sungalee S, Mamessier E, Morgado E, et al. Germinal center reentries of BCL2-overexpressing B cells drive follicular lymphoma progression. J Clin Invest 2014;124:5337-5351.

29. Wang S, Tzankov A, Xu-Monette ZY, et al. Clonally related composite follicular lymphoma and mantle cell lymphoma with clinicopathologic features and biological implications. Hum Pathol 2013;44:2658-2667.

30. Winkelmann N, Rose-Zerilli M, Forster J, et al. Low frequency mutations independently predict poor treatment free survival in early stage chronic lymphocytic leukemia and monoclonal B-cell lymphocytosis. Haematologica 2015;100:237-239.

31. Xochelli A, Kalpadakis C, Gardiner A, et al. Clonal B-cell lymphocytosis exhibiting immunophenotypic features consistent with a marginal zone origin: is this a distinct entity? Blood 2014;123:1199-1206.

32. Xochelli A, Oscier D, Stamatopoulos K. Clonal B-cell lymphocytosis of marginal zone origin. Best Pract Res Clin Haematol 2017;30:77-83.

7 CLINICAL WORKUP, STAGE, AND PROGNOSTIC FACTORS OF LYMPHOMA

This chapter briefly reviews the clinical issues involved in the workup and treatment of lymphoma patients. Knowledge of these issues facilitates communication and optimal multidisciplinary care. This chapter is not intended to be complete and the reader is referred to clinical textbooks for more detailed information.

CLINICAL WORKUP

The great diversity of lymphomas and their highly variable presentations make it challenging to apply a uniform approach for all patients. In Table 7-1, a list of most of the essential clinical, laboratory, and imaging studies to thoroughly evaluate lymphoma patients is provided.

As for any patient with an illness, a careful clinical history is essential. The clinical history needs to include queries for lymphoma risk factors, such as autoimmune diseases or viral infection, exposure to environmental risk factors (e.g., certain occupations have higher lymphoma risk), and assessment of the overall health (performance) status of the patient. Although most patients with lymphoma present with painless lymphadenopathy, involvement of various organs by lymphoma may be manifested by organ-related symptoms. For example, neurologic symptoms can be a manifestation of brain involvement by lymphoma or a lymphoma mass could cause obstruction of an airway, blood flow, or urine flow. B-type symptoms have prognostic importance; these include fever (temperature higher than 38°C), drenching night sweats, and unexplained weight loss (over 10 percent of body weight).

A thorough physical examination requires examination of all lymph node groups. Assessment of the central nervous system, Waldeyer ring, lungs, liver, and spleen is essential. The skin should be examined for lesions. Helpful laboratory studies include a complete blood count and differential count and a chemistry

---

Table 7-1

SUGGESTED WORKUP FOR PLANNING THERAPY FOR A LYMPHOMA PATIENT[a]

1. History with queries for B-type symptoms, localized pain, or obstructive symptoms

2. Physical examination searching for lymphadenopathy, palpable masses, abdominal organomegaly, or focal neurologic signs

3. Computed tomographic (CT) scans of the neck, chest, abdomen, and pelvis

4. 18F-fluorodeoxyglucose (FDG)-positron emission tomographic (PET)/CT whole body scan for lymphomas for which FDG uptake is reliable for staging disease[b]

5. Hematologic tests: complete blood count and differential count

6. Chemistry tests: serum creatinine, bilirubin, alkaline phosphatase, lactate dehydrogenase, beta-2-microglobulin, serum protein electrophoresis, calcium

7. Serologic testing: for virus infection (HIV[c], hepatitis, HTLV-1)

8. Results of diagnostic biopsy

9. Bone marrow aspiration and biopsy

10. Cytologic analysis of fluid specimens if indicated (e.g., CSF, effusions)

[a]Modified from Table 1 in reference 5.
[b]For some types of low-grade lymphoma (e.g., chronic lymphocytic lymphoma/small lymphocytic lymphoma [CLL/SLL], lymphoplasmacytic lymphoma/Waldenstrom macroglobulinemia, mycosis fungoides) FDG-PET is not reliable for staging.
[c]HIV = human immunodeficiency virus; HTLV-1 = human T-cell lymphotropic virus 1; CSF = cerebrospinal fluid.

Table 7-2

ANN ARBOR STAGING SYSTEM[a]

Stage I Involvement of a single lymph node region (I) or a single extralymphatic organ or site (E)

Stage II Involvement of two or more lymph node regions on the same side of the diaphragm (II) or localized involvement of an extralymphatic organ or site and one or more lymph node regions on the same side of the diaphragm (IIE)

Stage III Involvement of lymph node regions on both sides of the diaphragm (III), which may also be accompanied by involvement of the spleen (IIIS) or by localized involvement of an extralymphatic organ or site (IIIE)

Stage IV Diffuse or disseminated involvement of one or more extralymphatic organs or tissues, with or without associated lymph node involvement[b]

[a]Reported by Carbone et al. (2) and subsequently modified at the Cotswolds meeting (13) in which bulky disease was designated by an X, clinical versus pathologic stage were defined, and criteria for reporting response were added. The stages above are modified by the letter B if fever, drenching night sweats, or unexplained loss of >10 percent of body weight are present in the preceding 6 months. Absence of these systemic symptoms is designated by the letter A.
[b]Biopsy-documented involvement of stage IV sites is also denoted by letter suffixes: marrow = M+, lung = L+, liver = H+, pleura = P+, bone = O+, skin and subcutaneous tissue = D+.

panel. Liver or kidney function tests may point to organ involvement by lymphoma. An elevated serum calcium or alkaline phosphatase level suggests bone involvement. Serum protein electrophoresis and immunofixation are helpful for evaluating patients with plasma cell myeloma and B-cell lymphomas with extensive plasmacytic differentiation, such as Waldenstrom macroglobulinemia. Serum lactate dehydrogenase (LDH) and beta-2-microglobulin levels have prognostic value. Since some infections correlate with certain types of lymphoma, serologic studies to assess for evidence of infection, particularly certain viruses, are helpful.

A biopsy is essential to establish the diagnosis of lymphoma and an excisional biopsy is preferred if possible. Following diagnosis, a number of staging studies are required to complete the workup. Radiologic imaging studies help demonstrate the full extent of disease. Computerized tomography (CT), magnetic resonance imaging (MRI), and 18F-fluorodeoxyglucose-positron emission tomography (FDG-PET) all have a place in staging lymphomas. Bone marrow aspiration and biopsy are usually indicated. If the central nervous system is suspected to be involved, lumbar puncture with morphologic examination of cerebrospinal fluid is indicated. Other types of staging studies are based on suspected sites of involvement.

The integration of these data with the pathologic diagnosis creates a whole picture that allows the treating physician to develop a plan for therapy. The overall therapeutic goal is to personalize the treatment plan as much as possible to maximize the chances of cure while minimizing treatment-related toxicities.

STAGE

Hodgkin Lymphomas

The Ann Arbor staging system (2), published in 1971, was initially developed for patients with Hodgkin lymphoma (HL), a primarily nodal disease that spreads in a contiguous fashion. By the 1960s, therapeutic advances allowing more targeted delivery of radiation therapy highlighted the need for a staging system that documented more precisely the sites of disease. In addition, advances in combined chemotherapy required a better assessment of prognosis to allow for a better informed choice of radiation therapy versus chemotherapy.

As shown in Table 7-2, the Ann Arbor system (2) divides patients with HL into four stages: stage I is used to designate localized disease and stage IV is used to designate widespread or disseminated disease; stage II designates two or more sites of disease on the same side of the diaphragm and stage III designates disease on both sides of the diaphragm. The system also allows for specifying specific sites of disease, such as the spleen (S), bone marrow (M), or other specific sites. "E" is used to designate extranodal sites of disease and either "A" or "B" to designate the absence (A) or presence (B) of fever, night sweats, or weight loss.

The Ann Arbor stage, combined with the histologic type of HL, was the mainstay for predicting prognosis and designing the most appropriate therapy for a number of years. Patients with stage I disease had the best prognosis whereas patients with high-stage disease had a worse prognosis. In 1989, the Ann Arbor system was updated at a consensus conference in Cotswolds, England. The concept of bulky disease was incorporated with the designation X, newer radiologic techniques (e.g., computerized tomography) for staging were incorporated, and definitions for response to therapy were codified (13).

Although the Ann Arbor system remains valuable, the therapeutic approach for HL patients has undergone a dramatic evolution in the past few decades. The role of radiation therapy has been reduced and chemotherapy regimens have greatly improved. Currently, approximately 90 percent of HL patients with early stage disease and 70 to 80 percent of patients with advanced stage disease are cured with standard therapy, with the most commonly used regimen being doxorubicin, bleomycin, vinblastine, and dacarbazine (ABVD) (3). As a result, staging has assumed lesser importance in the management of patients with HL (1,9). In addition, the way in which patients are staged has continued to change with further evolution of radiologic imaging techniques.

Non-Hodgkin Lymphomas

Although not designed for patients with non-Hodgkin lymphoma (NHL), the Ann Arbor system was applied subsequently to these patients and shown to have prognostic value. The Ann Arbor system, however, has obvious drawbacks for NHL patients and therefore is less useful for guiding therapeutic decisions.

One major drawback is that NHLs are highly heterogeneous and encompass a large number of different diseases. Although patients with many types of NHL present initially with lymphadenopathy, as is the case for patients with HL, 30 to 40 percent of NHL patients have extranodal sites of involvement, usually bone marrow, liver, spleen, gastrointestinal tract, and Waldeyer ring. Secondly, some types of NHL present primarily as extranodal disease. The Ann Arbor system is generally less helpful for staging these patients because the system does not adequately stratify such patients into different stages or prognostic

subsets. A third drawback of the Ann Arbor system for staging NHL patients is that the system is based on a false premise. It was designated for HL, a disease that commonly spreads in a contiguous manner. This premise does not apply to patients with NHL in whom dissemination is not orderly and widespread disease is common at the time of initial diagnosis.

Although the Ann Arbor staging system for patients with either HL or NHL remains helpful, in many ways the original roles for this system in predicting prognosis and guiding therapy have been reduced. Currently, many other factors are useful for assessing the prognosis of lymphoma patients, such as patient age, tumor bulk, patient performance status, serum levels of LDH or beta-2-microglobulin, results of improved imaging techniques (e.g., PET or CT/PET scans), and tumor-associated biomarkers, including immunophenotypic, cytogenetic, and molecular data.

Other Staging Systems for Non-Hodgkin Lymphomas. The limitations of the Ann Arbor system, as applied to patients with NHL, are perhaps most pronounced for those with extranodal lymphoma. Childhood NHLs are an example of a group of lymphomas that are commonly extranodal, such as Burkitt lymphoma and lymphoblastic lymphoma. Patients with Burkitt lymphoma commonly present with a mass of the gastrointestinal tract, most often the ileocecal region, whereas patients with T-lymphoblastic lymphoma often present with a mediastinal mass. When using the Ann Arbor system, such patients are not adequately stratified into prognostic groups and the stages IE and IV groups are over represented.

Murphy et al. (15) devised a staging system to better capture the unique aspects of the presentation of childhood lymphomas to allow better prognostication. This system was used for about three decades, but recently an expert panel modified the Murphy system (Table 7-3) (19). The newly proposed system incorporates the many advances in staging and improved prognostication since the Murphy system was developed.

An example of an extranodal lymphoma in adults that highlights the limitations of the Ann Arbor system is extranodal natural killer (NK)/T-cell lymphoma of nasal type. These tumors most often arise in the nasopharynx and for these patients local tumor invasion, either

Table 7-3

INTERNATIONAL PEDIATRIC NON-HODGKIN LYMPHOMA STAGING SYSTEM[a]

Stage I[b]
Single tumor (nodal or extranodal including skin or bone) with exclusion of mediastinum and abdomen

Stage II
Single extranodal tumor with regional lymph node involvement
Two or more nodal areas on same side of diaphragm
Primary gastrointestinal (GI) tract tumor (usually in ileocecal region), with or without involvement of mesenteric lymph nodes only, that is completely resectable (if malignant ascites or tumor extends into adjacent organs the tumor is regarded as stage III)

Stage III
Two or more extranodal tumors (including skin or bone) above and below the diaphragm
Two or more nodal areas above and below the diaphragm
Any intrathoracic tumor (mediastinum, hilum, lungs, pleura, thymus)
Intra-abdominal and retroperitoneal disease, including liver, spleen, kidney, and/or ovary localization, regardless of degree of resection (except primary GI tumor [usually in ileocecal region] with or without involvement of associated mesenteric lymph nodes that is completely resectable)
Any paraspinal or epidural tumor, regardless of other disease sites
Single bone lesion with concomitant involvement of extranodal site and/or nonregional nodal sites

Stage IV
Any of the above findings with initial involvement of central nervous system (stage IV CNS) or bone marrow (stage IV BM) or both (stage IV combined) based on conventional methods

[a]This classification is a modification of the system developed by Murphy at al. (15).
[b]For each stage, the type of examination and degree of BM and CNS involvement should be specified.

into bone or skin, is important for determining prognosis. Kim et al. (11) suggested grouping patients with extranodal NK/T-cell lymphoma of nasal type into stages based on limited (stage I/II) upper airway disease without tumor invasion versus extensive disease. The patient group with extensive disease can be further subdivided into three subsets: stage I/II upper airway disease with local, contiguous invasion; stage III/IV upper airway disease; and non-upper airway (extranasal) disease (11).

PROGNOSTIC FACTORS

Prognostic Scoring Systems for Lymphoma Patients

Although pathologic diagnosis and stage are important, it has become clear that these two variables do not capture the full spectrum of tumor behavior. To better stratify lymphoma patients into prognostic groups, a number of systems have been developed that traditionally have incorporated clinical and laboratory findings to better assign prognosis. A complete discussion of these systems is beyond the scope of this chapter. Here, we briefly discuss a few of the most commonly used.

Hodgkin Lymphoma. Patients with nodular lymphocyte-predominant HL are commonly divided into two prognostic subsets: early (stage IA) and more advanced (1,9). Patients with early stage disease are potential candidates for involved field radiation therapy or watchful waiting, particularly for young, actively growing patients. Chemotherapy is usually chosen for patients with advanced-stage disease (1,9).

Patients with classic HL are commonly grouped into three prognostic categories: early stage favorable (stage I and IIA), early stage unfavorable, and advanced stage (1,9). The factors used to decide favorable versus unfavorable in patients with early stage disease differ in different systems but include one or more of the following factors: age (over 40 or 50 years), bulky mass (often mediastinal), B symptoms, elevated erythrocyte sedimentation rate, and multiple (more than two) nodal sites of disease. In general, the number of cycles of chemotherapy and the dose of involved field radiation therapy can be reduced in patients with early stage favorable disease

For patients with advanced classic HL, one popular scoring system to predict prognosis was proposed by Hasenclever et al. (8). This system includes seven features: serum albumin

Table 7-4

INTERNATIONAL PROGNOSTIC INDEX[a]

Prognostic Factor	Criterion	Points
Age	≤60 years versus > 60 years	1
Performance status	0-1 versus 2-4	1
LDH	Normal range versus above normal	1
Extranodal sites:	0-1 versus ≥2	1
Stage (Ann Arbor)	I and II versus III and IV	1

[a]The IPI was initially reported in 1993 (16).

Table 7-5

FOLLICULAR LYMPHOMA INTERNATIONAL PROGNOSTIC INDEX (FLIPI)[a]

Prognostic Factor	Criterion	Points
Age	≤60 years versus > 60 years	1
Number of nodal sites	0-4 versus >4	1
LDH	Normal range versus above normal	1
Hemoglobin	≥120 g/L versus <120 g/L	1
Stage (Ann Arbor)	I and II versus III and IV	1

[a]The FLIPI was initially reported by Solal-Celigny et al. (20).

less than 4 g/dL, hemoglobin less than 10.5 g/dL, male sex, Ann Arbor stage IV disease, age 45 years or older, white blood cell count over 15,000/mm[3,] and lymphocytes less than 600/mm[3] or less than 8 percent of total leukocyte count. Each factor is designated with one point. Patients with scores of 0-1, 2-3, and 4 or more are considered to have good, fair, and poor risk disease, respectively (8). Patients with high scores are candidates for more aggressive treatment regimens or clinical trials.

Non-Hodgkin Lymphoma. A number of prognostic scoring systems have been proposed for different types of NHL. One of the better established systems is the International Prognostic Index (IPI) (Table 7-4), which was developed for patients with diffuse large B-cell lymphoma (DLBCL). In this system, each of five variables is assigned one point (the mnemonic APLES is helpful for remembering these variables): age over 60 years, performance status of 2 or more, high (above normal range) serum LDH level, 2 or more extranodal sites, and advanced (III or IV) Ann Arbor stage (17). An IPI score of 0 or 1 is associated with excellent 5-year survival whereas scores of 4 or 5 correlate with substantially poorer survival. Patients with an IPI of 2 or 3 have an intermediate survival. For patients older than 60 years of age, a modified IPI, also known as the elderly (E) IPI, can be used based on three variables: performance status, serum LDH, and stage (16).

Although an essential part of the clinical assessment of DLBCL patients for approximately two decades, the IPI was developed using a group of patients treated with CHOP (cyclophospha-

mide, hydroxydoxorubicin, vincristine, and prednisone) as standard therapy. In the rituximab (R)-CHOP therapy era, the IPI has lost some of its power for discriminating risk groups, particularly higher-risk patients. A recent study based on raw data from the National Comprehensive Cancer Network (NCCN) proposed a new system, the NCCN-IPI (22), in which age and serum LDH levels are stratified and the definition of extranodal sites is refined. For age, there are three groups: 40 to 60 years (1 point), 60 to 75 years (2 points), and over 75 years (3 points). An elevated serum LDH level is divided into two groups: elevated but less than 3 times normal range (1 point) or more than 3 times normal range (2 points). The extranodal sites of involvement of prognostic importance are bone marrow, central nervous system, liver, gastrointestinal tract, and lung. This new system results in a maximum score of 8 points and is reported to be more powerful than the traditional IPI for predicting the prognosis of DLBCL patients (22). Additional time is needed to determine whether the NCCN-IPI will replace the traditional IPI.

The IPI has become a model for assessing the prognosis of patients with other common types of NHL. The Follicular Lymphoma International Prognostic Index (FLIPI) has been developed to better stratify the prognosis of patients with advanced follicular lymphoma (Table 7-5). The mnemonic NoLASH is helpful for remembering the five variables: number of nodal sites of disease (0-4 versus more than 4), serum LDH (normal versus elevated), age (under 60 versus over 60 years), Ann Arbor stage (I/II versus II/IV), and hemoglobin (120 g/L or more versus less than 120

Table 7-6

CLINICAL GROUPS OF NON-HODGKIN LYMPHOMAS[a]

Type	B Cell	T Cell

Indolent	CLL/SLL[b]
	Lymphoplasmacytic/WM
	Follicular, grades 1-3A
	Marginal zone lymphomas
	    Extranodal
	    Nodal
	    Splenic
		Mycosis fungoides
		Cutaneous ALCL
		Breast implant-associated ALCL

Aggressive	Mantle cell
	Follicular, grade 3B
	Diffuse large cell[c]
	High-grade B-cell lymphoma
		Peripheral T-cell NOS
		Angioimmunoblastic
		Extranodal NK/T-cell, nasal-type
		Subcutaneous panniculitis-like
		    Enteropathy-associated
		    Hepatosplenic
		    Systemic ALCL
		        ALK+
		        ALK-

Acute leukemia-like	Lymphoblastic Burkitt Double-hit lymphomas[d]	Lymphoblastic
Viral	Primary effusion (HHV-8+)	Adult T-cell leukemia/lymphoma (HTLV-1+)

[a]Grouping based on natural history, presentation, immunophenotype, and genetic features and using the terminology of the 2008 World Health Organization classification. Modified from Table 3 in reference 5.
[b]CLL/SLL = chronic lymphocytic leukemia/small lymphocytic lymphoma; WM = Waldenstrom macroglobulinemia; NOS = not otherwise specified; HHV-8 = human herpesvirus type 8; HTLV-1 = human T-cell lymphotropic virus type 1; ALCL = anaplastic large cell lymphoma; ALK = anaplastic lymphoma kinase.
[c]Includes all variants and subtypes of diffuse large B-cell lymphoma.
[d]Designated high-grade B-cell lymphoma with *MYC* and *BCL2* and/or *BCL6* rearrangements in current WHO system (21a).

g/L) (20). Each variable equals one point and the FLIPI separates follicular lymphoma patients into three statistically significant prognostic subsets more effectively than the traditional IPI: low (good), intermediate, and high (poor).

The number of prognostic systems for specific types of NHL has proliferated. Specific systems have been designed for chronic lymphocytic leukemia/small lymphocytic lymphoma (CLL/SLL), mantle cell lymphoma, marginal zone lymphoma, Burkitt lymphoma, and different types of T-cell and NK/T-cell lymphomas (4,6,10,18,21). These systems are mostly based on standard clinical and laboratory features (e.g., age, serum LDH or hematologic parameters, and tumor burden), but some systems include immunophenotypic, conventional cytogenetic, and molecular data to a variable degree. The reader is referred to the original publications for a description of these systems (4,6,19,18,21).

Prognostic Biomarkers

Although the IPI and similar systems have been helpful in stratifying lymphoma patients, it is clear that many of the variables used in these systems, such as age, stage, or serum enzyme levels are surrogates for the biology of the lymphoma. Not surprisingly then, these systems are imperfect in their ability to predict prognosis. The goal, therefore, is to better understand the biology of specific types of lymphoma and identify markers that better predict prognosis. Ideally, these markers would predict prognosis more reliably than current systems and, in some instances, could be used as therapeutic targets (20a). In general, a biomarker is based on the features of the neoplastic cells themselves (e.g., a specific chromosomal translocation) or is related to the tumor microenvironment.

It is beyond the scope of this chapter to discuss the numerous biomarkers that have been proposed for the many types of HL and NHL.

Many of the most relevant biomarkers as related to specific lymphoma types are discussed in subsequent chapters. Two examples of biomarkers that have achieved some utility are IGH somatic mutation status and ZAP70 expression in CLL/SLL (6) and germinal center versus activated B-cell type in DLBCL. Nevertheless, the incorporation of these (and many other) markers into standard prognostic scoring systems has proved challenging. For example, the use of gene expression signatures for the prognostication of DLBCL patients has not yet entered into routine practice, in large part because of the complexity of bioinformatic analysis. Immunohistochemistry markers have been employed as a surrogate for gene expression profiling, but these algorithms have not been robust. It is likely that smaller gene sets that can be analyzed from fixed, paraffin-embedded tissue will be helpful (and are in development). Creating a composite prognostic model that combines newer, biologic markers with standard prognostic systems is also likely to be statistically complex (22). A recent advance is the establishment of event-free survival at 24 months (EFS24), a reliable endpoint to assess therapy in patients with DLBCL (14).

Non-Hodgkin Lymphomas Divided into Prognostic Groups

The various types of NHL in the World Health Organization (WHO) classification can be divided into groups with similar prognoses. For example, Connors (5) subdivided NHLs into four groups: indolent, aggressive, acute leukemia-like, and viral-associated. Patients with indolent (also often referred to as low-grade) lymphomas commonly present with advanced-stage disease which is not curable using standard chemotherapy regimens (Table 7-6). These patients, however, often respond to short courses of systemic therapy and can have long intervals with minimal (or no) symptoms. The most common indolent lymphomas include low-grade follicular lymphoma, marginal zone lymphomas, and CLL/SLL. The 10-year overall survival rate for patients indolent lymphomas ranges from 60 to 80 percent, with older (over 60 years of age) patients having lower rates.

There are some types of indolent lymphoma, however, that require special mention because therapy is different. Many patients with extra-nodal marginal zone lymphoma of the stomach are cured by antibiotics, with or without radiation therapy, the latter often used for patients with advanced disease. Splenectomy often removes the bulk of disease in patients with splenic marginal zone lymphoma and corrects peripheral blood cytopenias. Mycosis fungoides and cutaneous anaplastic large cell lymphoma are indolent T-cell lymphomas of the skin that often respond to therapies directed to the skin. Breast implant-associated anaplastic large cell lymphoma is another recently described type of T-cell lymphoma that is often clinically indolent if patients are treated by implant removal and capsulectomy.

Aggressive NHLs include DLBCL, mantle cell lymphoma, and most peripheral T/NK-cell lymphomas. For these patients, aggressive chemotherapy regimens are needed and there is a chance of cure, particularly for patients with DLBCL. Using the standard R-CHOP chemotherapy regimen, approximately 60 percent of patients with DLBCL are cured.

There are three lymphomas in the aggressive NHL category that merit special mention based on their prognosis. Most patients with mantle cell lymphoma have a poor prognosis and treatment approaches are not standardized. Regimens originally designed for acute lymphoblastic leukemia have been used to treat mantle cell lymphoma patients. Some patients with mantle cell lymphoma have a neoplasm that behaves in a more indolent manner and can be managed more conservatively. Nasal T/NK cell lymphoma responds poorly to standard chemotherapy. Patients with localized disease need high-dose radiotherapy and patients with systemic disease do particularly poorly.

Patients with anaplastic lymphoma kinase (ALK)-positive anaplastic large cell lymphoma have a better prognosis than those with other types of T-cell lymphoma. The prognosis of patients with ALK-negative anaplastic large cell lymphoma is worse than for patients with ALK-positive tumors, but still better than for patients with other types of T/NK-cell lymphoma. In addition, ALK and CD30 expression, the latter in both ALK-positive and ALK-negative tumors, can be targeted with recently developed therapeutic agents.

Acute leukemia-like lymphomas include Burkitt lymphoma and both T- and B-lymphoblastic lymphoma/leukemia. Patients with these tumors usually have rapidly progressive disease, a high likelihood of bone marrow involvement, a leukemic phase in the blood, and a higher risk of central nervous system involvement. Patients with acute leukemia-like lymphomas require high-dose chemotherapy regimens and often hematopoietic stem cell transplantation. A more recent addition to this category is the double-hit high-grade B-cell lymphoma in which *MYC* rearrangement is associated with rearrangement of another oncogene, most often *BCL2*. Although these tumors may resemble DLBCL or Burkitt lymphoma, patients with double-hit lymphomas respond poorly to R-CHOP therapy (12).

The fourth category of NHLs includes two tumors associated with viral infection: adult T-cell leukemia/lymphoma associated with human T-cell lymphotropic virus 1 (HTLV-1) and primary effusion lymphoma associated with human herpesvirus 8 (HHV-8). The end stage of adult T-cell leukemia/lymphoma is similar to other acute leukemia-like lymphomas and requires rapid, progressive therapy although the prognosis is poor. Primary effusion lymphoma is also an aggressive disease that requires chemotherapy. These tumors are typically negative for CD20 and rituximab does not have a major role in therapy (5).

GRADING

The term grade as is used in hematopathology practice can have two different meanings: tumor grade and cytologic grade. *Tumor grade* is defined here as the assignment of an overall grade to a lymphoma based on the expected behavior of most tumors in the specific lymphoma category. Tumor grading was a part of some NHL classification systems in the past (e.g., Kiel classification), but is not a part of the WHO system. Nonetheless, pathologists and clinicians alike group different types of NHL into categories with similar prognoses, in effect, tumor grading. The system used by Connors (5) described above and in Table 7-6 is not far from the low-, intermediate-, and high-grade categories that were used in the Working Formulation (17).

Tumor grading is also used more informally in daily practice. As acknowledged in the WHO system, patients with a specific lymphoma type can exhibit a range in clinical behaviors, from less to more aggressive, that likely correspond with disease evolution or progression. Similarly, tumors within a specific lymphoma type can show a spectrum of morphologic features, from low- to high-grade, which correlates loosely with disease progression. Pathologists recognize this histologic spectrum and commonly refer to tumors with a high mitotic rate, a starry sky pattern, or a high proliferation rate as being high grade. These findings can have clinical or genetic correlates. In DLBCLs, for example, tumors with high-grade features are more likely to carry *MYC* abnormalities than their lower-grade counterparts (12). Therefore, identifying the morphologic features of these tumors as high grade may have some value in identifying lymphomas that should be sent for high-expense, ancillary genetic testing.

Cytologic grade uses the cytologic features of a neoplasm to predict likely prognosis. The best established cytologic grading system has been developed for follicular lymphoma, based on an average count number of centroblasts in 10 high-power microscopic fields (7). Grades 1 and 2 are thought to predict an indolent clinical course for patients with follicular lymphoma, whereas grade 3, particularly grade 3B, describes a poorer prognosis. This grading system is discussed in more detail in the chapter on follicular lymphoma.

REFERENCES

1. Ansell SM. Hodgkin lymphoma: 2016 update on diagnosis, risk-stratification, and management. Am J Hematol 2016;91:434-442.
2. Carbone P, Kaplan H, Musshoff K, Smithers DW, Tubiana M. Report of the Committee on Hodgkin's staging. Cancer Res 1971;31:1860-1861.
3. Canellos GP, Rosenberg SA, Friedberg JW, Lister TA, Devita VT. Treatment of Hodgkin lymphoma: a 50-year perspective. J Clin Oncol 2014;32:163-168.
4. Castillo JJ, Winer ES, Olszewski AJ. Population-based prognostic factors for survival in patients with Burkitt lymphoma: an analysis from the Surveillance, Epidemiology, and End Results database. Cancer 2013;119:3672-3679.
5. Connors JM. Non-Hodgkin lymphoma: the clinician's perspective—a view from the receiving end. Mod Pathol 2013;26(Suppl 1):S111-118.
6. Haferlach C, Dicker F, Weiss T, et al. Toward a comprehensive prognostic scoring system in chronic lymphocytic leukemia based on a combination of genetic parameters. Genes Chromosomes Cancer 2010;49:851-859.
7. Harris NL, Nathwani BN, Swerdlow SH, et al. Follicular lymphoma. In: Swerdlow SH, Campo E, Harris NL, et al, eds. WHO Classification of tumours of haematopoitic and lymphoid tissues. Lyon: IARC Press; 2008:220-226.
8. Hasenclever D, Diehl V. A prognostic score for advanced Hodgkin's disease. N Engl J Med 1998;339:1506-1514.
9. Hoppe RT, Advani RH, Ai WZ, et al. Hodgkin lymphoma, version 2.2012 featured updates to the NCCN guidelines. J Natl Compr Canc Netw 2012;10:589-597.
10. Hoster E, Klapper W, Hermine O, et al. Confirmation of the mantle-cell lymphoma International Prognostic Index in randomized trials of the European Mantle-Cell Lymphoma Network. J Clin Oncol 2014;32:1338-1346.
11. Kim TM, Heo DS. Extranodal NK / T-cell lymphoma, nasal type: new staging system and treatment strategies. Cancer Sci 2009;100:2242-2248.
12. Lin P, Medeiros LJ. The impact of MYC rearrangements and "double hit" abnormalities in diffuse large B-cell lymphoma. Curr Hematol Malig Rep 2013;8:243-252.
13. Lister TA, Crowther D, Sutcliffe SB, et al. Report of a committee convened to discuss the evaluation and staging of patients with Hodgkin's disease: Cotswolds Meeting. J Clin Oncol 1989;7:1630-1636.
14. Maurer MJ, Ghesquieres H, Jais JP, et al. Event-free survival at 24 months is a robust end point for disease-related outcome in diffuse large B-cell lymphoma treated with immunochemotherapy. J Clin Oncol 2014;32:1066-1073.
15. Murphy SB, Fairclough DL, Hutchison RE, Berard CW. Non-Hodgkin's lymphomas of childhood: an analysis of the histology, staging, and response to treatment of 338 cases at a single institution. J Clin Oncol 1989;7:186-193.
16. [No authors listed]. A predictive model for aggressive non-Hodgkin's lymphoma. The International Non-Hodgkin's Lymphoma Prognostic Factors Project. N Engl J Med 1993;329:987-994.
17. [No authors listed]. National Cancer Institute sponsored study of classifications of non-Hodgkin's lymphomas: summary and description of a working formulation for clinical usage. The Non-Hodgkin's Lymphoma Pathologic Classification Project. Cancer 1982;49:2112-2135.
18. Piccaluga PP, Fuligni F, De Leo A, et al. Molecular profiling improves classification and prognostication of nodal peripheral T-cell lymphomas: results of a phase III diagnostic accuracy study. J Clin Oncol 2013;31:3019-3025.
19. Rosolen A, Perkins SL, Pinkerton CR, et al. Revised International Pediatric Non-Hodgkin Lymphoma Staging System. J Clin Oncol 2015;33:2112-2118.
20. Solal-Celigny P, Roy P, Colombat P, et al. Follicular lymphoma international prognostic index. Blood 2004;104:1258-1265.
20a. Sun R, Medeiros LJ, Young RH. Diagnostic and predictive biomarkers for lymphoma diagnosis and treatment in the era of precision medicine. Mod Pathol 2016;29:1118-1142.
21. Tsimberidou AM, Wen S, O'Brien S, et al. Assessment of chronic lymphocytic leukemia and small lymphocytic lymphoma by absolute lymphocyte counts in 2.126 patients: 20 years of experience at The University of Texas M.D. Anderson Cancer Center. J Clin Oncol 2007;25:4648-4656.
21a. Swerdlow SH, Campo E, Pileri SA, et al. The 2016 revision of the World Health Organization classification of lymphoid neoplasms. Blood 2016;127:2375-2390.
22. Zhou Z, Sehn LH, Rademaker AW, et al. An enhanced International Prognostic Index (NCCN-IPI) for patients with diffuse large B-cell lymphoma treated in the rituximab era. Blood 2014;123:837-842.

8 EPIDEMIOLOGY OF HODGKIN AND NON-HODGKIN LYMPHOMAS

OVERALL STATISTICS

Approximately 300,000 new cases of lymphoma (of all types) develop worldwide per year (39). The incidence of lymphoma varies greatly according to the specific type and the geographic location in the world. This variation is likely attributable to both genetic and socioeconomic factors.

The United States has one of the highest incidence rates of lymphoma in the world. In 2015, it was estimated that 80,900 persons would develop lymphoma: 71,850 (88.8 percent) cases of non-Hodgkin lymphoma (NHL) and 9,050 (11.2 percent) cases of Hodgkin lymphoma (HL) (36). Lymphomas as a group represent 4.9 percent of all cancers. Males develop NHL more often than females. In 2015, 39,850 NHLs were estimated in men and 32,000 in women; NHL was the sixth most common cancer in both sexes (36). The overall age-adjusted incidence rate for developing NHL in the United States was 23.2 per 100,000 men and 16.1 per 100,000 women (36) (at the time of this writing 2015 estimates were available; 2016 data were recently published in reference 39a). These figures are similar in other developed countries including western Europe, Canada, Australia, and New Zealand (5,29,38,41).

In the United States in 2015 the estimated number of persons dying from NHL was 19,790 (36). The 5-year overall survival rate for patients with NHL has greatly improved over the past 40 years, from 47 percent in the interval of 1975 to 1977 to 71 percent in the interval of 2002 to 2007. Five-year survival rates are higher in Caucasians than African Americans (72 versus 63 percent). In the United States, approximately 500,000 individuals have had or are currently living with lymphoma (5).

Over the second half of the 20th century, the overall incidence of HLs decreased by approximately 15 percent (24). In contrast, the overall incidence of NHLs increased dramatically, av-eraging about 3 percent annually (5,15,29,38). These trends are true for the United States and other industrialized nations. There are some explanations for the increased incidence of NHLs. The average lifespan of the general population has increased and aging appears to be an important risk factor for NHL. Other explanations include improved reporting of lymphomas; changes in criteria for diagnosing NHLs, particularly for those NHLs involving extranodal sites (15); the human immunodeficiency virus/acquired immunodeficiency syndrome epidemic (35); and the increased prevalence of other types of immunodeficiency such as organ transplantation or as a result immunodysregulatory diseases (e.g., rheumatoid arthritis) and the associated use of immunosuppressive or immune-modulating therapeutic agents (2). It is currently thought, however, that these factors explain no more than half of the rapid increase in the incidence of NHLs from 1950 to 2000 (17).

In the late 1990s and the first decade of the 21st century, the incidence curves for NHLs in the United States and many other developed countries plateaued and are projected to remain stable (fig. 8-1). The reasons for this are poorly understood; however, the incidence of NHLs continues to rise in other countries, for example, Japan (8).

RELATIVE FREQUENCY OF LYMPHOMAS

The most common type of HL is nodular sclerosis, currently representing over 60 percent of all the cases, with a higher frequency of up to about 80 percent in more affluent populations (fig. 8-2). Although the overall incidence of HL has decreased, the relative frequency of the nodular sclerosis type has increased. This is the result of a true increase in the incidence of nodular sclerosis HL as well as reclassification of other types of classic HL. Currently, mixed cellularity HL is the second most frequent type, approximately 25 percent, followed by nodular lymphocyte-predominant HL, 5 percent; lymphocyte-rich classic HL, 5 percent; and lymphocyte-depleted HL, 1 percent (18,24).

Throughout the world, B-cell NHLs are far more frequent than T-cell NHLs. Approximately 90 percent of all NHLs are of B-cell lineage (5,18,29). Diffuse large B-cell lymphoma (DLBCL) is the most common type of NHL worldwide, but there are differences between

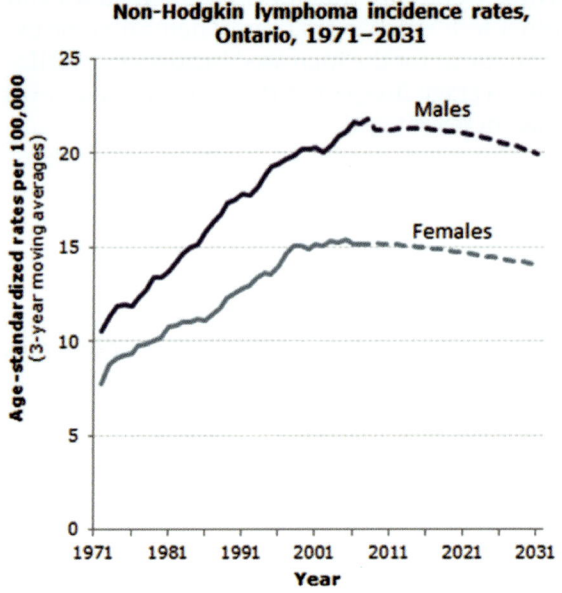

Non-Hodgkin lymphoma incidence rates, Ontario, 1971–2031

Source: Cancer Care Ontario (Ontario Cancer Registry, 2010)
Dashed lines are estimates.

Figure 8-1

INCIDENCE OF NON-HODGKIN LYMPHOMA (NHL)

Over the 20th century, the incidence of NHLs increased dramatically, but the trend leveled off and is projected to remain stable. (Data from Cancer Care Ontario, www.cancercare.on.ca/cancerfacts. Reprinted with permission.)

geographic regions for other NHL types (discussed subsequently). In the United States and Europe, DLBCL represents 31 percent of all cases of NHL, followed by follicular lymphoma (about 22 percent). Other somewhat frequent types of NHL include chronic lymphocytic leukemia/small lymphocytic lymphoma (CLL/SLL), 9 percent; extranodal marginal zone lymphoma of mucosa-associated lymphoid tissue (MALT lymphoma), 7.6 percent; and mantle cell lymphoma, 6 percent (fig. 8-3). All other types of B-cell NHL occur at lower frequencies, 1 to 3 percent, or are rare (18,27).

Natural killer (NK) and T-cell NHLs represent approximately 10 percent of NHLs (fig. 8-4) (18). Among NK/T-cell lymphomas, approximately 26 percent are peripheral T-cell lymphomas not otherwise specified, which represent about 2 to 3 percent of all NHLs (18,42). Other more frequent types of NK/T-cell lymphoma, in order of frequency, are: angioimmunoblastic T-cell lymphoma, 18.5 percent; extranodal NK/T-cell lymphomas, 10.4 percent, adult T-cell leukemia/lymphoma, 9.6 percent; anaplastic lymphoma kinase (ALK)-positive anaplastic large cell lymphoma, 6.6 percent; and ALK- anaplastic large cell lymphoma, 5.5 percent. All other types of NK/T-cell lymphoma are uncommon or rare (18,42).

AGE

The incidence of lymphoma increases with age: it is low in children and young adults, higher in adults of middle-age, and highest in persons over 70 years of age (5,29,36). The incidence of both nodal and extranodal NHL increases with age as well, and this trend remains

Figure 8-2

RELATIVE FREQUENCIES OF HODGKIN LYMPHOMA (HL)

The pie chart shows the relative frequencies of HL. (Data from reference 24.)

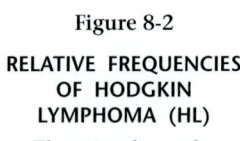

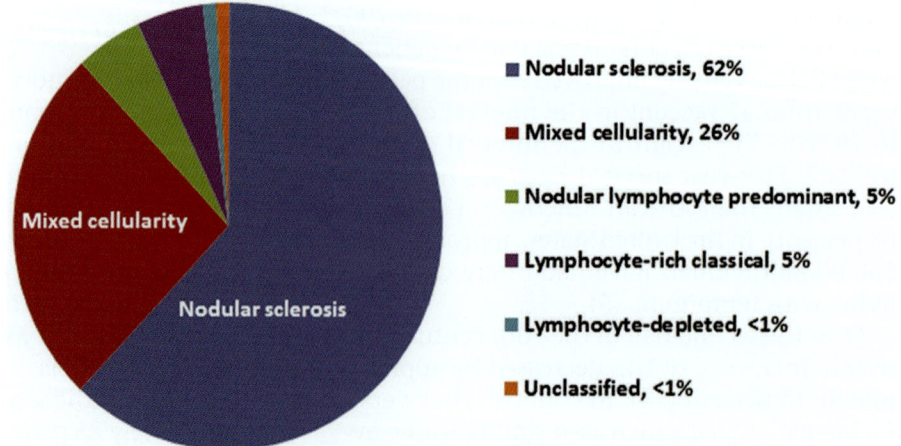

- Nodular sclerosis, 62%
- Mixed cellularity, 26%
- Nodular lymphocyte predominant, 5%
- Lymphocyte-rich classical, 5%
- Lymphocyte-depleted, <1%
- Unclassified, <1%

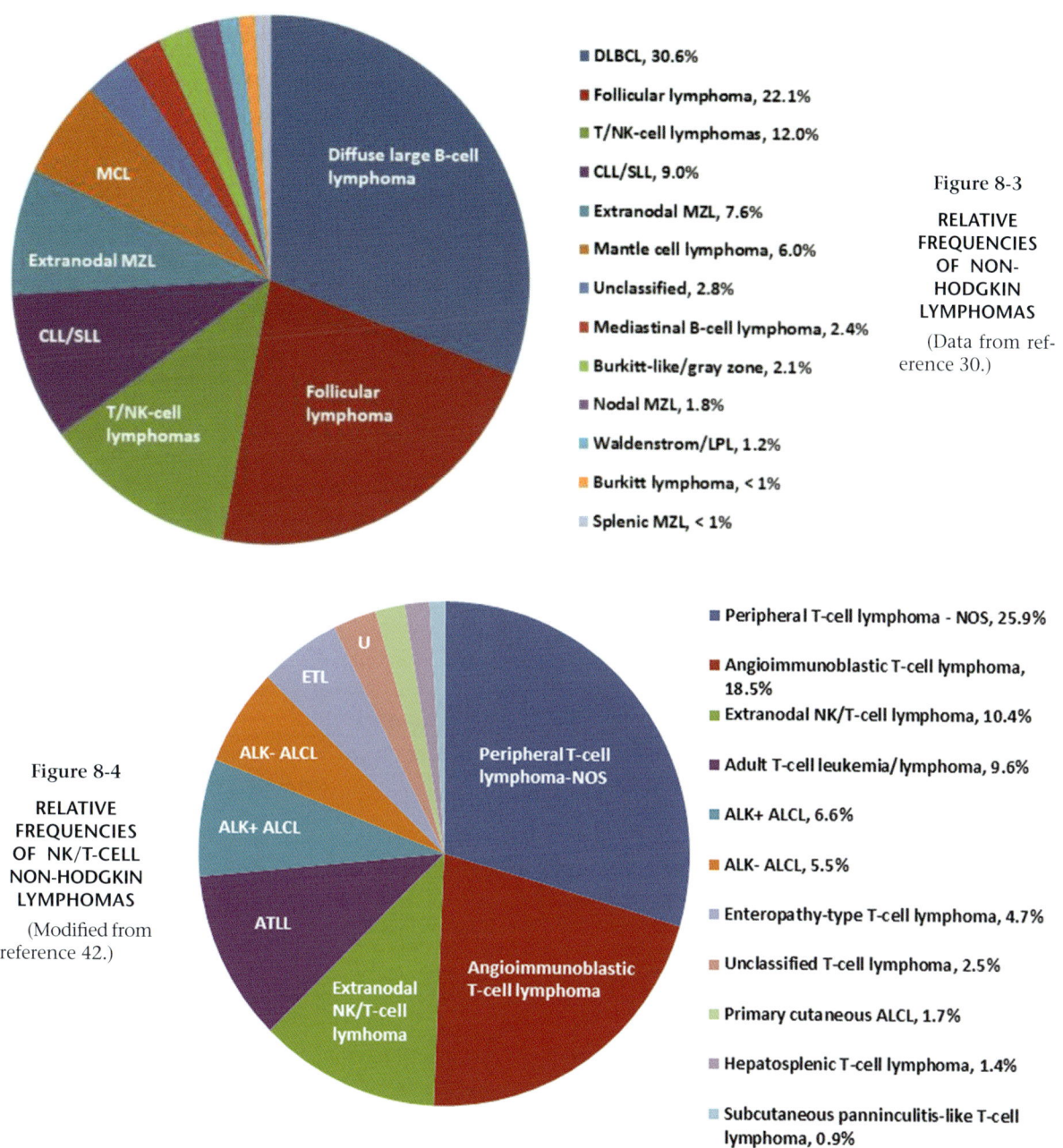

Figure 8-3

RELATIVE FREQUENCIES OF NON-HODGKIN LYMPHOMAS

(Data from reference 30.)

- DLBCL, 30.6%
- Follicular lymphoma, 22.1%
- T/NK-cell lymphomas, 12.0%
- CLL/SLL, 9.0%
- Extranodal MZL, 7.6%
- Mantle cell lymphoma, 6.0%
- Unclassified, 2.8%
- Mediastinal B-cell lymphoma, 2.4%
- Burkitt-like/gray zone, 2.1%
- Nodal MZL, 1.8%
- Waldenstrom/LPL, 1.2%
- Burkitt lymphoma, < 1%
- Splenic MZL, < 1%

Figure 8-4

RELATIVE FREQUENCIES OF NK/T-CELL NON-HODGKIN LYMPHOMAS

(Modified from reference 42.)

- Peripheral T-cell lymphoma - NOS, 25.9%
- Angioimmunoblastic T-cell lymphoma, 18.5%
- Extranodal NK/T-cell lymphoma, 10.4%
- Adult T-cell leukemia/lymphoma, 9.6%
- ALK+ ALCL, 6.6%
- ALK- ALCL, 5.5%
- Enteropathy-type T-cell lymphoma, 4.7%
- Unclassified T-cell lymphoma, 2.5%
- Primary cutaneous ALCL, 1.7%
- Hepatosplenic T-cell lymphoma, 1.4%
- Subcutaneous panninculitis-like T-cell lymphoma, 0.9%

true for men and women and for different races (fig. 8-5). The median age of patients when they develop NHL is the fifth or sixth decade. The age of onset of lymphoma is lower in developing countries (32).

For patients with HL, the nodular lymphocyte-predominant type affects both young and older patients with almost equal frequency (24). In contrast, classic HL has a bimodal age incidence rate, with peaks in adolescents/young adults, and in older adults (24). This distribution can be explained by the different types of classic HL. Nodular sclerosis HL is most common in adolescents and young adults and its incidence fades as patients get older. The mixed cellularity type of HL tends to develop in young children, 5 to 10 years of age, or in middle-aged or older adults. Lymphocyte-depleted HL is rare in younger adults

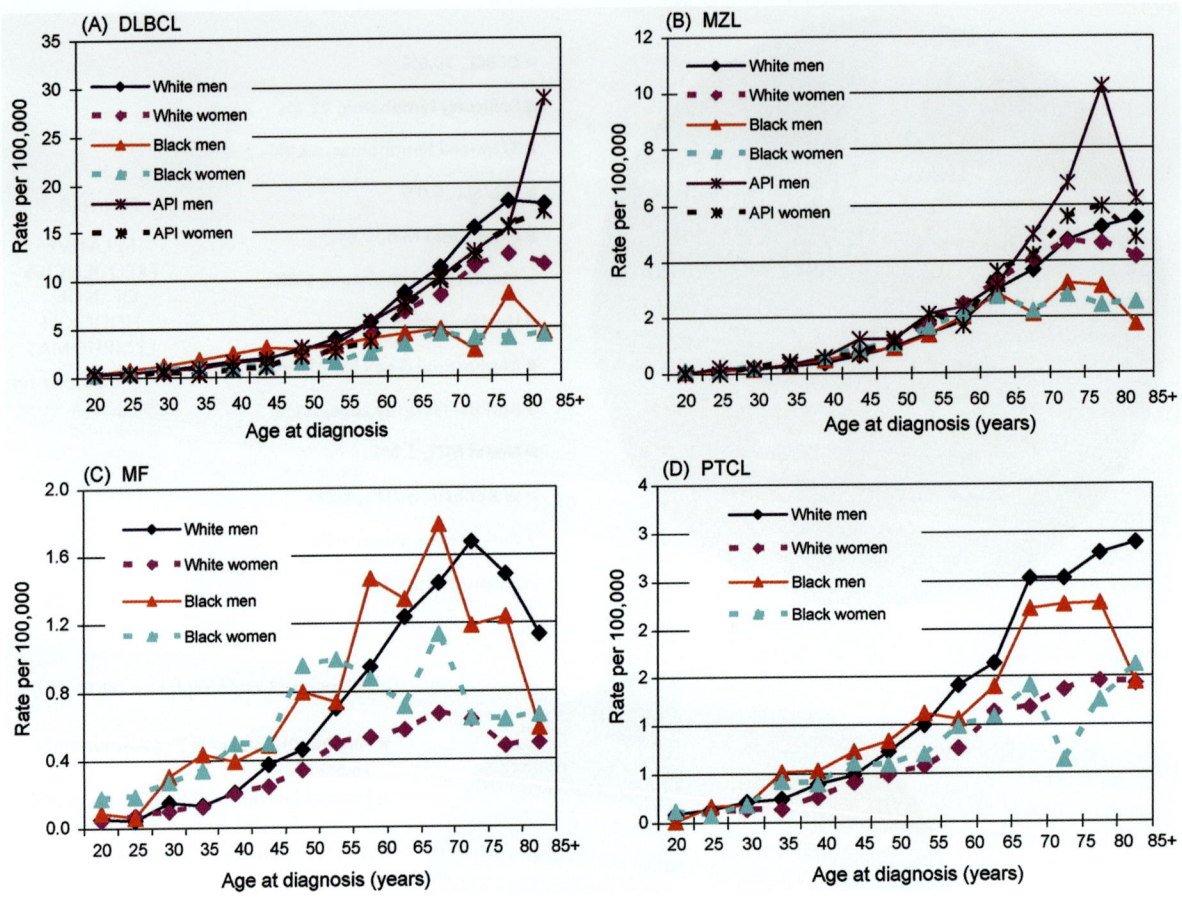

Figure 8-5

INCIDENCE OF NON-HODGKIN LYMPHOMA

Surveillance, epidemiology, and end results (SEER) data showing that the incidence of extranodal NHL increases with age. This trend is true for men and women and for all races. In this figure, four types of NHL are shown: diffuse large B-cell lymphoma (DLBCL), marginal zone lymphoma (MZL), mycosis fungoides (MF), and peripheral T-cell lymphoma (PTCL). (Fig. 2 from Wu XC, Andrews P, Chen VW, Groves FD. Incidence of extranodal non-Hodgkin lymphomas among whites, blacks, and Asians/Pacific Islanders (API) in the United States: anatomic site and histology differences. Cancer Epidemiol 2009;33:345.

and most patients are over 40 years of age at diagnosis. It is rare for any type of HL to develop in infants or children less than 3 years of age.

The most common types of NHL in the elderly include DLBCL (fig. 8-5), CLL/SLL, mantle cell lymphoma, and plasma cell myeloma (27). Other less common types that affect the elderly include nodal and splenic marginal zone lymphoma, Waldenstrom macroglobulinemia/ lymphoplasmacytic lymphoma, and angioimmunoblastic T-cell lymphoma. Patients with Waldenstrom macroglobulinemia have one of the highest median ages at the time of diagnosis (27). The peak age of patients and the incidence of extranodal marginal zone lymphomas varies

according to the anatomic site of origin. The incidence of cutaneous marginal zone lymphoma continues to rise with age whereas gastric, ocular adnexal, salivary gland, and thyroid marginal zone lymphomas occur more often in middle-aged patients (20). The median age of patients with follicular lymphoma is the sixth decade (18). The median age of patients who develop primary mediastinal B-cell lymphoma is approximately 35 years (27).

A few types of NHL more commonly arise in children and young adults. These include ALK-positive anaplastic large cell lymphoma, B- and T-lymphoblastic lymphoma/leukemia, DLBCL, and Burkitt lymphoma (16).

SEX AND RACE

Most types of HL and NHL occur more often in men than women (27,29,37). Overall, the male to female ratio is approximately 1.2 to 1.0. This ratio holds true from birth to death. Approximately 1 in 43 men and 1 in 52 women will develop lymphoma over their lifetime. Men are also slightly more likely to die from lymphoma than women, paralleling the incidence rate (36).

In patients with HL, nodular lymphocyte-predominant exhibits the most marked male predominance, with a male to female ratio of 3 to 1 (24,27). The lymphocyte-rich classic, mixed cellularity, and lymphocyte-depleted types of HL have a male to female ratio in the range of 2 to 1. Nodular sclerosis HL does not have a marked sex preference but may be slightly more common in females (24,39a).

In NHL patients, a male predominance is most prominent for Burkitt lymphoma and hairy cell leukemia, in which the male to female ratio is over 3 to 1 (15,27). Other NHLs that arise predominantly in men include mantle cell lymphoma, DLBCL, plasma cell myeloma, Waldenstrom macroglobulinemia, and most T-cell lymphomas. Lymphoblastic lymphomas of either B- or T-cell lineage occur more often in boys than girls (27). Follicular lymphoma affects the sexes fairly equally or there is a slight female predominance (18). Most types of extranodal marginal zone lymphoma are more common in men, but thyroid and salivary gland marginal zone lymphomas are associated with Sjögren syndrome and Hashimoto thyroiditis, respectively, and occur more often in women (20). Young women more commonly develop primary mediastinal large B-cell lymphoma with a male to female ratio of 1 to 2 (27).

Race is an important risk factor in lymphomas. In general, Caucasians have the highest incidence followed by Hispanics, African Americans and other blacks, Asians/Pacific Island inhabitants, and native Americans (5,27). Most epidemiologic studies, by grouping minority populations to allow statistical analysis, understate the genetic variation in these populations. In a study of recent immigrants to England, there were marked differences in the incidence and types of NHL between various minority groups, for example, blacks of African versus Carribean descent (37). More epidemiologic studies of minority populations are needed.

For HL, Caucasians have the highest frequency of classic HL (5,27). In contrast, nodular lymphocyte-predominant HL is more common in African-Americans. All types of HL are less common in Asians than in whites or blacks.

For NHL, the following types are far more common in whites, with a white to black ratio of over 2 to 1: follicular lymphoma, mantle cell lymphoma, Waldenstrom macroglobulinemia, DLBCL, marginal zone lymphomas, and hairy cell leukemia (27). Salivary gland marginal zone lymphoma has been linked with Hispanic ethnicity (20). African Americans have a greater frequency of plasma cell myeloma and a lower frequency of CLL/SLL and follicular lymphoma (36). T-cell lymphomas are more common in blacks; African-Americans have a higher frequency of mycosis fungoides whereas blacks of Carribean descent have a higher frequency of T-cell lymphoma related to human T-cell lymphoma virus 1 (HTLV-1) infection (18,36). Extranodal NK/T-cell lymphomas are more common in Asians than whites or blacks. Follicular lymphoma, CLL/SLL, and plasma cell myeloma are uncommon or rare in Asians (15,27,36).

GEOGRAPHIC VARIATION

There are major differences in the frequency and incidence of lymphomas in different areas of the world (fig. 8-6). There is a clear association with socioeconomic status: lymphomas are more common in developed nations than developing countries (5,29,32). There is also evidence that lymphomas are more common in urban areas as compared with rural areas (29). These factors likely explain the high incidence of lymphomas in the United States and other industrialized nations. An important caveat is that lymphomas are likely under-reported in developing nations.

HLs represent approximately 10 percent of all lymphomas in industrialized nations. The frequency of HL appears to be higher in Pakistan (37) and may be higher in the Middle East as a study from Iraq (46) reported that 24 percent of all lymphomas were HL. This report, however, needs confirmation because the workup of the cases in the study from Iraq was incomplete. HLs are uncommon in the study from Asia.

Nodular sclerosis is the most common type of HL in Europe, the United States, and other

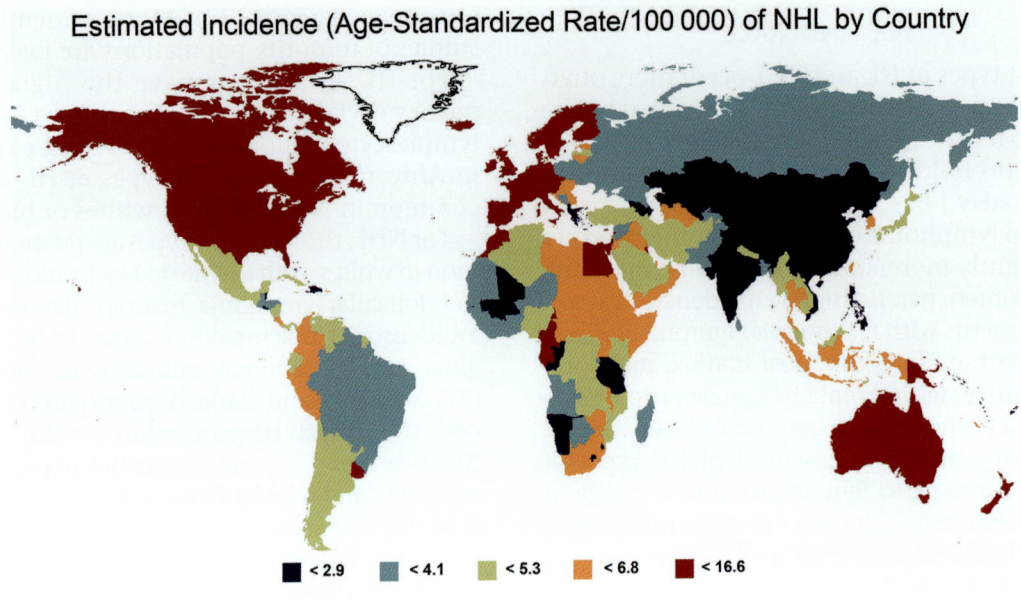

Estimated Incidence (Age-Standardized Rate/100 000) of NHL by Country

| ■ < 2.9 | ■ < 4.1 | ■ < 5.3 | ■ < 6.8 | ■ < 16.6 |

Figure 8-6

AGE-ADJUSTED INCIDENCE RATES

Global map showing age-adjusted incidence rates per country. (Image adapted from Ferlay J, Shin HR, Bray F, et al. GLOBOCAN 2008 Cancer Incidence and Mortality Worldwide: IARC CancerBase No. 10. Lyon: International Agency for Research on Cancer.)

industrialized nations. Mixed cellularity, in contrast, is much more common in developing countries such as Central America, Africa, and China (44). There seems to be less geographic variation for nodular lymphocyte-predominant HL.

The incidence of NHL is high in the United States and other developed nations and lower in Asian nations such as Japan, Taiwan, China, and Mongolia (5,8). The frequency of DLBCL is highest in the Middle East and Asia and lower in the United States and Europe (5,17a,29,38). Intestinal involvement by DLBCL, likely related to so-called Mediterranean lymphoma, is also common in the Middle East. DLBCL appears to be more frequent in South America than North America (10,19). Epstein-Barr (EBV)-positive DLBCL, as defined in the World Health Organization (WHO) classification, is far more common in Asia and Central America than it is in the United States and Europe (18). Among B-cell NHLs, CLL/SLL and follicular lymphoma are most common in Europe, the United States, and other developed nations, and are less common in the Middle East and Asia (5,45). CLL/SLL is particularly rare in Asia. South America also has a lower frequency of follicular lymphoma

compared with North America, with the possible exception of Argentina, which appears to have a frequency more in keeping with the United States and other industrialized countries (21). Mantle cell lymphomas are common in Northern Italy and Switzerland, representing 8 to 10 percent of all cases of NHL (1,18). Mantle cell lymphoma is less common in other areas of Europe and North America and is uncommon in Asia.

The most common type of extranodal marginal zone lymphoma in the United States and Europe arises in the stomach, followed in descending order of frequency by the ocular adnexal region, lung, skin, and salivary glands (20). Overall, extranodal marginal zone lymphomas appear to be more frequent in the Chile (7). In one study, primary mediastinal large B-cell lymphoma was most common in Switzerland (1). Endemic Burkitt lymphoma is well known for its near constant relationship with EBV and its distinctive geographic distribution along the equator in Africa, New Guinea, and Northern Brazil, which corresponds to regions with a high prevalence of malaria infection (23). In contrast, sporadic Burkitt lymphoma is a rare disease in Europe and the United States, representing 1 percent or less of all NHL cases, and only about 20 percent of these cases are EBV positive (18,23). Patients with human immunodeficiency virus (HIV) infection in developed countries have a higher frequency of Burkitt lymphoma and a higher frequency of EBV infection compared with sporadic cases (23,35).

The frequency of NK- and T-cell NHLs also shows marked geographic variation. EBV-positive NK/T-cell lymphomas are most common in Asia, particularly Southern China and Hong Kong (5,42,44). These tumors are uncommon in the United States, Canada, western Europe, Australia, and New Zealand (18,41,42). In the United States, Hispanics and Asians have a higher frequency of extranodal NK/T-cell lymphoma of nasal type than whites (18). Nasal type extranodal NK/T-cell lymphoma is more common in Central and South America, particularly in Native Americans (7,32). Peripheral T-cell lymphoma, not otherwise specified, is the most common type of T-cell NHL in most geographic regions, although its frequency is variable as determined by the frequency of more specific types. Angioimmunoblastic T-cell lymphoma is most common in Northern Europe and the United States and less frequent in Asia (42).

Adult T-cell leukemia/lymphoma is related to HTLV-1 infection and therefore its frequency is highest in endemic geographic regions. In southern Japan 8 to 10 percent of the general population is seropositive for HTLV-1 and this region has the highest frequency of adult T-cell leukemia/lymphoma (18). This tumor type is also common in the Caribbean basin and the coasts of South America (7,31a). The geographic regions with a substantial frequency of HTLV-1 infection may be related to the slave trade of earlier centuries because HTLV-1 is thought to have initially arisen in Africa.

RISK FACTORS FOR HODGKIN LYMPHOMAS

There is a genetic component in the pathogenesis of HL: both classic HL and nodular lymphocyte-predominant HL are known to run in families (14,43). Data are beginning to emerge linking genetic findings with an increased incidence of HL. Genetic polymorphisms involving the interleukin 6 (*IL6*) gene have been associated with HL (22). In a family with a history of classic HL, a reciprocal t(2;3)(q11.2;p21.3) involving the *KLHDC8B* gene has been identified (34).

In a family with nodular lymphocyte-predominant HL, a truncating germline mutation in the *NPAT* (nuclear protein ataxia-telangiectasia) gene was identified (33). To date, however, data on specific genes that may be involved in HL predisposition are sparse.

There are also environmental factors involved in the risk of classic HL. Epidemiologic evidence suggests that the risk of HL, particularly the mixed cellularity type, is linked with EBV infection. Patients with a history of infectious mononucleosis have an increased risk of HL, and EBV antibodies in serum have been shown in patients who subsequently developed HL (28). Primary EBV infection could explain a small peak in the incidence of mixed cellularity HL in young children and reactivation of EBV infection could explain the increased incidence in adults (24). HIV infection is also associated with an increased risk of HL, commonly of mixed cellularity type, and usually also associated with EBV infection (24,35).

For nodular sclerosis HL, EBV is present in approximately 20 percent of cases and therefore the virus seems less likely to have a major role in pathogenesis. Instead, there are epidemiologic studies showing that social factors correlate with increased risk, including small family size, early birth order, fewer siblings or neighborhood playmates, and higher level of parental education (16). These findings are somewhat similar to the paralytic polio model and raise the possibility of a viral cause for nodular sclerosis HL, although there is no direct data to support this hypothesis at this time.

Cigarette smoking has been linked with increasing risk of mixed cellularity HL as well as EBV-positive cases of HL (19). Exposure to ultraviolet radiation has been suggested to decrease the risk of EBV-positive HL, possibly via the induction of regulatory T cells (25). The older age of patients with lymphocyte-depleted HL at the time of diagnosis suggests that this type is an end-stage related to the progression of other HL types.

RISK FACTORS FOR NON-HODGKIN LYMPHOMAS

A number of risk factors have been proposed for patients with NHL and recent studies from the International Lymphoma Epidemiology Consortium (InterLymphoma) have shown

Table 8-1

**EPIDEMIOLOGIC RISK FACTORS FOR
NON-HODGKIN LYMPHOMAS (NHLS)**

Established
  Heredity
  Infectious agents
  Immunosuppression
  Autoimmune disease

Suggestive
  Genetic polymorphisms
  Exposure to agricultural agents
  Exposure to hair dyes
  Exposure to immunomodulator therapies

Not Established
  Diet
  Alcohol use
  Tobacco use
  Ultraviolet radiation
  Blood transfusions
  Drugs (nonimmunosuppressive)

that etiology varies, in part, based on the type of NHL. A summary of some of the better studied risk factors are shown in Table 8-1. Heredity plays a role. This conclusion seems clear based on known differences in the incidence of NHL between races and the fact that NHLs run in families (43). There are also some data showing that chromosomal regions and genetic polymorphisms are linked to specific types of NHL. For example, genetic polymorphisms of the interleukin 10 (*IL-10*) and tumor necrosis factor superfamily 10 (*TNFSF-10*) genes are more common in patients with CLL/SLL and Waldenstrom macroglobulinemia (4,22). Chromosomal locus 6p21.32 has been linked with follicular lymphoma, single nucleotide polymorphisms of the *BCL2L11* gene have been linked with B-cell NHLs, and CLL/SLL is associated with a number of single nucleotide polymorphisms (3,11). This is an area of active research and the reader is referred to many recent studies in the literature.

Factors clearly associated with an increased risk of NHL include infectious agents (see chapter 9), immunosuppression, and autoimmune diseases (2). Various bacterial organisms have been linked with extranodal marginal zone lymphomas at different sites. Viruses, such as HTLV-1, either cause lymphoma directly, or induce conditions such as immunosuppression and chronic antigenic stimulation that foster increased

NHL risk. Acquired immunodeficiency syndrome (AIDS), for example, is associated with over a 100-fold increased incidence of NHL, usually high-grade B-cell tumors (35). Hepatitis C virus infection has been linked with DLBCL and marginal zone lymphomas (26). Immunosuppression, unrelated to viral infections, also can result in abnormal immune regulation and is known to be associated with an increased risk of lymphomas (13). Autoimmune diseases are also associated with increased risk of lymphoma (2). Various immunomodulator agents used to treat autoimmune diseases appear to increase lymphoma risk, although it is difficult to separate the relative contributions of the primary disease versus the therapeutic agents (2).

Epidemiologic data suggest that farmers and other agricultural workers have an increased risk of NHL, particularly DLBCL and follicular lymphoma, and exposure to herbicides and pesticides is thought a likely explanation (5,6,12). This risk appears be particularly true for lymphomas associated with t(14;18)(q32;q21) (9). Unfortunately, it is difficult to quantify exposure to a specific chemical as often there are confounding factors such as exposure to multiple chemicals, animal pathogens, and sunlight, making it difficult to specifically ascertain risk. Prolonged exposure to hair dyes is associated with increased risk of NHLs, especially indolent B-cell lymphomas (47). In 1979, however, the United States Food and Drug Administration issued a warning and subsequently manufacturers changed their formulations to remove potential carcinogens.

A number of other factors have been suggested as increasing or decreasing NHL risk. A higher body mass index appears to be a risk factor for certain types of lymphoma, such as DLBCL and follicular lymphoma (26). Atopic disorders may have a protective effect against a number of NHL types (26). Meat (versus fish) consumption, alcohol use, and tobacco use have been suggested as increasing risk, but there is no consensus in the literature (3,13,31). It is possible that alcohol could have a protective effect from NHLs, but this is not clearly established (26,40). Despite the prominent role of tobacco use in the pathogenesis of many cancers, its role in NHL risk appears to be mild at most (11). Cigarette smoking appears to increase the risk of follicular lymphoma (26). Ultraviolet radiation has been suggested to decrease NHL risk in some studies (25,26). Blood transfusions have been correlated with increased risk of NHL, potentially due to transmission of an oncogenic virus, engraftment of lymphoma cells from the donor, or transfusion-associated immunosuppression (13). Nevertheless, the role of blood transfusion in the risk of NHL is currently not established.

Some therapeutic agents cause an immunodysregulatory state that clinically mimics lymphoma, but usually this state resolves once the therapy is discontinued. For example, dilantin therapy can cause rapid onset of widespread lymphadenopathy that histologically may resemble DLBCL, peripheral T-cell lymphoma, or angioimmunoblastic T-cell lymphoma. Some have hypothesized that these patients could be at increased risk of NHL (3,5,13). Few long-term studies, however, are currently available to support this hypothesis.

REFERENCES

1. Anderson JR, Armitage JO, Weisenburger DD. Epidemiology of the non-Hodgkin's lymphomas: distributions of the major subtypes differ by geographic locations. Non-Hodgkin's Lymphoma Classification Project. Ann Oncol 1998;9:717-720.
2. Baecklund E, Smedby KE, Sutton LA, Askling J, Rosenquist R. Lymphoma development in patients with autoimmune and inflammatory disorders—what are the driving forces? Semin Cancer Biol 2014;24:61-70.
3. Blinder V, Fisher SG; Lymphoma Research Foundation, New York. The role of environmental factors in the etiology of lymphoma. Cancer Invest 2008;26:306-316.
4. Berndt SI, Skibola CF, Joseph V, et al. Genome-wide association study identifies multiple risk loci for chronic lymphocytic leukemia. Nat Genet 2013;45:868-876.
5. Boffeta PI. Epidemiology of adult non-Hodgkin lymphoma. Ann Oncol 2011;22(Suppl 4): iv27-iv31.
6. Brauner EV, Sorensen M, Gaudreau E, et al. A prospective study of organochlorines in adipose tissue and risk of non-Hodgkin lymphoma. Environ Health Perspect 2012;120:105-111.
7. Cabrera ME, Martinez V, Nathwani BN, et al. Non-Hodgkin lymphoma in Chile: a review of 207 consecutive adult cases by a panel of five expert hematopathologists. Leuk Lymphoma 2012;53:1311-1317.
8. Chihara D, Ito H, Matsuo K. Comparison of the incidence and trends of hematologic malignancies between Japan and the United States. Rinsho Ketsueki 2015;56:368-374.
9. Chiu BC, Dave BJ, Blair A, Gapstur SM, Zahm SH, Weisenburger DD. Agricultural pesticide use and risk of t(14;18)-defined subtypes of non-Hodgkin lymphoma. Blood 2006;108:1363-1369.
10. Combariza JF, Lombana M, Torres AM, Castellanos AM, Arango M. General features and epidemiology of lymphoma in Colombia. A multicentric study. Ann Hematol 2015;94:975-980.
11. Conde L, Halperin E. Akers NK, et al. Genome-wide association study of follicular lymphoma identified a risk locus at 6p21.32. Nat Genet 2010;42:661-664.
12. Eriksson M, Hardell L, Carlberg M, Akerman M. Pesticide exposure as risk factor for non-Hodgkin lymphoma including histopathological subgroup analysis. Int J Cancer 2008;123:1657-1663.
13. Fisher S, Fisher RI. The epidemiology of non-Hodgkin's lymphoma. Oncogene 2004;23:6524-6534.
14. Goldin LR, Pfeiffer RM, Gridley G, et al. Familial aggregation of Hodgkin lymphoma and related tumors. Cancer 2004;100:1902-1908
15. Greiner TC, Medeiros LJ, Jaffe ES. Non-Hodgkin lymphoma. Cancer 1995;75(1 Suppl):370-380.
16. Gutensohn NM. Social class and age at diagnosis of Hodgkin's disease: new epidemiologic evidence for the "two disease hypothesis." Cancer Treat Rep 1982;66:689-695.
17. Hartge P, Devesa SS. Quantification of the impact of known risk factors on time trends in non-Hodgkin lymphoma incidence. Cancer Res 1992;52:5566S-5569S.
17a. Intragumtornchai T, Bunworasate U, Wudhikarn K, et al. Non-Hodgkin lymphoma in South East Asia: An analysis of the histopathology, clinical features, and survival from Thailand. Hematol Oncol 2017. [Epub ahead of print]
18. Jaffe ES, Harris NL, Stein H, et al. Introduction and overview of the classification of the lymphoid neoplasms. In: Swerdlow SH, Campo E, Harris NL, et al., eds. WHO classification of tumours of haematopoietic and lymphoid tissues. Lyon: IARC Press; 2008;165-166.
19. Kamper-Jorgensen M, Rostgaard K, Glaser SL, et al. Cigarette smoking and risk of Hodgkin lymphoma and its subtypes: a pooled analysis from the International Lymphoma Epidemiology Consortium (InterLymph). Ann Oncol 2013;24:2245-2255.
20. Khalil MO, Morton LM, Devesa SS, et al. Incidence of marginal zone lymphoma in the United States, 2001-2009 with a focus on primary anatomic site. Br J Haematol 2014;165:67-77.

21. Laurini JA, Perry AM, Boilesen E, et al. Classification of non-Hodgkin lymphoma in Central and South America: a review of 1028 cases. Blood 2012;120:4795-4801.

22. Liang XS, Caporaso N, McMaster ML, et al. Common genetic variants in candidate genes and risk of familial malignancies. Br J Haematol 2009;146;418-423.

23. Magrath I. Epidemiology: clues to the pathogenesis of Burkitt lymphoma. Br J Haematol 2012;156:744-756.

24. Medeiros LJ, Greiner TC. Hodgkin's disease. Cancer 1995;75(1 Suppl):357-369.

25. Monnereau A, Glaser SL, Schupp CW, et al. Exposure to UV radiation and risk of Hodgkin lymphoma: a pooled analysis. Blood 2013;122:3492-3499.

26. Morton LM, Slager SL, Cerhan JR, et al. Etiologic heterogeneity among non-Hodgkin lymphoma subtypes: the InterLymph Non-Hodgkin Lymphoma Subtypes Project. J Natl Cancer Inst Monogr 2014;Aug2014:130-144.

27. Morton LM, Wang SS, Devesa SS, Hartge P, Weisenburger DD, Linet MS. Lymphoma incidence patterns by WHO subtype in the United States, 1992-2001. Blood 2006;107:265-276.

28. Mueller N, Evans A, Harris NL, et al. Hodgkin's disease and Epstein-Barr virus. Altered antibody pattern before diagnosis. N Engl J Med 1989;320: 689-695.

29. Muller AMS, Ihorst G, Mertelsmann R, Englehardt M. Epidemiology of non-Hodgkin's lymphoma (NHL); trends, geographic distribution, and etiology. Ann Hematol 2005;84:1-12.

30. [No authors listed.] A clinical evaluation of the International Lymphoma Study Group classification of Non-Hodgkin's lymphoma. The Non-Hodgkin's Lymphoma Classification Project. Blood 1997;89:3909-3918.

31. Olberding NJ, Aschebrook-Kilfoy B, Caces DB, Smith SM, Weisenburger DD, Chiu BC. Dietary patterns and the risk of non-Hodgkin lymphoma. Public Health Nutr 2014;17:1531-1537.

31a. Oliveira PD, de Carvalho RF, Bittencourt AL. Adult T-cell leukemia/lymphoma in South and Central America and the Caribbean: systematic search and review. Int J STD AIDS 2017;28:217-228.

32. Perry AM, Diebold J, Nathwani BN, et al. Non-Hodgkin lymphoma in the developing world: review of 4539 cases from the International Non-Hodgkin Lymphoma Classification Project. Haematologica 2016;101:1244-1250.

33. Saarinen S, Aavikko M, Aittomaki K, et al. Exome sequencing reveals germline NPAT mutation as a candidate risk factor for Hodgkin lymphoma. Blood 2011;118:493-498.

34. Salipante SJ, Mealiffe ME, Wechsler J, et al. Mutations in a gene encoding a midbody kelch protein in familial and sporadic classical Hodgkin lymphoma lead to binucleated cells. Proc Natl Acad Sci U S A 2009;106:14920-14925.

35. Shiels MS, Engels EA, Linet MS, et al. The epidemic of non-Hodgkin lymphoma in the United States: disentangling the effect of HIV, 1992-2009. Cancer Epidemiol Biomarkers Prev 2013;22:1069-1078.

36. Siegel RL, Miller KD, Jemal A. Cancer statistics, 2015. CA Cancer J Clin 2015;65:5-29.

37. Shirley MH, Sayeed S, Barnes I, Finlayson A, Ali R. Incidence of haematological malignancies by ethnic group in England, 2001-7. Br J Haematol 2013;163:465-477.

38. Shankland KR, Armitage JO, Hancock BW. Non-Hodgkin lymphoma. Lancet 2012;380:848-857.

39. Stewart BW, Kleihues P. World Cancer Report. IARC Press, 2003.

39a. Teras LR, DeSantis CE, Cerhan JR, Morton LM, Jemal A, Flowers CR. 2016 US lymphoid malignancy statistics by World Health Organization subtypes. CA Cancer J Clin 2016 [Epub ahead of print]

40. Tramacere I, Pelucchi C, Bonifazi M, et al. Alcohol drinking and non-Hodgkin lymphoma risk: a systematic review and a meta-analysis. Ann Oncol 2012;23:2791-2798.

41. Van Leeuwen MT, Turner JJ, Joske DJ, et al. Lymphoid neoplasm incidence by WHO subtype in Australia 1982-2006. Int J Cancer 2014;135:2146-2156.

42. Vose J, Armitage J, Weisenburger D; International T-Cell Lymphoma Project. International peripheral T-cell and natural killer/T-cell lymphoma study: pathology findings and clinical outcomes. J Clin Oncol 2008;26:4124-4130.

43. Wang SS, Slager SL, Brennan P, et al. Family history of hematopoietic malignancies and risk of non-Hodgkin lymphoma (NHL): a pooled analysis of 10,211 cases and 11,905 controls from the International Lymphoma Epidemiology Consortium (InterLymph). Blood 2007;109:3479-3488.

44. Wang XM, Bassig BA, Wen JJ, et al. Clinical analysis of 1629 newly diagnosed malignant lymphomas in current residents of Sichuan province, China. Hematol Oncol 2016;34:193-199.

45. Wu XC, Andrews P, Chen VW, Groves FD. Incidence of extranodal non-Hodgkin lymphomas among whites, blacks, and Asians/Pacific Islanders in the United States: anatomic site and histology differences. Cancer Epidemiol 2009;33:337-346.

46. Yaqo RT, Hughson MD, Sulayvani FK, Al-Allawi NA. Malignant lymphoma in northern Iraq: a retrospective analysis of 270 cases according to the World Health Organization classification. Indian J Cancer 2011;48:446-451.

47. Zahm SH, Weisenburger DD, Babbitt PA, Saal RC, Vaught JB, Blair A. Use of hair coloring products and the risk of lymphoma, multiple myeloma, and chronic lymphocytic leukemia. Am J Public Health 1992;82:990-997.

INFECTIOUS ORGANISMS AND LYMPHOMAS

In the first decade of the 20th century, two Danish scientists, Vilhelm Ellerman and Oluf Bang, suggested a role for a virus in the transmission of avian erythroblastosis (54). Shortly thereafter, Francis Peyton Rous performed experiments that further suggested viral transmission of sarcomas in chickens. Over the remainder of the 20th century, the role of viruses and other infectious agents in oncogenesis became well established. Viruses are involved in the pathogenesis of hepatocellular carcinoma (hepatitis B), cervical carcinoma (human papillomaviruses), Kaposi sarcoma (human herpesvirus 8), and Merkel cell carcinomas (Merkel cell polyomavirus) (54). Viruses, as well as bacterial and parasitic infections, also have a role in lymphomagenesis. In this chapter, we focus on the association between infectious agents and lymphomas.

Infectious agents can induce or contribute to lymphomagenesis via direct or indirect mechanisms (fig. 9-1). Some infectious agents (mainly viruses) have direct oncogenic effects. They infect lymphocytes and participate directly in the neoplastic transformation of a cell either in the form of nuclear episomes or integration of the cellular DNA. Epstein-Barr virus (EBV), human herpesvirus 8 (HHV-8), and human T-cell lymphotropic virus type 1 (HTLV-1) are examples of lymphotropic viruses. These viruses activate cellular proto-oncogenes or inhibit tumor suppressor genes which eventually leads to dysregulation of the cellular signaling pathways involved in cell proliferation and survival.

Some infectious agents have indirect oncogenic effects. They do not infect lymphocytes directly, but cause immunodeficiency or induce chronic antigenic stimulation, prolonging lymphocyte lifespan and thereby increasing the likelihood of the occurrence of genetic abnormalities. Eventually a genetic "hit" arises that provides a growth advantage and, combined with other factors, leads to lymphoma. Human immunodeficiency virus (HIV), hepatitis C virus, and various bacterial organisms are examples of microorganisms that primarily induce lymphomagenesis indirectly (although they also have direct effects).

Figure 9-1

DIRECT AND INDIRECT LYMPHOMAGENESIS

Schematic showing direct and indirect mechanisms that viruses employ in lymphomagenesis. HTLV-I, human T-cell lymphotropic virus type 1; HIV, human immunodeficiency virus; HCV, hepatitis virus type C; EBV, Epstein-Barr virus; HHV-8, human herpesvirus type 8.

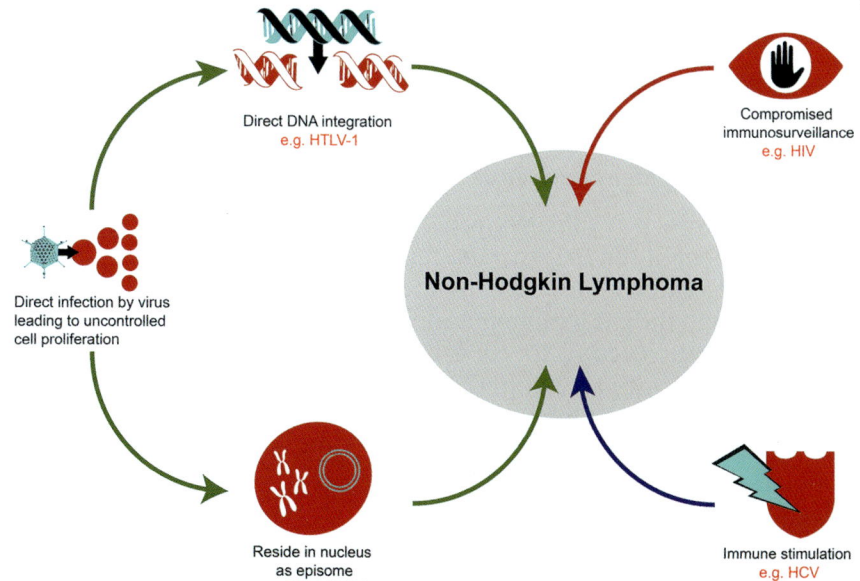

Direct DNA integration
e.g. HTLV-1

Compromised immunosurveillance
e.g. HIV

Direct infection by virus leading to uncontrolled cell proliferation

Non-Hodgkin Lymphoma

Reside in nucleus as episome
e.g. EBV, HHV-8

Immune stimulation
e.g. HCV

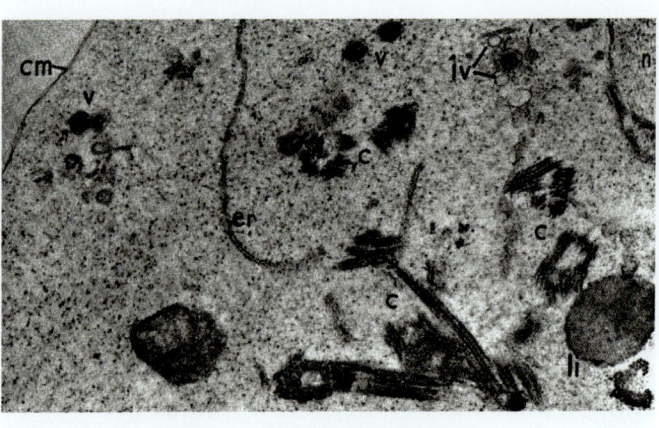

Figure 9-2

EPSTEIN-BARR VIRUS

Top: Original electron micrograph (X42,500) showing part of a lymphoblast from a Burkitt lymphoma that contains virus particles, as published by Epstein, Achong, and Barr in 1964. V, indicates the presence of virions; IV, immature virus particles; C, crystals; cm, cytoplasmic cell membrane (in the top left corner); n, nucleus (right corner); li, large lipid body; and er, endoplasmic reticulum. Numerous ribosomes are present throughout the cytoplasm. (Figure 1 from Epstein MA, Achong G, Barr YM. Virus particles in cultured lymphoblasts from Burkitt's lymphoma. Lancet 1964;283:702.)

Bottom: Schematic diagram of the circular EBV episome (a double-stranded circular form of the genome). There is clustering of open reading frames (ORF) for Epstein-Barr nuclear antigen (EBNA) and latent membrane proteins (LMP). Green arrows denote the direction of transcription during latency III. The short red arrow indicates the direction of transcription for EBNA1, activated during latency 1 and II. TR, terminal repeats; OriP (in orange), the origin for latent infection EBV episome replication, has plasmid maintenance and DNA replication activity. LMP1 transcription has an opposite direction to the other gene transcripts. LMP2A and -B can be only transcribed when EBV exists as an episome because of the gene span across the TR. In latency III, EBNA1 transcription begins from Cp (C promoter) or Wp (W promoter), whereas it starts from Qp (Q promoter) in latency I or II.

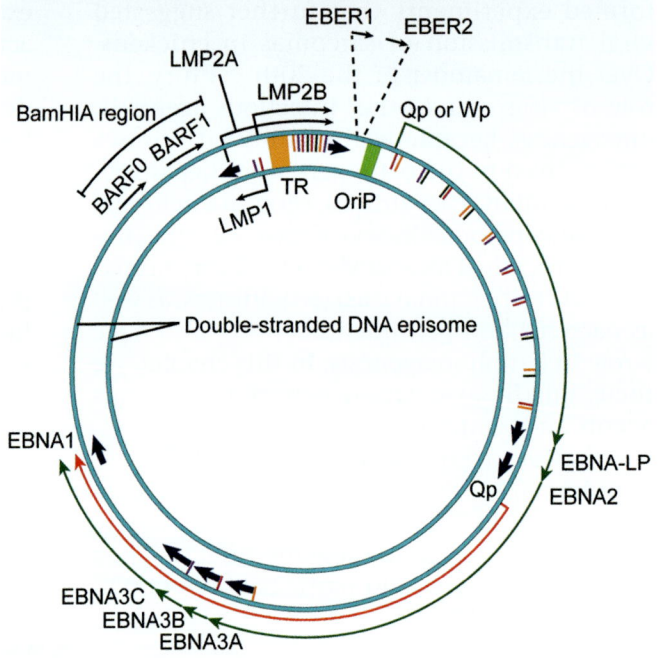

ORGANISMS WITH DIRECT ONCOGENIC EFFECTS

Epstein-Barr Virus

EBV, also known as *human herpesvirus 4 (HHV-4)*, is a member of the *Herpesviridae* family. EBV was the first human tumor virus discovered, cultured from a Burkitt lymphoma and observed by electron microscopy in 1964 by Epstein, Achong, and Barr (fig. 9-2, top) (27). EBV is one of the most common viruses to infect humans and approximately 90 percent of the world's population is seropositive for EBV. The viral infection has lytic and latent phases.

EBV has linear double-stranded DNA, an icosadeltahedral capsid, 162 capsomers, and an envelope. The EBV genome is about 172,000 base pairs and contains about 85 genes (7). The open reading frames (ORFs) are organized into separate lytic and latent sections. The ORFs for the latent membrane protein (LMP) and Epstein-Barr nuclear antigen (EBNA) proteins are clustered separately within the episome (fig. 9-2, bottom).

Primary EBV infection is often asymptomatic and usually occurs in childhood, but EBV causes infectious mononucleosis in 30 to 50 percent of adolescents and young adults. The virus is transmitted by saliva, as nearly all seropositive persons actively shed virus in the saliva. EBV can infect several cell types, including epithelial cells, monocytes, and B, T, and natural killer

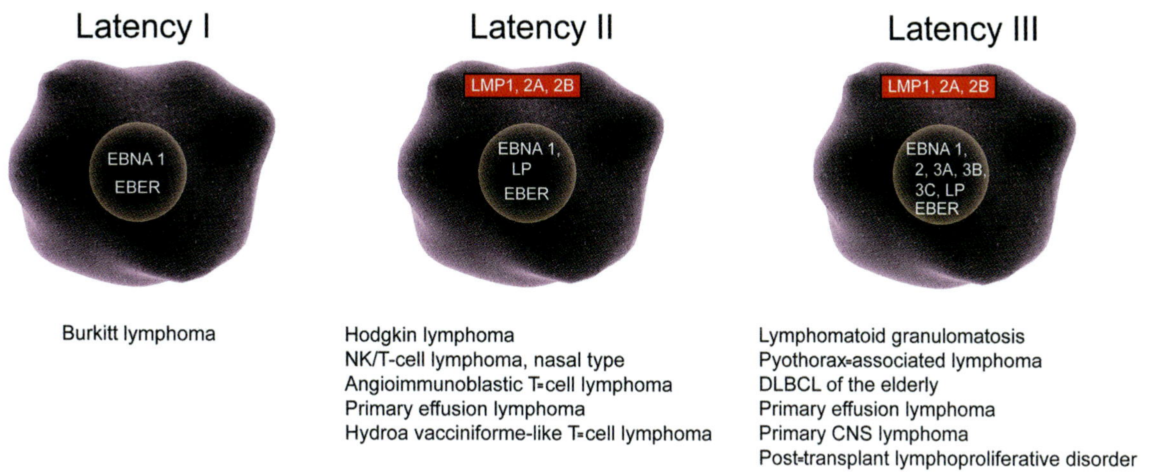

Figure 9-3

PATTERNS OF EBV GENE EXPRESSION IN DIFFERENT TYPES OF LATENCY

Below each latency program type are the lymphoma subtypes associated with them. For example, in latency type I, only EBV nuclear antigen 1 (EBNA1) and EBV small encoded RNA (EBER) are expressed and this program is characteristic of Burkitt lymphoma. (LMP = latent membrane protein; LP = leader protein.)

(NK) cells, but the virus has a special predilection for B cells. Infection of B cells occurs within the lymphoid organs of the oropharynx and is mediated by CD21 (formerly called CR2) and the viral glycoproteins (gp)350 and gp42. CD21 is also the receptor for the C3d component of complement. Normal mature and immature T cells express low and high levels of CD21, respectively; NK cells acquire CD21 by synaptic transfer from B cells (31,73,75). The virus is cleared by cytotoxic CD8-positive T cells.

The life cycle of EBV, and herpesviruses in general, is biphasic, with phases of lytic replication and latency. Lytic replication, or productive infection, results in the production of EBV virions. At the time of primary infection, there is brief and usually confined replication of the virus in epithelial cells. During lytic replication, viral DNA polymerase is responsible for copying the viral EBV genome. Other lytic proteins include gp350 and gp110. Unlike lytic replication for many other viruses, EBV lytic replication does not inevitably lead to the death of the host cells because EBV virions are produced by cell budding. Viral replication is spontaneously activated in a small percentage of latently infected B cells and in plasma cells (39). The commonly used antiviral agent acyclovir is only effective against lytic-replicating viruses and has no activity on latent infection.

Latency does not result in the production of virions but rather represents a viral strategy for eluding recognition of infected cells by the immune system. A resting memory B cell is the site of persistence of EBV within the body. The virus persists inside the nucleus of B cells as an episome and is copied by cellular DNA polymerase. EBV rarely integrates into cellular DNA and only has been reported in EBV-associated B-cell lymphomas, but not in classic Hodgkin lymphoma (HL) or T-cell lymphomas (57). In latent EBV infection, only 10 viral genes are expressed in vitro and there are three main latency programs (latency types III, II, and I) (26,75,76). These programs were initially discovered in cell lines but also relate to the biology of EBV in vivo. Different latency programs are found in different types of lymphomas (fig. 9-3).

EBV latency within B cells usually progresses from type III to II to I. Upon infecting a resting naive B cell, EBV enters type III latency (in which all latency genes are expressed). The set of proteins and RNAs produced in type III latency transforms the B cell into a proliferating blast. Later, the virus restricts its gene expression and enters into type II latency with expression of EBNA1, LMP1, and LMP2. During type II latency, B cells differentiate into memory B cells. Finally, EBV restricts gene expression even further and enters into type I latency (in which only EBNA1 and Epstein-Barr encoded RNA [EBER]

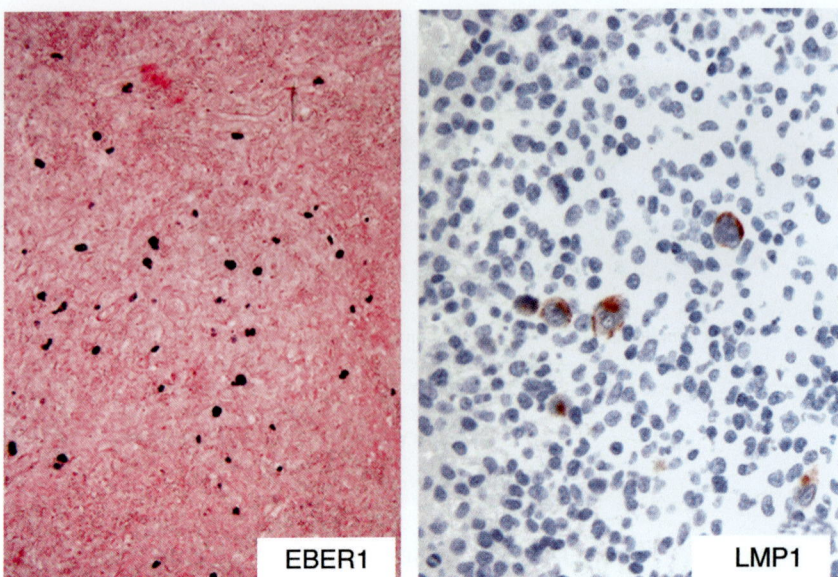

Figure 9-4

EBV LATENCY TYPE II IN CLASSIC HODGKIN LYMPHOMA

The Hodgkin and Reed-Sternberg cells express EBER1 and EBV latent membrane protein type 1 (LMP1) as detected by in situ hybridization and immunohistochemistry, respectively.

are expressed). Expression of EBNA1 allows the EBV genome to replicate when the host memory B cell divides.

EBV-Associated Lymphomas

EBV is associated with the development of classic HL and B- and NK/T-cell non-Hodgkin lymphomas (NHLs). Most EBV-related NHLs are of B-cell lineage and include Burkitt lymphoma, lymphomatoid granulomatosis, pyothorax-associated lymphoma, a small subset of diffuse large B cell lymphomas (DLBCL), and immunodeficiency-associated lymphomas.

Classic Hodgkin Lymphoma. Several lines of evidence strongly point to an association between EBV infection and classic HL (see chapters 38–41). Patients with a history of infectious mononucleosis have an increased risk of HL (38): the virus is present in approximately 40 percent of HL cases in industrialized nations, and in more than 90 percent of pediatric cases in Central America. The virus is most common in the mixed cellularity type of HL (up to 75 percent of cases).

When present, EBV is found in virtually all of the Reed-Sternberg and Hodgkin cells (78,82), and is present in monoclonal form (57,84). These findings suggest that EBV infection is an early event, present before neoplastic transformation. EBV-positive HL cases are characterized by a type II latency program (with expression of EBNA1 and LMP1 and -2) (fig. 9-4).

The role of EBV in the pathogenesis of classic HL is only partially understood. LMP-1 is a transmembrane protein that activates CD40, a molecule involved in activating the NF-κB pathway and other signals that provide survival and proliferative signals to tumor cells (29). However, other cofactors acting in concert with EBV infection are required to give rise to HL. One example of the abundant data that support this statement is that the risk of subsequent HL in a patient who develops infectious mononucleosis is very low, on the order of 1 case per 1,000 persons, suggesting that EBV infection alone is insufficient to cause HL (38).

Burkitt Lymphoma. Burkitt lymphoma (BL) is classified into three types that differ in geographic distribution and EBV association: endemic, sporadic, and immunodeficiency-associated (see chapter 25) (50). EBV has been detected in 95 percent of patients with endemic BL (equatorial belt of Africa, Brazil, New Guinea, and other countries), 20 to 30 percent of sporadic cases (industrialized nations), and 30 to 40 percent of the immunodeficiency-related cases (50). The tumor cells carry monoclonal EBV, suggesting that viral infection precedes neoplastic transformation. EBV-positive BL is usually characterized by a type I latency program; the tumors express EBNA1 and EBER1 (84). LMP1 is not expressed in BL (fig. 9-5).

Other infectious agents are associated with BL. There is an association with HIV infection.

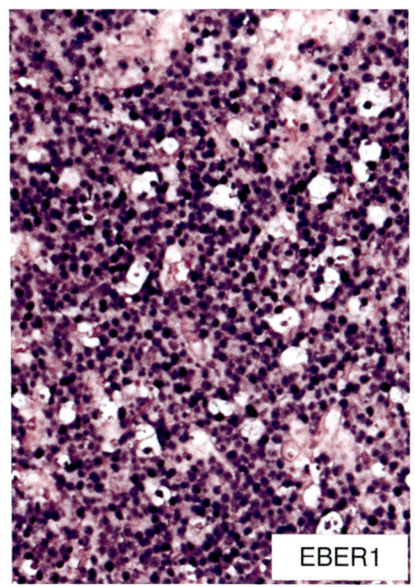
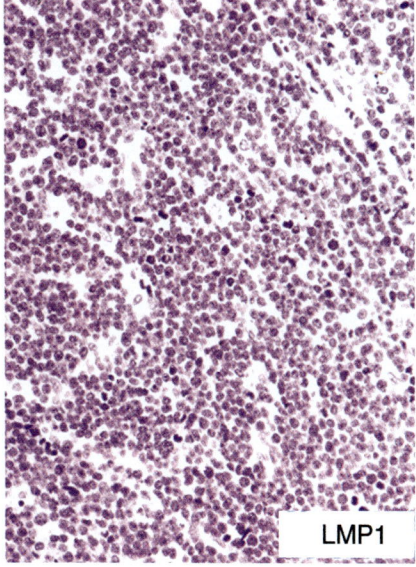

EBER1

LMP1

Figure 9-5

EBV LATENCY TYPE I IN BURKITT LYMPHOMA

The tumor cells express EBER1 (as detected by in situ hybridization) and are characteristically negative for LMP1 (immunohistochemistry), indicating type I latency.

This relationship is clear in industrialized nations, but the role of HIV infection in the pathogenesis of endemic BL in Africa is uncertain. In areas endemic for infection by *Plasmodium falciparum* (malaria), parasitic infection induces B-cell hyperplasia, activates memory B cells, and predisposes patients to BL. Moreover, malarial infection may have a direct role in the genesis of the chromosomal translocations associated with BL (50).

Plasmablastic Lymphoma. Plasmablastic lymphoma (PBL), a neoplasm with morphologic and immunophenotypic features of plasmablasts, was originally described in patients with HIV infection (see chapter 23) (21). This neoplasm typically arises in extranodal sites and is commonly diagnosed in the setting of immunodeficiency (49,79); it is also seen in patients without known immunodeficiency including the elderly. EBV is positive in about 75 percent of cases and HHV-8 is negative (fig. 9-6). EBV expression is usually restricted to EBERs (latency type I) but LMP-1 is expressed in some cases (21,33,79).

DLBCL Associated with Chronic Inflammation. Pyothorax-associated lymphoma is the prototype of this lymphoma category in the World Health Organization (WHO) classification (71a). Pyothorax-associated lymphoma occurs primarily in the pleura of patients with longstanding pleural inflammation that results from therapeutic artificial pneumothorax (the most significant risk factor) or tuberculosis

pleuritis (5). Pyothorax-associated lymphoma is associated with latent EBV but not HHV-8 infection. Most cases have been reported in Japan; these tumors are rare in Western countries. Pyothorax-associated lymphoma is characterized by a type III latency program with expression of EBNA1, EBNA2, LMP1 and EBER1 (5).

A microscopic tumor with morphologic and immunophenotypic features similar to pyothorax-associated lymphoma has been reported in restricted body spaces with chronic inflammation or suppurative conditions such as joints or pseudocysts (11,17). It is unclear whether these tumors should be grouped with pyothorax-associated lymphoma or whether they deserve their own unique category (11).

Lymphomatoid Granulomatosis. Lymphomatoid granulomatosis (LYG) is an extranodal EBV-positive B-cell lymphoproliferative disorder that typically involves the lungs; virtually all patients have pulmonary disease at some point during their clinical course (44,63). Other organs may be involved including skin, kidney, central nervous system, adrenal gland, and gastrointestinal tract. Lymphadenopathy and splenomegaly are uncommon. Morphologically, lung lesions are characterized by multifocal angiocentric and angiodestructive lesions composed predominantly of reactive T cells with a variable number of EBV-positive neoplastic B cells. EBV infection in LYG commonly shows a type III latency program (75).

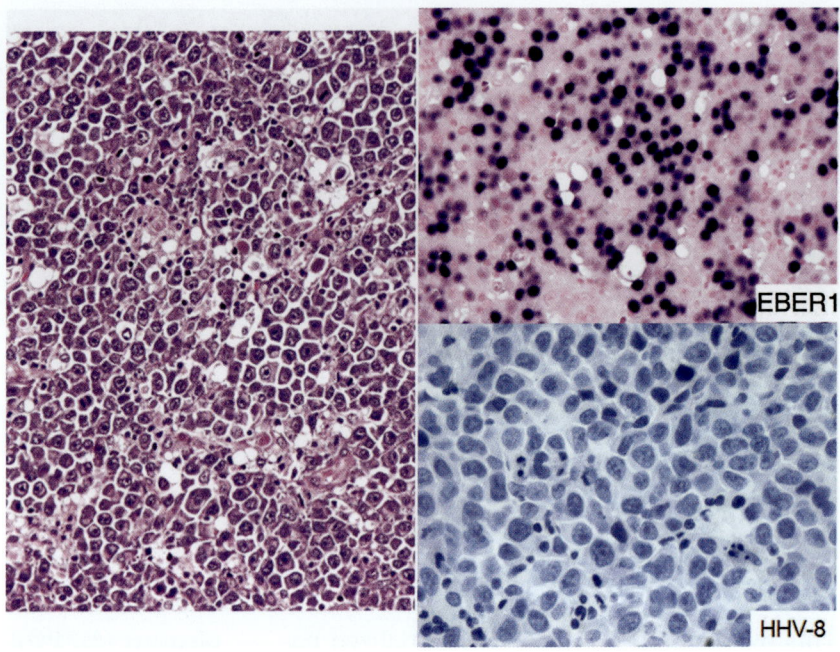

Figure 9-6

PLASMABLASTIC LYMPHOMA

The tumor cells are intermediate to large, with eccentric vesicular nuclei and distinct nucleoli (H&E stain). They express EBER1 (as detected by in situ hybridization) and are negative for human herpesvirus 8 (HHV-8).

In situ hybridization for EBER1 is positive in a variable number of the large neoplastic B cells (fig. 9-7), as is LMP-1. LYG lesions are graded by the number of EBV-positive neoplastic B cells and the extent of the necrosis (63). Grade 1 lesions are highly polymorphic, with few large cells and minimal, if any, necrosis. These lesions show less than 5 EBER1-positive cells per high-power field. Grade 2 lesions have a greater number of large cells, often in small clusters; show areas of necrosis; and have 5 to 20 EBER1-positive cells per high-power field. Grade 3 lesions have many large cells, often forming large aggregates and often associated with extensive necrosis; typically, there are more than 20 EBER1-positive cells per high-power field. These lesions resemble EBV-positive large B-cell lymphoma, but with prominent inflammatory cells in the background. The B-cell proliferation rate, as shown by Ki-67, correlates with the grade. Patients with grade 3 LYG are treated similarly to patients with DLBCL not otherwise specified, but the prognosis of LYG patients is poorer. Patients with low-grade LYG are managed more conservatively (67).

EBV-Positive DLBCL. This tumor in the WHO classification is defined as an EBV-positive DLBCL in a patient without any known immunodeficiency or prior lymphoma (71a). Previously, an age cutoff of 50 years was included in the disease definition, but this cutoff was arbitrary; similar tumors occur in younger patients. EBV-positive DLBCL often involves extranodal sites and the clinical course of patients is usually aggressive (58,71a). Large atypical cells forming prominent aggregates are easily observed and there is extensive necrosis. Polymorphic and monomorphic variants have been described, with a similar prognosis. EBV-positive DLBCL usually has a type III latency program (fig. 9-8), although some cases lack EBNA2 expression (latency type II). Currently, there are no consensus criteria for the percentage of EBV-positive cells required to establish the diagnosis.

Primary DLBCL of the Central Nervous System. Most DLBCLs arising in the brain occur in elderly patients and EBV is absent. Immunosuppressed patients, however, usually those who are HIV positive, can develop EBV-positive DLBCL of the brain (12). Primary DLBCL of the central nervous system has been reported to have a type III latency program with expression of LMP-1 and EBNA-2 (12).

Post-Transplant Lymphoproliferative Disorders. This is a heterogeneous group that occurs as a consequence of depressed T-cell function (due to immunosuppressive therapy) in the setting of solid organ or stem cell hematopoietic allografts (see chapter 47). Post-transplant lymphoproliferative disorders (PTLDs) are

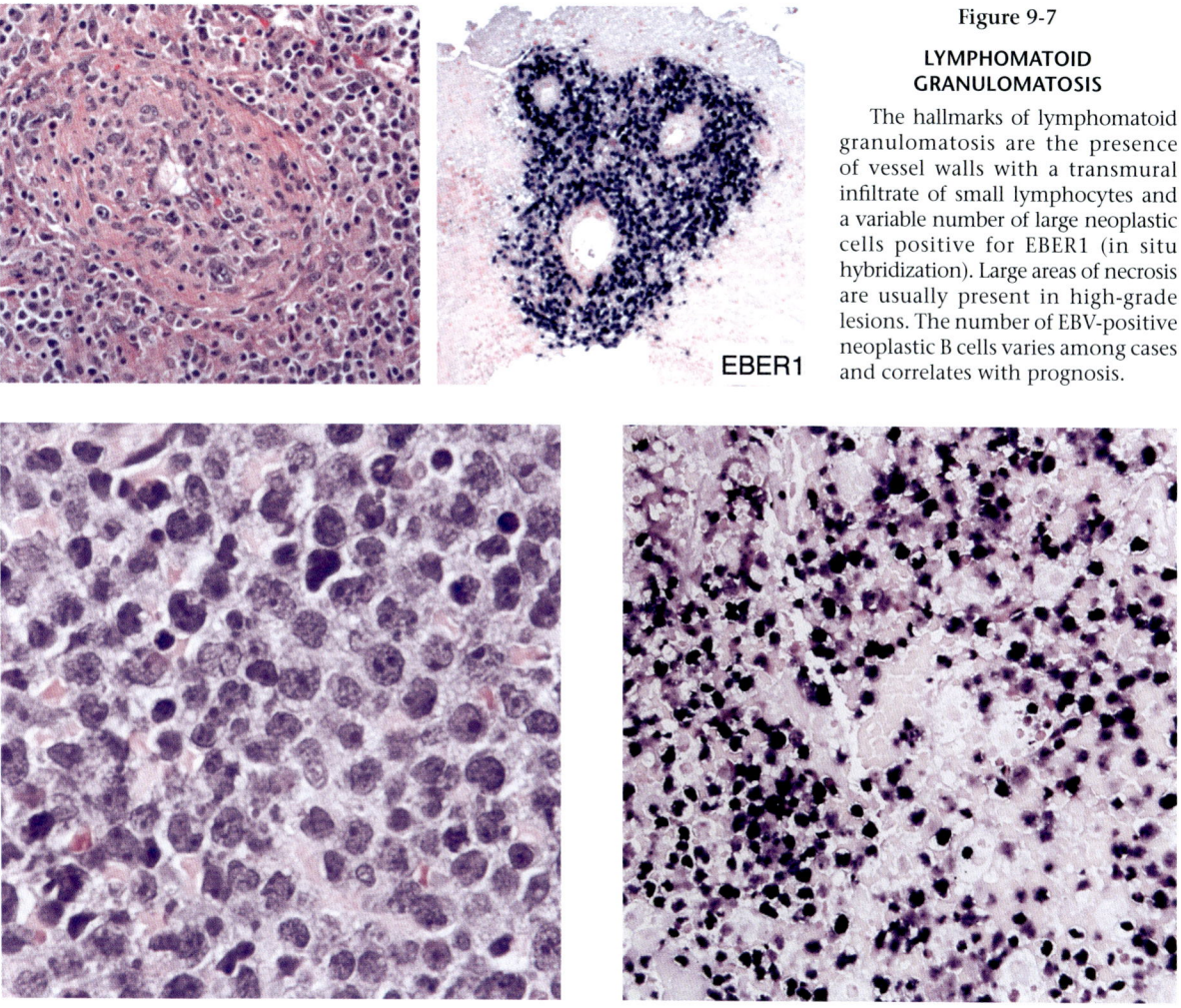

Figure 9-7

LYMPHOMATOID GRANULOMATOSIS

The hallmarks of lymphomatoid granulomatosis are the presence of vessel walls with a transmural infiltrate of small lymphocytes and a variable number of large neoplastic cells positive for EBER1 (in situ hybridization). Large areas of necrosis are usually present in high-grade lesions. The number of EBV-positive neoplastic B cells varies among cases and correlates with prognosis.

EBER1

Figure 9-8

EBV-POSITIVE DIFFUSE LARGE B-CELL LYMPHOMA (DLBCL)

This case involved the thigh of a 58-year-old man. Many tumor cells express EBER1 (left: H&E stain; right: in situ hybridization).

usually of B-cell origin, but 10 to 15 percent are of NK/T-cell origin. Classic HL also arises rarely after transplantation. PTLDs are associated with EBV infection in about 70 percent of cases (28). EBV-associated PTLDs occur early after the transplant, with almost 100 percent occurring within a year. EBV-negative PTLDs are more common in adults and tend to occur later (3 to 5 years after transplant). EBV-positive PTLDs typically display a type III latency pattern (fig. 9-9).

Iatrogenic (Immunomodulator) Lymphoproliferative Disorders. Iatrogenic lymphoproliferative disorders occur in patients receiving immunosuppressive therapy for autoimmune, immunodysregulatory diseases such as rheumatoid arthritis, systemic lupus erythematosus, dermatomyositis, or rarely psoriasis (see chapter 44) (42,43,61). Implicated drugs include methotrexate, azathioprine, tacrolimus, and cyclosporine. There are data also suggesting that tumor necrosis factor (TNF)-α antagonists and other recently developed immunomodulator agents are associated with increased lymphoma risk (36).

The best known examples in this disease category are lymphoproliferative disorders (LPDs) that arise in patients with rheumatoid arthritis treated with methotrexate. Approximately half of the methotrexate-associated LPDs

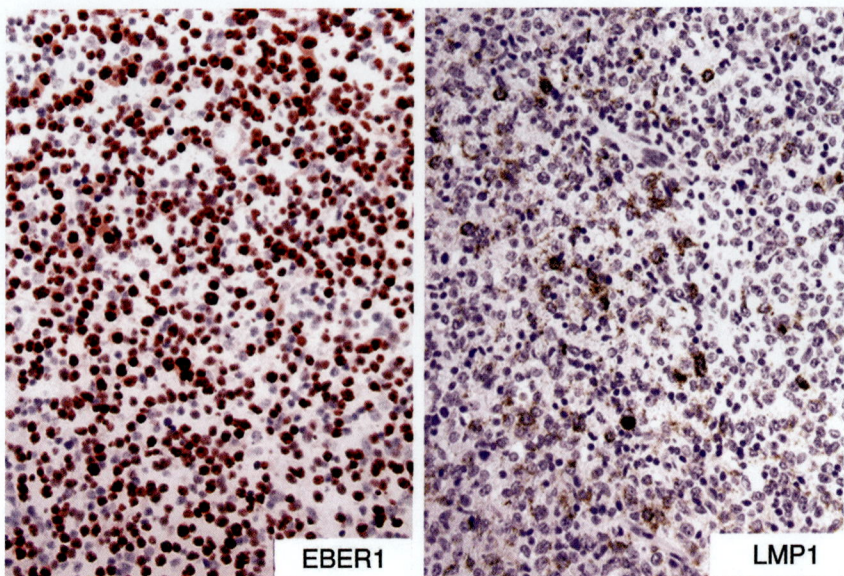

Figure 9-9

POST-TRANSPLANT LYMPHOPROLIFERATIVE DISORDER

This 29-year-old man underwent a kidney transplant 24 years ago. He was on immunosuppressive agents since that time. He developed cervical lymphadenopathy. The lymph node biopsy showed DLBCL that, based on the clinical history, was also monomorphous post-transplant lymphoproliferative disorder. The tumor cells are positive for EBER1 and LMP1.

are EBV-positive and these lesions commonly arise in extranodal sites. The most common histologic variant type is DLBCL in about one third of cases (42), followed by HL and polymorphic post-transplant lymphoproliferative disease (PTLD); other morphologic variants are uncommon (42,43). Patients with inflammatory bowel disease, and particularly Crohn disease, who are treated with a TNF-α inhibitor may have an increased risk of hepatosplenic T-cell lymphoma, but this issue is controversial (82a,85).

First-line therapy of iatrogenic lymphoproliferative disorders is typically reduction or, if possible, discontinuation of the immunosuppressive agent. Spontaneous regression of LPDs has been documented in some patients (42,43). Other patients require lymphoma-specific therapies.

EBV-Associated NK/T-Cell Lymphomas. EBV-associated NK/T-cell lymphomas include extranodal NK/T-cell lymphoma of nasal type (see chapter 35) and angioimmunoblastic T-cell lymphoma (see chapter 31). The WHO classification also recognizes systemic EBV-positive T-cell lymphoma of childhood and hydroa vacciniforme-like T-cell lymphoproliferative disorder.

Nasal-type extranodal NK/T-cell lymphomas usually involve the nasal/upper aerodigestive tract, often in middle-aged men (35,48). This neoplasm is far more prevalent in Asian and Hispanic than Caucasian populations in the United States and Europe. These neoplasms often have an angiocentric and angiodestructive growth pattern. EBV is detected in all cases and these tumors commonly have a type II latency program which includes expression of LMP1, EBNA-1, and EBER (35,48).

Angioimmunoblastic T-Cell Lymphoma. This tumor represents 15 to 20 percent of all peripheral T-cell lymphomas (see chapter 31). Angioimmunoblastic T-cell lymphoma (AITL) commonly affects middle-aged and elderly patients. It is characterized by B-type symptoms, rash, arthralgias, generalized peripheral lymphadenopathy, hepatosplenomegaly, and pleural effusions (22). Common laboratory abnormalities include hemolytic anemia and polyclonal hypergammaglobulinemia.

Although AITL is a T-cell lymphoma, it is common for B cells to be present in the background. The malignant T cells are usually negative for EBV, but the B cells and particularly B immunoblasts in the background are infected by EBV (81). Rarely, EBV-positive large B cells evolve into EBV-positive DLBCL or mimic HL. These EBV-positive B cells usually express a type II latency program, positive for LMP1 and/or EBNA-2.

Systemic EBV-Positive T-Cell Lymphoma of Childhood. This disease is life-threatening in children and young adults, and is characterized by a monoclonal proliferation of EBV-positive T cells with an activated cytotoxic phenotype. The disease is more prevalent in Asian and

Hispanic populations (64,71). It is systemic and nearly always accompanied by a fulminant hemophagocytic syndrome. The infiltrating T cells have minimal cytologic atypia and are positive for CD8, cytotoxic markers, and predominantly T-cell receptor alpha/beta (64). EBER1 is positive in the most of the lymphoid cells and EBV is usually present in monoclonal form (71).

Hydroa Vacciniforme-Like T-Cell Lymphoproliferative Disorder. This lesion is a monoclonal EBV-associated cutaneous lymphoma of NK/T cells (10,15a,16,18). These tumors affect primarily sun-exposed skin areas (face and arms) and are characterized by recurrent papulovesicular eruptions that generally progress to ulcers and then scarring. This neoplasm is more prevalent in Asian and Hispanic populations. The tumor cells are predominantly CD8-positive T cells with a cytotoxic immunophenotype (16). EBER1 is positive in most of the lymphoma cells and the virus is usually present in monoclonal form (10,15a).

Human Herpesvirus 8

Human herpesvirus 8 (HHV-8), also known as *Kaposi sarcoma-associated herpesvirus*, is an oncogenic herpes double-stranded DNA lymphotropic virus with four known major subtypes (A, B, C, and D) (24,47,54,69). HHV-8 is endemic in sub-Saharan Africa with a seroprevalence of 50 to 70 percent (subtypes B and A5) and the Mediterranean region with a seroprevalence of 20 to 30 percent (subtype C). In North America there is a 1 to 3 percent infection rate (subtype A) among asymptomatic blood donors (24).

HHV-8 has tropism for B cells, monocytes, dendritic cells, and epithelial and endothelial cells. Integrin α3β1 (CD49c/29) and DC-SIGN (dendritic cell-specific intercellular adhesion molecule 3-grabbing nonintegrin; CD209) can function as receptors for HHV-8 (1,65). The virus is transmitted through saliva and replicates in oropharyngeal cells. Viral transmission by blood transfusion or transplanted organs has been documented.

HHV-8 has linear double-stranded DNA of approximately 165 kb in size and encodes 87 ORFs and at least 17 microRNAs (fig. 9-10) (54). HHV-8, like other herpesviruses, exhibits a biphasic life cycle with predominant lifelong latent infection and a typically short-lived lytic replication cycle. A striking feature of HHV-8 is

that some of the ORFs (at least 14) encode genes with homology to cellular genes and seem to be "pirated" copies of human genes (56). It is believed that HHV-8 acquired these genes from human host cells and these genes provide HHV-8 with growth and immune evasion advantages (53,54). These viral (v) homolog genes include genes that encode for IL-6 (designated vIL6), vBCL2, vcyclin D, viral G protein-coupled receptor, interferon regulatory factor (vIRF), and Flice inhibitory protein (vFLIP), among others.

Primary HHV-8 infection can cause fever and a maculopapular rash (4), but in most patients, infection goes undetected and the virus persists in a latent state. The lytic phase of HHV-8 infection is characterized by expression of most of the viral genes in an orderly fashion and the production of infectious virion particles. Lytic proteins include K1, vBCL2, vIRFs, vIL6, viral-encoded chemokines, viral-encoded G protein-coupled receptor, and K15.

In the latent phase, HHV-8 does not integrate into cellular DNA and instead exists in the nucleus as an episome (47,54). The major latency phase-associated viral proteins are latency-associated nuclear antigen (LANA), vcyclin, vFLIP, viral encoded microRNA (miRNA), and kaposins (54). LANA maintains the viral episome and also interferes with important host antitumorigenic cellular pathways. LANA inhibits p53 and stabilizes β-catenin, leading to regulation of the Wnt signaling pathway (9,32). Viral-encoded cyclin D is a constitutive activator of cyclin-dependent kinase 6 (CDK6) which drives cellular proliferation and promotes viral replication. vFLIP binds to inhibitor of κB kinase-γ (IKKγ) leading to the direct activation of NF-κB (7). Kaposins contribute to the production of proinflammatory cytokines (51). One characteristic feature of HHV-8 latent infection is that infected cells downregulate cell surface markers, contributing to evasion of host immunity.

The rare lymphomas caused by HHV-8 mostly occur in patients with immunodeficiency. HHV-8 infection is associated with primary effusion lymphoma, multicentric Castleman disease (MCD), and MCD-associated large B-cell lymphoma (14,25,70). It is suspected, however, that HHV-8-associated lymphomas are under-reported in immunocompetent patient populations (47).

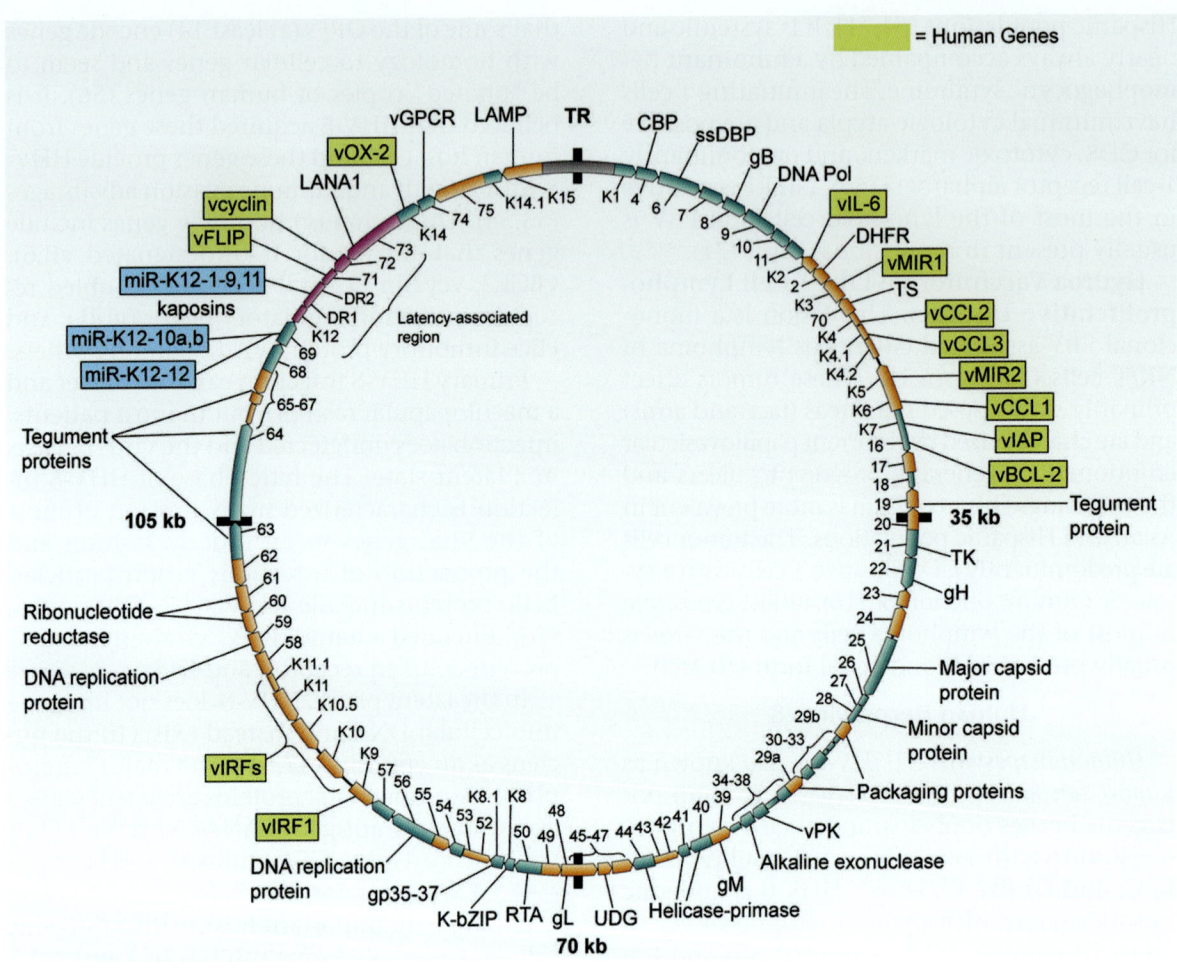

Figure 9-10

HUMAN HERPESVIRUS 8 EPISOME

Schematic diagram of the HHV-8 episome. The circular episome represents a fusion of the terminal repeats (TR) at each end of the linear genome. The episome contains open reading frames (ORFs) which code for viral proteins as well as the set of microRNAs (purple boxes). Some of the ORFs (yellow boxes) are homologous to cellular genes and seem to be "pirated" copies of human genes.

Human Herpesvirus-8–Associated Lymphomas

Primary Effusion Lymphoma. *Primary effusion lymphoma* (PEL), also known as *body cavity-based lymphoma*, is a HHV-8-associated large B-cell neoplasm that most often involves body cavities (pleural, pericardial, or peritoneal cavity) causing effusions without identifiable tumor masses (14,55). PEL is a rare type of lymphoma that occurs most frequently in HIV-infected patients (see chapter 43). PEL represents approximately 4 percent of all acquired immunodeficiency syndrome (AIDS)-related lymphomas but only 0.3 percent of all aggressive lymphomas in HIV-negative patients (47,55). It has been described in older individuals from HHV-8 endemic geographic areas, similar to the population at risk for HIV-negative classic Kaposi sarcoma (47).

HHV-8-positive lymphomas indistinguishable from PEL present on rare occasion as a solid tumor mass and are designated as extracavitary or solid variants of PEL (15,46,60). Pan et al. (60) recently suggested the term Kaposi sarcoma herpesvirus (KSHV)-associated large B-cell lymphoma for these tumors. Extranodal sites are most common, particularly the gastrointestinal tract (fig. 9-11), but lymph nodes are also involved.

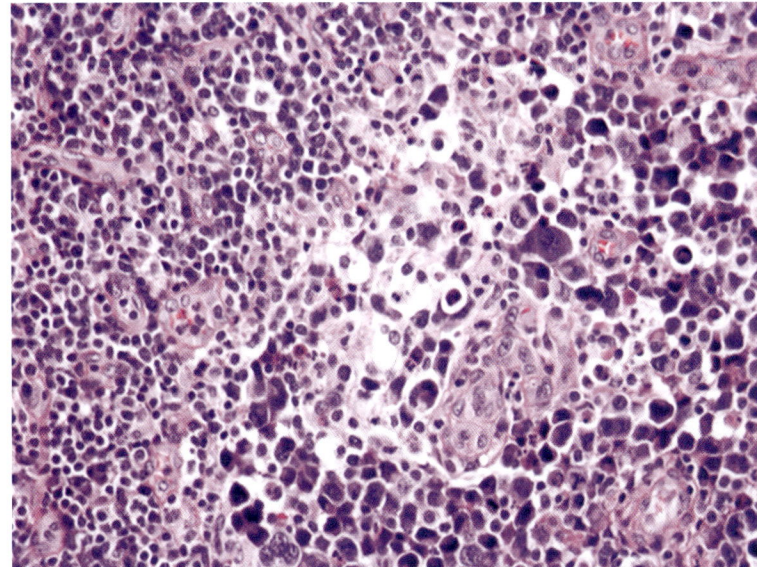

Figure 9-11

EXTRACAVITARY/SOLID VARIANT OF PRIMARY EFFUSION LYMPHOMA (PEL)

The neoplasm has an intrasinusoidal pattern and is composed of large atypical lymphoid cells with anaplastic features (H&E stain).

Figure 9-12

PRIMARY EFFUSION LYMPHOMA IN PLEURAL FLUID

The tumor cells are intermediate in size with irregular nuclear contours and dispersed nuclear chromatin. They are positive for EBER1 and HHV-8.

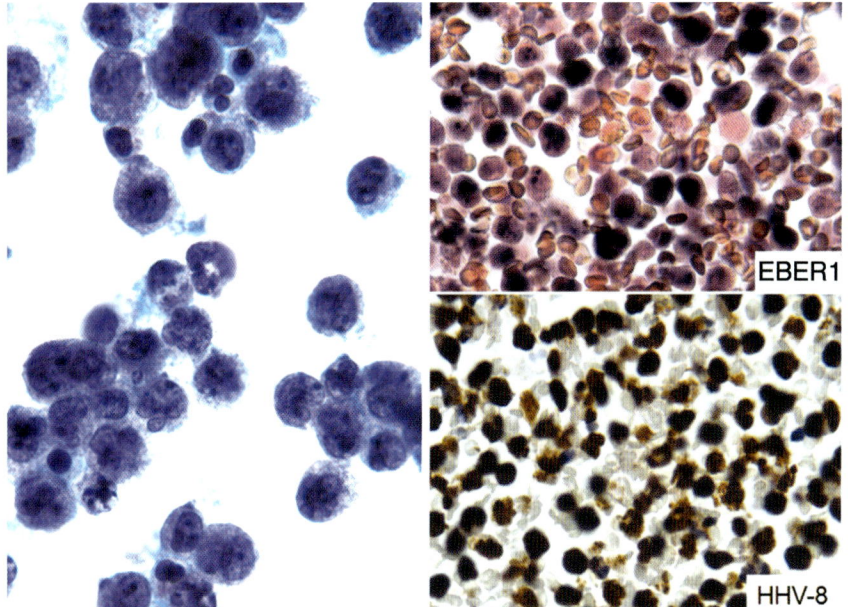

EBER1

HHV-8

PEL is frequently (over 90 percent) coinfected by EBV (fig. 9-12) (40). PEL is usually characterized by a type II EBV latency program with expression of EBNA1, LMP1, LMP2A, and EBER1 (72).

Rare cases reported as PEL are HHV-8 negative (2). Although morphologically similar, these tumors have some distinctive features. It seems prudent to exclude these HHV-8-negative cases from the PEL category.

HHV-8-Associated Multicentric Castleman Disease and Associated Large B-Cell Lymphoma. HHV-8-associated MCD is a rare lymphoproliferative disorder observed most often in patients with HIV. It is characterized by constitutional symptoms, cytopenias, lymphadenopathy, splenomegaly, and a waxing and waning clinical course. Patients have a poor prognosis and the disease is often lethal (59).

The pathogenesis of HHV-8-associated MCD is thought to be related to the production of angiogenic cytokines, including IL-6 and vascular endothelial growth factor (47). Many patients with MCD have concurrent Kaposi sarcoma and are at risk of developing HHV-8-associated lymphomas. The latter include PEL and a rare type of HHV-8-positive large B-cell lymphoma with plasmablastic features (see chapter 22).

The lymph nodes affected by HHV-8-associated MCD have many morphologic features of the hyaline vascular and plasma cell variant of Castleman disease, with regressed germinal centers and increased vascularization. These lymph nodes, however, commonly have a lymphocyte-depleted appearance and the boundary between germinal centers and mantle zones is blurred (3). HHV-8-infected plasmablasts are present in the mantle zones.

HHV-8-positive plasmablasts are positive for CD20 (variable), CD138, IgM, and lambda, and are negative for EBV. HHV-8 can be detected by immunohistochemistry using antibodies against LANA. Rarely, HHV-8 plasmablasts undergo additional genetic "hits," become monoclonal, and replace the lymph node to become HHV-8-associated large B-cell lymphoma (47).

HHV-8- and EBV-Associated Germinotropic Lymphoproliferative Disorder. This is a rare disorder occurring in immunocompetent adults who present with localized lymph node enlargement (23). A distinctive feature of this disease is the presence of a large number of plasmablasts involving germinal centers (germinotropism). The plasmablasts are positive for MUM1/IRF4, LANA1, and EBER1, and are negative for CD20, CD79a, BCL2, CD10, and BCL6 (19). Most patients reported with this rare disease have had an indolent clinical course but rare patients subsequently have developed a high-grade lymphoma positive for HHV-8 and EBV (19).

Human T-Cell Lymphotropic Virus Type 1

Human T-cell lymphotropic virus type 1 (HTLV-1) was the first retrovirus shown to cause a human malignancy, adult T-cell leukemia/lymphoma (ATLL) (77,83). HTLV-1 is a human RNA retrovirus member of the delta retrovirus family. Its genome is a single strand of RNA which in the host is converted to a provirus (double strand of DNA) that integrates into the host genome (83). Integration results in deregulated expression or function of a proto-oncogene.

HTLV-1 can infect many different cell types including T and B cells, dendritic cells, macrophages, and fibroblasts; CD4-positive T-regulatory cells [CD25(+), FOXP3(+)], however, are

particularly susceptible to immortalization by HTLV-1. The oncogenic capability of the virus is thought to be mediated by the expression of two genes encoding HTLV-1 transactivator protein (TAX) and HLTV-1 basic leucine zipper factor (HBZ), in a two phase process (fig. 9-13). In the first phase, TAX transactivates viral RNA, thereby activating a number of genes, including those of the NF-κB pathway as well as genes that inhibit apoptosis and increase genetic instability. In the second phase, HBZ drives cell proliferation and clonal expansion (68,83).

Currently, there are 20 million people infected with HTLV-1 worldwide (77). There are four HTLV-1 subtypes: subtype A is cosmopolitan and found in many geographic areas; subtype B is prevalent in Central Africa; subtype C is found in Papua New Guinea and the Solomon Islands; and subtype D has been identified in Central African Pygmies. The prevalence of HTLV-1 infection is high in endemic areas, 30 to 40 percent of all persons in some areas of southern Japan. In Europe and the United States, however, the prevalence is low, about 1 percent, and attributable primarily to immigrants from endemic regions (77,83). HTLV-1 is transmitted by blood exposure, through sexual contact, and from mother to child via breastfeeding. HTLV-1 infection is thought to occur at a young age and there is a long interval from infection to onset of ATLL (20 to 40 years).

HTLV-1-Associated Lymphoma. The most common and aggressive form of lymphoma caused by HTLV-1 infection is ATLL (see chapter 32). The number of persons who are HTLV-1 carriers greatly exceeds the number of patients who develop ATLL, and neoplastic transformation occurs decades after initial infection. It therefore appears that a number of genetic "hits" are required for ATLL to develop.

There are multiple clinical forms of ATLL: acute leukemia-like, lymphomatous, chronic, and smoldering (77). An indolent form that only affects skin also has been suggested. For patients with indolent disease, there is a tendency for the disease to eventually progress to the acute form, with an aggressive clinical course and poor prognosis. Patients with acute ATLL have marked leukocytosis, eosinophilia, skin lesions, hypercalcemia with or without lytic bone lesions, systemic lymphadenopathy, and often

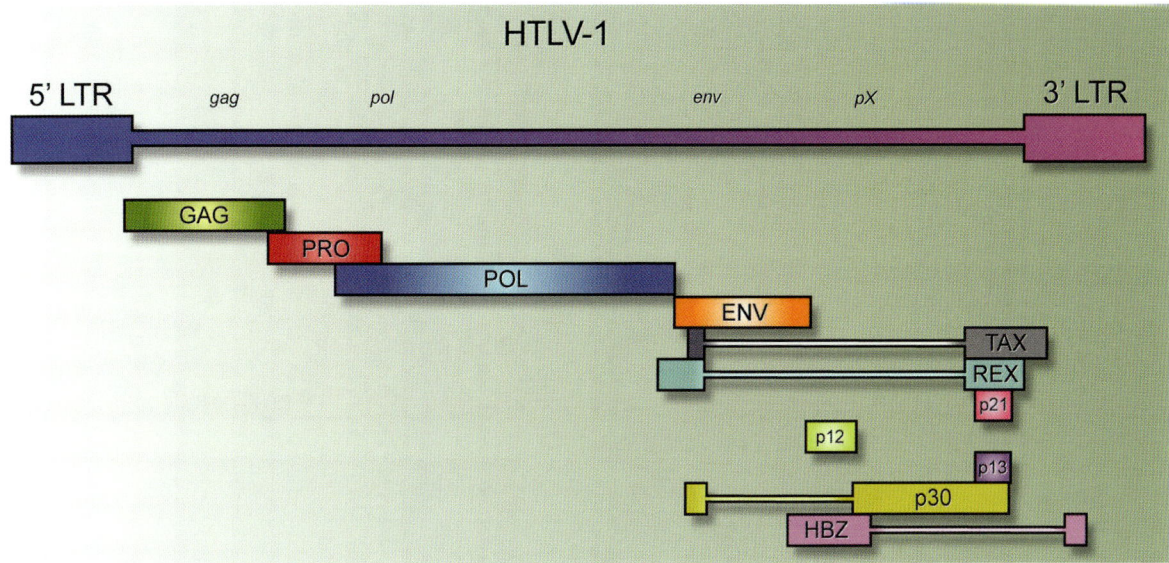

Figure 9-13

HTLV-1 PROVIRAL GENOME

The HTVL-1 genome is flanked by two long terminal repeats (LTR) as seen in other retroviruses, and contains the typical retroviral genes (*GAG, POL,* and *ENV*). A region called pX contains at least four partially overlapping genes encoding for the accessory proteins (p12, p13, p30), the post-transcriptional regulator *REX*, and the transacting transcriptional activator *TAX. TAX* is the counterpart of TAT in HIV. Another gene named *HBZ* has been recently discovered on the minus strand and seems to be essential for the maintenance of the leukemic stage.

hepatosplenomegaly (77). Involved lymph nodes exhibit a broad spectrum of appearances, resembling peripheral T-cell lymphoma unspecified, angioimmunoblastic T-cell lymphoma, anaplastic large cell lymphoma, or classic HL. In a blood smear, the leukemic cells often have a distinctive "flower-like" appearance (fig. 9-14).

INDIRECT ONCOGENIC EFFECTS

Bacteria

Extranodal marginal zone lymphomas (MZL) of mucosa-associated lymphoid tissue (also known as MALT lymphomas) (see chapter 15) are examples of the indirect oncogenic effects of infectious agents, although direct effects also may be involved. The infectious agent is a source of chronic antigenic stimulation, which prolongs the B-lymphocyte lifespan, indirectly increasing the likelihood of genetic abnormalities that result from genetic instability. In the case of gastric MZL, the inflammatory infiltrate (e.g., neutrophils) associated with the lymphoma also may have a direct effect by generating reactive oxygen species that cause genetic damage (74).

The best example and prototype of oncogenic bacterial infection in extranodal MZL pathogenesis is *Helicobacter pylori* and its effect on gastric MZL (discussed below). Other bacteria suspected of having a role in extranodal MZL pathogenesis are *Borrelia burgdorferi, Chlamydophila psittaci,* and *Campylobacter jejuni. B. burgdorferi* has been identified in 10 to 40 percent of cases of cutaneous MZL, primarily in Europe, but rarely in the United States. *C. psittaci* has been reported in 50 to 80 percent of ocular adnexal MZLs in Italy, Austria, Germany, and Korea, but much less commonly in nonendemic regions (74). Immunoproliferative small intestinal disease, once known as Mediterranean lymphoma, has been linked with *C. jejuni* infection.

Gastric Marginal Zone Lymphoma Associated with *Helicobacter Pylori*. Most extranodal sites involved by MZL, such as the stomach, are normally devoid of lymphoid tissue. The chronic antigenic stimulation of *H. pylori* infection results in the stomach acquiring lymphoid tissue with reactive lymphoid follicles and germinal centers, within which MZL can arise (74). B cells, when exposed to chronic

141

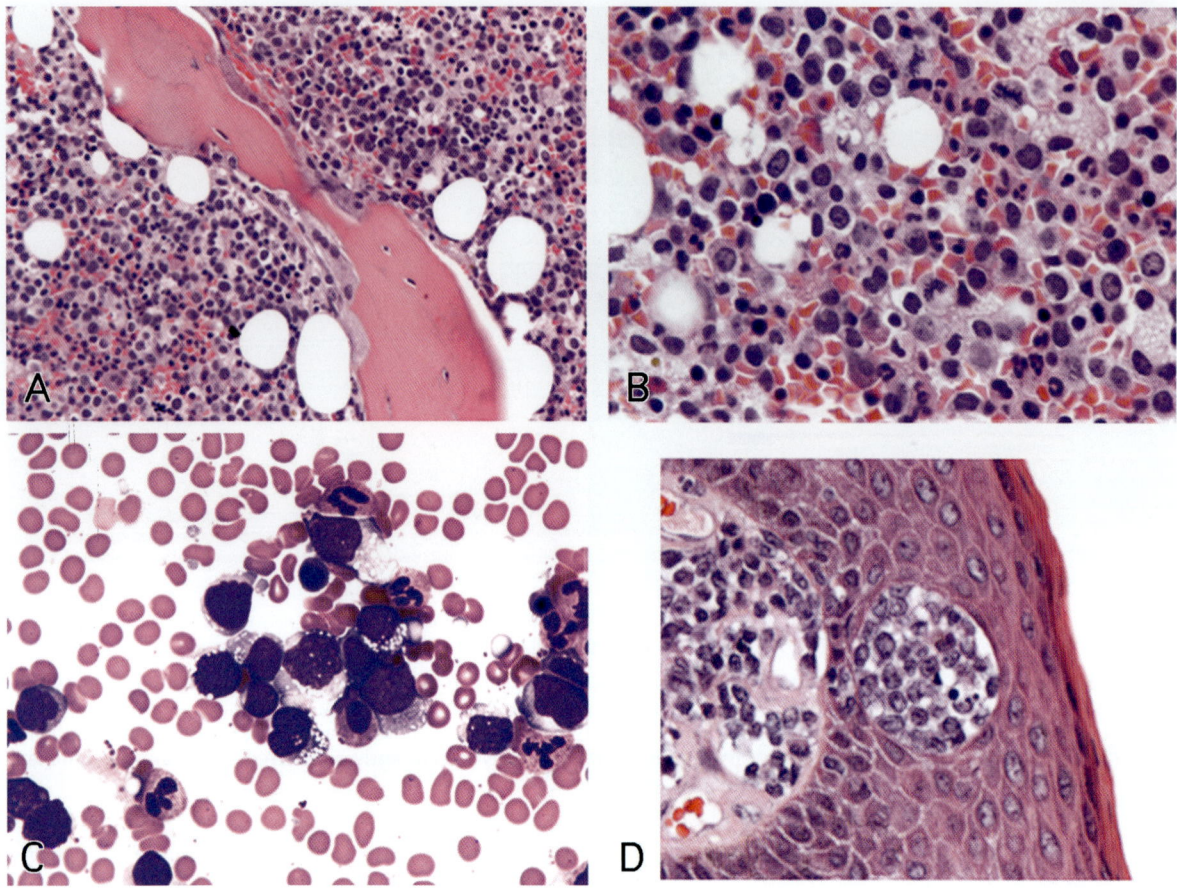

Figure 9-14

ADULT T-CELL LEUKEMIA/LYMPHOMA (ATLL)

A–C: Bone marrow biopsy (A,B) and peripheral blood (C) specimens from a patient with ATLL. The patient presented with hypercalcemia, retroperitoneal lymphadenopathy, and skin lesions. The bone marrow shows bone resorption and an interstitial lymphoid infiltrate composed of small to intermediate-sized lymphoid cells. The peripheral blood shows medium to large atypical lymphoid cells, some with irregular nuclear contours. The tumor cells were positive for CD2, CD3, CD4, and CD25 and negative for CD56 (H&E stain).

D: The skin lesion consists of an extensive dermal infiltrate with focal epidermotropism and Pautrier-like microabscesses (H&E stain).

antigenic stimulation, may accumulate genetic lesions through genomic instability within the germinal center microenvironment as a result of somatic hypermutation and class switch recombination.

H. pylori are Gram-negative, spiral-shaped, curved rods reidentified in 1982 by the Australian physicians Marshall and Warren (74). Each microorganism is 3 μm long with a diameter of 0.5 μm and has 4 to 6 unipolar flagella that help the bacterium colonize the stomach. *H. pylori* produces adhesins that bind to cell membrane-associated lipids as well as carbohydrates that help the organisms adhere to the gastric

epithelial cells. The organisms are microaerophilic and produce oxidase, catalase, and urease.

The survival of *H. pylori* in the acidic stomach environment is dependent on urease. Urease breaks down urea (normally secreted into the stomach) to carbon dioxide and ammonia. The ammonia produced is toxic to the epithelial cells, and, along with the other *H. pylori* products, including proteases, vacuolating cytotoxin A (VacA), and certain phospholipases, damages the gastric mucosa and induces an inflammatory response (fig. 9-15).

Humans are the main reservoir of *H. pylori* and it is estimated that 50 percent of the world's

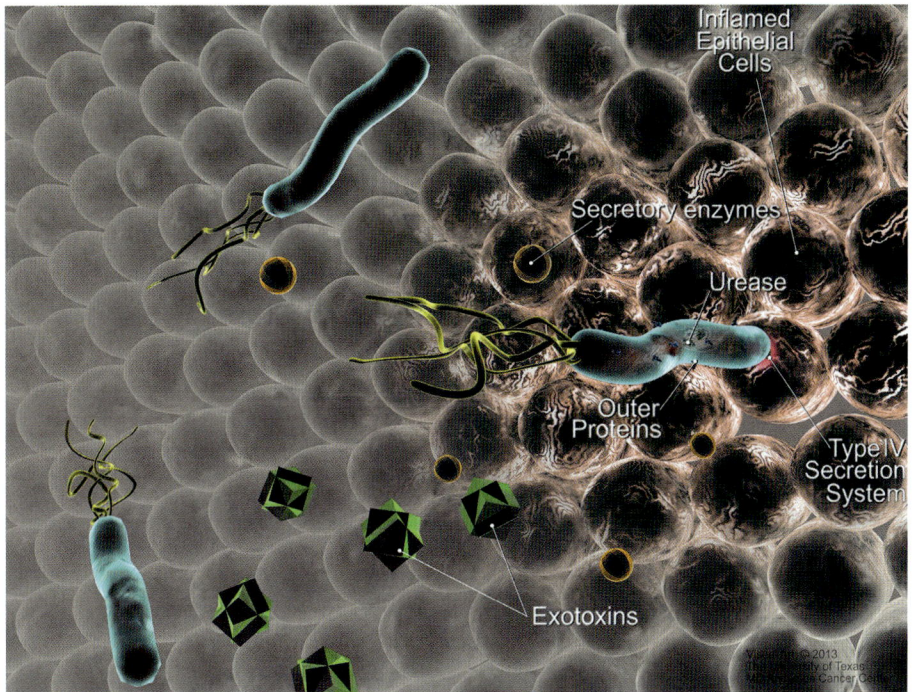

Inflamed
Epithelial
Cells

Secretory enzymes

Urease

Outer
Proteins

Type IV
Secretion
System

Exotoxins

© 2013
The University of Texas
MD Anderson Cancer Center

Figure 9-15

HELICOBACTER PYLORI

Helicobacter pylori are curved rods about 3 µm long with unipolar flagella. Urease activity and motility mediated by the flagella are important for the survival of the organism in niches adjacent to the gastric epithelial cells. Other virulence factors of *H. Pylori* that contribute to damage of gastric cells are shown in the schematic diagram. The adhesion of bacteria to epithelial cells induces an inflammatory response resulting in the recruitment of neutrophils, followed by B and T lymphocytes, and plasma cells, and the development of mucosa-associated lymphoid tissue (MALT).

population is infected, making it the most widespread infection in the world. Infection by *H. pylori* is usually acquired in early childhood and persists for life. The exact route of transmission is unknown, but person to person transmission by either fecal-to-oral or oral-to-oral exposure is likely the main route of infection.

Almost 90 percent of patients with gastric MZL are infected with *H. pylori* (fig. 9-16) and the risk of gastric MZL in *H. pylori*-infected individuals is 3- to 6-fold higher than in those who are not infected (45). *H. pylori* gastritis is thought to be the initial (or very early) step in the pathogenesis of most cases of gastric MZL. Bacterial infection is thought to cause chronic gastric inflammation and constant antigenic stimulation, leading to an increase of B cells. In addition, activated neutrophils generate radical oxygen species and genotoxins that contribute to DNA damage in B cells and lead to mutations/ genetic rearrangements and dysregulation of critical oncogenic pathways (41).

Treatment with antibiotics can eradicate *H. pylori* and disrupt these processes, resulting in regression of gastric MZL in many patients (80). Some patients, however, do not respond and further genetic evolution can result in progression to gastric DLBCL.

The role of antibiotic therapy in the treatment of patients with other types of extranodal MZL is less well established. Immunoproliferative small intestinal disease was the first lymphoma type shown to respond to antibiotic therapy, although early reports were more anecdotal. Doxycycline has cleared ocular adnexal MZL in an appreciable patient subset. In one international clinical trial, *C. psittaci* was identified in almost 90 percent of ocular adnexal MZLs: approximately half of patients responded to doxycycline therapy and 15 percent had complete regression of disease after treatment with the antibiotic alone (30). There are also cases of cutaneous MZL associated with *B. burgdoferi* infection that have regressed completely following antibiotic therapy (66).

Hepatitis C-Associated Lymphomas

Hepatitis C virus (HCV) is a small (about 9,600 nucleotide) encapsulated, positive strand RNA member of the *Flaviviridae* family (20,62). During replication, HCV produces a negative RNA strand, but does not create DNA, and therefore it seems unlikely that HCV integrates into host cell DNA. HCV is best known for its role as the major etiologic agent of non-A and -B chronic hepatitis, however, it can cause a broad spectrum of extrahepatic manifestations

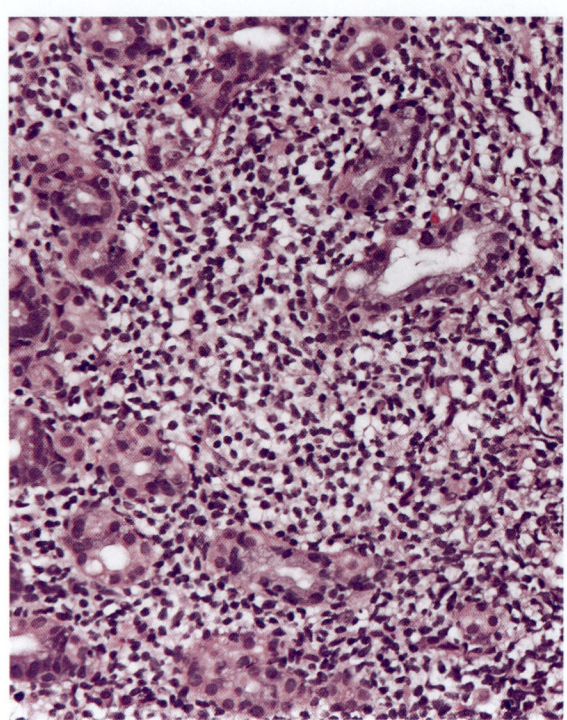 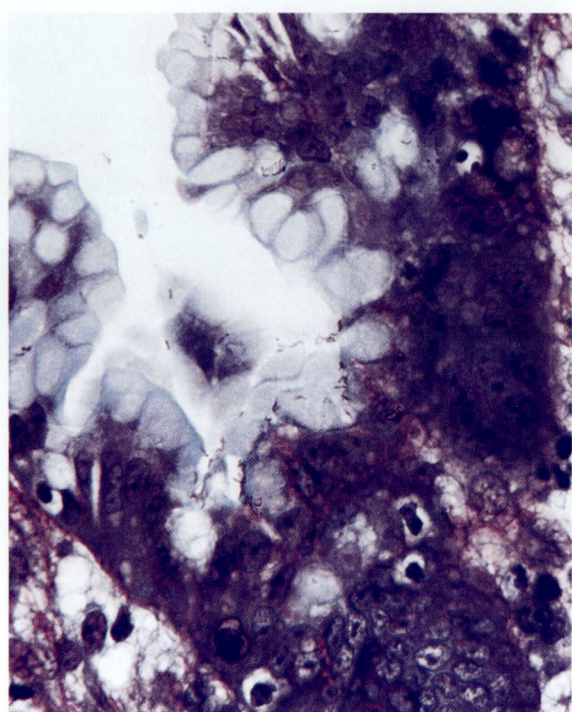

Figure 9-16

GASTRIC MALT LYMPHOMA ASSOCIATED WITH *HELICOBACTER PYLORI* INFECTION

Left: The lymphoma is composed of small lymphoid cells with slightly irregular nuclear contours. These cells infiltrate gastric epithelium to form lymphoepithelial lesions (H&E stain).

Right: *H. pylori* is identified by Giemsa stain (shown here) or by immunohistochemical methods in paraffin-embedded tissue sections. The organisms reside beneath the mucus on the luminal surface of the epithelium.

including type II mixed cryoglobulinemia and lymphoma (20). The lymphoma subtypes most frequently associated with HCV are MZL, DLBCL, and follicular lymphoma, but other lymphoma types and CD5-negative monoclonal B-cell lymphocytosis also have been reported (20,52).

There is epidemiologic evidence supporting an association between chronic HCV infection and malignant lymphoma. NHLs are more common in areas with a high frequency of HCV infection. More convincing evidence for a causal relationship is the observation in some patients of lymphoma regression after HCV eradication by antiviral therapy (6,37).

The mechanisms by which HCV contributes to lymphomagenesis are poorly understood. One hypothesis that seems likely is that persistent external antigenic stimulation of lymphocyte receptors by viral antigens (HCV E2 envelope protein) leads to chronic B-cell proliferation and activation (analogous to *H.*

pylori-associated gastric MALT lymphoma) (20,62). The association between HCV infection, type II mixed cryoglobulinemia, and lymphoma lend support to a multistep model in which HCV induces protracted stimulation of antigen-specific B-cell clones, leading to mixed cryoglobulinemia, and then overt lymphoma. Immunodeficiency, when present, may be a cofactor. Analysis of immunoglobulin variable region genes in NHLs in HCV-positive patients have shown a high frequency of mutations, indicating antigen exposure and further suggesting a role for antigen selection. In addition, tissue sections of HCV-associated lymphomas show virus in only a small subset of tumor cells, but virus is more common in stromal cells. This observation further suggests that HCV, through its effects on the microenvironment, causes chronic antigenic stimulation (20). Nevertheless, HCV is a lymphotropic virus and could have direct oncogenic effects in B cells (62).

More studies are needed and these hypotheses are not mutually exclusive.

Hepatitis B and G viruses are also lymphotropic and have been suggested as potential causes of lymphoma (20). There is some epidemiologic evidence to support the association with lymphoma, such as a higher prevalence of hepatitis G viral infection in patients with lymphoma, but more studies are needed.

Human Immunodeficiency Virus

HIV is a lymphotropic virus that, in contrast to other retroviruses, does not cause leukemia even though it replicates rapidly and inserts semi-randomly into host CD4-positive T cells and macrophages (13). HIV is thought to lack the capability to cause leukemia because infected cells are usually killed quickly, before neoplastic transformation can occur.

Two mechanisms are thought to underlie lymphomagenesis in patients with HIV infection. First, HIV is a cause of chronic antigen stimulation resulting in clonal B-cell expansion (34). About 50 percent of lymphomas arising in the context of HIV are likely due to persistent antigenic stimulation. The other half arise when immunodeficiency allows reactivation of oncogenic lymphotropic viruses, such as EBV and HHV-8, resulting in lymphomagenesis. In most HIV-associated lymphomas, HIV is not integrated into the lymphoma cell genome (unlike HTLV-1).

HIV-Associated Lymphomas. The development of NHL in a patient with HIV infection is a defining feature of AIDS (see chapter 43). Classic HL is not considered to be an AIDS-defining disease at this time. The overall incidence of lymphomas in AIDS patients, although far higher than in their immunocompetent counterparts, has decreased in the era of highly active retroviral therapy (HAART). The incidence of HL, however, has increased in the HAART era (13).

HIV-related lymphoproliferative disorders represent a broad spectrum of diseases that are a substantial cause of morbidity and mortality. Patients with HIV may develop high- or low-grade NHLs, with DLBCL being the most common followed by Burkitt lymphoma. In addition, HIV-infected patients develop reactive lymphoproliferative conditions, such as localized or disseminated lymphoid hyperplasia and progressive lymphadenopathy. HHV-8–associated primary effusion lymphoma and multicentric Castleman disease also occur most commonly in the setting of AIDS. In general, AIDS-related NHLs are frequently extranodal and clinically aggressive (13,34). Similarly, HIV-positive patients with classic HL have more aggressive disease with a higher frequency of extranodal involvement. Mixed cellularity HL is most common in the HIV setting.

EBV infection is common in HIV-associated lymphomas: it occurs in almost 100 percent of DLBCLs involving the CNS, about 80 percent of classic HLs, and a subset of DLBCLs. Nevertheless, about 50 percent of all lymphomas that arise in HIV patients are EBV negative. The latent EBV proteins EBNA1, LMP1, and LMP2A are usually expressed in the Reed-Sternberg and Hodgkin cells of HL.

REFERENCES

1. Akula SM, Pramod NP, Wang FZ, Chandran B. Integrin alpha3beta1 (CD 49c/29) is a cellular receptor for Kaposi's sarcoma-associated herpesvirus (KSHV/HHV-8) entry into the target cells. Cell 2002;108:407-419.
2. Alexanian S, Said J, Lones M, Pullarkat ST. KSHV/HHV8-negative effusion-based lymphoma, a distinct entity associated with fluid overload states. Am J Surg Pathol 2013;37:241-249.
3. Amin HM, Medeiros LJ, Manning JT, Jones D. Dissolution of the lymphoid follicle is a feature of the HHV8+ variant of plasma cell Castleman's disease. Am J Surg Pathol 2003;27:91-100.
4. Andreoni M, Sarmati L, Nicastri E, et al. Primary human herpesvirus 8 infection in immunocompetent children. JAMA 2002;287:1295-1300.
5. Aozasa K. Pyothorax-associated lymphoma. J Clin Exp Hematop 2006;46:5-10.
6. Arcaini L, Bruno R. Hepatitis C virus infection and antiviral treatment in marginal zone lymphomas. Curr Clin Pharmacol 2010;5:74-81.

7. Baer R, Bankier AT, Biggin MD, et al. DNA sequence and expression of the B95-8 Epstein-Barr virus genome. Nature 1984;310:207-211.

8. Bagneris C, Ageichik AV, Cronin N, et al. Crystal structure of a vFlip-IKKgamma complex: insights into viral activation of the IKK signalosome. Mol Cell 2008;30:620-631.

9. Ballestas ME, Chatis PA, Kaye KM. Efficient persistence of extrachromosomal KSHV DNA mediated by latency-associated nuclear antigen. Science 1999;284:641-644.

10. Barrionuevo C, Anderson VM, Zevallos-Giampietri E, et al. Hydroa-like cutaneous T-cell lymphoma: a clinicopathologic and molecular genetic study of 16 pediatric cases from Peru. Appl Immunohistochem Mol Morphol 2002;10:7-14.

11. Boroumand N, Ly TL, Sonstein J, Medeiros LJ. Microscopic diffuse large B-cell lymphoma (DLBCL) occurring in pseudocysts: do these tumors belong to the category of DLBCL associated with chronic inflammation? Am J Surg Pathol 2012;36:1074-1080.

12. Camilleri-Broet S, Martin A, Moreau A, et al. Primary central nervous system lymphomas in 72 immunocompetent patients: pathologic findings and clinical correlations. Groupe Ouest Est d'etude des Leucenies et Autres Maladies du Sang (GOELAMS). Am J Clin Pathol 1998;110:607-612.

13. Carbone A, Cesarman E, Spina M, Gloghini A, Schulz TF. HIV-associated lymphomas and gamma-herpesviruses. Blood 2009;113:1213-1224.

14. Cesarman E, Chang Y, Moore PS, Said JW, Knowles DM. Kaposi's sarcoma-associated herpesvirus-like DNA sequences in AIDS-related body-cavity-based lymphomas. N Engl J Med 1995;332:1186-1191.

15. Chadburn A, Hyjek E, Mathew S, Cesarman E, Said J, Knowles DM. KSHV-positive solid lymphomas represent an extra-cavitary variant of primary effusion lymphoma. Am J Surg Pathol 2004;28:1401-1416.

15a. Chen CC, Chang KC, Medeiros LJ, Lee JY. Hydroa vacciniforme and hydroa vacciniforme-like T-cell lymphoma: an uncommon event for transformation. J Cutan Pathol 2016;43:1102-1111.

16. Chen HH, Hsiao CH, Chiu HC. Hydroa vacciniforme-like primary cutaneous CD8-positive T-cell lymphoma. Br J Dermatol 2002;147:587-591.

17. Cheuk W, Chan AC, Chan JK, Lau GT, Chan VN, Yiu HH. Metallic implant-associated lymphoma: a distinct subgroup of large B-cell lymphoma related to pyothorax-associated lymphoma? Am J Surg Pathol 2005;29:832-836.

18. Cho KH, Kim CW, Heo DS, et al. Epstein-Barr virus-associated peripheral T-cell lymphoma in adults with hydroa vacciniforme-like lesions. Clin Exp Dermatol 2001;26:242-247.

19. Courville EL, Sohani AR, Hasserjian RP, Zukerberg LR, Harris NL, Ferry JA. Diverse clinicopathologic features in human herpesvirus 8-associated lymphomas lead to diagnostic problems. Am J Clin Pathol 2014;142:816-829.

20. Datta S, Chatterjee S, Policegoudra RS, Gogoi HK, Singh L. Hepatitis viruses and non-Hodgkin's lymphoma: A review. World J Virol 2012;1:162-173.

21. Delecluse HJ, Anagnostopoulos I, Dallenbach F, et al. Plasmablastic lymphomas of the oral cavity: a new entity associated with the human immunodeficiency virus infection. Blood 1997;89:1413-1420.

22. Dogan A, Attygalle AD, Kyriakou C. Angioimmunoblastic T-cell lymphoma. Br J Haematol 2003;121:681-691.

23. Du MQ, Diss TC, Liu H, et al. KSHV- and EBV-associated germinotropic lymphoproliferative disorder. Blood 2002;100:3415-3418.

24. Dukers NH, Rezza G. Human herpesvirus 8 epidemiology: what we do and do not know. AIDS 2003;17:1717-1730.

25. Dupin N, Diss TL, Kellam P, et al. HHV-8 is associated with a plasmablastic variant of Castleman disease that is linked to HHV-8-positive plasmablastic lymphoma. Blood 2000;95:1406-1412.

26. Eligio P, Delia R, Valeria G. EBV chronic infections. Mediterr J Hematol Infect Dis 2010;2: e2010022.

27. Epstein MA, Achong BG, Barr YM. Virus particles in cultured lymphoblasts from Burkitt's lymphoma. Lancet 1964;1:702-703.

28. Evens AM, Roy R, Sterrenberg D, Moll MZ, Chadburn A, Gordon LI. Post-transplantation lymphoproliferative disorders: diagnosis, prognosis, and current approaches to therapy. Curr Oncol Rep 2010;12:383-394.

29. Everly DN, Jr., Mainou BA, Raab-Traub N. Induction of Id1 and Id3 by latent membrane protein 1 of Epstein-Barr virus and regulation of p27/Kip and cyclin-dependent kinase 2 in rodent fibroblast transformation. J Virol 2004;78:13470-13478.

30. Ferreri AJ, Govi S, Pasini E, et al. Chlamydophila psittaci eradication with doxycyxline as first-line targeted therapy for ocular adnexae lymphoma: final results of an international phase II trial. J Clin Oncol 2012;20:2988-2994.

31. Fischer EM, Mouhoub A, Maillet F, et al. Expression of CD21 is developmentally regulated during thymic maturation of human T lymphocytes. Int Immunol 1999;11:1841-1849.

32. Fujimuro M, Wu FY, ApRhys C, et al. A novel viral mechanism for dysregulation of beta-catenin in Kaposi's sarcoma-associated herpesvirus latency. Nat Med 2003;9:300-306.

33. Gaidano G, Cerri M, Capello D, et al. Molecular histogenesis of plasmablastic lymphoma of the oral cavity. Br J Haematol 2002;119:622-628.

34. Grulich AE, Wan X, Law MG, et al. B-cell stimulation and prolonged immune deficiency are risk factors for non-Hodgkin's lymphoma in people with AIDS. AIDS 2000;14:133-140.

35. Gualco G, Domeny-Duarte P, Chioato L, Barber G, Natkunam Y, Bacchi CE. Clinicopathologic and molecular features of 122 Brazilian cases of nodal and extranodal NK/T-cell lymphoma, nasal type, with EBV subtyping analysis. Am J Surg Pathol 2011;35:1195-1203.

36. Hasserjian RP, Chen S, Perkins SL, et al. Immunomodulator agent-related lymphoproliferative disorders. Mod Pathol 2009;22:1532-4.

37. Hermine O, Lefrere F, Bronowicki JP, et al. Regression of splenic lymphoma with villous lymphocytes after treatment of hepatitis C virus infection. N Engl J Med 2002;347:89-94.

38. Hjalgrim H, Askling J, Sorensen P, et al. Risk of Hodgkin's disease and other cancers after infectious mononucleosis. J Natl Cancer Inst 2000;92:1522-1528.

39. Hochberg D, Souza T, Catalina M, Sullivan JL, Luzuriaga K, Thorley-Lawson DA. Acute infection with Epstein-Barr virus targets and overwhelms the peripheral memory B-cell compartment with resting, latently infected cells. J Virol 2004;78:5194-5204.

40. Horenstein MG, Nador RG, Chadburn A, et al. Epstein-Barr virus latent gene expression in primary effusion lymphomas containing Kaposi's sarcoma-associated herpesvirus/human herpesvirus-8. Blood 1997;90:1186-1191.

41. Hussain SP, Hofseth LJ, Harris CC. Radical causes of cancer. Nat Rev Cancer 2003;3:276-285.

42. Ichikawa A, Arakawa F, Kiyasu J, et al. Methotrexate/iatrogenic lymphoproliferative disorders in rheumatoid arthritis: histology, Epstein-Barr virus, and clonality are important predictors of disease progression and regression. Eur J Haematol 2013;91:20-28.

43. Kamel OW, van de Rijn M, Weiss LM, et al. Brief report: reversible lymphomas associated with Epstein-Barr virus occurring during methotrexate therapy for rheumatoid arthritis and dermatomyositis. N Engl J Med 1993;328:1317-1321.

44. Katzenstein AL, Carrington CB, Liebow AA. Lymphomatoid granulomatosis: a clinicopathologic study of 152 cases. Cancer 1979;43:360-373.

45. Kim SS, Ruiz VE, Carroll JD, Moss SF. Helicobacter pylori in the pathogenesis of gastric cancer and gastric lymphoma. Cancer Lett 2011;305:228-238.

46. Kim Y, Leventaki V, Bhaijee F, Jackson CC, Medeiros LJ, Vega F. Extracavitary/solid variant of primary effusion lymphoma. Ann Diagn Pathol 2012;16:441-446.

47. Laurent C, Meggetto F, Brousset P. Human herpesvirus 8 infections in patients with immunodeficiencies. Hum Pathol 2008;39:983-989.

48. Li S, Feng X, Li T, et al. Extranodal NK/T-cell lymphoma, nasal type: a report of 73 cases at MD Anderson Cancer Center. Am J Surg Pathol 2013;37:14-23.

49. Loghavi S, Alayed K, Aladily TN, et al. Stage, age, and EBV status impact outcomes of plasmablastic lymphoma patients: a clinicopathologic analysis of 61 patients. J Hematol Oncol 2015;8:65.

50. Magrath I. Epidemiology: clues to the pathogenesis of Burkitt lymphoma. Br J Haematol 2012;156:744-756.

51. McCormick C, Ganem D. The kaposin B protein of KSHV activates the p38/MK2 pathway and stabilizes cytokine mRNAs. Science 2005;307:739-741.

52. Mollejo M, Menárguez J, Guisado-Vasco P, et al. Hepatitis C virus-related lymphoproliferative disorders encompass a broader clinical and morphological spectrum than previously recognized: a clinicopathological study. Mod Pathol 2014;27:281-293.

53. Moore PS, Chang Y. Kaposi sarcoma-associated herpesvirus immunoevasion and tumorigenesis: two sides of the same coin? Annu Rev Microbiol 2003;57:609-639.

54. Moore PS, Chang Y. Why do viruses cause cancer? Highlights of the first century of human tumour virology. Nat Rev Cancer 2010;10:878-889.

55. Nador RG, Cesarman E, Chadburn A, et al. Primary effusion lymphoma: a distinct clinicopathologic entity associated with the Kaposi's sarcoma-associated herpes virus. Blood 1996;88:645-656.

56. Neipel F, Albrecht JC, Fleckenstein B. Cell-homologous genes in the Kaposi's sarcoma-associated rhadinovirus human herpesvirus 8: determinants of its pathogenicity? J Virol 1997;71:4187-4192.

57. Ohshima K, Suzumiya J, Kanda M, Kato A, Kikuchi M. Integrated and episomal forms of Epstein-Barr virus (EBV) in EBV associated disease. Cancer Lett 1998;122:43-50.

58. Ok CY, Papathomas TG, Medeiros LJ, Young SK. EBV-positive diffuse large B-cell lymphoma of the elderly. Blood 2013;122:328-340.

59. Oksenhendler E, Carcelain G, Aoki Y, et al. High levels of human herpesvirus 8 viral load, human interleukin-6, interleukin-10, and C reactive protein correlate with exacerbation of multicentric castleman disease in HIV-infected patients. Blood 2000;96:2069-2073.

60. Pan ZG, Zhang QY, Lu ZB, et al. Extracavitary KSHV-associated large B-cell lymphoma. A distinct entity or a subtype of primary effusion lymphoma? Study of 9 cases and review of an additional 43 cases. Am J Surg Pathol 2012;36:1129-1140.

61. Paul C, Le Tourneau A, Cayuela JM, et al. Epstein-Barr virus-associated lymphoproliferative disease during methotrexate therapy for psoriasis. Arch Dermatol 1997;133:867-871.

62. Peveling-Oberhag J, Arcaini L, Hansmann ML, Zeuzem S. Hepatitis C-associated B-cell non-Hodgkin lymphomas. Epidemiology, molecular signature and clinical management. J Hepatol 2013;59:169-177.

63. Pittaluga S, Wilson WH, Jaffe ES. Lymphomatoid granulomatosis. In: Swerdlow SH, Campo E, Harris NL, et al., eds. WHO classification of tumours of haematopoietic and lymphoid tissues. Lyon: IARC Press; 2008:247-249.

64. Quintanilla-Martinez L, Kumar S, Fend F, et al. Fulminant EBV(+) T-cell lymphoproliferative disorder following acute/chronic EBV infection: a distinct clinicopathologic syndrome. Blood 2000;96:443-451.

65. Rappocciolo G, Hensler HR, Jais M, et al. Human herpesvirus 8 infects and replicates in primary cultures of activated B lymphocytes through DC-SIGN. J Virol 2008;82:4793-4806.

66. Roggero E, Zucca E, Mainetti C, et al. Eradication of Borrelia burgdorferi infection in primary marginal zone B-cell lymphoma of the skin. Hum Pathol 2000;31:263-268.

67. Roschewski M, Wilson WH. Lymphomatoid granulomatosis. Cancer J 2012;18:469-474.

68. Satou Y, Yasunaga J, Yoshida M, Matsuoka M. HTLV-I basic leucine zipper factor gene mRNA supports proliferation of adult T cell leukemia cells. Proc Natl Acad Sci U S A 2006;103:720-725.

69. Schulz TF. Epidemiology of Kaposi's sarcoma-associated herpesvirus/human herpesvirus 8. Adv Cancer Res 1999;76:121-160.

70. Soulier J, Grollet L, Oksenhendler E, et al. Kaposi's sarcoma-associated herpesvirus-like DNA sequences in multicentric Castleman's disease. Blood 1995;86:1276-1280.

71. Su IJ, Wang CH, Cheng AL, Chen RL. Hemophagocytic syndrome in Epstein-Barr virus-associated T-lymphoproliferative disorders: disease spectrum, pathogenesis, and management. Leuk Lymphoma 1995;19:401-406.

71a. Swerdlow SH, Campo E, Pileri SA, et al. The 2016 revision of the World Health Organization classification of lymphoid neoplasms. Blood 2016;127:2375-2390.

72. Szekely L, Chen F, Teramoto N, et al. Restricted expression of Epstein-Barr virus (EBV)-encoded, growth transformation-associated antigens in an EBV- and human herpesvirus type 8-carrying body cavity lymphoma line. J Gen Virol 1998;79(Pt 6):1445-1452.

73. Tabiasco J, Vercellone A, Meggetto F, Hudrisier D, Brousset P, Fournié JJ. Acquisition of viral receptor by NK cells through immunological synapse. J Immunol 2003;170:5993-5998.

74. Thieblemont C, Bertoni F, Copie-Bergman C, Ferreri AJ, Ponzoni M. Chronic inflammation and extra-nodal marginal zone lymphomas of MALT-type. Sem Cancer Biol 2014;24:33-42.

75. Thorley-Lawson DA, Babcock GJ. A model for persistent infection with Epstein-Barr virus: the stealth virus of human B cells. Life Sci 1999;65:1433-1453.

76. Tierney RJ, Steven N, Young LS, Rickinson AB. Epstein-Barr virus latency in blood mononuclear cells: analysis of viral gene transcription during primary infection and in the carrier state. J Virol 1994;68:7374-7385.

77. Tsukasaki K, Tobinai K. Biology and treatment of HTLV-1 associated T-cell lymphomas. Best Pract Res Clin Hematol 2013;26:3-14.

78. Vasef MA, Kamel OW, Chen YY, Medeiros LJ, Weiss LM. Detection of Epstein-Barr virus in multiple sites involved by Hodgkin's disease. Am J Pathol 1995;147:1408-1415.

79. Vega F, Chang CC, Medeiros LJ, et al. Plasmablastic lymphomas and plasmablastic plasma cell myelomas have nearly identical immunophenotypic profiles. Mod Pathol 2005;18:806-815.

80. Weber DM, Dimopoulos MA, Anandu DP, Pugh WC, Steinbach G. Regression of gastric lymphoma of mucosa-associated lymphoid tissue with antibiotic therapy for Helicobacter pylori. Gastroenterology 1994;107:1835-1838.

81. Weiss LM, Jaffe ES, Liu XF, Chen YY, Shibata D, Medeiros LJ. Detection and localization of Epstein-Barr viral genomes in angioimmunoblastic lymphadenopathy and angioimmunoblastic lymphadenopathy-like lymphoma. Blood 1992;79:1789-1795.

82. Weiss LM, Movahed LA, Warnke RA, Sklar J. Detection of Epstein-Barr viral genomes in Reed-Sternberg cells of Hodgkin's disease. N Engl J Med 1989;320:502-506.

82a. Yabe M, Medeiros LJ, Daneshbod Y, et al. Hepatosplenic T-cell lymphoma arising in patients with immunodysregulatory disorders: a study of 7 patients who did not receive tumor necrosis factor-α inhibitor therapy and literature review. Ann Diagn Pathol 2017;26:16-22

83. Yoshida M. Discovery of HTLV-1, the first human retrovirus, its unique regulatory mechanisms, and insights into pathogenesis. Oncogene 2005;24:5931-5937.

84. Young LS, Rickinson AB. Epstein-Barr virus: 40 years on. Nat Rev Cancer 2004;4:757-768.

85. Zeidan A, Sham R, Shapiro J, Baratta A, Kouides P. Hepatopslenic T cell lymphoma in a patient with Crohn's disease who received infliximab therapy. Leuk Lymphoma 2007;48:1410-1413.

10 B-LYMPHOBLASTIC LEUKEMIA/LYMPHOMA

B-lymphoblastic leukemia/lymphoma is a neoplasm derived from precursor lymphocytes (or lymphoblasts) committed to B-cell lineage (2). These neoplasms are specified as either B-acute lymphoblastic leukemia (ALL) or lymphoblastic lymphoma (LBL). Patients with ALL have extensive bone marrow disease, usually with peripheral blood involvement. A cutoff of 25 percent lymphoblasts has been used traditionally to define extensive bone marrow disease and supports the designation of ALL. Patients with LBL present with a mass lesion with absent or low-level (less than 25 percent) involvement of bone marrow and minimal, if present, involvement of peripheral blood.

GENERAL FEATURES

There are approximately 6,000 new cases of ALL in the United States per year, 90 percent of which are of B-cell lineage (15). Approximately 60 to 70 percent of B-ALL cases occur in patients under 20 years of age, most of whom are young children (15). Boys slightly outnumber girls in a ratio of 1.3 to 1.0. Presentation as B-LBL is uncommon. Patients who present with B-LBL tend to be older with a median age of 20 years (17).

The World Health Organization (WHO) classification combines B-ALL and B-LBL into the same category, implying that these tumors are very similar; it is presumed that molecular data derived from the study of B-ALL cases apply to B-LBL cases (2). This assessment seems likely, but is largely unproven as few B-LBL cases have been assessed at the molecular level. Furthermore, the different presentations of B-ALL and B-LBL suggest that there may be some differences in pathogenesis.

The etiology of B-ALL/LBL is incompletely understood. Cases of B-ALL show a wide number and variety of genetic abnormalities at the cytogenetic and molecular level, indicating that B-ALL has a multifactorial pathogenesis (12,22). It is thought that B-ALL/LBL is derived from a precursor B cell that undergoes a primary genetic event, such as a chromosomal translocation or other mutation, followed by the acquisition of many other secondary genetic abnormalities. For some types of B-ALL, it appears that the initial genetic "hit" occurs in utero and that secondary genetic hits occur after birth (15). To illustrate this concept we focus on B-ALL associated with t(12;21)(p13;q22)/*ETV6-RUNX1* because abundant data support this model, and the pathogenesis of hyperdiploid B-ALL and infant leukemia associated with the 11q23/*MLL* rearrangement also seem to fit within this model (11,21).

ETV6-RUNX1 (formerly known as *TEL-AML1*) is one of the most common translocations detected in neonatal blood spots or Guthrie cards (11,22). This finding indicates that *ETV6-RUNX1* often arises in utero. However, only 1 percent of children with *ETV6-RUNX1* in neonatal blood spots subsequently develop B-ALL. In monozygotic twins in whom one twin develops B-ALL associated with *ETV6-RUNX1*, the other twin also carries *ETV6-RUNX1* at a low level even though they are disease free. These findings suggest that generation of the *ETV6-RUNX1* fusion gene is an initial event, necessary but not sufficient for leukemogenesis. Typically, in utero blood samples show the fusion gene at a low level and other abnormalities are uncommon, while cases of fully developed B-ALL commonly show additional cytogenetic and molecular abnormalities (discussed subsequently), which represent the additional genetic "hits" needed for B-ALL to develop after birth (11).

Studies of B-ALL cases have suggested that secondary genetic hits are acquired in a manner known as nonlinear branching clonal evolution (11). In other words, although all leukemic cells share common genetic abnormalities, different leukemic subclones have distinctive additional genetic mutations.

The events involved in the acquisition of these additional abnormalities are incompletely understood. Inherited genetic susceptibility/instability likely plays a role, as does exogenous

Table 10-1

GENETIC ABNORMALITIES IN B-ACUTE LYMPHOBLASTIC LYMPHOMA (ALL) RECOGNIZED IN THE WORLD HEALTH ORGANIZATION CLASSIFICATION WITH ASSOCIATED FINDINGS

Molecular Abnormality	Impaired Function	Frequency in Children	Frequency in Adults	Immunophenotypic Correlations	Prognosis
t(9;22)(q34;q11.2)/ *BCR-ABL1*	Signal transduction	3-5%	25-33%	CD10+, CD25+, CD34+, CD38-/↓, myeloid markers+	Unfavorable
t(variable;11q23)/ *KMT2A* rearranged	B-cell development	2-3%	3-7%	CD10-, CD15+, CD34-, CD33+	Unfavorable
t(12;21)(p13;q22)/ *ETV6-RUNX1*	B-cell development	25%	Rare	CD10+, CD13+, CD19+, CD34+ , CD56+	Favorable
Hyperploidy (51-65 chromosomes)	Unknown	20-30%	7%	CD10+, CD19+, CD34+, CD22↑, CD45-	Favorable
Hypodiploid (<44 chromosomes)	Unknown	3%	3%	Not distinctive	Unfavorable
t(5;14)(q31;q32)/ *IL3-IGH*	IL3 overexpression and eosinophilia	1-2%	1%	Not distinctive	Standard
t(1;19)(q23;p13.3)/ *TCF3-PBX1*	B-cell development	4-5%	2-3%	CD9+, CD10+, CD22+, CD34-, cytoplasmic IgM+	Standard

factors such as an infectious agent that could expand the *ETV6-RUNX1*-positive cell population, thereby fostering additional genetic events. Perhaps compromised immunosurveillance plays a role. Papaemmanuil et al. (26) have shown that the pattern of these secondary genetic changes suggests that aberrant activity of the recombination activating genes (RAGs) is involved.

Relapsed B-ALL can be derived from either major or minor subclones detected at the time of initial diagnosis. In one study that used next-generation sequencing methods to study *IGH* gene rearrangements in B-ALL, up to 4,000 unique *IGH* gene sequences were identified, each present at a low frequency of less than 0.1 percent, suggesting that B-ALL is highly heterogeneous at initial diagnosis, with one major or dominant clone and numerous other low-level clones (9). Therapy may therefore eradicate the predominant clone but select for a therapy-resistant clone that can lead to relapse. Other studies have shown that relapsed B-ALL cases can have a pattern of genetic abnormalities distinct from the initial leukemia, suggesting that the relapse is a new primary tumor arising from a common "preleukemic" precursor cell (4). The constellation of genetic changes in B-ALL results in impaired differentiation and uncontrolled proliferation, akin to

the class I and class II mutations postulated in acute myeloid leukemia.

The current WHO classification divides B-ALL into seven subgroups according to the common or distinctive molecular associated lesions (Table 10-1) (3). The frequency of these abnormalities is highly variable and differs in children versus adults (fig. 10-1). This approach to B-ALL classification has use, particularly for common abnormalities such as *BCR-ABL1*. However, as the list of genetic abnormalities associated with B-ALL continues to grow, and additional actionable drug targets are identified in the future, the current subgroups in the WHO classification already may be incomplete. Furthermore, a complete list of B-ALL subsets associated with recurrent genetic abnormalities or drug targets may eventually become excessive and impractical for use in a classification scheme.

A small subset (5 to 10 percent) of patients with B-ALL has a history of receiving cytotoxic therapy for another tumor. These patients have a more aggressive clinical course than do patients with de novo disease and a higher risk of abnormal cytogenetic findings. For patients who have received alkylating agents or topoisomerase II inhibitors, cases of B-ALL associated with t(4;11)(q21;q23) or hypodiploidy with loss

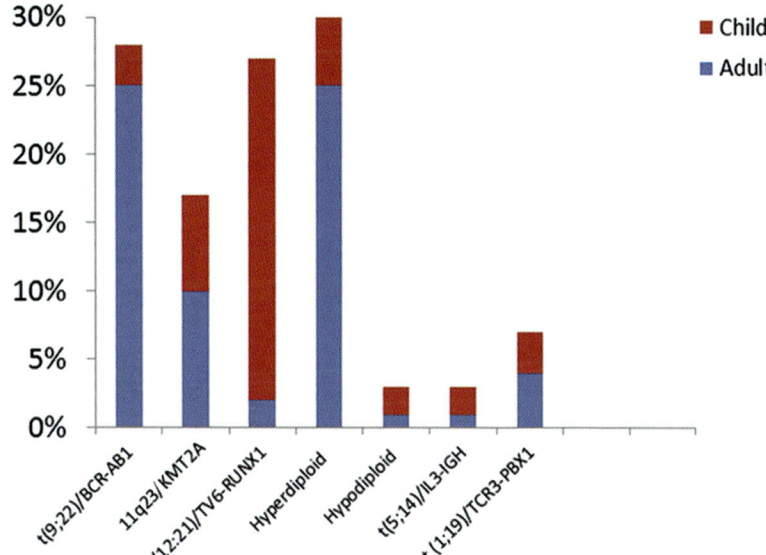

Figure 10-1

CYTOGENETIC SUBTYPES OF B-LYMPHOBLASTIC LEUKEMIA/LYMPHOMA

Frequency of cytogenetic subtypes of B-lymphoblastic leukemia/lymphoma recognized specifically in the World Health Organization (WHO) classification scheme. Children (red) and adults (blue) have different frequencies of these abnormalities.

of chromosomes 5, 7, or 17 have many features suggestive of a therapy-related neoplasm (33). An alternative view is that these tumors are related more to genetic predisposition rather than prior exposure to chemotherapy (8).

CLINICAL FEATURES

Patients with B-ALL have a variable clinical presentation (7,15,27). Symptoms include fever, malaise, arthralgias, bone pain, headache, vomiting, or altered mental status. Some patients are asymptomatic. Physical examination and imaging studies commonly show lymphadenopathy, hepatosplenomegaly, and involvement of other extramedullary sites. So-called sanctuary sites, the central nervous system and the testes in males, may be involved, and therapy must be tailored to specifically eradicate disease at these sites. A large mediastinal mass at presentation is rare, but involvement of the mediastinum can occur as part of widespread disease.

Most patients with B-ALL have hematologic abnormalities. Normochromic normocytic anemia with a low reticulocyte count and thrombocytopenia are common. The leukocyte count with circulating lymphoblasts is elevated in approximately half of patients. Eosinophilia occurs in a small patient subset, often associated with t(5;14)(q31;q32) (2,18).

Patients with B-LBL, by contrast, most often present with localized or migratory pain (17,19).

B-LBL shows a tropism for extranodal sites and some patients present with stage IE disease. The most common sites of involvement are skin, bones (lytic lesions), and soft tissue. Regional lymph nodes are often detected in patients with extranodal disease, but only 10 to 20 percent present primarily with lymphadenopathy. The gastrointestinal tract is often involved. If patients are appropriately treated, only a small number of localized B-LBLs will evolve into B-ALL. Most patients with B-LBL have a normal complete blood count; the lactate dehydrogenase (LDH) serum level is elevated in approximately 25 percent.

HISTOLOGIC FINDINGS

The histologic findings of B-ALL and B-LBL are virtually identical. In peripheral blood and bone marrow aspirate smears lymphoblasts are small to medium size, larger than reactive lymphocytes and often equivalent in size to granulocytes (fig. 10-2A,B) (2,20,36). Lymphoblasts have a high nucleus to cytoplasm ratio, with immature chromatin and a distinct nucleolus. Lymphoblasts have a range of morphologic features, recognized in the French-American-British (FAB) classification as L1 or L2. So-called L2 lymphoblasts are larger, with a prominent nucleolus and more abundant cytoplasm (36). The cytoplasm of the lymphoblasts is usually devoid of granules, but in 5 to 10 percent of cases lymphoblasts have coarse azurophilic granules

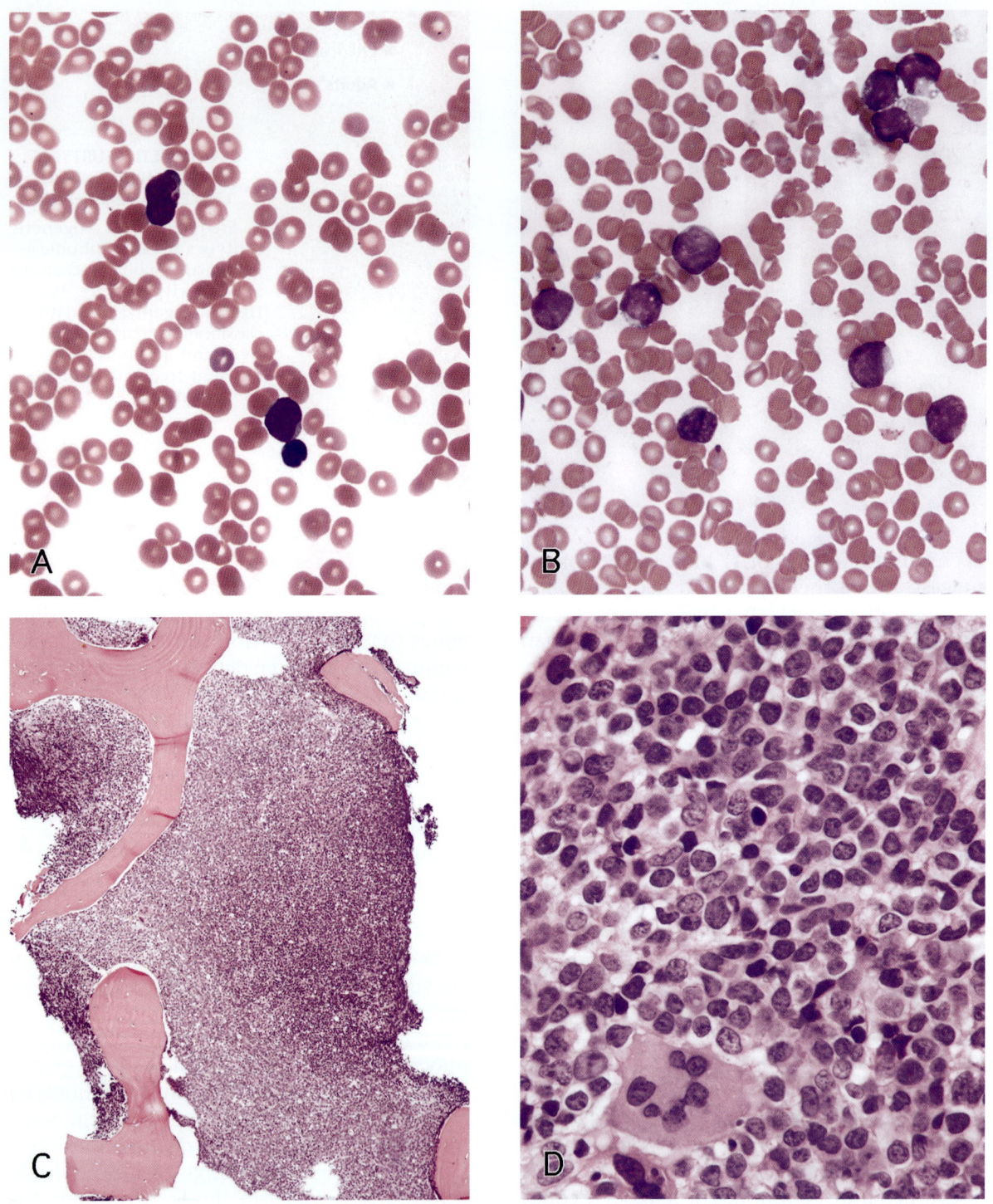

Figure 10-2

BCR-ABL1-POSITIVE B-ACUTE LYMPHOBLASTIC LEUKEMIA (ALL)

A: A peripheral blood smear shows two lymphoblasts in a background of pancytopenia.

B: A bone marrow aspirate smear shows many lymphoblasts.

C,D: The bone marrow biopsy specimen shows a hypercellular medullary space packed by numerous lymphoblasts crowding out normal hematopoiesis (A,B: Wright-Giemsa stain; C,D: hematoxylin and eosin [H&E] stain).

that are usually sparse. These granules are more commonly seen in *BCR-ABL1*-positive ALL and in patients with Down syndrome. Cytoplasmic vacuoles may be present. The cytoplasm of the lymphoblasts also occasionally exhibits a distinctive shape, resembling a handle and described as "hand mirror" cells.

In bone marrow biopsy specimens, B-ALL often diffusely replaces the bone marrow medullary space, crowding out normal hematopoietic cells (fig. 10-2C,D) (18,20,36). In some cases, B-ALL involves the bone marrow in an interstitial pattern. Reticulin fibrosis, resulting in a "dry tap," occurs in a subset of patients. Coagulative necrosis may be present and rarely is so extensive that the workup is compromised and another biopsy is required. Rare B-ALL patients initially present with a hypoplastic or aplastic bone marrow mimicking aplastic anemia.

In lymph nodes, B-ALL/LBL replaces the architecture in a diffuse pattern (17,19). The lymphoblasts commonly invade through the capsule into perinodal adipose tissue, and a single file pattern of infiltration can be observed (fig. 10-3). In some patients, lymph node biopsy specimens show partial involvement by B-ALL/LBL, with preferential sparing of medullary sinuses and follicles (fig. 10-4). A well-developed starry sky pattern is present in approximately 10 percent of cases, although a focal starry sky pattern is present in up to half. Foci of coagulative necrosis, crush artifact, and the Azzopardi effect (blood vessel walls with encrusted DNA that appears as basophilic material), may be observed.

A variety of extranodal sites are involved by B-LBL. In some cases, the neoplastic cells are compartmentalized by sclerosis or normal tissue structures, imparting a nodular appearance. In skin, B-LBL replaces the dermis and often extends into subcutaneous tissue (fig. 10-5). A grenz zone between tumor and epidermis is common. In soft tissue sites, a single file pattern of infiltration by lymphoblasts may be particularly prominent (fig. 10-6). In liver, the tumor can fill the portal tracts or infiltrate sinuses in a leukemic pattern (fig. 10-7). In lytic bone lesions, B-LBL fills the medullary space and destroys bone; the tumor can extend into contiguous soft tissues.

In hematoxylin and eosin (H&E)-stained tissue sections of B-ALL/LBL, lymphoblasts are typically smaller than reactive histiocytes and have a high nucleus to cytoplasm ratio, minimal visible cytoplasm, and finely stippled ("dusty") chromatin with inconspicuous nucleoli. The small nucleoli are better appreciated in B5 or Zenker fixatives than buffered formalin fixation. Lymphoblasts can have round or, less often, convoluted nuclear contours (fig. 10-8). Mitotic figures and apoptotic cells are common.

CYTOLOGIC FINDINGS

In fine-needle aspiration smears and touch imprints that are air dried and stained with Wright-Giemsa or other Romanowsky stains, the features of B-ALL/LBL are similar to those observed in blood and bone marrow aspirate smears (fig. 10-9, left). In Pap-stained smears, there is a considerable range in size, from small blastic cells with more condensed chromatin and indistinct nucleoli to larger blastic cells with fine chromatin and variably prominent nucleoli (fig. 10-9, right). The nuclei are lobulated, convoluted, or round. Mitotic figures are readily identified. The cells often contain a narrow rim of basophilic cytoplasm which may contain vacuoles. In aspirate smears, B and T lymphoblasts are morphologically similar and cannot be distinguished.

IMMUNOPHENOTYPIC FINDINGS

B-ALL/LBL is a neoplasm derived from lymphoblasts of B-cell lineage and is thought to represent a "frozen" state of differentiation as a result of neoplastic transformation. Others have arbitrarily divided B-ALL/LBL cases into stages based on a continuum of differentiation: pro-B, common B, and pre-B (2).

Cytochemistry has a minor role in the diagnosis of B-ALL and is rarely used to diagnose B-LBL. Myeloperoxidase is almost always negative and helps to exclude acute myeloid leukemia. Rare cases of B-ALL, however, express low density myeloperoxidase, usually present in a small subset of lymphoblasts (18,36). Similarly, Sudan black B is positive in a small subset of B-ALL cases. Cases of B-ALL with cytoplasmic granules may be positive for periodic acid–Schiff (PAS) or nonspecific esterase but these findings are not clinically important.

Although flow cytometry has replaced immunofluorescence as an immunophenotypic technique, immunofluorescence still can be applied

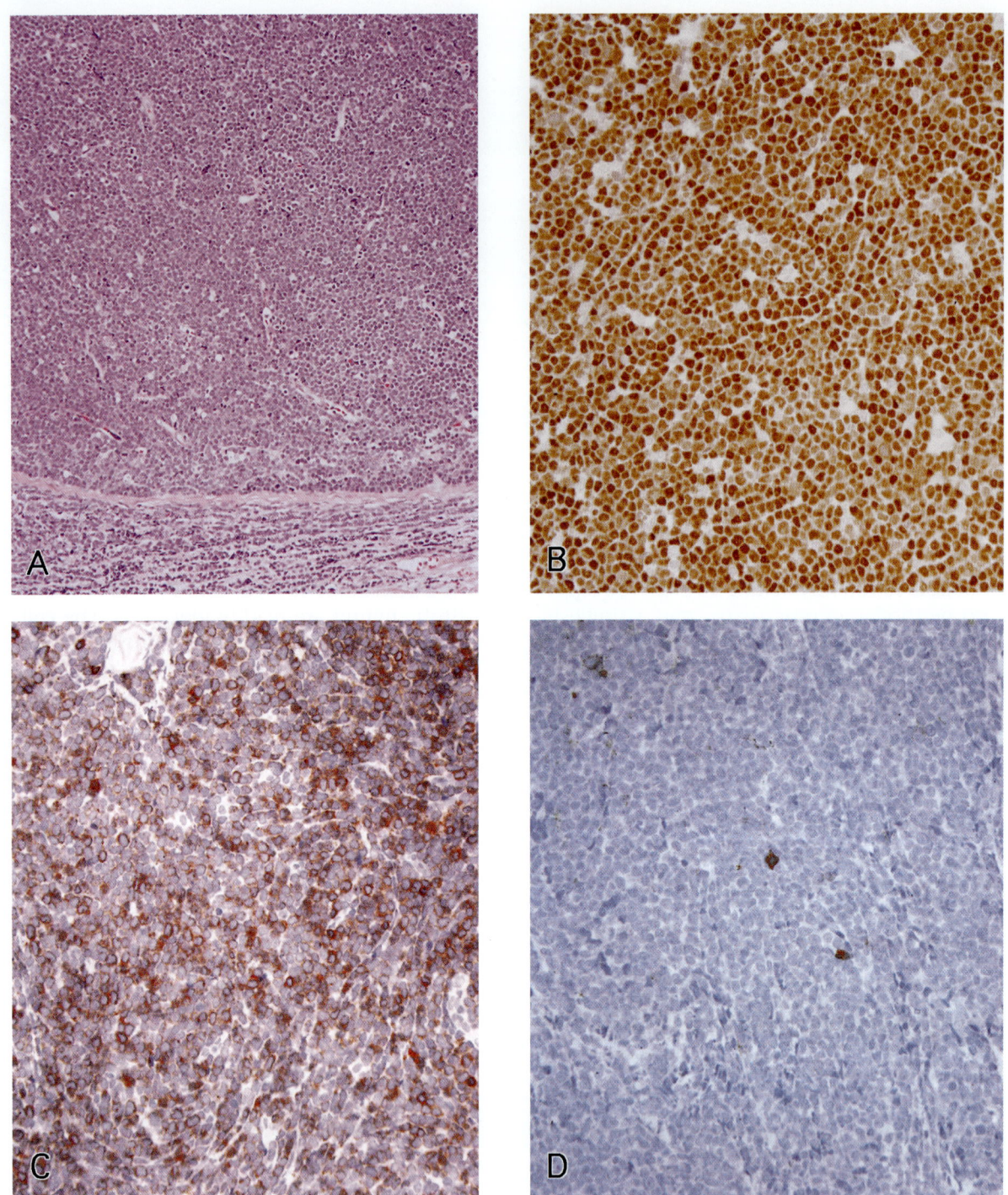

Figure 10-3

B-LYMPHOBLASTIC LYMPHOMA (LBL) EXTENSIVELY REPLACING LYMPH NODE

A: The neoplasm has a diffuse pattern and extends through the capsule into perinodal tissues, where a single file pattern of infiltration is appreciated (H&E stain).

B-D: Immunohistochemistry shows that the neoplasm is positive for TdT (B) and CD79a (C) but not CD20 (D). CD20 is often negative in B-LBL as the antigen is expressed relatively late in differentiation, around the time of immunoglobulin kappa light chain gene rearrangement.

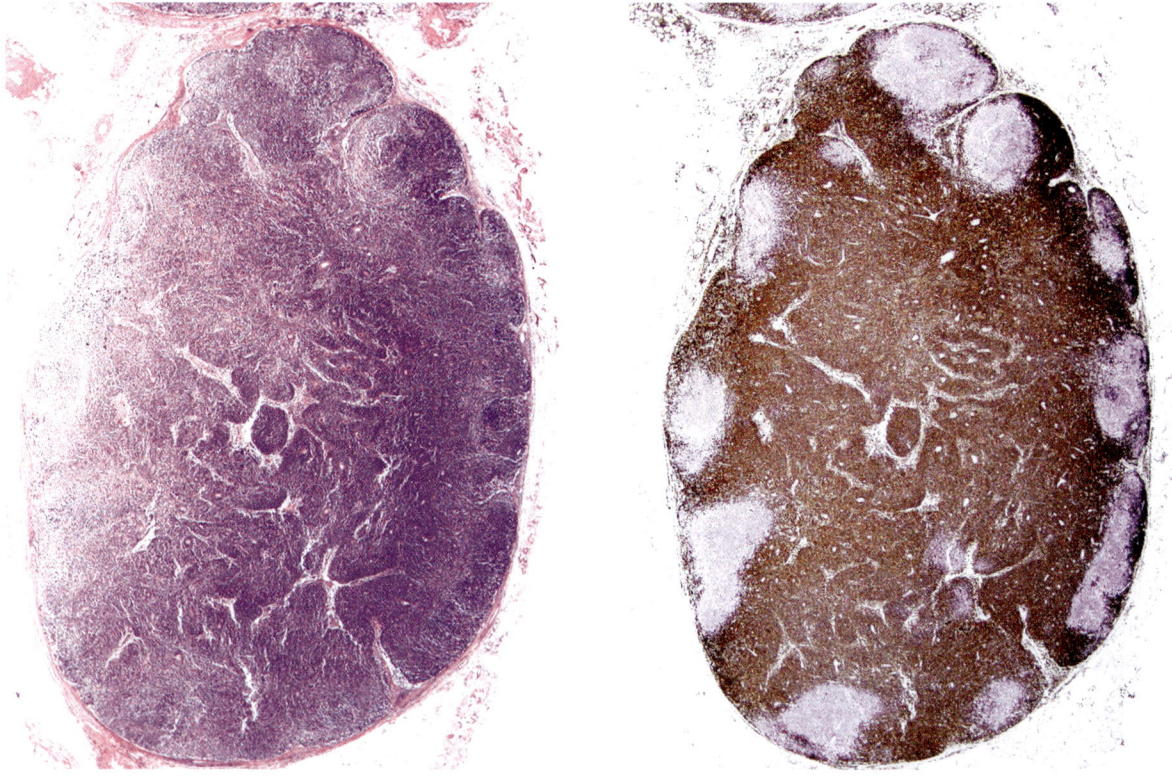

Figure 10-4

B-LYMPHOBLASTIC LYMPHOMA PARTIALLY REPLACING LYMPH NODE

Left: At this power, it is apparent that the medullary sinuses are spared. The follicles are also spared (better seen in right figure) (H&E stain).

Right: By immunohistochemistry, the neoplasm is brightly TdT positive with sparing of the follicles.

to blood or bone marrow aspirate smears or touch imprints. Immunofluorescence is helpful in scant specimens where the number of cells is low (e.g., cerebrospinal fluid). Assessment of TdT is perhaps the most popular application of immunofluorescence in the workup of B-ALL. Lymphoblasts have a finely granular pattern of staining (14).

If fresh tissue is available, flow cytometry immunophenotypic analysis is the best approach for assessing B-ALL/LBL as it allows the use of large antibody panels and has optimal sensitivity (2,32,36). CD19 and cytoplasmic CD79a are expressed in almost all cases of B-ALL/LBL (32,36). CD19 is expressed at the time of *IGH* gene rearrangement. CD10 (also known as common acute lymphoblastic leukemia antigen, or CALLA) and TdT are expressed at the common B stage. CD20 is expressed later, at the time of IG kappa light chain gene rearrangement. Cytoplasmic IgM is expressed at the pre-B-cell stage.

As B-ALL/LBL is an immature tumor, typically IGH and light chains are not expressed (as these markers correlate with a mature B-cell stage). Rare cases of B-ALL, however, express surface IgM only (so-called transitional B-ALL) and even more rarely, B-ALLs express surface IG (34).

Many other markers have been assessed by flow cytometry in B-ALL/LBL and virtually all cases have an aberrant immunophenotype (32). Most B-ALL/LBLs are positive for CD38 (often decreased) and HLA-DR. Most cases, particularly tumors corresponding to an early B-cell stage, are positive for CD34 (fig. 10-10). Conversely, CD45 is negative at an early stage of B-cell differentiation and since CD45 is commonly used in gating strategies, this is a potential pitfall in analysis (2,31,32,36). Myeloid antigens, such as CD13 and CD33, are often expressed in B-ALL/LBL; this expression usually correlates with an early stage of differentiation (31,32). Rare cases of B-ALL/LBL are

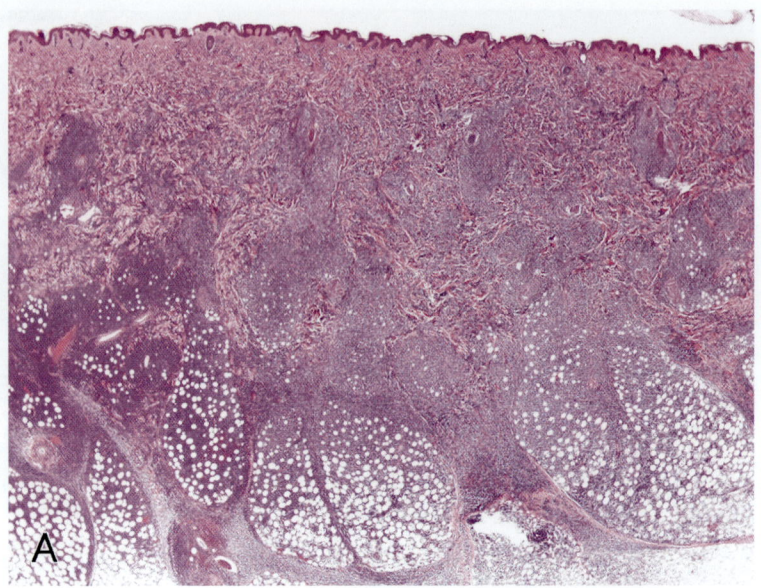

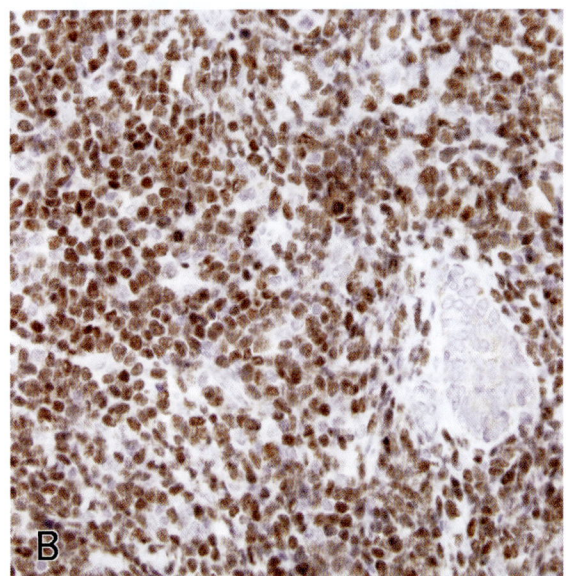

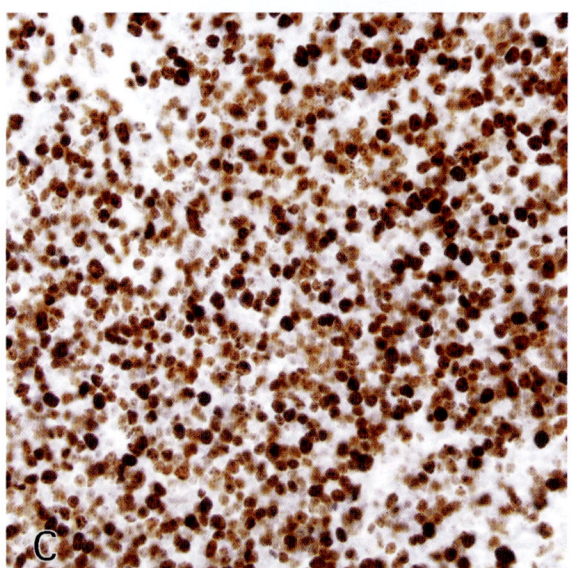

positive for myeloperoxidase (usually negative by cytochemistry). One study has reported a higher rate of relapse in pediatric patients with myeloperoxidase positive B-ALL (23a). CD3 (surface and cytoplasmic) and T-cell receptors are negative. Other pan-T-cell antigens (CD2, CD5, CD7) are expressed aberrantly in about 10 percent of B-ALL cases (32).

The varied immunophenotypes observed in B-ALL/LBL by flow cytometry include not only the presence or absence of antigen expression, but also varied intensity of the antigens that are expressed. For example, CD38 and CD45 are commonly expressed at a lower intensity and CD10 is expressed at a higher intensity in B-ALL/LBL compared with hematogones (normal B-cell precursors) (31,32). The aberrant B-ALL/LBL immunophenotypes are tumor specific and useful for monitoring residual disease, which impacts prognosis (1)

There are some correlations between immunophenotype and molecular abnormalities. Cases of B-ALL/LBL associated with *BCR-ABL1* often express myeloid antigens, such as CD13 and CD33, and are often CD25(+). Cases of B-ALL/LBL associated with t(4;11)(q21;q23) are

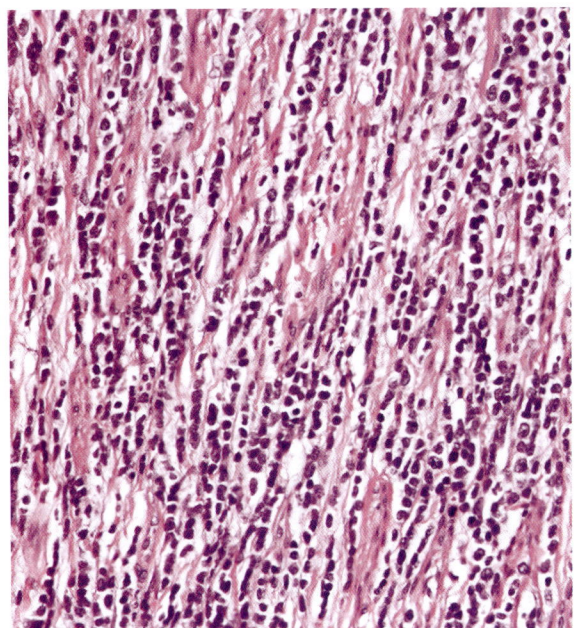

Figure 10-6

**B-LYMPHOBLASTIC LYMPHOMA
INVOLVING SOFT TISSUE**

There is a prominent single file pattern of infiltration (H&E stain).

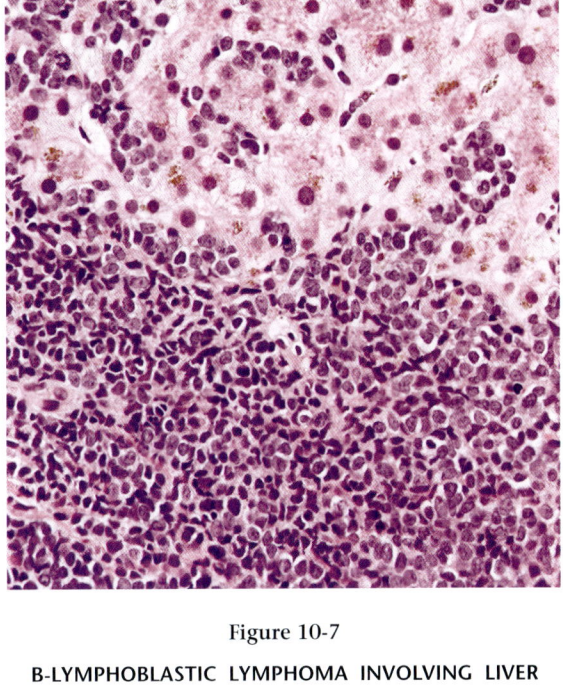

Figure 10-7

B-LYMPHOBLASTIC LYMPHOMA INVOLVING LIVER

This needle biopsy specimen shows that the neoplasm distends a portal tract and also infiltrates sinusoids. Uninvolved liver is at top (H&E stain).

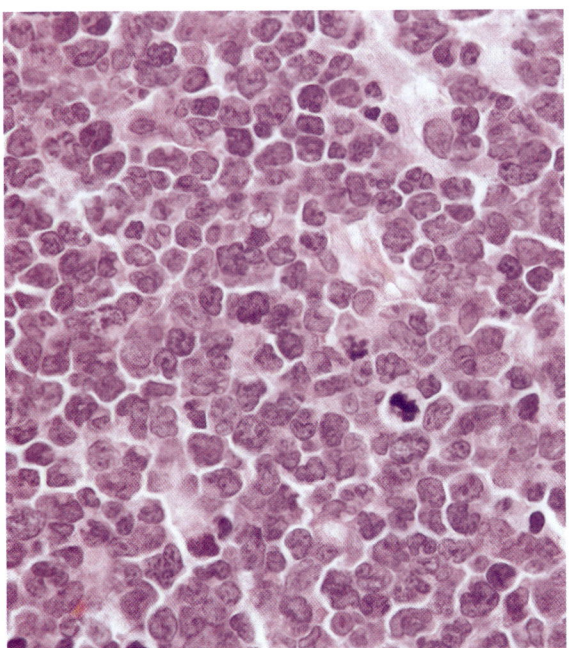

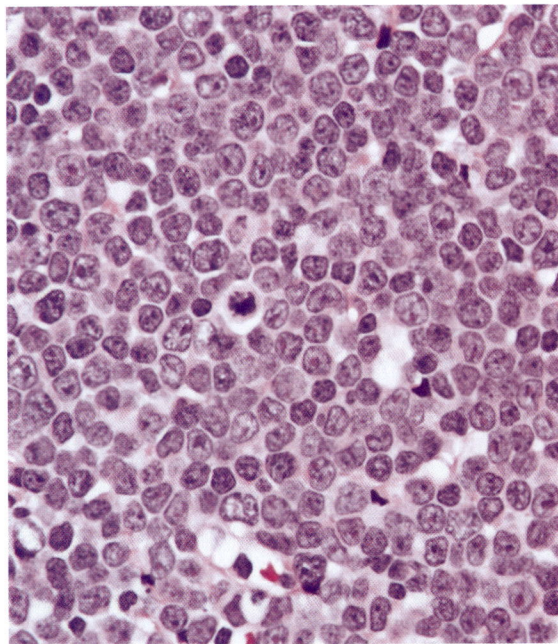

Figure 10-8

B-LYMPHOBLASTIC LYMPHOMA INVOLVING LYMPH NODE

The lymphoblasts can have convoluted (left) or nonconvoluted (right) nuclear contours. Mitotic figures are also easily appreciated in these tumors (H&E stain).

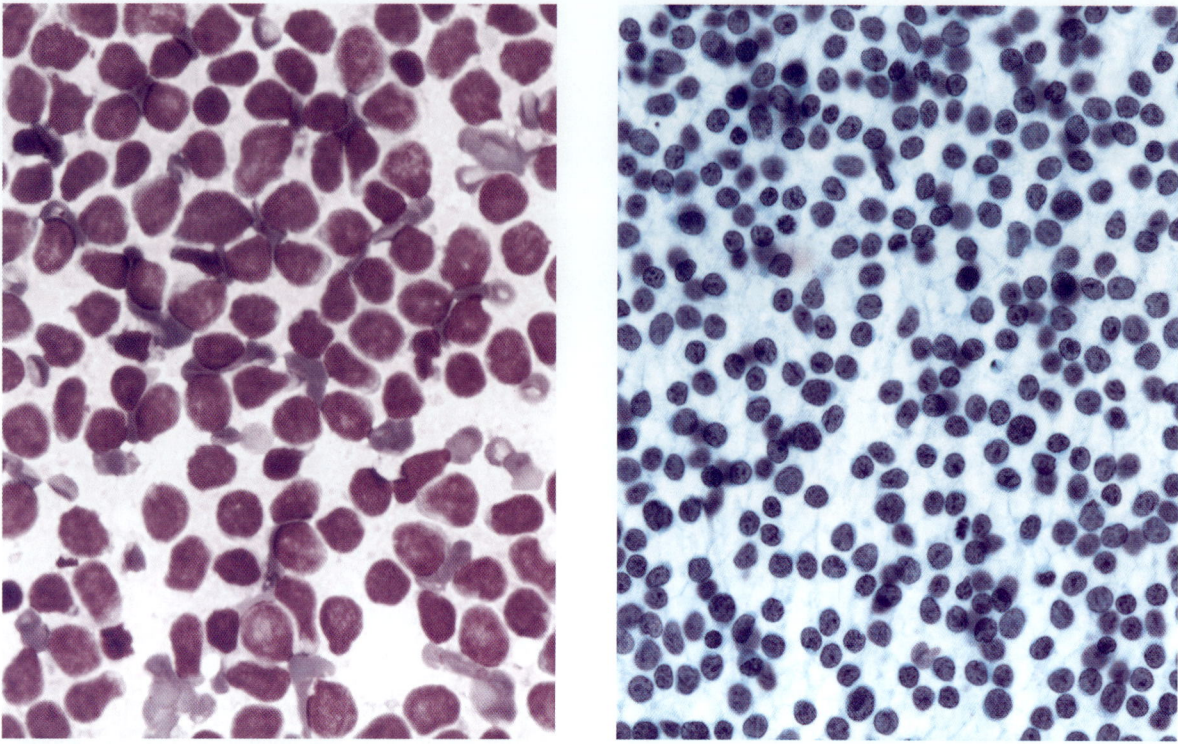

Figure 10-9

B-LYMPHOBLASTIC LYMPHOMA INVOLVING LYMPH NODE

Left: An air-dried aspirate smear shows intermediate-sized cells with fine chromatin and occasional nucleoli (Diff-Quik stain).

Right: A Papanicolaou-stained smear of the same case shows round to irregular nuclei and scant cytoplasm.

CD19(+), often CD15(+), and are CD10(-) and CD20(-). B-ALL/LBL associated with t(1;19) are commonly cytoplasmic IgM(+), CD9(+), CD10(+), CD19(+), and CD34(-) (12).

Immunohistochemical analysis using fixed paraffin-embedded tissue sections is valuable in characterizing the immunophenotype of B-ALL/LBL (2,36). Immunohistochemistry is less sensitive than flow cytometry and therefore dim antigen expression as detected by flow cytometry may be negative by immunohisto-chemistry. Antibodies specific for CD10, CD19, CD20, CD22, CD79a, and PAX5 are available for the immunohistochemical assessment of B-cell lineage. PAX5 is the most sensitive marker and positive in virtually all cases (fig. 10-5B); CD19, CD22, and CD79a are also sensitive markers (fig. 10-3C), although CD79a has the disadvantage of reacting with an appreciable subset of T-ALL/LBL cases. CD20 is positive in 40 to 50 percent of cases and therefore is not well suited to screen

for lineage (fig.10-3D) (25). TdT is positive and expressed brightly in most cases of B-ALL/LBL (figs. 10-3B, 10-4, right). CD34 and CD45/LCA are positive in some cases, but at a lower frequency than observed by flow cytometry.

The expression levels of CD20, CD34, and CD45 are variable in different tumor cells, suggesting that the cells are "frozen" in maturation in an asynchronous fashion. CD43 is a T-cell–associated marker but it is commonly positive in B-ALL/LBL. The T-cell–specific antigens CD3, CD5, and CD7, and T-cell receptors are negative in B-ALL/LBL. In many cases of B-ALL/LBL, some neoplastic cells express MYC, but in cases associated with t(9;22)/*BCR-ABL1* MYC-positive cells may be numerous. BCL6 is positive in about 15 percent of cases and this finding has therapeutic implications (discussed subsequently). B-ALL/LBL cases have a variable, but usually high, proliferation rate as shown by Ki-67 expression (fig. 10-5C). CCND1 is negative.

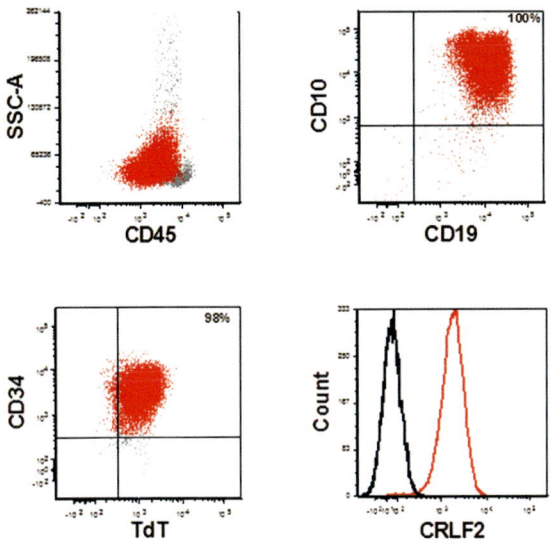

Figure 10-10

B-ACUTE LYMPHOBLASTIC LEUKEMIA: FLOW CYTOMETRY

The neoplastic cells are positive for CD10, CD19, CD34, and TdT. In addition, CRLF2 is expressed, a marker of BCR-ABL1-like B-ALL. (Courtesy of Dr. J. L. Jorgensen, Houston, TX.)

MOLECULAR GENETIC FINDINGS

B-ALL and B-LBL are characterized by monoclonal *IG* rearrangements. *IGH* rearrangement occurs first and is present in all cases of B-ALL. *IGH* rearrangement is followed by *IGK* and, if unsuccessful, followed by *IGL* gene rearrangement (2,36). *IGK* is rearranged in 50 to 60 percent of cases and *IGL* is rearranged in a smaller subset. T-cell receptor gene rearrangements are also common in B-ALL, and occur in a hierarchical fashion: *TRD* followed by *TRG*, *TRB*, and then *TRA*.

Conventional cytogenetic analysis performed almost exclusively on B-ALL divides cases into biologic and prognostic groups that inform therapeutic decisions (12). In many of the more common types of B-ALL, chromosomal translocations disrupt two genes and form novel chimeric fusions. The IG genes are rarely involved in B-ALL-associated translocations (less than 5 percent), although a large number of *IGH*-associated translocations have been described (Table 10-2) (6). In these translocations, the IG locus typically is juxtaposed with an intact gene, leading to overexpression. Other types of B-ALL are characterized by abnormalities in chromosome number, either too many or too few.

The WHO classification (3) recognizes seven categories that correspond to common or distinctive cytogenetic abnormalities (Table 10-1). B-ALL associated with t(9;22)(q34;q11.2)/*BCR-ABL1* is one of the common categories, affecting 3 to 5 percent of children and approximately 30 percent of adults (7,15,23). These neoplasms have traditionally been associated with a poor prognosis, although recent trials using tyrosine kinase inhibitors have resulted in improved survival.

In cases of childhood B-ALL associated with t(9;22)(q34;q11.2), the *BCR-ABL1* p190 isoform is usually formed. In adults, half of B-ALL cases are associated with the p190 and the other half the p210 isoform (as is common in chronic myeloid leukemia).

Other cytogenetic subsets of B-ALL include better and poorer prognostic groups (12,20,36). Patients with B-ALL associated with t(12;21)/*ETV6-RUNX1* and patients with hyperdiploidy (over 50 chromosomes) have a better prognosis. By contrast, patients with a hypodiploid karyotype (less than 45 chromosomes) and an *MLL* gene rearrangement have a poorer prognosis. Two categories of B-ALL recognized specifically in the WHO system are associated with standard risk: t(5;14)/*IL3-IGH* and t(1;19) *TCF3 (E2A)-PBX1* (3).

Ongoing research in B-ALL has shown the importance of other cytogenetic abnormalities. Intrachromosomal amplification of chromosome 21, defined as at least three copies of the chromosome region including *RUNX1* is associated with a poorer prognosis. *RB1* gene mutations and *cytokine receptor-like factor 2* (*CRLF2*) translocations are more common in this type of B-ALL. Other cytogenetic abnormalities in B-ALL are abnormalities or deletions of chromosome 9p that correlate with *CDKN2A/B* alterations (2,30). A rare type of B-ALL in young adults that carries t(14;19)(q32;p13.1)/*IGH-EPOR* is associated with a poor prognosis (16).

Gene expression profiling studies have shown clusters of B-ALL cases that correspond, in large part, to subsets known to be associated with chromosomal translocations (35). In addition, gene expression profiling studies have expanded the number of cases in individual categories

Table 10-2

IGH TRANSLOCATIONS IN B-ALL WITH ASSOCIATED FINDINGS[a]

Target Gene	Chromosomal Location	Presumed Mechanisms of Transformation	Associations
IL3	5q31	IL3 activation results in reactive eosinophilia	Hypereosinophilia
CRLF2	Xp22.3; Yp11.3	STAT5 pathway	½ of patients with Down syndrome; *JAK2* mutation common; poor prognosis
EPOR	19p13	STAT5 pathway	
ID4	6p21	Unknown	
CCAAT enhancer-binding protein (*CEBP*) delta	8q11	Unknown	1/3 of patients have Down syndrome; *BCR-ABL1* rare
CEBP alpha	19p13	Unknown	Also mutated in acute myeloid leukemia
CEBP epsilon	14q11	Unknown	
CEBP beta	20q13	Unknown	
CEBP gamma	19q13	Unknown	Very rare
IGF2BP1	17q21	Enhanced translation of oncogenic proteins	
MIR125B	11q24	Downregulation of p53	
BCL9	1q21	Deregulated WNT pathway	
hTERT	5p15	Unknown	Translocations also found in mature B-cell lymphomas
LHX4	1q21	Unknown	Involved in development of pituitary gland
DUX4	10q26	Unknown	Rare; cell line only
BCL2	18q21	Unknown	Rare; cell line only

[a]Blank spaces represent areas where knowledge is not well developed.

recognized previously by conventional cytogenetic analysis. In other words, some B-ALLs have a gene signature characteristic of a particular translocation, even though conventional cytogenetics is negative for the specific translocation. An important example of this phenomenon is *BCR-ABL1*-like ALL (discussed below).

Array comparative genomic hybridization, single nucleotide polymorphism (SNP) arrays, and next-generation sequencing methods have been applied to the study of B-ALL, particularly pediatric cases. Approximately 50 or so recurrent submicroscopic alterations, mostly deletions or amplifications, have been recognized (Table 10-3). Childhood B-ALL cases have a small number of genetic lesions compared with solid tumors, about 6 to 8 alterations per tumor (21). Adult B-ALL cases have been less well studied than childhood cases, but the number of genetic alterations is greater. Genetic alterations also correlate with cytogenetic findings (30). For ex-

ample, cases of 11q23/*KMT2A*-rearranged B-ALL often have only one (or very few) alteration(s), other than the *KMT2A* rearrangement itself. In contrast, cases of B-ALL associated with t(9;22)/*BCR-ABL1* and t(12;21)/*ETV6-RUNX1* usually have numerous genetic "hits."

Deletions and copy number changes for specific genes also occur in B-ALL. These changes can compromise gene function through deletion or can result in the formation of dominant negative isoforms (15a,22,30). Genetic alterations in B-ALL compromise a number of cell functions, such as lymphocyte development (e.g., *IZKF1*, *PAX5*, and *EBF1*), cell cycle control (e.g., *PTEN*, *RB1*, *CDKN2A/B*), transcriptional regulation (e.g., *ETV6* and *ERG*), and lymphocyte signaling (e.g., *CD200* and *TOX*). Of these, *PAX5* mutations are very common, occurring in up to one third of B-ALL cases; *IZKF1* mutations occur in about 15 percent of B-ALLs in children, with a higher frequency in adults as these mutations

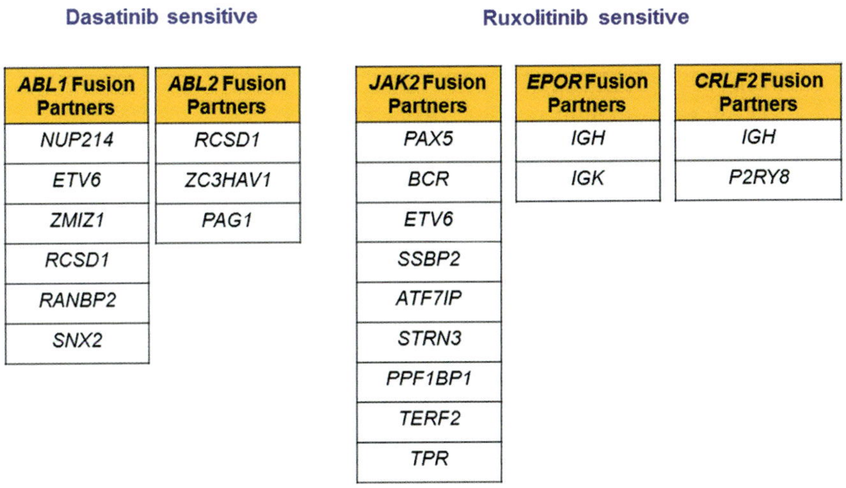

Dasatinib sensitive   **Ruxolitinib sensitive**

ABL1 Fusion Partners	ABL2 Fusion Partners
NUP214	RCSD1
ETV6	ZC3HAV1
ZMIZ1	PAG1
RCSD1	
RANBP2	
SNX2	

JAK2 Fusion Partners	EPOR Fusion Partners	CRLF2 Fusion Partners
PAX5	IGH	IGH
BCR	IGK	P2RY8
ETV6		
SSBP2		
ATF7IP		
STRN3		
PPF1BP1		
TERF2		
TPR		

Figure 10-11

**GENES COMMONLY INVOLVED
BCR-ABL1-LIKE B-ALL**

The figure includes the genes commonly involved in fusions and their many gene partners; genes are grouped according to potential therapy with either dasatinib (BCR/ABL and SRC family tyrosine kinase inhibitors) or ruxolitinib (JAK inhibitor).

are common in *BCR-ABL1*-positive B-ALL (22); *CDKN2A/B* mutations are more common in older children and adults and are also more common in *BCR-ABL1*-positive B-ALL and *TCF3-PBX1* B-ALL (30). *JAK* mutations occur in approximately 10 percent of B-ALLs overall, but are more common in children with Down syndrome. *JAK* mutations are also associated with translocations involving *CRLF2*, present in 10 to 15 percent of B-ALL cases overall, but in over 50 percent of B-ALL cases in the context of Down syndrome. Other common mutations involve *CREBBP* (about 20 percent of relapsed cases), *TP53* (about 10 percent of cases), and *IL7R* (about 7 percent of cases). These alterations predominantly cause loss-of-function mutations (15a,22,30).

To date, few molecular studies have been performed on cases that present as B-LBL, most likely because these cases are uncommon and often the diagnosis is unsuspected. As a result fresh cells or frozen cells are not available for molecular assessment. In 2001, Maitra et al. (19) reviewed the literature and identified eight B-LBL cases that had been karyotyped. Three of the eight had additional chromosome 21 material, either as polysomy or add(21q22). No cases with t(9;22), t(1;19), or t(4;11) were identified; fluorescence in situ hybridization (FISH) or other molecular methods were not performed on these cases. Sadrzadeh et al. (29) reported a case of B-LBL associated with *BCR-ABL1* presenting as a lytic lesion involving the left parietal skull.

BCR-ABL1-Like or Philadelphia Chromosome-Like B-ALL

Gene expression profiling and other high-throughput studies have led to the recognition and characterization of *BCR-ABL1*-like B-ALL (28). *BCR-ABL1*-like B-ALL represents about 15 percent of all cases of B-ALL. This frequency increases with age, being about 10 percent in young children and almost 30 percent in young adults with B ALL (28). *BCR-ABL1*-like B-ALL is defined as a tumor that does not carry t(9;22)/ *BCR-ABL1*, but has a gene expression profile that clusters closely with *BCR-ABL1*-positive B-ALL cases. STAT5B activation is a common feature. *BCR-ABL1*-like B-ALL is highly heterogeneous at the molecular level and therapies differ accordingly (see below). The recognition of *BCR-ABL1*-like B ALL is clinically important because affected patients have a poorer prognosis than other B-ALL patients and because early data indicate that these tumors can be treated with tyrosine kinase inhibitors (fig. 10-11) (28).

Morphologically and immunophenotypically, *BCR-ABL1*-like B-ALL is similar to other cases of B-ALL (13,28). One difference is CRLF2 is expressed in *BCR-ABL1*-like B-ALL, which can be used as a surrogate for this disease (fig. 10-11) (16a). Conventional cytogenetic analysis has shown that *BCR-ABL1*-like B-ALL cases do not carry any of the major cytogenetic abnormalities recognized by the WHO classification. At the molecular level, however, these tumors are subdivided into two major groups: half the cases

Table 10-3

GENETIC ABNORMALITIES IN B-ALL AND PROGNOSIS[a]

Molecular Abnormality	Impaired Function	Frequency in Children	Frequency In Adults	Associations	Prognosis
BCR-ABL1-like	Activation of kinase signaling	10%	20-30%	Two subgroups: 1) *CRLF2* fusion genes; 2) fusion genes involving *ABL1, ABL2,* and others; *IZKF1* mutations common	Unfavorable
Intrachromosomal amplification of *AMP21*	Unknown	2%	Rare	No distinctive features	Unfavorable
Del(7p13) or mutation/*IKZF1*	B-cell development	15%	~25%	~75% of *BCR-ABL1* ALL	Unfavorable
Del(9p13), rearrangement or mutation/*PAX5*	B-cell development	~20%	20-30%	Mutations are not associated with outcome	Variable
Del(9p21) or mutation/*CDKN2A/B*	Tumor suppressor	20-35%	~40%	Associated with *BCR-ABL1* and *TCF3-PBX1* ALL	Variable
JAK mutations (other than V617F)	Signal transduction	10%		10% of high risk *BCR-ABL1*-negative ALL; 20-35% of Down syndrome ALL cases	Unfavorable
RAS pathway mutations	Signal Transduction	50% in certain subsets		Common in hyperdiploid and MLL-rearranged ALL cases	Variable
CREBBP mutation	Histone acetylation	~20% at relapse		Associated with relapse, high hyperploidy, and steroid resistance	Unfavorable

[a]Blank spaces represent areas where knowledge is not well developed.

are characterized by overexpression of CRLF2 as a result of two gene fusions *(IGH-CRLF2* or *P2RY8-CRLF2)*. These tumors also commonly have *JAK2,* or less often, *EPOR* or other mutations in the JAK-STAT pathway and patients can be treated with JAK2 inhibitors. A second subset of *BCR-ABL1*-like B-ALL cases is associated with gene fusions that involve *ABL1, ABL2, CSFR1,* or *PDGFRβ,* and these patients may respond to ABL1 inhibitors such as dasatinib (28).

IZKF1, PAX5, and *CDKN2A/B* mutations are also common in *BCR-ABL1*-like B-ALL (13,23). In addition to the rearrangements and translocations of *CRLF2* described, other poorly characterized abnormalities also lead to CRLF2 overexpression (13).

B-ALL with Functional Pre-B-Cell Receptor Signaling

In most cases of B-ALL, the neoplastic cells lack a functional B-cell receptor; however, about 15 percent exhibit tonic pre-B-cell receptor (BCR) signaling. These tumors represent a distinct subset of B-ALL that includes B-ALL cases associated with *TCF3-PBX1* as well as cases with

del(6q21)/*PRDM1* (10). Pre-BCR signaling activates downstream tyrosine kinases (e.g., SYK, ZAP-70), which eventually result in activation of the PI3K-AKT and other pathways. Recognition of this disease subset is important because early (mostly preclinical) studies have shown that ibrutinib (a Bruton tyrosine kinase inhibitor) and idelalisib (a PI3Kδ inhibitor) have good activity against the leukemic cells, opening up a novel therapeutic approach for these B-ALL patients (10).

Recognition of cases of B-ALL with functional pre-BCR signaling can be achieved by assessing for expression of BCL6, which is activated by pre-BCR signaling. In most pathology laboratories, assessing BCL6 by immunohistochemistry is convenient and sensitive (10).

DIFFERENTIAL DIAGNOSIS

The differential diagnosis of B-ALL/LBL involves other blastic hematopoietic neoplasms.

T-Lymphoblastic Leukemia/Lymphoma. B- and T-ALL/LBL are morphologically similar. T-LBL cases commonly present as a mediastinal mass in adolescents and young adults. T-ALL cases are common in young children and the elderly. Immunophenotypic assessment is essential as these tumors have an immature T-cell immunophenotype.

Burkitt Lymphoma. These tumors usually present as an extranodal mass, but a primarily leukemic form also occurs. Burkitt lymphoma in tissue biopsy specimens has a prominent starry sky pattern, and the lymphoma cells are intermediately sized (larger than lymphoblasts), with thick nuclear membranes and multiple small nucleoli. Apoptosis and mitotic figures are numerous. In smears, Burkitt lymphoma cells have prominent cytoplasmic vacuoles (so-called L3 in FAB classification). These tumors have a mature germinal center B-cell immunophenotype [surface Ig(+), CD10(+), BCL6(+)].

Diffuse Large B-Cell Lymphoma. Diffuse large B-cell lymphoma is composed of large cells with vesicular nuclei. These tumors have a mature B-cell immunophenotype [surface Ig(+), TdT(-)].

Mantle Cell Lymphoma, Blastoid Variant. These tumors resemble B-ALL/LBL cytologically, but mantle cell lymphoma has a mature B-cell immunophenotype [surface Ig(+), CD5(+), CD20(+)] and is associated with t(11;14)(q13;q32) and cyclin D1 expression.

Acute Myeloid Leukemia and Myeloid Sarcoma. Myeloid neoplasms may resemble B-ALL/LBL, particularly cases with minimal differentiation (so-called M0 in the FAB classification). A complete immunophenotypic panel is required for this differential diagnosis because B-ALL/LBL can express myeloid antigens (but usually not myeloperoxidase).

Blastic Plasmacytoid Dendritic Cell Neoplasm (BPDCN). These tumors exhibit blastic morphology and some cells express TdT, usually variably. However, BPDCNs are positive for CD4, CD56, CD123, TCL1, and CD303, and do not express B-cell antigens.

Ewing Sarcoma/Peripheral Neuroectodermal Tumor (ES/PNET). In young patients with B-ALL/LBL who present with a lytic lesion involving bone the diagnosis of ES/PNET may be considered. CD99 can be expressed by B-ALL/LBL and this result can contribute to misinterpretation as ES/PNET (5). Complete immunophenotyping is required as ES/PNET lacks evidence of a B-cell lineage and is associated with distinctive translocations involving the *EWS* gene family.

TREATMENT AND PROGNOSIS

The therapy for patients with B-ALL/LBL is risk-adapted, multiagent chemotherapy (7,15, 27). Improvements in the prognosis of B-ALL patients can be attributed, in large part, to better risk stratification, allowing more tailored therapy. A leukocyte count of 50 x 10^9/L or more, central nervous system involvement, and patient age of 10 years or older are considered high-risk clinical features. Poor risk clinical features correlate with genetic alterations of *IKZF1* and *CDKN2A/B* (22,30). Further stratification is based on the presence and type of cytogenetic abnormalities. Patients with a hypodiploid karyotype, 11q23/*KMT2A* rearrangement, and t(9;22)/*BCR-ABL1*-positive tumors have a worse prognosis (Table 10-1) and receive more aggressive therapy. Recently, genetic studies have identified additional disease subsets, such as *BCR-ABL1*-like B-ALL, a poor risk subset and B-ALL with functional pre-BCR signaling, in which prognosis is currently being defined (Table 10-3).

Risk stratification also evolves with therapeutic advances. For example, traditionally, patients with *BCR-ABL1*-positive B-ALL were considered to be a high-risk, poor prognosis group, but the introduction of tyrosine kinase inhibitor therapy has improved prognosis and therefore patients with these tumors are currently considered closer to standard risk disease. These agents are also effective against *BCR-ABL1*-like B-ALL. Ibrutinib and idelalisib appear to have a role for cases of B-ALL with a functional pre-BCR.

Using current standardized treatment protocols, children with B-ALL have high complete remission and cure rates, up to 90 and 80 percent, respectively (15,27). The chemotherapy regimens used for adults with B-ALL were initially developed for children and later adapted. The prognosis of adults with B-ALL is less good, with complete remission and cure rates of 60 and 40 percent, respectively (7). In patients with relapse, novel therapies such as chimeric antigen receptor (CAR) T cells, and blinatumomab (antibody construct with specificity for CD19 and CD3) appear to be promising (24,37).

Less is known about patients with B-LBL as few cases have been reported in the literature and these patients have not been treated systematically (17,19). In one study at MD Anderson Cancer Center, aggressive chemotherapy resulted in complete remission in all 13 patients assessed, with long-term remission in 9 patients and a median survival of 5 years (17). Data regarding therapy are sparse for B-LBL patients, however, and a more systemic approach for treatment and risk stratification is needed.

REFERENCES

1. Bar M, Wood BL, Radich JP, et al. Impact of minimal residual disease, detected by flow cytometry, on outcome of myeloablative hematopoietic cell transplantation for acute lymphoblastic leukemia. Leuk Res Treatment 2014;2014:421723

2. Borowitz MJ, Chan JK. B lymphoblastic leukaemia/lymphoma. In: Swerdlow SH, Campo E, Harris NL, et al., eds. WHO classification of tumours of haematopoietic and lymphoid tissues. Lyon: IARC Press; 2008:168-170.

3. Borowitz MJ, Chan JK. B lymphoblastic leukaemia/lymphoma with recurrent genetic abnormalities. In: Swerdlow SH, Campo E, Harris NL, et al., eds. WHO classification of tumours of haematopoietic and lymphoid tissues. Lyon: IARC Press; 2008:171-175.

4. Davidsson J, Paulsson K, Lindgren D, et al. Relapsed childhood high hyperdiploid acute lymphoblastic leukemia: presence of preleukemic ancestral clones and the secondary nature of microdeletions and RTK-RAS mutations. Leukemia 2010;24:924-931.

5. Dworzak MN, Fritsch G, Fleischer C, et al. CD99 (MIC2) expression in paediatric B-lineage leukaemia/lymphoma reflects maturation-associated patterns of normal B-lymphopoiesis. Br J Haematol 1999;105:690-695.

6. Dyer MJ, Akasaka T, Capasso M, et al. Immunoglobulin heavy chain locus chromosomal translocations in B-cell precursor acute lymphoblastic leukemia: rare clinical curios or potent genetic drivers? Blood 2010;115:1490-1499.

7. Faderl S, O'Brien S, Pui CH, et al. Adult acute lymphoblastic leukemia: concepts and strategies. Cancer 2010;116:1165-76.

8. Ganzel C, Devlin S, Douer D, Rowe JM, Stein EM, Tallman MS. Secondary acute lymphoblastic leukaemia is constitutional and probably not related to prior therapy. Br J Haematol 2015;170:50-55.

9. Gawad C, Pepin F, Carlton V, et al. Massive evolution of the immunoglobulin heavy chain locus in children with precursor B-cell acute lymphoblastic leukemia. Blood 2012;120:4407-4417.

10. Geng H, Hurtz C, Lenz KB, et al. Self-enforcing feedback activation between BCL6 and pre-B cell receptor signaling defines a distinct subtype of acute lymphoblastic leukemia. Cancer Cell 2015;27:409-425.

11. Greaves M. Darwin and evolutionary tales in leukemia. The Ham-Wasserman lecture. Hematology Am Soc Hematol Educ Program 2009;3-12.

12. Harrison CJ. Cytogenetics of paediatric and adolescent acute lymphoblastic leukaemia. Br J Haematol 2009;144:147-156.

13. Harvey RC, Mulligan CG, Chen IM, et al. Rearrangement of CLRF2 is associated with mutation of JAK kinases, alteration of IKZF1, Hispanic/Latin ethnicity, and a poor outcome in pediatric B-progenitor acute lymphoblastic leukemia. Blood 2010;115:5312-5321.

14. Hurford MT, Altman AJ, DiGiuseppe JA, Sherburne BJ, Rezuke WN. Unique pattern of nuclear TdT immunofluorescence distinguishes normal precursor B cells (hematogones) from lymphoblasts of precursor B-lymphoblastic leukemia. Am J Clin Pathol 2008;129:700-705.

15. Inaba H, Greaves M, Mulligan CG. Acute lymphoblastic leukaemia. Lancet 2013;381:1943-1955.

15a. Iacobucci I, Mulligan CG. Genetic basis of acute lymphoblastic leukemia. J Clin Oncol 2017;35:975-983.

16. Jaso JM, Yin CC, Lu VW, et al. B acute lymphoblastic leukemia with t(14;19)(q32;p13.1) involving IGH/EPOR: a clinically aggressive subset of disease. Mod Pathol 2014;27:382-389.

16a. Konoplev S, Lu X, Konopleva M, et al. CRLF2-positive B-cell acute lymphoblastic leukemia in adult patients: a single-institution experience. Am J Clin Pathol 2017;147:357-363.

17. Lin P, Jones D, Dorfman DM, Medeiros LJ. Precursor B-cell lymphoblastic lymphoma: A predominantly extranodal tumor with a low propensity for leukemic involvement. Am J Surg Pathol 2000;24:1480-1490.

18. Loghavi S, Kutok JL, Jorgensen JL. B acute lymphoblastic leukemia/lymphoblastic lymphoma. Am J Clin Pathol 2015;144:393-418.

19. Maitra A, McKenna RW, Weinberg AG, Schneider NR, Kroft SH. Precursor B-cell lymphoblastic lymphoma: A study of nine cases lacking blood and bone marrow involvement and a review of the literature. Am J Clin Pathol 2001;115:868-875.

20. McGregor S, McNeer J, Gurbuxani S. Beyond the 2008 World Health Organization classification: the role of the hematopathology laboratory in the diagnosis and management of acute lymphoblastic leukemia. Semin Diagn Pathol 2012;29:2-11.

21. Mori H, Colman SM, Xiao Z, et al. Chromosome translocations and covert leukemic clones are generated during normal fetal development. Proc Natl Acad Sci U S A 2002;99:8242-8247.

22. Mullighan CG. Molecular genetics of B-precursor acute lymphoblastic leukemia. J Clin Invest 2012;122:3407-3415.

23. Mullighan CG, Miller CB, Radtke I, et al. BCR-ABL1 lymphoblastic leukaemia is characterized by the deletion of Ikaros. Nature 2008;453:110-114.

23a. Oberley MJ, Li S, Orgel E, Phei Wee C, Hagiya A, O'Gorman MR. Clinical significance of isolated myeloperoxidase expression in pediatric B-lymphoblastic leukemia. Am J Clin Pathol 2017;147:374-381.

24. Oluwole OO, Davila ML. At the bedside: clinical review of chimeric antigen receptor (CAR) T cell therapy for B cell malignancies. J Leukoc Biol 2016;100:1265-1272.

25. Oschlies I, Burkhardt B, Chassagne-Clement C, et al. Diagnosis and immunophenotype of 188 pediatric lymphoblastic lymphomas treated within a randomized prospective trial: experiences and preliminary recommendations from the European Childhood Lymphoma Pathology Panel. Am J Surg Pathol 2011;35:836-844.

26. Papaemmanuil R, Rapado I, Li Y, et al. RAG-mediated recombination is the predominant driver of oncogenic rearrangement in ETV6-RUNX1

acute lymphoblastic leukemia. Nat Genet 2014;46:116-125.

27. Pui CH, Robison LL, Look AT. Acute lymphoblastic leukemia. Lancet 2008;371:1030-1043.

28. Roberts KG, Li Y, Payne-Turner D, et al. Targetable kinase-activating lesions in Ph-like acute lymphoblastic leukemia. N Engl J Med 2014;371:1005-1015

29. Sadrzadeh H, Huck AE, Chen YB, Hasserjian RP, Fathi AT. Philadelphia chromosome (Ph) positive B-cell lymphoblastic lymphoma isolated to bone. Leuk Lymphoma 2013;54:2052-2054.

30. Schwab CJ, Chilton L, Morrison H, et al. Genes commonly deleted in childhood B-cell precursor acute lymphoblastic leukemia: association with cytogenetics and clinical features. Haematologica 2013;98:1081-1088.

31. Sedek L, Bulsa J, Sonsala A, et al. The immunophenotype of blast cells in B-cell precursor acute lymphoblastic leukemia: how different are they from their normal counterparts. Cytometry B Clin Cytom 2014;86B:329-339.

32. Seegmiller AC, Kroft SH, Karandikar NJ, McKenna RW. Characterization of immunophenotypic aberrancies in 200 cases of B acute lymphoblastic leukemia. Am J Clin Pathol 2009;132:940-949.

33. Tang G, Zuo Z, Thomas DA, et al. Precursor B-acute lymphoblastic leukemia occurring in patients with a history of prior malignancies: is it therapy-related? Haematologica 2012;97:919-925.

34. Vasef MA, Brynes RK, Murata-Collins JL, Arber DA, Medeiros LJ. Surface immunoglobulin light chain-positive acute lymphoblastic leukemia of FAB L1 or L2 type: a report of 6 cases in adults. Am J Clin Pathol 1998;110:143-149.

35. Yeoh EJ, Ross ME, Shurtleff SA, et al. Classification, subtype discovery, and prediction of outcome in pediatric acute lymphoblastic leukemia by gene expression profiling. Cancer Cell 2002;1:133-143.

36. Zhou Y, You MJ, Young KH, et al. Advances in the molecular pathobiology of B-lymphoblastic leukemia. Hum Pathol 2012;43:1347-1362.

37. Zugmaier G, Gökbuget N, Klinger M, et al. Long-term survival and T-cell kinetics in relapsed/refractory ALL patients who achieved MRD response after blinatumomab treatment.Blood 2015;126:2578-2584.

11 CHRONIC LYMPHOCYTIC LEUKEMIA/ SMALL LYMPHOCYTIC LYMPHOMA

Chronic lymphocytic leukemia/small lymphocytic lymphoma (CLL/SLL) is a neoplasm composed of small, round B lymphocytes and a variable number of larger cells with more prominent nucleoli, known as prolymphocytes in the peripheral blood, and referred to as prolymphocytes and paraimmunoblasts in lymph nodes. The cells of CLL/SLL have a characteristic immunophenotype: positive for surface immunoglobulin (dim), CD5, CD19, CD20 (dim), CD23, and CD200. The disease is highly heterogeneous at the molecular level and there is no unifying molecular abnormality.

The designation CLL is used to describe involvement of the peripheral blood with an elevated absolute lymphocyte count of over 5 x 10^9/L (31). Bone marrow, lymph nodes, and other tissue sites are also involved. The SLL designation is used to connote tissue involvement by a neoplasm that is currently indistinguishable from CLL at the morphologic, immunophenotypic, and genetic level, but arising in a patient without absolute lymphocytosis (31). Approximately 15 percent of all patients present with a SLL clinical picture (50).

GENERAL FEATURES

CLL is the most common form of leukemia in adults in North America and Europe, but is rare in Asia. In the United States, it is estimated that there will be 18,960 new cases of CLL in 2016 (28b). The annual incidence of CLL is approximately 4 cases per 100,000 individuals and increases with advancing age (28b,45).

The etiology of CLL is not well understood. The International Lymphoma Epidemiology Consortium reported five factors associated with an increased risk: first-degree family history of hematologic malignancy, hepatitis C infection, occupation as a farmer (or living on a farm), employment as a hairdresser, and increased height (46). These risk factors suggest that genetic and environmental factors are involved in pathogenesis. Stereotypy of surface immunoglobulin in a subset of CLL cases also suggests a role for antigen drive or selection in pathogenesis (51).

Biologic studies to determine the pathogenesis of CLL/SLL in the past have focused on CLL cells obtained from the blood. Presumably, blood CLL lymphocytes have been studied because of the convenience and ease of obtaining them in large numbers. However, CLL cells undergo apoptosis in vitro, showing the importance of the in vivo tumor microenvironment in CLL cell growth and survival. Proliferation centers (also known as pseudofollicular growth centers, or pseudofollicles) in lymph nodes are thought to be essential in CLL/SLL pathogenesis.

CLINICAL FEATURES

The median age of patients with CLL/SLL at the time of first diagnosis is 65 years (31,37); some cases present in younger individuals. The disease is more common in men, with a male to female ratio of 1.8 to 1.0. Approximately 30 percent of patients have B-type symptoms. The physical examination often reveals lymphadenopathy, which can be modest or marked, but is usually painless (37). Hepatomegaly or splenomegaly is common. Patients may report an increased frequency of infections. Bone marrow involvement is common: 75 percent of patients with SLL and virtually all patients with CLL (31). Some CLL patients are asymptomatic, with minimal or no physical findings, and the diagnosis is established incidentally by the detection of lymphocytosis in a complete blood count performed for unrelated reasons.

Laboratory studies show that most patients with CLL/SLL present with an absolute lymphocytosis that is usually between 10-150 x 10^9/L in the peripheral blood: the absolute lymphocyte count is over 50 x 10^9/L in about two thirds of patients (37). Cytopenias are common in patients with advanced stage disease, usually as a result of

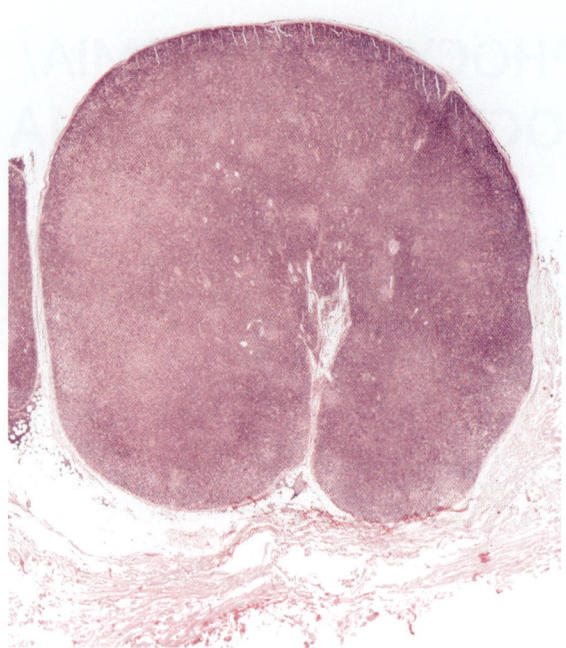
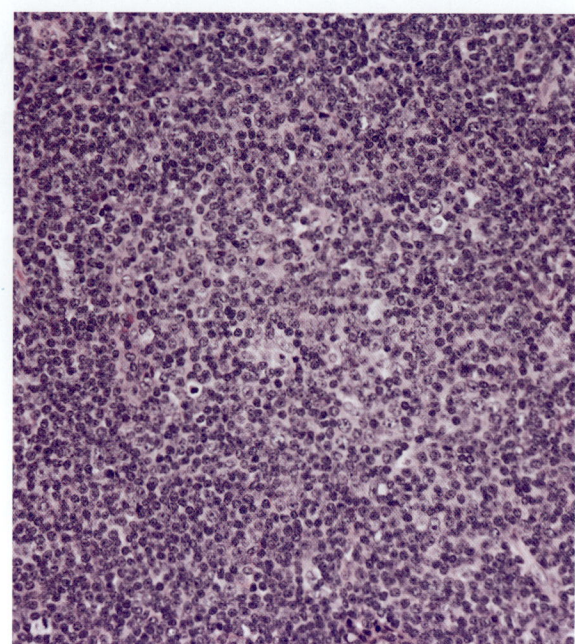

Figure 11-1

CHRONIC LYMPHOCYTIC LEUKEMIA/SMALL LYMPHOCYTIC LYMPHOMA (CLL/SLL) INVOLVING A SMALL LYMPH NODE

Left: Interspersed between the dark areas composed of small lymphocytes are subtle, vaguely nodular and pale areas known as proliferation centers.

Right: The proliferation centers contain intermediate-sized and larger cells with round nuclei and variably prominent nucleoli known as prolymphocytes and paraimmunoblasts (hematoxylin and eosin [H&E] stain).

high tumor burden in the bone marrow (31). Autoimmune cytopenias occur in 5 percent of patients (58), hypogammaglobulinemia occurs in about one quarter (36), and 2 to 3 percent, have an elevated serum immunoglobulin paraprotein level (57).

Serum lactate dehydrogenase (LDH) and β-2-microglobulin levels are increased in about one third of patients and this increase correlates with more aggressive disease. High serum thymidine kinase 1 levels are present in about 25 percent of patients (23,37). Visco et al. (53) reported that about 60 percent of CLL patients have detectable Epstein-Barr virus (EBV) DNA in peripheral blood mononuclear cells. Higher levels of LDH, β-2-microgloblin, thymidine kinase 1, and EBV DNA correlate with a poorer prognosis.

HISTOLOGIC FINDINGS

Lymph Nodes

In the lymph nodes, CLL/SLL is usually characterized by diffuse effacement of the architecture by a population of small lymphoid cells with clumped nuclear chromatin, round nuclear contours, and scant cytoplasm (31). Interspersed between the dark areas imparted by the neoplastic small lymphocytes are vaguely nodular and pale areas known as proliferation centers (or pseudofollicles) (figs. 11-1, 11-2). Proliferation centers contain larger cells with round nuclei and prominent nucleoli that represent a spectrum of prolymphocytes and paraimmunoblasts in addition to small round lymphocytes. Proliferation centers can be highly variable in size and cellular content (figs. 11-1, 11-2) (31).

In lymph nodes that are incompletely replaced by CLL/SLL, reactive lymphoid follicles may be present and, in some cases, these follicles are surrounded by the tumor. In cases in which CLL/SLL cells seem to completely replace the mantle and marginal zone cells, but spare residual germinal centers, these germinal centers have been referred to as being "naked." Naked germinal centers are rare in other types of non-Hodgkin lymphoma with the exception

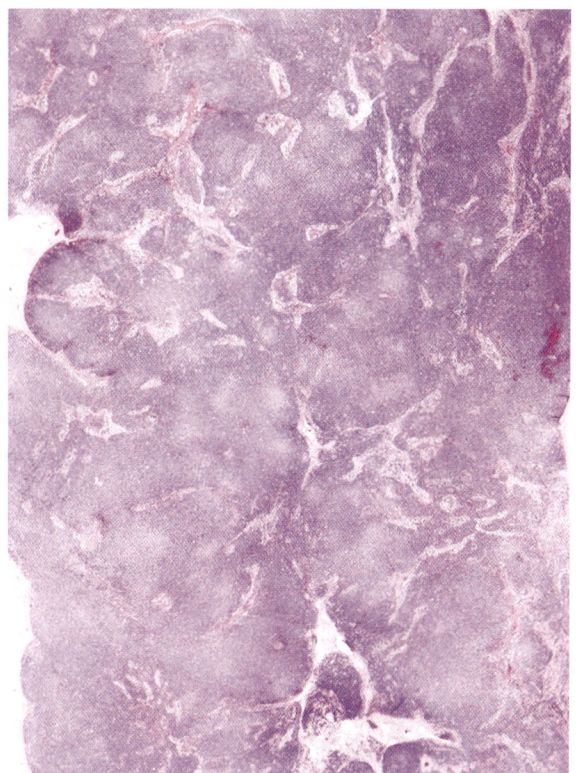 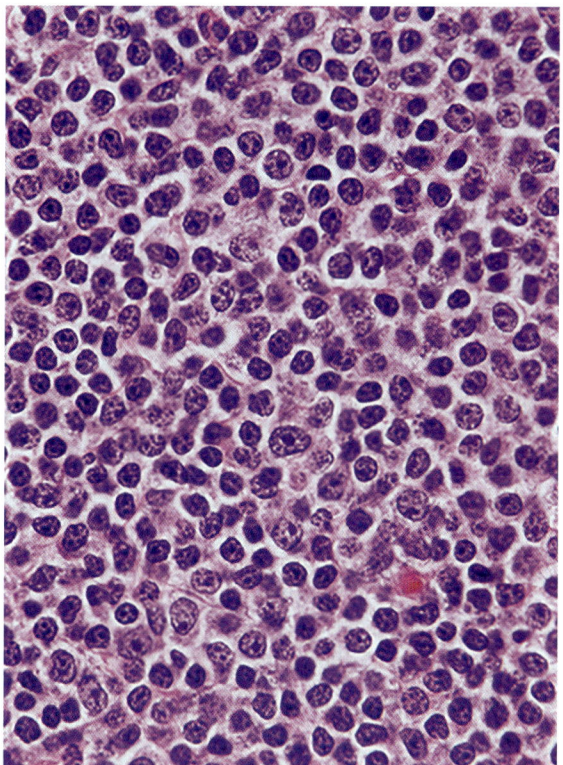

Figure 11-2

CLL/SLL INVOLVING LYMPH NODE

Left: The proliferation centers in this case are more prominent and easier to appreciate than the tumor shown in figure 11-1.
Right: Oil magnification of a proliferative center (H&E stain).

of mantle cell lymphoma. In other cases, CLL/SLL cells replace the marginal and outer mantle zone cells, but spare the inner mantle zone, a so-called perifollicular growth pattern (48).

In 5 to 10 percent of cases, CLL/SLL preferentially involves the interfollicular areas of the lymph nodes (fig. 11-3) (12,18). The interfollicular areas are expanded and proliferation centers may surround reactive follicles, mimicking a marginal zone pattern (12,18). In other cases, proliferation centers are less evident, and para-immunoblasts are dispersed and intermingled among small lymphocytes in the interfollicular area. Rare cases of CLL/SLL involving lymph nodes and other tissue sites exhibit plasmacytoid differentiation, including increased cytoplasm with eccentrically located nuclei or nuclear pseudoinclusions (Dutcher bodies). These features may be subtle or prominent, and may be identified in most or only a small subset of the tumor cells (fig. 11-4).

Peripheral Blood

In the peripheral blood, involvement by CLL/SLL is characterized by an absolute lymphocytosis (31). Other blood cells, such as erythrocytes, platelets, and granulocytes, may be of normal number but are often decreased. In most cases, the neoplastic lymphocytes are small (slightly larger than erythrocytes), with a high nuclear to cytoplasmic ratio (fig. 11-5). The nuclei are round, with condensed, "block-like" or "soccer ball" chromatin and inconspicuous nucleoli. The cytoplasm is scant and lightly basophilic. A few (less than 5 percent) prolymphocytes, which are medium-sized cells with larger round nuclei containing prominent central nucleoli and abundant pale cytoplasm, are often present. Cells intermediate between small lymphocytes and prolymphocytes are also observed. Cells with smudged nuclei and stripped cytoplasm (smudge cells) are often seen in blood smears. In some cases, CLL cells show plasmacytoid differentiation

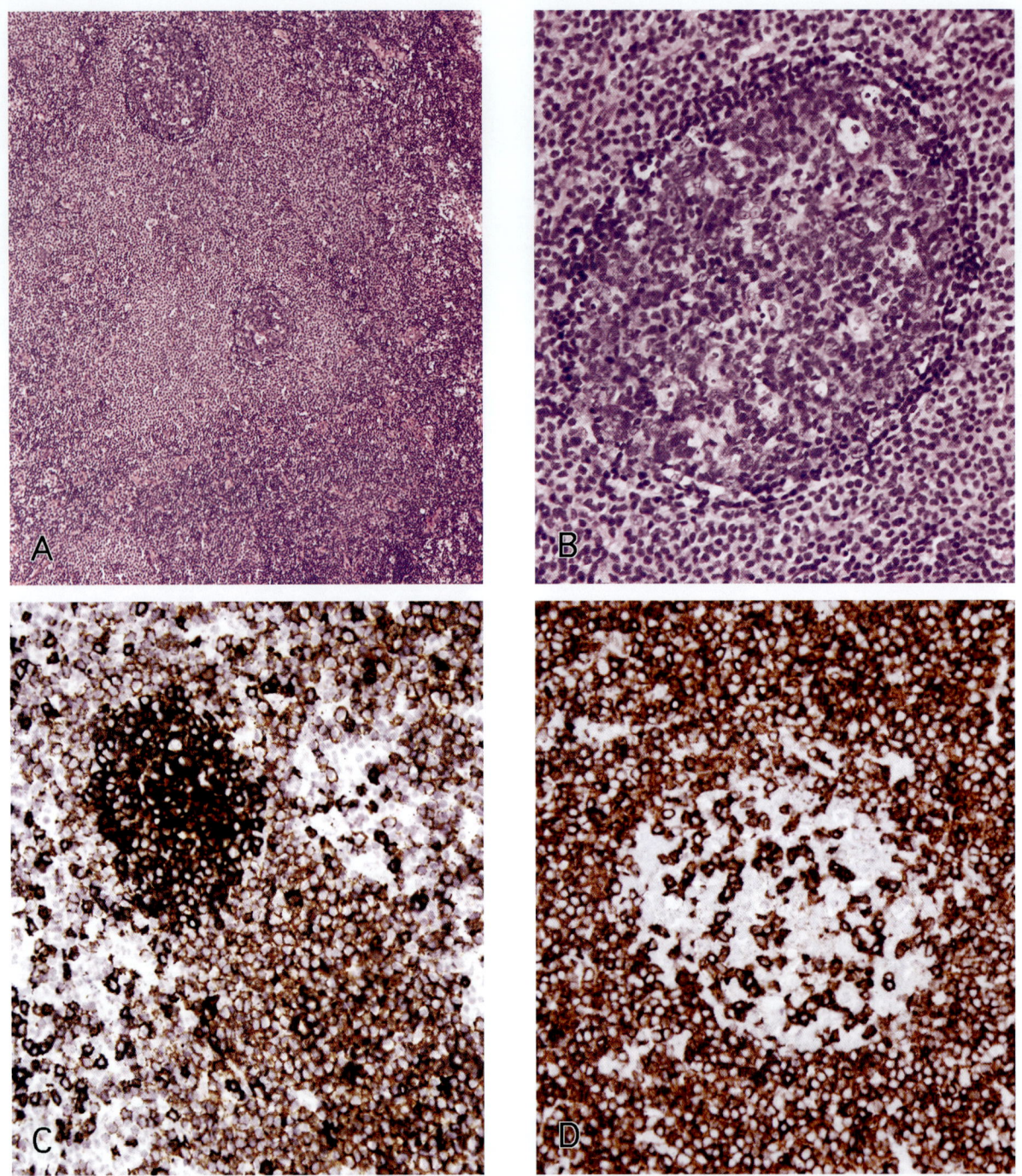

Figure 11-3

INTERFOLLICULAR VARIANT OF CLL/SLL

A: In this field, reactive follicles are present and interfollicular areas are expanded by CLL/SLL. Pale proliferation centers are prominent and surround the follicles, imparting a marginal zone lymphoma-like appearance.

B: High magnification of a reactive follicle with a prominent germinal center and small mantle zone surrounded by CLL/SLL.

C: This tumor is positive for CD20, which is dim in small cells and brighter in proliferation centers (lower right). A reactive follicle is also shown (upper left) and is strongly positive.

D: The CLL/SLL cells are positive for CD5; the central reactive follicle is negative. (A,B: H&E stain; C,D: immunohistochemistry with hematoxylin counterstain).

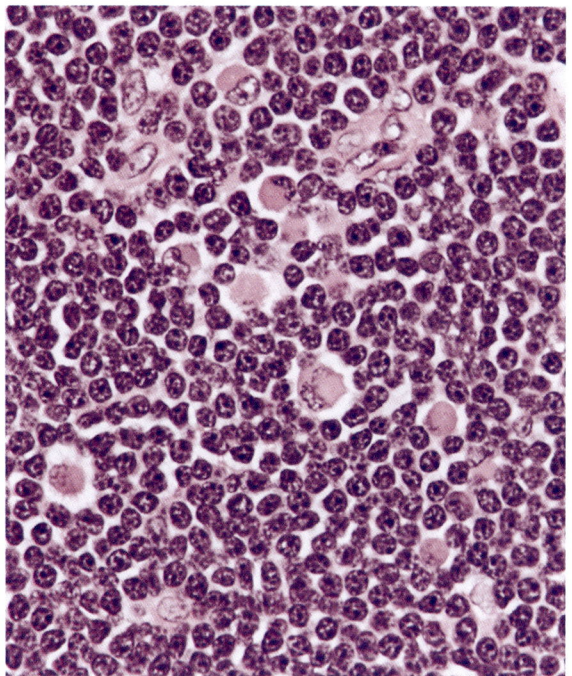

Figure 11-4

CLL/SLL INVOLVING LYMPH NODE

A small (less than 5 percent) subset of cells shows extensive plasmacytoid differentiation, in this case manifested by eosinophilic, Russell body-like cytoplasm. This neoplasm had an immunophenotype typical of CLL/SLL (H&E stain).

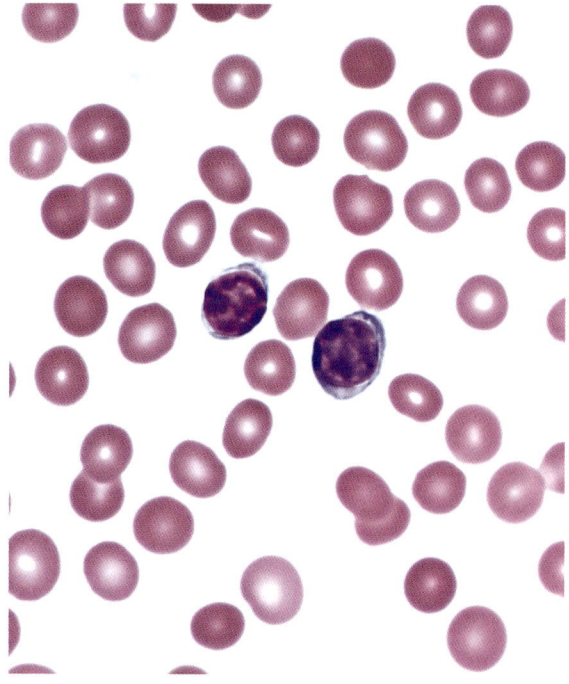

Figure 11-5

CLL INVOLVING PERIPHERAL BLOOD

Two small lymphocytes with block-like chromatin are seen. Pancytopenia is present (Wright-Giemsa stain).

(fig. 11-6), often correlating with the presence of a low level of serum paraprotein (57).

The lymphocytes may show atypical morphologic features. Over 10 percent of small lymphocytes show irregular nuclear contours (fig. 11-7) or plasmacytoid features, or have an increased number of prolymphocytes. These atypical morphologic features correlate with an atypical immunophenotype or cytogenetic findings, and less closely with prognosis (see below) (9,33).

Bone Marrow

Bone marrow smears of CLL/SLL contain cells with cytologic features resembling those seen in the peripheral blood (fig. 11-8). The bone marrow aspirates show variable numbers of intermediate-sized lymphoid cells with abundant cytoplasm. Bone marrow core biopsy sections may show a diffuse, nodular, or interstitial pattern of involvement by CLL/SLL or a combination of these (fig. 11-9) (34). In the diffuse pattern, there is

extensive replacement of the normal hematopoietic cells and adipose elements of the bone marrow by a diffuse proliferation of CLL/SLL cells. Proliferation centers may be observed in the bone marrow when involvement by CLL/SLL is diffuse (fig. 11-9A). In the nodular pattern, the neoplastic cells form aggregates distributed in discrete nodular foci (fig. 11-9B). The nodules in CLL/SLL are rarely paratrabecular and the presence of a paratrabecular pattern should lead to reconsideration of a diagnosis of CLL/SLL. In the interstitial pattern, the overall architecture of the bone marrow is preserved, and often the neoplastic cells are intermingled with adipocytes and normal hematopoietic cell elements without the formation of discrete aggregates (fig. 11-9C).

Other Sites

In the spleen, CLL/SLL shows a propensity for involving the white pulp, although the red pulp is often involved to a lesser extent. Proliferation centers are observed with extensive disease, but are usually less prominent than in the lymph nodes. In the liver, CLL/SLL preferentially

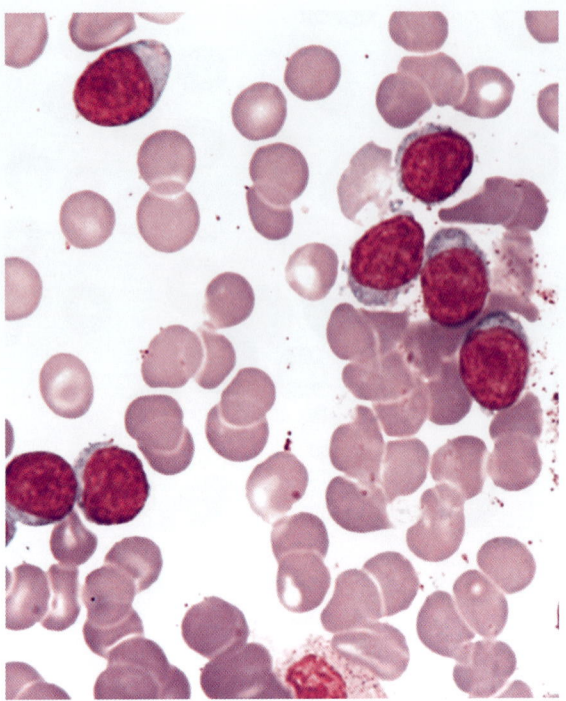

Figure 11-6

CLL INVOLVING PERIPHERAL BLOOD

The lymphocytes show plasmacytoid differentiation. The patient had a low level IgM paraprotein (Wright-Giemsa stain).

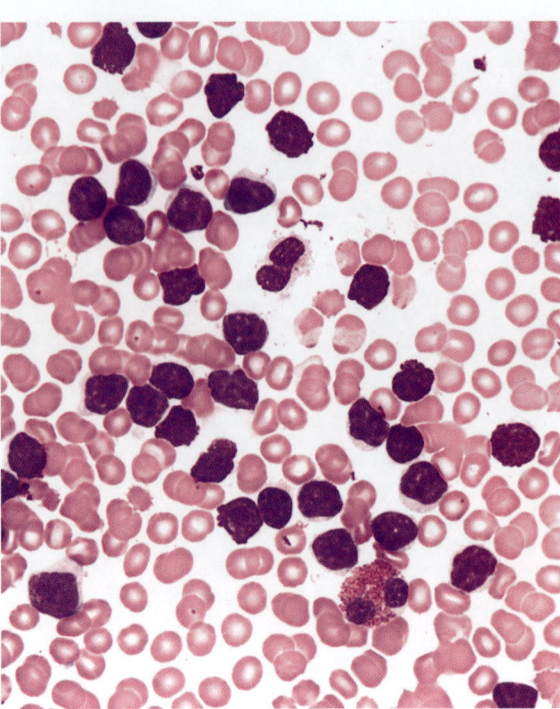

Figure 11-8

CLL/SLL INVOLVING BONE MARROW

Bone marrow aspirate smear shows many small lymphocytes. (Wright-Giemsa stain)

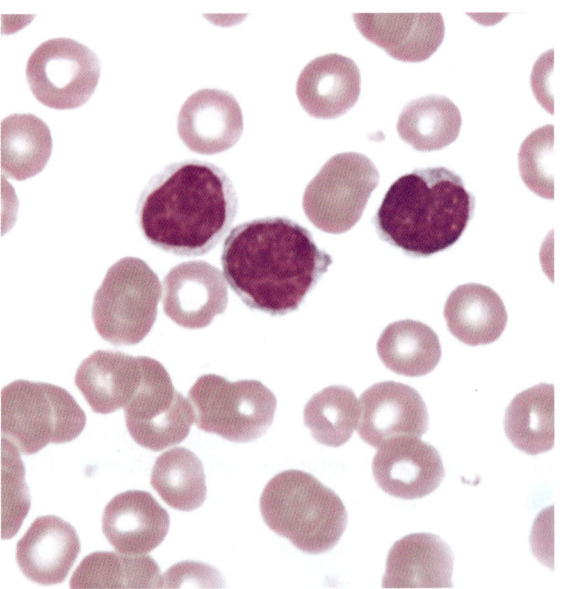

Figure 11-7

CLL WITH ATYPICAL MORPHOLOGIC FEATURES

Two lymphocytes in this field have nuclear clefts or folds. Flow cytometry also showed atypical immunophenotypic features (Wright-Giemsa stain).

involves the portal tracts. In skin, CLL/SLL typically involves the superficial and deep dermis (fig. 11-10). In older patients who undergo surgery for other reasons, CLL/SLL may be detected incidentally, for example, in femoral head specimens as part of hip replacement surgery.

CYTOLOGIC FINDINGS

In aspirate smears of CLL/SLL, most of the neoplastic cells are small, with round nuclei containing mature condensed chromatin and scant cytoplasm. A variable number of prolymphocytes or paraimmunoblasts is present (fig. 11-11). If the needle happens to localize in a proliferation center, larger cells predominate and there is a risk of considering the diagnosis of large cell lymphoma. Adequate sampling and immunophenotypic analysis help avoid this error.

IMMUNOPHENOTYPIC FINDINGS

Flow cytometric immunophenotypic analysis of CLL/SLL cells reveals expression of surface IgM/D (dim) with light chain restriction (30,31).

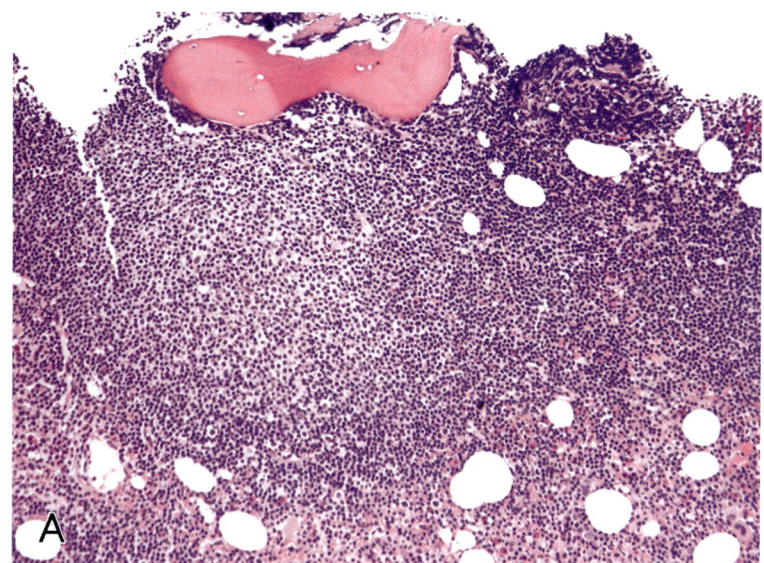

Figure 11-9

CLL/SLL INVOLVING BONE MARROW

A: CLL/SLL partially and diffusely replaces the bone marrow medullary space. A proliferation center is present.

B: Nodules of CLL/SLL cells in bone marrow.

C: The CLL/SLL pattern is interstitial in this bone marrow (A–C: H&E stain).

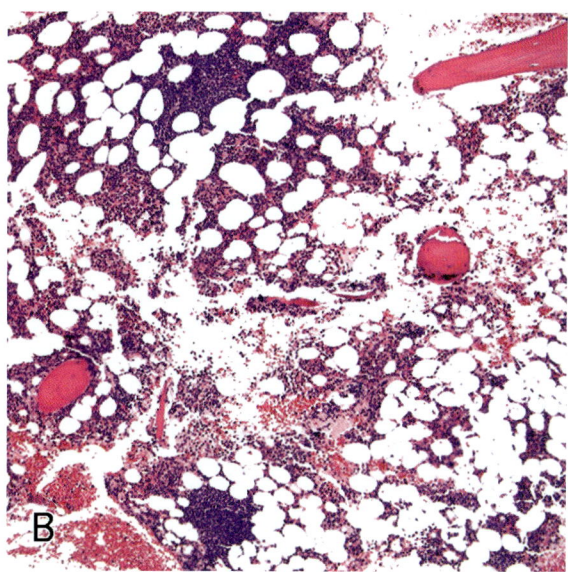

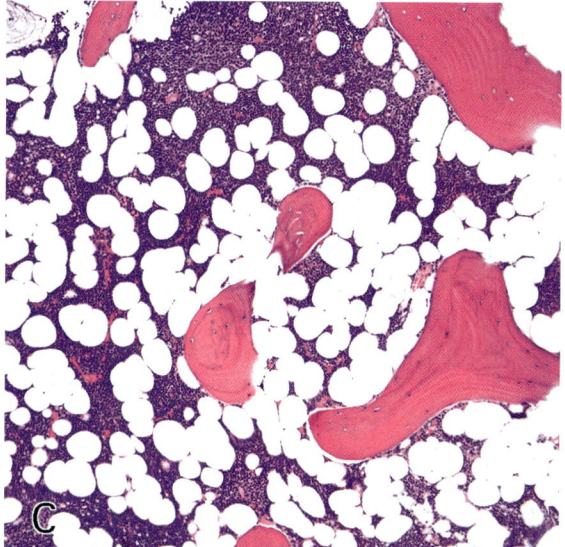

In addition, the neoplastic cells express CD19, CD20 (characteristically dim), CD22, CD23 (fig. 11-12, top), CD43, CD79a, CD200, and HLA-DR. CD3 and CD10 are negative. CD11c, CD79b, and FMC7 are typically negative, but these markers can be expressed individually or together in 10 to 20 percent of cases. About one third of CLL/SLL cases are positive for CD49d, which is associated with a poorer prognosis (4).

Some CLL cases exhibit an atypical immunophenotype (fig. 11-12, bottom) characterized by moderate or bright intensity surface immunoglobulin, weak or absent reactivity for CD23, and expression of CD11c, CD79b, and FMC7

(9,27). CD5 expression can be dim in atypical CLL, but absence of CD5 is rare (and should prompt consideration of another diagnosis).

The immunohistochemical findings in CLL/SLL recapitulate those observed by flow cytometry (figs. 11-3, 11-13). In general, immunohistochemistry is less sensitive and therefore dim antigen expression noted by flow cytometry may be negative. Lymphoid-enhancer-binding factor 1 (LEF1) is a highly specific marker of CLL/SLL, with a sensitivity reported to range from 70 to 100 percent (28,47). LEF1 is usually negative in other types of small B-cell lymphoma (but is positive in about one third of diffuse large B-cell

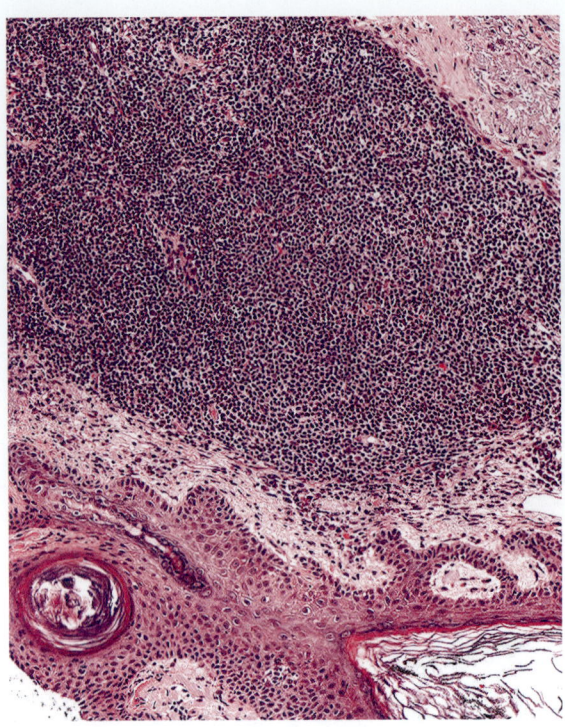

Figure 11-10

CLL/SLL INVOLVING SKIN

Skin is also a site that can be involved by CLL/SLL. Typically, the superficial dermis and deep dermis are involved (H&E stain).

lymphomas). CLL/SLL is usually positive for PAX5 and BCL2, and negative for BCL6, MUM1/IRF4, cyclin D1 (see below), and SOX11. The proliferation rate in CLL/SLL in small cell areas (excluding proliferation centers) as assessed by Ki-67 is usually low, in the range of 5 to 10 percent.

In tissue sections of CLL/SLL in which proliferation centers are recognized, the cells within these centers differ, in part, from the small lymphocytes. As the name implies, many of the cells in the proliferation centers are positive for Ki-67. Proliferation center cells also express a variety of activation and other markers not expressed by the remaining small cell areas, including CD25, CD71, MUM1/IRF4, and MYC (fig. 11-14). CD23 expression is usually brighter in proliferation center cells than in surrounding small lymphocytes (44). Follicular dendritic cell networks (CD21 and CD23 positive) may be present in proliferation centers, although they are often thinner and more delicate than the follicular dendritic cells present in reactive germinal centers (44,48). T cells are

more numerous in proliferation centers than in the surrounding areas of the neoplasm. In some cases, dim expression of cyclin D1 is observed in the larger cells of proliferation centers (fig. 11-15) (17). In these cases, SOX11 is negative and there is no evidence of t(11;14)(q13;q32/*CCND1-IGH* in proliferation center lymphocytes.

Zeta chain-associated protein kinase of 70 kD (ZAP70) and CD38 expression correlate (although not entirely) with unmutated immunoglobulin variable gene (*IGV*) status (see below) and have been used as surrogates for mutational status and prognostication in CLL patients (8,15,24,40,56). Typically, these markers are assessed in blood specimens by flow cytometry, but ZAP70 and CD38 also are assessed by immunohistochemistry, most often in bone marrow core or lymph node biopsy specimens in patients without lymphocytosis (1).

MOLECULAR GENETIC FINDINGS

Conventional cytogenetic analysis of CLL/SLL cases (mostly CLL) shows an abnormal karyotype in approximately one third (11). This is a result of CLL cells growing poorly in cytogenetic cell cultures. The presence of an abnormal karyotype, i.e., simply tumor growth in culture, correlates with a poorer prognosis. A wide number of abnormalities have been described in CLL cases including complex karyotypes. The most common abnormalities are discussed below in the paragraph on fluorescence in situ hybridization (FISH) analysis since this method is more sensitive for the detection of these abnormalities.

About 5 percent of CLL cases have an abnormal karyotype associated with chromosomal translocations involving *IGH*. The t(14;19) (q32;q13)/*IGH-BCL3* is associated with atypical morphologic features or immunophenotype, and is commonly associated with trisomy 12, a complex karyotype, and unmutated *IGH* variable genes (*IGHV*) (25). The t(14;18)(q32;q21)/*IGH-BCL2* also occurs in CLL patients, who also have trisomy 12 and mutated *IGHV;* these patients tend to be younger (49). *MYC* translocations, usually the result of t(8;14)(q24.1;q32), are rare in CLL and are associated with an increased number of prolymphocytes in the blood, complex karyotypes, and a poorer prognosis (21). The t(11;14) (q13;q32)/*IGH-CCND1* does not occur in CLL as a founding event, but rare cases of CLL are reported

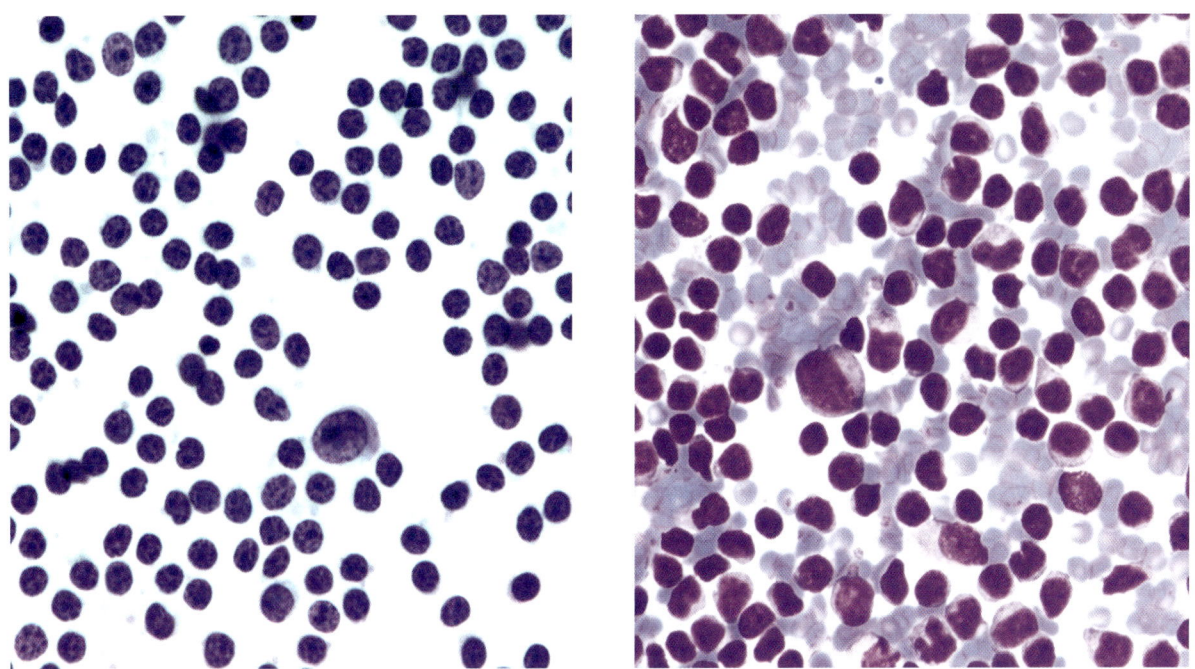

Figure 11-11

CLL/SLL IN ASPIRATE SMEAR

Left, Right: Fine-needle aspiration smears of CLL/SLL show a dispersed population of small round lymphocytes with clumped chromatin and rare paraimmunoblasts (left: Papanicolaou stain; right: Diff-Quik stain).

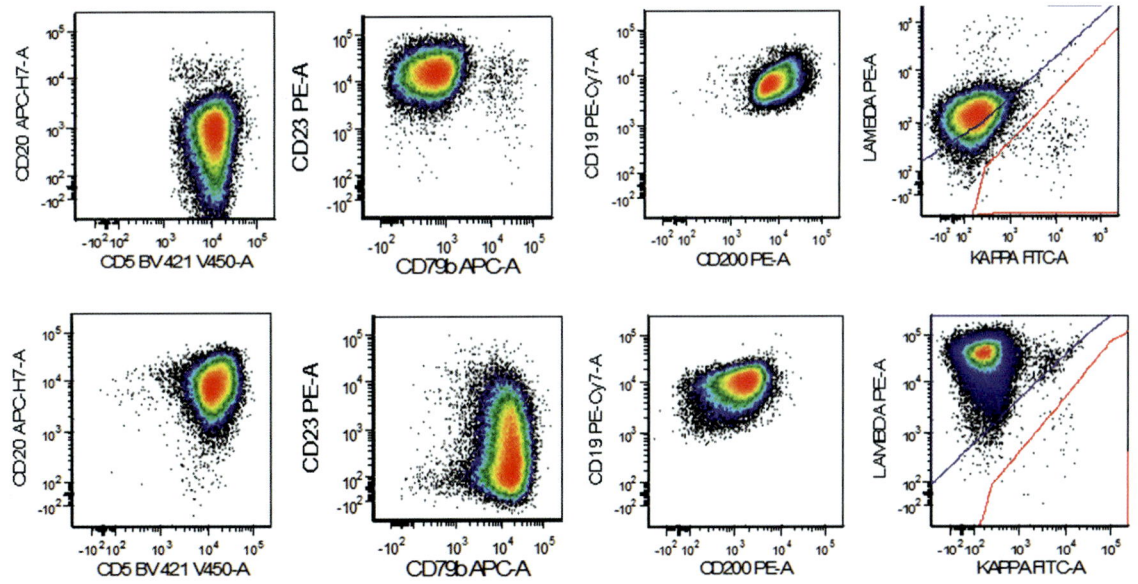

Figure 11-12

IMMUNOPHENOTYPIC FINDINGS

Upper panel: A case of typical CLL: CD19(+), CD20(dim +), CD5(+), CD23(+), CD79b (very dim +/negative), lambda(dim +), CD200 (bright and uniform +).

Lower panel: A case of atypical CLL with trisomy 12: CD19(+), CD20(bright +), CD5(+), CD23(partial +), CD79b(bright +), lambda(bright +), CD200(+). (Courtesy of Dr. Sa A. Wang, Houston, TX.)

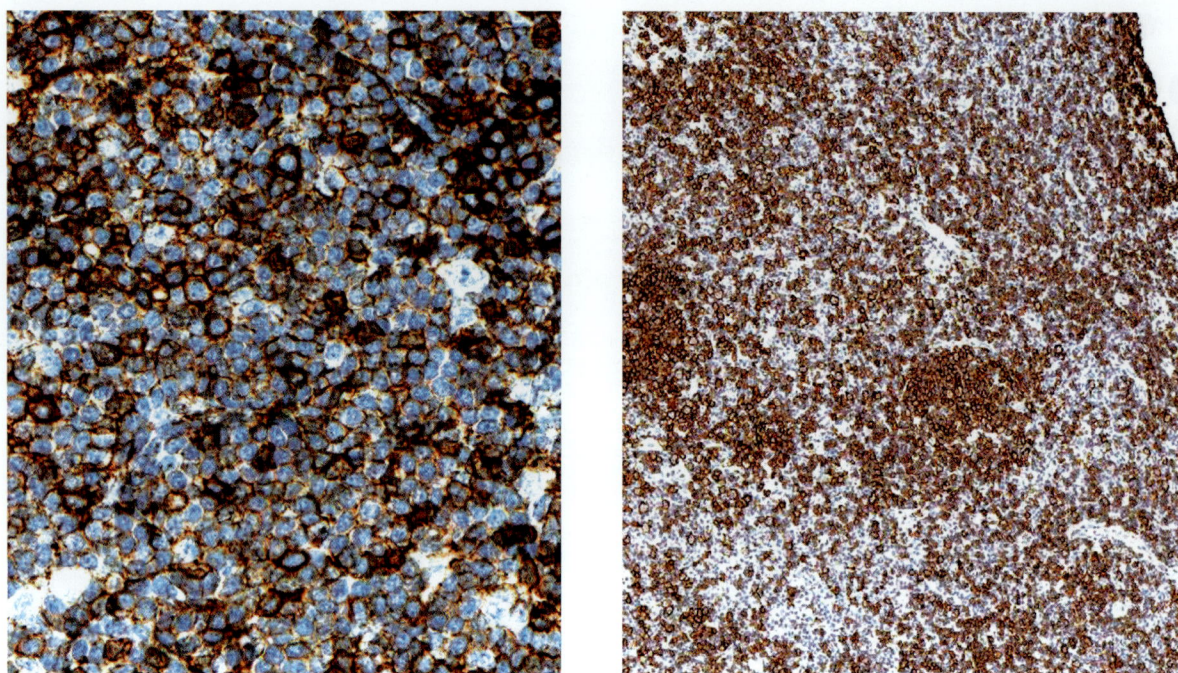

Figure 11-13

CLL/SLL INVOLVING LYMPH NODE

Immunohistochemistry is positive for CD43 (left) and CD23 (right) (immunohistochemistry with hematoxylin counterstain).

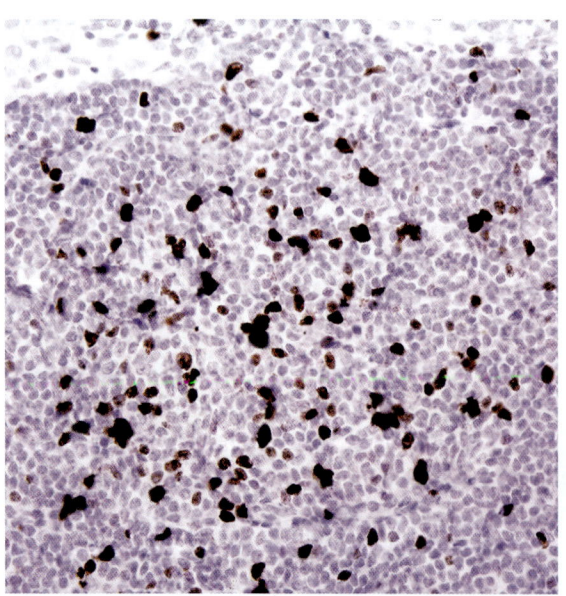

Figure 11-14

PROLIFERATION CENTER

The MIB-1 (Ki-67) antibody shows increased positive (proliferating) cells within a central proliferation center (immunohistochemistry with hematoxylin counterstain). (This is the same case as shown in figure 11-1).

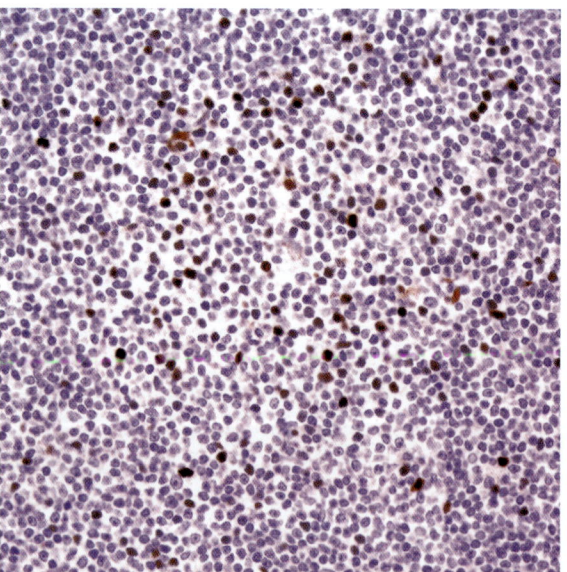

Figure 11-15

PROLIFERATION CENTER

Anti-cyclin D1 antibody shows dimly positive cells within a central proliferation center (immunohistochemistry with hematoxylin counterstain). (This is same case as shown in figure 11-1).

in which t(11;14)/*IGH-CCND1* was acquired after therapy resulting in cyclin D1 overexpression (32).

FISH analysis reveals that up to 80 percent of CLL cases have chromosomal abnormalities. The most common recurrent cytogenetic abnormality is a deletion involving the 13q14.3 locus, which occurs in 50 percent of cases. This deletion targets miR-16-1 and miR-15a (5,11,24). Approximately 25 percent of CLLs exhibit trisomy 12, which often is present in only a subset of lymphocytes, suggesting it is a later event in pathogenesis (27). Other important recurrent abnormalities include del(11q22-23) and del(17p13) in approximately 20 percent and 5 to 10 percent of cases, respectively. Del(11q) and del(17p) correlate with *ATM* and *TP53* mutations, respectively, and a poorer prognosis (11,24,43).

Deletion of a gene locus by FISH is a gross abnormality that is inherently less precise than analysis of specific genes at these loci. For example, in one large study (59), *TP53* mutations were detected in 8.5 percent of all CLL cases assessed, but del(17p) occurred in only 4.5 percent of these cases. In this study, del(17p) correlated with the *TP53* mutation, but FISH underestimated the number of mutated cases and del(17p) occurred in a small subset of cases without an identifiable mutation. The *TP53* mutation was a stronger prognostic marker than del(17p) in this study group. Not surprisingly, FISH detection of del(17p) also correlates imperfectly with p53 expression (7).

Monoclonal IG rearrangements are consistently identified in CLL/SLL. T-cell receptor gene rearrangements are rare. The *IGV* segments of both the *IGH* and light chain genes are somatically hypermutated in 50 to 60 percent of cases, and unmutated in the rest (10,20). IG mutational status defines clinically distinct subgroups of CLL; patients with mutated CLL have a better prognosis than patients with unmutated cases. In many studies in the literature only *IGHV* has been assessed for mutations.

Gene expression profiling studies have shown that both mutated and unmutated cases of CLL/SLL exhibit a transcriptional program suggestive of memory B cells (42,55). These studies were performed mostly on blood lymphocytes, which may not entirely reflect cell programs in CLL/SLL. Mittal et al. (29) compared the gene expression profile of CLL cells in lymph nodes versus blood. Lymph node CLL cells overexpressed

molecules associated with B-cell receptor (BCR) signaling, the NF-κB pathway, B-cell activating factor (BAFF), and an immunosuppression signature, suggesting that the lymph nodes are the primary site of CLL/SLL growth. In contrast, blood CLL cells overexpressed various chemokines thought to be involved in lymphocyte migration to lymph nodes or bone marrow (29). Cordoba et al. (6) studied lymph nodes involved by CLL/SLL and showed two subtypes, one characterized by overexpression of NF-κB and cytokine genes and one characterized by cell cycle genes.

As has been reviewed by Lazarian et al. (24a), a number of genes are mutated in CLL/SLL, mostly at low frequency, some of which are disease drivers or have prognostic significance. Some of the most important genes include: *TP53, NOTCH1, SF3B1,* and *ATM* (24a), *TP53* mutations occur in about 10 percent of CLL/SLL cases, correlate with poorer prognosis, and influence patient management (24a). *NOTCH1* and *ATM* mutations have been reported in 5 to 10 percent of CLL cases. *NOTCH1* mutations usually occur in exon 34 and result in a stop codon and a truncated, more stable, NOTCH1 protein (13,38). *FBXW7*, which encodes a negative regulator of NOTCH1, also is mutated infrequently in CLL. *NOTCH1* mutations have been correlated with unmutated *IGHV*, trisomy 12, and a poorer prognosis (52). NOTCH1 also can be activated in CLL independently of gene mutations and can transactivate MYC (13). *SF3B1*, involved in pre-mRNA splicing, is mutated in 10 to 15 percent of CLL cases (54). Other mutated genes (in 5 percent or fewer cases) include *CHD2, BRAF, ZMYM3, MAPK1, POT1, DDX3X, BIRC3, XPO1,* and *MYD88* (13,22,38,54). Mutated and unmutated CLL cases have different gene mutation profiles.

TRANSFORMATION

A subset of CLL/SLL patients develop diffuse large B-cell lymphoma (DLBCL), termed Richter syndrome, or much less often, classic Hodgkin lymphoma (2,31). The overall frequency of DLBCL in CLL/SLL patients ranges from 2 to 10 percent (31,35). A report from the Mayo Clinic described an overall risk of developing DLBCL of 2 to 3 percent and about 0.5 percent per year (35). In 70 to 80 percent of patients, the CLL/SLL and DLBCL are clonally related and therefore the DLBCL is a form of histologic transformation

(26,31). Patients with clonally related DLBCL have a worse prognosis than patients with clonally unrelated DLBCL, which, presumably, is a second tumor that may be related to inherent genetic risk, host immunosuppression, or possibly coincidence.

The risk of Richter syndrome is increased in patients with high tumor stage, high-risk cytogenetic abnormalities, unmutated *IGV*, and expression of ZAP70 or CD38. Some types of therapy also increase the risk of Richter transformation. At a genetic level, DLBCL arising as part of Richter syndrome is genetically distinct from de novo DLBCL (14).

In a subset of CLL/SLL patients who undergo biopsy for suspicion of Richter syndrome, the tissue biopsy shows features of so-called accelerated phase CLL/SLL. In these cases, some evidence suggests transformation, such as large proliferation centers that appear to be almost merging with each other, an increased mitotic rate, high Ki-67 expression, and necrosis; however, criteria for DLBCL are not met. Of these findings, an increased Ki-67 rate is unusual in CLL/SLL and when present is a likely indication of an early phase of transformation to DLBCL.

Although the accelerated phase of CLL/SLL has been recognized for years, there have been no consensus criteria for the recognition of this phase. Gine et al. (16) suggested three criteria: expanded proliferation centers broader than a low power (20X) microscopic field, a high mitotic rate within proliferation centers (over 2.4 mitotic figures per proliferation center), and a high proliferation index within the proliferation centers (greater than 40 percent). As acknowledged by the authors, this study has a bias in that patients underwent biopsy for suspicion of transformation. Therefore, these criteria need to be validated, but may prove useful for identifying CLL/SLL patients with accelerated phase disease.

Rare patients with CLL progress to a clinically aggressive phase characterized by high levels of lymphocytosis with numerous prolymphocytes in the blood. This form of transformation is known as *prolymphocytoid transformation of CLL*. In the absence of increased prolymphocytes in the blood, prolymphocytes can be increased in the lymph nodes and the term *prolymphocytoid transformation* has been used in this context (fig. 11-16). Prolymphocytoid transformation in lymph nodes is not well defined in the litera-

ture. These cases clinically and morphologically overlap with DLBCL and likely represent another manifestation of Richter syndrome or accelerated phase CLL/SLL.

DIFFERENTIAL DIAGNOSIS

Monoclonal B-Cell Lymphocytosis (MBL). Two variants of MBL are described: "low count" and "high count" (see chapter 6). The latter is relevant to the differential diagnosis. "High count" or clinical CLL-like MBL is characterized by a low-level B-cell lymphocytosis in the blood of less than 5×10^9/L (41). Bone marrow involvement has been reported, usually at a low level in a nodular pattern, and clinical evidence of lymphadenopathy or B-type symptoms are absent. MBL (1 to 2 percent per year) progresses to CLL. In many ways, patients with clinical CLL-like MBL and Rai stage 0 CLL overlap and the differential diagnosis is based on clinical and laboratory data (see chapter 6).

B-Cell Prolymphocytic Leukemia (B-PLL). Patients with B-PLL have a de novo disease characterized by over 55 percent prolymphocytes in the blood and an aggressive clinical course. B-PLL became a very rare disease once it was recognized that other small B-cell neoplasms may progress to a B-PLL-like clinical picture, including CLL/SLL, mantle cell lymphoma, and rarely, splenic marginal zone lymphoma. Approximately half of all cases with a B-PLL-like picture arise from CLL.

Mantle Cell Lymphoma. Some patients with mantle cell lymphoma present in an indolent, usually leukemic, phase that mimics CLL. CLL/SLL and mantle cell lymphoma are B-cell tumors that express CD5, but mantle cell lymphoma is usually negative for CD23 and positive for FMC7 (the converse of CLL). Mantle cell lymphoma also carries the t(11;14)(q13;q32), overexpresses cyclin D1, and expresses SOX11 in most cases (a subset of clinically indolent mantle cell lymphomas are negative for SOX11).

Other Small B-Cell Lymphomas. Other small B-cell lymphoproliferative disorders may involve the peripheral blood, bone marrow, or tissues, such as follicular lymphoma [cleaved nuclei, CD10(+), BCL6(+)], marginal zone B-cell lymphoma [usually CD5(-), bright surface immunoglobulin], and lymphoplasmacytic lymphoma/Waldenstrom macroglobulinemia [serum

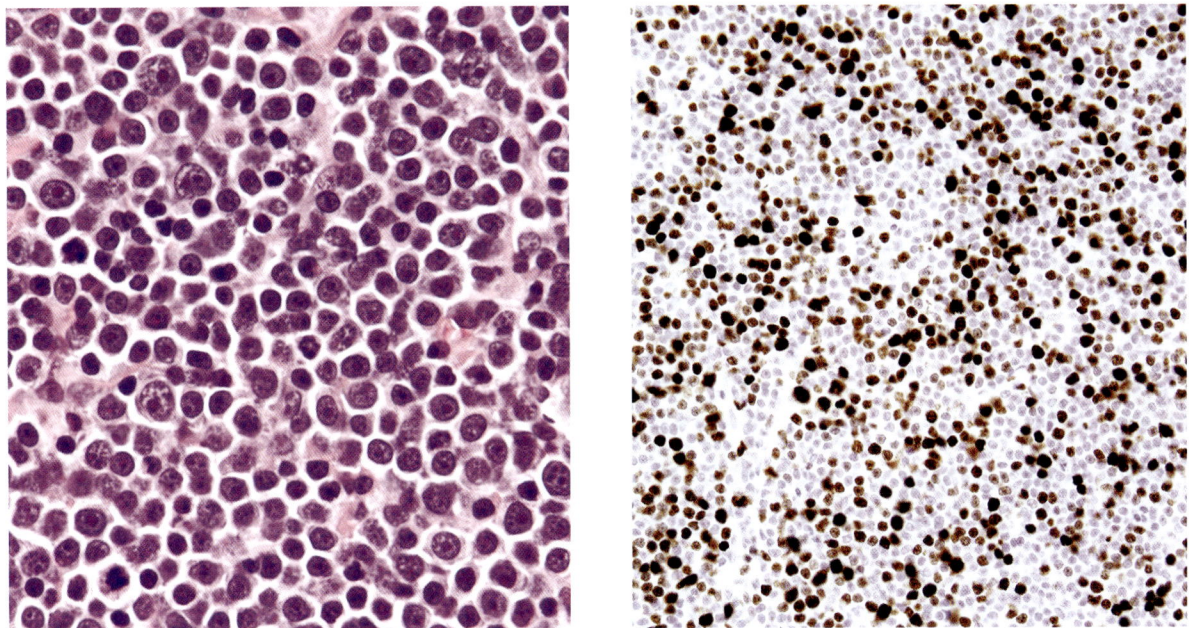

Figure 11-16

CLL/SLL WITH INCREASED PROLYMPHOCYTES IN LYMPH NODE

This patient had clinical evidence of aggressive disease, unlike the initial CLL phase.
Left: This field shows many nucleolated cells consistent with increased prolymphocytes (Wright-Giemsa stain).
Right: The MIB-1 (Ki-67) antibody shows numerous positive cells, indicative of a proliferation rate that is much higher than usually seen in CLL/SLL (immunohistochemistry with hematoxylin counterstain).

IgM paraprotein, usually CD5(-), *MYD88* mutation(+)]. The distinctive immunophenotype and the presence of proliferation centers in lymph nodes are key features for establishing the diagnosis of CLL/SLL.

TREATMENT AND PROGNOSIS

The treatment of CLL/SLL patients is highly dependent on the disease stage and other prognostic factors. Traditionally, the clinical stage was determined by the Binet or Rai staging schemes (Tables 11-1, 11-2) (3,39). More recently, biologic parameters are emerging as important prognostic markers. An atypical immunophenotype determined by flow cytometry correlates with a poorer prognosis (4,30). CD49d expression correlates with higher tumor lymphocyte doubling time and a poorer prognosis (4). Assessment of ZAP70 and CD38 expression are surrogates for unmutated IG variable genes, which correlate with a poorer prognosis (8,10,20,24,56).

As determined by FISH, isolated del(13q14.3) is associated with a more favorable outcome (5,11). Del(11q) correlates with *ATM* mutations

and is associated with bulky lymphadenopathy and a poorer prognosis (11,24,43). Del(17p) or *TP53* mutation identifies a group of CLL patients with a particularly poor outcome (11,59). Patients with del(17p) or *TP53* mutation, even if they have low-stage disease or few other risk factors, may be entered into clinical trials designed to evaluate early intervention strategies.

The German Chronic Lymphocytic Leukemia Study Group (37) has developed a prognostic score for CLL patients that uses eight weighted variables: del(17p) (6 points), serum thymidine kinase 1 greater than 10 U/L (2 points), serum β-2-microglobulin greater than 3.5 mg/L (2 points) or 1.7 to 3.5 mg/L (1 point), unmutated *IGHV* (1 point), Eastern Cooperative Oncology Group (ECOG) performance status greater than 0 (1 point), del(11q) (1 point), male (1 point), and age over 60 years (1 point) (37). The scores divide patients into four prognostic groups: 0-2 (low-risk) with 95 percent 5-year survival; 3-5 (intermediate risk) with 82 percent 5-year survival; 6-10 (high risk) with 68 percent 5-year survival; and 11-14 (very high risk) with 19

Table 11-1

BINET CLASSIFICATION

Stage	Clinical and Laboratory Features	Median Survival (months)
A	Hemoglobin ≥10 g/dL; platelets ≥100x10⁹/L; <three anatomic sites involved[a]	>120
B	Hemoglobin ≥10 g/dL; platelets ≥100x10⁹/L; ≥three anatomic sites involved	61
C	Hemoglobin <10 g/dL; platelets <100x10⁹/L; or both, regardless of the anatomic sites involved	32

[a]Anatomic sites include cervical, axillary, and inguinal lymph nodes (unilateral or bilateral), spleen, and liver.

Table 11-2

RAI CLASSIFICATION

Stage	Clinical and Laboratory Features	Median Survival (months)
0	Lymphocytosis in blood and bone marrow only	>120
I	Lymphocytosis and lymphadenopathy	95
II	Lymphocytosis and hepatomegaly or splenomegaly, or both; enlarged lymph nodes may or may not be present	72
III	Lymphocytosis and anemia (Hb <11 g/dL); lymph nodes, spleen, and liver may or may not be enlarged	30
IV	Lymphocytosis and thrombocytopenia (platelets <100 x 10⁹/L); anemia and organomegaly may or may not be present	30

percent 5-year survival. Although this system is highly promising, validation is needed.

For patients with low-stage disease and no adverse biologic markers, watchful waiting (observation) until there is a change in disease status is often a good approach. For patients with advanced disease requiring therapy, the fludarabine, cyclophosphamide, and rituximab (FCR) regimen is effective. In recent years, a number of novel agents have been developed that are being used in clinical trials, and targeted therapies are being developed (19,55). Newer therapies of promise include anti-CD20 antibodies (e.g., obinutuzumab/GA101), inhibitors of the B-cell receptor signaling and PI3 kinase pathways (e.g., ibrutinib inhibits Bruton tyrosine kinase and idelalisib inhibits the PI3 kinase p110δ isoform), BCL2 inhibitors (e.g., venetoclax), and immunomodulator agents (e.g., lenalidomide).

REFERENCES

1. Admirand JH, Rassidakis GZ, Abruzzo LV, Valbuena JR, Jones D, Medeiros LJ. Immunohistochemical detection of ZAP-70 in 341 cases of non-Hodgkin and Hodgkin lymphoma. Mod Pathol 2004;17:954-961.
2. Agbay RL, Jain N, Loghavi S, Medeiros LJ, Khoury JD. Histologic transformation of chronic lymphocytic leukemia/small lymphocytic lymphoma. Am J Hematol 2016;91:1036-1043.
3. Binet JL, Auquier A, Dighiero G, et al. A new prognostic classification of chronic lymphocytic leukemia derived from a multivariate survival analysis. Cancer 1981;48:198-206.
4. Bulian P, Shanafelt TD, Fegan C, et al. CD49d is the strongest flow cytometry-based predictor of overall survival in chronic lymphocytic leukemia. J Clin Oncol 2014;32:897-904.
5. Calin GA, Ferracin M, Cimmino A, et al. A microRNA signature associated with prognosis and progression in chronic lymphocytic leukemia. N Engl J Med 2005;353:1793-1801.

6. Cordoba R, Sanchez-Beato M, Herreros B, et al. Two distinct molecular subtypes of chronic lymphocytic leukemia give new insights on the pathogenesis of the disease and identify novel therapeutic targets. Leuk Lymphoma 2016;57:134-142.
7. Cordone I, Masi S, Mauro FR, et al. p53 expression in B-cell chronic lymphocytic leukemia: a marker of disease progression and poor prognosis. Blood 1998;91:4342-4349.
8. Crespo M, Bosch F, Villamor N, et al. ZAP-70 expression as a surrogate for immunoglobulin-variable-region mutations in chronic lymphocytic leukemia. N Engl J Med 2003;348:1764-1775.
9. Criel A, Michaux L, de Wolf-Peeters C. The concept of typical and atypical chronic lymphocytic leukaemia. Leuk Lymphoma 1999;33:33-45.
10. Damle RN, Wasil T, Fais F, et al. Ig V gene mutation stutus and CD38 expresion as novel prognostic indicators in chornic lymphocytic leukemia. Blood 1999;94:1840-1847.
11. Dohner H, Stilgenbauer S, Benner A, et al. Genomic aberrations and survival in chronic lymphocytic leukemia. N Engl J Med 2000;343:1910-1916.
12. Ellison DJ, Nathwani BN, Cho SY, Martin SE. Interfollicular small lymphocytic lymphoma: the diagnostic significance of pseudofollicles. Hum Pathol 1989;20:1108-1118.
13. Fabbri G, Holmes AB, Viganotti M, et al. Common nonmutational *NOTCH1* activation in chronic lymphocytic leukemia. Proc Natl Acad Sci U S A 2017;114:E2911-E2919.
14. Fabbri G, Khiabanian H, Holmes AB, et al. Genomic lesions associated with chronic lymphocytic leukemia transformation to Richter syndrome. J Exp Med 2013;210:2273-2282.
15. Ghia P, Guida G, Stella S, et al. The pattern of CD38 expression defines a distinct subset of chronic lymphocytic leukemia (CLL) patients at risk of disease progression. Blood 2003;101:1262-1269.
16. Gine E, Martinez A, Villamor N, et al. Expanded and highly active proliferation centers identify a histological subtype of chronic lymphocytic leukemia ("accelerated" chronic lymphocytic leukemia) with aggressive clinical behavior. Haematologica 2010;95:1526-1533.
17. Gradowski JF, Sargent RL, Craig FE, et al. Chronic lymphocytic leukemia/small lymphocytic lymphoma with cyclin D1 positive proliferation centers do not have CCND1 translocations or gains and lack SOX11 expression. Am J Clin Pathol 2012;138:132-139.
18. Gupta D, Lim MS, Medeiros LJ, Elenitoba-Johnson KS. Small lymphocytic lymphoma with perifollicular, marginal zone, or interfollicular distribution. Mod Pathol 2000;13:1161-1166.
19. Hallek M. Signaling the end of chronic lymphocytic leukemia: new frontline treatment strategies. Blood 2013;122:3723-3734.
20. Hamblin TJ, Davis Z, Gardiner A, Oscier DG, Stevenson FK. Unmutated Ig V(H) genes are associated with a more aggressive form of chronic lymphocytic leukemia. Blood 1999;94:1848-1854.
21. Huh YO, Lin KI, Vega F, et al. MYC translocation in chronic lymphocytic leukaemia is associated with increased prolymphocytes and a poor prognosis. Br J Haematol 2008;142:36-44.
22. Jebaraj BM, Kienle D, Buhler A, et al. BRAF mutations in chronic lymphocytic leukemia. Leuk Lymphoma 2013;54:1177-1182.
23. Konoplev SN, Fritsche HA, O'Brien S, et al. High serum thymidine kinase 1 level predicts poorer survival in patients with chronic lymphocytic leukemia. Am J Clin Pathol 2010;134:472-477.
24. Krober A, Bloehdorn J, Hafner S, et al. Additional genetic high-risk features such as 11q deletion, 17p deletion, and V3-21 usage characterize discordance of ZAP-70 and VH mutation status in chronic lymphocytic leukemia. J Clin Oncol 2006;24:969-975.
24a. Lazarian G, Guièze R, Wu CJ. Clinical implications of novel genomic discoveries in chronic lymphocytic leukemia. J Clin Oncol 2017;35: 984-993.
25. Martin Subero JI, Ibbotson R, Klapper W, et al. A comprehensive genetic and histopathologic analysis identified two subgroups of B-cell malignancies carrying a t(14;19)(q32;q13) or variant BCL3-translocation. Leukemia 2007;21:1532-1544.
26. Matolcsy A, Inghirami G, Knowles DM. Molecular genetic demonstration of the diverse evolution of Richter's syndrome (chronic lymphocytic leukemia and subsequent large cell lymphoma). Blood 1994;83:1363-1372.
27. Matutes E, Oscier D, Garcia-Marco J, et al. Trisomy 12 defines a group of CLL with atypical morphology: correlation between cytogenetic, clinical and laboratory features in 544 patients. Br J Haematol 1996;92:382-388.
28. Menter T, Dirnhofer S, Tzankov A. LEF1: a highly specific marker for the diagnosis of chronic lymphocytic leukaemia/small lymphocytic B cell lymphoma. J Clin Pathol 2015;68:473-478.
28b. Miller KD, Siegel RL, Lin CC, et al. Cancer treatment and survivorship statistics, 2016. CA Cancer J Clin 2016;66:271-289.
29. Mittal AK, Chaturvedi NK, Rai KJ, et al. Chronic lymphocytic leukemia cells in a lymph node microenvironment depict molecular signature associated with an aggressive disease. Mol Med 2014;20:290-301.
30. Moreau EJ, Matutes E, A'Hern RP, et al. Improvement of the chronic lymphocytic leukemia scoring system with the monoclonal antibody SN8 (CD79b). Am J Clin Pathol 1997;108:378-382.
31. Muller-Hermelink HK, Montserrat E, Catovsky D, et al. Chronic lymphocytic leukemia/small lymphocytic lymphoma. In: Swerdlow SH, Campo E, Harris NL, et al., eds. WHO classification of tumours of haematopoietic and lymphoid tissues. Lyon: IARC Press; 2008:180-182.
32. Nishida Y, Takeuchi K, Tsuda K, et al. Acquisition of t(11;14) in a patient with chronic lymphocytic leukemia carrying both t(14;19)(q32;q13.1) and +12. Eur J Haematol 2013;91:179-182.

33. Oscier DG, Matutes E, Copplestone A, et al. Atypical lymphocyte morphology: an adverse prognostic factor for disease progression in stage A CLL independent of trisomy 12. Br J Haematol 1997;98:934-939.

34. Pangalis GA, Roussou PA, Kittas C, Kokkinou S, Fessas P. B-chronic lymphocytic leukemia. Prognostic implication of bone marrow histology in 120 patients experience from a single hematology unit. Cancer 1987;59:767-771.

35. Parikh SA, Kay NE, Shanafelt TD. How we treat Richter syndrome. Blood 2014;123:1647-1657.

36. Parikh SA, Leis JF, Chaffee KG, et al. Hypogammaglobulinemia in newly diagnosed chronic lymphocytic leukemia: Natural history, clinical correlates, and outcomes. Cancer 2015;121:2883-2891.

37. Pflug N, Bahlo J, Shanafelt TD, et al. Development of a comprehensive prognostic index for patients with chronic lymphocytic leukemia. Blood 2014;124:49-62.

38. Puente XS, Pinyol M, Quesada V, et al. Whole-genome sequencing identifies recurrent mutations in chronic lymphocytic leukaemia. Nature 2011;475:101-105.

39. Rai KR, Sawitsky A, Cronkite EP, Chanana AD, Levy RN, Pasternack BS. Clinical staging of chronic lymphocytic leukemia. Blood 1975;46:219-234.

40. Rassenti LZ, Huynh L, Toy TL, et al. ZAP-70 compared with immunoglobulin heavy-chain gene mutation status as a predictor of disease progression in chronic lymphocytic leukemia. N Engl J Med 2004;351:893-901.

41. Rawstron AC, Green MJ, Kuzmicki A, et al. Monoclonal B lymphocytes with the characteristics of "indolent" chronic lymphocytic leukemia are present in 3.5% of adults with normal blood counts. Blood 2002;100:635-639.

42. Rosenwald A, Alizadeh AA, Widhopf G, et al. Relation of gene expression phenotype to immunoglobulin mutation genotype in B cell chronic lymphocytic leukemia. J Exp Med 2001;194:1639-1647.

43. Schaffner C, Stilgenbauer S, Rappold GA, Döhner H, Lichter P. Somatic ATM mutations indicate a pathogenic role of ATM in B-cell chronic lymphocytic leukemia. Blood 1999;94:748-753.

44. Schmid C, Isaacson PG. Proliferation centres in B-cell malignant lymphoma, lymphocytic (B-CLL): an immunophenotypic study. Histopathology 1994;24:445-451.

45. Siegel RL, Miller KD, Jemal A. Cancer statistics, 2015. CA Cancer J Clin 2015;65:5-29.

46. Slager SL, Benavente Y, Blair A, et al. Medical history, lifestyle, family history, and occupational risk factors for chronic lymphocytic leukemia/small lymphocytic lymphoma: the Interlymph Non-Hodgkin Lymphoma Subtypes Project. J Natl Cancer Inst Monogr 2014;2014:41-51.

47. Tandon B, Peterson L, Gao J, et al. Nuclear overexpression of lymphoid-enhancer-binding factor 1 identified chronic lymphocytic leukemia/small lymphocytic lymphoma in small B-cell lymphomas. Mod Pathol 2011;24:1433-1443.

48. Tandon B, Swerdlow SH, Hasserjian RP, Surti U, Gibson SE. Chronic lymphocytic leukemia/small lymphocytic lymphoma: another neoplasm related to the B-cell follicle? Leuk Lymphoma 2015;56:3378-3386.

49. Tang G, Banks HS, Sargent RL, Medeiros LJ, Abruzzo LV. Chronic lymphocytic leukemia with t(14;18)(q32;q21). Hum Pathol 2013;44:598-605.

50. Tsimberidou AM, Wen S, O'Brien S, et al. Assessment of chronic lymphocytic leukemia and small lymphocytic lymphoma by absolute lymphocyte counts in 2,126 patients: 20 years of experience at The University of Texas MD Anderson Cancer Center. J Clin Oncol 2007;25:4648-4656.

51. Vardi A, Agathangelidis A, Sutton LA, Ghia P, Rosenquist R, Stamatopoulos K. Immunogenetic studies of chronic lymphocytic leukemia: revelations and speculations about ontogeny and clinical evaluation. Cancer Res 2014;74:4211-4216.

52. Villamor N, Conde L, Martínez-Trillos A, et al. NOTCH1 mutations identify a genetic subgroup of chronic lymphocytic leukemia patients with high risk of transformation and poor outcome. Leukemia 2013;27:1100-1106.

53. Visco C, Falisi E, Young KH, et al. Epstein-Barr virus DNA load in chronic lymphocytic leukemia is an independent predictor of clinical course and survival. Oncotarget 2015;6:18653-18663.

54. Wang L, Lawrence MS, Wan Y, et al. SF3B1 and other novel cancer genes in chronic lymphocytic leukemia. N Engl J Med 2011;365:2497-2506.

55. Wierda WG, Zelenetz AD, Gordon LI, et al. NCCN guidelines insights: chronic lymphocytic leukemia/small lymphocytic leukemia, version 1.2017. J Natl Compr Canc Netw 2017;15:293-311.

56. Wiestner A, Rosenwald A, Barry TS, et al. ZAP-70 expression identifies a chronic lymphocytic leukemia subtype with unmutated immunoglobulin genes, inferior clinical outcome, and distinct gene expression profile. Blood 2003;101:4944-4951.

57. Yin CC, Lin P, Carney DA, et al. Chronic lymphocytic leukemia/small lymphocytic lymphoma associated with IgM paraprotein. Am J Clin Pathol 2005;123:594-602.

58. Zent CS, Ding W, Reinalda MS, et al. Autoimmune cytopenia in chronic lymphocytic leukemia/small lymphocytic lymphoma: changes in clinical presentation and prognosis. Leuk Lymphoma 2009;50:1261-1268.

59. Zenz T, Eichhorst B, Busch R, et al. TP53 mutation and survival in chronic lymphocytic leukemia. J Clin Oncol 2010;28:4473-4479.

12 MANTLE CELL LYMPHOMA

GENERAL FEATURES

Mantle cell lymphoma (MCL) is a type of B-cell non-Hodgkin lymphoma that is characterized by t(11;14)(q13;q32) (48). Most tumors are composed of a monotonous population of small CD5-positive B cells, but there are unusual morphologic and immunophenotypic variants that fit within the MCL category. The t(11;14) involves the *CCND1* gene at chromosome 11q13 and the *IGH* locus at chromosome 14q32, and results in dysregulated expression of cyclin D1.

MCL accounts for 3 to 10 percent of non-Hodgkin lymphomas, with some geographic variation in frequency (48). These tumors were originally recognized by Karl Lennert in 1973 and were shortly thereafter included in the Kiel classification as *centrocytic lymphoma* (24). They were also recognized by others using designations such as mantle zone lymphoma or intermediately differentiated lymphocytic lymphoma. Although overlap between these tumors was thought likely, the recognition of chromosome 11q13/*BCL1* locus breakpoints at a high frequency in these tumors (27,58) and cloning of the *CCND1* (41) resulted in an increased understanding that culminated in a consensus proposal to designate these tumors as mantle cell lymphomas in 1992 (1). This term was quickly accepted and has been used in lymphoma classifications since, including the current World Health Organization (WHO) classification.

CLINICAL FEATURES

MCL arises predominantly in older adults. The median patient age is in the seventh decade in many studies (4,23,48), but a recent study from France reported a median age of 72 years (26). In this study, the age-standardized incidence of MCL is 1.1 and 0.26 per 100,000 in men and women, respectively (26). The male to female ratio in most studies ranges from 3 to almost 4 to 1. Most patients with MCL present with peripheral lymph-adenopathy and 75 to 85 percent have advanced stage disease, either Ann Arbor stage III or IV (26); the bone marrow is involved in 60 to 70 percent of patients.

Morphologic evidence of MCL is present in blood in over 75 percent of patients, and this frequency is higher when flow cytometry immunophenotypic analysis is used to identify lymphoma cells (4,7). Usually patients have a normal leukocyte count with a low percentage of lymphoma cells; 5 to 10 percent of MCL patients have high leukocyte counts with numerous circulating lymphoma cells and a predominantly leukemic presentation (47). Some patients who present with disease limited to blood and bone marrow exhibit an indolent clinical course (35,43). Hepatosplenomegaly occurs in up to 50 to 60 percent of patients, some of whom have prominent splenomegaly.

MCL has a particular tropism for the gastrointestinal tract, with microscopic involvement in up to 90 percent of patients if endoscopy is performed on all newly diagnosed cases (40). Usually patients have low-volume disease in the gastrointestinal tract and are asymptomatic. About 20 percent have gastrointestinal tract symptoms and present with abdominal pain, diarrhea, hematochezia, chylous ascites, or acute abdomen due to small intestinal obstruction or perforation. These patients usually have extensive disease in the gastrointestinal tract. Many patients present with polyps of MCL distributed throughout the gastrointestinal tract, but with relative sparing of the esophagus and anus (48). This syndrome is known as *multiple lymphomatous polyposis*.

A variety of extranodal sites can be involved by MCL, including the ocular adnexal region, Waldeyer ring, lungs, genitourinary tract, skin, and brain (23). Although most often a manifestation of widely disseminated nodal disease, approximately 25 percent of patients present primarily with extranodal sites of involvement,

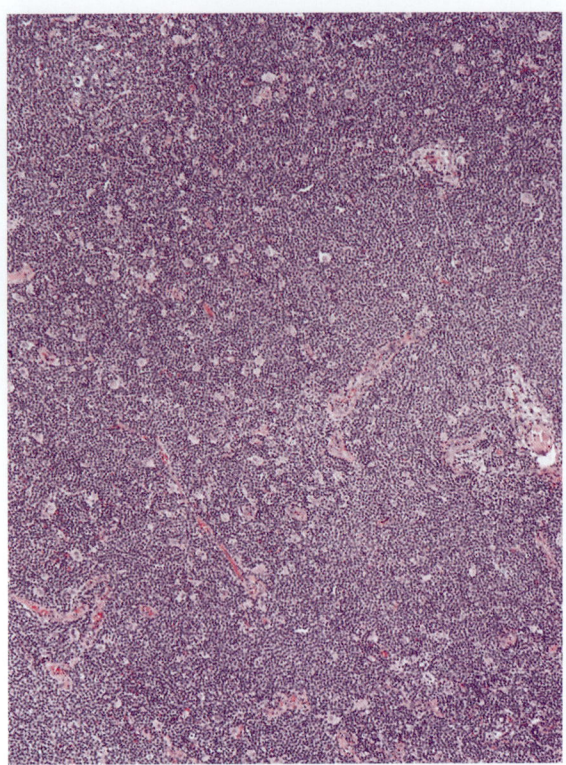

Figure 12-1

MANTLE CELL LYMPHOMA: DIFFUSE PATTERN

A lymph node biopsy specimen is involved by mantle cell lymphoma (MCL) with a diffuse pattern (hematoxylin and eosin [H&E] stain).

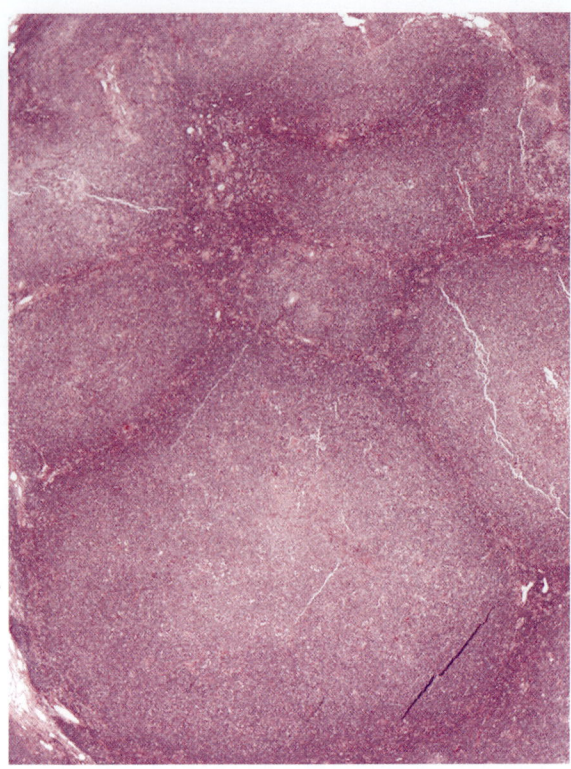

Figure 12-2

MANTLE CELL LYMPHOMA: NODULAR PATTERN

A lymph node biopsy specimen shows MCL with a nodular pattern (H&E stain).

which are sometimes localized. The central nervous system is involved by MCL in less than 5 percent of patients, and MCL can involve either the brain parenchyma or leptomeninges. Most often, patients with MCL involving the central nervous system have a high serum lactate dehydrogenase (LDH) level consistent with high tumor burden or highly proliferative or blastoid tumors (8).

A number of clinical and laboratory findings have been proposed for the prognostication of MCL patients. Perhaps the most popular is the MCL International Prognostic Index (MIPI) which incorporates age, Eastern Cooperative Oncology Group (ECOG) performance status, serum LDH level, and the total leukocyte count into a mathematical formula (19). The calculated result can be used to subdivide MCL patients into three prognostic groups: low, intermediate, and high risk, which correlate with overall survival. About half of MCL patients have a high-risk MIPI score (19,26). The Ki-67 index also can be

incorporated to create a biologic MIPI (bMIPI) and a convenient point system has been used to develop a simplified MIPI (sMIPI) for bedside use (19). An elevated absolute monocyte count and β-2-microglobulin level also have been suggested as complements to the MIPI for identifying MCL patients with a poorer prognosis (54).

HISTOLOGIC FINDINGS

Lymph Nodes

MCL involves lymph nodes in three architectural patterns (48,49,63). The diffuse pattern is the most common (75 to 80 percent of cases). In this pattern, the neoplastic cells completely efface the lymph node and obliterate the normal architecture (fig. 12-1). A nodular pattern occurs in approximately 20 percent of cases. In this pattern, the neoplastic cells form vague nodules that obliterate follicles and germinal centers (fig. 12-2). Some cases show dense sclerosis surrounding

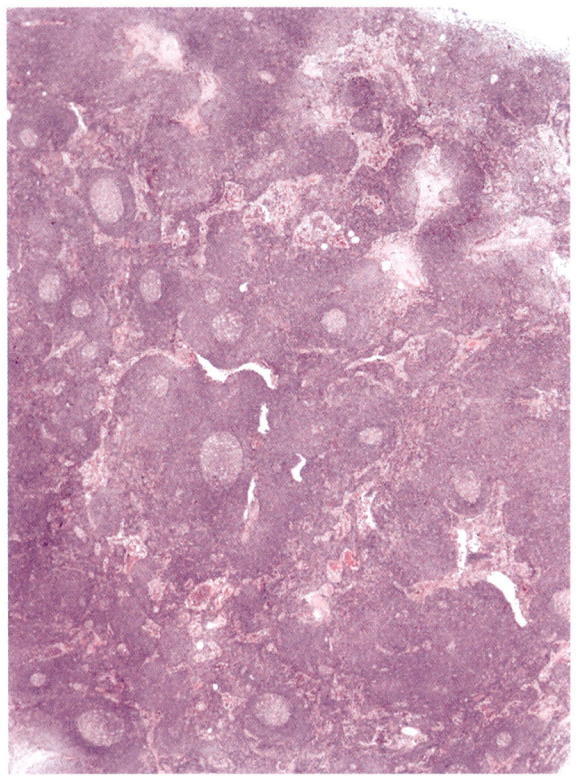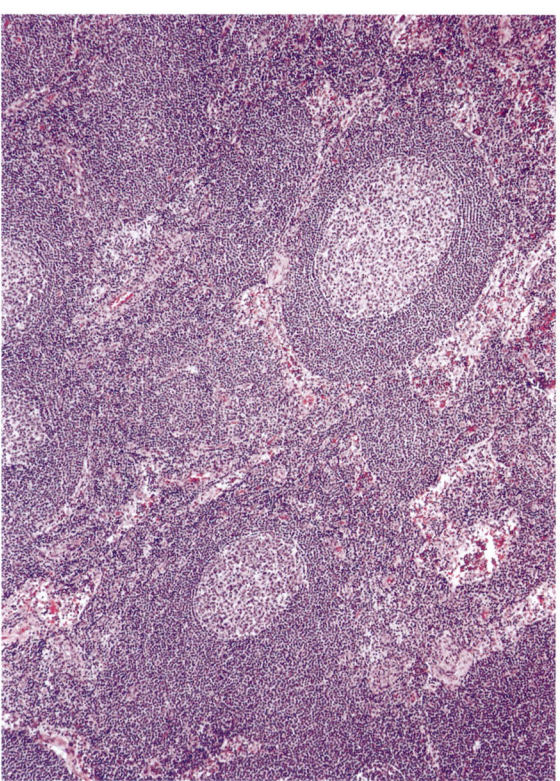

Figure 12-3

MANTLE CELL LYMPHOMA: MANTLE ZONE PATTERN

A lymph node biopsy specimen is partially involved by MCL with a pure (over 90 percent) mantle zone pattern. In both figures the mantle zones surrounding reactive germinal centers are expanded by a monotonous population of MCL cells (H&E stain).

the tumor nodules. The mantle zone pattern is the least common. A pure mantle zone pattern occurs in about 1 percent of all cases of MCL, although a partial mantle zone pattern, combined with either the diffuse or nodular pattern, is more common. In the mantle zone pattern, the neoplastic cells expand and broaden the mantle zones of follicles, with central reactive germinal centers that can be expanded or attenuated (fig. 12-3).

Other morphologic features common in cases of MCL and helpful for its recognition include: epithelioid histiocytes, naked germinal centers, and sclerotic blood vessels (48). None of these features is specific for MCL. Epithelioid histiocytes are usually singly scattered and have well-developed eosinophilic cytoplasm without intracytoplasmic cell fragments (tingible bodies) and therefore are also known as pink histiocytes (fig. 12-4). Pink histiocytes occur in about 75

percent of cases of MCL and are most commonly found in tumors with a diffuse pattern. Naked germinal centers occur in about one third of cases of MCL. Naked germinal centers lack a surrounding mantle zone cuff; in other words, tumor cells surround and abut upon the cells of the germinal center (fig. 12-5). Sclerotic blood vessels are common in MCL, seen in over two thirds of cases (fig. 12-6). In classic or typical MCL, the mitotic rate is low and areas of geographic necrosis are uncommon.

Cytologically, classic MCL is composed of a monomorphic population of small to intermediate-sized lymphocytes. The nuclei have mature chromatin with irregular nuclear contours; cytoplasm is scant (figs. 12-4, 12-6). Importantly, large cells, such as the centroblasts in follicular lymphoma, large cells and plasma cells in marginal zone lymphoma, and paraimmunoblasts in chronic lymphocytic leukemia/small lymphocytic

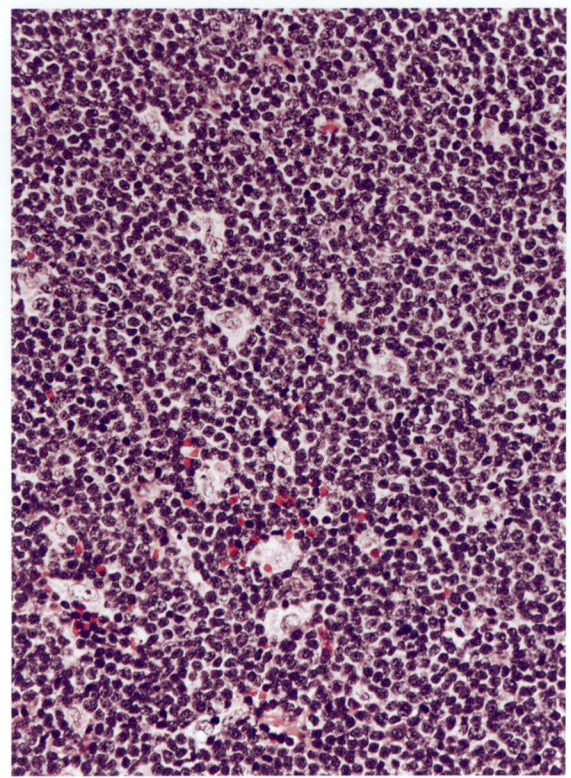

Figure 12-4

EPITHELIOID HISTIOCYTES

In this field (same case as shown in fig. 12-1), many reactive histiocytes with eosinophilic cytoplasm are scattered throughout the tumor. Pink histiocytes occur in up to 75 percent of cases of MCL (H&E stain).

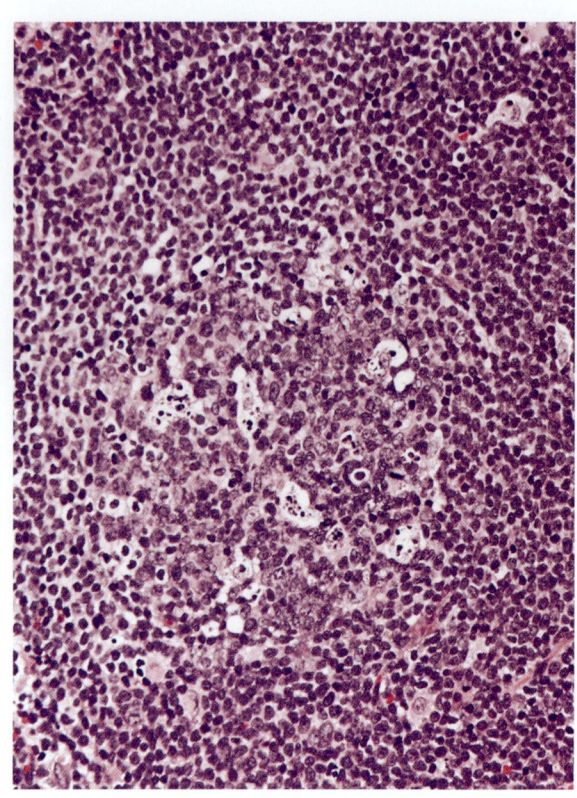

Figure 12-5

NAKED GERMINAL CENTER

A naked germinal center is surrounded by MCL cells. The term "naked" is used because the mantle zone surrounding the reactive germinal center is replaced by MCL (H&E stain).

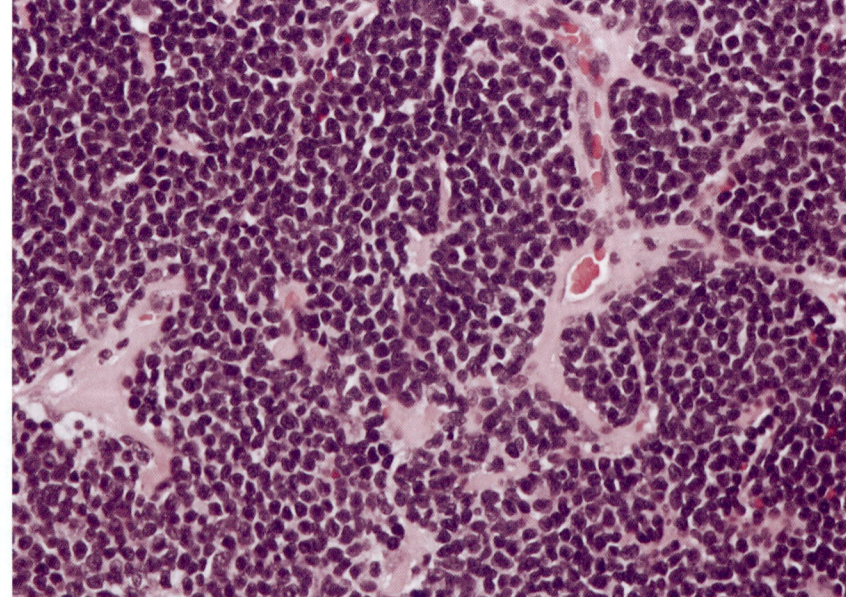

Figure 12-6

SCLEROTIC BLOOD VESSELS

Sclerotic blood vessels are common in MCL and are usually observed in areas of tumor with a diffuse pattern (H&E stain).

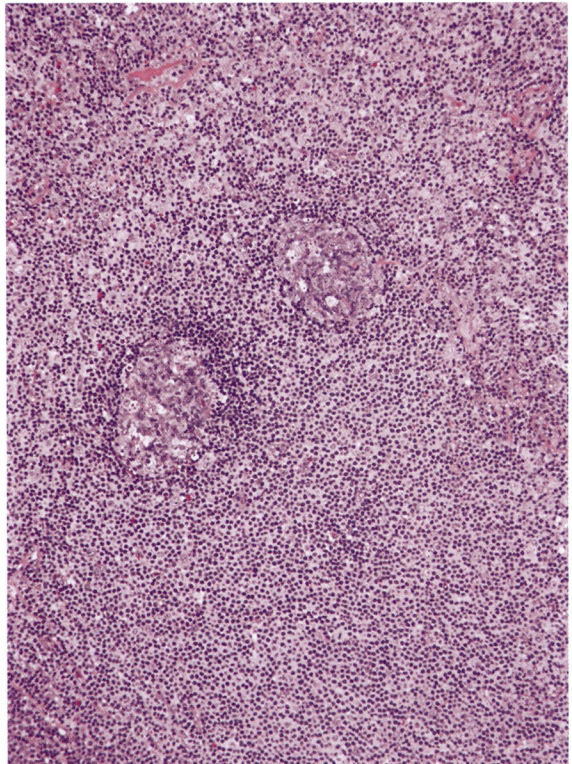

Figure 12-7

MARGINAL ZONE-LIKE MANTLE CELL LYMPHOMA

The MCL neoplastic cells have abundant pale (monocytoid) cytoplasm. Some reactive follicles retain mantle zone cuffs, mimicking marginal zone lymphoma. Nevertheless, the neoplastic cells expressed cyclin D1 and carried *CCND1-IGH* shown by fluorescence in situ hybridization (FISH) (H&E stain).

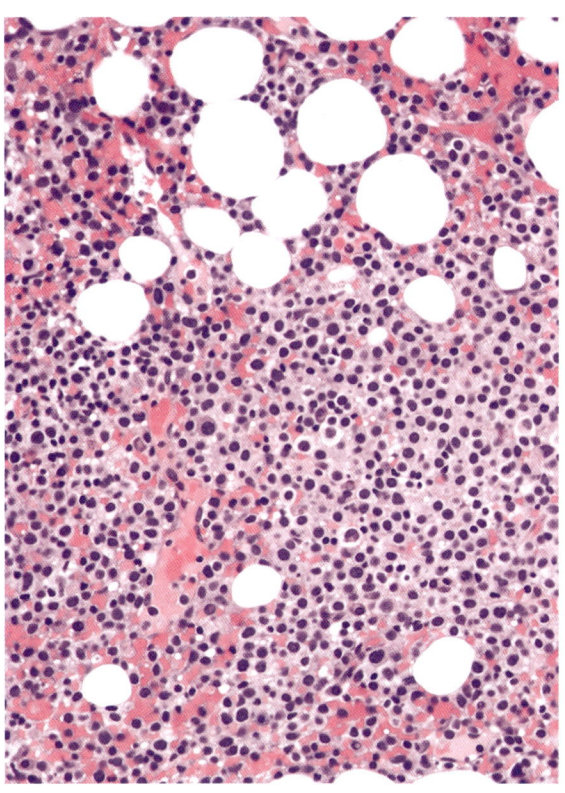

Figure 12-8

MARGINAL ZONE-LIKE MANTLE CELL LYMPHOMA

A case of MCL involving bone marrow in an interstitial and diffuse pattern. The neoplastic cells have abundant monocytoid cytoplasm, mimicking hairy cell leukemia or marginal zone lymphoma, but strongly expressed cyclin D1 and carried the t(11;14)(q13;q32) (H&E stain).

lymphoma (CLL/SLL) are absent. Proliferation centers are absent. In rare cases of MCL, monotypic plasma cells carry the t(11;14)(q13;q32) and represent a component of the tumor; these plasma cells are often in the center of tumor nodules or within reactive germinal centers (61).

Indolent Variants of MCL

A small subset of MCL patients have neoplasms that are often clinically indolent. These tumors show unusual morphologic features characterized by small, round or oval cells. They have an appropriate immunophenotype including cyclin D1 expression and carry t(11;14)(q13;q32). However, SOX11 is more often negative in indolent MCL.

CLL/SLL-Like MCL. Five to 10 percent of patients with MCL present exclusively with blood and bone marrow involvement. The lymphoma cells are round in smears, resembling, in large part, CLL (35,47). Many of these patients are initially misdiagnosed as having CLL and receive minimal therapy for a few years before the disease becomes more aggressive with development of lymphadenopathy and a more aggressive clinical course.

Marginal Zone-Like MCL. Rare cases of MCL are characterized by small cells with abundant pale or monocytoid cytoplasm; plasmacytoid differentiation also can be present (figs. 12-7, 12-8). Patients with these tumors present with only blood and bone marrow involvement, with lymphadenopathy or extranodal sites of disease, or both. In one study, these tumors commonly involved the gastrointestinal tract.

In Situ Mantle Cell Neoplasia. In these tumors, MCL cells are located in the mantle zones

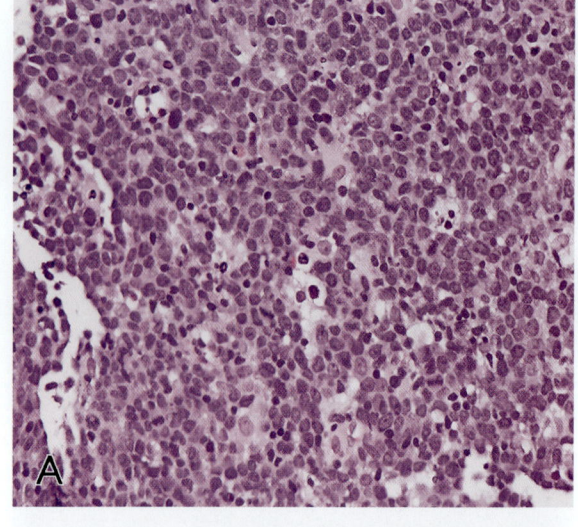

Figure 12-9

BLASTOID VARIANT OF MANTLE CELL LYMPHOMA

A: In this lymph node, the neoplastic cells have immature chromatin and a high mitotic rate (H&E stain).

B,C: The neoplastic cells have a high proliferation rate as shown by Ki-67 (B) and express p53 (C) (immunohistochemistry with hematoxylin counterstain).

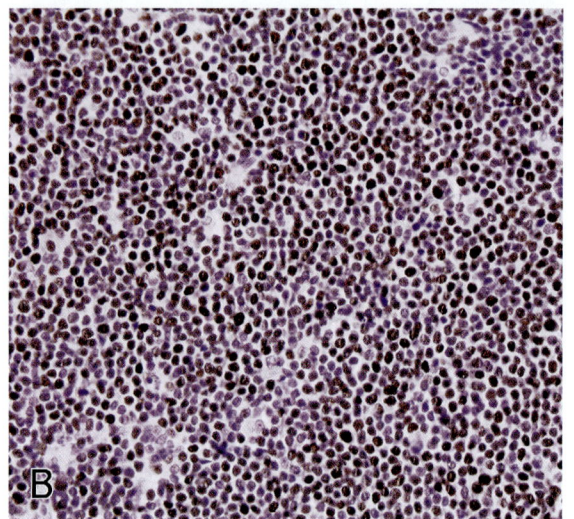

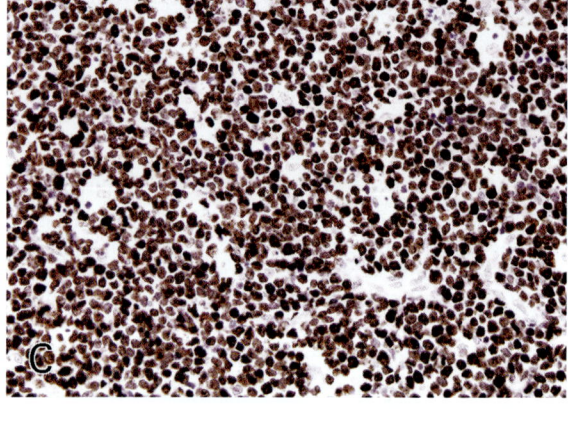

surrounding reactive germinal centers. Generally, there is no expansion or only minimal expansion of mantle zones. Often, cyclin D1 expression is required to appreciate the presence of disease (see chapter 6).

Histologically Aggressive Variants of MCL

Approximately 10 percent of patients with MCL have histologically aggressive variants of disease, designated as blastoid or pleomorphic, and often associated with an aggressive clinical course. Unlike classic MCL, blastoid and pleomorphic MCL variants have a high mitotic rate and some show foci of necrosis (48,49). Otherwise, these variants have an immunophenotype similar to classic MCL, including cyclin D1 overexpression, and carry t(11;14)(q13;q32).

Blastoid Variant. This variant of MCL is composed of cells that resemble, in part, lymphoblasts with finely reticulated and dispersed nuclear chromatin (fig. 12-9). Some blastoid tumors have a starry sky pattern and abundant apoptosis (fig. 12-10). Most often, blastoid MCL cases arise de novo.

Pleomorphic Variant. This variant of MCL is composed predominantly of pleomorphic cells that exhibit a spectrum of sizes, from intermediate-sized to large, with large irregular nuclei and sometimes prominent nucleoli with occasional multinucleation (fig. 12-11).

Pleomorphic MCL can arise de novo or occur in patients with a history of classic MCL who over time and following therapy acquire pleomorphic cytologic features (fig. 12-12). These

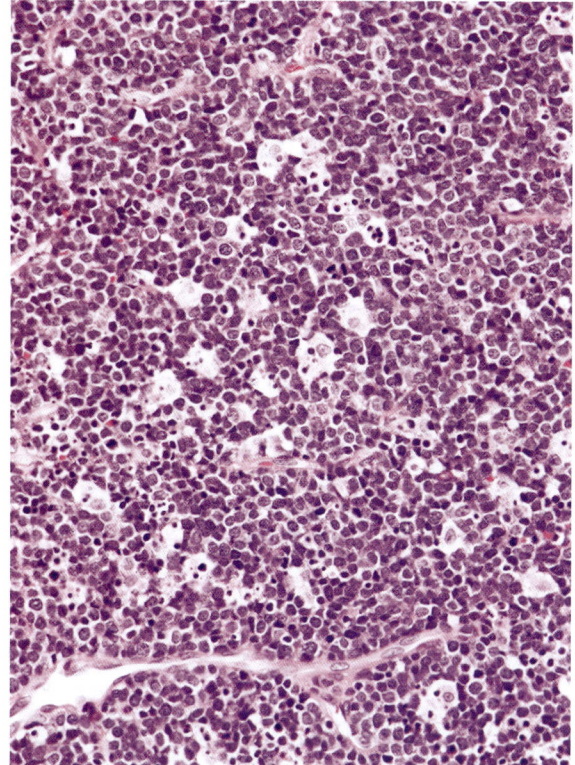

Figure 12-10

BLASTOID VARIANT OF MANTLE CELL LYMPHOMA

A prominent starry sky pattern is present. The possibility of Burkitt lymphoma was considered but the tumor expressed cyclin D1 and carried *CCND1-IGH*. A *MYC* rearrangement was also shown by FISH (H&E stain).

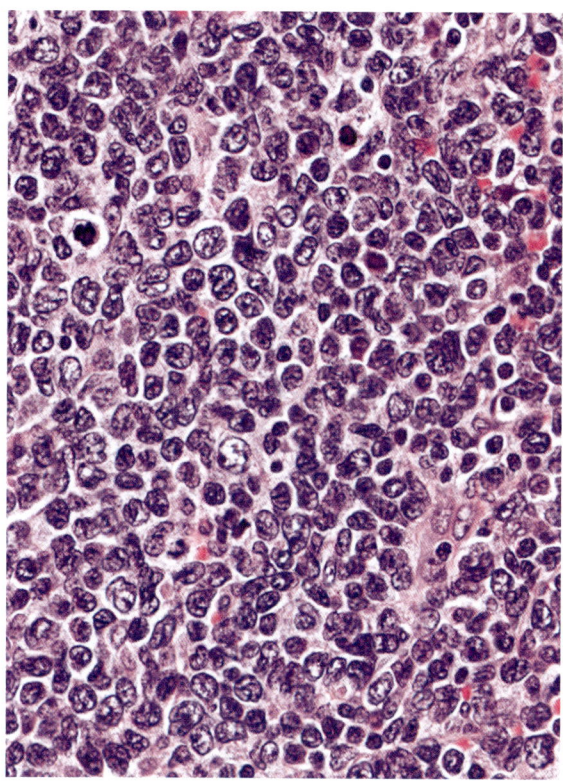

Figure 12-11

PLEOMORPHIC VARIANT OF MANTLE CELL LYMPHOMA

The neoplastic cells in this lymph node are intermediate to large, and the larger cells have some centroblastic features. Nevertheless, cyclin D1 was strongly expressed and t(11;14) was present (H&E stain).

morphologic features are likely a manifestation of disease progression, and probably relate to clonal evolution. In the few cases assessed, patients with both classic and pleomorphic MCL share clonal identity, supporting the idea of histologic progression (60).

Prolymphocytoid Variant. A few MCL patients present with or progress to a clinical picture that resembles B-cell prolymphocytic leukemia, with more than 55 percent prolymphocytoid cells in the blood (46). These cells are of intermediate size, with prominent central nucleoli (fig. 12-13). This variant is recognized by the presence of some typical MCL cells in the blood smear and nuclear prolymphocytoid contours that are usually more irregular than the prolymphocytes of de novo B-cell prolymphocytic leukemia or CLL/SLL in prolymphocytoid differentiation.

MCL Associated with Other Lymphoma Types (Composite Lymphoma)

In 2012, Papathomas et al. (36) reviewed the literature and identified 26 cases of composite lymphoma with a MCL component. The recognition of these tumors is facilitated greatly by immunohistochemical analysis for cyclin D1. The most common type of lymphoma associated with MCL is follicular lymphoma, present in about 30 percent of all cases. Other lymphoma types associated with MCL include CLL/SLL, classic Hodgkin lymphoma, plasma cell myeloma, and rare cases of marginal zone lymphoma, plasmablastic lymphoma, and Burkitt lymphoma. Most often the MCL and other lymphoma types are not clonally related, but a clonal relationship has been shown in about 15 percent of cases.

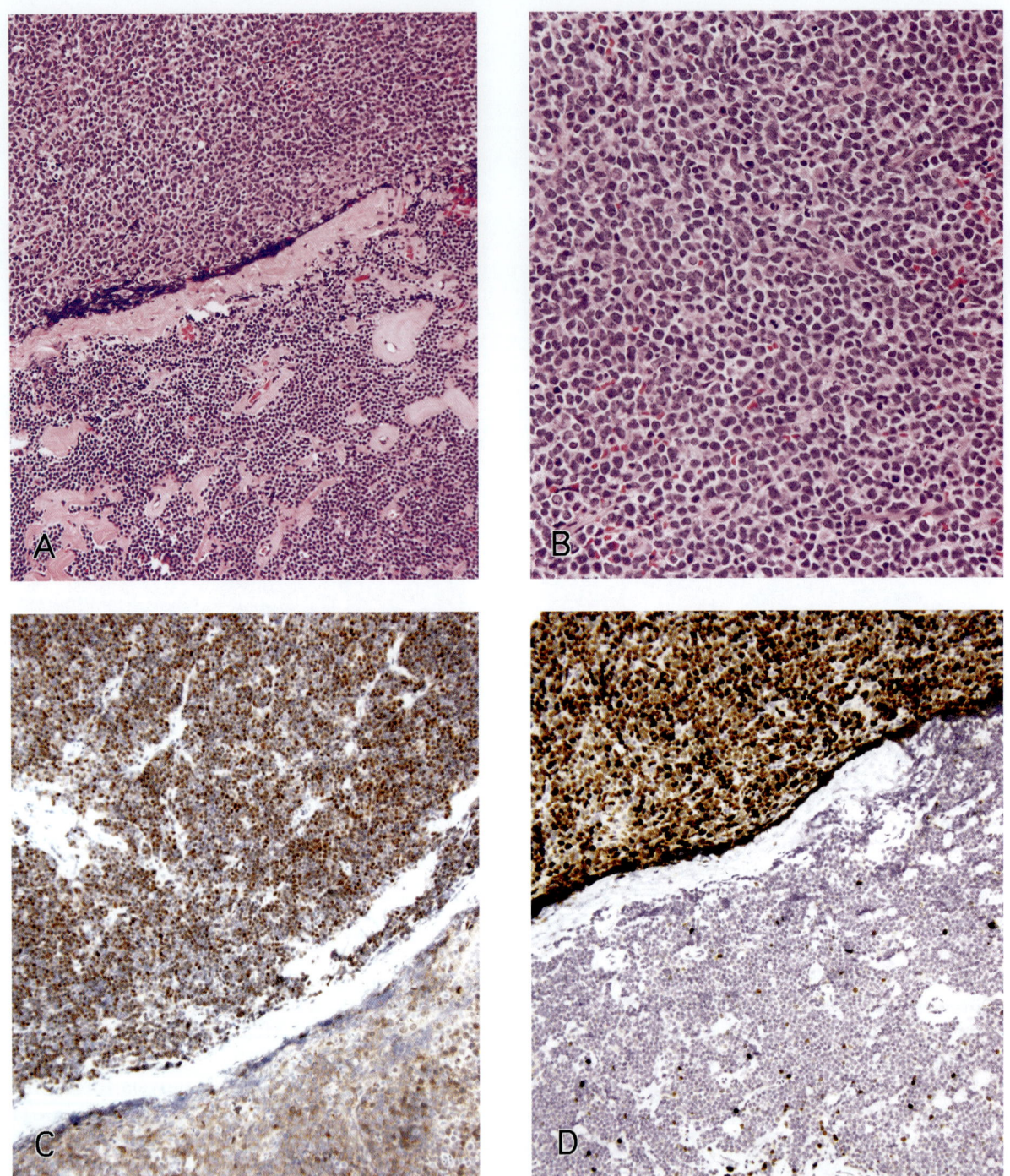

Figure 12-12

CLASSIC AND PLEOMORPHIC VARIANT OF MANTLE CELL LYMPHOMA

This biopsy specimen showed involvement by MCL with classic and pleomorphic variant components.

A: Pleomorphic variant MCL is at the top and classic MCL at the bottom of the field (A,B: H&E stain).

B: High magnification of the component of pleomorphic variant MCL. The cells are intermediate to large with more open chromatin and increased mitotic figures.

C,D: Both components are positive for cyclin D1 (C) but only the pleomorphic variant had a high proliferation rate shown by Ki-67 (D) (C,D: immunohistochemistry with hematoxylin counterstain).

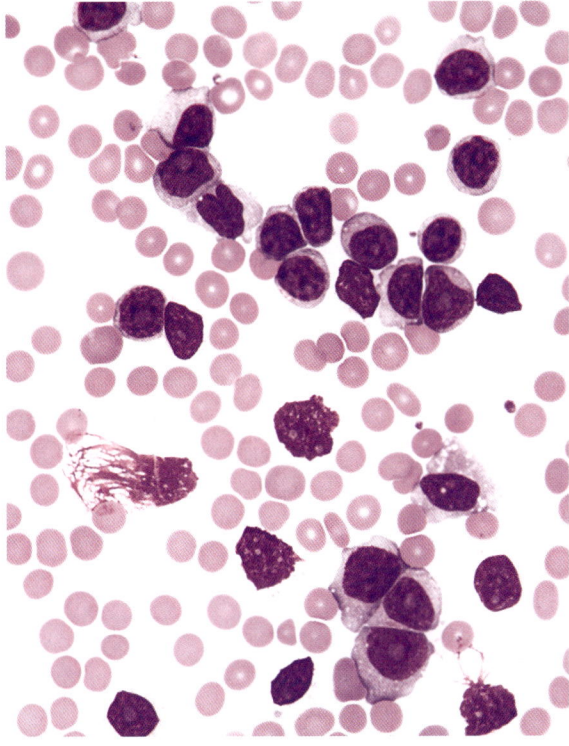

Figure 12-13

**PROLYMPHOCYTOID VARIANT
OF MANTLE CELL LYMPHOMA**

The blood smear shows many intermediate-sized and larger cells with prominent central nucleoli, perinuclear accentuation, and moderate cytoplasm, resembling prolymphocytes. A few smaller lymphoid cells, more in keeping with classic MCL cells, are present in the background. Flow cytometry showed a classic immunophenotype [CD5(+), CD20(+), CD23(-)] and conventional cytogenetics showed t(11;14)(q13;q32) (Wright-Giemsa stain).

Gastrointestinal Tract

The ileocecal region is usually most extensively involved by MCL, where the lymphoma can form a large mass (40,48). In endoscopic gastrointestinal tract biopsy specimens, MCL initially infiltrates the submucosa and surrounds reactive germinal centers, forming a mantle zone pattern or infiltrating the submucosa in a nodular or diffuse growth pattern. Small polyps can be captured in endoscopy biopsy specimens (fig. 12-14). The neoplastic cells exhibit classic or pleomorphic nuclear features. MCL also involves the appendix; although usually a part of a resection specimen for extensive disease, MCL may be detected incidentally in an appendectomy specimen (fig. 12-15).

Bone Marrow and Peripheral Blood

Bone marrow involvement is common in patients with MCL. In bone marrow biopsy sections, the pattern is often mixed and predominantly nonparatrabecular, with a minor paratrabecular component. Nodular and partial mantle zone patterns also occur (57). In patients with indolent MCL who present with disease limited to blood and bone marrow, the pattern of bone marrow infiltration is often interstitial. Lymphoma cells in bone marrow aspirates and peripheral blood smears show more variation in size and nuclear contours than often appreciated in routinely stained bone marrow biopsy specimens (figs. 12-16, 12-17). Lymphoma cells in the blood can be numerous, but more often they are uncommon or rare, and searching may be required for identification (4,7).

Spleen and Liver

When involved by MCL, the spleen can be close to normal in size or massive. Usually the white pulp is preferentially involved by MCL and this is most easily appreciated in smaller spleen specimens. The white pulp is replaced by tumor with a diffuse or vaguely nodular growth pattern. In spleens with extensive disease both white and red pulp are extensively replaced (fig. 12-18).

MCL initially involves the portal tracts of the liver (fig. 12-19). In leukemic cases a sinusoidal pattern is observed.

CYTOLOGIC FINDINGS

Aspirate smears of classic MCL show a monomorphous population of small to medium-sized lymphocytes with scant cytoplasm (fig. 12-20). The nuclear contours range from slightly to markedly irregular and indented, the chromatin is evenly distributed, and nucleoli are inconspicuous.

In the blastoid variant of MCL, aspirate smears may show a monomorphous population of immature, blast-like cells (fig. 12-21) or a mixture of small atypical and large blastic cells. Apoptotic bodies are common, as are mitotic figures.

In the pleomorphic variant of MCL, the lymphoma cells are more variable in size and nuclear contours (fig. 12-22). In some cases, the cells can more or less resemble centroblasts with vesicular chromatin and can be misinterpreted as large B-cell lymphoma (without knowledge of cyclin D1 expression).

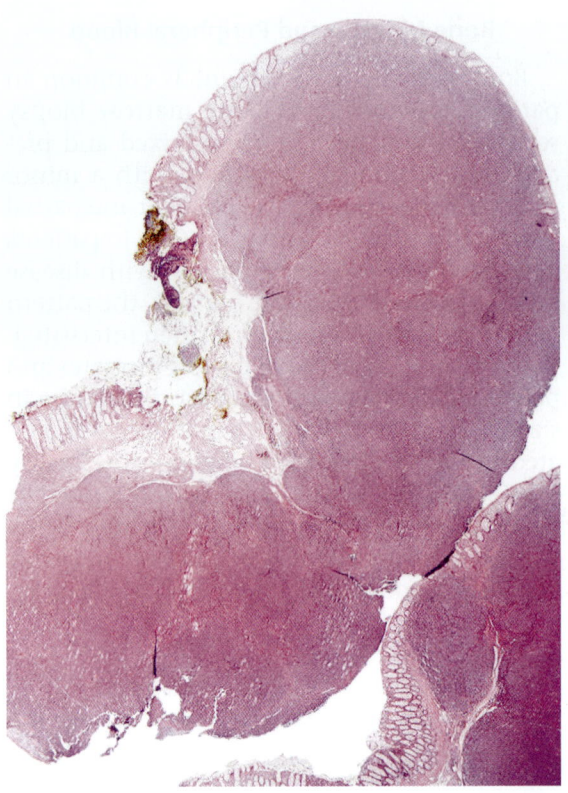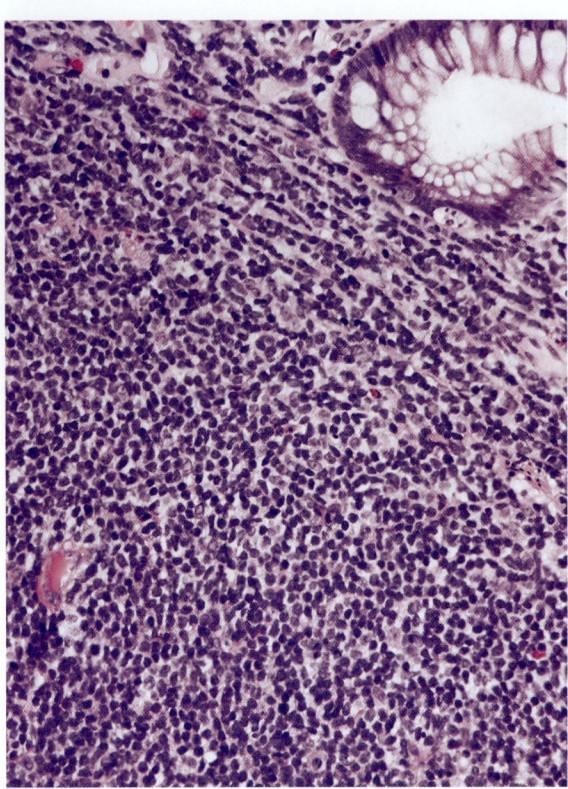

Figure 12-14

MANTLE CELL LYMPHOMA INVOLVING GASTROINTESTINAL TRACT

This case of MCL extensively involved the gastrointestinal tract.
Left: The endoscopist captured a polyp composed of MCL with a vaguely nodular pattern.
Right: High magnification shows the classic cytologic features. No lymphoepithelial lesions were identified (left, right: H&E stain).

Figure 12-15

MANTLE CELL LYMPHOMA INVOLVING GASTROINTESTINAL TRACT

An appendix removed as part of a right colectomy specimen shows involvement by MCL. The neoplasm predominantly involves the submucosa (H&E stain).

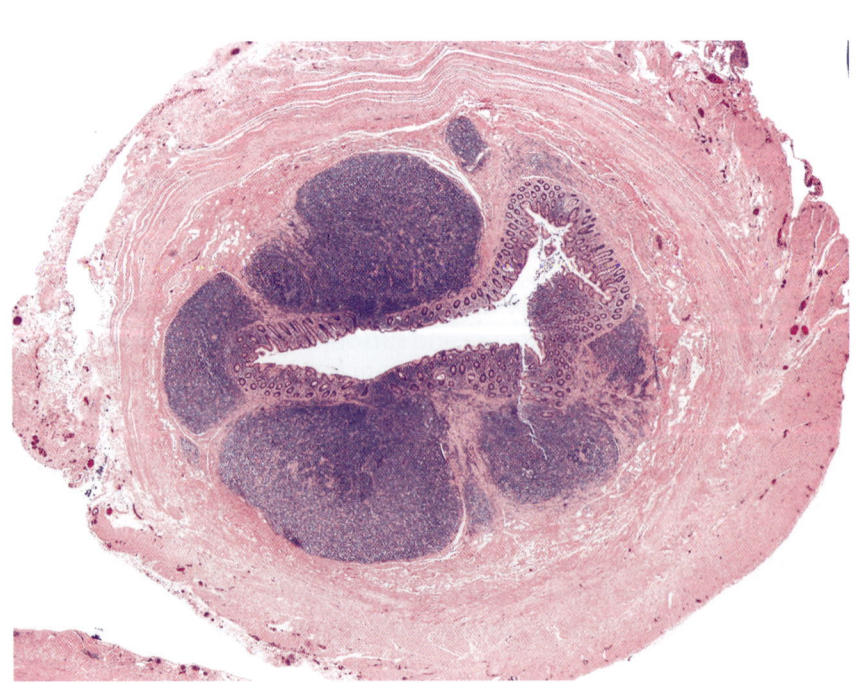

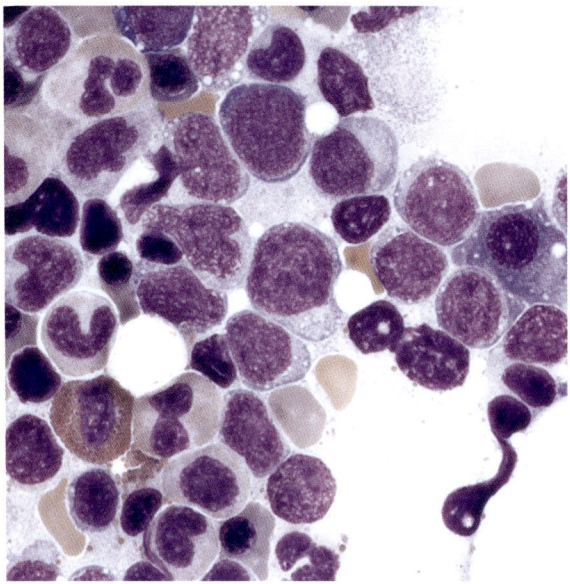

Figure 12-16

**MANTLE CELL LYMPHOMA
INVOLVING BONE MARROW**

Aspirate smear of MCL in which some of the cells have irregular nuclear contours and more open chromatin suggestive of the pleomorphic variant (Wright-Giemsa stain).

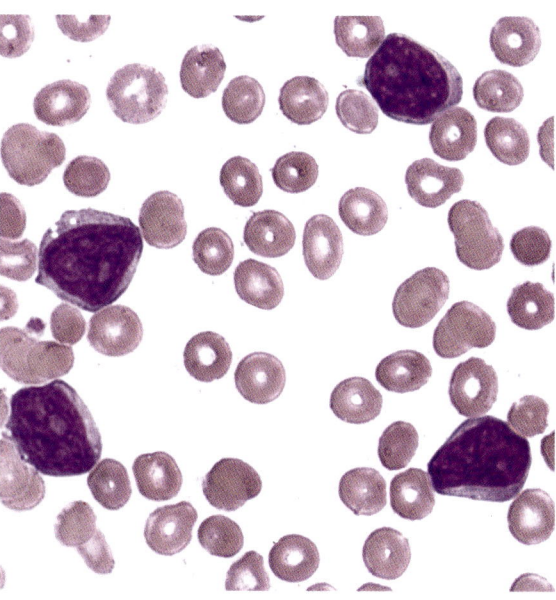

Figure 12-17

MANTLE CELL LYMPHOMA INVOLVING BLOOD

The cells have the classic cytologic features (Wright-Giemsa stain).

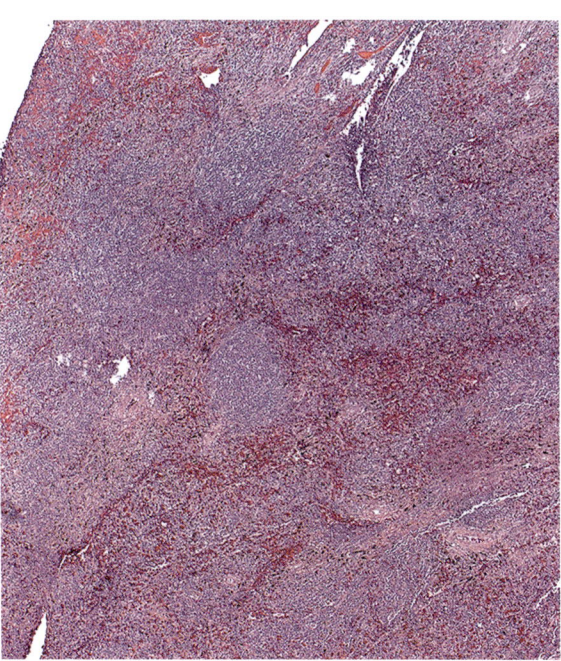

Figure 12-18

MANTLE CELL LYMPHOMA INVOLVING SPLEEN

This splenectomy specimen shows extensive involvement by MCL. The tumor involved white and red pulp, with preferential involvement of the white pulp (H&E stain).

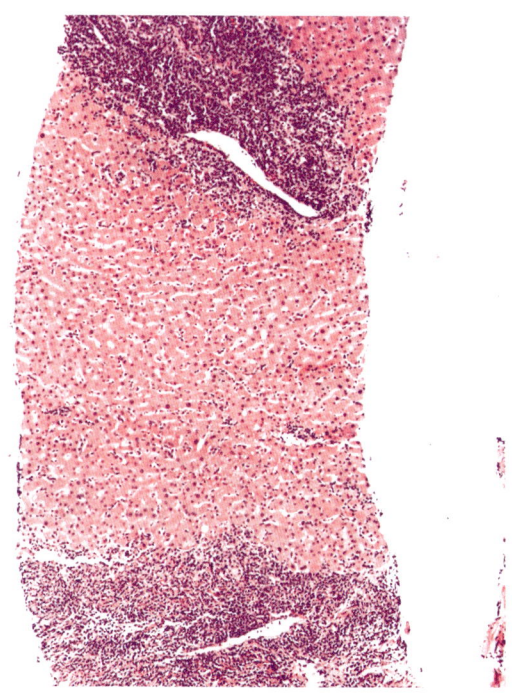

Figure 12-19

MANTLE CELL LYMPHOMA INVOLVING LIVER

A needle biopsy of liver shows extensive involvement of the portal tracts by MCL (H&E stain).

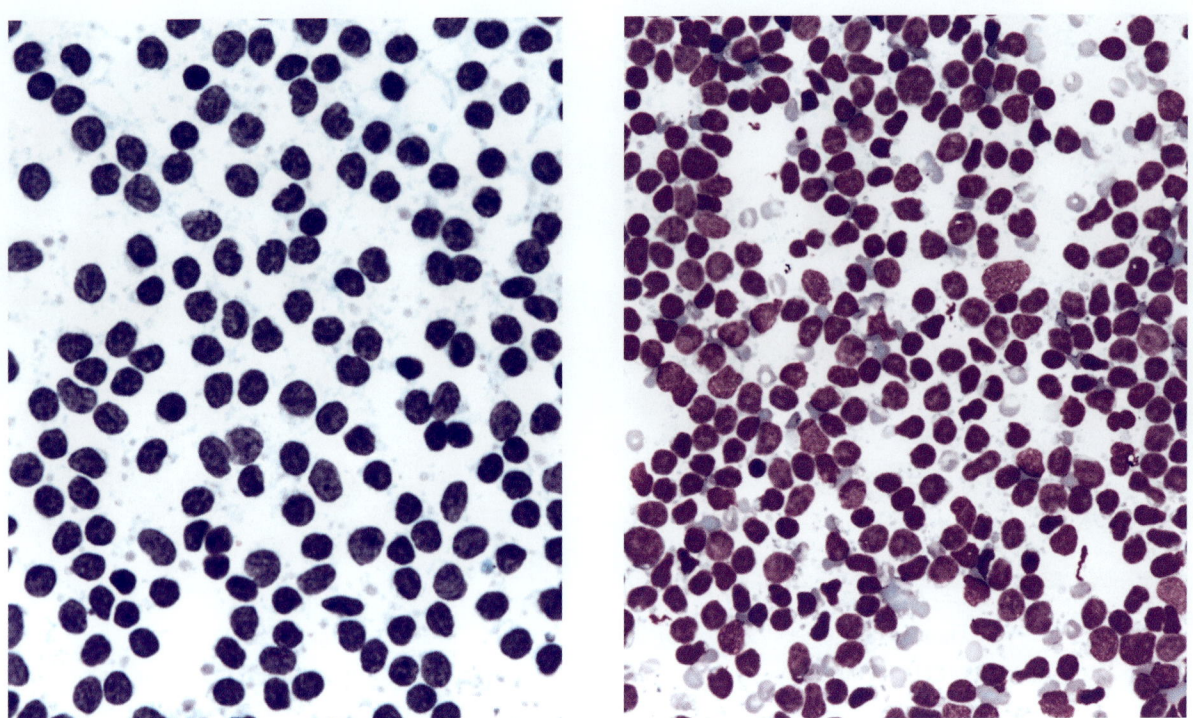

Figure 12-20

MANTLE CELL LYMPHOMA: CYTOLOGY

Aspirate smears of MCL with classic cytology show small lymphocytes with irregular nuclei. Large cells (such as paraimmunoblasts) are absent (left: Papanicolaou stain; right: Diff-Quik stain).

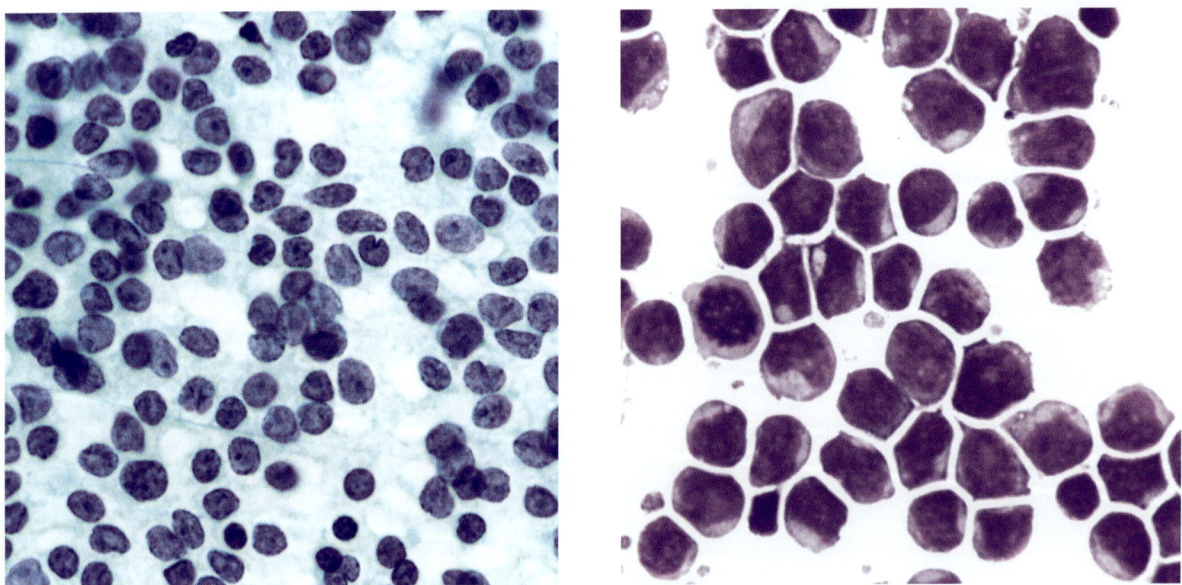

Figure 12-21

MANTLE CELL LYMPHOMA: CYTOLOGY

Aspirate smears of a case of the blastoid variant of MCL show intermediate-sized cells with blastic chromatin and conspicuous nucleoli (left: Papanicolaou stain; right: Diff-Quik stain).

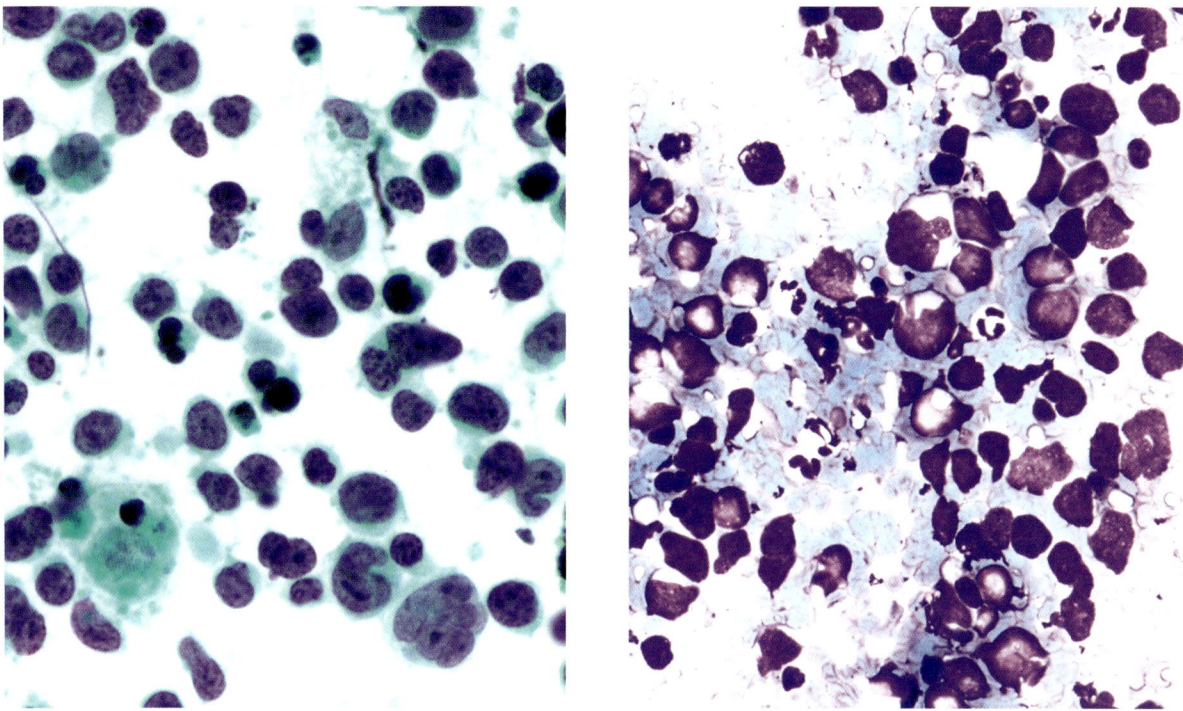

Figure 12-22

MANTLE CELL LYMPHOMA: CYTOLOGY

Aspirate smears of the pleomorphic variant of MCL show medium to large size cells with variably convoluted nuclei (left: Papanicolaou stain; right: Diff-Quik stain).

Fine-needle aspiration material can be sent for flow cytometry immunophenotyping and possibly conventional cytogenetics or fluorescence in situ hybridization (FISH) analysis for *CCND1-IGH*/t(11;14)(q13;q32) (5). Immunohistochemical analysis can be performed on smears, but immunostaining for cyclin D1 yields more optimal results using unstained tissue sections cut from a cell block.

IMMUNOPHENOTYPIC FINDINGS

Flow cytometry is well suited to the study of MCL. The neoplastic cells express IgM and usually IgD with monotypic immunoglobulin light chain restriction. More than 60 percent of MCL cases show immunoglobulin lambda light chain restriction (unlike most B-cell lymphomas in which kappa is predominant). MCL cells express pan-B-cell antigens including CD19, CD20, CD22, CD79a, and PAX5. FMC7 is usually positive as is CD79b (fig. 12-23). Almost all cases of MCL express CD5 and most also express CD43. MCL is negative for CD2, CD3, CD10, CD11c,

and CD34. Most cases are negative for CD23 but approximately 10 percent dimly express CD23. CD200 is also usually negative in MCL but about 5 percent of cases are positive. Cyclin D1 expression is difficult to assess reliably by flow cytometry.

Immunohistochemistry is very helpful for assessing MCL cases. Most importantly, cyclin D1 is physiologically expressed in normal B lymphocytes, but at a low level usually not detectable by immunohistochemical analysis. In MCL, however, cyclin D1 expression is markedly upregulated and can be detected by immunohistochemistry in almost all cases (fig. 12-24). Cyclin D1 expression is best assessed using formalin-fixed, paraffin-embedded tissue sections. A positive result shows crisp staining within in the tumor cell nuclei. Typically, the intensity of cyclin D1 varies in the tumor cells, likely correlating with the cell cycle. Cytoplasmic staining for cyclin D1 is not a true positive and may be an artifact or may be physiologic, although this is poorly understood.

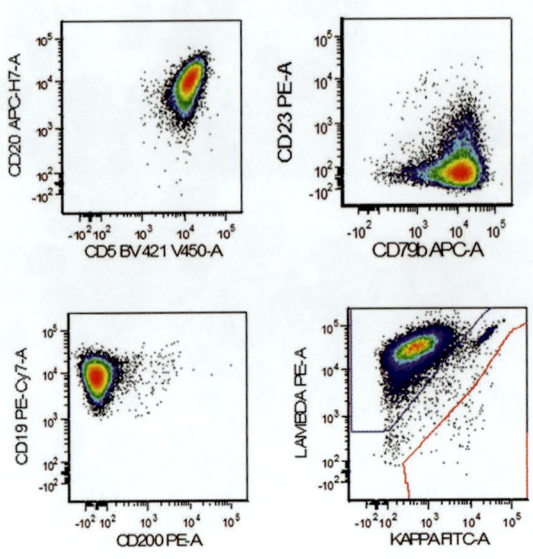

Figure 12-23

MANTLE CELL LYMPHOMA: FLOW CYTOLOGY

The neoplastic cells are positive for monotypic lambda, CD5, CD19, CD20, CD23 (partial), and CD79b and are negative for CD200. Approximately 10 percent of MCL cases express dim or partial CD23 and most are negative for CD200.

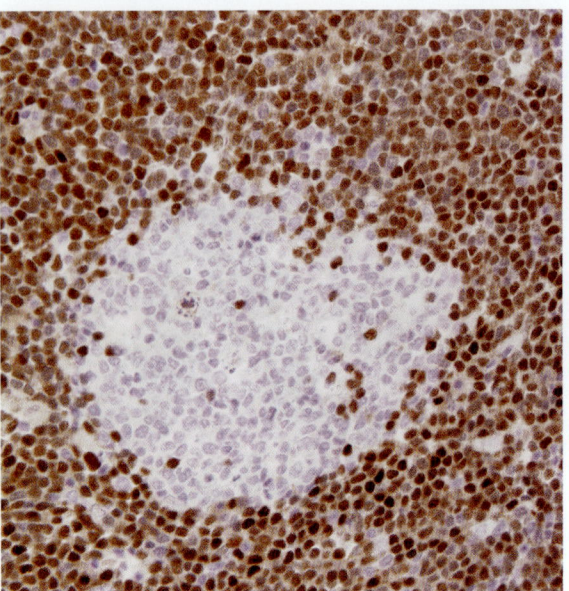

Figure 12-24

MANTLE CELL LYMPHOMA: CYCLIN D1

A cyclin D1 immunostain was performed on a case of MCL with classic features. The neoplastic cell nuclei express cyclin D1 with variable intensity. A benign germinal center in the field is negative for cyclin D1 (immunohistochemistry with hematoxylin counterstain).

Immunohistochemical analysis shows that rare cases of MCL overexpress cyclin D1 but do not have evidence of t(11;14) by routine FISH. In our experience, these tumors often have an unusual breakpoint or a variant translocation that is not detected by standard FISH testing. Additional FISH probe sets or conventional cytogenetic analysis can show 11q13/*CCND1* translocations, supporting the diagnosis of MCL.

SOX11 is a transcription factor with many functions including PAX5 regulation. In MCL, SOX11 is thought to block terminal B-cell differentiation (53). SOX11 also contributes to MCL growth by stimulating angiogenesis. SOX11 is expressed in a nuclear pattern in about 90 percent of cases of MCL (fig. 12-25) (11,30). Overall, SOX11 expression is present in most cases of MCL with classic morphology or aggressive morphologic variants, but is negative in clinically indolent variants of MCL. SOX11 expression also correlates with absent or low-level mutations of the *IGH* variable region genes in MCL (32). SOX11 is not entirely specific since it has been reported in other types of B-cell lymphoma, such as a subset of cases of Burkitt or B-lymphoblastic lymphoma (11,30).

Immunohistochemistry is valuable for assessing prognostic variables in MCL. p53 expression correlates with *TP53* mutation status and has been reported to correlate with aggressive morphologic variants and inferior survival (see fig. 12-9C) (48). Ki-67 expression is highly variable in MCL cases; patients with tumors with a high Ki-67 rate have a poorer prognosis (see fig. 12-9B). There is no clear consensus for the optimum Ki-67 cutoff to delineate the poorer prognosis group, but 30 or 40 percent seems to be used most often. The prognostic effect of high Ki-67 expression within MCL remains for patients treated with a variety of chemotherapy regimens (9,14,19,20). Ki-67 is a more powerful prognostic predictor than the presence of blastoid or pleomorphic morphology (19).

MYC is highly overexpressed in cases of MCL associated with 8q24/*MYC* translocations (fig. 12-26), however, a subset of MCL cases that do not carry *MYC* abnormalities also overexpress MYC. In our experience, MYC expression is more variable in cases without 8q24/*MYC* translocations.

Many of the other antigens assessed by flow cytometry are also assessed by immunohistochemistry, although this method is less sensitive. Immunoglobulin light chain expression is usually negative in routinely processed tissue sections because the tumor cells lack cytoplasmic immunoglobulin; however, light chains can be assessed in fine-needle aspiration specimens and touch imprints (fig. 12-27). All cases of MCL express BCL2. About 40 percent of MCLs are positive for MUM1/IRF4 and 10 percent for DBA.44. Cases of MCL with a nodular pattern are associated with irregular follicular dendritic cell networks that are usually positive for CD21 (fig. 12-28). MCL is almost always negative for CD23 and about 5 percent are negative for CD5. A few cases, usually tumors that have blastoid or pleomorphic features, express CD10 or BCL6 (fig. 12-29).

MOLECULAR GENETIC FINDINGS

Conventional cytogenetic analysis has shown t(11;14)(q13;q32) in almost all cases of MCL (10,34). Therefore, t(11;14) is thought to be a primary event in MCL pathogenesis. Nevertheless, t(11;14) is uncommonly (about 5 percent) a sole abnormality; additional chromosomal

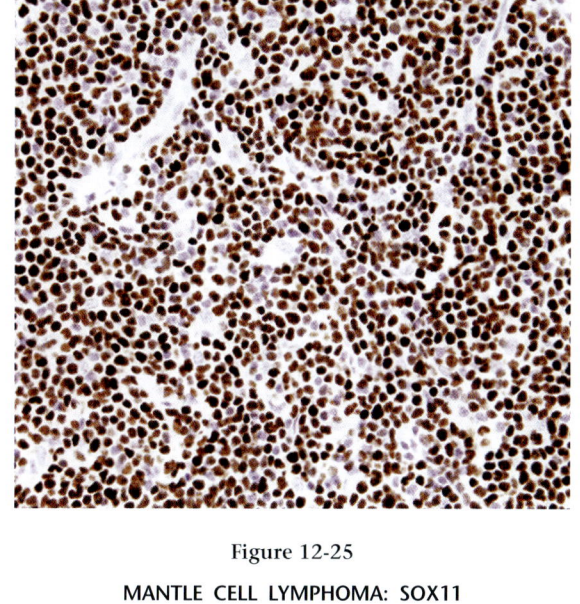

Figure 12-25

MANTLE CELL LYMPHOMA: SOX11

A SOX11 immunostain was performed on a case of MCL with classic features. The neoplastic cells exhibit a nuclear pattern of reactivity (immunohistochemistry with hematoxylin counterstain).

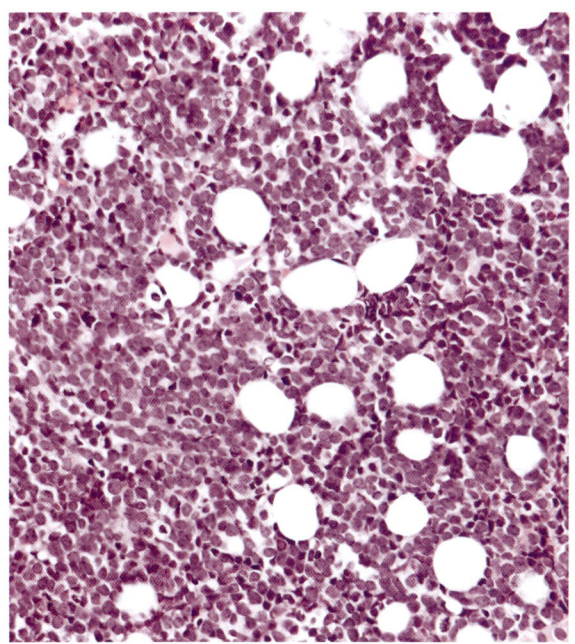

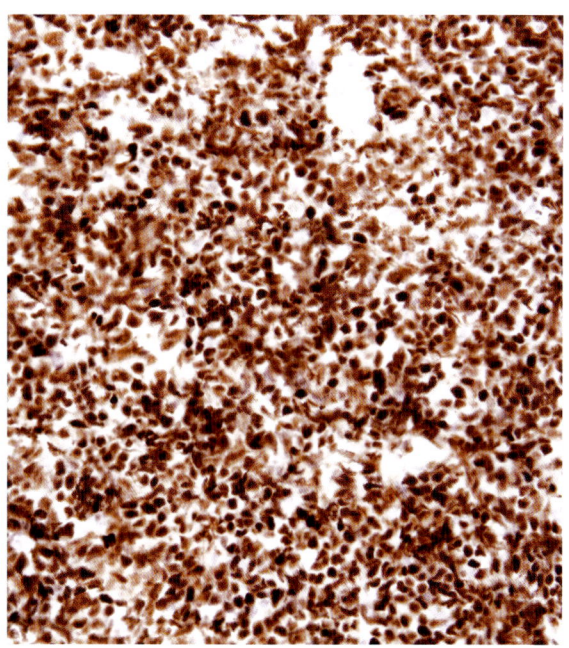

Figure 12-26

BLASTOID VARIANT OF MANTLE CELL LYMPHOMA WITH *MYC* TRANSLOCATION

Left: In this bone marrow specimen, the neoplastic cells had immature nuclear chromatin and a high mitotic rate, and resembled, in part, acute lymphoblastic leukemia. However, the neoplastic cells expressed cyclin D1 (not shown) and were associated with t(11;14)(q13;q32) and *MYC* translocation (H&E stain).

Right: The neoplastic cells are strongly positive for MYC (immunohistochemistry with hematoxylin counterstain).

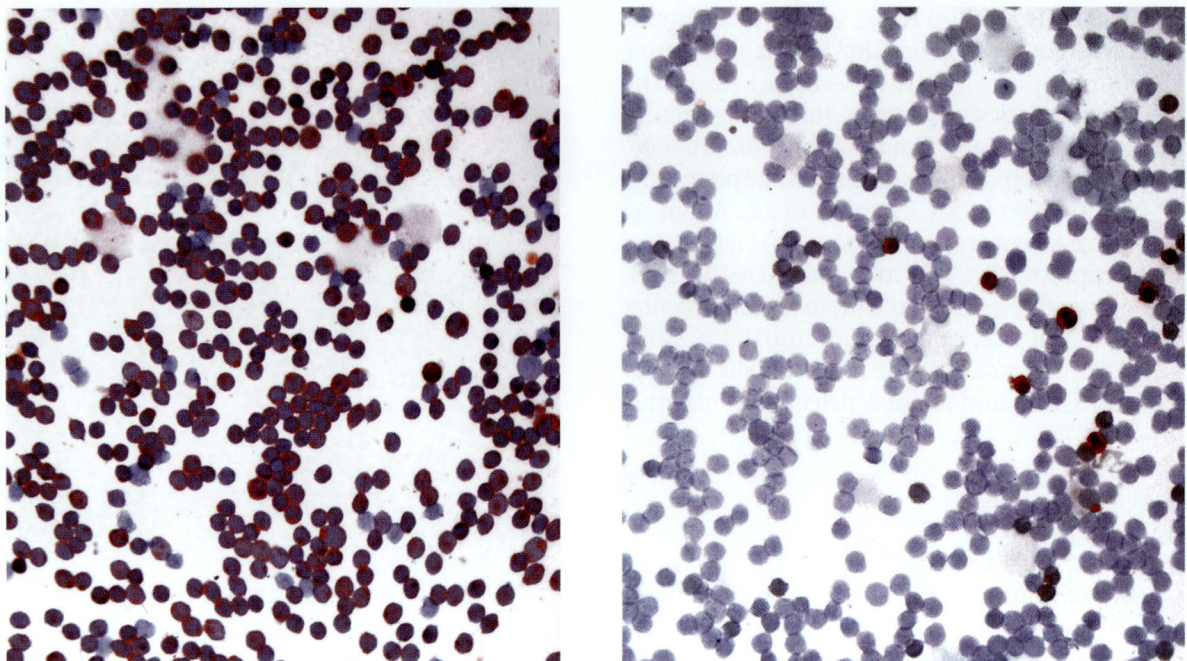

Figure 12-27

MANTLE CELL LYMPHOMA: LIGHT CHAINS ON SMEARS

Immunohistochemistry for lambda (left) and kappa (right) light chains in a case of MCL performed on a fine-needle aspiration cytology preparation (immunohistochemistry with hematoxylin counterstain).

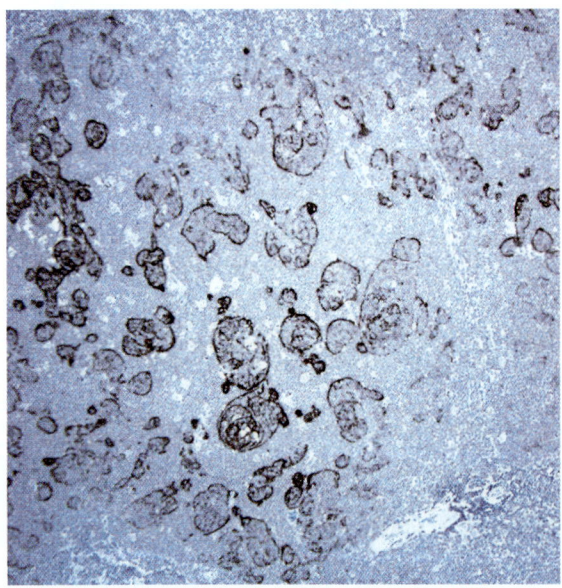

Figure 12-28

MANTLE CELL LYMPHOMA: CD21 IN NODULES

A case of MCL with a nodular pattern studied for CD21 by immunohistochemical analysis highlighted irregular networks of follicular dendritic cells (immunohistochemistry with hematoxylin counterstain).

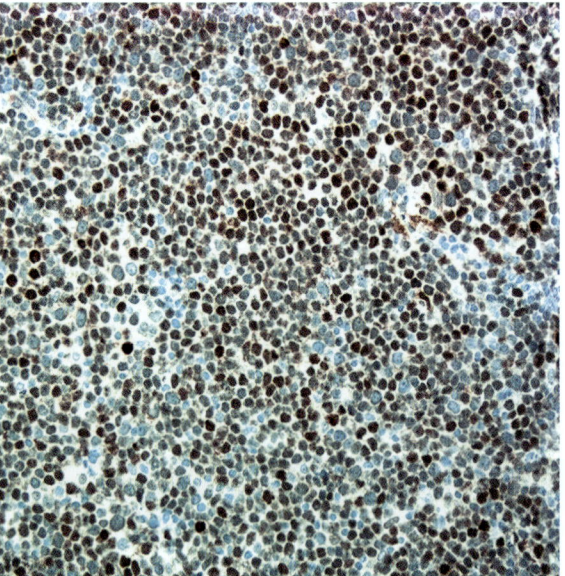

Figure 12-29

MANTLE CELL LYMPHOMA: BCL6

An immunostain for BCL6 shows weak reactivity in a case of blastoid MCL. Cases of blastoid and pleomorphic variant MCL express CD10 or BCL6 in a small subset of cases (immunohistochemistry with hematoxylin counterstain).

Table 12-1

DIFFERENTIAL DIAGNOSIS OF MANTLE CELL LYMPHOMA (MCL)

Differential Diagnosis	Similarities with MCL	Distinguishing Features
Chronic lymphocytic leukemia/small lymphocytic lymphoma (CLL/SLL)	Proliferation of small neoplastic cells CD5 expression	Prolymphocytes and paraimmunoblasts in CLL/SLL CD23 and CD200 expression in CLL/SLL Bright CD20, surface Ig and cyclin D1 expression in MCL t(11;14) in MCL
Follicular lymphoma (FL)	Nodular growth pattern	CD10/BCL6 expression in FL CD5/cyclin D1 expression in MCL t(11;14) in MCL
Marginal zone B-cell lymphoma (MZL)	Prominent monocytoid features in marginal zone-like MCL	Mixture of monocytoid B cells, large cells, and plasmacytoid cells in MZL CD5[a]/cyclin D1 expression in MCL t(11;14) in MCL
B-lymphoblastic lymphoma (B-LBL)	Blast-like features in blastoid MCL High mitotic rate in blastoid MCL	TdT[b] expression in B-LBL Surface Ig, CD5 and cyclin D1 expression in MCL t(11;14) in MCL
Burkitt lymphoma	Starry sky pattern in aggressive variants of MCL High mitotic rate in blastoid MCL	CD5, cyclin D1 and BCL2 expression in MCL t(11;14) in MCL
Diffuse large B-cell lymphoma (DLBCL)	Cytologic atypia and cell size in pleomorphic variant MCL	CD5, SOX11, and cyclin D1 in MCL[c] t(11;14) in MCL

[a]Marginal zone lymphoma can rarely express CD5.

[b]TdT = terminal deoxynucleotidyl transferase.

[c]DLBCL occasionally expresses CD5 and rare cases with cyclin D1 expression have been reported but co-expression of both markers is characteristic of MCL.

The pleomorphic variant of MCL can resemble diffuse large B-cell lymphoma (DLBCL). DLBCL is negative for CD5 and cyclin D1, unlike MCL, but a small subset of DLBCL cases expresses CD5 or cyclin D1, or rarely both. SOX11 is negative in DLBCL but usually positive in MCL. Most pathologists consider evidence of t(11;14) supportive of MCL over DLBCL, although this opinion is not universally held as Juskevicius et al. (21) reported a case of DLBCL that was negative for CD5 and SOX11 but carried t(11;14)(q13;q32).

Other Cyclin D1-Positive B-Cell Neoplasms. A number of B-cell neoplasms in addition to MCL express cyclin D1. These tumors include about 50 percent of hairy cell leukemias in which cyclin D1 is usually dim, about 30 percent of plasma cell myelomas (50,52), about 5 percent of DLBCLs, and rare cases of CLL/SLL in which dim cyclin D1 expression is observed within proliferation centers. The clinicopathologic features and immunophenotype of these tumors are usually distinctive and easily distinguished from MCL. Plasma cell myeloma with cyclin D1 expression is often associated with polysomy of chromosome 11 (50). The explanation for cyclin D1 expression in other lymphomas is not clear (29).

TREATMENT AND PROGNOSIS

The therapeutic approach to patients with MCL has undergone substantial evolution in recent years. Ten to 15 years ago, R-CHOP (rituximab, cyclophosphamide, hydroxydaunorubicin, vincristine, prednisone) chemotherapy was considered suboptimal treatment for patients with MCL. More aggressive chemotherapy regimens were used, including sequential R-CHOP/R-DHAP, dose-adjusted EPOCH-R, or R-HyperCVAD (39) with autologous stem cell transplantation in some patients (reviewed in reference 6). The recognition of the clinical heterogeneity of MCL, however, has led to a more tailored therapeutic approach (6,55). A number of other therapies are being evaluated based on the availability of therapeutic agents and the results of high-throughput studies of

MCL that have shown a number of potential targets (6). These agents include bendamustine, bortezomib, immunomodulatory agents (e.g., lenalidomide), BCL2 inhibitors (e.g., venetoclax), and mTOR inhibitors (e.g., temsirolimus). Bortezomib has been substituted for vincristine in the R-CHOP regimen, known as VR-CAP, with good response but increased toxicity (38). Two agents that appear to be very promising are idelalisib (a PI3Kδ inhibitor) and ibrutinib (a Bruton tyrosine kinase inhibitor) (22,56). For patients with clinically indolent MCL without symptoms observation may be employed.

Most MCL patients have a poor prognosis with a median survival period of 3 to 5 years (26,39,48,55). Overall survival in patients with high-risk MIPI scores is about half that of patients with low/intermediate-risk scores (26). Patients with the blastoid variant of MCL usually have an aggressive clinical course with shorter survival time (3a,48,49). Similarly, MCLs with high proliferative index (Ki-67) or a high proliferative signature defined by gene expression array analysis exhibit a very aggressive clinical course (49). There are patients who have more clinically indolent disease with a longer survival period (35); these patients often present primarily with non-nodal disease, sometimes with a leukemic picture or prominent splenomegaly (32,43).

REFERENCES

1. Banks PM, Chan J, Cleary ML, et al. Mantle cell lymphoma. A proposal for unification of morphologic, immunologic, and molecular data. Am J Surg Pathol 1992;16:637-640.
2. Bea S, Ribas M, Hernandez JM, et al. Increased number of chromosomal imbalances and high-level DNA amplifications in mantle cell lymphoma are associated with blastoid variants. Blood 1999;93:4365-4374.
3. Bea S, Valdés-Mas R, Navarro A, et al. Landscape of somatic mutations and clonal evolution in mantle cell lymphoma. Proc Natl Acad Sci U S A 2013;110:18250-18255.
3a. Bhatt VR, Loberiza FR Jr, Smith LM, et al. Clinicopathologic features, management and outcomes of blastoid variant of mantle cell lymphoma: a Nebraska Lymphoma Study Group Experience. Leuk Lymphoma 2016;57:1327-1334.
4. Bosch F, Lopez-Guillermo A, Campo E, et al. Mantle cell lymphoma: presenting features, response to therapy, and prognostic factors. Cancer 1998;82:567-575.
5. Caraway NP, Gu J, Lin P, Romaguera JE, Glassman A, Katz R. The utility of interphase fluorescence in situ hybridization for the detection of the translocation t(11;14)(q13;q32) in the diagnosis of mantle cell lymphoma on fine-needle aspiration specimens. Cancer 2005;105:110-118
6. Chen Y, Wang M, Romaguera J. Current regimens and novel agents for mantle cell lymphoma. Br J Haematol 2014;167:3-18.

7. Cohen PL, Kurtin PJ, Donovan KA, Hanson CA. Bone marrow and peripheral blood involvement in mantle cell lymphoma. Br J Haematol 1998;101:302-310.
8. Conconi A, Franceschetti S, Lobetti-Bodoni C, et al. Risk factors of central nervous system relapse in mantle cell lymphoma. Leuk Lymphoma 2013;54:1908-1914.
9. Determann O, Hoster E, Ott G, et al. Ki-67 predicts outcome in advanced-stage mantle cell lymphoma patients treated with anti-CD20 immunochemotherapy: results from randomized trials of the European MCL Network and the German Low Grade Lymphoma Study Group. Blood 2008;111:2385-2387.
10. Espinet B, Salaverria I, Bea S, et al. Incidence and prognostic impact of secondary cytogenetic aberrations in a series of 145 patients with mantle cell lymphoma. Genes Chromosomes Cancer 2010;49:439-451.
11. Ek S, Dictor M, Jerkeman M, Jirström K, Borrebaeck CA. Nuclear expression of the non B-cell lineage Sox11 transcription factor identifies mantle cell lymphoma. Blood 2008;111:800-805.
12. Fernandez V, Salamero O, Espinet B, et al. Genomic and gene expression profiling defines indolent forms of mantle cell lymphoma. Cancer Res 2010;70:1408-1418.
13. Fu K, Weisenburger DD, Greiner TC, et al. Cyclin D1-negative mantle cell lymphoma: a clinicopathologic study based on gene expression profiling. Blood 2005;106:4315-4321.

14. Garcia M, Romaguera JE, Inamdar KV, Rassidakis GZ, Medeiros LJ. Proliferation predicts failure-free survival in mantle cell lymphoma patients treated with rituximab plus hyperfractionated cyclophosphamide, vincristine, doxorubicin, and dexamethasone alternating with rituximab plus high-dose methotrexate and cytarabine. Cancer 2009;115:1041-1048.

15. Gesk S, Klapper W, Martin-Subero JI, et al. A chromosomal translocation in cyclin D1-negative/cyclin D2-positive mantle cell lymphoma fuses the CCND2 gene to the IGK locus. Blood 2006;108:1109-1110.

16. Halldorsdottir AM, Lundin A, Murray F, et al. Impact of TP53 mutation and 17p deletion in mantle cell lymphomas. Leukemia 2011;25:1904-1908.

17. Halldorsdottir AM, Sander B, Goransson H, et al. High-resolution genomic screening in mantle cell lymphoma—specific changes correlate with genomic complexity, the proliferation signature and survival. Genes Chromosomes Cancer 2011;50:113-121.

18. Hao S, Sanger W, Onciu M, Lai R, Schlette EJ, Medeiros LJ. Mantle cell lymphoma with 8q24 chromosomal abnormalities: a report of 5 cases with blastoid features. Mod Pathol 2002;15:1266-1272.

19. Hoster E, Rosenwald A, Berger F, et al. Prognostic value of Ki-67 index, cytology, and growth pattern in mantle-cell lymphoma: results from randomized trials of the European Mantle Cell Lymphoma Network. J Clin Oncol 2016;34:1386-1394.

20. Hsi ED, Jung SH, Lai R, et al. Ki67 and PIM1 expression predict outcome in mantle cell lymphoma treated with high dose therapy, stem cell transplantation and rituximab: a Cancer and Leukemia Group B 59909 correlative science study. Leuk Lymphoma 2008;49:2081-2090.

21. Juskevicius D, Ruiz C, Dirnhofer S, Tzankov A. Clinical, morphologic, phenotypic, and genetic evidence of cyclin D1-positive diffuse large B-cell lymphomas with CYCLIN D1 gene rearrangements. Am J Surg Pathol 2014;38:719-727.

22. Kahl BS, Spurgeon SE, Furman RR, et al. A phase 1 study of the PI3Kδ inhibitor idelalisib in patients with relapsed/refractory mantle cell lymphoma (MCL). Blood 2014;123:3398-3405.

23. Kang BW, Sohn SK, Moon JH, et al. Clinical features and treatment outcomes in patients with mantle cell lymphoma in Korea: study by the Consortium for Improving Survival of Lymphoma. Blood Res 2014;49:15-21.

24. Klapper W, Koch K, Mechler U, Borck C, Fuhry E, Siebert R. Lymphoma 'type K.'-in memory of Karl Lennert (1921-2012). Leukemia 2013;27:519-521.

25. Komatsu H, Yoshida K, Seto M, et al. Overexpression of PRAD1 in a mantle zone lymphoma patient with a t(11;22)(q13;q11) translocation. Br J Haematol 1993;85:427-429.

26. Leux C, Maynadie M, Troussard X, et al. Mantle cell lymphoma epidemiology: a population-based study in France. Ann Hematol 2014;93:1327-1333.

27. Medeiros LJ, Van Krieken JH, Jaffe ES, Raffeld M. Association of bcl-1 rearrangements with lymphocytic lymphoma of intermediate differentiation. Blood 1990;76:2086-2090.

28. Metcalf RA, Zhao S, Anderson MW, et al. Characterization of D-cyclin proteins in hematolymphoid neoplasms: lack of specificity of cyclin-D2 and D3 expression in lymphoma subtypes. Mod Pathol 2010;23:420-433.

29. Miranda RN, Briggs RC, Kinney MC, Veno PA, Hammer RD, Cousar JB. Immunohistochemical detection of cyclin D1 using optimized conditions is highly specific for mantle cell lymphoma and hairy cell leukemia. Mod Pathol 2000;13:1308-1314.

30. Mozos A, Royo C, Hartmann E, et al. SOX11 expression is highly specific for mantle cell lymphoma and identifies the cyclin D1-negative subtype. Haematologica 2009;94:1555-1562.

31. Navarro A, Clot G, Prieto M, et al. microRNA expression profiles identify subtypes of mantle cell lymphoma with different clinicobiological characteristics. Clin Cancer Res 2013;19:3121-3129.

32. Navarro A, Clot G, Royo C, et al. Molecular subsets of mantle cell lymphoma defined by the IGHV mutational status and SOX11 expression have distinct biologic and clinical features. Cancer Res 2012;72:5307-5316.

33. O'Malley DP, Lee JP, Bellizzi AM. Expression of LEF1 in mantle cell lymphoma. Ann Diagn Pathol 2017;26:57-59.

34. Onciu M, Schlette E, Medeiros LJ, Abruzzo LV, Keating M, Lai R. Cytogenetic findings in mantle cell lymphoma cases with a high level of peripheral blood involvement have a distinct pattern of abnormalities. Am J Clin Pathol 2001;116:886-892.

35. Ondrejka SL, Lai R, Smith SD, Hsi ED. Indolent mantle cell leukemia: clinicopathologic variant characterized by isolated lymphocytosis, interstitial bone marrow involvement, kappa light chain restriction, and good prognosis. Haematologica 2011;96:1121-1127.

36. Papathomas TG, Venizelos I, Dunphy CH, et al. Mantle cell lymphoma as a component of composite lymphoma: clinicopathologic parameters and biologic implications. Hum Pathol 2012;43:467-480.

37. Quintanilla-Martinez L, Slotta-Huspenina J, Koch I, et al. Differential diagnosis of cyclin D2+ mantle cell lymphoma based on fluorescence in situ hybridization and quantitative real-time-PCR. Haematologica 2009;94:1595-1598.

38. Robak T, Huang H, Jin J, et al. Bortezomib-based therapy for newly diagnosed mantle-cell lymphoma. N Engl J Med 2015;372:944-953.

39. Romaguera JE, Fayad L, Rodriguez MA, et al. High rate of durable remissions after treatment of newly diagnosed aggressive mantle-cell lymphoma with rituximab plus hyper-CVAD alternating with rituximab plus high-dose methotrexate and cytarabine. J Clin Oncol 2005;23:7013-7023. Erratum in J Clin Oncol 2006;24:724.

40. Romaguera JE, Medeiros LJ, Hagemeister FB, et al. Frequency of gastrointestinal involvement and its clinical significance in mantle cell lymphoma. Cancer 2003;97:586-591. Erratum in: Cancer 2003;97:3131.

41. Rosenberg CL, Wong E, Petty EM, et al. PRAD1, a candidate BCL1 oncogene: mapping and expression in centrocytic lymphoma. Proc Natl Acad Sci U S A 1991;88:9638-9642.

42. Rosenwald A, Wright G, Wiestner A, et al. The proliferation gene expression signature is a quantitative integrator of oncogenic events that predicts survival in mantle cell lymphoma. Cancer Cell 2003;3:185-197.

43. Royo C, Navarro A, Clot G, et al. Non-nodal type of mantle cell lymphoma is a specific biological and clinical subgroup of the disease. Leukemia 2012;26:1895-1898.

44. Rubio-Moscardo F, Climent J, Siebert R, et al. Mantle-cell lymphoma genotypes identified with CGH to BAC microarrays define a leukemic subgroup of disease and predict patient outcome. Blood 2005;105:4445-4454.

45. Salaverria I, Royo C, Carvajal-Cuenca A, et al. CCND2 rearrangements are the most frequent genetic events in cyclin D1(-) mantle cell lymphoma. Blood 2013;121:1394-1402.

46. Schlette E, Bueso-Ramos C, Giles F, Glassman A, Hayes K, Medeiros LJ. Mature B-cell leukemias with more than 55% prolymphocytes. A heterogeneous group that includes an unusual variant of mantle cell lymphoma. Am J Clin Pathol 2001;115:571-581.

47. Schlette E, Lai R, Onciu M, Doherty D, Bueso-Ramos C, Medeiros LJ. Leukemic mantle cell lymphoma: clinical and pathologic spectrum of twenty-three cases. Mod Pathol 2001;14:1133-1140.

48. Swerdlow SH, Campo E, Seto M, et al. Mantle cell lymphoma. In: Swerdlow SH, Campo E, Harris NL, et al., eds. WHO classification of tumours of haematopoietic and lymphoid tissues. Lyon: IARC Press; 2008:229-232.

49. Tiemann M, Schrader C, Klapper W, et al. Histopathology, cell proliferation indices and clinical outcome in 304 patients with mantle cell lymphoma (MCL): a clinicopathological study from the European MCL Network. Br J Haematol 2005;131:29-38.

50. Troussard X, Avet-Loiseau H, Macro M, et al. Cyclin D1 expression in patients with multiple myeloma. Hematol J 2000;1:181-185.

51. Vaandrager JW, Schuuring E, Zwikstra E, et al. Direct visualization of dispersed 11q13 chromosomal translocations in mantle cell lymphoma by multicolor DNA fiber fluorescence in situ hybridization. Blood 1996;88:1177-1182.

52. Vasef MA, Medeiros LJ, Yospur LS, Sun NC, McCourty A, Brynes RK. Cyclin D1 protein in multiple myeloma and plasmacytoma: an immunohistochemical study using fixed, paraffin-embedded tissue sections. Mod Pathol 1997;10:927-932.

53. Vegliante MC, Palomero J, Pérez-Galán P, et al. SOX11 regulates PAX5 expression and blocks terminal B-cell differentiation in aggressive mantle cell lymphoma. Blood 2013;121:2175-2185.

54. Von Hohenstaufen KA, Conconi A, de Campos CP, et al. Prognostic impact of monocyte count at presentation in mantle cell lymphoma. Br J Haematol 2013;162:465-473.

55. Vose JM. Mantle cell lymphoma: 2017 update on diagnosis, risk-stratification, and clinical management. Am J Hematol 2017;92:806-813.

56. Wang ML, Rule S, Martin P, et al. Targeting BTK with ibrutinib in relapsed or refractory mantle-cell lymphoma. N Engl J Med 2013;369:507-516.

57. Wasman J, Rosenthal NS, Farhi DC. Mantle cell lymphoma. Morphologic findings in bone marrow involvement. Am J Clin Pathol 1996;106:196-200.

58. Williams ME, Westermann CD, Swerdlow SH. Genotypic characterization of centrocytic lymphoma: frequent rearrangement of the chromosome 11 bcl-1 locus. Blood 1990;76:1387-1391.

59. Wlodarska I, Dierickx D, Vanhentenrijk V, et al. Translocations targeting CCND2, CCND3, and MYCN do occur in t(11;14)-negative mantle cell lymphomas. Blood 2008;111:5683-5690.

59a. Wu C, de Miranda NF, Chen L, et al. Genetic heterogeneity in primary and relapsed mantle cell lymphomas: Impact of recurrent CARD11 mutations. Oncotarget 2016;7:38180-38190.

60. Yin CC, Medeiros LJ, Cromwell CC, et al. Sequence analysis proves clonal identity in five patients with typical and blastoid mantle cell lymphoma. Mod Pathol 2007;20:1-7.

61. Young KH, Chan WC, Fu K, et al. Mantle cell lymphoma with plasma cell differentiation. Am J Surg Pathol 2006;30:954-961.

62. Zhang J, Jima, D, Moffitt AB, et al. The genomic landscape of mantle cell lymphoma is related to the epigenetically determined chromatin state of normal B cells. Blood 2014;123:2988-2996.

63. Zhou DM, Chen G, Zheng XW, Zhu WF, Chen BZ. Clinicopathologic features of 112 cases with mantle cell lymphoma. Cancer Biol Med 2015;12:46-52.

13 FOLLICULAR LYMPHOMA

GENERAL FEATURES

Follicular lymphoma (FL) is a neoplasm derived from follicle (germinal) center B cells, centrocytes, and centroblasts, present in varying proportions. Although a follicular pattern is characteristic of these neoplasms, coexistent diffuse areas are common, and rare cases have an entirely diffuse pattern (22).

FL was one of the first types of non-Hodgkin lymphoma to be recognized because of its follicular pattern and because the cytologic features resemble its normal counterpart, reactive follicles in lymph node. Older designations for FL include *Brill-Symmers disease* (named after authors of early papers describing FL), *nodular lymphoma* (Rappaport classification), *centroblastic/centrocytic lymphoma* (Kiel classification), and *follicular center lymphoma* (REAL classification) (see chapter 4). In excisional lymph node biopsy specimens, the diagnosis is often easy to establish because numerous tumor follicles replace the lymph node architecture. As a result, the importance of the pattern in FL is easy to overemphasize, but it is the cytologic composition of FL that is essential to its diagnosis, particularly in small biopsy specimens. It is helpful to remember the designation centroblastic/centrocytic lymphoma used for FL in the Kiel classification.

Although FL is one of the most common types of non-Hodgkin lymphoma in the United States and Europe, it is uncommon in Asia and underdeveloped nations (4,6,52). The age-standardized incidence rate for FL is 2 to 3 per 100,000 person-years in Western nations (47,67). In the United States, FL represents approximately 20 percent of all cases of non-Hodgkin lymphoma and is second only to diffuse large B-cell lymphoma (4,22,52). About 80 percent of all cases of FL are systemic nodal tumors that occur in adults, and most are associated with t(14;18)(q32;q21)/*IGH-BCL2*. This group of tumors is the major focus of this chapter. In recent years, small subsets of tumors designated as FL

have been recognized that differ from common FL in terms of clinical presentation, molecular findings, and pathogenesis. These FL subsets are discussed separately in this chapter.

The etiology of FL is unknown. The International Lymphoma Epidemiology Consortium (InterLymph) has identified a number of factors that likely influence the incidence of FL. Factors that increase the risk of FL include a first-degree family history of non-Hodgkin lymphoma, high body mass index as a young adult, and employment as a spray painter (12). In women, cigarette smoking and Sjögren syndrome also are associated with an increased risk of FL. Factors associated with a lower risk of FL include atopic disorders; prior blood transfusion; sun exposure; employment as a baker, miller, or teacher; and in women, alcohol consumption (12). Education level and height also have correlated positively with the presence of t(14;18)(q32;q21)/*IGH-BCL2*, suggesting that lifestyle factors may be involved in the incidence of FL.

Role of t(14;18)(q32;q21)/*IGH-BCL2* in Pathogenesis

t(14;18)(q32;21), which juxtaposes *BCL2* with the enhancer region of *IGH* on the derivative chromosome 14, is an early event in FL pathogenesis and is thought to be a founder genetic abnormality (63,74). The likely sequence of events has been reviewed by others and is only briefly summarized here (63).

t(14;18)(q32;q21)/*IGH-BCL2* is thought to result from a mistake in the physiologic recombinase-mediated V-D-J rearrangement that occurs in B-cell precursors of the bone marrow. The juxtaposition of *BCL2* adjacent to the *IGH* promoter leads to inappropriate expression of BCL2, an anti-apoptotic protein. B cells with t(14;18)/*IGH-BCL2* circulate in the blood and are able to enter, proliferate within, and exit germinal centers of secondary lymphoid organs, particularly lymph nodes

(63,74). Overexpression of BCL2 is thought to provide the cell with a survival advantage, allowing the cell to escape apoptosis in germinal centers. While in the germinal centers, the B cells carrying t(14;18)/*IGH-BCL2* come under the influence of activation-induced cytosine deaminase (AID), which is responsible for physiologic somatic hypermutation and class switch recombination, allowing opportunities for the development of additional mistakes that can result in adverse gene mutations (63,74). The sum of these events is thought to eventually lead to overt FL. In addition, this sequence of events indicates that the presence of t(14;18)/*IGH-BCL2* in the blood of apparently healthy persons is a molecular biomarker and risk factor for the subsequent development of FL, although the interval from detection to onset of FL is usually very long.

CLINICAL FEATURES

The median age of patients with FL is the sixth decade (22,52,66). FL is more common in women, with a male to female ratio of 1.0 to 1.7 (52). B-type symptoms occur in 10 to 20 percent of patients and most patients have nonbulky disease.

At time of initial diagnosis, most patients with FL have disseminated disease with involvement of peripheral or visceral lymph nodes (22,66). Mesenteric lymph nodes, uncommonly involved by other types of low-grade B-cell lymphoma, are commonly involved in patients with FL. The spleen and liver are involved in 50 to 60 percent and 50 percent of patients, with FL respectively. Bone marrow involvement occurs in about 40 percent of patients (22,52). Approximately 80 percent of FL patients present with advanced-stage disease (Ann Arbor stage III or IV) and 20 percent have localized disease (Ann Arbor stage I or II) (52).

Overall, laboratory abnormalities are uncommon in patients with FL. Anemia occurs in 10 to 15 percent of patients; leukopenia or thrombocytopenia are less common. A small subset (less than 5 percent) of FL patients present in a leukemic phase, with lymphocytosis; this is associated with a poor prognosis (68). Serum lactate dehydrogenase (LDH) or beta-2-microglobulin levels are elevated in about 15 percent of patients, usually not markedly so.

Recent studies have identified additional laboratory tests that correlate with prognosis. Mir et al. (46) reported that elevated serum levels of interleukin-2 receptor (IL-2R), IL-1RA, and CXCL9 are associated with poorer event-free survival. Others have reported that an elevated absolute monocyte count (over 0.63 x 10⁹/L) predicts a poorer prognosis (44).

For the purpose of prognostication, the International Prognostic Index (IPI), as used for patients with diffuse large B-cell lymphoma, has been modified for patients with FL and is known as the Follicular Lymphoma International Prognostic Index (FLIPI). This index combines clinical and laboratory abnormalities and is discussed in more detail in the section on prognosis (see below).

Patients with FL can undergo histologic transformation to a clinically aggressive, higher-grade lymphoma, usually diffuse large B-cell lymphoma (see chapter 5). The risk of transformation is 2 to 3 percent per year. The clinical features associated with histologic transformation include new onset of B-type symptoms, high serum LDH level, hypercalcemia, rapid growth of lymph nodes, and new onset of extranodal sites of disease. High standardized uptake values (SUV) using [18^F] fluorodeoxyglucose positron emission tomography (FDG-PET) can be helpful for predicting histologic transformation.

HISTOLOGIC FINDINGS

Lymph Nodes

The lymph node architecture is partially or completely effaced by lymphoma with a follicular (or nodular) pattern (22,49). The neoplastic follicles are numerous and may be somewhat spaced out, but more often are crowded together in a back-to-back distribution (figs. 13-1–13-3). Neoplastic follicles tend to be round and uniform (unlike reactive follicles) and may be either sharply defined or vague. Commonly, lymphoma cells are also present between the follicles (interfollicular areas), further contributing to the poor circumscription of neoplastic follicles. In some cases, the follicles are partially surrounded by residual mantle zones (fig. 13-4). When involvement is extensive, the lymphoma may obliterate trabecular and medullary sinuses. Follicles also can extend outside the lymph node capsule into perinodal adipose tissue (fig. 13-5).

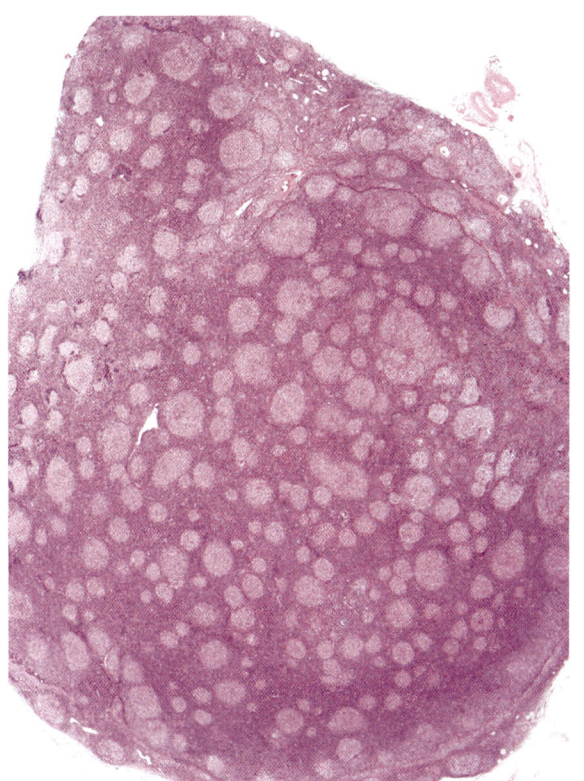 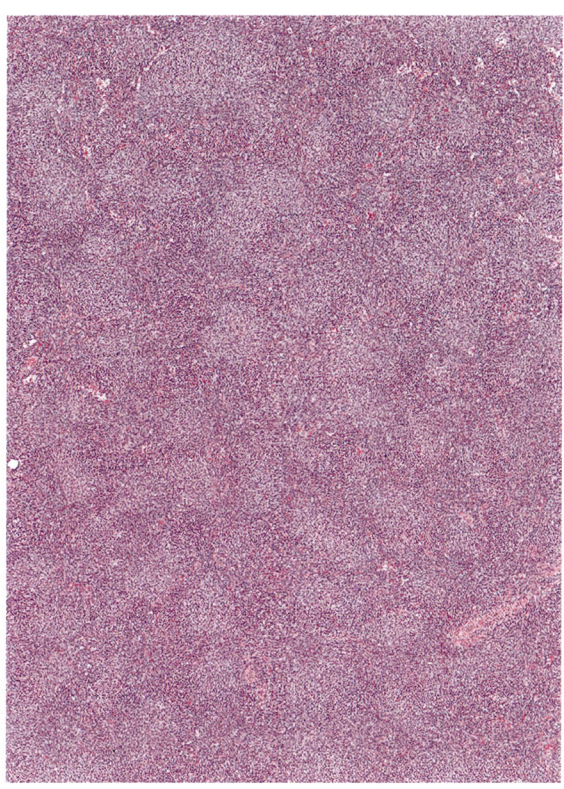

Figure 13-1

FOLLICULAR LYMPHOMA (FL) INVOLVING LYMPH NODE

Left: The neoplastic follicles are well defined, round, of similar size, and randomly distributed in the cortex and medulla of the lymph node. Unlike many cases of FL, the follicles are not back-to-back.

Right: In this case, the borders of the follicles are vague and not sharply defined. There is also less space between the follicles although they are not arranged in a back-to-back fashion (hematoxylin and eosin [H&E] stain).

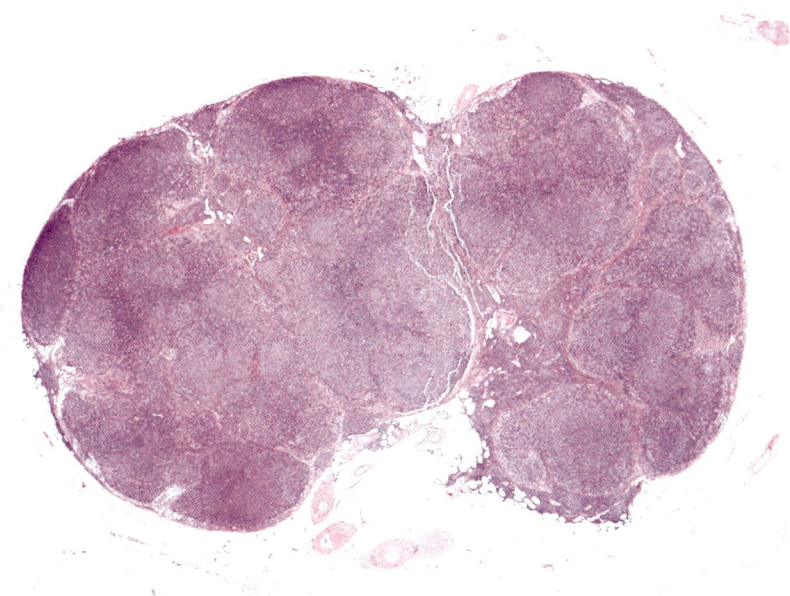

Figure 13-2

FOLLICULAR LYMPHOMA: BACK-TO-BACK FOLLICLES

In this lymph node, the neoplastic follicles are larger and arranged in a back-to-back fashion in some areas, replacing lymph node parenchyma (H&E stain).

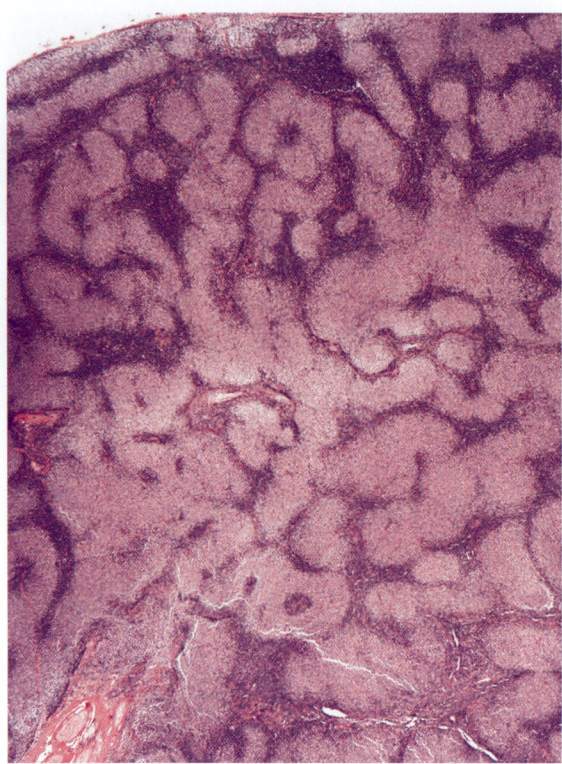

Figure 13-3

FOLLICULAR LYMPHOMA INVOLVING LYMPH NODE: LARGE FOLLICLES

In this case of FL most of the lymph node architecture is replaced by large follicles with serpiginous shapes (H&E stain).

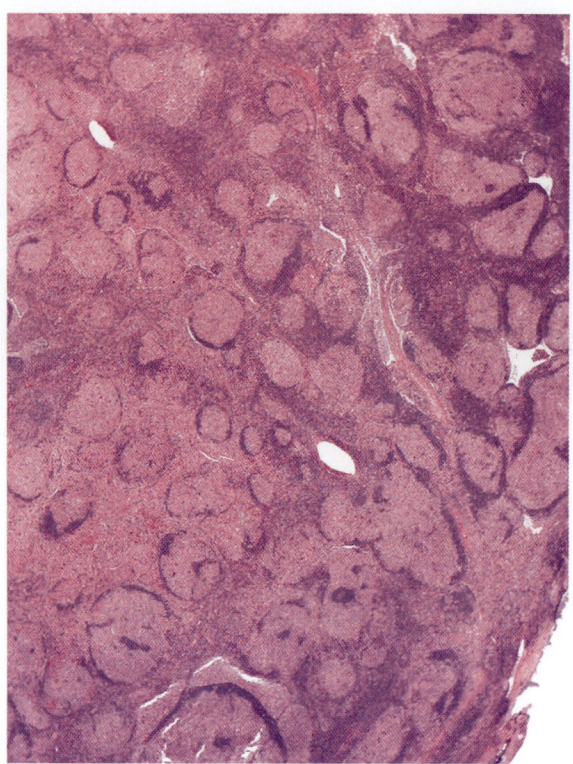

Figure 13-4

FOLLICULAR LYMPHOMA INVOLVING LYMPH NODE

The FL extensively replaces the lymph node. In this case the follicles are partially surrounded by residual mantle zones (H&E stain).

In some cases, neoplastic follicles are large and merge with neighboring follicles to yield confluent neoplastic follicles that may form geographic patterns or small diffuse areas.

Some cases of FL have unusual associated findings. Sclerosis may be prominent in lymph nodes involved by FL. The sclerosis is located within the neoplastic follicles, often associated with blood vessels (fig. 13-6, left), or is present as dense collagenous bands that surround the follicles (fig. 13-6, right). There may be a Lennert-like epithelioid histiocytic reaction (fig. 13-7). In rare cases of FL, the follicles are small and show regressive changes, sharing some features with the follicles observed in the hyaline-vascular variant of Castleman disease (fig. 13-8).

FLs are typically composed of centrocytes (small and large cleaved B cells) and larger centroblasts (large noncleaved B cells) (22,49). Centrocytes are small or medium-sized cells (large centrocytes) and have cleaved nuclei, inconspicuous nucleoli, and scant cytoplasm. Centroblasts are approximately 2 to 3 times the size of a mature lymphocyte nucleus. Centroblasts are characterized by vesicular chromatin with 1 to 3 small nucleoli, often situated near the nuclear membrane. In FL, centrocytes or centroblasts may predominate, or these cell types may be mixed. A few FL cases show plasmacytic differentiation with a component (usually small) of monotypic plasma cells or Dutcher bodies in centrocytes and centroblasts. In low-grade FL, the mitotic rate is usually low, but in high-grade FL the mitotic rate may be moderate or brisk.

The follicles of FL also contain many reactive T cells, follicular dendritic cells, and histiocytes, but tingible body macrophages are usually few and a starry sky appearance is absent. Other types of inflammatory cells, such as granulocytes or plasma cells, are usually rare.

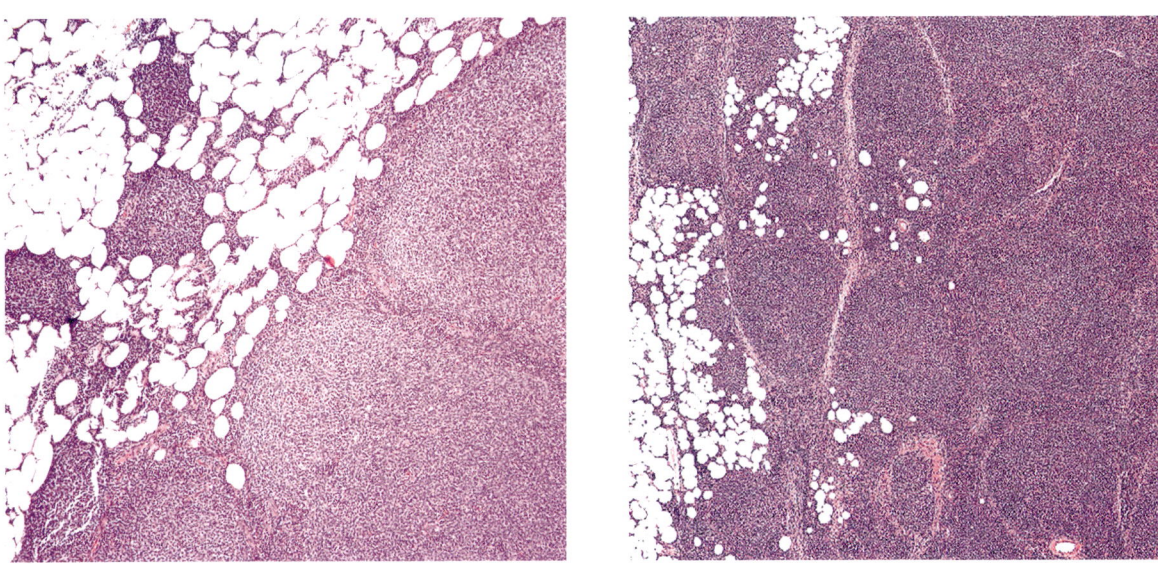

Figure 13-5

FOLLICULAR LYMPHOMA INVOLVING LYMPH NODE AND PERINODAL ADIPOSE TISSUE

Left: Small tumor follicles are present in the adipose tissue (left side of field), with the lymph node also shown (right side of field) (left, right: H&E stain).

Right: In a different case, there is more extensive involvement of perinodal adipose tissue (left of field) by FL.

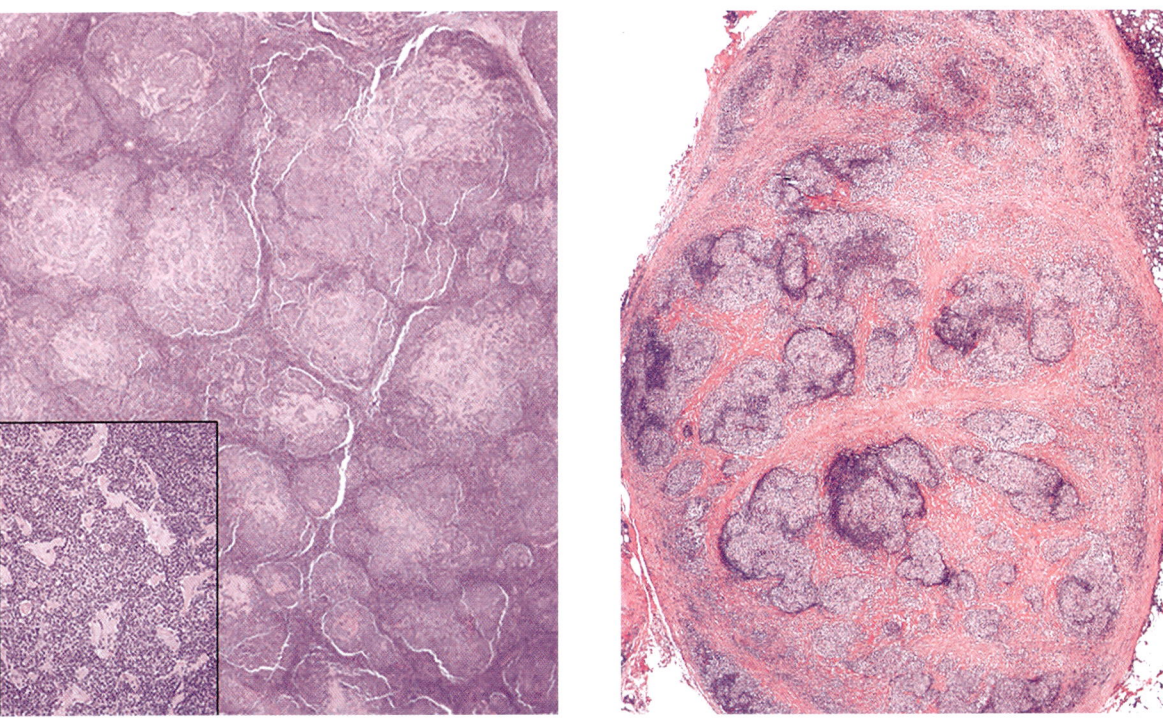

Figure 13-6

FOLLICULAR LYMPHOMA WITH EXTENSIVE SCLEROSIS INVOLVING LYMPH NODE

Left: Within the large tumor follicles, eosinophilic sclerosis is appreciated. Inset. At higher magnification, the sclerosis is predominantly associated with blood vessels in the follicles (left, right: H&E stain).

Right: Another case of FL in which sclerosis is present as broad, collagenous bands that surround follicles.

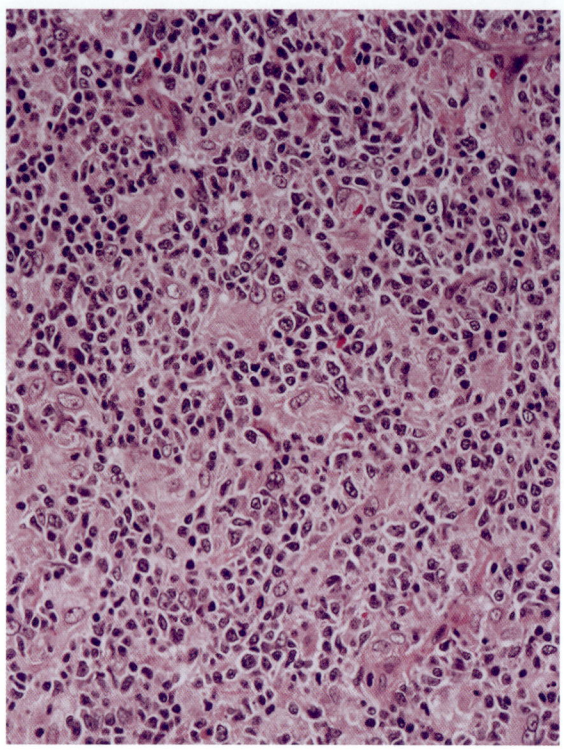

Figure 13-7

**FOLLICULAR LYMPHOMA
WITH EPITHELIOID HISTIOCYTES**

In this FL case there were numerous epithelioid histiocytes. High magnification of one follicle is shown (H&E stain).

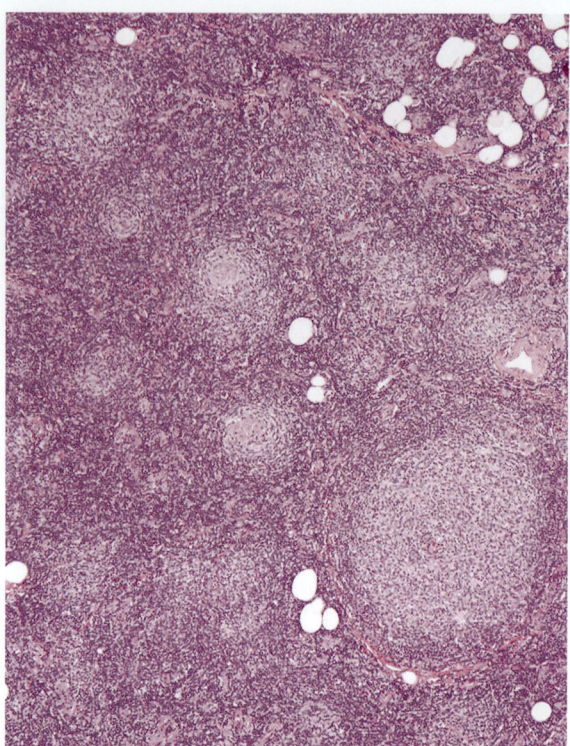

Figure 13-8

FOLLICULAR LYMPHOMA: CASTLEMAN-LIKE CHANGES

Some of the neoplastic follicles are small and exhibit regressive changes as is seen in the hyaline-vascular variant of Castleman disease. A larger, more typical neoplastic follicle is also present in this field (H&E stain).

Grading

Currently, there is no optimal grading system for FL. There is wide consensus in the literature that cases of FL show a spectrum of cytologic findings or grades, from neoplasms that are composed mostly of centrocytes with a low mitotic rate (low grade) to neoplasms with many centroblasts and an elevated mitotic rate (high grade). There is also agreement that high histologic grade correlates with aggressive clinical behavior and a higher likelihood for progression to diffuse large B-cell lymphoma.

Several approaches have been undertaken to grade FL in the past; all have utilized the proportion of centroblasts as a key grading index. The World Health Organization (WHO) adopted the system proposed initially by Risa Mann and Costan Berard in 1983, in which the number of centroblasts in 10 representative neoplastic follicles are counted and expressed per high-power

(400x) power field (hpf) (42). Cases with 0 to 5 centroblasts/hpf are classified as grade 1 (fig. 13-9), 6 to 15 are classified as grade 2, and over 15 as grade 3.

This system, however, has undergone substantial modifications for current use. First, microscopes have changed substantially since 1983. In particular, field of view oculars are often larger on current day microscopes. In the WHO classification, a correction factor is suggested (22). For microscopes with a 20-mm field of view ocular, the WHO suggests counting 8 hpfs and dividing by 10. For microscopes with a 22-mm field of view ocular, the WHO suggests counting 7 hpfs and dividing by 10 or counting 10 hpfs and dividing by 15. Also, it is recommended that low-grade cases of FL be reported as grade 1 to 2 because there is no clear difference in prognosis for patients with FL who have grade 1 versus

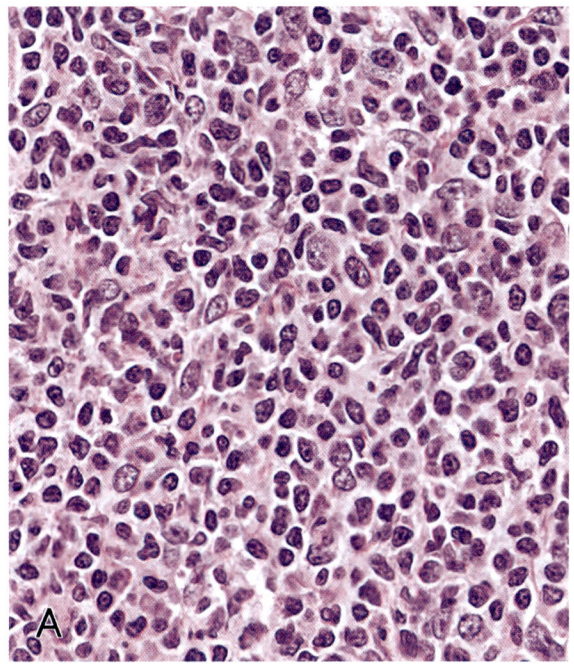

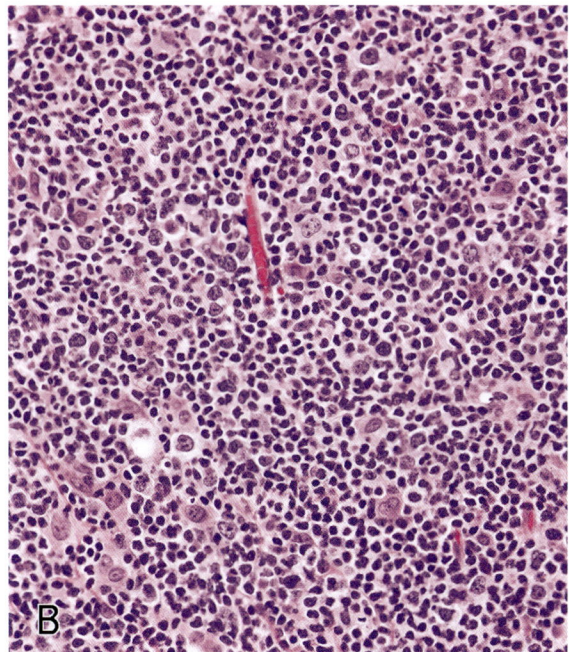

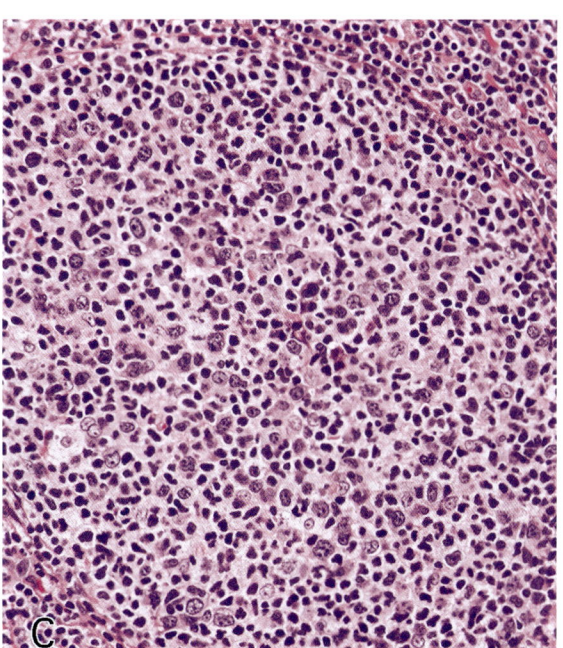

Figure 13-9

GRADES OF FOLLICULAR LYMPHOMA

Examples of different grades of FL involving lymph node: grades 1 (A), 2 (B), and 3A (C) (A–C: H&E stain).

grade 2 neoplasms. Lastly, the grade 3 category is split into 3A and 3B. Grade 3A neoplasms contain a mixture of centrocytes and centroblasts (fig. 13-9C) whereas grade 3B cases do not have, or have very few, centrocytes (22).

The current grading system has limitations that result in suboptimal reproducibility, for which there are a number of possible explana-

tions. First, a lymph node biopsy specimen involved by FL usually contains many more follicles than can be assessed by the examination of 10 hpfs. Therefore, sampling bias is a likely factor affecting reproducibility. Secondly, in FL the follicles often show a range in their cytologic composition and a mixture of grades 1, 2, and 3A follicles may coexist. It is unclear whether

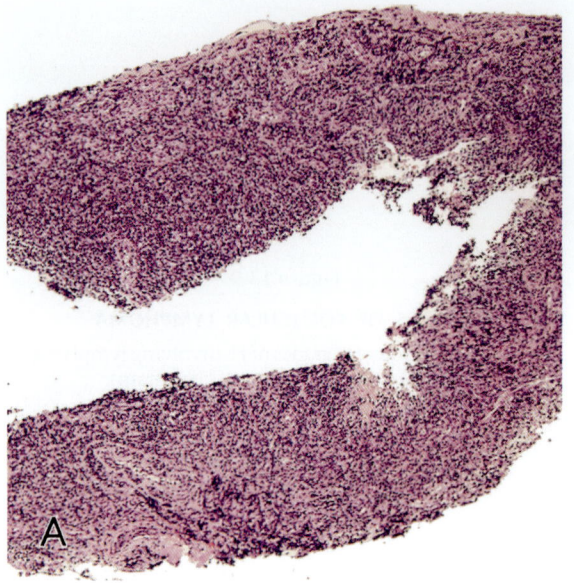

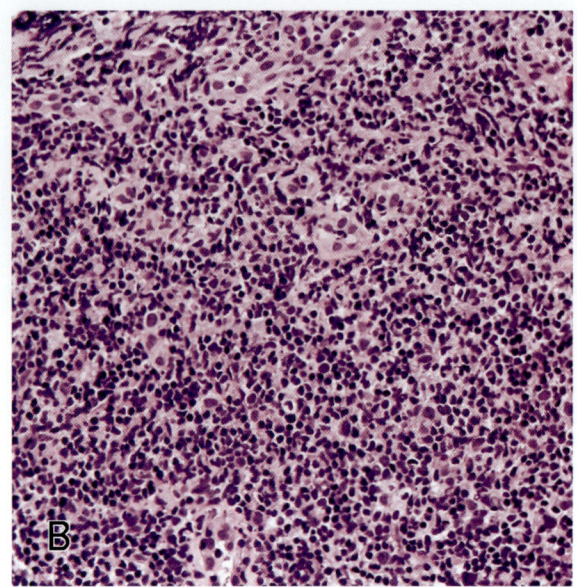

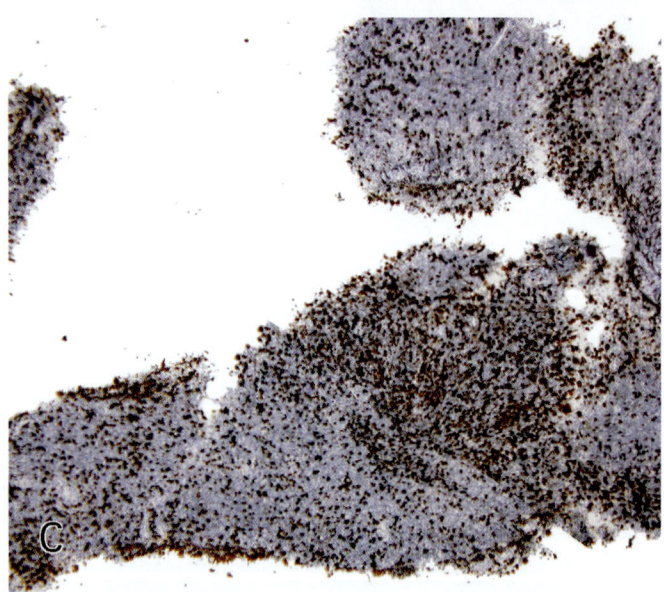

Figure 13-10

LOW-GRADE FOLLICULAR LYMPHOMA WITH HIGH KI-67

A,B: At both low and higher magnification the neoplasm is composed predominantly of centrocytes, with fewer centroblasts, supporting a low grade (H&E stain).

C: Ki-67 is highly expressed in one area of the neoplasm (corresponding to field shown in B), more in keeping with a high-grade neoplasm (immunohistochemistry with hematoxylin counterstain).

an observer should designate the grade based on the predominant follicles or the highest grade follicles. Lastly, the grading system implies that counting is performed in a rigorous fashion; however, not all observers share the same degree of enthusiasm for counting and some (if not many) pathologists estimate or "ballpark" the centroblast count.

Another limitation of the current grading system is the emphasis on counting centroblasts to the exclusion of other findings that correlate with clinical aggressiveness and therefore could be included as high-grade criteria. Cases of FL

composed predominantly of large centrocytes have been shown to behave aggressively (16), but centrocytes are not accounted for using the current grading system. In addition, some of FLs have a number of centroblasts, supporting grade 1 or 2, but the proliferation rate may be very high, more in keeping with grade 3 FL (fig. 13-10). In one study, Wang et al. (80) showed that about 20 percent of low-grade FLs have a high proliferation (Ki-67) rate and may behave more aggressively, more in keeping with grade 3 FL. Rarely, cases of FL are composed predominantly of small centrocytes and yet the nuclei are

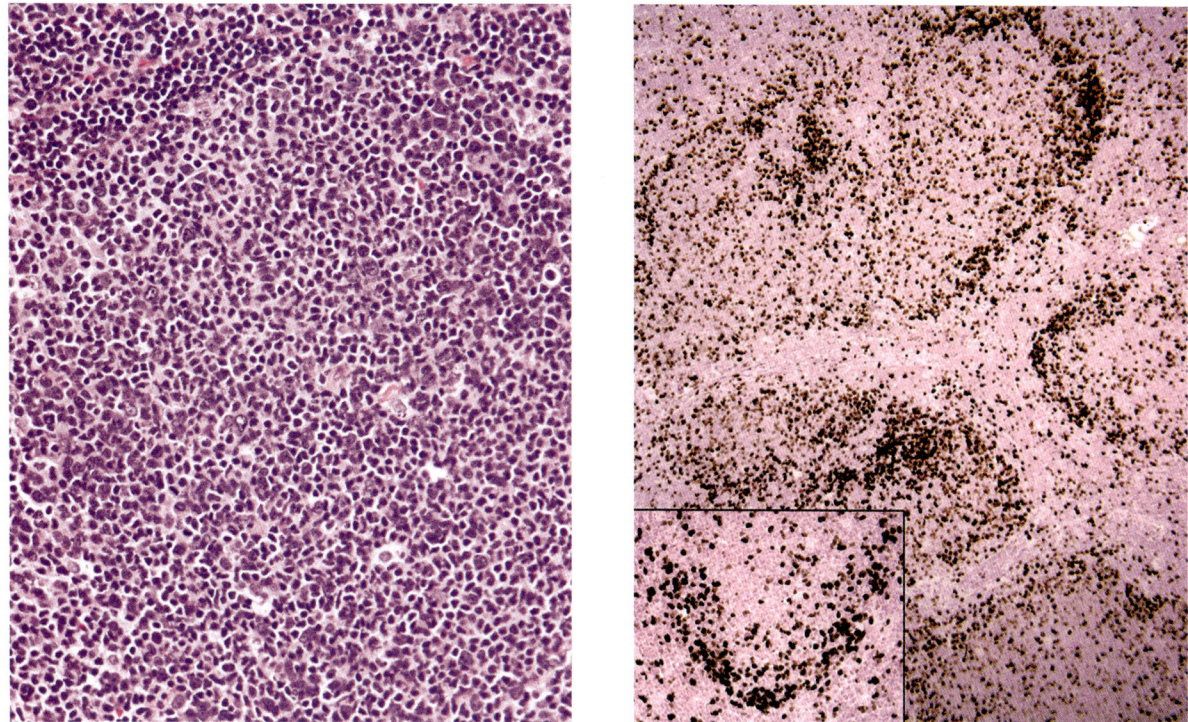

Figure 13-11

LOW-GRADE FOLLICULAR LYMPHOMA WITH POLARIZED FOLLICLES

Left: This follicle shows polarization. The light and dark zones are appreciated (H&E stain).

Right: Ki-67 expression in this case highlights the polarization in many follicles, with the cells in the dark zones being more highly proliferative than the cells in the light zones. Inset: one polarized follicle at high magnification (immunohistochemistry with hematoxylin counterstain).

highly immature or blastoid, so-called blastoid FL (50). It seems reasonable to suggest that the grading system of FL be expanded to include at least some of these other findings. It also may be time to consider image analysis for the counting of centroblasts as a part of the routine grading of FL cases.

Role for Ki-67 in Grading? The grading system currently recommended in the WHO classification does not incorporate Ki-67 results. Nevertheless, we believe the proliferation rate as assessed by Ki-67 can be helpful. For small biopsy specimens in which the FL cells are not well preserved and cell size is difficult to appreciate, reactivity for Ki-67 helps one discern the number of centroblasts more reliably. For cases in which the grade of FL is borderline, for example grade 2 versus grade 3A, a high Ki-67 result supports a higher-grade neoplasm.

There are also limitations to using Ki-67 to grade FL. In a some cases, Ki-67 results are not uniform throughout the neoplasm and therefore sampling bias is possible. In other cases, the follicles have a brisk proliferation rate while interfollicular regions involved by lymphoma have a very low Ki-67 rate. Should only the follicles be assessed or should an overall average value for Ki-67 be provided? If the interfollicular areas are much more numerous than the follicles, we try to estimate an average for the entire neoplasm; however, we only assess the follicles if they are predominant. (We acknowledge we have no data to support this approach.)

Another potential issue in cases of FL occurs when the neoplastic follicles are well polarized: the dark zone equivalents of the follicles have a much higher rate proliferation than the light zones (fig. 13-11). In some follicles, due to the level of the cut, only the dark zone of the neoplastic follicle appears in the tissue section; this finding should not be over interpreted as a neoplastic follicle with a high proliferation rate.

Reporting of Pattern and Coexistence of Diffuse Large B-cell Lymphoma (DLBCL). The WHO classification recommends reporting the pattern of FL cases as follows: follicular (over 75 percent), follicular and diffuse (25 to 75 percent), focally follicular (less than 25 percent), and diffuse (no follicular areas) (22). For patients with low-grade FL, the tumor pattern does not have prognostic importance. The WHO classification therefore accepts low-grade FL with an entirely diffuse pattern. However, since FL with an entirely diffuse pattern is rare, the WHO classification emphasizes that sampling issues may be involved, particularly in the era of needle biopsy, for the diagnosis of lymphoma (22).

The situation is different for cases of FL with a partial diffuse pattern composed of large cells. The WHO classification recommends that any area of diffuse pattern composed of 15 or more centroblasts/hpf should be reported as DLBCL (22). For example, a case of grade 3 FL in which 80 percent of the tumor has a follicular pattern and 20 percent a diffuse pattern should be designated as FL, grade 3, follicular pattern (80 percent) and DLBCL (20 percent). This approach is supported by data that show a diffuse pattern predicts poorer outcome (21). In addition, the presence of a component of DLBCL is useful for guiding the clinician in planning therapy. This approach should not be misinterpreted as the presence of two tumors (or composite lymphoma).

Although the above recommendations are generally useful, it seems reasonable to be judicious in the designation of areas of DLBCL in cases of FL. Any area of grade 3B with a diffuse pattern, even if small (e.g., about 10 percent), is best designated as DLBCL, but we have some reservations about a small area of grade 3A tumor being designated as DLBCL. Cases of FL usually show a spectrum of findings, often with a mixture of low-grade and grade 3A follicles and small diffuse areas. It is important not to "overcall" the presence DLBCL when the diffuse area is grade 3A and the overall findings are those of a low-grade neoplasm, especially if the clinical findings also fit with low-grade FL.

Grade 3B FL. As mentioned above, grade 3B FL is defined as a neoplasm with a purely follicular pattern that is composed of centroblasts without any (or at least very few) centrocytes (fig. 13-12). Some have suggested that grade 3B FL is better considered a follicular variant of DLBCL (7,25,58). This view is justified by the fact that patients with grade 3B FL often have aggressive disease that can involve nodal or extranodal sites, similar to DLBCL. In addition, following therapy there is a plateau of survival in patients with FL grade 3B, more in keeping with DLBCL and unlike other grades of FL (79). Other findings in grade 3B FL that are more similar to DLBCL include common positivity for MUM1/IRF4, a low frequency of CD10 and BCL2 expression, and a low frequency of t(14;18)(q32;q21)/*IGH-BCL2* (25,30,58). Grade 3B FLs express BCL6 and other germinal center B-cell associated markers (e.g., LMO2).

Morphologic Variants of Follicular Lymphoma

In Situ Follicular Neoplasia. In this lesion, the lymph node architecture is normal and follicles are of normal size, with an appearance that can be difficult to distinguish from normal follicles. Immunohistochemical analysis, however, shows that the follicles are composed of germinal center B cells that are positive for CD10 and BCL2 (see chapter 6).

Partial Involvement by Follicular Lymphoma. In some lymph node biopsy specimens, morphologically enlarged and abnormal tumor follicles are interspersed with reactive follicles and the lymph node architecture is partially preserved (fig. 13-13). The neoplastic follicles resemble those observed in typical cases of FL. In one large study of FL cases, about 10 percent of biopsy specimens showed partial involvement and this finding correlated with low-stage disease (2). This pattern of partial involvement also is associated with a simpler karyotype, fewer gene mutations, and a better prognosis (22).

Floral Variant. This variant was first described by Osborne and Butler in 1987 (56). The neoplastic follicles are irregular in shape and are surrounded by prominent mantle zones that penetrate into the center of the follicles (33,56). The darker mantle zones outline paler neoplastic follicle centers, imparting a lobular shape and resembling the petals of a flower, hence, the moniker floral variant (fig. 13-14). Most FLs that exhibit floral variant morphology are grade 3 neoplasms (20). These neoplasms have an immunophenotype that supports the diagnosis of FL and express monotypic surface immunoglobulin; some are CD5 positive

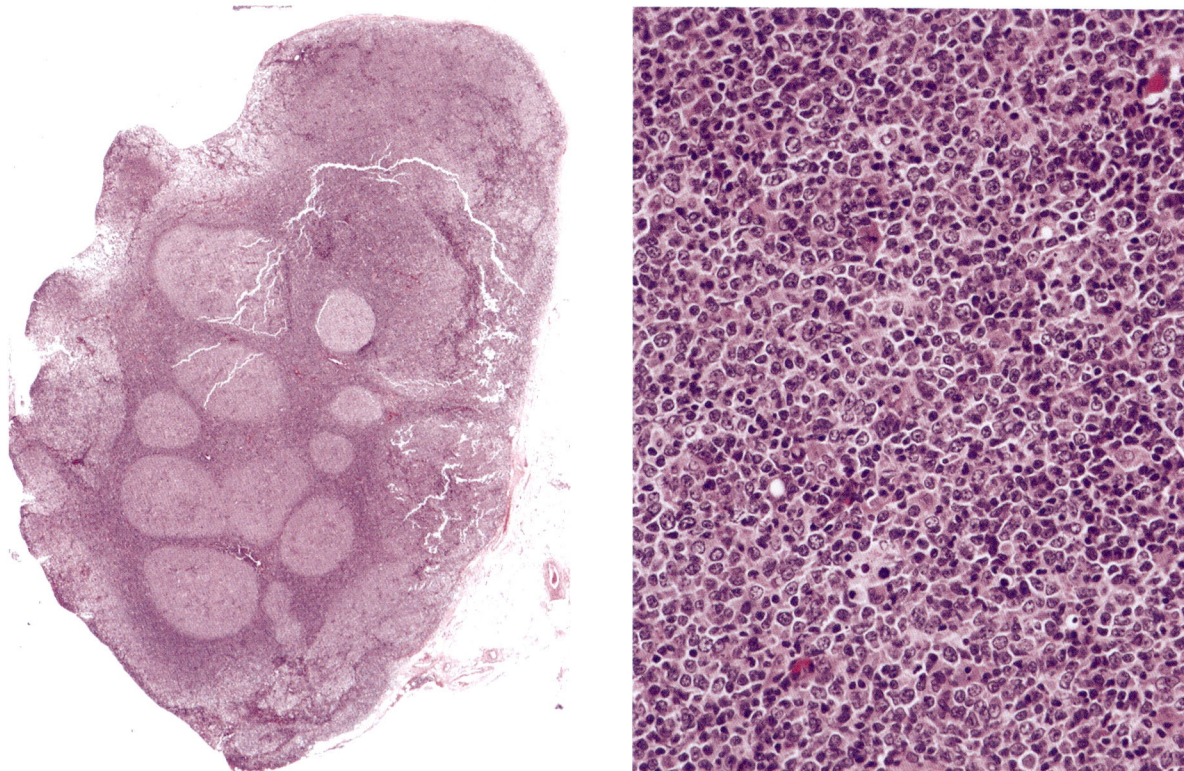

Figure 13-12

FOLLICULAR LYMPHOMA, GRADE 3B, INVOLVING LYMPH NODE

Left: The neoplasm is composed of large follicles that partially replace the lymph node parenchyma.
Right: The neoplasm is composed almost entirely of centroblasts (left, right: H&E stain).

(20,76). This morphologic variant is important to recognize because it closely resembles progressive transformation of germinal centers, a benign entity (20,33,56).

Follicular Lymphoma with Monocytoid (Marginal Zone) B-Cell Differentiation. In a study by Nathwani et al. (48), 9 percent of cases of FL had a prominent (defined as greater than 5 percent) perifollicular component of monocytoid B cells that correlated with high-stage disease and a poorer prognosis (fig. 13-15). Monocytoid B cells are usually clonally related to the neoplastic FL cells and do not represent evidence of composite lymphoma (61).

Follicular Lymphoma with Abundant Extracellular Periodic Acid–Schiff (PAS)-Positive Material. Some cases of FL are associated with eosinophilic material, also known as proteinaceous precipitate, within the neoplastic follicles (62). In rare cases, this material is extensive, making it difficult to recognize

the lymphoma cells (fig. 13-16) (13,62). This extracellular material is immunohistochemically positive for markers similar to those of FL including IgM, CD10, and CD19. Electron microscopic examination has shown that this material is composed of membranous structures, membrane-bound vesicles, and electron-dense bodies (13). This variant has no known unique clinical or pathogenetic features, and its importance lies in recognizing this tumor as a rare morphologic variant of common FL.

Signet Ring Cell Variant. Signet ring cell FL is a rare morphologic variant characterized by lymphoma cells with clear, vacuolated cytoplasm. The vacuoles often distend the cytoplasm, pushing the nucleus to an eccentric location and indenting it. Signet ring lymphoma cells are present within follicles and interfollicular areas (fig. 13-17). The vacuoles are thought to be composed of intracytoplasmic immunoglobulin deposits (14). This morphologic appearance should be

Figure 13-13

FOLLICULAR LYMPHOMA PARTIALLY INVOLVING LYMPH NODE

This needle biopsy specimen shows partial involvement by low-grade FL. The large follicles (right of field) were strongly positive for CD10 and BCL2 (not shown) but other follicles were negative for BCL2. The pattern of partial involvement is associated with lower clinical stage and less genomic complexity compared with common cases of FL (H&E stain).

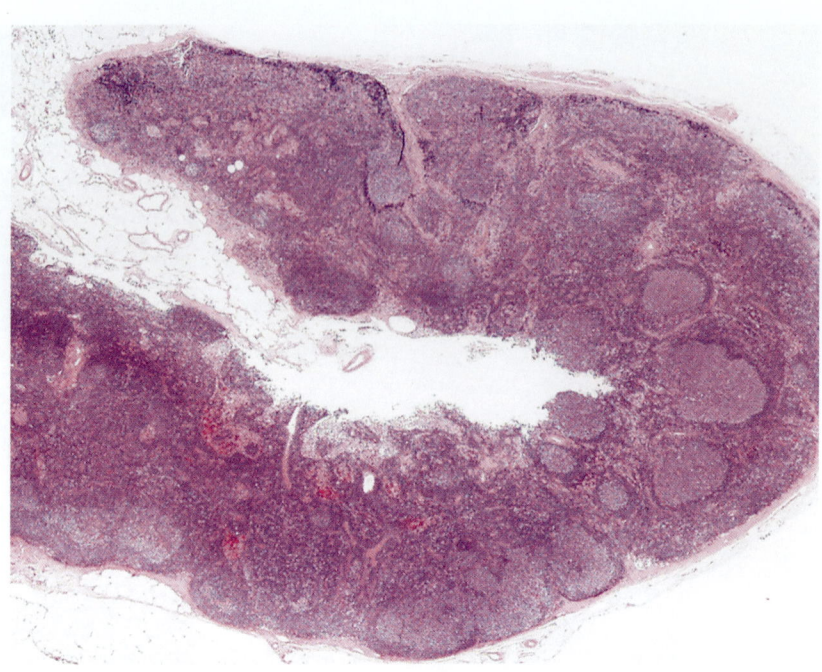

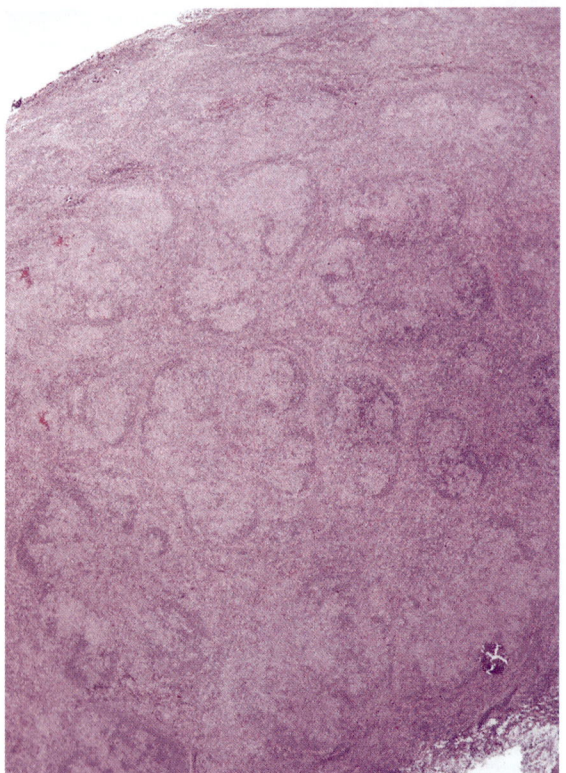
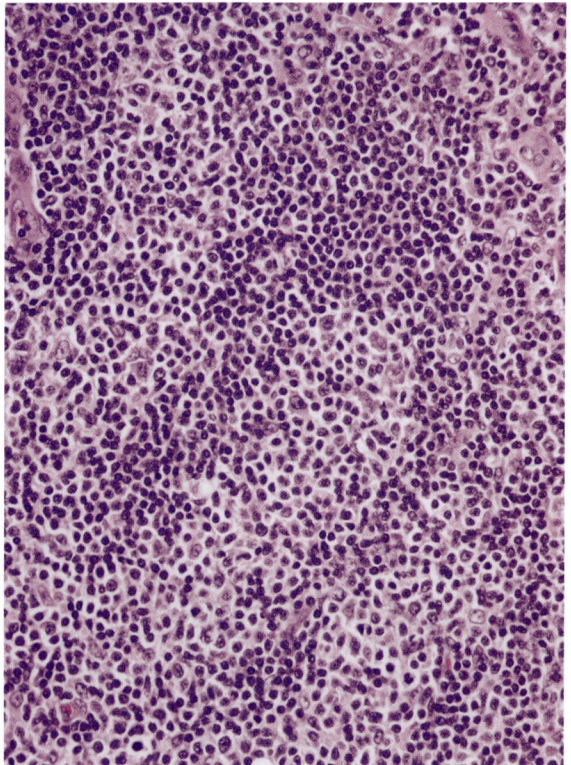

Figure 13-14

FLORAL VARIANT OF FOLLICULAR LYMPHOMA

Left: At low power, the neoplastic follicles are large and appear lobulated, resembling, in part, the petals of a flower.
Right: At high magnification, the pale FL cells are infiltrated by darker mantle zone lymphocytes (left, right: H&E stain).

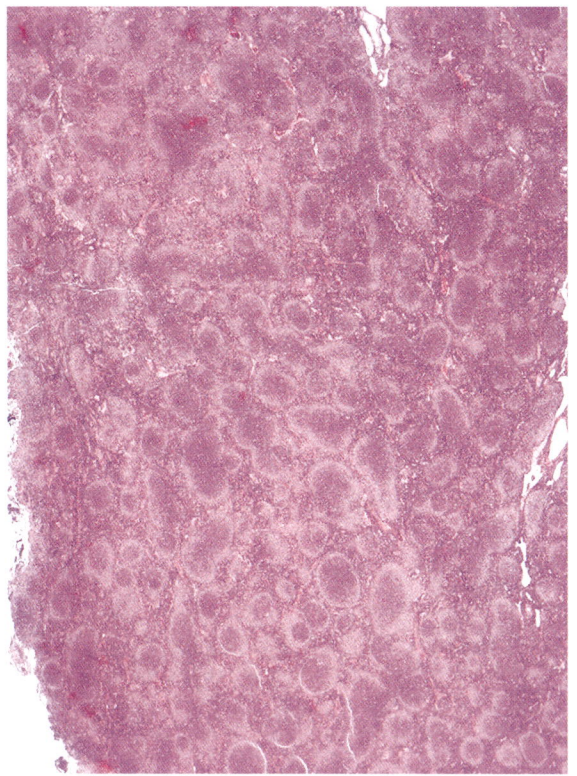 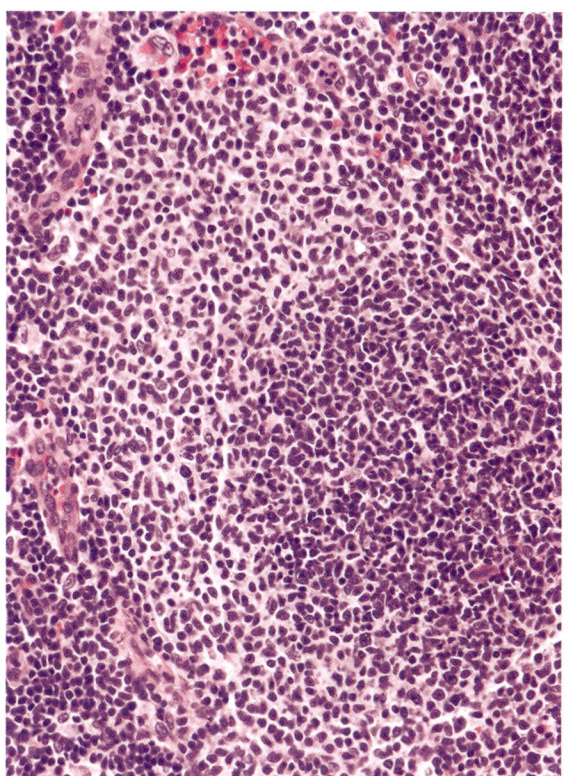

Figure 13-15

FOLLICULAR LYMPHOMA WITH MONOCYTOID (MARGINAL ZONE) DIFFERENTIATION

Left: The lymph node is replaced by numerous follicles of FL. The periphery of most of the neoplastic follicles is surrounded by paler rims of cells corresponding to monocytoid/marginal zone differentiation.

Right: Higher magnification shows marginal zone cells with abundant pale cytoplasm. Marginal zone differentiation is reported to correlate with poorer prognostic features (left, right: H&E stain).

recognized to avoid misdiagnosis as metastatic signet ring cell adenocarcinoma. In contrast with adenocarcinoma cells, the vacuoles in signet ring FL cells do not have a targetoid appearance and are negative for mucin.

Liver and Spleen

The liver and spleen are commonly involved in patients with FL (22). In the liver, FL preferentially involves the portal tracts (fig. 13-18). Large nodules replace hepatic parenchyma in patients with extensive disease. In the spleen, FL preferentially involves the white pulp, and two patterns have been described (22,26). Most often, the white pulp is expanded, forming variably enlarged nodules of lymphoma (fig. 13-19). Less often, the white pulp is involved, with relative preservation of the splenic architecture (26).

Bone Marrow

The bone marrow may be focally or extensively involved by FL (22,27). The most characteristic pattern of involvement is paratrabecular in which the lymphoma cells are closely aligned along, and often partially surround, the borders of trabecular bone (fig. 13-20). The paratrabecular pattern is present in 80 to 90 percent of patients (27). Nonparatrabecular nodules or an interstitial pattern also occurs, often associated with a paratrabecular pattern, and uncommonly, the medullary space is diffusely replaced by FL. A pure follicular pattern of FL is observed in the bone marrow in about 5 percent of patients (77).

Peripheral Blood

FL cells are commonly present in the blood at low levels. These cells are observed in the blood smear, or by flow cytometry or molecular

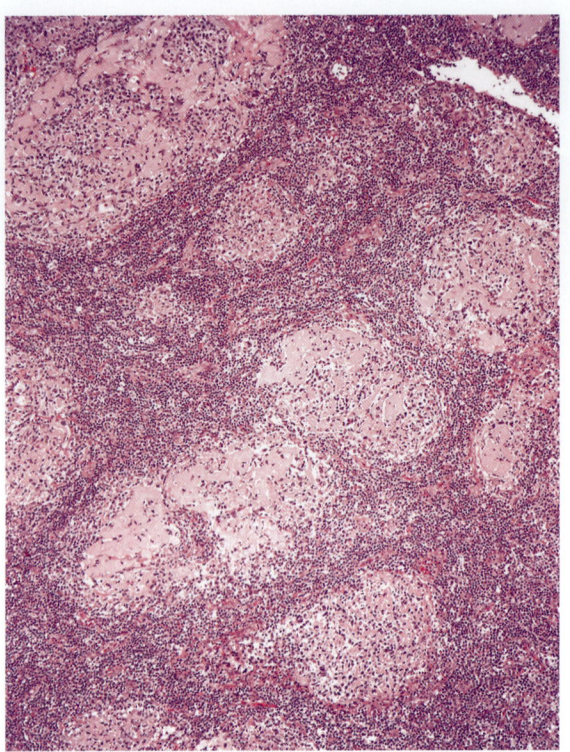
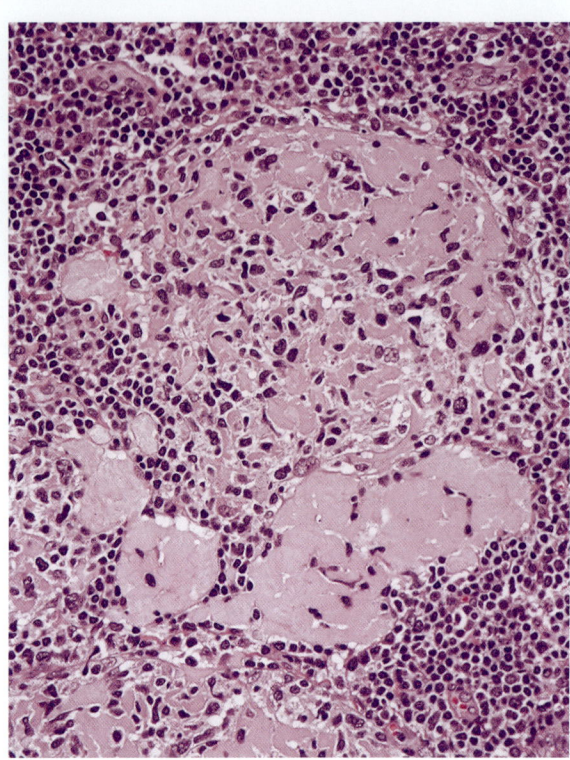

Figure 13-16

FOLLICULAR LYMPHOMA WITH ABUNDANT EXTRACELLULAR EOSINOPHILIC MATERIAL (OR PRECIPITATE)

Left: The follicles are numerous in the cortex and medulla of the lymph node and many are composed mostly of the eosinophilic material.

Right: Higher magnification shows a follicle with abundant eosinophilic material and a few lymphoma cells. The eosinophilic material was positive for CD20 and IgM and negative for Congo red stain, in this case in keeping with the opinion that the eosinophilic material is related to the contents of the lymphoma cells (left, right: H&E stain).

methods. Some patients with FL present with an absolute lymphocytosis that can be very high, referred to in the older literature as lymphosarcoma cell leukemia (22,68). The FL cells are typically small to intermediate-sized, with cleaved nuclei containing mature clumped chromatin and scant cytoplasm; these are referred to as buttock cells (fig. 13-21).

SPECIFIC TYPES OF FOLLICULAR LYMPHOMA

CD5-Positive Follicular Lymphoma

CD5 is expressed by about 5 percent of FL cases. Patients with CD5-positive FL are adults, with an age range from 31 to 86 years; men are more often affected (37). The disease usually involves lymph nodes, but almost half of patients have bone marrow involvement and 25 percent have other extranodal sites of disease.

Histologically, all grades of FL are represented, with most patients having grade 1 or 2 disease (fig. 13-22). A diffuse pattern is commonly associated with CD5-positive FL. These neoplasms are positive for pan-B-cell antigens, CD10 (about 70 percent), BCL2, and BCL6, and two thirds of patients carry t(14;18)/*IGH-BCL2*. Importantly, patients with CD5-positive FL have a higher rate of subsequent transformation to DLBCL and a poorer progression-free survival rate than patients with typical CD5-negative FL (37).

Duodenal-Type Follicular Lymphoma

Duodenal-type FL usually involves the second portion of the duodenum. Patients may have gastrointestinal complaints that prompt endoscopy, but commonly, the disease is detected incidentally during endoscopy performed for other reasons (see fig. 13-8). Patients with

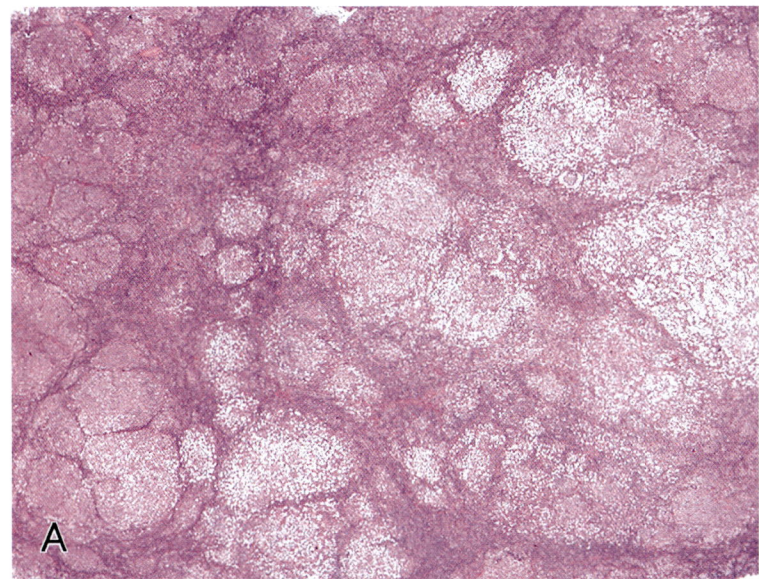

Figure 13-17

**FOLLICULAR LYMPHOMA
WITH PROMINENT SIGNET
RING CELL FEATURES**

A: At this magnification, the pale follicles are those with the greatest number of signet ring lymphoma cells.

B: High magnification demonstrates the signet ring features (A,B: H&E stain).

C: Fine-needle aspiration smear of a lymph node shows cells with cytoplasmic vacuoles indenting the nuclei, resembling signet ring cells. The vacuoles are clear and do not have targetoid mucin, unlike signet ring cell adenocarcinoma (C: Diff-Quik stain).

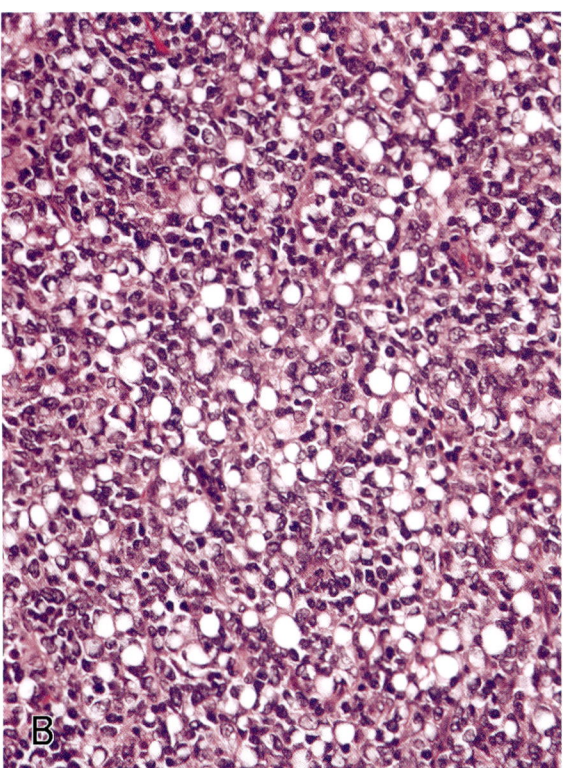

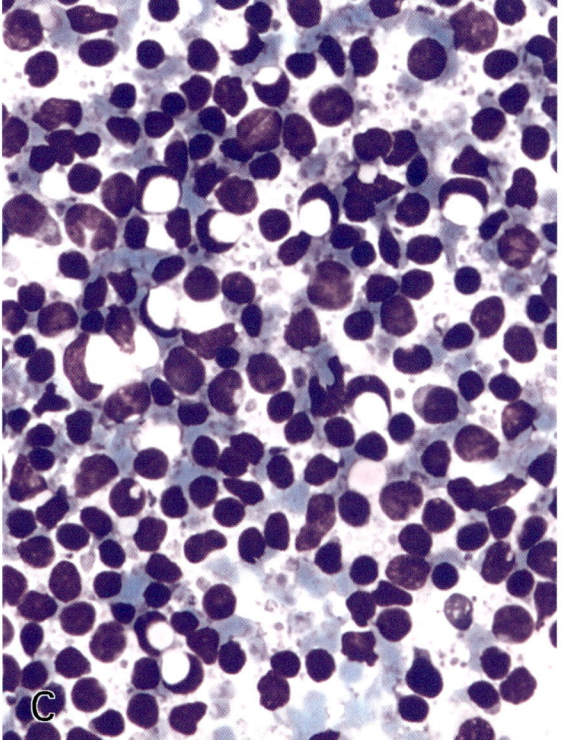

duodenal-type FL usually have small, submucosal nodules and the disease is localized (fig. 13-23) (69,71,82).

Morphologically, these neoplasms closely mimic low-grade FL in lymph nodes. The lymphoma cells are usually positive for CD10, BCL6, and BCL2, and carry t(14;18)/*IGH-BCL2* (69,71).

Duodenal-type FL is clinically indolent and many patients can be followed without therapy (watchful waiting). Radiation therapy also is employed (23). It is important to distinguish duodenal-type FL from systemic FL secondarily involving the intestine; the latter is more likely to involve areas of small intestine other than the

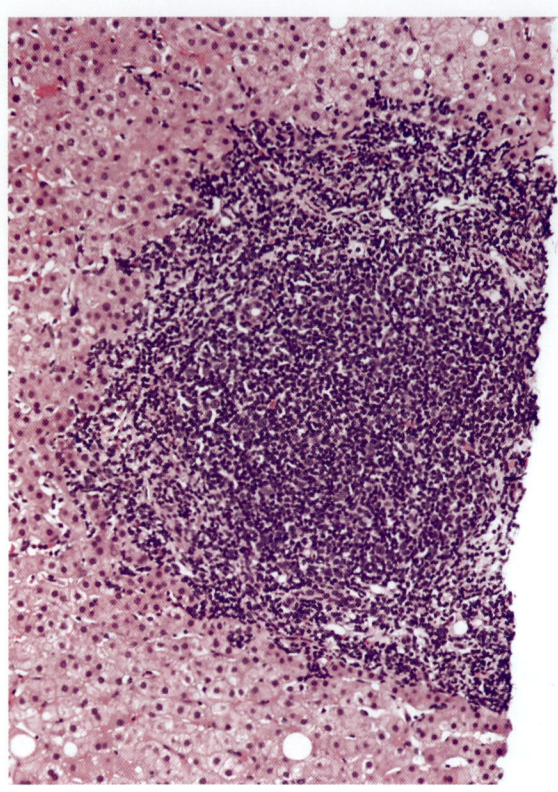

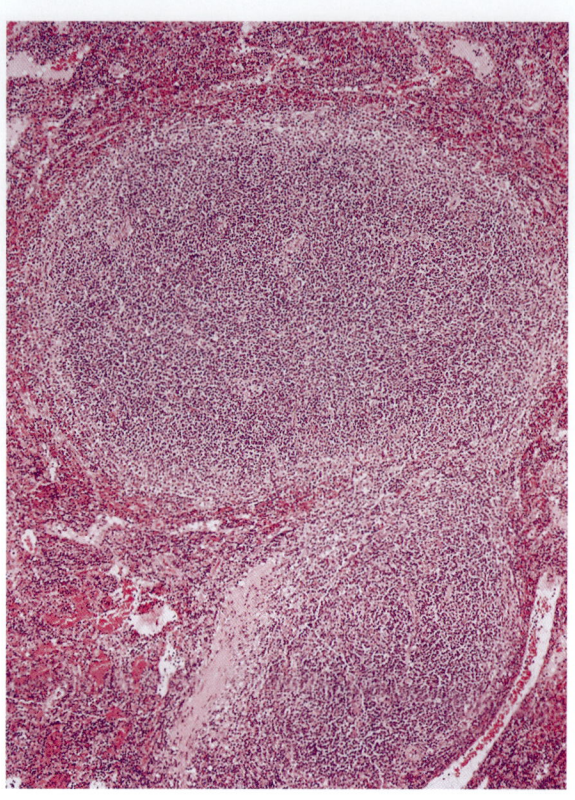

Figure 13-18

FOLLICULAR LYMPHOMA INVOLVING LIVER

A wedge biopsy specimen of the liver shows a portal tract expanded by FL (H&E stain).

Figure 13-19

FOLLICULAR LYMPHOMA INVOLVING SPLEEN

The white pulp is greatly expanded by FL (H&E stain).

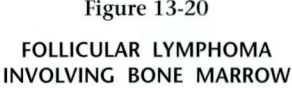

Figure 13-20

FOLLICULAR LYMPHOMA INVOLVING BONE MARROW

A bone marrow biopsy specimen is extensively involved by FL. The lymphoma has a predominantly paratrabecular pattern (H&E stain).

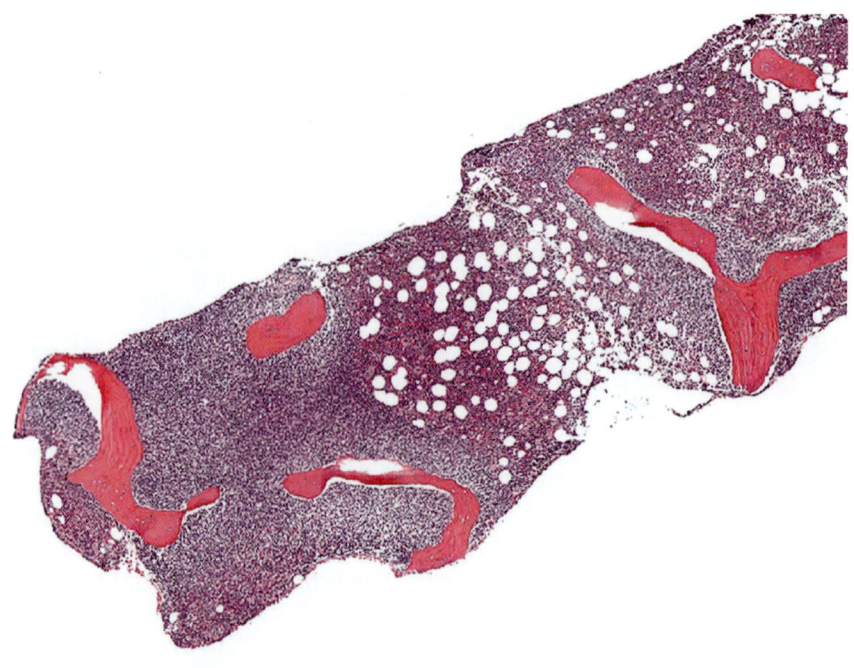

second part of the duodenum and the disease is often more aggressive.

Follicular Lymphoma in Children

FL is rare in children and young adolescents. In this age group, FL represents 1 to 2 percent of all B-cell non-Hodgkin lymphomas. Childhood FL is divided into two groups: one group closely resembles FL in adults and is therefore considered to be adult type FL occurring in children; the other is distinctive and is considered to be unique. As this second group of tumors rarely occurs in adults, the designation *pediatric-type FL* is used in the WHO classification.

Pediatric-type FLs occur predominantly in boys of a median age in the second decade, but occur as early as 4 or 5 years of age (39,40,75). Pediatric-type FL usually involves head and neck lymph nodes and most patients have localized (stage I) disease. Histologically, the lymph node architecture is partially or completely effaced by large, expansile, and serpiginous follicles usually composed predominantly of centroblasts (grade

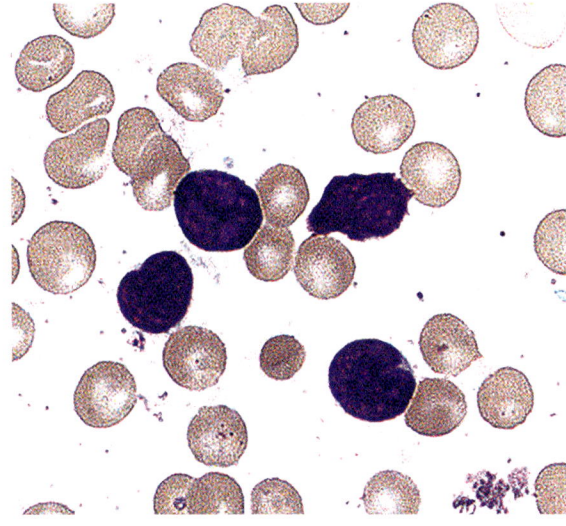

Figure 13-21

FOLLICULAR LYMPHOMA INVOLVING PERIPHERAL BLOOD

The lymphoma cells have a high nucleus-cytoplasm ratio, irregular nuclear contours, and minimal cytoplasm (Wright stain).

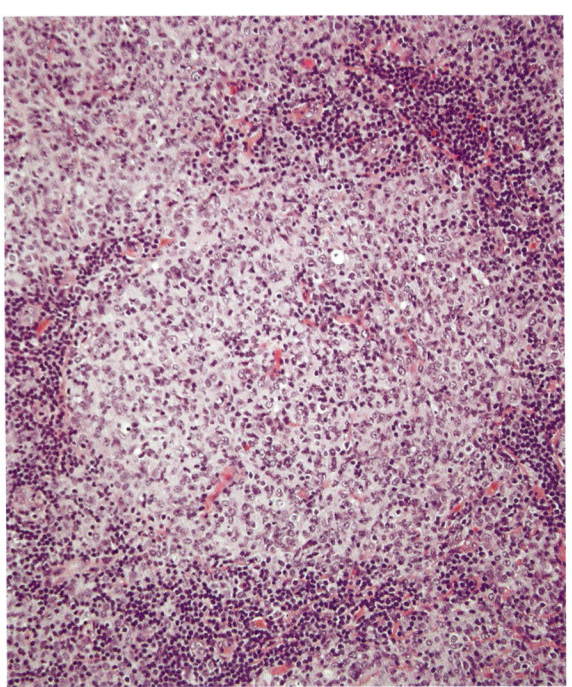
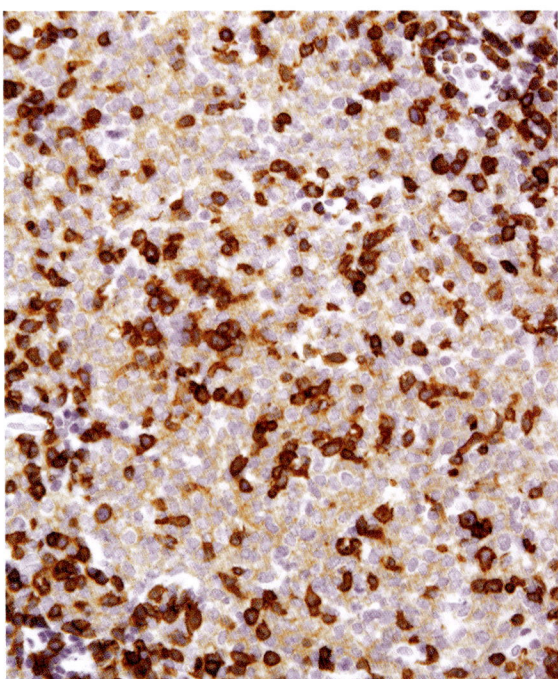

Figure 13-22

CD5-POSITIVE FOLLICULAR LYMPHOMA INVOLVING LYMPH NODE

This case of CD5-positive FL had a follicular and diffuse pattern and was positive for *IGH-BCL2* (not shown).

Left: A neoplastic follicle is present in the center of field (H&E stain).

Right: The lymphoma cells are weakly positive for CD5. CD5 expression was also shown by flow cytometry immunophenotypic analysis (immunohistochemistry with hematoxylin counterstain). (Courtesy of Dr. C. C. Yin, Houston, TX.)

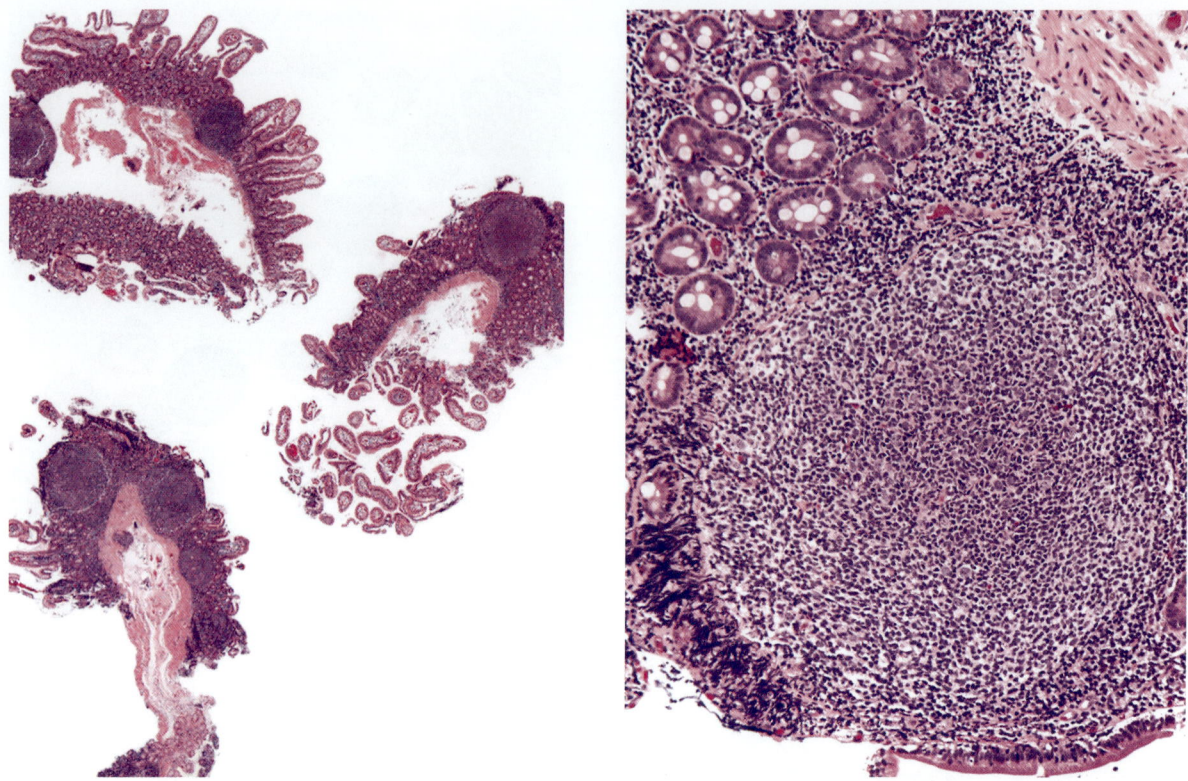

Figure 13-23

DUODENAL-TYPE FOLLICULAR LYMPHOMA

Left: At low power magnification, six neoplastic follicles in the duodenal mucosa are appreciated in these small tissue fragments.

Right: High magnification of one follicle shows a grade 1 FL (left, right: H&E stain).

3); diffuse areas are uncommon (fig. 13-24) (40). Pediatric-type FL is usually positive for pan-B-cell antigens, CD10, and MUM1/IRF4, but is negative or only weakly positive for BCL2 (about 20 percent of cases). The t(14;18)/*IGH-BCL2* is not present. The presence of monoclonal immunoglobulin rearrangements, usually detected by polymerase chain reaction (PCR) methods, is helpful for establishing the diagnosis. Loss of heterozygosity of chromosome 1p36 and mutations of *TNFRSF14* and *MAP2K1* are common in pediatric type FL (40a,45).

Patients with pediatric-type FL usually have a clinically indolent disease and the prognosis is excellent without further therapy following complete excision (40,75). Watchful waiting with close clinical follow-up is a reasonable first approach in patient management.

It seems likely that cases of pediatric-type FL, because of their indolent clinical behavior,

have been described in the literature as reactive lesions. In retrospect, at least a some cases described by Osborne and Butler (57) as reactive lymph node hyperplasia with giant follicles were likely pediatric-type FL. Similarly, some cases of reactive follicular hyperplasia with a monotypic B-cell population identified by flow cytometry immunophenotyping, as described by Kussick et al. (34), were likely pediatric-type FL.

Follicular Lymphoma with *IRF4* Rearrangement

A small subset of cases of FL is characterized by MUM1/IRF4 expression, and usually translocations that involve *IRF4* at chromosome 6p25.3 and *IGH* at chromosome 14q32 (65). As these neoplasms can be follicular or entirely diffuse, they are designated in the current WHO classification as *large B-cell lymphoma with IRF4 rearrangement* (75). Here we focus on tumors with a follicular pattern.

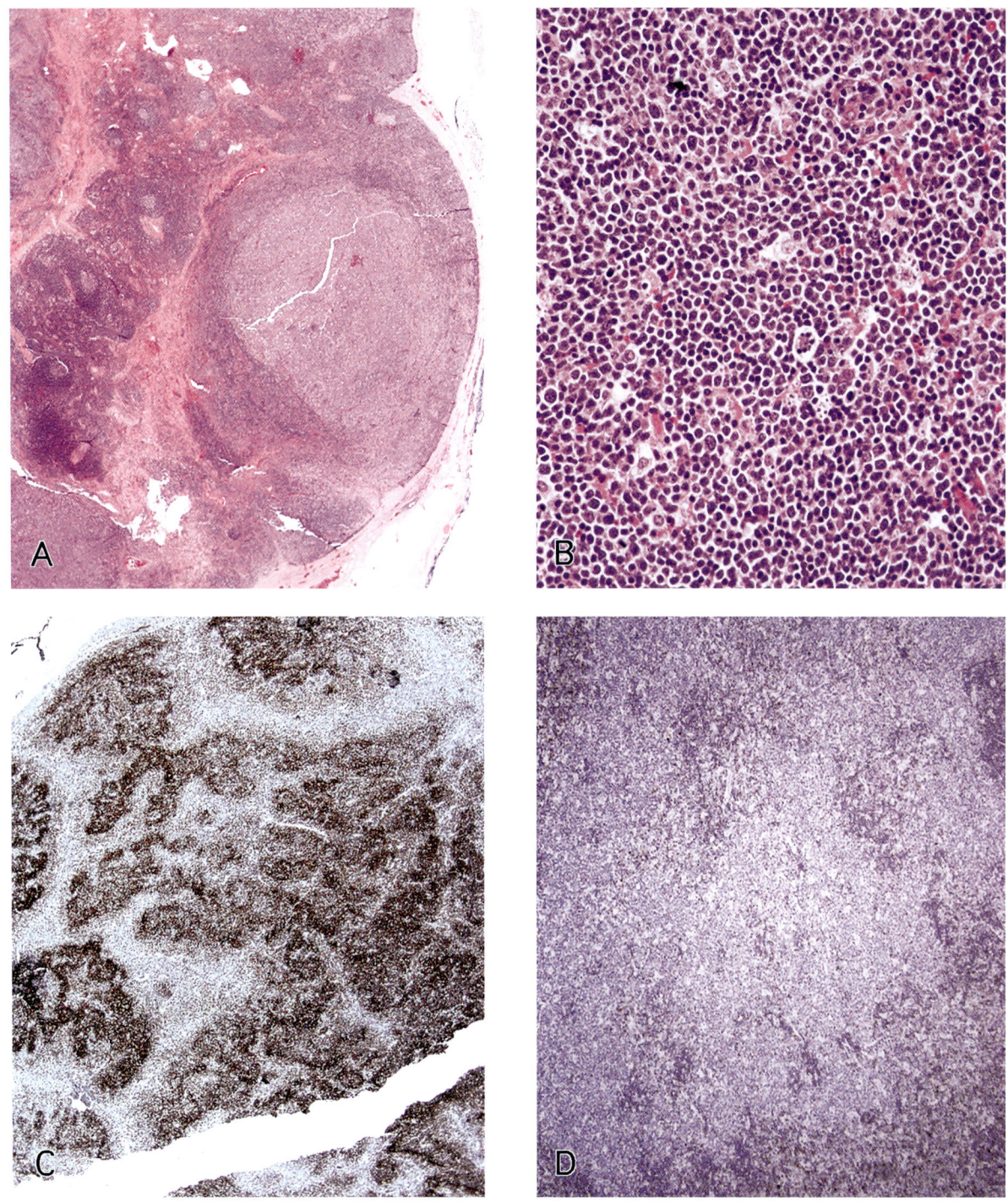

Figure 13-24

PEDIATRIC-TYPE FOLLICULAR LYMPHOMA INVOLVING LYMPH NODE

A: In this case of FL from a 15-year-old boy, a large follicle partially replaces the lymph node parenchyma.

B: High magnification of a neoplastic follicle shows many large cells and apoptotic cells (A,B: H&E stain).

C: The follicles have a high proliferation rate as shown by Ki-67 expression.

D: The follicles are negative for BCL2, as is common in pediatric-type FL (C,D: immunohistochemistry with hematoxylin counterstain).

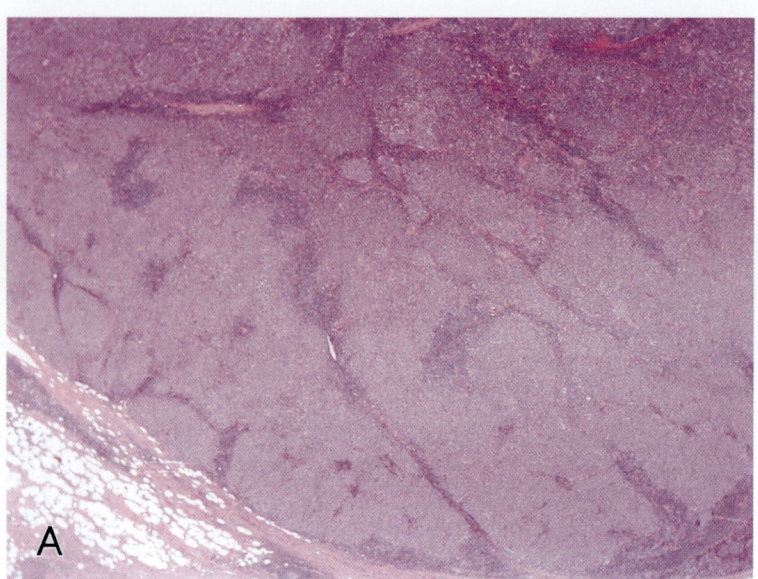

Figure 13-25

FOLLICULAR LYMPHOMA ASSOCIATED WITH *IRF4* TRANSLOCATION

A. The lymph node is almost completely replaced by lymphoma characterized by large expansile follicles and diffuse areas (A,B: H&E stain).

B. High magnification of the lymphoma cells.

C: The lymphoma cells are positive for MUM1/IRF4 and BCL6 (not shown) and negative for BCL2 (not shown) (immunohistochemistry with hematoxylin counterstain).

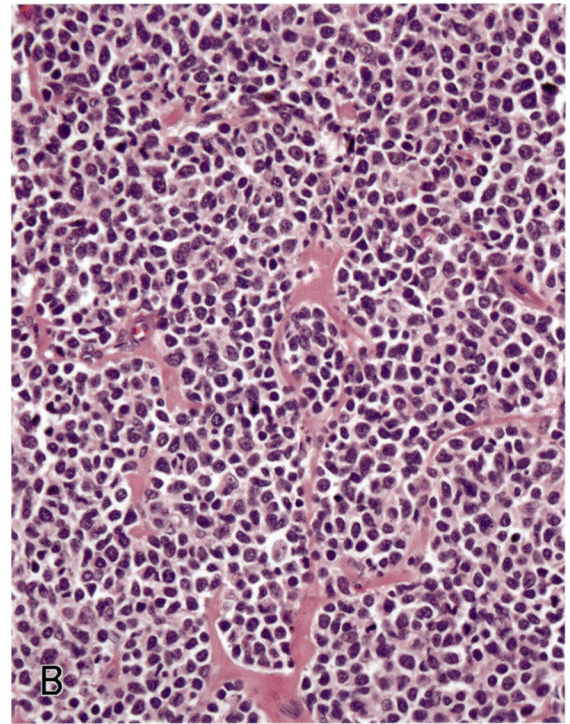

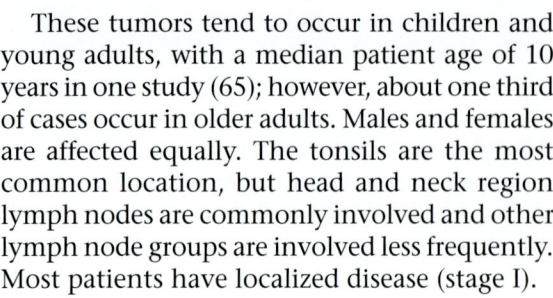

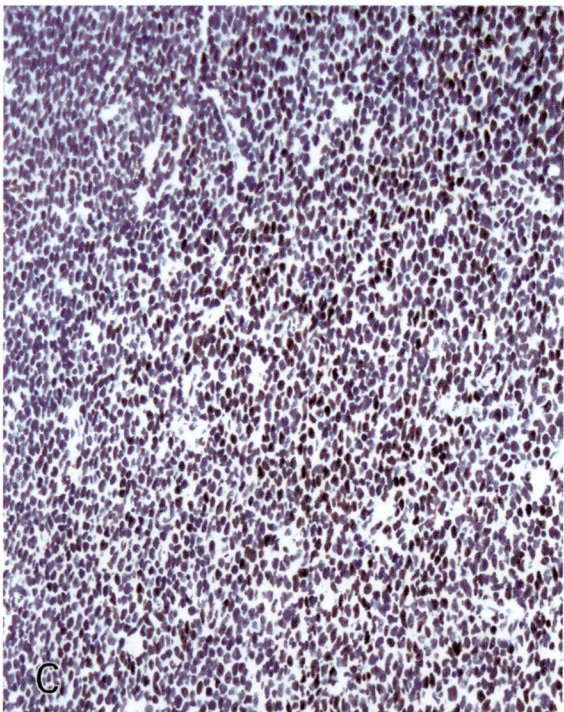

These tumors tend to occur in children and young adults, with a median patient age of 10 years in one study (65); however, about one third of cases occur in older adults. Males and females are affected equally. The tonsils are the most common location, but head and neck region lymph nodes are commonly involved and other lymph node groups are involved less frequently. Most patients have localized disease (stage I).

Histologically, the tonsil or lymph node is replaced by large and expansile follicles composed of centroblasts with attenuated mantle zones (fig. 13-25). Diffuse areas are common. These neoplasms are positive for MUM1/IRF4, pan-B-cell antigens, CD10, BCL2, and BCL6, and have a high proliferation (Ki-67) rate. Nevertheless, patients commonly have indolent disease and watchful waiting is used for localized disease.

The t(6;14)(p25.3;q32) is often cryptic by conventional cytogenetic analysis, but can be recognized by FISH. In addition to *IRF4* translocations, a number of other genetic changes have been identified in these neoplasms by comparative genomic hybridization including gains of Xq28, 11q22.3-qter, and 7q32.1-qter and losses of 6q13-16.1, 15q14-22.3, and 17p (64). *TP53* mutations occur in some cases with loss of 17p.

Follicular Lymphoma of the Testis

Most patients with FL of the testis are children or adolescents who present with a testicular mass and localized disease (5,38). These neoplasms have a follicular or follicular and diffuse pattern, and are commonly grade 3 (fig. 13-26). The immunophenotype of FL of the testis is distinctive, positive for CD10, but often BCL2 negative. The t(14;18)/*IGH-BCL2* is not present. Patients with testicular FL usually have clinically indolent disease and surgical excision alone is adequate therapy.

Follicular Lymphoma with del1p36/*TNFRSF14* Abnormalities

Cases of FL associated with chromosome 1p36/*TNFRSF14* abnormalities have been described (45,72). These neoplasms tend to occur in younger patients and usually involve the inguinal region, although rare cases involve other peripheral lymph node groups.

These neoplasms have a follicular pattern, but diffuse areas are also often present and many neoplasms are entirely diffuse (72). Most of these tumors are of low histologic grade. Follicular lymphomas with del1p36/*TNFRSF14* abnormalities are positive for pan-B-cell antigens as well as CD10 and BCL2 (particularly in diffuse areas); CD23 is usually expressed by the lymphoma cells. Most cases do not carry t(14;18), but carry deletions of chromosome 1p36 or mutations of *TNFRSF14*. *STAT6* mutations are also common (72).

Primary Cutaneous Follicular Lymphoma

The designation used for these tumors in the WHO classification is *primary cutaneous follicle center cell lymphoma*. Primary cutaneous FL is confined to the skin and typically involves the deep dermis. These tumors have a purely follicular, follicular and diffuse, or entirely

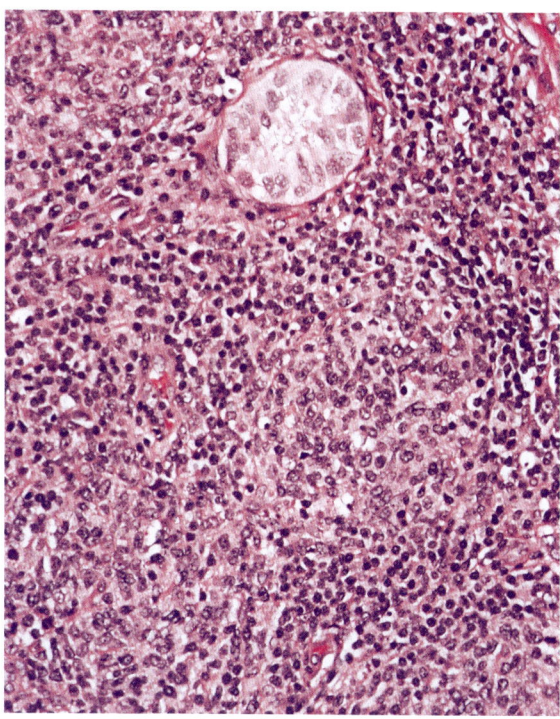

Figure 13-26

FOLLICULAR LYMPHOMA OF THE TESTIS

This 6-year-old boy presented with a testicular mass, but was otherwise asymptomatic. The neoplastic follicles surround a seminiferous tubule in the field (H&E stain).

diffuse pattern and can be of any grade (fig. 13-27). Unlike nodal FL, primary cutaneous FL is commonly negative for BCL2 and t(14;18)/*IGH-BCL2* (78).

The clinical course for patients with primary cutaneous FL is usually indolent and therefore systemic chemotherapy is rarely indicated. For this reason, the authors of the WHO classification recommend that these neoplasms not be graded. However, other extranodal cases of FL are often graded, despite their excellent prognosis, and it seems reasonable to handle cases of primary cutaneous FL like other cases of FL. In addition, staging information is often not available when the skin biopsy specimen is assessed.

Epstein-Barr Virus-Positive Follicular Lymphoma

Mackrides et al. (41) described 10 cases of Epstein-Barr virus (EBV)-positive FL in patients in the United States. These tumors represented 2.6 percent of all cases of FL surveyed in this study.

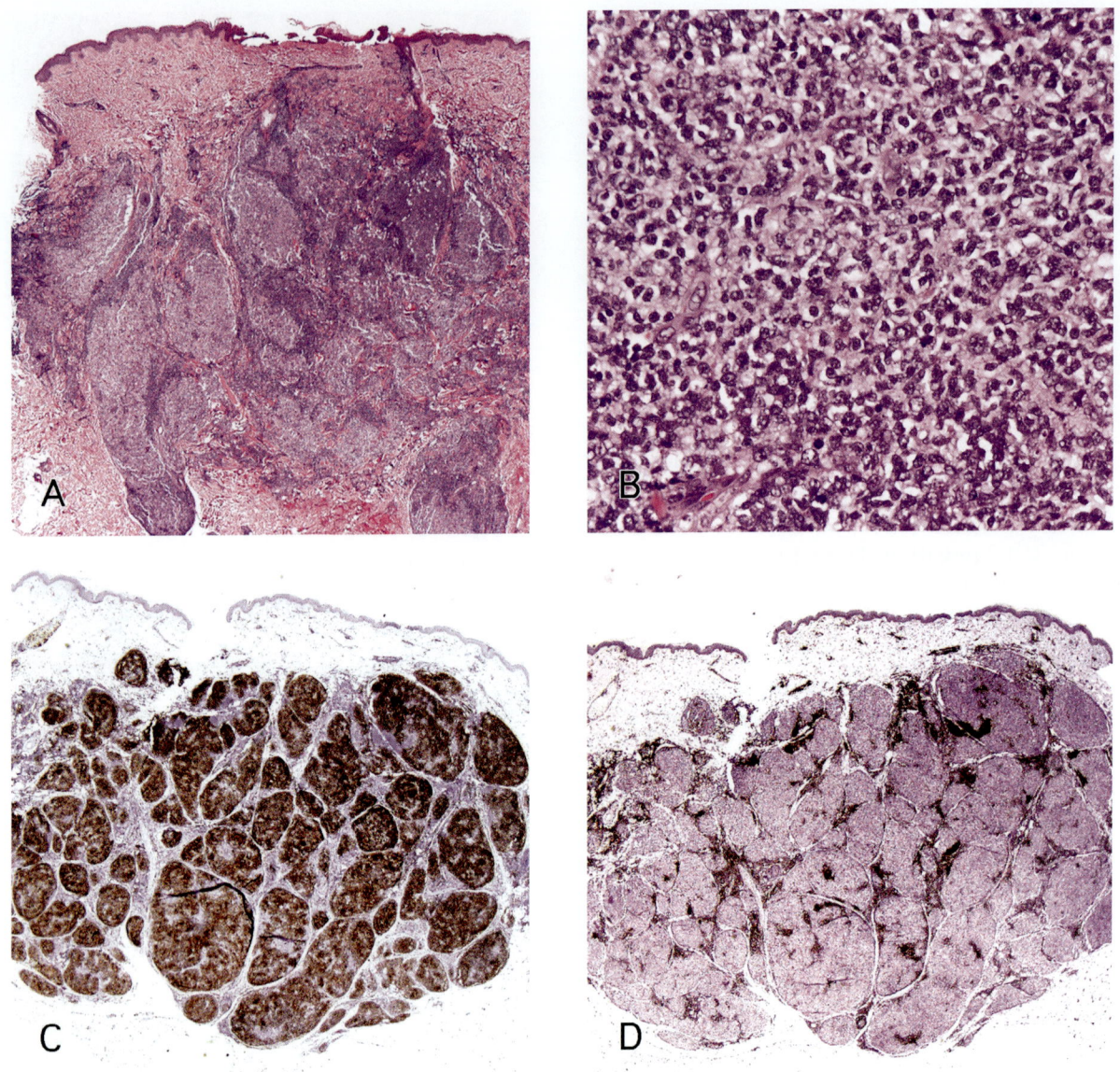

Figure 13-27

PRIMARY CUTANEOUS FOLLICULAR LYMPHOMA

A: Numerous neoplastic follicles are present in the dermis and extend more deeply.

B: The follicles are composed mostly of centrocytes (A,B: H&E stain).

C,D: The lymphoma cells are positive for CD10 (C) and negative for BCL2 (D). Patients with primary cutaneous FL usually have clinically indolent disease, regardless of the cytologic grade, and are commonly negative for BCL2 (immunohistochemistry with hematoxylin counterstain).

The patients were elderly, and 9 patients did not have any evidence of immunodeficiency. Most patients with staging information available had high-stage disease; most cases were grade 3 (either 3A or 3B). Over 75 percent of the lymphoma cells were positive for EBV-encoded RNA1 (EBER1) by in situ hybridization. The follow-up period in this study was short. In our own limited experience, only a subset of the tumor follicles in these cases of FC is EBER1 positive (fig. 13-28). Additional studies of EBV-positive FL are needed to better define this potential entity.

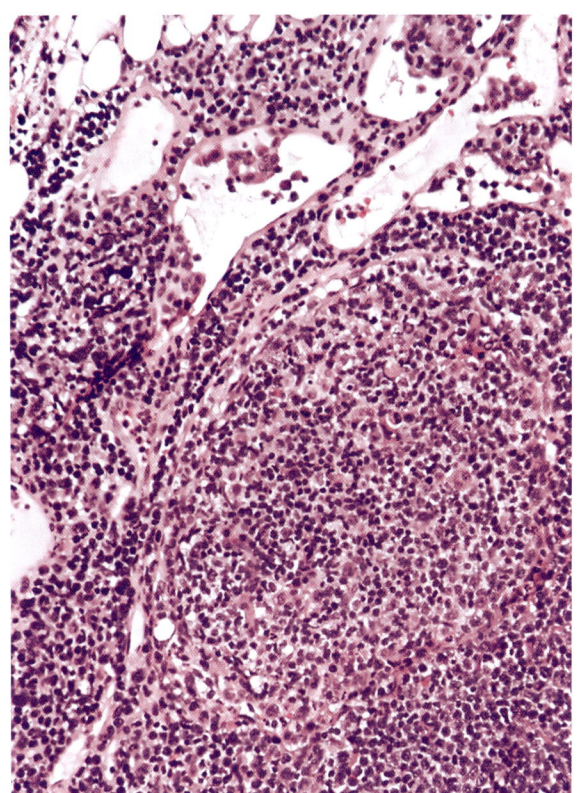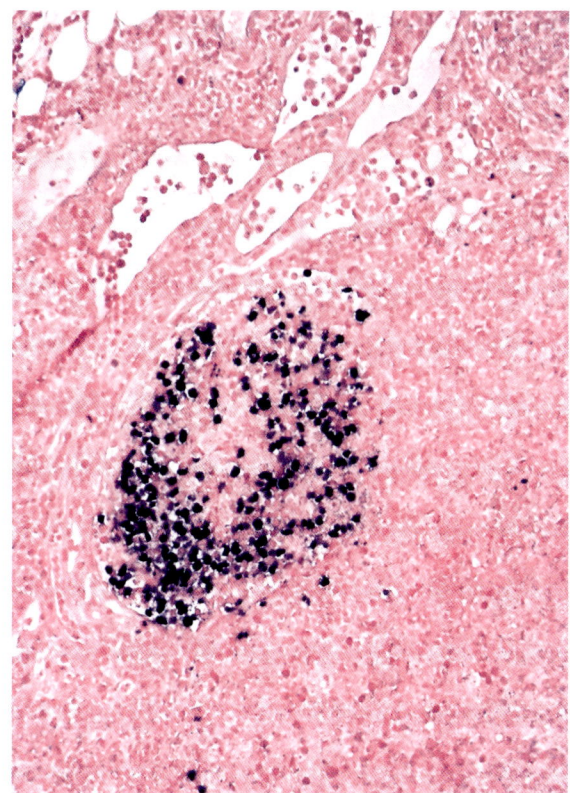

Figure 13-28

FOLLICULAR LYMPHOMA ASSOCIATED WITH INFECTION BY EPSTEIN-BARR VIRUS (EBV)

In this lymph node biopsy specimen, approximately 5 percent of the follicles had numerous cells positive for EBV, with few positive cells elsewhere in the neoplasm.

Left: One neoplastic follicle is shown (H&E stain).

Right: Many cells in this follicle (left) were positive for EBV-encoded RNA1 (EBER1) (in situ hybridization with eosin counterstain).

CYTOLOGIC FINDINGS

Fine-needle aspirate smears of FL show variable numbers of centrocytes and centroblasts. The somewhat cohesive aggregates of lymphoma cells associated with follicular dendritic cells are suggestive of follicles. These aggregates are not diagnostic of FL since they are observed in reactive follicular hyperplasia as well as other lymphoma types with a nodular pattern.

There is no standard approach for grading FL cases in cytology specimens. A two-tier grading system, as proposed by others (83) and in keeping with the current WHO classification which recommends combining cases of FL 1 and 2 together as low-grade, is used (22). Aspirates of low-grade FL show primarily small centrocytes while high-grade FLs contain many large centrocytes and centroblasts, often associated with mitotic figures

and apoptotic cells (fig. 13-29). Importantly, not all cases of FL can be classified in cytology smears. For instance, it may be difficult to distinguish high-grade FL from DLBCL of follicular center origin. Also, rare cases of FL have signet ring cell features that should not be mistaken for metastatic signet ring cell carcinoma.

IMMUNOPHENOTYPIC FINDINGS

FL cells typically express pan-B-cell markers including CD19, CD20 (fig. 13-30, left), CD22, CD79a, CD79b, and PAX5 (22). Additionally, FL cells express CD45/LCA, CD200, and surface immunoglobulin (Ig), most often IgM and less often IgG or IgA. Cytoplasmic Ig is usually negative, but positive in a small subset of cases of FL with plasmacytoid differentiation. Many germinal center B-cell antigens such as CD10

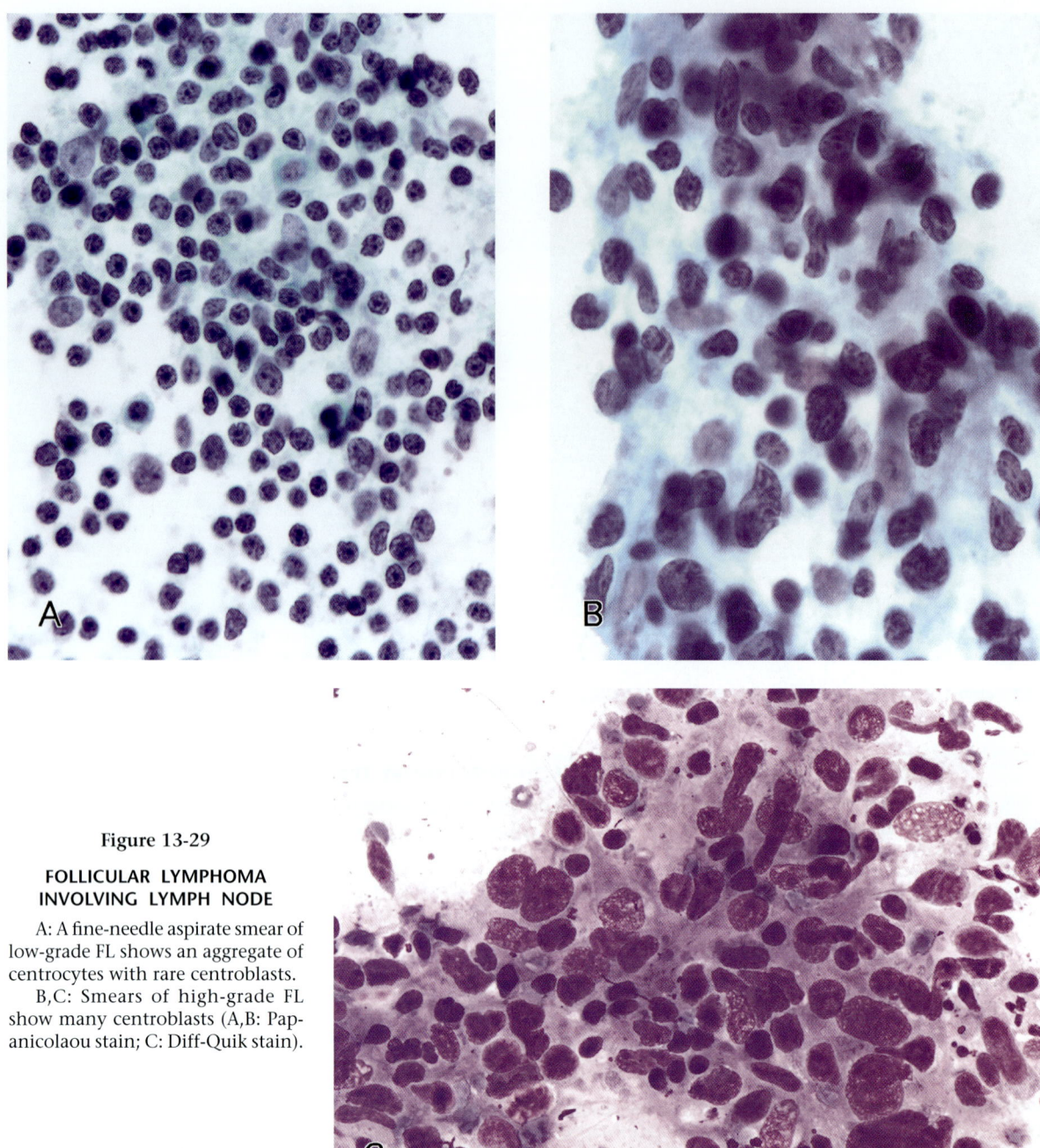

Figure 13-29

FOLLICULAR LYMPHOMA INVOLVING LYMPH NODE

A: A fine-needle aspirate smear of low-grade FL shows an aggregate of centrocytes with rare centroblasts.

B,C: Smears of high-grade FL show many centroblasts (A,B: Papanicolaou stain; C: Diff-Quik stain).

(fig. 13-30, right), BCL6, LMO2, and GCET2/HGAL, are expressed. Expression of CD10 and BCL6 seems to be modulated by the microenvironment, being positive in follicles but often dim or negative in the interfollicular regions. There are small subsets of cases of FL that are negative for CD10 and BCL6. Marafioti et al. (43) have reported that STMN1/stathmin is a sensitive germinal center B-cell marker. A small percentage of FL cases, usually grade 3, has a subset of cells positive for CD30 (fig. 13-31); rarely, many FL cells are CD30 positive. Most cases of low-grade FL have a low proliferation rate, often 30 percent or less shown by Ki-67 expression. Grade 3 cases have a range of Ki-67–positive cells (between 30 and 80 percent),

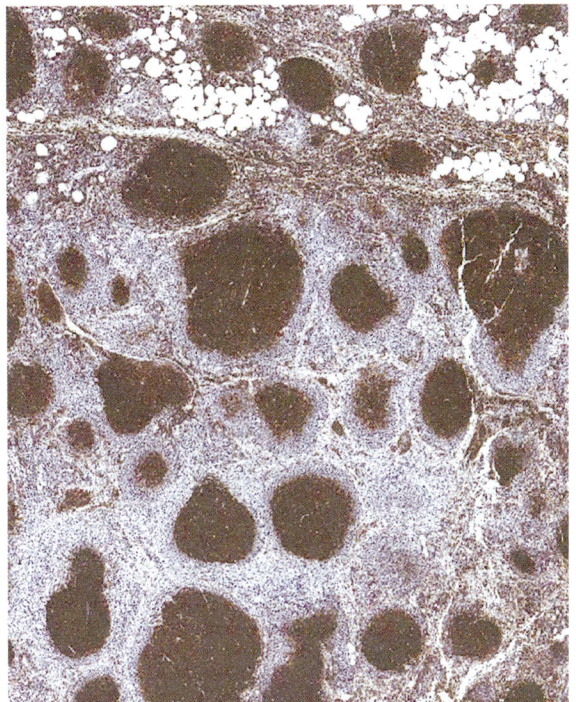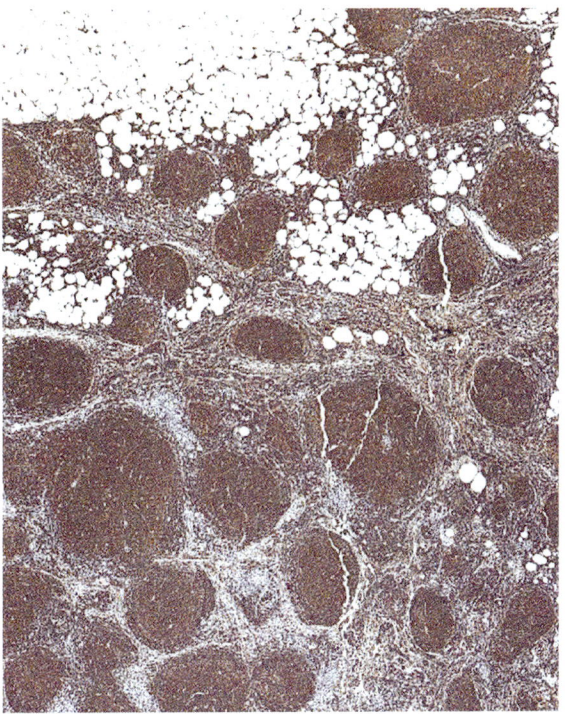

Figure 13-30

FOLLICULAR LYMPHOMA IMMUNOHISTOCHEMISTRY

Most cases of nodal FL are positive for CD20 (left) and CD10 (right) (left, right: immunohistochemistry with hematoxylin counterstain).

with grade 3B neoplasms usually having higher proliferation rates than grade 3A neoplasms.

At least 80 percent of cases of FL are positive for BCL2, unlike the germinal centers in reactive follicles (fig. 13-32) (1,7,43). Some BCL2-negative cases are explained by the presence of mutations in the BCL2 epitope recognized by the most commonly used anti-BCL2 antibody, clone 124 (70). These cases are positive using other anti-BCL2 antibodies, for example, clone E17, which recognizes a different epitope of BCL2 (fig. 13-32) (1,70). Nevertheless, a subset of cases of FL is truly negative for BCL2 (22,43).

Cases of FL are negative for pan-T-cell antigens including CD2, CD3, CD5 (minor subset positive), CD7, and CD43 (minor subset positive), and T-cell receptors (22). They are also usually negative for markers of follicular dendritic cells (see below) and are negative for CD1a, CD4, CD8, CD11c, myeloid-associated antigens, CD34, CD68, and CD163. Many reactive T cells (CD4 more than CD8) and histiocytes are intermixed within FL follicles.

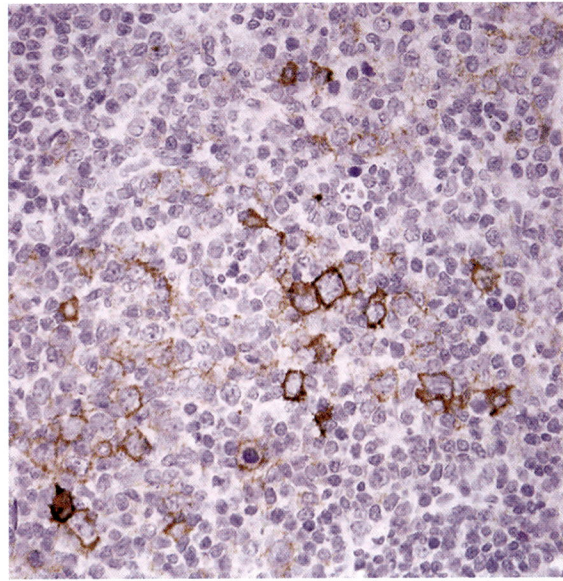

Figure 13-31

FOLLICULAR LYMPHOMA IMMUNOHISTOCHEMISTRY

Some centroblasts in a case of FL involving lymph node are positive for CD30 (immunohistochemistry with hematoxylin counterstain).

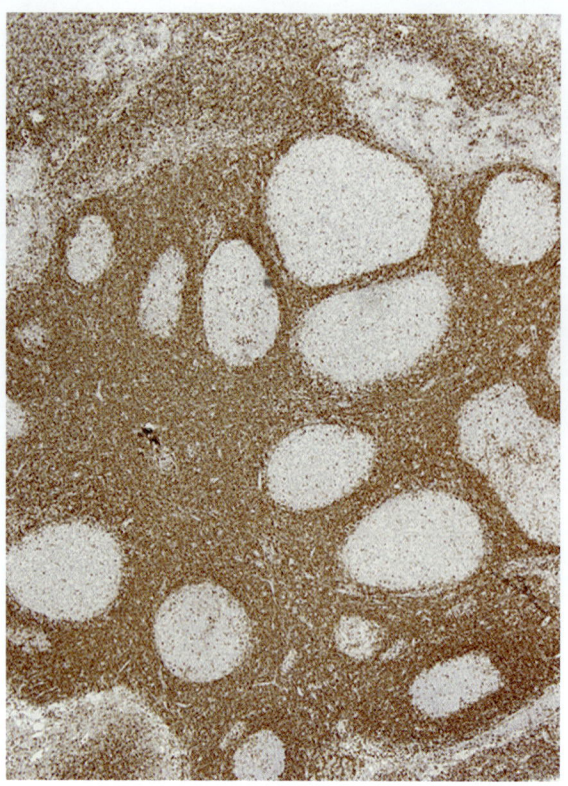 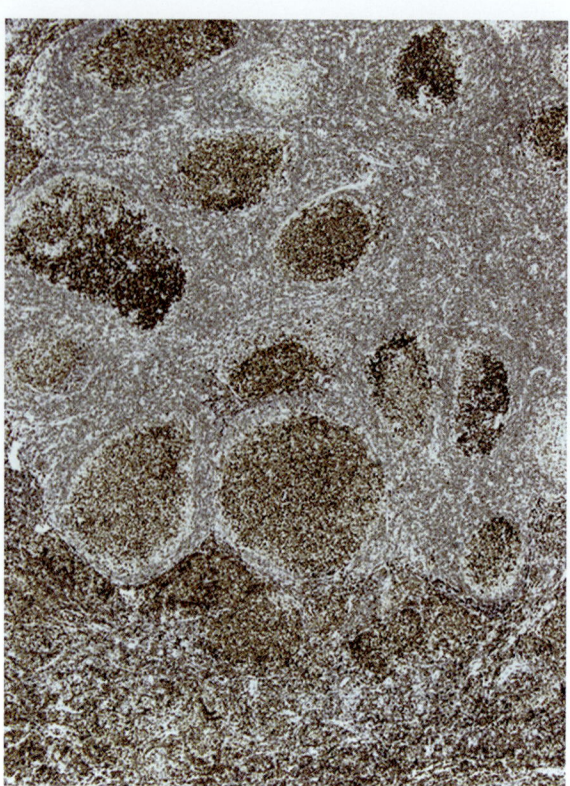

Figure 13-32

FOLLICULAR LYMPHOMA IMMUNOHISTOCHEMISTRY

BCL2 expression was assessed using two different antibodies.

Left: The most commonly used anti-BCL2 antibody reactive with amino acids 41-54 (clone 124) does not highlight the neoplastic follicles.

Right: In contrast, a rabbit monoclonal antibody reactive with amino acids 50-150 (E17) is positive for BCL2. This result may be explained by the presence of a *BCL2* mutation within the epitope recognized by the 124 antibody (left, right: immunohistochemistry with hematoxylin counterstain). (Courtesy of Dr. J. D. Khoury, Houston, TX.)

Antibodies specific for antigens expressed by follicular dendritic cells (FDCs), such as CD21 (fig. 13-33), CD23, CD35, CXCL13, clusterin, D2-40, and others highlight networks of FDCs in the neoplastic follicles. Although these networks are present in all follicles, not all FDCs express all of these antigens in FL. As shown by Chang et al. (10), CXCL13 tends to highlight FDCs in the follicles of all (or almost all) cases of FL; in contrast, FDCs may be negative for CD21, CD23, or CD35; CD23 was most often absent in their study. These data suggest that FDCs in neoplastic FLs undergo either differentiation or dedifferentiation (after benign follicles are colonized by lymphoma cells) and that not all FDCs in follicles of FL have a mature immunophenotype. Neoplastic follicles with a greater number of T cells more often have FDCs with a mature immunophenotype (10).

These findings also raise an issue regarding the definition of a neoplastic follicle in cases of FL. Is morphologic appreciation of a clearly nodular pattern adequate or does the presence of FDCs in a nodule need to be proven to conclude that it is indeed a follicle? In our opinion, morphologic assessment is usually adequate for this purpose. Although using CD21 immunohistochemical staining to prove a follicular pattern is helpful, this approach does have some limitations (as stated above).

MOLECULAR GENETIC FINDINGS

Conventional cytogenetic analysis of typical nodal FL shows a recurrent chromosomal

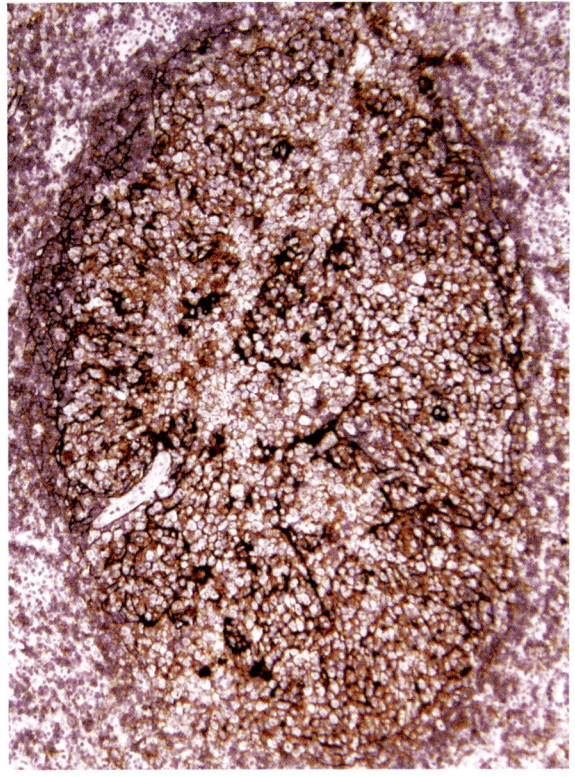

Figure 13-33

**FOLLICULAR LYMPHOMA
IMMUNOHISTOCHEMISTRY**

Nodal FL was assessed using an anti-CD21 antibody which highlights an extensive network of follicular dendritic cells within a neoplastic follicle (immunohistochemistry with hematoxylin counterstain).

translocation, t(14;18)(q32;q21), in 80 to 90 percent of cases, involving *IGH* and *BCL2* (24). Rare cases of FL with t(2;18)(p11;q21) or t(18;22) (q21;q11) juxtaposing *BCL2* with the κ or λ locus, respectively, have been reported. Leich et al. (35) have reported that t(14;18)/*IGH-BCL2* is less common in patients with low-stage disease. The t(14;18)/*IGH-BCL2* is also less common in children and in some types of extranodal FL, such as primary cutaneous FL (40,78).

The t(14;18)/*IGH-BCL2* is rarely an isolated finding in FL. Additional and often multiple cytogenetic alterations are common. In a study of FLs by Hoglund et al. (24), 28 chromosomal alterations at a frequency of 5 percent or greater were identified: del(6q11-27) was the most frequent (30 percent), followed by trisomy 7 or 12 or X; del(1p32-36); del(17p11-13); and gains

of 1p11-q44, der(18), and trisomy 18. About six additional karyotypic abnormalities are present in FL, with some having up to 14 additional chromosomal alterations.

Studies using high resolution methods such as comparative genomic hybridization and single nucleotide polymorphism (SNP) analysis have confirmed and extended the karyotypic data. Using SNP arrays, Bouska et al. (8) found gains of regions on chromosomes 2, 5, 6p, 7, 8, 12, 17q, 18, 21, and X as well as losses of 6q and 17p.

The t(14;18) results in *BCL2* being juxtaposed with *IGH*, resulting in an *IGH-BCL2* fusion gene. *BCL2* has three exons and at least four breakpoint cluster regions, allowing detection of *IGH-BCL2* by PCR methods. In most cases, the breakpoint in *BCL2* occurs in the major breakpoint region (MBR) between the second and third exons. PCR assays are routinely available to detect the MBR as well as a minor cluster region (MCR), which involves 5 to 10 percent of FL cases. An intermediate cluster region (ICR) also is involved in 10 to 20 percent of cases (3), although this breakpoint is not routinely assessed in many laboratories.

Using probes specific for *BCL2* and *IGH*, FISH is an alternative method for detecting t(14;18)/*IGH-BCL2* in cases of FL and can be applied to fixed, paraffin-embedded tissue sections. The large *BCL2* probes available detect virtually all of the breakpoints and therefore this method has greater diagnostic sensitivity than PCR when tumor tissue is analyzed (17). FISH is less helpful, however, for the analysis of liquid specimens with a low percentage of lymphoma cells and, unlike PCR, is not useful in assessing for minimal residual disease.

BCL6 abnormalities have been identified in cases of FL. Translocations involving *BCL6*, most often t(3;14)(q27;q32)/*BCL6-IGH*, have been identified in 10 to 15 percent of cases of FL (28,35). Somatic mutations of *BCL6* also occur commonly, usually in the first intron (28). Cases of FL with *BCL6* translocations express BCL6, and are more often negative for CD10 and BCL2. *MYC* translocations occur in 2 to 6 percent of cases of FL, usually in only a small subset of lymphoma cells (35).

Monoclonal rearrangements of the IG genes, with ongoing somatic mutations in the variable gene segments, occur in FL. The presence of somatic mutations may preclude the annealing of PCR primers and lead to false positive PCR results when analyzing for either IG clonality or *IGH-BCL2*. For this reason, the use of multiple primer sets and analysis of the *IGH* and *IGK* genes as well as *IGH-BCL2* are ideal for the molecular assessment of clonality in FL cases. The T-cell receptor genes are usually in the germline configuration.

A number of gene mutations have been identified in FL (Table 13-1). In most instances, these mutations are secondary events that occur in B cells that carry t(14;18)/*IGH-BCL2* (36,53,60). Many mutations are involved in epigenetic regulation of the genome, such as *KMT2D/MLL2* (about 80 percent of FL cases), *MEF2B*, linker histone genes, and *EZH2*. *EZH2*, a catalytic component of the polycomb repressive complex 2 that functions to trimethylate lysine 27 on histone H3, is mutated in up to 20 percent of FL cases (53,60).

The ephrin receptor A7 (*EPHA7*), located on chromosome 6q16, is physiologically involved in neuronal development, but also is a tumor suppressor gene in FL. *EPHA7* is mutated in about 70 percent of all cases (55). *CREBBP* (about 65 percent of cases) and *EP300* (about 15 percent) are often mutated in FL. These genes are non-histone acetyltransferases that function as transcriptional coactivators of DNA-binding transcription factors (53,59). The RB pathway is inactivated in up to 50 percent of cases of FL (54). The major alterations include gains of chromosome 12 (encompassing *CDK4*, deletions of the *RB1* locus) and deletions of p16/*CDKN2A*. *TNFRSF14* mutations occur in 20 to 50 percent of all cases. Mutations in the B-cell receptor and CXCR4 signaling pathways have been identified in about 40 percent of FLs (33a).

A number of other mutations in FL have been reported at a lower frequency, and likely are later events in pathogenesis. The NF-κB pathway is dysregulated in FL (53,60). *TNFAIP3* encodes A20, a negative regulator of NF-κB, and its mutation leads to activation of this pathway. *CARD11* mutations have been reported in about 10 percent of cases (53,60). The JAK-STAT pathway is dysregulated as a result of mutations in *STAT6* or *SOCS1* in 10 to 20 percent of cases (53,81). B-cell development is altered in 10 to 15 percent of cases with *EBF1* mutations (53). *NOTCH* is

Table 13-1
GENETIC ABNORMALITIES IN FOLLICULAR LYMPHOMA

Gene Mutated	Frequency
t(14;18)(q32;q21)/*IGH-BCL2*	80-90%
KMT2D (MLL2)	80-90%
BCL2	~75%
EPHA7	~ 70%
CREBBP	60-70%
BCL6	~ 50%
TNFRSF14	30-50%
CREBBP	~ 30%
EZH2	~20%
MEF2B	~ 15%
ARID1A	~15%
BCL6 translocations	~15%
EP300	~ 15%
CARD11	~10%
STAT6	~10%
TNFAIP3/A20	5-25%
FAS	5-10%
FOXO1	5-10%
TP53	~ 5%

mutated in about 5 percent of cases (31). The FAS pathway is mutated in 5 to 10 percent of cases, resulting in impairment of apoptosis.

Follicular Lymphoma Microenvironment

As is true for many types of lymphoma, the tumor microenvironment plays a role in FL cell survival. Many benign cells are present within FLs, including a number of T-cell subsets, macrophages, FDCs, and stromal cells. It seems clear that FL cells and reactive cells in the follicular microenvironment exhibit extensive crosstalk and that the host response plays a role in FL cell survival. For example, FL cells are known to have mannosylated B-cell receptors, and macrophages in the tumor microenvironment have mannose receptors (37a). This interaction may help explain microenvironmental support of the growth of FL cells. T cells in the FL microenvironment are particularly heterogeneous and include T-follicular helper cells, CD8-positive cytolytic T cells, and T-regulatory cells as well as others. A

Table 13-2

FEATURES THAT DISTINGUISH FOLLICULAR HYPERPLASIA FROM FOLLICULAR LYMPHOMA

Feature	Follicular Hyperplasia	Follicular Lymphoma
Architecture	Preserved	Effaced
Number of follicles	Lower	Higher
Follicle size	Variable	Uniform
Follicle shape	Irregular	Regular
Mantle zones	Well developed	Poorly developed or absent
Polarization of follicle	Present	Often absent
Cytologic composition	Mixed	More uniform
Histiocytes	Many, often with starry sky pattern	Few
Mitotic figures	Many	Few (except grade 3)
Apoptotic cells	Often many	Few (except grade 3)
BCL2 expression	Negative	Positive
Monotypic Ig (flow)	Absent	Present
t(14;18)(q32;q21)	Absent	Present (~80%)

recent study has shown CD8-positive cells that recognize specific driver mutations in FL (51).

The microenvironment also plays a role in the prognosis of patients with FL. The seminal study by the Leukemia and Lymphoma Molecular Profiling Group of a large number of cases of FL showed two expression signatures that correlated with a better or worse survival period, ranging from 3.9 to 13.6 years (15). The signature designated immune response 1, associated with a better prognosis, encompassed many T-cell–associated genes as well as genes associated with monocytes. Immune response 2, associated with a poorer prognosis, represented a different set of genes associated with T cells and monocytes as well as genes associated with dendritic cells (15). Although helpful in terms of discovery, this approach is not practical and attempts to dissect out various reactive cell subsets involved in prognosis have been contradictory to date.

DIFFERENTIAL DIAGNOSIS

Reactive Follicular Hyperplasia. A number of morphologic features are helpful for distinguishing reactive follicular hyperplasia from FL (Table 13-2). In general, the number of follicles is lower in follicular hyperplasia than in FL (49). A high number of follicles accounts for the back-to-back distribution of follicles observed in typical cases of FL. Benign lymph node fol-

licles are usually restricted to, or are much more numerous in, the cortex and follicles are more often irregularly shaped or elliptical. In contrast, in FL follicles are more randomly distributed in the cortex and medulla, and the follicles are more uniform and rounder.

Reactive follicles have germinal centers with well-formed light and dark zones, also known as polarity. The light and dark zones are often lost in neoplastic follicles. Mantle zones are well developed in reactive follicles and are often accentuated at one pole of the follicle. In FL, mantle zones are commonly less well developed or absent and there is no accentuation.

Reactive follicles are composed of a heterogeneous population of cells including centrocytes, centroblasts, and tingible body macrophages that impart a "starry-sky" appearance; these histiocytes contain phagocytized apoptotic and karyorrhectic debris within their cytoplasm. Mitotic figures are also numerous. In contrast, in FL the cellular composition is more monotonous, tingible body macrophages are uncommon or absent, and mitotic figures are fewer in low-grade FL. For biopsy specimens that show a mixture of features, immunophenotypic and molecular analyses usually resolve this differential diagnosis easily, as FL is positive for monotypic surface Ig and BCL2 and carries monoclonal *IG* rearrangements and t(14;18)/*IGH-BCL2*.

Follicular Hyperplasia with a Monoclonal B-Cell Population. There are rare cases in which a lymph node biopsy specimen is benign and reactive using histologic criteria and yet flow cytometry or molecular analysis shows a monotypic B-cell population. In a study of six cases reported by Kussick et al. (34), the monotypic B-cell population was over 20 percent as assessed by flow cytometry immunophenotypic analysis. Most often, these patients are adolescents or young adults. Using immunohistochemistry, the germinal centers are negative for BCL2. Some of these cases, in retrospect, may be examples of pediatric-type FL.

Progressive Transformation of Germinal Centers (PTGC). Unlike FL, with the exception of the floral variant, the follicles of PTGC are usually large, 3 to 5 times the normal size of reactive follicles, and are composed of small mantle zone lymphocytes within germinal centers. In most cases of PTGC, the lymph node architecture is not replaced, unlike FL. In PTGC, the germinal center B-cells are negative for BCL2 and there is no evidence of a monotypic B-cell population by immunophenotypic analysis. Molecular studies show no evidence of monoclonal *IG* rearrangements or t(14;18)/*IGH-BCL2*.

Castleman Disease, Hyaline-Vascular Variant. In this variant of Castleman disease, the follicles are large, but widely spaced. The follicle germinal centers are depleted of lymphocytes and have distinctive hyaline-vascular lesions. Mantle zones show "onion skin" type features. These features differ greatly from those of most cases of FL. However, rare cases of FL have neoplastic follicles with some degree of lymphocyte depletion and bear some resemblance to Castleman disease follicles. In these cases, immunophenotypic and molecular studies resolve the differential diagnosis by showing evidence of monoclonality in FL.

Nodular Lymphocyte-Predominant Hodgkin Lymphoma (NLPHL). Both FL and NLPHL have a nodular pattern. In NLPHL, however, the nodules tend to be larger, with vague outlines, and are composed of many small round lymphocytes, epithelioid histiocytes, and scattered LP cells. Centrocytes and centroblasts are absent. The small lymphocytes and LP cells in NLPHL are negative for surface IG and CD10, and do not carry t(14;18)/*IGH-BCL2*, unlike FL.

Mantle Cell Lymphoma. In most cases of mantle cell lymphoma, the lymphoma cells are small and monotonous, and centroblasts are not present, unlike FL. Ancillary testing is helpful as the cells of mantle cell lymphoma are usually positive for CD5 and SOX11, negative for CD10 and BCL6, and carry t(11;14)(q13;q32)/*CCND1-IGH*, unlike cases of FL.

Nodal Marginal Zone Lymphoma. Nodal marginal zone lymphomas may have a marginal zone distribution, colonize follicles, or have a diffuse pattern, and are often composed of cells with abundant, pale cytoplasm. Plasmacytoid differentiation is common and mature monotypic plasma cells may be present. They are also commonly associated with reactive follicular hyperplasia. These lymphomas express BCL2, but usually are negative for CD10, BCL6, and other germinal center B-cell–associated markers; a subset is positive for MNDA and IRTA1; and they do not carry t(14;18)/*IGH-BCL2*. A major diagnostic dilemma is distinguishing t(14;18)-negative FL from nodal marginal zone lymphoma colonizing follicles. This differential diagnosis is discussed in more detail in chapter 14.

TREATMENT AND PROGNOSIS

Patients with an initial diagnosis of FL are generally subdivided into three groups for the planning of therapy: those with low-stage disease, advanced-stage disease with low tumor burden, and advanced-stage disease with a high tumor burden (19,29). The presence or absence of symptoms also influences therapeutic decisions.

Localized disease with a low disease burden occurs in 10 to 20 percent of patients. There is no consensus treatment for this subset. Involved field radiotherapy with curative intent is most often recommended, but for older patients, careful monitoring without therapy (watchful waiting) is used, particularly if the patient is asymptomatic. Patients with advanced-stage disease and low tumor burden also can undergo watchful waiting. If a patient is opposed to watchful waiting, single agent rituximab is a potential option.

Patients with advanced-stage disease and high tumor burden are most often treated with rituximab plus chemotherapy. The most commonly used chemotherapy regimen in the past has been rituximab, cyclophosphamide, doxorubicin, vincristine, and prednisone (R-CHOP), but other traditional chemotherapy regimens have been used and most recently, bendamustine plus rituximab has become a popular front-line regimen (19,29). Lenalidomide combined with rituximab also appears to be promising (29). Patients who relapse after therapy are candidates for combination chemotherapy and radioimmunotherapy, or selected patients may undergo stem cell transplantation (19,29).

In the past decade, the overall prognosis of FL patients has improved, with a median survival period of 10 to 12 years (19,29). This improved prognosis is attributable, in large part, to the use of anti-CD20 monoclonal antibody therapy. Other factors, such as earlier detection because of improved diagnostic tools and stage migration (recognition of minimal disease at sites previously thought to negative by morphologic examination alone) also may be involved.

A powerful predictor of poorer overall survival in patients with FL is a short (less than 2 years) length of remission after treatment with standard immunochemotherapy (9). In terms of predicting prognosis upfront, before therapy, the Follicular Lymphoma International Prognostic Index (FLIPI) and FLIPI-2 have gained

acceptance as tools for prognostication (18,73). The FLIPI, based on a large database of FL patients treated in the pre-rituximab era, separates FL patients into three prognostic groups and uses five independent predictive factors: age over 60 years, hemoglobin less than 12 g/dL, serum LDH greater than normal, Ann Arbor stage III/IV, and number of involved nodal areas greater than 4 (73). Higher scores correlate with a poorer prognosis. The FLIPI-2 system, based on FL patients treated in the rituximab era, employs a slightly different system with the following components: age over 60 years, hemoglobin less than 12 g/dL, bone marrow involvement, beta-2-microglobulin greater than normal, and longest diameter of largest involved lymph node over 6 cm (18).

Specific gene mutations have been correlated with prognosis (11,53,60). The m7-FLIPI has been proposed for prognostication of patients with FL. In this system, the FLIPI is combined with the mutation status of seven genes: *EZH2, ARID1A, MEF2B, EP300, FOXO1, CREBBP,* and *CARD11* (60). This system appears to refine prognostic groups of FL patients and seems to better identify high-risk patients, but this system will need to be validated by other groups.

REFERENCES

1. Adam P, Baumann R, Schmidt J, et al. The BCL2 E17 and SP66 antibodies discriminate 2 immunophenotypically and genetically distinct subgroups of conventionally BCL2-"negative" grade 1/2 follicular lymphomas. Hum Pathol 2013;44:1817-1826.
2. Adam P, Katzenberger T, Eifert M, et al. Presence of preserved reactive germinal centers in follicular lymphoma is a strong histopathologic indicator of limited disease stage. Am J Surg Pathol 2005;29:1661-1664.
3. Albinger-Hegyi A, Hochreutener B, Abdou MT, et al. High frequency of t(14;18)-translocation breakpoints outside of major breakpoint and minor cluster regions in follicular lymphoma: improved polymerase chain reaction protocols for their detection. Am J Pathol 2002;160:823-832.
4. Anderson JR, Armitage JO, Weisenburger DD. Epidemiology of the non-Hodgkin's lymphomas: distributions of the major subtypes differ by geographic locations. Non-Hodgkin's Lymphoma Classification Project. Ann Oncol 1998;9:717-720.
5. Bacon CM, Ye H, Diss TC, et al. Primary follicular lymphoma of the testis and epididymis in adults. Am J Surg Pathol 2007;31:1050-1058.
6. Biagi JJ, Seymour JF. Insights into the molecular pathogenesis of follicular lymphoma arising from geographic variation. Blood 2002;99:4265-4275.
7. Bosga-Bouwer AG, van den Berg A, Haralambieva E, et al. Molecular, cytogenetic, and immunophenotypic characterization of follicular lymphoma grade 3B; a separate entity or part of the spectrum of diffuse large B-cell lymphoma or follicular lymphoma? Hum Pathol 2006;37:528-533.
8. Bouska A, McKeithan TW, Deffenbacher KE, et al. Genome-wide copy-number analyses reveal genomic abnormalities involved in transformation of follicular lymphoma. Blood 2014;123:1681-1690.
9. Casulo C, Byrtek M, Dawson KL, et al. Early relapse of follicular lymphoma after rituximab plus cyclophosphamide, doxorubicin, vincristine, and prednisone defines patients at high risk for death: an analysis from the National LymphoCare Study. J Clin Oncol 2015;33:2516-2522.

10. Chang KC, Huang X, Medeiros LJ, Jones D. Germinal centre-like versus undifferentiated stromal immunophenotypes in follicular lymphoma. J Pathol 2003;201:404-412.

11. Cheung KJ, Johnson NA, Affleck JG, et al. Acquired TNFRSF14 mutations in follicular lymphoma are associated with worse prognosis. Cancer Res 2010;70:9166-9174.

12. Chihara D, Nastoupil LJ, Williams JN, Lee P, Koff JL, Flowers CR. New insights into the epidemiology of non-Hodgkin lymphoma and implications for therapy. Expert Rev Anticancer Ther 2015;15:531-544.

13. Chittal SM, Caveriviere P, Voigt JJ, et al. Follicular lymphoma with abundant PAS-positive extracellular material. Immunohistochemical and ultrastructural observations. Am J Surg Pathol 1987;11:618-624.

14. Coffing BN, Lim MS. Signet ring cell lymphoma in a patient with elevated CA-125. J Clin Oncol 2011;29:e416-418.

15. Dave SS, Wright G, Tan B, et al. Prediction of survival in follicular lymphoma based on molecular features of tumor-infiltrating immune cells. N Engl J Med 2004;351:2159-2169.

16. El-Behery RA, Laurini JA, Weisenburger DD, et al. Follicular large cleaved cell lymphoma is a distinctive morphological and clinical variant of follicular lymphoma. Mod Pathol 2013;26(Suppl 2):327A-328A.

17. Espinet B, Bellosillo B, Melero C, et al. FISH is better than BIOMED-2 PCR to detect IgH/BCL2 translocation in follicular lymphoma at diagnosis using paraffin-embedded tissue. Leuk Res 2008;32:737-742.

18. Federico M, Bellei M, Marcheselli L, et al. Follicular lymphoma international prognostic index 2: a new prognostic index for follicular lymphoma developed by the International Follicular Lymphoma Prognostic Factor Project. J Clin Oncol 2009;27:4555-4562.

19. Freedman A. Follicular lymphoma: 2015 update on diagnosis and management. Am J Hematol 2015;90:1172-1178.

20. Goates JJ, Kamel OW, LeBrun DP, Benharroch D, Dorfman RF. Floral variant of follicular lymphoma. Immunological and molecular studies support a neoplastic process. Am J Surg Pathol 1994;18:37-47.

21. Hans CP, Weisenburger DD, Vose JM, et al. A significant diffuse component predicts for inferior survival in grade 3 follicular lymphomas, but cytologic subtypes do not predict survival. Blood 2003;101:2363-2367.

22. Harris NL, Swerdlow SH, Jaffe ES, et al. Follicular lymphoma. In: Swerdlow SH, Campo E, Harris NL, Jaffe ES, Pileri SA, Stein H, Thiele J, Vardiman JW, eds. WHO classification of tumours of haematopoietic and lymphoid tissues. Lyon: IARC Press; 2008:220-228.

23. Harada A, Oguchi M, Terui Y, et al. Radiation therapy for localized duodenal low-grade follicular lymphoma. J Radiat Res 2016;57:412-417.

24. Höglund M, Sehn L, Connors JM, et al. Identification of cytogenetic subgroups and karyotypic pathways of clonal evolution in follicular lymphomas. Genes Chromosomes Cancer 2004;39:195-204.

25. Horn H, Schmelter C, Leich E, et al. Follicular lymphoma grade 3B is a distinct neoplasm according to cytogenetic and immunohistochemical profiles. Haematologica 2011;96:1327-1334.

26. Howard MT, Dufresne S, Swerdlow SH, Cook JR. Follicular lymphoma of the spleen: multiparameter analysis of 16 cases. Am J Clin Pathol 2009;131:656-662.

27. Iancu D, Hao S, Lin P, et al. Follicular lymphoma in staging bone marrow specimens: correlation of histologic findings with the results of flow cytometry immunophenotypic analysis. Arch Pathol Lab Med 2007;131:282-287.

28. Jardin F, Gaulard P, Buchonnet G, et al. Follicular lymphoma without BCL-6 rearrangement: a lymphoma subtype with distinct pathological, molecular and clinical characteristics. Leukemia 2002;16:2309-2317.

29. Kahl BS, Yang D. Follicular lymphoma: evolving therapeutic strategies. Blood 2016;127:2055-2063.

30. Karube K, Guo Y, Suzumiya J, et al. CD10-MUM1+ follicular lymphoma lacks BCL2 gene translocation and shows characteristic biologic and clinical features. Blood 2007;109:3076-3079.

31. Karube K, Martínez D, Royo C, et al. Recurrent mutations of NOTCH genes in follicular lymphoma identify a distinctive subset of tumours. J Pathol 2014;234:423-430.

32. Kelly RS, Roulland S, Morgado E, et al. Determinants of the t(14;18) translocation and their role in t(14;18)-positive follicular lymphoma. Cancer Causes Control 2015;26:1845-1855.

33. Kojima M, Yamanaka S, Yoshida T, et al. Histological variety of floral variant of follicular lymphoma. APMIS 2006;114:626-632.

33a. Krysiak K1, Gomez F, White BS, et al. Recurrent somatic mutations affecting B-cell receptor signaling pathway genes in follicular lymphoma. Blood 2017;129:473-483.

34. Kussick SJ, Kalnoski M, Braziel RM, Wood BL. Prominent clonal B-cell populations identified by flow cytometry in histologically reactive lymphoid proliferations. Am J Clin Pathol 2004;121:464-472.

35. Leich E, Hoster E, Wartenberg M, et al. Similar clinical features in follicular lymphomas with and without breaks in the BCL2 locus. Leukemia 2016;30:854-860.

36. Li H, Kaminski MS, Li Y, et al. Mutations in linker histone genes HIST1H1 B, C, D, and E; OCT2 (POU2F2); IRF8; and ARID1A underlying the pathogenesis of follicular lymphoma. Blood 2014;123:1487-1498.

37. Li Y, Hu S, Zuo Z, et al. CD5-positive follicular lymphoma: clinicopathologic correlations and outcome in 88 cases. Mod Pathol 2015;28:787-798.

37a. Linley A, Krysov S, Ponzoni M, Johnson PW, Packham G, Stevenson FK. Lectin binding to surface Ig variable regions provides a universal persistent activating signal for follicular lymphoma cells. Blood 2015;126:1902-1910.

38. Lones MA, Raphael M, McCarthy K, et al. Primary follicular lymphoma of the testis in children and adolescents. J Pediatr Hematol Oncol 2012;34:68-71.

39. Lorsbach RB, Shay-Seymore D, Moore J, et al. Clinicopathologic analysis of follicular lymphoma occurring in children. Blood 2002;99:1959-1964.

40. Louissaint A Jr, Ackerman AM, Dias-Santagata D, et al. Pediatric-type nodal follicular lymphoma: an indolent clonal proliferation in children and adults with high proliferation index and no BCL2 rearrangement. Blood 2012;120:2395-2404.

40a. Louissaint A Jr, Schafernak KT, Geyer JT, et al. Pediatric-type nodal follicular lymphoma: a biologically distinct lymphoma with frequent MAPK pathway mutations. Blood 2016;128:1093-1100.

41. Mackrides N, Campuzano-Zuluaga G, Maque-Acosta Y, et al. Epstein-Barr virus-positive follicular lymphoma. Mod Pathol 2017;30:519-529.

42. Mann RB, Berard CW. Criteria for the cytologic subclassification of follicular lymphomas: a proposed alternative method. Hematol Oncol 1983;1:187-192.

43. Marafioti T, Copie-Bergman C, Calaminici M, et al. Another look at follicular lymphoma: immunophenotypic and molecular analyses identify distinct follicular lymphoma subgroups. Histopathology 2013;62:860-875.

44. Marcheselli L, Bari A, Anastasia A, et al. Prognostic roles of absolute monocyte and absolute lymphocyte counts in patients with advanced-stage follicular lymphoma in the rituximab era: an analysis from the FOLL05 trial of the Fondazione Italiana Linfomi. Br J Haematol 2015;169:544-551.

45. Martin-Guerrero I, Salaverria I, Burkhardt B, et al. Recurrent loss of heterozygosity in 1p36 associated with TNFRSF14 mutations in IRF4 translocation negative pediatric follicular lymphomas. Haematologica 2013;98:1237-1241.

46. Mir MA, Maurer MJ, Ziesmer SC, et al. Elevated serum levels of IL-2R, IL-1RA, and CXCL9 are associated with a poor prognosis in follicular lymphoma. Blood 2015;125:992-998.

47. Morton LM, Wang SS, Devesa SS, Hartge P, Weisenburger DD, Linet MS. Lymphoma incidence patterns by WHO subtype in the United States, 1992-2001. Blood 2006;107:265-276.

48. Nathwani BN, Anderson JR, Armitage JO, et al. Clinical significance of follicular lymphoma with monocytoid B cells. Non-Hodgkin's Lymphoma Classification Project. Hum Pathol 1999;30:263-268.

49. Nathwani BN, Winberg CD, Diamond LW, Bearman RM, Kim H. Morphologic criteria for the differentiation of follicular lymphoma from florid reactive follicular hyperplasia: a study of 80 cases. Cancer 1981;48:1794-1806.

50. Natkunam Y, Warnke RA, Zehnder JL, Jones CD, Milatovich-Cherry A, Cornbleet PJ. Blastic/blastoid transformation of follicular lymphoma: immunohistologic and molecular analyses of five cases. Am J Surg Pathol 2000;24:525-534.

51. Nielsen JS, Sedgwick CG, Shahid A, et al. Toward personalized lymphoma immunotherapy: identification of common driver mutations recognized by patient CD8+ T cells. Clin Cancer Res 2016;22:2226-2236.

52. No authors listed. A clinical evaluation of the international Lymphoma Study Group classification of non-Hodgkin's lymphoma. The Non-Hodgkin's Lymphoma Classification Project. Blood 1997;89:3909-3918.

53. Okosun J, Bodor C, Wang J, et al. Integrated genomic analysis identifies recurrent mutations and evolution patterns driving the initiation and progression of follicular lymphoma. Nat Genet 2014;46:176-181.

54. Oricchio E, Ciriello G, Jiang M, et al. Frequent disruption of the RB pathway in indolent follicular lymphoma suggests a new combination therapy. J Exp Med 2014;211:1379-1391.

55. Oricchio E, Nanjangud G, Wolfe AL, The Eph-Receptor A7 is a soluble tumor suppressor for follicular lymphoma. Cell 2011;147:554-564.

56. Osborne BM, Butler JJ. Follicular lymphoma mimicking progressive transformation of germinal centers. Am J Clin Pathol 1987;88:264-269.

57. Osborne BM, Butler JJ, Variakojis D, Kott M. Reactive lymph node hyperplasia with giant follicles. Am J Clin Pathol 1982;78:493-499.

58. Ott G, Katzenberger T, Lohr A, et al. Cytomorphologic, immunohistochemical, and cytogenetic profiles of follicular lymphoma: 2 types of follicular lymphoma grade 3. Blood 2002;99:3806-3812.

59. Pasqualucci L, Dominguez-Sola D, Chiarenza A, et al. Inactivating mutations of acetyltransferase genes in B-cell lymphoma. Nature 2011;471:189-195.

60. Pastore A, Jurinovic V, Kridel R, et al. Integration of gene mutations in risk prognostication for patients receiving first-line immunochemotherapy for follicular lymphoma: a retrospective analysis of a prospective clinical trial and validation in a population-based registry. Lancet Oncol 2015;16:1111-1122.

61. Robetorye RS, Bohling SD, Medeiros LJ, Elenitoba-Johnson KS. Follicular lymphoma with monocytoid B-cell proliferation: molecular assessment of the clonal relationship between the follicular and monocytoid B-cell components. Lab Invest 2000;80:1593-1599.

62. Rosas-Uribe A, Variakojis D, Rappaport H. Proteinaceous precipitate in nodular (follicular) lymphomas. Cancer 1973;31:532-542.

63. Roulland S, Faroudi M, Mamessier E, Sungalee S, Salles G, Nadel B. Early steps of follicular lymphoma pathogenesis. Adv Immunol 2011;111:1-46.

64. Salaverria I, Martin-Guerrero I, Burkhardt B, et al. High resolution copy number analysis of IRF4 translocation-positive diffuse large B-cell and follicular lymphomas. Genes Chromosomes Cancer 2013;52:150-155.

65. Salaverria I, Philipp C, Oschlies I, et al. Translocations activating IRF4 identify a subtype of germinal center-derived B-cell lymphoma affecting predominantly children and young adults. Blood 2011;118:139-147.

66. Salles GA. Clinical features, prognosis and treatment of follicular lymphoma. Hematology Am Soc Hematol Educ Program 2007;216-225.

67. Sant M, Allemani C, Tereanu C, et al. Incidence of hematologic malignancies in Europe by morphologic subtype: results of the HAEMACARE project. Blood 2010;116:3724-3734.

68. Sarkozy C, Baseggio L, Feugier P, et al. Peripheral blood involvement in patients with follicular lymphoma: a rare disease manifestation associated with poor prognosis. Br J Haematol 2014;164:659-667.

69. Sato Y, Ichimura K, Tanaka T, et al. Duodenal follicular lymphomas share common characteristics with mucosa-associated lymphoid tissue lymphomas. J Clin Pathol 2008;61:377-381.

70. Schraders M, de Jong D, Kluin P, Groenen P, van Krieken H. Lack of Bcl-2 expression in follicular lymphoma may be caused by mutations in the BCL2 gene or by absence of the t(14;18) translocation. J Pathol 2005;20:329-335

71. Shia J, Teruya-Feldstein J, Pan D, et al. Primary follicular lymphoma of the gastrointestinal tract: a clinical and pathologic study of 26 cases. Am J Surg Pathol 2002;26:216-224.

72. Siddiqi IN, Friedman J, Barry-Holson KQ, et al. Characterization of a variant of t(14;18) negative nodal diffuse follicular lymphoma with CD23 expression, 1p36/TNFRSF14 abnormalities, and STAT6 mutations. Mod Pathol 2016;29:570-581.

73. Solal-Celigny P, Roy P, Colombat P, et al. Follicular lymphoma international prognostic index. Blood 2004;104:1258-1265.

74. Sungalee S, Mamessier E, Morgado E, et al. Germinal center reentries of BCL2-overexpressing B cells drive follicular lymphoma progression. J Clin Invest 2014;124:5337-5350.

75. Swerdlow SH, Campo E, Pileri SA, et al. The 2016 revision of the World Health Organization classification of lymphoid neoplasms. Blood 2016;127:2375-2390.

76. Tiesinga JJ, Wu CD, Inghirami G. CD5+ follicle center lymphoma. Immunophenotyping detects a unique subset of "floral" follicular lymphoma. Am J Clin Pathol 2000;114:912-921.

77. Torlakovic E, Torlakovic G, Brunning RD. Follicular pattern of bone marrow involvement by follicular lymphoma. Am J Clin Pathol 2002;118:780-786.

78. Vergier B, Belaud-Rotureau MA, Benassy MN, et al. Neoplastic cells do not carry bcl2-JH rearrangements detected in a subset of primary cutaneous follicle center B-cell lymphomas. Am J Surg Pathol 2004;28:748-755.

79. Wahlin BE, Yri OE, Kimby E, et al. Clinical significance of the WHO grades of follicular lymphoma in a population-based cohort of 505 patients with long follow-up times. Br J Haematol 2012;156:225-233.

80. Wang SA, Wang L, Hochberg EP, Muzikansky A, Harris NL, Hasserjian RP. Low histologic grade follicular lymphoma with high proliferation index: morphologic and clinical features. Am J Surg Pathol 2005;29:1490-1496.

81. Yildiz M, Li H, Bernard D, et al. Activating STAT6 mutations in follicular lymphoma. Blood 2015;125:668-679.

82. Yoshino T, Miyake K, Ichimura K, et al. Increased incidence of follicular lymphoma in the duodenum. Am J Surg Pathol 2000;24:688-693.

83. Young NA. Grading follicular lymphoma on fine-needle aspiration specimens - a practical approach. Cancer 2006;108:1-9.

14 NODAL MARGINAL ZONE LYMPHOMA

GENERAL FEATURES

Nodal marginal zone lymphoma (MZL) is a primary neoplasm of mature B cells originating in lymph nodes. Marginal zone lymphoma involving lymph nodes (usually regional) in patients with extranodal or splenic MZL is excluded from this category (9).

This entity was originally described and named *monocytoid B-cell lymphoma* by Sheibani et al. (30), who thought the neoplastic cells resembled the monocytoid B cells commonly observed in lymph nodes of patients with infection by *Toxoplasma* species or human immunodeficiency virus (HIV). Subsequently, the name was changed to nodal marginal zone lymphoma, which is used in the World Health Organization (WHO) classification (9).

In retrospect, the designation nodal marginal zone lymphoma has some limitations. Nodal MZL is a distinctive biologic entity that is clearly different from extranodal and splenic MZL, despite their very similar names. In addition, the cell of origin of nodal MZL is not precisely defined. This group of tumors appears to be heterogeneous at the molecular level and may arise from more than one cell type in the lymph node marginal zone (10). Origin from monocytoid B cells in a some cases is not excluded.

Nodal MZL is uncommon, with an incidence of less than 1 in 100,000 adults per year and representing 1 to 2 percent of all lymphoid neoplasms (3,19,26,33). Its etiology is poorly understood. An association with hepatitis C virus infection has been observed and is common in some geographic locations (8,22,32). Associations with HIV infection and autoimmune diseases are known (1,2). Nodal marginal zone hyperplasia in children, a possible precursor of pediatric nodal MZL, is associated with *Haemophilus influenzae* infection (20).

Biased use of immunoglobulin heavy chain variable regions has been reported, suggesting a role for antigen selection (10,21). In aggregate, these data implicate a role for chronic inflammation in lymphomagenesis, as has been reviewed by others (33).

CLINICAL FEATURES

Nodal MZL occurs predominantly in individuals in the seventh decade of life, and the disease is slightly more common in men or is equally distributed among the sexes (1,19,32a). Cases that are reported in children are typically localized at presentation and show a male predominance, with a male to female ratio of 5.4 to 1.0 (13,27a).

Most often, patients present with painless localized or generalized enlargement of peripheral lymph nodes (2,3). Head and neck lymph nodes are most frequently involved and the disease is rarely bulky (33). The bone marrow is involved in approximately one third of patients and leukemic involvement occurs in a small subset of patients (3,26,32a). Elevated serum lactate dehydrogenase and/or beta-2-microglobulin levels occur in 20 to 30 percent of patients (23). A serum paraprotein, most often of IgM type and usually at a low level, is present in approximately 10 to 15 percent of patients (1,27a,33).

HISTOLOGIC FINDINGS

Lymph Nodes

Nodal MZL involves the lymph nodes in a diffuse, interfollicular, or nodular pattern (figs. 14-1–14-3) (4,8,29,30,34). In some cases, there is a marginal zone pattern (fig. 14-2), characterized by neoplastic cells expanding the lymph node marginal zones and growing outward into interfollicular areas and inward into follicle centers. Reactive follicles are common and may be expanded and hyperplastic. In some cases, the follicles are well preserved, with reactive germinal centers and an intact lymphoid cuff (fig. 14-4); in other cases, the lymphoid follicles are regressed and lack well-formed germinal centers.

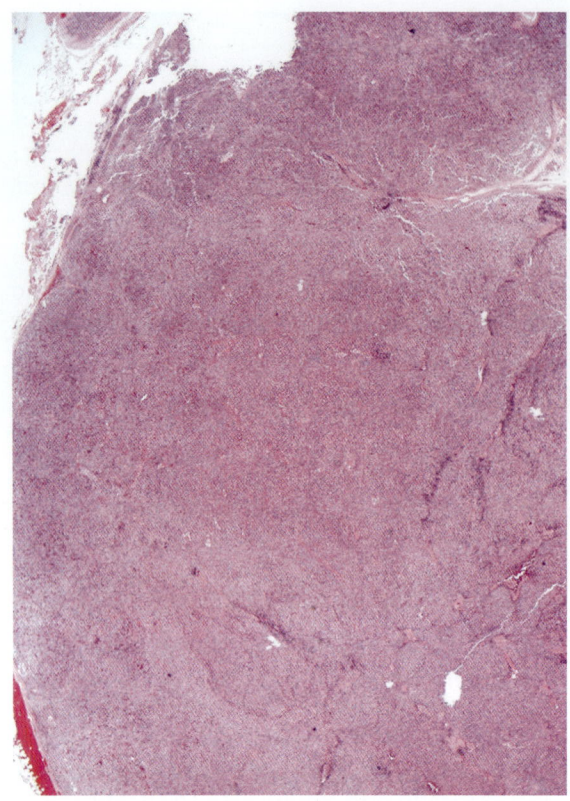

Figure 14-1

NODAL MARGINAL ZONE LYMPHOMA DIFFUSELY REPLACING LYMPH NODE

The neoplasm has a pale appearance at low power magnification because the cells have abundant cytoplasm (hematoxylin and eosin [H&E] stain).

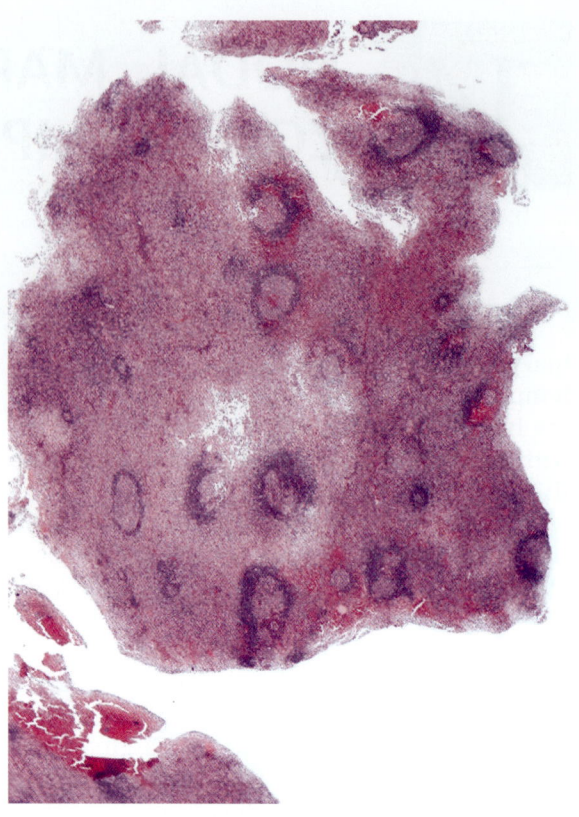

Figure 14-2

NODAL MARGINAL ZONE LYMPHOMA: MARGINAL ZONE AND INTERFOLLICULAR PATTERN

The lymphoma spares reactive follicles with hyperplastic germinal centers and variably formed mantle zones (H&E stain).

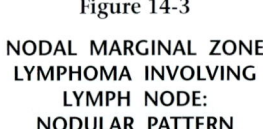

Figure 14-3

NODAL MARGINAL ZONE LYMPHOMA INVOLVING LYMPH NODE: NODULAR PATTERN

A: The prominent nodular pattern mimics follicular lymphoma.

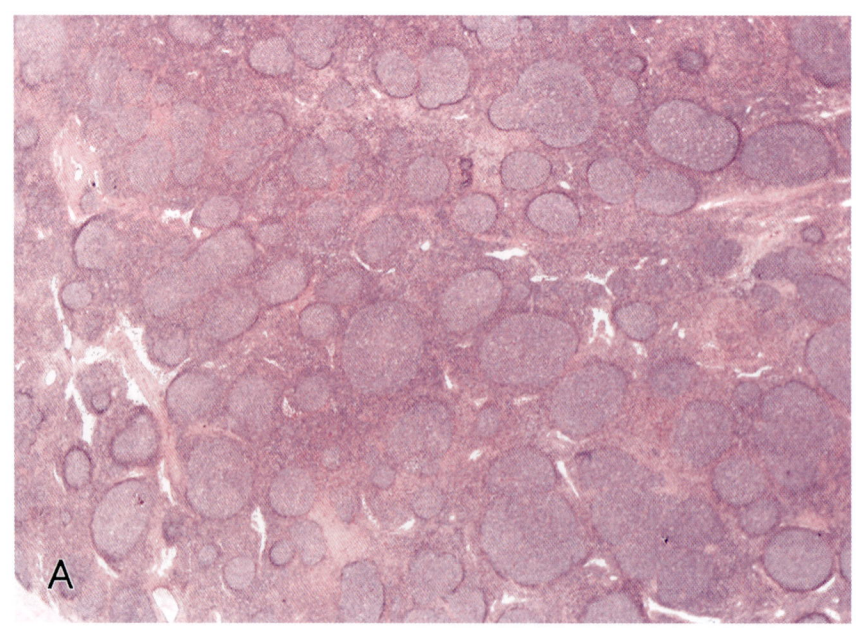

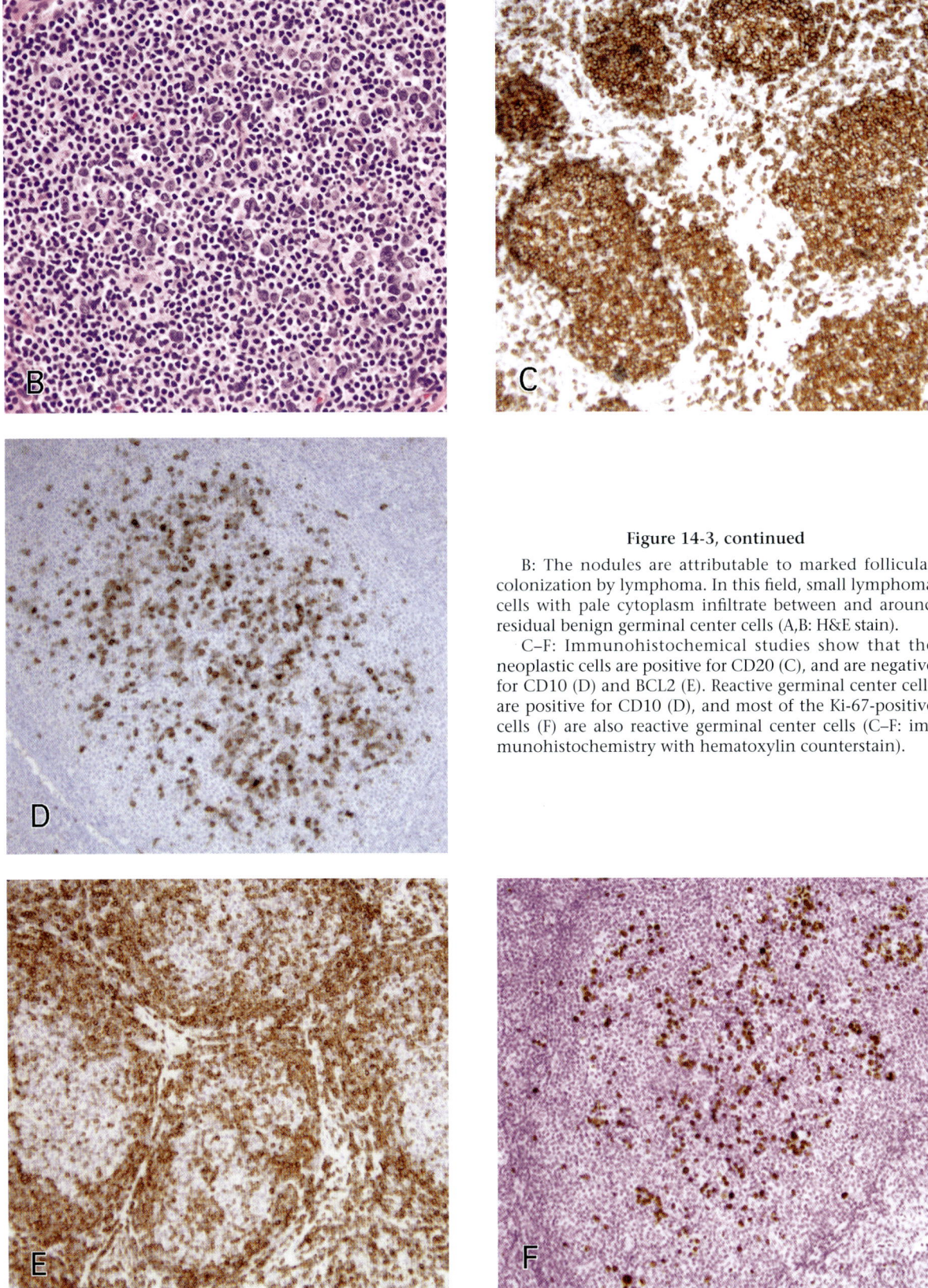

Figure 14-3, continued

B: The nodules are attributable to marked follicular colonization by lymphoma. In this field, small lymphoma cells with pale cytoplasm infiltrate between and around residual benign germinal center cells (A,B: H&E stain).

C–F: Immunohistochemical studies show that the neoplastic cells are positive for CD20 (C), and are negative for CD10 (D) and BCL2 (E). Reactive germinal center cells are positive for CD10 (D), and most of the Ki-67-positive cells (F) are also reactive germinal center cells (C–F: immunohistochemistry with hematoxylin counterstain).

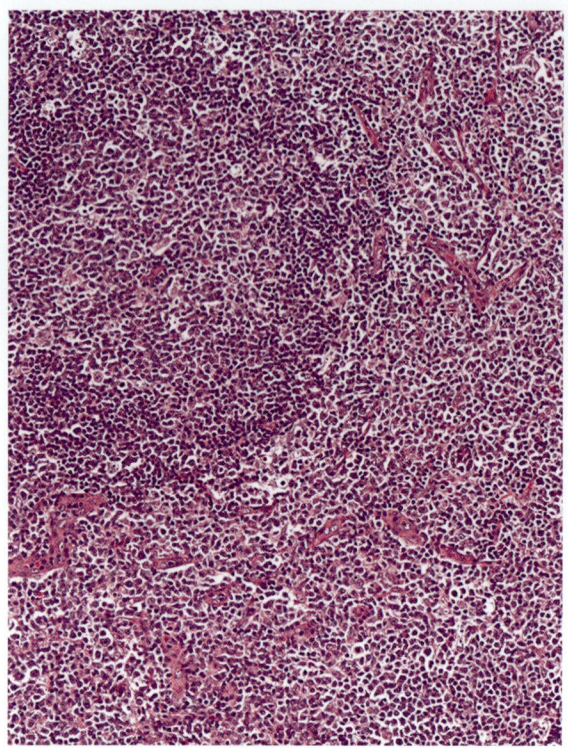

Figure 14-4

**NODAL MARGINAL ZONE
LYMPHOMA INVOLVING LYMPH NODE**

Nodal MZL partially replaces the lymph node, sparing a reactive follicle composed of a reactive germinal center and a mostly intact, but thin mantle zone (H&E stain).

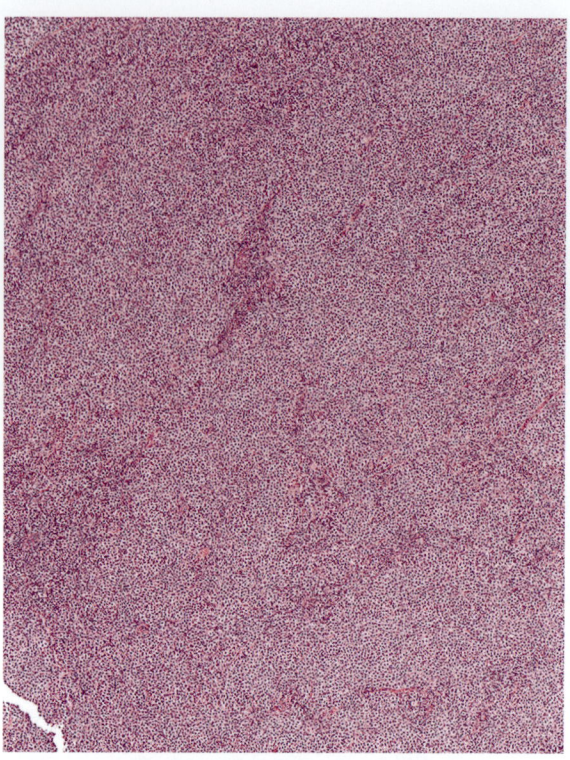

Figure 14-5

**NODAL MARGINAL ZONE LYMPHOMA ALMOST
COMPLETELY REPLACING LYMPH NODE**

The lymphoma has a diffuse and vaguely nodular pattern (H&E stain).

Commonly, neoplastic cells infiltrate the follicles, known as follicular colonization, and disrupt the follicular architecture (fig. 14-3 A,B). In some cases, vague nodules coalesce to form ill-defined sheets and aggregates (fig. 14-5).

Nodal MZLs show a spectrum of cytologic findings (4,27a,29,30,34). In most cases the neoplastic cell population is polymorphous, with a mixture of centrocyte-like cells, small lymphocytes, monocytoid lymphocytes, and large cells (blasts) (fig. 14-6). Plasmacytoid differentiation (fig. 14-7) is common and observed in the form of plasmacytoid lymphocytes and plasma cells. (In some cases, plasma cells are prominent, simulating plasmacytoma.)

In 10 to 20 percent of cases, the neoplastic cells are predominantly small and monocytoid (fig. 14-8) (4,30). These cells have central nuclei, abundant pale cytoplasm, and well-defined cell membranes. Monocytoid cells are often abundant in cases with well-defined follicles. Large

cells are also present but are usually a minority cell population in predominantly monocytoid cases. Sheets of large cells are not present in nodal MZL unless transformation to large B-cell lymphoma has occurred.

In children, a variant of nodal MZL has been described in which large nodules composed of enlarged tumor-infiltrated follicles are present. These nodules, in part, resemble progressively transformed germinal centers (fig. 14-9) (13,32). This variant has been designated as *pediatric nodal MZL* in the WHO classification (32).

Bone Marrow

Nodal MZL can involve the bone marrow, usually in a mixed paratrabecular and non-paratrabecular pattern (16). The cell population mirrors that observed in lymph nodes except that the number of large cells is often fewer. Antibodies reactive with CD21 and CD23 highlight irregular follicular dendritic cell networks

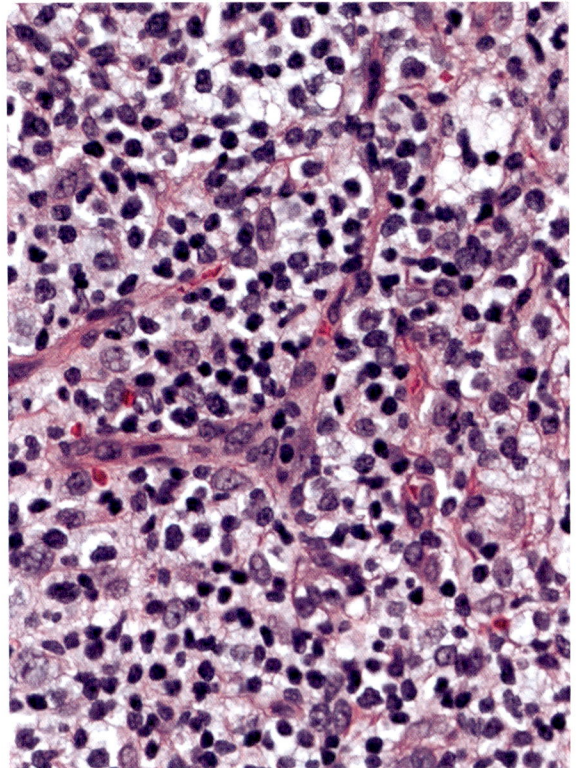

Figure 14-6

**NODAL MARGINAL ZONE LYMPHOMA
INVOLVING LYMPH NODE**

This nodal MZL is composed of a polymorphous mixture of small irregular lymphocytes (centrocyte-like cells), monocytoid cells, and scattered large blasts (H&E stain).

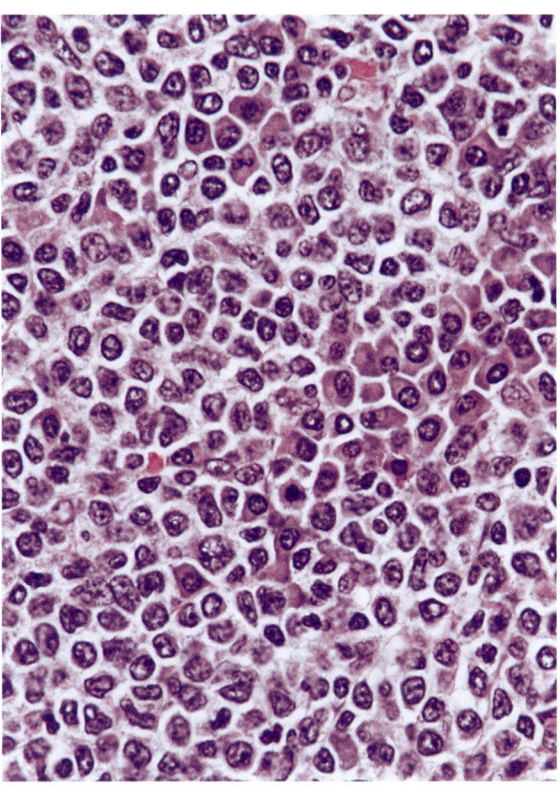

Figure 14-7

**NODAL MARGINAL ZONE LYMPHOMA
INVOLVING LYMPH NODE**

Many small irregular lymphocytes, plasmacytoid lymphocytes, and plasma cells are seen (H&E stain).

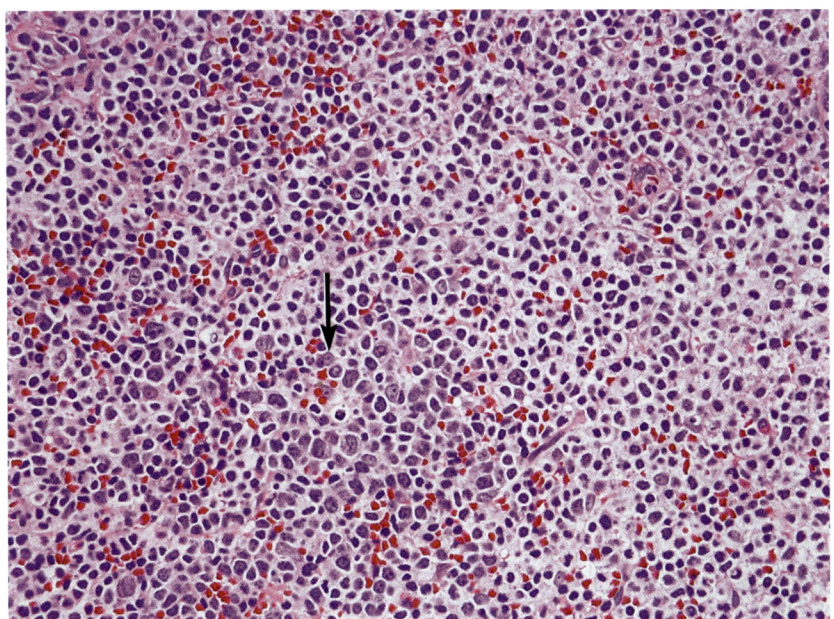

Figure 14-8

**NODAL MARGINAL ZONE
LYMPHOMA INVOLVING
LYMPH NODE**

A population of monocytoid lymphocytes with pale/clear cytoplasm is seen. A "naked" germinal center without a mantle zone cuff (arrow) is also present in this field (H&E stain). (This image corresponds to the case shown in fig. 14-1.)

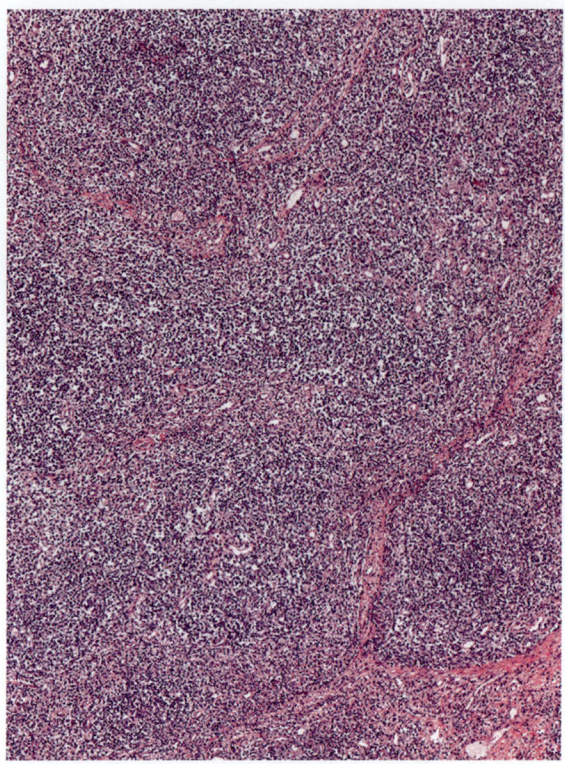

Figure 14-9

**NODAL MARGINAL ZONE LYMPHOMA
ARISING IN A CHILD (PEDIATRIC VARIANT)**

The lymphoma is characterized by large nodules composed of tumor-infiltrated follicles which form structures that resemble, in part, progressively transformed germinal centers (H&E stain).

associated with the lymphoma aggregates. Rarely, a sinusoidal pattern is present.

CYTOLOGIC FINDINGS

The infiltrate in nodal MZL is characterized by cells with irregularly shaped nuclei, slightly clumped chromatin, inconspicuous nucleoli, and pale to clear cytoplasm. Some cells with abundant pale to clear cytoplasm resemble monocytoid B cells; although commonly a minority population these cells can be numerous (fig. 14-10A,B). The infiltrate also may contain plasmacytoid lymphocytes and plasma cells. A variable number of large transformed cells is also consistently present and may represent up to 20 percent of the neoplastic cell population (fig. 14-10C). The delicate pale cytoplasm of monocytoid cells can be disrupted during the smearing of aspirates.

IMMUNOPHENOTYPIC FINDINGS

Nodal MZL is easily assessed by flow cytometry immunophenotypic analysis. The neoplastic cells express monotypic surface immunoglobulin light chain, CD11c (common), CD19, CD20, CD22, CD79a, and FMC7 (common). CD38 and CD43 are positive in approximately 50 percent of cases. IgD is usually negative, but may be expressed in a minority of cases. The neoplastic cells are negative for pan-T-cell markers as well as CD10 and CD21. CD5 is usually negative but is expressed in 10 to 15 percent of cases (8,17). CD23 is partially or fully expressed in 10 to 20 percent of tumors (4,8).

Immunohistochemistry has a valuable role in assessing nodal MZL. The lymphoma cells are usually positive for pan-B-cell antigens, including CD20 (figs. 14-3C, 14-11), CD79A, PAX5, and OCT2. The neoplastic cells commonly express MUM1 and BCL2 (fig. 14-3E). Myeloid cell nuclear differentiation antigen (MNDA), TBX21/T-bet, and immunoglobulin superfamily receptor translocation-associated 1 (IRTA-1) are expressed in approximately 75 percent of nodal MZLs (4,14,24). Purely monocytoid cases of nodal MZL are less often positive for T-bet or IRTA-1 (4). About 25 percent of cases are positive for DBA.44 (8).

In situ hybridization for Epstein-Barr virus (EBV)-encoded RNA (EBER1) is uncommonly (less than 10 percent) positive (4,8). EBV latent membrane protein is usually negative. Ki-67 usually shows a low proliferation rate, ranging from 10 to 30 percent. Most cases of nodal MZL are negative for SOX11, but moderate to bright SOX11 expression has been reported rarely (37). Nodal MZLs are usually negative for CD1a, CD3, CD10 (fig. 14-3D), CD21, CD23, CD30 (usually), CD279 (PD-1), cyclin D1, ALK, annexin A1, p53, LMO2, GCET1, HGAL/GCET2, BCL6, and nuclear BCL10.

Evidence of underlying follicular remnants is revealed by antibodies specific for follicular dendritic cells, such as CD21, CD23 (fig. 14-12), or clusterin, among others. Importantly, a small subset of nodal MZL cases, especially cases that show follicular colonization and increased large cells, express (usually dim) germinal center B-cell antigens, most often BCL6, LMO2, and CD10 (35,36). Reactive T cells may be numerous and many PD-1-positive T cells have been

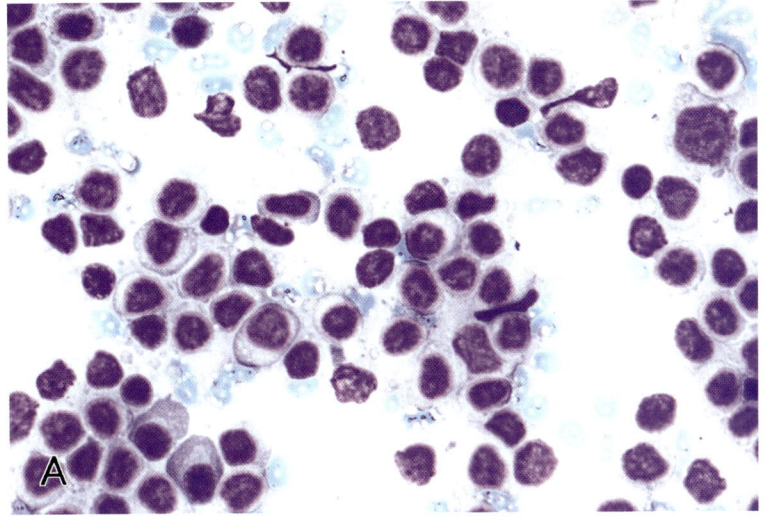

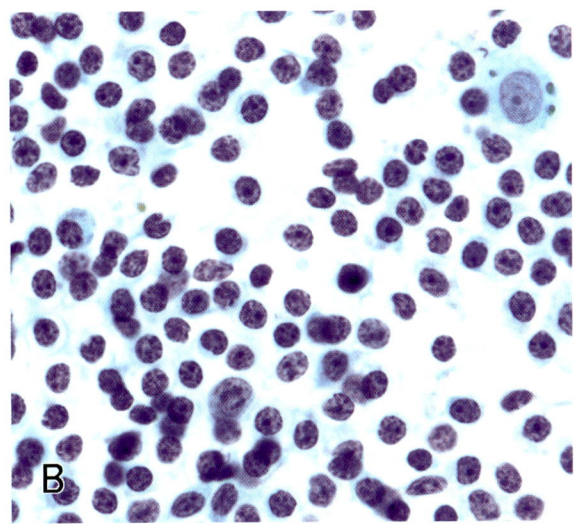

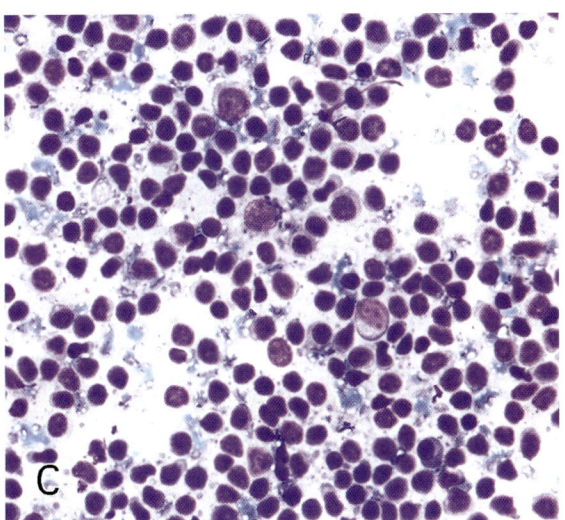

Figure 14-10

NODAL MARGINAL ZONE LYMPHOMA CYTOLOGY

Each image shows variable proportions of small lymphocytes, monocytoid lymphocytes, plasmacytoid cells, histiocytes, and larger blasts. The air-dried smears highlight monocytoid and plasmacytoid cells (A,C: Diff-Quik stain; B: Papanicolaou stain).

Figure 14-11

NODAL MARGINAL ZONE LYMPHOMA: CD20

Nodal MZL cells brightly express CD20 and other pan-B-cell antigens. Many follicles also can be appreciated in this field (immunohistochemistry with hematoxylin counterstain).

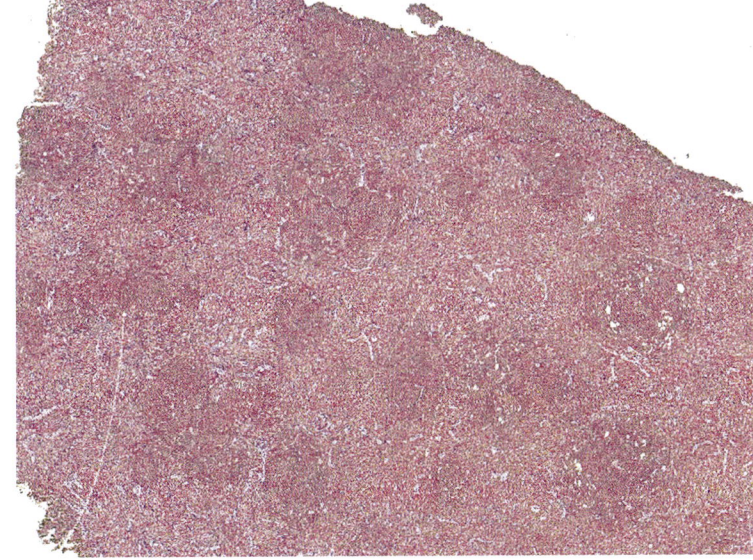

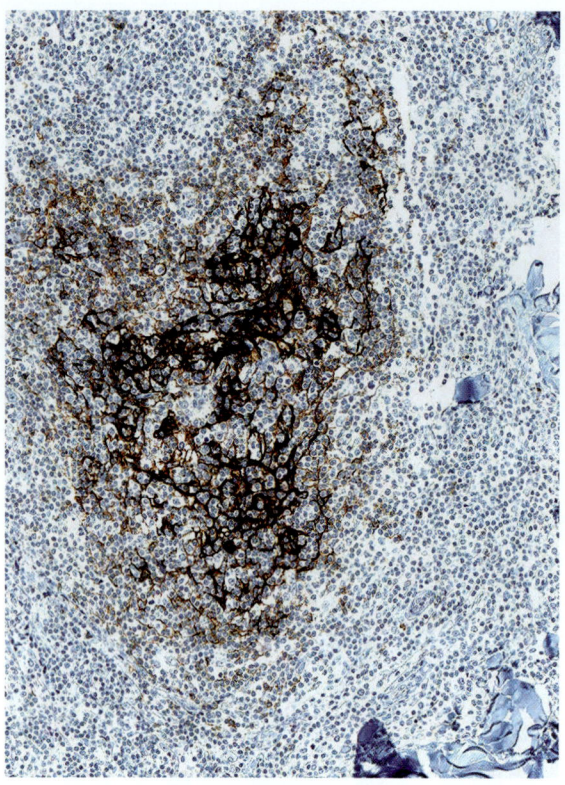

Figure 14-12

**NODAL MARGINAL ZONE
LYMPHOMA: FDC NETWORK**

A residual follicle in the center of the field is highlighted by the CD23 antibody. A partially disrupted follicular dendritic cell (FDC) network within nodules is common in nodal MZL (immunohistochemistry with hematoxylin counterstain).

observed in a subset of cases (4). Histiocytes are also numerous in some cases.

MOLECULAR GENETIC FINDINGS

Conventional cytogenetic analysis has shown a number of abnormalities in nodal MZL, but no recurrent specific chromosomal translocations have been reported (7). One case with a t(11;14)(q23;q32)/*DDX6-IGH* was reported (31), as were trisomies of chromosomes 3, 7, 12, and 18 (6,11,34). Trisomy of chromosome 3 is the most common (11,33).

Comparative genomic hybridization analysis of nodal MZL has shown frequent gains of chromosomal loci 1q, 2p, 3p, 3q, 6p, 6q, and 18q, and losses of 1q and 6q (5,20). Trisomy 3 occurs in about 25 percent of cases of nodal

MZL and gains of 18q23/NFATC1 occur in up to 50 percent of cases (33). Krijgsman et al. (21) reported that cases of nodal MZL and BCL2-negative follicular lymphoma share many DNA alterations. Genome-wide DNA profiling studies have shown that the DNA copy number changes seen in nodal MZLs share many abnormalities with extranodal MZLs (5). Unlike splenic MZLs, deletions of 7q are rare in nodal MZL (21,28). Chromosomal translocations that are known to occur in a subset of extranodal MZLs have not been identified in nodal MZLs.

As has been reviewed by Thieblemont et al. (33), a number of recent studies and abstracts have better defined the spectrum of molecular changes in nodal MZL. Gene expression profiling and microRNA analysis have shown differences in the profiles of nodal MZL versus follicular lymphoma. Overall, the NF-κB, B-cell receptor, toll-like receptor, and NOTCH pathways are important. In particular, sequencing methods have shown mutations of *KMT2D/MLL2* (about 35 percent), *TNFAIP3/A20* (about 33 percent), protein tyrosine phosphatase receptor delta (PTPRD; about 20 percent), *NOTCH2* (about 20 percent), and *KLF2* (17 percent) in nodal MZL (30a). *PTPRD* appears to be specific for nodal MZL. There is also evidence of activation of chromatin remodeling/transcriptional regulation (about 70 percent of cases), JAK-STAT, cell cycle, and immune escape pathways (33).

Nodal MZLs carry rearranged immunoglobulin genes. The T-cell receptor genes are usually in the germline configuration. The immunoglobulin variable region genes demonstrate variable levels of somatic hypermutation (10,22,25). Mutations in other genes, such as *BCL6* and *PAX5,* are infrequent.

DIFFERENTIAL DIAGNOSIS

Marginal Zone Hyperplasia. Normal lymph nodes usually do not show a histologically recognizable marginal zone, with the exception of mesenteric lymph nodes. In some circumstances, however, lymph nodes are enlarged, and histologic examination shows expanded marginal zones (15). Marginal zone hyperplasia occurs in lymph nodes with preserved overall architecture and is commonly associated with other reactive features including prominent follicular hyperplasia, reactive microgranulomas, and reactive immunoblastic (CD30-positive) hyperplasia.

Table 14-1

**FEATURES OF NODAL MARGINAL ZONE LYMPHOMA (MZL)
WITH FOLLICULAR COLONIZATION VERSUS FOLLICULAR LYMPHOMA**

Feature	Nodal MZL	Follicular Lymphoma
Distribution of follicles	Usually confined to lymph node	Extend into perinodal fat
Growth pattern	Tumor begins outside follicle and grows in	Tumor begins in follicle and grows out
Cytology	Often rounder cells +/- plasmacytoid differentiation	Centrocytes and centroblasts Plasmacytoid differentiation is rare
Cell cytoplasm	Pale (pink)	Darker (blue)
CD10, BCL6, LMO2, HGAL/GCET2	Germinal centers + Tumor cells -	Tumor cells +
BCL2	Germinal centers - Tumor cells +	Tumor cells usually + except some grade 3 cases)
Ki-67	Germinal centers high Tumor low	Usually low (unless grade 3)
IGH-BCL2	Absent	Present

The histologic features most helpful in distinguishing marginal zone hyperplasia from nodal MZL include marginal zone B cells confined to marginal zones and absence of marginal zone cells outside the lymph node capsule. Features that suggest nodal MZL over hyperplasia are numerous monocytoid B cells and prominent follicular colonization. Nevertheless, there may be morphologic overlap between extreme marginal zone hyperplasia and nodal MZL in which immunophenotypic analysis and/or molecular studies are needed (4).

Progressive Transformation of Germinal Centers (PTGC). The pediatric variant of nodal MZL can morphologically mimic PTGC (13). Pediatric patients with nodal MZL have a clinically indolent disease that can mimic a benign process. Immunophenotypic and molecular studies demonstrate that nodal MZL is a monotypic B-cell lymphoma with monoclonal immunoglobulin gene rearrangements.

Other Types of Marginal Zone Lymphoma. Nodal MZL can closely mimic other types or MZL involving lymph nodes. Immunophenotypic markers and genetic studies are generally not helpful, although expression of IgD or del(7q) suggests the possibility of splenic MZL involving lymph node. Nodal MZL, in large part, is a diagnosis of exclusion and a rigorous search for extranodal or splenic sites of disease is required.

Mantle Cell Lymphoma. Most cases of mantle cell lymphoma are composed of a monotonous population of small, irregular lymphoid cells that have a blue hue at low power, but rare cases with monocytoid features have been described. Expression of CD5 and cyclin D1, and the t(11;14)(q13;q32), do not occur in nodal MZL (see chapter 12). SOX11, although commonly expressed in mantle cell lymphoma, has been reported in a small subset of nodal MZLs (37).

Follicular Lymphoma. Follicular lymphomas usually have a well-developed follicular pattern and the follicles commonly extend through the lymph node capsule into perinodal adipose tissue. Immunophenotypic analysis shows that the lymphoma cells are positive for germinal center B-cell markers such as CD10, BCL6, LMO2, and HGAL/GCET2, supporting the diagnosis of follicular lymphoma. Conventional cytogenetic or fluorescence in situ hybridization (FISH) studies showing t(14;18)(q32;q21)/*IGH-BCL2* also support follicular lymphoma.

The major diagnostic challenge is distinguishing nodal MZL from t(14;18)-negative follicular lymphoma, particularly grade 3 cases, which extensively colonize follicles (fig. 14-3). In general, follicular lymphoma begins in the germinal center and grows outward whereas nodal MZL begins in the marginal zone and grows into and colonizes germinal centers (Table 14-1).

Although immunophenotypic studies are helpful because nodal MZL cases are usually negative for germinal center B-cell markers, some reports found that these antigens can be expressed by nodal MZL cells (usually only a few and dimly) when these cells are present within the follicular microenvironment (35,36). In addition, both nodal MZL and follicular lymphoma express BCL2 and follicular lymphomas can downregulate CD10 and BCL6 when the cells leave the follicular microenvironment. In nodal MZL, antibodies specific for follicular dendritic cells often show irregularly shaped and disrupted follicular dendritic cell networks, unlike many cases of follicular lymphoma; however, irregular follicular dendritic cell networks are observed in some cases of follicular lymphoma.

Van den Brand et al. (35,36) have focused on this issue and they have made some helpful suggestions. They emphasize that cases of nodal MZL that colonize follicles often do so variably and therefore some follicle centers may show a mixture of nodal MZL cells (BCL2 positive, Ki-67 low) and reactive germinal center B cells (BCL2 negative and Ki-67 high). This occurs less frequently in cases of follicular lymphoma. They also developed an algorithm that uses an antibody panel approach. The panel includes four germinal center B-cell markers (CD10, BCL6, LMO2, and HGAL/GCET2) as well as MNDA and IRTA-1 (36). Lastly, the authors acknowledge that sometimes it is not possible to distinguish nodal MZL with extensive follicular colonization from follicular lymphoma (36).

Lymphoplasmacytic Lymphoma/Waldenstrom Macroglobulinemia. Clinical and laboratory data are helpful for distinguishing lymphoplasmacytic lymphoma from nodal MZL. Patients with bone marrow involvement and a serum IgM paraprotein, particularly if the paraprotein is at a high level, most likely have Waldenstrom macroglobulinemia. Histologic findings that support nodal MZL include large reactive follicles, a marginal zone pattern of involvement, and prominent monocytoid B cells. *MYD88* mutations are present in most cases of Waldenstrom macroblobulinemia and are rare in nodal MZLs (see chapter 16).

Angioimmunoblastic T-Cell Lymphoma. At low power magnification, nodal MZL and angioimmunoblastic T-cell lymphoma share some similarities. Both tumors infiltrate lymph nodes in an interfollicular pattern and may be composed of many cells with clear or pale cytoplasm. This differential diagnosis is resolved by immunophenotypic or molecular analysis (see chapter 31).

TREATMENT AND PROGNOSIS

Currently, there is no consensus regarding the optimal treatment of patients with nodal MZL (12,18,32a,33). For patients with localized disease, radiation therapy or watchful waiting is advocated. For patients with disseminated disease but with a low tumor burden, watchful waiting is often the initial approach. A spectrum of therapeutic approaches has been used for patients with disseminated, high burden disease. The R-CHOP (rituximab, cyclophosphamide, doxorubicin, vincristine, and prednisone) regimen has been used most often in the past, but other more recently used regimens include R-bendamustine and R plus FC (fludarabine and cyclophosphamide, also known as FCR).

There is no optimal clinical stratification system analogous to the International Prognostic Index (IPI) or follicular lymphoma IPI (FLIPI) that can be used to guide the therapy of nodal MZL patients. The clinically indolent disease course is similar to that of other types of low-grade B-cell lymphoma involving lymph nodes and nongastric extranodal MZL, but is worse than that of splenic MZL (18,23,32a,). Reported 5-year survival rates for patients after a diagnosis of nodal MZL have ranged from 60 percent to almost 90 percent (23,27,33).

REFERENCES

1. Abella E, Besses C, Barranco C, Pedro C, Buch J, Espinet B. Nodal marginal zone lymphoma in AIDS patients: a causal association? AIDS 2002;16:2232-2234.
2. Arcaini L, Paulli M, Burcheri S, et al. Primary nodal marginal zone B-cell lymphoma: clinical features and prognostic assessment of a rare disease. Br J Haematol 2007;136:301-304.
3. Berger F, Felman P, Thieblemont C, et al. Non-MALT marginal zone B-cell lymphomas: a description of clinical presentation and outcome in 124 patients. Blood 2000;95:1950-1956.
4. Bob R, Falini B, Marafioti T, Paterson JC, Pileri S, Stein H. Nodal reactive and neoplastic proliferation of monocytoid and marginal zone B cells: an immunoarchitectural and molecular study highlighting the relevance of IRTA1 and T-bet as positive markers. Histopathology 2013;63:482-498.
5. Braggio E, Dogan A, Keats JJ, et al. Genomic analysis of marginal zone and lymphoplasmacytic lymphomas identified common and disease-specific abnormalities. Mod Pathol 2012;25:651-660.
6. Brynes RK, Almaguer PD, Leathery KE, et al. Numerical cytogenetic abnormalities of chromsomes 3, 7, and 12 in marginal zone lymphoma. Mod Pathol 1996;9:995-1000.
7. Callet-Bauchu E, Baseggio L, Felman P, et al. Cytogenetic analysis delineates a spectrum of chromosomal changes that can distinguish non-MALT marginal zone B-cell lymphomas among mature B-cell entities: a description of 103 cases. Leukemia 2005;19:1818-1823.
8. Camacho FI, Algara P, Mollejo M, et al. Nodal marginal zone lymphoma: a heterogeneous tumor. A comprehensive analysis of a series of 27 cases. Am J Surg Pathol 2003;27:762-771.
9. Campo E, Pileri SA, Jaffe ES, et al. Nodal marginal zone lymphoma. In: Swerdlow SH, Campo E, Harris NL, Jaffe ES, Pileri SA, Stein H, Thiele J, Vardiman JW, eds. WHO classification of tumours of haematopoietic and lymphoid tissues. Lyon: IARC Press; 2008;218-219.
10. Conconi A, Bertoni F, Pedrinis E, et al. Nodal marginal zone lymphomas may arise from different subsets of marginal zone B lymphocytes. Blood 2001;98:781-786.
11. Dierlamm J, Wlodarska I, Michaux L, et al. Genetic abnormalities in marginal zone B-cell lymphoma. Hematol Oncol 2000;18:1-13.
12. Dreyling M, Thieblemont C, Gallamini A, et al. ESMO consensus conferences: guideleines on malignant lymphoma. part 2. marginal zone lymphoma, mantle cell lymphoma, peripheral T-cell lymphoma. Ann Oncol 2013;24:857-877.
13. Elenitoba-Johnson KS, Kumar S, Lim MS, Kingma DW, Raffeld M, Jaffe ES. Marginal zone B-cell lymphoma with monocytoid B-cell lymphocytes in pediatric patients without immunodeficiency. A report of two cases. Am J Clin Pathol 1997;107:92-98.
14. Falini B, Agnostelli C, Bigerna B, et al. IRTA1 is selectively expressed in nodal and extranodal marginal zone lymphomas. Histopathology 2012;61:930-941.
15. Hunt JP, Chan JA, Samoszuk M, et al. Hyperplasia of mantle/marginal zone B cells with clear cytoplasm in peripheral lymph nodes. A clinicopathologic study of 35 cases. Am J Clin Pathol 2001;116:550-559.
16. Inamdar KV, Medeiros LJ, Jorgensen JL, Amin HM, Schlette EJ. Bone marrow involvement by marginal zone B-cell lymphomas of different types. Am J Clin Pathol 2008;129:714-722.
17. Jaso JM, Yin CC, Wang SA, et al. Clinicopathologic features of CD5-positive nodal marginal zone lymphoma. Am J Clin Pathol 2013;140:693-700.
18. Kahl B, Yang D. Marginal zone lymphomas: management of nodal, splenic, and MALT NHL. Hematology Am Soc Hematol Educ Program 2008:359-364.
19. Khalil MO, Morton LM, Devesa SS, et al. Incidence of marginal zone lymphoma in the United States, 2001-2009 with a focus on primary anatomic site. Br J Haematol 2014;165:67-77.
20. Kluin PM, Langerak AW, Beverdam-Vincent J, et al. Pediatric nodal marginal zone B-cell lymphadenopathy of the neck: a Haemophilus influenzae driven immune disorder? J Pathol 2015;236:302-314.
21. Krijgsman O, Gonzalez P, Ponz OB, et al. Dissecting the gray zone between follicular lymphoma and marginal zone lymphoma using morphological and genetic features. Haematologica 2013;98:1921-1929.
22. Marasca R, Vaccari P, Luppi M, et al. Immunoglobulin gene mutations and frequent use of VH1-69 and VH4-34 segments in hepatitis C virus-positive and hepatitis C-negative nodal marginal zone B-cell lymphoma. Am J Pathol 2001;159:253-261.
23. Mazloom A, Medeiros LJ, McLaughlin PW, et al. Marginal zone lymphomas: factors that affect the final outcome. Cancer 2010;116:4291-4298.

24. Metcalf RA, Monabati A, Vyas M, et al. Myeloid cell nuclear differentiation antigen is expressed in a subset of marginal zone lymphomas and is useful in the differential diagnosis with follicular lymphoma. Hum Pathol 2014;45:1730-1736.

25. Miranda RN, Cousar JB, Hammer RD, Collins RD, Vnencak-Jones CL. Somatic mutation analysis of IgH variable regions reveals that tumor cells of most parafollicular (monocytoid) b-cell lymphoma, splenic marginal zone lymphoma, and some hairy cell leukemia are composed of memory B lymphocytes. Hum Pathol 1999;30:306-312.

26. Nathwani BN, Anderson JR, Armitage JO, et al. Marginal zone B-cell lymphoma: a clinical comparison of nodal and mucosa-associated lymphoid tissue types. Non-Hodgkin's Lymphoma Classification Project. J Clin Oncol 1999; 17:2486-2492.

27. Olszewski AJ, Castillo JJ. Survival of patients with marginal zone lymphomas: analysis of the Surveillance, Epidemiology, and End Results database. Cancer 2013;119:629-638.

27a. Pileri S, Ponzoni M. Pathology of nodal marginal zone lymphomas. Best Pract Res Clin Haematol 2017;30:50-55.

28. Rinaldi A, Mian M, Chigrinova E, et al. Genome-wide DNA profiling of marginal zone lymphomas identifies subtype-specific lesions with an impact on the clinical outcome. Blood 2011;117:1595-1604.

29. Salama ME, Lossos IS, Warnke RA, Natkunam Y. Immunoarchitectural patterns in nodal marginal zone lymphoma. A study of 51 cases. Am J Clin Pathol 2009:132:39-49.

30. Sheibani K, Sohn CC, Burke JS, Winberg CD, Wu AM, Rappaport H. Monocytoid B-cell lymphoma. A novel B-cell neoplasm. Am J Pathol 1986;124:310-318.

30a. Spina V, Khiabanian H, Messina M, et al. The genetics of nodal marginal zone lymphoma. Blood 2016;128:1362-1373.

31. Stary S, Vinatzer U, Müllauer L, Raderer M, Birner P, Streubel B. t(11;14)(q23;q32) involving IGH and DDX6 in nodal marginal zone lymphoma. Genes Chromosomes Cancer 2013;52:33-43.

32. Swerdlow SH, Campo E, Pileri SA, et al. The 2016 revision of the World Health Organization classification of lymphoid neoplasms. Blood 2016;127:2375-2390.

32a. Tadmor T, Polliack A. Nodal marginal zone lymphoma: clinical features, diagnosis, management and treatment. Best Pract Res Clin Haematol 2017;30:92-98.

33. Thieblemont C, Molina T, Davi F. Optimizing therapy for nodal marginal zone lymphoma. Blood 2016;127:2064-2071.

34. Traverse-Glehen A, Felman P, Callet-Bauchu E, et al. A clinicopathological study of nodal marginal zone B-cell lymphoma. A report on 21 cases. Histopathology 2006;48:162-173.

35. Van den Brand M, Mathijssen JJ, Garcia-Garcia M, et al. Immunohistochemical differentiation between follicular lymphoma and nodal marginal zone lymphoma-combined performance of multiple markers. Haematologica 2015;100:e358-e360.

36. van den Brand M, van Krieken JH. Recognizing nodal marginal zone lymphoma: recent advances and pitfalls. A systematic review. Haematologica 2013;98:1003-1013.

37. Zhang LN, Cao X, Lu TX, et al. Polyclonal antibody targeting SOX11 cannot differentiate mantle cell lymphoma from B-cell non-Hodgkin lymphomas. Am J Clin Pathol 2013;140:795-800.

15 EXTRANODAL MARGINAL ZONE LYMPHOMA OF MUCOSA-ASSOCIATED LYMPHOID TISSUE

GENERAL FEATURES

Extranodal marginal zone lymphoma (MZL) of mucosa-associated lymphoid tissue (MALT), also known as *MALT lymphoma*, is a neoplasm of mature B cells that arises at extranodal sites (14). The neoplastic cell infiltrate is polymorphous and composed of atypical small B lymphocytes that exhibit a variable mixture of monocytoid, centrocyte-like, or plasmacytoid features, associated with a small number of larger transformed cells.

In 1983, Isaacson and Wright (15) described two patients with low-grade B-cell lymphoma of the stomach and coined the name B-cell lymphoma of MALT. Thirty years later, in large part through the efforts of Isaacson and many colleagues, it is clear that extranodal lymphomas differ greatly from nodal lymphomas in their clinicopathologic features, immunophenotype, and pathogenesis (14). These efforts also resulted in the realization that many extranodal lesions that had been classified as so-called pseudolymphoma were, in fact, lymphomas with potential for dissemination (29). In retrospect, the term B-cell lymphoma of MALT is a misnomer since these tumors do not always arise in association with mucosa.

Extranodal MZLs are clinically indolent tumors that are derived from B cells that presumably correspond to an extranodal equivalent of nodal marginal zone B cells. While extranodal MZLs arise uncommonly in anatomic sites that normally are composed of MALT tissue (e.g., Waldeyer ring, Peyer patches), most arise at anatomic sites that have acquired persistent lymphoid hyperplasia (or MALT) as a result of chronic B-cell activation (25,47).

The chronic B-cell activation of extranodal MZL is caused by infectious agents, autoimmune diseases, and possibly other causes. Gastric MZL arises in a background of persistent lymphoid hyperplasia that is often acquired in response to chronic *Helicobacter pylori* infection. The proliferation of gastric MZL cells in *H. pylori*–infected patients is dependent on the presence of T cells activated by *H. pylori* antigen. *Chlamydia psittaci*, *Borelia* species, and *Achromobacter xylosoxidans* are implicated in the pathogenesis of ocular adnexal, cutaneous, and lung MZLs, respectively; immunoproliferative small intestinal disease (previously known as Mediterranean lymphoma) is associated with *Campylobacter jejuni* infection (1,11,14,22,26). There is also an association between extranodal MZL and hepatitis C infection, with most studies originating in Europe and especially Italy; some patients respond to anti-viral therapy (3,33). B-cell activated autoimmune disorders linked to extranodal MZLs include Sjögren syndrome, which often precedes MZL of the salivary gland, and Hashimoto thyroiditis, which almost always precedes MZL of the thyroid gland (14,17).

Extranodal MZLs show some regional differences in incidence. A high incidence of gastric MZL is reported in northern Italy where *H. pylori* infection is very common, although the frequency has been dropping over the past decade (9,47). Ocular adnexal MZLs associated with *C. psittaci* infection are more frequent in Italy, Austria, Germany, and Korea and less common in France, Japan, and China (47). Cutaneous MZLs associated with *Borrelia* infection are more common in Europe. Whether *B. burgdorferi* or *B. garinii* organisms are involved is uncertain but there is evidence to implicate *B. burgdorferi*. *B. garinii*, however, is unique to Europe and therefore may explain the geographic distribution of these tumors. Immunoproliferative small intestinal disease is more prevalent in the Middle East and in the Cape region of South Africa (34).

CLINICAL FEATURES

Extranodal MZLs account for approximately 7 percent of all B-cell non-Hodgkin lymphomas. The disease is most frequently seen in adults in the seventh decade of life, with a median patient age of 61 years (14,16,31). There is a slight female predominance, with a male to female ratio of 1.0 to 1.2. The predominance of women is more pronounced in patients with extranodal MZL associated with autoimmune disease.

The stomach is the most frequent anatomic site, representing up to half of all extranodal MZLs in various studies (28,41). Other commonly involved sites, in descending order of frequency, include salivary glands (mostly the parotid gland), ocular adnexa, skin, lung, and intestine. Virtually any other extranodal site can be involved, with the more common (of the rare sites) being soft tissue, Waldeyer ring, thyroid gland, breast, and kidney (28,41).

Extranodal MZLs can involve lymph nodes, most often regional lymph nodes. Approximately 20 percent of patients with extranodal MZL have regional lymph node involvement at the time of diagnosis (8,16,23). Some patients with extranodal MZL present initially with lymphadenopathy, usually at a single regional lymph node (23,41); rarely is the lymphadenopathy widespread. The frequency of lymph node involvement is higher in patients with neoplasms that have increased large cells or that have transformed into diffuse large B-cell lymphoma (23). Bone marrow infiltration by extranodal MZL occurs in 10 to 15 percent of patients, more commonly in patients with nongastric MZLs (8,16,41). Leukemic involvement is unusual.

Extranodal MZL presents as localized disease (stage I or IIE) in 65 to 76 percent of patients (8,16,28,41). Disseminated disease occurs in up to a third of patients, more often in those with nongastric MZL (8,41). The frequency of high-stage disease is influenced by the rigor of the staging workup. Raderer et al. (38), after performing an extensive staging workup in over 100 patients, reported that about 25 percent of patients with gastric MZL and almost 50 percent with nongastric MZL have high-stage disease. In their study, disease stage did not influence prognosis. In other studies, extranodal MZL patients have had multiple extranodal sites of lymphoma, often involving the same organ system (8,16,24); these multiple sites may not be clonally related, suggesting multiple concurrent primary tumors (24).

The staging of MZL involving paired extranodal organs, with no other sites of disease, is controversial. In the World Health Organization (WHO) classification, bilateral paired organ involvement by extranodal MZL is not considered evidence of disseminated disease (14). Extranodal MZLs are thought to express homing receptors that account for their patterns of dissemination and paired organ involvement is thought to be a manifestation of this phenomenon.

Laboratory studies in patients with extranodal MZL show evidence of anemia or hypoalbuminemia in approximately 10 percent of patients. Serum beta-2-microglobulin levels are elevated in up to one third and lactate dehydrogenase (LDH) levels are elevated in less than 10 percent (28). A serum paraprotein (M-spike) is detected in up to 30 percent of patients with extranodal MZL, usually in tumors with prominent plasmacytoid differentiation. A monoclonal IgA paraprotein is common in patients with immunoproliferative small intestinal disease (34).

Depending on the study, 5 to 20 percent of patients with extranodal MZL transform to diffuse large B-cell lymphoma, either detected at initial diagnosis or during clinical follow-up (14,25). Transformation is associated with a more aggressive clinical course and poorer prognosis.

HISTOLOGIC FINDINGS

Extranodal Sites

Extranodal MZLs are characterized by a polymorphous infiltrate that consists of a variable mixture of small lymphoid cells with irregular nuclear contours (so-called centrocyte-like cells), small lymphocytes with pale cytoplasm and small nuclei with inconspicuous nucleoli (monocytoid cells), plasmacytoid lymphocytes, plasma cells, and occasional large lymphoid cells (figs. 15-1–15-3). Dutcher (fig. 15-4) and Russell bodies may be numerous. Many cases of extranodal MZL have a biphasic appearance, with paler areas corresponding to monocytoid (figs. 15-2, 15-5) or plasmacytoid differentiation and darker areas composed mostly of small lymphocytes. Cases associated with t(11;18)(q21;q21) (see below) tend to be more monotonous, with relatively less monocytoid or plasmacytoid differentiation. Reactive follicles are very common, usually surrounded by tumor cells. In some cases, a narrow

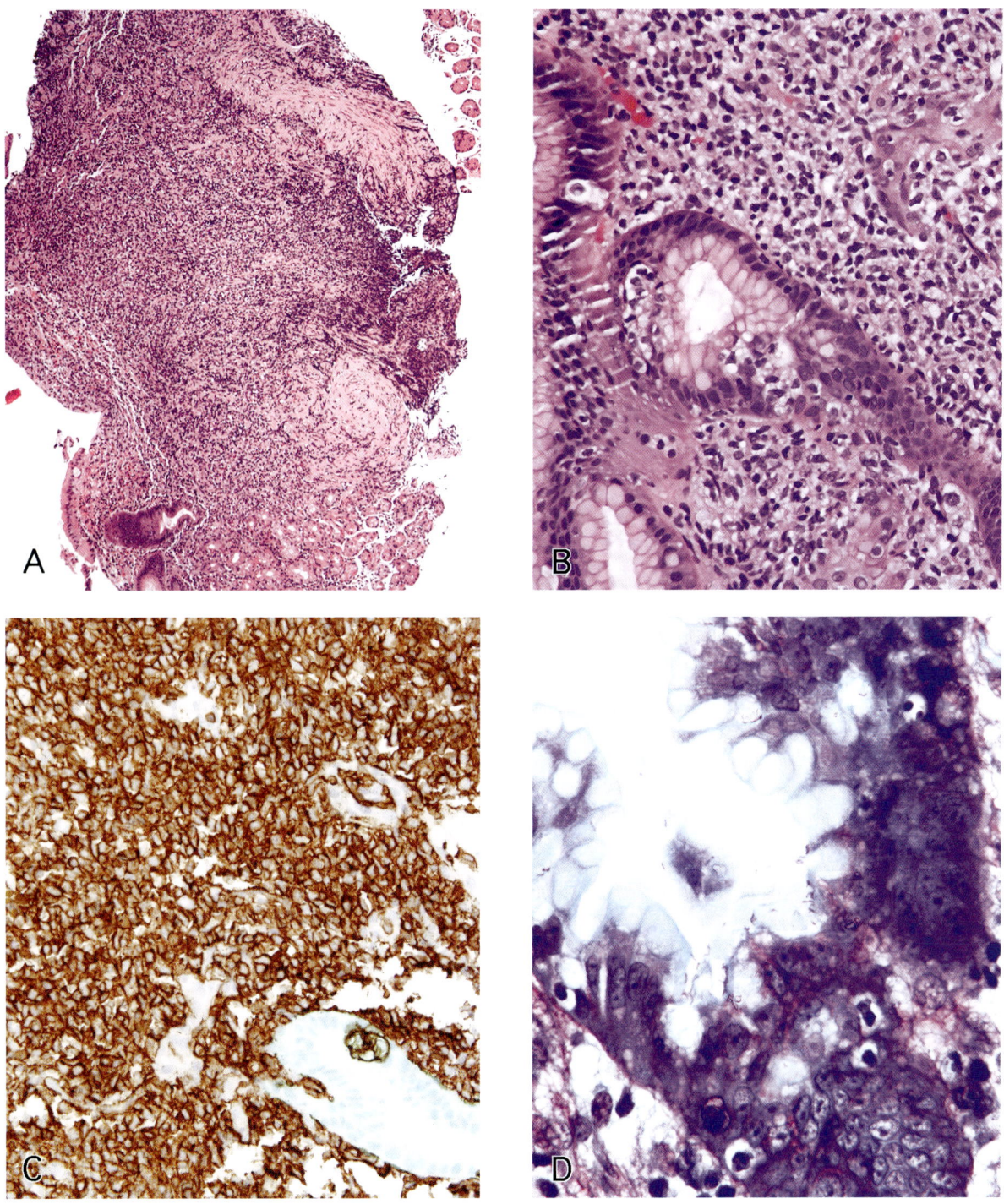

Figure 15-1

EXTRANODAL MARGINAL ZONE LYMPHOMA (MZL) OF STOMACH

A: The neoplasm replaces much of the gastric fundic-type mucosa.

B: The neoplastic cells have abundant pale (monocytoid) cytoplasm and lymphoepithelial lesions are shown (A,B: hematoxylin and eosin [H&E] stain).

C: The lymphoma cells are positive for CD20. This antibody also highlights B cells in lymphoepithelial lesions.

D: Many *Helicobacter pylori* organisms are present on the luminal surface (Giemsa stain).

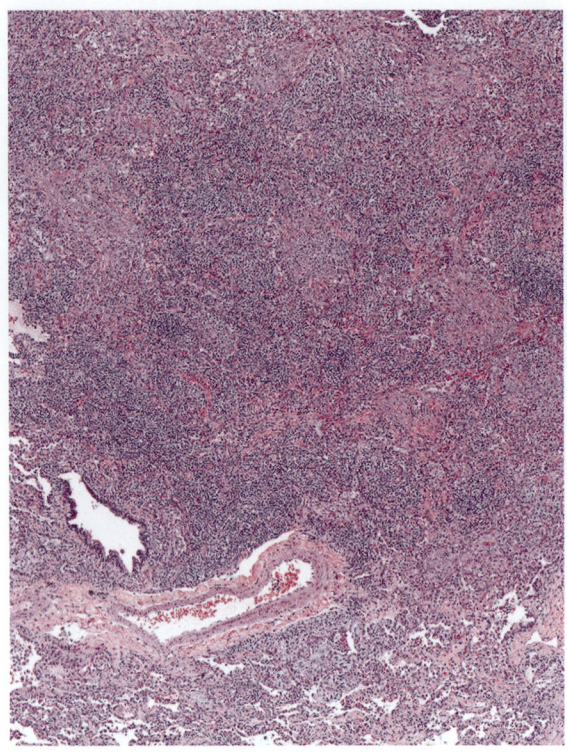

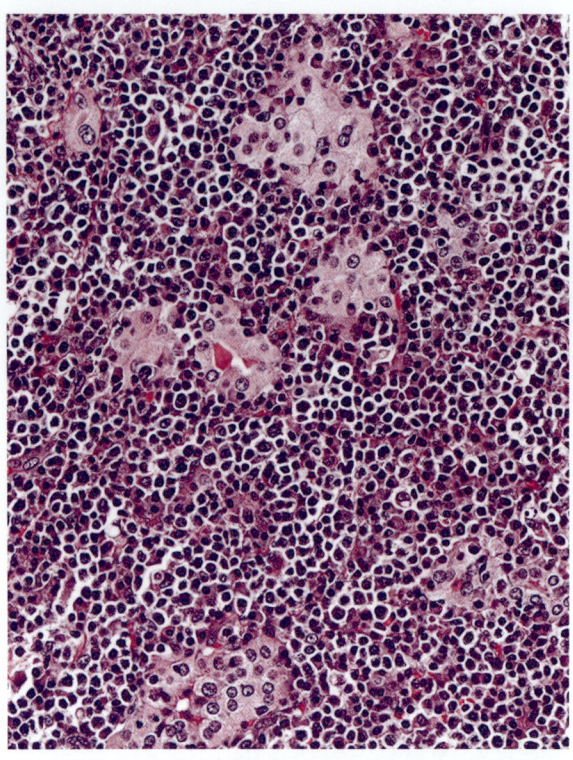

Figure 15-2

**EXTRANODAL MARGINAL ZONE
LYMPHOMA OF LUNG**

The neoplasm has paler and darker areas, imparting a biphasic appearance at low-power magnification. Alveolar parenchyma is at the bottom of the field (H&E stain).

Figure 15-3

**EXTRANODAL MARGINAL ZONE
LYMPHOMA OF THYROID GLAND**

This patient had Hashimoto thyroiditis. The associated oncocytic change in the thyroid epithelium is typical of Hashimoto thyroiditis, a disease associated with a high risk of extranodal MZL of the thyroid gland (H&E stain).

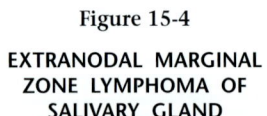

Figure 15-4

**EXTRANODAL MARGINAL
ZONE LYMPHOMA OF
SALIVARY GLAND**

Numerous intranuclear pseudo-inclusions (Dutcher bodies) are present (H&E stain).

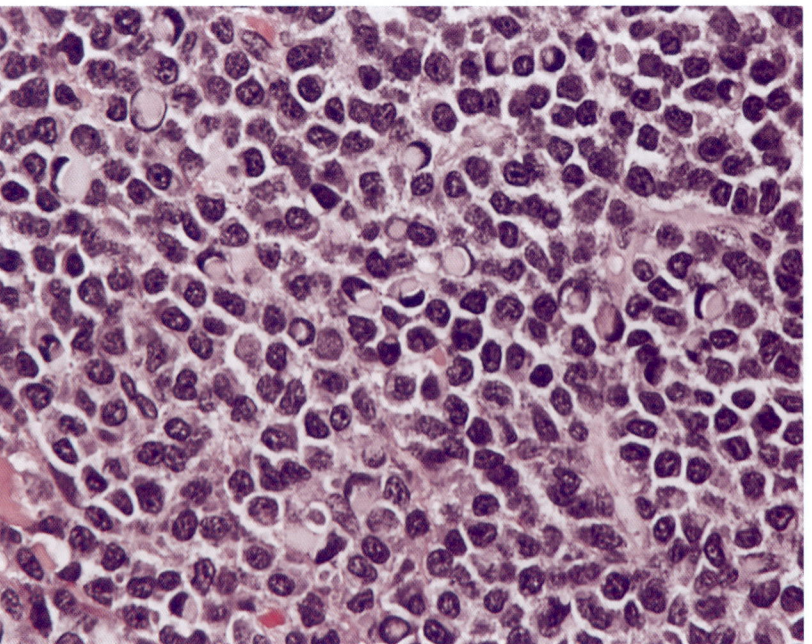

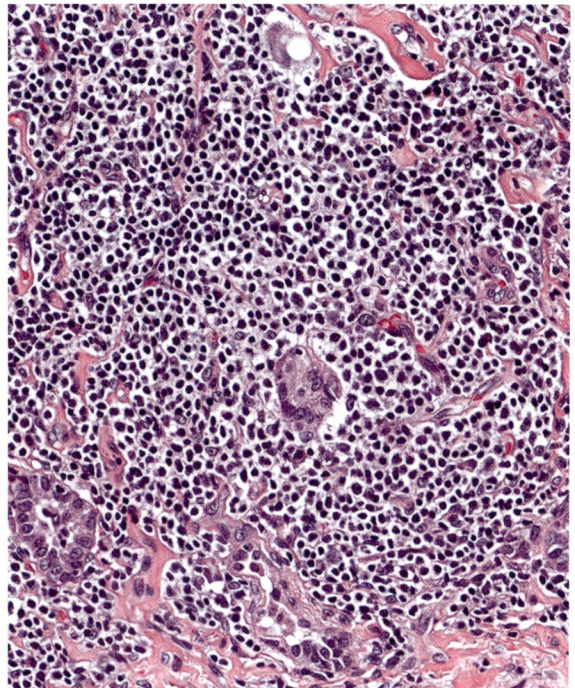

Figure 15-5

EXTRANODAL MARGINAL ZONE LYMPHOMA

Many tumor cells with abundant cytoplasm impart a monocytoid appearance (H&E stain).

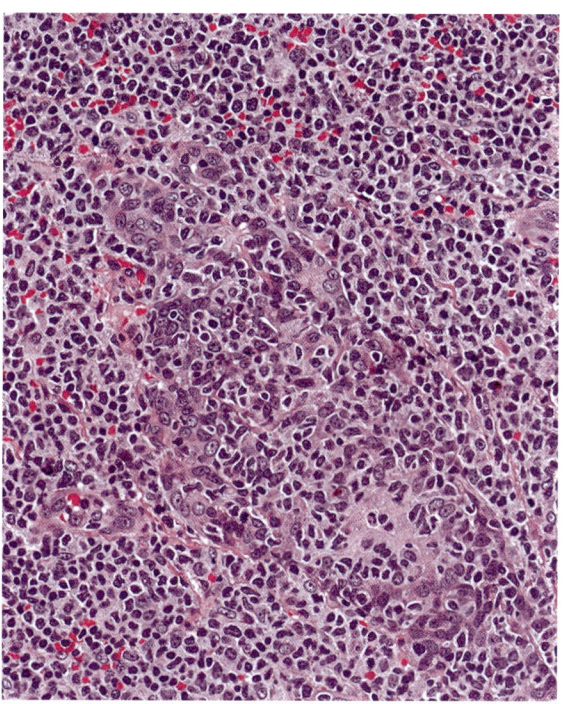

Figure 15-7

EXTRANODAL MARGINAL ZONE LYMPHOMA OF SALIVARY GLAND

Many neoplastic cells infiltrate the epithelium to form lymphoepithelial lesions (H&E stain).

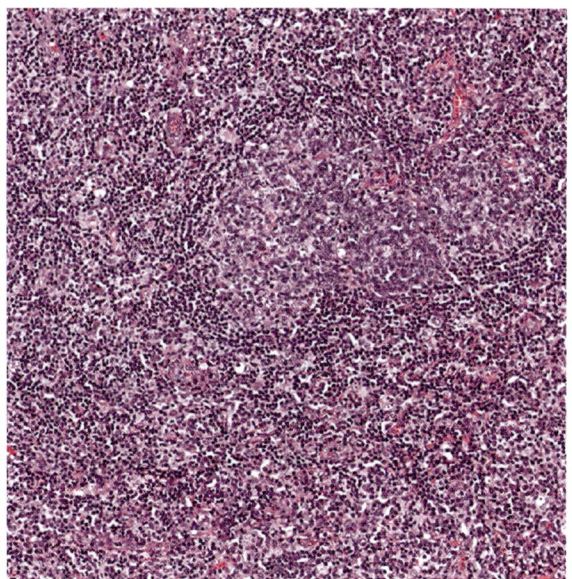

Figure 15-6

EXTRANODAL MARGINAL ZONE LYMPHOMA

A reactive follicle is surrounded by lymphoma. There is a narrow rim of mantle zone between the germinal center and the tumor cells (H&E stain).

rim of mantle zone cells separates the tumor from the reactive germinal center (fig. 15-6). In other cases, the neoplastic cells infiltrate the germinal centers of follicles, preserving the overall follicular appearance, so-called follicular colonization. Amyloid deposition occurs in some patients; the amyloid may be associated with the neoplastic lymphocytes at the time of initial diagnosis or in relapsed disease (46).

The glandular epithelium found at some extranodal sites may be infiltrated and destroyed by tumor cells, resulting in lymphoepithelial lesions (figs. 15-1B, 15-7). A lymphoepithelial lesion is an aggregate of three or more neoplastic B cells that have infiltrated glandular epithelium, often distorting or destroying local glandular structures. Although lymphoepithelial lesions are common in extranodal MZLs, they also occur in benign MALT tissue. In the stomach, numerous lymphoepithelial lesions suggest the diagnosis of extranodal MZL, but their presence is not helpful in the lung, salivary gland, or thyroid gland.

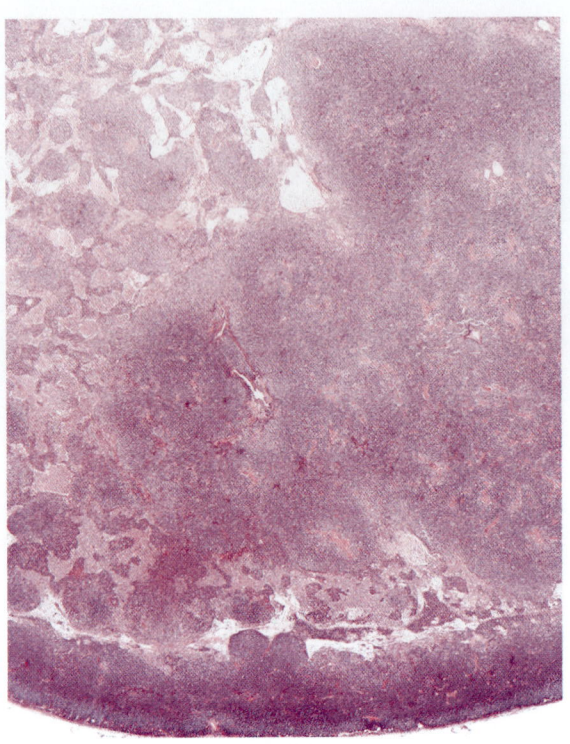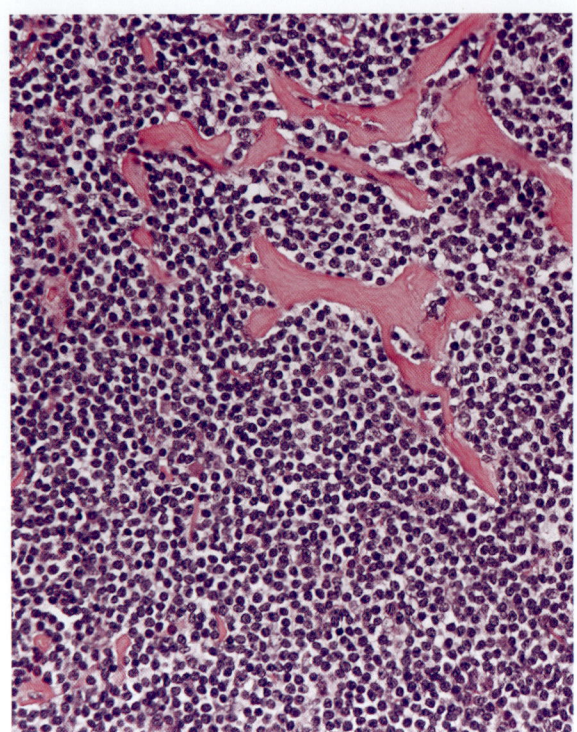

Figure 15-8

EXTRANODAL MARGINAL ZONE LYMPHOMA PARTIALLY INVOLVING LYMPH NODE

This patient had a history of breast MZL and this lymph node is from the oxilla.
Left: This field shows areas of architectural replacement and other uninvolved areas with open sinuses.
Right: The neoplasm is composed of numerous small lymphoid cells (left, right: H&E stain).

Lymph Nodes

Extranodal MZL can efface the lymph node architecture in a sinusoidal, perifollicular, interfollicular, nodular, or diffuse pattern (figs. 15-8, 15-9) (23). In patients with low-grade extranodal MZL, often lymph nodes are partially involved by lymphoma in a sinusoidal or perifollicular pattern. Usually only a few regional lymph nodes are involved. In patients with increased large cells or a component of large B-cell lymphoma, an interfollicular or diffuse pattern is more common and multiple regional lymph node are often involved (23). The nodular pattern in lymph nodes usually corresponds to follicular colonization of reactive germinal centers by extranodal MZL cells, which can be prominent in some cases (fig. 15-10).

Bone Marrow

Extranodal MZLs involve the bone marrow in a paratrabecular and nonparatrabecular pattern (fig. 15-11) (13). The lymphoid aggregates are commonly associated with follicular dendritic cells (CD21 or CD23 positive). A sinusoidal pattern is rarely observed in extranodal MZL (unlike splenic MZL).

CYTOLOGIC FINDINGS

Cytologic smears of extranodal MZL show a heterogeneous population of cells, including clusters of centrocyte-like and monocytoid cells (fig. 15-12). Scattered larger transformed centroblasts are usually present. Plasma cell differentiation is evident in some cases (7).

IMMUNOPHENOTYPIC FINDINGS

Extranodal MZLs are most often diagnosed in small biopsy specimens, such as a gastrointestinal tract biopsy specimen. The lymphoma cells express CD19, CD20, CD22, CD79a, PAX5, and BCL2, and are negative for pan-T-cell antigens, CD10, CD21, CD23, and cyclin D1 (10,17).

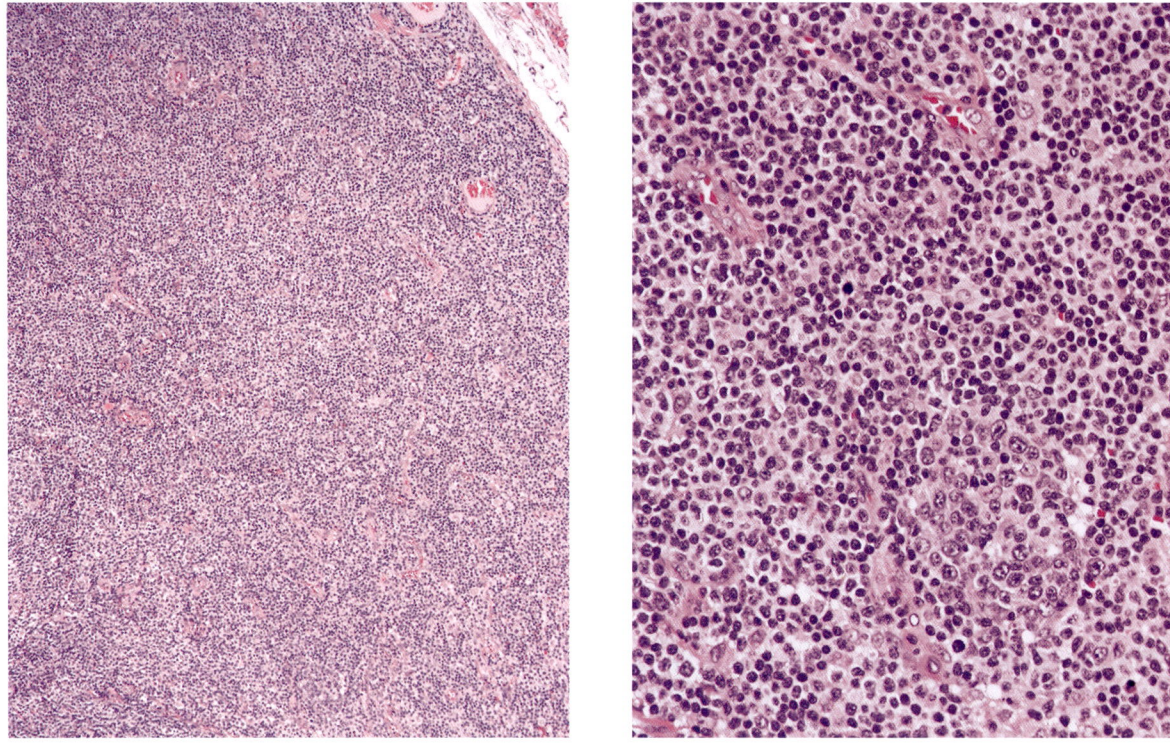

Figure 15-9

EXTRANODAL MARGINAL ZONE LYMPHOMA INVOLVING REGIONAL LYMPH NODE

Left: Most of the lymph node is replaced by lymphoma.
Right: The lymphoma cells are monocytoid, with abundant pale cytoplasm. A residual germinal center is present in this field (left, right: H&E stain).

MNDA and IRTA-1 are reported to be expressed by most cases of extranodal MZL, although different studies show a higher or lower frequency of positive cases (10,21). CD43 is expressed in many cases; CD5 is rarely expressed (CD5-positive cases appear to disseminate more often than CD5-negative cases) (18). Although BCL6 is a germinal center B-cell marker and negative in most cases of extranodal MZL, it can be dimly expressed in a small subset of cases, more often in cases with transformation to diffuse large B-cell lymphoma (25). If flow cytometry is performed, the lymphoma cells express monotypic immunoglobin (IG); in paraffin sections one third of cases have monotypic cytoplasmic IG.

MOLECULAR GENETIC FINDINGS

The IG genes show monoclonal rearrangements in extranodal MZLs. In half of the cases, the IG variable gene segments are somatically hypermutated, suggesting a postgerminal center or memory B-cell derivation. The T-cell receptor genes are usually in the germline configuration. Trisomy of chromosomes 3 and 18 occurs in 40 to 60 percent of cases. Trisomy 3 may be more common in tumors with monocytoid features (6). Trisomy of chromosomes 7 and 12 is less common, but tends to occur in cases with translocations (6,25). BCL6 translocations, commonly in the form of *IGH-BCL6*, have been reported in a small subset of cases (44). Array comparative genomic hybridization has shown a high frequency of gains of chromosomal loci 3p, 6p, and 18p, and loss of 6q23 (*TNFAIP3*) (39). Preliminary microRNA studies have suggested the importance of upregulation of mir-142-5p, miR-150, and miR-155 in gastric MZLs (12,40). Mutations of *TP53* and *TP16* are uncommon, and when present, are associated with transformation to diffuse large B-cell lymphoma.

Recurrent chromosomal aberrations are present in 30 to 40 percent of cases of extranodal

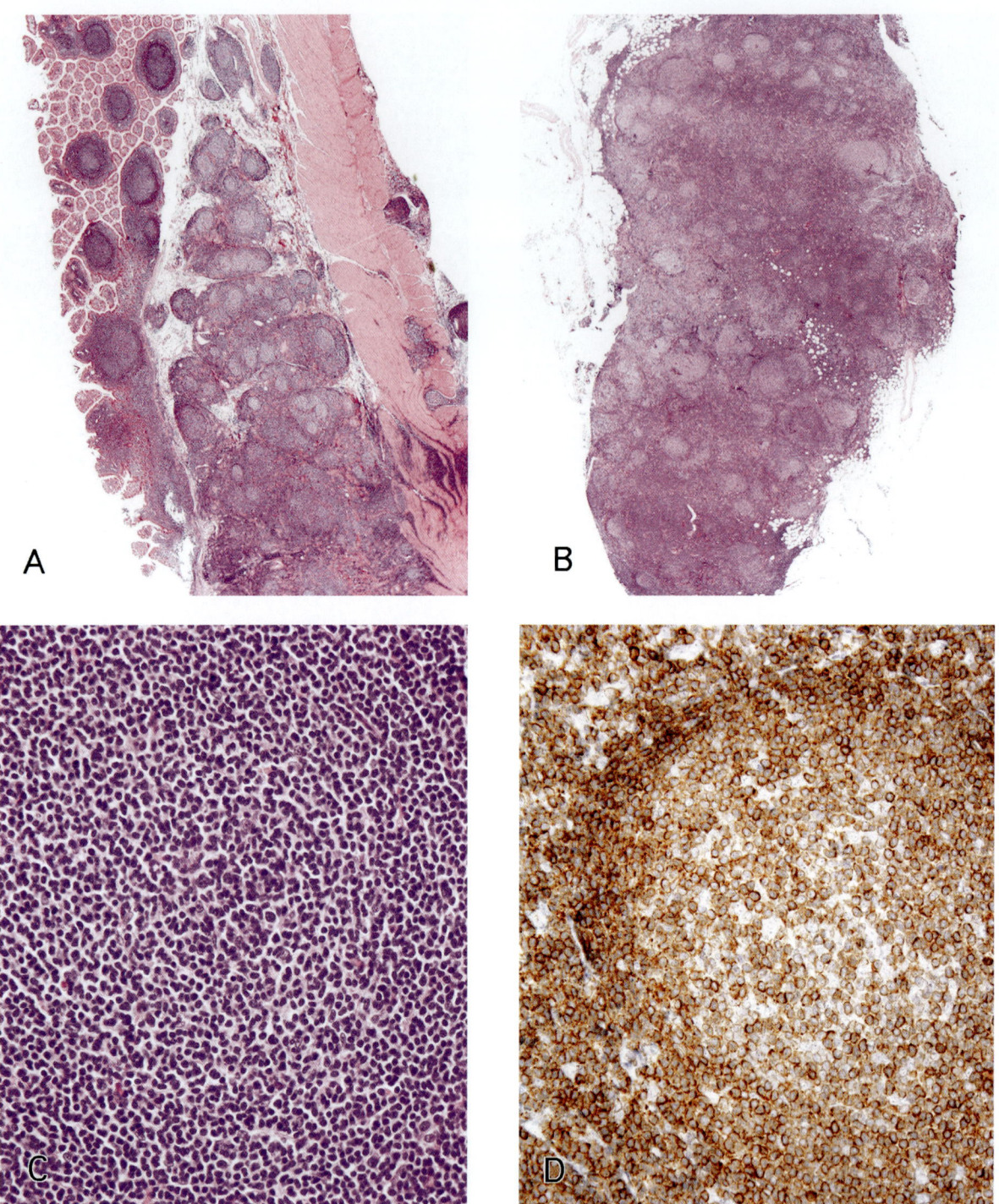

Figure 15-10

**EXTRANODAL MARGINAL ZONE LYMPHOMA PARTIALLY
INVOLVING REGIONAL LYMPH NODE OF SMALL INTESTINE**

A: Low-power magnification of the small intestine shows many nodules of lymphoma with extensive follicular colonization (A–C: H&E stain).

B: A regional lymph node is involved by lymphoma with a pattern similar to the small intestine.

C: High-power magnification of lymphoma in the lymph node.

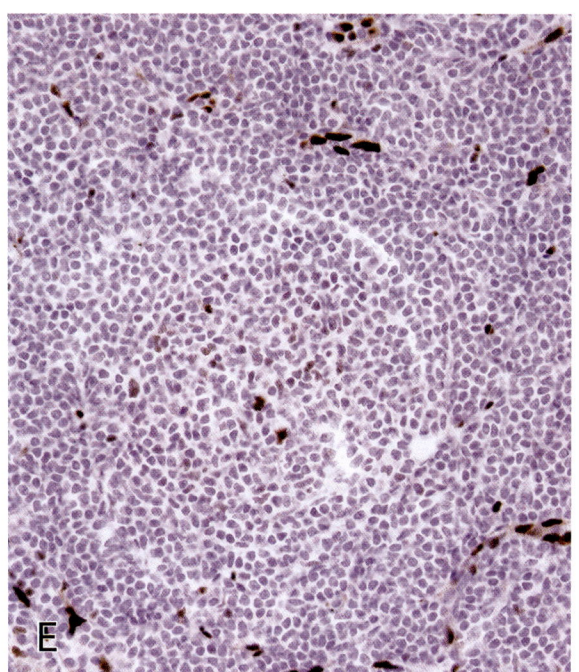

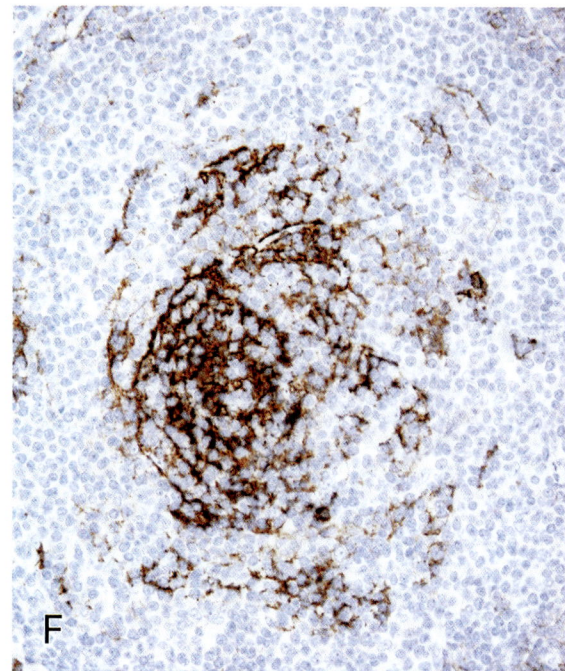

Figure 15-10, continued

D–F: Immunohistochemical studies show that the lymphoma cells are positive for CD20 (not shown) and BCL2 (D), and negative for CD10 (not shown), LMO2 (E), and CD23 (F). The LM02 antibody highlights residual germinal center B cells. The CD23 antibody highlights residual follicular dendritic cells (D–F: immunohistochemistry with hematoxylin counterstain).

MZL (Table 15-1). Each translocation, by itself, is thought to be insufficient to cause lymphoma and other genetic abnormalities are required for lymphomagenesis. Some of these translocations activate the NF-κB pathway, which is thought to be important in the pathogenesis of extranodal MZLs (9a,47). The first translocation described in extranodal MZLs was t(11;18)(q21p21), which results in a chimeric gene, *BIRC3-MALT1. BIRC3* (also known as *cIAP2* and *API2*) encodes an anti-apoptotic protein and is fused to *MALT1,* which encodes a paracaspase inhibitor protein. The t(11;18)/*API2-MALT1* induces the cleavage of *LIMA1,* resulting in a LIM domain-only (LMO) fragment that drives oncogenesis (30). *LIMA1* is a known tumor suppressor gene and its cleavage occurs as a result of *MALT1* paracaspase activity (30). t(11;18)/*BIRC3-MALT1* is present most often in extranodal MZLs arising in the lung and stomach, and less often at other anatomic sites.

Other translocations in extranodal MZLs juxtapose different genes with the *IGH* locus (14,42). t(14;18)(q32;q21), which leads to transcriptional deregulation of an intact *MALT1,*

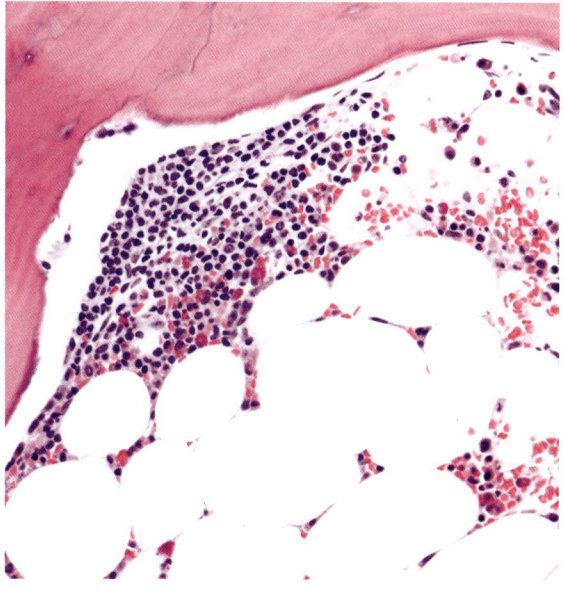

Figure 15-11

EXTRANODAL MARGINAL ZONE LYMPHOMA INVOLVING BONE MARROW

Bone marrow involvement in this case showed a paratrabecular pattern. This patient had an ocular adnexal MZL (H&E stain).

259

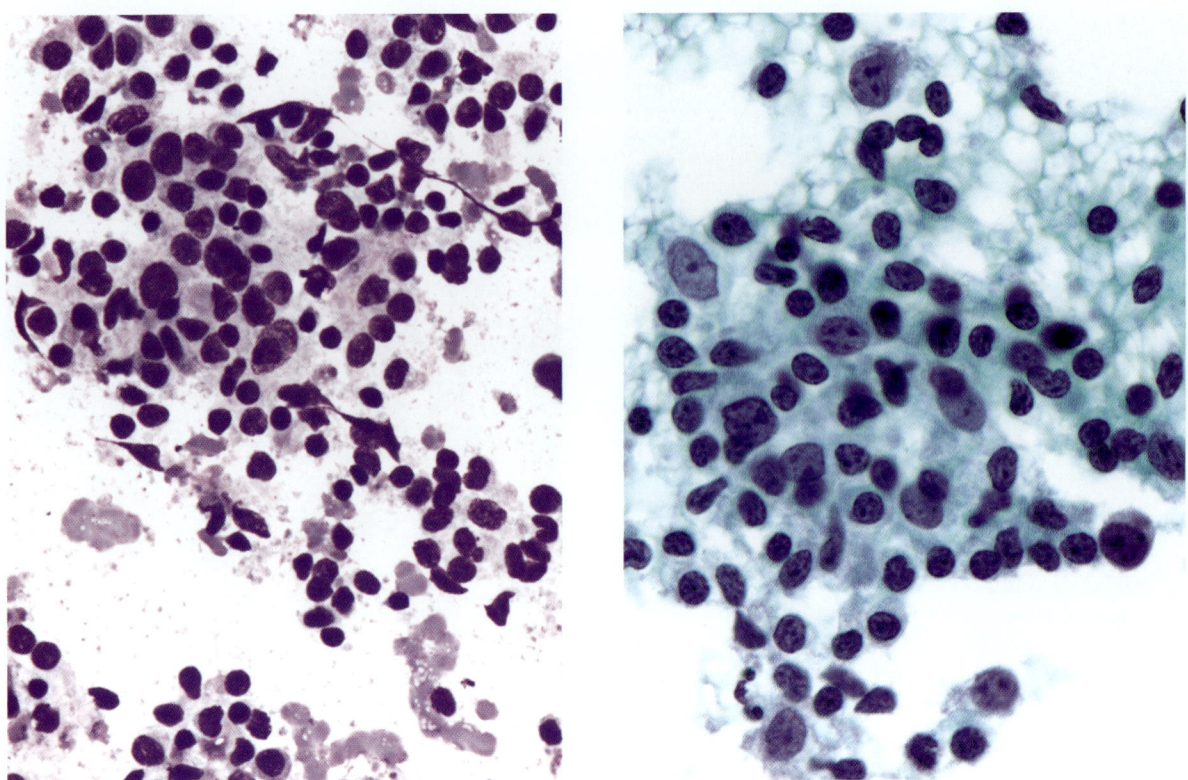

Figure 15-12

EXTRANODAL MARGINAL ZONE LYMPHOMA

Aspirate smears show polymorphous lymphocytes and scattered monocytoid cells that can mimic a reactive process (left: Diff-Quik stain; right: Papanicolaou stain).

tends to occur in extranodal MZLs of the liver, skin, and ocular adnexa, whereas t(3;14)(p14.1;q32), which leads to transcriptional deregulation of *FOXP1*, occurs more often in extranodal MZLs of the thyroid gland, skin, and ocular adnexa. Other translocations are infrequent: t(1;14)(p22;q32) leads to transcriptional deregulation of *BCL10* and occurs most often in the lung or gastrointestinal tract; t(X;14)(p11;q32) is associated with autoimmune disease and involves *GPR34* which encodes a G-protein-coupled receptor involved in cell growth, including the ERK pathway (2,4); and GPR34 overexpression occurs in a subset of extranodal MZLs without t(X;14), suggesting a unique molecular subset of MZLs (2). Additional rare transformations juxtapose *CNN3* (1p21), *KDM4C* (9p24) or *TENM2* (5q34) with *IGH* (42). These translocations tend to be mutually exclusive in extranodal MZLs. Mutations in *TNFAIP3*, which encodes A20 protein and is a negative regulator of the NF-κB pathway, also have been reported, usually mutually exclusive with chromosomal translocations (32).

Recurrent mutations have been detected in MALT lymphomas, including regulators of NF-κB (e.g., *TNFAIP3*, *MYD88*) in approximately 60 percent, *KMT2D/MLL2* in 20 percent, and *NOTCH* (1 and 2) in about 10 percent (18a).

Immunohistochemical assessment for the presence and pattern of BCL10 has been suggested as useful for predicting the presence of some translocations in extranodal MZLs (14). Strong nuclear expression of BCL10 correlates with t(1;14)/*IGH-BCL10* and moderate expression correlates with either t(14;18)/*IGH-MALT1* or t(11;18)/*API2-MALT1*. However, the pattern of BCL10 expression cannot reliably predict the presence of these translocations as nuclear BCL10 expression is observed in lymphomas without these translocations; in other words, it can be falsely positive (45).

Table 15-1

CYTOGENETIC ABNORMALITIES IN EXTRANODAL MARGINAL ZONE LYMPHOMA

Abnormality	Genes	Overall Frequency	Preferred Anatomic Sites	Comments
t(11;18)(q21;q21)	*API2 (BIRC3)* and *MALT1*	20-30%	Lung Stomach Ocular adnexa	First translocation described in EMZL
t(14;18)(q32;q21)	*IGH* and *MALT1*	10-15%	Liver Skin Ocular adnexa	
t(3;14)(p14.1;q32)	*FOXP1* and *IGH*	~10%	Thyroid gland Ocular adnexa Skin	
t(1;14)(p22;q32)	*BCL10* and IGH	~5%	Lung Small intestine Stomach	
3q27 rearrangements	*BCL6*	<5%	Stomach Small intestine Lung Salivary gland Skin	*BCL6-IGH* most common
t(X;14)(p11.2;q32)	*GPR34* and *IGH*	2-3%	Lung Parotid gland	Associated with autoimmune disease
t(1;2)(p22;p12)	*BCL10* and *IGK*	~1%	Stomach	
t(1;14)(p21;q32)	*CNN3* and *IGH*	Rare	Parotid gland	
t(5;14)(q34;q32)	*TENM2* and *IGH*	Rare	Skin Ocular adnexa	
t(9;14)(p24;q32)	*KDM4C* and *IGH*	Rare	Parotid gland Ocular adnexa	
t(6;7)(q25;q11)	Unknown	Rare	Ocular adnexa	
Del(6p23)	*TNFAIP3*/A20	10-20%	Ocular adnexa Thyroid gland Salivary gland	A20 is a global inhibitor of NF-κB; mutations usually occur in translocation-negative cases
Trisomy 3 and 18	Unknown	40-60%	Intestine Salivary gland Skin Ocular adnexa	Trisomy 3 may be more common in cases with monocytoid features
Trisomy 7 and 12	Unknown	~30%		Associated with translocations in EMZL

DIFFERENTIAL DIAGNOSIS

Reactive Lesions. Reactive lymph nodes, particularly those with a lymphoplasmacytic infiltrate, can mimic extranodal MZL. Sheets of monocytoid B cells or centrocyte-like cells support lymphoma. Numerous nuclear pseudoinclusions of cytoplasm (Dutcher bodies) also support lymphoma. Marginal zone cells can colonize follicles, but preserve the follicular pattern. In this circumstance BCL2 and BCL6 are helpful markers: BCL2 is negative and BCL6 is positive in reactive germinal centers and the converse is true in extranodal MZL colonizing follicles. Sheets of B cells, monotypic immunoglobulin light chain expression, or evidence of monoclonality by cytogenetics or molecular methods supports lymphoma.

Other Types of MZL. In lymph nodes, extranodal MZL may closely resemble nodal or splenic MZL. A careful search for extranodal sites of disease or splenomegaly is mandatory. In general, extranodal MZLs tend to involve

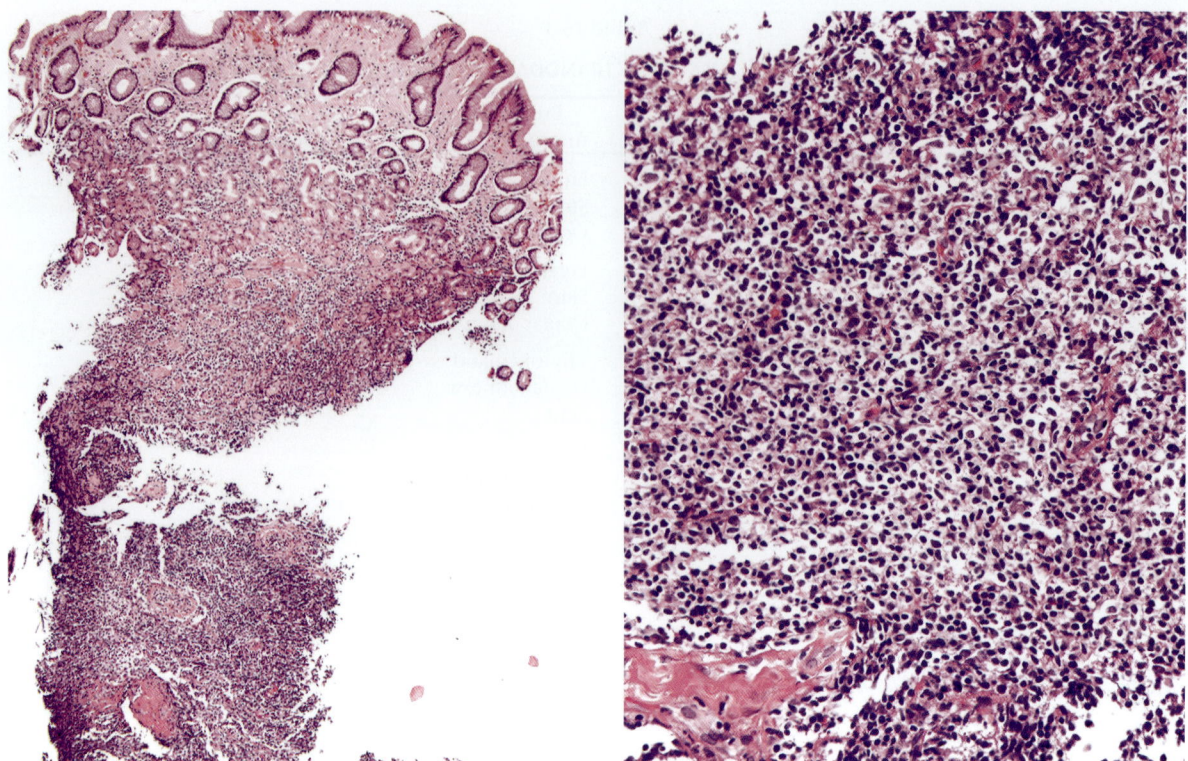

Figure 15-13

GASTRIC EXTRANODAL MARGINAL ZONE LYMPHOMA

The lymphoma, in a 67-year-old man, was associated with a *MYD88* mutation and did not completely respond to either antibiotic therapy or radiation therapy.
Left: Low magnification shows MZL (top of field) located deep to the superficial mucosa and lumen of the stomach.
Right: The lymphoma cells have abundant pale cytoplasm and monocytoid features and few large cells (left, right: H&E stain).

regional lymph nodes draining the extranodal site of disease. In addition, extranodal MZLs often have numerous monocytoid B cells. Patients with splenic MZL often present with complete blood count abnormalities, splenomegaly, and bone marrow involvement, unlike patients with extranodal MZL.

Lymphoplasmacytic Lymphoma. Over 90 percent of patients with lymphoplasmacytic lymphoma (LPL) have a serum IgM paraprotein and bone marrow disease and therefore are more specifically classified as having Waldenstrom macroglobulinemia (WM) (see chapter 16). Some patients with LPL or WM present with extranodal sites of disease, and morphologically these lesions resemble, in part, extranodal MZL.

The clinical history of a serum paraprotein and bone marrow disease supports the diagnosis of LPL/WM. In general, the cells of LPL/WM tend to be more monotonous, Dutcher bodies

are more frequent, and sinuses (in regional lymph nodes) more often patent compared with extranodal MZL. The presence of a *MYD88* L265P mutation is also very helpful, because this finding occurs in over 90 percent of cases of WM and is uncommon in other types of low-grade B-cell lymphoma including extranodal MZL. Nevertheless, we (and others) have observed rare patients with lesions that closely resemble extranodal MZL but carry a *MYD88* mutation. Some of these patients have a serum paraprotein. If such a patient has an IgM paraprotein and bone marrow involvement, we classify the lesion as LPL/WM involving an extranodal site. If the paraprotein is not IgM and there is no bone marrow disease, we classify the lesion as extranodal MZL (fig. 15-13).

Follicular Lymphoma. When extranodal MZL colonizes follicles, the neoplasm may resemble follicular lymphoma, particularly grade 3 tumors. IRTA-1 and MNDA are helpful markers as both are expressed by extranodal MZL, but are rarely expressed by follicular lymphoma. Both extranodal MZL and follicular lymphoma often express BCL2, but residual benign germinal center cells in follicles colonized by extranodal MZL are negative for BCL2, positive for BCL6, and have a high proliferation rate as shown by Ki-67 expression.

Mantle Cell Lymphoma. Mantle cell lymphoma is usually more monomorphic in its appearance than extranodal MZL. In addition, mantle cell lymphoma is positive for CD5, SOX11, and cyclin D1. Rare cases of extranodal MZL, however, are CD5 positive (18), and some cases of mantle cell lymphoma are negative for SOX11. The presence of t(11;14)(q13;q32)/ *CCND1-IGH* supports the diagnosis of mantle cell lymphoma.

Chronic Lymphocytic Leukemia/Small Lymphocytic Lymphoma (CLL/SLL). In 5 to 10 percent of CLL/SLL cases the neoplasm has an interfollicular pattern in which the tumor surrounds reactive germinal centers (see chapter 11). In some cases, prominent proliferation centers wrap around germinal centers, mimicking monocytoid B cells in a marginal zone pattern. Immunophenotyping shows the characteristic immunophenotype of CLL/SLL: dim surface immunoglobulin and CD20, CD5(+), and CD23(+).

Angioimmunoblastic T-Cell Lymphoma. Patients with angioimmunoblastic T-cell lymphoma (AITL) commonly have extranodal sites of disease, such as the skin. In addition, biopsy specimens of AITL often show many reactive B cells intermixed with the neoplastic T cells. At extranodal sites, the number of B cells may suggest the misdiagnosis of extranodal MZL (19). The clinical history is important for this differential diagnosis because patients with extranodal MZL often have localized disease and patients with AITL almost always have generalized lymphadenopathy. Ancillary studies are also useful: extranodal MZLs are usually negative for Epstein-Barr virus (EBV) infection and carry monoclonal *IG* rearrangements; in contrast, cases of AITL involving the skin have a T-follicular helper cell immunophenotype [(CD10(+), BCL6(+), PD-1(+)], are commonly EBV positive, and carry monoclonal *TCR* rearrangements.

Transformation to Diffuse Large B-Cell Lymphoma. Extranodal MZL transforms to

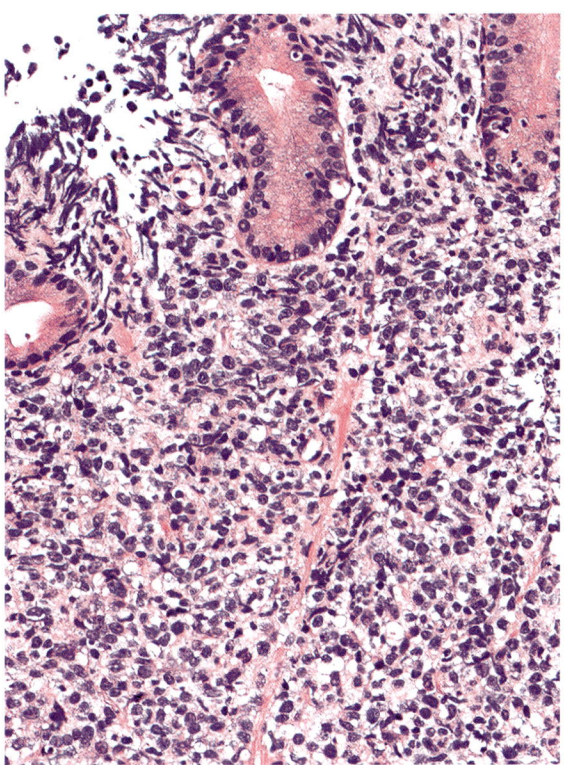

Figure 15-14

GASTRIC EXTRANODAL MARGINAL ZONE LYMPHOMA TRANSFORMED TO DIFFUSE LARGE B-CELL LYMPHOMA

This patient had a history of gastric MZL and subsequently the neoplasm transformed to diffuse large B-cell lymphoma. The lymphoma cells are mostly intermediate-sized or large (H&E stain).

diffuse large B-cell lymphoma in some patients. The risk of transformation is about 5 percent at 15 years and is more common in patients with advanced-stage disease (30a). Scattered large cells are usually evident in all extranodal MZLs and are numerous in some cases. The clinical impact of increased large cells is not well established, but in the stomach, increased large cells (not in sheets) correlates with a poorer response to antibiotic therapy. Nevertheless, the current consensus is to require the presence of sheets of large cells to establish the diagnosis of transformation to diffuse large B-cell lymphoma (fig. 15-14) (14).

TREATMENT AND PROGNOSIS

In a discussion of therapy, it is useful to divide patients with extranodal MZL into gastric and nongastric groups. There is little consensus regarding the therapeutic approach with the exception of gastric MZL. Antibiotic therapy is recommended as first-line therapy for patients with gastric MZL, and particularly for patients with localized disease (47). Eighty to 90 percent of gastric MZLs are associated with *H. pylori* infection and 60 to 70 percent of patients respond with complete remission following combined antibiotic therapy (43). In addition, a small subset of patients with *H. pylori*-negative gastric MZL also responds to antibiotic therapy (37,47). It can take up to a year for a gastric MZL to completely resolve following antibiotic therapy (43). Antibiotic therapy is often ineffective in patients with gastric MZL associated with a chromosomal translocation, most often t(11;18)(q21;q21) (27). In these patients, if the disease is localized, radiation therapy can be highly effective. For patients with advanced-stage disease, various treatment strategies have been applied, analogous to those used for other types of low-grade B-cell lymphoma (20). In general, patients with early-stage disease have a better prognosis than patients with late-stage disease (35,47). Asymptomatic patients with low tumor burden are managed by watchful waiting. Single agent rituximab and various combination chemotherapy regimens have been used for symptomatic or high tumor burden patients with gastric MZL (20,35,47).

Patients with nongastric extranodal MZL, in large part, do not respond to antibiotic therapy but there are some exceptions. Approximately 50 percent of patients with ocular adnexal MZLs associated with *C. psittacci* may respond to doxycycline (11,47). Immunoproliferative small intestinal disease may respond to antibiotics, as can a small subset of patients with cutaneous MZL associated with *Borrelia* species (5,47). For most patients with nongastric MZL, radiation therapy is effective for localized disease. Patients with high-stage disease are managed similarly to those with other types of low-grade B-cell lymphoma (20), either watchful waiting or various single agents or combinations of agents.

Patients with extranodal MZL of gastric or nongastric type may have multiple sites of disease, and are often asymptomatic, and therefore careful staging is necessary (47). Nevertheless, the disease is indolent and survival is long term. In a study of salivary gland MZLs, the median overall survival period was 18.3 years (17). Some have applied the Follicular Lymphoma International Prognostic Index (FLIPI) or other systems for prognostication to these patients (28,47). Younger patient age and localized disease are associated with a better prognosis, as is a history of Sjogren syndrome in patients with salivary gland MZL (17). Relapse of extranodal MZL is common and prolonged clinical follow-up is required (36,47). Transformation to diffuse large B-cell lymphoma portends a poorer prognosis.

REFERENCES

1. Adam P, Czapiewski P, Colak S, et al. Prevalence of Achromobacter xylosoxidans in pulmonary mucosa-associated lymphoid tissue lymphoma in different regions of Europe. Br J Haematol 2014;164:804-810.
2. Ansell SM, Akasaka T, McPhail E, et al. t(X;14)(p11;q32) in MALT lymphoma involving GPR34 reveals a role for GPR34 in tumor cell growth. Blood 2012;120:3949-3957.
3. Arcaini L, Vallisa D, Rattotti S, et al. Antiviral treatment in patients with indolent B-cell lymphomas associated with HCV infection: a study of the Fondazione Italiana Linfomi. Ann Oncol 2014;25:1404-1410.
4. Baens M, Finalet Ferreiro J, Tousseyn T, et al. t(X;14)(p11.4;q32;33) is recurrent in marginal zone lymphoma and up-regulates GPR34. Haematologica 2012;97:184-188.
5. Ben-Ayed F, Halphen M, Najjar T, et al. Treatment of alpha chain disease. Results of a prospective study in 21 Tunisian patients by the Tunisian-French Intestinal Lymphoma Study Group. Cancer 1989;63:1251-1256.
6. Brynes RK, Almaguer PD, Leathery KE, et al. Numerical cytogenetic abnormalities of chromosomes 3, 7, and 12 in marginal zone lymphomas. Mod Pathol 1996;9:995-1000.
7. Crapanzano JP, Lin O. Cytologic findings of marginal zone lymphoma. Cancer 2003;99:301-309.
8. De Boer JP, Hiddink RF, Raderer M, et al. Dissemination patterns in non-gastric MALT lymphoma. Haematologica 2008;93:201-206.
9. Doglioni C, Wotherspoon AC, Moschini A, de Boni M, Isaacson PG. High incidence of primary gastric lymphoma in northeastern Italy. Lancet 1992;339:834-835.
9a. Du MQ. MALT lymphoma: genetic abnormalities, immunological stimulation and molecular mechanism. Best Pract Res Clin Haematol 2017;30:13-23.
10. Falini B, Agostinelli C, Bigerna B, et al. IRTA1 is selectively expressed in nodal and extranodal marginal zone lymphomas. Histopathology 2012;61:930-941.
11. Ferreri AJ, Ponzoni M, Guidoboni M, et al. Bacteria-eradicating therapy with doxycycline in ocular adnexal MALT lymphoma: a multicenter prospective trial. J Natl Cancer Inst 2006;98:1375-1382.
12. Gebauer N, Kuba J, Senft A, Schillert A, Bernard V, Thorns C. MicroRNA-150 Is up-regulated in extranodal marginal zone lymphoma of MALT Type. Cancer Genomics Proteomics 2014;11:51-56.
13. Inamdar KV, Medeiros LJ, Jorgensen JL, Amin HM, Schlette EJ. Bone marrow involvement by marginal zone B-cell lymphomas of different types. Am J Clin Pathol 2008;129:714-722.
14. Isaacson PG, Chott A, Nakamura S, et al. Extranodal marginal zone lymphoma of mucosa-associated lymphoid tissue (MALT lymphoma). In: Swerdlow SH, Campo E. Harris NL, et al. WHO Classification of Tumours of Haematopoietic and Lymphoid Tissue, Lyon, IARC 2008; 214-217.
15. Isaacson P, Wright DH. Malignant lymphoma of mucosa-associated lymphoid tissue. A distinctive type of B-cell lymphoma. Cancer 1983;52:1410-1416.
16. Ishii Y, Tomita N, Suzuki T, et al. Dissemination pattern of extranodal marginal zone lymphoma of mucosa-associated lymphoid tissue. Leuk Lymphoma 2015;56:2750-2752.
17. Jackson AE, Mian M, Kalpadakis C, et al. Extranodal marginal zone lymphoma of mucosa-associated lymphoid tissue of salivary glands: a multicenter, international experience of 248 patients (IELSG 41). Oncologist 2015;20:1149-1153.
18. Jaso J, Chen L, Li S, et al. CD5-positive mucosa-associated lymphoid tissue (MALT) lymphoma: a clinicopathologic study of 14 cases. Hum Pathol 2012;43:1436-1443.
18a. Johansson P, Klein-Hitpass L, Grabellus F, et al. Recurrent mutations in NF-κB pathway components, KMT2D, and NOTCH1/2 in ocular adnexal MALT-type marginal zone lymphomas. Oncotarget 2016;7:62627-62639.
19. Kaffenberger B, Haverkos B, Tyler K, Wong HK, Porcu P, Gru AA. Extranodal marginal zone lymphoma-like presentations of angioimmunoblastic T-cell lymphoma: a T-cell lymphoma masquerading as a B-cell lymphoproliferative disorder. Am J Dermatopathol 2015;37:604-613.
20. Kahl B, Yang D. Marginal zone lymphomas: management of nodal, splenic, and MALT NHL. Hematology Am Soc Hematol Educ Program 2008:359-364.
21. Kanellis G, Roncador G, Arribas A, et al. Identification of MNDA as a new marker for nodal marginal zone lymphoma. Leukemia 2009;23:1847-1857.
22. Kim TM, Kim KH, Lee MJ, et al. First-line therapy with doxycycline in ocular adenexal mucosa-associated lymphoid tissue lymphoma: a retrospective analysis of clinical predictors. Cancer Sci 2010;101:1199-1203
23. Ko YH, Han JJ, Noh JH, Ree HJ. Lymph nodes in gastric B-cell lymphoma: pattern of involvement and early histological changes. Histopathology 2002;40:497-504.

24. Konoplev S, Lin P, Qiu X, Medeiros LJ, Yin CC. Clonal relationship of extranodal marginal zone lymphomas of mucosa-associated lymphoid tissue involving different sites. Am J Clin Pathol 2010;134:112-118.

25. Kuper-Hommel MJ, van Krieken JH. Molecular pathogenesis and histologic and clinical features of extranodal marginal zone lymphomas of mucosa-associated lymphoid tissue type. Leuk Lymphoma 2012;53:1032-1045.

26. Lecuit M, Abachin E, Martin A, et al. Immunoproliferative small intestinal disease associated with Campylobacter jejuni. N Engl J Med 2004;350:239-248.

27. Liu H, Ruskon-Fourmestraux A, Lavergne-Slove A, et al. Resistance of t(11;18) positive gastric mucosa-associated lymphoid tissue lymphoma to Helicobacter pylori eradication therapy. Lancet 2001;357:39-40.

28. Mazloom A, Medeiros LJ, McLaughlin PW, et al. Marginal zone lymphomas: factors that affect the final outcome. Cancer 2010;116:4291-4298.

29. Medeiros LJ, Harmon DC, Linggood RM, Harris NL. Immunohistologic features predict clinical behavior of orbital and conjunctival lymphoid infiltrates. Blood 1989;74:2121-2129.

30. Nie Z, Du MQ, McAllister-Lucas LM, et al. Conversion of the LIMA1 tumour suppressor into an oncogenic LMO-like protein by API2-MALT1 in MALT lymphoma. Nat Commun 2015;6:5908.

30a. Maeshima AM, Taniguchi H, Toyoda K, et al. Clinicopathological features of histological transformation from extranodal marginal zone B-cell lymphoma of mucosa-associated lymphoid tissue to diffuse large B-cell lymphoma: an analysis of 467 patients. Br J Haematol 2016;174:923-931.

31. No authors listed. A clinical evaluation of the International Lymphoma Study Group classification of non-Hodgkin's lymphoma. The Non-Hodgkin's Lymphoma Classification Project. Blood 1997;89:3909-3918.

32. Novak U, Rinaldi A, Kwee I, et al. The NF-{kappa}B negative regulator TNFAIP3 (A20) is inactivated by somatic mutations and genomic deletions in marginal zone lymphomas. Blood 2009;113:4918-4921.

33. Paulli M, Arcaini L, Lucioni M, et al. Subcutaneous 'lipoma-like' B-cell lymphoma associated with HCV infection: a new presentation of primary extranodal marginal zone B-cell lymphoma of MALT. Ann Oncol 2010;21:1189-1195.

34. Price SK. Immunoproliferative small intestinal disease: a study of 13 cases with alpha heavy-chain disease. Histopathology 1990;17:7-17.

35. Raderer M, Kiesewetter B, Ferreri AJ. Clinicopathologic characteristics and treatment of marginal zone lymphoma of mucosa-associated lymphoid tissue (MALT lymphoma). CA Cancer J Clin 2016;66:153-171.

36. Raderer M, Streubel B, Woehrer S, et al. High relapse rate in patients with MALT lymphoma warrants lifelong follow-up. Clin Cancer Res 2005;11:3349-3352.

37. Raderer M, Wohrer S, Kiesewetter B, et al. Antibiotic treatment as sole management of Helicobacter pylori-negative gastric MALT lymphoma: a single center experience with prolonged follow up. Ann Hematol 2015;94:969-973.

38. Raderer M, Wohrer S, Streubel B, et al. Assessment of disease dissemination in gastric compared with extragastric mucosa-associated lymphoid tiossue lymphoma using extensive staging: a single-center experience. J Clin Oncol 2006;24:3136-3141.

39. Rinaldi A, Mian M, Chigrinova E, et al. Genome-wide DNA profiling of marginal zone lymphomas identifies subtype-specific lesions with an impact on the clinical outcome. Blood 2011;117:1595-1604.

40. Saito Y, Suzuki H, Tsugawa H, et al. Overexpression of miR-142-5p and miR-155 in gastric mucosa-associated lymphoid tissue (MALT) lymphoma resistant to Helicobacter pylori eradication. PLoS One 2012;7:e47396.

41. Thieblemont C, Berger F, Dumontet C, et al. Mucosa-associated lymphoid tissue lymphoma is a disseminated disease in one third of 158 patients analyzed. Blood 2000;95:802-806.

42. Vinatzer U, Gollinger M, Müllauer L, Raderer M, Chott A, Streubel B. Mucosa-associated lymphoid tissue lymphoma: novel translocations including rearrangements of ODZ2, JMJD2C, and CNN3. Clin Cancer Res 2008;14:6426-6433.

43. Wotherspoon AC, Doglioni C, Diss TC, et al. Regression of primary low-grade B-cell gastric lymphoma of mucosa-associated lymphoid tissue type after eradication of Helicobacter pylori. Lancet 1993;342:575-577.

44. Ye H, Remstein ED, Bacon CM, Nicholson AG, Dogan A, Du MQ. Chromosomal translocations involving BCL6 in MALT lymphoma. Haematologica 2008;93:145-146.

45. Yeh KH, Kuo SH, Chen LT, et al. Nuclear expression of BCL10 or nuclear factor kappa B helps predict Helicobacter pylori-independent status of low-grade gastric mucosa-associated lymphoid tissue lymphomas with or without t(11;18)(q21;q21). Blood 2005;106:1037-1041.

46. Zhang Q, Pocrnich C, Kurian A, et al. Amyloid deposition in extranodal marginal zone lymphoma of mucosa-associated lymphoid tissue: a clinicopathologic study of 5 cases. Pathol Res Pract 2016;212:185-189.

47. Zucca E, Bertoni F. The spectrum of MALT lymphoma at different sites: biological and therapeutic relevance. Blood 2016;127:2082-2092.

16 LYMPHOPLASMACYTIC LYMPHOMA AND WALDENSTROM MACROGLOBULINEMIA

GENERAL FEATURES

Lymphoplasmacytic lymphoma (LPL) is defined as a neoplasm of B lineage composed of small B lymphocytes, plasmacytoid B lymphocytes, and plasma cells (47). The neoplastic cells are most commonly found in the peripheral blood and bone marrow; lymph nodes and spleen are involved in a small subset of patients. LPL is frequently associated with a paraprotein, most often of IgM type, but as currently defined, a paraprotein is not required to establish the diagnosis of LPL (47). *Waldenstrom macroglobulinemia* (WM) is defined as a B-cell lymphoma that is consistent with LPL that involves the bone marrow and is accompanied by an IgM monoclonal paraprotein of any concentration (37,47).

Inherent in the above definition of WM is the fact that this diagnosis requires the presence of LPL in the bone marrow. This being true, an argument can be made that the diagnosis of LPL/WM is redundant if the patient is known to have bone marrow involvement and a serum IgM paraprotein. Furthermore, using current diagnostic criteria, about 95 percent of all cases in the category of LPL/WM are, in fact, WM and studies of LPL in the medical literature published to date are, for the most part, composed of patients with WM. We therefore suggest that combining LPL and WM as "LPL/WM" makes it difficult to explore the differences between these two entities, the former diagnosis based on pathologic criteria and the latter based on clinical and pathologic criteria. For these reasons, WM is the major focus of this chapter and, from this point forward, WM and LPL of non-WM type are specified separately. When the term WM is used here it needs to be understood that the patient has LPL (in addition to WM).

The pathogenesis of WM is incompletely understood. A familial predisposition is observed in approximately 20 percent of patients (2,36,49). Other risk factors identified by the InterLymph Non-Hodgkin Lymphoma Subtypes Project include: history of autoimmune disease, serologic evidence of hepatitis C infection, history of hay fever, higher body weight, long duration of cigarette smoking, and occupation as a medical doctor (52). The autoimmune diseases most often associated with WM are Sjogren syndrome and systemic lupus erythematosus (46,52). Patients with WM associated with hepatitis C infection have been reported most often in Italy and may have mixed (type II) cryoglobulinemia (1,41).

Patients with IgM type monoclonal gammopathy of uncertain significance (MGUS) have a greater than 200-fold increased risk of WM (21,22). IgM MGUS is therefore thought to be the precursor of WM. Progression from IgM MGUS to smoldering WM and then full-blown WM has been documented in many patients, supporting the concept that IgM MGUS is a precursor lesion (21). The discovery of myeloid differentiation primary response 88 (*MYD88*) mutations in most cases of WM and at least 50 percent of IgM MGUS cases also supports a precursor role (51,53). In line with this idea, the cell of origin of WM is thought to be an IgM-secreting memory B cell.

The annual incidence of WM is 3 to 4 cases per million persons per year, accounting for about 1 percent of lymphomas in the United States and Europe (47,52). In the United States there are approximately 1,500 cases of WM per year. The disease is even less common in Asia.

CLINICAL FEATURES

WM occurs most frequently in adult Caucasian patients in the seventh decade of life and is uncommon in African Americans. The male to female ratio of 1.2 to 1.0 (47). Autoimmune diseases and other paraneoplastic phenomena can occur in WM patients, including a rare syndrome of diffuse urticaria known as *Schnitzler syndrome*.

Approximately 70 percent of WM patients are symptomatic at the time of diagnosis (36,46). The asymptomatic group includes patients with so-called smoldering WM, defined as the presence of minimal (about 10 percent) bone marrow disease and an IgM paraprotein in a patient without end organ damage. Symptomatic WM patients have clinical signs and symptoms that can be attributed to one or more of the following disease features: 1) serum hyperviscosity; 2) IgM autoantibodies; 3) effects of paraprotein deposition into tissues; and 4) infiltration of tissues by lymphoma (36,47).

The most common symptoms in patients with WM are malaise and lethargy; these are frequently associated with cytopenias as a result of bone marrow infiltration by lymphoma. B-type symptoms (fever, night sweats, and weight loss) occur in up to 25 percent of patients. Lymphadenopathy and hepatosplenomegaly occur in 10 to 20 percent of patients at time of diagnosis, but are more common with disease progression (36,46).

Hyperviscosity syndrome is perhaps the best known complication of WM, occurring in 10 to 15 percent of patients (13,46) and was described by Waldenstrom himself in his original paper (54). Hyperviscosity results from the unique physical characteristics of IgM, which, when secreted in serum, forms 925-kD pentamers with 10 antigen-combining sites. As a result, IgM paraprotein is a large and complex structure that is restricted to the intravascular space. Other factors, such as level of hydration and erythrocyte mass, are also involved. The shear forces associated with hyperviscosity result in rupture of unsupported venous channels and vascular obstruction. Visual changes due to retinal compromise, headache, dizziness, and oronasal bleeding are also common symptoms in patients with hyperviscosity syndrome (13).

Patients with WM show a wide range of IgM paraprotein levels, from 0.1 to over 8.0 g/dL (or rarely, higher) (13,25,38). There is a strong correlation between higher paraprotein levels, particularly over 6.0 g/dL, and hyperviscosity syndrome (13). Normal patients have a serum viscosity in the range of 1.4 to 1.8 centipoise (cp). In contrast, patients with hyperviscosity syndrome usually have a serum viscosity of at least 4 to 5 cp. This degree of hyperviscosity requires a paraprotein level of at least 5 g/dL (13). Serum levels of IgG and IgA are often decreased in WM patients.

Other problems associated with an IgM paraprotein correlate less with serum IgM levels.

Disorders in coagulation are associated with IgM binding of platelets, clotting factors, or fibrin. IgM-associated cryoglobinemia occurs in up to 20 percent of patients (1,41) and approximately 5 percent have symptoms related to cryoglobulins. IgM-related neuropathy can result from antibody reactivity or tissue deposition, and occurs 10 to 30 percent of patients (36,46). Kidney failure, gastrointestinal symptoms, or bullous skin disease can result from IgM deposition into tissues. Anti-IgM recognizes erythrocytes that express I antigen, resulting in cold agglutinin hemolytic anemia in 5 to 10 percent of patients that have been reported as having WM (see Differential Diagnosis).

As WM is defined, all patients have bone marrow involvement. About 20 percent present with or subsequently develop lymphadenopathy and 10 to 15 percent have splenomegaly or hepatomegaly. A wide variety of other anatomic sites may be involved, often associated with disease progression (4). Approximately 5 percent of patients have extramedullary disease, most often involving the lungs, soft tissue, central nervous system, kidneys, and bones (4). Extramedullary involvement by WM at time of initial diagnosis is associated with poor prognostic features and a shorter survival period (4,8). Involvement of the central nervous system, so-called *Bing-Neel syndrome*, is also associated with a poorer prognosis.

HISTOLOGIC FINDINGS

Lymph Nodes and Other Tissues

The most common patterns of involvement by WM in lymph nodes are medullary, interfollicular, and paracortical, and the disease may be subtle and associated with patent sinuses (figs. 16-1, 16-2) (24,46,47). Residual follicles are small or hyperplastic (figs. 16-1C, 16-2, right). The neoplasm also may diffusely replace the lymph node architecture. Follicular colonization can occur, but is uncommon. Monocytoid cells can be seen in WM, but these cells are not (or rarely) prominent.

Eosinophilic intranuclear pseudoinclusions (known as Dutcher bodies) (fig. 16-3) and cytoplasmic inclusions (Russell bodies) are commonly present and can be numerous. Dutcher and Russell bodies are commonly positive for the periodic acid–Schiff (PAS) reaction. Mast cells are

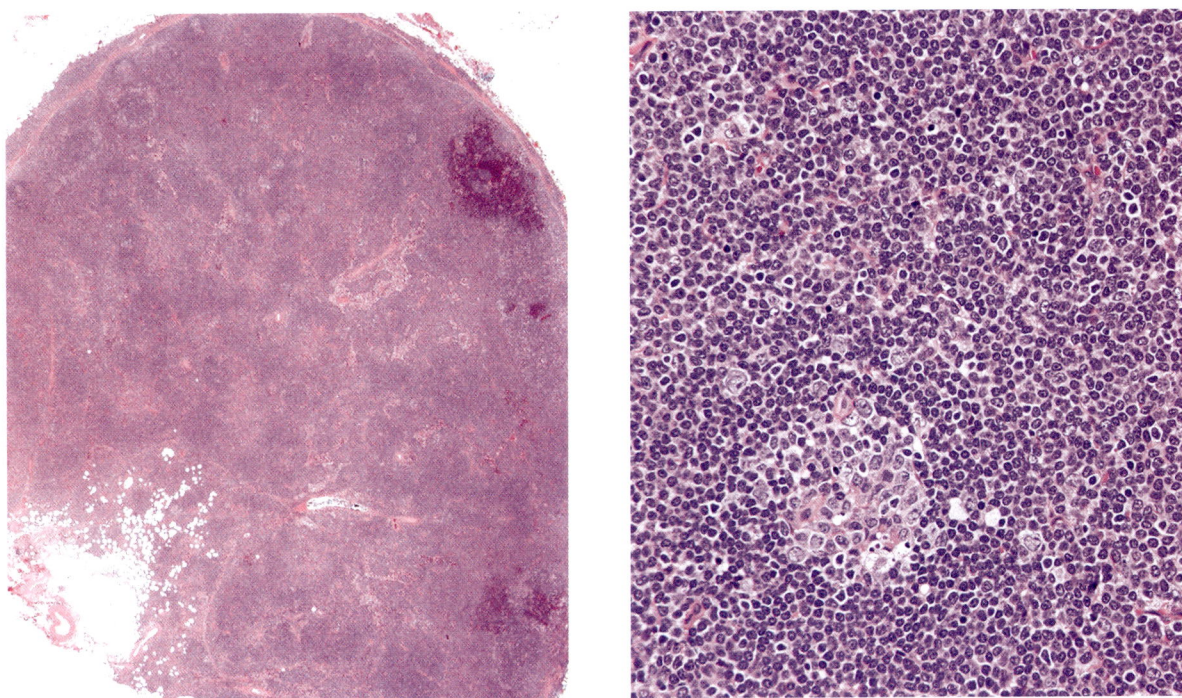

Figure 16-1

WALDENSTROM MACROGLOBULINEMIA INVOLVING LYMPH NODE

Left: The neoplasm involves the interfollicular and medullary regions of the lymph node (lower left), and some sinuses are patent. The overall purplish hue is attributable to cells with plasmacytoid differentiation.

Right: The neoplasm surrounds and spares a small reactive germinal center in this field (left, right: hematoxylin and eosin [H&E] stain).

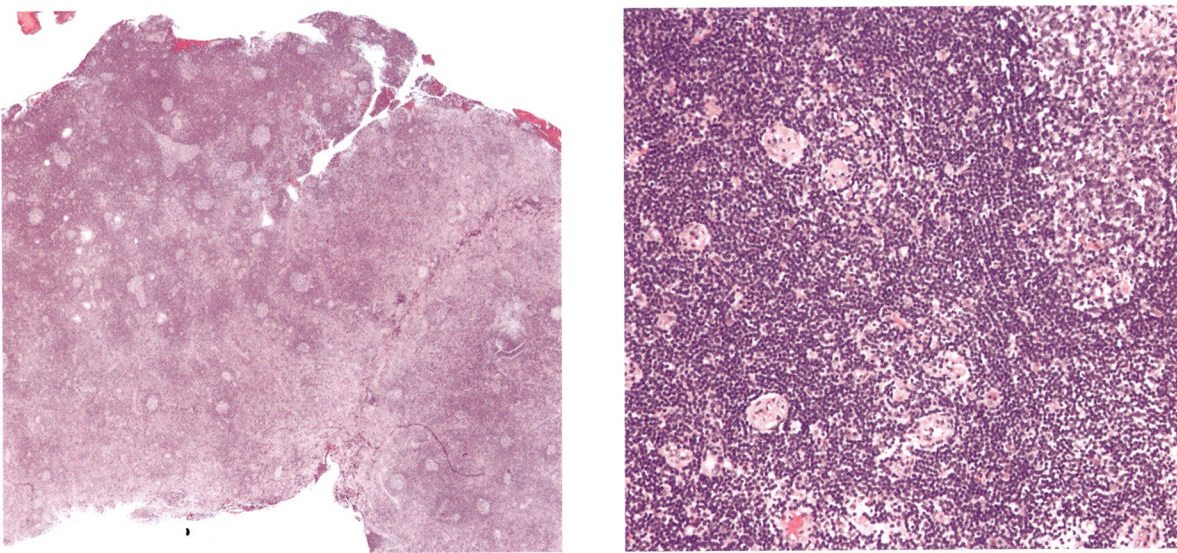

Figure 16-2

WALDENSTROM MACROGLOBULINEMIA INVOLVING LYMPH NODE

Left: The lymphoma infiltrates between reactive follicles. A purplish hue is seen at this magnification.
Right: Higher magnification shows a prominent reactive follicle (upper right) (left, right: H&E stain).

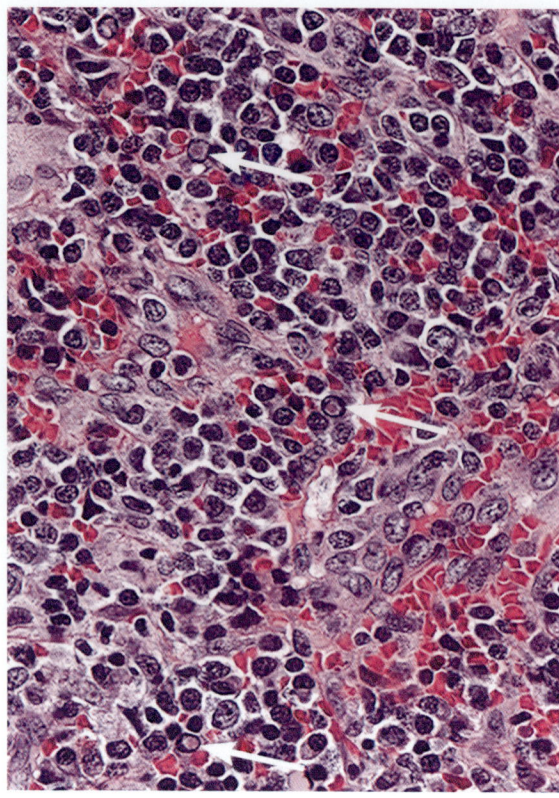

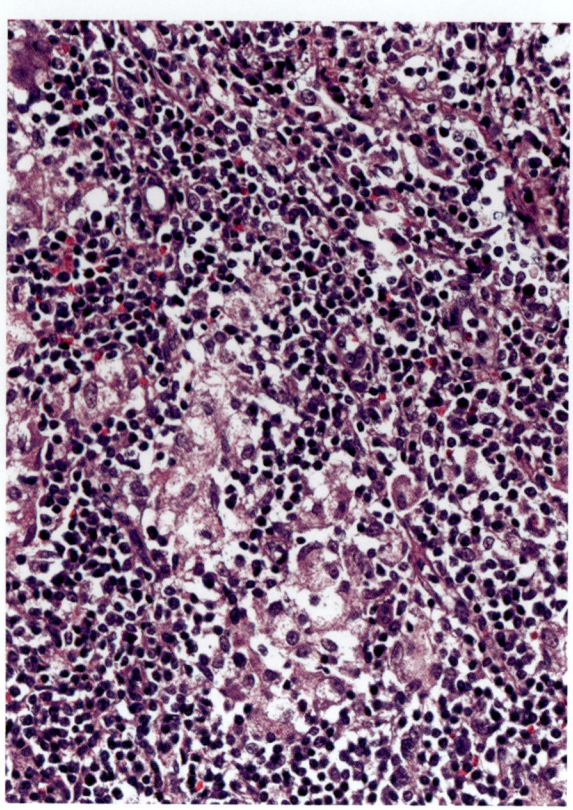

Figure 16-3

**WALDENSTROM MACROGLOBULINEMIA
INVOLVING LYMPH NODE**

Some of the neoplastic cells have intranuclear pseudo-inclusions of cytoplasm known as Dutcher bodies (arrows) (H&E stain).

Figure 16-4

**WALDENSTROM MACROGLOBULINEMIA
INVOLVING LYMPH NODE**

A sinus is distended by histiocytes (H&E stain).

increased in many cases. The patent sinuses may have histiocytes (fig. 16-4) containing pink amorphous (PAS positive) material (immunoglobulin) or hemosiderin deposits. Amyloid deposits are uncommon but can be observed (fig. 16-5).

The neoplastic cells of WM show a spectrum of features including small round lymphocytes with minimal cytoplasm, plasmacytoid cells with moderate or more abundant cytoplasm, and mature plasma cells (Marschalko type). Occasional (less than 5 percent) scattered large cells may be present.

In lymph nodes WM can exhibit a cytologic spectrum (24). The lymphoplasmacytoid variant (fig. 16-6A) is characterized by numerous small lymphocytes with minimal plasmacytoid differentiation; the lymphoplasmacytic variant (fig. 16-6B) is characterized a mixture of small lymphocytes and mature plasma cells; and the polymorphous type (fig. 16-6C) is characterized by an increased number of larger cells, at least 5 percent. The lymphoplasmacytoid and lymphoplasmacytic variants do not have prognostic importance and knowledge of these variants is mostly helpful in facilitating the recognition of WM. In contrast, the polymorphous variant of WM correlates with a higher frequency of abnormalities detected by conventional cytogenetics and may represent an early step in the evolution of WM to diffuse large B-cell lymphoma (DLBCL) (27).

Cases of LPL of non-WM type involving lymph nodes are less well characterized and distinguishing these tumors from MZLs can be arbitrary in some cases (47). In general, the features of LPL of non-WM type involving lymph nodes resemble those described above for WM (fig. 16-7) (7).

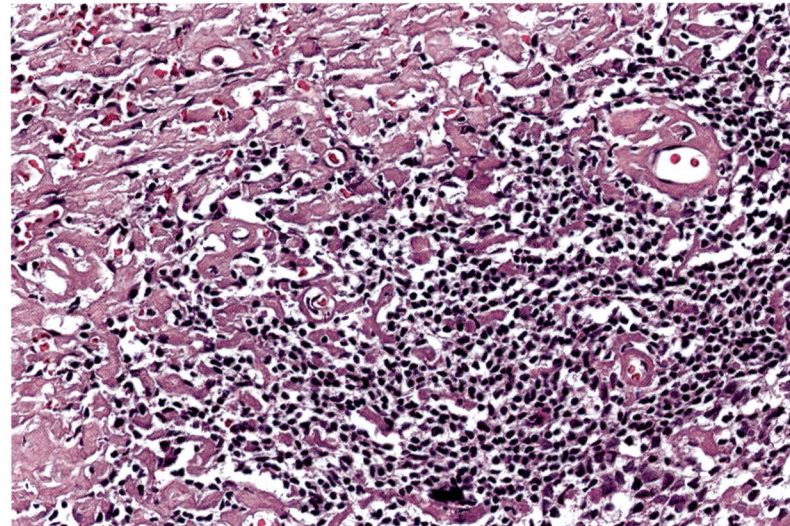

Figure 16-5

**WALDENSTROM
MACROGLOBULINEMIA
ASSOCIATED WITH AMYLOID**

The neoplasm is associated with amyloid around blood vessels and between lymphoid cells (H&E stain).

Figure 16-6

**WALDENSTROM MACROGLOBULINEMIA:
MORPHOLOGIC VARIANTS**

Three morphologic variants of WM are shown: lymphoplasmacytoid (A); lymphoplasmacytic variant with more numerous mature plasma cells (B); and polymorphous with increased large cells in the range of 5 percent (C) (A–C: H&E stain).

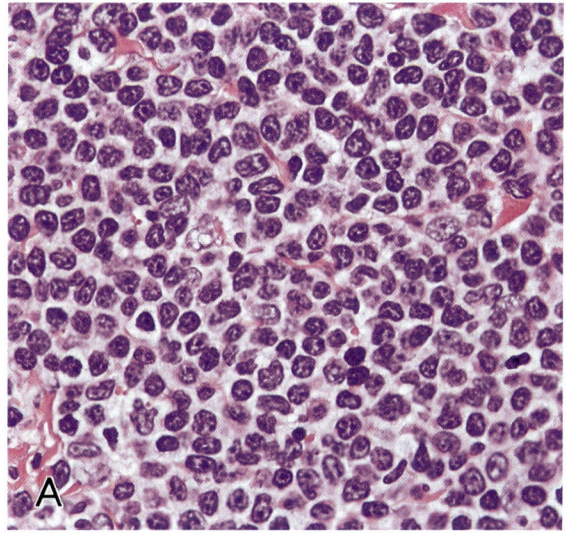

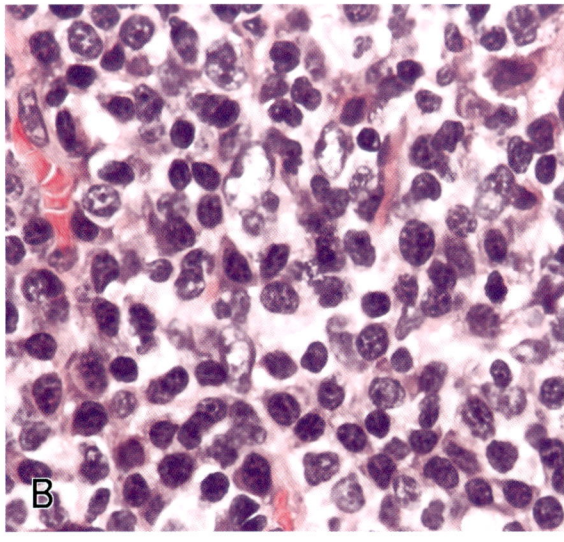

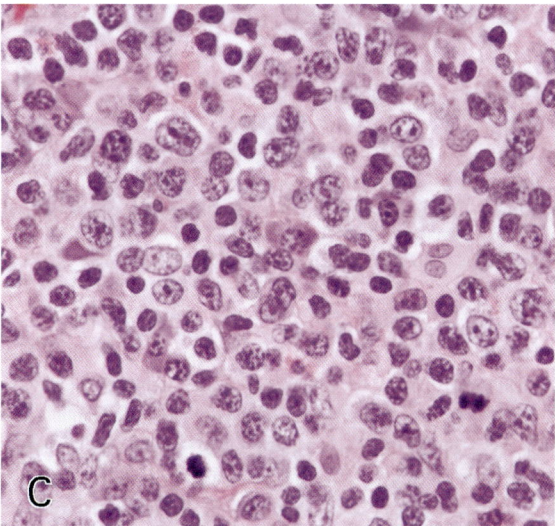

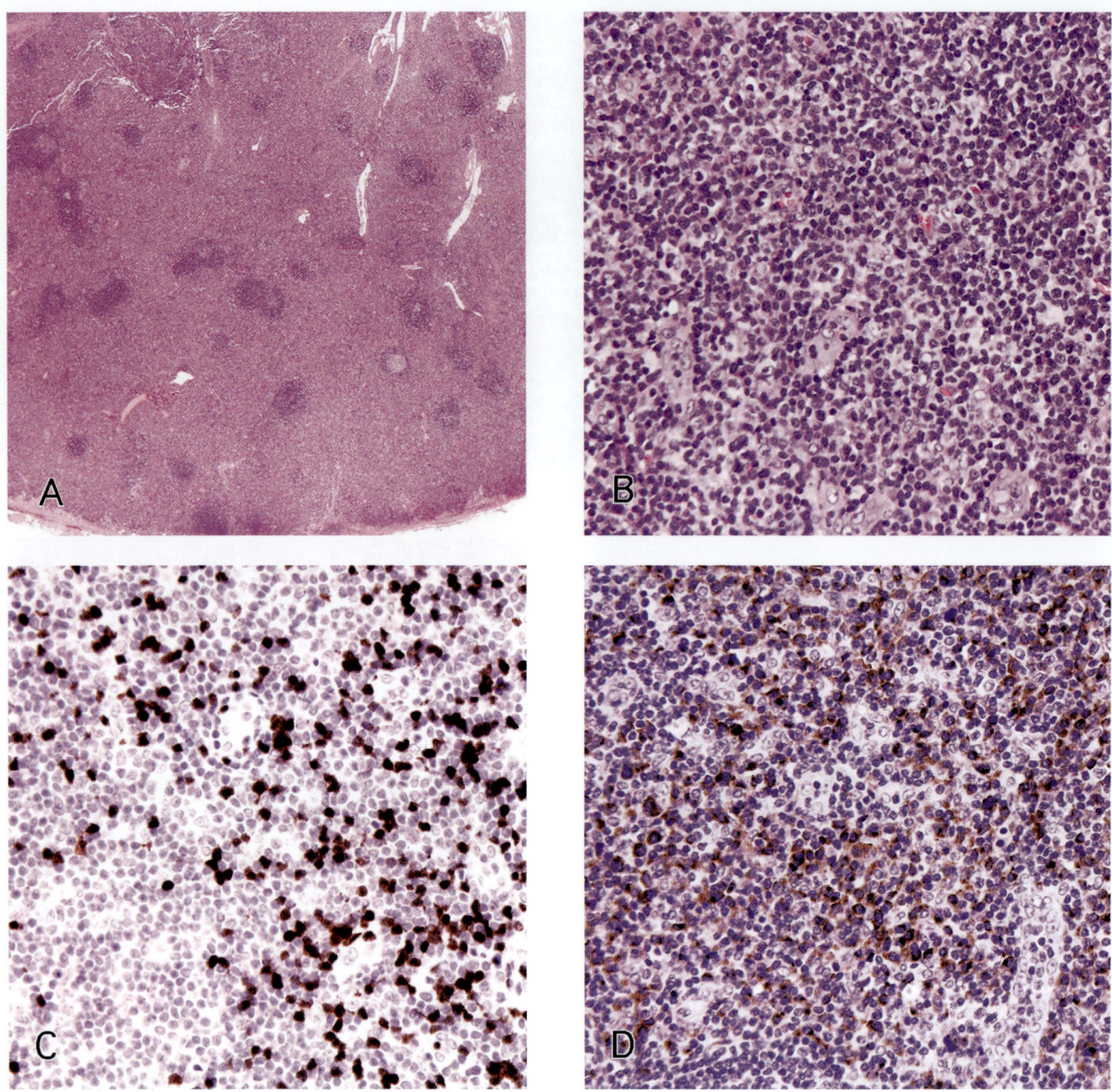

Figure 16-7

LYMPHOPLASMACYTIC LYMPHOMA OF NON-WM TYPE INVOLVING LYMPH NODE

A: At low power magnification, the neoplasm extensively replaces the lymph node while sparing many follicles (A,B: H&E stain).

B: The neoplastic cells are a mixture of small lymphocytes, plasmacytoid lymphocytes, and plasma cells.

C: The neoplastic lymphocytes express PAX5 (C,D: immunohistochemistry with hematoxylin counterstain).

D: Plasmacytoid lymphocytes and plasma cells express cytoplasmic monotypic immunoglobulin kappa.

Peripheral Blood

Patients with WM usually do not have leukocytosis, but some exhibit low-level lymphocytosis. The lymphocytes often show plasmacytoid features. Platelets and erythrocytes are often decreased as a result of bone marrow infiltration and replacement by lymphoma. Erythrocytes can exhibit rouleaux, in which erythrocytes adhere to each other and resemble "a stack of coins" (fig. 16-8). This phenomenon is explained by elevated serum levels of IgM paraprotein, which interferes with the zeta potential of erythrocytes.

Bone Marrow

WM most often involves the bone marrow in an interstitial or diffuse pattern, but a nodular pattern also occurs (fig. 16-9). A paratrabecular pattern of involvement in WM also has been reported, but in our opinion when this pattern is observed marginal zone lymphoma (particularly splenic type) needs to be excluded. Scattered or more numerous reactive mast cells are often intermixed with the neoplastic cells, which are more easily appreciated when highlighted immunohistochemically (fig. 16-10). Dutcher and Russell bodies (fig. 16-11) may be prominent in bone marrow biopsy specimens.

In bone marrow aspirate smears, the neoplastic cells show a range of cell types, including small B lymphocytes, plasmacytoid lymphocytes, plasma cells, and rare larger cells (fig. 16-12). The three variants of WM in lymph node (see above) were described by Bartl et al. (6) in bone marrow. Mast cells are metachromatic in Romanowsky stains and are often most numerous and entangled within the particles. Amyloid deposits can be identified in smears and/or biopsy specimens.

CYTOLOGIC FINDINGS

In cytologic preparations of WM, the cellular infiltrate closely mimics the findings in bone marrow, including small mature lymphocytes, plasmacytoid lymphocytes, and plasma cells (fig. 16-13). Dutcher bodies may be numerous (fig. 16-14) and Russell bodies also are observed. Dutcher bodies are rare in benign infiltrates but the number of Russell bodies is not well correlated with malignancy. Mast cells are highlighted by the Diff-Quik or other Romanowsky stains and can provide an early clue to the diagnosis (fig. 16-15).

IMMUNOPHENOTYPIC FINDINGS

The cells of WM are most commonly analyzed in the bone marrow by flow cytometric immunophenotypic analysis (19,30). There are two cell populations in WM that need to be analyzed: lymphocytes and plasmacytoid lymphocytes/plasma cells. Lymphocytes express monotypic surface immunoglobulin light chain, IgM, CD19, CD20, CD22, and CD79a. CD25, CD27, and FMC7 are usually positive and CD45 may be variably positive. Approximately half of WM cases express CD11c or CD23 dimly.

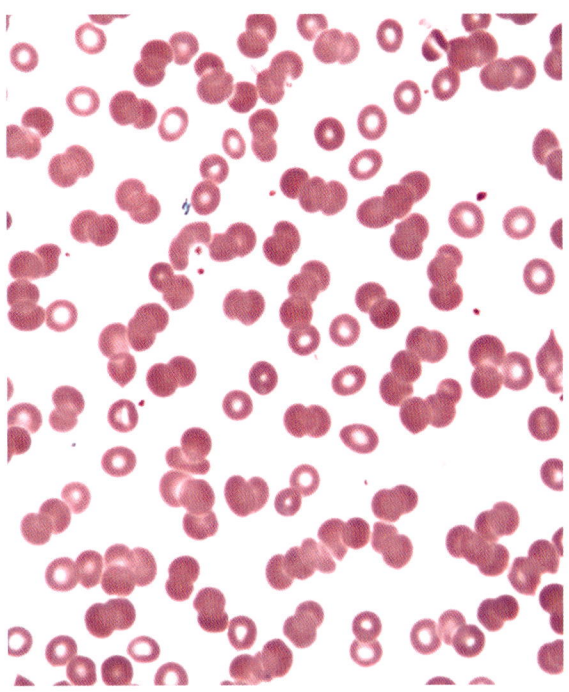

Figure 16-8

ROULEAUX IN A PATIENT WITH WALDENSTROM MACROGLOBULINEMIA

Rouleaux formation in a blood smear is attributable to increased IgM paraprotein (Wright-Giemsa stain).

Most cases are negative for CD5 or CD10, but rare WM cases are positive, usually dimly. WM cells are characteristically IgD negative, and uniformly negative for CD2, CD3, CD7, and CD103. The plasmacytic cells of WM express cytoplasmic IgM, monotypic cytoplasmic light chain, CD38, and CD138. CD19 is often expressed by the plasmacytoid cells. LPL cases not meeting the criteria for WM in bone marrow closely resemble WM except that these cases express IgG or IgA.

Immunohistochemical analysis also is used to assess WM cases using many of the antibodies available by flow cytometry. The lymphocytes express a variety of B-cell antigens including CD19, CD20 (fig. 16-16), CD22, CD79A, and PAX5. Typically, dim expression of CD5, CD10, and CD23 that can be observed by flow cytometry is absent by immunohistochemistry. Plasmacytoid cells express CD19, CD79A, cytoplasmic IgM and light chain, and plasma cell-associated antigens (fig. 16-16). Approximately 75 percent of cases of WM are positive for TCL-1, which is

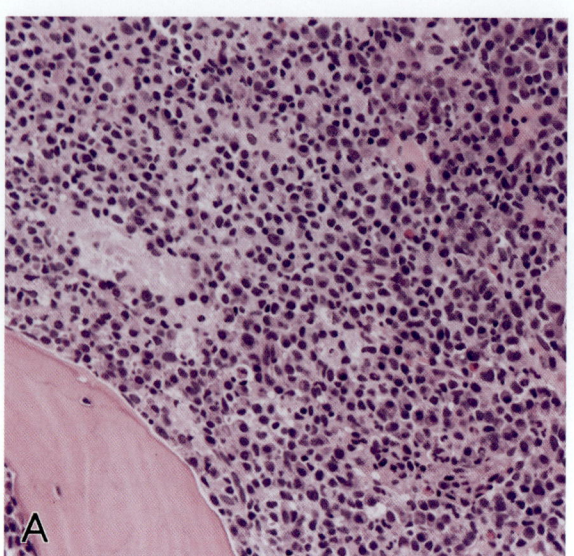

Figure 16-9

**WALDENSTROM MACROGLOBULINEMIA
INVOLVING BONE MARROW**

Patterns of bone marrow involvement by WM include:
diffuse (A); interstitial (B); and/or nodular (C) (A–C: H&E
stain).

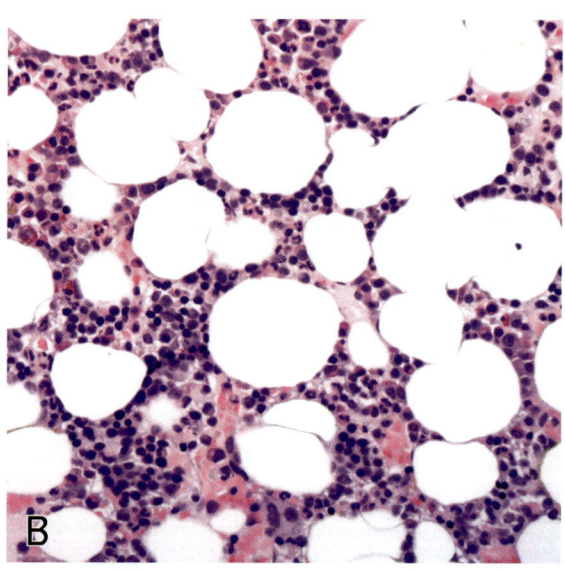

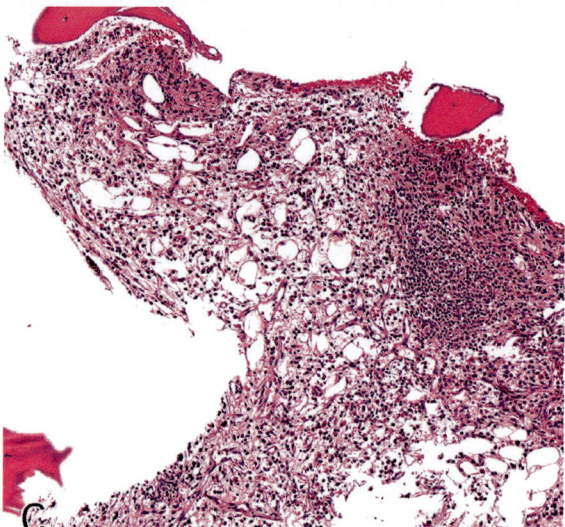

associated with a poorer prognosis (23). Most
cases have a low proliferation rate as assessed
by Ki-67. Cyclin D1 is negative and there is no
evidence of Epstein-Barr virus. Lymphocytes
and plasma cells often do not respond to therapy equally. Plasma cells may persist whereas
lymphocytes may be absent in post-therapy
bone marrow specimens (5,11).

MOLECULAR GENETIC FINDINGS

Cases of WM and LPL of non-WM type show
monoclonal *IGH* and light chain rearrangements
and the T-cell receptor genes are in the germline configuration. In WM, the *IGH* variable
gene segments show somatic hypermutation,

without ongoing mutations, and no evidence
of isotype switching. In addition, there appears
to be preferential usage the VH3 and JH4 gene
segments (44). These results suggest that WM
arises from IgM-positive memory B cells which
normally are located in the bone marrow.

Deletions of chromosome 6q21-25 have
been reported in 30 to 60 percent of bone
marrow-based WM cases, but seem to be less
frequent in tissue-based WM (9,27,33,45). A large
review of 174 WM cases (32) showed the following frequency of cytogenetic abnormalities listed
in descending order: del(6q), 30 percent; trisomy
18, 15 percent; del(13q), 13 percent; del(17p),
8 percent; trisomy 4, 8 percent; and del(11q), 7

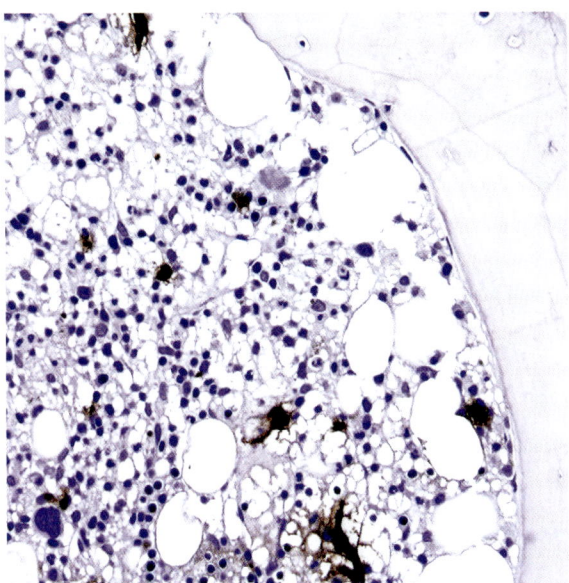

Figure 16-10

**WALDENSTROM MACROGLOBULINEMIA:
MAST CELLS**

Tryptase highlights scattered mast cells in a bone marrow biopsy specimen involved by WM (immunohistochemistry with hematoxylin counterstain).

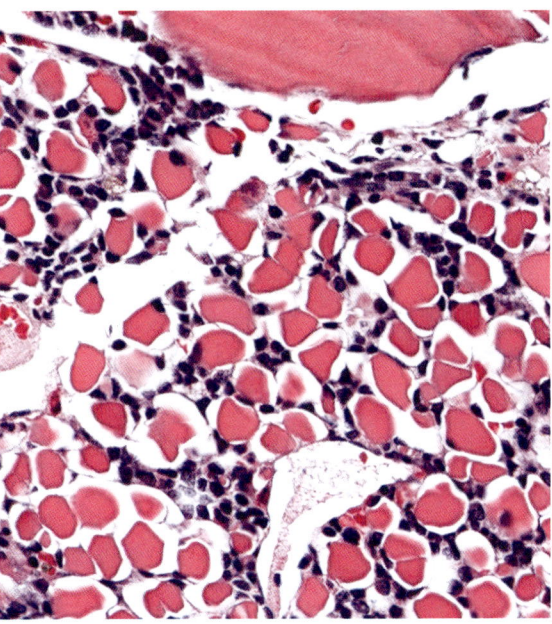

Figure 16-11

**WALDENSTROM MACROGLOBULINEMIA
INVOLVING BONE MARROW BIOPSY**

The plasma cell component exhibits numerous cells with cytoplasm distended by immunoglobulin (Russell bodies) (H&E stain).

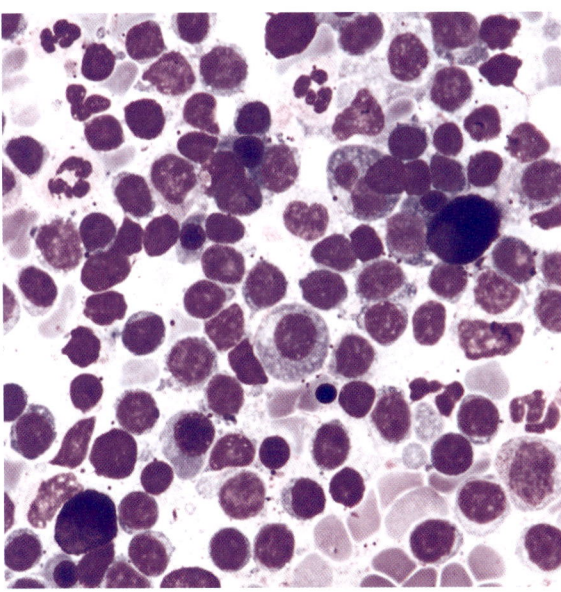

Figure 16-12

**WALDENSTROM MACROGLOBULINEMIA:
BONE MARROW ASPIRATE SMEAR**

Many lymphocytes, plasmacytoid lymphocytes, and scattered metachromatic, purple mast cells are present (Wright-Giemsa stain).

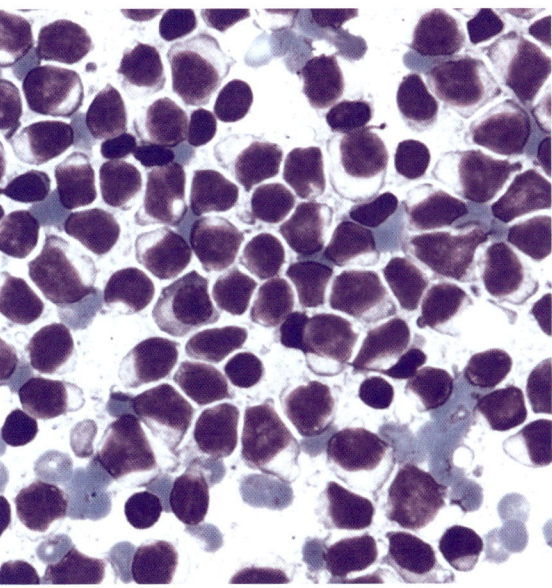

Figure 16-13

**WALDENSTROM MACROGLOBULINEMIA:
LYMPH NODE ASPIRATE SMEAR**

There are many small lymphocytes and plasmacytoid cells seen in this fine-needle aspirate (Diff-Quik stain).

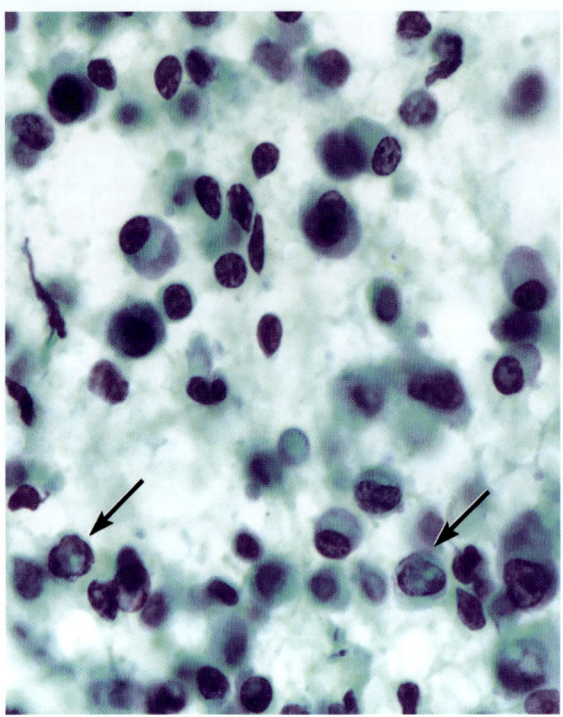

Figure 16-14

**WALDENSTROM MACROGLOBULINEMIA:
LYMPH NODE ASPIRATE**

In this fine-needle aspirate, scattered plasmacytoid cells with Dutcher bodies (arrows) are seen (Papanicolaou stain).

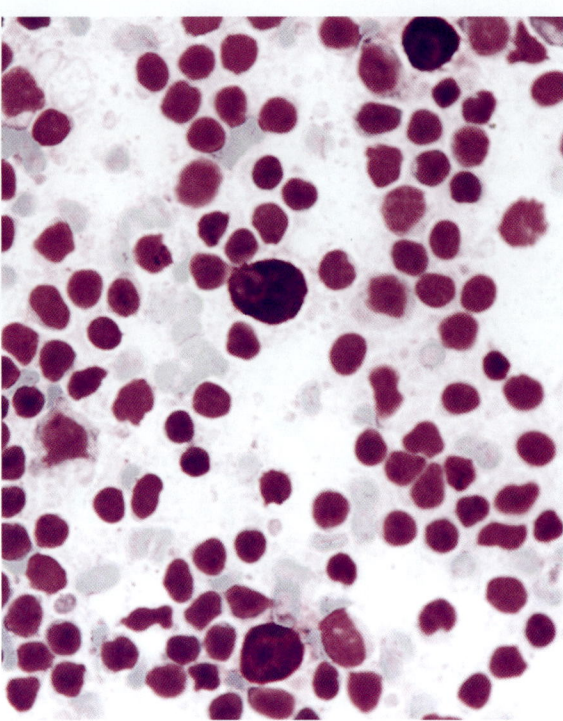

Figure 16-15

**WALDENSTROM MACROGLOBULINEMIA
INVOLVING LYMPH NODE**

A scrape preparation of a freshly cut lymph node involved by WM. The observation of mast cells can be an early indication of the diagnosis, even before histologic sections are examined (H&E stain).

percent. *IGH* translocations and trisomy 12 were rare, each less than 5 percent. Deletion of 17p and trisomy 12 correlated with a poorer prognosis.

The t(9;14)(p13;q32)/*IGH-PAX5* was reported to be highly associated with WM in the third edition of the World Health Organization (WHO) classification published in 2001. It was shown in subsequent studies, however, that this translocation is rare and not specific for WM (10,15,27,34). Other translocations, such as t(8;14)(q24;q32/*MYC-IGH*, t(11;14)(q13;q32)/ *CCND1-IGH*, and t(14;18)(q32;q21)/*IGH-BCL2*, are characteristically absent in WM (27,32).

Studies using gene expression profiling and RNA sequence analysis have shown that WM cells overexpress VDJ recombination genes, CXCR4 pathway genes, and some BCL2 family members (16a). *MYD88* mutations occur in up to 90 percent of WM cases (12,18,39,51,53). MYD88 is an adaptor protein involved in the interleukin-1 (IL-1) and toll-like receptor pathways and encoded by a gene located at chromo-

some 3p22.2. Following IL-1/toll-like receptor stimulation, MYD88 is recruited to the activated complex which then forms a complex with IL-1R-associated kinase (IRAK-1). Subsequently, the complex activates tumor necrosis factor receptor-associated factor 6 and eventually NF-κB. The most common *MYD88* mutation, L265P, is a somatic T to C change that results in an amino acid change from leucine to proline (51). Uncommon non-L265P mutations also have been described. *MYD88* mutation results in activation of pathways that include Bruton tyrosine kinase and other molecules and results in constitutive NF-κB activation and enhanced cell survival (51,56).

CC-X-C chemokine receptor type 4 (*CXCR4*) mutations have been reported in 30 to 40 percent of WM cases and correlate with greater tumor burden, more aggressive disease, and hyperviscosity syndrome (16,39,48). Other

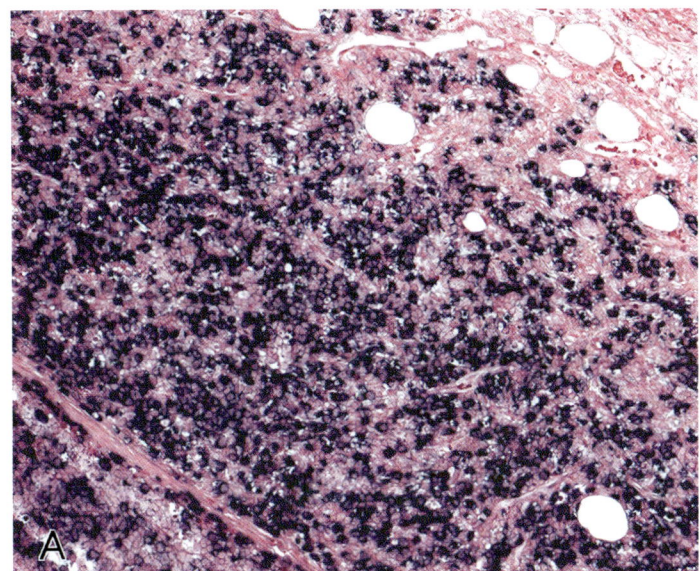

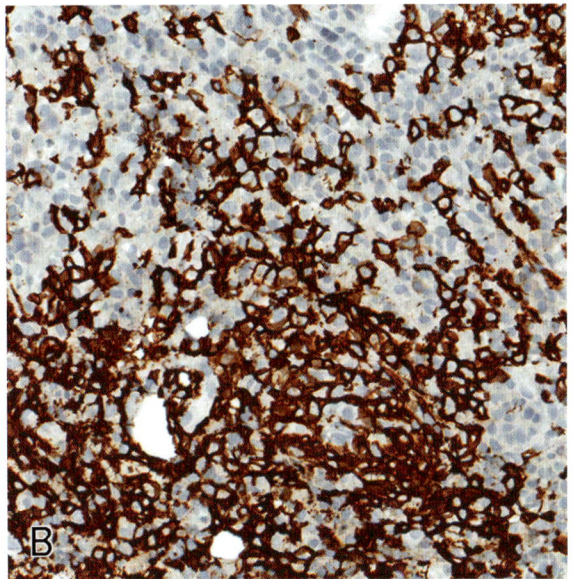

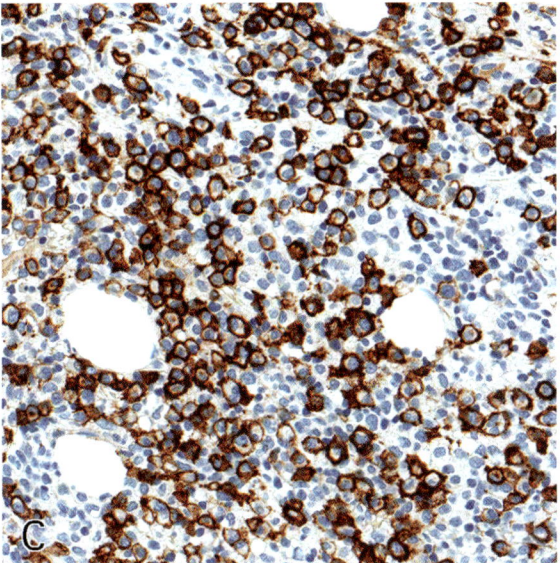

Figure 16-16

WALDENSTROM MACROGLOBULINEMIA INVOLVING LYMPH NODE

A: The cytoplasm of the neoplastic cells shows monotypic immunoglobulin Kappa RNA.

B,C: Subsets of neoplastic cells express CD20 (B) or CD138 (C) (A: in situ hybridization; B,C. immunohistochemistry with hematoxylin counterstain).

mutations reported in WM include: AT-rich interactive domain IA (*ARID1A*) in 17 percent; *CD79B* in 7 percent; *KMT2D/MLL2* in 7 percent; *TP53* in 7 percent; and *MYBBP1A* in 7 percent (16). A number of deletions and other copy number abnormalities have been shown in WM including *ARID1B* (about 70 percent), *LYN* (about 70 percent), and *HIVEP2* (about 80 percent).

Are *MYD88* Mutations Specific for WM? Although highly characteristic of cases of WM, *MYD88* mutations are not specific for WM. *MYD88* mutations have been reported in cases of DLBCL, including about 30 percent of cases

of DLBCL, NOS, and in a higher percentage of cases of primary DLBCL of the central nervous system, DLBCL of the testis, and primary cutaneous DLBCL of leg type.

In one study (18a), about 40 percent of cases of LPL of non-WM type had *MYD88* mutation and other small B-cell lymphomas also have been reported to carry the *MYD88* mutation including splenic MZL (10 to 20 percent), nodal MZL (about 5 percent), extranodal MZL (less than 5 percent), chronic lymphocytic leukemia/small lymphocytic lymphoma (CLL/SLL) (less than 5 percent), and rarely, mantle cell lymphoma (28,35). These findings also raise questions about the current criteria used to distinguish these entities from WM (51–53,55).

DIFFERENTIAL DIAGNOSIS

IgM Monoclonal Gammopathy. Patients with IgM MGUS have a serum IgM paraprotein and a few plasma cells in the bone marrow, but they lack bone marrow or tissue infiltration by WM (21,31). *MYD88* mutations have been reported with a variable frequency in IgM MGUS cases, depending on the method used for detection, with a likely overall frequency of at least 50 percent (up to 80 percent in some studies) (55). It is unclear whether *MYD88* L265P mutation is a founding mutation in a specific subtype of IgM MGUS that goes on to progress to WM or whether *MYD88* L265P mutation is a later event in the pathogenesis of both IgM MGUS and WM. Deletions of chromosome 6q are rare in IgM MGUS (32).

Splenic Marginal Zone Lymphoma. Patients with splenic MZL can present with an elevated IgM paraprotein, sometimes at a high level. In most patients, the bone marrow is involved by lymphocytes and lymphoplasmacytic cells in a nodular and often paratrabecular pattern. If the splenomegaly is not appreciated clinically, these patients may be misclassified as having WM. The presence of a paratrabecular pattern of involvement in the bone marrow is helpful; in our experience, a paratrabecular pattern is more common in splenic MZL than in WM. The lymphoid aggregates of splenic MZL are commonly associated with CD21- and CD23-positive follicular dendritic cells, uncommon in WM aggregates in the bone marrow (17). The presence of *MYD88* mutation in cases of splenic MZL has been shown to correlate with IgM paraprotein and bone marrow infiltration (28).

Nodal Marginal Zone B-Cell Lymphoma. Current pathologic criteria are suboptimal for distinguishing all cases of WM from nodal MZL in lymph nodes (46,47). In general, the tumor cell population in WM is composed of small and monotonous cells and the neoplasm often spares sinuses. In contrast, in nodal MZL the neoplastic cells are more heterogeneous, may show a marginal zone pattern, and often colonize follicles. Nevertheless, monocytoid B cells and follicular colonization uncommonly are present in WM.

The presence of bone marrow involvement and an IgM paraprotein support WM over nodal MZL, but these findings are not absolute (38). Focal bone marrow involvement is common in patients with nodal MZL, and rarely, these patients have a low level of serum paraprotein.

Distinguishing LPL of non-WM type from nodal MZL is more problematic as there is clearly morphologic overlap between these neoplasms. The presence of a serum paraprotein of IgG or IgA supports LPL of non-WM type, but is not an absolute criterion. Preferential medullary or interfollicular involvement, patent sinuses and obvious plasmacytic differentiation, including Dutcher and Russell bodies, and *MYD88* mutations support LPL of non-WM type, whereas marked monocytoid differentiation, prominent reactive follicular hyperplasia, a marginal zone pattern, and disrupted follicular dendritic cell meshworks (CD21 or CD23 positive) support nodal MZL.

Extranodal Marginal Zone Lymphoma. Extranodal involvement is uncommon in patients with WM at initial diagnosis, and therefore this differential diagnosis is rarely a practical problem. However, extranodal involvement by WM can occur in a small subset of patients, usually as a manifestation of disease progression, and can closely mimic extranodal MZL morphologically (4). The history of WM and the presence of IgM paraprotein and *MYD88* mutation support WM.

Plasma Cell Myeloma. Plasma cell myeloma, unlike WM, is entirely plasmacytic and lacks a component of neoplastic B lymphocytes. Numerous mast cells in the bone marrow support WM over plasma cell myeloma. Patients with plasma cell myeloma commonly have an IgG or IgA paraprotein (rarely, IgM) and have evidence of lytic bone lesions or renal failure. *IGH* translocations, common in plasma cell myeloma, are rare in WM. Conversely, *MYD88* mutations are absent in plasma cell myeloma (including IgM cases) and in IgG MGUS (55).

Gamma Heavy Chain Disease. Gamma heavy chain disease is defined by an abnormally truncated IgG monoclonal protein that lacks the sites required for binding the light chains secreted into the serum. Morphologically, these neoplasms tend to be composed of small B lymphocytes, plasma cells, and scattered large lymphoid cells, and therefore have morphologic features similar to MZLs or LPL of non-WM type. In the 2008 WHO classification, gamma heavy chain disease was considered to be a clinically aggressive variant of LPL of non-WM type (47). In the revised WHO classification gamma heavy chain disease is considered separate from LPL of non-WM type, based on studies that have shown that gamma heavy chain disease is not associated with *MYD88* mutation (15).

Primary Cold Agglutinin-Associated Lymphoproliferative Disease. Patients with primary cold-agglutinin lymphoproliferative disease often present with hemolytic anemia as a result of serum antibodies composed of IgM, often associated with kappa light chain, that react with erythrocytes that express I antigen (42). Most patients have bone marrow involvement by non-paratrabecular nodules of small B lymphocytes that express IgM, IgD, and pan-B-cell antigens and that are usually negative for CD5 and CD23. Patients with primary cold agglutinin-associated lymphoproliferative disease usually do not have lymphadenopathy or splenomegaly. In the past, many of these cases were classified as WM, but this disease is not associated with *MYD88* mutations and therefore primary cold-agglutinin lymphoproliferative disease is a distinct disease separate from WM (42).

TREATMENT AND PROGNOSIS

WM is usually a clinically indolent, but incurable disease, with a median survival period of about 5 years and a disease-specific survival period of 10 years (3). Many patients, especially asymptomatic patients, can be observed. For symptomatic patients, systems that employ clinical and laboratory data (e.g., age, cytopenias) have been developed to guide therapy (reviewed by Morel in reference 29). The Mayo Clinic group also has proposed guidelines for treating WM patients (www.mSMART.org) (3).

Symptomatic patients require therapy but there is no consensus approach at this time.

Firstline therapies include single agent rituximab or various chemotherapeutic agents, alone or in combination, such as alkylating agents (e.g., chlorambucil, cyclophosphamide) and purine nucleoside analogs (e.g., cladribine or fludarabine). A number of less established or novel agents have been employed or are in development for WM patients (reviewed in references 10a and 43). Some of these agents include bortezomib, immunomodulators (e.g., thalidomide, lenalidomide), newer monoclonal antibodies (e.g., ofatumumab) everolimus, ibrutinib, CXCR4 inhibitors (e.g., plerixafor), and other agents. Ibrutinib has been shown to be active in patients with WM (50). As has been reviewed elsewhere (16b), *MYD88* and *CXCR4* mutation status as well as other genetic abnormalities can be used for risk stratification and to guide therapy in WM patients. In particular, ibrutinib is effective in patients with *MYD88* mutation, but less so if *CXCR4* mutation is present (16b). Plasmapheresis is reserved for patients with manifestations of hyperviscosity syndrome or symptoms of antibody-related damage.

The therapy for patients with LPL of non-WM type is less well defined. Patients often are treated similarly to WM patients or they may be treated like patients with other types of low-grade B-cell lymphoma. The risk of symptoms related to hyperviscosity is low and therefore plasmapheresis is rarely required.

Transformation to DLBCL occurs in about 10 percent of patients with WM (see chapter 5) (8a,26). A clonal relationship has been shown in some cases. Rare patients with WM develop classic Hodgkin lymphoma, peripheral T-cell lymphoma, and other lymphoid neoplasms. The clonal relationship between these tumors and WM is largely unknown. EBV appears to be involved in a subset of cases. Underlying immunosuppression related to therapy also may be involved although a coincidental relationship cannot be excluded.

REFERENCES

1. Agnello V, Chung RT, Kaplan LM, et al. A role for hepatitis C virus infection in type II cryoglobulinemia. N Engl J Med 1992;327:1490-1495.

2. Altieri A, Bermejo JL, Hemminki K. Familial aggregation of lymphoplasmacytic lymphoma with non-Hodgkin lymphoma and other neoplasms. Leukemia 2005;19:2342-2343.

3. Ansell SM, Kyle RA, Reeder CB, et al. Diagnosis and management of Waldenström macroglobulinemia: Mayo stratification of macroglobulinemia and risk-adapted therapy (mSMART) guidelines. Mayo Clin Proc 2010;85:824-833.

4. Banwait R, Aljawai Y, Cappuccio J, et al. Extramedullary Waldenstrom macroglobulinemia. Am J Hematol 2015;90:100-104.

5. Barakat FH, Medeiros LJ, Wei EX, Konoplev S, Lin P, Jorgensen JL. Residual monotypic plasma cells in patients with Waldenstrom macroglobulinemia after therapy. Am J Clin Pathol 2011;135:365-373.

6. Bartl R, Frisch B, Mahl G, et al. Bone marrow histology in Waldenström's macroglobulinemia. Clinical relevance of subtype recognition. Scand J Haematol 1983;31:359-375.

7. Cao X, Medeiros LJ, Xia Y, et al. Clinocopathologic features and outcomes of lymphoplasmacytic lymphoma patients with monoclonal IgG or IgA paraprotein expression. Leuk Lymphoma 2016;57:1104-1115.

8. Cao X, Ye Q, Orlowski RZ, et al. Waldenstrom macroglobulinemia with extramedullary involvement at initial diagnosis portends a poorer prognosis. J Hematol Oncol 2015;8:74.

8a. Castillo JJ, Gustine J, Meid K, Dubeau T, Hunter ZR, Treon SP. Histological transformation to diffuse large B-cell lymphoma in patients with Waldenström macroglobulinemia. Am J Hematol 2016;91:1032-1035.

9. Chang H, Qi C, Trieu Y, et al. Prognostic relevance of 6q deletion in Waldenström's macroglobulinemia: a multicenter study. Clin Lymphoma Myeloma 2009;9:36-38.

10. Cook JR, Aguilera NI, Reshmi-Skarja, et al. Lack of PAX5 rearrangements in lymphoplasmacytic lymphomas: reassessing the reported association with t(9;14). Hum Pathol 2004;35:447-454.

10a. Dimopoulos MA, Kastritis E, Ghobrial IM. Waldenström's macroglobulinemia: a clinical perspective in the era of novel therapeutics. Ann Oncol 2016;27:233-240.

11. de Tute RM, Rawstron AC, Owen RG. Immunoglobulin M concentration in Waldenström macroglobulinemia: correlation with bone marrow B cells and plasma cells. Clin Lymphoma Myeloma Leuk 2013;13:211-213.

12. Gachard N, Parrens M, Soubeyran I, et al. IGHV gene features and MYD88 L265P mutation separate the three marginal zone lymphoma entities and Waldenstrom macroglobulinemia/lymphoplasmacytic lymphomas. Leukemia 2013;27:183-189.

13. Gustine JN, Meid K, Dubeau T, et al. Serum IgM level as predictor of symptomatic hyperviscosity in patients with Waldenström macroglobulinaemia. Br J Haematol 2017;177:717-725.

14. Hamada T, Yonetani N, Ueda C, et al. Expression of the PAX5/BSAP transcription factor in haematological tumour cells and further molecular characterization of the t(9;14)(p13;q32) translocation in B-cell non-Hodgkin's lymphoma. Br J Haematol 1998;102:691-700.

15. Hamadeh F, MacNamara SP, Bacon CM, Sohani AR, Swerdlow SH, Cook JR. Gamma heavy chain disease lacks the MYD88 L265P mutation associated with lymphoplasmacytic lymphoma. Haematologica 2014;99:e154-155.

16. Hunter Z, Xu L, Yang G, et al. The genomic landscape of Waldenstom's macroglobulinemia is characterized by highly recurring MYD88 and WHIM-like CXCR4 mutations, and small somatic deletions associated with B-cell lymphomagenesis. Blood 2014;123:1637-1646.

16a. Hunter ZR, Xu L, Yang G, et al. Transcriptome sequencing reveals a profile that corresponds to genomic variants in Waldenström macroglobulinemia. Blood 2016;128:827-838.

16b. Hunter ZR, Yang G, Xu L, Liu X, Castillo JJ, Treon SP. Genomics, signaling, and treatment of Waldenström macroglobulinemia. J Clin Oncol 2017. [Epub ahead of print]

17. Inamdar KV, Medeiros LJ, Jorgensen JL, Amin HM, Schlette EJ. Bone marrow involvement by marginal zone B-cell lymphomas of different types. Am J Clin Pathol 2008;129:714-722.

18. Jiménez C, Sebastián E, Chillón MC, et al. MYD88 L265P is a marker highly characteristic of, but not restricted to, Waldenström's macroglobulinemia. Leukemia 2013;27:1722-1728.

18a. King RL, Gonsalves WI, Ansell SM, et al. Lymphoplasmacytic lymphoma with a non-IgM paraprotein shows clinical and pathologic heterogeneity and may harbor MYD88 L265P mutations. Am J Clin Pathol 2016;145:843-851.

19. Konoplev S, Medeiros LJ, Bueso-Ramos CE, Jorgensen JL, Lin P. Immunophenotypic profile of lymphoplasmacytic lymphoma/Waldenström macroglobulinemia. Am J Clin Pathol 2005;124:414-420.

20. Kristinsson SY, Koshiol J, Goldin LR, et al. Genetic and immune-related factors in the pathogenesis of lymphoplasmacytic lymphoma/Waldenstrom's macroglobulinemia. Clin Lymphoma, Myeloma 2009;9:23-26.

21. Kyle RA, Dispenzieri A, Kumar S, Larson D, Therneau T, Rajkumar SV. IgM monoclonal gammopathy of undetermined significance (MGUS) and smoldering Waldenstrom's macroglobulinemia (SWM). Clin Lymphoma Myeloma Leuk 2011;11:74-76.

22. Kyle RA, Rajkumar SV, Therneau TM, Larson DR, Plevak MF, Melton LJ 3rd. Prognostic factors and predictors of outcome of immunoglobulin M monoclonal gammopathy of undetermined significance. Clin Lymphoma 2005;5:257-260.

23. Lemal R, Bard-Sorel S, Montrieul L, et al. TCL1 expression patterns in Waldenstrom macroglobulinemia. Mod Pathol 2016;29:83-88.

24. Lin P, Bueso-Ramos C, Wilson CS, Mansoor A, Medeiros LJ. Waldenstrom macroglobulinemia involving extramedullary sites: morphologic and immunophenotypic findings in 44 patients. Am J Surg Pathol 2003;27:1104-1113.

25. Lin P, Hao S, Handy BC, Bueso-Ramos CE, Medeiros LJ. Lymphoid neoplasms associated with IgM paraprotein: a study of 382 patients. Am J Clin Pathol 2005;123:200-205

26. Lin P, Mansoor A, Bueso-Ramos C, Bueso-Ramos CE, Medeiros LJ. Diffuse large B-cell lymphoma occurring in patients with lymphoplasmacytic lymphoma/Waldenstrom macroglobulinemia. Am J Clin Pathol 2003;120:246-253.

27. Mansoor A, Medeiros LJ, Weber DM, et al. Cytogenetic findings in lymphoplasmacytic lymphoma/Waldenstrom macroglobulinemia. Chromosomal abnormalities are associated with the polymorphous subtype and an aggressive clinical course. Am J Clin Pathol 2001;116:543-549.

28. Martinez-Lopez A, Curiel-Olmo S, Mollejo M, et al. MYD88 (L265P) somatic mutation in marginal zone B-cell lymphoma. Am J Surg Pathol 2015;39:644-651.

29. Morel P, Merlini G. Risk stratification in Waldenström macroglobulinemia. Expert Rev Hematol 2012;5:187-199.

30. Morice WG, Chen D, Kurtin PJ, Hanson CA, McPhail ED. Novel immunophenotypic features of marrow lymphoplasmacytic lymphoma and correlation with Waldenström's macroglobulinemia. Mod Pathol 2009;22:807-816.

31. Morra E, Cesana C, Klersy C, et al. Predictive variables for malignant transformation in 452 patients with asymptomatic IgM monoclonal gammopathy. Semin Oncol 2003;30:172-177.

32. Nguyen-Khac F, Lambert J, Chapiro E, et al. Chromosomal aberrations and their prognostic value in a series of 174 untreated patients with Waldenström's macroglobulinemia. Haematologica 2013;98:649-54.

33. Ocio EM, Schop RF, Gonzalez B, et al. 6q deletion in Waldenstrom macroglobulinemia is associated with features of adverse prognosis. Br J Haematol 2007;136:80-86.

34. Offit K, Parsa NZ, Jhanwar SC, Filippa D, Wachtel M, Chaganti RS. Clusters of chromosome 9 aberrations are associated with clinico-pathologic subsets of non-Hodgkin's lymphoma. Genes Chromosomes Cancer 1993;7:1-7.

35. Ondrejka SL, Lin JJ, Warden DW, Durkin L, Cook JR, Hsi ED. MYD88 L265P somatic mutation: its usefulness in the differential diagnosis of bone marrow involvement by B-cell lymphoproliferative disorders. Am J Clin Pathol 2013;140:387-394.

36. Owen RG, Pratt G, Auer RL, et al. Guidelines on the diagnosis and management of Waldenström macroglobulinaemia. Br J Haematol 2014;165:316-333.

37. Owen RG, Treon SP, Al-Katib A, et al. Clinicopathological definition of Waldenstrom's macroglobulinemia: consensus panel recommendations from the Second International Workshop on Waldenstrom's Macroglobulinemia. Semin Oncol 2003;30:110-115.

38. Pangalis GA, Kyrtsonis MC, Kontopidou FN, et al. Differential diagnosis of Waldenstrom's macroglobulinemia and other B-cell disorders. Clin Lymphoma 2005;5:235-240.

39. Poulain S, Roumier C, Decambron A, et al. MYD88 L265P mutation in Waldenstrom macroglobulinemia. Blood 2013;121:4504-4511.

40. Poulain S, Roumier C, Venet-Caillault A, et al. Genomic landscape of CXCR4 mutations in Waldenstrom macroglobulinemia. Clin Cancer Res 2016;22:1480-1488.

41. Pozzato G, Mazzaro C, Crovatto M, et al. Low-grade malignant lymphoma, hepatitis C virus infection, and mixed cryoglobulinemia. Blood 1994;84:3047-3053.

42. Randen U, Troen G, Tierens A, et al. Primary cold agglutinin-associated lymphoproliferative disease: a B-cell lymphoma of the bone marrow distinct from lymphoplasmacytic lymphoma. Haematologica 2014;99:497-504.

43. Sahin I, Leblebjian H, Treon SP, Ghobrial IM. Waldenstrom macroglobulinemia: from biology to treatment. Exp Rev Hematol 2014;7:157-168.

44. Sahota SS, Forconi F, Ottensmeier CH, et al. Typical Waldenstrom macroglobulinemia is derived from a B-cell arrested after cesssation of somatic mutation but prior to isotype switch events. Blood 2002;100:1505-1507.

45. Schop RF, Kuehl WM, Van Wier SA, et al. Waldenström macroglobulinemia neoplastic cells lack immunoglobulin heavy chain locus translocations but have frequent 6q deletions. Blood 2002;100:2996-2300.

46. Shaheen SP, Talwalkar SS, Lin P, Medeiros LJ. Waldenström macroglobulinemia: a review of the entity and its differential diagnosis. Adv Anat Pathol 2012;19:11-27.

47. Swerdlow SH, Berger F, Pileri SA, Harris NL, Jaffe ES, Stein H. Lymphoplasmacytic lymphoma. In: Swerdlow SH, Campo E, Harris NL, Jaffe ES, Pileri SA, Stein H, Thiele J, Vardiman JW, eds. World Health Organization classification of tumours. Tumors of haematopoietic and lymphoid tissues. Lyon: IARC Press; 2008:194-195.

48. Treon SP, Cao Y, Xu L, Yang G, Liu X, Hunter ZR. Somatic mutations in MYD88 and CXCR4 are determinants of clinical presentation and overall survival in Waldenstrom's macroglobulinemia. Blood 2014;123:2791-2796.

49. Treon SP, Hunter ZR, Aggarwal A, et al. Characterization of familial Waldenstrom's macroglobulinemia. Ann Oncol 2006;17:488-494.

50. Treon SP, Tripsas CK, Meid K, et al. Ibrutinib in previously treated Waldenstrom's macroglobulinemia. N Engl J Med 2015;372:1430-1440.

51. Treon SP, Xu L, Yang G, et al. MYD88 L265P somatic mutation in Waldenström's macroglobulinemia. N Engl J Med 2012;367:826-833.

52. Vajdic CM, Landgren O, McMaster ML, et al. Medical history, lifestyle, family history, and occupational risk factors for lymphoplasmacytic lymphoma/Waldenstrom's macroglobulinemia: the InterLymph Non-Hodgkin Lymphoma Subtypes Project. J Natl Cancer Inst 2014;48:87-97.

53. Varettoni M, Arcaini L, Zibellini S, et al. Prevalence and clinical significance of the MYD88 (L265P) somatic mutation in Waldenstrom's macroglobulinemia and related lymphoid neoplasms. Blood 2013;121:2522-2528.

54. Waldenström J. Incipient myelomatosis or essential hyperglobulinemia with fibrinogenopenia: a new syndrome? Acta Med Scand 1944;117:216-247.

55. Xu L, Hunter ZR, Yang G, et al. MYD88 L265P in Waldenstrom macroglobulinemia, immunoglobulin M monoclonal gammopathy, and other B-cell lymphoproliferative disorders using conventional and quantitative allele-specific polymerase chain reaction. Blood 2013;121:2051-2058

56. Yang G, Zhou Y, Liu X, et al. A mutation in MYD88 (L265P) supports the survival of lymphoplasmacytic cells by activation of Bruton tyrosine kinase in Waldenström macroglobulinemia. Blood 2013;122:1222-1232.

17 DIFFUSE LARGE B-CELL LYMPHOMA, NOT OTHERWISE SPECIFIED

GENERAL FEATURES

Diffuse large B-cell lymphoma (DLBCL) is defined in the World Health Organization (WHO) classification as a neoplasm composed of large lymphoid cells of B-cell lineage arranged in a diffuse pattern (96). A large cell in this context is defined as a cell with a nucleus equal to or greater than a macrophage nucleus or more than two times the size of a normal lymphocyte. The designation DLBCL encompasses a heterogeneous group of clinically aggressive B-cell lymphomas, within which are more specific subsets (Table 17-1). The designation not otherwise specified (NOS) is applied to cases of DLBCL that cannot be more specifically classified; they represent the largest subgroup of DLBCL.

DLBCL is the most common type of non-Hodgkin lymphoma worldwide. In Europe, the incidence rate is 3.57 per 100,000 per year for women and 4.06 per 100,000 per year for men (overall, 3.81 per 100,000 per year) (93). In the United States, DLBCL represents approximately 30 percent of all cases of non-Hodgkin lymphoma or about 30,000 new cases per year (7), the fifth most common cancer in the United States. In developing nations, DLBCL represents

Table 17-1

WORLD HEALTH ORGANIZATION CLASSIFICATION OF DIFFUSE LARGE B-CELL LYMPHOMA[a]

Diffuse large B-cell lymphoma (DLBCL), not otherwise specified (NOS)
  Morphologic variants
  Gene expression signatures (GCB[b] versus ABC)
  Immunohistochemical subgroups
    CD5+
    GCB versus non-GCB

DLBCL subtypes
  T-cell/histiocyte-rich large B-cell lymphoma
  Primary DLBCL of the central nervous system
  Primary cutaneous DLBCL, leg type
  EBV-positive DLBCL, NOS

Other lymphomas composed of large B cells
  Primary mediastinal (thymic) large B-cell lymphoma
  Intravascular large B-cell lymphoma
  DLBCL associated with chronic inflammation
  Lymphomatoid granulomatosis
  ALK-positive large B-cell lymphoma
  Plasmablastic lymphoma
  HHV8 positive DLBCL, NOS
  Primary effusion lymphoma

Borderline (gray zone)
  High-grade B-cell lymphoma, NOS
  High-grade B-cell lymphoma with *MYC* and *BCL2* and/or *BCL6* rearrangement
  B-cell lymphoma, unclassifiable, with features intermediate between DLBCL and classic Hodgkin lymphoma

[a]Based primarily on the 2008 version of the WHO classification, with some modifications based on the 2016 revision (96a). Provisional entities are not included.
[b]GCB = germinal center B cell; ABC = activated B-cell-like; EBV = Epstein-Barr virus; ALK = anaplastic lymphoma kinase; HHV = human herpesvirus.

Figure 17-1

**GERMINAL CENTER
ILLUSTRATION**

A schematic of a germinal center and a physiologic hyperplastic germinal center are shown (bottom left of the field). In the schematic, a naïve B cell enters the dark zone of the germinal center where it undergoes T-cell–dependent stimulation and somatic hypermutation (SHM). Cells that encode for high affinity antibodies selectively survive and move to the germinal center light zone, where they undergo class switch recombination (CSR) under the influence of follicular dendritic cells (FDCs) and T-follicular helper cells (TFH) before they emerge from the germinal center as plasma cells or memory B cells.

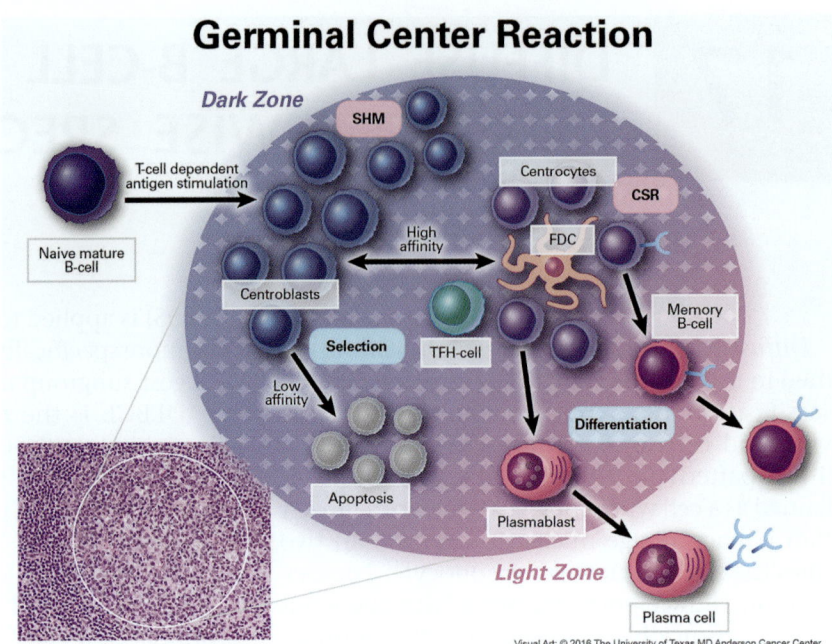

Germinal Center Reaction

Visual Art: © 2016 The University of Texas MD Anderson Cancer Center

a greater percentage of all cases of non-Hodgkin lymphoma, up to 40 percent.

It seems likely that most cases of DLBCL, NOS (henceforth referred to simply as DLBCL) arise from B cells within germinal centers of the secondary follicles of lymph nodes or other lymphoid tissues. The germinal center is the site of physiologic somatic hypermutation of the immunoglobulin (IG) variable region genes as well as *IGH* class switch recombination (fig. 17-1). Both of these processes require double-strand DNA breaks, allowing for mistakes to occur that result in chromosomal translocations, gene mutations, and other abnormalities. In support of this interpretation, in some chromosomal translocations an oncogene is brought under inappropriate control of IG regulatory elements. Evidence of heptamer-nonomer recognition motifs involved in physiologic DNA rearrangement has been identified near the oncogene in a few of these translocations.

The etiology of DLBCL is unknown, but epidemiologic data suggest a multifactorial etiology. Immunodeficiency is a clear risk factor and inheritance also plays a role since some cases run in families. The International Lymphoma Epidemiology Consortium (19) has identified a number of other factors associated with an increased DLBCL risk: B-cell activating diseases (e.g., rheumatoid arthritis), hepatitis C infec-

tion, higher body mass index, cigarette smoking (linked to DLBCL arising in the central nervous system, skin, or testis), living on a farm and hair dye use (both linked to primary mediastinal B-cell lymphoma), inflammatory bowel disease (linked to DLBCL of gastrointestinal tract), and a variety of occupations including crop farmer (women), seamstress/embroiderer (women), hairdresser (women), and driver/equipment handler (men). Factors associated with a decreased risk of DLBCL include: higher socioeconomic status, any atopic disorder, increased recreational sun exposure, low body mass index, hormone therapy in women beginning at age 50 years or older, oral contraceptive use before 1970 (women), history of blood transfusion (men), and alcohol consumption (men).

In line with its multifactorial etiology, DLBCL is also a highly heterogeneous disease at the morphologic, immunophenotypic, and genetic levels. Although patients with DLBCL currently receive a standard immunochemotherapy regimen (see Treatment section) regardless of the known biologic differences, this approach is already being (and will be further) modified as new targets in DLBCL are identified and targeted therapies become more readily available. At this time, the diagnosis of DLBCL, by itself, is only the first step. An immunophenotypic and molecular workup is needed to identify prognostic and predictive markers as well as targets for the rational design of therapy. In other words, a precision medicine approach is currently applied to the management of DLBCL patients, currently most often in the relapse setting, but eventually there will be a number of frontline therapeutic strategies based on tumor biology (100).

CLINICAL FEATURES

Patients with DLBCL have a wide age range that includes children and the elderly, but the median age is in the early part of the seventh decade (6,80,96). Although uncommon in children overall, DLBCL represents 25 to 30 percent of all lymphomas that occur in children. The male to female ratio is 1.2 to 1.0. Approximately one third of patients have systemic B-type symptoms. Patients typically present with a single or several rapidly enlarging masses involving lymph nodes or extranodal sites, and about 70 percent have extranodal disease during their disease course (7). Body cavity effusions occur in 30 to 40 percent of patients (18). The bone marrow is involved in less than 25 percent of patients (see below). About 50 percent of patients have stage I or II disease and the other half has widely disseminated disease (7,80,96).

Thirty to 40 percent of patients present exclusively with extranodal disease. The gastrointestinal tract is the most common extranodal site, particularly the stomach or ileocecal region, but other sites include skin, bone, spleen, testis, Waldeyer ring, salivary glands, thyroid glands, kidneys, liver, and adrenal glands (96). Symptoms and signs at the time of presentation depend on the anatomic site of disease and the extent of involvement, since the tumor may compress adjacent tissues or obstruct tubular organs (7).

Laboratory abnormalities are common. About one third of patients have elevated serum lactate dehydrogenase (LDH) or beta-2-microglobulin levels that are indirect manifestations of tumor burden. Organ-specific laboratory abnormalities depend on the site of disease. For example, elevated liver function tests may accompany extensive liver involvement by DLBCL and pancytopenia(s) may occur in patients with extensive bone marrow involvement.

Infrequently, patients with DLBCL present with a leukemic phase of disease with leukocytosis. These patients commonly have B-type

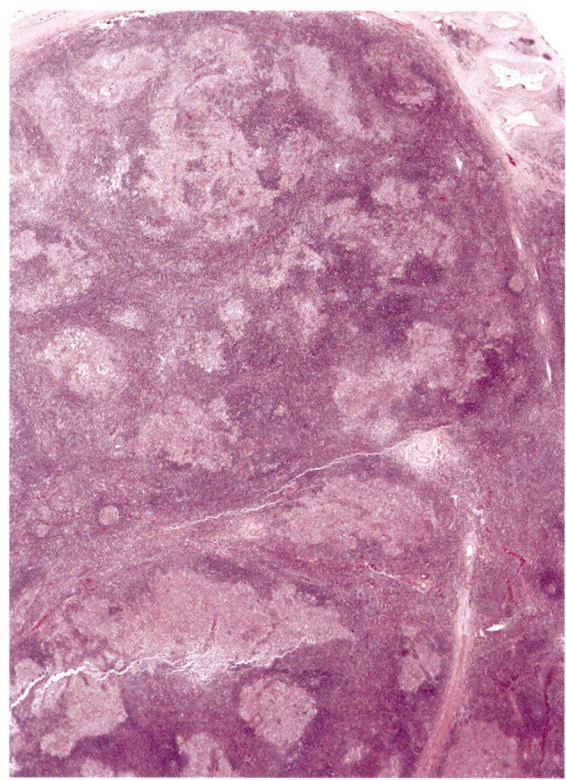

Figure 17-2

DIFFUSE LARGE B-CELL LYMPHOMA (DLBCL)

DLBCL partially replaces the lymph node parenchyma (hematoxylin and eosin [H&E] stain).

symptoms, a high serum LDH level, and a high International Prognostic Index (IPI) score. In these patients the bone marrow is virtually always involved by DLBCL; other extranodal sites commonly involved include spleen, lungs, liver, and bones (70).

HISTOLOGIC FINDINGS

Lymph Node

DLBCL can partially or completely replace the lymph node parenchyma. In cases with partial replacement, the lymphoma may have a paracortical distribution, sparing some follicles, or rarely, has a predominantly sinusoidal growth pattern (figs. 17-2, 17-3). In cases with complete lymph node replacement, no recognizable lymph node structures are appreciated (fig. 17-4). Mitotic figures and apoptotic cells are present. About 10 percent of cases of DLBCL have a prominent starry sky pattern (fig. 17-5),

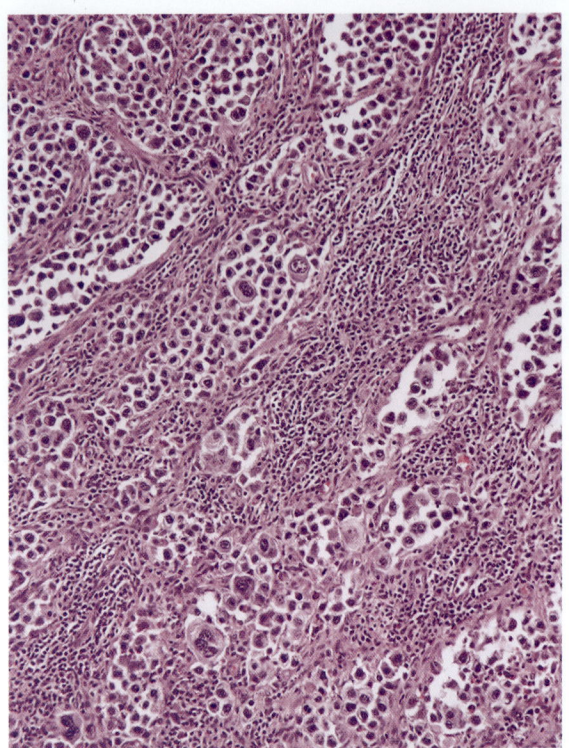

Figure 17-3

DIFFUSE LARGE B-CELL LYMPHOMA

The sinusoids of the lymph node are preferentially involved (H&E stain).

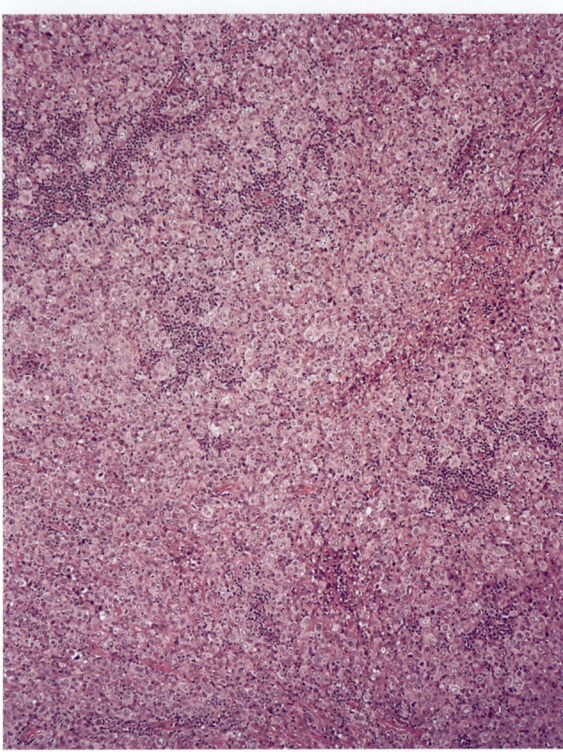

Figure 17-4

DIFFUSE LARGE B-CELL LYMPHOMA

The lymph node parenchyma is almost completely replaced in a diffuse pattern. Small areas of uninvolved lymph node with many reactive small lymphocytes are also present (H&E stain).

which correlates with a high number of mitoses and apoptotic cells (fig. 17-6) and a high proliferation (Ki-67) rate. Coagulative necrosis may be present and in a small subset of cases, the tumor is completely necrotic, likely the result of tumor infarct. The neoplastic cells are associated with a background of small reactive T lymphocytes and macrophages. Epithelioid granulomas (fig. 17-7) are associated with the lymphoma cells in some cases, and rarely, eosinophils are numerous in the background (fig. 17-8).

As defined above, the lymphoma cells are large, with moderate to more abundant cytoplasm that is basophilic, amphophilic, eosinophilic, or pale or clear (fig. 17-9). There are a number of cytologic variants of DLBCL, including centroblastic, immunoblastic, and anaplastic, as well as other rare variants.

The *centroblastic variant* of DLBCL is most common and represents 75 to 85 percent of all cases (96). A centroblast has a vesicular nucleus, fine chromatin, 2 to 4 small nucleoli often in close

proximity to the nuclear membrane, and minimal to moderate cytoplasm (figs. 17-9, 17-10). The *immunoblastic variant* represents about 10 percent of cases of DLBCL. The classic immunoblast is larger than a centroblast; it is an ovoid cell with moderate to abundant cytoplasm and a central or eccentric nucleus with a prominent, basophilic, rectangular-shaped nucleolus. Some nucleoli have string-like chromatin attached to the nuclear membrane ("spider legs") (figs. 17-11). A Giemsa stain helps distinguish a centroblast from an immunoblast since the cytoplasm of an immunoblast has a deeper blue color.

Although these descriptions of a centroblast and an immunoblast seem straightforward, in practice, designating cases of DLBCL as the centroblastic or immunoblastic variant can be challenging and result in suboptimal intraobserver and interobserver reproducibility. Some cases of DLBCL are composed of a mixture of centroblasts and immunoblasts. In small needle

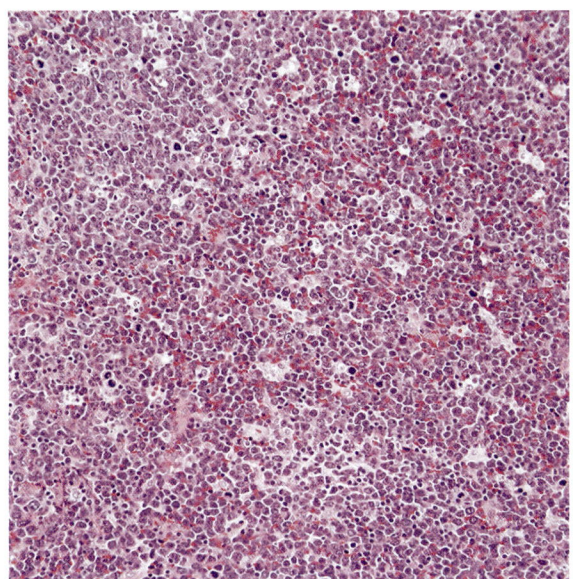

Figure 17-5

DIFFUSE LARGE B-CELL LYMPHOMA

The lymph node parenchyma is diffusely replaced with a starry sky pattern. The "stars" are reactive histiocytes admixed within a sheet of large lymphoma cells. The starry sky pattern is characteristic of a rapidly growing lymphoma (H&E stain).

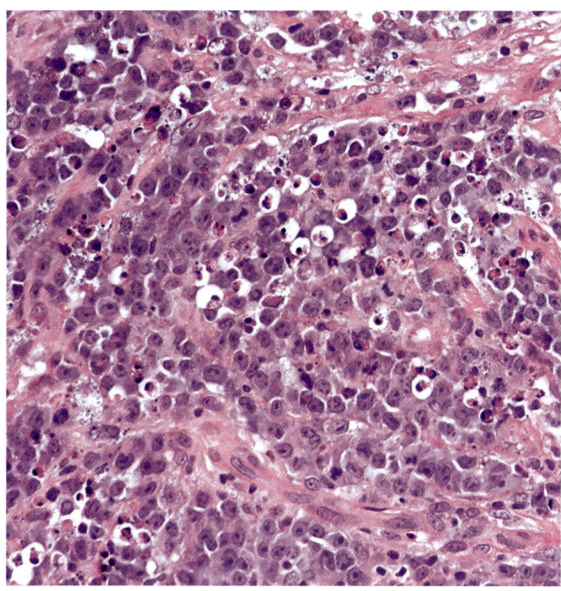

Figure 17-6

DIFFUSE LARGE B-CELL LYMPHOMA

Numerous apoptotic cells are present. Mitotic figures also can be appreciated in this field (center) (H&E stain).

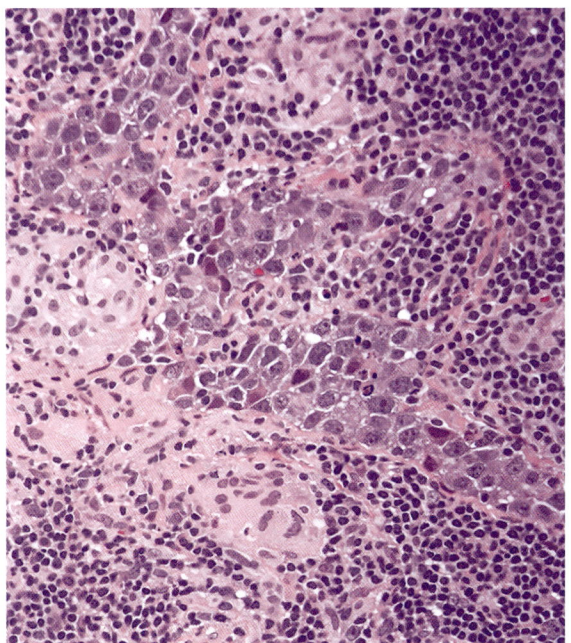

Figure 17-7

DIFFUSE LARGE B-CELL LYMPHOMA

The lymph node shows DLBCL in a sinusoidal distribution associated with epithelioid granulomas (H&E stain).

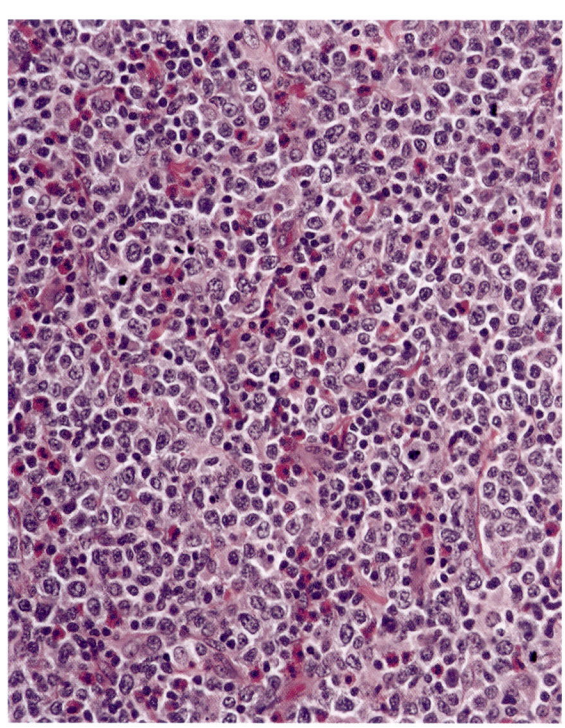

Figure 17-8

DIFFUSE LARGE B-CELL LYMPHOMA

Numerous eosinophils are seen in the background (H&E stain).

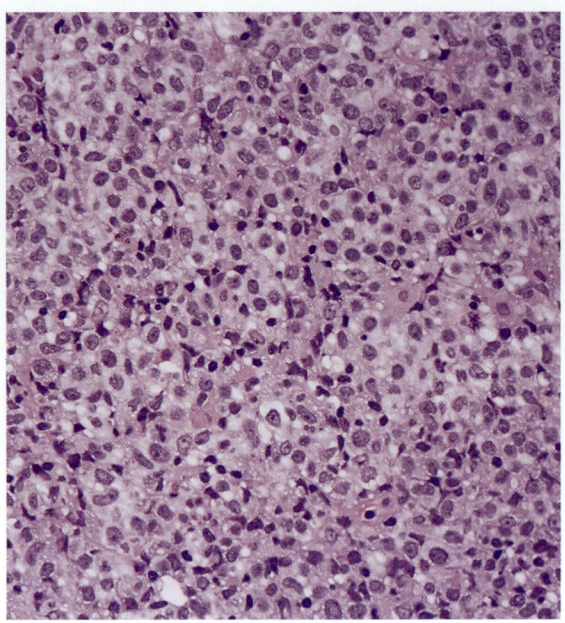

Figure 17-9

DIFFUSE LARGE B-CELL LYMPHOMA, CENTROBLASTIC VARIANT

The lymphoma cells have abundant pale cytoplasm (H&E stain).

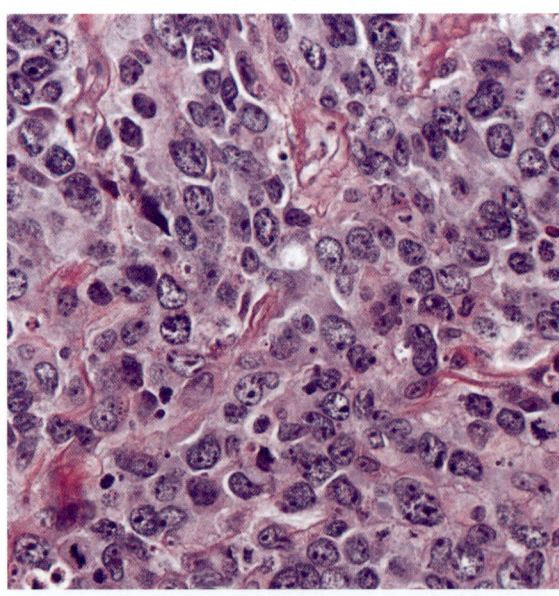

Figure 17-10

DIFFUSE LARGE B-CELL LYMPHOMA, CENTROBLASTIC VARIANT

The lymphoma cell nuclei in the centroblastic variant of DLBCL are vesicular (cleared out), with usually 2 or 3 small nucleoli, of which one is more central and others are in close proximity to the nuclear membrane (H&E stain).

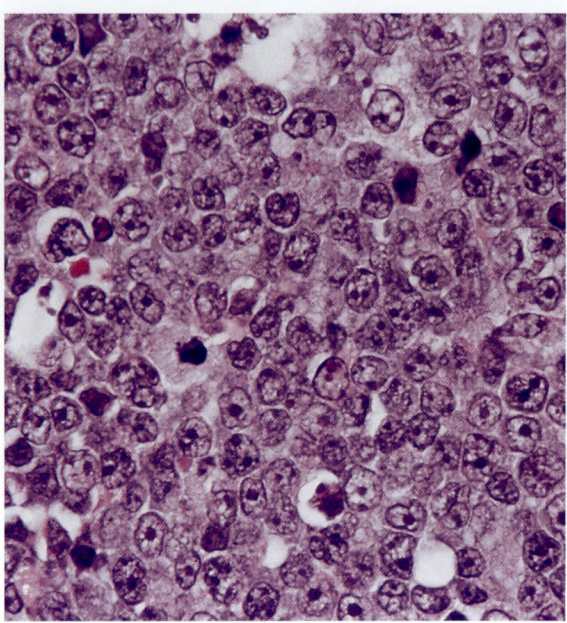

Figure 17-11

DIFFUSE LARGE B-CELL LYMPHOMA, IMMUNOBLASTIC VARIANT

As defined in the World Health Organization (WHO) classification, the lymphoma cells are larger than centroblasts and over 90 percent have a single prominent nucleolus (H&E stain).

biopsy specimens, the lymphoma cells may be poorly preserved, making it difficult to discern their cytologic features. Nevertheless, there are unequivocal cases of the centroblastic or immunoblastic variant DLBCL and, as the morphology correlates with some important biologic differences (see below), these morphologic variants should be specified when possible.

The current WHO classification suggests that cases of the immunoblastic variant should be composed of 90 percent or more immunoblasts (96); this approach is derived from an earlier definition by Englehard et al. (33). This is obviously an arbitrary cutoff, but the message seems to be that the immunoblastic variant should be pure. Horn et al. (41) suggested an alternative definition for the immunoblastic variant: these tumors should contain fewer than 10 percent centroblasts and large centrocytes. This view is based on their observations that the immunoblastic variant commonly has medium-sized cells with plasmacytoid features and that only about 10 percent of the immunoblastic variant cases contain over 90 percent classic immunoblasts (fig. 17-12).

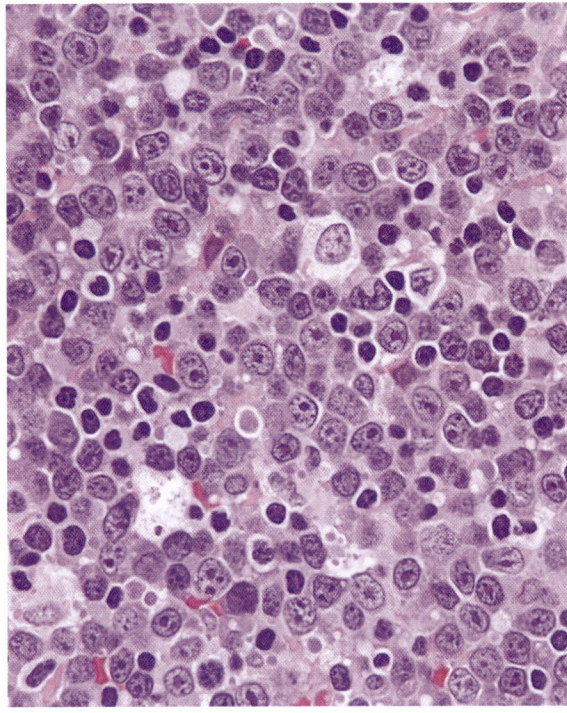

Figure 17-12

DIFFUSE LARGE B-CELL LYMPHOMA, IMMUNOBLASTIC VARIANT

Some cases of DLBCL with numerous immunoblasts, often associated with many plasmacytoid cells, do meet the 90 percent threshold as in the case shown. Horn et al. (41) proposed an alternative definition: numerous immunoblasts with less than 10 percent centroblasts and large centrocytes (H&E stain).

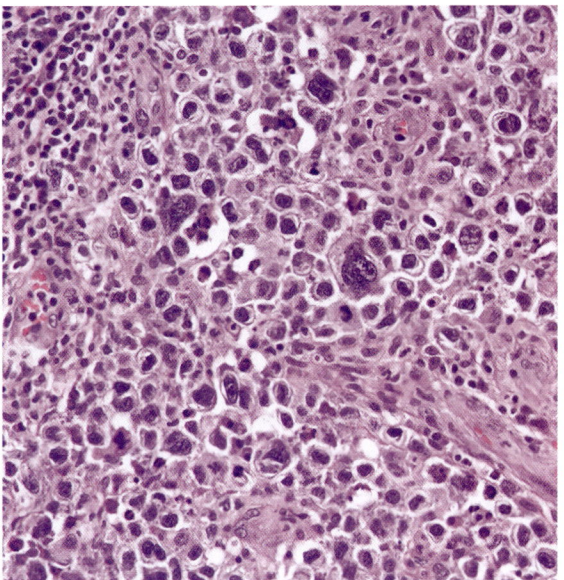

Figure 17-13

DIFFUSE LARGE B-CELL LYMPHOMA, ANAPLASTIC VARIANT

The lymphoma cells are pleomorphic and some cells are gigantic. This case showed a partial sinusoidal pattern and is the same case as shown in figure 17-3 (H&E stain).

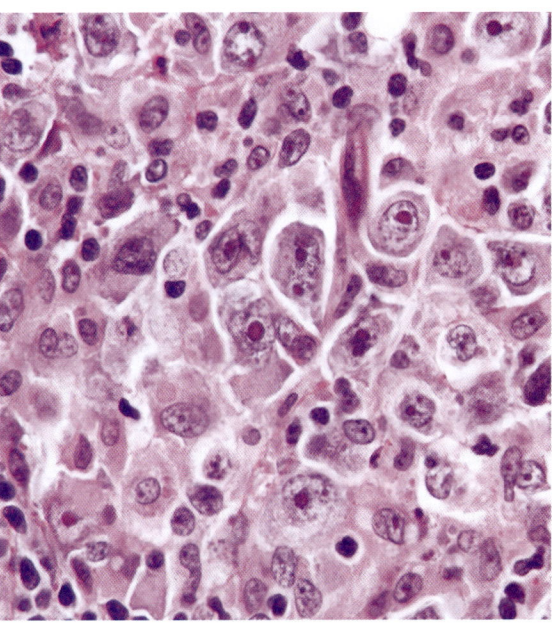

Figure 17-14

DIFFUSE LARGE B-CELL LYMPHOMA, ANAPLASTIC VARIANT

In this oil immersion image, the lymphoma cells have prominent, eosinophilic, Hodgkin-like nucleoli. These cells were positive for CD30 (not shown) (H&E stain).

The *anaplastic variant* of DLBCL represents 2 to 3 percent of cases of DLBCL. These tumors are characterized by large, pleomorphic and bizarre cells, including cells that resemble Reed-Sternberg or Hodgkin cells and cells that resemble the hallmark cells of anaplastic large cell lymphoma (figs. 17-13, 17-14). In some cases, the lymphoma cells have a predominantly sinusoidal distribution. These tumors commonly express CD30, but CD30 expression is not a prerequisite for designating a case of DLBCL as anaplastic (58a).

Other rare morphologic variants of DLBCL occur (96). In some cases, the lymphoma cells appear centroblastic, but the cells seem smaller than usual (so-called small cell centroblastic). The lymphoma cells may be polylobated (fig. 17-15) or have a prominent spindle shape with a fibroblast-like or sarcoma-like appearance (fig. 17-16). The lymphoma cells can resemble

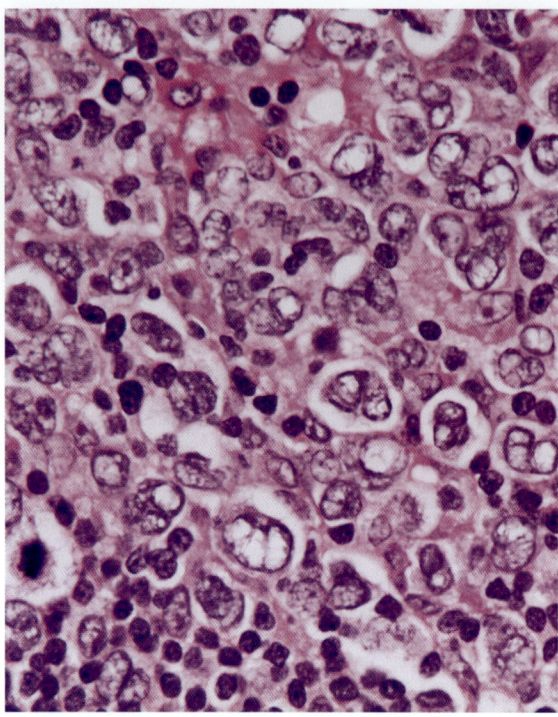

Figure 17-15

DIFFUSE LARGE B-CELL LYMPHOMA

The lymphoma cells have polylobated nuclei (H&E stain).

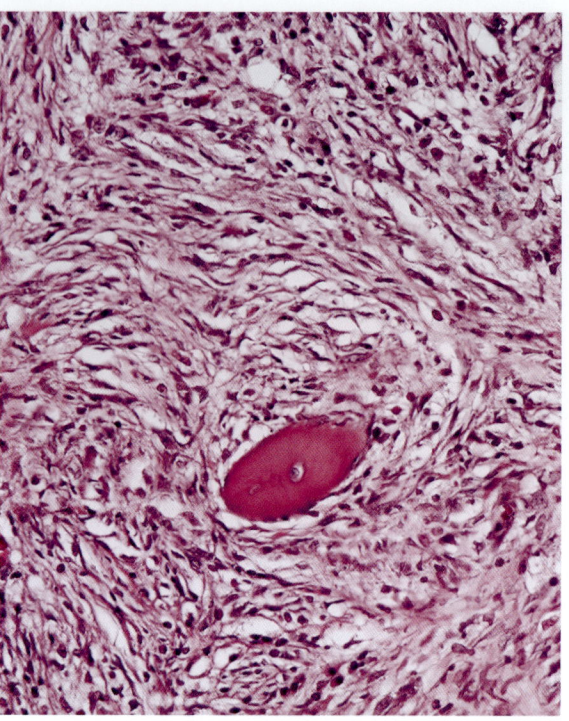

Figure 17-16

DIFFUSE LARGE B-CELL LYMPHOMA INVOLVING BONE

In this case the lymphoma cells have a prominent spindle shape and were positive for B-cell antigens by immunohistochemistry (not shown) (H&E stain).

signet ring cells with prominent cytoplasmic vacuolization (fig. 17-17) or be arranged in an alveolar-like pattern. The lymphoma cells may appear to form rosettes or be associated with a fibrillary matrix (almost neuroblastoma-like appearance). In rare cases, the lymphoma cells have microvillous projections, identified by electron microscopy. The stroma may exhibit a prominent myxoid appearance. Due to the rarity of these variants, there is virtually no data available correlating these morphologic variants with molecular features.

Bone Marrow

The bone marrow is involved in 10 to less than 25 percent of patients with DLBCL. The sensitivity of this range depends on the bone marrow workup employed. Flow cytometry immunophenotypic or immunohistochemical analysis improves the sensitivity of lymphoma detection. Involvement of the bone marrow is highly variable, and ranges from focal interstitial clusters of large lymphoma cells difficult to appreciate in

routinely stained sections, to sinusoidal involvement, to extensive and diffuse replacement of the medullary space (figs. 17-18, 17-19).

Low-grade lymphoma can involve the bone marrow of patients with DLBCL, so-called discordant disease, as reviewed by Brudno et al. (13). Discordant bone marrow involvement occurs in 5 to 10 percent of patients with DLBCL. In the most common scenario, patients with DLBCL in lymph nodes or other extranodal sites have low-grade B-cell lymphoma in the bone marrow, usually follicular lymphoma (fig. 17-20) (13). Molecular studies have shown that DLBCL and low-grade lymphoma are clonally related in about two thirds of cases (54).

Histologic discordance has prognostic importance and therefore must be noted. Patients with DLBCL who have low-grade lymphoma in the bone marrow have an overall survival rate in keeping with an absence of bone marrow disease, and substantially better than patients

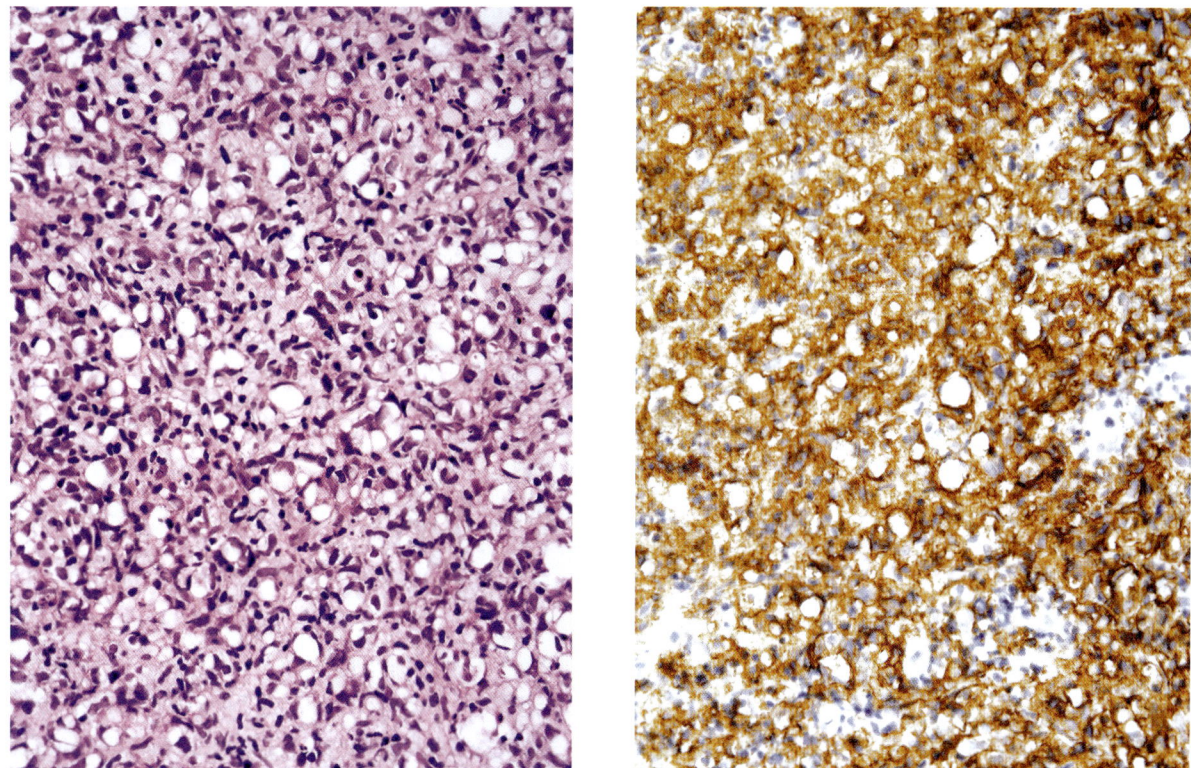

Figure 17-17

DIFFUSE LARGE B-CELL LYMPHOMA, INVOLVING LYMPH NODE

Left: The lymphoma cells have prominent cytoplasmic vacuoles, imparting a signet ring-like appearance (H&E stain).
Right: The lymphoma cells are positive for CD20 and negative for T-cell antigens (not shown) (immunohistochemistry with hematoxylin counterstain).

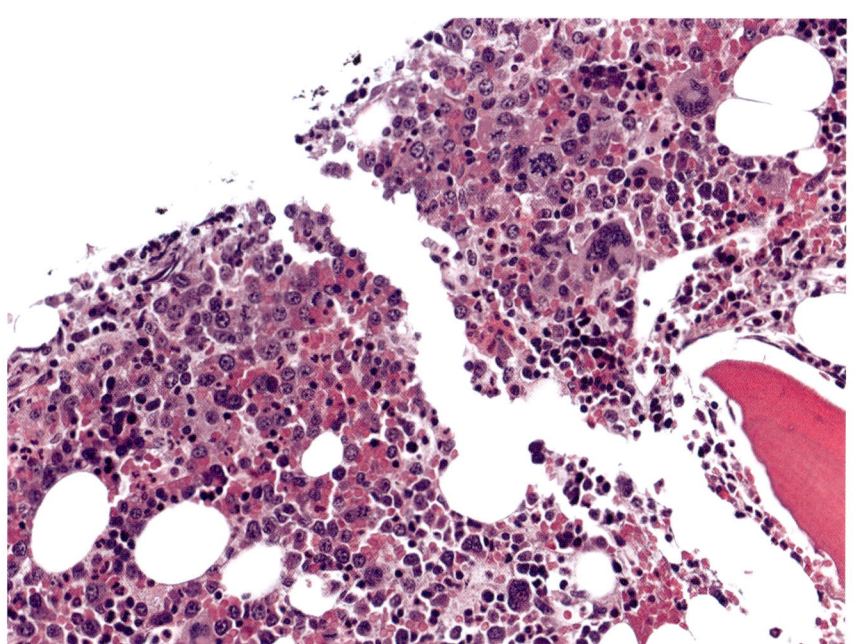

Figure 17-18

DIFFUSE LARGE B-CELL LYMPHOMA INVOLVING BONE MARROW

Involvement is focal, present as small aggregates of large lymphoma cells in an interstitial distribution (H&E stain).

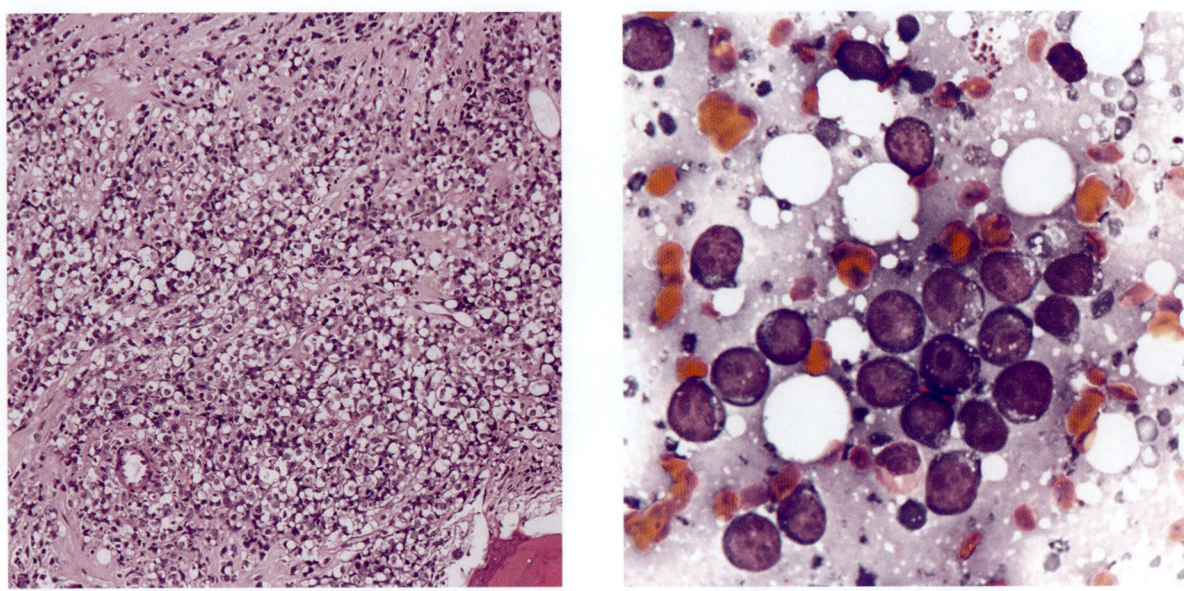

Figure 17-19

DIFFUSE LARGE B-CELL LYMPHOMA INVOLVING BONE MARROW

Left: The lymphoma cells diffusely replace the bone marrow medullary space and are associated with sclerosis. Trabecular bone is present at the bottom right corner of the field (H&E stain).

Right: A touch imprint shows large lymphoma cells with cytoplasmic vacuoles; some lymphoma cells have a prominent central nucleolus (Wright-Giemsa stain).

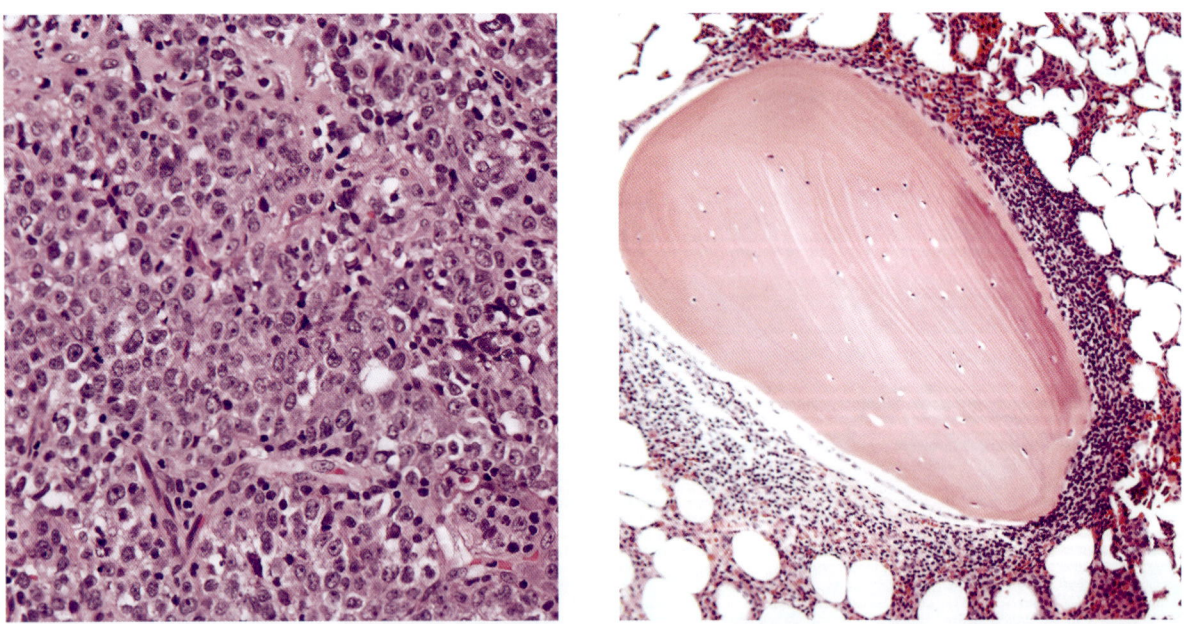

Figure 17-20

HISTOLOGIC DISCORDANCE

Left: DLBCL presented as a peritonsillar mass in a 56-year-old woman.

Right: Bone marrow biopsy showed paratrabecular aggregates of centrocytes consistent with follicular lymphoma. Histologic discordance occurs in 5 to 10 percent of patients with DLBCL and the presence of low-grade lymphoma in the bone marrow has minimal impact on prognosis (left, right: H&E stain).

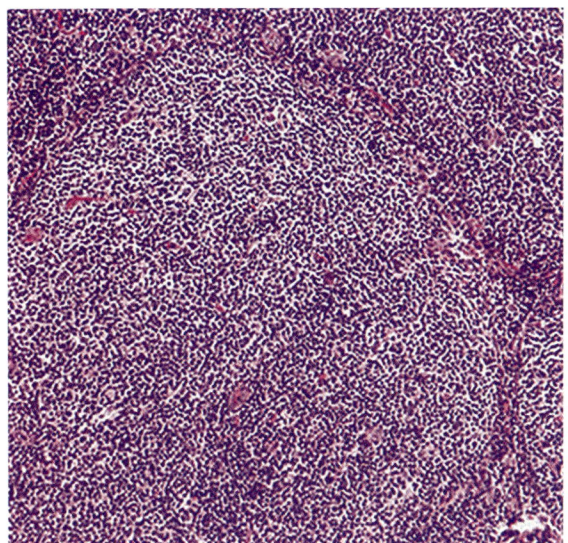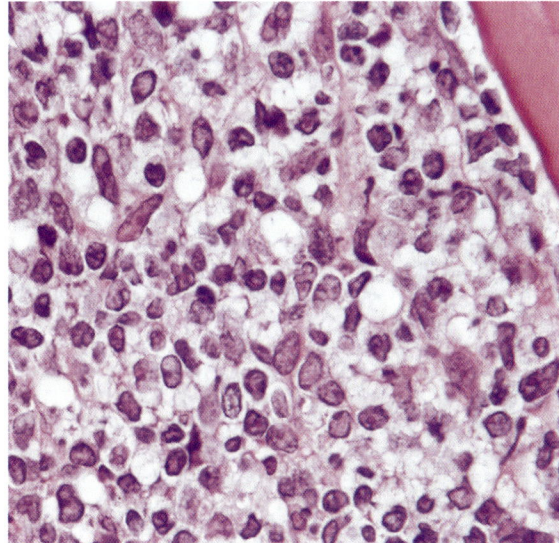

Figure 17-21

HISTOLOGIC TRANSFORMATION

Left: This lymph node biopsy from an elderly man who presented with lymphadenopathy and multiple sites of bone pain shows low-grade follicular lymphoma.

Right: The bone marrow biopsy shows large B-cell lymphoma. In this patient, the bone marrow was the first documented site of histologic transformation, an uncommon event in patients with follicular lymphoma (left, right: H&E stain).

with concordant DLBCL in bone marrow (13). The latter subset of patients has clinically aggressive disease and a simultaneous or subsequent increased risk of central nervous system involvement. In another uncommon manifestation of histologic discordance, patients with low-grade B-cell lymphoma may have DLBCL in the bone marrow. This occurs predominantly in patients with nodal follicular lymphoma (1 to 2 percent of patients) (fig. 17-21). The DLBCL in the bone marrow is usually clonally related to the nodal follicular lymphoma and is likely a manifestation of histologic transformation. Rarely, patients with other types of low-grade B-cell lymphoma develop DLBCL in the bone marrow in the absence of DLBCL at other anatomic sites.

Peripheral Blood

As stated above, rare patients with DLBCL present with a leukemic phase of disease (fig. 17-22). More often, in 5 to 10 percent of patients, the complete blood count or leukocyte count is normal but rare lymphoma cells are observed in the blood smear; the lymphoma cells are more common at the edges of the smear. Most patients with large lymphoma cells in the blood

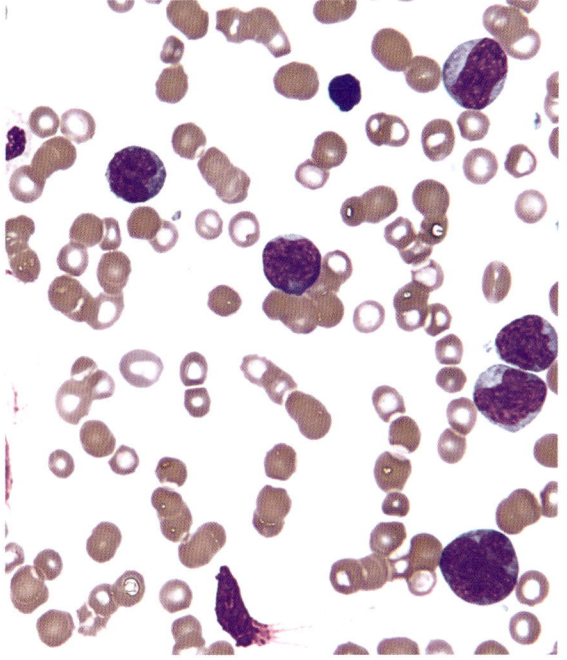

Figure 17-22

DIFFUSE LARGE B-CELL LYMPHOMA: LEUKEMIC PHASE

This patient with DLBCL presented in a leukemic phase, with leukocytosis and many large lymphoma cells in the blood smear (Wright-Giemsa stain).

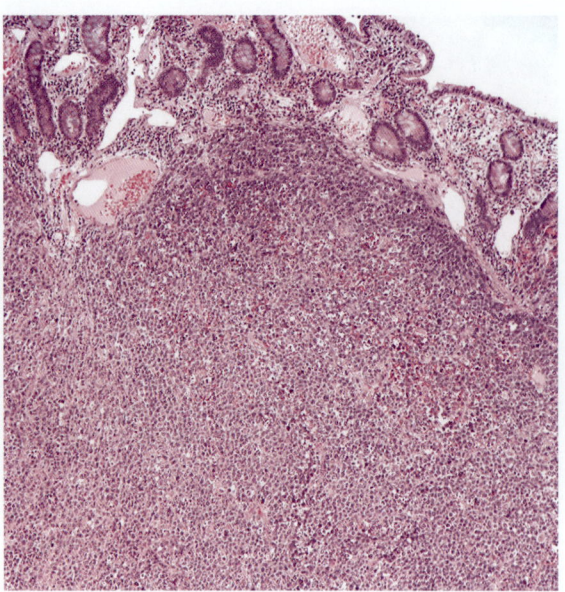 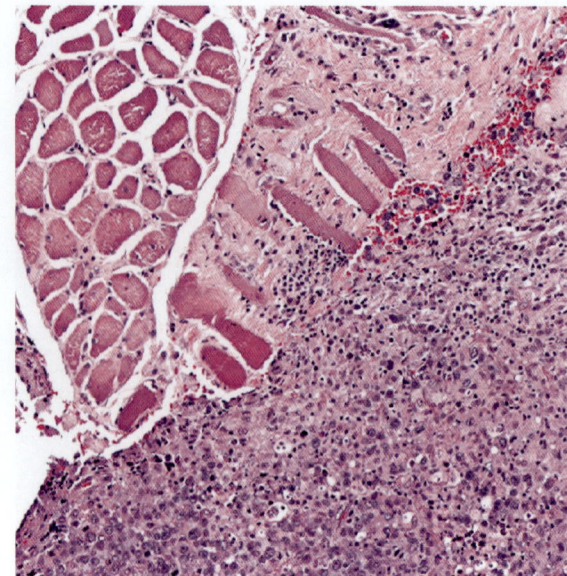

Figure 17-23

DIFFUSE LARGE B-CELL LYMPHOMA INVOLVING EXTRANODAL SITES

Left: DLBCL subtotally replaces the wall of the small intestine.
Right: DLBCL involves extranodal soft tissue. Skeletal muscle is present in the field (left, right: H&E stain).

smear, either in leukemic phase or low-level involvement, also have lymphoma in the bone marrow (7,70,96).

Other Extranodal Sites

Virtually any extranodal site can be involved by DLBCL. The neoplasm may arise primarily at an extranodal site or may be a manifestation of systemic dissemination of nodal DLBCL. The gastrointestinal tract is the most common primary extranodal site for DLBCL (figs. 17-23). In the gastrointestinal tract, as well as other sites, the DLBCL may be associated with extranodal marginal zone lymphoma of mucosa-associated lymphoid tissue (MALT lymphoma).

At extranodal sites, DLBCL may exhibit morphologic features that differ from those of nodal disease, possibly because of the different microenvironment of extranodal sites versus lymph nodes, although there also may be biologic mechanisms involved. In some biopsy specimens, the large B cells are compartmentalized by bands of tumor-associated sclerosis that impart an appearance of tumor cell cohesion. This appearance is common in primary mediastinal large B-cell lymphoma, but also occurs at other

extranodal sites. Some cases of DLBCL are associated with collagenous sclerosis and superficially resemble nodular sclerosis Hodgkin lymphoma at low power magnification (fig. 17-24).

When DLBCL involves adipose tissue, incomplete destruction of the normal stromal framework can impart a pseudonodular or cohesive appearance. Large B cells also commonly infiltrate between normal structures before these cells completely replace them. As a result, a prominent single cell pattern of infiltration may be observed. Unlike lymph nodes, the cells of DLBCL at extranodal sites are often not well rounded and may have a spindle cell appearance. The technique of needle biopsy, often used to assess an extranodal site, can distort lymphoma cells further, adding to a spindle cell shape.

The current WHO classification recognizes a number of large B-cell lymphomas that involve extranodal sites and have distinctive clinical, morphologic, or immunophenotypic features (96). Many of these tumors also involve the lymph nodes or spleen and are discussed in other chapters. Here, we briefly discuss the extranodal large B-cell lymphomas that are not mentioned in other chapters.

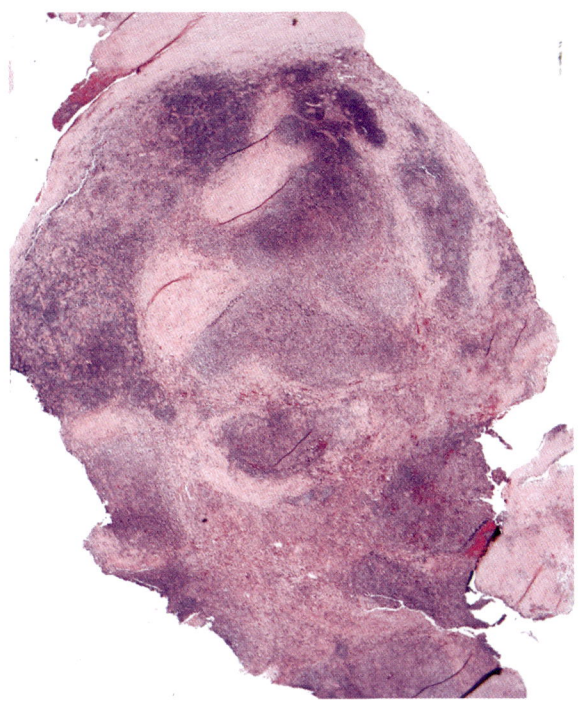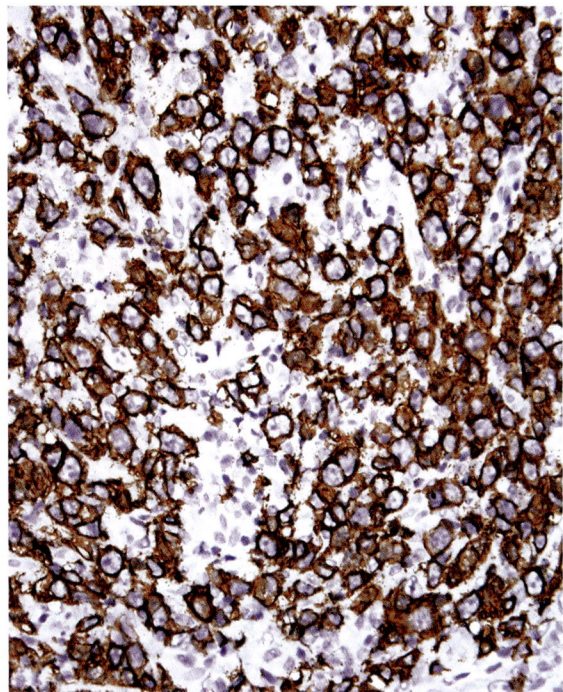

Figure 17-24

DIFFUSE LARGE B-CELL LYMPHOMA INVOLVING SOFT TISSUE

Left: The tumor is associated with abundant, collagenous sclerosis, and at low magnification has a superficial resemblance to nodular sclerosis Hodgkin lymphoma (H&E stain).

Right: The lymphoma cells have a B-cell immunophenotype, positive for CD20 (shown) and CD45/LCA, and negative for CD15 and CD30 (immunohistochemistry with hematoxylin counterstain).

OTHER EXTRANODAL LARGE B-CELL LYMPHOMAS

Primary DLBCL of the Central Nervous System

Primary DLBCL of the central nervous system (CNS) is defined as a large B-cell lymphoma that involves the brain parenchyma or intraocular regions; patients with systemic disease, immunodeficiency, dura-based disease, and specific subtypes such as intravascular large B-cell lymphoma are excluded (51). Primary DLBCL of the CNS represents less than 1 percent of all non-Hodgkin lymphomas.

The median patient age is about 60 years, with a slight male predominance. Patients commonly present with focal neurological symptoms or psychiatric manifestations. Most tumors arise in the brain parenchyma at a supratentorial location. The leptomeninges are involved in about 5 percent of patients. Intraocular involvement occurs in about 20 percent of patients with disease involving other areas of the brain, and most patients with disease first presenting as an intraocular tumor eventually develop disease elsewhere in the brain. The blood-brain barrier complicates therapeutic decisions because standard therapy for patients with DLBCL, R-CHOP (rituximab, cyclophosphamide, hydroxydaunorubicin, vincristine, and prednisone), does not adequately penetrate this barrier and therefore methotrexate is an important therapeutic agent (51).

Primary DLBCL of the CNS most often presents as a single mass but multiple lesions occur in about 30 percent of patients. Microscopic examination shows that these tumors are composed of large cells, commonly located in a perivascular distribution best observed at the margin of the lesion, and often associated with necrosis (fig. 17-25). The lymphoma cells are of B-cell lineage, positive for BCL2 (about 50 percent), BCL6 (60 to 80 percent), and MUM1/IRF4 (about 90 percent); uncommonly positive for

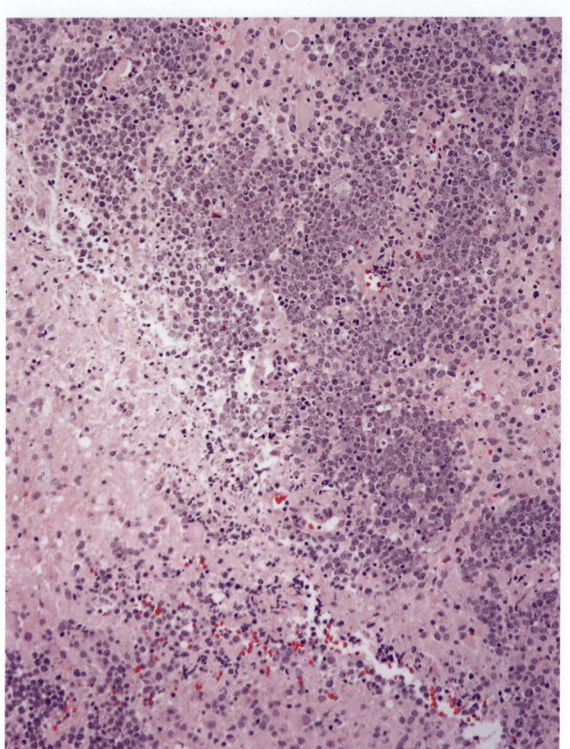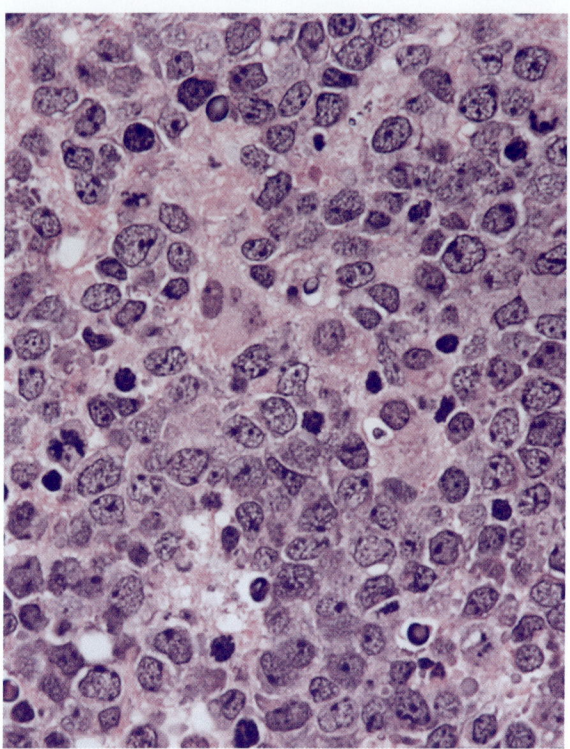

Figure 17-25

DIFFUSE LARGE B-CELL LYMPHOMA INVOLVING CENTRAL NERVOUS SYSTEM

Left: The lymphoma cells from a brain biopsy are arranged in a diffuse pattern and are associated with foci of necrosis.
Right: The lymphoma cells have centroblastic features (left, right: H&E stain).

CD10 (10 to 20 percent); and usually negative for Epstein-Barr virus (EBV) infection (51).

The genetic profile of these tumors is distinctive, with unique findings as well as findings that are shared with systemic cases of DLBCL (12,16,51). Cases of DLBCL of the CNS have a high load of ongoing somatic hypermutations of the immunoglobulin variable regions and biased use of VH4/34. *BCL6* translocations have been identified in 20 to 50 percent of cases. Array-based methods of analysis have shown gains of chromosomal loci 12q, 18q21, and 22q, and loss of 6p21/HLA class II. Other common chromosomal abnormalities include biallelic deletion of 8q12.2 (site of *TOX*, a high mobility group gene), 3p21.3 (protein kinase C delta; *PKCD*) and 9p21 (*CDKN2A/p16*). Copy number alterations of 9p24.1/*PD-L1/PD-L2* have been identified. *MYD88* mutations occur in about 80 percent of cases, CD79B is mutated in about 60 percent of cases, and *TP53* mutations occur in less than 5 percent of cases (12,16). Overall, these changes

implicate activation of the Toll-like and B-cell receptor pathways and immune escape in the pathogenesis of primary DLBCL of the CNS.

Intravascular Large B-Cell Lymphoma

Intravascular large B-cell lymphoma is an extranodal lymphoma characterized by the selective growth of large B cells within the lumens of blood vessels, particularly capillaries, with common sparing of large arteries and veins (71). Patients are usually older, with a median age of 67 years and a male to female ratio of close to 1 to 1 (71,81). Virtually any extranodal site can be involved, but brain, skin, and bone marrow are the most common. B-type symptoms and symptoms related to the specific organ involved are usual.

Histologically, large lymphoma cells of B-cell lineage are located within the lumens of small vessels (figs. 17-26, 17-27). A subset of cases is positive for either CD5 or CD10. The lymphoma cells commonly do not express homing receptors, possibly explaining their intravascular location.

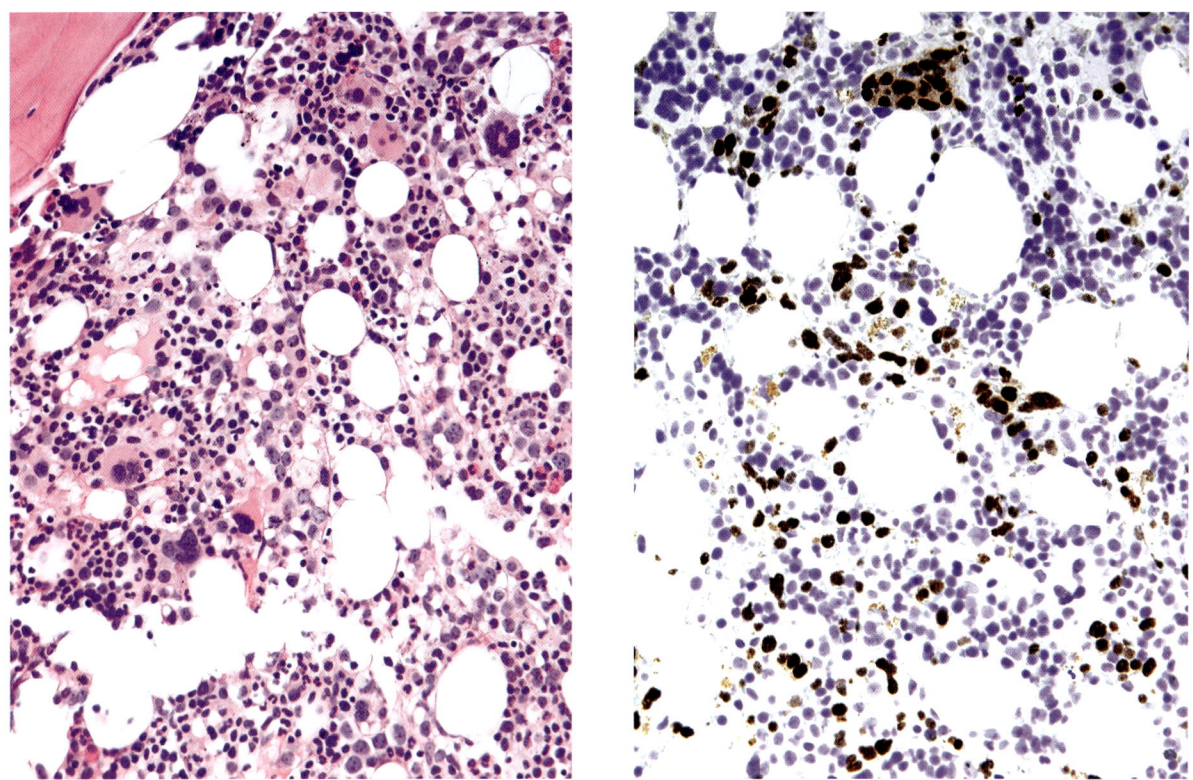

Figure 17-26

INTRAVASCULAR LARGE B-CELL LYMPHOMA

Left: Lymphoma cells distend bone marrow sinusoids but tend to blend with hematopoietic cells and potentially could be not identified (H&E stain).

Right: The anti-PAX5 antibody highlights the lymphoma cells (immunohistochemistry with hematoxylin counterstain).

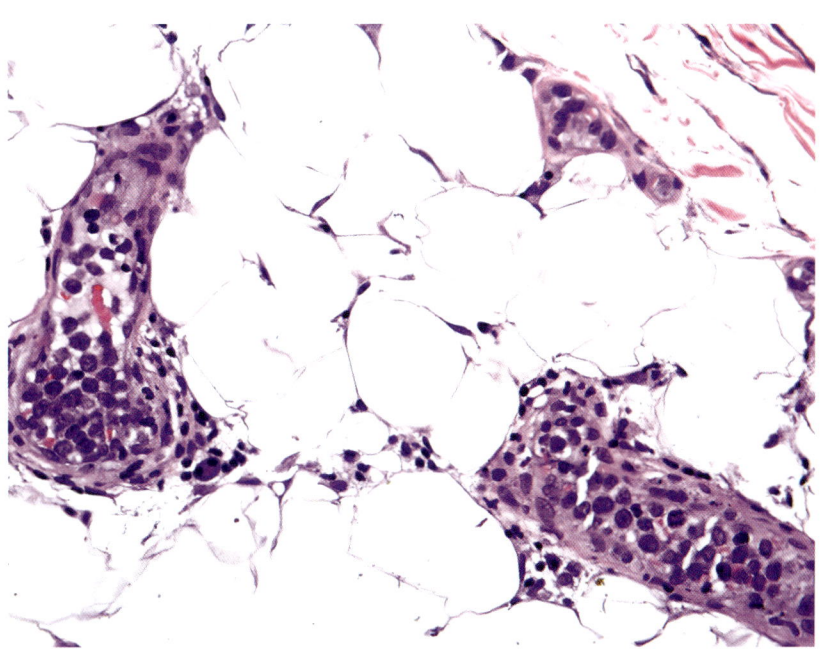

Figure 17-27

INTRAVASCULAR LARGE B-CELL LYMPHOMA

The lymphoma cells are seen within small blood vessels in the subcutaneous tissue. The epidermis and dermis of this specimen were normal (H&E stain).

At autopsy, the central lymph nodes are sometimes involved. The karyotype of the lymphoma cells is often complex, but otherwise little is known about the molecular pathogenesis of this lymphoma (71,81). A focal intravascular pattern can be observed in cases of DLBCL, but these tumors are not included in the category of intravascular large B-cell lymphoma.

Diffuse Large B-Cell Lymphoma Associated with Chronic Inflammation

Diffuse large B-cell lymphoma associated with chronic inflammation is an EBV-positive large B-cell lymphoma arising in the context of longstanding chronic inflammation (15). The prototype for this entity is *pyothorax-associated lymphoma* (PAL), a disease most common in Japan, but also observed uncommonly in Western nations. PAL is associated with the use of artificial pneumothorax as a surgical therapy for tuberculosis of the lungs.

Patients tend to be older and develop PAL years after the onset of pyothorax. The tumors in the thoracic cavity are bulky, usually in the pleura, with local invasion of lung and ribs. Patients present with fever, chest pain, and cough.

Histologically, necrosis or an angiocentric growth pattern is present and the neoplastic cells may have centroblastic or immunoblastic features. The lymphoma cells are large and express B-cell antigens; some cases show plasmacytoid differentiation and are positive for CD138 or IRF4/MUM1. In situ hybridization for EBER1 is positive. Patients require chemotherapy and often radiation therapy, but overall survival is poor (20 to 30 percent at 5 years).

There is a second, rare group of lymphomas that is included in this category in some studies. These cases of DLBCL are small tumors, often detected incidentally in cysts and pseudocysts, on cardiac valves, in chronic osteomyelitis, or near metallic implants of various types in apparently immunocompetent patients (15). The morphologic features and immunophenotype of these neoplasms are similar to those of DLBCL associated with chronic inflammation, but these lesions are often very small and completely excised and detected incidentally (fig. 17-28) (10,11a,15). It is unclear whether these patients require therapy or whether they can be managed in a more conservative manner. A small number of patients have done well after excision without chemotherapy (10,11a). On the basis of the very different presentation and prognosis of these tumors as compared with PAL, it has been suggested that they be identified separately and not included within the category of DLBCL associated with chronic inflammation (10,11a).

Primary Cutaneous DLBCL, Leg Type

Primary cutaneous DLBCL, leg type, is defined as DLBCL arising in the skin, most often on the lower leg of elderly patients, but non-leg sites also are affected (65). The median age is in the seventh decade, and women are more often affected, with a male to female ratio of at least 1 to 3. Patients present with skin tumors, often large and ulcerating, that histologically are composed of sheets of large round cells with centroblastic or immunoblastic features (fig. 17-29). Mitotic figures are usually numerous and there is no epidermotropism. The lymphoma cells are of B-cell lineage and positive for BCL2, BCL6, MUM1/IRF4, FOXP1 and p63, and are usually negative for CD10. DLBCL, leg type, is an aggressive disease with an overall survival rate of about 50 percent.

The molecular features are unique. Most tumors have an activated B-cell-like (ABC) profile, and translocations involving *MYC*, *BCL6*, and *IGH* are common (65). Amplification of 18q21.31-33, including *MALT1* and *BCL2*, and deletion of 9p21.3 involving *CDKN2A* and *CDKN2B* occur in over half of cases, and *MYD88* mutations are common (about 70 percent) (84).

Lymphomatoid Granulomatosis

Lymphomatoid granulomatosis (LYG) is an angiocentric and angiodestructive extranodal lymphoproliferative disease composed of EBV-positive B cells (85). These lesions usually begin in the lungs, but other involved extranodal sites include the brain, skin, liver, and kidneys. Patients with LYG are mostly adults, with a male to female ratio of 2 to 1. Patients usually present with respiratory and B-type symptoms. Imaging studies show bilateral, necrotizing nodules in the middle and lower lung lobes.

Histologically, LYG is both angiocentric and angiodestructive. It is composed of a mixture of atypical lymphoid cells associated with reactive lymphocytes, histiocytes, and plasma cells (fig. 17-30). Granulocytes are absent. Low-grade cases

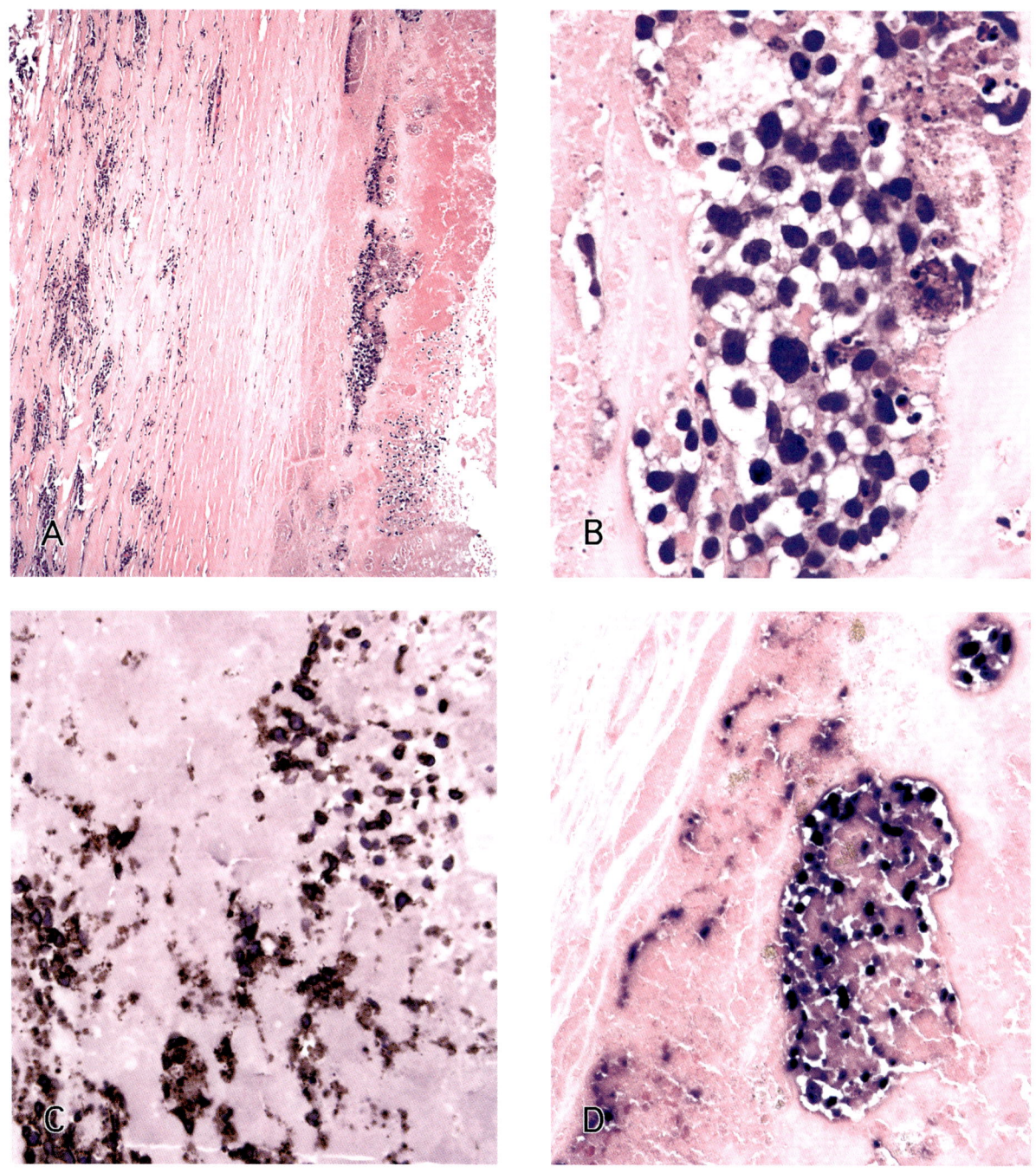

Figure 17-28

DIFFUSE LARGE B-CELL LYMPHOMA IN HYDROCELE

This case of DLBCL was detected incidentally within a paratesticular hydrocele. Some investigators include these tumors in the WHO category of diffuse large B-cell lymphoma associated with chronic inflammation, but patients tend to do very well, and the few patients not treated have also done well.

A: The lymphoma cells are present as groups of cells within the contents of the hydrocele (right). The wall and foci of chronic inflammation are also shown in this field (A,B: H&E stain).

B: High magnification of clusters of large lymphoma cells.

C,D: The lymphoma cells are positive for CD79A (C) and Epstein-Barr virus (EBV)-encoded RNA1 (D) (C: immunohistochemistry with hematoxylin counterstain; D: in situ hybridization with eosin counterstain).

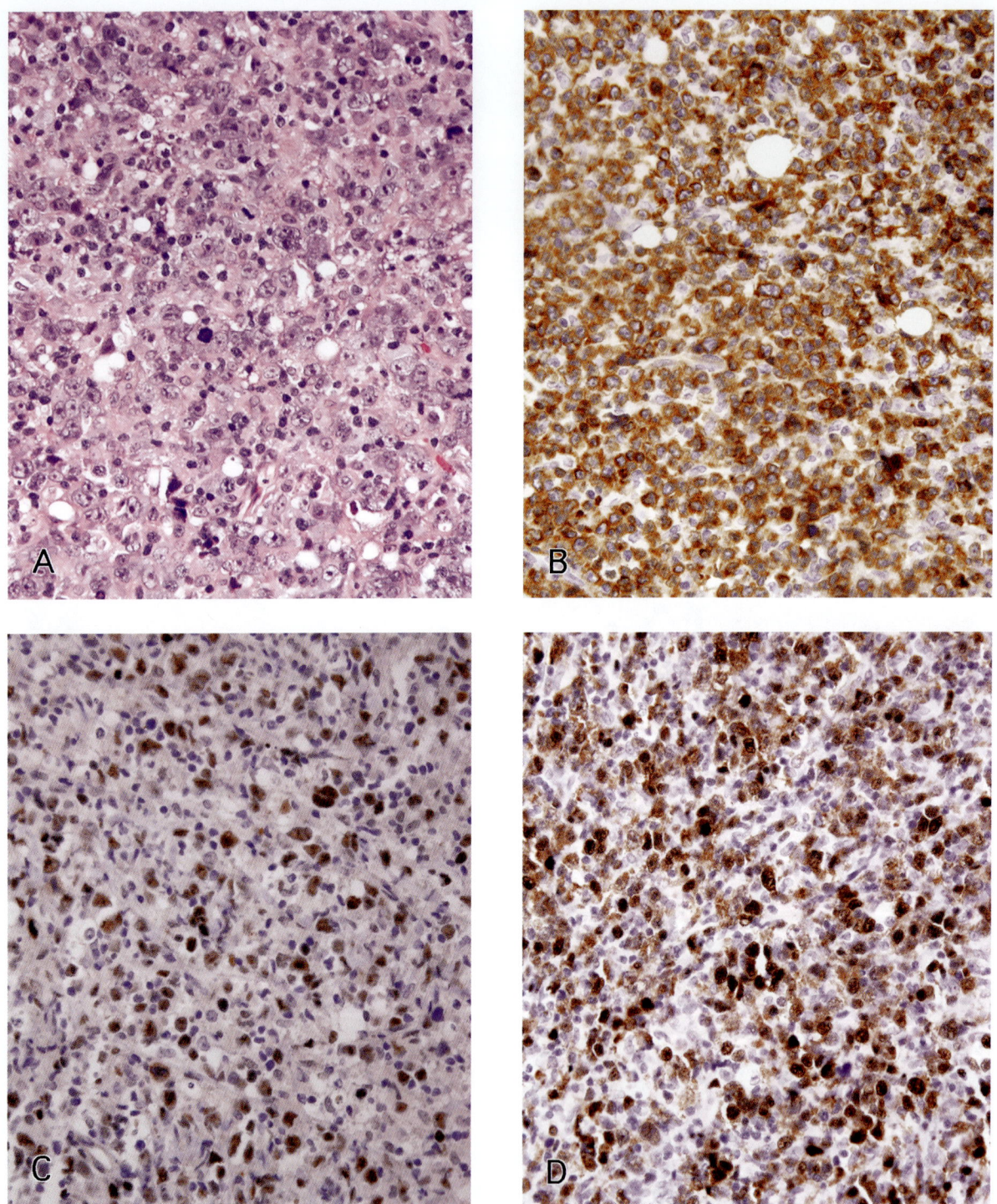

Figure 17-29

PRIMARY CUTANEOUS DIFFUSE LARGE B-CELL LYMPHOMA, LEG TYPE

A: The lymphoma has a diffuse pattern. The cells have immunoblastic features, with round nuclei and prominent nucleoli (H&E stain).

B–D: The lymphoma cells are positive for BCL2 (B), BCL6 (C), and MUM1/IRF4 (D) (B–D: immunohistochemistry with hematoxylin counterstain).

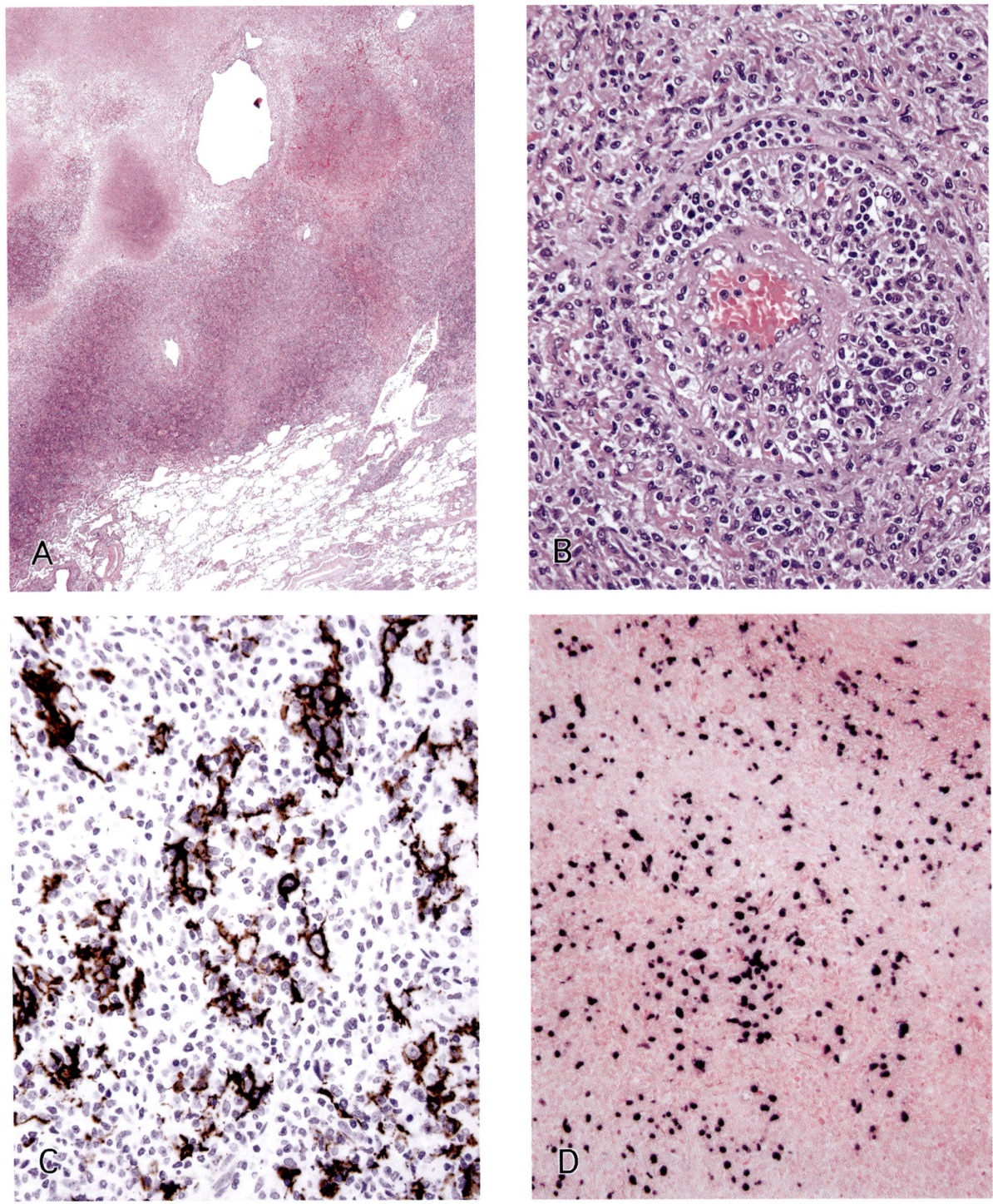

Figure 17-30

HIGH-GRADE LYMPHOMATOID GRANULOMATOSIS (DIFFUSE LARGE B-CELL LYMPHOMA)

A: The lung parenchyma is replaced by lymphoma with areas of coagulative necrosis (A,B: H&E stain).

B: The lymphoma cells preferentially involve and destroy blood vessels.

C,D: The large lymphoid cells are of B-cell lineage, positive for CD20 (C) and EBER1 (D) (C: immunohistochemistry with hematoxylin counterstain; D: in situ hybridization with eosin counterstain).

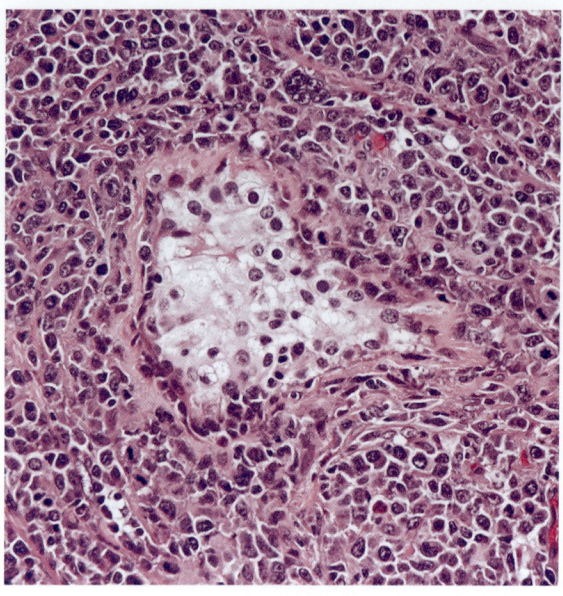

Figure 17-31

DIFFUSE LARGE B-CELL LYMPHOMA ARISING IN THE TESTIS

The lymphoma cells surround a seminiferous tubule (H&E stain).

have few large cells and do not meet the criteria for DLBCL. High-grade cases are composed of sheets of large cells and therefore meet criteria for DLBCL, but the background often has a more heterogeneous mixture of inflammatory cells compared with most cases of DLBCL (85). The neoplastic cells are of B-cell lineage, positive for EBV, and large cells are often CD30 positive [also CD45(+) and CD15(-)].

The overall survival period of patients with LYG is short, often less than 2 years (85). Rare cases of NK- or T-cell lymphoma involving the lungs can closely resemble LYG, but these tumors are not included in this category.

Diffuse Large B-Cell Lymphoma Arising at Other Extranodal Sites

It seems likely that other subsets of DLBCL arising at extranodal sites may be recognized separately in future lymphoma classification schemes. This statement is supported by the number of extranodal large B-cell lymphomas already recognized separately in the WHO classification (96a). It also seems reasonable to suggest that future studies will show different mechanisms of pathogenesis and potential ther-

apeutic targets for additional cases of DLBCL that arise at different extranodal sites.

One example of an extranodal DLBCL likely on its way to separate recognition is *DLBCL of the testis* (fig. 17-31). These tumors represent about 90 percent of all testicular lymphomas and less than 1 percent of all non-Hodgkin lymphomas. Testicular DLBCL affects older men of a median age in the seventh decade (30,118). A testicular mass, often painless, is the most common presentation. Approximately 75 percent of patients present with stage I and II disease, and bilateral involvement occurs in about 5 percent. Patients with testicular DLBCL often completely respond to standard therapy for DLBCL, but they have a high rate of relapse at other extranodal sites, including the contralateral testis, adrenal gland, and central nervous system. Testicular DLBCL uncommonly disseminates to the bone marrow. The prognosis of patients with DLBCL of the testis is poorer than that of patients with nodal DLBCL (118). As a result, the therapeutic approach requires chemotherapy, contralateral radiation therapy, and central nervous system prophylaxis.

Most cases of testicular DLBCL have a non-germinal center B-cell (non-GCB) or activated B-cell (ABC) (85 percent) immunophenotype. Expression of FOXP1 or TCL1 has been correlated with a poorer prognosis (30). At the molecular level, DLBCL of the testis has distinctive features. These tumors have a high frequency of somatic mutations of the *IGH* variable regions. The gene expression signature is unique, with deregulated expression of proliferation, adhesion, immune response genes, BCL6, and B-cell receptor signaling (30). *MYD88* mutations occur in about 80 percent of cases (implicating the Toll-like receptor pathway) and about half of these tumors have mutations in the B-cell receptor pathway. Biallelic *CDKN2A* loss is common. Gene fusions and copy number alterations of 9p24.1/*PD-L1/PD-L2* are common and translocations involving *CIITA* occur in about 10 percent of cases. These findings suggest that evasion of host immune response plays a role in pathogenesis and that immune checkpoint inhibitor therapy may be promising (16,98). Rearrangements of *FOXP1* (about 7 percent) have been shown and *TP53* mutations are rare (16,98).

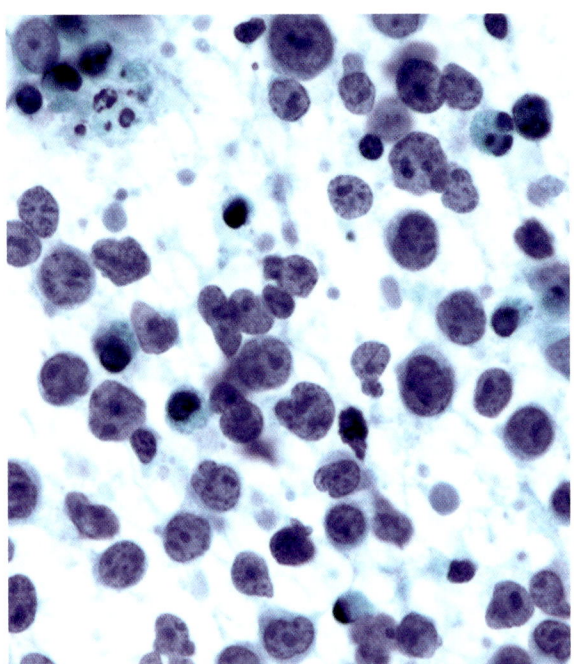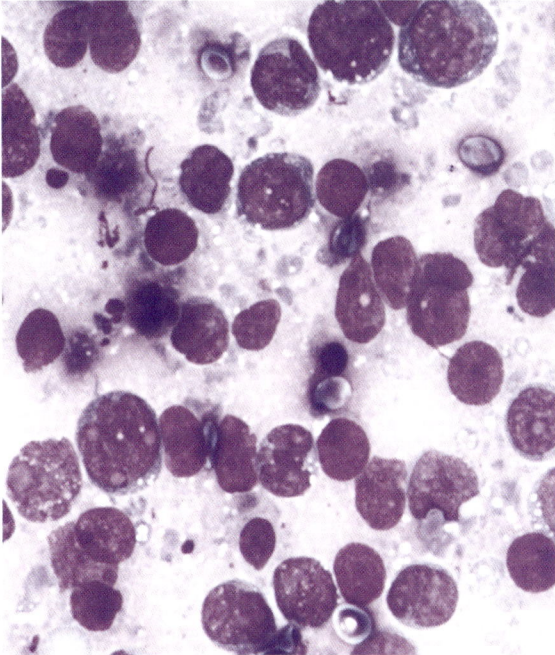

Figure 17-32

DIFFUSE LARGE B-CELL LYMPHOMA WITH CENTROBLASTIC FEATURES

Left, right: Both smears show a dispersed population of large cells with multiple nucleoli, apoptotic cells, and karyorrhectic debris. In the left figure, a tingible body macrophage is appreciated (upper left of field). In the right, some of the large cells have small cytoplasmic vacuoles (left: Papanicolaou stain; right: Diff-Quik stain).

CYTOLOGIC FINDINGS

In fine-needle aspirate specimens, the cells of DLBCL are large and resemble their appearance in tissue sections. The cells have centroblastic, immunoblastic, or anaplastic features (figs. 17-32–17-34). Cases of DLBCL with a high proliferation fraction often show mitotic figures, apoptotic cells, karyorrhectic debris, and cytoplasmic vacuoles (fig. 17-35). In cases with a starry sky pattern, numerous tingible-body macrophages are present in aspirate smears.

IMMUNOPHENOTYPIC FINDINGS

Flow cytometry immunophenotypic or immunohistochemical analysis can be employed to assess cases of DLBCL. The lymphoma cells are positive for pan-B-cell antigens and transcription factors including CD19, CD20, CD22, CD79A, PAX5, OCT2, and BOB.1. Most cases also express CD45/LCA and some are positive for CD5 (5 to 10 percent) (fig. 17-36), CD10 (40 to 60 percent), CD23 (about 15 percent), CD30 (15 to 25 percent overall and over 50 percent in anaplastic variant cases), CD38, CD40, CD44, CD200 (most cases bright), BCL2 (60 to 70 percent), BCL6 (60 to 80 percent), MUM1/IRF4 (40 to 70 percent), MYC (about 30 percent), P53 (20 to 40 percent), MYD88 (about 40 percent) and cyclin D1 (less than 5 percent) (fig. 17-37). MYD88 expression does not correlate with *MYD88* L265P mutation (19). Most cases of DLBCL express surface light chain and usually IgM, but some express IgA or IgG and others are negative for immunoglobulin.

The proliferation index of DLBCL cases, evaluated by Ki-67, is variable but typically in the range of 50 to 80 percent, with a lower end of 30 to 40 percent and many cases over 90 percent (fig. 17-36E). EBER1 is positive in 4 to 5 percent of DLBCL cases in Western nations, and when present in many cells, supports the diagnosis of EBV-positive DLBCL (see chapter 19).

The cells of DLBCL are negative for T-cell antigens including CD1a, CD2, CD3, CD4, CD7, CD8, and T-cell receptors. The lymphoma cells are also negative for myeloid-associated markers such as CD13, CD33, and myeloperoxidase;

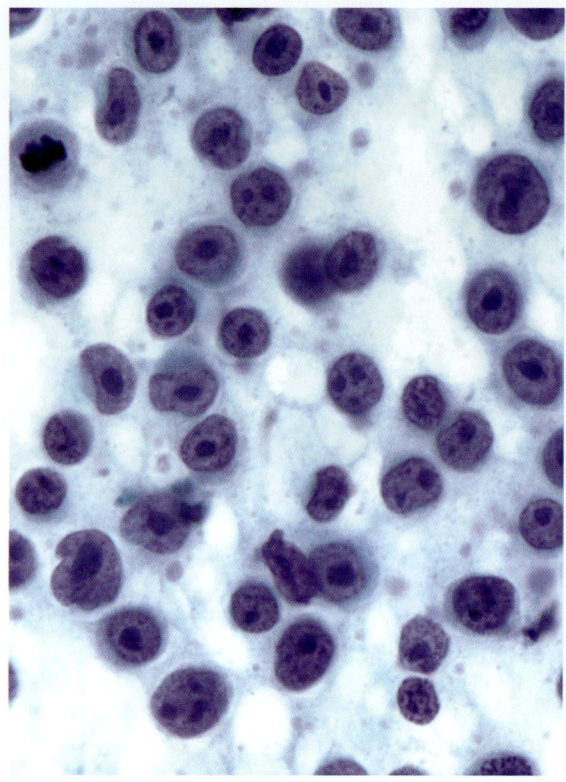

Figure 17-33

**DIFFUSE LARGE B-CELL LYMPHOMA
WITH IMMUNOBLASTIC FEATURES**

The lymphoma cells have round nuclei and prominent central nucleoli (Papanicolaou stain).

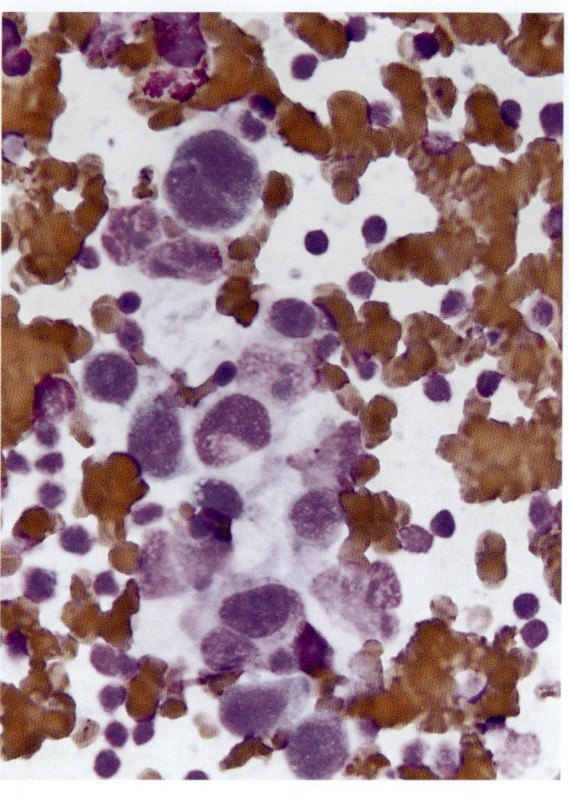

Figure 17-34

**DIFFUSE LARGE B-CELL LYMPHOMA
WITH ANAPLASTIC FEATURES**

The lymphoma cells are large and pleomorphic (Diff-Quik stain).

Figure 17-35

**DIFFUSE LARGE B-CELL
LYMPHOMA WITH VACUOLES**

The lymphoma cells have numerous cytoplasmic vacuoles (Wright-Giemsa stain).

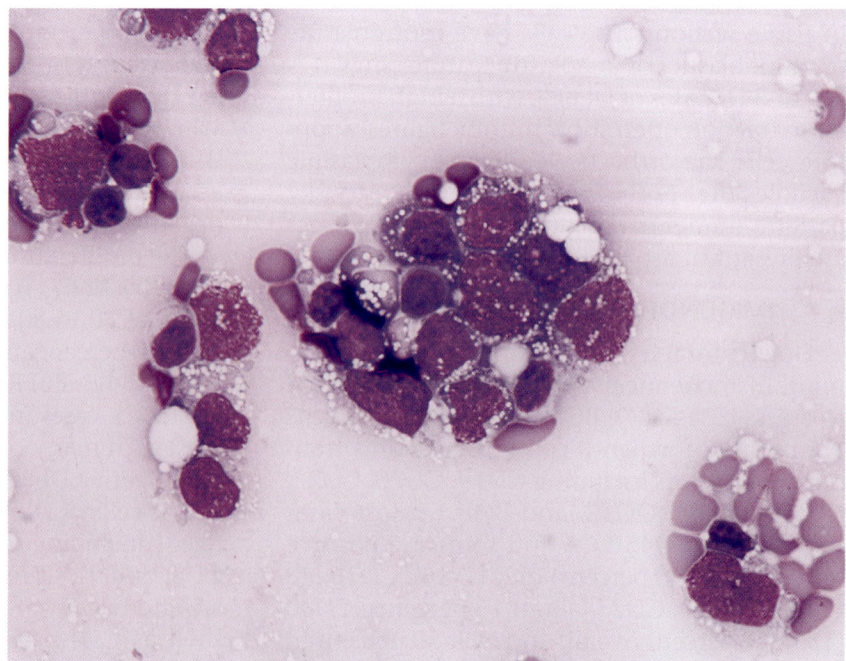

histiocyte-associated/accessory cells antigens including CD11c, CD14, CD15, CD21, CD35, CD68, CD163, and S-100 protein; keratins; sarcoma-associated markers; and CD31, CD34, SOX11, ALK, and TdT. Rare cases of DLBCL are CD3-positive; others are very rarely positive for keratin, usually with focal and variable expression, and only detectable using sensitive pancytokeratin antibodies (fig. 17-36F).

Assessment of some markers in DLBCL has therapeutic relevance. Perhaps the best example is CD20, which is the target of rituximab and therefore required as part of the workup of a case of DLBCL. CD30, expressed by a subset of DLBCL cases, is a target of brentuximab vedotin (fig. 17-38) and its assessment may be required, more often in the setting of relapsed disease. The application of high-throughput molecular methods to the analysis of DLBCL cases has elucidated many additional abnormalities involving cellular pathways for which novel therapeutic agents are in clinical trials or development. It seems highly likely that assessment of expression of additional proteins as potential therapeutic targets will need to be incorporated into the workup of DLBCL to guide therapy, either at the time of initial diagnosis or relapse. Typical endpoints of assessment include the presence or absence of various proteins as well as the detection of phosphorylated or mutated proteins using specific antibodies.

The expression of other markers in DLBCL has been reported to have prognostic relevance. Perhaps the best studied in the literature are immunohistochemical algorithms that function as surrogates for gene expression profiling (GEP) analysis. As reviewed by others (26), at least nine algorithms have been proposed, but for this chapter we focus on four systems that are used most often (fig. 17-39). The first system, proposed by Hans et al. (38), is the most popular: CD10, MUM1/IRF4, and BCL6 are used, each with a 30 percent or greater cutoff. CD10 expression supports GCB type; those cases that are CD10 negative but MUM1/IRF4 positive are classified as non-GCB type; and cases negative for CD10 and MUM1/IRF4 but BCL6 positive are GCB type (figs. 17-40, 17-41).

More recent systems proposed by Choi et al. (21) and Visco et al. (101) agree with GEP profiles with over 90 percent concordance (slightly better than the Hans system). The Choi et al. system uses five antibodies: GCET1 (cutoff, 80 percent or more), CD10 (30 percent or more), BCL6 (30 percent or more), MUM1/IRF4 (80 percent or more), and FOXP1 (80 percent or more). The Visco-Young system (96) uses three antibodies: CD10 (30 percent or more), FOXP1 (60 percent or more), and BCL6 (30 percent or more). The Tally method (66) is also used and, unlike other systems, this system does not require analysis of results in sequence. The Tally method uses five antibodies (each 1 point) and 30 percent or more cutoffs: CD10 and GCET1 support GCB type; FOXP1 and MUM1/IRF4 support non-GCB type; and if cell of origin is not resolved after using these four antibodies, LMO2 is used as a tiebreaker to support GCB type (66).

As shown by others (26), immunohistochemical algorithms show poor concordance with each other due to suboptimal interlaboratory reproducibility, both technical and interpretive. Reproducibility is hampered by differences in algorithm design (sequenced versus nonsequenced results) as well as different cutoffs, use of semi-quantification, and other technical issues. An example of discordance is the comparison of the Hans algorithm versus the Tally method. A DLBCL that is CD10(+), GCET1(-), FOXP1(+), MUM1/IRF4(+) and LMO2(-) would be considered GCB using the Hans algorithm, but non-GCB using the Tally method.

Based on the above discussion, a number of antibodies have been recommended for the workup of DLBCL by various groups. A panel is suggested in Table 17-2. A number of other

Table 17-2

IMMUNOPHENOTYPIC MARKERS RECOMMENDED FOR THE WORKUP OF DIFFUSE LARGE B-CELL LYMPHOMA[a]

Essential
  CD3, CD5, CD10, CD20, BCL2, BCL6, MUM1/IRF4, MYC

Useful (subset of cases)
  CD19, CD21, CD22, CD23, CD30, CD45/LCA, CD79A, CD138, Ki-67, PAX5, FOXP1, ALK, HHV8, EBER1 (in situ hybridization)

Optional
  CD68, cyclin D1, SOX11, other T-cell antigens

[a]Modified from data in reference 114; antibodies for cell of origin classification based on the Hans algorithm.

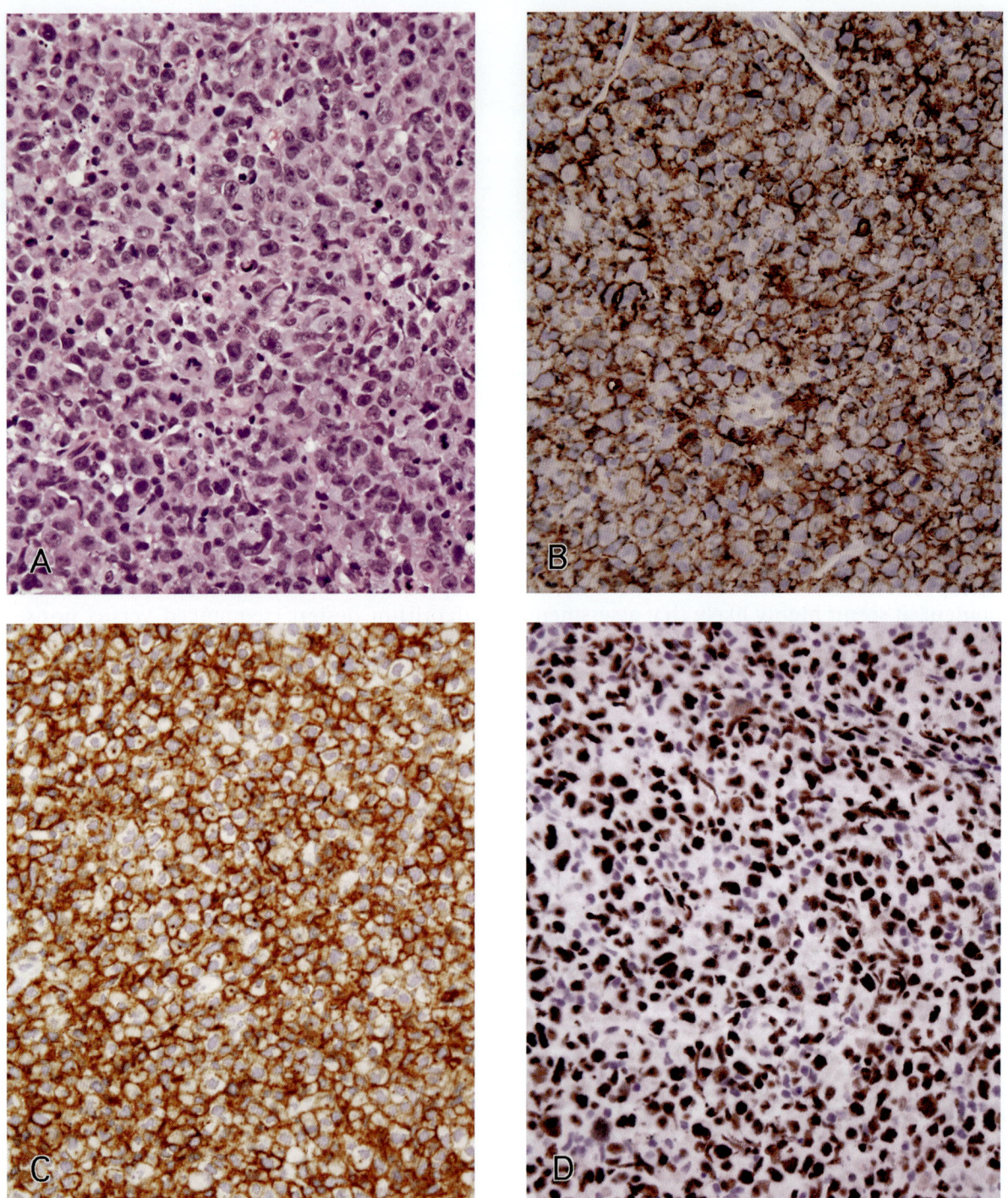

Figure 17-36

CD5-POSITIVE DIFFUSE LARGE B-CELL LYMPHOMA WITH A NON-GERMINAL CENTER B-CELL IMMUNOPHENOTYPE

A: The lymphoma cells are large with many mitotic figures and apoptotic cells, suggesting a rapidly growing tumor (H&E stain).

B–F: The lymphoma cells are positive for CD20 (B), CD5 (C), and FOXP1 (D); have a high Ki-67 rate (E); and show focal, weak cytoplasmic expression for the sensitive pankeratin antibody OSCAR (F). The lymphoma cells were negative for CD3, CD10, and other pankeratin antibodies (not shown) (B–F: immunohistochemistry with hematoxylin counterstain).

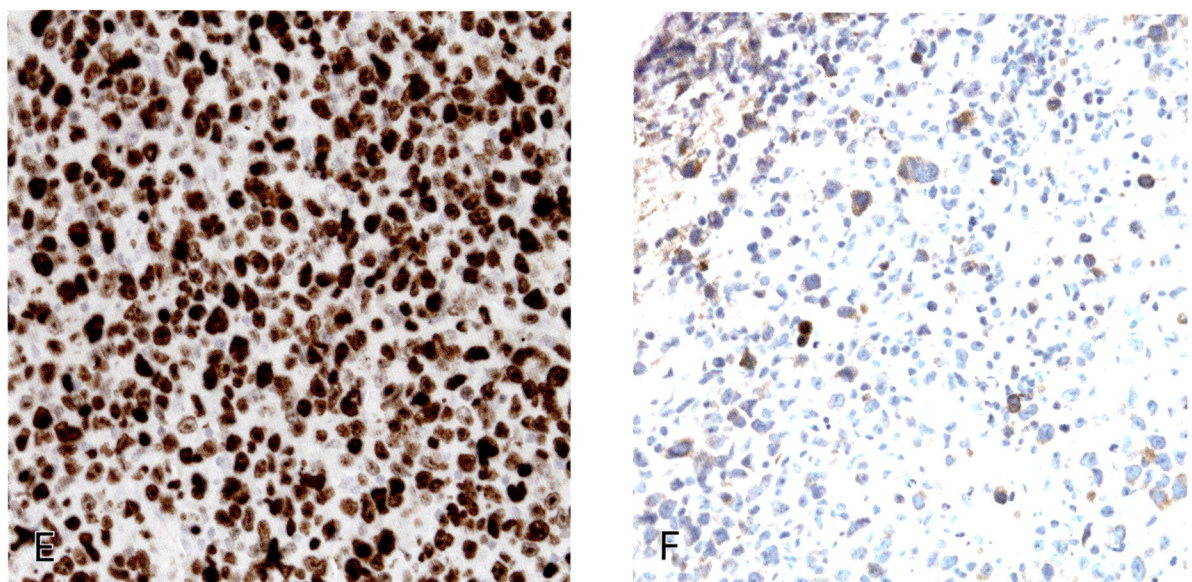

Figure 17-36, continued

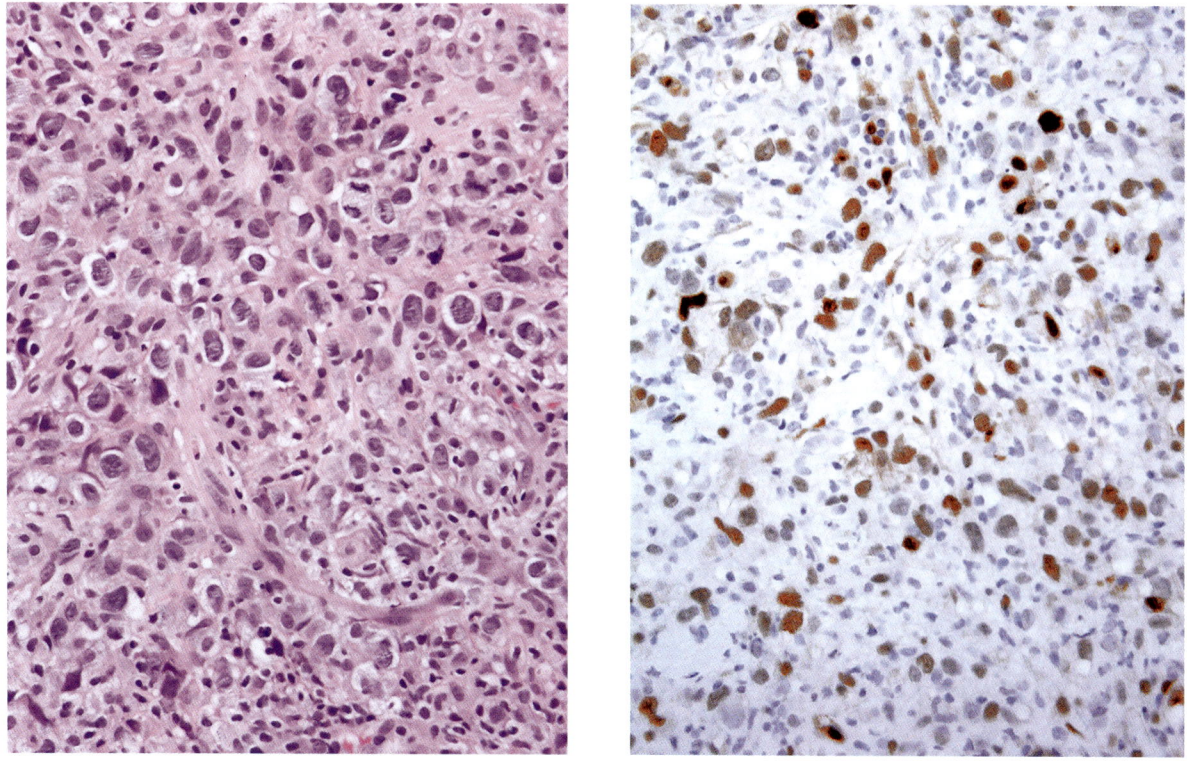

Figure 17-37

CYCLIN D1-POSITIVE DIFFUSE LARGE B-CELL LYMPHOMA WITH A NON-GCB IMMUNOPHENOTYPE

Left: The lymphoma cells are arranged in a diffuse pattern and are large (H&E stain).

Right: Cyclin D1 is expressed to a variable degree in some lymphoma cells. Unlike mantle cell lymphoma, where the lymphoma cells are usually uniformly positive for cyclin D1, variable expression is typical in DLBCL. This tumor showed no evidence of *CCND1-IGH* by fluorescence in situ hybridization (immunohistochemistry with hematoxylin counterstain).

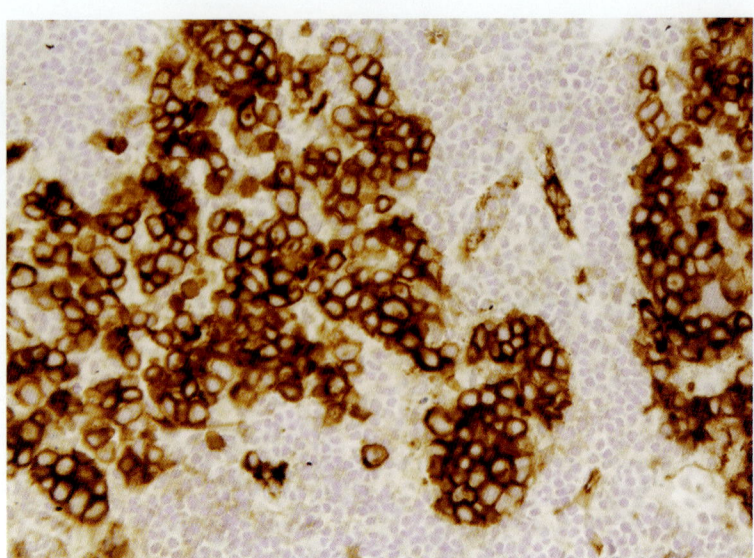

Figure 17-38

CD30-POSITIVE DIFFUSE LARGE B-CELL LYMPHOMA

This case of DLBCL with a sinusoidal pattern was strongly positive for CD30, suggesting that the tumor may respond to therapy targeting CD30 (immunohistochemistry with hematoxylin counterstain).

A. Hans*

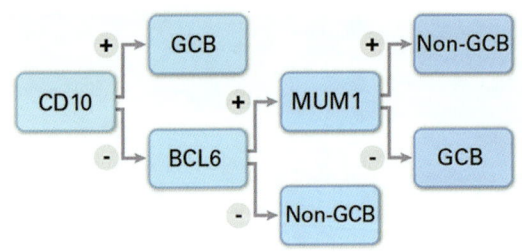

*30% cutoff for each antibody

B. Visco-Young

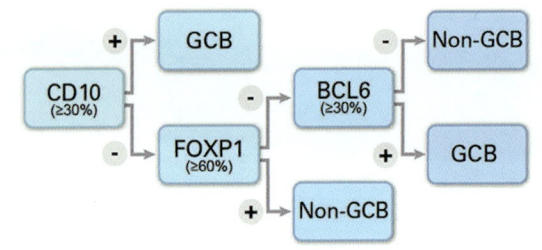

C. Choi

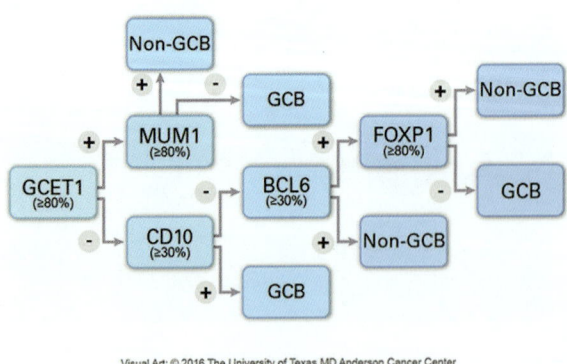

Visual Art: © 2016 The University of Texas MD Anderson Cancer Center

D. Tally

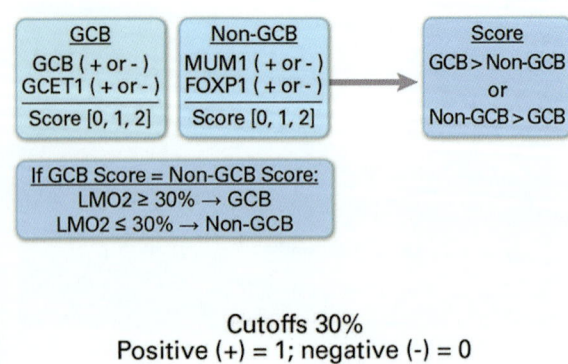

Cutoffs 30%
Positive (+) = 1; negative (−) = 0

Figure 17-39

IMMUNOHISTOCHEMICAL ALGORITHMS

Shown are four immunohistochemical algorithms commonly used for predicting the cell of origin in cases of DLBCL. (GCB = germinal of center B-cell immunophenotype; MUM1 = MUM1/IRF4.)

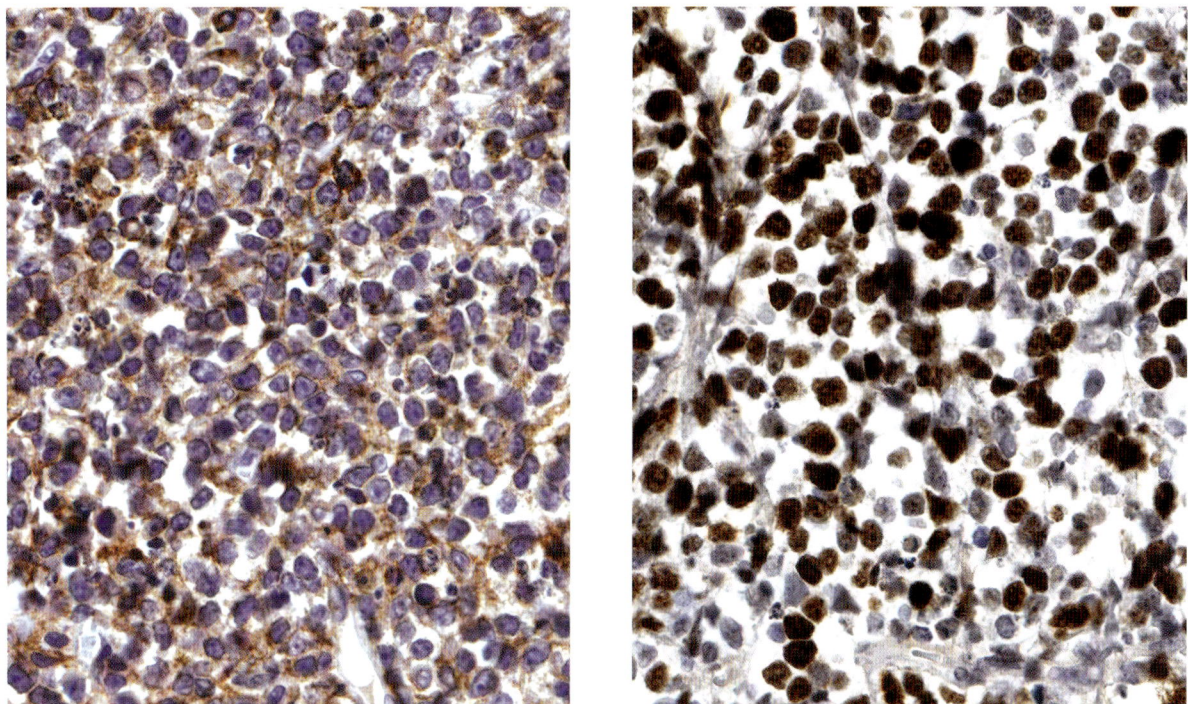

Figure 17-40

DIFFUSE LARGE B-CELL LYMPHOMA: HANS ALGORITHM

Left, right: This case of DLBCL was positive for CD10 (left) and BCL6 (right) and was negative for MUM1/IRF4 (not shown), supporting a GCB immunophenotype using the Hans algorithm (left, right: immunohistochemistry with hematoxylin counterstain).

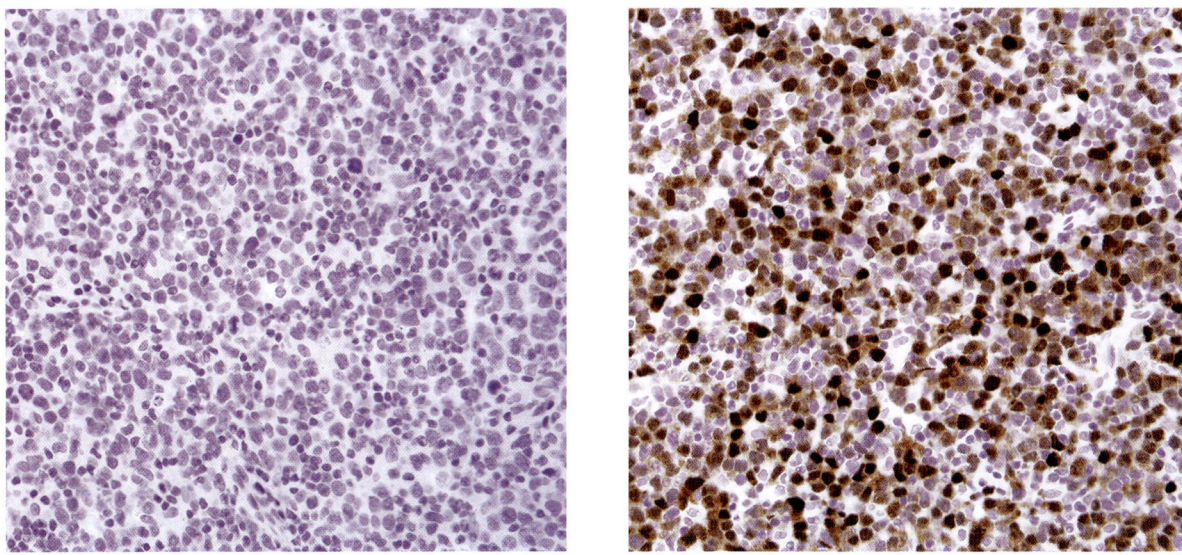

Figure 17-41

DIFFUSE LARGE B-CELL LYMPHOMA: HANS ALGORITHM

Left, right: This case of DLBCL was negative for CD10 (left) and positive for MUM1/IRF4 (right), supporting a non-GCB immunophenotype using the Hans algorithm (left, right: immunohistochemistry with hematoxylin counterstain).

Table 17-3

MARKERS AND PROGNOSIS IN PATIENTS WITH DIFFUSE LARGE B-CELL LYMPHOMA

Marker[a]	Prognostic Impact	Comments	Reference(s)
CD3 (high reactive cells)	Favorable		25
CD4 (high reactive cells)	Favorable		1
FOXP3 (high reactive cells)	Favorable		1,25
PD-1 (high reactive cells)	Favorable		1
CD8 (>5% reactive cells)	Favorable	DLBCL of bone	86
P21	Favorable		104
CD30	Favorable		43
CD40	Favorable		91
P63	Favorable	Activated B-cell type and wild type *TP53*	110
NF-κB/p52	Favorable	Correlates with CD30+ and BCL2-negative	79
MDM2	No impact		107
Cyclin D1	No impact		80
BCL2	No impact	Was adverse using CHOP therapy	45
BCL6	No impact	Was adverse using CHOP therapy	105
Cyclin E	No impact	Was adverse using CHOP therapy	36
EBV[b]	No impact	Adverse if associated with CD30+	78
STAT3	No independent impact	Correlates with ABC type and MYC expression	77
CD5	Adverse		3,108
Ki-67	Adverse, if high	Controversial; not all studies support	53
P53	Adverse, if high	≥50% positive cells correlates with *TP53* mutation	109
FOXP1	Adverse	Correlates with ABC type in DLBCL; also patients with testicular DLBCL	29,30
TCL1	Adverse	Patients with testicular DLBCL	30
MYC	Adverse, if high	Correlates with MYC translocation	106
MYC+BCL2	Adverse		44,49
Survivin	Adverse		62,116
MYD88	Adverse		20
MET	Adverse	Loss of expression is prognostic	52
RON	Adverse	Loss of expression is prognostic	52
PI3K/AKT	Adverse		27,40
CXCR4	Adverse		17
TNF-α	Adverse		72
BMI1	Adverse		99
PD-L1	Adverse		50
GRHL3	Adverse		61

[a]Marker assessed on neoplastic cells unless otherwise specified.
[b]EBV = Epstein-Barr virus.

Table 17-4

CHROMOSOMAL TRANSLOCATIONS AND GENES IN DIFFUSE LARGE B-CELL LYMPHOMA[a]

Translocation	Genes	Frequency
t(3;v)(q27;v)[b]	*BCL6* and other partners; *IGH* most common	30-40%
t(14;18)(q32;q21)	*IGH* and *BCL2*	20-30%
t(8;v)(q24;v)	*MYC* and other partners; *IGH* most common; *IGK* or *IGL* in ~10%; also non-IG partners	~10%
inv(3q)	*TBL1XR1-TP63*	~5%
t(6;v)(p25.3;v)	*IRF4* with IG locus; usually *IGH* but rarely light chain genes	4-5%
t(14;16)(q32;q24.1)	*IGH* and *IRF8*	2-3%
t(5;14)(q33;q32)	*IGH* and *EBF1*	1-2%
t(14;17)(q32;p13.1)	*IGH* and *TNFRSF13*	1-2%
t(9;14)(p13;q32)	*PAX5* and *IGH*	1%

[a]Other rare translocations have been described in DLBCL but apparently occur in <1%.
[b]v = variable (a number of potential gene partners occur); IG = immunoglobulin.

proteins that can be assessed by routine immunophenotypic methods have been reported to have prognostic significance in patients with DLBCL. A complete discussion of this topic is beyond the scope of this chapter, but a list of some of these markers is presented in Table 17-3.

MOLECULAR GENETIC FINDINGS

Chromosomal Abnormalities

Conventional cytogenetic analysis has shown a number of abnormalities in cases of DLBCL. In one study, the most common chromosomal abnormalities, excluding translocations (see below), were as follows: loss of 6q (39 percent), loss of 1p (27 percent), gain of 1q (18 percent), loss of 17p (16 percent), loss of 1q (about 16 percent), loss of 4q or 14q (each about 15 percent), breaks in 1q36 (about 12 percent), and loss of 10q (10 percent) (35). Spectral karyotyping and comparative genomic hybridization methods also have been applied to cases of DLBCL and have shown a greater number of abnormalities per case (9,73). In a study by Bea et al. (9), common sites of gain included 18q, Xq, 2q, 7q, and 12p, present in 14 to 20 percent of cases, and losses of 6q and 17p, each in 14 percent of cases.

A number of chromosomal translocations occur in DLBCL (Table 17-4). The most common involve *BCL6, BCL2, MYC,* or a combination of these genes. The 3q27/*BCL6* locus is targeted in 30 to 40 percent of DLBCL cases (76). The

14q32/*IGH* locus is the most frequent partner of *BCL6*, creating t(3;14)(q27;q32), but several other non-*IGH* partners of *BCL6* have been observed. *BCL6* translocations occur more commonly in the ABC type of DLBCL. The t(14;18)(q32;q21)/ *IGH-BCL2* is present in 20 to 30 percent of cases of DLBCL, almost exclusively in the GCB type (35,102). 8q24/*MYC* translocations occur in 10 to 15 percent of cases. 8q24/*MYC* can partner with *IGH* (or light chain genes) or non-IG gene partners. *MYC* translocations are associated with a poorer prognosis (see below); 5 to 10 percent of DLBCL cases carry a *MYC* translocation associated with a *BCL2* (most common) and/or *BCL6*, and rarely other oncogenes. These neoplasms are designated as double-hit or triple-hit lymphoma (see chapter 27) (59).

Other chromosomal translocations occur at a lower frequency. Translocations involving *IRF4* occur in 4 to 5 percent of DLBCL cases and are associated with younger patient age, involvement of the head and neck region including Waldeyer ring, and a favorable prognosis (92). *IRF4* translocated cases are almost always positive for MUM1/IRF4 and BCL6, with CD10 and CD5 positive in 67 percent and 30 percent of cases, respectively. The gene expression profile of these tumors is distinctive (92). An inversion of chromosome 3q leads to a *TBL1XR1-TP63* novel fusion gene in about 5 percent of cases of DLBCL, exclusively of GCB type, but associated with primary refractory disease when treated with standard therapy (95). Other transloca- tions are present in 1 to 3 percent of cases and involve *EBF1*, *IRF8*, *TNFRSF13*, and *PAX5* (11). Other rare translocations in DLBCL are not discussed here.

Gene Expression Profiling

Gene expression profiling analysis has high- lighted the heterogeneity of tumors included in the category of DLBCL. Alizadeh et al. (4) were the first to apply GEP methods to DLBCL. They divided cases into GCB and activated ABC groups as well as a small (10 to 15 percent) unclassifiable group. Importantly, they showed that for patients with DLBCL treated with CHOP therapy, those with a GCB type had a better survival rate than patients with an ABC type (4). Subsequently, this observation was confirmed in patients treated with the R-CHOP regimen (89). Over time, the GCB versus ABC model has become popular and many studies have shown its value for predicting prognosis. In addition, this model has biologic correlates as virtually all cases of DLBCL with t(14;18) or *MYC* translocations fall within the GCB group, whereas NF-κB activation is much more prominent in the ABC group.

This dichotomous approach may be too simplistic for the following reasons: 1) subsets of patients with GCB tumors do poorly, for example, patients with double-hit lymphomas; 2) some patients with ABC tumors (20 to 30 percent) respond well to therapy and are cured; 3) patients with DLBCL exhibiting loss of a MHC class II gene expression signature have a poorer outcome (88); and 4) most importantly, high-throughput methods of analysis of DLBCL cases have shown that the GCB and ABC groups are genetically heterogeneous categories, with a large number of single gene mutations, gene amplifications, gene/chromosomal deletions, chromosomal translocations and inversions, and copy number alterations that cast addition- al light on cell of origin classification.

There are other approaches to subdividing cases of DLBCL using GEP data. Monti et al. (67) created three groups, which were designated oxidative phosphorylation, B-cell receptor/ proliferation, and host response. The oxidative phosphorylation group includes tumors carry- ing t(14;18) as well as tumors with defects in apoptotic pathways. The B-cell receptor/pro- liferation group includes tumors that carry *BCL6* translocations and likely overlaps with the ABC subtype. The host response group has a T-cell and dendritic cell signature and likely includes cases of T-cell/histiocyte-rich large B-cell lymphoma (see chapter 18). In other studies, primary mediastinal B-cell lymphomas (see chapter 20) and DLBCL associated with *IRF4* translocations also have distinctive gene expression signatures (92).

More recently, another approach has been advocated by Dybkaer et al. (31). These authors used flow cytometry to sort B cells from normal tonsils and identified five B-cell–associated gene signatures (BAGS): naïve, centrocyte, centroblast, memory, and plasmablast B cells. Within the group of DLBCLs of GCB type, patients with tumors with a centrocytic BAGS had a better prognosis than patients whose tumors had a centroblastic BAGS. These subtypes were also associated with molecular differences: centrocytic tumors had a lower num- ber of genetic alterations, but higher frequency of *TP53* mutations whereas centroblastic tumors had much greater genomic complexity. Although this work needs confirmation by others, these data suggest that the GCB versus ABC model for DLBCL does not adequately capture the biologic spectrum of B-cell differentiation; this spectrum may have biologic and prognostic importance.

The tumor microenvironment is also impor- tant in DLBCL pathogenesis (5,25,56,60,67). Lenz et al. (56) divided gene expression sig- natures in DLBCL into three groups: germinal center B-cell, stromal-1, and stromal-2. The stromal-1 signature (prognostically favorable) is reflective of extracellular matrix deposition and histiocyte infiltration. The stromal-2 signature (unfavorable) reflects tumor blood vessel density. Specific gene mutations in cells of the microen- vironment likely affect the GEP profile or may more directly lead to increased signaling or loss of key signals to lymphoma cells.

Cells in the microenvironment also stim- ulate tumor cell pathways in the absence of genetic abnormalities. Epigenetic modulation of tumor cells and microenvironmental cells (e.g., methylation) are probably important in DLBCL pathogenesis and have been linked with resistance to chemotherapy (22).

MicroRNA alterations have been described in DLBCL and likely play an important role in

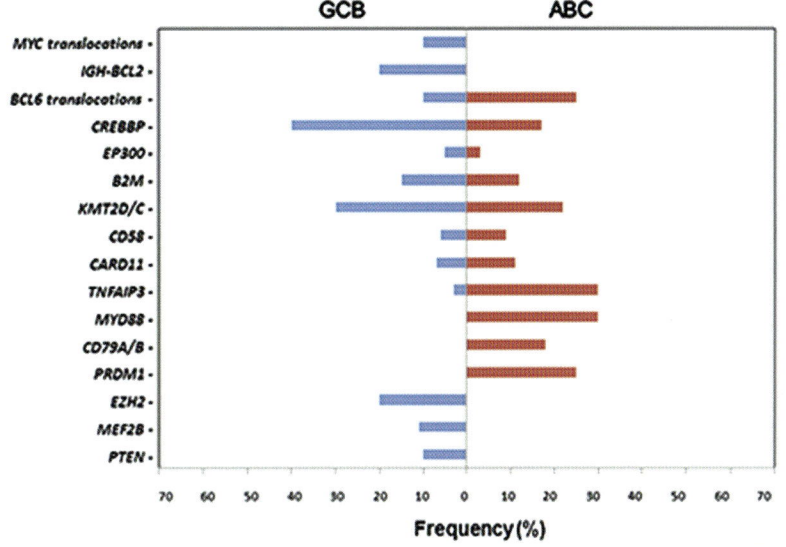

Figure 17-42

GENE MUTATIONS AND TRANSLOCATIONS IN DIFFUSE LARGE B-CELL LYMPHOMA

These are divided according to cell of origin classification.

Gene Mutations

activating or inhibiting the cell pathways involved in lymphomagenesis. These microRNAs have been assessed in the serum of DLBCL patients as well as in the tumors directly. Elevated serum levels of miR-15a, miR-16-1, miR-21, miR-29c, and miR-155 are common in patients with DLBCL whereas miR-34a is often downregulated (57,75). Elevated miR-155 levels adversely impact the response to therapy (46,75). The micro-RNA field is both preliminary and immense, and beyond the scope of this chapter, and the reader is referred to a review by Ni et al. (75).

Gene Mutations

It has been known for a number of years that gene mutations or deletions play a role in the pathogenesis of DLBCL. Using single gene methods, deletion of chromosome 9p21, including *CDK2NA/P16*, *CDK2NB/P15*, and *P14/ARF*, or other mechanisms of inactivation of these genes such as methylation, occurs in about one third of DLBCL cases (37). *TP53* mutations occur in about 20 percent of cases and in about 50 percent of anaplastic tumors (58a,113). The *MYD88* L265P mutation is present in 5 to 10 percent of cases of DLBCL overall and is very common in specific DLBCL types, including primary DLBCL of the CNS and primary cutaneous DLBCL, leg type (20).

Next-generation sequencing methods have been applied to the study of DLBCL cases. An average of 75 to 90 mutations per tumor affecting a number of genes in DLBCL has been reported. The frequency of abnormalities is higher in studies using whole genome versus exome sequencing methods (68). Data suggest that DLBCL undergoes multiple rounds of clonal expansion and that gene mutations occur at any time during this process (68).

Gene mutations in DLBCL are further divided into driver versus passenger mutations. Driver mutations tend to occur earlier in DLBCL pathogenesis and impair key cellular processes involved in lymphomagenesis. Some studies, however, have shown that driver mutations can occur as late events (68). Passenger mutations, in contrast, are not thought to have an important role in pathogenesis and may be innocent bystander events. It is also true that each case of DLBCL undergoes evolution over time, with intraclonal heterogeneity and selection for subclones that impart the greatest survival advantage.

Gene mutations in DLBCL are involved in many cellular processes and pathways, including histone modification (methylation and acetylation), cell growth and proliferation, metabolism, differentiation, apoptosis, survival, homing/migration, response to DNA damage, activation of B-cell receptor signaling and the toll-like receptor pathway (both of which result in NF-κB activation), angiogenesis, and immunoregulation (14,28,69,74,83,115). Gene alterations also correlate with cell of origin classification as defined by GEP analysis (fig. 17-42). Cases of GCB DLBCL more often have mutations involving histone modification (*EZH2, EP300, CREBBP, KMT2D*), B-cell homing (*GNA13, GNAI2, SIPR2*), and inactivation of *CDK2NA/P16* and *CDK2NB/P15*. In contrast, genetic abnormalities that result in activation of the NF-κB pathway are more common in the ABC type of DLBCL (*CD79A/B, CARD11, MALT1, BCL10, TNFAIP3, MYD88*). Mutations in immunosurveillance genes (*CD58, B2-microglobulin, TNFRSF14,* and *CIITA*) and *TP53* occur in either type of DLBCL (14,28,69,109).

Assessment of the antigen receptor genes in DLBCL shows monoclonal immunoglobulin gene rearrangements; the T-cell receptor genes are usually in the germline configuration. The *IGH* variable regions are hypermutated in 40 to 50 percent of cases (96). Other genes are aberrantly mutated via the somatic hypermutation machinery in subsets of DLBCL cases, including *BCL6, MYC, PAX5, CXCR4, CIITA,* and other genes (48). These mutations likely also alter the function of these genes and play a role in pathogenesis.

TRANSFORMED DLBCL

A number of low-grade lymphomas transform to DLBCL, including chronic lymphocytic leukemia/small lymphocytic lymphoma (CLL/SLL), follicular lymphoma, marginal zone lymphomas, lymphoplasmacytic lymphoma/Waldenstrom macroglobulinemia, and nodular lymphocyte-predominant Hodgkin lymphoma. These cases, at the time of transformation, are also included in the category of DLBCL. This topic is covered in chapter 5 and therefore only brief comments are included here.

Morphologically, biopsy specimens of transformed DLBCL may show evidence of the low-grade lymphoma or features suggestive of the possibility, such as a vague nodular appearance on low-power examination in a patient with a history of follicular lymphoma. Cytologically, the transformed lymphoma cells often show minor differences compared with the cells of de novo cases. For example, in transformed cases, the lymphoma cells often show more size variation and may not be as large as the cells in de novo tumors. In many cases, however, it is not possible to distinguish de novo from transformed DLBCL on the basis of morphologic or immunophenotypic findings. Importantly, at the biologic level, DLBCL cases that arise via transformation of low-grade lymphoma are dis-

tinctive. The gene mutation profiles differ, often greatly, from cases of DLBCL that arise de novo.

DIFFERENTIAL DIAGNOSIS

Reactive Conditions. The differential diagnosis of DLBCL includes conditions in which reactive immunoblastic proliferations are prominent.

Infectious Mononucleosis. Patients with infectious mononucleosis are often young and present with a history suggestive of a viral illness. Histologically, biopsy specimens involved by infectious mononucleosis usually show paracortical expansion by a mixture of plasma cells, plasmacytoid lymphocytes, immunoblasts, and histiocytes, unlike the common monotonous large lymphoid cell population in DLBCL. Serologic evidence of recent EBV infection or the presence of numerous EBER-positive cells by in situ hybridization is characteristic of infectious mononucleosis. In contrast, most cases of DLBCL are negative for EBV infection.

Kikuchi-Fujimoto Lymphadenitis. There are three histologic phases of Kikuchi-Fujimoto disease (KFD): proliferative, necrotizing, and histiocytic/granulomatous. The proliferative phase is most likely to be confused with DLBCL. In this phase, the lymph node shows a paracortical, often wedge-shaped infiltrate of numerous histiocytes, plasmacytoid dendritic cells, and immunoblasts, which superficially can resemble sheets of large lymphoma cells. Patients with KFD are usually young (15 to 30 years of age), more often women, and present with neck lymphadenopathy. Histologically, a helpful clue to the proliferative phase KFD is the presence of many apoptotic cells. In more advanced cases, eosinophilic zones of necrosis, without neutrophils, are present that can be surrounded by lipid-laden histiocytes. Immunohistochemical studies make this distinction straightforward: in KFD, the infiltrate is composed of many CD68-positive histiocytes, CD123-positive plasmacytoid dendritic cells, and CD30-positive immunoblasts. Intermixed T cells are often CD8 positive and express cytotoxic markers.

Drug Reactions. Drug-induced hypersensitivity reactions can result in localized or disseminated lymphadenopathy that clinically mimics lymphoma. A number of medications are associated with drug-induced hypersensitivity reactions and lymphadenopathy, such as seizure medications (e.g., dilantin, tegretol). Lymphadenopathy also occurs in patients treated with methotrexate or other immunomodulating agents. Drug-associated lymphadenopathy can develop suddenly, be localized or generalized, and often resolves once the drug is discontinued.

Morphologically, seizure medications often result in a paracortical proliferation of lymphocytes of varying sizes, including many immunoblasts. These cells are usually negative for EBV. In contrast, in patients receiving immunomodulating agents such as methotrexate, the lymph node often shows a paracortical proliferation of plasma cells, plasmacytoid lymphocytes, immunoblasts, and histiocytes and the cells are often positive for EBV. Unlike DLBCL, monotonous sheets of large B cells are usually absent and there is no evidence of a monoclonal B-cell population in drug-induced lymphadenopathy (see chapter 44).

Metastatic Tumors. Some cases of DLBCL predominantly involve the lymph node sinuses in a pattern reminiscent of metastatic carcinoma. In other cases, tumor-associated sclerosis compartmentalizes large B cells, superficially mimicking cohesion. Unlike carcinoma, however, the cells of DLBCL are not truly cohesive nor do they make glands or keratin.

Some cases of metastatic nasopharyngeal carcinoma, particularly the lymphoepithelial type, are particularly problematic because the tumor cells resemble large lymphoma cells and are associated with reactive T cells and histiocytes in the background. Immunohistochemical analysis usually clarifies the diagnosis because the neoplastic cells are strongly positive for keratins and other epithelial markers and metastatic nasopharyngeal carcinoma can be positive for EBER1.

Metastatic seminoma is another tumor that may be confused with DLBCL in lymph nodes. The tumor cells often have prominent nucleoli, resemble immunoblasts, and have a background of small lymphocytes and histiocytes. Immunohistochemical analysis is helpful because seminoma cells are positive for SOX17, SALL4, OCT3/4, CD117/KIT, and keratin and are negative for B-cell markers.

Other Hematolymphoid Neoplasms. DLBCL may be confused with a number of hematolymphoid neoplasms. The differential diagnosis of these diseases is discussed in chapters relating to them: B- and T-lymphoblastic leukemia/lymphoma (chapters 10 and 29), pleomorphic variant of mantle cell lymphoma (chapter 12), plasmablastic lymphoma (chapter 23), Burkitt lymphoma (chapter 25), ALK-positive and ALK-negative anaplastic large cell lymphoma (chapters 33 and 34), classic Hodgkin lymphoma, particularly the syncytial variant of nodular sclerosis (chapter 38) or lymphocyte depletion (chapter 41), myeloid/monocytic sarcoma (chapter 51), and histiocytic sarcoma (chapter 52).

TREATMENT

Current chemotherapy for patients with DLBCL began with the introduction of the CHOP regimen in the 1970s. Using CHOP, about 40 to 50 percent of patients with DLBCL were cured. Although other more intensive chemotherapy regimens were tried during the following 15 years, it became clear that no other regimen was superior to CHOP, which became the standard (34). Nevertheless, it was clear then that better therapy was needed.

A major advance was the development of rituximab and its combination with CHOP, which is currently the standard firstline therapy for patients with DLBCL (24). Most patients respond to R-CHOP therapy, but about 30 percent relapse eventually and another 10 percent have primary refractory disease. As a result, only approximately 60 percent of patients with DLBCL achieve durable remissions and are cured with R-CHOP therapy (100). For patients who fail R-CHOP, however, there is a low chance of cure with current salvage therapy. A common second line therapeutic approach is more dose-intense chemotherapy followed by autologous stem cell transplantation, but this approach is not suitable for older patients or those with comorbidities. Novel therapies are needed for patients with primary refractory or relapsed disease. Even for patients who can potentially be cured, replacing R-CHOP with therapeutic agents that are equally efficacious, but less toxic, is desirable.

More dose-intense chemotherapy regimens have been used for patients with DLBCL associated with poor prognostic factors (see below). Dose-adjusted etoposide, prednisone, vincristine, cyclophosphamide, hydroxydaunorubicin, and rituximab (DA-EPOCH-R) has been reported to be effective. French groups have employed rituximab, doxorubicin/adriamycin, cyclophosphamide, vindesine, bleomycin, and prednisone (R-ACVBP). At MD Anderson Cancer Center, the regimen of rituximab, cyclophosphamide, vincristine, doxorubicin, and dexamethasone alternating with methotrexate and cytarabine (R-hyperCVAD) has been used in the past to treat physically fit patients with *MYC*-rearranged DLBCL.

Based on the heterogeneity of DLBCL and increasingly available knowledge regarding the molecular abnormalities and potential therapeutic targets in these tumors, many novel agents are in development or in clinical trials and a few of these agents have been approved by the US Food and Drug Administration. Novel anti-CD20 antibodies as well as antibodies against CD19 or CD22 have been developed. CD30, expressed in 15 to 25 percent of cases of DLBCL, is a potential target for brentuximab vedotin (anti-CD30 linked to monomethyl auristatin E) (43,47).

Agents being tested primarily in patients with ABC type DLBCL include bortezomib (proteasome inhibitor), ibrutinib (Bruton tyrosine kinase inhibitor), fostamatinib (Syk inhibitor), idelalisib (PI3K delta inhibitor), and lenalidomide (an immunomodulator which acts on T and NK cells and also targets cereblon and its downstream molecules such as MUM1/IRF4). Early results using ibrutinib look particularly promising for patients with ABC type DLBCL (112). Inhibitors of *EZH2*, *BCL2*, or *BCL6* may be useful in patients with GCB DLBCL. Initially, novel agents will be added to already established regimens, but it seems likely that new combinations of agents will eventually replace traditional chemotherapy (100).

PROGNOSIS

Clinical Features

DLBCL is a clinically aggressive disease that is commonly fatal if not treated. The presentation of patients with DLBCL at initial diagnosis, however, is highly variable. Patients can present with asymptomatic disease or have B-type symptoms, the latter associated with a poorer prognosis. The disease can be of small size (nonbulky) or large (bulky) as well as localized or widespread; bulk

and high stage correlate with a poorer prognosis. Patients also present with nodal or extranodal disease, and some extranodal sites are associated with a poorer prognosis (32). Body cavity effusions correlate with a worse prognosis (18), as does bone marrow involvement (5-year overall survival of 10 percent) (32).

Laboratory findings are also highly variable in patients with DLBCL, with some patients having no abnormalities and others a wide range of abnormalities. Serum chemistry parameters shown to correlate with prognosis include LDH, beta-2-microglobulin, and calcium levels. Elevated levels of LDH or beta-2-microglobulin occur commonly in DLBCL patients and predict a poorer prognosis. Hypercalcemia is rare, but also correlates with poor survival. Hematologic parameters that correlate with a worse prognosis include a marked leukemic phase of disease, a low absolute lymphocyte count (ALC), and a high absolute monocyte count (AMC); the combination of low ALC and high AMC identifies a subset of DLBCL patients with a poorer prognosis (103).

To capture some of this clinical and prognostic heterogeneity, the IPI was developed to aid in predicting prognosis, and this system has guided treatment decisions for over 20 years. The IPI was developed using a large group of DLBCL patients who were treated with the CHOP regimen (6). The IPI is composed of five criteria, each representing 1 point, tabulated for an overall score that ranges from 0 to 5. The criteria of the IPI are: age (under 60 versus 60 years or older), performance status (less than 2 versus 2 or more), LDH (normal versus elevated), number of extranodal sites (less than 2 versus 2 or more) and stage (I/II versus III/IV). In the initial IPI study, an age-adjusted IPI was also proposed based on three variables: performance status, stage, and serum LDH level. The age-adjusted IPI is also in common use.

In clinical practice, patients with an IPI score of 0-1 have the best prognosis and a potential cure rate of 80 to 85 percent. Patients with a high IPI score, 3 or more, have a poorer prognosis and lower cure rate of 40 to 50 percent. Standard therapeutic approaches using chemotherapy, with or without radiation therapy, are often tailored, at least in part, based on the IPI score.

The IPI has undergone minor modifications over time to improve prognostic stratification, particularly because it was developed based on patients treated with CHOP and some prognostic stratification was lost in patients treated with the current standard therapy, R-CHOP. The National Comprehensive Cancer Network modified the IPI to better capture the spectrum of DLBCL patients by subdividing them by age into under 40, 40 to 60, 60 to 75, and over 75 years (117). In this system, serum LDH levels were further subdivided into three groups: normal, above normal but less than 3 times the upper normal limit, and 3 or more times normal. This system has been reported to better stratify the prognosis of patients with DLBCL. Although the IPI and newer versions have value and continue to be useful, a criticism of the IPI approach is that the variables are surrogates for the biology of DLBCL. The goal, therefore, is to more specifically determine parameters that reflect more directly the biology of each case of DLBCL.

Morphologic Features

Overall, the morphologic features of DL-BCL have not been shown to correlate with prognosis. There are two possible exceptions, however, the immunoblastic variant and a starry sky pattern.

Immunoblastic Variant. Ott et al. (82) reported that immunoblastic morphology predicts a poorer outcome in patients with DLBCL. The immunoblastic variant of DLBCL has a high frequency of the ABC subtype. In addition, about 30 to 40 percent of these cases carry *MYC* translocations that commonly partner with IG genes and are often the only cytogenetic abnormality (41). Therefore, immunoblastic morphology appears to include a poor prognosis subset of DLBCL with *MYC* translocations.

Starry Sky Pattern. The starry sky pattern is a characteristic morphologic finding in Burkitt lymphoma, but it also can occur in about 10 percent of cases of DLBCL. Tumors with a starry sky pattern have high mitotic and apoptotic rates. In patients with DLBCL, a starry sky pattern has been correlated a poorer prognosis (63,64). The starry sky pattern also correlates with other features in DLBCL that are associated with a poorer prognosis including a high proliferation (Ki-67) index, high MYC expression, *MYC* translocation, and double-hit lymphoma.

Gene Expression Profile

The separation of patients with DLBCL into GCB versus ABC groups based on the gene expression signature has been shown to have prognostic value in most studies. Patients with DLBCL of GCB type have a better clinical outcome than those with ABC type (4,89). In general, the GCB versus ABC model is best applied to patients with DLBCL, NOS. This model has some limitations for predicting the prognosis of patients with extranodal DLBCL as well as for patients with some specific types of DLBCL as defined in the WHO classification. The GEP signature is also misleading for patients with double-hit lymphoma, most of which are of GCB type, and these tumors have been moved out of the DLBCL category in the revised WHO classification (96a).

A study by Hong et al. (39) challenges the prognostic value of GEP itself. These authors acknowledged that GEP signatures have predictive value for prognosis, but believe that GEP provides little additional value to established factors of risk assessment, such as the IPI. This report has been controversial, but a recent study by Staiger et al. (95a) also did not show prognostic value.

Gene expression profiles of the tumor microenvironment also are predictive of prognosis. As mentioned above, Lenz et al. (56) have shown that gene expression signatures in DLBCL can be of stromal-1 or stromal-2 type: the stromal-1 signature is prognostically favorable and the stromal-2 signature is unfavorable. Other studies have shown that overrepresentation of specific genes characteristic of cells in the microenvironment are associated with either a better prognosis or refractory disease (60,91). Overall, genes associated with a better prognosis reflect a high content of inflammatory cells and, particularly, reactive T cells admixed within the tumor, but are not simply a surrogate for the number of reactive cells (5,60,91). Overexpression of *TNFRSF9/CD137*, mostly by a subset of T cells, is associated particularly with a better prognosis (5). Others have reported that a greater number of macrophages (CD68 positive) within the microenvironment is associated with a better prognosis in patients treated with immunochemotherapy (87).

Immunophenotypic Findings

Also controversial is the prognostic value of using immunohistochemical algorithms as surrogates for GEP. Various studies have supported and contradicted the prognostic value of this approach in R-CHOP-treated patients with DLBCL (42,66,97). The controversy may be attributable to the more simplistic approach of using a small number of markers to capture the complexity of gene expression profiles. In addition, it is recognized that GEP cannot classify the 10 to 15 percent of cases of DLBCL that are commonly incorporated into either GCB or non-GCB type using immunohistochemical algorithms. A study of stage I patients with DLBCL treated with R-CHOP showed that cell of origin classification, as determined using the Hans algorithm, did not have prognostic value (55). Overall, "the jury is still out" on the prognostic value of immunohistochemical algorithms (and possibly gene expression profiling itself).

CD5 Positivity. Approximately 5 percent of cases of DLBCL are CD5 positive (108,111). Patients tend to be elderly and present with nodal or extranodal disease. These tumors may have centroblastic or immunoblastic features, commonly with a high mitotic or proliferation rate, and most often an ABC or non-GCB immunophenotype (fig. 17-36). *BCL6* translocations occur in up to one quarter of cases, but *MYC* or *IGH-BCL2* translocations are rare. A number of studies have shown that patients with CD5-positive DLBCL have clinically more aggressive disease and a poorer prognosis (3,96b,108,111).

MYC Expression. Patients with DLBCL with many cells positive for MYC by immunohistochemistry have a poorer prognosis (106). There is also a correlation between high MYC expression and the presence of *MYC* translocation. Immunohistochemical assessment for MYC, however, is not a reliable screening tool for cases with *MYC* translocation. Regardless of the cutoff used for MYC overexpression, there are some cases of DLBCL in which the number of MYC-positive cells is below cutoff but they have a *MYC* translocation at the genetic level.

MYC and BCL2 Expression. Intuitively, one would hypothesize that the prognostic impact of a gene translocation is the result of protein overexpression, and some have sought to assess cases of DLBCL for simultaneous MYC and BCL2 expression as a surrogate for these translocations. The biologic picture, however, is more complicated. Twenty-five to 35 percent of cases of DLBCL overexpress MYC and BCL2, known as double positive or double-expressor lymphomas (48a,44,49). As this group is three times more common than genetically defined double-hit lymphomas (see below), immunohistochemical expression is not equivalent to genetic translocation. In addition, whereas most cases of genetically defined double-hit lymphomas have a GCB cell of origin, most cases of double-positive lymphoma have an ABC (or non-GCB) cell of origin. Obviously, mechanisms other than translocation are involved in the expression of MYC and BCL2, especially in tumors of ABC type (44,49).

Patients with double-positive DLBCL have a poorer prognosis than the remainder of patients with DLBCL (44,49,95a) and have an increased risk of CNS relapse (94). Patients with genetically defined double-hit lymphomas, however, have an even worse prognosis (59). Hu et al. (44) suggested that simultaneous MYC and BCL2 overexpression may explain the poorer prognosis of patients with the ABC type of DLBCL, independent of cell of origin classification. Alternatively, cell of origin classification and MYC/BCL2 overexpression may both have independent prognostic value.

Cytogenetic Findings

A complex karyotype (more than three abnormalities) is common in cases of DLBCL and is associated with a poorer prognosis (35). Loss of chromosome 17p is associated with a poorer prognosis in a number of studies, most likely explained by inactivation of *TP53* at 17p13.1 (9,35). *TP53* mutations have been shown to be associated with a poorer prognosis (see below).

Many studies have shown that a *MYC* translocation is associated with a poor prognosis in DLBCL. *MYC* can partner with IG (heavy or light chains) or non-IG genes, but *IG-MYC* translocations are particularly associated with a poorer prognosis in patients with DLBCL (23). Recent studies have shown that patients with DLBCL with the *MYC* translocation, with no evidence of *BCL2* or *BCL6* translocations, have a poor prognosis (8,42,59). The presence of a *MYC* translocation is often associated with other findings associated with a poor prognosis, including a complex karyotype and simultaneous *BCL2* and/or *BCL6* translocations (double-hit lymphoma).

The prognostic value of a *BCL2* translocation is less well established, and has not been shown to have prognostic impact overall in DLBCL. However, Visco et al. (102) reported that a *BCL2* translocation conveys a poorer prognosis in patients with GCB type of DLBCL. Horn et al. (42) also have shown *BCL2* translocations correlate with a poorer prognosis in younger, poor-prognosis DLBCL patients.

The prognostic importance of a *BCL6* translocation is poorly established. A group from Turkey suggested that *BCL6* translocations correlate with a poorer prognosis (2), but other studies have shown no prognostic impact.

Patients who have DLBCL associated with *MYC* and *BCL2* or *BCL6* translocations (double-hit lymphoma) have a very poor prognosis. This is true for both patients with *MYC/BCL2* double-hit lymphoma, the most common scenario, as well as patients with *MYC/BCL6*

double-hit lymphoma, although prognosis for the latter patient group is less well established. Double-hit lymphomas represent 5 to 10 percent of all cases of DLBCL and are designated as high-grade B-cell lymphoma in the revised WHO classification (96a). This topic is discussed separately in chapter 27.

Gene Mutations

The prognostic importance of most of the large number of mutations and other genetic abnormalities that occur in DLBCL has not been well studied. Some of these mutations correlate with cell of origin classification as well as prognosis, but it is unclear whether these two parameters are independent. In one study, *MYD88* L265P mutations occurred in 22 percent of cases of DLBCL and correlated with ABC type, extranodal involvement, and a poorer prognosis (90). The adverse prognostic impact of *TP53* mutations, particularly mutations that affect the DNA-binding domain, has been well established (109,113).

REFERENCES

1. Ahearne MJ, Bhuller K, Hew R, Ibrahim H, Naresh K, Wagner SD. Expression of PD-1 (CD279) and FoxP3 in diffuse large B-cell lymphoma. Virchows Arch 2014;465:351-358.
2. Akyurek N, Uner A, Benekli M, Barista I. Prognostic significance of MYC, BCL2, and BCL6 rearrangements in patients with diffuse large B-cell lymphoma treated with cyclophosphamide, doxorubicin, vincristine, and prednisone plus rituximab. Cancer 2012;118:4173-4183.
3. Alinari L, Gru A, Quinion C, et al. De novo CD5+ diffuse large B-cell lymphoma: adverse outcomes with and without stem cell transplantation in a large, multi-center, rituximab treated cohort. Am J Hematol 2016;91:395-399.
4. Alizadeh AA, Eisen MB, Davis RE, et al. Distinct types of diffuse large B-cell lymphoma identified by gene expression profiling. Nature 2000;403(6769):503-511.
5. Alizadeh AA, Gentles AJ, Alencar AJ, et al. Prediction of survival in diffuse large B-cell lymphoma based on expression of 2 genes reflecting tumor and microenvironment. Blood 2011;118:1350-1358.
6. A predictive model for aggressive non-Hodgkin's lymphoma. The International Non-Hodgkin's Lymphoma Prognostic Factors Project. N Engl J Med 1993;329:987-984. [no authors listed]
7. Armitage JO, Weisenburger DD. New approach to classifying non-Hodgkin's lymphomas: clinical features of the major histologic subtypes. Non-Hodgkin's Lymphoma Classification Project. J Clin Oncol 1998;16:2780-2795.
8. Aukema SM, Kreuz M, Kohler CW, et al. Biologic characterization of adult MYC-translocation positive mature B-cell lymphomas other than molecular Burkitt lymphoma. Haematologica 2014;99:726-735.
9. Bea S, Colomo L, Lopez-Guillermo A, et al. Clinicopathologic significance and prognostic value of chromosomal imbalances in diffuse large B-cell lymphomas. J Clin Oncol 2004;22:3498-3506.
10. Boroumand N, Ly TL, Sonstein J, Medeiros LJ. Microscopic diffuse large B-cell lymphoma (DLBCL) occurring in pseudocysts: do these tumors belong to the category of DLBCL associated with chronic inflammation? Am J Surg Pathol 2012;36:1074-1080.

11. Bouamar H, Abbas S, Lin AP, et al. A capture-sequencing strategy identifies IRF8, EBF1, and APRIL as novel IGH fusion partners in B-cell lymphoma. Blood 2013;122:726-733.

11a. Boyer DF, McKelvie PA, de Leval L, et al. Fibrin-associated EBV-positive large B-cell lymphoma: an indolent neoplasm with features distinct from diffuse large B-cell lymphoma associated with chronic inflammation. Am J Surg Pathol 2017;41:299-312.

12. Braggio E, Van Wier S, Ojha J, et al. Genome-wide analysis uncovers recurrent alterations in primary central nervous system lymphomas. Clin Cancer Res 2015;21:3986-3994.

13. Brudno J, Tadmor T, Pittaluga S, Nicolae A, Polliack A, Dunleavy K. Discordant bone marrow involvement in non-Hodgkin lymphoma. Blood 2016;127:965-970.

14. Challa-Malladi M, Lieu YK, Califano O, et al. Combined genetic inactivation of beta2-microglobulin and CD58 reveals frequent escape from immune recognition in diffuse large B cell lymphoma. Cancer Cell 2011;20:728-740.

15. Chan JK, Aozasa K, Gaulard P. DLBCL associated with chronic inflammation. In: Swerdlow SH, Campo E, Harris NL, Jaffe ES, Pileri SA, Stein H, Thiele J, Vardiman JW, eds. WHO classification of tumours of haematopoietic and lymphoid tissues. Lyon: IARC Press; 2008:245-246.

16. Chapuy B, Roemer MG, Stewart C, et al. Targetable genetic features of primary testicular and primary central nervous system lymphomas. Blood 2016:127:869-881.

17. Chen J, Xu-Monette ZY, Deng L, et al. Dysregulated CXCR4 expression promotes lymphoma cell survival and independently predicts disease progression in germinal center B-cell-like diffuse large B-cell lymphoma. Oncotarget 2015;6:5597-5614.

18. Chen YP, Huang HY, Lin KP, Medeiros LJ, Chen TY, Chang KC. Malignant effusions correlate with poorer prognosis in patients with diffuse large B-cell lymphoma. Am J Clin Pathol 2015;143:707-715.

19. Chihara D, Nastoupil LJ, Williams JN, Lee P, Koff JL, Flowers CR. New insights into the epidemiology of non-Hodgkin lymphoma and implications for therapy. Expert Rev Anticancer Ther 2015;15:531-544.

20. Choi JW, Kim Y, Lee JH, Kim YS. MYD88 expression and L265P mutation in diffuse large B-cell lymphoma. Hum Pathol 2013;44:1375-1381.

21. Choi WW, Weisenburger DD, Greiner TC, et al. A new immunostain algorithm classifies diffuse large B-cell lymphoma into molecular subtypes with high accuracy. Clin Cancer Res 2009;15:5494-5502.

22. Clozel T, Yang S, Elstrom RL, et al. Mechanism-based epigenetic chemosensitization therapy of diffuse large B-cell lymphoma. Cancer Discov 2013;3:1002-1019.

23. Copie-Bergman C, Cuillière-Dartigues P, Baia M, et al. MYC-IG rearrangements are negative predictors of survival in DLBCL patients treated with immunochemotherapy: a GELA/LYSA study. Blood 2015;126:2466-2474.

24. Coiffier B, Lepage E, Briere J. CHOP chemotherapy plus rituximab compared with CHOP alone in elderly patients with diffuse large B-cell lymphoma. N Engl J Med 2002;346:235-242.

25. Coutinho R, Clear A, Mazzola E, et al. Revisiting the immune microenvironment of diffuse large B-cell lymphoma using a tissue microarray and immunohistochemistry: robust semi-automated analysis reveals CD3 and FoxP3 as potential predictors of response to R-CHOP. Haematologica 2015;100:363-369.

26. Coutinho R, Clear A, Owen A, et al. Poor concordance among nine immunohistochemistry classifiers of cell-of-origin for diffuse large B-cell lymphoma: implications for treatment strategies. Clin Cancer Res 2013;19:6686-6695.

27. Cui W, Cai Y, Wang W, et al. Frequent copy number variations on PISK/AKT pathway and aberrant protein expression of PI3K subunits are associated with inferior survival in diffuse large B cell lymphoma. J Transl Med 2014;12:10.

28. Davis RE, Ngo VN, Lenz G, et al. Chronic active B-cell-receptor signalling in diffuse large B-cell lymphoma. Nature 2010;463:88-92.

29. Dekker JD, Park D, Shaffer AL, et al. Subtype-specific addiction of the activated B-cell subset of diffuse large B-cell lymphoma to FOXP1. Proc Natl Acad Sci U S A 2016;113:E577-886.

30. Deng L, Xu-Monette ZY, Loghavi S, et al. Primary testicular diffuse large B-cell lymphoma displays distinct clinical and biological features for treatment failure in rituximab era: a report from the International PTL Consortium. Leukemia 2016;30:361-372.

31. Dybkaer K, Bogsted M, Falgreen S, et al. Diffuse large B-cell lymphoma classification system that associates normal B-cell subset phenotypes with prognosis. J Clin Oncol 2015;33:1379-1388.

32. El-Galaly TC, Villa D, Alzahrani M, et al. Outcome prediction by extranodal involvement, IPI, R-IPI, and NCCN-IPI in the PET/CT and rituximab era: A Danish-Canadian study of 443 patients with diffuse-large B cell lymphoma. Am J Hematol 2015;90:1041-1046.

33. Engelhard M, Brittinger G, Huhn D, et al. Subclassification of diffuse large B-cell lymphomas according to the Kiel classification: distinction of centroblastic and immunoblastic lymphomas is a prognostic risk. Blood 1997;89:2291-2297.

34. Fisher RI, Gaynor ER, Dahlberg S, et al. Comparison of a standard regimen (CHOP) with three intensive chemotherapy regimens for advanced non-Hodgkin's lymphoma. N Engl J Med 1993;328:1002-1006.

35. Fishvik I, Aamot HV, Delabie J, et al. Karyotyping of diffuse large B-cell lymphomas: loss of 17p is associated with poor patient outcome. Eur J Haematol 2013;91:332-338.

36. Frei E, Visco C, Xu-Monette ZY, et al. Addition of rituximab to chemotherapy overcomes the negative prognostic impact of cyclin E expression in diffuse large B-cell lymphoma. J Clin Pathol 2013;66:956-961.

37. Guney S, Jardin F, Bertrand P, et al. Several mechanisms lead to the inactivation of the CDKN2A (P16), P14ARF, or CDKN2B (P15) genes in the GCB and ABC molecular DLBCL subtypes. Genes Chromosomes Cancer 2012;51:858-867.

38. Hans CP, Weisenburger DD, Greiner TC, et al. Confirmation of the molecular classification of diffuse large B-cell lymphoma by immunohistochemistry using a tissue microarray. Blood 2004;103:275-282.

38a. Herrera AF, Mei M, Low L, et al. Relapsed or refractory double-expressor and double-hit lymphomas have inferior progression-free survival after autologous stem-cell transplantation. J Clin Oncol 2017;35:24-31.

39. Hong F, Kahl BS, Gray R. Incremental value in outcome prediction with gene expression-based signatures in diffuse large B-cell lymphoma. Blood 2013;121:156-158.

40. Hong JY, Hong ME, Choi MK, et al. The impact of activated p-AKT expression on clinical outcomes in diffuse large B-cell lymphoma: a clinicopathological study of 262 cases. Ann Oncol 2014;25:182-188.

41. Horn H, Staiger AM, Vohringer M, et al. Diffuse large B-cell lymphomas of immunoblastic type are a major reservoir for MYC-IGH translocations. Am J Surg Pathol 2015;39:61-66.

42. Horn H, Ziepert M, Wartenberg M, et al. Different biological risk factors in young poor-prognosis and elderly patients with diffuse large B-cell lymphoma. Leukemia 2015;29:1564-1570.

43. Hu S, Xu-Monette ZY, Balasubramanyam A, et al. CD30 expression defines a novel subgroup of diffuse large B-cell lymphoma with favorable prognosis and distinct gene expression signature: a report from the International DLBCL Rituximab-CHOP Consortium Program Study. Blood 2013;121:2715-2724.

44. Hu S, Xu-Monette ZY, Tzankov A, et al. MYC/BCL2 protein coexpression contributes to the inferior survival of activated B-cell subtype of diffuse large B-cell lymphoma and demonstrates high-risk gene expression signatures: a report from The International DLBCL Rituximab-CHOP Consortium Program. Blood 2013;121:4021-4031.

45. Iqbal J, Meyer PN, Smith LM, et al. BCL2 predicts survival in germinal center B-cell-like diffuse large B-cell lymphoma treated with CHOP-like therapy anf rituximab. Clin Cancer Res 2011; 17:7785-7795.

46. Iqbal J, Shen Y, Huang X, et al. Global microRNA expression profiling uncovers molecular markers for classification and prognosis in aggressive B-cell lymphomas. Blood 2015;125:1137-1145.

47. Jacobsen ED, Sharman JP, Oki Y, et al. Brentuximab vedotin demonstrates objective responses in a phase 2 study of relapsed/refractory DLBCL with variable CD30 expression. Blood 2015;125:1394-1402.

48. Jiang Y, Soong TD, Wang L, Melnick AM, Elemento O. Genome-wide detection of genes targeted by non-Ig somatic hypermutation in lymphoma. PLoS One 2012;7:e40332.

49. Johnson NA, Slack GW, Savage KJ, et al. Concurrent expression of MYC and BCL2 in diffuse large B-cell lymphoma treated with rituximab plus cyclophosphamide, doxorubicin, vincristine, and prednisone. J Clin Oncol 2012;30:3452-3459.

50. Kiyasu J, Miyoshi H, Hirata A, et al. Expression of programmed cell death ligand 1 is associated with poor overall survival in patient with diffuse large B-cell lymphoma. Blood 2015;126:2193-2201.

51. Kluin PM, Deckert M, Ferry JA. Primary diffuse large B-cell lymphoma of the CNS. In: Swerdlow SH, Campo E, Harris NL, Jaffe ES, Pileri SA, Stein H, Thiele J, Vardiman JW, eds. WHO classification of tumours of haematopoietic and lymphoid tissues. Lyon: IARC Press; 2008:240-241.

52. Koh YW, Hwang HS, Jung SJ, et al. Receptor tyrosine kinases MET and RON as prognostic factors in diffuse large B-cell lymphoma patients receiving R-CHOP. Cancer Sci 2013;104:1245-1251.

53. Koh YW, Hwang HS, Park CS, Yoon DH, Suh C, Huh J. Prognostic effect of Ki-67 expression in rituximab, cyclophosphamide, doxorubicin, vincristine and prednisone-treated diffuse large B-cell lymphoma is limited to non-germinal center B-cell-like subtype in late-elderly patients. Leuk Lymphoma 2015;56:2630-2636.

54. Kremer M, Spitzer M, Mandl-Weber S, et al. Discordant bone marrow involvement in diffuse large B-cell lymphoma: comparative molecular analysis reveals a heterogeneous group of disorders. Lab Invest 2003;83:107-114.

55. Kumar A, Lunning MA, Zhang Z, Migliacci JC, Moskowitz CH, Zelenetz AD. Excellent outcomes and lack of prognostic impact of cell of origin for localized diffuse large B-cell lymphoma in the rituximab era. Br J Haematol 2015;171:776-783.

56. Lenz G, Wright G, Dave SS, et al. Stromal gene signatures in large-B-cell lymphomas. N Engl J Med 2008;359:2313-2323.

57. Li J, Fu R, Yang L, Tu W. miR-21 expression predicts prognosis in diffuse large B-cell lymphoma. Int J Clin Exp Pathol 2015;8:15019-15024.

58. Li L, Xu-Monette ZY, Ok CY, et al. Prognostic impact of c-Rel nuclear expression and REL amplification and crosstalk between c-Rel and the p53 pathway in diffuse large B-cell lymphoma. Oncotarget 2015;6:23157-23180.

58a. Li M, Liu Y, Wang Y, et al. Anaplastic variant of diffuse large B-cell lymphoma displays intricate genetic alterations and distinct biological features. Am J Surg Pathol 2017. [Epub ahead of print]

59. Li S, Weiss VL, Wang XJ, et al. High-grade B-cell lymphoma with MYC rearrangement and without BCL2 or BCL6 rearrangements is associated with high p53 expression and a poor prognosis. Am J Surg Pathol 2016;40:253-261.

60. Linderoth J, Eden P, Ehinger M, et al. Genes associated with the tumor microenvironment are differentially expressed in cured versus primary chemotherapy-refractory diffuse large B-cell lymphoma. Br J Haematol 2008;141:423-432.

61. Liu W, Ha M, Wang X, Yin N. Clinical significance of GRHL3 expression in diffuse large B cell lymphoma. Tumour Biol 2016;57:9557-9561.

62. Liu Z, Xu-Monette ZY, Cao X, et al. Prognostic and biological significance of survivin expression in patients with diffuse large B-cell lymphoma treated with rituximab-CHOP therapy. Mod Pathol 2015:28:1297-1314.

63. Maeshima AM, Taniguchi H, Fukuhara S, et al. Bcl-2, Bcl-6, and the International Prognostic Index are prognostic indications in patients with diffuse large B-cell lymphoma treated with rituximab-containing chemotherapy. Cancer Sci 2012;103:1898-1904.

64. McClure RF, Remstein ED, Macon WR, et al. Adult B-cell lymphomas with Burkitt-like morphology are phenotypically and genotypically heterogeneous with aggressive clinical behavior. Am J Surg Pathol 2005;29:1652-1660.

65. Meijer CJLM, Vergier B, Duncan LM, et al. Primary cutaneous DLBCL, leg type. In: Swerdlow SH, Campo E, Harris NL, Jaffe ES, Pileri SA, Stein H, Thiele J, Vardiman JW, eds. WHO classification of tumours of haematopoietic and lymphoid tissues. Lyon: IARC Press; 2008:242.

66. Meyer PN, Fu K, Greiner TC, et al. Immunohistochemical methods for predicting cell of origin and survival in patients with diffuse large B-cell lymphoma treated with rituximab. J Clin Oncol 2011;29:200-207.

67. Monti S, Savage KJ, Kutok JL, et al. Molecular profiling of diffuse large B-cell lymphoma identified robust subtypes including one characterized by host inflammatory response. Blood 2005;105:1851-1861.

68. Morin RD, Mungall K, Pleasance E, et al. Mutational and structural analysis of diffuse large B-cell lymphoma using whole genome sequencing. Blood 2013;122:1256-1265.

69. Morin RD, Mendez-Lago M, Mungall AJ, et al. Frequent mutation of histone-modifying genes in non-Hodgkin lymphoma. Nature 2011;476(7360):298-303.

70. Muringampurath-John D, Jaye DL, Flowers CR, et al. Characteristics and outcomes of diffuse large B-cell lymphoma presenting in leukaemic phase. Br J Haematol 2012;158:608-614.

71. Nakamura S, Ponzoni M, Campo E. Intravascular large B-cell lymphoma. In: Swerdlow SH, Campo E, Harris NL, Jaffe ES, Pileri SA, Stein H, Thiele J, Vardiman JW, eds. WHO classification of tumours of haematopoietic and lymphoid tissues. Lyon: IARC Press; 2008:252.

72. Nakayama S, Yokote T, Hirata Y, et al. TNF-α expression in tumor cells as a novel prognostic marker for diffuse large B-cell lymphoma, not otherwise specified. Am J Surg Pathol 2014;38:228-234.

73. Nanjangud G, Rao PH, Hegde A, et al. Spectral karyotyping identifies new rearrangements, translocations, and clinical associations in diffuse large B-cell lymphoma. Blood 2002;99:2554-2561.

74. Ngo VN, Young RM, Schmitz R, et al. Oncogenically active MYD88 mutations in human lymphoma. Nature 2011;470:115-119.

75. Ni H, Tong R, Zou L, Song G, Cho WC. MicroRNAs in diffuse large B-cell lymphoma. Oncology Letters 2016;11:1271-1280.

76. Offit K, Lo Coco F, Louie DC, et al. Rearrangement of the bcl-6 gene as a prognostic marker in diffuse large-cell lymphoma. N Engl J Med 1994;331:74-80.

77. Ok CY, Chen J, Xu-Monette ZY, et al. Clinical implications of phosphorylated STAT3 expression in de novo diffuse large B-cell lymphoma. Clin Cancer Res 2014; 20:5113-5123.

78. Ok CY, Li L, Xu-Monette ZY, et al. Prevalence and clinical implications of Epstein-Barr virus infection in de novo diffuse large B-cell lymphoma in Western countries. Clin Cancer Res 2014;20:2338-2349.

79. Ok CY, Xu-Monette ZY, Li L, et al. Evaluation of NF-κB subunit expression and signaling pathway activation demonstrates that p52 expression confers better outcome in germinal center B-cell-like diffuse large B-cell lymphoma in association with CD30 and BCL2 functions. Mod Pathol 2015;28:1202-1213.

80. Ok CY, Xu-Monette ZY, Tzankov A, et al. Prevalence and clinical implications of cyclin D1 expression in diffuse large B-cell lymphoma (DLBCL) treated with immunochemotherapy: a report from the International DLBCL Rituximab-CHOP Consortium Program. Cancer 2014;120:1818-1829.

81. Orwat DE, Batalis NI. Intravascular large B-cell lymphoma. Arch Pathol Lab Med 2012;136:333-338.

82. Ott G, Ziepert M, Klapper W, et al. Immunoblastic morphology but not the immunohistochemical GCB/nonGCB classifier predicts outcome in diffuse large B-cell lymphoma in the RICOVER-60 trial of the DSHNHL. Blood 2010;116:4916-4925.

83. Pasqualucci L, Dominguez-Sola D, Chiarenza A, et al. Inactivating mutations of acetyltransferase genes in B-cell lymphoma. Nature 2011;471:189-195.

84. Pham-Ledard A, Beylot-Barry M, Barbe C, et al. High frequency and clinical prognostic value of MYD88 L265P mutation in primary cutaneous diffuse large B-cell lymphoma, leg-type. JAMA Dermatol 2014;150:1173-1179.

85. Pittaluga S, Wilson WH, Jaffe ES. Lymphomatoid granulomatosis. In: Swerdlow SH, Campo E, Harris NL, Jaffe ES, Pileri SA, Stein H, Thiele J, Vardiman JW, eds. WHO classification of tumours of haematopoietic and lymphoid tissues. Lyon: IARC Press; 2008:247-249.

86. Rajnai H, Heyning FH, Koens L, et al. The density of CD8+ T-cell infiltration and expression of BCL2 predicts outcome of primary diffuse large B-cell lymphoma of bone. Virchows Arch 2014;464:229-239.

87. Riihijarvi S, Fishvik I, Taskinen M, et al. Prognosic influence of macrophages in patients with diffuse large B-cell lymphoma: a correlative study from as Nordic phase II trial. Haematologica 2015;100:238-245.

88. Rimsza LM, Roberts RA, Campo E, et al. Loss of MHC class II gene and protein expression in diffuse large B-cell lymphoma is related to decreased tumor immunosurveillance and poor patient survival regardless of other prognostic factors: a follow-up study from the Leukemia and Lymphoma Molecular Profiling Project. Blood 2004;103:4251-4258.

89. Rosenwald A, Wright G, Chan WC, et al. The use of molecular profiling to predict survival after chemotherapy for diffuse large-B-cell lymphoma. N Engl J Med 2002;346:1937-1947.

90. Rovira J, Karube K, Valera A, et al. MYD88 L265P mutations, but no other variants, identify a subpopulation of DLBCL patients of activated B-cell origin, extranodal involvement and poor outcome. Clin Can Res 2016;22:2755-2764.

91. Rydstrom K, Joost P, Ehinger M, et al. Gene expression profiling indicates that immunohistochemical expression of CD40 is a marker of an inflammatory reaction in the tumor stroma of diffuse large B-cell lymphoma. Leuk Lymphoma 2012;53:1764-1768.

92. Salaverria I, Philipp C, Oschlies I, et al. Translocations activating IRF4 identify a subgroup of germinal center-derived B-cell lymphoma affecting predominantly children and young adults. Blood 2011;118:139-147.

93. Sant M, Allemani C, Tereanu C, et al. Incidence of hematologic malignancies in Europe by morphologic subtype: results of the HAEMACARE project. Blood 2010;116:3724-3734.

94. Savage KJ, Slack GW, Motok A, et al. Impact of dual expression of MYC and BCL2 by immunohistochemistry on the risk of CNS relapse in DLBCL. Blood 2016;127:2182-2188.

95. Scott DW, Mungall KL, Ben-Neriah S, et al. TBL1XR1/TP63: a novel recurrent gene fusion in B-cell non-Hodgkin lymphoma. Blood 2012;119:4949-4952.

95a. Staiger AM, Ziepert M, Horn H, et al. Clinical impact of the cell-of-origin classification and the MYC/ BCL2 dual expresser status in diffuse large b-cell lymphoma treated within prospective clinical trials of the German High-grade Non-Hodgkin's Lymphoma Study Group. J Clin Oncol 2017. [Epub ahead of print]

96. Stein H, Warnke RA, Chan WC, et al. Diffuse large B-cell lymphoma, not otherwise specified. In: Swerdlow SH, Campo E, Harris NL, Jaffe ES, Pileri SA, Stein H, Thiele J, Vardiman JW (eds.): WHO Classification of Tumours of Haematopoietic and Lymphoid Tissues. IARC: Lyon 2008; 233-237.

96a. Swerdlow SH, Campo E, Pileri SA, et al. The 2016 revision of the World Health Organization classification of lymphoid neoplasms. Blood 2016;127:2375-2390.

96b. Thakral B, Medeiros LJ, Desai P, et al. Prognostic impact of CD5 expression in diffuse large B-cell lymphoma in patients treated with rituximab-EPOCH. Eur J Haematol 2017;98:415-421.

97. Thieblemont C, Briere J, Mounier N, et al. The germinal center/activated B-cell subclassification has a prognostic impact for response to salvage therapy in relapsed/refractory diffuse large B-cell lymphoma: a bio-CORAL study. J Clin Oncol 2011;29:4079-4087.

98. Twa DD, Mottok A, Chan FC, et al. Recurrent genomic rearrangements in primary testicular lymphoma. J Pathol 2015;236:136-141.

99. van Galen JC, Muris JJ, Oudejans JJ, et al. Expression of the polycomb-group gene BMI1 is related to an unfavourable prognosis in primary nodal DLBCL. J Clin Pathol 2007;60:167-172.

100. Vermaat JS, Pals ST, Younes A, et al. Precision medicine in diffuse large B-cell lymphoma: hitting the target. Haematologica 2015;100:989-993.

101. Visco C, Li Y, Xu-Monette ZY, et al. Comprehensive gene expression profiling and immunohistochemical studies support application of immunophenotypic algorithm for molecular subtype classification in diffuse large B-cell lymphoma: a report from the International DLBCL Rituximab-CHOP Consortium Program Study. Leukemia 2012;26:2103-2113.

102. Visco C, Tzankov A, Xu-Monette ZY, et al. Patients with diffuse large B-cell lymphoma of germinal center origin with BCL2 translocations have poor putcome, irrespective of MYC status: a report from an International DLBCL rituximab-CHOP Consortium Program Study. Haematologica 2013;98:255-263.

323

103. Wilcox RA, Ristow K, Habermann TM, et al. The absolute monocyte and lymphocyte prognostic score predicts survival and identifies high-risk patients in diffuse large B-cell lymphoma. Leukemia 2011;25:1502-1509.

104. Winter JN, Li S, Aurora V, et al. Expression of p21 protein predicts clinical outcome in DLBCL patients older than 60 years treated with R-CHOP but not CHOP: a prospective ECOG and Southwest Oncology Group correlative study on E4494. Clin Cancer Res 2010;16:2435-2442.

105. Winter JN, Weller EA, Horning SJ, et al. Prognostic significance of Bcl-6 protein expression in DLBCL treated with CHOP or R-CHOP: a prospective study. Blood 2006;107:4207-4213.

106. Xu-Monette ZY, Dabaja BS, Wang X, et al. Clinical features, tumor biology, and prognosis associated with MYC rearrangement and Myc overexpression in diffuse large B-cell lymphoma patients treated with rituximab-CHOP. Mod Pathol 2015;28:1555-1573.

107. Xu-Monette ZY, Møller MB, Tzankov A, et al. MDM2 phenotypic and genotypic profiling, respective to TP53 genetic status, in diffuse large B-cell lymphoma patients treated with rituximab-CHOP immunochemotherapy: a report from the International DLBCL Rituximab-CHOP Consortium Program. Blood 2013;122:2630-2640.

108. Xu-Monette ZY, Tu M, Jabbar KJ, et al. Clinical and biological significance of de novo CD5+ diffuse large B-cell lymphoma in Western countries. Oncotarget 2015;6:5615-5633.

109. Xu-Monette ZY, Wu L, Visco C, et al. Mutational profile and prognostic significance of TP53 in diffuse large B-cell lymphoma patients treated with R-CHOP: report from an International DLBCL Rituximab-CHOP Consortium Program Study. Blood 2012;120:3986-3996.

110. Xu-Monette ZY, Zhang S, Li X, et al. p63 expression confers significantly better survival outcomes in high-risk diffuse large B-cell lymphoma and demonstrates p53-like and p53-independent tumor suppressor function. Aging (Albany NY) 2016;8:345-365.

111. Yamaguchi M, Nakamura N, Suzuki R, et al. De novo CD5+ diffuse large B-cell lymphoma: results of a detailed clinicopathological review in 120 patients. Haematologica 2008;93:1195-1202.

112. Younes A, Thieblemont C, Morschhauser F, et al. Combination of ibrutinib with rituximab, cyclophosphamide, doxrubicin, vincristine, and prednisone (R-CHOP) for treatment-naïve patients with CD20-positive B-cell non-Hodgkin lymphoma: a non-randomised, phase 1b study. Lancet Oncol 2014;15:1019-1026.

113. Young KH, Weisenburger DD, Dave BJ, et al. Mutations in the DNA-binding codons of TP53, which are associated with decreased expression of TRAIL receptor-2 predict for poor survival in diffuse large B-cell lymphoma. Blood 2007;110:4396-4405.

114. Zelenetz AD, Gordon LI, Wierda WG, et al. Diffuse large B-cell lymphoma Version 1.2016. J Natl Compr Canc Netw 2016;14:196-231.

115. Zhang J, Dominguez-Sola D, Hussein S, et al. Disruption of KMT2D perturbs germinal center B cell development and promotes lymphomagenesis. Nat Med 2015;21:1190-1198.

116. Zhang Y, Wang J, Sui X, et al. Prognostic and clinicopathological value of survivin in diffuse large B-cell lymphoma: a meta-analysis. Medicine (Baltimore) 2015;94:e1432.

117. Zhou Z, Sehn LH, Rademaker AW, et al. An enhanced International Prognostic Index (NCCN-IPI) for patients with diffuse large B-cell lymphoma treated in the rituximab era. Blood 2014;123:837-842.

118. Zucca E, Conconi A, Mughal TI, et al. Patterns of outcome and prognostic factors in primary large-cell lymphoma of the testis in a survey by the International Extranodal Lymphoma Study Group. J Clin Oncol 2003;21:20-27.

18 T-CELL/HISTIOCYTE-RICH LARGE B-CELL LYMPHOMA

GENERAL FEATURES

T-cell/histiocyte-rich large B-cell lymphoma (THRLBCL) is an aggressive form of non-Hodgkin lymphoma characterized by a diffuse pattern and a minority (less than 10 percent) population of large B cells within a background population of reactive T cells and/or histiocytes (7). In the World Health Organization (WHO) classification, THRLBCL is considered a subtype of diffuse large B-cell lymphoma, not otherwise specified (DLBCL-NOS) (7,16a).

The term T-cell-rich B-cell lymphoma was coined by Ramsay et al. (16) in 1988. In this study, the authors emphasized the prominent reactive T-cell population that could obscure the small neoplastic large B-cell population. Subsequently, Delabie et al. (6) described histiocyte-rich B-cell lymphoma, a tumor rich in nonepithelioid histiocytes and reactive T cells, with a small number of large neoplastic B cells. Delabie et al. emphasized the poor prognosis of patients with histiocyte-rich B-cell lymphoma (6). The current WHO classification includes both of these tumor types under the designation T-cell/histiocyte-rich large B-cell lymphoma (7,16a). It is recognized in the WHO classification that this entity is heterogeneous clinically and these tumors are also likely to be heterogeneous at the molecular level.

CLINICAL FEATURES

THRLBCL accounts for less than 5 percent of cases of DLBCL-NOS. It occurs predominantly in men, with a male to female ratio of 1.3-1.7 to 1.0 (1,3,9,17). Patients with THRLBCL are younger than patients with DLBCL-NOS, with a median age in the fourth or fifth decade (3,9). Children rarely develop THRLBCL. B symptoms occur, in 50 to 60 percent of patients (3,17). Patients may present with peripheral lymphadenopathy or extranodal sites of disease. Liver, spleen, and bone marrow involvement are common (3,8,9,16). Over 50 percent of patients present with advanced-stage (Ann Arbor III-IV) disease (1,9,17) and the International Prognostic Index (IPI) score is intermediate or high (usually 2 or more) (7,9).

Some patients with THRLBCL have a history or concurrent evidence of NLPHL. The term *THRLBCL-like transformation* has been used for this occurrence in the revised WHO classification (16a) and these tumors often resemble the so-called histiocyte-rich B-cell lymphoma as described by Delabie et al (6).

HISTOLOGIC FINDINGS

Lymph Node

THRLBCL almost always diffusely effaces the architecture of lymph nodes or other tissue sites (2,3,7,14); Treetipsatit et al. (18), however, have described an uncommon vaguely nodular variant. THRLBCL is polymorphous and characterized by scattered, neoplastic, large atypical lymphoid cells, representing a small percentage of all cells in the lesion, in a background of numerous reactive cells (figs. 18-1–18-3). An arbitrary cutoff of less than 10 percent large B cells is recommended; often the large B cells represent about 1 percent of all cells in the tumor. These large B cells can resemble centroblasts, immunoblasts, and less often, lymphocyte-predominant (LP) and Reed-Sternberg and Hodgkin (RS+H) cells (fig. 18-4). The remaining cells in the tumor are reactive cells, mostly small T lymphocytes or histiocytes in varying proportions. Eosinophils or plasma cells are rare or absent.

Spleen and Liver

THRLBCL involves the splenic white pulp in a multifocal and multinodular pattern (fig. 18-5) (8). These tumors preferentially involve the portal tracts of the liver (fig. 18-6). The histologic composition of extranodal sites of disease is similar to that observed within lymph nodes.

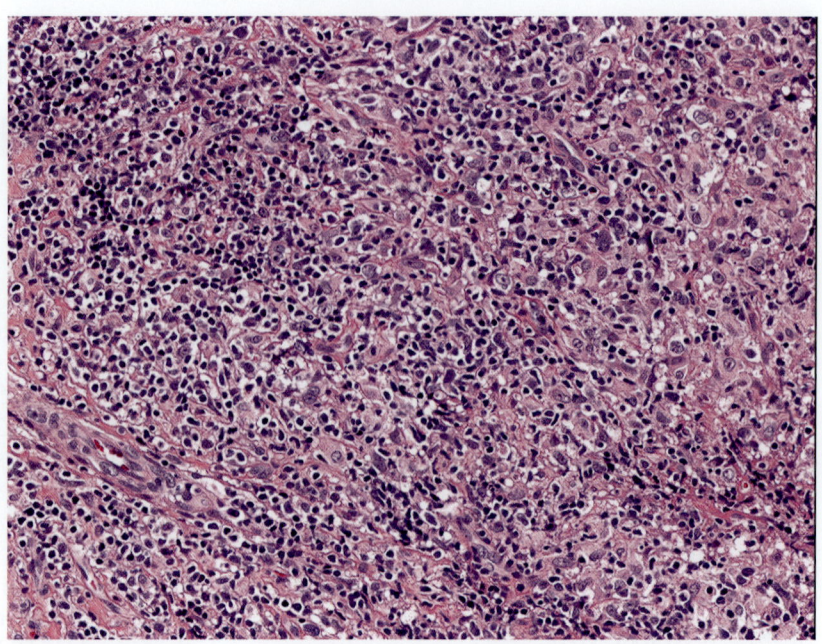

Figure 18-1

T-CELL/HISTIOCYTE-RICH LARGE B-CELL LYMPHOMA INVOLVING LYMPH NODE

There is diffuse effacement of the normal lymph node architecture by a polymorphous infiltrate composed of predominantly small lymphocytes, histiocytes, and few large atypical B cells (hematoxylin and eosin [H&E] stain).

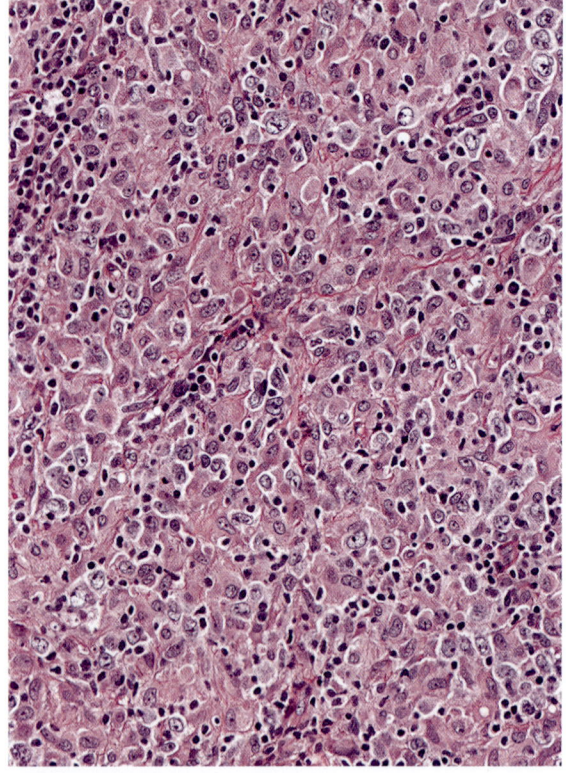

Figure 18-2

T-CELL/HISTIOCYTE-RICH LARGE B-CELL LYMPHOMA INVOLVING LYMPH NODE

There is diffuse effacement of the normal architecture by sheets of epithelioid histiocytes, with only occasional large neoplastic B cells (H&E stain).

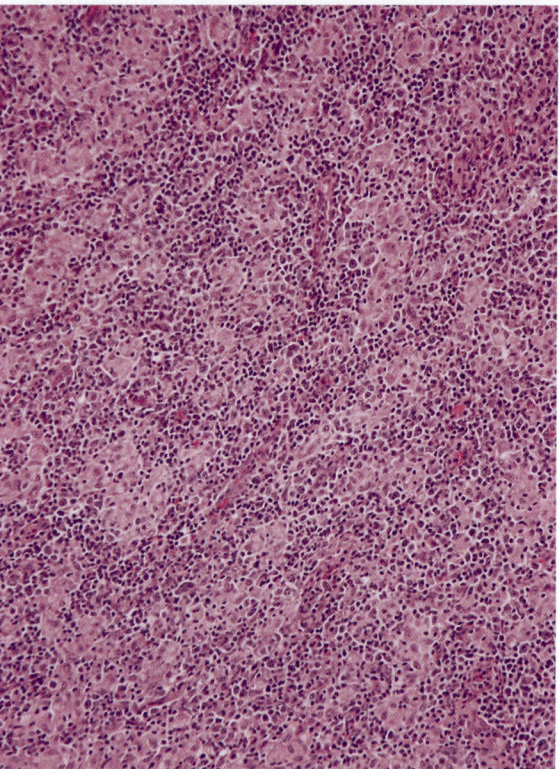

Figure 18-3

T-CELL/HISTIOCYTE-RICH LARGE B-CELL LYMPHOMA INVOLVING LYMPH NODE

There is diffuse effacement of the normal architecture by tumor with a Lennert-like histiocytic reaction and occasional large neoplastic B cells (H&E stain).

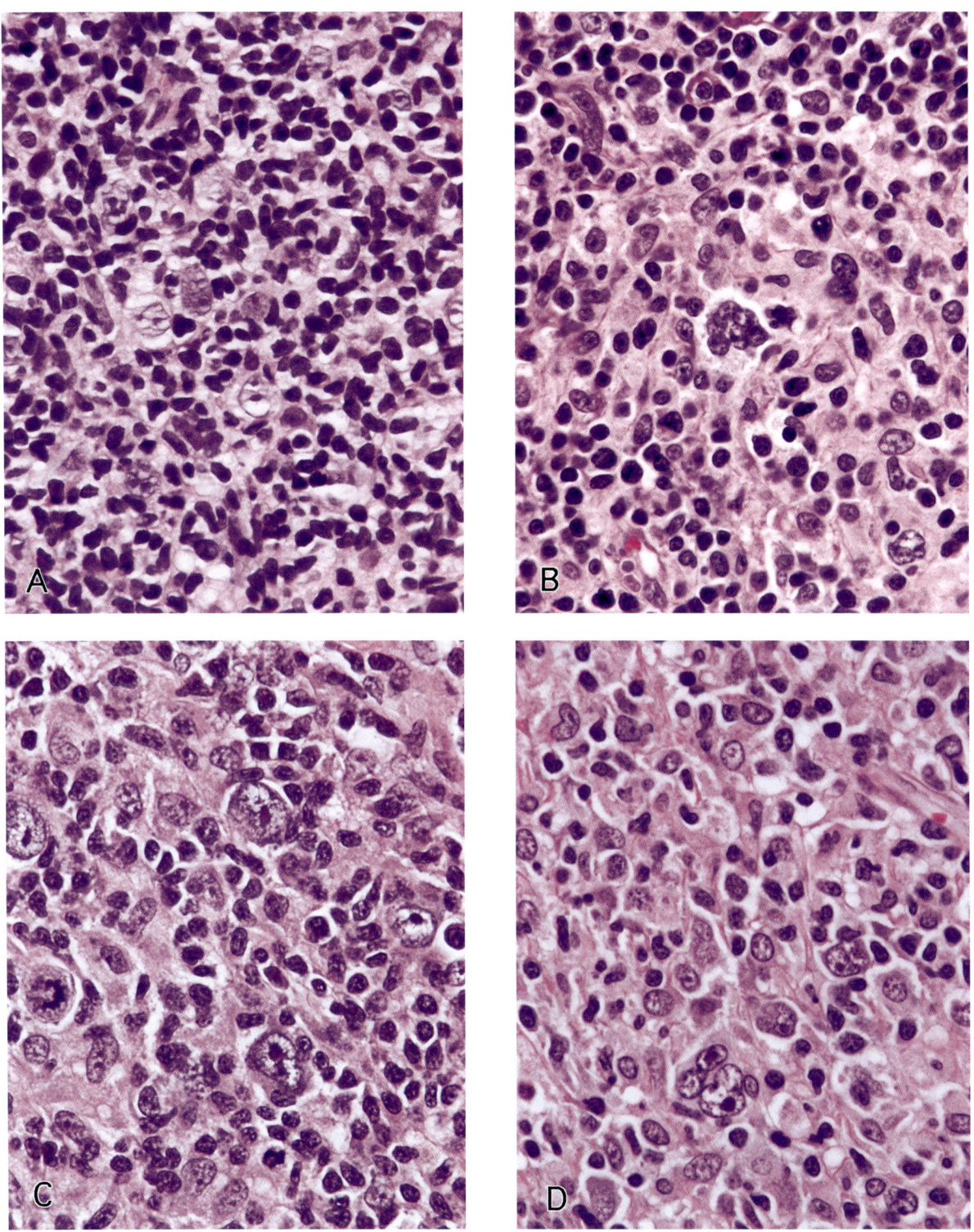

Figure 18-4

CYTOLOGIC SPECTRUM OF LARGE NEOPLASTIC B CELLS IN T-CELL/HISTIOCYTE-RICH LARGE B-CELL LYMPHOMA

A–D: The large B cells can resemble centroblasts (A), LP cells (B), Hodgkin cells (C), and Reed-Sternberg-like cells (D) (A–D: H&E stain).

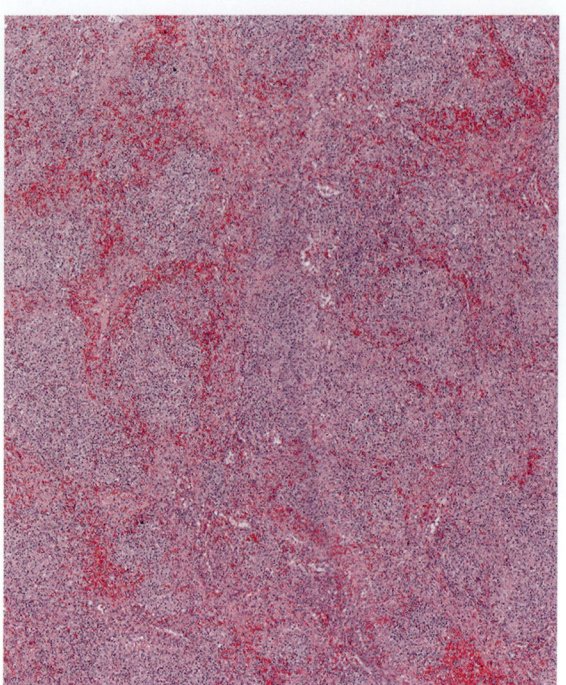
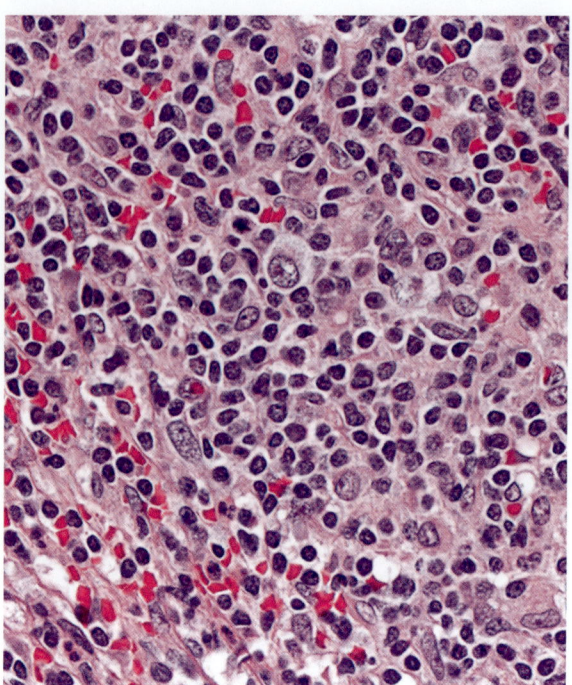

Figure 18-5

T-CELL/HISTIOCYTE-RICH LARGE B-CELL LYMPHOMA INVOLVING SPLEEN

Left: Widespread involvement of the white and red pulp of the spleen by T-cell/histiocyte-rich large B-cell lymphoma (TCHRLBL) shows a micronodular growth pattern.

Right: The nodules are composed of a polymorphous lymphoid infiltrate of small reactive lymphoid cells and histiocytes surrounding occasional large atypical B cells (H&E stain).

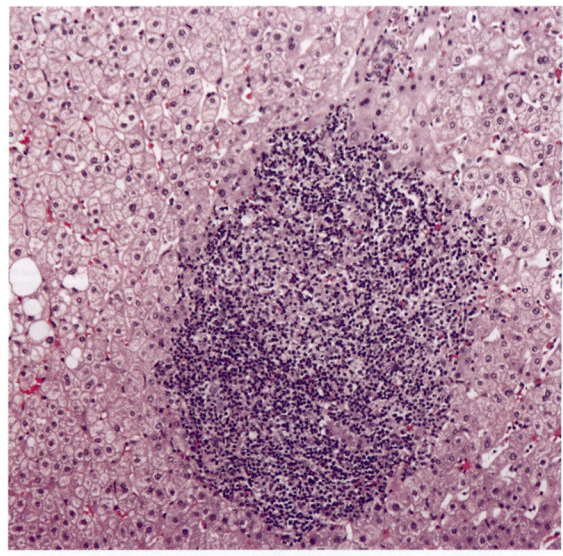

Figure 18-6

T-CELL/HISTIOCYTE-RICH LARGE B-CELL LYMPHOMA INVOLVING LIVER

The portal tract in a liver biopsy specimen is expanded by TCHRLBCL (H&E stain).

Bone Marrow

Bone marrow involvement by THRLBCL is focal or extensive. Focal involvement consists of nodules in a nonparatrabecular pattern. Extensive involvement diffusely replaces the medullary space (fig. 18-7). As in lymph nodes, the large B cells represent less than 10 percent of the bone marrow cell population. In patients treated with systemic chemotherapy, lesions in the bone marrow can persist as collections of reactive T cells and histiocytes for a variable time interval, despite the clearance of the large B cells.

CYTOLOGIC FINDINGS

In aspirate smears, THRLBCL is composed predominantly of small reactive lymphocytes with scattered large transformed cells (fig. 18-8). The large transformed cells contain large vesicular or hyperchromatic nuclei with irregular contours, and variably sized nucleoli. As stated above, the large transformed cells usually

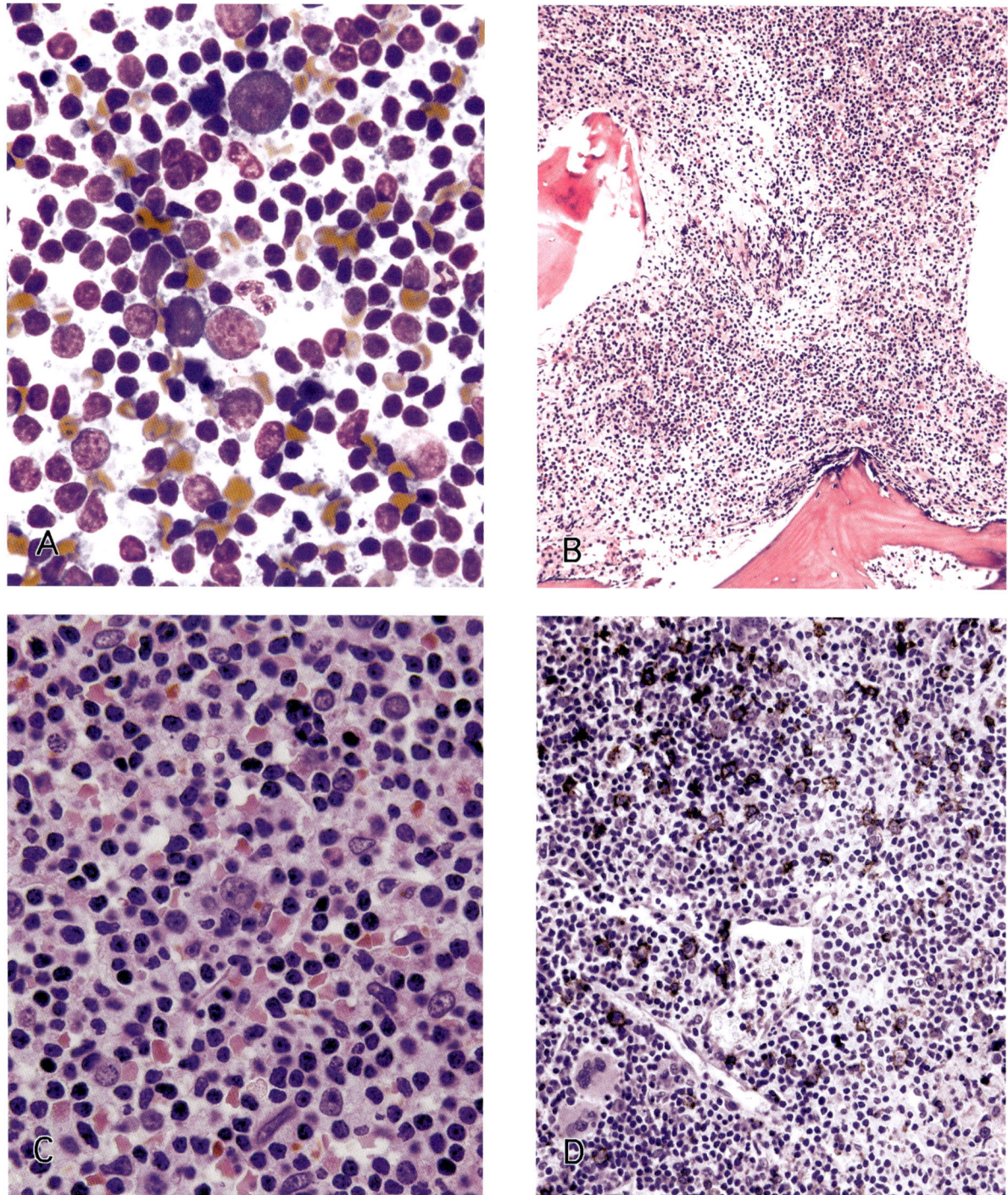

Figure 18-7

T-CELL/HISTIOCYTE-RICH LARGE B-CELL LYMPHOMA EXTENSIVELY REPLACING BONE MARROW

A: The bone marrow aspirate smear shows scattered large neoplastic cells surrounded by hematopoietic cells (Wright-Giemsa stain).

B: The medullary space in the biopsy specimen is extensively replaced by lymphoma (B,C: H&E stain).

C: At high power magnification, many small lymphocytes and scattered large neoplastic cells are seen.

D: The large cells (and a few small cells) are positive for CD20 (immunohistochemistry with hematoxylin counterstain).

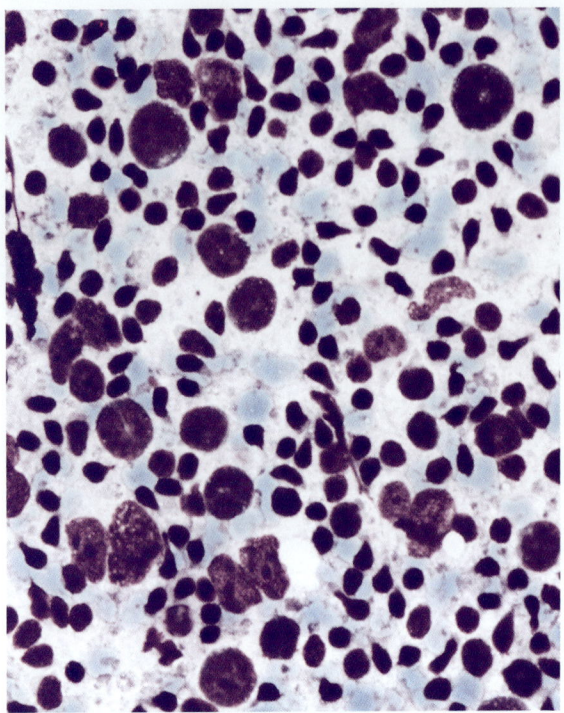

Figure 18-8

**T-CELL/HISTIOCYTE-RICH LARGE
B-CELL LYMPHOMA: CYTOLOGY**

Fine-needle aspirate smear shows neoplastic cells with large nuclei, often containing nucleoli, and scant basophilic cytoplasm, in a background of small lymphocytes (Diff-Quik stain).

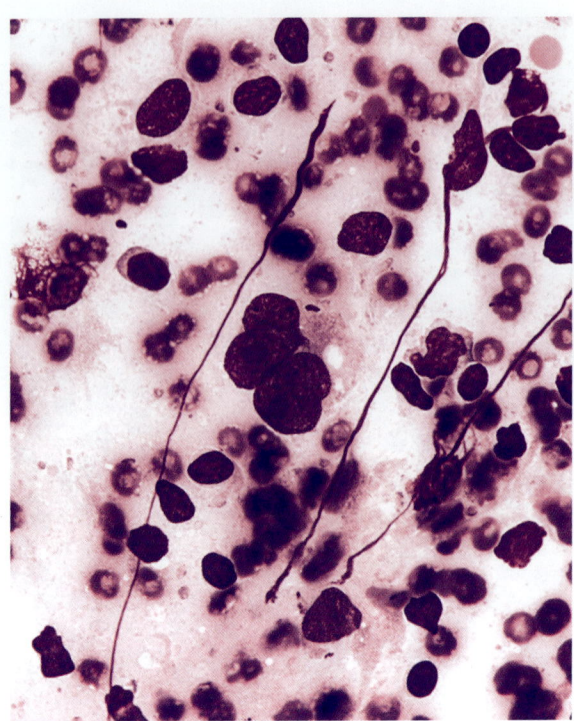

Figure 18-9

**T-CELL/HISTIOCYTE-RICH LARGE
B-CELL LYMPHOMA: CYTOLOGY**

Scrape preparation of a lymph node involved by TCHRLBCL shows a Reed-Sternberg-like nucleus (Wright-Giemsa stain).

resemble centroblasts or immunoblasts, but also can resemble RS+H (fig. 18-9) or LP cells.

IMMUNOPHENOTYPIC FINDINGS

The small percentage of large neoplastic B cells in THRLBCL can make it difficult to assess these cells using standard flow cytometry immunophenotypic methods. Flow cytometry, however, can analyze the reactive cells in these lesions. Wu et al. (20) reported a background T-cell infiltrate that is CD3(+), CD4(+), CD7(bright+), and CD45(bright+), in THRLBCL. Small B cells are few.

Using immunohistochemistry, the large neoplastic cells express pan-B-cell markers including: CD19, CD20 (fig. 18-10), CD22, CD79a, PAX5, OCT-2 (fig. 18-11), and BOB.1 (fig. 18-12). In a substantial subset of cases the large B cells express BCL6 (fig. 18-13) and MUM1/IRF4, with BCL6 more frequent. The lymphoma cells usually express CD45/LCA, variably express BCL2

and epithelial membrane antigen (EMA) (about 50 percent of cases), and are positive for REL in approximately one third of cases (11). In about 50 percent of cases, the neoplastic cells express PD-L1 or PD-L2. The large B cells are negative for CD10, CD15, CD138, IgD, and pan-T-cell antigens. In most cases they are negative for CD30; up to 10 percent of cases may be positive (7,14).

The reactive T cells are positive for pan-T-cell markers such as CD3 (fig. 18-10, right). Many T cells express PD-1/CD279, and, in most cases, CD8-positive T cells are numerous and often express cytotoxic molecules such as TIA-1 and granzyme B. Rarely, T cells form rosettes around the large B cells. The histiocytes are positive for CD68 and other histiocyte-associated markers (e.g., lysozyme, CD163). Histiocytes are also positive for metal-binding proteins, such as metallothionein 2A, an unusual finding in histiocytes associated with other types of lymphoma (12). There are no follicular dendritic

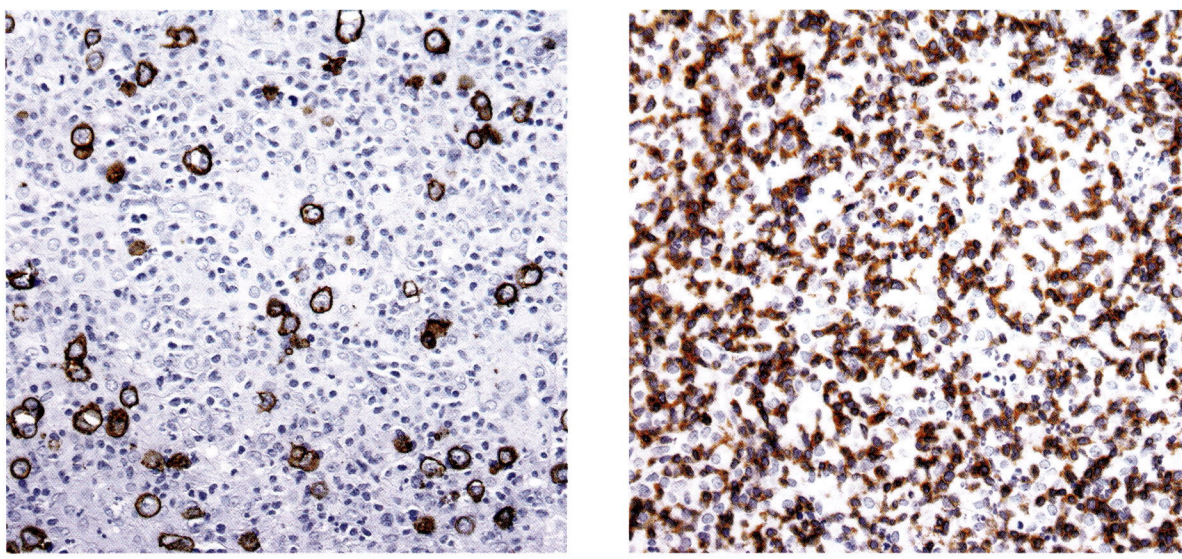

Figure 18-10

T-CELL/HISTIOCYTE-RICH LARGE B-CELL LYMPHOMA: IMMUNOHISTOCHEMISTRY

Immunohistochemical analysis of a case of TCHRLBL shows that the large neoplastic cells are positive for CD20 (left) and negative for CD3 (right). Many small reactive lymphocytes are positive for CD3 (immunohistochemistry with hematoxylin counterstain).

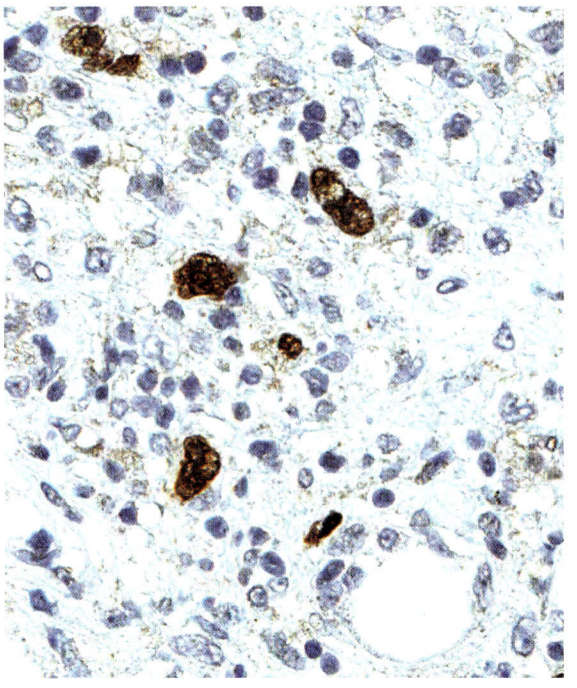

Figure 18-11

**T-CELL/HISTIOCYTE-RICH
LARGE B-CELL LYMPHOMA: OCT2**

The large neoplastic cells are positive for the B-cell transcription factor, OCT2 (immunohistochemistry with hematoxylin counterstain).

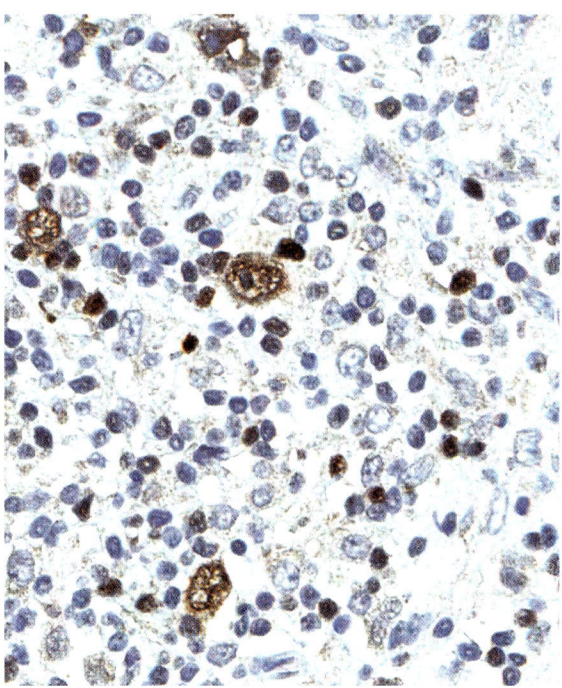

Figure 18-12

**T-CELL/HISTIOCYTE-RICH
LARGE B-CELL LYMPHOMA: BOB.1**

The large neoplastic cells are positive for the B-cell transcription co-factor BOB.1 (immunohistochemistry with hematoxylin counterstain).

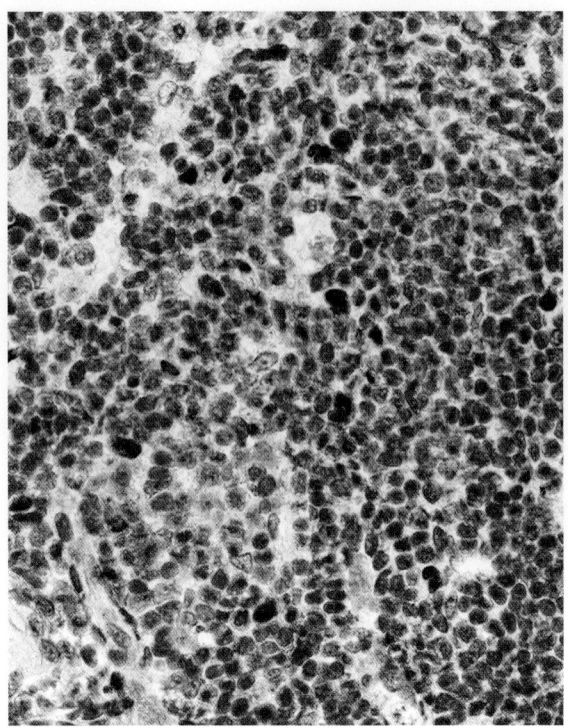

Figure 18-13

**T-CELL/HISTIOCYTE-RICH
LARGE B-CELL LYMPHOMA: BCL6**

The large neoplastic cells are positive for BCL6, suggestive of germinal center B-cell derivation (immunohistochemistry with hematoxylin counterstain).

cell networks and therefore antibodies that react with follicular dendritic cells (e.g., CD21, CD23) are negative. Epstein-Barr virus (EBV)-latent membrane protein type 1 and in situ hybridization for EBV encoded RNA1 (EBER1) are usually negative.

Reactive B cells are few (or absent) in most cases of THRLBCL. These B cells express pan-B-cell antigens and may be positive for IgD. In cases in which B cells are more numerous, the possibility of THRLBCL-like transformation should be considered.

MOLECULAR GENETIC FINDINGS

Conventional cytogenetic analysis of THRLBCL cases has shown no consistent abnormalities. Comparative genomic hybridization performed on whole tissue sections of microdissected large B cells has shown chromosomal imbalances (10,11). There are a number of genomic imbalances in THRLBCL, including gains of 2p16.1/

REL and losses of 2p11.2 and 9p11.2. These genetic changes are similar to those of NLPHL, although the number of genomic abnormalities is greater in THRLBCL (11). These data also suggest that THRLBCL and NLPHL are closely related and may be part of a spectrum (11).

Copy number alterations of chromosome 9p24.1 involving the PD-L1/*CD274* and PD-L2/*PDCD1LG2* loci have been detected by fluorescence in situ hybridization (FISH) in 50 to 60 percent of cases. These copy number alterations correlate with the expression of PD-L1 and PD-L2 detected by immunohistochemistry.

Assessment of clonality in THRLBCL using single cell polymerase chain reaction (PCR) has shown that the neoplastic B cells carry monoclonal immunoglobulin gene rearrangements and the variable regions segments have a high level of somatic hypermutations (5). The T-cell receptor genes are in the germline configuration. Clonality results may be falsely negative when PCR or Southern blot analysis is applied to whole tissues because the large neoplastic B cells may be too few.

Gene expression profiling studies of whole tissues have shown that the signature of THRLBCL is dominated by T cells and histiocytes within the microenvironment (12,15,19). Van Loo et al. (19) reported upregulation of a variety of molecules (e.g., CCL8, gamma interferon, Toll-like receptors) that may be responsible for recruiting T lymphocytes, histiocytes, and dendritic cells to the tumor. The net effect is a microenvironment that may protect the neoplastic cells from host immune attack. Gene expression profiling of single neoplastic cells from cases of THRLBCL have shown a signature similar to that of the LP cells of NLPHL (19).

DIFFERENTIAL DIAGNOSIS

Nodular Lymphocyte-Predominant Hodgkin Lymphoma. A nodular growth pattern supports the diagnosis of NLPHL over THRLBCL. Importantly, the definition of nodularity in NLPHL includes the architectural pattern and the composition of the nodules. Antibodies specific for follicular dendritic cells are helpful in recognizing nodular areas. Small, reactive B lymphocytes are also present and usually numerous in the nodules of NLPHL and are rare or absent in THRLBCL. NLPHL, however, can exhibit areas of a diffuse

Table 18-1

FEATURES OF T-CELL/HISTIOCYTE-RICH LARGE B-CELL LYMPHOMA (THRLBCL) VERSUS NODULAR LYMPHOCYTE-PREDOMINANT HODGKIN LYMPHOMA (NLPHL)

	THRLBCL	NLPHL
Pattern	Diffuse	Nodular (at least partial)
Large B cells	< 10%	< 10%
Cytology of large B cells	Highly variable	LP
Immunophenotype of large B cells		
Pan-B-cell antigens	+	+
CD15	-	-
CD30	-/+	< 10% +
CD45/LCA	+	+
BCL6	+/-	+
MUM1/IRF4	+/-	-/+
Pan-T-cell antigens	-	-
Microenvironment		
Small B cells	Absent or rare	Numerous
CD4+ T cells	Few	Numerous
CD8+ T cells	Numerous	Few
Cytotoxic T cells	Numerous	Few
Histiocytes	Can be numerous	Few
CD21+ follicular dendritic cells	Absent	Numerous

pattern where small reactive B cells are fewer (Table 18-1).

Classic Hodgkin Lymphoma. THRLBCL can resemble classic Hodgkin lymphoma, particularly the lymphocyte-rich classic and mixed cellularity types. Immunophenotypic analysis is helpful as the RS+H cells of classic Hodgkin lymphoma are positive for CD15 and CD30 and are negative for CD45/LCA; they also uncommonly express CD20 and rarely express CD20 strongly.

Diffuse Large B-Cell Lymphoma, Not Otherwise Specified. These tumors have a much greater number of large neoplastic B cells, usually present in large sheets. The arbitrary cutoff for large B cells of 10 percent or more supports DLBCL (see chapter 17).

Peripheral T-Cell Lymphoma. The large number of T cells in THRLBCL raises the possibility of T-cell lymphoma, while the presence of many PD1-positive cells suggests the possibility of angioimmunoblastic T-cell lymphoma (chapters 30 and 31). The T cells in THRLBCL are reactive, however, do not exhibit cytologic atypia and are polyclonal at the molecular level.

Histiocytic Sarcoma. The presence of numerous histiocytes in THRLBCL may suggest the possibility of a histiocytic tumor such as histiocytic sarcoma. Histiocytic sarcoma more often involves extranodal sites. The neoplastic histiocytes of histiocytic sarcoma often show cytologic atypia and granulocytes can be present in the background. A population of large neoplastic B cells is not present in histiocytic sarcoma.

TREATMENT AND PROGNOSIS

The frontline therapy for patients with THRLBCL is the same as for patients with DLBCL-NOS: rituximab, cyclophosphamide, doxorubicin, vincristine, and prednisone (R-CHOP) (1,3,7,13). The identification of copy number alterations of PD-L1 and PD-L2 as well as overexpression of these molecules suggest a role for PD1 inhibitors.

As mentioned above, patients commonly present with B-type symptoms and advanced-stage disease. However, when matched for stage and other prognostic features, the survival of patients with THRLBCL is not significantly different from that of patients with DLBCL-NOS (1,3,4,13). Patients who initially have THRLBCL can relapse with a tumor that resembles either THRLBCL or typical DLBCL-NOS. Less often, the converse occurs: a patient with DLBCL-NOS relapses with a tumor that resembles THRLBCL.

REFERENCES

1. Abramson JS. T-cell/histiocyte-rich B-cell lymphoma: biology, diagnosis, and management. Oncologist 2006;11:384-392.
2. Achten R, Verhoef G, Vanuytsel L, De Wolf-Peeters C. T-cell/histiocyte-rich large B-cell lymphoma: a distinct clinicopathologic entity. J Clin Oncol 2002;20:1269-1277.
3. Aki H, Tuzuner N, Ongoren S, et al. T-cell-rich B-cell lymphoma: a clinicopathologic study of 21 cases and comparison with 43 cases of diffuse large B-cell lymphoma. Leuk Res 2004;28:229-236.
4. Bouabdallah R, Mounier N, Guettier C, et al. T-cell/histiocyte-rich large B-cell lymphomas and classical diffuse large B-cell lymphomas have similar outcome after chemotherapy: a matched-control analysis. J Clin Oncol 2003;21:1271-1277.
5. Brauninger A, Kuppers R, Spieker T, et al. Molecular analysis of single B cells from T-cell-rich B-cell lymphoma shows the derivation of the tumor cells from mutating germinal center B cells and exemplifies means by which immunoglobulin genes are modified in germinal center B cells. Blood 1999;93:2679-2687.
6. Delabie J, Vandenberghe E, Kennes C, et al. Histiocyte-rich B cell lymphoma. A distinct clinicopathologic entity possibly related to lymphocyte predominant Hodgkin's disease, paragrnuloma type. Am J Surg Pathol 1992;16:37-48.
7. De Wolf-Peeters C, Delabie J, Campo E, Jaffe ES, Delsol G. T cell/histiocyte-rich large B-cell lymphoma. In: Swerdlow SH, Campo E, Harris NL, Jaffe ES, Pileria SA, Stein H, Thiele J, Vardiman JW, eds. WHO classification of tumours of haematopoietic and lymphoid tissues. Lyon: IARC Press; 2008:238-239.
8. Dogan A, Burke JS, Goteri G, Stitson RN, Wotherspoon AC, Isaacson PG. Micronodular T-cell/histiocyte-rich large B-cell lymphoma of the spleen: histology, immunophenotype, and differential diagnosis. Am J Surg Pathol 2003;27:903-911.
9. El Weshi A, Akhtar S, Mourad WA, et al. T-cell/histiocyte-rich B-cell lymphoma: clinical presentation, management and prognostic factors: report on 61 patients and review of the literature. Leuk Lymphoma 2007;48:1764-1773.
10. Franke S, Wlodarska I, Maes B, et al. Comparative genomic hybridization pattern distinguishes T-cell/histiocyte-rich B-cell lymphoma from nodular lymphocyte predominance Hodgkin's lymphoma. Am J Pathol 2002;161:1861-1867.
11. Hartmann S, Doring C, Vucic E, et al. Array comparative hybridization reveals similarities between nodular lymphocyte predominant Hodgkin lymphoma and T cell/histiocyte rich large B cell lymphoma. Br J Haematol 2015;169:415-422.
12. Hartmann S, Tousseyn T, Doring C, et al. Macrophages in T cell/histiocyte rich large B cell lymphoma strongly express metal-binding proteins and show a bi-activated phenotype. Int J Cancer 2013;133:2609-2618.
13. Kim YS, Ji JH, Ko YH, Kim SJ, Kim WS. Matched-pair analysis comparing the outcomes of T cell/histiocyte-rich large B cell lymphoma and diffuse large B cell lymphoma in patients treated with rituximab-CHOP. Acta Haematol 2014;131:156-161.
14. Lim MS, Beaty M, Sorbara L, et al. T-cell/histiocyte-rich large B-cell lymphoma: a heterogeneous entity with derivation from germinal center B cells. Am J Surg Pathol 2002;26:1458-1466.
15. Monti S, Savage KJ, Kutok JL, et al. Molecular profiling of diffuse large B-cell lymphoma identifies robust subtypes including one characterized by host inflammatory response. Blood 2005;105:1851-1861.
16. Ramsay AD, Smith WJ, Isaacson PG. T-cell-rich B-cell lymphoma. Am J Surg Pathol 1988;12:433-443.
16a. Swerdlow SH, Campo E, Pileri SA, et al. The 2016 revision of the World Health Organization classification of lymphoid neoplasms. Blood 2016;127:2375-2390.
17. Tousseyn T, De Wolf-Peeters C. T cell/histiocyte-rich large B-cell lymphoma: an update on its biology and classification. Virchows Arch 2011;459:557-563.
18. Treetipsatit J, Metcalf RA, Warnke RA, Natkunam Y. Large B-cell lymphoma with T-cell-rich background and nodules lacking follicular dendritic cell meshworks: description of an insufficiently recognized variant. Hum Pathol 2015;46:74-83.
19. Van Loo P, Tousseyn T, Vanhentenrijk V, et al. T-cell/histiocyte-rich large B-cell lymphoma shows transcriptional features suggestive of a tolerogenic host immune response. Haematologica 2010;95:440-448.
20. Wu D, Thomas A, Fromm JR. Reactive T cells by flow cytometry distinguish Hodgkin lymphomas from T cell/histiocyte-rich large B cell lymphoma. Cytometry B Clin Cytom 2016;90:424-432.

19 EPSTEIN-BARR VIRUS-POSITIVE DIFFUSE LARGE B-CELL LYMPHOMA

GENERAL FEATURES

Epstein-Barr virus (EBV)-positive diffuse large B-cell lymphoma (DLBCL) is a neoplasm composed of large B cells, many of which are EBV positive, in a patient without a history of lymphoma or immunodeficiency (17). There is no consensus cutoff for the number of EBV-positive neoplastic cells, but a substantial number of positive cells is required and EBV-positive reactive cells in the microenvironment are excluded. Other forms of EBV-positive B-cell lymphoma that occur in the context of other clinicopathologic syndromes (e.g., lymphomatoid granulomatosis) are also excluded from this disease category.

EBV positive DLBCL was first described in Asia and initially designated as senile EBV-associated B-cell lymphoproliferative disorder or age-related EBV-associated B-cell lymphoproliferative disorder (22–24). Although most common in Asia, these neoplasms were also reported in the United States, Europe, and other industrialized nations (4,7,20). In the 2008 World Health Organization (WHO) classification, the designation *EBV-positive DLBCL of the elderly* was included

as a provisional entity (17). An age cutoff of 50 years was used to define elderly in the WHO classification, but this cutoff was clearly arbitrary. Subsequently, it became evident that these neoplasms can occur in substantially younger patients (4,9,13,18,21,27). Therefore, in the 2016 revision of the WHO classification, the designation "of the elderly" is eliminated (26a).

A number of findings support the concept that EBV is essential for lymphomagenesis. EBV is present in monoclonal form. Latent membrane protein type 1 (LMP1) resides on the cell surface and can mimic CD40 signaling (fig. 19-1). In addition, LMP2a has been shown to enhance MYC-driven proliferation and can mimic B-cell receptor signaling (5,15). EBV infection results in the activation of many cellular pathways including NF-κB, PI3K/AKT, and JAK-STAT as has been reviewed by Ok et al. (21).

Immunodeficiency is also thought to be involved in pathogenesis. Although affected patients have no known explanation for the immunodeficiency, one speculation for older patients is that these tumors are linked to the

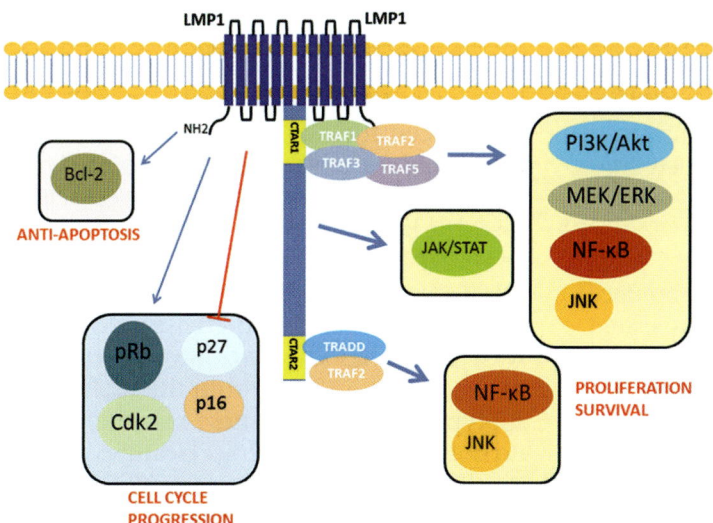

Figure 19-1

EPSTEIN-BARR VIRUS (EBV)-MEDIATED ONCOGENIC SIGNALING PATHWAYS IN EPSTEIN-BARR VIRUS-POSITIVE DIFFUSE LARGE B-CELL LYMPHOMA (DLBCL)

EBV latent membrane protein type 1 (LMP1) on the cell surface can activate many cellular pathways. LMP1 also has effects on the cell cycle and inhibition of apoptosis. CTAR, C-terminal activation region; TRAF, tumor necrosis factor receptor-associated factor; TRADD, tumor necrosis factor receptor type 1-associated death domain; PI3K, phosphatidylinositol 3-kinase; MEK, MAPK/ERK kinase; JNK, c-Jun N-terminal kinase; AP-1, activator protein 1. (Courtesy of Dr. C. Y. Ok, Houston, TX.)

immunological decline that occurs as a result of aging (23). There are also data that EBV reactivation is more common in older patients. The reasons for immunodeficiency in younger patients are unknown. Some have suggested that a low-grade inflammatory state promotes lymphomagenesis, perhaps via generation of free radical oxygen species (21).

CLINICAL FEATURES

EBV-positive DLBCL represents 7 to 11 percent of DLBCL cases in Asian countries (8,24–27) but is rare in industrialized nations where it represents 2 to 4 percent of all DLBCL cases (7,8,20). These tumors also are common in Central and South America: EBV-positive DLBCL is reported to represent 7 percent of all DLBCL cases in Mexico (8) and up to 15 percent of all DLBCL cases in Peru (4). Affected patients have a median age in the eighth decade in most studies, with an age range from 50 to 92 years (3,6,22,25–27); patients are younger in Mexico (8) and in industrialized nations (20). As mentioned above, a small subset of patients is younger than 50 years (4,9,13,18). The male to female ratio in different studies is even or there is a slight male predominance.

B-type symptoms are present in 40 to 50 percent of patients (3,21,26,27). Serum lactate dehydrogenase (LDH) levels are elevated and the International Prognostic Index (IPI) is high in 50 to 60 percent of patients (3,24). Lymphadenopathy is present in 70 to 80 percent of patients and about 40 percent present with disease limited to lymph nodes. In one study, lymphadenopathy was more common in Mexico than in Germany (8). Extranodal disease is common, with or without lymphadenopathy, and can involve a wide variety of sites including skin, soft tissue, Waldeyer ring, bone, lung and pleura, gastrointestinal tract, liver, spleen, and bone marrow (20,24,27).

HISTOLOGIC FINDINGS

All cases of EBV-positive DLBCL diffusely efface normal tissue structures and are often associated with foci of geographic necrosis (fig. 19-2). Mitotic figures may be numerous. Epithelioid histiocytes are individually sprinkled within the neoplastic infiltrate or distributed in small clusters.

The broad spectrum of histologic findings is subdivided into polymorphic and monomor-

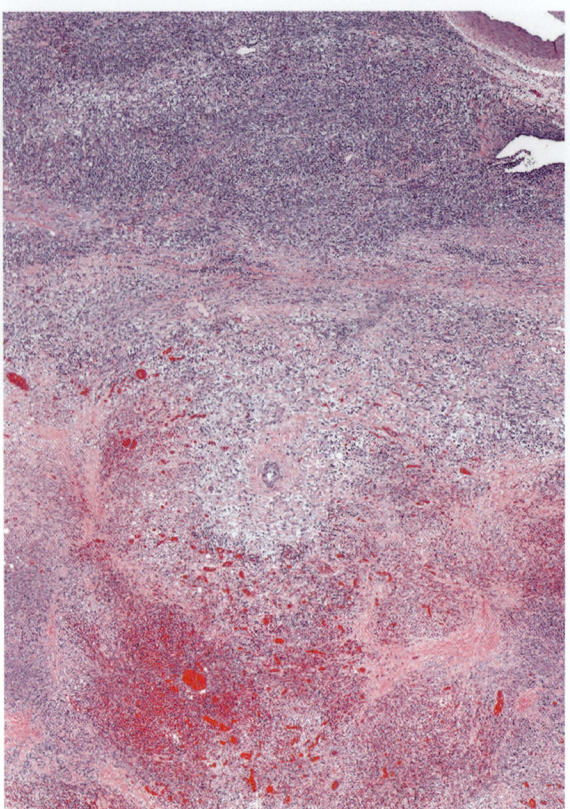

Figure 19-2

**EPSTEIN-BARR VIRUS-POSITIVE DIFFUSE
LARGE B-CELL LYMPHOMA**

This tumor destroyed the lymph node architecture resulting in large areas of geographic necrosis. Viable tumor cells are present at the edge of the necrosis (hematoxylin and eosin [H&E] stain).

phic (large cell lymphoma) subtypes. In some tumors, both subtypes are present or distinction between the two seems arbitrary. Polymorphic lesions (fig. 19-3) have a broad range of B cells, including centroblasts or immunoblasts, admixed with many reactive cells including small lymphocytes, histiocytes, and fewer plasma cells. In some cases the large cells resemble Reed-Sternberg-like or Hodgkin-like cells (fig. 19-4). Monomorphic lesions are composed of sheets of large cells and resemble DLBCL, not otherwise specified. Cases with plasmablastic features have been recognized in the elderly and fit within the monomorphic subtype (11). To date, these morphologic types do not correlate with clinical features or prognosis; their value lies in awareness of the spectrum for establishing the diagnosis.

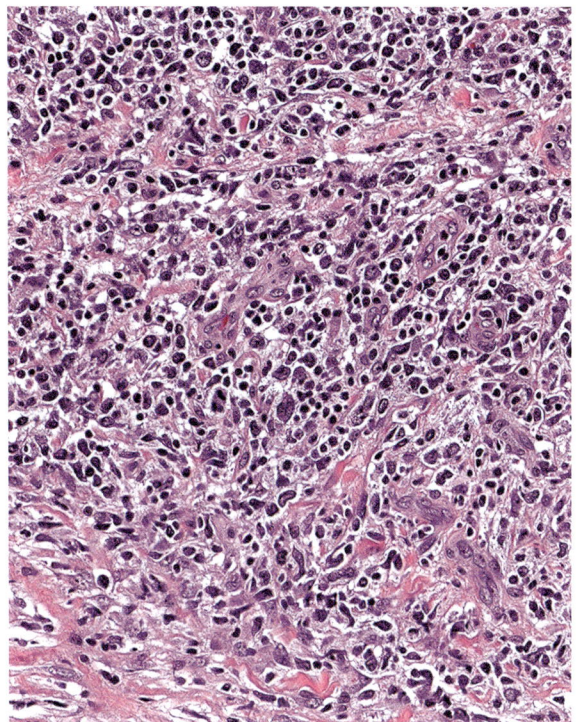

Figure 19-3

POLYMORPHOUS SUBTYPE OF EPSTEIN-BARR VIRUS-POSITIVE DIFFUSE LARGE B-CELL LYMPHOMA

Numerous small to intermediate-sized lymphoid cells and scattered large cells are present (H&E stain).

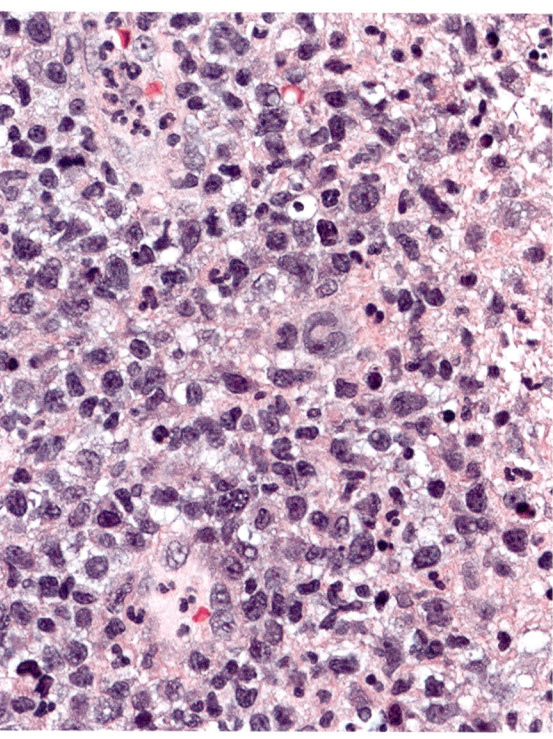

Figure 19-4

POLYMORPHOUS SUBTYPE OF EPSTEIN-BARR VIRUS-POSITIVE DIFFUSE LARGE B-CELL LYMPHOMA

The large neoplastic cells include some multinucleated cells with the morphologic features similar to Reed-Sternberg and Hodgkin cells (H&E stain).

CYTOLOGIC FINDINGS

Fine-needle aspirate smears of the polymorphous subtype of EBV-positive DLBCL show a heterogeneous population of lymphoid cells that includes scattered reactive small lymphocytes, larger atypical transformed cells, and multinucleated Reed-Sternberg-like and Hodgkin-like cells (fig. 19-5). A variable number of histiocytes and plasma cells may be present. In the monomorphic subtype, a sheet-like proliferation of transformed cells resembling centroblasts, immunoblasts, plasmablasts, or a mixture of these cells is present, with fewer reactive cells.

IMMUNOPHENOTYPIC FINDINGS

The neoplastic cells are mature B cells that express pan-B-cell antigens such as CD19, CD20 (fig. 19-6), CD22, CD79a, and PAX5. Sixty to 70 percent of cases have a nongerminal center B-cell immunophenotype: positive for MUM1/IRF4 and negative for CD10 and BCL6 (3,6,16,21,24,27).

The neoplastic cells usually express CD45/LCA. Antibodies specific for Ki-67 show a variable, but often high-proliferation rate, in part dependent on the number of large transformed cells. BCL2 is commonly positive and CD30 is also often positive (fig. 19-7). Cases with plasmacytoid differentiation may show cytoplasmic monotypic immunoglobulin light chain and are negative for CD20. Pan-T-cell antigens, histiocyte-associated antigens, CD15, and cyclin D1 are negative. A high proportion of reactive cytotoxic (TIA-1-positive) T cells may be present in the background of these neoplasms (27).

Epstein-Barr Virus

In situ hybridization for EBV-encoded RNA1 (EBER1) commonly shows evidence of EBV infection in the large neoplastic cells (fig. 19-8), and most (70 to 90 percent) EBV-positive cases are also positive for EBV latent membrane protein type

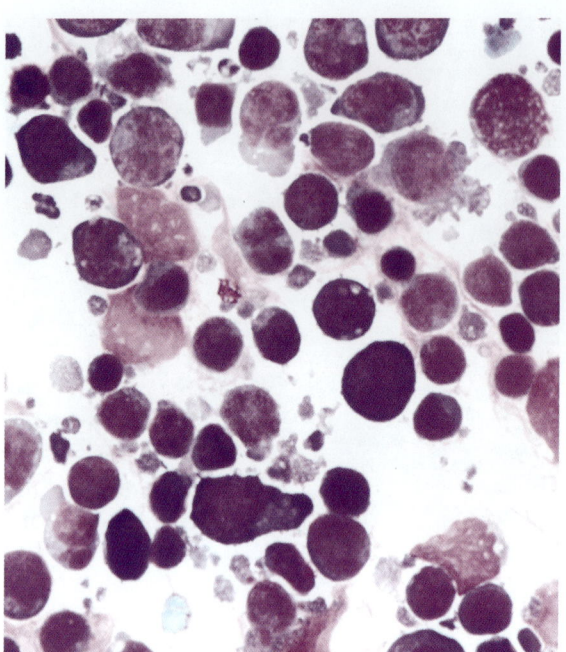
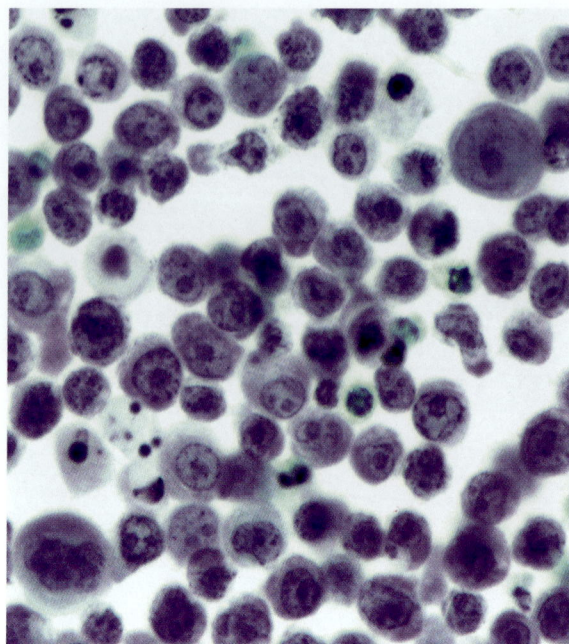

Figure 19-5

EPSTEIN-BARR VIRUS-POSITIVE DIFFUSE LARGE B-CELL LYMPHOMA

The large lymphoma cells vary in size, with irregular nuclear contours, prominent nucleoli, and variable amounts of cytoplasm (left: Diff-Quik stain; right: Papanicolaou stain).

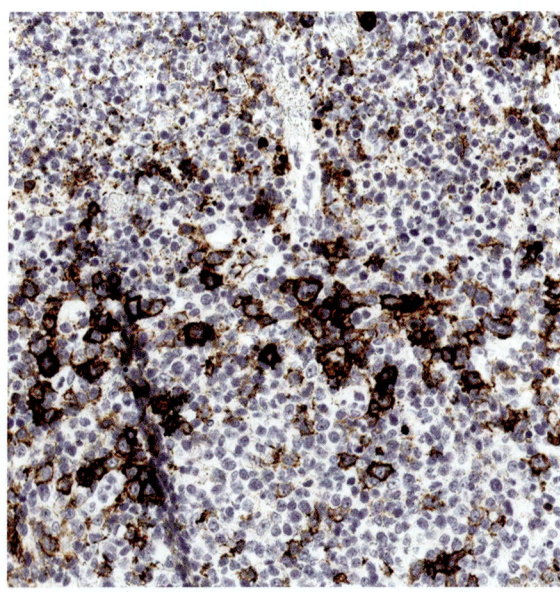

Figure 19-6

POLYMORPHOUS SUBTYPE OF EPSTEIN-BARR VIRUS-POSITIVE DIFFUSE LARGE B-CELL LYMPHOMA

The neoplastic cells express CD20 (immunohistochemistry with hematoxylin counterstain).

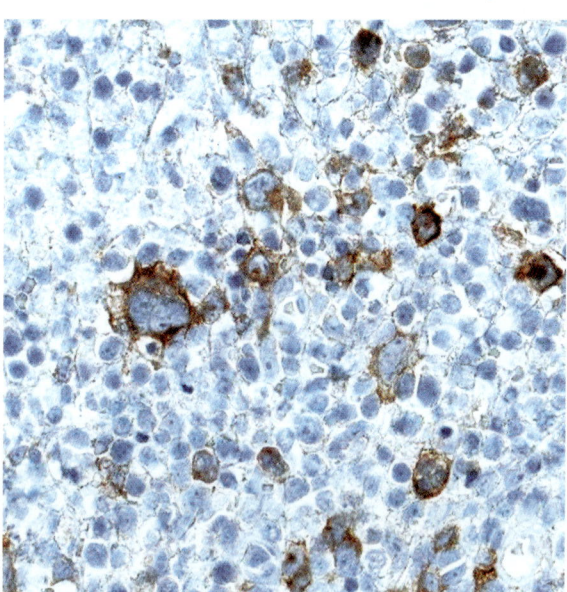

Figure 19-7

EPSTEIN-BARR VIRUS-POSITIVE DIFFUSE LARGE B-CELL LYMPHOMA

CD30 is commonly and often variably expressed in EBV-positive DLBCL. In this field a multinucleated Reed-Sternberg-like cell is present (center left) (immuno-histochemistry with hematoxylin counterstain).

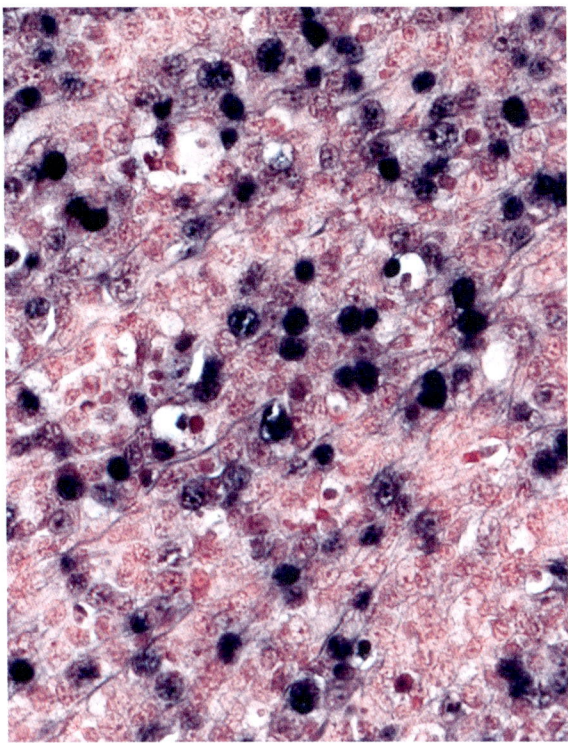

Figure 19-8

**EPSTEIN-BARR VIRUS-POSITIVE
DIFFUSE LARGE B-CELL LYMPHOMA**

This case of EBV-positive DLBCL contains numerous EBV-encoded RNA1 (EBER1)-positive cells (in situ hybridization with eosin counterstain).

1 (8,18,20,27). EBNA2 is positive in a minority of cases, up to 25 percent (8,27). There is some variation in EBV type. In a study from Mexico, approximately half of cases had type B EBV with a 30-base pair deletion in EBV LMP1. Type A EBV is more common in industrialized nations (8).

Various cutoffs for the percentage of EBV-positive tumor cells have been used for diagnosis of EBV-positive DLBCL. Cutoffs commonly seen in the literature are 20 percent, 30 percent, or 50 percent (3,20,25,26). The number of EBV-positive cases as a percentage of all DLBCL cases is lower in studies that use a higher threshold of EBV-positive cells (21). In Asia, a type III latency pattern of EBV infection is most common (27); in industrialized nations, however, the latency pattern of EBV infection is more variable. The type III pattern is present in about 40 percent of cases, but 60 percent of cases are almost evenly split between type I and type III latency patterns (20).

MOLECULAR GENETIC FINDINGS

Most cases of EBV-positive DLBCL carry monoclonal *IGH* rearrangements (6). The *TRG* and *TRB* genes are usually in the germline configuration. Minor T-cell clones are present in a small subset of cases (6,16). Few cases have been studied by conventional cytogenetics, but chromosomal aberrations are uncommon. Gebauer et al. (6) identified *BCL6* translocations in 15 percent of cases. *MYC* translocations are rare (5 percent or less) and translocations involving *BCL2*, *MDM2*, and *CCND1* do not occur. One case with a t(9;14)(p13;q32)/*PAX5-IGH* has been reported (19).

Few cases have been assessed systematically for gene mutations. Overall, gene mutations appear to be infrequent. *CARD11* mutations were identified in 2 of 26 (8 percent) cases in one study (6). One case with a germinal center B-cell immunophenotype had an *EZH2* mutation. There is no evidence of *CD79B*, MYD88, or *TP53* mutations (6,20).

Many copy number alterations have been detected in EBV-positive DLBCL (27). The most common sites of gain include 1q23.2-23.3, 1q32, 5p15.3, 8q22.3, 8q24.1-24.2, and 9p24.1/PD-L2 (27). Areas of loss include 6q27, 7q11.2, and 7q36.2-36.3 (27). One study has shown that EBV-positive DLBCL has a distinctive microRNA (miR) profile, with upregulation of five miRs and downregulation of one miR (1). In this study, upregulation of miR-146b and miR-222 were most specific for EBV-positive DLBCL. In another study, EBV-miR-BHRF1-2 has been shown to target *PRDM1*/Blimp1 (14).

Gene expression profiling and other methods have shown that EBV-positive DLBCL is distinctly different than EBV-negative DLBCL (10,16,20). EBV-positive DLBCL is characterized by genes involved in the activation of the NF-κB and JAK-STAT pathways as well as genes involved in cell metabolism, cell cycle progression, cell proliferation, resistance to chemotherapy, and host immune response (10,20,27).

DIFFERENTIAL DIAGNOSIS

Epstein-Barr Virus-Positive Lymphoproliferative Disorders Occurring in the Context of Immunodeficiency. The clinical findings, histologic features, and immunophenotype of EBV-positive DLBCL may closely resemble cases of DLBCL arising in the immunodeficiency setting. It is therefore essential to exclude other causes of immunodeficiency, either congenital or acquired.

DLBCL, Not Otherwise Specified (NOS). The monomorphic type of EBV-positive DLBCL can be morphologically identical to either DLBCL, NOS or rarely, plasmablastic lymphoma. Demonstration of EBV infection in a substantial subset of tumor cells, in the appropriate clinical context, is required to distinguish EBV-positive DLBCL.

Some cases of DLBCL-NOS have EBV present in reactive cells. These tumors do not meet the criteria for EBV-positive DLBCL, but the presence of virus in bystander cells has been reported to correlate with poorer prognosis (18a).

T-Cell/Histiocyte-Rich Large B-Cell Lymphoma. The polymorphic subtype of EBV-positive DLBCL can resemble THRLBCL. Unlike EBV-positive DLBCL, THRLBCL less often has geographic necrosis and the background infiltrate is less heterogeneous. The large neoplastic cells of THRLBCL are negative for EBV.

Intrafollicular Epstein-Barr Virus–Positive Large B-Cell Lymphoma. This is a rare newly described entity in which EBV-positive large B cells colonize germinal centers (12). Patients are older, over 60 years of age, and do not have evidence of immunodeficiency. The lymphoma cells can resemble centroblasts or Reed-Sternberg- and Hodgkin-like cells. The neoplastic cells have a nongerminal center B-cell immunophenotype, express MYC and STAT3, and BCL2 is weak or absent. There are no rearrangements of *MYC*, *BCL2*, or *BCL6*. The small number of patients studied responded poorly to therapy (12).

Classic Hodgkin Lymphoma. The polymorphic subtype of EBV-positive DLBCL resembles classic Hodgkin lymphoma, particularly the mixed cellularity and lymphocyte depletion types, which are usually EBV positive. In some cases, the polymorphic type of EBV-positive DLBCL has cells that resemble Reed-Sternberg or Hodgkin cells that express CD30. Immunohistochemical analysis is helpful as the neoplastic cells of EBV-positive DLBCL usually express pan-B-cell markers (brightly) and CD45/LCA, and are negative for CD15 (2). Molecular studies of whole tissue sections commonly show monoclonal *IGH* rearrangements in EBV-positive DLBCL, but not in classic Hodgkin lymphoma.

Angioimmunoblastic-Like T-Cell Lymphoma (AITL). The polymorphic subtype of EBV-positive DLBCL may resemble AITL. Most AITL cases have a heterogeneous cell population and EBV-positive large cells are common. However, cases of AITL often have many eosinophils and the T-cell population is usually more numerous and atypical, unlike EBV-positive DLBCL. CD10, BCL6, and PD1 expression by the neoplastic T cells and monoclonal T-cell receptor gene rearrangements support AITL.

TREATMENT AND PROGNOSIS

In Asia, EBV-positive DLBCL is commonly characterized by an aggressive clinical course. The median overall survival period has been reported to be about 2 years (24–27). In contrast, in industrialized nations, the presence of EBV in DLBCL has less influence on prognosis (7,8,20). Nevertheless, the combination of CD30 expression and EBV infection in DLBCL is associated with a poor prognosis (20). Cell of origin classification does not correlate independently with prognosis in patients with EBV-positive DLBCL (20,27).

REFERENCES

1. Andrade TA, Evangelista AF, Campos AH, et al. A microRNA signature in EBV+ diffuse large B-cell lymphoma of the elderly. Oncotarget 2014;5: 11813-11826.

2. Asano N, Yamamoto K, Tamaru J, et al. Age-related Epstein-Barr virus (EBV)-associated B-cell lymphoproliferative disorders: comparison with EBV-positive classic Hodgkin lymphoma in elderly patients. Blood 2009;113:2629-2636.

3. Battle-Lopez A, Gonzalez de Villambrosia S, Nuñez J, et al. Epstein-Barr virus-associated diffuse large B-cell lymphoma: diagnosis, difficulties and therapeutic options. Expert Rev Anticancer Ther 2016;16:411-421.

4. Beltran BE, Morales D, Quiñones P, Medeiros LJ, Miranda RN, Castillo JJ. EBV-positive diffuse large B-cell lymphoma in young immunocompetent individuals. Clin Lymphoma Myeloma Leuk 2011;11:512-516.

5. Fish K, Chen J, Longnecker R. Epstein-Barr virus latent membrane protein 2A enhances MYC-driven cell cycle progression in a mouse model of B lymphoma. Blood 2014;123:530-540.

6. Gebauer N, Gebauer J, Hardel TT, et al. Prevalence of targetable oncogenic mutations and genomic alterations in Epstein-Barr virus-associated diffuse large B-cell lymphoma of the elderly. Leuk Lymphoma 2015;56:1100-1106.

7. Gibson SE, Hsi ED. Epstein-Barr virus-positive B-cell lymphoma of the elderly at a United States tertiary medical center: an uncommon aggressive lymphoma with a nongerminal center B-cell phenotype. Hum Pathol 2009;40:653-661.

8. Hofscheier A, Ponciano A, Bonzheim I, et al. Geographic variation in the prevalence of Epstein-Barr virus-positive diffuse large B-cell lymphoma of the elderly: a comparative analysis of a Mexican and a German population. Mod Pathol 2011;24:1046-1054.

9. Hong JY, Yoon DH, Suh C, et al. EBV-positive diffuse large B-cell lymphoma in young adults: is this a distinct disease entity? Ann Oncol 2015;26:548-555.

10. Kato H, Karube K, Yamamoto K, et al. Gene expression profiling of Epstein-Barr virus-positive diffuse large B-cell lymphoma of the eldely reveals alterations of characteristic oncogenetic pathways. Cancer Sci 2014;105:537-544.

11. Liu F, Asano N, Tatematsu A, et al. Plasmablastic lymphoma of the elderly: a clinicopathological comparison with age-related Epstein-Barr virus-associated B cell lymphoproliferative disorder. Histopathology 2012;61:1183-1197.

12. Lorenzi L, Lonardi S, Essatari MH, et al. Intra-follicular Epstein-Barr virus positive large B cell lymphoma. A variant of "germinotropic" lymphoproliferative disorder. Virchows Arch 2016;468:441-440.

13. Lu TX, Liang JH, Miao Y, et al. Epstein-Barr virus positive diffuse large B-cell lymphoma predict poor outcome, regardless of the age. Sci Rep 2015;5:12168.

14. Ma J, Nie K, Redmond D, et al. EBV-miR-BHRF1-2 targets PRDM1/Blimp1: potential role in EBV lymphomagenesis. Leukemia 2016;30:594-604.

15. Mancao C, Hammerschmidt W. Epstein-Barr virus latent membrane protein 2A is a B-cell receptor mimic and essential for B-cell survival. Blood 2007;110:3715-3721.

16. Montes-Moreno S, Odqvist L, Diaz-Perez JA, et al. EBV-positive diffuse large B-cell lymphoma of the elderly is an aggressive post-germinal center B-cell neoplasm characterized by prominent nuclear factor-kB activation. Mod Pathol 2012;25:968-982.

17. Nakamura S, Jaffe ES, Swerdlow SH. EBV positive diffuse large B-cell lymphoma of the elderly. In: Swerdlow SH, Campo E, Harris NL, Jaffe ES, Pileria SA, Stein H, Thiele J, Vardiman JW, eds. WHO Classification of tumours of haematopoietic and lymphoid tissues. Lyon: IARC Press; 2008:243-244.

18. Nicolae A, Pittaluga S, Abdullah S, et al. EBV-positive large B-cell lymphomas in young patients: a nodal lymphoma with evidence for a tolerogenic immune environment. Blood 2015;126:863-872.

18a. Ohashi A, Kato S, Okamoto A, et al. Reappraisal of Epstein-Barr virus (EBV) in diffuse large B-cell lymphoma (DLBCL): comparative analysis between EBV-positive and EBV-negative DLBCL with EBV-positive bystander cells. Histopathology 2017;71:89-97.

19. Ohno H, Nishikori M, Haga H, Isoda K. Epstein-Barr virus-positive diffuse large B-cell lymphoma carrying a t(9;14)(p13;q32) translocation. Int J Hematol 2009;89:704-708.

20. Ok CY, Li L, Xu-Monette ZY, et al. Prevalence and clinical implications of Epstein-Barr virus infection in de novo diffuse large B-cell lymphoma in western countries. Clin Cancer Res 2014;20:2338-2349.

21. Ok CY, Papathomas TG, Medeiros LJ, Young KH. EBV-positive diffuse large B-cell lymphoma of the elderly. Blood 2013;122:328-340.

22. Oyama T, Ichimura K, Suzuki R, et al. Senile EBV+ B-cell lymphoproliferative disorders: a clinicopathologic study of 22 patients. Am J Surg Pathol 2003;27:16-26.

23. Oyama T, Yamamoto K, Asano N, et al. Age-related EBV-associated B-cell lymphoproliferative disorders constitute a distinct clinicopathologic group: a study of 96 patients. Clin Cancer Res 2007; 13:5124-5132.

24. Park S, Lee J, Ko YH, et al. The impact of Epstein-Barr virus status on clinical outcome in diffuse large B-cell lymphoma. Blood 2007;110:972-978.

25. Shimoyama Y, Asano N, Kojima M, et al. Age-related EBV-associated B-cell lymphoproliferative disorders: diagnostic approach to a newly recognized clinicopathological entity. Pathol Int 2009;59:835-843.

26. Shimoyama Y, Yamamoto K, Asano N, Oyama T, Kinoshita T, Nakamura S. Age-related Epstein-Barr virus-associated B-cell lymphoproliferative disorders: special references to lymphomas surrounding this newly recognized clinicopathologic disease. Cancer Sci 2008;99:1085-1091.

26a. Swerdlow SH, Campo E, Pileri SA, et al. The 2016 revision of the World Health Organization classification of lymphoid neoplasms. Blood 2016;127:2375-2390.

27. Yoon H, Park S, Ju H, et al. Integrated copy number and gene expression profiling analysis of Epstein-Barr virus-positive diffuse large B-cell lymphoma. Genes Chromosomes Cancer 2015;54:383-396.

PRIMARY MEDIASTINAL LARGE B-CELL LYMPHOMA

GENERAL FEATURES

Primary mediastinal large B-cell lymphoma (PMBL) is a distinctive type of B-cell lymphoma that arises in the mediastinum (7). In the literature, these tumors also are referred to as *primary mediastinal B-cell lymphoma, thymic B-cell lymphoma*, and *clear cell lymphoma*.

The putative cell of origin of PBML is thought to be a thymic medullary B cell, also referred to as a thymic asteroid B cell in the literature (12,32). An alternative hypothesis proposed for the cell of origin, based on expression of germinal center-associated antigens and *IGH* variable region mutations in PMBL, is a germinal center B cell that migrates to the thymus gland.

The pathogenesis of PMBL is complex, but two major mechanisms have prominent roles: activation of the JAK-STAT pathway and escape from host immunosurveillance. The latter is accomplished by reduction of immune antigens on the surface of the lymphoma cells and by impairment of the host T-cell response against the lymphoma cells (see Molecular Genetic Findings).

The current standard criteria for the diagnosis of PMBL include a combination of clinical findings (young patient age and prominent mediastinal mass), histologic recognition of large cell lymphoma, and a B-cell immunophenotype, often with expression of CD23, CD30 (weak, variable), MAL, nuclear c-Rel, CD200, and other markers. These criteria, however, are not entirely specific and some cases of nodal diffuse large B-cell lymphoma (DLBCL) that present in mediastinal lymph nodes may be misinterpreted as PMBL. In one gene expression profiling study performed over a decade ago, about a quarter of cases originally included in the study cohort as PMBL based on standard clinical and pathologic assessment were eventually excluded on the basis of their gene expression profiles (25). In addition, standard criteria for a diagnosis of PBML are not entirely sensitive. It may be difficult to recognize PMBL in patients with unusual features, such as older age or a patient who presents with widely disseminated disease. Yuan et al. (37) suggested that rare cases of DLBCL can have a gene expression profile typical of PMBL, even though the patient does not have a mediastinal mass. Additional tools are needed to refine the category of PMBL as well as improve the sensitivity and specificity of diagnosis.

CLINICAL FEATURES

PMBL is an uncommon tumor that accounts for about 2 percent of all non-Hodgkin lymphomas (2,4,7). It is predominantly a disease of young adults. The median patient age at the time of diagnosis is 30 to 35 years and the male to female ratio is 1 to 2 (1,2,4,15,35,38). However, this sex predominance is less pronounced for blacks as compared with whites (17a).

Most patients present initially with a bulky anterior-superior mediastinal mass (fig. 20-1), sometimes accompanied by local compression effects that can result in cough, dyspnea, or superior vena cava syndrome (1,17a,35,38). The tumor may directly extend into the lungs, pleura, or pericardium; involvement of serosal surfaces may be accompanied by effusions. Involvement of the recurrent laryngeal nerve may cause hoarseness. Supraclavicular or cervical lymph nodes may be involved (1,2,4,17a,35,38).

Particularly at the time of recurrence, PMBL can widely disseminate, with a propensity for involvement of extranodal sites including kidneys, adrenal glands, liver, ovary, breast, and the central nervous system. The bone marrow is rarely involved by PMBL at the time of presentation and is an unusual site of dissemination (4,7).

HISTOLOGIC FINDINGS

Mediastinum

In a biopsy specimen from the mediastinum, identification of remnants of thymic tissue is helpful in supporting a thymic origin and

343

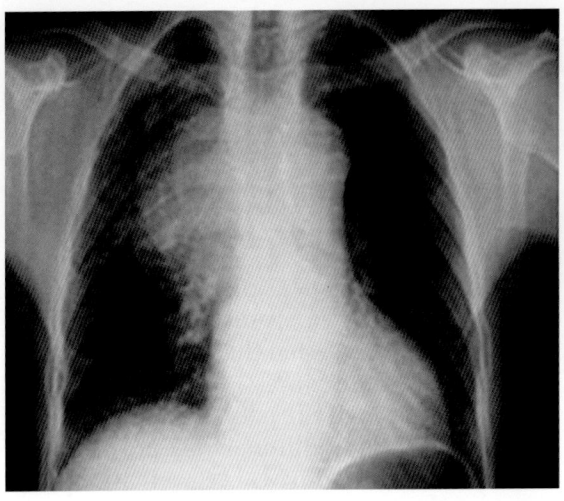

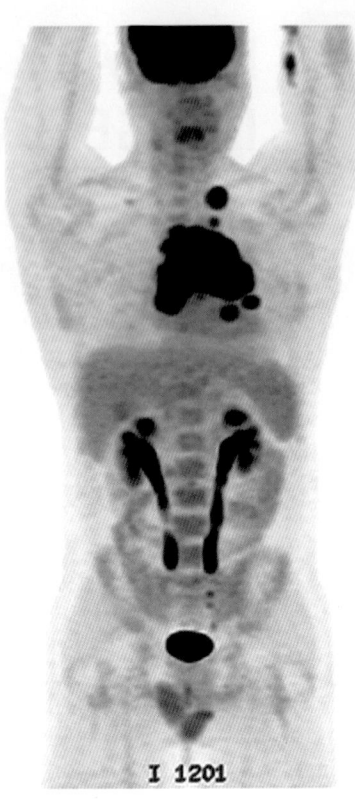

Figure 20-1

PRIMARY MEDIASTINAL LARGE B-CELL LYMPHOMA

Above: Plain chest film shows a large mediastinal mass.

Right: The positron emission tomography (PET) scan shows a large mediastinal mass and small peripheral lymph nodes that are 18-fluorodeoxyglucose (FDG) avid. These results indicate that the tumor is metabolically active and rapidly growing. (The kidneys also uptake 18-FDG normally as it is excreted in urine.)

I 1201

the diagnosis of PMBL over another type of lymphoma involving mediastinal lymph nodes (fig. 20-2, left). PMBL is characterized by a diffuse proliferation of neoplastic cells that are compartmentalized into aggregates or lobules by interstitial fibrosis (figs. 20-2, right; 2-3) (7,20,21). The fibrosis is typically delicate and usually does not form broad bands of sclerosis (unlike nodular sclerosis Hodgkin lymphoma), although broad sclerotic bands are present in a small subset of cases (fig. 20-2, left). Mitotic figures and apoptotic cells (fig. 20-2, right) are usually numerous and some cases exhibit small or large foci of coagulative necrosis (fig. 20-4). A starry sky pattern is uncommon.

The neoplastic cells are usually large but can be of intermediate size. They often have abundant pale or clear cytoplasm (fig. 20-5) and the cytoplasmic membranes may be indistinct. In formalin-fixed tissue, retraction artifact of the tumor cell cytoplasm may be prominent (fig. 20-6). In most cases, the lymphoma cells have round or ovoid nuclei with vesicular chromatin, but less frequently, exhibit hyperchromasia. In some cases, the neoplastic cell nuclei may be pleomorphic (fig. 20-7) or contain multilobated or "cloverleaf" forms (fig. 20-8). In some cases the neoplastic cells resemble Hodgkin or, less often, Reed-Sternberg cells (20). The recognition of these histologic features in needle biopsy specimens can be challenging because of crush artifact.

Lymph Nodes

In biopsy specimens of cervical or supraclavicular lymph nodes, the neoplastic cells usually diffusely replace the parenchyma (fig. 20-9). Unlike the findings in extranodal tissue specimens, the neoplastic cells often appear more oval or round, and less often are associated with fine sclerosis. Pleomorphism is often less prominent. Otherwise, the cytologic findings in the lymph nodes resemble those observed at extranodal sites. Mitotic figures and apoptotic cells are common.

CYTOLOGIC FINDINGS

There is a range of cellularity, from high to low. In cellular specimens, the neoplastic cells are large and usually dispersed, but the tumor cells may be present in loose aggregates (fig. 20-10).

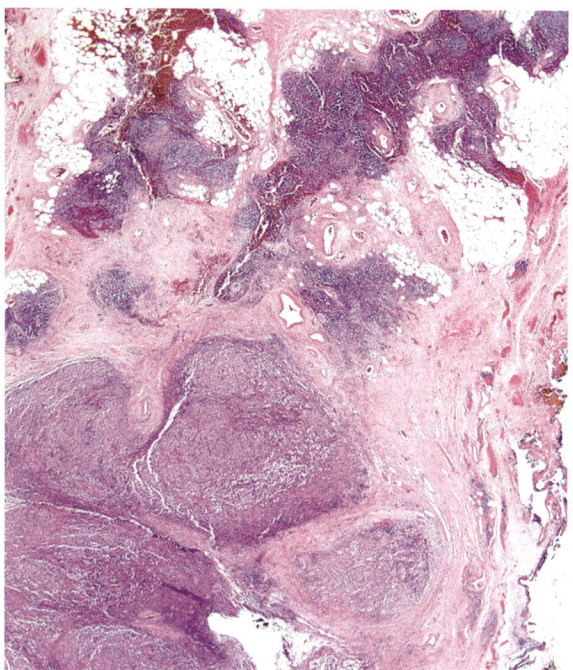 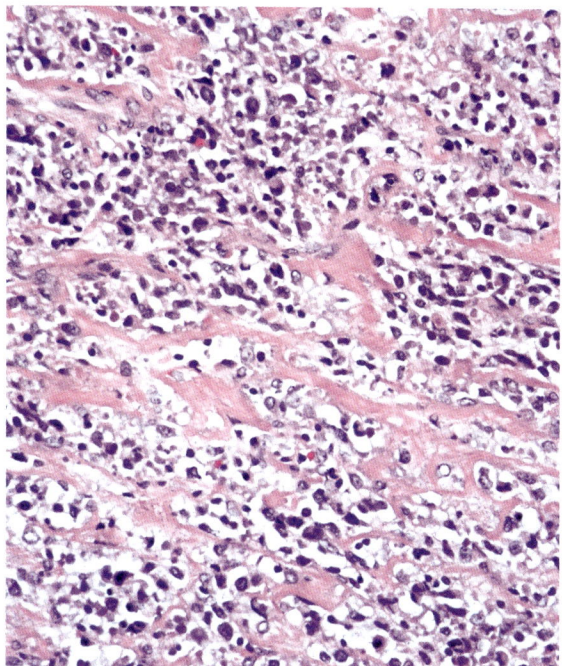

Figure 20-2

PRIMARY MEDIASTINAL LARGE B-CELL LYMPHOMA

Left: At the top of the field, normal thymus tissue is present, indicating that the lymphoma (bottom of field) involves and likely arose in the thymus gland. Broad sclerotic bands course through the PMBL.

Right: Fibrotic bands course through the tumor, which was composed of large cells with pale cytoplasm. The cells also show single cell necrosis and apoptosis (left, right: hematoxylin and eosin [H&E] stain).

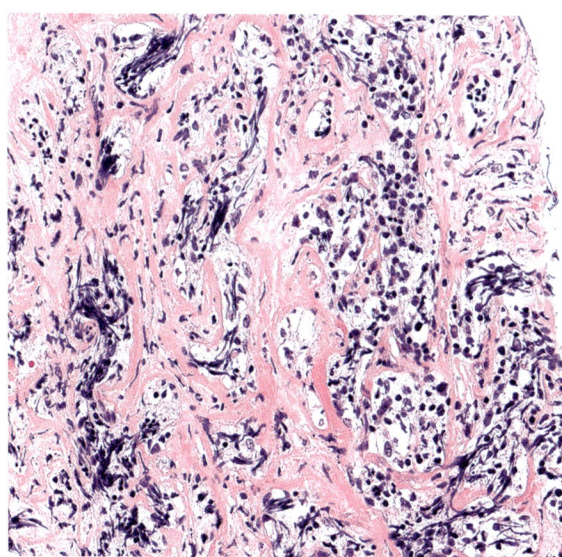 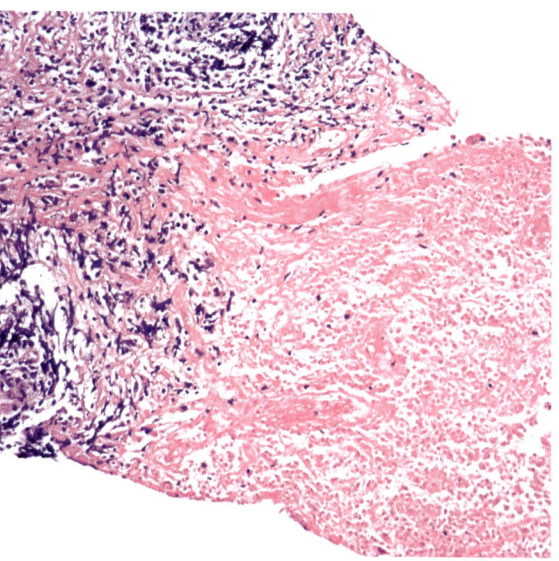

Figure 20-3

PRIMARY MEDIASTINAL LARGE B-CELL LYMPHOMA

Large lymphoma cells are compartmentalized into lobules by interstitial fibrosis. A few background small reactive lymphocytes are also present (H&E stain).

Figure 20-4

PRIMARY MEDIASTINAL LARGE B-CELL LYMPHOMA WITH NECROSIS

There is a large area of coagulative necrosis in this specimen (H&E stain).

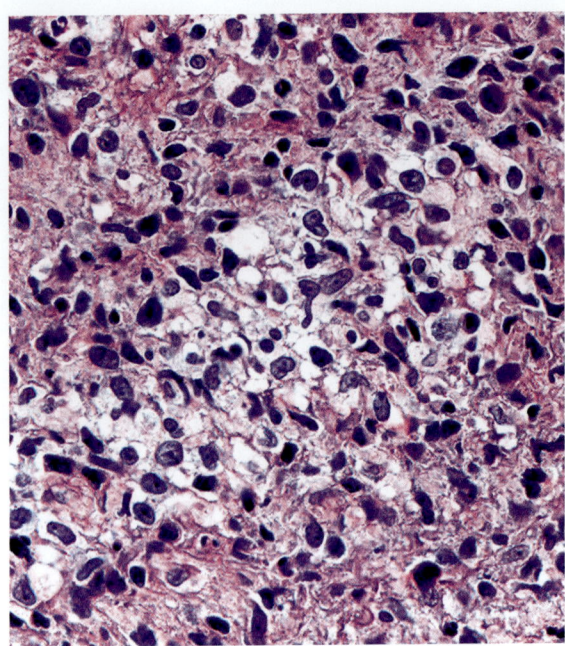

Figure 20-5

PRIMARY MEDIASTINAL LARGE B-CELL LYMPHOMA

The neoplastic cells have abundant clear cytoplasm and their nuclear contours are highly variable (H&E stain).

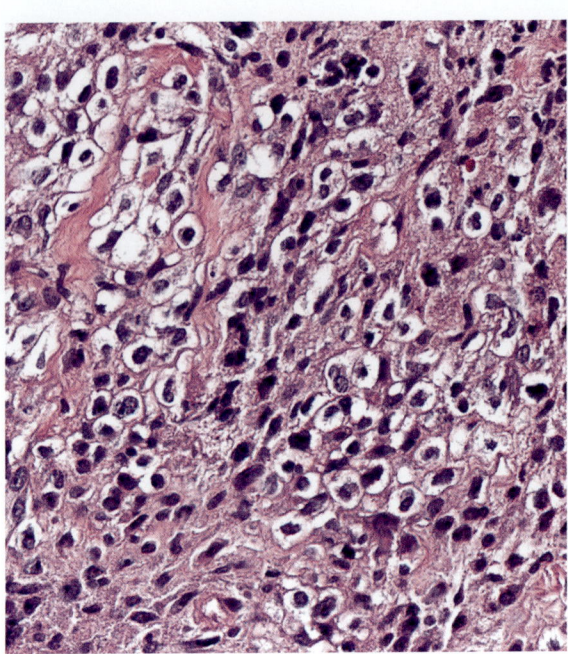

Figure 20-6

PRIMARY MEDIASTINAL LARGE B-CELL LYMPHOMA

The neoplastic cells are associated with abundant sclerosis and show marked retraction artifact of the cytoplasm (H&E stain).

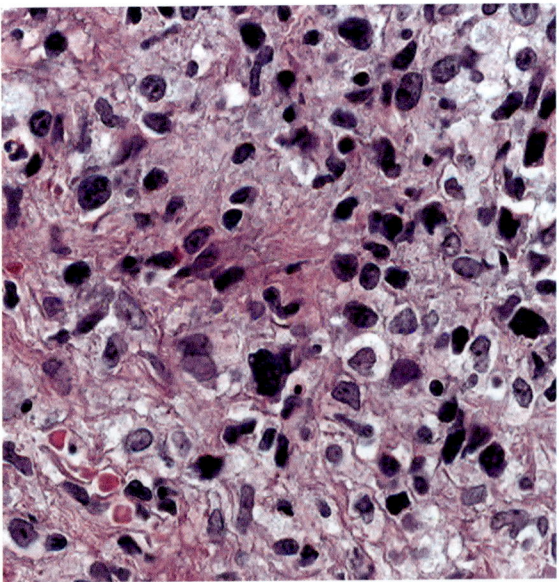

Figure 20-7

PRIMARY MEDIASTINAL LARGE B-CELL LYMPHOMA

The neoplastic cells have pale cytoplasm and nuclei with highly irregular contours, including polylobated and multinucleated forms (H&E stain).

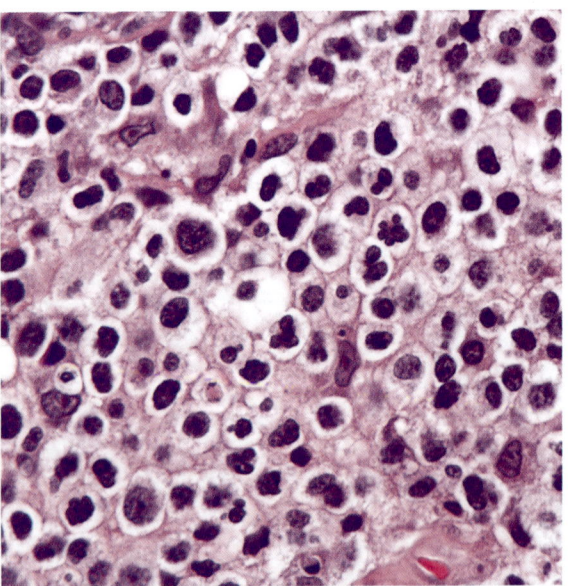

Figure 20-8

PRIMARY MEDIASTINAL LARGE B-CELL LYMPHOMA

The neoplastic cells exhibit a range in size, from intermediate-sized to large, with pale or retracted cytoplasm. Some tumor cell nuclei also show multilobation and "cloverleaf" forms (H&E stain).

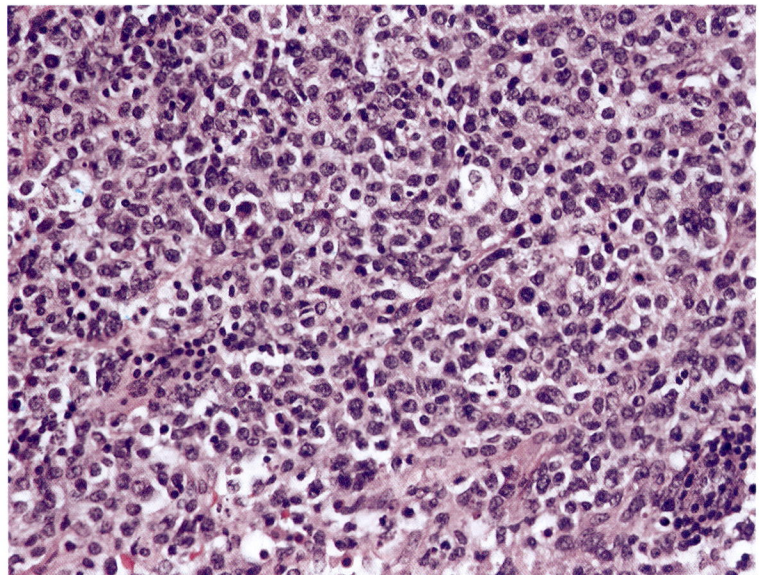

Figure 20-9

**PRIMARY MEDIASTINAL
LARGE B-CELL LYMPHOMA
INVOLVING LYMPH NODE**

A small lymph node involved by PMBL was at the periphery of a large mass in the mediastinum (same case as shown in fig. 20-2). The neoplastic cells diffusely efface the lymph node. Unlike the extranodal portion of this specimen, the neoplastic cells are not associated with fine sclerosis and show minimal cytoplasmic retraction artifact (H&E stain).

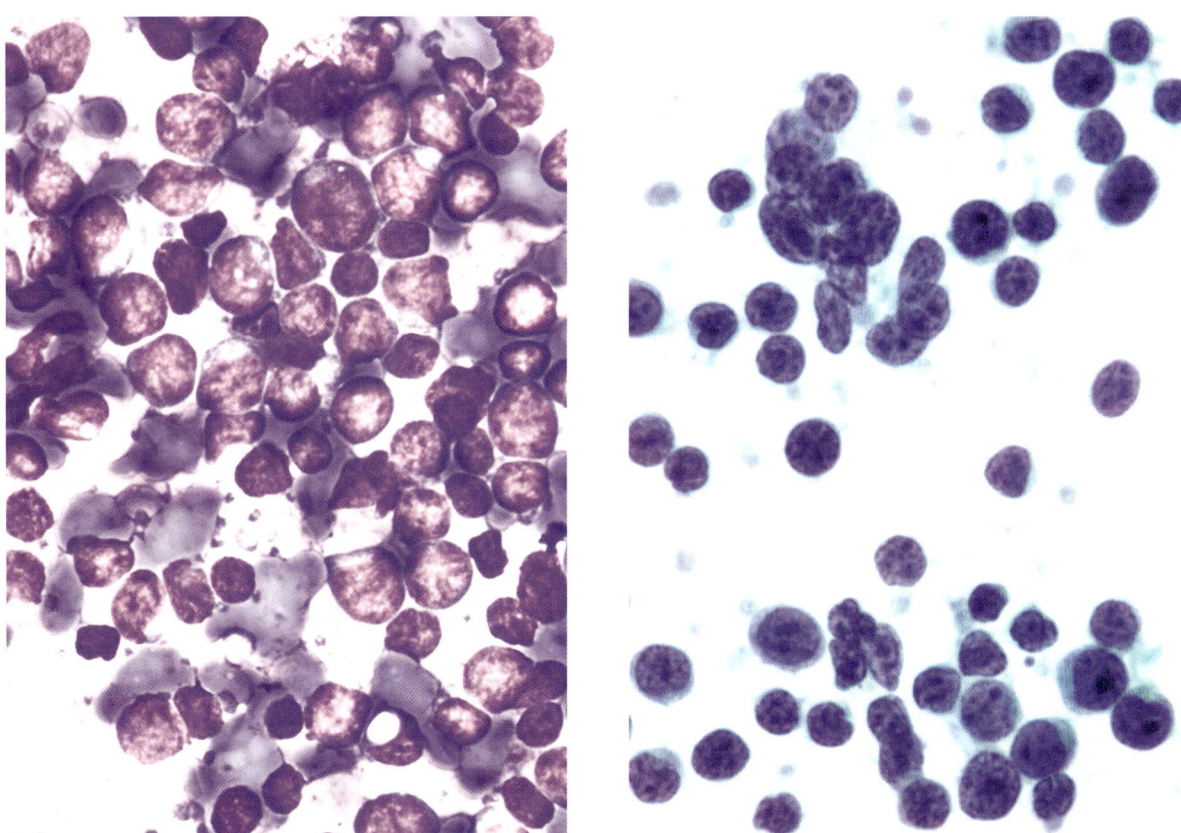

Figure 20-10

PRIMARY MEDIASTINAL LARGE B-CELL LYMPHOMA: CYTOLOGY

Left: This fine-needle aspiration smear shows medium to large tumor cells with round nuclei and nucleoli (Diff-Quik stain).

Right: The neoplastic cells occur singly or in loose aggregates (Papanicolaou stain).

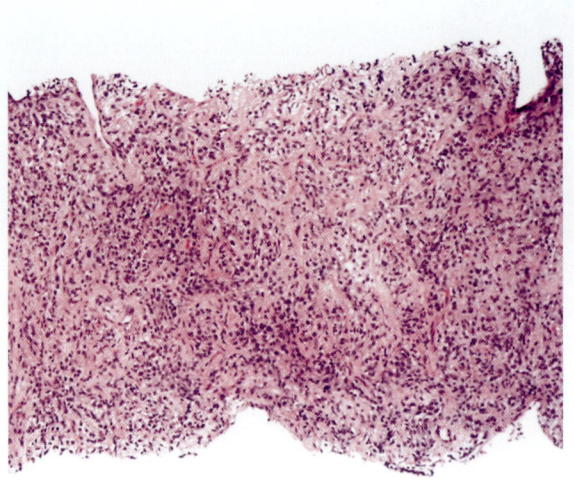
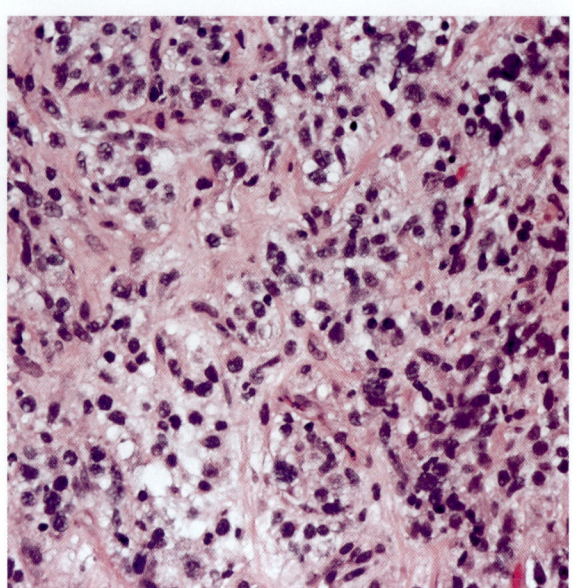

Figure 20-11

PRIMARY MEDIASTINAL LARGE B-CELL LYMPHOMA: NEEDLE BIOPSY

Left: This needle core biopsy specimen is completely replaced by lymphoma in a diffuse pattern.

Right: Large tumor cells with pale to clear cytoplasm are compartmentalized into groups by delicate fibrosis (left, right: H&E stain).

Lymphoglandular bodies may be numerous. Hypocellular smears are common and most likely attributable to the fibrosis associated with the tumor. In some cases, microscopic tissue fragments are aspirated that are well suited for analysis in a cell block specimen. In tissue sections of cell block or small needle biopsy specimens (fig. 20-11), however, it is common for the neoplastic cells to be somewhat distorted or crushed, thereby appearing elongated or spindled (30).

IMMUNOPHENOTYPIC FINDINGS

The neoplastic cells of PMBL express the pan-B-cell antigens CD19, CD20 (fig. 20-12), CD22, and CD79a, and also commonly express (with at least moderate intensity) the B-cell transcription factors PAX5, BOB.1, Oct-2, and PU.1 (14,17,21). Variable and often patchy expression of CD30 is observed in about 80 percent of cases (fig. 20-12E) (11,21). The neoplastic cells are commonly positive for MUM1/IRF4 (75 percent of cases), CD23 (about 70 percent), programmed cell death ligand 2 (PD-L2) (70 percent), MAL (about 70 percent), and CD200 (5,7,7a,29). BCL2, BCL6, PD-L1, TRAF1, and nuclear expression of c-REL are commonly expressed. Coexpression of

TRAF1 and nuclear c-REL is almost completely specific, but insensitive (about 50 percent of cases) for PMBL (24). The proliferation index is moderate to high as assessed by Ki-67 (fig. 20-12F).

MYC is expressed in 20 to 30 percent of PBMLs, and expression does not correlate with *MYC* rearrangements. CD10 expression has been reported in a minor subset of PBML cases (about 15 percent). PMBLs are commonly negative for immunoglobulin (14,21); HLA class I and II molecules are not expressed or are only weakly expressed by the neoplastic cells in most cases (23).

Cases of PMBL are negative for pan-T-cell antigens, CD34, TdT, cyclin D1, human herpesvirus (HHV)-8, Epstein-Barr virus (EBV), and most myeloid-associated antigens. FOXO1 is often negative in PMBL, unlike reactive B cells (36). CD15 is usually negative; rare cases of PMBL with CD15 expression have been reported (4).

MOLECULAR GENETIC FINDINGS

Cases of PMBL carry monoclonal immunoglobulin gene rearrangements, and the T-cell receptor genes are usually in the germline

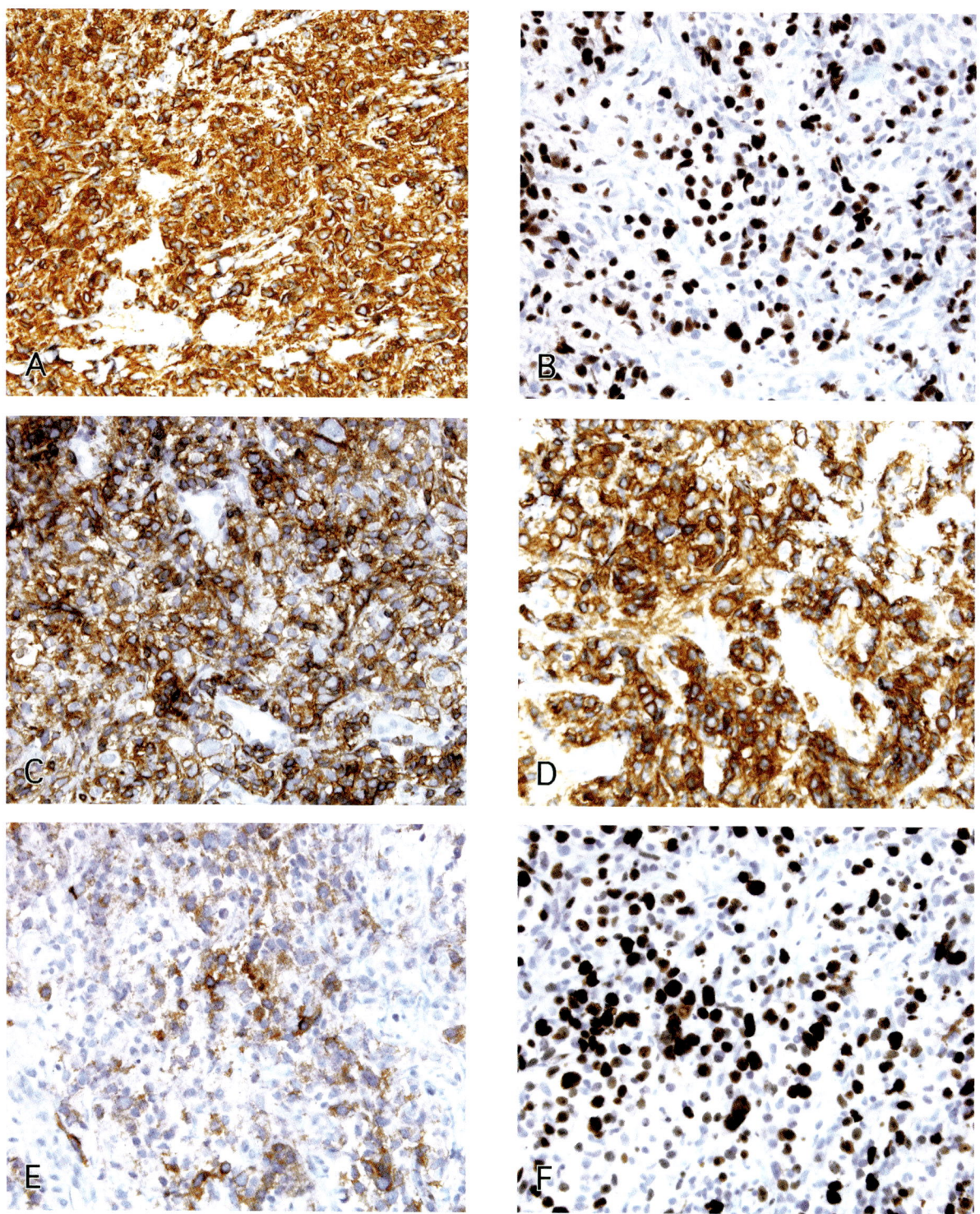

Figure 20-12

PRIMARY MEDIASTINAL LARGE B-CELL LYMPHOMA: IMMUNOHISTOCHEMISTRY

The neoplastic cells are brightly positive for CD20 (A), PAX5 (B), CD45/LCA (C), and CD23 (D); some tumor cells are variably and weakly positive for CD30 (E). The Ki-67 (proliferation) rate is moderate, about 40 to 50 percent (F) (immunohistochemistry with hematoxylin counterstain). (Same case as fig. 20-11.)

Table 20-1

COMMON GENETIC ABERRATIONS IN PRIMARY MEDIASTINAL LARGE B-CELL LYMPHOMA

Gene	Pathway or Function	Frequency
Translocation/Rearrangement		
CIITA	HLA class II/antigen presentation	~40%
PDL1/PDL2	Induction of T-cell exhaustion/apoptosis	~20%
BCL6	B-cell differentiation	Sporadic
Copy number gain/amplification		
REL	NF-κB PATHWAY	60-70%
PDL1/PDL2	Induction of T-cell exhaustion/apoptosis	~40%
JAK2	JAK-STAT pathway	~60%
JMJD2C	Histone modification	~60%
Gene mutations		
SOCS1	JAK-STAT pathway	50-60%
STAT6	JAK-STAT pathway	~40%
TNFAIP3	NF-κB pathway	~40%
MYC	Multipurpose transcription factor	20-30%
PTPN1	JAK-STAT pathway	~20%
NFKBIE (deletion)	NF-κB pathway	~20%
TP53	P53 pathway	~15%
TP16 (hypermethylation)	Cell cycle	~10%

configuration. The *IG* variable regions have a high degree of somatic hypermutations, but no ongoing mutations, suggesting that these cells traversed the germinal center as a part of their development (16).

Using conventional cytogenetic analysis, fluorescence in situ hybridization (FISH), whole exome sequencing, and other methods, many molecular abnormalities have been shown in PMBL (Table 20-1). Gains of the chromosomal loci 2p, 9p, 12q, and Xq are common (3,28,33). In 75 percent of cases, the common region of 9p gain is localized to 9p24.1, the location of *JAK2* (29,33). Gains of chromosome 2p15 involving *REL* occur in about half of PMBL cases (19,33,34). Rearrangements or gene fusions involving the major histocompatibility complex class II transactivator (*CIITA*) at chromosome 16p13 occur in 30 to 40 percent of cases (19,31). The rearrangement impairs expression of MHC class II molecules and therefore reduces tumor cell immunogenicity. *PD-L1/CD274* and *PD-L2/PDCD1LG2* at chromosome 9p24.1 are rearranged in about 20 percent of PMBL cases and this locus also shows amplification in a subset of tumors (8,31,33). Expression of PD-L1 or PD-L2 impairs the host T-cell response.

Rearrangements of *BCL6/3q27* have been reported inconsistently in a small subset of PMBL cases. Rearrangements of *MYC/8q24* are uncommon and there is no evidence of t(11;14)(q13;q32)/*CCND1-IGH*. t(14;18)(q32;q21/*IGH-BCL2* has been reported uncommonly in PMBL; the presence of t(14;18) raises the possibility of DLBCL, not otherwise specified (NOS), presenting initially in mediastinal lymph nodes.

Gene expression profiling studies have shown a distinctive signature for PMBL that distinguishes these tumors from cases of DL-BCL-NOS. High expression of specific genes located on 9p24, such as *JAK2*, *PD-L1*, *PD-L2*, and *SMARCA2*, is common and fairly distinctive for PMBCL (25,27). High expression of *MAL* and *FIG1* also reliably distinguishes PMBL from other forms of DLBCL (27).

Authors have reported similarities in the gene expression profile of PMBL and nodular sclerosis Hodgkin lymphoma (25,27). The degree of similarity is reported to be 30 to 40 percent. A major difference is in the expression of B-cell receptor signaling pathway genes, which is much higher in PMBL than nodular sclerosis Hodgkin lymphoma.

A variety of gene mutations and other abnormalities have been reported in PMBL (Table 20-1). Common genetic abnormalities in the JAK-STAT pathway include *JAK2* amplification (60 percent) and mutations of *SOCS1* (50 percent), *STAT6* (40 percent), and *PTPN1* (20 percent) (9,18,34). *SOCS11* and *PTPN1* function as tumor suppressors, and mutations inactivate these genes, thereby facilitating JAK-STAT activation. *REL/2p15* amplification (60 to 70 percent), *TNFAIP3* mutations (about 40 percent), and *NFKBIE* deletions (about 20 percent) are common molecular abnormalities that activate the NF-κB pathway (17a,38). *TNFAIP3* encodes for A20 protein, a negative regulator of the NF-κB pathway. Other genetic mutations reported in PMBL include: *MYC* (20 to 30 percent), *TP53* (about 15 percent), and less often *BCL6*. *TP16* is inactivated by hypermethylation or rarely mutation or 9p locus deletion in about 10 percent of cases.

DIFFERENTIAL DIAGNOSIS

Diffuse Large B-Cell Lymphoma, Not Otherwise Specified (DLBCL-NOS). DLBCL-NOS can involve mediastinal lymph nodes and present as a mediastinal mass. Affected patients are older and the mass is smaller than in patients with PMBL. Using standard clinical, morphologic, and immunophenotypic criteria, particularly in a fine-needle aspiration or needle biopsy specimens, it may be difficult to distinguish PMBL from DLBCL-NOS involving mediastinal lymph nodes (see above). Histologic evidence of lymphoma involving the thymus gland supports PMBL. Evidence of expression of CD23, CD30, MAL, TRAF1, nuclear REL, PD-L1 or PD-L2, and CD200 also supports PMBL although these markers are not entirely specific. It seems likely that molecular markers, some near to being available for routine clinical diagnosis, will be helpful in this differential diagnosis.

Nodular Sclerosis Hodgkin Lymphoma. Hodgkin lymphoma can involve the thymus or mediastinal lymph nodes. Cases with many Reed-Sternberg and Hodgkin cells, so-called grade 2 or syncytial variant cases, in particular, share morphologic features with PMBL. Features that support nodular sclerosis Hodgkin lymphoma include well-developed sclerotic bands and a typical immunophenotype: CD15(+), CD30(+), and CD45/LCA(-). Unlike PMBL, B-cell antigens and transcription factors are not expressed or only weakly expressed in most cases of Hodgkin lymphoma. Evidence of EBV, seen in approximately 20 percent of nodular sclerosis Hodgkin lymphomas, is unusual in PMBL.

B-Cell Lymphoma, Unclassifiable, with Features Between Diffuse Large B-Cell Lymphoma and Classic Hodgkin Lymphoma. These tumors, also known as gray zone lymphomas, exhibit a spectrum of features. Some of these tumors morphologically mimic classic Hodgkin lymphoma, but the immunophenotype is much more similar to PMBL (e.g., bright CD20). Other gray zone lymphomas may morphologically mimic PMBL, but have some immunophenotypic features similar to classic Hodgkin lymphoma (positive for CD15 and CD30, and negative for CD45/LCA). Morphologic features that are either Hodgkin-like or non-Hodgkin-like are not mutually exclusive; a mixture of morphologic features in an individual gray zone lymphoma is common.

Thymic Tumors. Some thymomas and thymic carcinomas are composed of many large epithelioid cells that may resemble, in part, PMBL. Epithelial variants of thymoma and thymic carcinomas are cohesive tumors and carcinomas commonly show atypia, necrosis, and a high mitotic rate. Immunohistochemical studies show that the neoplastic cells express keratins and other epithelial markers and are negative for CD20 and other B-cell markers.

Mediastinal Germ Cell Tumors. These tumors occasionally mimic lymphoma. In particular, embryonal carcinoma can be composed of sheets of large cells that express CD30. These tumors, however, express germ cell markers (e.g., OCT 3/4) and are negative for CD20 and other B-cell markers.

TREATMENT AND PROGNOSIS

The prognosis of patients with PMBL has been controversial. Early studies indicated a poor prognosis, likely attributable to tumor bulk. More recent studies suggest that patients with PMBL have a prognosis that is similar to, and in some studies better, than patients with DLBCL-NOS (17a,22,26,27,38). Negative predictors of survival in patients with PMBL include a serum lactate dehydrogenase (LDH) level two times above the upper limit of normal, poor performance status, male sex, and advanced-stage disease (35,38). To date, the genetic abnormalities in PBML have had little impact on prognostication or choice of therapy. In a preliminary analysis, *CIITA* rearrangements correlated with a poorer prognosis (31).

The optimal therapy for patients with PMBCL is evolving. Over the years, patients have been treated with variable success using the CHOP or R-CHOP chemotherapy regimens, and R-CHOP with radiation therapy has been the recent standard of care (1,6,10,15,17a,35,38). Radiation therapy is considered an integral component of the treatment regimen, in large part because these tumors are often bulky, and this approach has been effective treatment (22). However, there is a desire to get away from radiation therapy because of the long-term sequelae, such as an increased risk of breast carcinoma in women (6).

More recently, the rituximab, etoposide, vincristine, cyclophosphamide, and doxorubicin (R-EPOCH) chemotherapy regimen, an infusional regimen that is dose adjusted, has been shown to be highly effective for patients with PMBL (6). Proponents of this approach have emphasized that the use of rituximab and the success of the R-EPOCH regimen obviates the need for radiation therapy (6). Other authors believe that radiation is still required for optimal outcome (13). The role of radiation therapy in the treatment of patients with PMBL is still evolving and additional clinical trials are needed to further address the value of the R-EPOCH regimen as well as the role of radiation therapy in the treatment of PMBL patients.

REFERENCES

1. Ahn HJ, Yoon DH, Kim S, et al. Primary mediastinal large B-cell lymphoma: a single-center experience in Korea. Blood Res 2014;49:36-41.
2. Barth TF, Leithauser F, Joos S, Bentz M, Möller P. Mediastinal (thymic) large B-cell lymphoma: where do we stand? Lancet Oncol 2002;3:229-234.
3. Bentz M, Barth TF, Bruderlein S, et al. Gain of chromosome arm 9p is characteristic of primary mediastinal B-cell lymphoma (MBL): comprehensive molecular cytogenetic analysis and presentation of a novel MBL cell line. Genes Chromosomes Cancer 2001;30:393-401.
4. Cazals-Hatem D, Lepage E, Brice P, et al. Primary mediastinal large B-cell lymphoma. A clinicopathologic study of 141 cases compared with 916 nonmediastinal large B-cell lymphomas, a GELA ("Groupe d'Etude des Lymphomes de l'Adulte") study. Am J Surg Pathol 1996;20:877-888.
5. Dorfman DM, Shahsafaei A, Alonso MA. Utility of CD200 immunostaining in the diagnosis of primary mediastinal large B cell lymphoma: comparison with MAL, CD23, and other markers. Mod Pathol 2012;25:1637-1643.
6. Dunleavy K, Wilson WH. Primary mediastinal B-cell lymphoma and mediastinal gray zone lymphoma: do they require a unique therapeutic approach? Blood 2015;125:33-39.
7. Gaulard P, Harris NL, Pileri SA, et al. Primary mediastinal (thymic) large B-cell lymphoma. In: Swedlow SH, Campo E, Harris NL, Jaffe ES, Pileri SA, Stein H, Thiele J, Vardiman JW, eds.. WHO classification of tumours of haematopoietic and lymphoid tissues. Lyon: IARC Press; 2008;250-251.
7a. Gentry M, Bodo J, Durkin L, Hsi ED. Performance of a commercially available MAL antibody in the diagnosis of primary mediastinal large B-cell lymphoma. Am J Surg Pathol 2017;41:189-194.
8. Green MR, Monti S, Rodig SJ, et al. Integrative analysis reveals selective 9p24.1 amplification, increased PD-1 ligand expression, and further induction via JAK2 in nodular sclerosing Hodgkin lymphoma and primary mediastinal large B-cell lymphoma. Blood 2010;116:3268-3277.
9. Gunawardana J, Chan FC, Telenius A, et al. Recurrent somatic mutations of PTPN1 in primary mediastinal B cell lymphoma and Hodgkin lymphoma. Nat Genet 2014;46:329-335.
10. Hamlin PA, Portlock CS, Straus DJ, et al. Primary mediastinal large B-cell lymphoma: optimal therapy and prognostic factor analysis in 141 consecutive patients treated at Memorial Sloan Kettering from 1980 to 1999. Br J Haematol 2005;130:691-699.
11. Higgins JP, Warnke RA. CD30 expression is common in mediastinal large B-cell lymphoma. Am J Clin Pathol 1999;112:241-247.
12. Isaccson PG, Norton AJ, Addis BJ. The human thymus contains a novel population of B lymphocytes. Lancet 1987;2:1488-1491.
13. Jackson MW, Rusthoven CG, Jones BL, Kamdar M, Rabinovitch R. Improved survival with combined modality therapy in the modern era for primary mediastinal B-cell lymphoma. Am J Hematol 2016;91:476-480.
14. Kanavaros P, Gaulard P, Charlotte F, et al. Discordant expression of immunoglobulin and its associated molecule mb-1/CD79a is frequently found in mediastinal large B cell lymphomas. Am J Pathol 1995;146:735-741.

15. Lazzarino M, Orlandi E, Paulli M, et al. Treatment outcome and prognostic factors for primary mediastinal (thymic) B-cell lymphoma: a multicenter study of 106 patients. J Clin Oncol 1997;15:1646-1653.

16. Leithauser F, Bauerle M, Huynh MQ, Möller P. Isotype-switched immunoglobulin genes with a high load of somatic hypermutation and lack of ongoing mutational activity are prevalent in mediastinal B-cell lymphoma. Blood 2001;98:2762-2770.

17. Mansouri L, Noerenberg D, Young E, et al. Frequent NFKBIE deletions are associated with poor outcome in primary mediastinal B-cell lymphoma. Blood 2016;128:2666-2670.

17a. Martelli M, Ferreri A, Di Rocco A, Ansuinelli M, Johnson PW. Primary mediastinal large B-cell lymphoma. Crit Rev Oncol Hematol 2017;113:318-327.

18. Mestre C, Rubio-Moscardo F, Rosenwald A, et al. Homozygous deletion of SOCS1 in primary mediastinal B-cell lymphoma detected by CGH to BAC microarrays. Leukemia 2005;19:1082-1084.

19. Mottok A, Woolcock B, Chan FC, et al. Genomic alterations in CIITA are frequent in primary mediastinal large B cell lymphoma and are associated with diminished MHC class II expression. Cell Rep 2015;13:1418-1431.

20. Paulli M, Strater J, Gianelli U, et al. Mediastinal B-cell lymphoma: a study of its histomorphologic spectrum based on 109 cases. Hum Pathol 1999;30:178-187.

21. Pileri SA, Gaidano G, Zinzani PL, et al. Primary mediastinal B-cell lymphoma: high frequency of BCL-6 mutations and consistent expression of the transcription factors OCT-2, BOB.1, and PU.1 in the absence of immunoglobulins. Am J Pathol 2003;162:243-253.

22. Pinnix CC, Dabaja B, Ahmed MA, et al. Single-institution experience in the treatment of primary mediastinal B cell lymphoma treated with immunochemotherapy in the setting of response assessment by 18fluorodeoxyglucose positron emission tomography. Int J Radiat Biol Phys 2015;92:113-121.

23. Roberts R, Wright G, Rosenwald A, et al. Loss of major histocompatibility class II gene and protein expression in primary mediastinal large B-cell lymphoma is highly coordinated and related to poor patient survival. Blood 2006;108:311-318.

24. Rodig S, Savage KJ, LaCasce AS, et al. Expression of TRAF1 and nuclear c-Rel distinguishes primary mediastinal large cell lymphoma from other types of diffuse large B-cell lymphoma. Am J Surg Pathol 2007;31:106-112.

25. Rosenwald A, Wright G, Leroy K, et al. Molecular diagnosis of primary mediastinal B cell lymphoma identifies a clinically favorable subgroup of diffuse large B cell lymphoma related to Hodgkin lymphoma. J Exp Med 2003;198:851-862.

26. Savage KJ, Al-Rajhi N, Voss N, et al. Favorable outcome of primary mediastinal large B-cell lymphoma in a single institution: the British Columbia experience. Ann Oncol 2006;17:123-130.

27. Savage KJ, Monti S, Kutok JL, et al. The molecular signature of mediastinal large B-cell lymphoma differs from that of other diffuse large B-cell lymphomas and shares features with classical Hodgkin lymphoma. Blood 2003;102:3871-3879.

28. Scarpa A, Taruscio D, Scardoni M, et al. Nonrandom chromosomal imbalances in primary mediastinal B-cell lymphoma detected by arbitrarily primed PCR fingerprinting. Genes Chromosomes Cancer 1999;26:203-209.

29. Shi M, Roemer MG, Chapuy B, et al. Expression of programmed cell death 1 ligand 2 (PD-L2) is a distinguishing feature of primary mediastinal (thymic) large B-cell lymphoma and associated with PDCD1LG2 copy gain. Am J Surg Pathol 2014;38:1715-1723.

30. Silverman JF, Raab SS, Park HK. Fine-needle aspiration cytology of primary large-cell lymphoma of the mediastinum: cytomorphologic findings with potential pitfalls in diagnosis. Diagn Cytopathol 1993;9:209-14.

31. Steidl C, Shah SP, Woolcock BW, et al. MHC class II transactivator CIITA is a recurrent gene fusion partner in lymphoid cancers. Nature 2011;471:377-381.

32. Taubenberger JK, Jaffe ES, Medeiros LJ. Thymoma with abundant L26-positive "asteroid" cells. A case report with an analysis of normal thymus and thymoma specimens. Arch Pathol Lab Med 1991;115:1254-1257.

33. Twa DD, Chan FC, Ben-Neriah S, et al. Genomic rearrangements involving programmed death ligands are recurrent in primary mediastinal large B-cell lymphoma. Blood 2014;123:2062-2065.

34. Twa DD, Steidl C. Structural genomic alterations in primary mediastinal large B-cell lymphoma. Leuk Lymphoma 2015;56:2239-2250.

35. van Besien K, Kelta M, Bahaguna P. Primary mediastinal B-cell lymphoma: a review of pathology and management. J Clin Oncol 2001;19:1855-1864.

36. Xie L, Ritz O, Leithäuser F, et al. FOXO1 downregulation contributes to the oncogenic program of primary mediastinal B-cell lymphoma. Oncotarget 2014;5:5392-5402.

37. Yuan J, Wright G, Rosenwald A, et al. Identification of primary mediastinal large B-cell lymphoma at nonmediastinal sites by gene expression profiling. Am J Surg Pathol 2015;39:1322-1330.

38. Zinzani PL, Piccaluga PP. Primary mediastinal DLBCL: evolving biologic understanding and therapeutic strategies. Curr Oncol Rep 2011;13:407-415.

21 ANAPLASTIC LYMPHOMA KINASE-POSITIVE LARGE B-CELL LYMPHOMA

GENERAL FEATURES

Anaplastic lymphoma kinase (ALK)-positive large B-cell lymphoma is a type of non-Hodgkin lymphoma characterized by a diffuse proliferation of monomorphic large B cells with immunoblastic or plasmablastic features that express ALK protein (6). ALK-positive large B-cell lymphoma is a rare tumor. In a review of the literature Sakamoto et al. (17) identified 112 cases and Pan et al. (15) subsequently reported an additional 26 cases.

The most distinctive feature of this type of B-cell lymphoma is the aberrant expression of ALK protein as a result of chromosomal abnormalities, most often translocations, involving the *ALK* locus at chromosome 2p23 (6). The most common abnormality is t(2;17)(p23;q23), which creates a chimeric *CLATHRIN-ALK* fusion gene (6,8). Other less common abnormalities involving *ALK* also have been reported.

CLINICAL FEATURES

The median age of affected patients is in the fourth decade, but there is a wide age range, from 9 to 85 years of age (1,10,15,17); 10 to 15 percent of patients are under 18 years of age. The male to female ratio is approximately 3 or 4 to 1. There is no association with any geographic region. Rare patients with human immunodeficiency virus (HIV) infection are reported (19). A patient with ulcerative colitis on immunosuppressive therapy who developed ALK-positive B-cell lymphoma has been reported (15a).

The lymph nodes are most often involved, with the cervical region involved in about two thirds of patients (15,17). However, other lymph node groups can be involved as well as a wide variety of extranodal sites (15,17). Reported extranodal sites include brain, Waldeyer ring (nasopharynx, tongue), gastrointestinal tract, liver, spleen, ovary, bones, and bone marrow (1,3,4,10,15,17). Patients with ALK-positive large B-cell lymphoma commonly present with stage III or IV disease (6,17).

HISTOLOGIC FINDINGS

ALK-positive large B-cell lymphoma is characterized by a monotonous proliferation of large lymphoid cells arranged in a diffuse pattern (fig 21-1) (1,6,10,15,16). The neoplastic cells have a propensity for sinusoidal infiltration (fig. 21-1, right). They have abundant amphophilic cytoplasm and contain single or multiple large nuclei, with round, central, and prominent nucleoli. These cells most often exhibit immunoblast-like features (21-2, left) but some show prominent plasmablastic features (fig. 21-2, right). Multinucleated giant cells are present in some cases. Mitotic figures and apoptotic cells are often numerous (fig. 21-3A). Necrosis may be present.

In bone marrow aspirate smears, the neoplastic cells are large, with abundant cytoplasm (fig. 21-4A). In bone marrow biopsy specimens, these neoplasms focally or diffusely replace the bone marrow medullary space (fig. 21-4B). A paratrabecular pattern is unusual.

CYTOLOGIC FINDINGS

In cytologic smears, the cells of ALK-positive large B-cell lymphoma resemble those described in histologic sections (13,17a). The cells are large, with large nuclei, prominent central nucleoli, and moderately abundant cytoplasm (fig. 21-5). The nucleus may be eccentric with a prominent perinuclear "hof." Scattered multinucleated giant cells may be found and are prominent in some cases. Mitotic figures, apoptotic bodies, and reactive small lymphocytes are present in the background.

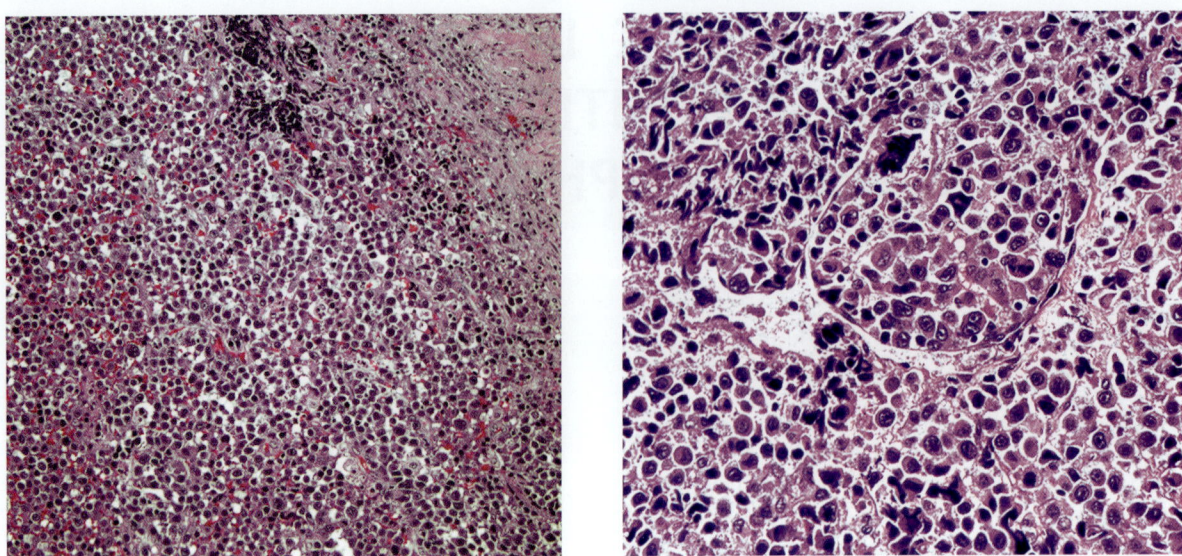

Figure 21-1

ANAPLASTIC LYMPHOMA KINASE-POSITIVE LARGE B-CELL LYMPHOMA

Left: There is diffuse effacement of the tissue by sheets of large atypical lymphoid cells.
Right: The sinusoids are involved by lymphoma (left, right: hematoxylin and eosin [H&E] stain).

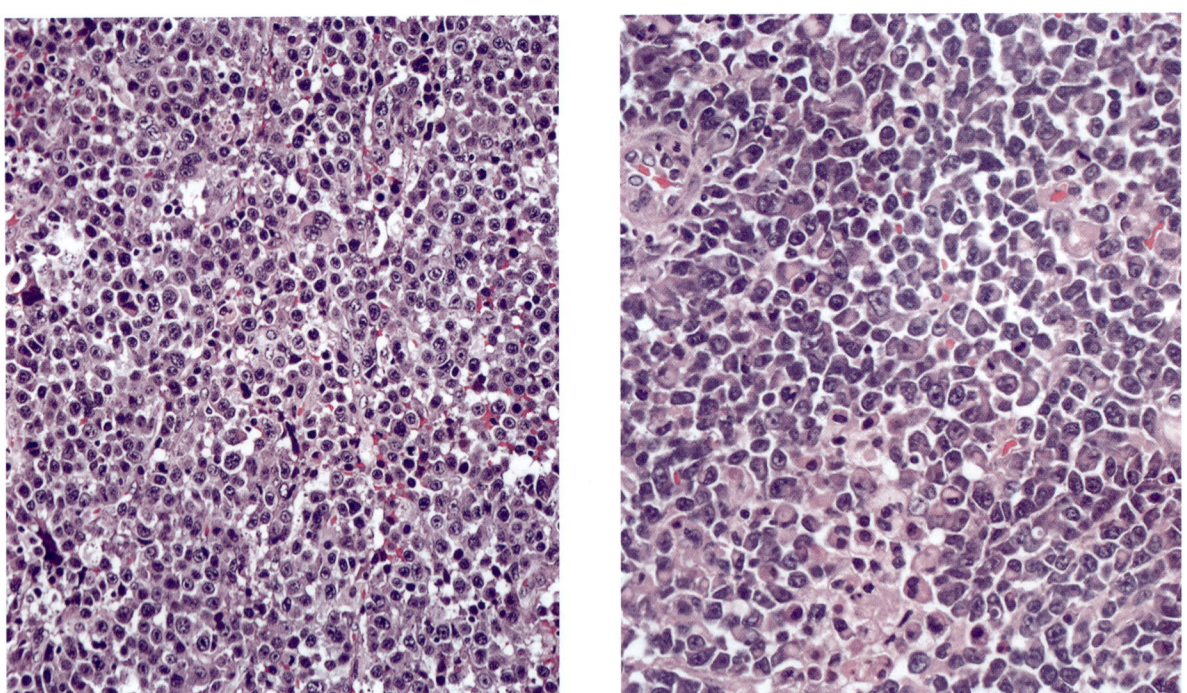

Figure 21-2

ANAPLASTIC LYMPHOMA KINASE-POSITIVE LARGE B-CELL LYMPHOMA: NUCLEAR FEATURES

Left: In this case the lymphoma cells show features of immunoblasts with prominent nuclear membranes and distinct central nucleoli.
Right: In contrast, this case has neoplastic cells with eccentrically located nuclei and abundant eosinophilic cytoplasm more in keeping with plasmablasts (left, right: H&E stain).

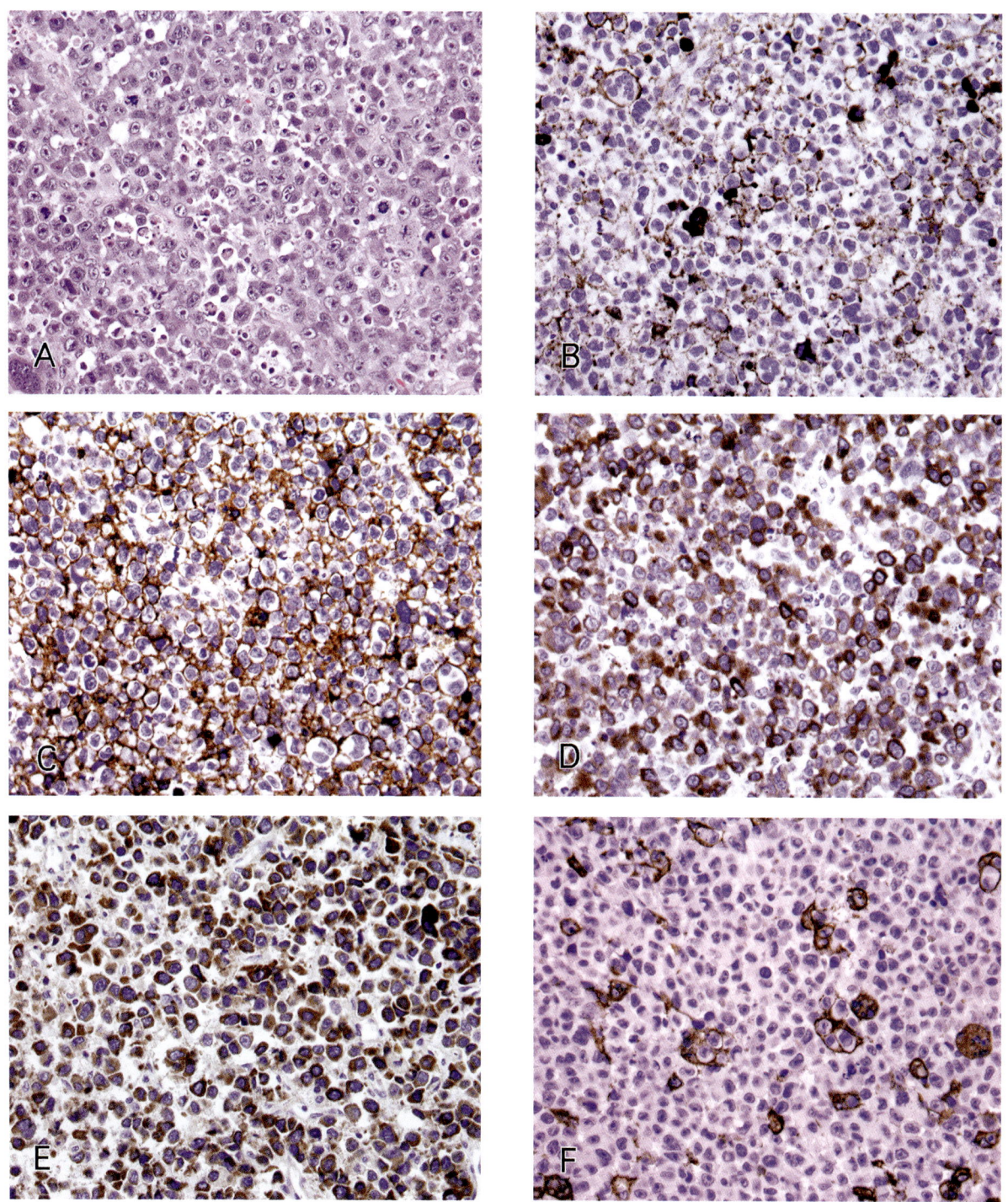

Figure 21-3

ANAPLASTIC LYMPHOMA KINASE-POSITIVE LARGE B-CELL LYMPHOMA: IMMUNOPHENOTYPE

A: The neoplastic cells have prominent nucleoli and abundant eosinophilic cytoplasm, consistent with plasmablastic features. The mitotic figures and apoptotic cells indicate that the tumor is highly proliferative (H&E stain).

B–F. Using immunohistochemistry, the neoplastic cells are positive for CD138 (B), CD45/LCA (C), CD79A (D), cytoplasmic IgA (E) and a small subset is positive for CD4 (F). Lymphocytes and histiocytes in F are also positive for CD4 (B–F: immunohistochemistry with hematoxylin counterstain).

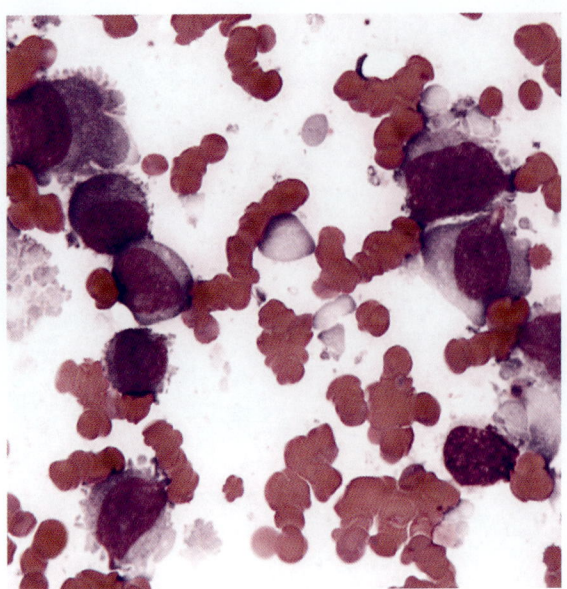 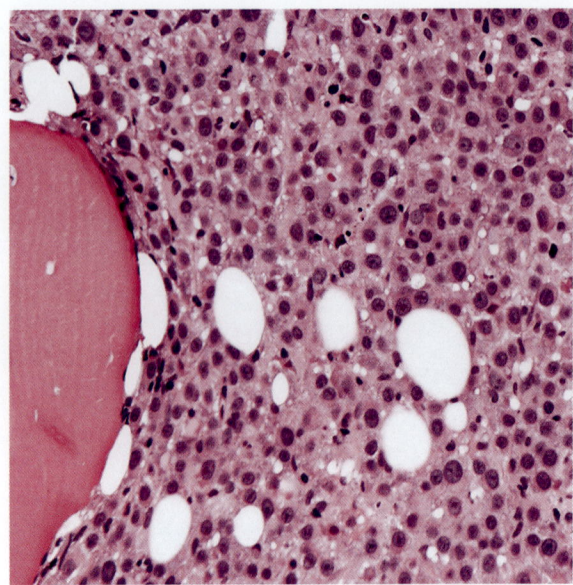

Figure 21-4

ANAPLASTIC LYMPHOMA KINASE-POSITIVE LARGE B-CELL LYMPHOMA INVOLVING BONE MARROW

Left: The aspirate smear shows large neoplastic cells with abundant cytoplasm and irregular borders (Wright-Giemsa stain).
Right: The tumor diffusely replaces the medullary space (H&E stain).

IMMUNOPHENOTYPIC FINDINGS

ALK-positive large B-cell lymphoma cells have a plasmablastic immunophenotype: positive for CD138 (fig. 21-3B) and negative for CD20. These tumors also express a variety of other markers associated with plasmacytoid differentiation including CD38, vs38c, epithelial membrane antigen (EMA), BLIMP1, XBP1, and IRF4/MUM1 (6,21). CD45/LCA (fig. 21-3C) and CD79A (fig. 21-3D) are expressed in some cases.

ALK-positive large B-cell lymphomas typically express cytoplasmic immunoglobulin. The light chain is more often lambda than kappa and the heavy chain is usually IgA (fig. 21-3E), but IgG can be expressed (6,10).

Valera et al. (21) have shown that most ALK-positive large B-cell lymphomas express nuclear and phosphorylated STAT3 (evidence of activation) and MYC. Beta-catenin in a cytoplasmic pattern may be expressed and may contribute to STAT3 activation (5).

There is focal reactivity for CD4 (fig. 21-3F), CD43, or CD57 in a subset of cases (6,10,16,19). In one small study, all three cases of ALK-positive large B-cell lymphoma assessed were positive for napsin A (9). Most cases are negative for CD30, but some may be weakly positive (19).

Some cases are positive for perforin, but TIA-1 and granzyme B have been negative in scattered reports (5,18,19). Cytokeratin can be expressed, usually weakly, in these tumors (11).

ALK-positive large B-cell lymphomas are negative for T-cell–specific antigens including CD5 as well as B-cell antigens including CD10, CD19, CD22, PAX5, and BCL6. In one report, OCT2 and BOB1 were positive in a tumor negative for CD19, CD20, and PAX5 (5). BCL2 is usually negative. CD56 and histiocyte-associated markers are usually negative. Cyclin D1 and human herpesvirus 8 (HHV-8) are negative. There is no evidence of Epstein-Barr virus (EBV) infection.

By definition, ALK-positive large B-cell lymphomas express ALK protein. ALK is usually expressed uniformly by the cells, either brightly or moderately (fig. 21-6), but rarely, ALK is expressed by only a subset of tumor cells. The pattern of ALK reactivity correlates well with the molecular abnormality involving the *ALK* locus (described below).

MOLECULAR GENETIC FINDINGS

Complex karyotypes have been reported in approximately half of ALK-positive large B-cell lymphoma cases that have been studied by

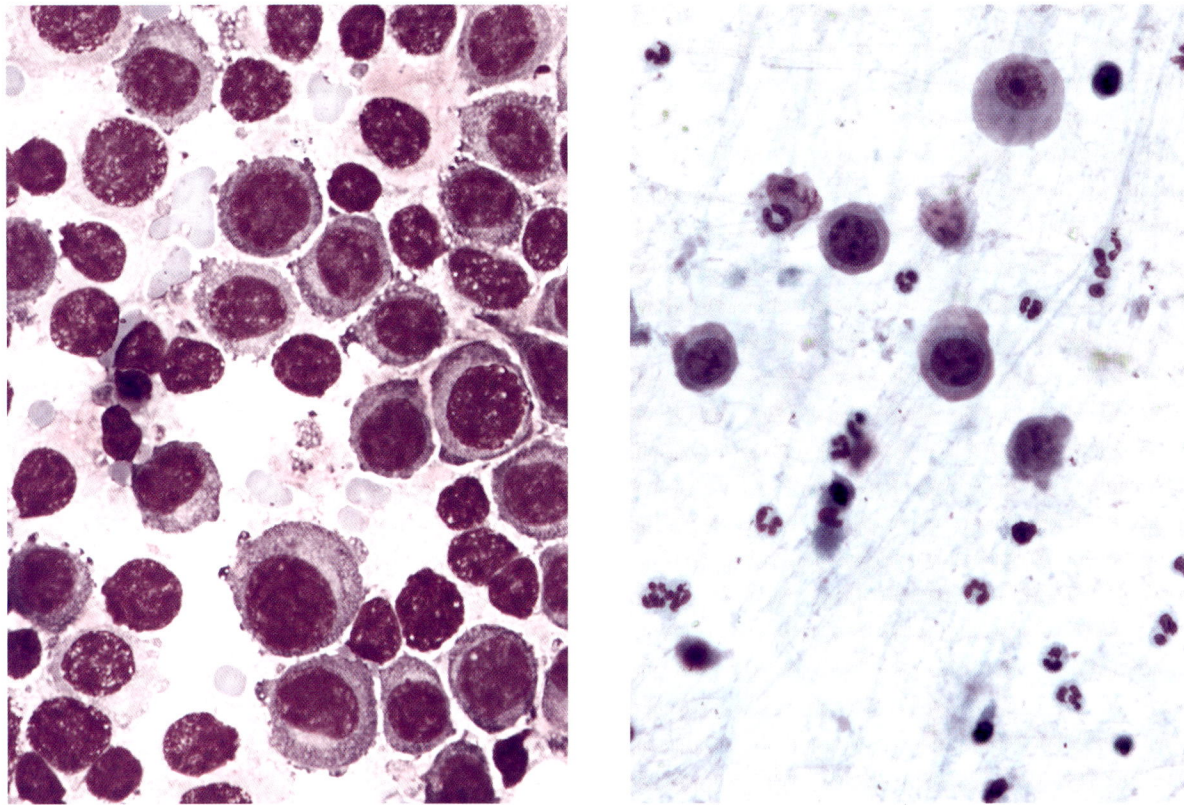

Figure 21-5

ANAPLASTIC LYMPHOMA KINASE-POSITIVE LARGE B-CELL LYMPHOMA: CYTOLOGIC FEATURES

The tumor cells are large, with round nuclei and abundant cytoplasm (left: Diff-Quik stain; right: Papanicolaou stain).

conventional cytogenetics. ALK-positive large B-cell lymphomas usually carry monoclonal immunoglobulin gene loci rearrangements (4,10) and are derived from post-germinal center B cells. The T-cell receptor genes are usually in the germline configuration. There is no evidence of t(11;14)(q13;q32)/*CCND1-IGH*, t(14;18) (q32;q21)/*IGH-BCL2*, or translocations involving *MYC* (6,21).

The most frequent translocation associated with ALK-positive large B-cell lymphoma is t(2;17)(p23;q23)/*CLTC-ALK* (Table 21-1) (6,8). A few cases carry t(2;5)(p23;q35), resulting in the chimeric *NPM-ALK* fusion (14,22). Other rare cases carry different translocations: t(2;5) (p23;q34.2)/*SDQTM1-ALK*, t(2;2)(p23;p13)/ *RANB2-ALK*, t(2;2)(p21;p23)/*EML4-ALK*, and rearrangements of *SEC31A* (5,12,20,22). Other abnormalities are also recognized, but are not fully characterized (18,19). In the initial paper describing ALK-positive large B-cell lymphoma,

full length ALK protein expression was reported (7). In retrospect, many of these cases were shown to carry *ALK* locus translocations (8) and did not express full length ALK.

ALK Expression Pattern and Molecular Abnormalities

The pattern of ALK reactivity correlates well with the *ALK* locus abnormality. Most cases of ALK-positive large B-cell lymphoma exhibit a coarse and granular (or fluffy) cytoplasmic pattern of expression (fig. 21-6) that correlates well with t(2;17)/*CLTC-ALK*. Clathrin is a component of the membrane of cytoplasmic microvesicles and is involved in intracellular transport. Some cases show nuclear and cytoplasmic ALK reactivity, reflecting the presence of t(2;5)(p23;q35)/ *NPM-ALK*. NPM can shuttle between the nucleus and cytoplasm taking ALK with it. In one case involving RANBP2, the pattern of ALK expression was that of the nuclear membrane associated

Table 21-1

ALK LOCUS ABNORMALITIES IN ALK-POSITIVE LARGE B-CELL LYMPHOMA

Cytogenetic Abnormality	ALK Partner	Pattern of ALK Immunoreactivity
t(2;17)(p23;q23)	Clathrin	Cytoplasmic and coarsely granular
t(2;5)(p23;q35)	Nucleophosmin	Nuclear and cytoplasmic
t(2;5)(p23;q34.2)	SQSTM1	Cytoplasmic
Often cryptic as part of a complex karyotype	SEC31A	Cytoplasmic
t(2;2)(p23;q13)	RANBP2	Membranous and perinuclear dot-like
t(2;2)(p21;p23)	EML4	Cytoplasmic and diffuse (nongranular)
Insertion of 3' *ALK* into 4q22-24	Unknown	Cytoplasmic
t(X;2)(q21;p23)	Unknown	Cytoplasmic
t(2;12)(p23;q24.1)	Unknown	Cytoplasmic

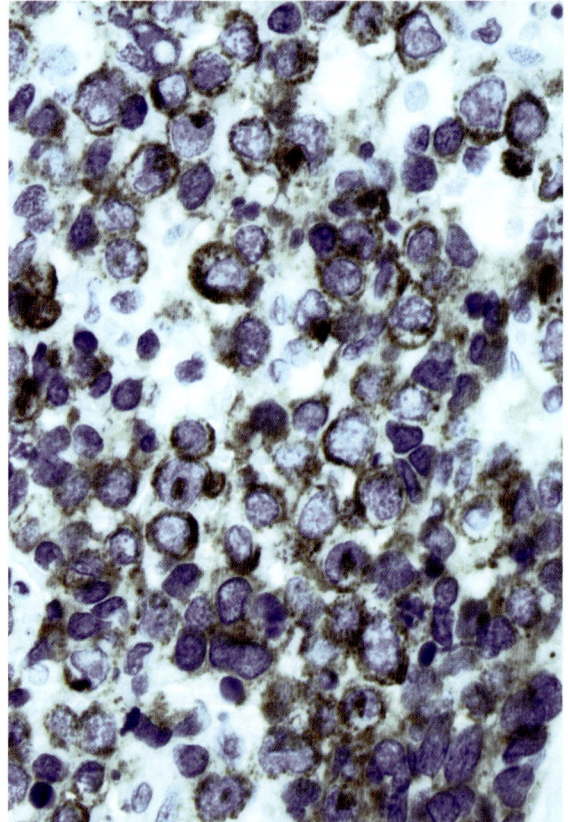

Figure 21-6

**ANAPLASTIC LYMPHOMA KINASE-POSITIVE
LARGE B-CELL LYMPHOMA ASSESSED FOR ALK**

Intermediate to strong, granular and cytoplasmic expression of ALK in the neoplastic cells is seen. This pattern most often correlates with t(2;17)/*CLATHRIN-ALK* (immunohistochemistry with hematoxylin counterstain).

with a perinuclear dot-like pattern (12). Other *ALK* locus aberrations reported have resulted in a cytoplasmic and finely granular or diffuse pattern of ALK expression.

DIFFERENTIAL DIAGNOSIS

Plasmablastic Lymphoma. Plasmablastic lymphoma also has plasmablastic morphology and an immunophenotype similar to that of ALK-positive large B-cell lymphoma. Plasmablastic lymphoma is commonly associated with immunodeficiency, particularly HIV infection, and usually involves extranodal sites. Approximately 70 percent of plasmablastic lymphomas have evidence of EBV infection and ALK is not expressed.

Primary Effusion Lymphoma (PEL), Extracavitary (Solid) Variant. PEL is another neoplasm with plasmablastic morphology and immunophenotype. These tumors are also associated with immunodeficiency, most often HIV, involve extranodal sites, and are often positive for EBV infection. Most helpful, PEL cases are positive for HHV8 infection. ALK is not expressed.

Plasmacytoma and Plasma Cell Myeloma. Plasma cell neoplasms usually have more fully developed plasmacytic differentiation at the morphologic level and appear more differentiated/ mature, with the exception of plasmablastic myeloma. The presence of a serum paraprotein, lytic bone lesions, and other manifestations of plasma cell myeloma are usually not observed in patients with ALK-positive large B-cell lymphoma. Plasma cell tumors do not express ALK.

Diffuse Large B-Cell Lymphoma (DLB-CL), Not Otherwise Specified. Some cases of ALK-positive large B-cell lymphoma resemble the immunoblastic variant of DLBCL. DLBCLs express a variety of B-cell antigens and express plasma cell-associated markers variably or not at all. ALK is not expressed.

ALK-Positive Anaplastic Large Cell Lymphoma. A sinusoidal pattern of infiltration, the presence of ALK expression, and *ALK* locus abnormalities are features shared by ALK-positive large B-cell lymphoma and ALK-positive anaplastic large cell lymphoma. The latter entity, however, has a T-cell or null-cell immunophenotype and carries monoclonal T-cell receptor gene rearrangements. The most common *ALK* translocation in ALK-positive anaplastic large cell lymphoma, t(2;5)/*NPM-ALK*, is rare in ALK-positive large B-cell lymphoma.

Poorly Differentiated Carcinoma. The immunophenotype of ALK-positive large B-cell lymphoma, in particular, expression of EMA, CD138, and rarely keratin in the absence CD45/LCA, can suggest an epithelial neoplasm. Expression of ALK and other plasma cell-associated markers is helpful to exclude carcinoma.

TREATMENT AND PROGNOSIS

ALK-positive large B-cell lymphoma is a highly aggressive tumor that responds poorly to conventional therapies. Some report a 5-year survival rate of 25 percent or worse in patients with high-stage disease. The median overall survival period is approximately 1 year (1,10,16,17).

To date, most patients have been treated with regimens designed for DLBCL, including autologous stem cell transplantation in a subset of patients, but there is no consensus regarding optimal therapy. Theoretically, ALK-positive large B-cell lymphoma would be suitable for small molecule inhibitors targeted against the ALK tyrosine kinase, such as crizotinib, and a few patients so treated have had a short term response (2,23).

Sakamoto et al. (17) suggested that the ALK pattern of expression may correlate with prognosis. In particular, patients with neoplasms that exhibit a nongranular pattern of reactivity (including *NPM-ALK* and other rare abnormalities) have a poorer prognosis than patients with neoplasms that exhibit a cytoplasmic coarse and granular ALK pattern (*CLTC-ALK* tumors).

REFERENCES

1. Beltran B, Castillo J, Salas R, et al. ALK-positive diffuse large B-cell lymphoma: report of four cases and review of the literature. J Hematol Oncol 2009;2:11.
2. Cerchietti L, Damm-Welk C, Vater I, et al. Inhibition of anaplastic lymphoma kinase (ALK) activity provides a therapeutic approach for CLTC-ALK-positive human diffuse large B cell lymphomas. PLoS One 2011;6:e18436.
3. Chen YP, Hung LY, Shan YS, Chang KC. ALK-positive large B-cell lymphoma presenting with jejunal intussusception. Eur J Haematol 2013;90:261.
4. Chikatsu N, Kojima H, Suzukawa K, et al. ALK+, CD30-, CD20- large B-cell lymphoma containing anaplastic lymphoma kinase (ALK) fused to clathrin heavy chain gene (CLTC). Mod Pathol 2003;16:828-832.
5. d'Amore ES, Visco C, Menin A, Famengo B, Bonvini P, Lazzari E. STAT3 pathway is activated in ALK-positive large B-cell lymphoma carrying SQSTM1-ALK rearrangement and provides a possible therapeutic target. Am J Surg Pathol 2013;37:780-786.
6. Delsol G, Campo E, Gascoyne RD. ALK-positive large B-cell lymphoma. In: Swerdlow SH, Campo E, Harris NL, et al., eds. WHO Classification of tumours of haematopoietic and lymphoid tissue. Lyon: IARC Press; 2008:254-255.
7. Delsol G, Lamant L, Mariame B, et al. A new subtype of large B-cell lymphoma expressing the ALK kinase and lacking the 2;5 translocation. Blood 1997;89:1483-1490.
8. Gascoyne RD, Lamant L, Martin-Subero Jl et al. ALK-positive diffuse large B-cell lymphoma is associated with clathrin-ALK rearrangements: report of 6 cases. Blood 2003;102:2568-2573.
9. Jain D, Mallick SR, Singh V, Singh G, Mathur SR, Sharma MC. Napsin A expression in anaplastic lymphoma kinase-positive diffuse large B-cell lymphoma: a diagnostic pitfall. Appl Immunohistochem Mol Morphol 2016;24:e34-40.

10. Laurent C, Do C, Gascoyne RD, et al. Anaplastic lymphoma kinase-positive diffuse large B-cell lymphoma: a rare clinicopathologic entity with poor prognosis. J Clin Oncol 2009;27:4211-4216.

11. Lee HW, Kim K, Kim W, Ko YH. ALK-positive diffuse large B-cell lymphoma: report of three cases. Hematol Oncol 2008;26:108-113.

12. Lee SE, Kang SY, Takeuchi K, Ko YH. Identification of RANBP2-ALK fusion in ALK positive diffuse large B-cell lymphoma. Hematol Oncol 2014;32:221-224.

13. Nakatsuka S, Oku K, Nagano T, et al. A case of anaplastic lymphoma kinase-positive large B-cell lymphoma: aspiration cytology findings. Diagn Cytopathol 2014;42:69-72.

14. Onciu, M, Behm FG, Downing JR, et al. ALK-positive plasmablastic B-cell lymphoma with expression of the NPM-ALK fusion transcript: report of 2 cases. Blood 2003;102:2642-2644.

15. Pan Z, Hu S, Li M, et al. ALK-positive large B-cell lymphoma: a clinicopathologic study of 26 cases with review of additional 108 cases in the literature. Am J Surg Pathol 2017;41:25-38.

15a. Quesada AE, Huh YO, Wang W, Medeiros LJ, Thakral B. Anaplastic lymphoma kinase (ALK)-positive large B-cell lymphoma in a patient treated with azathioprine for ulcerative colitis. Pathology 2016;48:513-515.

16. Reichard, KK, McKenna RW, Kroft SH. ALK-positive diffuse large B-cell lymphoma: report of four cases and review of the literature. Mod Pathol 2007;20:310-319.

17. Sakamoto K, Nakasone H, Togashi Y, et al. ALK-positive large B-cell lymphoma: identification of EML4-ALK and a review of the literature focusing on the ALK immunohistochemical staining pattern. Int J Hematol 2016;103:399-408.

17a. Sakr H, Cruise M, Chahal P, et al. Anaplastic lymphoma kinase positive large B-cell lymphoma: Literature review and report of an endoscopic fine needle aspiration case with tigroid backgrounds mimicking seminoma. Diagn Cytopathol 2017;45:148-155.

18. Shi M, Miron PM, Hutchinson L, et al. Anaplastic lymphoma kinase-positive large B-cell lymphoma with complex karyotype and novel ALK gene rearrangements. Hum Pathol 2011;42:1562-1567.

19. Stachurski D, Miron PM, Al-Homsi S, et al. Anaplastic lymphoma kinase-positive diffuse large B-cell lymphoma with a complex karyotype and cryptic 3' ALK gene insertion to chromosome 4q22-24. Hum Pathol 2007;38:940-945.

20. Takeuchi K, Soda M, Togashi Y, et al. Identification of a novel fusion, SQSTM1-ALK, in ALK-positive large B-cell lymphoma. Haematologica 2011;96:464-467.

21. Valera A, Colomo L, Martínez A, et al. ALK-positive large B-cell lymphomas express a terminal B-cell differentiation program and activated STAT3 but lack MYC rearrangements. Mod Pathol 2013;26:1329-1337.

22. Van Roosbroeck K, Cools J, Dierickx D, Thomas J. ALK-positive large B-cell lymphoma with cryptic SEC31A-ALK and NPM1-ALK fusions. Haematologica 2010;95:509-513.

23. Wass M, Behlendorf T, Schädlich B, et al. Crizotinib in refractory ALK-positive diffuse large B-cell lymphoma: a case report with a short-term response. Eur J Haematol 2014;92:268-270.

22 HUMAN HERPESVIRUS 8-POSITIVE LARGE B-CELL LYMPHOMAS AND ASSOCIATED DISEASES

Human herpesvirus 8 (HHV-8), also known as *Kaposi sarcoma-associated herpesvirus* (KSHV), is an oncogenic double-stranded DNA lymphotropic virus that is endemic in sub-Saharan Africa and the Mediterranean region (see chapter 9) (26). In North America, the prevalence of HHV-8 infection is low. Transmission of the virus usually occurs via saliva, but also occurs by blood transfusion and organ transplant (26,27).

The HHV-8 genome is composed of over 90 genes and both lytic and latent infection of human cells occur. Some lytic and latent HHV-8 genes are highly homologous to human genes and may co-opt various cellular pathways, including cell cycle progression and inhibition of apoptosis (reviewed in references 5 and 9a). Viral genes and cytokines, likely in concert with human genes and cytokines, that appear to be important in pathogenesis include: HHV-8 latency-associated nuclear antigen 1, viral (v) interleukin 6 (v-IL6), v-BCL2, v-interferon regulatory factor (v-IRF), IL-10, and vascular endothelial growth factor (VEGF) (5,9a).

Infection by HHV-8 is associated with a small group of lymphoid neoplasms and associated disorders (Table 22-1). Many of these diseases arise in patients with severe immunodeficiency, particularly those with human immunodeficiency virus (HIV) infection, but some patients with HHV-8-positive lymphoproliferative lesions do not have immunodeficiency (13). In the 2008 World Health Organization (WHO) classification, two categories of HHV-8-positive lymphoma were defined, designated as *primary effusion lymphoma* and *large B-cell lymphoma arising in HHV-8-associated multicentric Castleman disease* (15). Primary effusion lymphoma (including the extracavitary/solid variant) is discussed in detail in the chapter on HIV-associated lymphoproliferative diseases (see chapter 43). In this chapter, we focus of multicentric Castleman

disease and associated large plasmablastic/large B-cell proliferations, some of which fulfill the morphologic criteria for large B-cell lymphoma.

Since 2008, our knowledge of the spectrum of HHV-8-positive lymphoproliferative diseases has expanded. Other rare HHV-8-positive lymphomas are now recognized. This greater spectrum of HHV-8 positive lymphomas is more fully recognized in the 2016 WHO classification (28).

HHV-8-POSITIVE MULTICENTRIC CASTLEMAN DISEASE

General Features. *HHV-8-positive multicentric Castleman disease* (MCD) is a multiorgan inflammatory disease attributable to HHV-8 infection that involves dysregulation of inflammatory cytokines. Many patients with HHV-8-positive MCD have profound immunosuppression.

MCD, also known as in the literature as plasmablastic MCD, is a rare disorder. Fajgenbaum et al. (12) estimated that about 1,000 persons per year are affected in the United States. Most cases of MCD in patients with HIV infection are associated with HHV-8 infection. The incidence of HHV-8-positive MCD in HIV-positive patients appears to have increased

Table 22-1

HHV8-ASSOCIATED LYMPHOMAS AND ASSOCIATED DISEASES

Human herpesvirus 8 (HHV8)-positive multicentric Castleman disease (MCD)

Large B-cell lymphoma associated with HHV8-positive MCD

Primary effusion lymphoma (HHV8 positive) Extracavitary/solid variant

HHV8-positive germinotropic lymphoproliferative disorder

HHV8-positive diffuse large B-cell lymphoma, not otherwise specified since the advent of highly active antiretroviral therapy (HAART) (24)

Of the 10 percent of HIV-negative patients with HHV-8-positive MCD, some have another cause of immunodeficiency, such as an organ transplant, whereas others live in geographic regions endemic for HHV-8 infection (26). HHV-8-positive MCD (as well as HHV-8-negative cases), also can arise in patients with POEMS syndrome, a multisystemic disease named for its manifestations of polyneuropathy, organomegaly, endocrinopathy, monoclonal gammopathy, and skin changes (9).

Although not the focus of this chapter, a small percentage of cases of MCD, including rare HIV-positive patients, are not associated with HHV-8 infection. These cases have been referred to in the literature as *idiopathic MCD* or *HHV-8-negative MCD* (12,31). Patients with idiopathic MCD present with a clinical picture similar to that of HHV-8-positive MCD. The etiology of idiopathic MCD is unknown but autoimmunity, ectopic secretion of cytokines by presumably one or more abnormal cell types, and another etiologic virus have been hypothesized (12,31). A variant of idiopathic MCD has been described, known as *Castleman-Kojima disease,* or *TAFRO syndrome,* characterized by thrombocytopenia, ascites and other effusions, microcytic anemia, fever, renal dysfunction, and organomegaly (16,18).

Although MCD is not a lymphoma in the traditional sense, the underlying abnormality is associated with the secretion of numerous cytokines that drive the proliferation of plasma cells, B cells, histiocytes, and likely other cells. In addition, HHV-8-positive MCD is often an aggressive disease and can be a precursor of HHV-8-positive lymphoma.

Clinical Features. Most patients with HHV-8-positive MCD and HIV infection are severely immunocompromised. The median interval from HIV infection to the onset of HHV-8-positive MCD in one study was 2.5 years, but with a wide range (from under 1 to over 20 years) (2). HIV-positive patients with HHV-8-positive MCD are predominantly men, with a median age in the fourth or fifth decade.

Patients commonly complain of fever, night sweats, fatigue, weight loss, and edema. Physical examination shows systemic lymphadenopathy, hepatosplenomegaly, rash or cherry hemangio-

mas, effusions, and sometimes, central nervous system defects (2,3,25). Laboratory studies commonly show anemia, leukopenia, thrombocytopenia, hypoalbuminemia, polyclonal hypergammaglobulinemia, and other cytokine-induced or autoimmune manifestations. Serum studies often show elevated levels of HHV-8 and IL6. HIV-positive patients with HHV-8-positive MCD may have other disease manifestations of HHV-8 infection, most often Kaposi sarcoma and less often other rare types of HHV-8-associated lymphoma (3,13,25). Rarely, HHV-8-positive polyclonal plasmablasts reach high numbers in the peripheral blood, mimicking a leukemic phase of lymphoma (20).

KSHV-Associated Inflammatory Cytokine Syndrome. A small subset of patients with both HHV-8 and HIV infection present with a high viral load of HHV-8, elevated serum levels of IL6 and IL10, and many of the symptoms and laboratory abnormalities observed in patients with HHV-8-positive MCD (23). However, these patients do not have prominent lymphadenopathy or splenomegaly, and therefore do not have all the features required for MCD. The designation KSHV-associated inflammatory cytokine syndrome (KISC) has been used for this disorder (23) which may be a prodromal form of HHV-8-positive MCD (3).

Histologic Findings. *Lymph Node.* Although the histologic findings in patients with HHV-8-positive MCD are most often of the plasma cell variant, a spectrum of findings may be seen and focal hyaline-vascular lesions can occur (1,6). Although rare cases of HHV-8-positive MCD have been classified as the hyaline-vascular variant or mixed type in the literature, we believe that most of these cases are a part of the disease spectrum of HHV-8-positive MCD.

The interfollicular regions in lymph nodes involved by HHV-8-positive MCD are expanded by marked plasmacytosis and vascular proliferation (fig. 22-1). Many follicles are hyperplastic, but some are small, with involuted or regressed germinal centers and increased vascularization. The germinal centers are surrounded by mantle zone lymphocytes that can appear as linear layers (so-called onion skin). A characteristic finding in HHV-8-positive MCD is the blurring of the boundaries between germinal centers and mantle zones. In addition, the mantle zones and

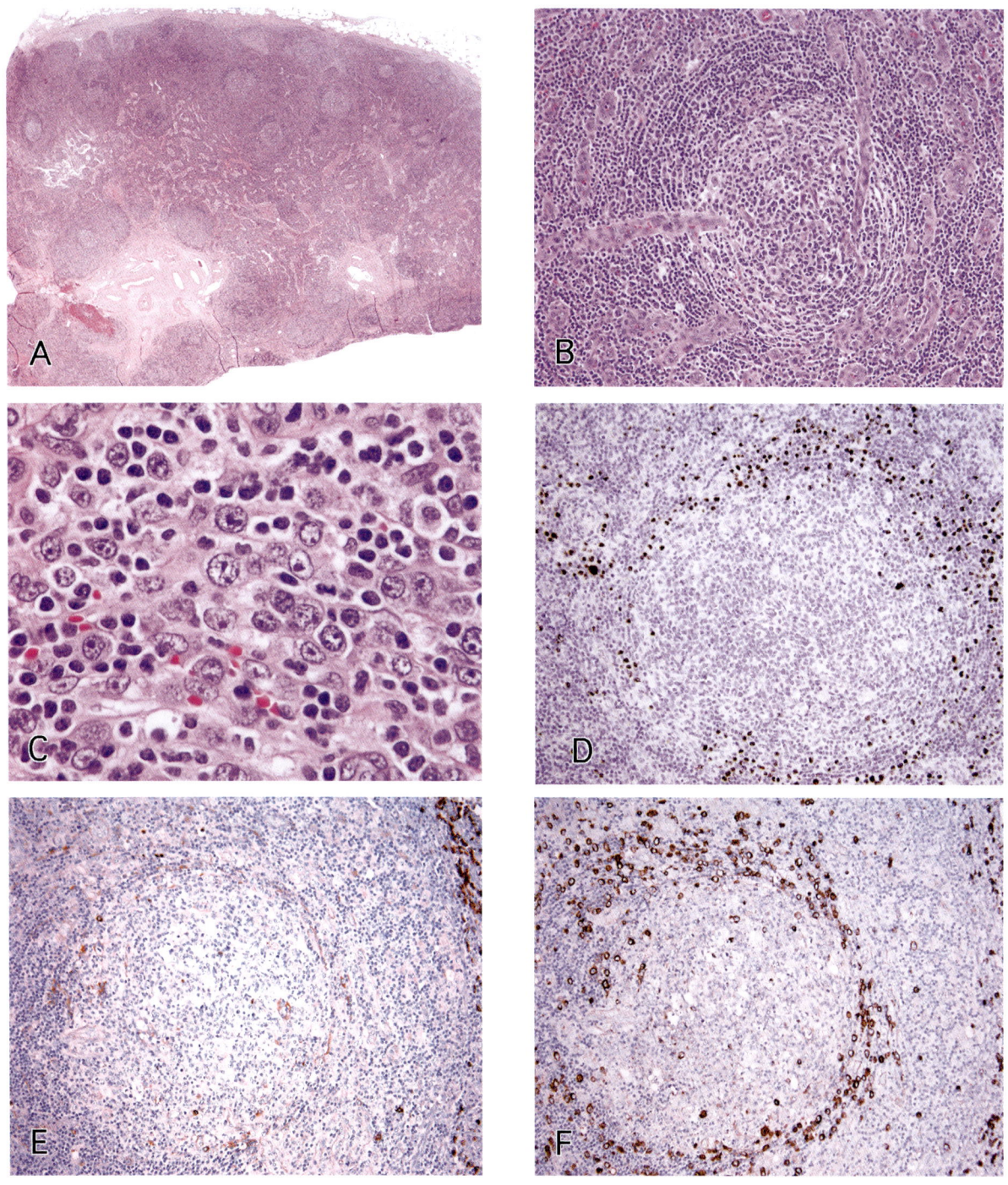

Figure 22-1

HHV-8-POSITIVE MULTICENTRIC CASTLEMAN DISEASE (MCD) INVOLVING LYMPH NODE

This patient had human immunodeficiency virus (HIV) infection.

A–D: Low-power magnification (A) shows partial involvement characterized by prominent follicles and interfollicular expansion. Hyaline-vascular features are present (B), large plasmablasts in a mantle zone are shown (C), and many plasmablasts are positive for HHV-8 (D).

E,F: The plasmablasts are negative for kappa and positive for lambda light chains and are beginning to cluster to form a so-called microlymphoma (hematoxylin and eosin [H&E] stain). (Courtesy of Dr. B. Kemp, Houston, Texas.)

interfollicular regions contain large cells with plasmacytoid (or immunoblastic) features, also known as plasmablasts (1,6). These plasmablasts are usually singly scattered but they can form small clusters in the mantle zones and interfollicular regions.

In HIV-positive patients, lymph nodes involved by HHV-8-positive MCD often have an overall lymphocyte-depleted appearance. In HHV-8-positive MCD arising in patients with POEMS syndrome, interfollicular sheets of plasma cells are very prominent (and can be monotypic) and there is less overall lymphocyte depletion than in cases in HIV-positive patients (fig. 22-2).

In a subset of cases of HHV-8-positive MCD, the plasmablasts become more numerous and form small nodules that involve and immediately surround the follicles (figs. 22-1, 22-3). These nodules are known as "microlymphomas" and may correlate with disease progression (8,11,13). Rarely do microlymphomas develop into clinically important large B-cell lymphoma and usually they have no prognostic significance (6,15). When large plasmablasts substantially extend outside the follicles into the interfollicular regions, the possibility of overt large B-cell (plasmablastic) lymphoma arising within HHV-8-positive MCD is suggested (see below) (14).

Bone Marrow. The bone marrow in patients with HHV-8-positive MCD can be normocellular or hypercellular (14a,30). The most common finding is an interstitial, reactive plasmacytosis that can be mild or more prominent (about 25 percent). The plasma cells can form small clusters in biopsy specimens, but large nodules or sheets of plasma cells are absent. Polymorphous and reactive lymphoid aggregates occur in approximately a third of patients. These aggregates are most often nonparatrabecular. Bone marrow hematopoietic cells do not show morphologic evidence of dysplasia.

Immunophenotypic Findings. The presence of scattered HHV-8-positive plasmablasts is most conveniently shown by immunohistochemistry using an antibody specific for HHV-8 latency-associated nuclear antigen 1 (LANA-1) (fig. 22-3C). HHV-8 reactivity is located in the nucleus and has a granular pattern. In lymph nodes, HHV-8-positive plasmablasts are most frequent in the mantle zones (1,6). In bone marrow,

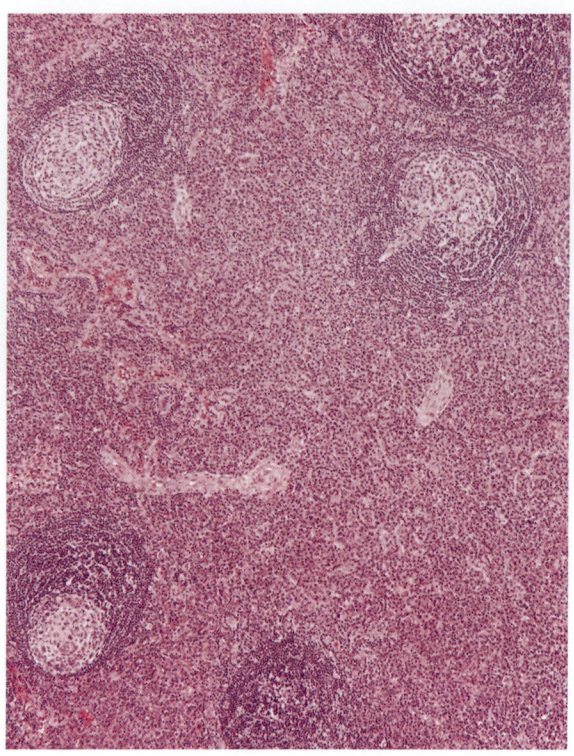

Figure 22-2

HHV-8-POSITIVE MULTICENTRIC CASTLEMAN DISEASE INVOLVING LYMPH NODE

This patient had POEMS syndrome. The interfollicular regions are markedly expanded by plasma cells that express monotypic lambda light chain (not shown). Follicles have expanded mantle zones ("onion skin") and one follicle with a small hyaline vascular lesion is present in this field (H&E stain).

HHV-8-positive cells are single and scattered in an interstitial distribution (30).

The HHV-8-positive plasmablasts are positive for cytoplasmic monotypic lambda light chain (fig. 22-3D), IgM, CD19, and CD27. CD38, CD45/LCA, and CD79A are often negative, but may be variably expressed in a subset of cases (6,10,14). In one reported case, plasmablasts expressed MYC (21). Plasmablasts are usually negative for CD10, CD20, CD30, CD138, BCL6, PAX5, T-cell antigens, and Epstein-Barr virus (EBV) infection (14).

Reactive plasma cells express polytypic cytoplasmic light chains, often express IgA, are positive for CD38 and CD138, and rare cells express EBV-encoded RNA1 (EBER1). Scattered plasmablasts in bone marrow or other organs share similar immunophenotypic features. In a small subset of

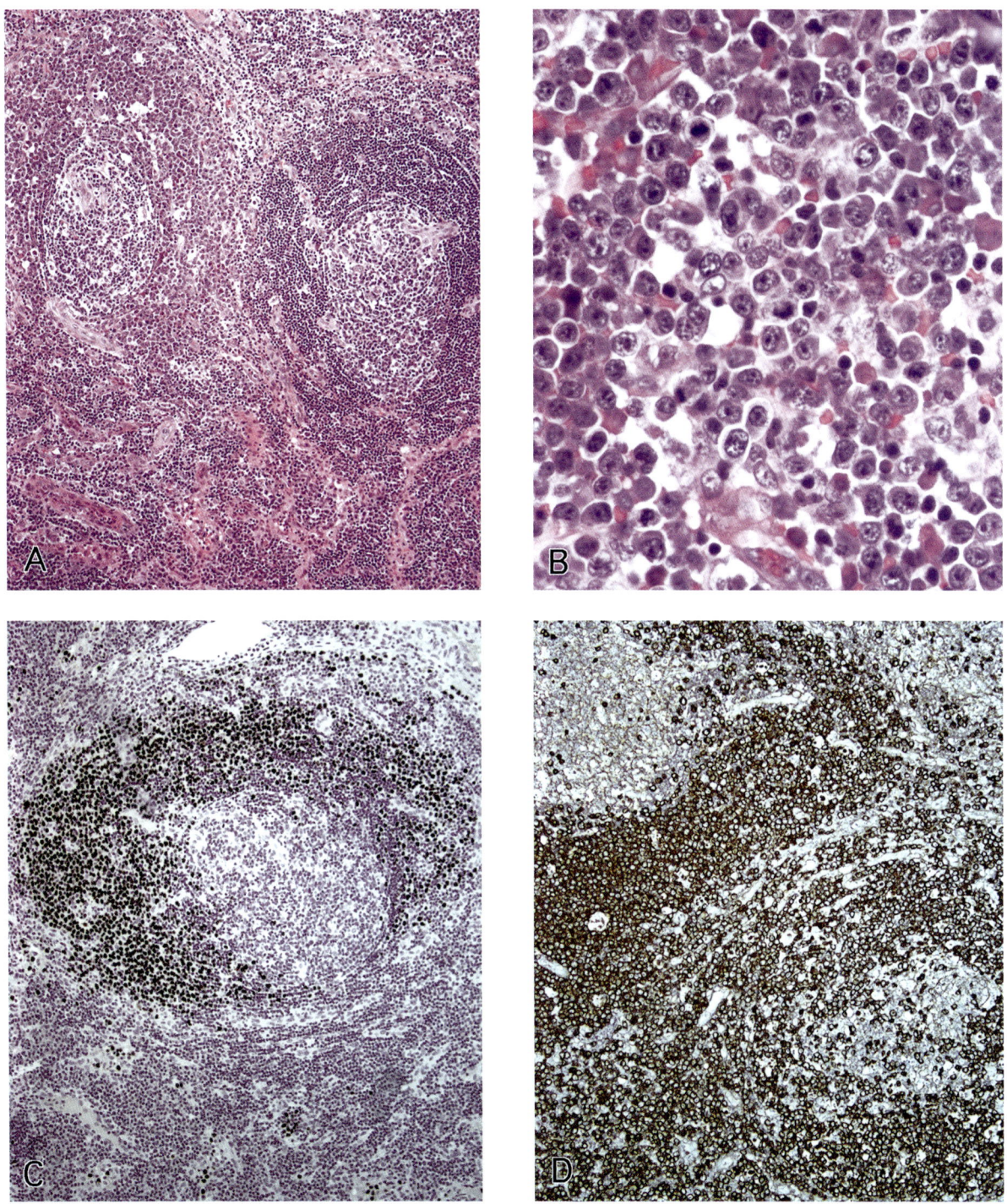

Figure 22-3

HHV-8-POSITIVE MULTICENTRIC CASTLEMAN DISEASE WITH MANY PLASMABLASTS

A: Two regressed follicles with hyaline-vascular type changes are shown. The left follicle shows a broad mantle zone composed of large plasmablastic cells with dense amphophilic cytoplasm (A,B: H&E stain).

B: High magnification of a mantle zone composed of plasmablasts with abundant amphophilic cytoplasm and prominent nucleoli.

C,D: The plasmablasts are positive for HHV-8 latent nuclear antigen 1 in a nuclear pattern (C) and show lambda light chain restriction (D) (immunohistochemistry with hematoxylin counterstain).

cases, small monotypic plasma cell populations are identified in the bone marrow (30).

Molecular Genetic Findings. Little is known regarding the molecular or cytogenetic findings in HHV-8-positive MCD including cases with microlymphomas. In most cases there is no evidence of monoclonal *IGH* or T-cell receptor gene rearrangements (10,15). This is true even in cases with lambda light chain restriction. Analysis of HHV-8 terminal repeat regions has shown that the viral episomes are usually polyclonal (17). By analyzing the highly polymorphic human androgen receptor α (*HUMARA*) gene in whole tissue specimens, Chang et al. (7) showed a small number of MCD cases in which the pattern was monoclonal. Analysis for antigen receptor gene rearrangements in the same cases showed polyclonal results, suggesting that stromal cells in MCD may be monoclonal. In a few cases assessed by fluorescence in situ hybridization (FISH) there was no evidence of aneuploidy or t(8;14)(q24;q32)/*MYC-IGH* (21).

Treatment and Prognosis. Most recommendations regarding the therapeutic approach to patients with HHV-8-positive MCD are based on the treatment of HIV-positive patients (25). There is no consensus optimal treatment approach. Many patients are treated with rituximab and various chemotherapy regimens. Monoclonal antibodies against IL6 have shown promise; of these, the chimeric anti-IL6 antibody siltuximab is approved by the US Food and Drug Administration. These antibodies are not curative, but symptomatic patients have responded. Antibodies against interleukin 1, bortezomib (to inhibit the NF-kB pathway), immunosuppression using cyclosporine A and steroids, and immunomodulator agents have been employed with some benefit.

The clinical course of patients with HHV-8-positive MCD can wax and wane. Relapses are common. The prognosis of HIV-positive patients with HHV-8-positive MCD is closely related to the overall degree of immunosuppression. With recent improvements in therapy, including HAART, Bower et al. (2) reported a 5-year survival rate of 78 percent. HIV-positive patients with HHV-8-positive MCD have a high risk of developing Kaposi sarcoma and non-Hodgkin lymphomas, including HHV-8-positive lymphomas. The risk of classic Hodgkin lymphoma also is increased in these patients. Therapy that includes rituximab may decrease the risk of developing second lymphomas (25).

LARGE B-CELL LYMPHOMA ARISING IN HHV-8-POSITIVE MULTICENTRIC CASTLEMAN DISEASE

General Features. In the 2008 WHO classification, *large B-cell lymphoma arising in HHV-8-positive MCD* was defined as a monoclonal proliferation of HHV-8-positive lymphoid cells resembling plasmablasts that express IgM and arise in the context of MCD (15). Although these lesions meet the morphologic criteria for lymphoma composed of plasmablasts or large B cells, criteria useful for predicting aggressive clinical behavior are not well defined.

The onset of HHV-8-positive large B-cell lymphoma is usually associated with constitutional symptoms, cytopenias, rapidly enlarging lymph nodes, and splenomegaly (11,15). Often this development coincides with worsening immunosuppression. Kaposi sarcoma and other HHV-8-associated lesions also occur in these patients (19).

Histologic Findings. Overt HHV-8-positive large B-cell lymphoma (LBCL) likely represents progression of a microlymphoma. It is histologically characterized by involvement of the interfollicular regions and then progressive effacement of the lymph node architecture by an infiltrate of large HHV-8-positive cells that resemble plasmablasts or less often immunoblasts (fig. 22-4) (14,15). Mitotic figures are often numerous and necrosis can be present. Some cases exhibit pleomorphism (14).

HHV-8-positive LBCL can disseminate widely, but common sites include the spleen, lungs, liver, and gastrointestinal tract. The bone marrow may be involved and rare patients present primarily with cutaneous disease. A leukemic phase can develop, usually as a terminal event (20).

Cytologic Findings. The lymphoma cells arising in HHV-8-positive MCD are large and commonly exhibit abundant eosinophilic cytoplasm and eccentric vesicular nuclei containing one or two prominent nucleoli (fig. 22-5).

Immunophenotypic Findings. HHV-8-positive LBCL cells are positive for IgM, lambda, and often CD45/LCA and MUM1/IRF4 (10,11,14,15). The tumor cells are usually negative for pan-B-cell

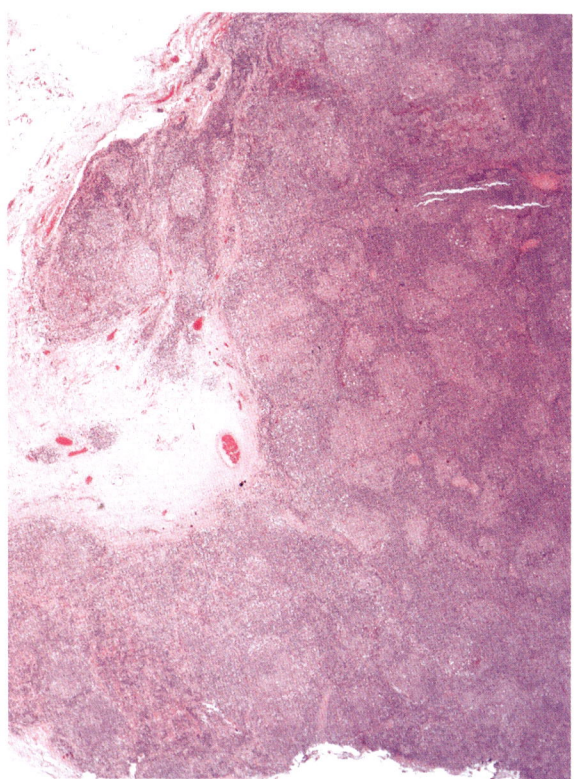 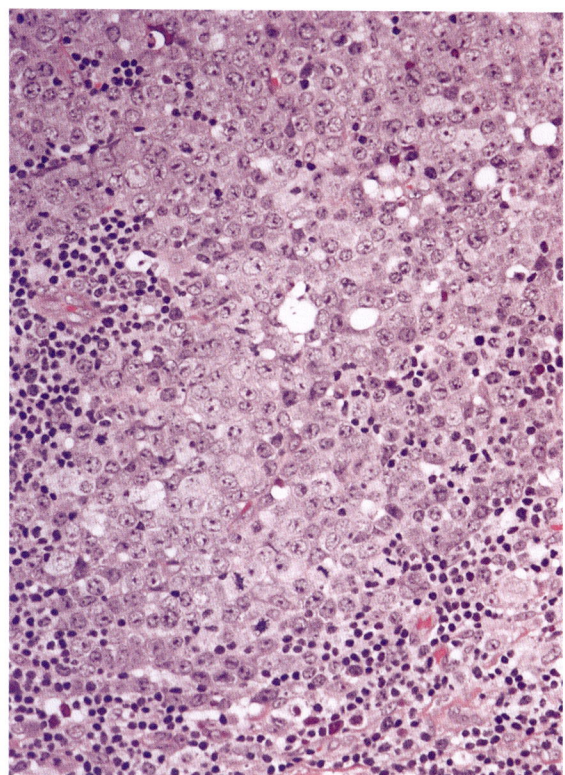

Figure 22-4

HHV-8-POSITIVE LARGE B-CELL LYMPHOMA ARISING IN A PATIENT WITH MULTICENTRIC CASTLEMAN DISEASE

Left: Low-power view of lymph node shows many enlarged nodules, some beginning to fuse, and diffusely replacing normal architecture.

Right: There are sheets of large neoplastic cells that resemble plasmablasts or immunoblasts (left, right: H&E stain).

antigens, but CD20 or CD79a are expressed in some cases. CD30, CD38, and CD138 are usually negative, but can be expressed in a small subset of cases. The cells are negative for EBV, pan-T-cell antigens, CD21, and CD23 (14). Follicular dendritic cells (CD21 or CD23 positive) are often intermixed with the neoplastic cells (14).

Molecular Genetic Findings. HHV-8-positive LBCL is usually characterized by monoclonal *IGH* rearrangements. The variable regions of the *IGH* genes are often unmutated (11). HHV-8 is present in monoclonal form (17). Little other cytogenetic or molecular data are available. If present, cytogenetic abnormalities or oncogene mutations (e.g., *TP53*) or rearrangements (e.g., *MYC*) suggest aggressive clinical behavior.

Treatment and Prognosis. The prognosis of patients with HHV-8-positive LBCL is poor. This disease is highly aggressive and the severe immunosuppression in many of these patients

contributes to a very short median survival period, often only a few months (13,15).

HHV-8-POSITIVE GERMINOTROPIC LYMPHOPROLIFERATIVE DISORDER

This is a rare disease with no more than 10 to 15 cases reported in the literature. Patients with *HHV-8-positive germinotropic lymphoproliferative disorder* (GLD) are HIV-negative, immunocompetent adults. Most patients are men, who present with localized lymphadenopathy. Almost all patients reported have had an indolent clinical course (15,22,29), but rare patients initially diagnosed with HHV-8-positive GLD subsequently have developed widespread disease and required chemotherapy (8).

The distinctive morphologic feature of HHV-8-positive GLD is the presence of numerous plasmablasts preferentially involving germinal centers (germinotropism) (fig. 22-6). We have

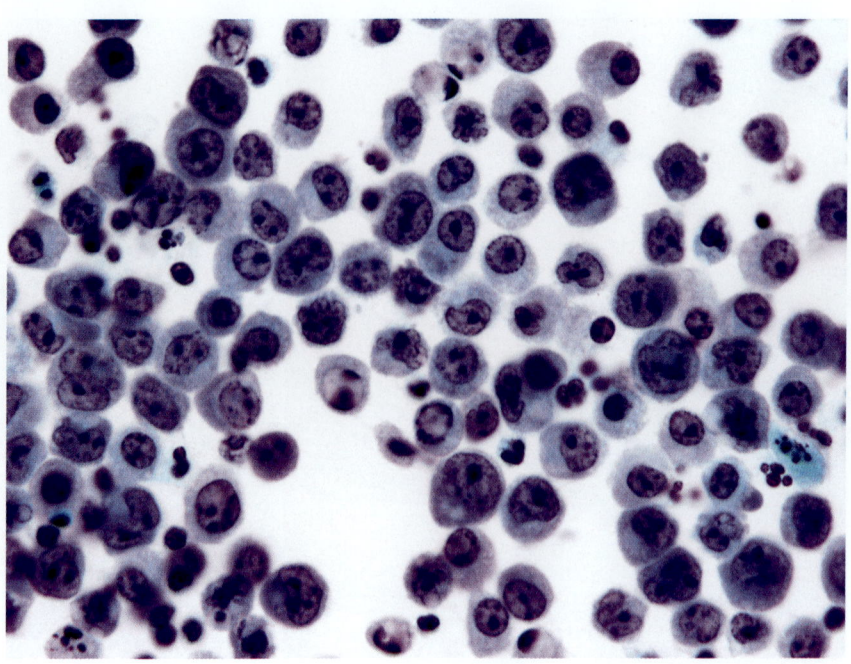

Figure 22-5

LARGE B-CELL LYMPHOMA ARISING IN AN HIV-POSITIVE PATIENT WITH HHV-8-ASSOCIATED MULTICENTRIC CASTLEMAN DISEASE

Most of the neoplastic cells in the pleural effusion are large with eccentrically located nuclei and prominent nucleoli (Papanicolaou stain).

observed one case in which the plasmablasts seemed to involve mantle or marginal zones as well as germinal centers. In some cases, Reed-Sternberg-like or Hodgkin-like cells are present (8,29). The plasmablasts are positive for cytoplasmic monotypic light chain (kappa or lambda), often IgA, CD38, MUM-1/IRF4, HHV-8 (fig. 22-6C), and EBER1 (fig. 22-6D), and are negative for CD10, CD20, CD79a, BCL2, and BCL6 (8,15). One case reported was positive for PD-L1 and NOTCH1 (25a). Most cases lack monoclonal immunoglobulin gene rearrangements.

HHV-8-POSITIVE DIFFUSE LARGE B-CELL LYMPHOMA, NOT OTHERWISE SPECIFIED

Rare cases of *HHV-8-positive large B-cell lymphoma* have been described in patients who do not fit within the entities described above (4,8,14). Patients are adults who are negative for HIV infection and have no apparent evidence of immunodeficiency. These patients present with lymphadenopathy, splenomegaly, or extranodal sites of disease and may have localized or advanced stage disease (4).

Histologically, the lymph nodes are diffusely replaced by a neoplasm composed of plasmablasts or cells with more anaplastic features (4). A sinusoidal pattern also has been described and one unique case had an intravascular distribution of disease (4,8).

Immunohistochemical studies have shown that the lymphoma cells have a plasmablastic immunophenotype, positive for CD138 (can be variable), VS38c, and/or MUM1/IRF4 (fig. 22-7) and negative for pan-B-cell markers (4). The lymphoma cells are also positive for HHV-8 and EBER1, and have a high proliferation rate as shown by Ki-67 expression. CD45/LCA may be partially positive and aberrant expression of CD3 (cytoplasmic) or CD43 can be observed.

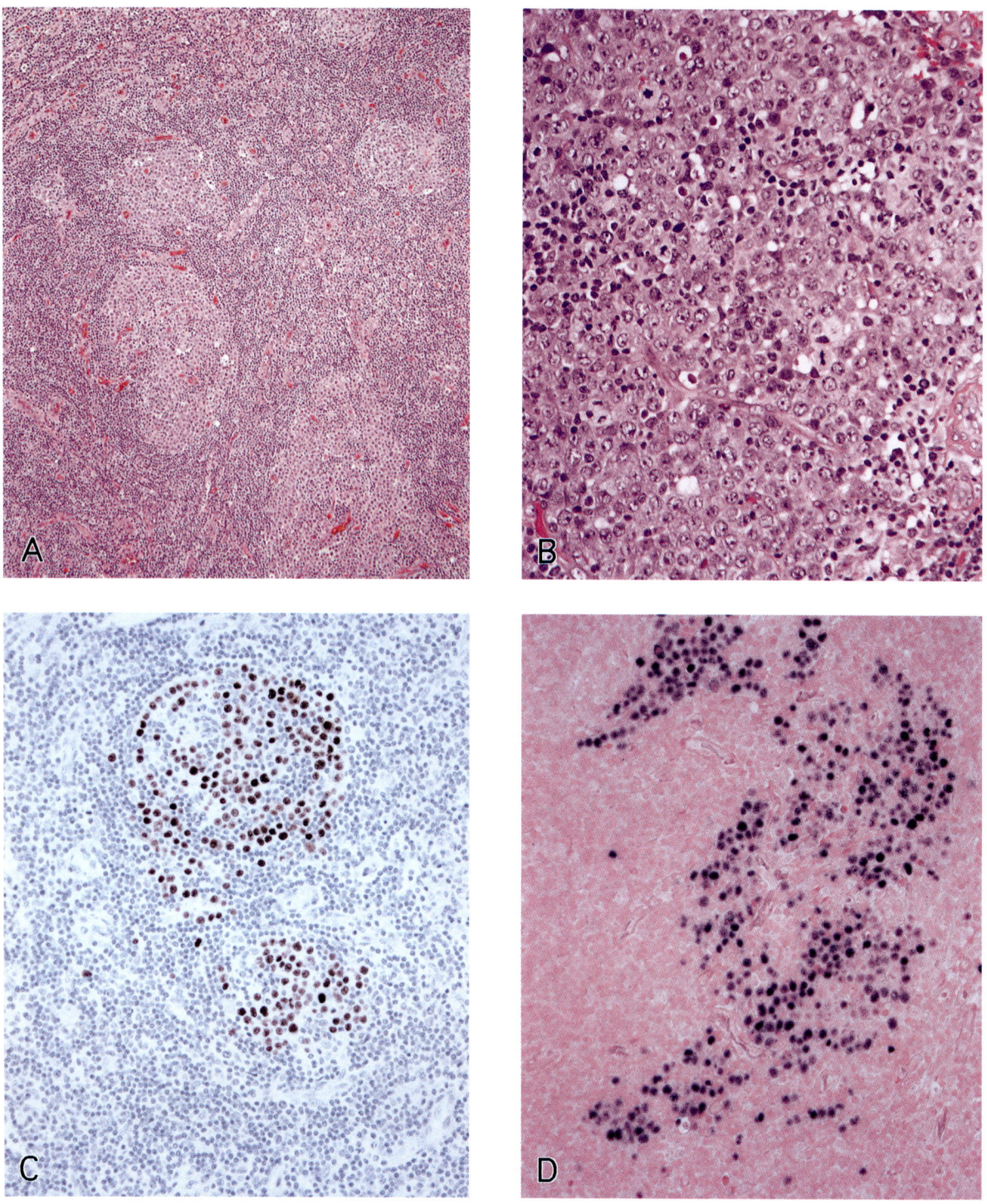

Figure 22-6

HHV-8-POSITIVE GERMINOTROPIC LYMPHOPROLIFERATIVE DISORDER INVOLVING LYMPH NODE

A: At low-power magnification, multiple nodules of plasmablasts replace germinal centers (A,B: H&E stain).

B: Higher magnification of one nodule. The plasmablasts are large with abundant eosinophilic cytoplasm.

C,D: The plasmablasts are positive for HHV-8 (C) and EBV-encoded RNA1 (EBER1) (D) (C: immunohistochemistry with hematoxylin counterstain; D: in situ hybridization with eosin counterstain).

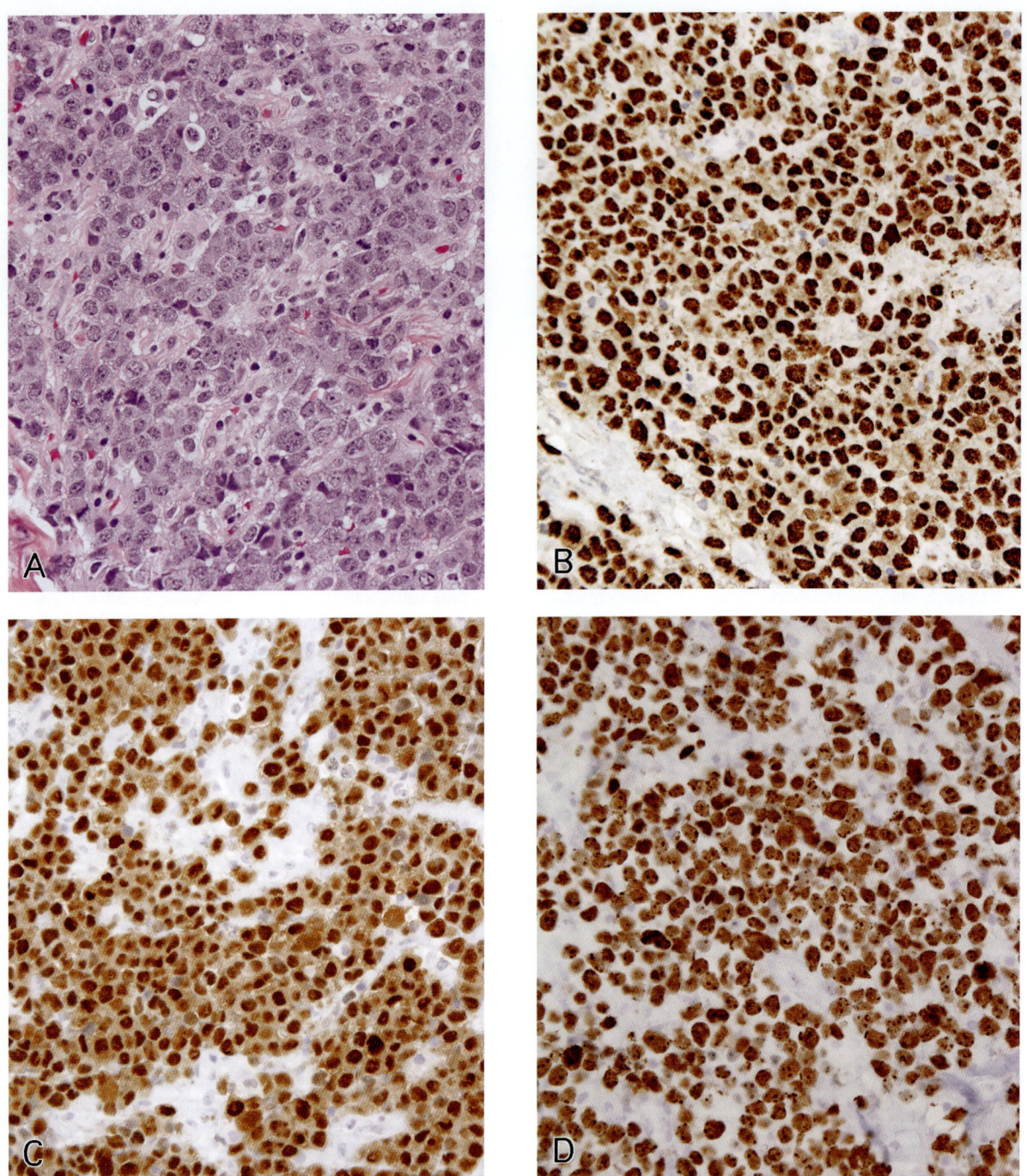

Figure 22-7

HHV-8-POSITIVE DIFFUSE LARGE B-CELL LYMPHOMA, NOT OTHERWISE SPECIFIED

A 67-year-old woman with no evidence of HIV infection, body cavity effusions, or travel history presented with widespread lymphadenopathy and underwent excisional lymph node biopsy. The diagnosis of HHV-8-positive diffuse large B-cell lymphoma, not otherwise specified, was established.

A: Lymphoma cells are arranged in sheets and have abundant cytoplasm, consistent with plasmablastic features. They replace the lymph node parenchyma (H&E stain).

B–E: The lymphoma cells are positive for HHV-8 (B), MUM1/IRF4 (C), Ki-67 (D), and cytoplasmic CD3 (E) (C–E: immunohistochemistry with hematoxylin counterstain).

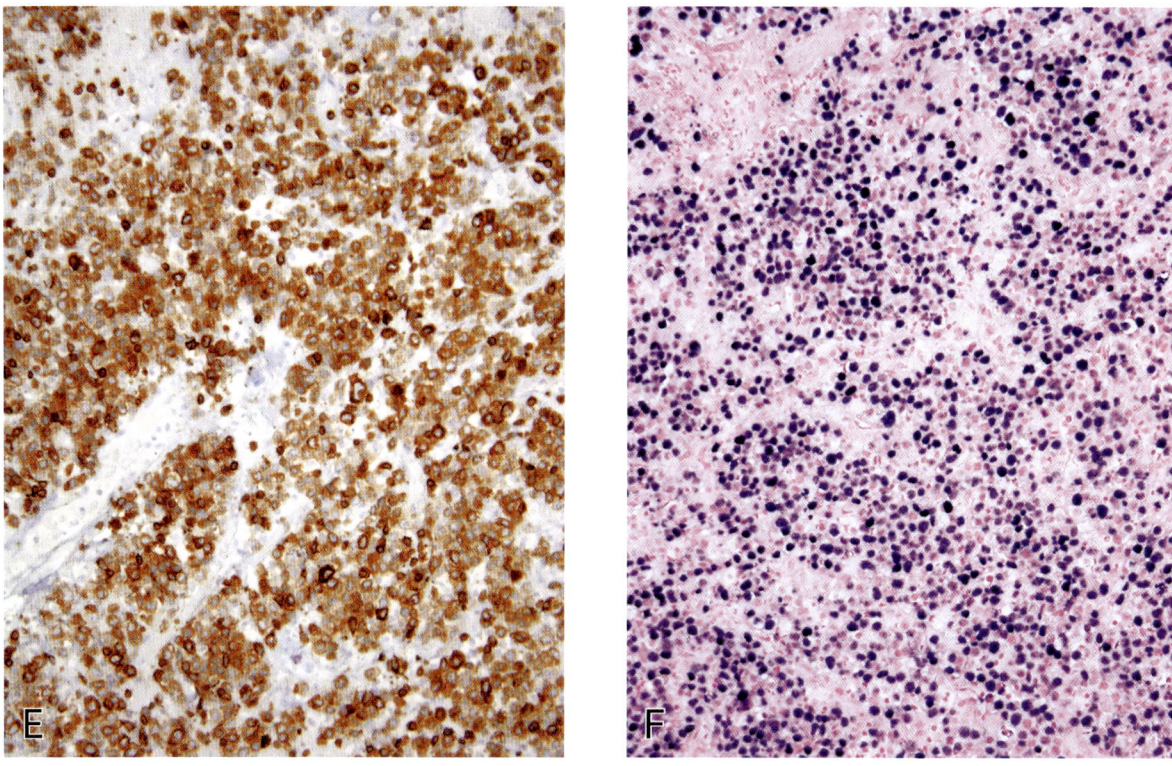

Figure 22-7, continued

F: In situ hybridization shows that the lymphoma cells are positive for EBER1 (in situ hybridization with eosin counterstain).

REFERENCES

1. Amin HM, Medeiros LJ, Manning JT, Jones D. Dissolution of the lymphoid follicle is a feature of the HHV8+ variant of plasma cell Castleman's disease. Am J Surg Pathol 2003;27:91-100.
2. Bower M, Dalla Pria A, Coyle C, Nelson M, Naresh K. Diagnostic criteria schemes for multicentric Castleman disease in 75 cases. J Acquir Immune Defic Syndr 2014;65:e80-82.
3. Carbone A, De Paoli P, Gloghini A, Vaccher E. KSHV-associated multicentric Castleman disease: a tangle of different entities requiring multitarget treatment strategies. Int J Cancer 2015;137:251-261.
4. Carbone A, Gloghini A, Vaccher E, Marchetti G, Gaidano G, Tirelli U. KSHV/HHV-8 associated lymph node based lymphomas in HIV seronegative subjects. Report of two cases with anaplastic morphology and plasmablastic immunophenotype. J Clin Pathol 2005;58:1039-1045.
5. Cesarman E. Gammaherpesviruses and lymphoproliferative disorders. Annu Rev Pathol 2014;9:349-372.
6. Chadburn A, Hyjek EM, Tam W, et al. Immunophenotypic analysis of the Kaposi sarcoma herpesvirus (KSHV; HHV-8) - infected B cells in HIV+ multicentric Castleman disease (MCD). Histopathology 2008;53:513-524.
7. Chang KC, Wang YC, Hung LY, et al. Monoclonality and cytogenetic abnormalities in hyaline vascular Castleman disease. Mod Pathol 2014;27:823-831.
8. Courville EL, Sohani AR, Hasserjian RP, Zukerberg LR, Harris NL, Ferry JA. Diverse clinicopathologic features in human herpesvirus 8-associated lymphomas lead to diagnostic problems. Am J Clin Pathol 2014;142:816-829.

9. Dispenzieri A. POEMS syndrome: update on diagnosis, risk-stratification, and management. Am J Hematol 2015;90:951-962.

9a. Dittmer DP, Damania B. Kaposi sarcoma-associated herpesvirus: immunobiology, oncogenesis, and therapy. J Clin Invest 2016;126:3165-3175.

10. Du MQ, Liu H, Diss TC, et al. Kaposi sarcoma-associated herpesvirus infects monotypic (IgM lambda) but polyclonal naive B cells in Castleman disease and associated lymphoproliferative disorders. Blood 2001;97:2130-2136.

11. Dupin N, Diss TL, Kellam P, et al. HHV-8 is associated with a plasmablastic variant of Castleman disease that is linked to HHV-8-positive plasmablastic lymphoma. Blood 2000;95:1406-1412.

12. Fajgenbaum DC, Uldrick TS, Bagg A, et al. International, evidence-based consensus diagnostic criteria for HHV-8-negative/idiopathic multicentric Castleman disease. Blood 2017;129:1646-1657.

13. Gloghini A, Dolcetti R, Carbone A. Lymphomas occurring specifically in HIV-infected patients: from pathogenesis to pathology. Sem Cancer Biol 2013;23:457-467.

14. Hsi ED, Lorsbach RB, Fend F, Dogan A. Plasmablastic lymphoma and related disorders. Am J Clin Pathol 2011;136:183-194.

14a. Ibrahim HA, Balachandran K, Bower M, Naresh KN. Bone marrow manifestations in multicentric Castleman disease. Br J Haematol 2016;172:923-929.

15. Isaacson PG, Campo E, Harris NL. Large B-cell lymphoma arising in HHV8-associated multicentric Castleman disease. In: Swerdlow SH, Campo E, Harris NL, Jaffe ES, Pileri SA, Stein H, Thiele J, Vardiman JW, eds. WHO classification of tumours of haematopoietic and lymphoid tissues. Lyon: IARC Press; 2008:258-259.

16. Iwaki N, Fajgenbaum DC, Nabel CS, et al. Clinicopathologic analysis of TAFRO syndrome demonstrates a distinct subtype of HHV-8-negative multicentric Castleman disease. Am J Hematol 2016;91:220-226.

17. Judde JG, Lacoste V, Brière J, et al. Monoclonality or oligoclonality of human herpesvirus 8 terminal repeat sequences in Kaposi's sarcoma and other diseases. J Natl Cancer Inst 2000;92:729-736.

18. Masaki Y, Kawabata K, Takai K, et al. Proposed diagnostic criteria, disease severity classification, and treatment strategy for TAFRO syndrome, 2015 version. Int J Hematol 2016;103:686-692.

19. Oksenhendler E, Boulanger E, Galicier L, et al. High incidence of Kaposi sarcoma-associated herpesvirus-related non-Hodgkin lymphoma in patients with HIV infection and multicentric Castleman disease. Blood 2002;99:2331-2336.

20. Oksenhendler E, Boutboul D, Beldjord K, et al. Human herpesvirus 8+ polyclonal IGM? B-cell lymphocytosis mimicking plasmablastic leukemia/lymphoma in HIV-infected patients. Eur J Haematol 2013;91:497-503.

21. Pagni F, Bosisio FM, Sala E, et al. The plasmablasts in Castleman disease. Am J Clin Pathol 2013;139:555-559.

22. Papoudou-Bai A, Hatzimichael E, Kyriazopoulou L, Briasoulis E, Kanavaros P. Rare variants in the spectrum of human herpesvirus 8/Epstein-Barr virus-copositive lymphoproliferations. Hum Pathol 2015;46:1566-1571.

23. Polizzotto MN, Uldrick TS, Wyvill KM, et al. Clinical features and outcomes of patients with symptomatic Kaposi sarcoma herpesvirus (KSHV)-associated inflammation: prospective characterization of KSHV inflammatory cytokine syndrome (KICS). Clin Infect Dis 2016;62:730-738.

24. Powles T, Stebbing J, Bazeos A, et al. The role of immune suppression and HHV8 in the increasing incidence of HIV-associated multicentric Castleman's disease. Ann Oncol 2009;20:775-779.

25. Reddy D, Mitsuyasu R. HIV-associated multicentric Castleman disease. Curr Opin Oncol 2011; 23:475-481.

25a. Ronaghy A, Wang HY, Thorson JA, et al. PD-L1 and Notch1 expression in KSHV/HHV-8 and EBV associated germinotropic lymphoproliferative disorder: case report and review of the literature. Pathology 2017;49:430-435.

26. Schulz TF. Epidemiology of Kaposi's sarcoma-associated herpesvirus/human herpesvirus 8. Adv Cancer Res 1999;76:121-160.

27. Speicher DJ, Sehu MM, Mollee P, Shen L, Johnson NW, Faoagali JL. Successful treatment of iatrogenic multicentric Castleman's disease arising due to recrudescence of HHV-8 in a liver transplant patient. Am J Transplant 2014;14:1207-1213.

28. Swerdlow SH, Campo E, Pileri SA, et al. The 2016 revision of the World Health Organization (WHO) classification of lymphoid neoplasms. Blood 2016;127:2375-2390.

29. Taris M, de Mascarel A, Riols M, et al. [KSHV/EBV associated germinotropic lymphoproliferative disorder: a rare entity, case report and review of the literature.] Ann Pathol 2014;34:373-377. [French]

30. Venkataraman G, Uldrick TS, Aleman K, et al. Bone marrow findings in HIV-positive patients with Kaposi sarcoma herpesvirus-associated multicentric Castleman disease. Am J Clin Pathol 2013;139:851-861.

31. Yu L, Tu M, Cortes J, et al. Clinical and pathological characteristics of HIV- and HHV-8-negative Castleman disease. Blood 2017;129:1658-1668.

23 PLASMABLASTIC LYMPHOMA

GENERAL FEATURES

Plasmablastic lymphoma (PBL) is an aggressive lymphoma in which the neoplastic cells are large and resemble immunoblasts, plasmablasts, or centroblasts and exhibit an immunophenotype characteristic of plasma cells (20). Mature plasma cells also can be present. PBLs often arise in immunocompromised patients and are commonly positive for Epstein-Barr virus (EBV).

Although lymphomas with features of PBL had been reported decades earlier (2), our current understanding of PBL as a morphologic entity began with a study by Delecluse et al. (7) who reported 16 patients with PBL involving the oral cavity. Of these, 15 patients were positive for human immunodeficiency virus (HIV) and 9 of 15 tumors tested were positive for EBV-encoded RNA (EBER1) (fig. 23-1).

Currently, a wider clinical spectrum of patients with PBL is recognized and includes HIV-negative patients with other forms of immunodeficiency, such as organ transplantation (either solid organ or hematopoietic stem cell) and autoimmune diseases. In addition, patients with HIV-negative PBL can be immunocompetent. PBL occurs in elderly patients without apparent immunodeficiency, possibly related to age-associated immune compromise, and these cases may be a morphologic variant of EBV-positive diffuse large B-cell lymphoma (DLBCL) (11).

The overall frequency of PBL is low, but higher in HIV-positive than HIV-negative patients. In studies from Germany and Italy, 18 of 302 (6 percent) and 18 of 231 (7.8 percent) lymphomas in HIV-positive patients, respectively, were plasmablastic lymphomas (5,19). There are some data to suggest that the frequency of PBL has increased in the era of highly active antiretroviral therapy (HAART), although increased recognition of this type of lymphoma cannot be excluded (5).

Approximately 30 percent of PBL cases occur in HIV-negative patients and at least half of these patients have no obvious evidence of immunodeficiency (3,4,13,14,16). As reviewed by Liu et al. (13), over 100 cases of PBL in HIV-negative patients have been reported. Patients who have undergone transplantation represent about one third of all HIV-negative patients and PBL associated with autoimmune diseases, most often inflammatory bowel diseases, represent the smallest subset of patients with PBL (3,4,16).

Literature reviews of all reported cases of PBL (4,12,13,16), totaling well over 300 cases, show clear differences in the clinical features, immunophenotype, and molecular findings in patients with HIV-positive PBL, HIV-negative PBL arising in the setting of transplantation, and PBL arising in immunocompetent patients. These findings suggest that PBL, as currently defined, is a heterogeneous entity. These three subsets of PBL likely have a different pathogenesis and the therapeutic approach to PBL patients may eventually reflect these differences.

CLINICAL FEATURES

HIV-Positive PBL

The median age of HIV-positive patients at time of initial diagnosis of PBL is in the fourth or fifth decade in most studies, with a wide age range up to approximately 70 years (3,5,14,19,21a). Children with HIV infection also develop PBL. Vaubell et al. (23) identified 11 of 153 (7 percent) cases of PBL in children, with a median age of 12 years (range, 5 to 18 years). Males are more frequently affected, with a male to female ratio of 3 or 4 to 1 (3,5,13,14,16,19,21a). There is no known racial or ethnic predisposition for developing PBL.

The interval from the diagnosis of HIV infection to the onset of PBL is variable, with a median interval of 2.5 to 5.0 years (3–5). The median CD4-positive cell count is often in the low normal range, but typically lower in patients with more advanced stage disease. EBV DNA levels in serum are often elevated in patients with

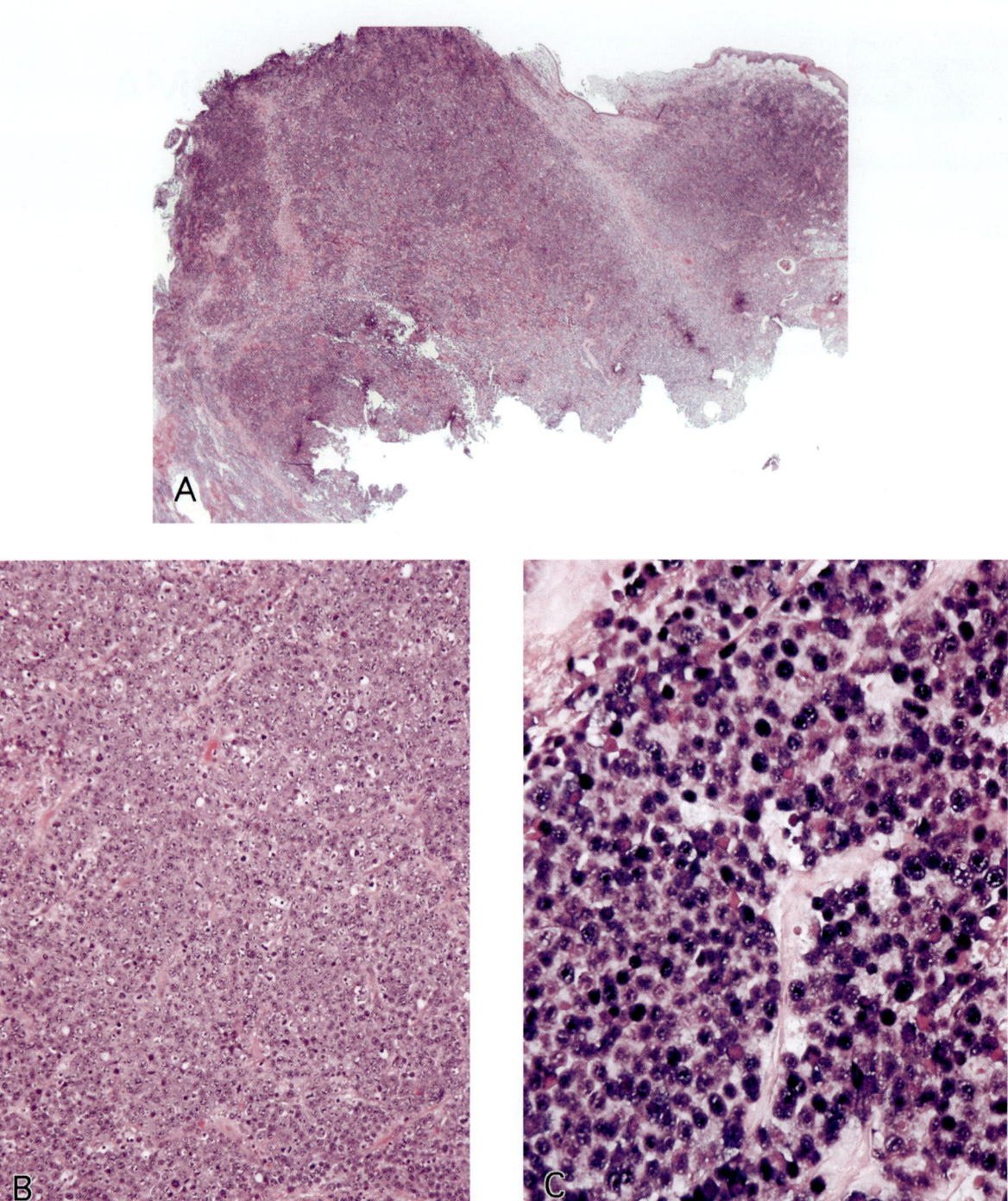

Figure 23-1

**PLASMABLASTIC LYMPHOMA (PBL) INVOLVING GINGIVA
IN HUMAN IMMUNODEFICIENCY VIRUS (HIV)-POSITIVE PATIENT**

This case closely mimics the initial description of PBL by Delecluse et al. (7).

A: At low power, the squamous epithelium is at the right top edge of the field (A,B: hematoxylin and eosin [H&E] stain).

B: Diffuse replacement by PBL with a partial starry sky pattern.

C: Numerous cells are positive for Epstein-Barr virus (EBV)-encoded RNA1 (EBER1) (in situ hybridization with eosin counterstain).

EBV-positive tumors. Systemic B-type symptoms occur in one third of patients (4).

Most patients present with extranodal sites of disease. The oral cavity is involved in approximately 50 percent of patients and other extranodal head and neck sites include the nasal sinuses, nasopharynx, and orbit (3–5,7). Extranodal sites not involving the head and neck region include: skin, bones, soft tissue, central nervous system, mediastinum, lung, pleura, liver, gastrointestinal tract (small intestine, colon, anus), genitourinary tract, ovary, spermatic cord, and testis (2–5,13,14). Bone marrow is involved in about one third of patients (3). Lymph nodes may be involved, however, HIV-positive patients rarely present primarily with lymphadenopathy. Most HIV-positive patients with PBL present with advanced-stage disease (stages III to IV) and a high International Prognostic Index (IPI) (3–5).

Immunocompetent Patients with PBL

This subset of patients has no clinical or laboratory evidence of immunodeficiency and most are HIV negative. The median age of patients at diagnosis of PBL is the sixth decade, with many over 65 years of age (3–5,16); PBL is rare in HIV-negative children.

In immunocompetent patients, PBL occurs most often in men, and the male to female ratio is lower than in HIV-positive patients. Extranodal sites are commonly involved, but the oral cavity is involved in only about 10 percent of patients (4,16). B-type symptoms occur in about 50 percent of patients. Lymph node involvement is more common in immunocompetent patients compared with immunodeficient patients. A subset of immunocompetent patients present primarily with lymphadenopathy. The frequency of advanced-stage disease, bone marrow involvement, and elevated IPI scores is similar to that of HIV-positive patients (4,16).

Transplantation-Associated PBL

PBL has been reported in patients following most types of solid organ transplantation, but the frequency is higher in patients who have heart or kidney transplants (16). Approximately one quarter of PBL patients have received an autologous hematopoietic stem cell transplant. Patients are most often older adults, with a marked male predominance. In a study by Morscio et al. (16), the median age was 63 years (range, 6 to 76 years) and all 12 patients were men. Extranodal sites are usually involved, similar to other PBL patients, with common involvement of skin, gastrointestinal tract, and oral cavity. Some patients present primarily with lymphadenopathy.

Autoimmune Diseases Associated with PBL

PBL arising in the setting of autoimmune disease is the least frequent of the clinical variants. These cases are usually included with HIV-negative PBL in various reports and few cases are reported in adequate detail. Patients are usually 30 to 50 years of age, and there is a male predominance. In our experience, albeit limited and restricted to an academic center, inflammatory bowel diseases are common forms of autoimmune disease associated with PBL. Patients may have a history of either Crohn disease or ulcerative colitis and PBL can present as an intestinal mass (fig. 23-2).

HISTOLOGIC FINDINGS

At extranodal sites (figs. 23-3, 23-4) and lymph nodes (fig. 23-5) PBL usually extensively replaces normal parenchyma. In lymph nodes, a sinusoidal pattern may be observed in areas of partial involvement (fig. 23-5, left). The tumor cells are most often arranged in diffuse sheets and have a cohesive appearance. In some cases, cells are arranged in nests surrounded by delicate fibrous bands or form pseudoalveolar structures. A starry sky pattern is common, often diffusely throughout the tumor (fig. 23-4), but the pattern can be focal. Areas of coagulative necrosis occur. Mitotic figures and single cell apoptosis are usually abundant (fig. 23-2, right).

At high-power magnification, the neoplastic cells are large or consist of intermediate-sized and large cells, and often have abundant cytoplasm and a polygonal shape. The cells often exhibit either immunoblastic or plasmablastic features with prominent nucleoli and basophilic or amphophilic cytoplasm (fig. 23-6). In 10 to 20 percent of cases of PBL, the cells resemble centroblasts, with smaller nucleoli. In some tumors, the neoplastic cells exhibit more overt evidence of plasmacytic differentiation (i.e., maturation), with more abundant cytoplasm and large eccentric nuclei. Plasmacytic differentiation is more

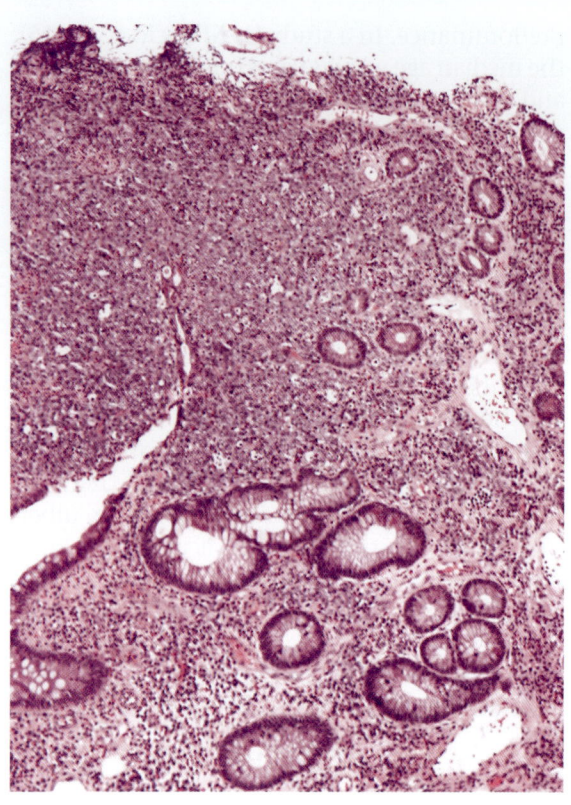
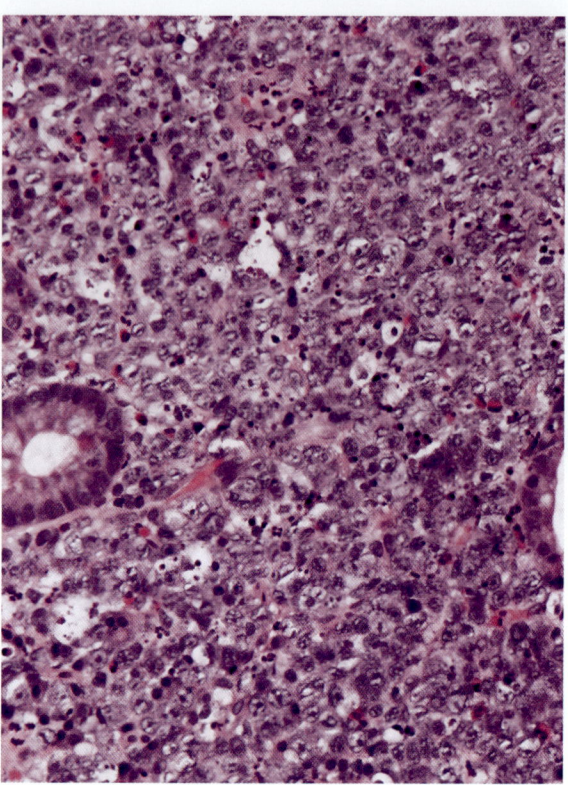

Figure 23-2

PLASMABLASTIC LYMPHOMA INVOLVING RECTUM

The patient had a longstanding history of ulcerative colitis and was HIV-negative.
Left: In this field, PBL partially replaces colonic mucosa and has a partial starry sky pattern.
Right: At high power, the neoplastic cells are large and there is abundant apoptosis (left, right: H&E stain).

common in HIV-negative patients. In some cases of PBL, a mixture of cell types is present or bizarre multinucleated cells are observed (fig. 23-7). Electron microscopic evaluation has shown abundant concentric rings of rough endoplasmic reticulum in the tumor cell cytoplasm, in keeping with prominent plasmablastic or plasmacytic differentiation (9).

CYTOLOGIC FINDINGS

In aspirate smears, numerous mitotic figures, apoptotic cells, or both, are consistently observed (10,25). The neoplastic cells are usually large, but in some cases, a spectrum of intermediate-sized to large cells are appreciated (fig. 23-8). The cytologic types of neoplastic cells identified in histologic sections are also seen in smears. Neoplastic cells with a perinuclear hof or clearing may be observed (25). Binucleated and large bizarre multinucleated cells also may be seen.

IMMUNOPHENOTYPIC FINDINGS

Immunophenotypic studies are essential to the recognition of PBL since these tumors have a plasmablastic immunophenotype, defined as expression of plasmacytic markers and absence of CD20 (figs. 23-9, 23-10) (20). Immunohistochemistry is often more convenient than flow cytometry because these tumors are often extranodal and may not be routinely submitted for flow cytometry. In addition, it is useful to assess both cytoplasmic and surface antigens as part of the workup of PBL.

The neoplastic cells of PBL are usually (95 percent) positive for CD38, CD138 (fig. 23-9A), MUM1/IRF4 (fig. 23-10A), PRDM1/BLIMP1, XBP1, and VS38c. Epithelial membrane antigen (EMA) and CD31 are commonly, but variably, expressed (14,15,24). Although individual plasmacytic markers may be negative, it is rare for a tumor to be negative for more than one marker,

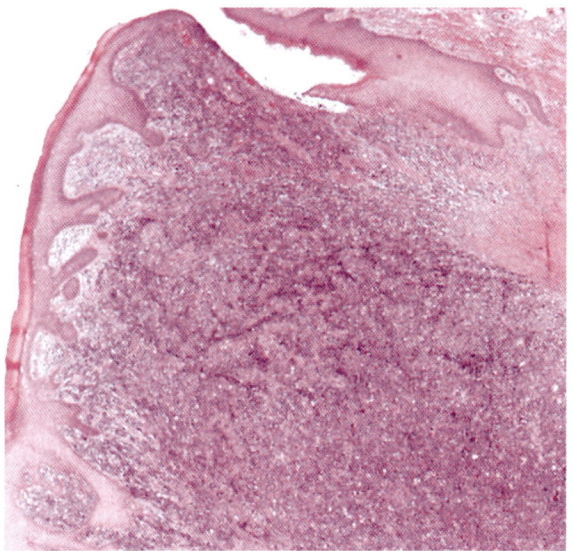

Figure 23-3

**PLASMABLASTIC LYMPHOMA INVOLVING
SKIN OF HIV-POSITIVE PATIENT**

The neoplasm was primarily located in the dermis (H&E stain).

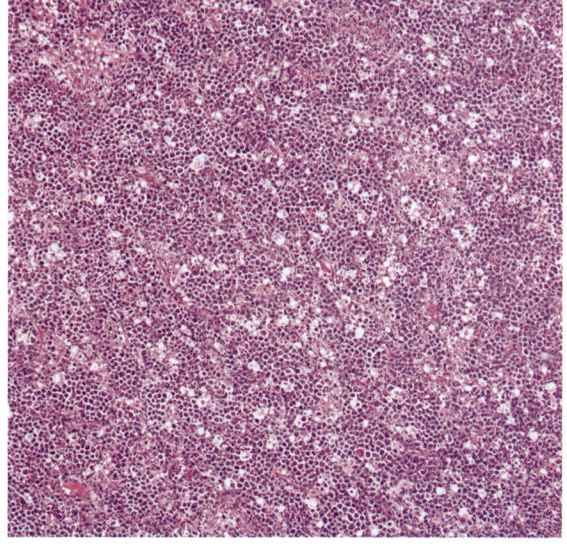

Figure 23-4

PLASMABLASTIC LYMPHOMA INVOLVING OVARY

The neoplasm has a prominent starry sky pattern. This patient was HIV-positive and presented with extensive abdominal disease and underwent resection of the ovaries, uterus, appendix, and a portion of the mesentery (H&E stain).

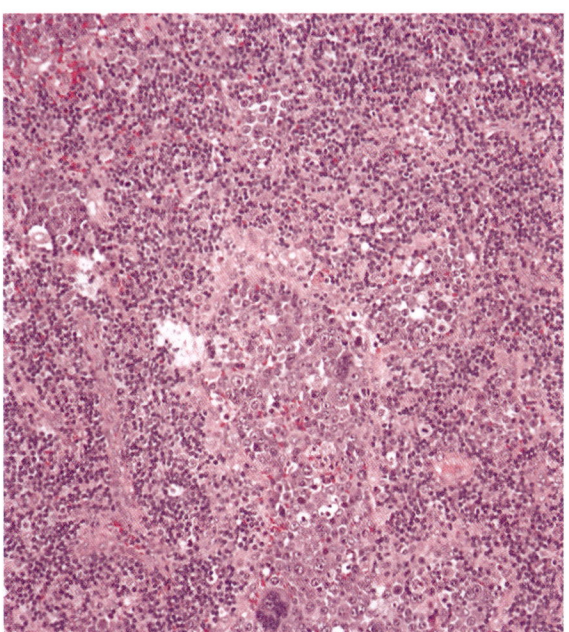

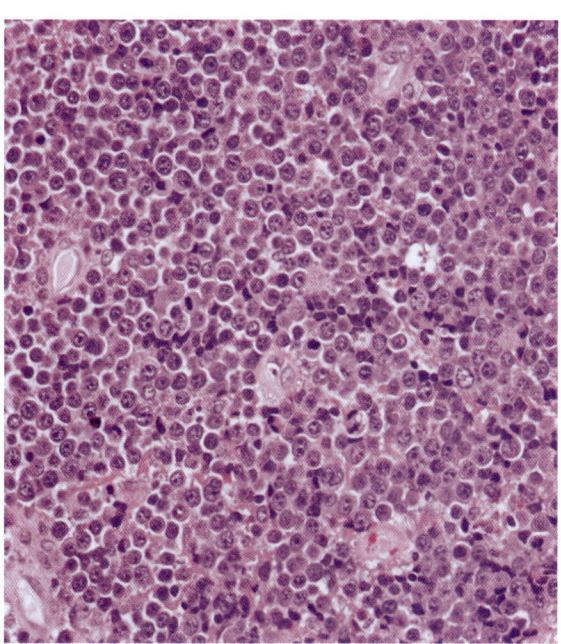

Figure 23-5

PLASMABLASTIC LYMPHOMA INVOLVING PERICOLONIC LYMPH NODES

A 64-year-old man without immunodeficiency had a large PBL. The tumor carried a *MYC* rearrangement as shown by fluorescence in situ hybridization (FISH). The pericolonic lymph nodes are shown.
Left: The tumor partially involves this lymph node in a sinusoidal pattern.
Right: Another pericolonic lymph node is diffusely effaced by PBL (left, right: H&E stain).

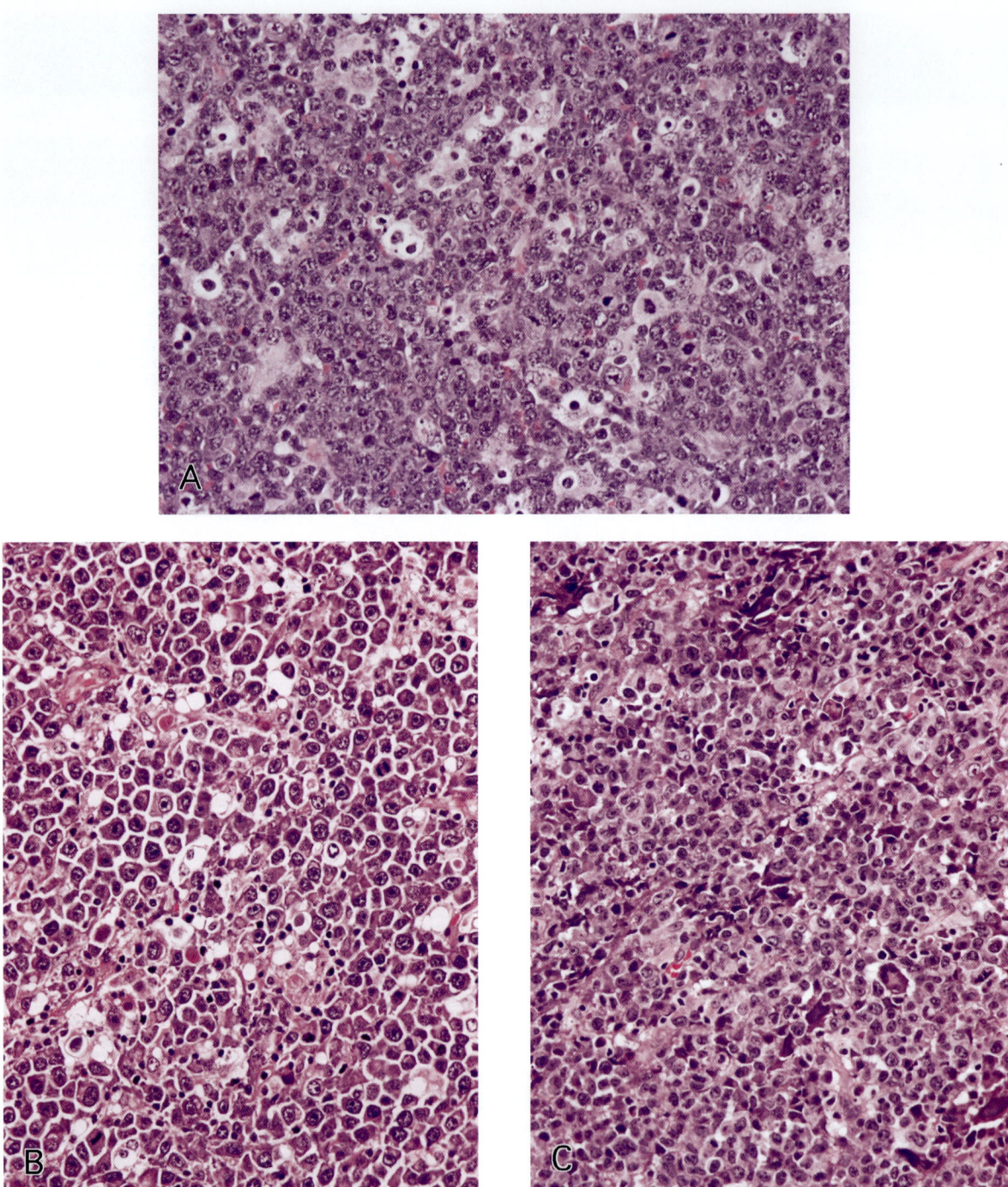

Figure 23-6

SPECTRUM OF DIFFERENTIATION IN PLASMABLASTIC LYMPHOMA

A: This case from the nasopharynx shows mostly immunoblastic features although some cells have increased cytoplasm, suggesting minimal plasmacytic differentiation.

B: A different case from the ovary (same as fig. 23-4) shows many plasmablastic cells as well as cells with more obvious plasmacytic differentiation.

C: This case from the skin (same as fig. 23-3) shows a mixture of centroblasts and cells with more cytoplasm suggestive of plasmacytic differentiation (A–C: H&E stain).

although we have seen rare cases negative for both CD38 and CD138.

Cytoplasmic immunoglobulin light chain (fig. 23-9C,D) is also commonly expressed, in up to 75 percent of PBL cases. Kappa light chain is expressed most frequently and IgG expression is common (fig. 23-11). CD79a is observed in 50 to 75 percent of cases and is often expressed variably (fig. 23-9B). CD30 is expressed commonly, but often variably. CD56 and BCL2 are positive in subsets of cases. CD45/LCA may be expressed, usually dimly. Cyclin D1 may be positive, often variably, in a small subset of cases. The pan-B-cell antigens CD19, CD20 (fig. 23-10, right), CD22, and PAX5 are typically negative in PBLs, although rarely, one of more of these markers is expressed dimly by some cells. CD10 is expressed (often dimly) and PD-L1 is positive, each in about 20 percent of cases. MYC is expressed in PBL, often variably; high MYC expression levels correlate imperfectly with the

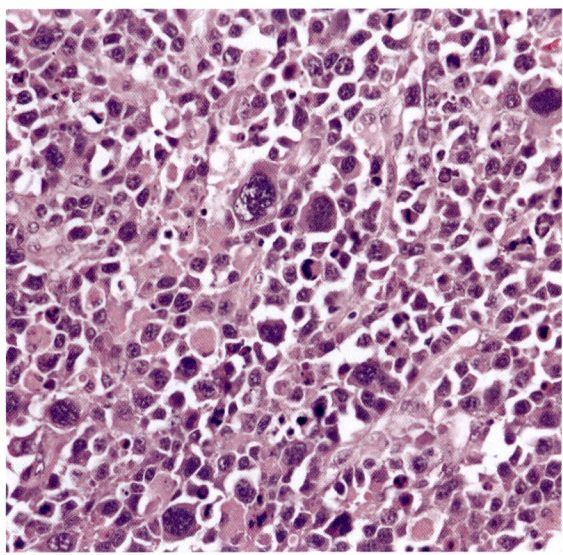

Figure 23-7

PLASMABLASTIC LYMPHOMA

Many multinucleated cells are present (H&E stain).

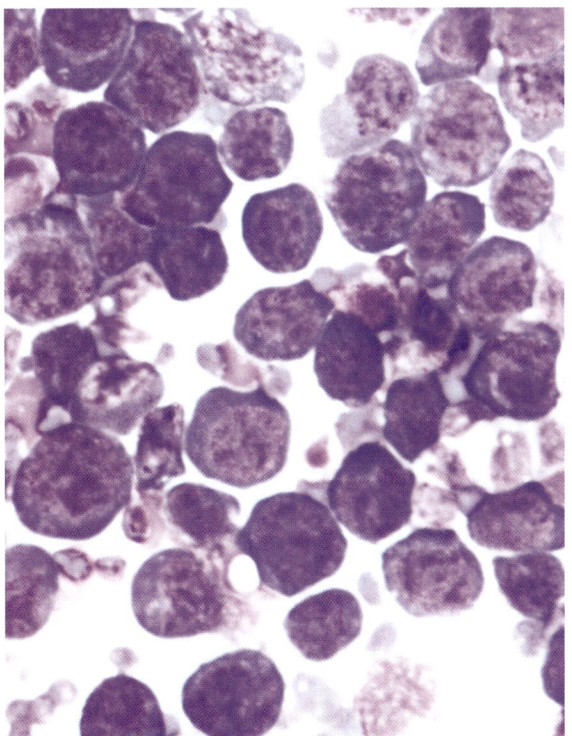
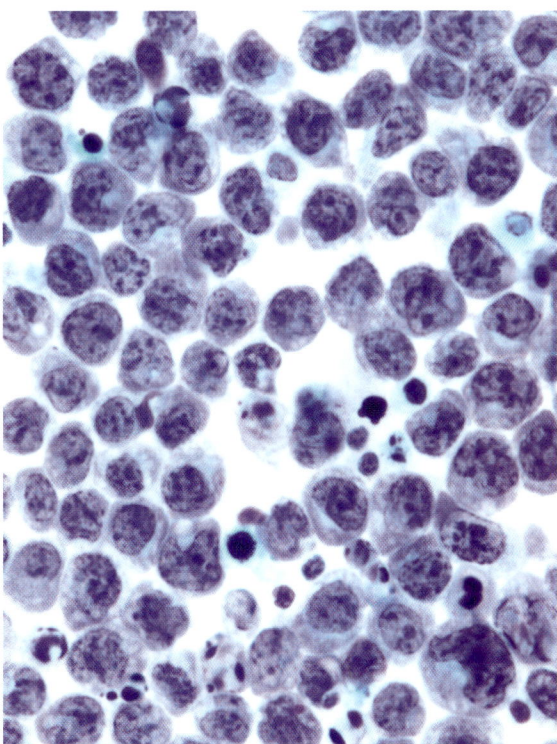

Figure 23-8

PLASMABLASTIC LYMPHOMA

The neoplastic cells in this fine-needle aspirate smear are large, with eccentrically located nuclei, nucleoli, and variable amounts of basophilic cytoplasm. Binucleated cells and mitotic figures are also present (left: Diff-Quik stain; right: Papanicolaou stain). (Courtesy of Dr. J. Stewart, Houston, TX.)

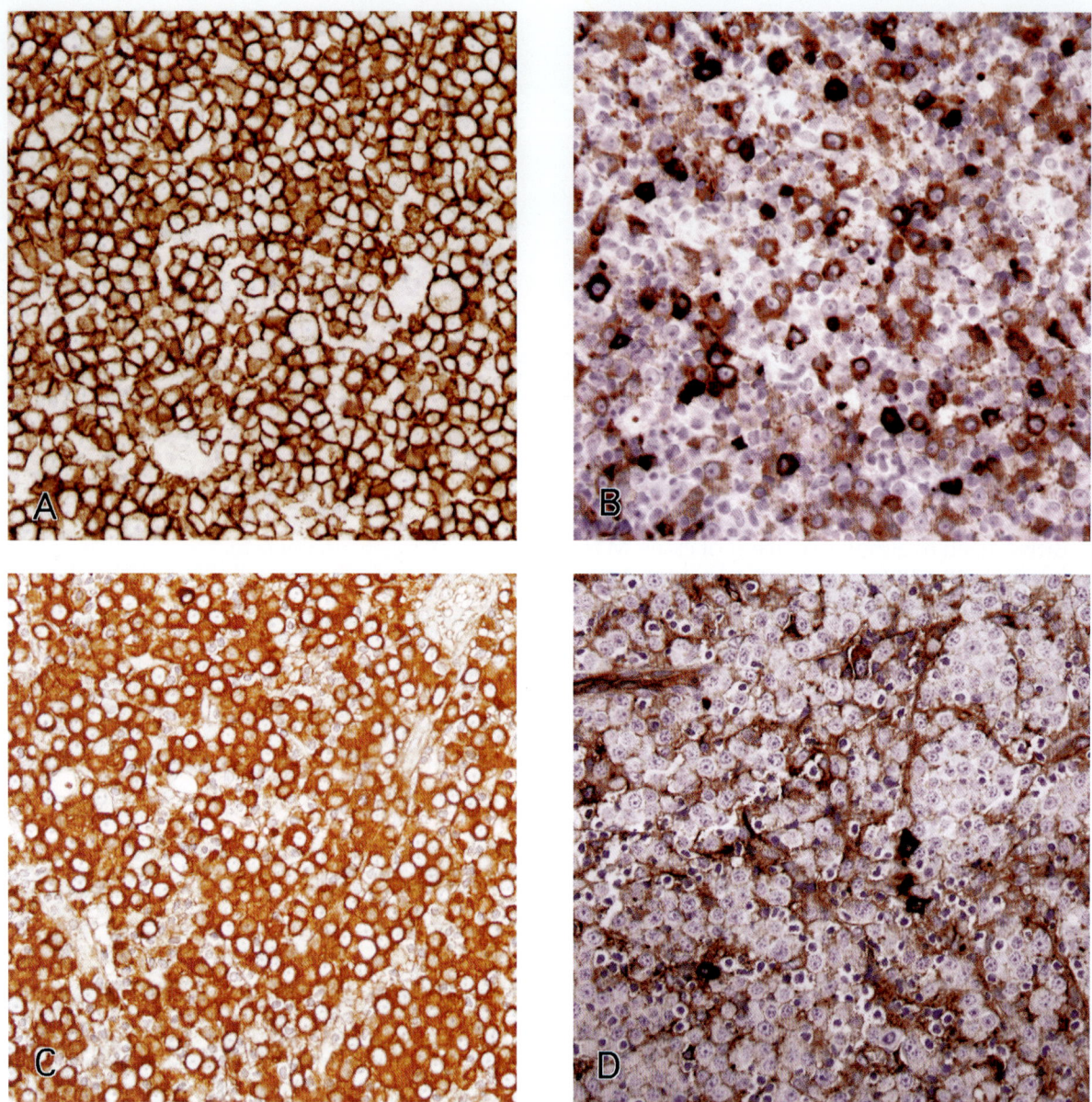

Figure 23-9

**PLASMABLASTIC LYMPHOMA INVOLVING NASAL CAVITY OF
IMMUNOCOMPETENT PATIENT: IMMUNOHISTOCHEMISTRY**

The neoplastic cells are positive for CD138 (A), CD79A (subset) (B), and cytoplasmic lambda (C) and are negative for cytoplasmic kappa (D). (A–D: immunohistochemistry with hematoxylin counterstain).

presence of *MYC* rearrangements (fig. 23-12). The neoplastic cells are negative for BCL6.

Cases of PBL are almost always negative for pan-T-cell antigens, but rare aberrant expression of usually only one T-cell antigen has been reported (21). PBLs are negative for human herpesvirus 8 (HHV8) and anaplastic lymphoma kinase (ALK).

The proliferative index, as measured by Ki-67 reactivity, is usually over 75 percent and often over 90 percent (fig. 23-13). Overall, EBER1 as assessed by in situ hybridization is identified in about 70 percent of cases of PBL (fig. 23-14). EBV latent membrane protein type 1 is present in a small subset of EBER1-positive cases.

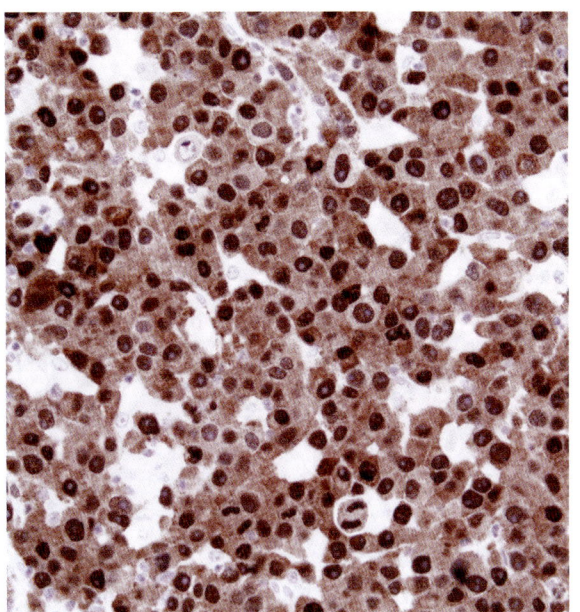 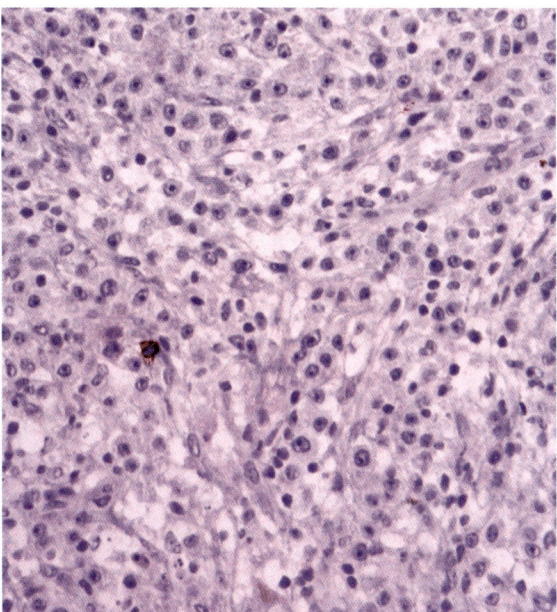

Figure 23-10

PLASMABLASTIC LYMPHOMA INVOLVING OVARY: IMMUNOHISTOCHEMISTRY

The tumor is positive for MUM1/IRF4 (left) and negative for CD20 (right). CD38 and CD138 were positive and CD45/LCA was negative (not shown) (left, right: immunohistochemistry with hematoxylin counterstain). (Same case as shown in fig. 23-3.)

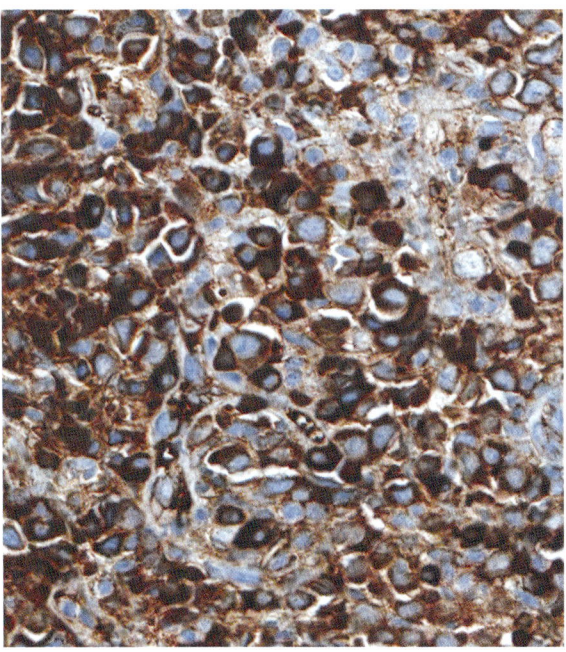 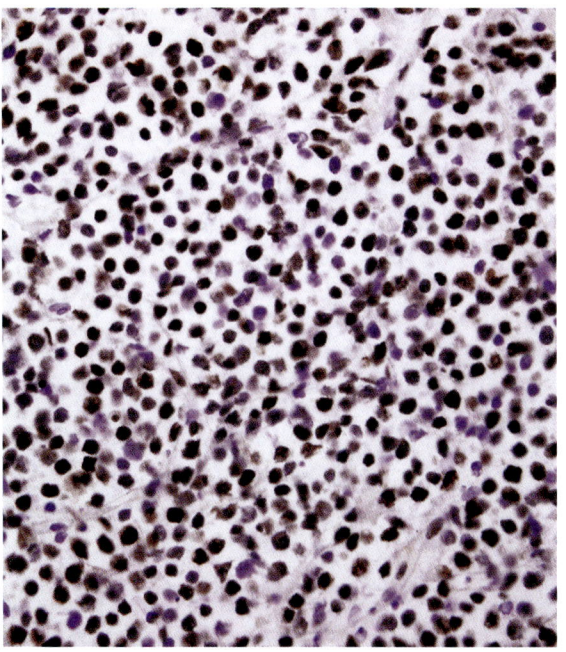

Figure 23-11

PLASMABLASTIC LYMPHOMA: IgG

IgG is commonly expressed in PBL, as shown in this case with abundant cytoplasmic IgG (immunohistochemistry with hematoxylin counterstain).

Figure 23-12

PLASMABLASTIC LYMPHOMA: MYC

MYC is overexpressed by almost all of the cells in this case of PBL (same case as shown in fig. 23-1). FISH showed *MYC* rearrangement (not shown) (immunohistochemistry with hematoxylin counterstain).

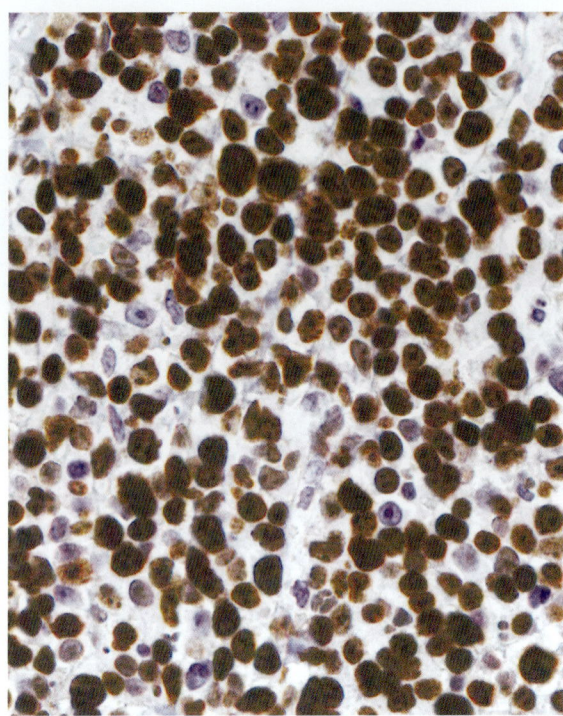

Figure 23-13
PLASMABLASTIC LYMPHOMA: KI-67

Ki-67 is usually high in cases of PBL, indicating a high proliferation rate. The case showed a proliferation rate of about least 90 percent (immunohistochemistry with hematoxylin counterstain).

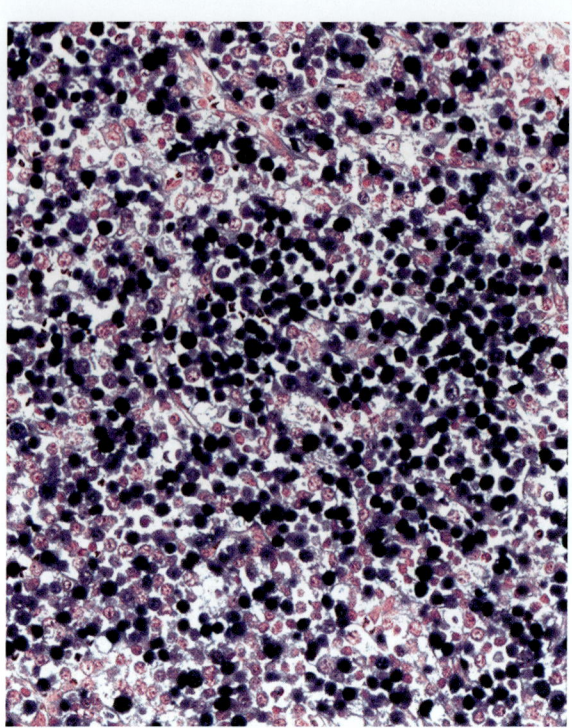

Figure 23-14
PLASMABLASTIC LYMPHOMA: EBER1

Numerous cells are positive for EBV encoded RNA1 (EBER1) (in situ hybridization with eosin counterstain).

There are some immunophenotypic differences between clinically defined PBL subsets. CD10 (42 percent of cases) and CD45/LCA (70 percent) are more commonly expressed in post-transplant PBLs (16). CD56 is more frequently expressed in HIV-associated PBL than in other groups (24). BCL2 is often expressed in PBLs in immunocompetent patients and is detected less often in PBLs arising in HIV-positive or post-transplant patients. In one study, immunohistochemical expression of p53 was common in PBL arising in immunocompetent patients and rare in post-transplant PBLs (16).

MOLECULAR GENETIC FINDINGS

Conventional cytogenetic analysis of PBLs often shows a complex karyotype. Translocations involving chromosome 8q24/*MYC* are common (22). Comparative genomic hybridization analysis has shown gains in multiple chromosomal loci.

PBLs exhibit monoclonal rearrangements of the immunoglobulin genes, with unmutated or mutated variable region sequences (8). *MYC* rearrangements, often partnered with *IGH*, are present in approximately 50 percent of PBLs. *MYC* rearrangements are more common in PBLs arising in HIV-positive patients and in EBV-positive cases; they are uncommon in PBLs that arise following transplantation (16). In one study, *PRDM1* mutations were identified in half of the PBL cases assessed (15a). Translocations involving *CCND1*, *BCL2*, *BCL6*, *MALT1*, and *PAX5* are rare or absent in PBLs (22).

A few gene expression profiling studies of PBL have been reported. Morscio et al. (16) published five cases and Chapman et al. (6) reported on 15 cases. The results show a gene signature more similar to plasma cell neoplasms than DLBCL, with downregulation of B-cell receptor signaling molecules and upregulation of a number of plasma cell–associated molecules, such as CD138, CD300, CD320, and XBP1 (6,16). BAX and mitochondrial gene products are also overexpressed in PBL cases (6).

Plasmablastic Lymphoma
Fits within a Spectrum of B-Cell Differentiation

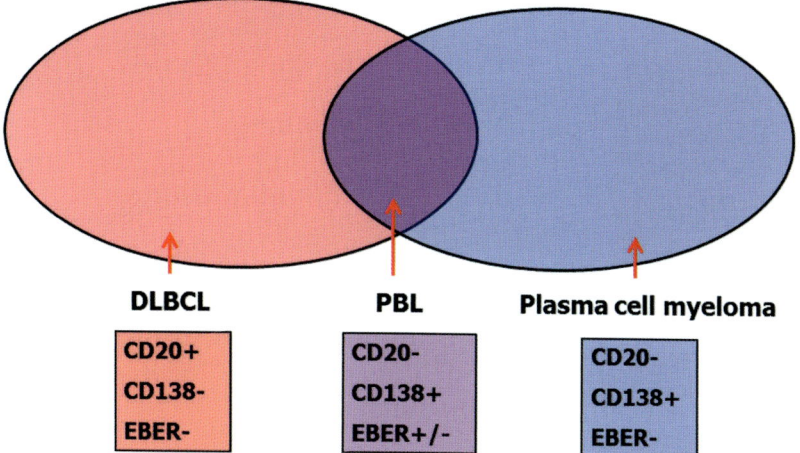

Figure 23-15

OVERLAP BETWEEN DIFFUSE LARGE B-CELL LYMPHOMA (DLBCL), PLASMA CELL MYELOMA, AND PLASMABLASTIC LYMPHOMA (PBL)

The schematic shows PBL in the overlap area. The presence of EBV infection and immunodeficiency are very helpful for recognizing PBL, however, there are cases of PBL with evidence of neither and these cases are difficult to distinguish from DLBCL and anaplastic plasma cell myeloma.

DIFFERENTIAL DIAGNOSIS

Plasma Cell Myeloma. Patients with plasma cell myeloma usually present with a paraprotein in serum, urine, or both, as well as lytic bone lesions, hypercalcemia, kidney failure, and other evidence of end-organ damage. Patients with PBL, in contrast, rarely have serum or urine paraprotein, lytic bone lesions, or other end-organ damage; nevertheless, some PBL patients do have a serum paraprotein (usually low level) or lytic bone lesions. Most cases of plasma cell myeloma show overt evidence of plasmacytic differentiation and are easy to recognize as plasma cell myeloma; those with plasmablastic features are the diagnostic challenge. PBL is more common in patients with HIV infection or other immunocompromised states.

The immunophenotype of PBL and plasma cell myeloma can be very similar, but EBV infection is common in PBL and rarely reported in plasma cell myeloma (24). One study suggested that CD117 is helpful, being negative in PBL but often positive in plasma cell myeloma (14a). In some immunocompetent patients with EBV-negative tumors, distinguishing PBL from plasmablastic plasma cell myeloma is a gray area (fig. 23-15).

Extramedullary Plasmacytoma. These tumors involve extranodal sites, similar to PBL. Usually, patients with extramedullary plasma-cytoma are immunocompetent. Histologically, substantial atypia is lacking and the mitotic rate is low, unlike PBL. As is the case for plasma cell myeloma, the immunophenotype of PBL and plasmacytoma can be very similar, but the proliferation rate in plasmacytoma is usually much lower than PBL. EBV infection is common in PBL and rare in plasmacytoma (see chapter 24).

Diffuse Large B-Cell Lymphoma (DLBCL), Not Otherwise Specified (NOS). Some cases of PBL morphologically resemble DLBCL. Immunophenotypic studies are essential for this differential diagnosis since the cells of DLBCL strongly express pan-B-cell antigens (CD19, CD20, CD22, and PAX5) and are usually negative for CD138, PRDM1/BLIMP1, and XBP1. Rarely, cases of DLBCL with a typical immunophenotype also exhibit areas with morphologic and immunophenotypic features of plasmablastic differentiation and resemble, in part, PBL (fig. 23-16) (15). These cases are better grouped with DLBCL because the plasmablastic areas are likely a secondary phenomenon related to EBV infection or other mechanisms.

ALK-Positive Large B-Cell Lymphoma. This tumor exhibits morphologic features of plasmablasts and expresses plasma cell-associated markers, closely mimicking PBL. Immunohistochemistry for ALK or cytogenetic and fluorescence in situ hybridization (FISH) studies showing 2p23/*ALK*

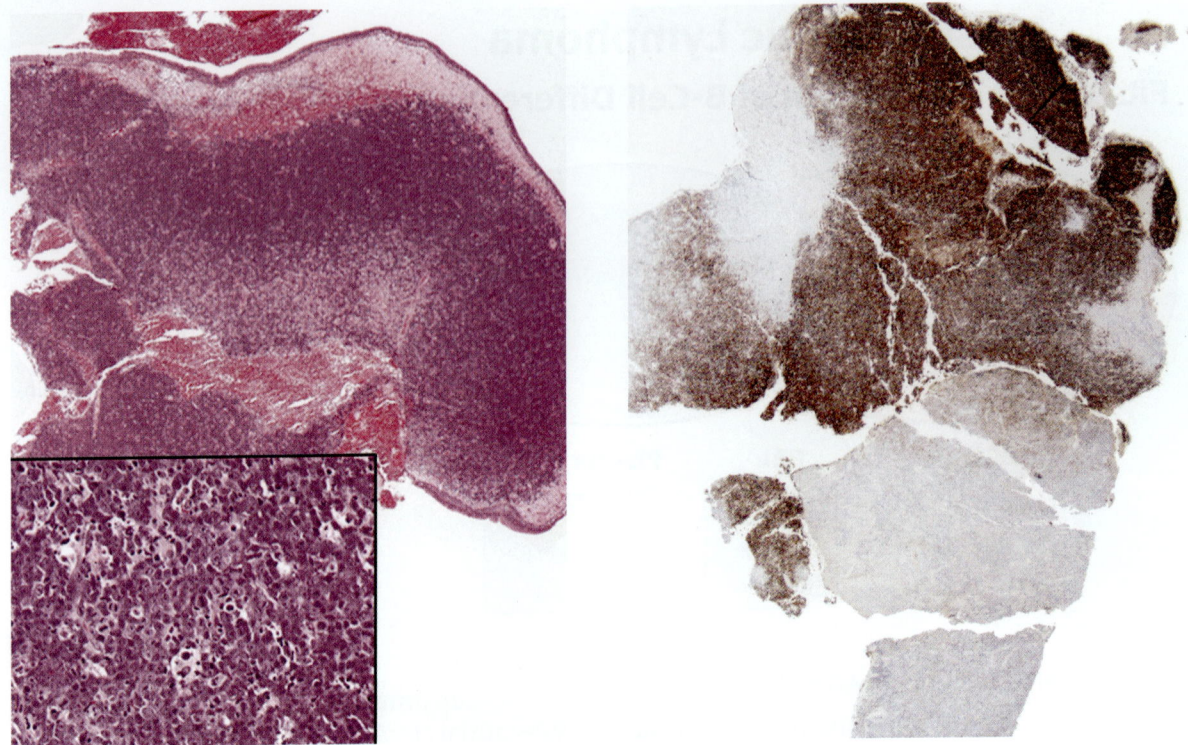

Figure 23-16

DIFFUSE LARGE B-CELL LYMPHOMA INVOLVING MAXILLARY SINUS OF AN IMMUNOCOMPETENT PATIENT WITH PLASMABLASTIC AREAS

Left: At low-power magnification, the neoplasm replaced sinus mucosa and was composed of large (inset) CD20-positive cells that were negative for EBV (H&E stain).

Right: An immunostain for CD138 showed areas that resembled PBL [CD138(+), CD20(-)] whereas the remainder of the tumor had a typical B-cell immunophenotype (immunohistochemistry with hematoxylin counterstain). (Courtesy of Dr. B. Kemp, Houston, TX.)

rearrangements are essential for recognizing ALK-positive large B-cell lymphoma.

Primary Effusion Lymphoma, Solid Variant (HHV8-Positive). These rare tumors occur in the setting of immunodeficiency, particularly HIV infection, and can resemble PBL at the morphologic and immunophenotypic levels. Importantly, these tumors are infected by EBV and HHV8.

Plasmablastic Transformation of Low-Grade Lymphoma or Plasma Cell Myeloma. Rarely, patients with low-grade B-cell lymphomas such as chronic lymphocytic leukemia/small cell lymphoma (CLL/SLL) or follicular lymphoma transform to a high-grade tumor that closely resembles PBL (discussed in chapter 5). These tumors may or may not be positive for EBV infection. Similarly, patients with plasma cell myeloma may undergo histologic transformation to

a neoplasm that resembles PBL. These secondary forms of PBL have a pathogenesis distinct from de novo PBL and are not included in the category of PBL in the WHO classification (20).

TREATMENT AND PROGNOSIS

There is no consensus regarding the optimal treatment regimen for patients with PBL (1,3,5). As these tumors are CD20 negative, there is no role for rituximab. Patients with PBL who have been treated with the cyclophosphamide, doxorubicin, vincristine, and prednisone (CHOP) chemotherapy regimen have had a poor prognosis. For patients with HIV infection, some suggest that more aggressive chemotherapy regimens may be helpful (17). The value of HAART in allowing patients to undergo aggressive therapy also has been emphasized for this patient population (3,17,19). Others, however, have reviewed the literature and have not found the data for aggressive chemotherapy regimens compelling (3,4). In a case report, bortezomib added to a chemotherapy regimen resulted in complete remission (26). There are advocates for using autologous hematopoietic stem cell transplantation, although this approach is currently under investigation (1).

The overall prognosis for PBL patients is poor regardless of HIV status. Most patients have an aggressive clinical course and survive 2 to 3 years or less after diagnosis (3–5,13,14,16,21a). Patients with localized (stage I) PBL may have a better response to therapy and longer survival (3,18). Patients with *MYC*-rearranged PBL appear to have a poorer prognosis. Additional factors associated with a worse prognosis in PBL patients include: age over 60 years, advanced clinical stage, and bone marrow involvement, however, only stage was significant in a multivariate analysis (3,4).

REFERENCES

1. Al-Malki MM, Castillo JJ, Sloan JM, Re A. Hematopoietic cell transplantation for plasmablastic lymphoma: a review. Biol Blood Marrow Transplant 2014;20:1877-1884.
2. Banks PM, Keller RH, Li CY, White WL. Malignant lymphoma of plasmablastic identity. A neoplasm with both "immunoblastic" and plasma cellular features. Am J Med 1978;64:906-909.
3. Castillo JJ, Bibas M, Miranda RN. The biology and treatment of plasmablastic lymphoma. Blood 2015;125:2323-2330.
4. Castillo JJ, Winer ES, Stachurski D, et al. Clinical and pathological differences between human immunodeficiency virus-positive and human immunodeficiency virus-negative patients with plasmablastic lymphoma. Leuk Lymphoma 2010;51:2047-2053.
5. Cattaneo C, Re A, Ungari M, et al. Plasmablastic lymphoma among human immunodeficiency virus-positive patients: results of a single center's experience. Leuk Lymphoma 2015;56:267-269.
6. Chapman J, Gentles AJ, Sujoy V, et al. Gene expression analysis of plasmablastic lymphoma identifies downregulation of B cell receptor signaling and additional unique transcriptional programs. Leukemia 2015;29:2270-2273.
7. Delecluse HJ, Anagnostopoulos I, Dallenbach F, et al. Plasmablastic lymphomas of the oral cavity: a new entity associated with the human immunodeficiency virus infection. Blood 1997;89:1413-1420.
8. Gaidano G, Cerri M, Capello D, et al. Molecular histogenesis of plasmablastic lymphoma of the oral cavity. Br J Haematol 2002;119:622-628.
9. Goedhals J, Beukes CA, Cooper S. The ultrastructural features of plasmablastic lymphoma. Ultrastruct Pathol 2006;30:427-433.
10. Lin O, Gerhard R, Zerbini MC, Teruya-Feldstein J. Cytologic features of plasmablastic lymphoma. Cancer 2005;105:139-144.
11. Liu F, Asano N, Tatematsu A, et al. Plasmablastic lymphoma of the elderly: a clinicopathological comparison with age-related Epstein-Barr virus-associated B cell lymphoproliferative disorder. Histopathology 2012;61:1183-1197.
12. Liu JJ, Zhang L, Ayala E, et al. Human immunodeficiency virus (HIV)-negative plasmablastic lymphoma: a single institutional experience and literature review. Leuk Res 2011;35:1571-1577.
13. Liu M, Liu B, Liu B, et al. Human immunodeficiency virus-negative plasmablastic lymphoma: A comprehensive analysis of 114 cases. Oncol Rep 2015;33:1615-1620.
14. Loghavi S, Aladily TN, Alayed K, et al. Stage, age, and EBV status impact outcomes of plasmablastic lymphoma patients: a clinicopathologic analysis of 61 patients. J Hematol Oncol 2015;8:65.
14a. Marks E, Shi Y, Wang Y. CD117 (KIT) is a useful marker in the diagnosis of plasmablastic plasma cell myeloma. Histopathology 2017;71:81-88.
15. Montes-Moreno S, Gonzalez-Medina AR, Rodriguez-Pinilla SM, et al. Aggressive large B-cell lymphoma with plasma cell differentiation: immunohistochemical characterization of plasmablastic lymphoma and diffuse large B-cell lymphoma with partial plasmablastic phenotype. Haematologica 2010;95:1342-1349.
15a. Montes-Moreno S, Martinez-Magunacelaya N, Zecchini-Barrese T, et al. Plasmablastic lymphoma phenotype is determined by genetic alterations in MYC and PRDM1. Mod Pathol 2017;30:85-94.

16. Morscio J, Dierickx D, Nijs J, et al. Clinicopathologic comparison of plasmablastic lymphoma in HIV-positive, immunocompetent, and post-transplant patients: Single-center series of 25 cases and meta-analysis of 277 reported cases. Am J Surg Pathol 2014;38:875-886.

17. Noy A, Lensing SY, Moore PC, et al. Plasmablastic lymphoma is treatable in the HAART era. A 10 year retrospective by the AIDS Malignancy Consortium. Leuk Lymphoma 2016;57:1731-1734.

18. Pinnix CC, Shah JJ, Chuang H, et al. Doxorubicin-based chemotherapy and radiation therapy produces favorable outcomes in limited-stage plasmablastic lymphoma: a single institution review. Clin Lymphoma Myeloma Leuk 2016;16:122-128.

19. Schommers P, Hentrich M, Hoffmann C, et al. Survival of AIDS-related diffuse large B-cell lymphoma, Burkitt lymphoma, and plasmablastic lymphoma in the German HIV Lymphoma Cohort. Br J Haematol 2015;168:806-810.

20. Stein H, Harris NL, Campo E. Plasmablastic lymphoma. In: Swerdlow SH, Campo E, Harris NL, Jaffe ES, Pileri SA, Stein H, Thiele J, Vardiman JW, eds. WHO Classification of Tumours of Haematopoietic and Lymphoid Tissues. Lyon: IARC Press; 2008:256-257.

21. Sun J, Medeiros LJ, Lin P, Lu G, Bueso-Ramos CE, You MJ. Plasmablastic lymphoma involving the penis: a previously unreported location of a case with aberrant CD3 expression. Pathology 2011;43:54-57.

21a. Tchernonog E, Faurie P, Coppo P, et al. Clinical characteristics and prognostic factors of plasmablastic lymphoma patients: analysis of 135 patients from the LYSA group. Ann Oncol 2017;28:843-848.

22. Valera A, Balague O, Colomo L, et al. IG/MYC rearrangements are the main cytogenetic alteration in plasmablastic lymphomas. Am J Surg Pathol 2010;34:1686-1694.

23. Vaubell JI, Sing Y, Ramburan A, et al. Pediatric plasmablastic lymphoma: a clinicopathologic study. Int J Surg Pathol 2014;22:607-616.

24. Vega F, Chang CC, Medeiros LJ, et al. Plasmablastic lymphomas and plasmablastic plasma cell neoplasms have nearly identical immunophenotypic profiles. Mod Pathol 2005;18:806-815.

25. Wang J, Hernandez OJ, Sen F. Plasmablastic lymphoma involving breast: a case diagnosed by fine-needle aspiration and core needle biopsy. Diagn Cytopathol 2008;36:257-261.

26. Yan M, Dong Z, Zhao F, et al. CD20-positive plasmablastic lymphoma with excellent response to bortezomib combined with rituximab. Eur J Hematol 2014;93:77-80.

24 PLASMACYTOMA

GENERAL FEATURES

Plasmacytoma is a neoplasm composed entirely of monoclonal plasma cells in a patient without radiologic or laboratory evidence of plasma cell (multiple) myeloma at the time of diagnosis. Plasmacytomas are traditionally subdivided into two subsets: *solitary plasmacytoma of bone* (also known as *solitary osseous plasmacytoma*), a lesion confined to bone, and *extramedullary (nonosseous) plasmacytoma* (16,21,25).

Although not the focus of this chapter, the World Health Organization (WHO) classification recognizes a number of plasma cell neoplasms (Table 24-1) (21). Plasma cell myeloma is the most common malignant tumor derived from plasma cells. The incidence of plasma cell myeloma is 5.35 per 100,000 person-years (6). The median age of patients with plasma cell myeloma is in the seventh decade, and the neoplasm is more common in men than women (ratio of 3 to 1). Plasma cell myeloma occurs more often in African-Americans than whites (6). Patients with plasma cell myeloma usually present with a monoclonal paraprotein in serum and urine, often at a high level; hypercalcemia, renal failure, anemia, and lytic bone lesions (so-called CRAB); and damage to other organs as a result of monoclonal protein (21,25). Lymph node involvement is uncommon, or at least is rarely biopsied, at the time of initial diagnosis of plasma cell myeloma.

Plasmacytoma is a rare tumor that is approximately 16 times less frequent than plasma cell myeloma, with an incidence of 0.34/100,000 person-years (6). Plasmacytomas represent about 6 percent of all plasma cell neoplasms (21,26). The median age of patients with plasmacytoma is 60 to 70 years, the male to female ratio is over 2 to 1, and plasmacytoma (like myeloma) is more common in African Americans (6).

Solitary plasmacytoma of bone represents approximately two thirds of all cases of plasmacytoma. Patients present with a single bone lesion. Sampling of the posterior iliac crest bone marrow is either negative or shows little involvement by neoplastic plasma cells. Involvement of the iliac crest, best detected by a sensitive method such as flow cytometry immunophenotyping, correlates with a poorer prognosis (24). Approximately 75 percent of cases arise in the axial skeleton, most frequently in the vertebrae, ribs, skull, and pelvis (13,26). Approximately 25 percent of cases involve the appendicular skeleton, most frequently the femur or humerus (13,26). Patients with involvement of the appendicular skeleton are often a few years older than patients with axial skeleton disease (6).

In the Surveillance, Epidemiology, and End Results (SEER) database, the median age of patients with extramedullary plasmacytoma (EMP, all sites) occurs in the sixth decade, with a male to female ratio of 2.6 to 1.0 (6). African-Americans have a higher risk of EMP than whites; Asians have the lowest risk (6). EMP presents at a wide variety of anatomic sites. The upper

---

Table 24-1

PLASMA CELL NEOPLASMS RECOGNIZED IN THE WORLD HEALTH ORGANIZATION CLASSIFICATION

Monoclonal gammopathy of uncertain/unknown significance (MGUS): IgM and IgG/A

Heavy chain diseases: μ, γ, α

Plasmacytoma
Solitary lesion of bone
Extramedullary (extraosseous)

Plasma cell myeloma
Variants
Asymptomatic/smoldering
Nonsecretory
Plasma cell leukemia

Monoclonal immunoglobulin deposition diseases
Primary amyloidosis
Systemic light and heavy chain deposition diseases

Osteosclerotic myeloma/POEMS[a] syndrome

[a]POEMS = polyneuropathy, organomegaly, endocrinopathy, monoclonal gammopathy, and skin changes.

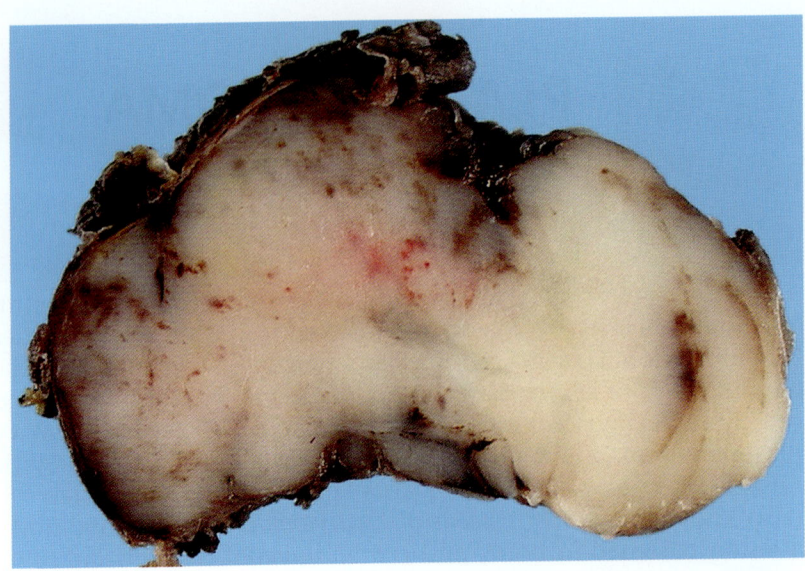

Figure 24-1

SOLITARY PLASMACYTOMA INVOLVING SUBMANDIBULAR GLAND

This case was unusual because the plasma cells were positive for Epstein-Barr virus (EBV). (Courtesy of Dr. F. Petersson, Hong Kong.)

aerodigestive tract is most commonly involved (70 to 80 percent of patients) (26). The head and neck region is another common location (fig. 24-1) (9). Ten to 20 percent of patients with EMP arising at these two sites have regional lymph node involvement, usually the cervical lymph nodes. Other anatomic sites involved by EMP include the central nervous system, breast, gastrointestinal tract, bladder, testis, and skin. Rarely, EMP arises in lymph nodes.

The focus of this chapter is on plasma cell tumors that involve the lymph nodes, particularly, EMP arising in lymph nodes. EMP draining to regional lymph nodes as well plasma cell myeloma involving lymph nodes are also briefly covered. Two immunoglobulin deposition diseases commonly associated with plasma cell neoplasms, amyloidosis and crystal-storing histiocytosis, are also discussed.

CLINICAL FEATURES

EMP arising in lymph node (*nodal plasmacytoma*) represents less than 10 percent of all cases of EMP and about 0.1 percent of all plasma cell neoplasms (17,22). By definition, the bone marrow is not involved in patients with nodal plasmacytoma. Compared with EMP overall, the median age of patients with nodal plasmacytoma is younger and the male to female ratio may be lower, but is at least 1.5 to 1.0 (17,22). Little data correlating nodal plasmacytoma with race are available. Most patients with nodal plasmacytoma have an unremarkable medical history and

are asymptomatic. Usually only a single lymph node or, less often, a group of lymph nodes, is involved. Nevertheless, rare patients with bilateral or generalized lymphadenopathy are reported. The lymph node size is variable, often small, but some patients present with large lymph nodes, up to 10 cm (22). Cytopenias are uncommon.

For EMP patients overall, almost half have a serum (or urine) paraprotein and the level of the serum paraprotein correlates with the risk of dissemination (26). Rare patients have high serum paraprotein levels (28). Patients with nodal plasmacytoma have a lower frequency (20 percent) and lower level of serum paraprotein, often IgA or IgG, than EMP overall (13,29). They also have a very low risk of disease dissemination to other lymph nodes or bone marrow, and progression to plasma cell myeloma is rare.

A study by Shao et al. (27) differs somewhat from other studies. These authors reported 12 patients with EMP associated with IgA secretion, including 9 patients with nodal plasmacytoma. The patients were young, with a median age in the fourth decade, and included 2 adolescents and 1 child. Two thirds of these patients had a history of an autoimmune disorder and half had low-level IgA paraprotein in serum. None developed plasma cell myeloma. The authors raise the possibility that IgA-positive cases of EMP represent a distinct clinicopathologic subset.

Patients with regional lymph node involvement by EMP have symptoms related to the extranodal tumor mass. For example, nasal obstruction, epistaxis, and rhinorrhea are commonly associated with EMP of the upper respiratory tract. Patients with EMP draining to regional lymph nodes have lymphadenopathy that may be prominent, but are otherwise asymptomatic.

HISTOLOGIC FINDINGS

In nodal plasmacytoma, the lymph node architecture is partially or completely effaced by sheets of plasma cells (fig 24-2). In cases with subtotal involvement, the plasma cells initially involve the medulla and paracortical regions and spare residual lymphoid follicles (17,22). In cases with total effacement, the neoplasm has a diffuse pattern and can extend into perinodal soft tissue. In regional lymph nodes draining EMP, the plasma cells involve the lymph node partially, in sinusoids, medulla, or interfollicular regions, consistent with a pattern suggestive of drainage (fig. 24-3).

In both nodal plasmacytoma and regional lymph nodes draining EMP, the findings may be similar. The plasma cells are usually well differentiated, mature (or Marschalko type) cells, with eccentrically situated nuclei with alternating segments of dark and lighter areas of chromatin condensation, so-called clock-faced chromatin (fig. 24-4). Nucleoli are absent or inconspicuous. The plasma cell cytoplasm is abundant and amphophilic, and may contain multiple eosinophilic globules that compress the nucleus to the periphery of the cells (Russell bodies). Immunoglobulin also may protrude into nuclei, which on cross section appear as eosinophilic pseudoinclusions (Dutcher bodies). Amyloid deposits, often associated with a foreign body giant cell reaction, may be present (fig. 24-3C). In some cases, more common in EMP draining to lymph nodes, the plasma cells exhibit some degree of nuclear polymorphism, usually mild or moderate (fig. 24-3B). Necrosis is uncommon and the mitotic rate is low.

Plasma cell myeloma also involves lymph nodes, partially or completely replacing lymph node architecture. Cases of plasma cell myeloma that disseminate to lymph nodes often exhibit moderate to severe cytologic atypia, with a high nucleus to cytoplasm ratio, prominent nucleoli, and increased mitotic activity (figs. 24-5, 24-6).

CYTOLOGIC FINDINGS

Neoplastic plasma cells in cytologic preparations show a range of differentiation. In most cases of EMP, they are well differentiated. Aspirate smears typically show a dispersed population of cells characterized by eccentrically located round nuclei with clumped clock-faced chromatin, inconspicuous to absent nucleoli, and abundant cytoplasm (fig. 24-7A). The plasmacytoid features are more easily appreciated on Romanowsky-based stains than Papanicolaou or hematoxylin and eosin (H&E) stains. The Giemsa or Diff-Quik stain highlights the abundant basophilic cytoplasm with a prominent perinuclear Golgi area, also known as a perinuclear hof (fig. 24-7B). Plasma cells show some variation in size and maturity. Binucleated and occasionally multinucleated cells are also seen. Poorly differentiated plasma cells, as often seen in plasma cell myeloma, have high nuclear to cytoplasmic ratios with large nuclei, vesicular chromatin, prominent nucleoli, and often less cytoplasm (fig. 24-7C, 24-7D). Mitotic figures and apoptotic bodies are often observed.

IMMUNOPHENOTYPIC FINDINGS

As nodal plasmacytoma is rare, most ancillary data available are derived from studies of as EMP involving all anatomic sites (16). The plasma cells of EMP demonstrate cytoplasmic monotypic immunoglobulin (Ig) light chain restriction (figs. 24-5C, 24-5D). The cells usually express IgG or IgA, evidence of class-switched Ig heavy chain. IgD and IgE are rarely expressed and IgM almost never expressed by EMP.

The plasma cells are positive for CD38, CD79A (usually), CD138 (fig. 24-2C), VS38, EMA, MUM1/IRF4, XBP1, and BLIMP1 and are typically negative for pan-B-cell antigens such as CD19 and CD20. EMPs are usually negative for CD56, but a small subset of cases is positive (in contrast to plasma cell myeloma, which is often CD56 positive). BCL2 is often positive, but usually weak (16). The few cases assessed for MYC expression have had few positive cells or were negative (3). EMPs, including nodal plasmacytomas, are usually negative for CD43, cyclin D1, p21, and p53 (16,17). The proliferation fraction in EMP is generally low, ranging from 5 to 30 percent Ki-67-positive cells.

Epstein-Barr Virus in Extramedullary Plasmacytoma

Almost all cases of EMP are negative for Epstein-Barr virus (EBV) infection and no

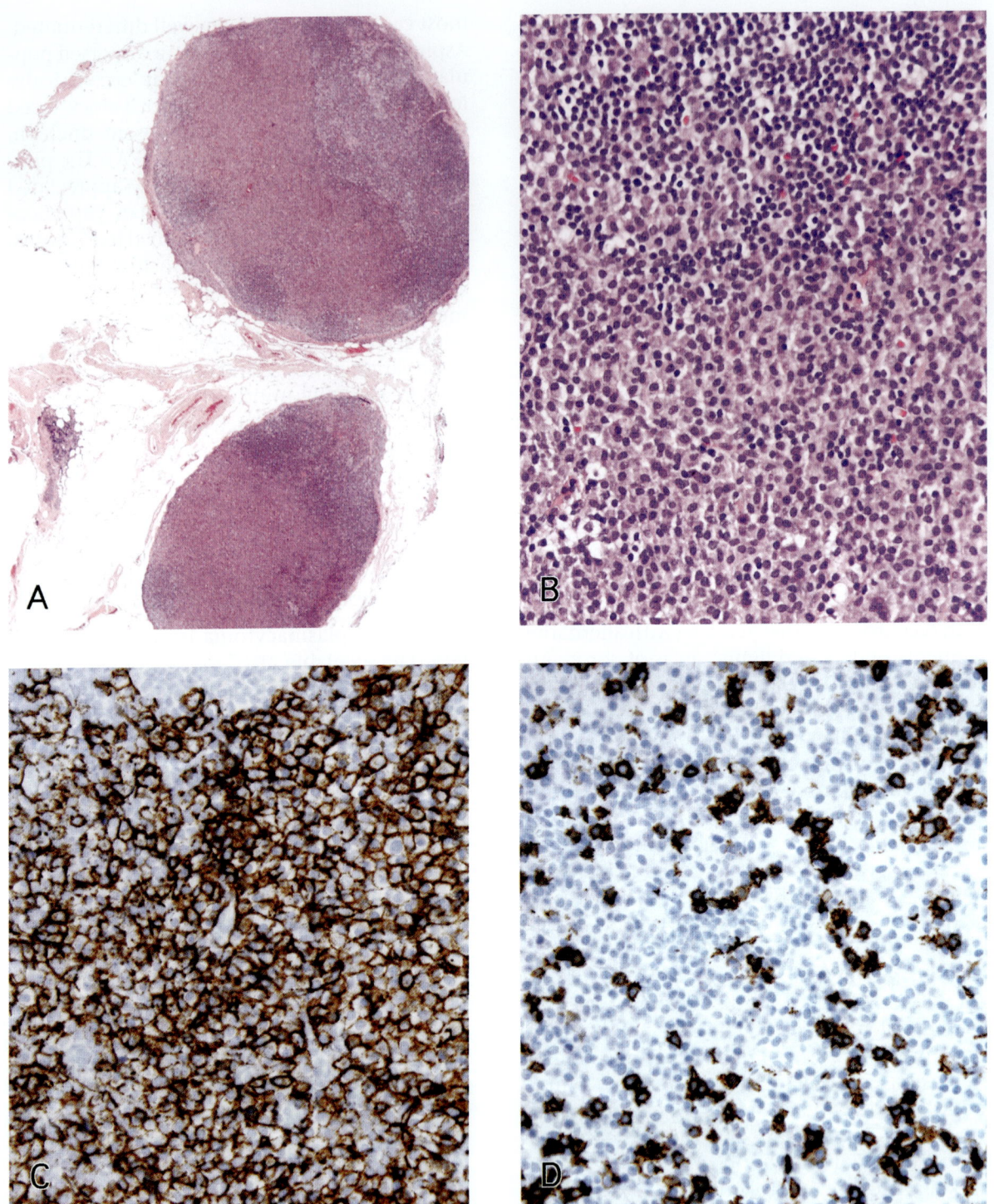

Figure 24-2

SOLITARY PLASMACYTOMA INVOLVING AXILLARY LYMPH NODE

A: The plasma cells partially replace the lymph node (A,B: hematoxylin and eosin [H&E] stain).

B: The plasma cells are small and monomorphous (uninvolved lymph node at top of field).

C,D: Immunohistochemical analysis shows that the plasma cells are positive for CD138 (C) and negative for CD20 (D) (C,D: immunohistochemistry with hematoxylin counterstain).

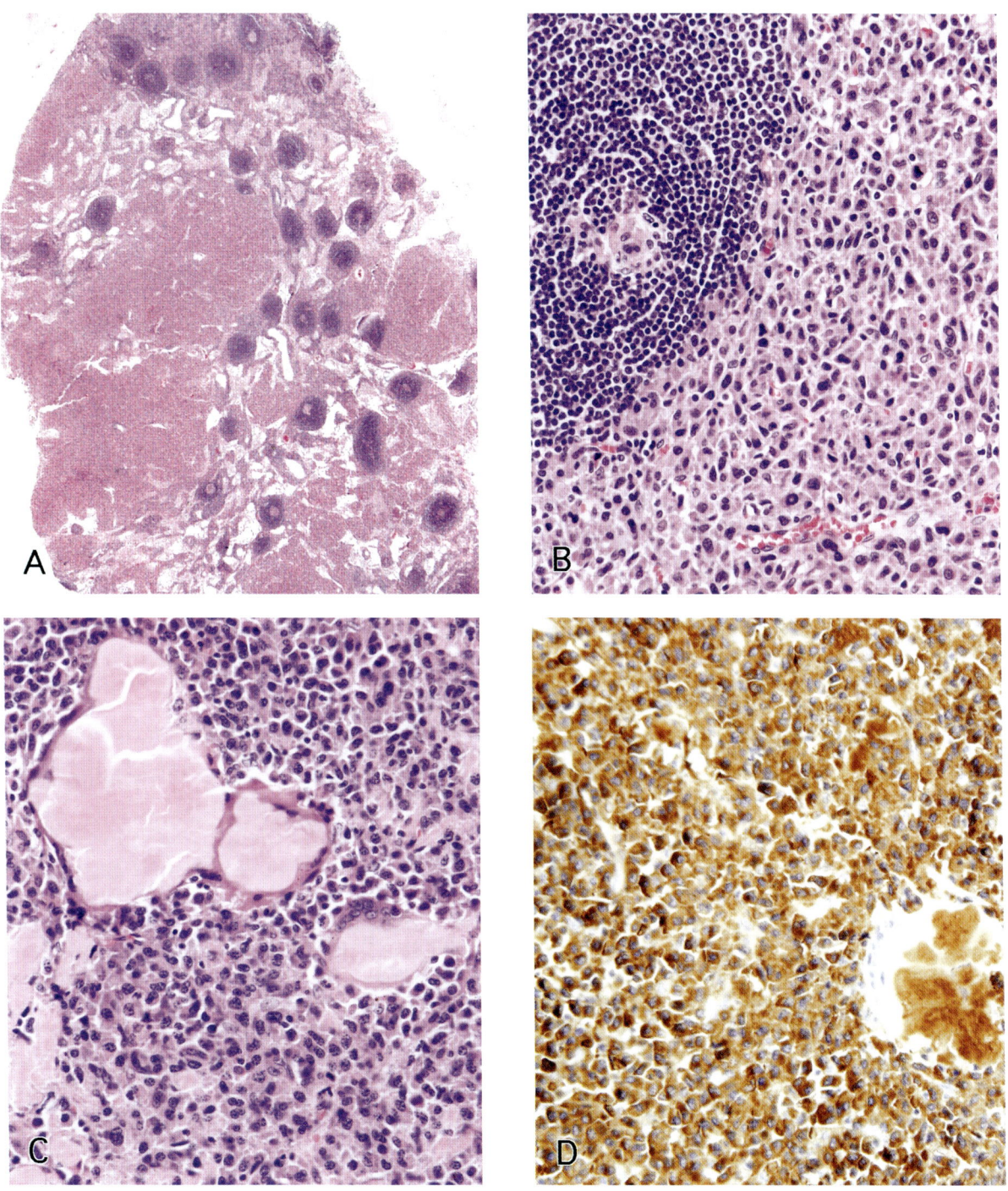

Figure 24-3

MESENTERIC LYMPH NODE DRAINING AN EXTRAMEDULLARY PLASMACYTOMA OF INTESTINE

A: The lymph node parenchyma is partially involved by eosinophilic collections of mature plasma cells. Patent sinuses and residual lymphoid follicles (appearing blue) are also present in this field (A–C: H&E stain).

B: High-power view of the plasma cells and a residual lymphoid follicle (top left of field).

C: Amyloid deposits surrounded by foreign body giant cells are associated with the plasma cells in this lymph node.

D: Immunohistochemical analysis shows that the plasma cells and amyloid are positive for kappa light chain (immunohistochemistry with hematoxylin counterstain).

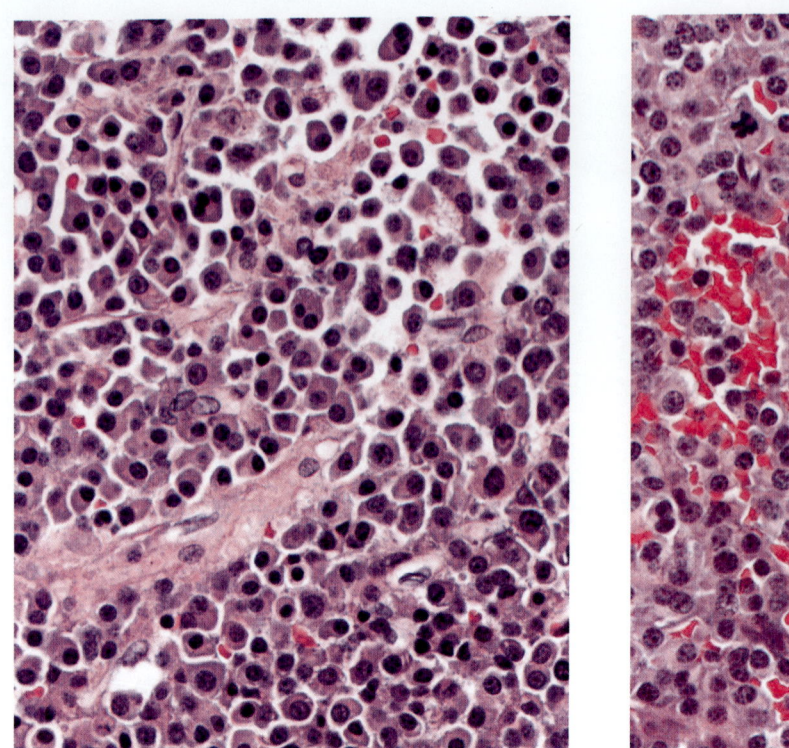
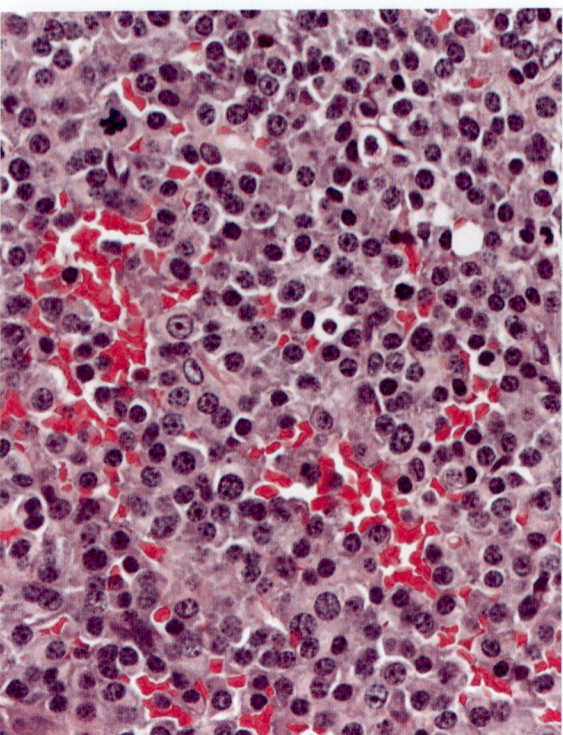

Figure 24-4

CYTOLOGIC SPECTRUM OF EXTRAMEDULLARY PLASMACYTOMA

Left: Well-differentiated, Marschalko-type plasma cells are seen. The plasma cells have "clock-face" chromatin and some cells have a perinuclear hof (clear zone). Binucleated forms are also present in this field.

Right: Moderately differentiated plasma cells. A subset of the cells has distinct nucleoli and a mitotic figure (top left) is present in this field (left, right: H&E stain).

EBV-positive cases of nodal plasmacytoma have been reported (17). Nevertheless, a few cases of extranodal EBV-positive plasmacytoma involving the head and neck region and the gastrointestinal tract have been reported (18,30,31). Loghavi et al. (18) identified seven cases in the literature and added four cases from the United States. The latter four cases involved the nasal cavity, esophagus, or mediastinum. These tumors were localized and patients had a good prognosis following therapy. Morphologically, these tumors were composed of mature-appearing plasma cells that were EBV-encoded RNA (EBER) positive. The tumor cells were associated with a prominent cytotoxic, CD8-positive T-cell infiltrate (fig. 24-8). All four patients were apparently immunocompetent.

The other few cases of EBV-positive plasmacytoma have been reported in the United States and Asia, although some reported cases had limited clinicopathologic data. Tomita et al. (30)

reported two cases of EBV-positive gastrointestinal tract plasmacytoma that were positive for EBV latent membrane protein type 1, EBER1, and EBNA2; polymerase chain reaction analysis showed EBV type A. Yan et al. (31) described four cases of EBER1-positive plasmacytoma that did not show evidence of translocations involving *MYC* and *CCND1* and there was no evidence of del(13q14).

MOLECULAR GENETIC FINDINGS

The genetic findings of EMP are poorly understood and no studies have focused on nodal plasmacytoma. Cases of EMP carry monoclonal immunoglobulin rearrangements. The T-cell receptor genes are usually in the germline configuration. Few cases of EMP assessed by conventional cytogenetics have been reported, but there are some studies that used fluorescence in situ hybridization (FISH).

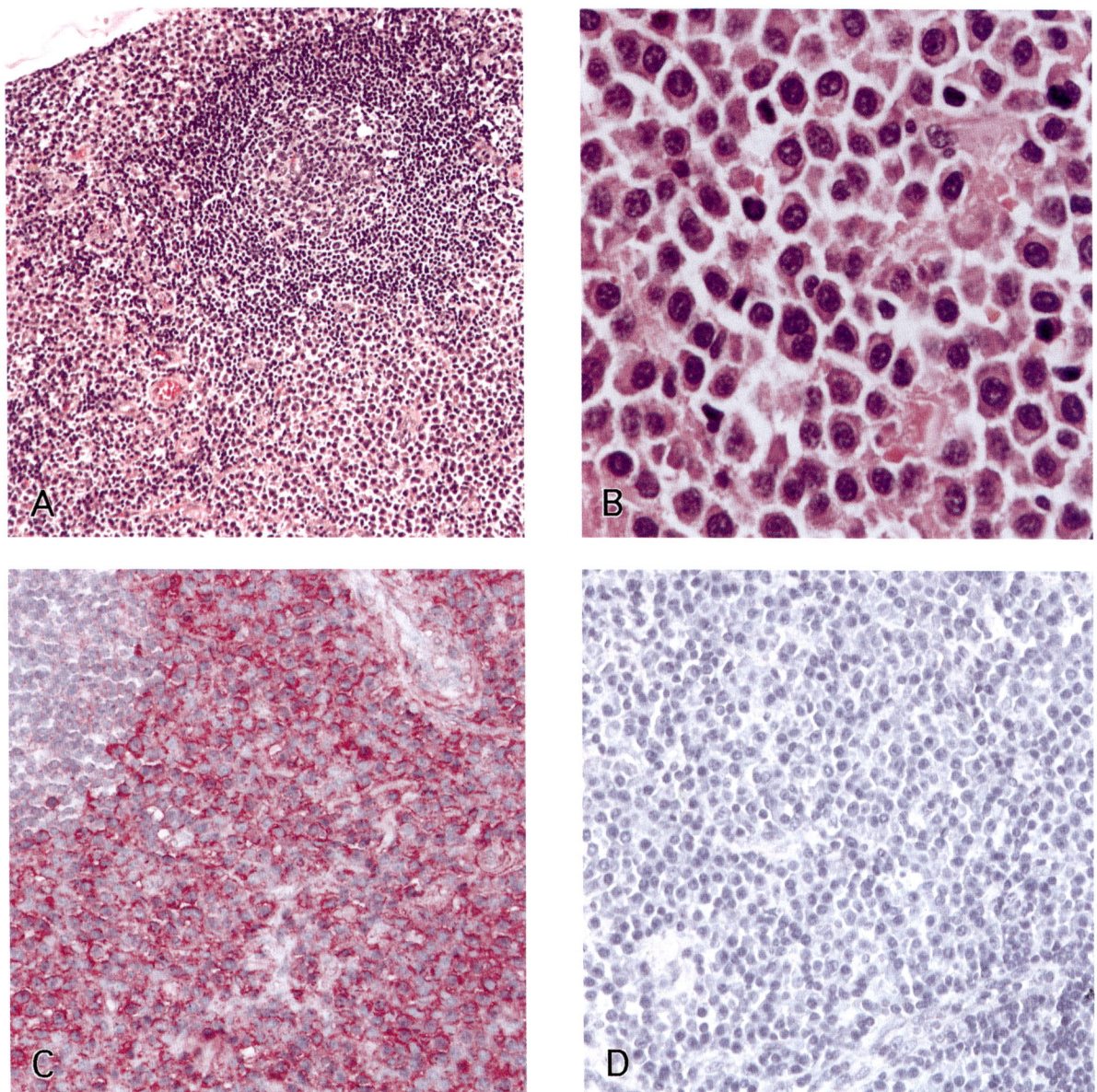

Figure 24-5

PLASMA CELL MYELOMA INVOLVING LYMPH NODE

This tumor was detected almost simultaneously with involvement of the bone marrow.

A: The plasma cells replace most of the lymph node but spare a lymphoid follicle.

B: The plasma cells are moderately differentiated, with hyperchromatic nuclear features and some distinct nucleoli (A,B: H&E stain).

C,D: Immunohistochemical analysis shows that the plasma cells are positive for kappa (C) and negative for lambda light chains (D) (C,D: immunohistochemistry with hematoxylin counterstain).

In general, EMP cases share genetic abnormalities with plasma cell myeloma, but EMP cases usually have fewer abnormalities (2,3). Bink et al. (3) showed genetic abnormalities in 14 of 38 (37 percent) of cases of EMP. The most common finding was polysomy of one or more odd numbered chromosomes, particularly chromosomes 1, 5, 9, and 11. Deletion of chromosome 13q14 and t(4;14)(p16;q32)/*IGH-FGFR3* were also identified in subsets of cases. These features are

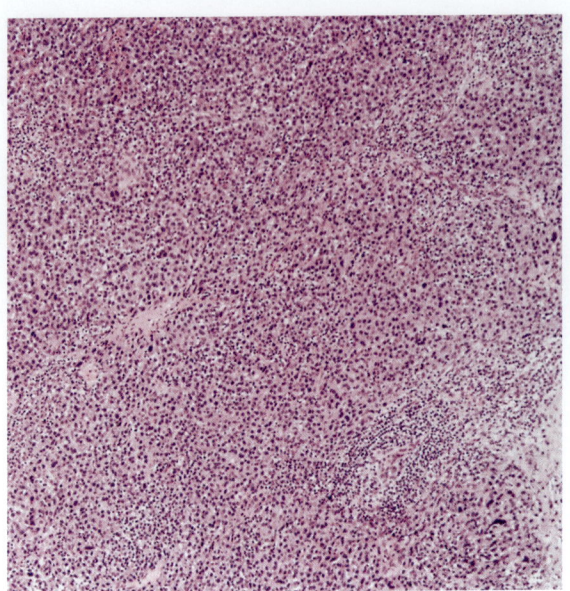
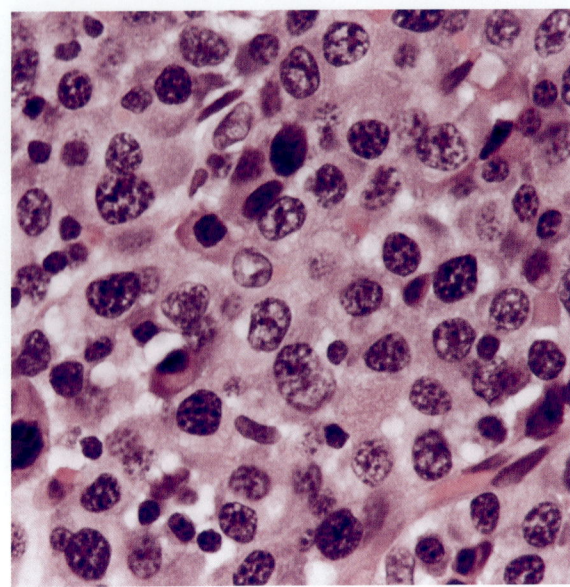

Figure 24-6

PLASMA CELL MYELOMA INVOLVING LYMPH NODE

This patient had a history of plasma cell myeloma. Lymph node involvement occurred at the time of relapse.

Left: The plasma cells almost completely replace the lymph node parenchyma, with only some foci of residual lymphoid tissue.

Right: The plasma cells are highly pleomorphic and atypical (left, right: H&E stain).

similar to some plasma cell myelomas. In this study, EMP, unlike plasma cell myeloma, did not carry translocations such as t(11;14)(q13;q32)/ *CCND1-IGH*, t(14;16)(q32;q23)/*IGH-MAF*, or t(8;14)(q24;q32)/*MYC-IGH* and there were no breaks in the MALT lymphoma-associated genes such *MALT1*, *BCL6*, or *FOXP1*. Five nodal plasmacytomas were included in this study: 4 cases showed polysomy and 2 showed del(13q14); no cases showed *IGH* breaks. One case of plasmacytoma associated with t(4;14)(p16;q32)/ *FGFR3-IGH* has been reported (19). Deletion of 17p13/*TP53* is rare in EMP (2).

Little data are available using gene expression profiling methods to assess EMP. Hedvat et al. (12), however, used gene expression profiling to assess plasma cell myeloma and plasma cell leukemia cases. The authors also included 6 cases of plasmacytoma: 3 solitary plasmacytoma of bone and 3 EMP (2 nodal). A large number of genes were differentially expressed between systemic plasma cell tumors and plasmacytoma, including genes involved in angiogenesis (e.g., *PECAM1* encoding, CD31) and cell adhesion. The authors suggested that genes in these pathways

allow plasma cell myeloma to grow outside of the bone marrow microenvironment and are likely to be involved in dissemination. It is unclear whether these data can be applied to nodal plasmacytoma, but these pathways may be active in cases of plasma cell myeloma that disseminate to lymph nodes.

DIFFERENTIAL DIAGNOSIS

Plasma Cell Variant of Castleman Disease. In cases of plasma cell variant Castleman disease, particularly cases associated with POEMS syndrome or human herpesvirus 8 (HHV8)-positive multicentric disease Castleman disease, monotypic plasma cell populations may be prominent. Recognition of the histologic features of Castleman disease, such as hyaline-vascular lesions or evidence of HHV8 infection, distinguishes these cases from nodal plasmacytoma.

Monoclonal Plasma Cells of Uncertain Significance in Lymph Node. Rarely, a monotypic population of plasma cells is identified in lymph nodes in a patient without evidence of plasma cell myeloma or lymphoma. This is most common in patients with autoimmune disease.

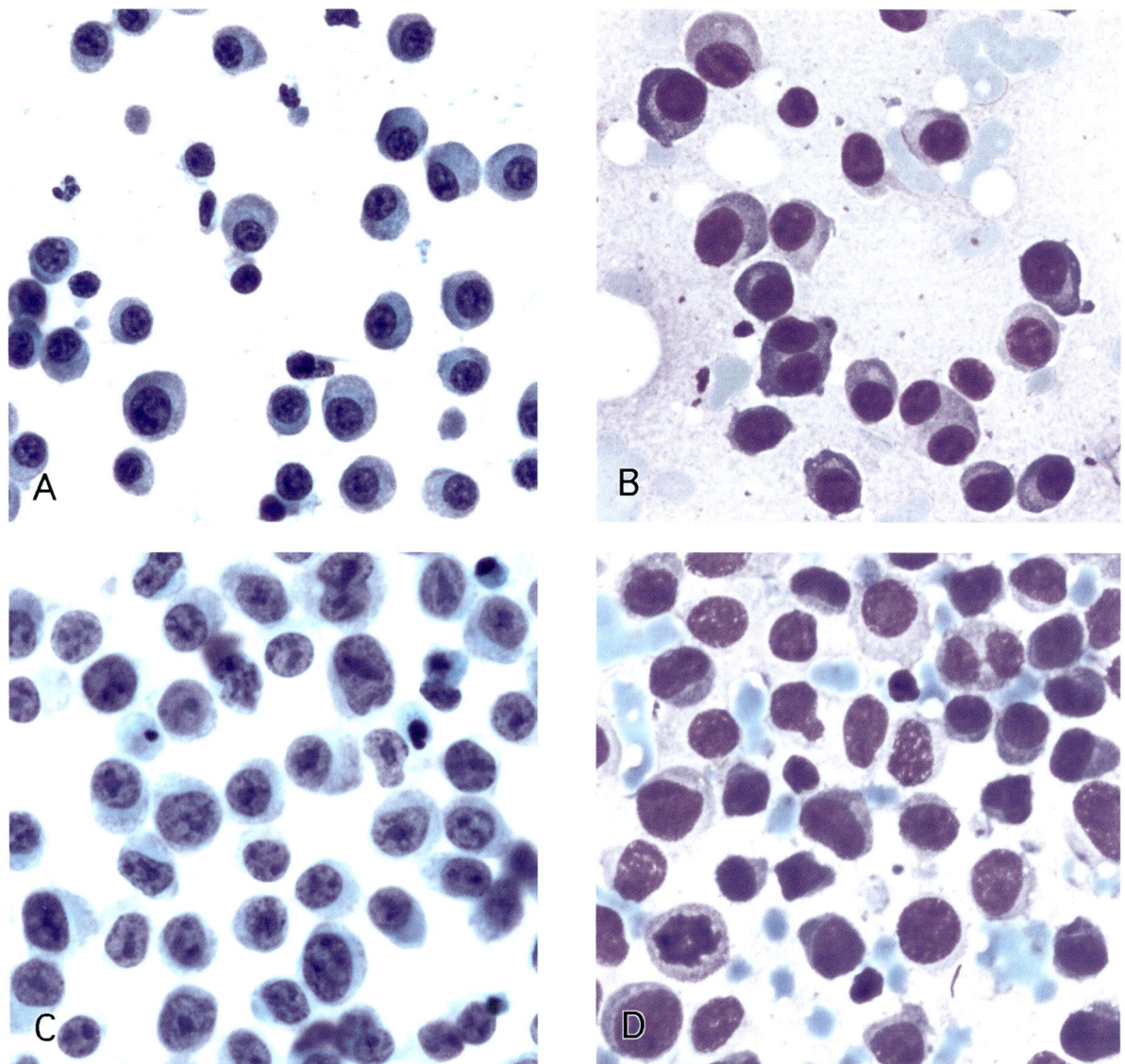

Figure 24-7

SPECTRUM OF NEOPLASTIC PLASMA CELLS WITHIN CYTOLOGIC SMEARS

A,B: Well-differentiated plasma cells with clock-faced chromatin, eccentrically located nuclei, and abundant cytoplasm with perinuclear hofs are seen. The distinctive chromatin is best observed in the Pap stain (A), whereas the Diff-Quik stain (B) highlights the basophilic cytoplasm and the perinuclear hofs.

C,D: This plasma cell myeloma involved an extramedullary site. These cells show round to irregular nuclei, prominent nucleoli, and scant cytoplasm (A,C: Papanicolaou stain; B,D: Diff-Quik stain).

Typically, the monotypic plasma cells do not form sheets that replace the lymph node, as is the case in plasmacytoma.

Extranodal Marginal Zone Lymphoma (MZL). The extranodal location and sometimes close resemblance of EMP and extranodal MZL may suggest that these two diseases are closely related. However, cases of EMP lack rearrangements of *MALT1*, *FOXP1*, and other extranodal MZL-associated genes (3). The diagnosis of extranodal MZL is supported by the presence of a component of B-cell lymphoma, even if small, which is absent in nodal plasmacytoma (see chapter 15).

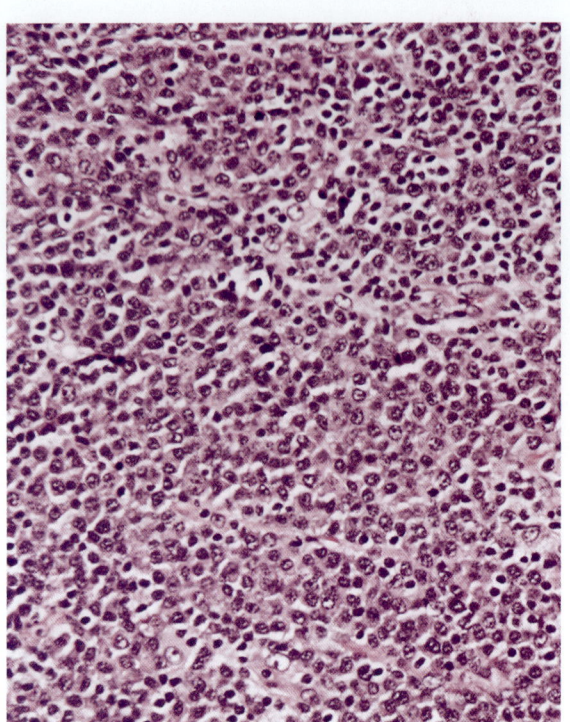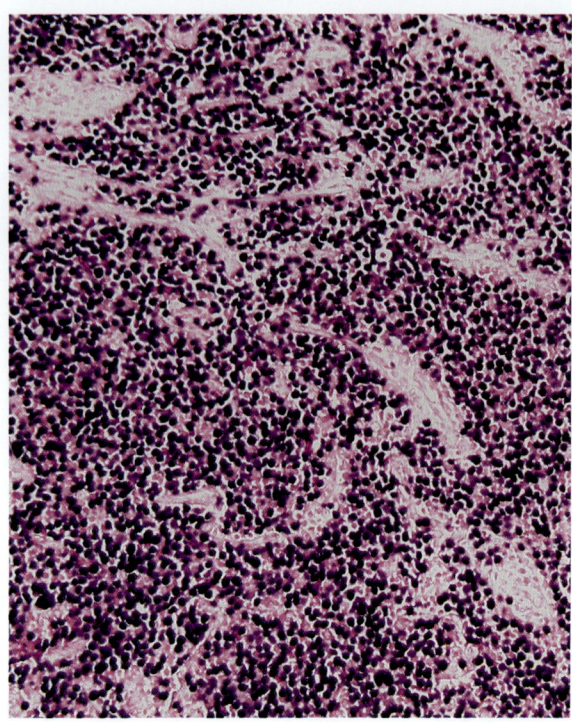

Figure 24-8

EPSTEIN-BARR VIRUS-POSITIVE PLASMACYTOMA IN AN IMMUNOCOMPETENT PATIENT INVOLVING ESOPHAGUS

Left: The neoplasm is composed of sheets of mature plasma cells without atypia. An infiltrate of small lymphocytes (CD8-positive, not shown) is also present within the tumor (left, right: H&E stain).
Right: Virtually all the plasma cells are positive for EBV-encoded RNA1 (EBER1).

Lymphoplasmacytic Lymphoma. Most patients with lymphoplasmacytic lymphoma also have Waldenstrom macroglobulinemia. Therefore, an IgM paraprotein in serum, bone marrow involvement, and both B-cell and plasma cell components are present. The immunophenotype of the plasma cells in Waldenstrom macroglobulinemia is distinctive (CD19 positive) and these neoplasms are also commonly associated with *MYD88* gene mutations (see chapter 16).

Plasmablastic Lymphoma. Plasmablastic lymphoma cases fit into two general groups. The oral cavity variant commonly arises in patients with immunodeficiency and is commonly associated with EBV infection. Histologically, these tumors are monotonous, and somewhat cohesive, and commonly the cells resemble immunoblasts, unlike plasmacytoma. The second group of cases of plasmablastic lymphoma is etiologically more heterogeneous. These tumors may be more plasmacytic in their appearance and therefore show more overlap with plasma-cytoma. Unlike plasmacytoma, however, all cases of plasmablastic lymphoma are histologically aggressive, with cytologic atypia, a brisk mitotic rate, a high proliferation rate, and often a starry sky pattern (see chapter 23).

TREATMENT AND PROGNOSIS

EMP is usually responsive to local radiotherapy, but regional recurrences are observed in up to 25 percent of patients (26). Often, these patients also undergo surgical excision or receive other therapies. Plasmacytoma arising in the upper respiratory tract or head and neck region spreads to cervical lymph nodes in up to 15 percent of patients (22). For all cases of EMP (lymph nodes and other sites), the 10-year survival rate is high, 70 to 80 percent (10,15,26). Ten to 20 percent of patients with EMP progress to plasma cell myeloma. Dissemination and survival depends on the anatomic site of the EMP as well as the morphologic findings (10,15,26). The clinical course of patients with nodal plasmacytoma is particularly indolent, with a low rate of dissemination and a high survival rate, about 90 percent at 10 years, compared with other anatomic sites of origin of EMP (6,17,22).

Patients with plasma cell myeloma, although a heterogeneous group, have a much poorer prognosis than patients with EMP. When patients with plasma cell myeloma develop lymphadenopathy, the disease has evolved to the point that the bone marrow microenvironment is no longer required for growth. Lymph node involvement in patients with plasma cell myeloma is therefore often associated with progressive disease and poor survival.

MONOCLONAL IMMUNOGLOBULIN DEPOSITION DISEASES

Amyloidosis

Patients with *primary* or *secondary amyloidosis* can develop lymphadenopathy and splenomegaly. Most patients with primary amyloidosis have a plasma cell or lymphoid neoplasm responsible for the secretion of abnormal Ig light chains which are deposited into tissues, also known as AL-type amyloid (8,21). Monoclonal gammopathy of uncertain significance is the most common, followed by plasma cell myeloma and then B-cell lymphomas with plasmacytic differentiation (8,21). The median age of patients with primary amyloidosis is in the seventh decade and the male to female ratio is 2 to 1.

Patients with secondary amyloidosis usually have an autoimmune disease, chronic infection, or a neoplasm that is associated with reactive or secondary amyloid, also known as AA-type amyloid. Amyloid deposition occurs more commonly in lymph nodes of patients with end-stage renal failure, in 22 percent of patients in one study (11). The amyloid in these cases is usually beta-2-microglobulin.

Patients with amyloidosis present with symptoms and signs attributable to amyloid deposition into tissues. The lymph nodes may be involved, the frequency of which varies in different studies, but these patients represent a minor subset of patients with amyloidosis. Rarely, patients present with prominent lymphadenopathy involving one or multiple lymph nodes (20). In studies, from the Mayo Clinic and

the Kiel registry, patients presenting with lymph node involvement by amyloidosis represented far less than 1 percent of all cases of amyloidosis (7,23). However, Fu et al. (8) studied about 3,000 patients with amyloidosis and 1.6 percent presented with lymphadenopathy. The cervical or supraclavicular lymph nodes are the most commonly involved by amyloid deposition. Rarely, amyloidosis presents as an isolated enlargement of a lymph node (or other sites) without systemic disease (1).

Histologically, amyloid deposits preferentially involve blood vessels, lymph node follicles, and sinuses (fig. 24-9), or diffusely replace the lymph node parenchyma; often the pattern is mixed (22,23). Amyloid deposits in lymph nodes are eosinophilic, amorphous, and acellular and may be associated with a multinucleated giant cell reaction. Amyloid deposits are pink when stained by Congo red and show apple-green birefringence using polarized light (fig. 24-9) (1,21,23).

The AL and AA types of amyloid are usually distinguished by immunohistochemistry using antibodies specific for Ig light chains. AL-type amyloid is composed of one type of light chain whereas AA amyloid is polytypic. A study using mass spectrometry showed that amyloid in lymph nodes is usually, but not always, Ig derived and composed of a mixture of Ig light and heavy chains (7). A number of apoproteins are commonly associated with amyloid deposits and may have a role in pathogenesis (7).

Crystal-Storing Histiocytosis

Crystal-storing histiocytosis (CSH) is defined as the presence of crystalline material within the cytoplasm of histiocytes. In approximately 90 percent of all cases of CSH reported, the crystalline material is immunoglobulin (IG) and is associated with underlying hematologic neoplasms including plasma cell myeloma, plasmacytoma, monoclonal gammopathy of undetermined significance, and B-cell lymphomas associated with plasmacytoid differentiation: lymphoplasmacytic lymphoma/Waldenstrom macroglobulinemia and marginal zone B-cell lymphomas (5,14). Cases of CSH not associated with IG crystals are not further discussed here but a proposed classification has been published by Dogan et al. (5).

Approximately 100 cases of CSH have been reported in the literature (5,14,19). The median

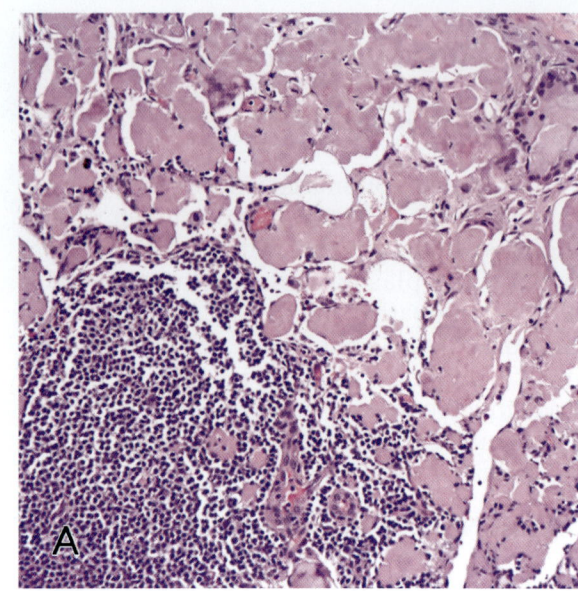

Figure 24-9

AMYLOID INVOLVING LYMPH NODE

In this biopsy specimen, amyloid deposits preferentially involve lymph node sinuses.

A: A sinus is expanded by amorphous and eosinophilic amyloid deposits. A foreign body-type giant cell is also present (top right) in the field (H&E stain).

B,C: The amyloid deposits are positive for Congo red (B) and show apple-green birefringence under polarized light (C) (B: Congo red stain; C: Congo red stain viewed under polarized light).

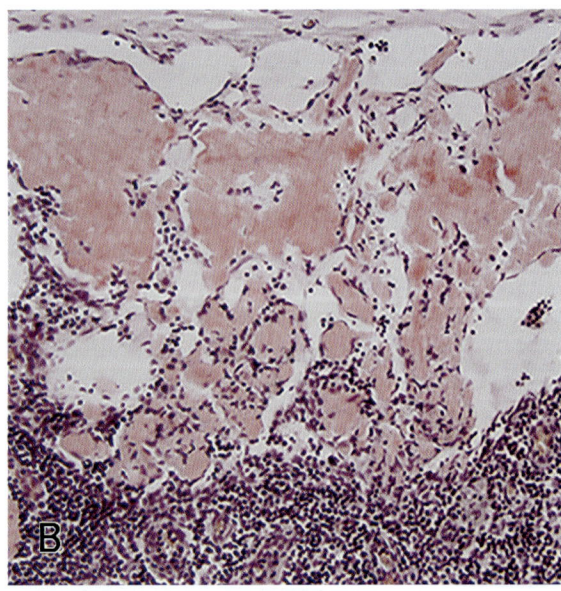

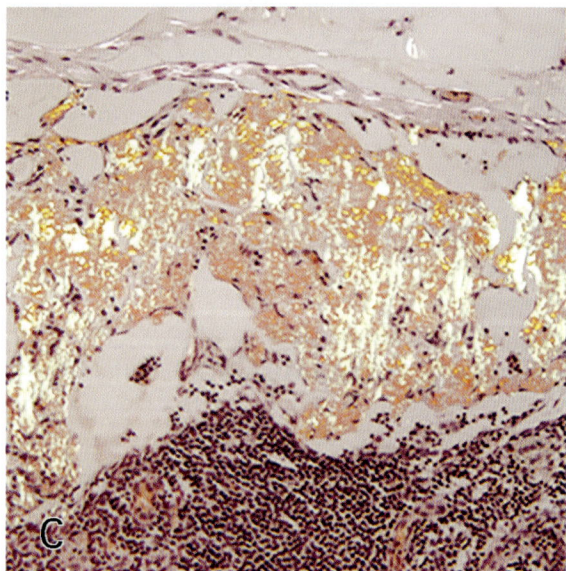

patient age is approximately 60 years, with a wide age range, 17 to 81 years (5). Approximately 60 percent of patients have localized CSH and the rest have generalized CSH (5). The head and neck region is the most common region involved by CSH, but almost any site can be involved (5,14). In patients with generalized CSH, the bone marrow is almost always involved. Lymph nodes are involved by CSH in about 10 percent of localized and 40 to 50 percent of generalized CSH cases (5,14).

Histologically, CSH is characterized by eosinophilic histiocytes stuffed with crystalline material that are present in aggregates or sheets; the histiocytes partially or completely replace normal architecture (fig. 24-10). The histiocytes do not show cytologic atypia and mitotic figures are absent or rare. In many cases, the cytoplasmic crystals blend in with the cytoplasm, and if the cells are not assessed at high magnification, may be subtle. In many cases, the biopsy specimen is also involved by the underlying plasma cell neoplasm or B-cell lymphoma.

The histiocytes of CSH express lineage-appropriate antigens, such CD11c, CD68, and CD163 and are negative for B-cell and T-cell antigens

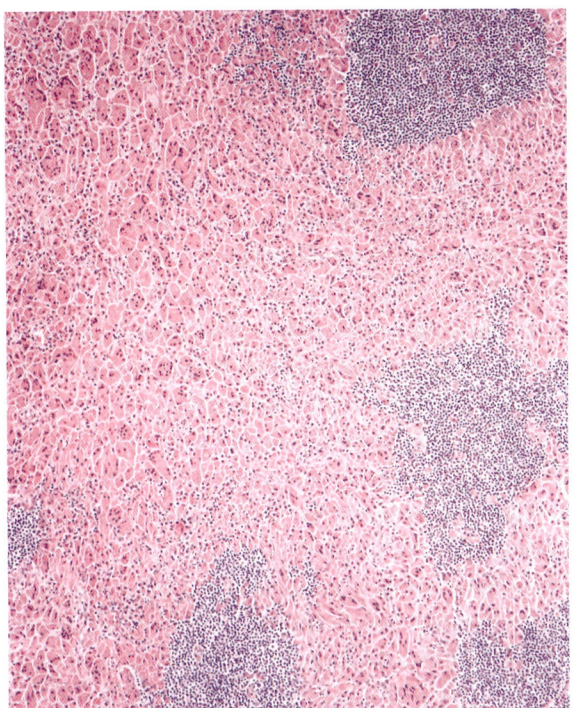 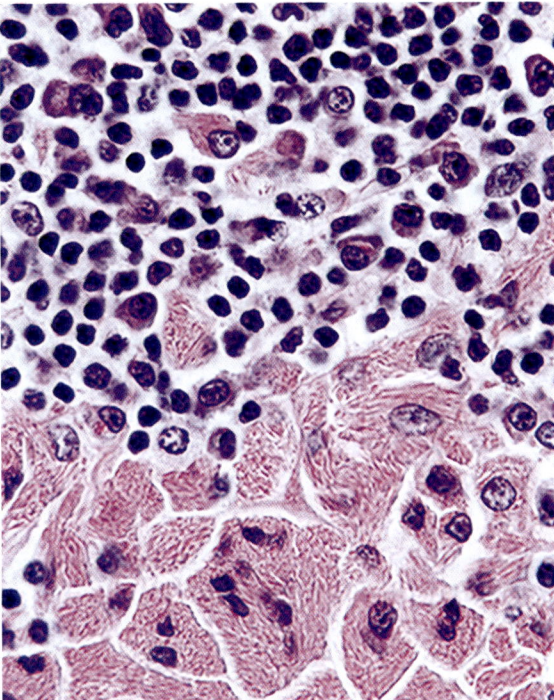

Figure 24-10

CRYSTAL-STORING HISTIOCYTOSIS ASSOCIATED WITH LYMPHOPLASMACYTIC LYMPHOMA/WALDENSTROM MACROGLOBULINEMIA INVOLVING LYMPH NODE

Left: Sheets of eosinophilic histiocytes and aggregates of darker lymphocytes and plasmacytoid lymphocytes replace nodal parenchyma.

Right: Using oil magnification, eosinophilic immunoglobulin crystals distend the cytoplasm of histiocytes (right of field) (left, right: H&E stain).

(14). The crystals are reactive with antibodies specific for immunoglobulin heavy and light chains. In the literature, most cases of CSH are associated with kappa light chain, but a recent study by Kanagal-Shammana et al. (14) showed a less marked predominance of kappa-positive cases, with only 50 percent kappa versus 40 percent lambda positive. Mass spectrometry has shown that the crystals are composed of IG heavy and light chain variable region fragments.

The etiology and mechanism of CSH are unknown. Abnormalities in secreted IG by the neoplastic cells as well as the inability of histiocytes to process immunoglobulins have been suggested.

REFERENCES

1. Biewend ML, Menke DM, Calamia KT. The spectrum of localized amyloidosis: a case series of 20 patients and review of the literature. Amyloid 2006;13:135-142.
2. Billecke L, Murga Penas EM, May AM, et al. Cytogenetics of extramedullary manifestations in multiple myeloma. Br J Haematol 2013;161:87-94.
3. Bink K, Haralambieva E, Kremer M, et al. Primary extramedullary plasmacytoma: similarities with and differences from multiple myeloma revealed by interphase cytogenetics. Haematologica 2008;93:623-626.
3a. de Waal EG, Leene M, Veeger N, et al. Progression of a solitary plasmacytoma to multiple myeloma. A population-based registry of the northern Netherlands. Br J Haematol 2016;175:661-667.
4. Dayton VD, Williams SJ, McKenna RW, Linden MA. Unusual extramedullary hematopoietic neoplasms in lymph nodes. Hum Pathol 2017;62:13-22.

5. Dogan S, Barnes L, Cruz-Vetrano WP. Crystal-storing histiocytosis: report of a case, review of the literature (80 cases) and a proposed classification. Head and Neck Pathol 2012;6:111-120.

6. Dores GM, Landgren O, McGlynn KA, Curtis RE, Linet MS, Devesa SS. Plasmacytoma of bone, extramedullary plasmacytoma, and multiple myeloma: incidence and survival in the United States, 1992-2004. Br J Haematol 2009;144:86-94.

7. D'Souza A, Theis J, Quint P, et al. Exploring the amyloid proteome in immunoglobulin-derived lymph node amyloidosis using laser capture microdissection/tandem mass spectrometry. Am J Hematol 2013;88:577-580.

8. Fu J, Seldin DC, Berk JL, et al. Lymphadenopathy as a manifestation of amyloidosis: a case series. Amyloid 2014;21:256-260.

9. Gerry D, Lentsch EJ. Epidemiologic evidence of superior outcomes for extramedullary plasmacytoma of the head and neck. Otolaryngol Head Neck Surg 2013;148:974-981.

10. Ghodke K, Shet T, Epari S, Sengar M, Menon H, Gujral S. A retrospective study of correlation of morphologic patterns, MIB1 proliferation index, and survival analysis in 134 cases of plasmacytoma. Ann Diagn Pathol 2015;19:117-123.

11. Guz G, Ozdemir BH, Sezer S, et al. High frequency of amyloid lymphadenopathy in uremic patients. Renal Failure 2000;22:613-621.

12. Hedvat CV, Comenzo RL, Teruya-Feldstein J, et al. Insights into extramedullary tumour growth revealed by expression profiling of human plasmacytomas and multiple myeloma. Br J Haematol 2003;122:728-744.

13. International Myeloma Working Group. Criteria for the classification of monoclonal gammopathies, multiple myeloma and related disorders. Br J Haematol 2003;121:749-757.

14. Kanagal-Shamanna R, Xu-Monette ZY, Miranda RN, et al. Crystal-storing histiocytosis: a clinicopathological study of 13 cases. Histopathology 2016;68:482-491.

15. Katoditrou E, Terpos E, Symeonidis AS, et al. Clinical features, outcome, and prognostic factors for survival and evolution to multiple myeloma of solitary plasmacytomas: a report of the Greek myeloma study group in 97 patients. Am J Hematol 2014;89:803-808.

16. Kremer M, Ott G, Nathrath M, et al. Primary extramedullary plasmacytoma and multiple myeloma: phenotypic differences revealed by immunohistochsmical analysis. J Pathol 2005;205:92-101.

17. Lin BT, Weiss LM. Primary plasmacytoma of lymph nodes. Hum Pathol 1997;28:1083-1090.

18. Loghavi S, Khoury JD, Medeiros LJ. Epstein-Barr virus-positive plasmacytoma in immunocompetent patients. Histopathology 2015;67:225-234.

19. Lv Y, Liu Y, Li X, Yan Q, Wang Z. Plasmacytoma with crystal-storing histiocytosis exhibiting FGFR3 and IgH translocation. Pathology 2015;47:82-85.

20. Matsuda M, Gono T, Shimojima Y, et al. AL amyloidosis manifesting as systemic lymphadenopathy. Amyloid 2008;15:117-124.

21. McKenna RW, Kyle RA, Kuehl WM, Grogan TM, Harris NL, Coupland RW. Plasma cell neoplasms. In: Swerdlow SH, Campo E, Harris NL, Jaffe ES, Pileri SA, Stein H, Thiele J, Vardiman JW, eds. World Health Organization Classification of tumours of haematopoietic and lymphoid tissues. Lyon: IARC Press; 2008:200-211.

22. Menke DM, Horny HP, Griesser H, et al. Primary lymph node plasmacytomas (plasmacytic lymphomas). Am J Clin Pathol 2001;115:119-126.

23. Newland JR, Linke RP, Lennert K. Amyloid deposits in lymph nodes: a morphologic and immunohistochemical study. Hum Pathol 1986;17:1245-1249.

24. Paiva B, Chandia M, Vidriales MB, et al. Multiparameter flow cytometry for staging solitary bone plasmacytoma: new criteria for risk of progression to myeloma. Blood 2014;124:1300-1303.

25. Rajkumar SV, Dimopoulos MA, Palumbo A, et al. International Myeloma Working Group updated criteria for the diagnosis of multiple myeloma. Lancet Oncol 2014;15:e538-e548.

26. Reed V, Shah J, Medeiros LJ, et al. Solitary plasmacytomas: outcome and prognostic factors after definitive radiation therapy. Cancer 2011;117:4468-4474.

27. Shao H, Xi L, Raffeld M, et al. Nodal and extranodal plasmacytomas expressing immunoglobulin A. An indolent lymphoproliferative disorder with a low risk of clinical progression. Am J Surg Pathol 2010;34:1425-1435.

28. Shek TW, Ma SK, Au WY. Nodal plasmacytoma with significant paraproteinaemia. Leuk Lymphoma 2001;40:235-238.

29. Soutar R, Lucraft H, Jackson G, et al. Guidelines on the diagnosis and management of solitary plasmacytoma of bone and solitary extramedullary plasmacytoma. Br J Haematol 2004;124:717-726.

30. Tomita Y, Ohsawa M, Hashimoto M, et al. Plasmacytoma of the gastrointestinal tract in Korea: higher incidence than in Japan and Epstein-Barr virus association. Oncology 1998;55:27-32.

31. Yan J, Wang J, Zhang W, Chen M, Chen J, Liu W. Solitary plasmacytoma associated with Epstein-Barr virus: a clinicopathologic, cytogenetic study and literature review. Ann Diagn Pathol 2017;27:1-6.

BURKITT LYMPHOMA

GENERAL FEATURES

Burkitt lymphoma (BL) is a highly aggressive lymphoma derived from germinal center B cells that commonly presents in extranodal sites, particularly the jaw, gastrointestinal tract, and gonads or as a "leukemic neoplasm." As stated in the World Health Organization (WHO) (20), there is a no "gold standard" for the diagnosis of BL. However, features that are characteristic of this neoplasm include: 1) sheets of monomorphic, intermediate-sized lymphoid cells arranged in a starry sky pattern; 2) very high rates of mitosis, apoptosis, and proliferation; and 3) chromosomal translocations involving *MYC*.

In 1957, Denis Burkitt, a surgeon by training who was working in Uganda, saw a 5-year-old boy with bilateral masses involving the maxillary and mandibular bones (22). Shortly thereafter, Burkitt searched the records of Mulago Hospital in Kampala, Uganda, and identified and described 38 children with "sarcoma" involving the jaws (5). Although others had previously observed and published jaw tumors in young children in Africa, Denis Burkitt was the first person to propose that these jaw tumors, regardless of other sites of disease, were the same neoplasm (22). Almost simultaneously, similar tumors were recognized in the coastal regions of Papua, New Guinea, and subsequently, in Europe, the United States, and other developed countries (21).

BL is currently known to have a worldwide distribution and is classified into three variants: endemic, sporadic, and immunodeficiency-related (20). These variants are morphologically similar, but they differ in geographic distribution, epidemiologic and molecular features, and association with Epstein-Barr virus (EBV) infection.

Endemic BL is the most common malignancy of childhood in equatorial Africa. Endemic BL is distributed over the so-called "malaria or lymphoma belt" (about 10° north and 10° south of the equator) of Africa. Endemic BL is associated with early exposure to EBV as well as climatic factors, such as high rainfall, temperature, and, to a lesser degree, altitude; these factors are linked to malaria infection (22). Within the lymphoma belt, endemic BL accounts for up to three quarters of childhood malignant neoplasms. Endemic BL in New Guinea also displays many of the epidemiologic characteristics of BL in equatorial Africa. Endemic BL also occurs in other equatorial countries, for example, Brazil has a similar incidence (29). The incidence of endemic BL is 5 to 10 per 100,000 persons per year (20).

The *sporadic variant of BL* is substantially less common than the endemic form, but has a worldwide distribution and is the most common form of BL in developed countries. Sporadic BL accounts for 30 to 50 percent of non-Hodgkin lymphomas in children in North America, Europe, and China, and about 1 percent of non-Hodgkin lymphomas in adults (15,20). Sporadic BL is not linked to malaria, and EBV is positive in a minority of cases. The incidence of sporadic BL is 0.01 per 100,000 persons per year (20).

Immunodeficiency-associated BL is associated with immunodeficiency of any cause, including human immunodeficiency virus (HIV) infection, following organ transplantation, or in patients with primary immunodeficiency syndromes. HIV infection, however, is by far the most common etiology associated with immunodeficiency-associated BL. This form of BL also has a worldwide distribution and approximately one third of HIV-associated BL cases are EBV positive (20).

Although these variants are a helpful framework, there is overlap. Both endemic and sporadic BLs occur in South America and North Africa. Immunodeficiency-associated BL, in addition to endemic BL, occurs within the lymphoma belt of Africa, and it can be difficult to distinguish between variants because these neoplasms have many overlapping features.

In general, immunodeficiency-associated BL occurs in older patients than endemic BL.

PATHOGENESIS

A chromosomal translocation that results in the juxtaposition of *MYC* with one of the *IG* loci is a key event in the pathogenesis of BL. *MYC* translocations are present in all three BL variants and in almost all cases. In addition, *MYC* translocation often occurs in the context of a simpler karyotype than observed in other types of aggressive B-cell lymphoma, particularly diffuse large B-cell lymphoma (DLBCL) (4,16). Dysregulation of *MYC* contributes to the aggressive biologic features of BL, including a very rapid doubling time and extremely rapid growth. In addition, *MYC* is the most frequently mutated gene in BL, in about 70 percent of cases (39). Nevertheless, *MYC* translocations or mutations alone are insufficient to cause BL and other cofactors likely contribute to lymphomagenesis.

A number of possible cofactors have been identified in endemic BL (discussed below). Other than EBV infection, cofactors that contribute to the pathogenesis of sporadic BL are unknown. In HIV-associated BL, chronic antigenic stimulation (e.g., HIV and EBV) and immunosuppression are likely involved in pathogenesis. However, BL in HIV-infected patients most often occurs in those with higher CD4-positive T-cell counts and less severe immunodeficiency than is characteristic of patients with full-blown acquired immunodeficiency syndrome (AIDS) (20), suggesting that other cofactors are involved in pathogenesis.

Cofactors Thought Likely to Be Involved in BL Pathogenesis

Epstein-Barr Virus Infection. EBV has been detected in 95 percent of cases of endemic BL, in 20 to 30 percent of sporadic cases (industrialized or developed countries), and in 30 to 40 percent of immunodeficiency-related cases. EBV is transmitted via body fluids, most often saliva, but also blood or semen. In Africa, mothers of infants often chew food before giving it to their children during the weaning process (22).

EBV-positive BL is usually characterized by a type I EBV latency program: EBNA1 and EBV-encoded RNA (EBER) are expressed, but not viral latent membrane protein type 1 (LMP1)

(44). The virus is carried in the tumor cells as a nuclear episome that is present in monoclonal form, but the contribution of EBV to the pathogenesis of BL is incompletely understood. EBV infects and immortalizes B lymphocytes, resulting in polyclonal activation and proliferation of B cells. Viral-induced B-cell proliferation is controlled by cytotoxic T cells and situations in which there is a decrease in the function or number of cytotoxic T cells could contribute to lymphomagenesis (44). It also has been shown that EBV molecules inhibit mechanisms of cellular apoptosis, by prolonging cell lifespan, likely enhancing the chance that transforming events can occur (44).

***Plasmodium Falciparum* Infection.** The role of malarial infection in the pathogenesis of endemic BL is supported by the geographic overlap of these diseases. In addition, nationwide malarial reduction programs have resulted in a decreased frequency of endemic BL (22).

The exact role of malarial infection in the pathogenesis of BL is incompletely understood. It is thought that the association between malaria and endemic BL arises from a combination of immunosuppression (inhibition of host cytotoxic T cells) and expansion and activation of B cells mediated by EBV infection, and likely malaria itself (1,17). Robbiani et al. (32) in a mouse model have shown that *Plasmodium* infection can induce a longlasting expansion of germinal center B cells, possibly by digesting erythrocytes with a byproduct, hemozoin, capable of stimulating Toll-like receptors on the B-lymphocyte surface. Activation-induced cytosine deaminase (AID) in germinal center B cells is upregulated, either by hemozoin or possibly direct infection, resulting in widespread chromosomal damage in these cells. Inactivation of *TP53* is also involved since its functional impairment seems to be required for *MYC* translocations to arise, probably as a result of mistakes in DNA joining and defective DNA repair (32).

Arbovirus Infection. Arboviruses are RNA viruses transmitted by insect vectors, such as mosquitoes (same insect vector as for malaria). Some epidemiologic studies have suggested that variations in the incidence of endemic BL over time do not match well with the incidence of malaria and could be better explained by the cyclical changes observed in the activity of

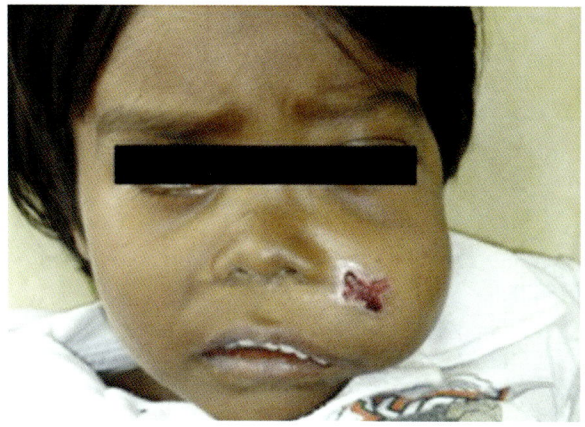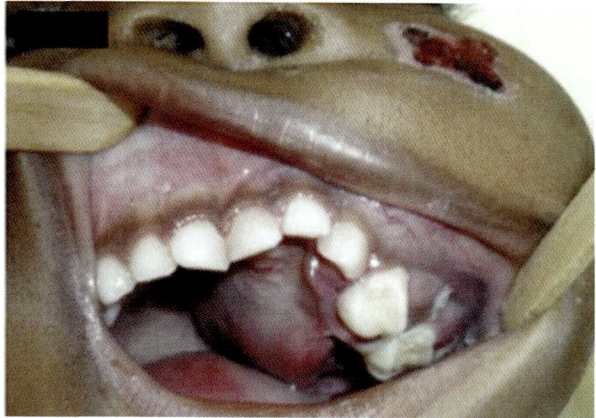

Figure 25-1

ENDEMIC BURKITT LYMPHOMA

A 3-year-old child from Brazil had Burkitt lymphoma (BL) involving the maxilla. (Fig. 1C from Rebelo-Pontes HA, de Abreu MC, Guimaraes DM, et al. Burkitt's lymphoma of the jaws in the Amazon region of Brazil. Med Oral Patol Cir Bucal 2014;19:e32.)

arboviruses (11,45). In addition, the age distribution of patients with endemic BL fits best with the pattern of acquisition of antibodies to arboviruses, rather than to malaria.

Use of Tumor-Promoting Plants. A common plant within the lymphoma belt is Euphorbia tirucalli. This bush is commonly used as a toy, hedge, and herbal remedy. This plant has been found more frequently in the houses of children with endemic BL compared with the houses of children without BL (45). This plant produces carcinogenic and EBV-promoting substances that activate latent EBV and can induce chromosomal translocations in B cells (45).

CLINICAL FEATURES

Patients with BL share many clinical features. The disease is more common in males and B-type symptoms are found in 40 to 50 percent of patients (15,20). Due to the rapid growth and dissemination of BL, patients often have symptoms only a few days or weeks before seeking medical attention. A bulky mass occurs in 20 to 40 percent of patients and at least two thirds of patients present with Ann Arbor stage III or IV disease. Patients with BL are at high risk for involvement of the central nervous system. Laboratory studies usually show high serum levels of lactate dehydrogenase (LDH) and beta-2-microglobulin, increased C-reactive protein, and elevated soluble interleukin-2. Anemia can be a result of bone marrow replacement by the lymphoma.

Endemic Variant

Patients in endemic regions who develop BL are usually children between the ages of 4 and 7 years. The male to female ratio is about 2 to 1 (5,29,47). About 50 percent of patients present with jaw or orbital tumors (fig. 25-1), but these patients often have evidence of disease elsewhere, in particular, involvement of the central nervous system, thyroid or salivary gland, breasts, gastrointestinal tract, omentum, kidneys, gonads, and long bones. The bone marrow is involved in some patients although a leukemic blood picture is rare. Lymph nodes are rarely involved.

Sporadic Variant

Patients with sporadic BL have a bimodal distribution of ages. The first peak in frequency occurs in young children and adolescents; the second peak occurs in younger adults, in the range of 30 to 45 years of age (6,15,21,37). The preference for males is even greater than in endemic BL, with a male to female ratio of 2.5–3.5 to 1.0.

An abdominal mass and particularly a bulky mass in the ileocecal region of the gastrointestinal tract is the usual presentation of sporadic BL. Abdominal masses can be associated with abdominal pain, distention, diarrhea, and rarely, intussusception. Many other extranodal sites are often involved, including the central nervous system and

Table 25-1

ST. JUDE/MURPHY STAGING SYSTEM FOR BURKITT LYMPHOMA (BL)

Stage	Description
I	Single tumor (extranodal) or a single anatomic area (nodal) with exclusion of mediastinum or abdomen
II	A single extranodal tumor with regional lymph node involvement Two single extranodal tumors on the same side of the diaphragm with or without regional lymph node involvement Primary gastrointestinal tumor with or without involvement of associated mesenteric lymph nodes (only) Two or more nodal areas on the same side of the diaphragm
IIR	Completely resected intra-abdominal disease
III	Two single extranodal tumors on opposite sides of the diaphragm All primary intrathoracic tumors (mediastinal, pleural, thymic) All paraspinal or epidural tumors, regardless of other tumor sites All extensive primary intra-abdominal disease Two or more nodal areas on opposite sides of the diaphragm
IIIA	Localized but nonresectable intra-abdominal disease
IIIB	Widespread multiorgan abdominal disease
IV	Any of the above with initial central nervous system and/or bone marrow involvement (< 25% replacement of marrow cells by tumor without circulating blasts)

bone marrow, but jaw tumors are rare. Rarely, patients with sporadic BL present with a leukemic blood picture, mimicking acute lymphoblastic leukemia; these patients have a high frequency of central nervous system involvement. Waldeyer ring and the mediastinum are also infrequently involved. Patients with sporadic BL can present with lymphadenopathy, more common in adults than children and adolescents (6,37).

Based on the common extranodal distribution of BL at time of presentation, as well as the fact that bulky extranodal disease may be surgically resected, the Ann Arbor staging system is not well suited for stratifying patients for risk-adapted therapy. Murphy (23) therefore designed an alternative staging system for pediatric lymphomas including sporadic BL that, in a modified form, is often used for children and adolescents (Table 25-1).

In Japan, Satou et al. (37) separately analyzed EBV-positive versus EBV-negative cases of sporadic BL. Patients with EBV-positive sporadic BL were often older (42 versus 13 years of age); had a higher frequency of involvement of the tonsils, adrenal glands, and cervical lymph nodes; and less frequently had gastrointestinal tract involvement.

Immunodeficiency-Associated Variant

The epidemiologic features of immunodeficiency-associated BL, in large part, are attributed to the epidemiologic features of AIDS patients. Men are affected more often than women, with a ratio as high as 4 or 5 to 1 in some studies (48). Most patients with HIV-associated BL are adults with a median age in the late 30s or early 40s. Most have advanced-stage disease, 20 to 30 percent have bulky disease, and extranodal involvement is common (48). In contrast with other BL variants, patients with HIV-associated BL commonly present with lymphadenopathy, have a relatively higher frequency of bone marrow and blood involvement, and may develop a leukemic phase (20).

HISTOLOGIC FINDINGS

Lymph Nodes

The morphologic features of the endemic, sporadic, and immunodeficiency-associated variants of BL are very similar (20,47). Lymph nodes are involved in some patients with sporadic or immunodeficiency-associated BL, but only infrequently in patients with endemic BL (figs. 25-2–25-5). The lymph node architecture is replaced by lymphoma in a diffuse growth pattern and a prominent starry sky pattern is almost always present (fig. 25-2) (15,20,47). The starry sky pattern is characterized by tingible body macrophages ("stars") in a background of neoplastic cells ("sky"). The tingible body

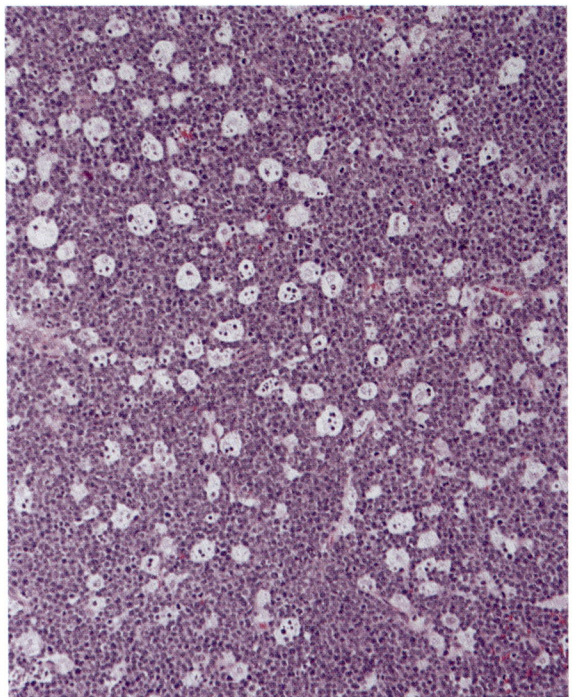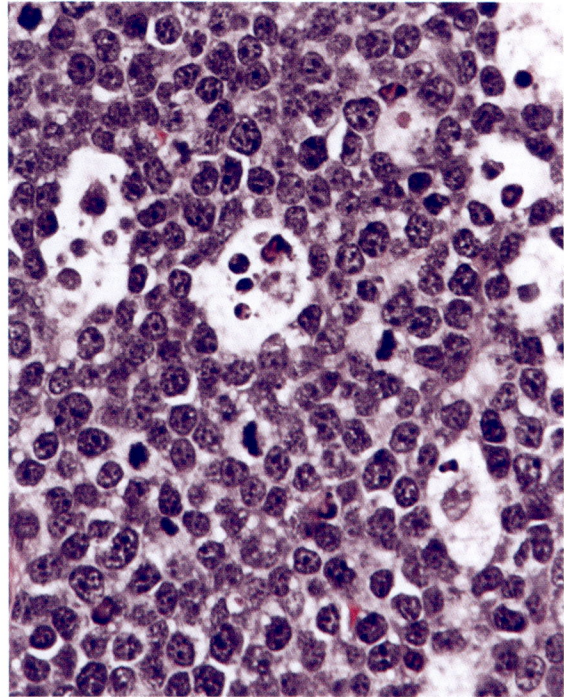

Figure 25-2

HUMAN IMMUNODEFICIENCY VIRUS (HIV)-ASSOCIATED BURKITT LYMPHOMA INVOLVING LYMPH NODE

Left: The neoplasm has a diffuse pattern with a prominent starry sky appearance.

Right: Oil magnification shows that the neoplastic cells are of intermediate size, slightly smaller than histiocyte nuclei, with multiple small nucleoli. Mitotic figures are numerous in this field and tingible body macrophages contain abundant apoptotic cell debris (left, right: hematoxylin and eosin [H&E] stain).

macrophages contain apoptotic tumor cells within their cytoplasm. Large areas of necrosis may be present. In a small subset of cases, lymphoid follicles are focally colonized by BL, imparting a nodular pattern (fig. 25-3).

Cytologically, the lymphoma cells are usually monomorphic, medium-sized cells that are of similar size to the nuclei of tingible body macrophages (20,47). The lymphoma cells have central, round nuclei with dispersed chromatin and 2 to 4 small basophilic nucleoli (fig. 25-2, right). BL cells also have a moderate amount of basophilic cytoplasm with many lipid vacuoles. Numerous apoptotic tumor cells and mitotic figures are present. In HIV-associated BL, the neoplastic cells may have eccentric nuclei and exhibit a more plasmacytoid appearance (fig. 25-4) (20).

In BL, the cells are densely packed and are often opposed to one another. The cytoplasmic borders of the lymphoma cells are "squared off" against each other. If cytoplasmic retraction is present, often a result of tissue fixation, the squared-off appearance is accentuated and has been likened to a "jig-saw puzzle" appearance (fig. 25-6).

The dense packing of tumor cells described above is, in part, explained by the low number of benign cells admixed within the neoplasm. In other words, the tumor microenvironment of BL is sparse. These tumors have few reactive T lymphocytes or histiocytes (other than tingible body macrophages) and there is minimal intercellular stroma or fibrosis. A small subset of BL cases, however, has been reported in which the lymphoma cells are associated with an intense granulomatous (sarcoid-like) reaction (13,37). This reaction pattern is associated with localized disease and a better prognosis (13).

Over the past two decades, with the availability of immunophenotypic and genetic data to incorporate into the diagnosis, there has been a trend away from using pure morphologic criteria for the diagnosis of BL. In the WHO classification it is emphasized that all available data are used

Figure 25-3

SPORADIC BURKITT LYMPHOMA INVOLVING LYMPH NODE

The neoplasm appears to have colonized and expanded a lymphoid follicle, imparting a nodular pattern (H&E stain).

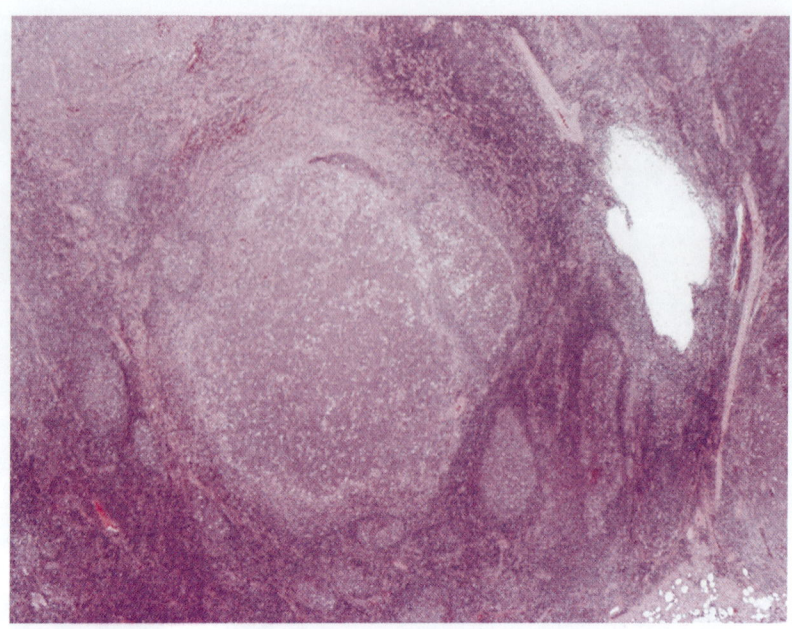

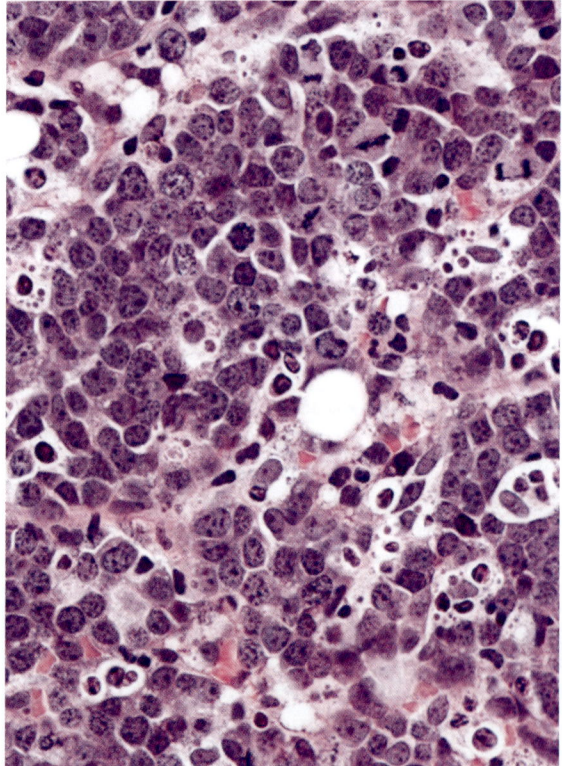

Figure 25-4

HIV-ASSOCIATED BURKITT LYMPHOMA INVOLVING LYMPH NODE

A starry sky pattern, intermediate-sized cells with many mitotic figures, and occasional tumor cells with eccentrically located nuclei and a plasmacytoid appearance are present (H&E stain).

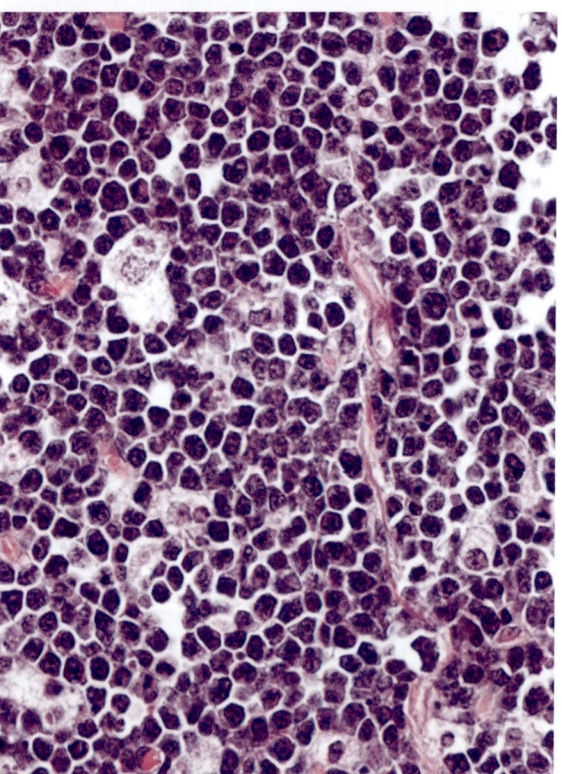

Figure 25-5

SPORADIC BURKITT LYMPHOMA

The cytoplasmic borders of the lymphoma cells are apposed and appear to be "squared off," accentuated by mild retraction artifact attributable to tissue fixation (H&E stain).

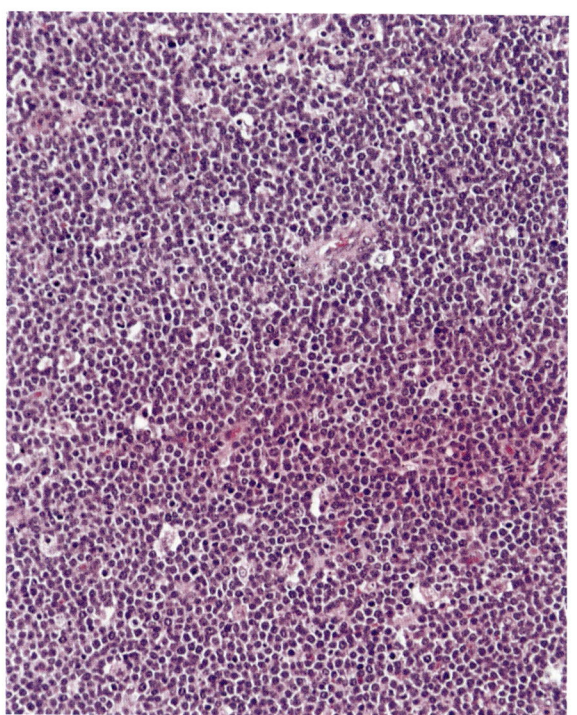 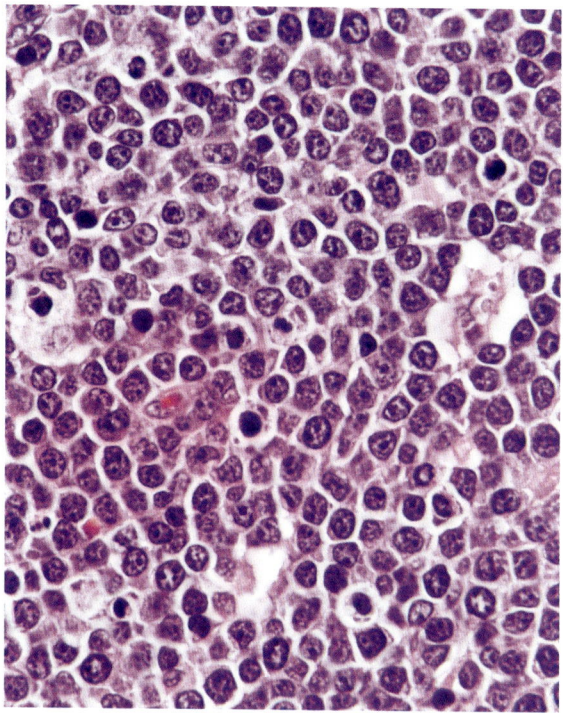

Figure 25-6

ENDEMIC BURKITT LYMPHOMA INVOLVING JAW

Left: At low-power magnification, this tumor from a child from Brazil, has a diffuse pattern with a starry sky appearance.

Right: The oil immersion magnification image shows that the neoplastic cells are of intermediate size, slightly smaller than histiocyte nuclei, with multiple small nucleoli. The space between the tumor cells is the result of retraction artifact which highlights the squared off borders of the tumor cell cytoplasm. Tingible body macrophages contain abundant apoptotic cell debris in this field (left, right: H&E stain). (Courtesy of Dr. C. Bacchi, Botucatu, Brazil.)

to establish the diagnosis of BL (20,40a). In the past, cases that had many features of BL but had greater variation in the size and shape of the lymphoma cells were considered as atypical BL or Burkitt-like lymphoma. These neoplasms are now recognized as BL if in accord with available ancillary data, usually immunophenotypic or cytogenetic results, and gene expression profiling studies have supported this approach (7,16).

Extranodal Sites

At all extranodal sites, BL has a histologic appearance that is similar to that observed in the lymph nodes. A diffuse growth pattern and a prominent starry sky pattern are characteristic features and the cytologic features are similar (figs. 25-6, 25-7). At extranodal sites, BL may infiltrate between muscle or collagen bundles in a single cell pattern and necrosis is often greater, particularly in biopsy specimens obtained from

a bulky mass. In addition, extranodal BL can surround benign lymph nodes, focally infiltrating them in some cases, clinically mimicking a nodal presentation.

Leukemic Presentation of BL. BL patients, particularly those with advanced disease and high tumor burden, can present in a "leukemic" phase characterized by lymphoma cells, often numerous, in the peripheral blood. Leukemic BL was once designated in the French-American-British (FAB) classification as the L3 type of acute lymphoblastic leukemia. This FAB term is now considered obsolete, replaced by *leukemic phase of Burkitt lymphoma*.

Patients with leukemic phase of BL are further subdivided into two groups: patients who also have a tumor mass versus patients with only leukemic involvement, so-called pure Burkitt leukemia (42). Adult patients with pure Burkitt leukemia tend to have a better prognosis than

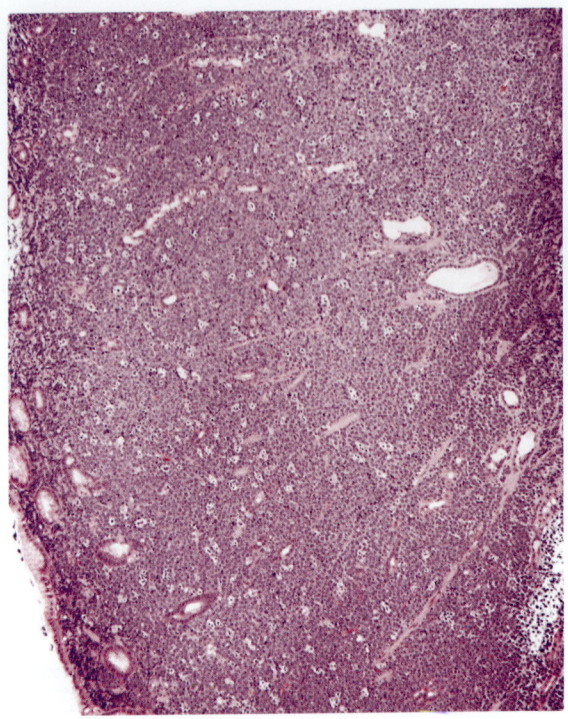 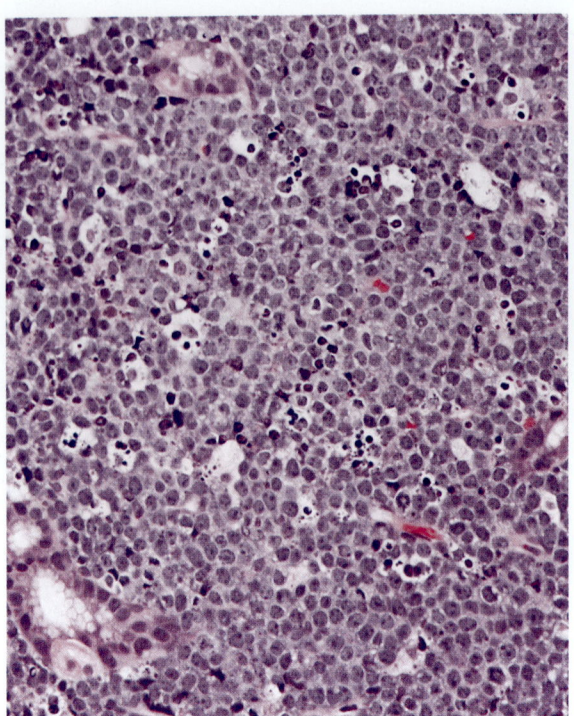

Figure 25-7

SPORADIC BURKITT LYMPHOMA INVOLVING STOMACH

Left: The mucosa is diffusely and almost completely replaced by lymphoma with a starry sky pattern.
Right: At this power, the tingible macrophages are associated with many apoptotic tumor cell nuclei (left, right: H&E stain).

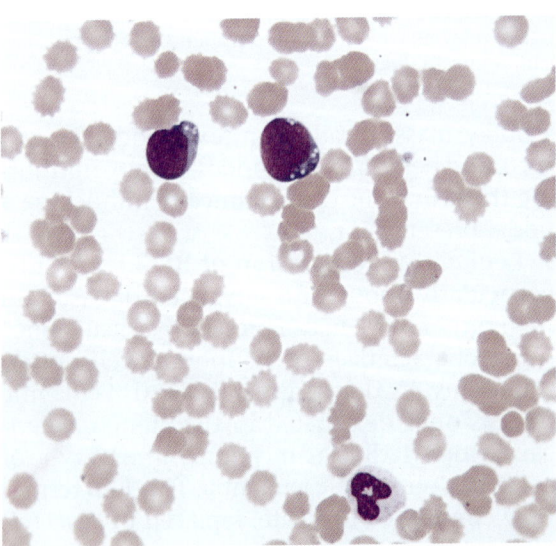

Figure 25-8

SPORADIC BURKITT LYMPHOMA INVOLVING PERIPHERAL BLOOD

The two lymphoma cells shown in this field have small nucleoli and multiple cytoplasmic vacuoles, and are slightly larger than the neutrophil in the field (Wright-Giemsa stain).

patients who have leukemic involvement and a tumor mass (42).

In Wright-Giemsa–stained blood (fig. 25-8) or bone marrow aspirate smears, BL cells have basophilic (almost royal blue) cytoplasm with numerous lipid vacuoles that appear as clear, punched-out spaces in the cell cytoplasm (fig. 25-9) (20,42). This highly vacuolated cytoplasm is not specific, but is highly characteristic of BL cells. The cytoplasmic vacuoles contain lipid that can be highlighted by oil red O stain.

CYTOLOGIC FINDINGS

Cytologic smears of BL show intermediate (medium)-sized cells with round nuclei and finely clumped chromatin containing 2 to 4 small nucleoli and moderate, deeply basophilic cytoplasm (fig. 25-10). As mentioned above, cytoplasmic lipid vacuoles are prominent in Romanowsky-stained slides. A high mitotic rate, many apoptotic cells, and variable numbers of tingible-body macrophages are almost always present.

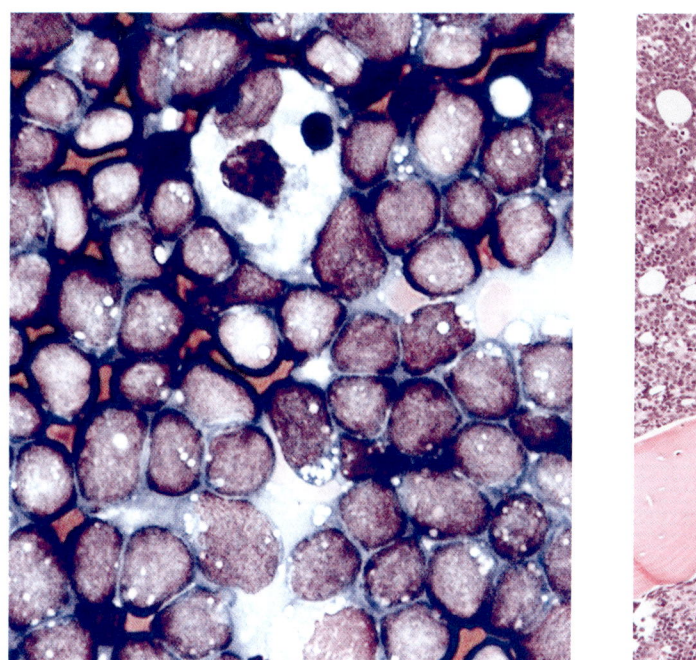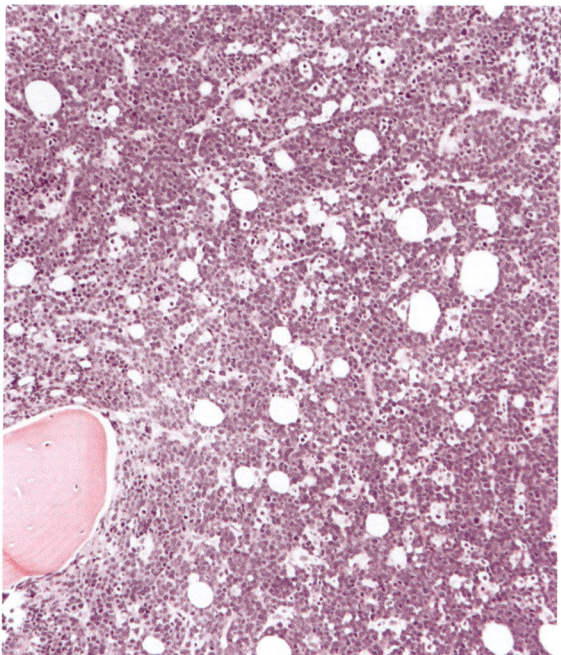

Figure 25-9

SPORADIC BURKITT LYMPHOMA INVOLVING BONE MARROW

Left: A touch imprint of a bone marrow biopsy specimen shows numerous lymphoma cells with many cytoplasmic vacuoles. A tingible body macrophage is also present in the upper part of the field (Wright-Giemsa stain).

Right: A bone marrow biopsy specimen shows diffuse replacement of the medullary space by lymphoma. The starry sky pattern can be prominent in bone marrow specimens extensively replaced by BL (H&E stain).

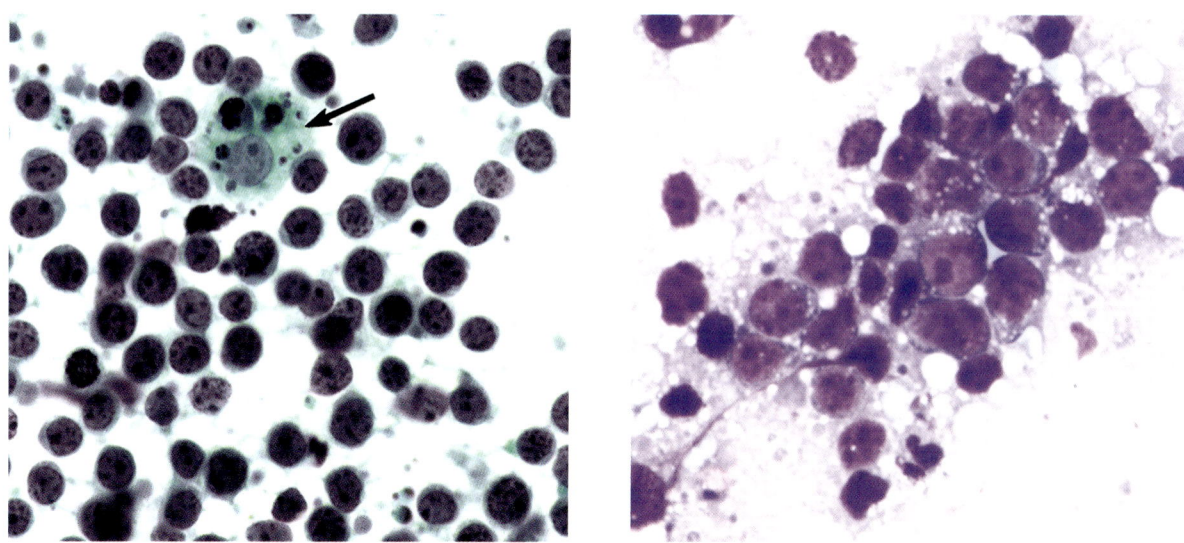

Figure 25-10

HIV-ASSOCIATED BURKITT LYMPHOMA INVOLVING LYMPH NODE

Left: The lymphoma cells in this lymph node aspirate smear are slightly smaller than a tingible body macrophage nucleus (arrow) and have round nuclei, coarse chromatin, and multiple small nucleoli. A mitotic figure and apoptotic bodies are also present in this field (Papanicolaou stain).

Right: A Diff-Quik stain highlights the basophilic cytoplasm and cytoplasmic vacuoles. Apoptotic bodies are also present.

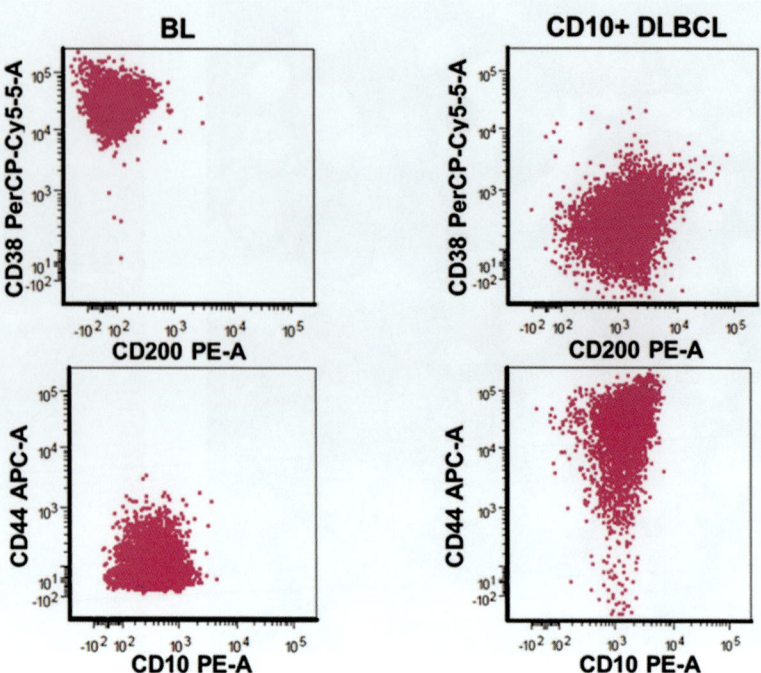

Figure 25-11

FLOW CYTOMETRIC RESULTS IN SPORADIC BURKITT LYMPHOMA VERSUS DIFFUSE LARGE B-CELL LYMPHOMA

The panel of CD10, CD38, CD44, and CD200 is helpful for diagnosis. In Burkitt lymphoma (BL), the lymphoma cells are positive for CD10 and CD38 (bright), dimly positive for CD44, and negative for CD200. A case of CD10-positive diffuse large B-cell lymphoma (DLBCL) is shown for comparison. (Courtesy of Dr. J. L. Jorgensen, Houston, TX.)

IMMUNOPHENOTYPIC FINDINGS

The immunophenotype of the endemic, sporadic, and immunodeficiency-associated variants is very similar (3,12,15,33,40). Using flow cytometry, BL cells are positive for monotypic surface light chain, with moderate to bright intensity, and pan-B-cell antigens including CD19, CD20, CD22, and CD79a. BL cells are also positive for CD10, brightly positive for CD38, and dimly positive or negative for CD44 and CD200 (fig. 25-11). In the literature, most cases of BL express IgM, but IgM can be negative in a subset of cases (possibly suggesting origin from different stages of B-cell differentiation). BL cells are negative for T-cell markers including CD2, CD3, CD4, CD5, CD7, CD8, and T-cell receptors as well as CD1a, CD23, CD138, and TdT.

Immunohistochemical analysis of BL is also essential for diagnosis (fig. 25-12). The lymphoma cells are positive for pan-B-cell markers including PAX5; germinal center B-cell-associated antigens, such as CD10 and BCL6 (fig. 25-13); but in our experience, can be negative for GCET1. TCL-1 is usually positive (33), and CD43 and FOXP1 are commonly expressed. MUM1/IRF4 is positive in about 40 percent of cases. CD21 is often expressed by the cells of endemic BL, but usually not in sporadic or immunodeficiency-associated BL.

MYC expression is high (fig. 25-14). Adipophilin, a marker of altered lipid metabolism, has been reported to be positive in over 90 percent of BL cases (2). BCL2 is usually negative (fig. 25-12C), but rare neoplastic cells express weak BCL2. In cases of relapsed BL after therapy, weak-moderate BCL2 expression is more common (fig. 25-15). The cells of BL have an extremely high proliferation fraction as shown by an anti-Ki-67 antibody; in most cases virtually all tumor cells are positive and proliferating (fig. 25-12D). BL cells are usually negative for LMO2 (6a) and invariably negative for ALK, HHV-8, and cyclin D1.

BL usually has a type I latency pattern of EBV infection and therefore immunohistochemical analysis for EBV latent membrane protein type 1 is usually negative. Immunohistochemistry for EBNA1 or in situ hybridization for EBER1 is required to demonstrate EBV infection (fig. 25-16).

MOLECULAR GENETIC FINDINGS

Conventional cytogenetic analysis of BL shows chromosomal translocations involving *MYC* in almost all cases (4,9,26). The t(8;14)(q24;q32) is very common, found in 80 to 85 percent of cases. The t(2;8)(p11;q24) and t(8;22)(q24;q11), also known as the variant translocations, occur in 10 to 15 percent of cases. Molecular analysis

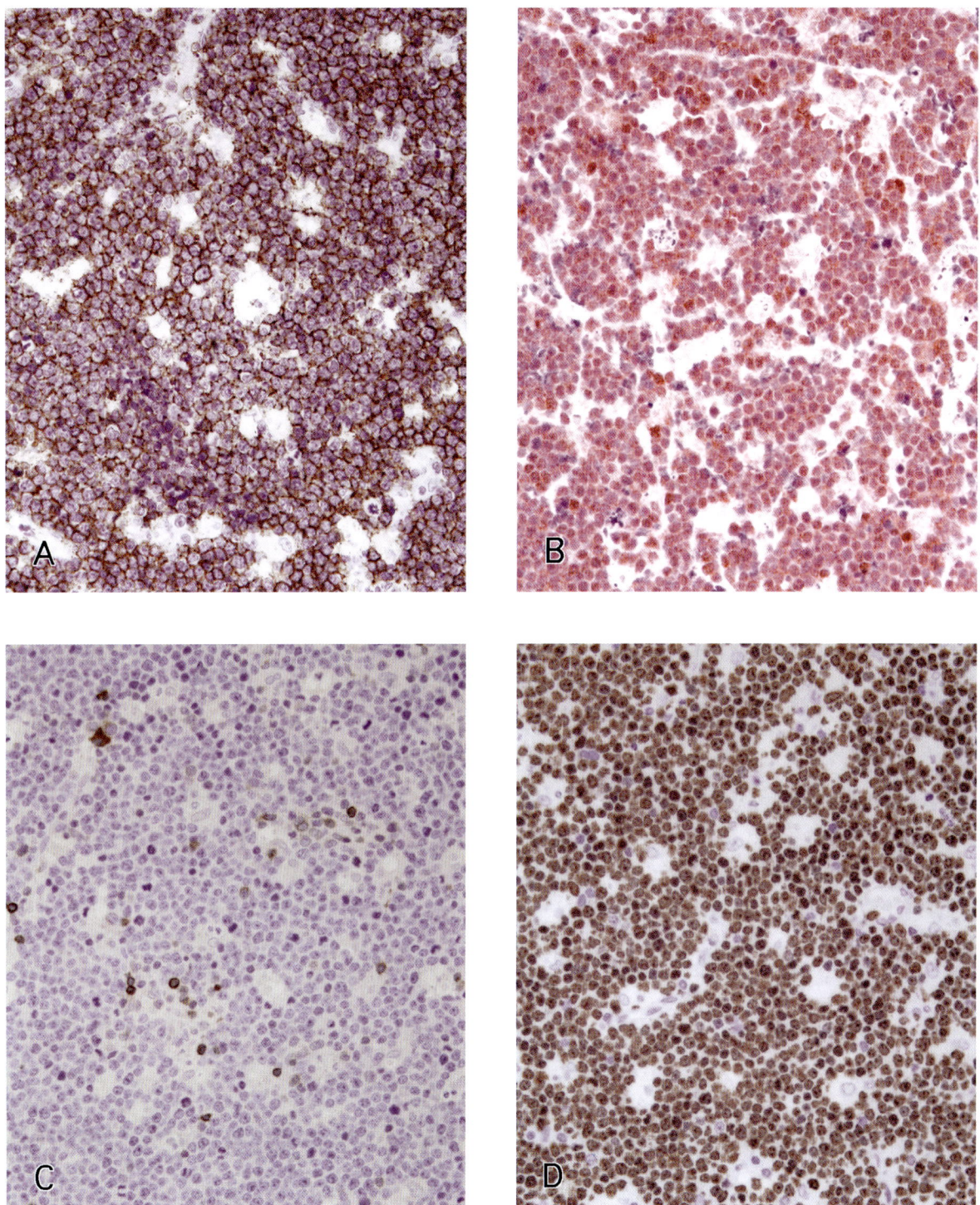

Figure 25-12

HIV-ASSOCIATED BURKITT LYMPHOMA INVOLVING LYMPH NODE

A–D: Immunohistochemical analysis shows that the neoplastic cells are positive for CD20 (A), TCL1 (B) and are negative for BCL2 (C). The lymphoma cells have a Ki-67 (proliferation) rate of almost 100 percent (D). These images are from the same case as shown in fig. 25-2 (immunohistochemistry with hematoxylin counterstain).

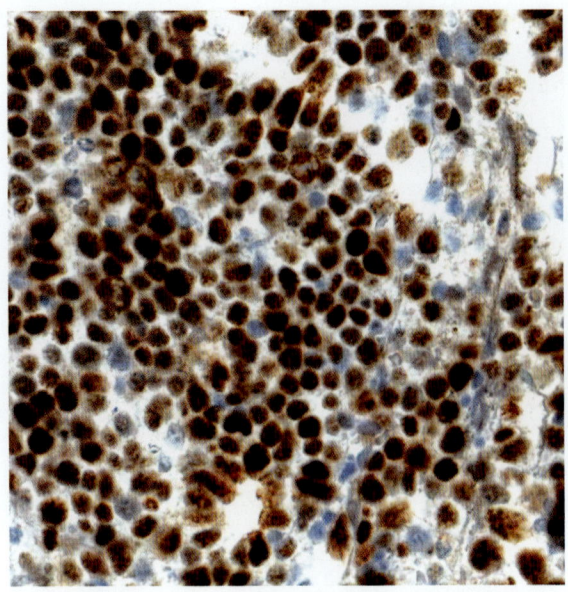

Figure 25-13

SPORADIC BURKITT LYMPHOMA: BCL6

Most cases of BL are strongly and uniformly positive for BCL6 (immunohistochemistry with hematoxylin counterstain).

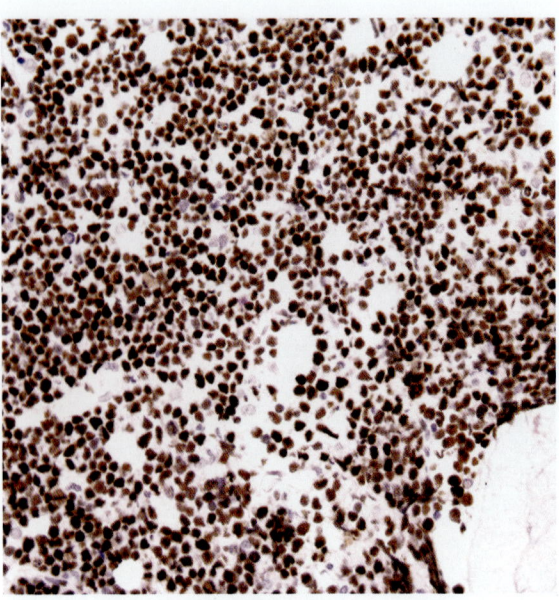

Figure 25-14

SPORADIC BURKITT LYMPHOMA: MYC

The lymphoma cells of BL strongly express MYC in almost all tumor cells. This is the same case shown in fig. 25-9 (immunohistochemistry with hematoxylin counterstain).

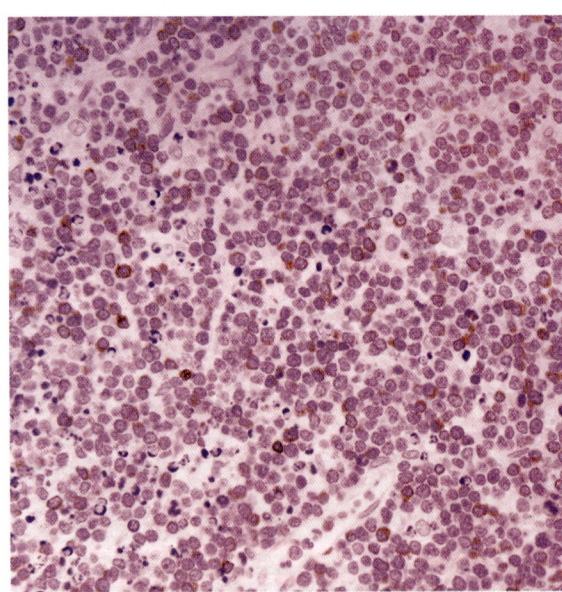

Figure 25-15

RELAPSED SPORADIC BURKITT LYMPHOMA POSITIVE FOR BCL2

This 29-year-old man had BL 7 months earlier with a typical immunophenotype including BCL2 negative. At relapse, BCL2 was positive (weak-moderate intensity) in many lymphoma cells (immunohistochemistry with hematoxylin counterstain).

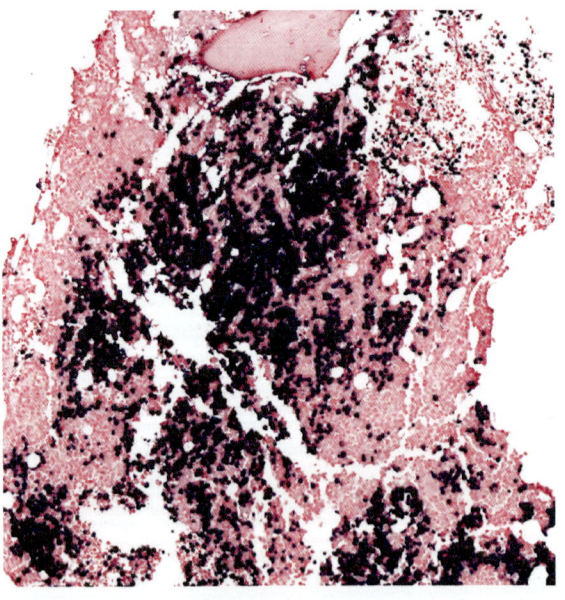

Figure 25-16

SPORADIC BURKITT LYMPHOMA INVOLVING BONE MARROW: EBER1

In situ hybridization shows that the lymphoma cells are positive for Epstein-Barr virus (EBV)-encoded RNA1 (EBER1) (in situ hybridization with eosin counterstain).

414

has shown that the t(8;14) juxtaposes *MYC* 5' to the *IGH* locus on the derivative chromosome 14. In contrast, t(2;8) and t(8;22) juxtapose the *IGK* and *IGL* light chain loci, respectively, 3' to the *MYC* gene on the derivative 8 chromosome. All translocations place *MYC* under the control of immunoglobulin gene enhancers and result in MYC being overexpressed.

The karyotype of BL is less complex than the karyotype of DLBCL and high-grade B-cell lymphoma, not otherwise specified (NOS) (4,16,40). In part, this may be attributable to patient age because BL patients are often children and younger adults, but age alone is not an adequate explanation. About 75 percent of cases of BL have a simple karyotype in which a *MYC* translocation is the sole abnormality or only a few additional chromosomal aberrations are present (4). The rest of the cases have a more complex karyotype and this may be attributable to tumor evolution and progression (4). These additional abnormalities, particularly involving chromosomes 1, 13, and 22 in children and chromosome 17p13 and 18q21 in adults are associated with a poorer prognosis (9,14,26,28).

Studies using array comparative genomic hybridization (CGH) to assess BL cases are in keeping with the concept that BL is cytogenetically simpler than DLBCL or high-grade B-cell lymphoma, NOS (16,35). Hummel et al. (16) showed that the median number of chromosomal imbalances in BL was only two, substantially less than that of other large B-cell lymphomas. The most common secondary aberrations that occur in BL are copy number gains involving chromosomes 1q, 7, and 12 and losses involving chromosomes 6q, 13q32-34, and 17p (4).

There are differences in the cytogenetic profiles of pediatric versus adult BL. Havelange et al. (14) reported 7q32q36 gain, 13q31.3q32.1 amplification, and 5q23.3 copy neutral loss of heterozygosity more often in childhood BL. In contrast, 17p13 and 18q21 copy neutral loss of heterozygosity were restricted to adult cases.

Although *MYC-IGH* translocations are identical at the cytogenetic level in the clinical variants of BL, this is not the case at the molecular level (24). Based on the location of the chromosome 8 breakpoint in relation to *MYC*, translocations have been designated as class I, II, or III. In class I, breakpoints occur in the first exon or intron of *MYC*; in class II, breakpoints occur immediately upstream of the gene; and in class III, breakpoints occur 5' at a distance from *MYC*. In sporadic and immunodeficiency (HIV)-associated BL, breakpoints occur immediately 5' (class II) or within (class I) the *MYC* gene. By contrast, in endemic BL the breakpoints are located far 5' (over 100 kb) to the *MYC* gene (class III).

The breakpoints on chromosome 14 also vary between variants. In sporadic BL and immuno-deficiency (HIV)-associated BL, the breakpoints occur commonly within the *IGH* switch or constant (C) regions, upstream of Cμ, Cγ, or Cα (24). By contrast, most breakpoints in endemic BL occur within the *IGH* joining (J) region. These differences suggest that endemic BL arises earlier in B-cell differentiation, as a mistake in normal V-D-J rearrangement, whereas sporadic and immunodeficiency-associated BL occur later in differentiation, at the time of *IG* heavy chain switching.

The number of breakpoints in BL variants has implications for their detection by polymerase chain reaction (PCR)-based methods or FISH when conventional cytogenetic analysis has not been performed. Fresh tissue is not required for PCR or FISH assays, a major advantage. The number of partners and many breakpoints, however, effectively exclude routine PCR-based assays to detect *MYC* translocations (although research PCR applications are more effective). Therefore, FISH is most often used because the large size of the *MYC* probes allows detection of virtually all 8q24 breakpoints (fig. 25-17). Using *MYC* break-apart probes, the partner cannot be identified. Alternatively, commercially available *IGH* and *MYC* probe sets can be used to detect *MYC-IGH*. Overall, FISH analysis of BL cases will detect *MYC* translocations in about 90 percent of cases. Technical reasons and misdiagnosis likely explain a subset of false negative cases, but there are some cases that meet the morphologic criteria for BL but lack *MYC* translocation.

About 5 percent of cases of BL do not carry *MYC* translocations (8,20). It is thought that alternate mechanisms of *MYC* activation are occurring in translocation-negative cases. De Falco et al. (8) have shown differential expression of four microRNAs between *MYC* translocation-positive and -negative cases. These authors also showed overexpression of DNA methyl transferase members and *MYCN*. Salaverria et

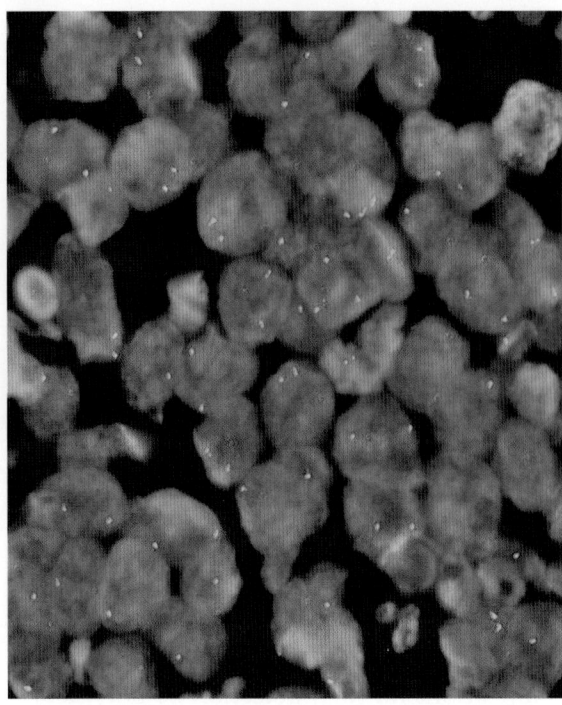

Figure 25-17

**FLUORESCENCE IN SITU HYBRIDIZATION
USING A *MYC*/8q24 BREAKAPART PROBE**

The yellow signals show an intact MYC locus whereas the green and red signals correspond to separation of the probes as a result of MYC translocation. The partner of MYC cannot be discerned using a breakapart strategy.

al. (34) described another small subset (about 3 percent) of cases that fulfilled traditional criteria for BL and supported by gene expression profiling, but lacking *MYC* translocations. These tumors had interstitial gains at chromosome 11q23.2-q23.3 and telomeric losses of 11q24.1-qter. The authors showed loss or mutation of the *ETS1* gene in about 25 percent of tumors and overexpression of *PAFAH1B2* (platelet-activating factor acetylhydrolase 1B subunit β). These neoplasms are designated provisionally as *Burkitt-like lymphoma with 11q aberration* in the 2016 update of the WHO classification (40a).

Next-generation sequencing and other methods of analysis of cases of sporadic BL have uncovered several mutations in BL (38,39). Perhaps most important, these studies have shown constitutive activation of *TCF3* in BL, via mutations of *ID3* and *TCF3*, mutated in 50 to 60 percent and 10 to 25 percent of cases, respectively. *ID3* is a direct transcriptional target of *MYC* and normally functions to control cell cycle progression and proliferation, in part via its role as a negative regulator of *TCF3*. Mutations in *ID3* inactivate the protein and result in constitutive upregulation of *TCF3*. Alternatively, *TCF3* itself is mutated, which prevents binding by ID3, also resulting in constitutive activation. TCF3 is a master regulator of germinal center B-cell differentiation. *TCF3* promotes tonic B-cell receptor (BCR) signaling, engaging the PI3 kinase pathway, and promotes cell cycle progression (39,41,43).

The PI3 kinase pathway is also important in BL pathogenesis. Next-generation sequencing analysis of BL has shown mutations in various genes of the PI3 kinase pathway. Mouse models, in which germinal center B cells are manipulated to show MYC and PI3 kinase activation, develop tumors that resemble sporadic BL (36). These data suggest that MYC and the PI3K pathway cooperate, probably with the ID3-TCF3 axis, in the pathogenesis of BL (41,46).

It has been known for some time that point mutations in *MYC* occur in about 70 percent of BLs; these mutations often involve the *MYC* transactivation domain (39). Next-generation sequencing of sporadic BL cases has shown a number of other gene mutations involved in cell cycle progression, including *CCND3* (35 to 40 percent), *CDKN2A/P16/INK4a* (18 percent), *TP53* (about 35 percent), nucleosome remodeling genes (e.g., *ARID1A* and *SMARCA4*), and focal adhesion family genes (e.g., *GNA13, RHOA*). Fewer sequencing studies have been performed on cases of endemic or immunodeficiency-associated BL, but some differences have been shown in the frequency of gene mutations.

Gene expression profiling studies indicate that most cases of BL exhibit a gene expression signature that is unique, resembling that of normal centroblasts in the germinal center dark zone, and distinct from DLBCL (7,16). The gene expression profile of children and adults with BL is very similar (7,16). BL shows high expression levels of *MYC* target and germinal center B-cell genes, and low levels of expression of NF-κB pathway and MHC class I genes. Gene expression profiling studies also have shown that the variants of BL have similar gene signatures (27).

There are some differences between the variants, however, particularly between endemic versus sporadic BL. EBV is much less common in sporadic BL and therefore appears to be less important in pathogenesis, reflected in gene and microRNA expression profiles. The frequencies of *TCF3* and *ID3* mutations are lower and the frequency of *IGH* variable region somatic mutations is higher in endemic BL than in sporadic BL (1). These results suggest that endemic BL is driven by external stimulation of B-cell receptor signaling, in keeping with the role of cofactors, as discussed above. In contrast, B-cell receptor signaling is driven by gene mutations and is tonic in sporadic BL (1). Proteomic analysis has shown differences between endemic and sporadic BL cases (10).

As BL is a mature B-cell tumor, virtually all cases carry monoclonal immunoglobulin rearrangements and the T-cell receptor genes are in the germline configuration. PCR-based assays to detect gene rearrangements can be performed, but it must be remembered that the *IGH* variable region genes are commonly somatically hypermutated (18). As a result, variable region primers may not anneal, yielding a false negative result.

DIFFERENTIAL DIAGNOSIS

Diffuse Large B-Cell Lymphoma. It is clinically important to distinguish BL from DLBCL because BL patients have much better survival rate when treated with intensive chemotherapy protocols. Unlike BL (described above), in DLBCL the cells are usually larger and exhibit greater nuclear pleomorphism. The presence of stromal fibrosis and numerous reactive T cells and histiocytes in the background is common in DLBCL, but unusual in BL. Ancillary studies are helpful in this differential diagnosis. Cases of DLBCL show variable positivity for BCL6, a subset of tumors strongly positive for BCL2, a proliferation rate (Ki-67) usually less than 90 percent, and a karyotype that can be complex. *MYC* translocations occur in about 10 percent of DLBCL cases. Chromosomal translocations involving *BCL6* are one of the most frequent genetic abnormalities in DLBCL. By contrast, in BL, the neoplastic cells uniformly express BCL6, BCL2 is negative, and Ki-67 is positive in over 95 percent (and often virtually all) lymphoma cells. Conventional cytogenetic analysis often shows a simpler karyotype and *MYC* translocations involve immunoglobulin loci in 85 to 90 percent of BL cases. Some DLBCL cases, however, have an immunophenotype identical to BL and a subset of these cases has *MYC* translocations.

High-Grade B-Cell Lymphoma, NOS. In the 2008 WHO classification, these neoplasms were designated as B-cell lymphoma, unclassifiable, with features intermediate between DLBCL and BL. In the 2016 update of the WHO classification, these tumors are designated as high-grade B-cell lymphoma, NOS (40a). Features that support the diagnosis of high-grade B-cell lymphoma, NOS over BL include the presence of a cytologic spectrum of medium-sized to large tumor cells, strong positivity for BCL2, variable expression of CD10 or BCL6, less than 90 percent Ki-67 positivity, and a complex karyotype. Cases may or may not carry *MYC* translocations that involve *IG* or non-*IG* partners. Rarely, cases of low-grade B-cell lymphoma undergo transformation to a tumor that can resemble BL. Most of these cases, however, are BCL2 positive and fit best in the high-grade B-cell lymphoma category.

Double- (and Triple-) Hit Lymphomas. Conventional cytogenetic or FISH analysis is required to identify this subset of aggressive B-cell lymphomas that are generally refractory to standard chemotherapy. The morphologic spectrum of double-hit lymphoma is wide; most cases resemble DLBCL or fit within the spectrum of high-grade B-cell lymphoma. Clues that a neoplasm that morphologically resembles BL may, in fact, be a double-hit lymphoma include: older patient age, nodal location, greater nuclear pleomorphism, and BCL2 positivity (see chapter 27). In the revised WHO classification, these neoplasms are designated as high-grade B-cell lymphoma with *MYC* and *BCL2* and/or *BCL6* rearrangements (40a).

Rarely, patients with low-grade B-cell lymphoma, most often follicular lymphoma, subsequently develop a neoplasm that closely mimics BL at the morphologic level. Only a few patients have been studied by molecular methods; the BL may be clonally unrelated or related to the underlying low-grade B-cell lymphoma. Clonally unrelated cases of BL are BCL2 negative and may be coincidental. Cases that are clonally related to low-grade B-cell lymphoma are obviously biologically different from de novo BL. Clonally related tumors often occur in patients who are generally older, BCL2 is often positive, and the cytogenetic makeup of these tumors is likely to be more complex than de novo BL. Both t(14;18)(q32;q21)/*IGH-BCL2* and *MYC* translocations may be present, supporting classification as double-hit lymphoma.

Lymphoblastic Lymphoma/Leukemia. Approximately 10 percent of cases of lymphoblastic lymphoma of either T- or B-cell lineage have a prominent starry sky pattern and superficially resemble BL. However, the cells of lymphoblastic lymphoma are smaller than BL cells, with finely granular or "dusty" chromatin, inconspicuous nucleoli, and less cytoplasm. This differential diagnosis is easily resolved by immunophenotypic analysis. About 90 percent of lymphoblastic lymphomas are of T-cell lineage. B-lymphoblastic lymphoma is more problematic as these tumors can resemble BL by involving extranodal sites, have a high proliferation (Ki-67) rate, and express CD10 or BCL6 in a subset of cases. Importantly, lymphoblastic lymphoma (T and B) has an immature immunophenotype with expression of TdT, CD34, or both antigens.

Blastoid Variant of Mantle Cell Lymphoma. Rare cases of blastoid mantle cell lymphoma exhibit a starry sky pattern or carry *MYC* translocations and therefore resemble BL. Unlike BL, however, mantle cell lymphoma is positive for CD5 and cyclin D1 and carries t(11;14)(q13;q32)/*CCND1-IGH*.

Peripheral T-Cell Lymphomas. Rare cases of anaplastic large cell lymphoma (ALK positive or negative) or peripheral T-cell lymphoma, not otherwise specified, exhibit a prominent starry sky pattern and resemble BL. These tumors, however, are of T-cell lineage and anaplastic large cell lymphomas express uniform and bright CD30, unlike BL.

Nonhematopoietic Tumors with Blastoid Appearance. A variety of nonhematopoietic tumors with a blastoid appearance can, at least superficially, resemble BL. Small cell carcinoma and Merkel cell carcinoma usually occur in older patients, unusual for BL. Small blue cell tumors of childhood, such as neuroblastoma, alveolar rhabdomyosarcoma, neuroblastoma, and Ewing sarcoma/peripheral neuroectodermal tumor, are more likely to be an issue in the differential diagnosis. Immunophenotypic analysis easily separates BL from the other childhood tumors because BL is positive for CD45/LCA and B-cell antigens, and is negative for epithelial markers/cytokeratins and most markers associated with sarcomas.

TREATMENT AND PROGNOSIS

Despite its rapid growth and aggressive clinical behavior, BL is highly sensitive to chemotherapy, as was shown initially by Burkitt himself (22). The overall strategy for the treatment of BL patients is high dose, relatively short course, multi-agent chemotherapy. The addition of rituximab to chemotherapy also has value (30). Central nervous system prophylaxis is required for most patients and potential tumor lysis syndrome must be averted (19).

In developed countries, the overall survival (cure) rate for patients with localized sporadic BL approaches 90 percent (19). For patients with advanced-stage disease, the overall survival rate is 60 to 80 percent. Children have a better prognosis than adults. Involvement of the central nervous system and a leukemic presentation are poor prognostic factors. Additional cytogenetic changes (karyotype or high-throughput analysis) likely correlate with a poorer prognosis and a recent study reported that overexpression of miR-17 correlates with poorer overall survival (31).

Patients with HIV infection who develop BL often have a very good response to combination chemotherapy, but the treatment is toxic and overall survival depends, in large part, on the status of the HIV infection. The prognosis of patients with endemic BL is often very poor because of inadequate resources in endemic areas; treating these patients is highly challenging. Nevertheless, attempts to bring modern chemotherapy regimens to equatorial Africa have been somewhat successful, with a 2-year overall survival rate of about 60 percent (25).

REFERENCES

1. Amato T, Abate F, Piccaluga P, et al. Clonality analysis of immunoglobulin gene rearrangement by next generation sequencing in endemic Burkitt lymphoma suggests antigen drive activation of BCR as opposed to sporadic Burkitt lymphoma. Am J Clin Pathol 2016;145:116-127.
2. Ambrosio MR, Piccaluga PP, Ponzoni M, et al. The alteration of lipid metabolism in Burkitt lymphoma identifies a novel marker: adipophilin. PLoS One 2012;7:e44315.
3. Barth TF, Muller S, Pawlita M, et al. Homogeneous immunophenotype and paucity of secondary genomic aberrations are distinctive features of endemic but not of sporadic Burkitt's lymphoma and diffuse large B-cell lymphoma with MYC rearrangement. J Pathol 2004;203:940-945.
4. Boerma EG, Siebert R, Kluin PM, Baudis M. Translocations involving 8q24 in Burkitt lymphoma and other malignant lymphomas: a historical review of cytogenetics in the light of todays knowledge. Leukemia 2009;23:225-234.
5. Burkitt D. A sarcoma involving the jaws in African children. Br J Surg 1958;46:218-223.
6. Castillo JJ, Winer ES, Olszewski AJ. Population-based prognostic factors for survival in patients with Burkitt lymphoma: an analysis from the Surveillance, Epidemiology, and End Results database. Cancer 2013;119:3672-3679.
6a. Colomo L, Vazquez I, Papaleo N, et al. LMO2-negative expression predicts the presence of MYC translocations in aggressive B-cell lymphomas. Am J Surg Pathol 2017;41:877-886.
7. Dave SS, Fu K, Wright GW, et al. Molecular diagnosis of Burkitt's lymphoma. N Engl J Med 2006;354:2431-2442.
8. De Falco G, Ambrosio MR, Fuligni F, et al. Burkitt lymphoma beyond MYC translocation: N-MYC and DNA methyltranferases dysregulation. BMC Cancer 2015;15:668.
9. De Souza MT, Hassan R, Liehr T, et al. Conventional and molecular cytogenetic characterization of Burkitt lymphoma with bone marrow involvement in Brazilian children and adolescents. Pediatr Blood Cancer 2014;61:1422-1426.
10. El-Mallawany NK, Day N, Ayello J, et al. Differential proteomic analysis of endemic and sporadic Epstein-Barr virus-positive and negative Burkitt lymphoma. Eur J Cancer 2015;51:92-100.
11. Geser A, Brubaker G, Draper CC. Effect of a malaria suppression program on the incidence of African Burkitt's lymphoma. Am J Epidemiol 1989;129:740-752.
12. Haralambieva E, Boerma EJ, van Imhoff GW, et al. Clinical, immunophenotypic, and genetic analysis of adult lymphomas with morphologic features of Burkitt lymphoma. Am J Surg Pathol 2005;29:1086-1094.
13. Haralambieva E, Rosati S, van Noesel C, et al. Florid granulomatous reaction in Epstein-Barr virus-positive nonendemic Burkitt lymphomas: report of four cases. Am J Surg Pathol 2004;28:379-383.
14. Havelange V, Pepermans X, Ameye G, et al. Genetic differences between paediatric and adult Burkitt lymphomas. Br J Haematol 2016;173:137-144.
15. Huang H, Liu ZL, Zeng H, et al. Clinicopathological study of sporadic Burkitt lymphoma in children. Chinese Med J 2015;128:510-514.
16. Hummel M, Bentink S, Berger H, et al. A biologic definition of Burkitt's lymphoma from transcriptional and genomic profiling. N Engl J Med 2006;354:2419-2430.
17. Illingworth J, Butler NS, Roetynck S, et al. Chronic exposure to Plasmodium falciparum is associated with phenotypic evidence of B and T cell exhaustion. J Immunol 2013;190:1038-1047.
18. Isobe K, Tamaru J, Nakamura S, Harigaya K, Mikata A, Ito H. VH gene analysis in sporadic Burkitt's lymphoma: somatic mutation and intraclonal diversity with special reference to the tumor cells involving germinal center. Leuk Lymphoma 2002;43:159-164.
19. Jacobson C, LaCasce A. How I treat Burkitt lymphoma in adults. Blood 2014;124:2913-2920.
20. Leoncini L, Raphael M, Stein H, Harris NL, Jaffe ES, Klein P. Burkitt lymphoma. In: Swerdlow SH, Campo E, Harris NL, Jaffe ES, Pileri SA, Stein H, Thiele J, Vardiman JW, eds. WHO Classification of tumours of haematopoietic and lymphoid tissues. Lyon: IARC Press; 2008:262-264.
21. Levine PH, Connelly RR, Berard CW, et al. The American Burkitt Lymphoma Registry: a progress report. Ann Intern Med 1975;83:31-36.
22. Magrath I. Denis Burkitt and the African lymphoma. Ecancermedicalscience 2009;3:159.
23. Murphy SB. Childhood non-Hodgkin's lymphoma. N Engl J Med 1978;299:1446-1448.
24. Neri A, Barriga F, Knowles DM, Magrath IT, Dalla-Favera R. Different regions of the immunoglobulin heavy-chain locus are involved in chromosomal translocations in distinct pathogenetic forms of Burkitt lymphoma. Proc Natl Acad Sci USA 1988;85:2748-2752.

25. Ngoma T, Adde M, Durosinmi M, et al. Treatment of Burkitt lymphoma in equatorial Africa using a simple three-drug combination followed by a salvage regimen for patients with persistent or recurrent disease. Br J Haematol 2012;158:749-762.

26. Onciu M, Schlette E, Zhou Y, et al. Secondary chromosomal abnormalities predict outcome in pediatric and adult high-stage Burkitt lymphoma. Cancer 2006;107:1084-1092.

27. Piccaluga PP, De Falco G, Kustagi M, et al. Gene expression analysis uncovers similarity and differences among Burkitt lymphoma subtypes. Blood 2011;117:3596-3608.

28. Poirel HA, Cairo MS, Heerema NA, et al. Specific cytogenetic abnormalities are associated with a significantly inferior outcome in children and adolescents with mature B-cell non-Hodgkin's lymphoma: results of the FAB/LMB 96 international study. Leukemia 2009;23:323-331.

29. Rebelo-Pontes HA, de Abreu MC, Guimaraes DM, et al. Burkitt's lymphoma of the jaws in the Amazon region of Brazil. Med Oral Patol Cir Bucal 2014;19:e32-e38.

30. Ribrag V, Koscielny S, Bosq J, et al. Rituximab and dose-dense chemotherapy for adults with Burkitt's lymphoma: a randomised, controlled, open-lable, phase 3 trial. Lancet 2016;387:2402-2411.

31. Robaina MC, Faccion RS, Mazzoccoli L, et al. muR-17-92 cluster components analysis in Burkitt lymphoma: overexpression of miR-17 is associated with poor prognosis. Ann Hematol 2016;95:881-891.

32. Robbiani DF, Deroubaix S, Feldhahn N, et al. Plasmodium infection promotes genomic instability and AID-dependent B cell lymphoma. Cell 2015;162:727-737.

33. Rodig SJ, Vergilio JA, Shahsafaei A, Dorfman DM. Characteristic expression patterns of TCL1, CD38, and CD44 identify aggressive lymphomas harboring a MYC translocation. Am J Surg Pathol 2008;32:113-122.

34. Salaverria I, Martin-Guerrero I, Wagener R, et al. A recurrent 11q aberration pattern characterizes a subset of MYC-negative high-grade B-cell lymphomas resembling Burkitt lymphoma. Blood 2014;123:1187-1193.

35. Salaverria I, Zettl A, Bea S, et al. Chromosomal alterations detected by comparative genomic hybridization in subgroups of gene expression-defined Burkitt's lymphoma. Haematologica 2008;93:1327-1334.

36. Sander S, Calado DP, Srinivasan L, et al. Synergy between PI3K signaling and MYC in Burkitt lymphomagenesis. Cancer Cell 2012;22:167-179.

36a. Satou A, Asano N, Kato S, et al. Prognostic impact of MUM1/IRF4 expression in Burkitt lymphoma (BL): a reappraisal of 88 BL patients in Japan. Am J Surg Pathol 2017;41:389-395.

37. Satou A, Asano N, Nakazawa A, et al. Epstein-Barr virus (EBV)-positive sporadic Burkitt lymphoma: an age-related lymphoproliferative disorder? Am J Surg Pathol 2015;39:227-235.

38. Schmitz R, Ceribelli M, Pittaluga S, Wright G, Staudt LM. Oncogenic mechanisms in Burkitt lymphoma. Cold Spring Harb Perspect Med 2014;4.

39. Schmitz R, Young RM, Ceribelli M, et al. Burkitt lymphoma pathogenesis and therapeutic targets from structural and functional genomics. Nature 2012;490:116-120.

40. Seegmiller AC, Garcia R, Huang R, Maleki A, Karandikar NJ, Chen W. Simple karyotype and bcl-6 expression predict a diagnosis of Burkitt lymphoma and better survival in IG-MYC rearranged high-grade B-cell lymphomas. Mod Pathol 2010;23:909-920.

40a. Swerdlow SH, Campo E, Pileri SA, et al. The 2016 revision of the World Health Organization classification of lymphoid neoplasms. Blood 2016;127:2375-2390.

41. Shortt J, Martin BP, Newbold A, et al. Combined inhibition of PI3K-related DNA damage response kinases and mTORC1 induces apoptosis in MYC-driven B-cell lymphomas. Blood 2013;121:2964-2974.

42. Song JY, Venkataraman G, Fedoriw Y, et al. Burkitt leukemia limited to the bone marrow has a better prognosis than Burkitt lymphoma with bone marrow involverment in adults. Leuk Lymphoma 2016;57:866-871.

43. Srinivasan L, Sasaki Y, Calado DP, et al. PI3 kinase signals BCR-dependent mature B cell survival. Cell 2009;139:573-586.

44. Thorley-Lawson DA, Gross A. Persistence of the Epstein-Barr virus and the origins of associated lymphomas. N Engl J Med 2004;350:1328-1337.

45. van den Bosch CA. Is endemic Burkitt's lymphoma an alliance between three infections and a tumour promoter? Lancet Oncol 2004;5:738-746.

46. Walsh K, McKinney MS, Love C, et al. PAK1 mediates resistance to PI3K inhibition in lymphomas. Clin Cancer Res 2013;19:1106-1115.

47. Wright DH. Burkitt's lymphoma: a review of the pathology, immunology, and possible etiologic factors. Pathol Annu 1971;6:337-363.

48. Xicoy B, Ribera JM, Müller M, et al. Dose-intensive chemotherapy including rituximab is highly effective but toxic in human immunodeficiency virus-infected patients with Burkitt lymphoma/leukemia: parallel study of 81 patients. Leuk Lymphoma 2014;55:2341-2348.

26   HIGH-GRADE B-CELL LYMPHOMA, NOT OTHERWISE SPECIFIED

GENERAL FEATURES

In the 2008 World Health Organization (WHO) classification, the term B-cell lymphoma, unclassifiable, with features intermediate between diffuse large B-cell lymphoma (DLBCL) and Burkitt lymphoma (BL) was introduced (11). This category was created because these neoplasms have morphologic features intermediate between DLBCL and BL, a B-cell immunophenotype, and often complex cytogenetic and/or molecular abnormalities. As was stated in the WHO classification at that time, this category was not considered a distinct disease entity, but was thought to be useful in allowing classification of cases that did not meet the criteria for BL or DLBCL (11).

There were two problems with this designation. First and most important, the criteria for this category were imprecisely defined and therefore challenging to apply at both the diagnostic and scientific levels. Secondly, the term was awkward to use in daily practice. As a result, these neoplasms were commonly referred to as "gray zone lymphomas," a convenient, but vague term that is also used for other B-cell lymphomas.

In the 2016 update of the WHO classification, these neoplasms will be designated as *high-grade B-cell lymphoma, not otherwise specified* (HGBL-NOS) (17). This term is used in the remainder of this chapter.

Although the designation for these neoplasms in the 2008 WHO classification may have given the impression that they represented a newly described entity, in fact, these neoplasms were a well-recognized challenge. In older classification schemes, they were referred to as *undifferentiated, non-Burkitt type* (updated Rappaport classification); *small noncleaved cell lymphoma, non-Burkitt* (Working Formulation); and *high-grade B-cell lymphoma, Burkitt-like* (Revised European American Lymphoma [REAL]).

The latter designation, because it is self-explanatory, was appealing and the new 2016 designation is similar to the REAL terminology.

In the 2016 WHO classification update, the designation of high-grade B-cell lymphoma is further modified as being either not otherwise specified or as being associated with *MYC* and either *BCL2* or *BCL6* translocations, also known as *double-hit B-cell lymphoma* (1) or more simply, *double-hit lymphoma*. Double-hit lymphomas are the subject of chapter 27.

CLINICAL FEATURES

HGBL-NOS is an uncommon group of neoplasms that represents about 1 percent of lymphomas in adults. In various studies the median age of patients is between 50 and 60 years (5,14,16). These neoplasms are uncommon in children. There is a male predominance of approximately 2 to 1.

Most patients present with high clinical stage disease (Ann Arbor stage III to IV), extranodal sites of disease, poor performance status, high serum lactate dehydrogenase (LDH) or beta-2-microglobulin levels, and a high International Prognostic Index (IPI) (5–7,14,16). The bone marrow (fig. 26-1) and central nervous system are common extranodal sites of involvement.

HISTOLOGIC FINDINGS

All cases of HGBL-NOS have a diffuse growth pattern and show morphologic evidence of aggressiveness, including a starry sky pattern, high apoptotic rate and high mitotic index (fig. 26-1) (5–7,12–14). These neoplasms have a mixture of cells, some the size of BL cells and others closer in size to DLBCL cells, with a greater degree of nuclear irregularity or pleomorphism than observed in BL (figs. 26-2, 26-3). Some cases closely resemble BL, but have atypical immunophenotypic features, in particular BCL2 overexpression (fig. 26-4), or atypical genetic features.

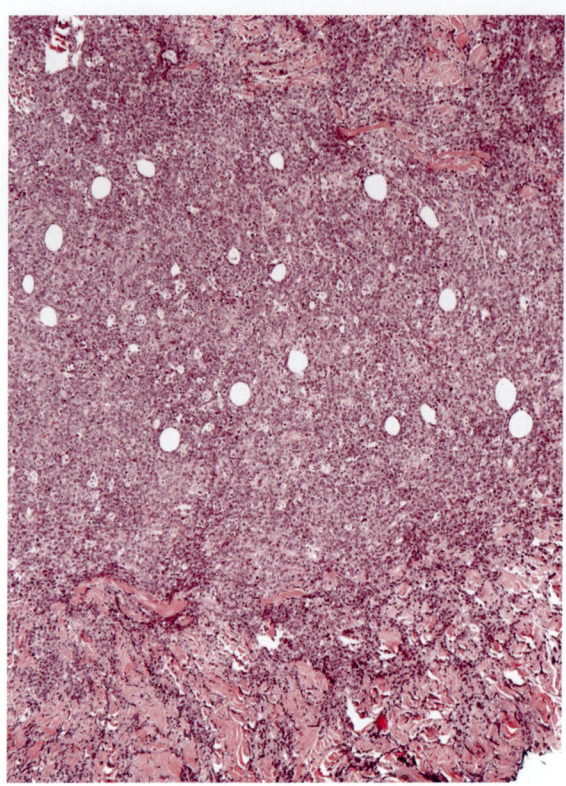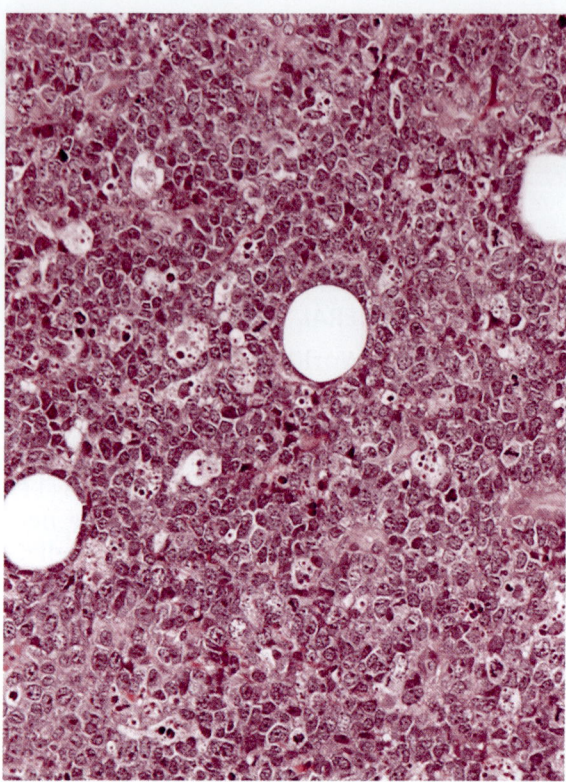

Figure 26-1

HIGH-GRADE B-CELL LYMPHOMA, NOT OTHERWISE SPECIFIED, INVOLVING SKIN

Left: The tumor is located in the dermis and has a diffuse pattern. A starry sky pattern can be easily seen at this power.
Right: High-power magnification shows tumor cells of intermediate to large size, some of which resemble centroblasts, among which are scattered starry sky histiocytes and numerous apoptotic cells (left, right: hematoxylin and eosin [H&E] stain).

Figure 26-2

HIGH-GRADE B-CELL LYMPHOMA, NOT OTHERWISE SPECIFIED, INVOLVING BONE MARROW

This field shows intermediate-sized and large cells with cytoplasmic vacuoles. (Wright-Giemsa stain)

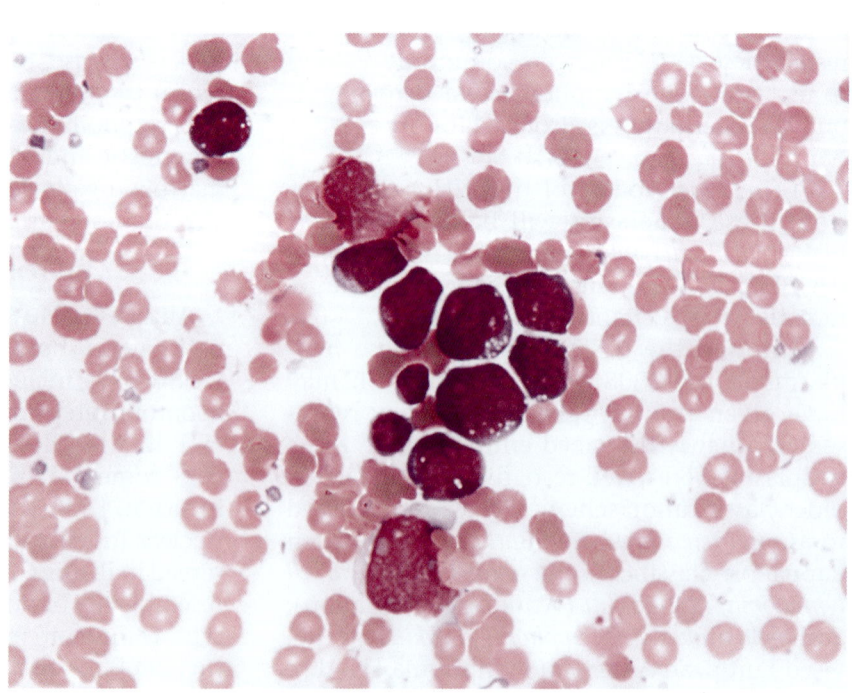

CYTOLOGIC FINDINGS

In bone marrow smears, touch imprints and fine-needle aspirate smears, cases of HGBL-NOS show intermediate-sized or intermediate to large cells, usually with a high mitotic rate and abundant apoptosis (figs. 26-2, 26-5). In some cases the neoplastic cells have cytoplasmic vacuoles (9). The nuclei of the neoplastic cells show variability from cell to cell, with irregular nuclear contours and prominent nucleoli. Cell blocks prepared from fine-needle aspiration specimens are helpful for diagnosis, since they are used for immunohistochemical studies and fluorescence in situ hybridization (FISH) to assess for rearrangements of *MYC* or other oncogenes (9).

IMMUNOPHENOTYPIC FINDINGS

All cases of HGBL-NOS are B-cell neoplasms that express pan-B-cell antigens including CD19, CD20, CD22, CD79a, and PAX5 (5,7,14,16). Using flow cytometry immunophenotyping, some cases exhibit dim or absent CD20 expression and also dim CD19 (19). Many cases of HGBL-NOS dimly express or completely lack surface immunoglobulin. T-cell antigens are negative or only rarely aberrantly expressed.

Cases of HGBL-NOS have either a germinal center B-cell or an activated B-cell immunophenotype, approximately in equal frequency (7). Lymphomas with a germinal center B-cell immunophenotype are positive for CD10 and BCL6. MUM1/IRF4 and CD138 are commonly expressed in neoplasms with an activated B-cell immunophenotype (6,7,14,16).

BCL2 is positive in 60 to 70 percent of HGBL-NOS cases when using the commonly available monoclonal anti-BCL2 antibody (clone 124). Mutations in *BCL2* explain a lack of BCL2 reactivity in a subset of cases (16). MYC is often highly expressed (7,13), CD38 is variably increased, and CD45/LCA is variably decreased. SOX11 is positive in a subset of cases (5). Ki-67 expression is typically high, in the range of 75 to over 99 percent, with the highest rates in tumors with a starry sky pattern that closely resemble BL (6,14,16).

Some cases of HGBL-NOS express both MYC and BCL2 and can be further designated as *double-positive lymphoma* (DPL) or *double-expressor lymphoma*. (This subset of neoplasms includes cases of diffuse large B-cell lymphoma as well

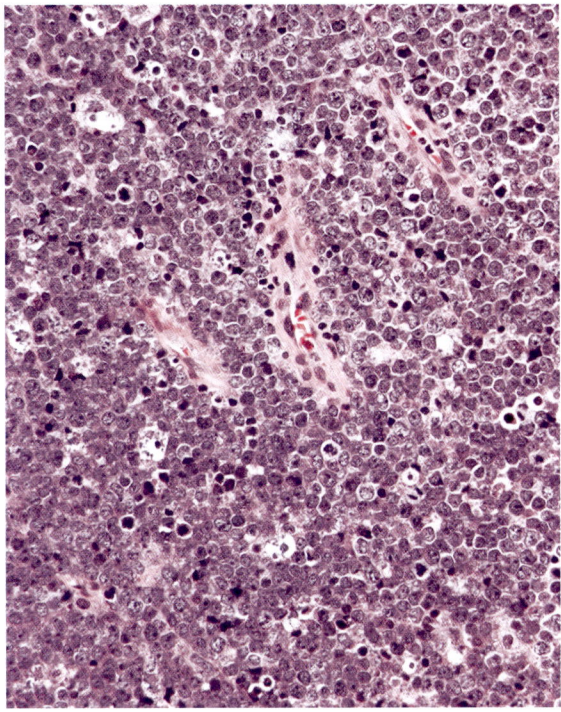

Figure 26-3

HIGH-GRADE B-CELL LYMPHOMA, NOT OTHERWISE SPECIFIED, INVOLVING LYMPH NODE

The tumor has a diffuse pattern and is composed of a mixture of intermediate-sized and larger cells. A starry sky pattern is present (H&E stain).

as HGBL-NOS.) DPL cases include neoplasms with a *MYC* translocation or amplification as well as lymphomas without *MYC* abnormalities. A *MYC* translocation in DPL is associated with a poorer prognosis. Some DPL cases carry *MYC* and *BCL2* translocations; these cases are double hit lymphomas and are discussed in chapter 27.

MOLECULAR GENETIC FINDINGS

Conventional cytogenetic analysis of HGBL-NOS commonly shows a complex karyotype with three or more abnormalities (4,14,16). Array-based comparative genomic hybridization has shown many gains and losses in these tumors (4). Gene expression profiling studies have shown a pattern of expression within the spectrum between DLBCL and BL, or very similar to BL (8,10).

Conventional cytogenetics and FISH studies of HGBL-NOS have shown that translocations involving chromosome 8q24/*MYC* occur in 30

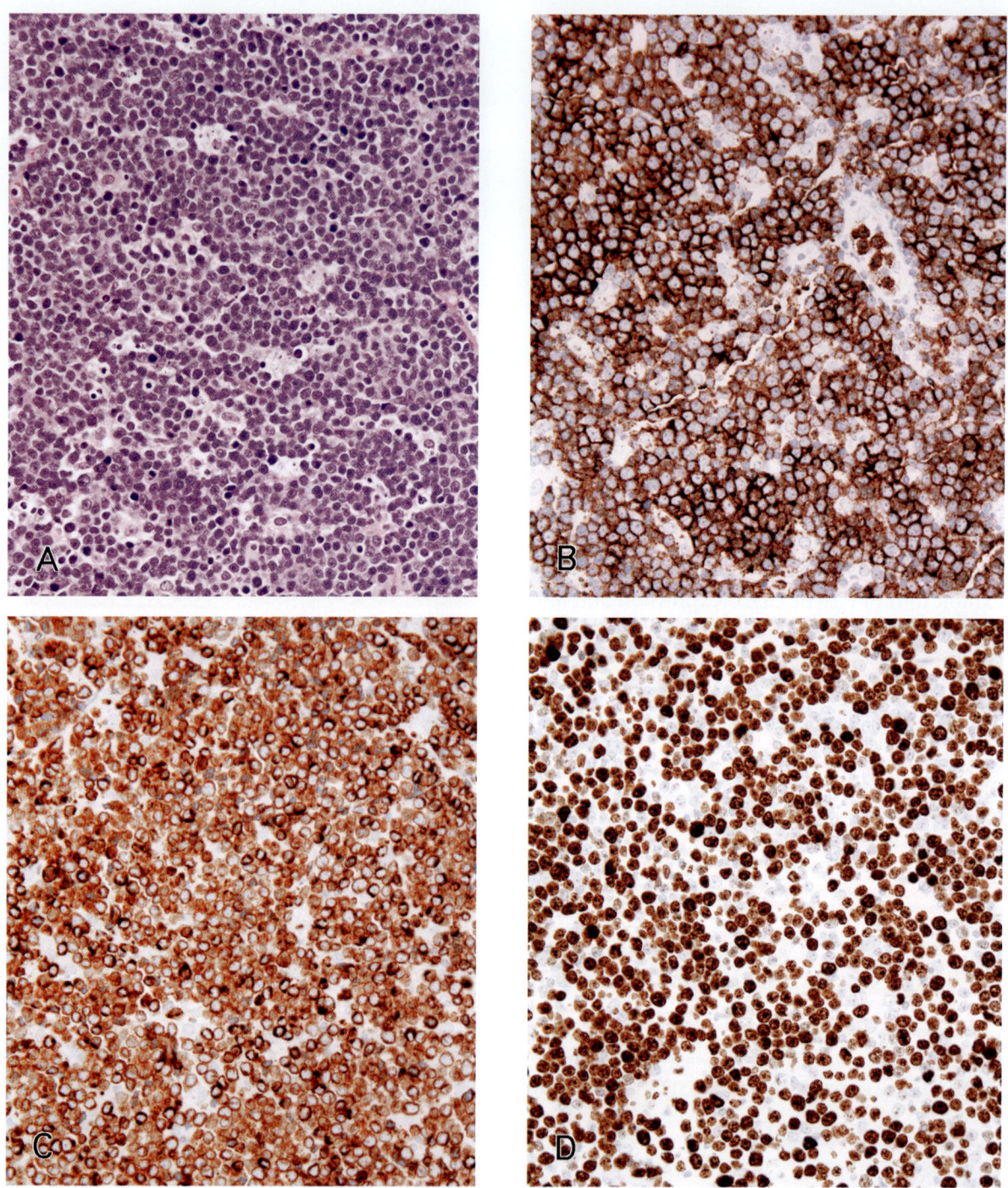

Figure 26-4

HIGH-GRADE B-CELL LYMPHOMA, NOT OTHERWISE SPECIFIED, INVOLVING LYMPH NODE

A: This tumor closely resembles Burkitt lymphoma since the neoplastic cells are monotonous, are intermediate in size, and a starry sky pattern is well developed (H&E stain).

B–D: Immunohistochemical analysis showed that the neoplastic cells are positive for CD10 (B), CD20 (not shown), BCL2 (C), and BCL6 (not shown), and virtually all cells are positive for Ki-67 (D). Strong expression of BCL2, as shown in this tumor, is atypical for Burkitt lymphoma and supports the diagnosis of HGBL-NOS. This tumor was shown to carry *MYC* rearrangement by fluorescence in situ hybridization (FISH) (B–D: immunohistochemistry with hematoxylin counterstain).

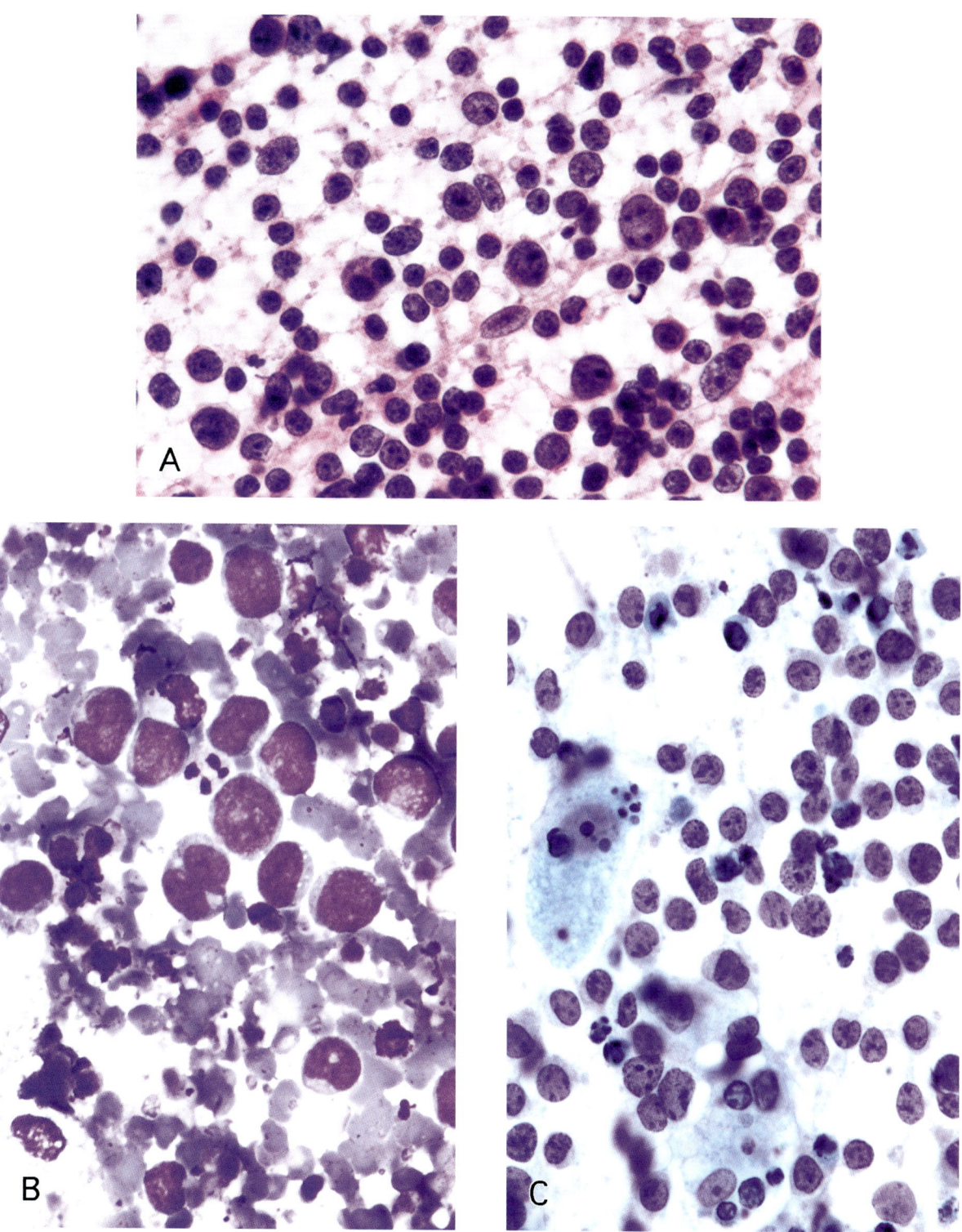

Figure 26-5

HIGH-GRADE B-CELL LYMPHOMA, NOT OTHERWISE SPECIFIED, INVOLVING LYMPH NODE

Touch imprints (A) and aspirate smears (B,C) show a range of cell sizes, including intermediately sized and larger cells (A: H&E stain; B: Diff-Quik stain; C: Papanicolaou stain).

to 40 percent of cases (11). Cases with *MYC* translocations can be divided into three groups: *MYC-IGH* (or light chain gene) translocations (cytogenetically simple or complex) and associated with the highest levels of MYC expression, *MYC* translocated with non-IG partners (usually cytogenetically complex), and double-hit lymphomas characterized by rearrangement of *MYC* and another oncogene (see below) (14). Cases in the first two groups, in other words *MYC* translocation alone, have been referred to in the literature as *single-hit lymphomas*. These tumors are often associated with high p53 expression (and presumably associated *TP53* abnormalities) (13).

Next-generation sequencing has been performed on a small number of HGBL-NOS cases to date. Momose et al. (15) assessed a series of 108 aggressive B-cell lymphomas for mutations in 10 genes, including 4 genes associated with BL (*ID3*, *TCF3*, *CCND3*, and *MYC*) and 6 genes associated with DLBCL (*BCL2*, *EZH2*, *CREBBP*, *EP300*, *MEF2B*, and *SGK1*). These authors showed that cases of HGBL-NOS had a mutational profile intermediate between BL and DLBCL. Specifically, mutations occurred in either *ID3* or *TCF3*, 67 percent; *BCL2*, 58 percent, *CCND3*, 29 percent; *CREBBP/EP300*, 29 percent; and *EZH2*, 12 percent. *MEF2B* and *SGK1* were rarely mutated in HGBL-NOS. *MYC* mutations were associated with *MYC* translocation.

As cases of HGBL-NOS are mature B-cell neoplasms, most carry monoclonal immunoglobulin gene rearrangements and the T-cell receptor genes are in the germline configuration. Low-level amplification of the *IGH* locus also has been shown by FISH in over half of HGBL-NOS cases (3). A small subset of cases has extra copies or true amplification of *MYC*, *BCL2*, and/or *BCL6*, as shown by FISH analysis (11).

Double-Hit Lymphomas

Thirty to 40 percent of the neoplasms that were included in the B-cell lymphomas, unclassifiable category as defined in the 2008 WHO classification fulfill criteria for double-hit lymphomas (11). These neoplasms are defined as having a translocation involving *MYC* as well as one or more translocations involving other oncogenes, such as *BCL2*, *BCL6*, or rarely *BCL3* (1). Triple-hit lymphomas with translocations

involving *MYC*, *BCL2*, and *BCL6* also have been reported. As stated above, these neoplasms are now designated as high-grade B-cell lymphoma with *MYC* and *BCL2* and/or *BCL6* rearrangements (see chapter 27).

DIFFERENTIAL DIAGNOSIS

Diffuse Large B-Cell Lymphoma. An obvious case of DLBCL is composed of large cells, clearly larger than the size of a benign histiocyte nucleus, with centroblastic or, less commonly, immunoblastic features. The proliferation (Ki-67) rate is usually in the range of 50 to 80 percent and a starry sky pattern is usually absent. Some cases are positive for CD10 and BCL6, and BCL2 is expressed in 60 to 70 percent of cases. *MYC* translocation occurs in 10 to 15 percent of DLBCL cases and is associated with a poorer prognosis (1,2,16,18).

Unlike DLBCL, HGBL-NOS is composed of a mixture of intermediate-sized and large cells with a starry sky pattern and a high proliferation rate. Tumors that resemble DLBCL morphologically but are associated with double-hit cytogenetics are specified in the revised WHO classification as double-hit lymphoma or high-grade B-cell lymphoma with *MYC* and *BCL2* and/or *BCL6* rearrangement (see chapter 27).

Burkitt Lymphoma. A typical case of BL is composed of intermediate-sized cells, about the size of a benign histiocyte nucleus, with a prominent starry sky pattern, a monotonous cell population, and a high (over 95 percent) proliferation rate. BL cases are typically CD10(+), BCL6(+), and BCL2(-), and carry *MYC* translocations with IG gene partners.

HGBL-NOS differs from BL in one of two ways. One subset shows a much greater range of cell sizes and more pleomorphism in the neoplastic cell population. The second subset of cases closely resembles BL, but is strongly BCL2 positive. In the latter subset, some cases have a proliferation rate below 90 percent, which is unusual in BL. The karyotype of HGBL-NOS cases is generally more complex than BL (10,11).

Other Aggressive B-Cell Lymphomas. The differential diagnosis of HGBL-NOS includes other B-cell neoplasms that show high-grade features and morphologic overlap with HGBL-NOS. These include DLBCL arising in a patient with chronic lymphocytic leukemia/small lymphocytic lymphoma (CLL/SLL), so-called Richter syndrome;

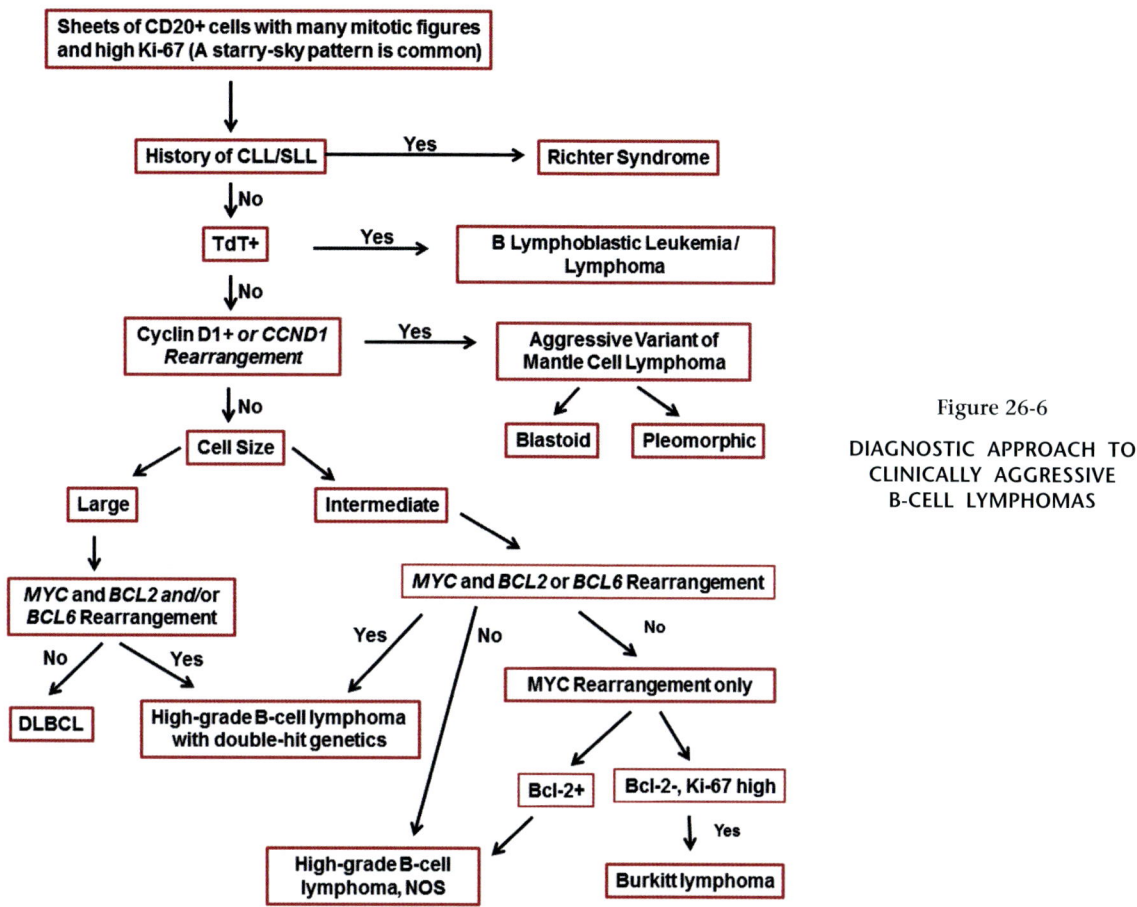

Figure 26-6

DIAGNOSTIC APPROACH TO
CLINICALLY AGGRESSIVE
B-CELL LYMPHOMAS

aggressive variants of mantle cell lymphoma and B-lymphoblastic lymphoma/leukemia. As discussed above, double-hit lymphomas with *MYC* and *BCL2* and/or *BCL6* rearrangements also need to be distinguished from HGBL-NOS. An algorithm is shown in figure 26-6 that provides guidance in this differential diagnosis.

TREATMENT AND PROGNOSIS

At the present time, there is no consensus regarding the best therapy for patients with HGBL-NOS. Neither standard frontline therapy for DLBCL, i.e., rituximab, cyclophosphamide, doxorubicin, vincristine, and prednisone (R-CHOP) nor more intensive regimens that

are often used for patients with BL or acute lymphoblastic leukemia have been curative (6,11,14,16). There may be a role for autologous stem cell transplantation although this is not well established. The median survival period of patients with HGBL-NOS is usually less than 2 years.

Patients who have low-stage disease or a low IPI score have had a better survival rate in some studies (16). Patients with HGBL-NOS associated with *MYC* translocation alone, i.e., single-hit lymphoma, appear to have a poor prognosis, similar to that of patients with double-hit lymphomas although *TP53* mutations also may be involved as a "second hit" in this context (13).

REFERENCES

1. Aukema SM, Siebert R, Schuuring E, et al. Double hit B-cell lymphomas. Blood 2011;117:2319-2331.

2. Barrans S, Crouch S, Smith A, et al. Rearrangement of MYC is associated with poor prognosis in patients with diffuse large B-cell lymphoma treated in the era of rituximab. J Clin Oncol 2010;28:3360-3365.

3. Bellone M, Zaslav AL, Ahmed T, Lee HL2, Ma Y1, Hu Y. IGH amplification in patients with B cell lymphoma unclassifiable, with features intermediate between diffuse large B cell lymphoma and Burkitt's lymphoma. Biomarker Research 2014;2:9

4. Boerma EG, Siebert R, Kluin PM, Baudis M. Translocations involving 8q24 in Burkitt lymphoma and other malignant lymphomas: a historical review of cytogenetics in light of today's knowledge. Leukemia 2009;23:225-234.

5. Burgesser MV, Gualco G, Diller A, Natkunam Y, Bacchi CE. Clinicopathological features of aggressive B-cell lymphomas including B-cell lymphoma, unclassifiable, with features intermediate between diffuse large B-cell and Burkitt lymphomas: a study of 44 patients from Argentina. Ann Diagn Pathol 2013;17:250-255.

6. Carbone A, Gloghini A, Aiello A, Testi A, Cabras A. B-cell lymphomas with features intermediate between distinct pathologic entities. From pathogenesis to pathology. Hum Pathol 2010;41:621-631.

7. Cook JR, Goldman B, Tubbs RR, et al. Clinical significance of MYC expression and/or "high-grade" morphology in non-Burkitt, diffuse aggressive B-cell lymphomas. A SWOC S9704 correlative study. Am J Surg Pathol 2014;38:494-501.

8. Dave SS, Fu K, Wright GW, et al. Molecular diagnosis of Burkitt's lymphoma. N Engl J Med 2006;354:2431-2442.

9. Elkins CT, Wakely PE. Cytopathology of "double hit" non-Hodgin lymphoma. Cancer Cytopathology 2011;119:263-271.

10. Hummel M, Bentink S, Berger H, et al. A biologic definition of Burkitt's lymphoma from transcriptional and genomic profiling. N Engl J Med 2006;354:2419-2430.

11. Kluin PM, Harris NL, Stein H, et al. B-cell lymphoma, unclassifiable, with features intermediate between diffuse large B-cell lymphoma and Burkitt lymphoma. In: Swerdlow SH, Campo E, Harris NL, Jaffe ES, Pileria SA, Stein H, Thiele J, Vardiman JW, eds. WHO Classification of tumours of haematpoietic and lymphoid tissues, 4th ed. Lyon: IARC Press; 2008:265-266.

12. Li S, Lin P, Fayad LE, et al. B-cell lymphomas with MYC/8q24 rearrangements and IGH@ BCL2/t(14;18)(q32;q21): an aggressive disease with heterogeneous histology, a germinal center cell immunophenotype, and poor outcome. Mod Pathol 2012;25:145-156.

13. Li S, Weiss VL, Wang XJ, et al. High-grade B-cell lymphoma with MYC rearrangement and without BCL2 and BCL6 rearrangements is associated with high p53 expression and a poor prognosis. Am J Surg Pathol 2016;40:253-261.

14. Lin P, Dickason TJ, Fayad LE, et al. Prognostic value of MYC rearrangement in cases of B-cell lymphoma, unclassifiable, with features intermediate between diffuse large B-cell lymphoma and Burkitt lymphoma. Cancer 2012;118:1566-1573.

15. Momose S, Weissbach S, Pischimarov J, et al. The diagnostic gray zone between Burkitt lymphoma and diffuse large B-cell lymphoma is also a gray zone of the mutational spectrum. Leukemia 2015;29:1789-1791.

16. Perry AM, Crockett D, Dave BJ, et al. B-cell lymphoma, unclassifiable, with features intermediate between diffuse large B-cell lymphoma and Burkitt lymphoma: study of 39 cases. Br J Hematol 2013;162:40-49.

17. Swerdlow SH, Campo E, Pileri SA, et al. The 2016 revision of the World Health Organization (WHO) classification of lymphoid neoplasms. Blood 2016;127:2375-2390.

18. Tzankov A, Xu-Monette ZY, Gerhard M, et al. Rearrangements of MYC gene facilitate risk stratification in diffuse large B-cell lymphoma patients treated with rituximab-CHOP. Mod Pathol 2014;27:958-971.

19. Wu D, Wood BL, Dorer R, Fromm JR. "Double-hit" mature B-cell lymphomas show a common immunophenotype by flow cytometry that includes decreased CD20 expression. Am J Clin Pathol 2010;134:258-265.

27 DOUBLE-HIT LYMPHOMAS

GENERAL FEATURES

Double-hit lymphoma (DHL) is a neoplasm of B-cell lineage that is characterized by a translocation involving *MYC* at chromosome 8q24, with a second translocation involving another oncogene, most often *BCL2*, less often *BCL6*, and rarely other oncogenes such as *BCL3*. *CCND1-IGH*/t(11;14)(q13;q32) also can occur with a *MYC* translocation and theoretically fits within the conceptual framework of DHL. Rare tumors have been reported with four translocations involving *MYC, BCL2, BCL6*, and *CCND1* (3). In the revised World Health Organization (WHO) classification, tumors with *CCND1* rearrangements are usually designated as aggressive (either pleomorphic or blastoid) variants of mantle cell lymphoma (28b).

The 2008 WHO classification recognized DHL, but did not specify this neoplasm as a distinctive entity (15). Instead, cases of DHL were placed in the category of B-cell lymphoma, unclassifiable (BLCU), with features intermediate between diffuse large B-cell lymphoma (DLBCL) and Burkitt lymphoma (BL). In the revised WHO classification, DHL cases are included in a category designated as high-grade B-cell lymphoma (HGBL), which will replace the designation BCLU (28b). Cases of HGBL will be further specified as having *MYC* rearrangement and *BCL2* and/or *BCL6* rearrangement (i.e., DHL).

Although cases of DHL have been described over the past 20 years, the concept of DHL became more widely accepted following the review by Aukema et al. published in 2011 (2). The designation DHL, however, is somewhat vague and allows for marked genetic heterogeneity. As specific genetic findings in DHL will likely be shown to be important for therapy or prognosis in the future, it seems prudent to further designate cases of DHL according to their genetic abnormalities (16,20).

DHLs are rare, representing 1 percent of all non-Hodgkin lymphomas and approximately 5 to 10 percent of all cases of DLBCL (1,12,20,23). DHLs represent a higher percentage of cases of DLBCL with aggressive morphologic features, such as a starry sky pattern or high proliferation rate, and DHLs represent 30 to 40 percent of cases previously designated as BCLU in the 2008 WHO classification (15). The most common type of DHL combines *MYC* and *BCL2* translocations (65 percent of all cases) (1,12,16,18). Tumors with translocations involving *MYC, BCL2*, and *BCL6*, so-called *triple-hit lymphomas*, represent about 20 percent of all cases, and the combination of *MYC* and *BCL6* is least common, in about 15 percent of all cases (16).

CLINICAL FEATURES

Clinical data are most abundant for patients with *MYC/BCL2* DHL. These tumors occur predominantly in adults with a wide age range, from young adults to the very elderly, with a median age in the seventh decade (12,18,23–25). The frequency of DHL increases with age and these tumors are rare in children. There is a male predominance, and about 20 percent of patients with *MYC/BCL2* DHL have a history of concurrent follicular lymphoma (18). Patients with *MYC/BCL2* DHL often present with poor performance status and commonly have elevated serum levels of lactate dehydrogenase (LDH) and beta-2-microglobulin. Patients present with lymphadenopathy, but extranodal sites of disease are also common (18,23,24,25). Most patients have advanced (III/IV) stage disease and a high International Prognostic Index (IPI) score (12,18,23,24). Bone marrow involvement is common and the central nervous system is involved in 10 to 20 percent of patients (12,23,25). Triple-hit lymphomas involving *MYC, BCL2*, and *BCL6* appear to behave similarly to *MYC/BCL2* DHL (16,31).

Patients with *MYC/BCL6* DHL are similarly older adults with a wide age range (17,27,29). Women are more frequently affected and the male to female ratio is close to 1. Most patients

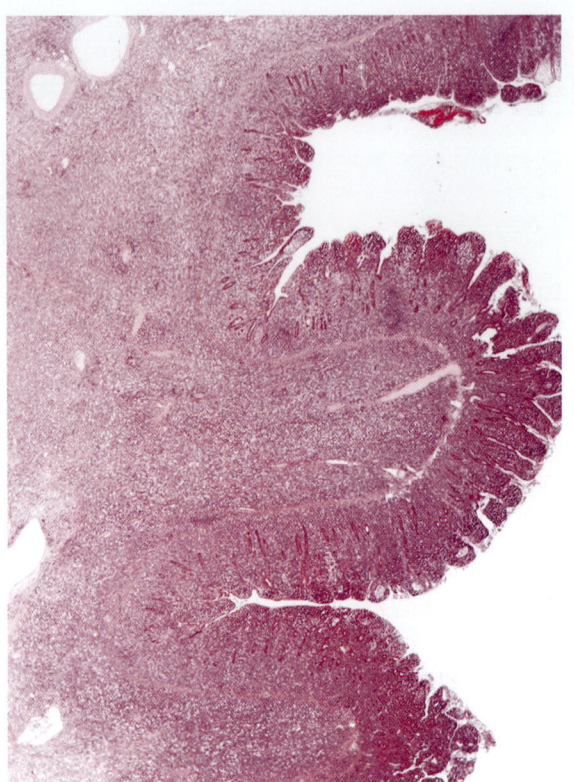
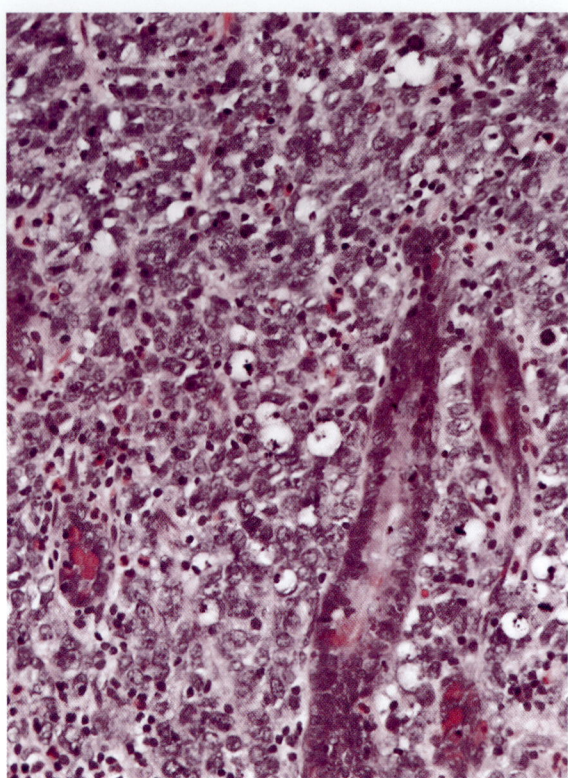

Figure 27-1

DOUBLE-HIT LYMPHOMA WITH *MYC* AND *BCL2* REARRANGEMENTS INVOLVING GASTROINTESTINAL TRACT

The morphologic features of this neoplasm were similar to those of diffuse large B-cell lymphoma (DLBCL).

Left: The neoplasm extensively and diffusely replaces the lamina propria of the small intestine. A starry sky pattern can be appreciated.

Right: The neoplastic cells are generally large with a high rate of apoptosis (left, right: hematoxylin and eosin [H&E] stain).

present with de novo disease. Extranodal presentations appear to be more common in this group of patients and one study suggested that liver involvement is more common (29). In most studies, patients with *MYC/BCL6* DHL have a high IPI score, high-stage disease, an aggressive clinical course, and poor survival, similar to patients with *MYC/BCL2* DHL (17,27,29). In one study, however, patients with *MYC/BCL6* DHL had a better prognosis than patients with *MYC/BCL2* DHL (34). In the latter study, patients with triple hit lymphoma were specifically excluded from analysis, a limitation of other studies.

Few cases of triple-hit lymphoma have been reported to date, mostly included in larger studies of DHL or in small case series. In a review of the literature in 2015 Wang et al. (31) identified 40 cases. Triple-hit lymphomas arise in older adults, with a median age in the seventh decade

(range, 50 to 82 years) (3,31). The male to female ratio is over 2 to 1. Some patients have a history of follicular lymphoma. Bone marrow involvement is common. Many patients have refractory disease and median survival is less than 1 year (31). Bacher et al. (3) described two patients with four genetic "hits" involving *MYC*, *BCL2*, *BCL6*, and *CCND1*; both patients died shortly after diagnosis.

HISTOLOGIC FINDINGS

MYC/BCL2 Double-Hit Lymphoma

MYC/BCL2 DHLs exhibit a spectrum of histologic findings (figs. 27-1–27-4) (12,13,18,24). Most cases have a diffuse growth pattern, usually with a starry sky appearance. A high apoptotic rate or areas of coagulative necrosis are common (fig. 27-3). Mitotic figures are usually easily identified.

The cellular composition of these tumors is variable. Many *MYC/BCL2* DHL cases resemble DLBCL (fig. 27-1). About 40 to 50 percent of cases are composed of intermediate-sized and larger cells with pleomorphism, designated in the 2016 revised WHO classification as HGBL (fig. 27-2) (12,15,18). A smaller subset of *MYC/BCL2* DHL closely mimics BL morphologically, but strongly expresses *BCL2* (precluding the diagnosis of BL) (figs. 27-2, 27-3).

There are other rare histologic patterns that occur in cases of *MYC/BCL2* DHL. Some tumors are composed of small blastoid cells resembling small centroblasts or lymphoblasts, but are TdT negative (13). Uncommonly, DHL morphologically resembles follicular lymphoma, usually grade 3B, but rarely also low-grade follicular lymphoma (18,21a). Rarely, *MYC/BCL2* DHL cases are composed of blastic cells that are TdT-positive and resemble B-lymphoblastic lymphoma (14,21). One highly unusual case that met the histologic criteria for composite lymphoma has been reported, with distinct components that resembled DLBCL and B-lymphoblastic lymphoma (22).

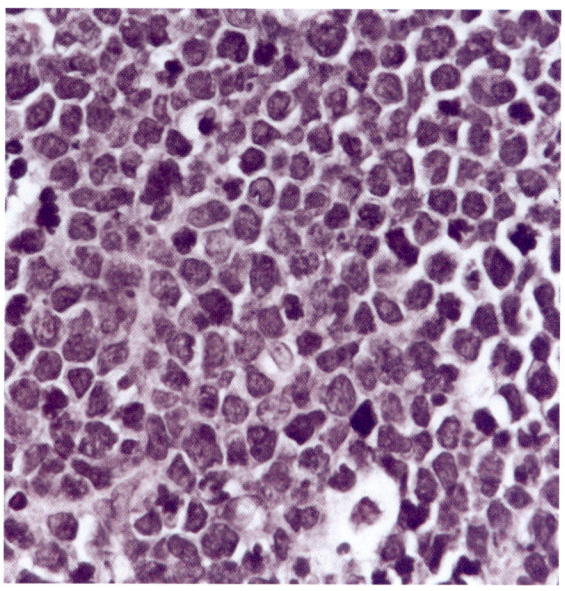

Figure 27-2

DOUBLE-HIT LYMPHOMA WITH *MYC* AND *BCL2* REARRANGEMENTS INVOLVING LYMPH NODE

The patient had a history of follicular lymphoma. The tumor has the morphologic features of a high-grade B-cell lymphoma (HGBL) (H&E stain).

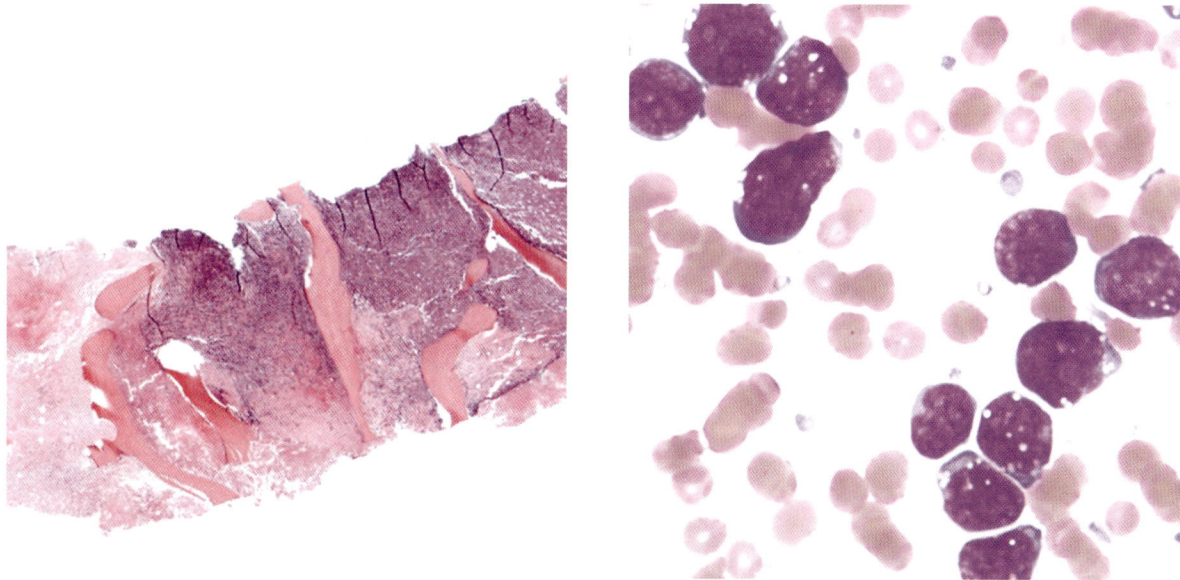

Figure 27-3

DOUBLE-HIT LYMPHOMA WITH *MYC* AND *BCL2* REARRANGEMENTS INVOLVING BONE MARROW

Left: The bone marrow biopsy specimen shows tumor with extensive coagulative necrosis (left of field).

Right: The bone marrow aspirate smear shows intermediately sized cells with multiple nucleoli and cytoplasmic vacuoles (left: H&E stain; right: Wright-Giemsa stain).

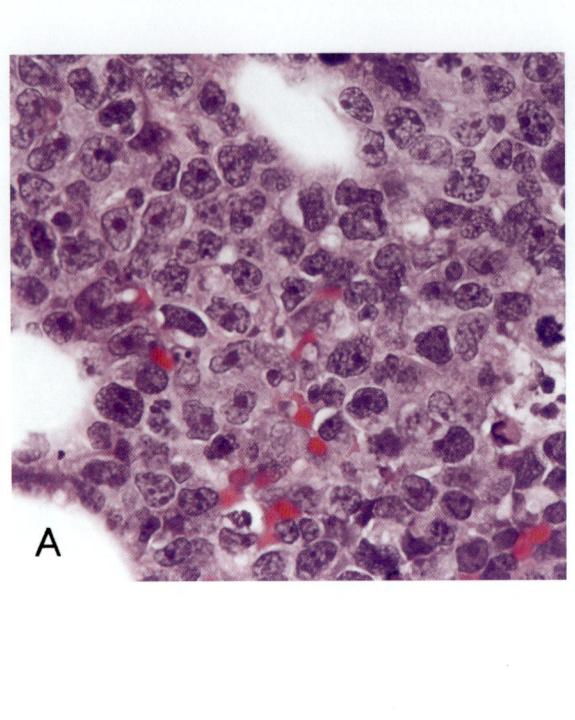

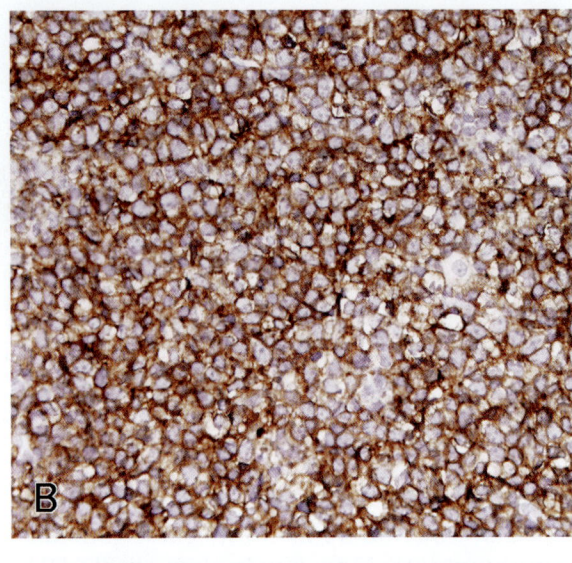

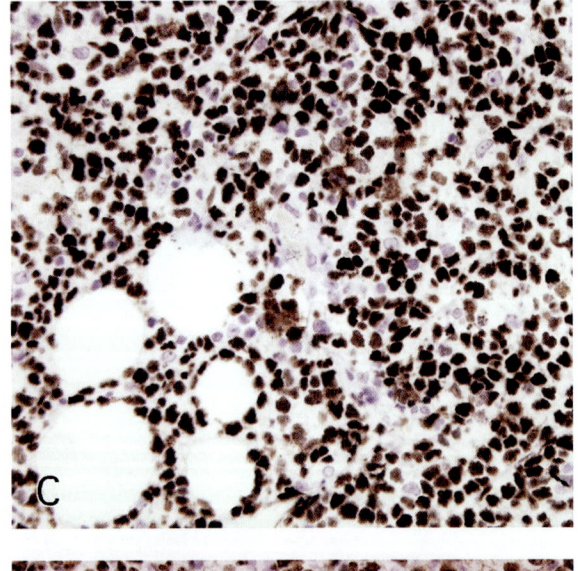

Figure 27-4

DOUBLE-HIT LYMPHOMA WITH *MYC* AND *BCL2* REARRANGEMENTS INVOLVING SOFT TISSUE

The neoplasm had the morphologic features of DLBCL.

A: The neoplastic cells are large, with cytologic features of immunoblasts and centroblasts (H&E stain).

B,C: Immunohistochemical analysis shows a germinal center immunophenotype positive for CD10 (B) and BCL6 (C).

D,E: The tumor is also positive for BCL2 (D) and has many proliferating (Ki-67-positive) cells (E) (B–E, immunohistochemistry with hematoxylin counterstain).

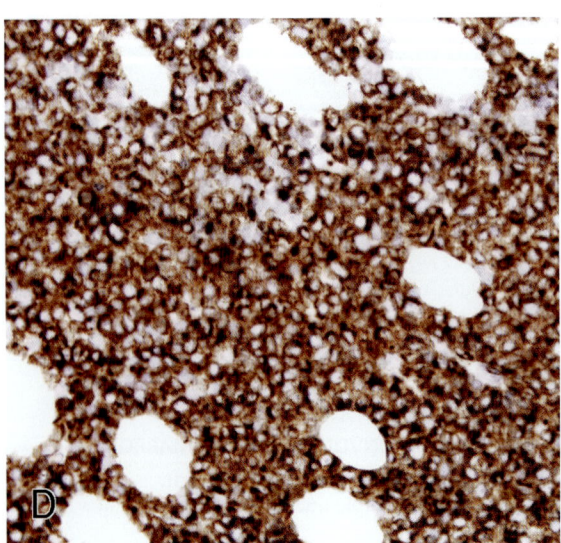

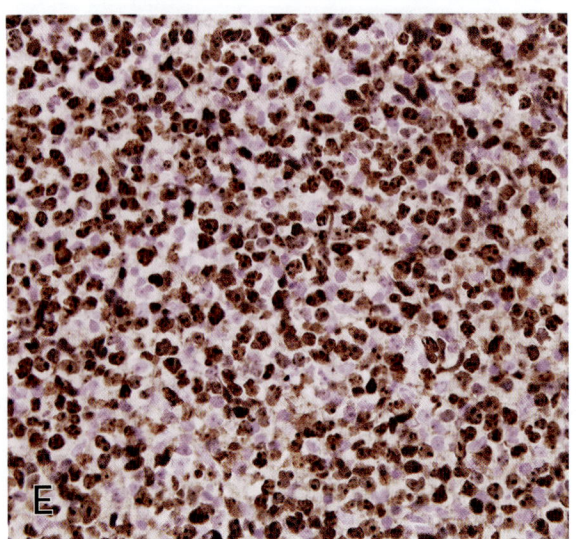

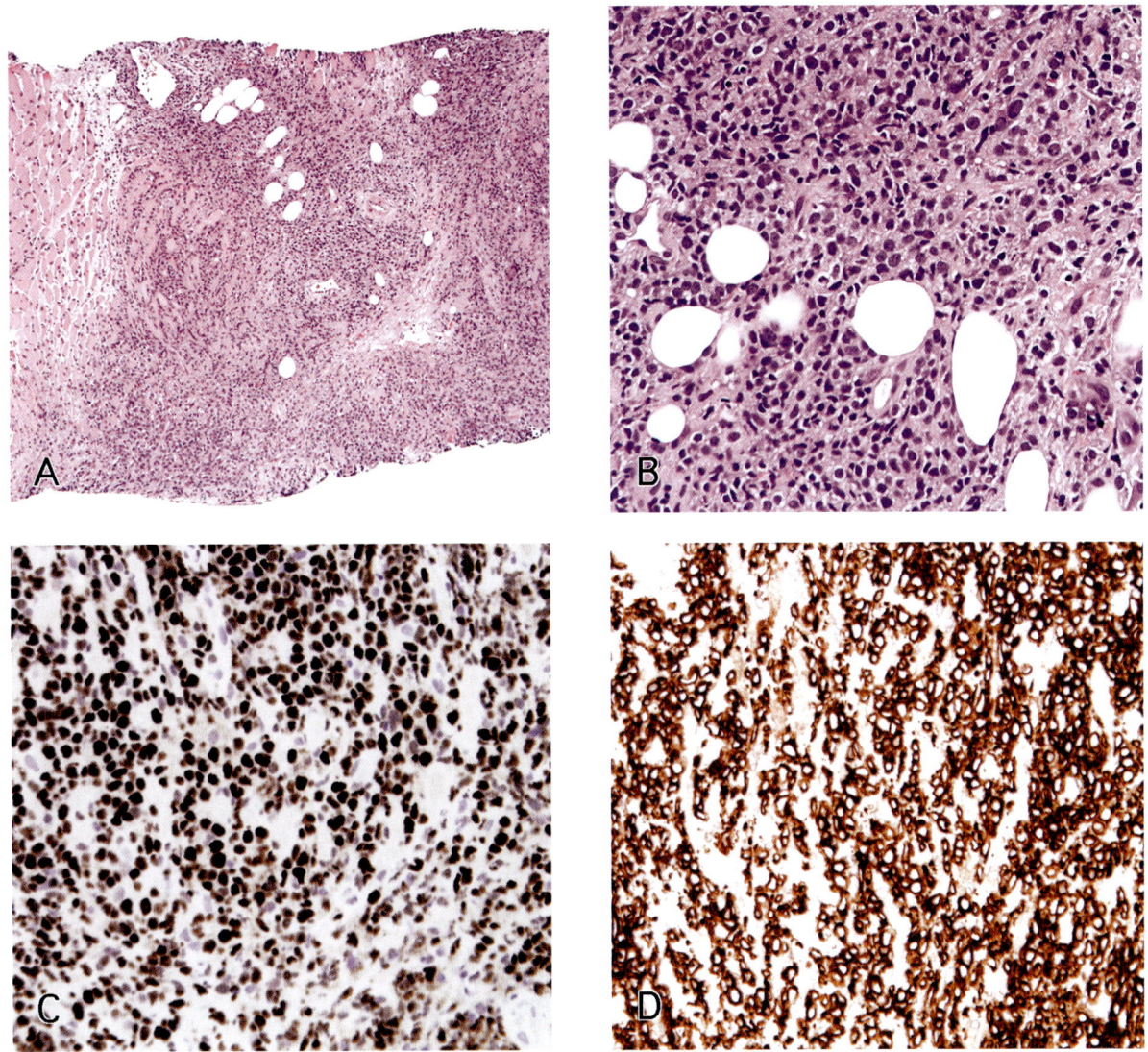

Figure 27-5

DOUBLE-HIT LYMPHOMA WITH *MYC* AND *BCL6* REARRANGEMENTS WITH MORPHOLOGIC FEATURES OF DLBCL

A: The neoplasm has a diffuse pattern and involves skeletal muscle (A,B: H&E stain).

B: Most of the neoplastic cells are large.

C,D: The neoplastic cells are strongly positive for BCL6 (C) and BCL2 (D) (C,D: immunohistochemistry with hematoxylin counterstain).

MYC/BCL6 Double-Hit Lymphoma

This subset of DHL is less well described. In four clinicopathologic studies, 39 cases have been reported (17,27,29,34). In addition, Pillai et al. (27) reviewed 13 cases in the Mitleman database. The most common histologic types are DLBCL and HGBL (fig. 27-5) with a subset designated as BL (27,29). A starry sky pattern is very common, and mitotic figures and apoptosis are abundant. Up to 25 percent of *MYC/BCL6* DHLs exhibited plasmacytic differentiation in one study (27).

MYC/BCL2/BCL6 Triple-Hit Lymphoma

In general, the morphologic findings of triple-hit lymphomas are less well characterized in the literature. Wang et al. (31) reported 11

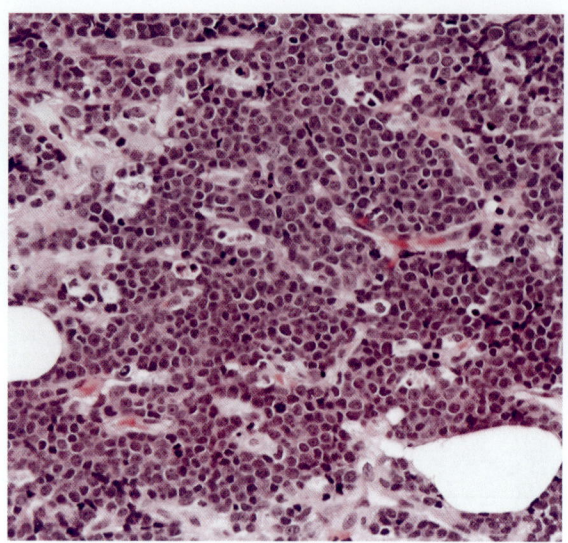

Figure 27-6

TRIPLE-HIT LYMPHOMA WITH REARRANGEMENTS OF *MYC*, *BCL2*, AND *BCL6*

The morphologic features of BCLU are seen (H&E stain).

cases: 5 (45 percent) were classified as BCLU (using 2008 WHO terminology) (fig. 27-6); 4 (36 percent) were DLBCL; 1 (9 percent) was DLBCL associated with concurrent follicular lymphoma; and 1 (9 percent) was morphologically low-grade follicular lymphoma (few centroblasts) that had a high mitotic rate. A starry sky pattern can be prominent, particularly in cases with BCLU morphologic features (31).

Bone Marrow

Some patients with *MYC/BCL2* DHL or *MYC/BCL6* DHL present with a leukemic picture and a packed bone marrow as well as low- or intermediate-level lymphocytosis in the peripheral blood. The lymphoma cells in these cases are intermediate or large in size and often have cytoplasmic vacuoles that can mimic BL cells (figs. 27-7, 27-8).

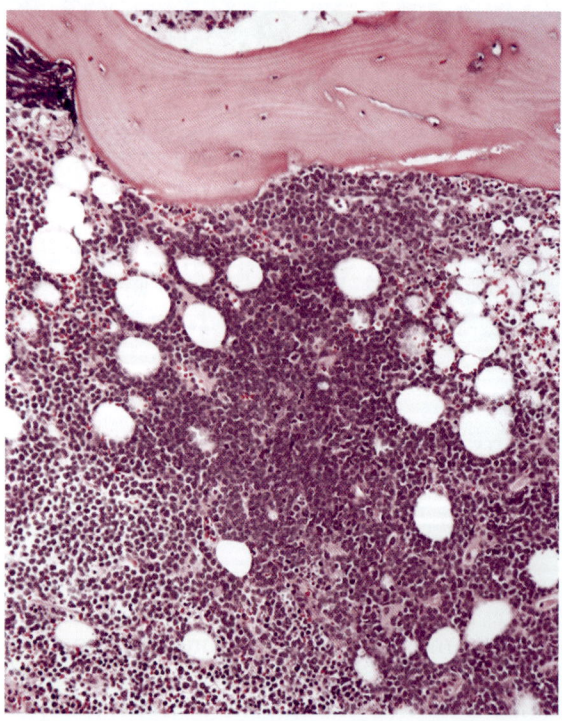
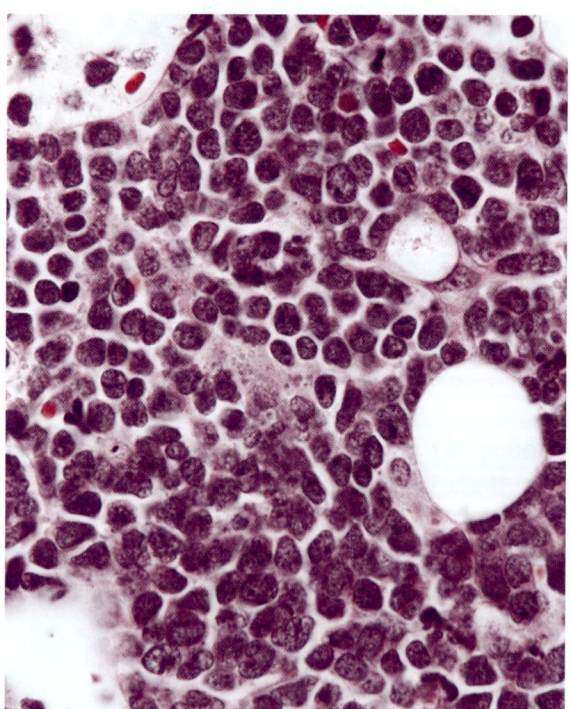

Figure 27-7

TRIPLE-HIT LYMPHOMA WITH REARRANGEMENTS OF *MYC*, *BCL2*, AND *BCL6*

The morphologic features are similar to those of acute lymphoblastic leukemia but the neoplastic cells expressed surface immunoglobulin and were negative for TdT.

Left: The neoplasm extensively replaces the medullary space.

Right: The neoplastic cells are small to intermediate size, with immature chromatin (left, right: H&E stain).

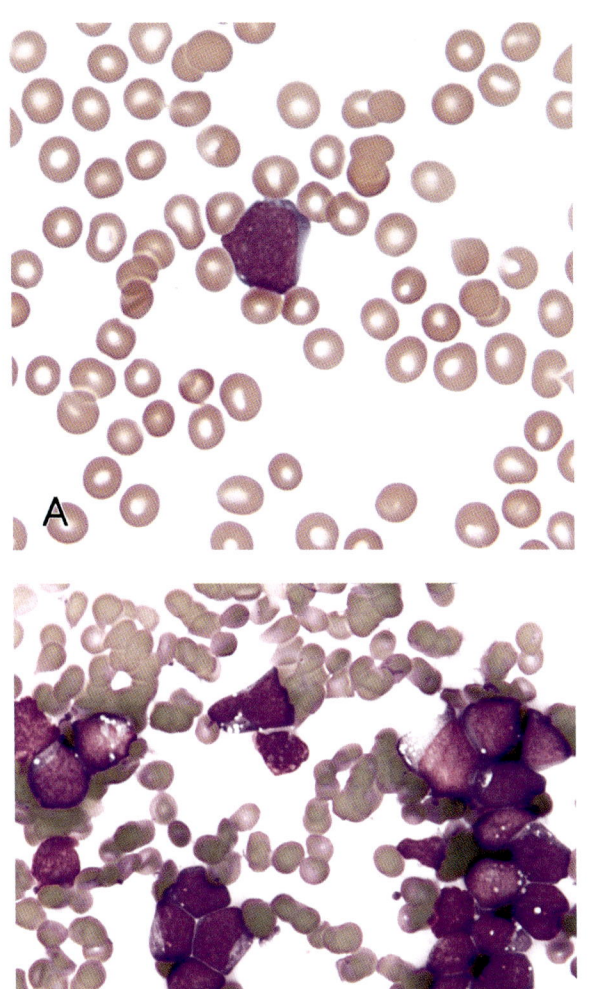

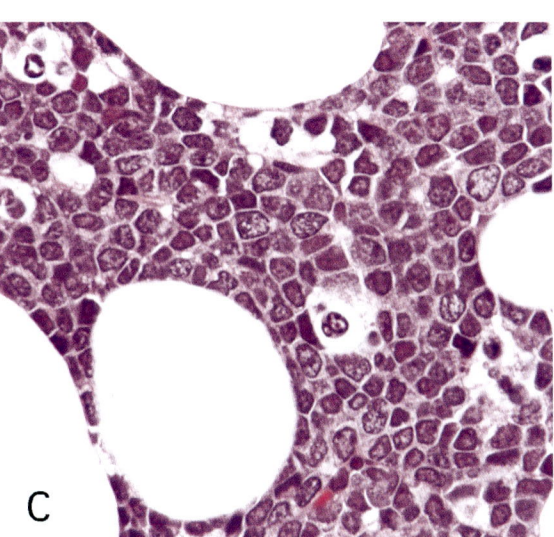

Figure 27-8

DOUBLE-HIT LYMPHOMA WITH *MYC* AND *BCL6* REARRANGEMENTS INVOLVING BONE MARROW

This neoplasm mimicked Burkitt lymphoma but was BCL2 positive and classified as HGBL.

A: A single large neoplastic cell within a peripheral blood smear is shown (A,B: Wright-Giemsa stain).

B: The neoplastic cells in the bone marrow aspirate smear are intermediate-sized, with many cytoplasmic vacuoles.

C: High-power magnification shows bone marrow extensively involved by lymphoma (H&E stain).

CYTOLOGIC FINDINGS

Fine-needle aspiration (FNA) specimens and touch imprints of DHL cases show a spectrum of findings (fig. 27-9). The neoplastic cells often show a mixture of intermediate-sized and larger cells, but either cell type can predominate. The cells are usually oval to round, but in one study some cases had cleaved nuclei (5). Tingible body macrophages, apoptotic cells, mitotic figures, and cytoplasmic vacuoles are common.

As has been emphasized by others, it is difficult to establish the diagnosis of DHL on the basis of cytologic findings alone. When FNA is used, it is helpful to prepare a cell block because this specimen is convenient for immunohisto-

chemistry and in situ hybridization analysis (5). Performing multiple aspirates to obtain fresh cells for flow cytometry immunophenotyping or conventional cytogenetic analysis is helpful

IMMUNOPHENOTYPIC FINDINGS

DHLs of either *MYC/BCL2* or *MYC/BCL6* type are B-cell tumors that express pan-B-cell antigens. Almost all cases of *MYC/BCL2* DHL have a germinal center B-cell (GCB) immunophenotype, positive for CD10 (fig. 27-4B) and BCL6 (fig. 27-4C) (12,18,20). Most cases of *MYC/BCL2* DHL also express BCL2 (fig. 27-4D); a few tumors negative for BCL2 have mutations that preclude reactivity with commonly used monoclonal antibodies, but are reactive with other, more recently developed

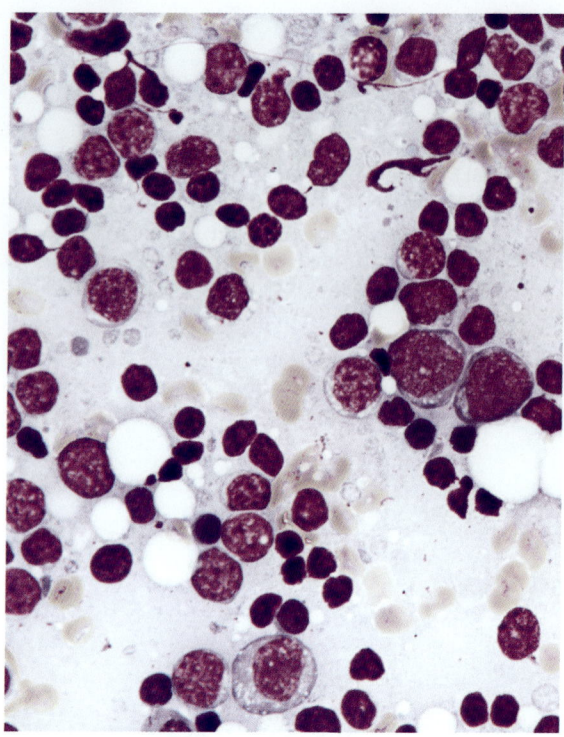

Figure 27-9

DOUBLE-HIT LYMPHOMA WITH *MYC* AND *BCL2* REARRANGEMENTS

This touch imprint shows a range of cell sizes, including intermediate-sized and large cells (Wright-Giemsa stain).

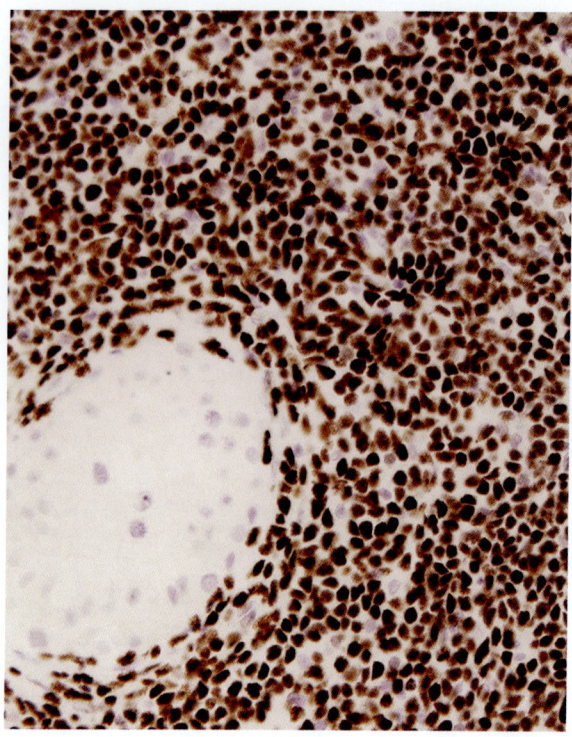

Figure 27-10

DOUBLE-HIT LYMPHOMA WITH *MYC* AND *BCL2* REARRANGEMENTS INVOLVING THE TESTIS

The neoplastic cells are strongly positive for MYC (immunohistochemistry with hematoxylin counterstain).

anti-BCL2 antibodies (12). *MYC/BCL2* DHL cases are usually negative for MUM1/IRF4 and FOXP1.

Compared with *MYC/BCL2* DHL, cases of *MYC/BCL6* DHL less often have a GCB immunophenotype (50 to 60 percent of cases) (17,27,29). These tumors are less often positive for CD10 (60 percent) and BCL6 (60 percent) (fig. 27-8C), more frequently express IRF4/MUM1 (75 percent), and are often BCL2 positive. The proliferation (Ki-67) rate in these tumors is usually very high, with a median of over 95 percent, in one study (27). CD23 can be weakly expressed in *MYC/BCL6* DHL. Other findings in these tumors are similar to those in *MYC/BCL2* DHLs.

MYC/BCL2/BCL6 triple-hit lymphomas are usually positive for CD20, but expression can be dim in a subset of tumors. Most have a GCB immunophenotype using various immunohistochemical algorithms. In one study, all tumors were positive for CD10, BCL2, and FOXP1 (31). BCL6 was positive in about 75 percent of tumors, and MUM1/IRF4 was positive in about half.

In both types of DHL and in triple-hit lymphomas, Ki-67 expression is high, with a range from 70 to over 99 percent, and tumors that resemble BCLU have the highest proliferation rate (12,18,31). MYC (fig. 27-10) is also highly expressed in DHLs (1,25). Double-hit and triple-hit lymphomas are negative for T-cell antigens, including CD5, and rarely show evidence of Epstein-Barr virus (EBV) infection.

Flow cytometry immunophenotypic analysis of *MYC/BCL2* and *MYC/BCL6* DHLs has shown that the neoplastic cells often show diminished expression of surface light chain and B-cell antigens, such as CD19, CD20, and CD22, compared with normal resting B cells (28,33). In one study, 9 of 19 (47 percent) cases were negative for surface light chain, and CD19 and CD20 as well as CD45 were underexpressed in 40 to 50 percent of cases (28). BCL2 levels are lower in *MYC/BCL6* DHL cases (28). The combination of decreased CD19 and CD20 in a CD10-positive high-grade B-cell lymphoma is highly suggestive of *MYC/BCL2* DHL (33).

Double-Positive or Double-Expressor Lymphoma

Double-positive or double-expressor lymphomas, henceforth abbreviated as DPL, overexpress MYC and BCL2, as assessed by immunohistochemistry. A number of studies have shown that patients with *MYC/BCL2* DPL have an aggressive clinical course and poor prognosis (9,10,30). To date, little data are available for patients with *MYC/BCL6* DPL and therefore this group is not further discussed.

Approximately 30 percent of DLBCLs overexpress MYC and BCL2 (9,10). This frequency is much higher than is true for classically defined DHL in DLBCL. In most studies, immunohistochemical cutoffs for MYC and BCL2 are used, often 40 or 50 percent and 60 or 70 percent positive cells, respectively. *MYC/BCL2* DPLs have either a GCB or activated/non-GCB immunophenotype, but the latter is more common. In one study, Hu et al. (10) suggested that MYC and BCL2 double overexpression is a more important prognostic factor than cell of origin classification (GCB versus non-GCB). This suggestion is currently controversial.

Classic *MYC/BCL2* DHL and *MYC/BCL2* DPL, although biologically related, are not prognostically equivalent, and patients with DHL have a poorer prognosis (32). The level of MYC expression is higher in DHL than in DPL (1). As most cases of classic *MYC/BCL2* DHL overexpress MYC, MYC immunostaining may be a convenient screen to decide which tumors should be analyzed by fluorescence in situ hybridization (FISH) or other molecular methods to assess for *MYC* translocations. However, MYC immunostaining, no matter what cutoff is chosen, will not "catch" all cases of *MYC/BCL2* DHL and is not specific. Therefore, FISH testing for MYC is required.

MOLECULAR GENETIC FINDINGS

Conventional cytogenetic analysis of DHLs usually shows a complex karyotype; array-based comparative genomic hybridization analysis shows multiple gains or losses of chromosomal material (1,3). Gains of chromosomes 8q and 12q are common in DHL. In 60 percent of *MYC/BCL2* DHL, the chromosome 8q24/*MYC* locus partners with *IGH* or less often *IGK* or *IGL*. In the other 40 percent of cases, 8q24/*MYC* partners with non-IG genes. Two of the more common non-IG partners are *PAX5* at chromosome 9p13 and *BCL6*. In most studies of DHL, *MYC* partners have not correlated with clinicopathologic characteristics or prognosis (1,18). Cases of DHL with *MYC-IGH* translocations have higher *MYC* transcript levels (1).

MYC/BCL6 DHL is often less complex than *MYC/BCL2* DHL at the cytogenetic level (27). In these tumors, *MYC* also can partner with either IG or non-IG loci without apparent clinical importance. *BCL6* also can partner with IG or non-IG gene loci, the latter including *MYC* in a subset of cases. In one study of triple-hit lymphomas, conventional cytogenetic analysis showed highly complex karyotypes and FISH showed deletions of *CDKN2A* in about half of cases (3).

The gene expression profile of DHLs is either intermediate between true DLBCL and BL, or is closer to BL (11). Little gene expression data comparing *MYC/BCL2* DHL and *MYC/BCL6* DHL cases are available. In one study, 120 genes were differentially expressed in *MYC/BCL2* DHL and *MYC/BCL6* DHL (1). *MYC* transcript levels were similar in both types of DHL.

TP53 mutations occur in about one third of *MYC/BCL2* DHLs but are rare in *MYC/BCL6* DHLs (4,7,28a). Others have suggested that *MYC* translocation combined with *TP53* mutation is another form of double-hit lymphoma (4). *ID3* mutations occur in about 25 percent of cases of DHL and are found at a similar frequency in both the *MYC/BCL2* and *MYC/BCL6* types (6). *IGH* mutations occur in 10 to 15 percent of DHLs and may be more common in the *MYC/BCL2* type (1). *MYC* mutations occur in less than 10 percent of DHLs of either *MYC/BCL2* or *MYC/BCL6* type, and *MYD88* mutations are rare (1,8).

Atypical *MYC/BCL2* Double-Hit Lymphoma

Uncommonly, an aggressive B-cell lymphoma is associated with cytogenetic abnormalities involving *MYC* with *BCL2*, but not necessarily translocations involving these genes (19). The three possible combinations in this category include: *MYC* translocation with extra copies of *BCL2*; extra copies of *MYC* with *BCL2* translocation; and extra copies of both *MYC* and *BCL2* without translocations. Preliminary studies have shown that patients with atypical *MYC/BCL2* DHL have an aggressive clinical course and poorer prognosis, similar to patients with classic *MYC/BCL2* DHL (18,19). Valera et al. (30) distinguished between *MYC* amplification and gains and found that only amplification is associated with a poorer prognosis. Currently, however, there is no a consensus that cases of atypical DHL are equivalent to cases of classic defined DHL (see below). Also, there is little data for cases that could be considered examples of atypical *MYC/BCL6* DHL.

Lymphomas with *BCL2* and *BCL6* Translocations

Some cases of DLBCL may carry transloca- tions that involve both *BCL2* and *BCL6*, but there is no evidence of a *MYC* translocation. Although these neoplasms have two "hits," they do not meet the criteria for DHL as defined by Aukema et al. (2). In our experience, patients with these tumors tend to be elderly and often present with extranodal disease. A GCB (60 to 70 percent) immunophenotype is more com- mon. The prognosis of this subset of patients is not well studied.

DIFFERENTIAL DIAGNOSIS

The differential diagnosis of DHL depends, in large part, on its morphologic appearance. In general, a histologically aggressive B-cell lym- phoma with a starry sky pattern, particularly if it is difficult to classify or is strongly BCL2 posi- tive, is a likely candidate to be a DHL. Similarly, highly proliferative lymphomas, as shown by Ki-67, are more likely to include cases of DHL.

Diffuse Large B-Cell Lymphoma. Most cases of DLBCL lack a starry sky pattern and have a proliferation rate of 50 to 80 percent. Further- more, many of these cases lack CD10 or BCL6 and do not express BCL2. Only a few DLBCL cases mimic DHL by having a starry sky pattern, a GCB immunophenotype, and strong BCL2 expression. For this subset of cases, cytogenetic or FISH analysis is needed to distinguish DLBCL from DHL. In the revised WHO classification, a tumor that resembles DLBCL but which carries double hit genetics should be classified as HGBL with *MYC* rearrangement and *BCL2* and/or *BCL6* rearrangement (28b).

Burkitt Lymphoma. BL is composed of a monomorphic population of neoplastic cells, typically has a high (over 90 percent) prolifera- tion rate, is negative for BCL2, and has a simple karyotype with a *MYC* translocation involving *IGH* in the light chain genes. In contrast, most cases of DHL show a range of cell sizes with more pleomorphism than BL, although some can closely mimic BL morphologically. DHLs are usually strongly BCL2 positive and have a com- plex karyotype, and 40 to 50 percent have *MYC* translocations that involve a non-IG partner.

TREATMENT AND PROGNOSIS

The therapeutic options for patients with DHL have been reviewed by Petrich et al. (26). Currently, there is no consensus regarding the best therapy for these patients. Patients who received intensive chemotherapy regimens have had a higher complete remission rate than patients who were treated with R-CHOP, but in most studies intensive chemotherapy did not result in improved overall survival, nor is there clear benefit associated with the use of autologous stem cell transplantation (9a,15a,26). However, a subset of patients have long-term complete remission, suggesting that there is a potential role for risk stratification (23,25). Fac- tors that appear to correlate with worse prognosis in patients with DHL differed between the two studies but included: poor performance status, bone marrow involvement, leukocytosis, elevat- ed serum LDH, advanced-stage disease, and in- volvement of the central nervous system (23,25).

There are also data that suggest that the part- ner of *MYC*, specifically *BCL2* versus *BCL6*, may be important for prognosis (16). In a multicenter study of cases of *MYC/BCL2* DHL, Petrich et al. (25) suggested that stem cell transplant may be beneficial if poor prognostic factors are ac- counted for in the analysis. The median survival period of most patients with DHL is short, in the range of 1 to 2 years (12,18,23–25). For patients who relapse after initial therapy, there are no effective therapeutic options at this time.

With the advent of routine FISH testing, oc- casional patients with DHL are detected who do not have poor prognostic features, so-called low- risk DHL (24). These patients are usually also treated with intensive therapies currently, but this patient subset needs further investigation.

REFERENCES

1. Aukema SM, Kreuz M, Kohler CW, et al. Biological characterization of adult MYC-translocation-positive mature B-cell lymphomas other than molecular Burkitt lymphoma. Haematologica 2014;99:726-735.
2. Aukema SM, Siebert R, Schuuring E, et al. Double hit B-cell lymphomas. Blood 2011;117:2319-2331.
3. Bacher U, Haferlach T, Alpermann T, Kern W, Schnittger S, Haferlach C. Several lymphoma-specific genetic events in parallel can be found in mature B-cell neoplasm. Genes Chromosomes Cancer 2011;50:43-50.
4. Clipson A, Barrans S, Zeng N, et al. The prognosis of MYC translocation positive diffuse large B-cell lymphoma depends on the second hit. J Pathol Clin Res 2015;1:125-133.
5. Elkins CT, Wakely PE. Cytopathology of "double hit" non-Hodgkin lymphoma. Cancer Cytopathology 2011;119:263-271.
6. Gebauer N, Bernard V, Feller AC, Merz H. ID3 mutations are recurrent events in double-hit B-cell lymphomas. Anticancer Res 2013;33:4771-4778.
7. Gebauer N, Bernard V, Gebauer W, Thorns C, Feller AC, Merz H. TP53 mutations are frequent events in double-hit B-cell lymphomas with MYC and BCL2 but not MYC and BCL6 translocations. Leuk Lymphoma 2015;56:179-185.
8. Gebauer N, Bernard V, Thorns C, Feller AC, Merz H. Oncogeneic MYD88 mutations are rare events in double-hit B-cell lymphomas. Acta Haematol 2015;133:113-115.
9. Green TM, Young KH, Visco C, et al. Immunohistochemical double-hit score is a strong predictor of outcome in patients with diffuse large B-cell lymphoma treated with rituximab plus cyclophosphamide, doxorubicin, vincristine, and prednisone. J Clin Oncol 2012;30:3460-3467.
9a. Herrera AF, Mei M, Low L, et al. Relapsed or refractory double-expressor and double-hit lymphomas have inferior progression-free survival after autologous stem-cell transplantation. J Clin Oncol 2017;35:24-31.
10. Hu S, Xu-Monette ZY, Tzankov A, et al. MYC/BCL2 protein coexpression contributes to the inferior survival of activated B-cell subtype of diffuse large B-cell lymphoma and demonstrates high-risk gene expression signatures: a report from The International DLBCL Rituximab-CHOP Consortium Program. Blood 2013;121:4021-4031.
11. Hummel M, Bentink S, Berger H, et al. A biologic definition of Burkitt's lymphoma from transcriptional and genomic profiling. N Engl J Med 2006;354:2419-2430.
12. Johnson NA, Savage KJ, Ludkowski O, et al. Lymphomas with concurrent BCL2 and MYC translocations: the critical factors associated with survival. Blood 2009;114:2273-2279.
13. Kanagal-Shamanna R, Medeiros LJ, Lu G, et al. High-grade B cell lymphoma, unclassifiable, with blastoid features: an unusual morphological subgroup associated frequently with BCL2 and/or MYC gene rearrangements and a poor prognosis. Histopathology 2012;61:945-954.
14. Kelemen K, Holden J, Johnson JL, Davion S, Robetorye RS. Immunophenotypic and cytogenetic findings of B-lymphoblastic leukemia/lymphoma associated with combined IGH/BCL2 and MYC rearrangement. Cytometry B Clin Cytom 2015 [Epub ahead of print].
15. Kluin PM, Harris NL, Stein H, et al. B-cell lymphoma, unclassifiable, with features intermediate between diffuse large B-cell lymphoma and Burkitt lymphoma. In: Swerdlow SH, Campo E, Harris NL, et al., eds. WHO classification of tumours of haematopoietic and lymphoid tissues, 4th ed. Lyon: IARC Press; 2008:265-266.
15a. Landsburg DJ, Falkiewicz MK, Maly J, et al. Outcomes of patients with double-hit lymphoma who achieve first complete remission. J Clin Oncol 2017;35:2260-2267.
16. Landsburg DJ, Petrich AM, Abramson JS, et al. Impact of oncogene rearrangement patterns on outcomes in patients with double-hit non-Hodgkin lymphoma. Cancer 2016;122:559-564.
17. Li S, Desai P, Lin P, et al. MYC/BCL6 double-hit lymphoma (DHL): a tumour associated with an aggressive clinical course and poor prognosis. Histopathology 2016;68:1090-1098.
18. Li S, Lin P, Fayad LE, et al. B-cell lymphomas with MYC/8q24 rearrangements and IGH@BCL2/t(14;18)(q32;q21): an aggressive disease with heterogeneous histology, a germinal center cell immunophenotype, and poor outcome. Mod Pathol 2012; 25:145-156.
19. Li S, Seegmiller AC, Lin P, et al. B-cell lymphomas with concurrent MYC and BCL2 abnormalities other than translocations behave similarly to MYC/BCL2 double-hit lymphomas. Mod Pathol 2015;28:208-217.
20. Lin P, Medeiros LJ. High-grade B-cell lymphoma/leukemia associated with t(14;18) and 8q24/MYC rearrangement: a neoplasm of germinal center immunophenotype with poor prognosis. Haematologica 2007;92:1297-1301.

21. Liu W, Hu S, Konopleva M, et al. De novo MYC and BCL2 double-hit B-cell precursor acute lymphoblastic leukemia (BCL-ALL) in pediatric and young adult patients associated with poor prognosis. Pediatr Hematol Oncol 2015;32:535-547.

21a.Miao Y, Hu S, Lu X, et al. Double-hit follicular lymphoma with MYC and BCL2 translocations: a study of 7 cases with a review of literature. Hum Pathol 2016;58:72-77.

22. Nanua S, Bartlett NL, Hassan A, et al. Composite diffuse large B-cell lymphoma and precursor B lymphoblastic lymphoma presenting as a double-hit lymphoma with MYC and BCL2 translocation. J Clin Pathol 2011;64:1032-1034.

23. Oki Y, Noorani M, Lin P, et al. Double hit lymphoma: the MD Anderson Cancer Center clinical experience. Br J Haematol 2014;166:891-901.

24. Pedersen MØ, Gang AO, Poulsen TS, et al. Double-hit BCL2/MYC translocations in a consecutive cohort of patients with large B-cell lymphoma—a single centre's experience. Eur J Haematol 2012;89:63-71.

25. Petrich AM, Gandhi M, Jovanovic B, et al. Impact of induction regimen and stem cell transplantation on outcomes in patients with double hit lymphoma: a large multicenter retrospective analysis. Blood 2014;124:2354-2361.

26. Petrich AM, Nabhan C, Smith SM. MYC-associated and double-hit lymphomas: a review of pathobiology, prognosis, and therapeutic approaches. Cancer 2014;120:3884-3895.

27. Pillai RK, Sathanoori M, Van Oss SB, Swerdlow SH. Double-hit B-cell lymphomas with BCL6 and MYC translocations are aggressive, frequently extranodal lymphomas distinct from BCL2 double-hit B-cell lymphomas. Am J Surg Pathol 2013;37:323-332.

28. Roth CG, Gillespie-Twardy A, Marks S, et al. Flow cytometric evaluation of double/triple hit lymphomas. Oncol Res 2016;23:137-146.

28a.Schiefer AI, Kornauth C, Simonitsch-Klupp I, et al. Impact of single or combined genomic alterations of TP53, MYC, and BCL2 on survival of patients with diffuse large B-cell lymphomas: a retrospective cohort study. Medicine (Baltimore) 2015;94:e2388.

28b.Swerdlow SH, Campo E, Pileri SA, et al. The 2016 revision of the World Health Organization classification of lymphoid neoplasms. Blood 2016;127:2375-2390.

29. Turakhia SK, Hill BT, Dufresne SD, Nakashima MO, Cotta CV. Aggressive B-cell lymphomas with translocations involving BCL6 and MYC have distinct clinical-pathologic characteristics. Am J Clin Pathol 2014;142:339-346.

30. Valera A, López-Guillermo A, Cardesa-Salzmann T, et al. MYC protein expression and genetic alterations have prognostic impact in diffuse large B-cell lymphoma treated with immunochemotherapy. Haematologica 2013;98:1554-1562.

31. Wang W, Hu S, Lu X, Young KH, Medeiros LJ. Triple-hit B-cell lymphoma with MYC, BCL2 and BCL6 translocations/rearrangements: clinicopathologic features of 11 cases. Am J Surg Pathol 2015;39:1132-1139.

32. Wang XJ, Medeiros LJ, Lin P, et al. MYC cytogenetic status correlates with expression and has prognostic significance in patients with MYC/BCL2 protein double-positive diffuse large B-cell lymphoma. Am J Surg Pathol 2015;39:1250-1258.

33. Wu D, Wood BL, Dorer R, Fromm JR. "Double-hit" mature B-cell lymphomas show a common immunophenotype by flow cytometry that includes decreased CD20 expression. Am J Clin Pathol 2010;134:258-265.

34. Ye Q, Xu-Monette ZY, Tzankov A, et al. Prognostic impact of concurrent MYC and BCL6 rearrangements and expression in de novo diffuse large B-cell lymphoma. Oncotarget 2016;19:2401-2406.

28

B-CELL LYMPHOMA, UNCLASSIFIABLE, WITH FEATURES INTERMEDIATE BETWEEN DIFFUSE LARGE B-CELL LYMPHOMA AND CLASSIC HODGKIN LYMPHOMA (GRAY ZONE LYMPHOMA)

GENERAL FEATURES

B-cell lymphomas, unclassifiable, with features intermediate between diffuse large B-cell lymphoma and classic Hodgkin lymphoma are of B-cell lineage and exhibit intermediate clinical, histologic, and immunophenotypic features (9). Currently, there are no uniform diagnostic criteria available by which these tumors are classified (13). Furthermore, these neoplasms are rare and clinical follow-up of patients has been short.

These neoplasms have been recognized and debated for a number of years. Terms used in the literature for these lymphomas include *large B-cell lymphoma with Hodgkin features, anaplastic large cell lymphoma, Hodgkin-related*, and the most popular and convenient term, although somewhat vague, *gray zone lymphoma* (6,12–14). These tumors were only formally recognized in the 2008 version of the World Health Organization (WHO) classification (9) and this category is retained in the 2016 revised WHO classification (14b). For simplicity, the designation gray zone lymphoma (GZL) will be used for the remainder of this chapter.

GZLs have been reported almost exclusively in developed nations, possibly because recognition of these tumors usually requires utilization of an extensive panel of antibodies assessed by immunohistochemistry. The etiology is unknown.

GZLs occur commonly in the mediastinum and therefore the designation *mediastinal GZL* is often used (6–9,13). They also have been reported at other sites (5,6,8,12,14). Although mediastinal tumors are more common in most studies, a recent report by Evens et al. (5) showed that 57 percent of GZL cases occurred at nonmediastinal sites. Based on the morphologic, immunophenotypic, and molecular heterogeneity of GZLs, it is possible (if not likely) that this category in

the WHO classification includes more than one biologic entity.

A patient can present with GZL de novo or at the time of relapse, following an initial diagnosis of either classic HL, usually of nodular sclerosis type, or primary mediastinal large B-cell lymphoma (PMBL). Rarely, a composite lymphoma composed of nodular sclerosis HL and PMBL can occur. These cases are in accord with the suggestion that nodular sclerosis HL, mediastinal gray zone lymphoma, and PMBL arise from a common precursor B-cell in the thymic medulla (1). Lineage plasticity (reprogramming of differentiation) is thought a possible explanation for the transition from one to another disease manifestation.

In the WHO classification, patients with composite classic HL and PMBL, or sequential HL and DLBCL or vice versa, are not included specifically in the category of GZL. It has been suggested, however, that composite or sequential tumors are closely related (1,7,9), and in some research studies and review articles, authors have included composite and sequential lymphomas in the GZL category (1,2,7).

CLINICAL FEATURES

GZLs affect men more often than women, with a wide age range, but with a median age in the fourth decade (5,7,12,14,15). In one large study, however, women were affected slightly more often (14a). The disease is rare in children (under 18 years of age). Patients commonly present with a large mediastinal mass and about half of patients have a mass 10 cm or larger (14a,15) that can be associated with regional lymphadenopathy or local invasion of contiguous structures. A large mediastinal mass may cause the patient

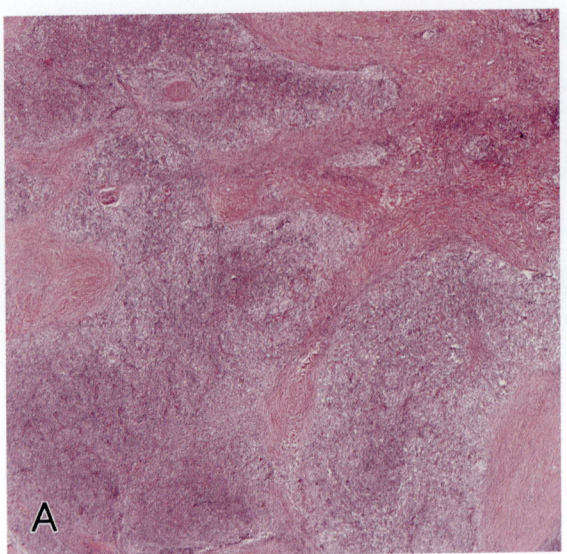
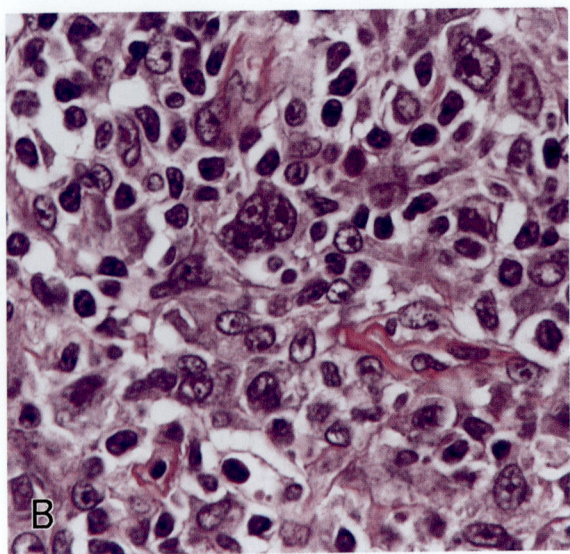

Figure 28-1

B-CELL LYMPHOMA, UNCLASSIFIABLE, WITH FEATURES INTERMEDIATE BETWEEN DIFFUSE
LARGE B-CELL LYMPHOMA AND CLASSIC HODGKIN LYMPHOMA

Morphologically, this neoplasm had features suggestive of classic Hodgkin lymphoma (HL) but the immunophenotype was more in keeping with B-cell non-Hodgkin lymphoma.

A: Low-power magnification shows nodules of cells surrounded by fibrous bands (A,B: hematoxylin & eosin [H&E] stain).

B: Cells with Reed-Sternberg-like and Hodgkin-like cells are present in a background of small lymphocytes and histiocytes. Granulocytes are rare in this case.

to develop respiratory distress or superior vena cava syndrome. Direct invasion of the pleura or lungs may be associated with prominent pleural effusions. Mediastinal GZL can disseminate, most often to bone marrow, liver, and spleen (9).

Patients with nonmediastinal GZL tend to be older, with a median age of 50 years (5). Nodal and a wide variety of extranodal sites may be involved. Compared to patients with mediastinal GZL, patients with nonmediastinal tumors more frequently have bone marrow involvement, multiple extranodal sites of involvement, and a higher stage of disease (5,8,12). In addition, non-mediastinal GZL cases are generally less bulky (5).

HISTOLOGIC FINDINGS

Gualco et al. (7) subdivided GZLs into four patterns, essentially expanding on what is written in the WHO classification (9). A similar approach was taken by Sarkozy et al. (14a). Although there are no known prognostic or scientific correlates with these patterns, they are useful for describing the spectrum of these tumors.

In pattern 1, the tumor morphologically resembles classic HL, but has immunophenotypic features more like DLBCL [i.e., CD45/LCA(+), B-cell antigens brightly (+)] (fig. 28-1). In pattern 2, the tumor morphologically resembles PMBL (or DLBCL) but has an immunophenotype more like nodular sclerosis HL [e.g., CD15(+), CD45/LCA(-)] (fig. 28-2). In pattern 3, the morphologic features overlap with areas that look more or less like HL or DLBCL. Pattern 4 designates cases of composite HL and DLBCL as well as sequential cases of HL and DLBCL or vice versa.

In tumors (or areas) that resemble classic HL, large, pleomorphic neoplastic cells are present that resemble Hodgkin or lacunar cell variants. Reed-Sternberg-like cells can be present, but are not numerous (1,7,9). The large cells are present in an inflammatory cell background that includes lymphocytes, histiocytes, and less often, eosinophils. In tumors (or areas) that resemble DLBCL, sheets of large neoplastic cells appear centroblastic or more pleomorphic, with a sparse inflammatory cell background. Reed-Sternberg- or Hodgkin-like cells may be present and necrosis is common. Fibrous bands are present in a third to half of cases, most often in cases that involve the mediastinum

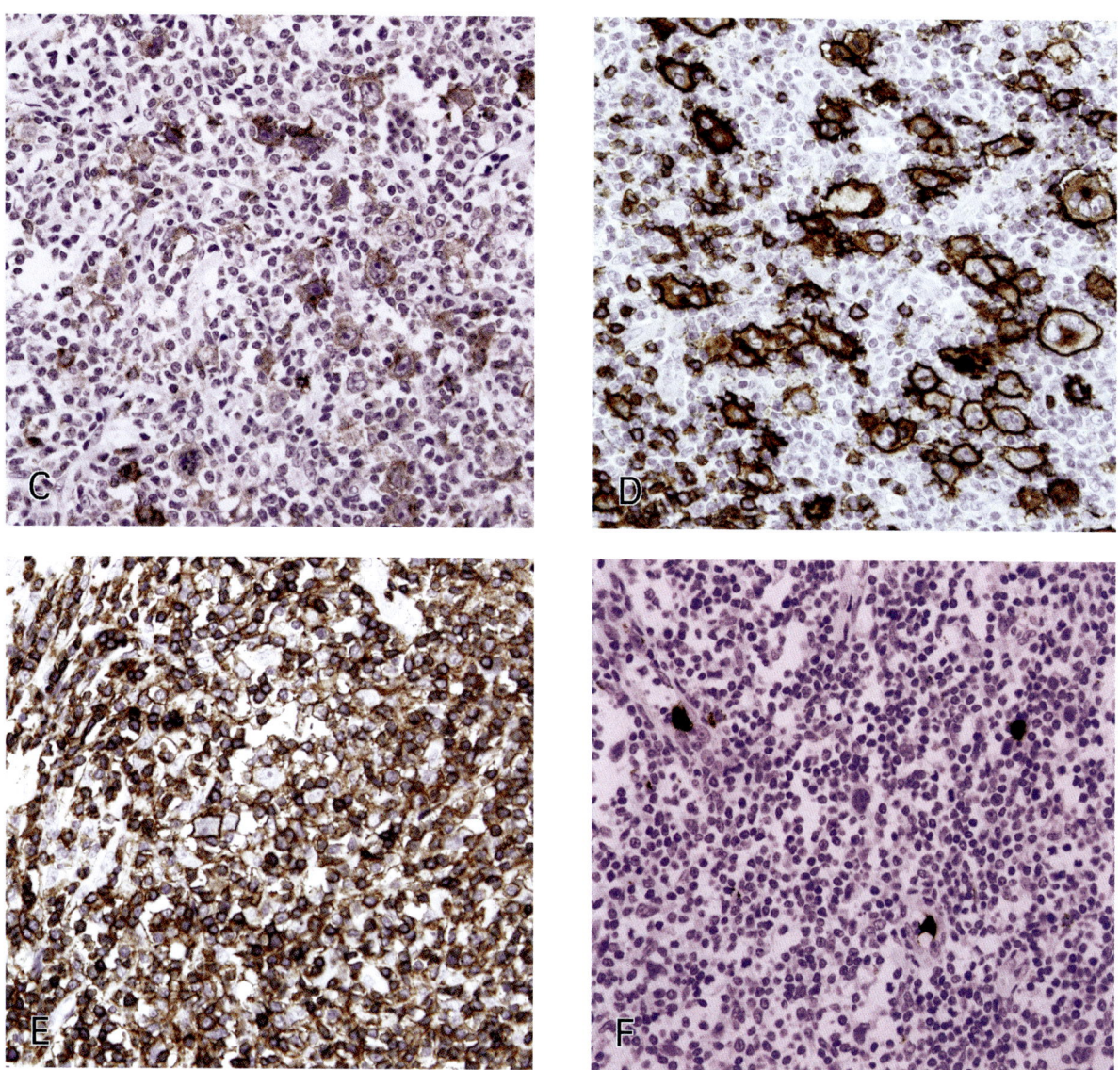

Figure 28-1, continued

C–F: Immunohistochemical studies show that the neoplastic cells are positive for CD30 (C), CD20 (D), and CD45/LCA (E), and are negative for CD15 (F) (C–F: immunohistochemistry with hematoxylin counterstain).

(1,7,9,12,14a), but the fibrous bands may not be well developed. Sinusoidal invasion may occur.

CYTOLOGIC FINDINGS

Little is written about using fine-needle aspiration (FNA) to establish the diagnosis of GZL. In one case reported, a polymorphous population of reactive and neoplastic cells was present (10). The neoplastic cells were large and had cytoplasmic vacuoles; classic Reed-Sternberg cells were not present. As stated by the authors, GZLs are difficult to diagnose on cytologic smears as the cells can resemble either HL or DLBCL (fig. 28-3).

In general, the diagnosis of GZL by using FNA seems to be an endeavor associated with a high risk of error. At the least an extensive battery of immunohistochemical studies needs to be performed on a cell block to support a GZL diagnosis (12). The diagnosis of GZL can be established in a core needle biopsy specimen more easily than by FNA. Again, a battery of immunostains is required to establish a diagnosis of GZL.

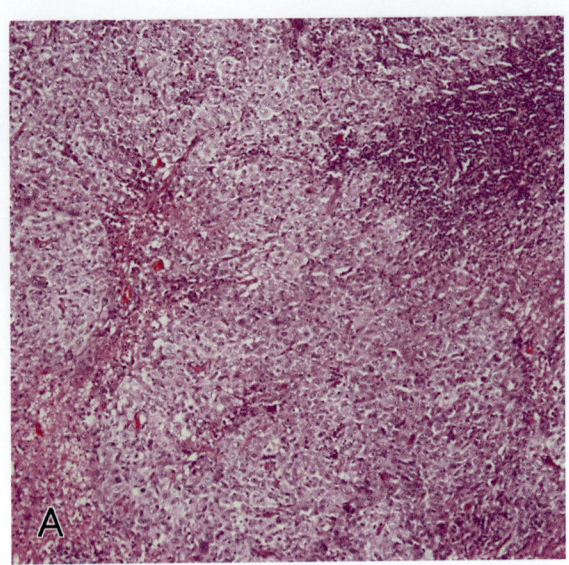
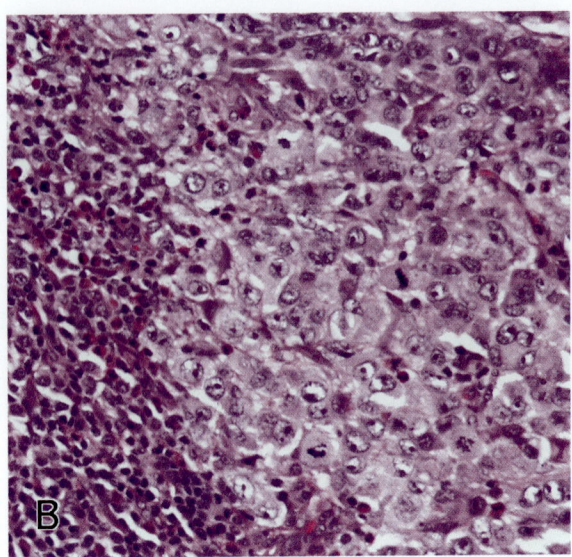

Figure 28-2

**B-CELL LYMPHOMA, UNCLASSIFIABLE, WITH FEATURES INTERMEDIATE BETWEEN
DIFFUSE LARGE B-CELL LYMPHOMA AND CLASSIC HODGKIN LYMPHOMA**

Morphologically, this neoplasm had features suggestive of diffuse large B-cell lymphoma (DLBCL) but immunohistochemical studies showed that the neoplastic cells expressed CD15 and CD30, similar to classic HL.

A: Low-power magnification shows sheets of large cells (A,B: H&E stain).

B: The neoplastic cells have features of centroblasts and immunoblasts. Many lymphocytes and eosinophils are at the edge of the tumor.

IMMUNOPHENOTYPIC FINDINGS

A key feature of GZL emphasized in the WHO classification is a discordance between the morphologic features and the immunophenotype (9,14b). This particularly applies to patterns 1 and 2 as described above. In tumors that resemble classic HL, the neoplastic cells are CD30(+), often CD45/LCA(+), and usually CD15(-). In addition, the tumor cells show evidence of B-cell differentiation, being positive for CD20 (often bright), CD79a, PAX5 (moderate to bright), and other B-cell transcription factors (fig. 28-1C–F). In tumors that resemble DLBCL, the neoplastic cells are usually strongly positive for B-cell antigens such as CD20 and CD79a, but are also positive for CD30 (bright) and often positive for CD15 (fig. 28-2C–F). It is rare for CD20 to be dim or absent in cases of GZL.

Overall, CD30 is expressed in almost all cases of GZL (1,4a,5–7,9). Most GZLs express B-cell antigens, including CD20, CD79a, OCT2, BOB.1, PAX5, and CD19 (assessed in a limited number of cases to date). CD15 is expressed in 50 to 80 percent of cases (1,5,6,9,15). CD23 is positive in many mediastinal cases (7). Cyclin E is positive

in approximately 85 percent and MUM-1/IRF4, BCL6, BCL2, and p63 are expressed in 50 to 60 percent of tumors (7,9). The proliferation rate, as assessed by Ki-67 expression, is usually high in GZLs and P53 is commonly expressed, but *TP53* is rarely mutated (6).

NF-κB pathway activation is common in GZLs and therefore evidence of activation such as c-REL/p65 expression, often in a nuclear pattern, or expression in phosphorylated form (indicating activation) is common (6,9). EMA is positive in approximately one quarter to one third of cases. MAL is expressed variably in a small subset of cases (9,13). Epstein-Barr virus (EBV) encoded RNA1 (EBER1) and less often latent membrane protein-type 1 (LMP-1) have been reported in about 15 percent of cases (4,4a,6,7,9,14b). CD43 is expressed in a small subset of cases; other T-cell antigens are usually negative. CD10 and ALK are negative in GZL (6,9).

Histiocytes and dendritic cells are commonly intermixed within GZL biopsy specimens and attempts have been made to correlate cell numbers with prognosis. In one small study of 24 patients with mediastinal GZL (15), tumors with high

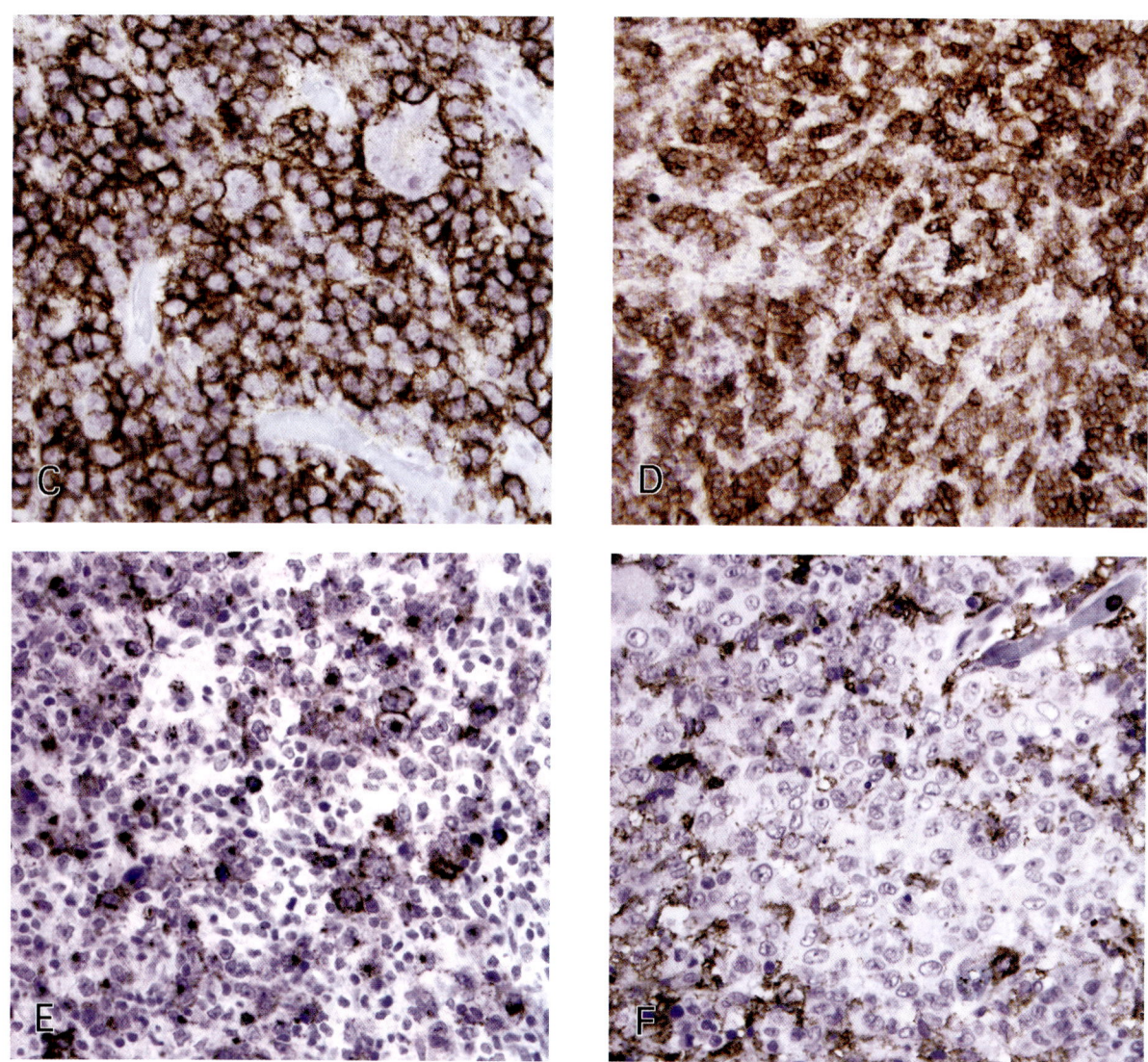

Figure 28-2, continued

C–F: Immunohistochemical studies show that the neoplastic cells are brightly positive for CD20 (C) and CD30 (D). Some of the neoplastic cells are positive for CD15 in a membranous and paranuclear pattern (E), and the neoplastic cells are negative for CD45/LCA (small lymphocytes and histiocytes positive) (F) (C–F: Immunohistochemistry with hematoxylin counterstain).

numbers of cells positive for dendritic cell-specific intercellular adhesion molecule-3-grabbing nonintegrin (DC-SIGN; CD209), which highlights dendritic cells and activated macrophages, were associated with poorer patient outcome. Using CD68 to highlight histiocytes was not as helpful for predicting prognosis in this study.

MOLECULAR GENETIC FINDINGS

Little cytogenetic or molecular information is available for GZL. The little data available are derived from cases involving the mediastinum.

Few cases reported have been assessed by conventional cytogenetic analysis. Eberle et al. (4) used fluorescence in situ hybridization (FISH) to assess 27 cases of GZL. This study showed abnormalities of chromosome 9q24.1/*JAK2/PDL2* (about 55 percent), 2p16.1/*BCL11A/REL* locus (about 33 percent), 16p13.13/*CIITA* locus (about 25 percent), and 8q24/*MYC* (about 25 percent). The *MYC* abnormalities were gains and not translocations. *BCL6* translocations and trisomy 3 have been reported in 2 of 9 and 1 of 9 cases, respectively (6). Others, however,

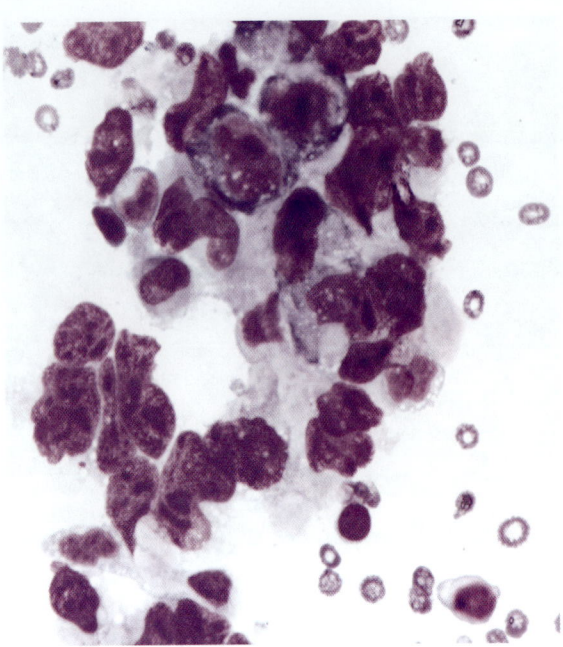 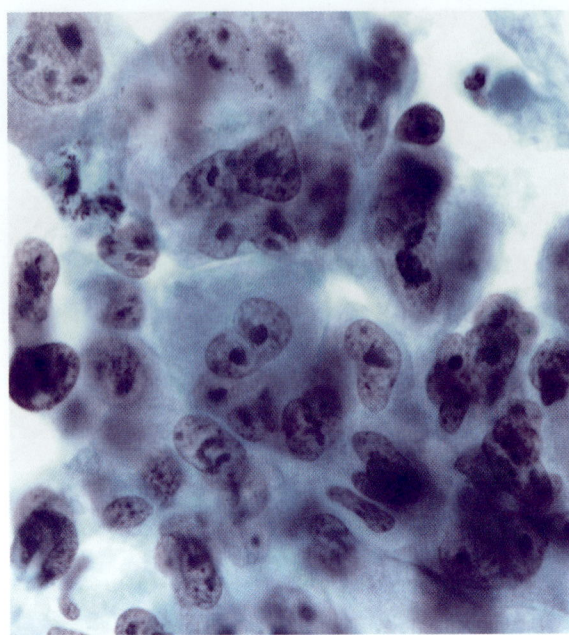

Figure 28-3

B-CELL LYMPHOMA, UNCLASSIFIABLE, WITH FEATURES INTERMEDIATE BETWEEN DIFFUSE LARGE B-CELL LYMPHOMA AND CLASSIC HODGKIN LYMPHOMA

Left, Right: Aspirate smears show large and pleomorphic tumor cells with irregular nuclear contours, variably sized nucleoli, and scant to moderately abundant cytoplasm (left: Diff-Quick stain; right: Papanicolaou stain.)

have not shown *BCL6* rearrangements in GZLs (7). There is no evidence of t(14;18)(q32;q21) or *BCL2* rearrangements in GZL cases (1,7,9).

The methylation profiles of mediastinal GZL, classic HL, and PMBL have been assessed (3). Cases of classic HL show marked hypermethylation, perhaps explaining the silencing of the B-cell differentiation program typical of Hodgkin and Reed-Sternberg cells in these tumors. In contrast, mediastinal GZL and PMBL show various degrees of hypomethylation, in particular, hypomethylation of *HOXA5* in virtually all cases of mediastinal GZL. The authors suggested that assessment of 22 methylation sites could be used to classify cases as classic HL, mediastinal GZL, or PMBL. This system correctly classified about 90 percent of the cases included in their study (3).

Gene expression profiling analysis has shown that the signatures of classic HL and PMBL can overlap. This finding, in part, lead to the development of the concept of mediastinal GZL. To date, molecular studies have not shown significant differences between tumors that morphologically more closely resemble HL or DLBCL or that appear to be a mixture of HL and DLBCL

(3,4,8). Monoclonal *IGH* gene rearrangements are common in GZL, particularly in cases with numerous large cells.

DIFFERENTIAL DIAGNOSIS

Nodular Sclerosis HL. The differential diagnosis of a mediastinal GZL can be problematic. In the differential diagnosis of nodular sclerosis HL versus GZL, features favoring the former include a typical or consistent morphologic appearance, with the Reed-Sternberg and Hodgkin cells showing CD15(+) and CD30(+) (strong and uniform), PAX5 weak, other B-cell antigens(-), and CD15/LCA(-). Evidence of EBV infection is uncommon, but more likely in HL than in GZL. Variable and often weak expression of B-cell antigens, such as CD20, can occur and does not exclude HL. Bright CD20 expression is acceptable for HL, but only if the clinicopathologic and other immunophenotypic findings otherwise fit with this diagnosis (13).

PMBL. In the differential diagnosis of GZL versus PMBL, most cases of GZL are CD15(+) (50 to 75 percent of cases), CD30(+), and CD20(+) (usually uniform and/or bright). Other B-cell antigens and transcription factors as well as CD45/LCA can be positive or negative in GZL, but variable expression of B-cell antigens and a negative result for CD45/LCA provide support for GZL. Cases of PMBL are usually strongly positive for CD19, CD20, CD79A, PAX5, and the B-cell transcription factors OCT2 and BOB.1. CD45/LCA is usually brightly positive and CD30 is expressed variably. PMBL is usually negative for CD15 and EBV. As CD15 expression is highly unusual in PMBL, its presence in an otherwise apparent case of B-cell lymphoma is an important signal to do a rigorous workup to exclude GZL.

O'Malley et al. (11) suggested a scoring system for distinguishing classic HL from B-cell lymphoma, with the latter category including cases of GZL as well as PMBL. This system uses eight antibodies as well as EBER1 and is shown in Table 28-1. Using this system, the maximal score favoring classic HL is +6 and the minimum score favoring B-cell lymphoma is -6. These authors reviewed 61 cases using this system and reported good predictive power. Most cases of classic HL had a score of 4 to 6, most cases of GZL fit within the -4 to +3 range, and cases of PMBL or DLBCL-NOS scored -6 to -3. Although this approach appears to be promising, it needs to be tested by others and validated.

Nonmediastinal GZLs. For nonmediastinal GZLs, many of which involve extranodal sites, usually DLBCL not otherwise specified (NOS), is the main entity in the differential diagnosis. The statements above for GZL versus PMBL also apply to GZL versus DLBCL-NOS.

TREATMENT AND PROGNOSIS

There is no consensus therapy for patients with GZL. Regimens used for patients with classic HL or PMBL have been employed. The standard chemotherapy regimen for patients with classic HL is adriamycin, bleomycin, vincristine, and dacarbazine (ABVD). This regimen seems suboptimal for patients with GZL (2,5,7) in most studies. The standard therapeutic approach for patients with PMBL is rituximab, cyclophosphamide, doxorubicin, vincristine, and prednisone (R-CHOP) with radiation therapy. In most studies, GZL patients treated in this manner have done better than those treated with ABVD (5,7). In a comparison of CHOP versus R-CHOP plus radiation therapy, rituximab provided a

Table 28-1

PROPOSED SCORING SYSTEM TO DISTINGUISH CLASSIC HODGKIN LYMPHOMA FROM B-CELL LYMPHOMA[a]

Antibody In Situ	Negative	Weak or Focal	Strong
CD15	0	+1	+1
CD30[b]	0	0	0
CD45/LCA	+1	-1	-1
CD20	+1	+1	-1
PAX5	0	+1	-1
CD79a	0	-1	-1
MUM1/IRF4	-1	0	0
EBER1	0	+1	+1
OCT2/BOB.1[c]	+1	+1	-1

[a]Maximum score for classic Hodgkin lymphoma: +6; minimum score for B-cell lymphoma: -6. +1 favors classic Hodgkin lymphoma; 0 is equivocal; -1 favors B-cell lymphoma (11).
[b]CD30 positivity has no result because a tumor is unlikely to be included in this differential diagnosis if CD30 negative.
[c]Negative/negative = +1; negative/positive or positive/negative = +1; positive/positive = -1.

survival benefit (5), but this was not confirmed by others (14a). There are concerns, however, about the long-term sequelae associated with radiation therapy, for example, breast carcinoma. Radiation therapy doses used currently are much lower than those used historically, but there is no long-term follow-up study proving that reduced dose radiation therapy is less toxic.

A newer approach to therapy has been proposed by Wilson et al. (15) at the National Cancer Institute who used infusional dose-adjusted etoposide, prednisone, vincristine, cyclophosphamide, doxorubicin, and rituximab (DA-EPOCH-R) to treat patients with GZL. With almost 5 years of clinical follow-up, overall and event-free survival were 74 percent and 62 percent, respectively. Thus, DA-EPOCH-R appears to be equal to or better than standard therapy and is becoming popular for the treatment of patients with GZL (1a,9a,15). As DA-EPOCH-R is also advocated as the best approach for patients with PMBL, the distinction between GZL versus PMBL is less critical for choosing the appropriate therapy, taking the pressure off the pathologist somewhat. However, there are associated treatment issues, such as using central nervous system prophylaxis, where the diagnosis of GZL versus PMBL still may have implications. For patients with GZL who relapse, salvage chemotherapy followed by autologous hematopoietic stem cell transplant has been suggested (9a).

Clinical findings correlate with prognosis in patients with GZL. High performance status and advanced-stage disease predict poorer survival (5,7,14a). In the study by Wilson et al. (15), a low absolute lymphocyte count in the blood,

high numbers of dendritic cells (DC-SIGN positive) in the tumor, and CD15 expression by the neoplastic cells (15) correlated with poorer prognosis. Mediastinal versus nonmediastinal site of disease did not significantly correlate with 2-year overall or progression-free survival in the study by Evens et al. (5).

REFERENCES

1. Carbone A, Gloghini A, Aiello A, Testi A, Cabras A. B-cell lymphomas with features intermediate between distinct pathologic entities. From pathogenesis to pathology. Hum Pathol 2010;41:621-631.

1a. Chihara D, Fowler NH, Oki Y, et al. Dose-adjusted EPOCH-R and mid-cycle high dose methotrexate for patients with systemic lymphoma and secondary CNS involvement. Br J Haematol 2016. [Epub ahead of print]

2. Dunleavy K, Wilson WH. Primary mediastinal B-cell lymphoma and mediastinal gray zone lymphoma: do they require a unique therapeutic approach? Blood 2015;125:33-39.

3. Eberle FC, Rodriguez-Canales J, Wei L, et al. Methylation profiling of mediastinal gray zone lymphoma reveals a distinctive signature with elements shared by classical Hodgkin's lymphoma and primary mediastinal large B-cell lymphoma. Haematologica 2011;96:558-566.

4. Eberle FC, Salaverria I, Steidl C, et al. Gray zone lymphoma: chromosomal aberrations with immunophenotypic and clinical correlations. Mod Pathol 2011;24:1586-1597.

4a. Elsayed AA, Satou A, Eladl AE, Kato S, Nakamura S, Asano N. Grey zone lymphoma with features intermediate between diffuse large B-cell lymphoma and classical Hodgkin lymphoma: a clinicopathological study of 14 Epstein-Barr virus-positive cases. Histopathology 2017;70:579-594.

5. Evens AM, Kanakry JA, Sehn LH, et al. Gray zone lymphoma with features intermediate between classical Hodgkin lymphoma and diffuse large B-cell lymphoma: characteristics, outcomes, and prognosticaltion among a large multicenter cohort. Am J Hematol 2015;90:778-783.

6. Garcia JF, Mollejo M, Fraga M, et al. Large B-cell lymphoma with Hodgkin's features. Histopathology 2005;47:101-110.

7. Gualco G, Natkunam Y, Bacchi CE. The spectrum of B-cell lymphoma, unclassifiable, with features intermediate between diffuse large B-cell lymphoma and classical Hodgkin lymphoma: a description of 10 cases. Mod Pathol 2012;25:661-674.

8. Iwaki N, Sato Y, Kurokawa T, et al. B-cell lymphoma, unclassifiable, with features intermediate between diffuse large B-cell lymphoma and classical Hodgkin lymphoma without me-

diastinal disease: mimicking nodular sclerosis classical Hodgkin lymphoma. Med Mol Morphol 2013;46:172-176.

9. Jaffe ES, Stein H, Swerdlow SH, Campo E, Pileri SA, Harris NL. B-cell lymphoma, unclassifiable, with features intermediate between diffuse large B-cell lymphoma and classical Hodgkin lymphoma. In: Swerdlow SH, Campo E, Harris NL, et al., eds. WHO classification of tumours of haematopoietic and lymphoid tissues. Lyon: IARC Press; 2008:267-268.

9a. Kritharis A, Pilichowska M, Evens AM. How I manage patients with grey zone lymphoma. Br J Haematol 2016;174:345-350.

10. Lynnhtun K, Varikatt W, Pathmanathan N. B cell lymphoma, unclassifiable, with features intermediate between diffuse large B cell lymphoma and classical Hodgkin lymphoma: Diagnosis by fine-needle aspiration cytology. Diagn Cytopathol 2014;42:690-693.

11. O'Malley DP, Fedoriw Y, Weiss LM. Distinguishing classical Hodgkin lymphoma, gray zone lymphoma, and large B-cell lymphoma: a proposed scoring system. Appl Immunohistochem Mol Morphol 2016;24:535-540.

12. Pileri S. Controversies on Hodgkin's disease and anaplastic large cell lymphoma. Haematologica 1994;79:299-310.

13. Quintanilla-Martinez L, Fend F. Mediastinal gray zone lymphoma. Haematologica 2011;96:496-499.

14. Rudiger T, Jaffe ES, Delsol G, et al. Workshop report on Hodgkin's disease and related ('grey zone' lymphoma). Ann Oncol 1998;9(Suppl 5):S31-S38.

14a. Sarkozy C, Molina T, Ghesquières H, et al. Mediastinal grey zone lymphoma: clinico-pathological characteristics and outcomes of 99 patients from the LYSA. Haematologica 2017;102:150-159.

14b. Swerdlow SH, Campo E, Pileri SA, et al. The 2016 revision of the World Health Organization classification of lymphoid neoplasms. Blood 2016;127:2375-2390.

15. Wilson WH, Pittaluga S, Nicolae A, et al. A prospective study of mediastinal gray-zone lymphoma. Blood 2014;124:1563-1569.

29

T-LYMPHOBLASTIC LEUKEMIA/LYMPHOMA

GENERAL FEATURES

T-lymphoblastic leukemia/lymphoma is a neoplasm that is derived from immature T lymphocytes (or T lymphoblasts). Involvement of peripheral blood and bone marrow constitutes a leukemic phase, and exclusive extramedullary involvement of lymph nodes or extranodal sites with a mass lesion is designated as lymphoma. Using conventional definitions, therefore, the term *T-acute lymphoblastic leukemia* (T-ALL) is used if there are over 25 percent blasts involving the bone marrow; if the neoplasm predominantly forms a mass lesion, the designation *T-lymphoblastic lymphoma* (T-LBL) is used (7).

T-ALL and T-LBL are uncommon diseases. According to data from the Surveillance, Epidemiology, and End Results (SEER) Program of the National Cancer Institute, there were 6,000 new cases of ALL in the United States in 2016 (34). This number includes both B- and T-ALL cases, and there is no obvious sex preference overall. By far, B-ALL is more common; T-ALL accounts for about 15 percent of all cases of ALL in children and 25 to 30 percent of all cases in adults (7,11), or about 1,000 new cases per year. Lymphoblastic lymphoma represents about 1 percent of all cases of non-Hodgkin lymphoma in the United States, of which about 90 percent are of T-cell lineage.

Although the World Health Organization (WHO) classification includes cases of T-ALL and T-LBL together, there are some biological differences between them, including gene expression and mutation profiles, that may explain differences in clinical presentation (6,33). At some point in the future, it may be more appropriate to separate T-ALL from T-LBL. In addition, at the genetic level T-ALL/LBL is highly heterogeneous, suggesting a multifactorial etiology (see below).

CLINICAL FEATURES

T-ALL tends to arise in children or the elderly. Virtually all patients present with involvement of the bone marrow and peripheral blood, and the total leukocyte count is often high. Most patients also have a mediastinal mass and about 10 percent have central nervous system (CNS) involvement at initial diagnosis (7,8,11,27).

T-LBL occurs predominantly in adolescents and young adults, and males are affected more often than females. Most T-LBL patients present with an anterior mediastinal mass, without a leukemic phase (7). Other sites of involvement by T-LBL include skin, breast, liver, spleen, tonsil, CNS, and gonads (7).

HISTOLOGIC FINDINGS

Lymph Nodes

In lymph nodes involved by T-ALL/LBL, the architecture is often diffusely effaced (fig. 29-1A) (29). In partially involved lymph nodes, the neoplastic cells are usually distributed in a paracortical manner, with expansion of the interfollicular region of the lymph node and sparing or compression of residual follicles (fig. 29-2). A starry sky appearance, imparted by histiocytes engulfing karyorrhectic nuclear material, may be present, often not well developed or focal, but this pattern is prominent in 10 to 20 percent of cases (fig. 29-1B) (29). The lymphoblasts of T-ALL/LBL have a high nucleus to cytoplasm ratio, stippled or slightly condensed chromatin, inconspicuous nucleoli, and scant cytoplasm (figs. 29-1C, 29-3) (5,7,16,24). The nuclei are convoluted or round. Mitotic figures are frequently seen. Rare cases of T-ALL/LBL are associated with eosinophilia (fig. 29-4) (1).

Other Tissue Sites

In the mediastinum, T-ALL/LBL often completely replaces the thymic parenchyma in a diffuse pattern, but in some cases residual Hassall corpuscles are present. Fibrous bands may surround large aggregates of lymphoblasts and impart a low-power nodular appearance (20). At

Figure 29-1

T-LYMPHOBLASTIC LYMPHOMA INVOLVING LYMPH NODE

A: At low-power magnification, the lymph node architecture is diffusely replaced by lymphoma. The lymphoma cells extend through the capsule into perinodal adipose tissue and a starry sky pattern can be appreciated at this power.

B: At higher magnification, a prominent starry sky pattern is seen. The "stars" are histiocytes that contain apoptotic nuclear debris in their cytoplasm.

C: Oil immersion magnification shows sheets of lymphoblasts that are smaller than histiocyte nuclei and have a high nucleus to cytoplasm ratio and immature chromatin (A–C: hematoxylin and eosin [H&E] stain).

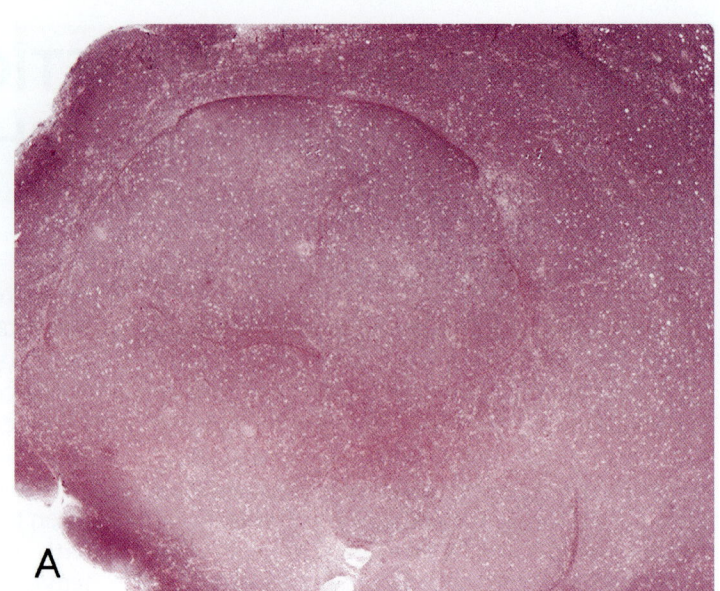

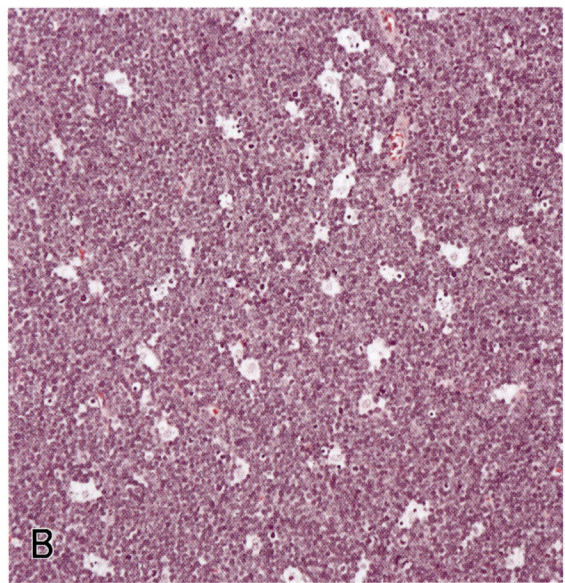

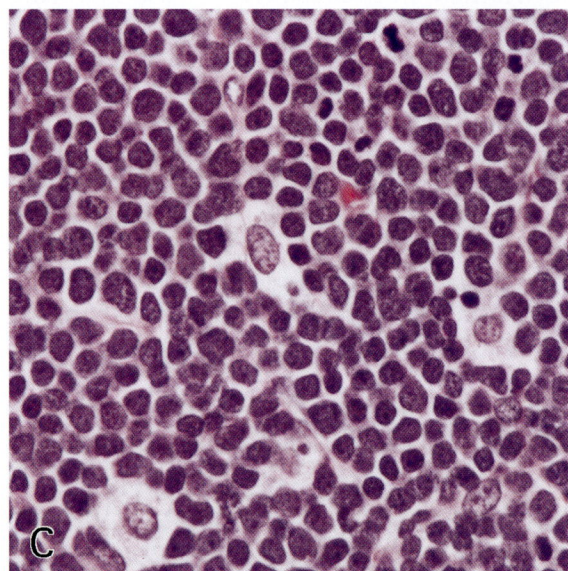

collagenous extranodal sites, lymphoblasts can infiltrate between collagen bundles and show a prominent single file pattern (fig. 29-5). In skin, T-ALL/LBL may involve the dermis in a patchy or extensive and diffuse pattern, and also can extend into deeper adipose tissue; the epidermis is usually spared (fig. 29-6). In the testis, lymphoblasts infiltrate between seminiferous tubules or completely efface the parenchyma (fig. 29-7).

Peripheral Blood and Bone Marrow

In peripheral blood (fig. 29-8) and bone marrow (fig. 29-9) aspirate specimens, T-ALL/LBL cells are small to medium-sized, but are larger than small reactive lymphocytes. Lymphoblasts have a high nucleus to cytoplasm ratio, with nuclei exhibiting a range of cytologic features (5,7). The chromatin is usually fine, with small nucleoli, and the nuclear contours are irregular (convoluted) or round. The cytoplasm is scant and slightly to deeply basophilic, and may contain vacuoles. In some cases, T lymphoblasts in smears exhibit chromatin condensation and therefore resemble, at least in part, reactive lymphocytes or the cells of a mature T-cell leukemia. In bone marrow biopsy specimens,

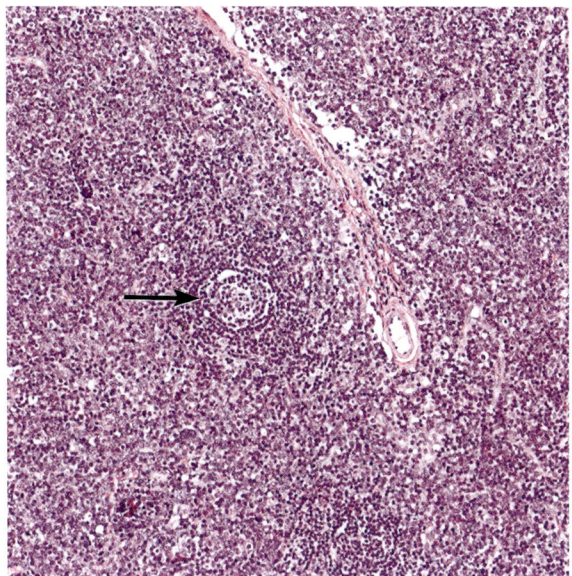

Figure 29-2

**T-LYMPHOBLASTIC LYMPHOMA
SUBTOTALLY REPLACING LYMPH NODE**

In the center of the field a small lymphoid follicle (arrow) is surrounded by lymphoblasts (H&E stain).

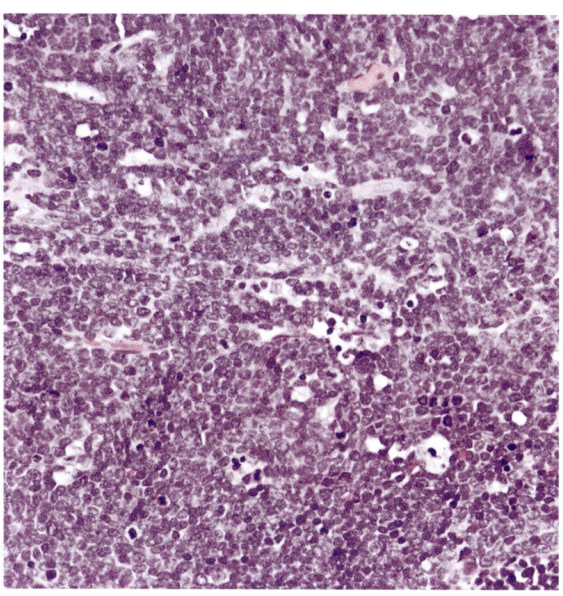

Figure 29-3

**T-LYMPHOBLASTIC LYMPHOMA
INVOLVING THE MEDIASTINUM**

The lymphoblasts have a high nucleus to cytoplasm ratio and immature chromatin. A focal starry sky pattern is present (H&E stain).

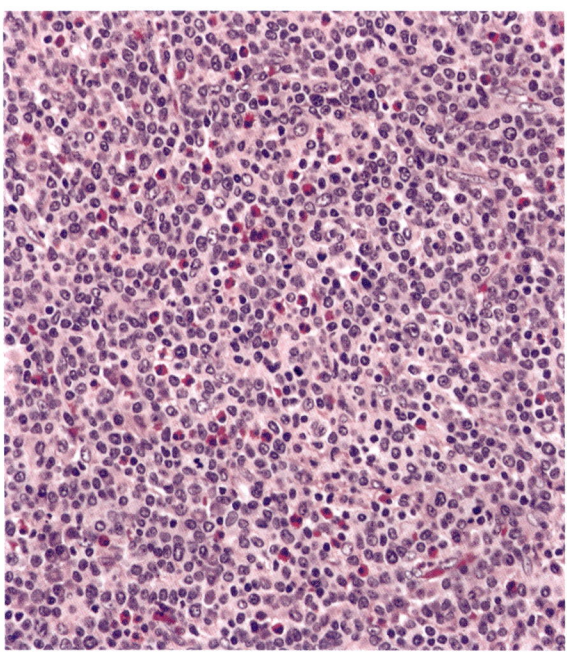

Figure 29-4

**T-LYMPHOBLASTIC LEUKEMIA/LYMPHOMA
ASSOCIATED WITH EOSINOPHILS**

In this case, many reactive eosinophils are present in the background. The patient also had eosinophilia in blood and bone marrow (H&E stain).

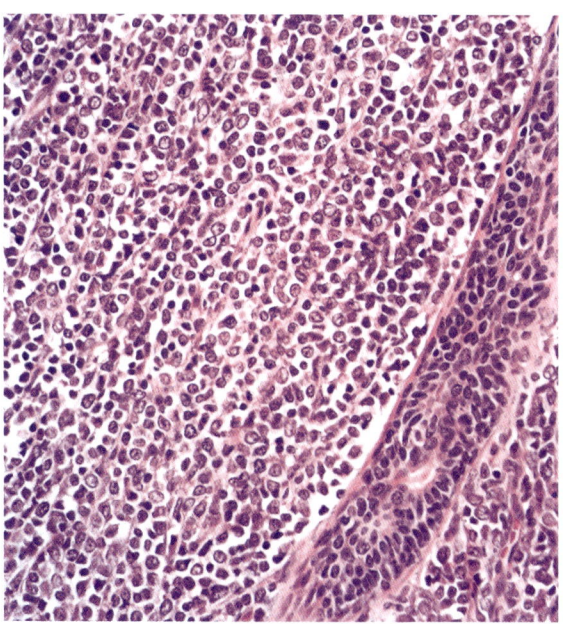

Figure 29-5

T-LYMPHOBLASTIC LYMPHOMA INVOLVING BREAST

A prominent single file pattern of infiltration is present. Without immunohistochemical studies, the possibility of lobular carcinoma might be considered (H&E stain).

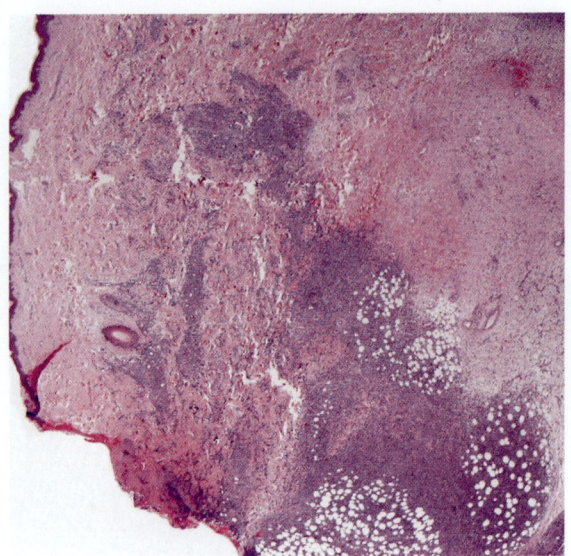
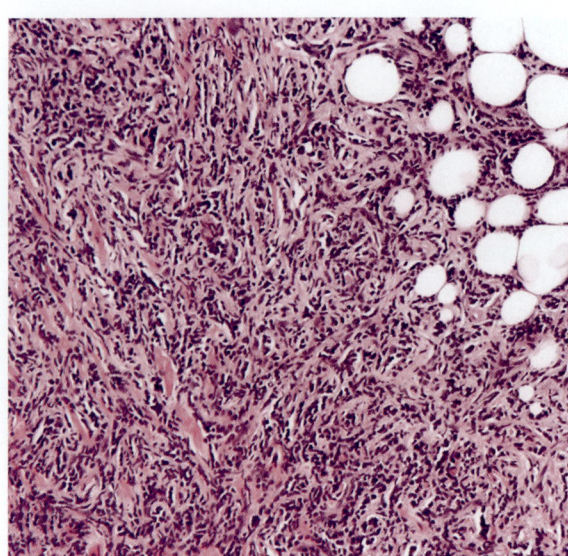

Figure 29-6

T-LYMPHOBLASTIC LYMPHOMA INVOLVING SKIN

This young man presented with only skin disease.

Left: The neoplasm Is located in the dermis and subcutaneous adipose tissue (left, right: H&E stain).

Right: In the dermis, the lymphoma cells are spindled (right) and were positive for CD34 (not shown). The diagnosis of dermatofibrosarcoma protuberans was considered initially. The patient subsequently developed blood and bone marrow involvement and the diagnosis of T-acute lymphoblastic leukemia (T-ALL) was established (immunohistochemistry with hematoxylin counterstain).

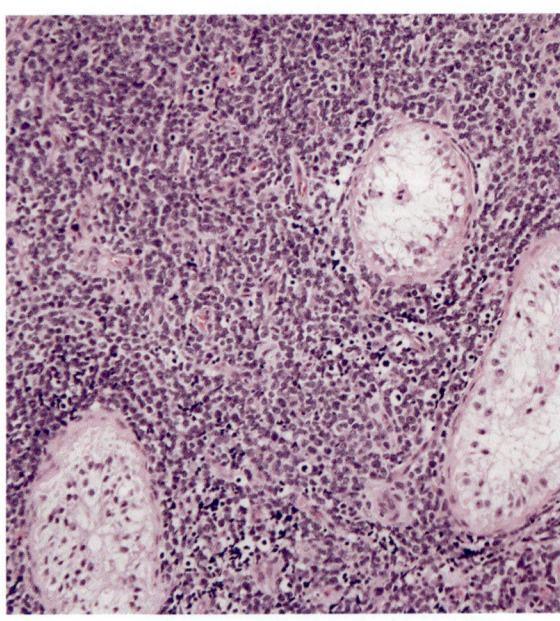

Figure 29-7

**T-ACUTE LYMPHOBLASTIC
LEUKEMIA INVOLVING TESTIS**

Lymphoblasts infiltrate between the seminiferous tubules of the testis (H&E stain).

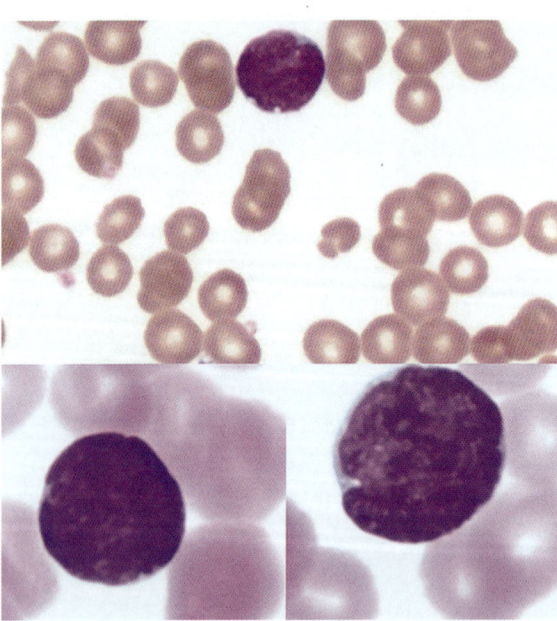

Figure 29-8

**T-ACUTE LYMPHOBLASTIC LEUKEMIA
INVOLVING PERIPHERAL BLOOD**

There is a high nuclear/cytoplasmic ratio with fine open chromatin small nucleoli, and irregular nuclear contours (Wright stain).

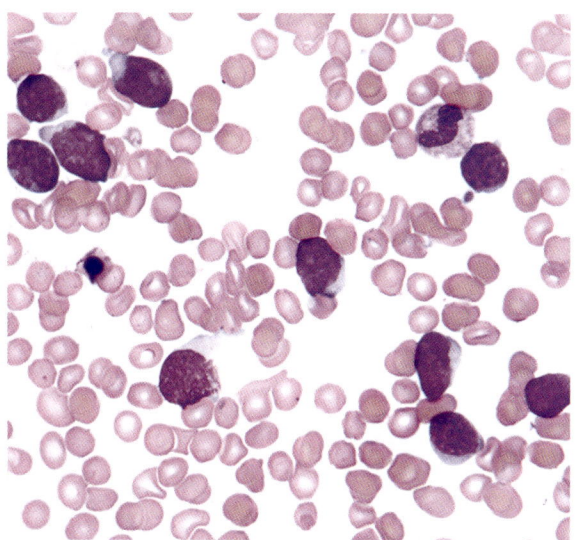
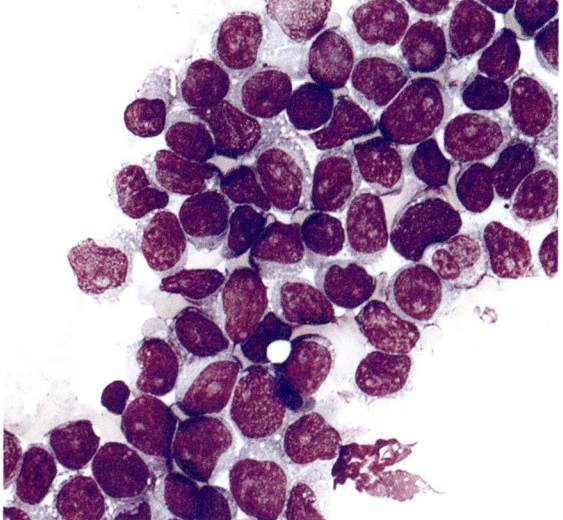

Figure 29-9

T-ACUTE LYMPHOBLASTIC LEUKEMIA INVOLVING BONE MARROW

Left: In this smear, the lymphoblasts show a range of cell sizes and have agranular cytoplasm. Most of the lymphoblasts have small indistinct nucleoli but a few larger lymphoblasts have a single, more prominent nucleolus.

Right: In this squash preparation from another patient, the lymphoblasts exhibit a range of cell sizes, from small to intermediate, with variably sized nucleoli and chromatin condensation (left, right: Wright stain).

the growth pattern is usually diffuse, but can be interstitial (fig. 29-10). The neoplastic cells show condensed nuclear chromatin and inconspicuous nucleoli.

CYTOLOGIC FINDINGS

Lymphoblasts of T-ALL/LBL exhibit a range of cytologic features but typically are of small to medium size, with a high nucleus to cytoplasm ratio (fig. 29-11) (24). The nuclei have round, slightly irregular or convoluted contours and may show finely dispersed or condensed chromatin. Nucleoli are visible although often not prominent. Mitotic figures are usually readily identified. Mature smaller lymphocytes are often scattered among the lymphoblasts. In Romanowsky stained smears, the lymphoblasts usually have minimal basophilic cytoplasm that may contain vacuoles (fig. 29-11, right).

IMMUNOPHENOTYPIC FINDINGS

Flow cytometry analysis is a very useful method to immunophenotype cases of T-ALL/LBL and is well suited to liquid specimens (fig. 29-12). The immunophenotype of neoplastic T lymphoblasts reflects their immature stage of differentiation. The concept of lymphoblasts being "frozen" in

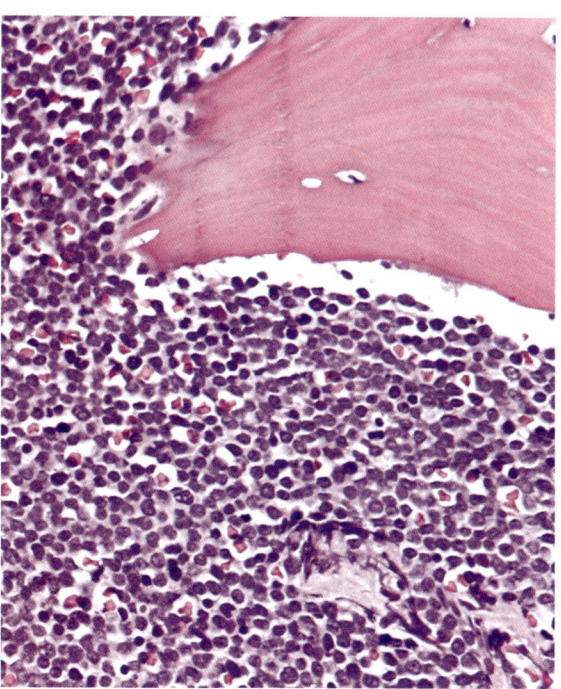

Figure 29-10

T-ACUTE LYMPHOBLASTIC LEUKEMIA INVOLVING BONE MARROW

A bone marrow biopsy specimen shows extensive and diffuse infiltration of the medullary space by T-ALL (H&E stain).

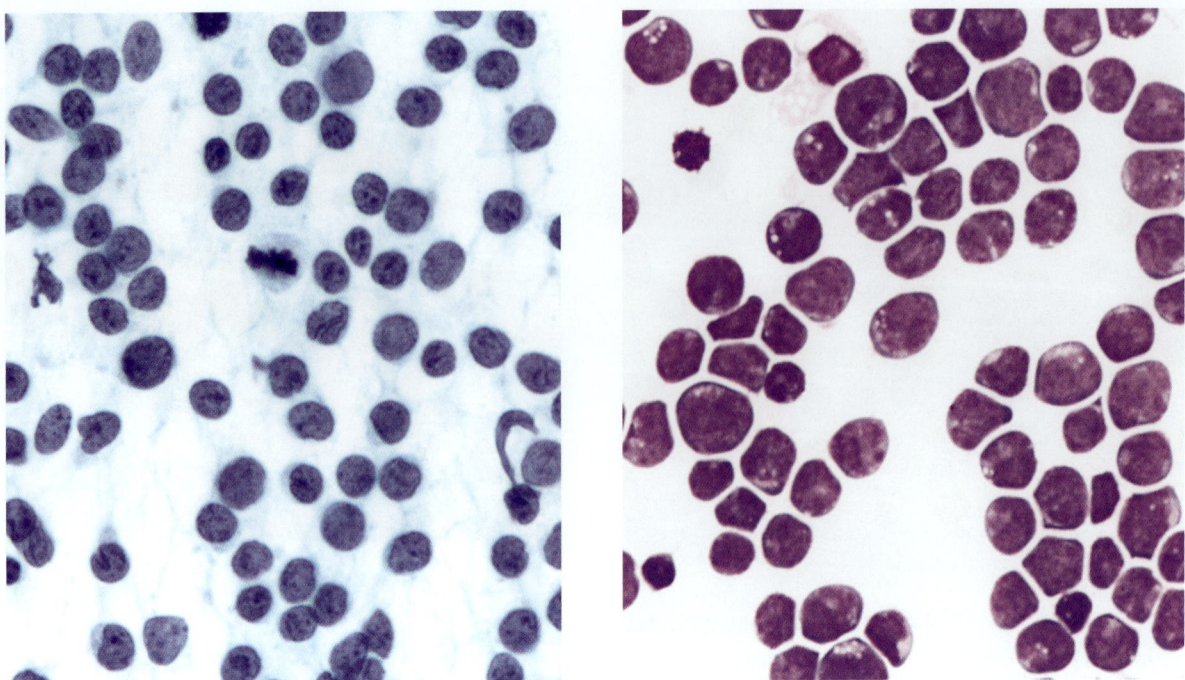

Figure 29-11

T-LYMPHOBLASTIC LYMPHOMA: CYTOLOGIC FEATURES

Left: Fixed smear obtained by fine-needle aspiration shows many lymphoblasts with immature chromatin and scattered mitotic figures (Pap stain).

Right: An air-dried smear shows fine nuclear chromatin with scant cytoplasm containing vacuoles (Diff-Quik stain).

place by neoplastic transformation is useful for understanding, although this concept is likely simplistic (7,23,31).

T lymphoblasts display a profile featuring variable reactivity for CD1a, CD2, CD3, CD4, CD5, CD7, CD8, and usually TdT. Cytoplasmic expression precedes surface expression. CD7 is the first T-cell–associated marker to be expressed, followed by CD2. Cytoplasmic CD3 is also expressed early in differentiation whereas surface CD3 is a much later event. CD4 and CD8 can be co-expressed and CD10 (common acute leukemia antigen [CALLA]) is expressed in 50 to 60 percent of cases (23). Approximately 10 percent of T-ALL/LBL cases express CD79A and a greater number express myeloid-associated antigens such as CD13, CD33, and CD117 (7,23,31,35). CD117 is associated with, but not equivalent to, the presence of activating mutations of *FLT3* (19). Approximately 10 percent of T-ALL/LBL cases do not express TdT (41). These tumors are highly immature and overlap, in part, with early T-cell precursor leukemia

(discussed subsequently). CD56 is expressed in about 10 percent of cases.

In 1995, the European Group for the Immunological Characterization of Leukemias proposed classification of T-ALL/LBL into four groups: pro-T [CD7(+)], pre-T [CD2(+) and CD5(+) and/or CD8(+)], cortical T [CD1a(+)], and mature T [surface CD3(+), CD1a(-)] (4). This approach has been a useful construct for conceptualizing T-ALL/LBL, assigning lineage, and guiding construction of diagnostic flow cytometry panels. The cortical immunophenotype is associated with a better prognosis (10). However, this approach is less helpful in understanding the heterogeneity and genetic basis of T-ALL.

In routinely processed tissue biopsy specimens, immunohistochemical analysis is helpful for diagnosis, with two caveats. First, immunohistochemistry is less sensitive than flow cytometry immunophenotyping. Second, immunohistochemistry detects cytoplasmic and surface antigens whereas standard flow cytometry methods (no cell permeabilization) only assess surface antigens. This

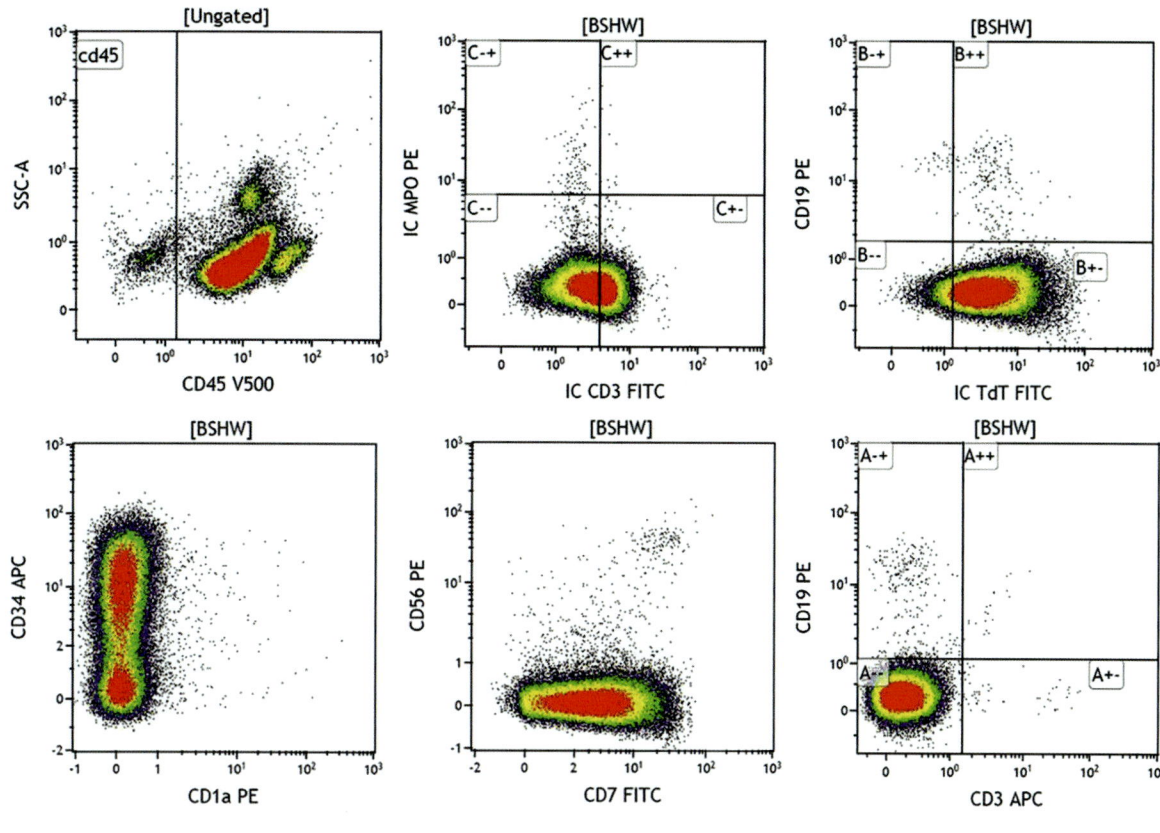

Figure 29-12

FLOW CYTOMETRIC IMMUNOPHENOTYPIC ANALYSIS OF T-ACUTE LYMPHOBLASTIC LEUKEMIA

The lymphoblasts are positive for CD3 (dim), CD7, CD34, and TdT, and are negative for CD1A, CD19, CD56, and myeloperoxidase (MPO).

can result in discrepancies between immunohistochemistry and flow cytometry when an antigen is expressed in the cytoplasm but is not yet expressed on the cell surface. The discordance between cytoplasmic CD3, which is expressed early in T-cell differentiation, and surface CD3, which is expressed much later, is perhaps most likely to cause diagnostic confusion.

Using immunohistochemistry, most of the antibodies that can be assessed by flow cytometry also can be assessed in tissue sections. Virtually all cases of T-ALL/LBL express CD7 (fig. 29-13A) and cytoplasmic CD3 (fig. 29-13B), and most express moderate-bright and nuclear TdT (fig. 29-13C) and have a brisk proliferation rate as shown by Ki-67 expression (fig. 29-13D). More mature cases (cortical thymocyte stage) express CD1A and CD10. Immature cases express CD34 and myeloid-associated antigens such as CD13 and CD33. To exclude B-cell lineage,

antibodies specific for CD19 and PAX5 are specific and sensitive. In contrast, anti-CD20 is not sensitive and CD79A is not specific.

MOLECULAR GENETIC FINDINGS

Leukemic transformation of immature thymocytes is a multistep process involving numerous genetic abnormalities that permit uncontrolled cell growth (2,13,28,37). Usually there is a primary genetic event, followed by a number of secondary genetic changes that are acquired in a nonlinear fashion.

Conventional cytogenetic studies have shown abnormalities in approximately 50 percent of cases of T-ALL/LBL (7,10,13,28); complex karyotypes occur in about 10 percent (27,28). Fluorescence in situ hybridization (FISH) analysis also has detected abnormalities in many cases in which conventional cytogenetics showed a diploid karyotype and has better defined various abnormalities.

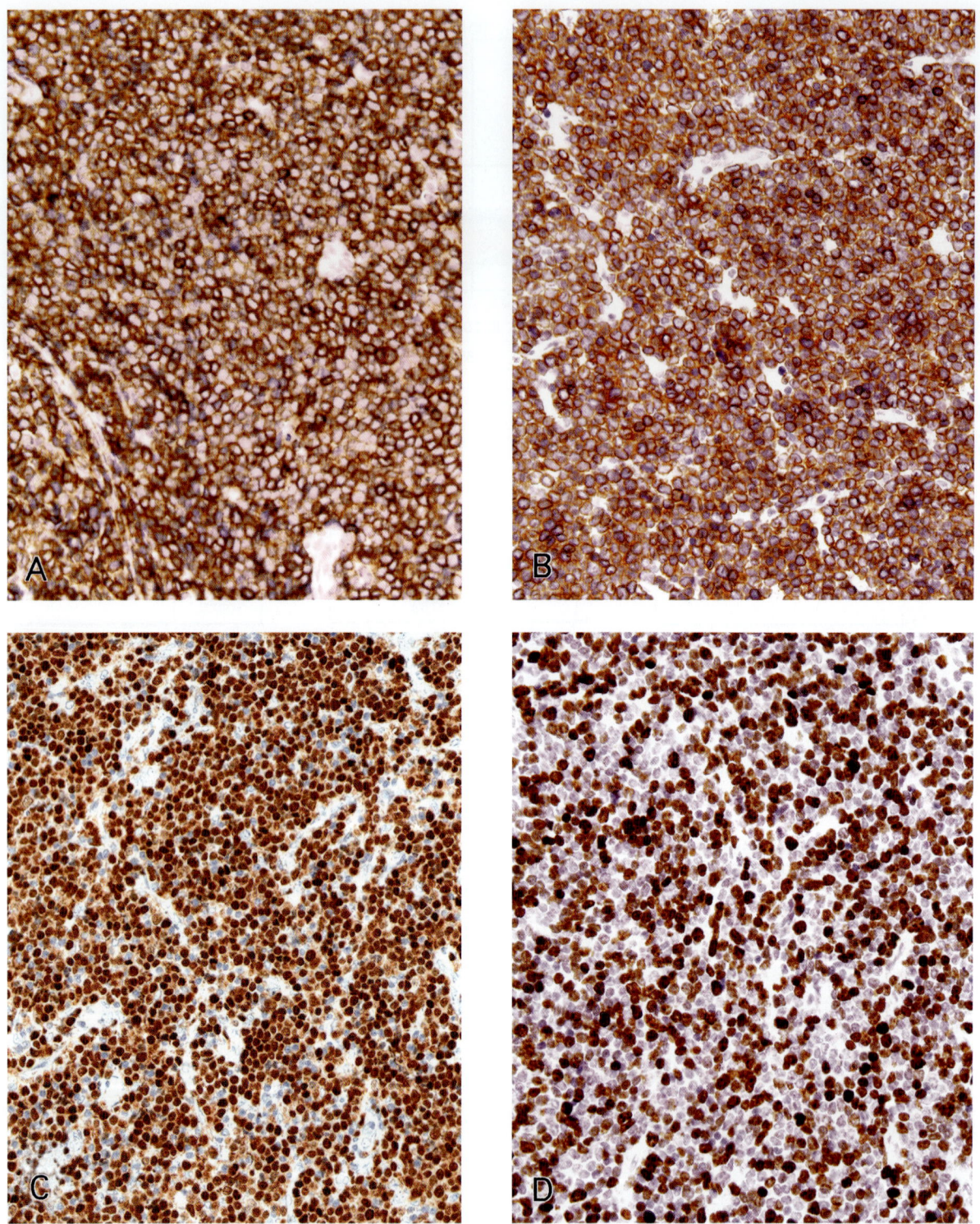

Figure 29-13

T-ACUTE LYMPHOBLASTIC LEUKEMIA/LYMPHOMA

A–D: The lymphoblasts are positive for CD7 (A), CD3(B), TdT (C), and Ki-67 (D) (immunohistochemistry with hematoxylin counterstain).

A wide range of genetic abnormalities is reported in T-ALL/LBL. Approximately 30 percent of cases carry chromosomal translocations that involve the chromosomal loci 14q11 and 7q34-35, the sites of the T-cell receptor loci *TRA/D* and *TRB*, respectively (25). The *TRG* at 7p14 is involved infrequently. A large number of genes can partner with the T-cell receptor genes in these translocations (Table 29-1). The recombinase enzymes are involved in these translocations since these enzymes recognize a recombination signal sequence that is near the oncogene partner. Mistakes in DNA repair are also involved (25).

The 11q23/*KMT2A* (also known as *MLL*) locus is involved in translocations in T-ALL/LBL. Other common abnormalities detected by conventional cytogenetics include deletions of chromosomal loci 6q, 9p, 13q, and 17p, and abnormalities of 11q (27,28). Using conventional cytogenetics or FISH, others have reported a very high frequency (up to 60 percent of cases) of chromosome 9p21/ *CDKN2A/B* deletions in T-ALL/LBL.

Molecular studies have focused more on cases of T-ALL than on T-LBL, in large part, because the cells are more easily obtained for research. There may be some differences in the molecular profile of T-ALL compared to T-LBL.

Monoclonal rearrangements of the TR loci are invariably detected in T-ALL/LBL. The *TRD* rearranges first, followed by *TRG*, *TRB*, and then *TRA* (14). Up to 20 percent of cases show rearrangements of *IGH*, so-called lineage infidelity (14). *IGK* or *IGL* rearrangements are rare in T-ALL/LBL.

Two types of translocations have been characterized in T-ALL/LBL. In one type, oncogenes are juxtaposed with the T-cell receptor genes resulting in upregulation (Table 29-1). In a second type, translocations (or cryptic deletions) result in the creation of novel fusion genes. The translocation partners include a variety of genes that affect basic cellular functions. The *KMT2A/MLL* locus is most often involved in translocations that result in chimeric fusion genes.

Gene expression profiling studies of T-ALL have shown at least four distinct molecular subsets, and early T-cell precursor leukemia (ETP-ALL) appears to represent a fifth subset (Table 29-2). These subsets correlate with known cytogenetic abnormalities, but there are also many cases of T-ALL that have the characteristic gene expression profile while lacking a cytogenetic

Table 29-1

TRANSLOCATIONS INVOLVING T-CELL RECEPTOR GENES AND THEIR PARTNERS IN T-ACUTE LYMPHOBLASTIC LEUKEMIA (ALL)/ LYMPHOBLASTIC LYMPHOMA (LBL)

TCR	Partner
TRB	*HOXA*
	TLX1
	LMO1
	LMO2
	MYB
	TAL1
	LEF1
	ILR2B
TCRA/D	*TLX1*
	LMO2
	TAL1
	MYC
	HOXA
	IGH
	NKX2-4
	GNAQ
	IGLV5-45

abnormality, thereby expanding the number of cases in each category (2,33,37).

Approximately 60 percent of T-ALLs harbor activating mutations of *NOTCH1*, which encodes for a protein that is critical for T-cell development (38). Inactivating mutations of *FBXW7*, which encodes for E3 ubiquitin ligase, are detected in 10 to 20 percent of T-ALL cases and are also a part of the *NOTCH1* pathway (39,43). *MYC* is important in T-ALL pathogenesis and a long-range *MYC* enhancer controlled by *NOTCH1*, designated as *NOTCH MYC* enhancer, also has been implicated in pathogenesis (18).

Next-generation sequencing analysis has shown that the genetic landscape of T-ALL is complex. A number of genes are mutated in different cases. Many of the more common mutations (more than 5 percent frequency) are listed in Table 29-3. The genetic profiles of pediatric versus adult T-ALL differ, suggesting that targeted therapy in the future will need to account for patient age. In children and young adult T-ALL, 106 putative driver genes have been identified in a recent study (26). In cases of adult immature T-ALL, a group that overlaps with ETP-ALL cases (see below), *ETV6* mutations and mutations of myeloid-specific genes such

Table 29-2

MUTUALLY EXCLUSIVE GENETIC SUBSETS OF T-ALL/LBL[a]

Subset	Frequency	Genes	Chromosomal Abnormalities	Prognosis
TAL/LMO	40-50%	*TAL1*	t(1;14)(p32;q11) t(1;7)(p32;q34) del(1p32)	Intermediate or good
		TAL2	t(7;9)(q34;q32)	
		LMO1	t(11;14)(p15;q11) t(7;11)(q34;p15)	
		LMO2	t(11;14)(p13;q11) t(7;11)(q34;p13) del(11p13)	
		LMO3	t(7;12)(q34;p12)	
TLX3	20%	*TLX3/HOX11L2*	t(5;14)(q35;q32)	Poor
TLX1	5-10%	*TLX1/HOX11*	t(10;14)(q24;q11) t(7;10)(q34;q24)	Good
HOXA	20%	*HOXA*	inv(7)(p15q34) t(7;7)(p15;q34) t(10;11)(p13;q14) t(11;19)(q23;p13) del(9q34)	Poor
MYB	<5%	*MYB*	t(6;7)(q23;q34)	Unknown
Early precursor T-ALL	10%	Many mutations	Identified by gene expression profiling	Poor

[a]Modified from Table 1 in reference 28.

as *IDH1, IDH2, DNMT3A, FLT3*, and *NRAS* have been reported (3,35,36).

In contrast to T-ALL, little genetic data are available for T-LBL. In a small study that used whole exome sequencing, cases of pediatric T-LBL had an appreciable frequency of mutations in seven genes: *NOTCH1, PHF6, MUC4, PRDM2, PAPPA, NFIL3*, and *ZNF91*; the latter three genes are rarely reported to be mutated in cases of T-ALL (6). In another study, *JAK2* was mutated in 2 of 16 (12.5 percent) cases of T-LBL (33a).

EARLY T-CELL ACUTE PRECURSOR LEUKEMIA

These tumors represent a relatively recently recognized type of T-ALL/LBL associated with a poorer prognosis, described initially in children (12) but also occurring in adults (17,21,30). Almost all reported cases to date have presented as T-ALL (fig. 29-14). These tumors are positive for cytoplasmic CD3, are negative or dimly positive for CD5 (fewer than 75 percent lymphoblasts), and express one or more myeloid- or stem cell-associated markers including CD11b, CD13, CD33, CD34, CD65, CD117, or HLA-DR in more

than 25 percent of lymphoblasts (12,21). Cases of ETP-ALL are negative for CD1a, CD4, CD8, and myeloperoxidase. This immunophenotype is also known as an early thymic phenotype.

Cases of ETP-ALL were originally recognized by gene expression profiling of childhood T-ALL cases and subsequently a surrogate immunophenotype was recognized (12). It needs to be remembered, however, that the immunophenotype is a surrogate and that immunophenotypic variations from the original definition may be discovered, especially in adults (39). Genetic studies of ETP-ALL have shown that these tumors have an unstable genome that is heterogeneous at the DNA level (40). There are some differences between ETP-ALL in children and adults (30). Overall, however, these tumors appear to be as similar to stem cells or early myeloid precursors as they are similar to T-cell precursors, and therefore may be derived from precursor cells in the thymus that recently immigrated from the bone marrow.

Up to 75 percent of cases of ETP-ALL have cytogenetic abnormalities, including a high frequency of deletions involving chromosomal

Table 29-3

RECURRENT (5% OR MORE) MOLECULAR ABNORMALITIES IN T-ALL/LBL[a]

Gene	Frequency	Mechanism	Cell Function	Prognosis
CDKN2A/2B	~60	9p21 deletion	cell cycle alteration	good
NOTCH1	60%	activation mutation	NOTCH1 pathway	good
PHF6	20-40%	inactivating mutation	chromatin remodeling	no impact
PTEN	20%	inactivating mutation or 10q23 deletion	tumor suppressor	no impact
FBXW7	10-20%	inactivating mutation	NOTCH1 pathway	unknown
RUNX1	10-20%	inactivating mutation	transcription factor	no impact
DNMT3A	15-20%	inactivating mutation	DNA methylation	poor
EZH2	10-15%	inactivating mutation	chromatin remodeling	poor
LEF1	10-15%	inactivating mutation	transcription factor	unknown
ETV6	13%	inactivating mutation	transcription factor	poor; associated with immature T-ALL cases
BCL11b	10%	inactivation mutation	transcription factor	no impact
WT1	10%	inactivation mutation	transcription factor	no impact
IL7R	10%	activating mutation	transcription factor	no impact
SUZ12	10%	inactivating mutation	chromatin remodeling	no impact
EED	10%	inactivating mutation	chromatin remodeling	no impact
NRAS	5-10%	activating mutation	signal transduction	no impact
JAK1	5-10% (~20% in adults)	activating mutation	signal transduction	no impact

[a]This list is likely not complete and frequencies vary in pediatric versus adult cases.

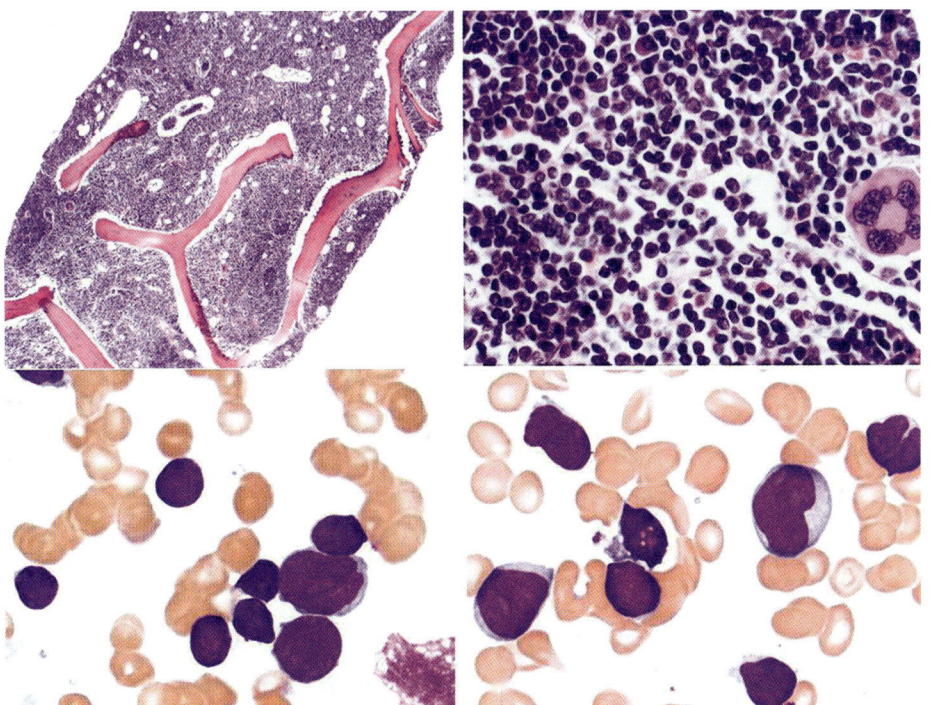

Figure 29-14

EARLY T-CELL PRECURSOR LEUKEMIA INVOLVING BONE MARROW

Biopsy specimen (top) and aspirate smear (bottom) from bone marrow (top, H&E stain; bottom, Wright-Giemsa stain).

loci 5q, 11q, and 13q (12,17). At the molecular level, genes in the JAK-STAT and RAS signaling pathways and genes involved in early hematopoietic cell development are frequently mutated (40). Compared with cases in children, cases in adults have a higher frequency of mutations of *DNMT3A, FAT1, FAT3,* and *KMT2D/MLL2* and a lower frequency of *EZH2* and *SUZ12* mutations (30). *NOTCH1* mutations are less common in ETP-ALL.

ETP-ALL Compared to Immature T-ALL

The poor prognosis of patients with ETP-ALL is generally accepted and clinically actionable, and therefore the designation of ETP-ALL needs to be used carefully. Although immunophenotypic variations from the original definition by Coustan-Smith et al. (12) are likely, as much as possible ETP-ALL needs to be defined strictly. Importantly, there are also T-ALL cases with an immature immunophenotype that express myeloid-associated markers such as CD13, CD33, and CD117 and are negative for CD1a and TdT (35). This group is broader but overlaps with ETP-ALL. EPT-ALL cases overlap with, but are not synonymous with another subset of immature T-ALL in adults, so-called *LYL1*-positive T-ALL, identified by gene expression profiling (17).

The prognosis of the larger group of immature T-ALL patients is less well established. Some have reported that patients with immature T-ALL have a poorer prognosis (27). It is unclear whether the poorer prognosis can be attributed to patients with ETP-ALL within this larger group or if an immature T-ALL immunophenotype conveys a poorer prognosis independently of ETP-ALL.

DIFFERENTIAL DIAGNOSIS

Indolent T-Lymphoblastic Proliferation. These lesions are rare and less than 20 cases have been reported at this writing. Indolent T-lymphoblastic proliferations often occur in association with other diseases including carcinomas of various types, follicular dendritic cell sarcoma, angioimmunoblastic T-cell lymphoma, Castleman disease, and myasthenia gravis.

Indolent T-lymphoblastic proliferations tend to be located in normal T-cell areas of lymphoid tissue without replacing normal architecture. The cells are morphologically similar to the cells of T-LBL, with a high mitotic rate, but unlike T-LBL, the cells of indolent T-lymphoblastic proliferation lack nuclear atypia, do not show evidence of an aberrant T-cell immunophenotype, and do not show monoclonal T-cell receptor gene rearrangements.

B-Lymphoblastic Leukemia/Lymphoma. Patients with T-LBL tend to be adolescents or young adults and patients who present with T-ALL are either much younger or elderly. Patients with T-ALL/LBL also commonly present with a mediastinal mass. In contrast, patients with B-LBL are usually young children and rarely have a mediastinal mass. At the morphologic level, B- and T-ALL/LBL are virtually identical. Immunophenotypic studies show a B- versus T-cell lineage. It is important to remember that molecular studies are less helpful for distinguishing B from T because of lineage infidelity, i.e., *IGH* rearrangements can occur in about 20 percent of T-ALL/LBL and T-cell receptor gene rearrangements occur commonly in B-ALL/LBL.

Burkitt Lymphoma. Most patients with Burkitt lymphoma present with an extranodal mass although rare patients present initially as acute leukemia. A mediastinal mass is uncommon in patients with Burkitt lymphoma, unlike patients with T-ALL/LBL.

Morphologically, Burkitt lymphoma has a prominent starry sky pattern and is composed of intermediately sized cells with multiple small nucleoli and thick nuclear membranes. In smears, Burkitt lymphoma cells usually have numerous cytoplasmic vacuoles. About 10 percent of cases of T-ALL/LBL have a prominent starry sky pattern and the presence of prominent cytoplasmic vacuoles is uncommon. Unlike Burkitt lymphoma, the cells of T-LBL are smaller, with finer chromatin. Burkitt lymphoma has a mature B-cell immunophenotype positive for surface immunoglobulin, pan-B-cell antigens, CD10, and BCL6; has a very high proliferation rate; and is negative for CD34, CD99, BCL2 and TdT. Cases of T-LBL can express BCL2, and have a high proliferation rate, but T-LBL is positive for pan-T-cell antigens, usually TdT positive and often positive for CD34 and CD99.

Diffuse Large B-Cell Lymphoma. DLBCL is composed of large cells with vesicular nuclei and often 2 to 3 prominent nucleoli. In most cases, T-LBL is morphologically distinct but there are rare cases composed of larger cells with distinct nucleoli (although usually not prominent, so-called L2 variant of T-LBL). Immunophenotypic studies are helpful because DLBCL has mature B-cell immunophenotype, quite distinct from T-LBL.

Mantle Cell Lymphoma, Blastoid Variant. Rare patients with mantle cell lymphoma, usually the blastoid variant, present with a leukemia blood picture that resembles T-ALL/LBL clinically and morphologically. Mantle cell lymphoma has a mature B-cell immunophenotype and is associated with t(11;14)(q13;q32) and cyclin D1 expression, unlike T-ALL/LBL.

Acute Myeloid Leukemia (AML)/Myeloid Sarcoma. In peripheral blood and bone marrow aspirate smears, it is well known that the blasts of AML and T-ALL/LBL can be morphologically similar. This is particularly true for cases of AML with minimal differentiation (M0 in FAB classification).

In hematoxylin and eosin (H&E)-stained tissue sections, some myeloid sarcoma cases resemble T-LBL. In about 50 percent of cases, however, the cells of myeloid sarcoma have abundant eosinophilic cytoplasm or are associated with maturing myeloid precursors such as eosinophilic myelocytes. In blood and bone marrow, flow cytometry with a complete panel is needed and helpful for the distinction. It is important to remember that a large subset of T-ALL cases express myeloid antigens, such as CD13 or CD33. In tissue specimens, immunohistochemical studies are helpful because myeloid sarcoma is positive for lysozyme, CD68, myeloperoxidase, and other myeloid-associated markers and is negative for pan-T- and pan-B-cell markers. Importantly, some markers of T-LBL, such as CD10, CD34, CD99, and TdT, are expressed in some myeloid sarcoma cases.

Blastic Plasmacytoid Dendritic Cell Neoplasm (BPDCN). BPDCN can exhibit blastic morphologic features and resemble T-LBL in tissue sections from lymph nodes, skin, or bone marrow. The cells of BPDCN can be in the size range of T-LBL and have immature chromatin; a subset of cases is positive for TdT. However, immunophenotypic studies readily distinguish the two. Unlike cases of T-LBL that have a T-cell immunophenotype and usually express TdT uniformly, the cells of BPDCN express TdT variably and have a unique immunophenotype. BPDCN is positive for CD4, CD56, CD123, TCL-1, and CD303/BDCA-2 and almost always nega-

tive for CD3. Unlike T-LBL, BPDCN is negative for T-cell receptor gene rearrangements.

Lymphocyte-Rich Thymoma. It can be difficult to distinguish T-LBL from lymphocyte-rich thymoma, particularly in small needle biopsy specimens (39). The major confounding factor is that the lymphocytes of thymoma are immature T cells that resemble lymphoblasts and have an immature immunophenotype with TdT expression similar to lymphoblasts. When the specimen is of adequate size, immunohistochemical studies show that thymoma is composed of thymic epithelial cells positive for keratin and p63, unlike T-LBL. Jegalian et al. (22) have described an antibody specific for NOTCH1 intracellular domain; all cases of T-LBL were positive and all cases of thymoma were negative in their study. Flow cytometry immunophenotypic studies are also helpful: T lymphoblasts are more uniform in their antigen expression and are usually identified in the blast gate, unlike the T cells of thymoma that show antigenic expression patterns supporting T-cell maturation. Monoclonal T-cell receptor gene rearrangements support T-LBL over thymoma.

TREATMENT AND PROGNOSIS

As has been reviewed by others (32,42), patients with T-ALL/LBL need to be treated with intensive chemotherapy regimens. The survival rate of patients with T-ALL, however, is substantially lower than of patients with B-ALL. In one large study, the 5-year overall survival rate for adults with T-ALL was 48 percent (27). Children fare better (8,11,15,32). Patients with T-LBL are treated similarly (15,42). Patients with T-ALL/LBL who relapse after therapy have a poor prognosis; stem cell transplantation has a role for high-risk prognostic groups. Investigational therapies are also being used in clinical trials, for example, α secretase inhibitors (NOTCH1); inhibitors of ABL1, JAK1, and JAK2; and histone deacetylase inhibitors (TAL1) (10).

In some, but not all studies, CNS disease has correlated with poorer prognosis. Immunophenotypic data has been correlated with prognosis, with conflicting results: CD2, CD33, CD34, CD56, and CD117 have been associated with a poorer response to therapy or survival only in some studies (10,35). There is general agreement that patients with ETP-ALL have a poorer prognosis. It may be true that patients with T-ALL that have an immature immunophenotype that expresses myeloid-associated antigens (e.g., CD13) and are negative for CD1a have a poorer prognosis (21). A complex karyotype also correlates with a worse prognosis.

The prognostic importance of various gene mutations in T-ALL/LBL is poorly understood.

NOTCH1 mutations were associated with a worse prognosis in adults with T-ALL/LBL, but not children in one study (35). In another study, *NOTCH1* mutations in pediatric T-LBL were associated with a better prognosis (9). Mutations of *DNMT3A*, *IDH1*, or *IDH2* have been correlated with poorer prognosis in adults with T-ALL (3,35).

REFERENCES

1. Abruzzo LV, Jaffe ES, Cotelingam JD, Whang-Peng J, Del Duca V Jr, Medeiros LJ. T-cell lymphoblastic lymphoma with eosinophilia associated with subsequent myeloid malignancy. Am J Surg Pathol 1992;16:236-245.

2. Aifantis I, Raetz E, Buonamic S. Molecular pathogenesis of T-cell leukaemia and lymphoma. Nat Rev Immunol 2008;8:380-390.

3. Aref S, El Menshawy N, El-Ghonemy MS, Zeid TA, El-Baiomy MA. Clinicopathologic effect of DNMT3A mutation in adult T-cell acute lymphoblastic leukemia. Clin Lymphoma Myeloma Leuk 2016;16:43-48.

4. Bene MC, Castoldi G, Knapp W, et al. Proposals for the immunological classification of acute leukemias. European Group for the Immunological Characterization of Leukemias (EGIL). Leukemia 1995;9:1783-1786.

5. Bennett JM, Catovsky D, Daniel MT, et al. Proposals for the classification of chronic (mature) B and T lymphoid leukaemias. French-American-British (FAB) Cooperative Group. J Clin Pathol 1989;42:567-584.

6. Bonn BR, Huge A, Rohde M, et al. Whole exome sequencing hints at a unique mutational profile of paediatric T-cell lymphoblastic lymphoma. Br J Haematol 2015;168:308-313.

7. Borowitz M, Chan JK. T lymphoblastic leukaemia/lymphoma. In: Swerdlow SH, Campo E. Harris NL, et al., eds. WHO classification of tumours of haematopoietic and lymphoid tissues. Lyon: IARC Press; 2008:176-178.

8. Burkhardt B, Reiter A, Landmann E, et al. Poor outcome for children and adolescents with progressive disease or relapse of lymphoblastic lymphoma: a report from the Berlin-Frankfurt-Muenster group. J Clin Oncol 2009;27:3363-3369.

9. Callens C, Baleydier F, Lengline E, et al. Clinical impact of NOTCH1 and/or FBXW7 mutations, FLASH deletion, and TCR status in pediatric T-cell lymphoblastic lymphoma. J Clin Oncol 2012;30:1966-1973.

10. Chiaretti S, Foa R. T-cell acute lymphoblastic leukemia. Haematologica 2009;94:160-162.

11. Chiaretti S, Vitale A, Cazzaniga G, et al. Clinicobiologic features of 5202 acute lymphoblastic leukemia patients enrolled in the Italian AIEOP and GIMEMA Protocols and stratified in age-cohorts. Haematologica 2013;98:1702-1710.

12. Coustan-Smith E, Mullighan CG, Onciu M, et al. Early T-cell precursor leukaemia: a subtype of very high-risk acute lymphoblastic leukaemia. Lancet Oncol 2009;10:147-156.

13. De Keersmaecker K, Marynen P, Cools J. Genetic insights in the pathogenesis of T-cell acute lymphoblastic leukemia. Haematologica 2005;90:1116-1127.

14. Felix CA, Poplack DG. Characterization of acute lymphoblastic leukemia of childhood by immunoglobulin and T-cell receptor gene patterns. Leukemia 1991;5:1015-25.

15. Fielding AK, Banerjee L, Marks DI. Recent developments in the management of T-cell precursor acute lymphoblastic leukaemia/lymphoma. Curr Hematol Malig Rep 2012;7:160-169.

16. Griffith RC, Kelly DR, Nathwani BN, et al. A morphologic study of childhood lymphoma of the lymphoblastic type. The Pediatric Oncology Group experience. Cancer 1987;59:1126-1131.

17. Haydu JE, Ferrando AA. Early T-cell precursor acute lymphoblastic leukaemia. Curr Opin Hematol 2013;20:369-373.

18. Herranz D, Ambesi-Impiombato A, Palomero T, et al. A NOTCH1-driven MYC enhancer promotes T cell development, transformation and acute lymphoblastic leukemia. Nat Med 2014;20:1130-1137.

19. Hoehn D, Medeiros LJ, Chen SS, et al. CD117 expression is a sensitive but nonspecific predictor of FLT3 mutation in T acute lymphoblastic leukemia and T/myeloid acute leukemia. Am J Clin Pathol 2012;137:213-219.

20. Ioachim HL, Finbeiner JA. Pseudonodular pattern of T-cell lymphoma. Cancer 1980;145:1370-1378.

21. Jain N, Lamb AV, O'Brien S, et al. Early T-cell precursor acute lymphoblastic leukemia/lymphoma (ETP-ALL/LBL) in adolescents and adults: a high-risk subtype. Blood 2016;127:1863-1869.

22. Jegalian AG, Bodo J, Hsi ED. NOTCH1 intracellular domain immunohistochsmistry as a diagnostic tool to distinguish T-lymphoblastic lymphoma from thymoma. Am J Surg Pathol 2015;39:565-572.

23. Khalidi HS, Chang KL, Medeiros LJ, et al. Acute lymphoblastic leukemia. Survey of immunophenotype, French-American-British classification, frequency of myeloid antigen expression, and karyotypic abnormalities in 210 pediatric and adult cases. Am J Clin Pathol 1999;111:467-476.

24. Koo CH, Rappaport H, Sheibani K, Pangalis GA, Nathwani BN, Winberg CD. Imprint cytology of non-Hodgkin's lymphomas. Based on a study of 212 immunologically characterized cases: correlation of touch imprints with tissue sections. Hum Pathol 1989;20(Suppl 1):1-137.

25. Le Noir S, Abdelali RB, Lelorch M, et al. Extensive molecular mapping of TCRα/δ- and TCRβ-involved chromosomal translocations reveals distinct mechanisms of oncogene activation in T-ALL. Blood 2012;120:3298-3309.

26. Liu Y, Easton J, Shao Y, et al. The genomic landscape of pediatric and young adult T-lineage acute lymphoblastic leukemia. Nat Genet 2017. [Epub ahead of print]

27. Marks DI, Paietta EM, Moorman AV, et al. T-cell acute lymphoblastic leukemia in adults: clinical features, immunophenotype, cytogenetics, and outcome from the large randomized prospective trial (UKALL XII/ECOG 2993). Blood 2009;114:5136-5145.

28. Meijerink JP. Genetic rearrangements in relation to immunophenotype and outcome in T-cell acute lymphoblastic leukemia. Best Pract Res Clin Haematol 2010;23:307-318.

29. Nathwani BN, Diamond LW, Winberg CD, et al. Lymphoblastic lymphoma: a clinicopathologic study of 95 patients. Cancer 1981;48:2347-2357.

30. Neumann M, Heesch S, Schlee C, et al. Whole-exome sequencing in adult ETP-ALL reveals a high rate of DNMT3A mutations. Blood 2013;121:4749-4752.

31. Oschlies I, Burkhardt B, Chassagne-Clement C, et al. Diagnosis and immunophenotype of 188 pediatric lymphoblastic lymphomas treated within a randomized prospective trial: experiences and preliminary recommendations from the European Childhood Lymphoma Pathology Panel. Am J Surg Pathol 2011;35:836-844.

32. Pui CH, Campana D, Pei D, et al. Treating childhood acute lymphoblastic leukemia without cranial irradiation. N Engl J Med 2009;360:2730-2741.

33. Raetz EA, Perkins SL, Bhojani D, et al. Gene expression profiling reveals intrinsic differences between T-cell acute lymphoblastic leukemia and T-cell lymphoblastic lymphoma. Pediatr Blood Cancer 2006;47:130-140.

33a. Roncero AM, López-Nieva P, Cobos-Fernández MA, et al. Contribution of JAK2 mutations to T-cell lymphoblastic lymphoma development. Leukemia 2016;30:94-103.

34. Teras LR, DeSantis CE, Cerhan JR, Morton LM, Jemal A, Flowers CR. 2016 US lymphoid malignancy statistics by World Health Organization subtypes. CA Cancer J Clin 2016;66:443-459.

35. Van Vlierberghe P, Ambesi-Impiombato A, De Keersmaecker K, et al. Prognostic relevance of integrated genetic profiling in adute T-cell acute lymphoblastic leukemia. Blood 2013;122:74-82.

36. Van Vlierberghe P, Ambesi-Impiombato A, Perez-Garcia A, et al. ETV6 mutations in early human T cell leukemias. J Exp Med 2011;208:2571-2579.

37. Van Vlierberghe P, Ferrando A. The molecular basis of T cell acute lymphoblastic leukemia. J Clin Invest 2012; 122:3398-3406.

38. Weng AP, Ferrando AA, Lee W, et al. Activating mutations of NOTCH1 in human T cell acute lymphoblastic leukemia. Science 2004;306:269-271.

39. You MJ, Medeiros LJ, Hsi ED. T-lymphoblastic leukemia/lymphoma. Am J Clin Pathol 2015;144: 411-422.

40. Zhang J, Ding L, Holmfeldt L, et al. The genetic basis of early T-cell precursor acute lymphoblastic leukemia. Nature 2012;481:157-163.

41. Zhou Y, Fan X, Routbort MJ, et al. Absence of terminal deoxynucleotidyl transferase expression identifies a subset of high-risk adult T-lymphoblastic leukemia/lymphoma. Mod Pathol 2013;26:1338-1345.

42. Zhu MY, Wang H, Huang CY, et al. A childhood chemotherapy protocol improves overall survival among adults with T-lymphoblastic lymphoma. Oncotarget 2016;7:38884-38891.

43. Zhu YM, Zhao WL, Fu JF, et al. NOTCH1 mutations in T-cell acute lymphoblastic leukemia: prognostic significance and implication in multifactorial leukemogenesis. Clin Cancer Res 2006;12:3043-3049.

30 PERIPHERAL T-CELL LYMPHOMA, NOT OTHERWISE SPECIFIED

GENERAL FEATURES

Peripheral T-cell lymphoma (PTCL), *not otherwise specified* (NOS) encompasses a heterogeneous group of aggressive nodal and extranodal neoplasms with a mature T-cell immunophenotype. These neoplasms do not correspond to any of the more clearly defined types of T-cell and NK-cell lymphomas specified in the World Health Organization (WHO) classification (21,28a).

The approach to the classification of PTCLs differs from that used for B-cell lymphomas; in particular, the classification is more fluid. Unlike some types of B-cell lymphoma that recapitulate structures in reactive lymph nodes (e.g., lymphoid follicles) that are helpful in recognizing the cell of origin, there are no normal structures in reactive lymph nodes that allow identification of T-cell subsets. As a result, T-cell non-Hodgkin lymphomas were not recognized before the advent of immunophenotypic analysis.

Currently, the identification of T-cell lineage remains the keystone of T-cell lymphoma classification and, in practice, once a neoplasm is identified as having a T-cell immunophenotype, diagnosis begins with PTCL-NOS. If a patient has distinctive clinical features or their tumors have distinctive pathologic, immunophenotypic, or genetic features, the neoplasm is then classified into a more specific T-cell lymphoma category as specified in the WHO classification. For example, evidence of human T-cell lymphoma virus (HTLV)-1 infection points to specific classification as adult T-cell lymphoma/leukemia whereas anaplastic lymphoma kinase (ALK) expression supports the diagnosis of anaplastic large cell lymphoma. The diagnosis of PTCL-NOS remains unchanged when the patient or tumor does not have distinctive features to support classification into a more specific T-cell lymphoma category.

As new knowledge becomes available, new types of T-cell lymphoma are defined and cases once classified as PTCL-NOS are moved into a more specific category. The converse also occurs to a lesser degree: when the definition of a specific type of T-cell lymphoma is refined, in some instances, tumors once designated as that specific entity are returned to the PTCL-NOS category. In other words, past and active research has led to the discovery of new markers or more reliable criteria that have changed and will continue to change the borders between PTCL-NOS and other better-characterized mature T-cell lymphomas. Currently, PTCL-NOS cases represent 25 to 30 percent of all T-cell lymphomas.

Advances in T-Cell and NK-Cell Immunity Contribute to Classification

Advances have led to the recognition that T-cell immunity can be divided into innate and adaptive immune responses. The innate immune system is an evolutionarily older, primitive defense system important in mucosal or skin immunity. It includes dendritic cells, NK cells, and $\gamma\delta$ T cells. $\gamma\delta$ T cells represent fewer than 5 percent of normal T cells and are particularly enriched in certain locations, such as splenic red pulp, intestinal mucosa, and other epithelial sites.

The adaptive immune system, by contrast, is evolutionarily more advanced. Antigen recognition is major histocompatability complex (MHC) restricted, and the adaptive system also has immune memory allowing for more efficient responses upon re-exposure to the same antigen. T cells that are a part of adaptive immune system are quite heterogeneous and functionally complex. α/β T cells are mostly involved in adaptive immunity. Effector T cells of the adaptive immune system include regulatory T cells (T_{reg}), follicular helper T cells (T_{FH}), cytotoxic T cells, and memory T cells. CD4-positive T cells act via cytokine production, whereas CD8-positive and double-negative T cells are primarily cytotoxic, acting via secretion of cytotoxic molecules directly affecting target cells.

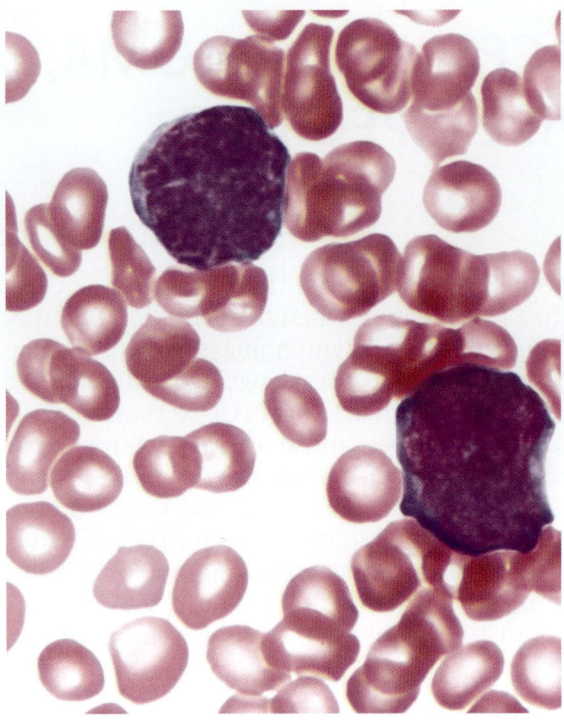

Figure 30-1

**PERIPHERAL T-CELL LYMPHOMA,
NOT OTHERWISE SPECIFIED (PTCL-NOS)**

Two lymphoma cells are present in a peripheral blood smear. Leukemic involvement is uncommon in PTCL-NOS patients (Wright-Giemsa stain).

Our improved understanding of T-cell immunity and NK cells has been applied to the study of T-cell lymphomas. Many types of T-cell lymphoma can be attributed to a cell of origin in either system. For example, γδ T-cell lymphomas and NK-cell lymphomas are likely derived from the innate immune system whereas most α/β T-cell lymphomas including PTCL-NOS are likely derived from the adaptive immune system. These studies also have shown similarities between NK and T cells, one of the reasons why NK-cell lymphomas are grouped with T-cell lymphomas in the WHO classification (21,28a).

CLINICAL FEATURES

PTCL-NOS is the most common type of T-cell lymphoma in North America and Europe, and the second most frequent type in Asia (1,31,33). In the United States, PTCL-NOS is more common in African-Americans than whites and has the lowest frequency in Native Americans (2).

The median age of patients in most studies is around 60 years, and approximately 70 percent of patients present with advanced-stage disease (III/IV) and B symptoms (1,21,31,33). About 85 percent of patients present with lymphadenopathy, but extranodal disease occurs in about 60 percent. Skin and lungs are common extranodal sites of disease. Liver and spleen are involved in 17 and 25 percent of the patients, respectively. Leukemic involvement is uncommon (fig. 30-1). Rarely, patients have a history of prior immunosuppressive therapy or an immune system disorder (33).

The International Prognostic Index (IPI) predicts overall survival and failure-free survival for patients with PTCL-NOS. A number of other scoring systems have been developed specifically for T-cell lymphomas (34). One system that predicts survival, designated as a prognostic index for T-cell lymphomas (PIT), includes patient age, performance status, serum lactate dehydrogenase (LDH) level, and bone marrow involvement (33,34). Other proposed systems incorporate one of more of these parameters as well as the presence of cytopenias, serologic or tumor-associated evidence of Epstein-Barr virus (EBV) infection, and high tumor Ki-67 (proliferation) index (5,33).

HISTOLOGIC FINDINGS

Cases of PTCL-NOS partially, or more often, diffusely replace the lymph node architecture (20,21,31). In cases with subtotal involvement, the neoplasm is preferentially located in the paracortex (figs. 30-2, 30-3). Uncommonly, PTCL-NOS has a vaguely nodular growth pattern. Postcapillary venules may be present although the degree of arborization of these vessels is substantially less than that observed in angioimmunoblastic T-cell lymphoma (fig. 30-4, left). Some PTCL-NOS cases are highly proliferative and have a partial or more fully developed starry sky pattern (fig. 30-4, right).

The overall cell population is often polymorphous and the lymphoma cells of PTCL-NOS show a broad cytologic spectrum (fig. 30-5). The neoplastic cells are typically medium-sized to large, with pleomorphic, irregular and vesicular nuclei. In many cases, a mixture of small and large cells is present. In some cases, large cells predominate and, less often, neoplasms are composed predominantly of small cells. The small cells can have abundant pale or clear cytoplasm and form

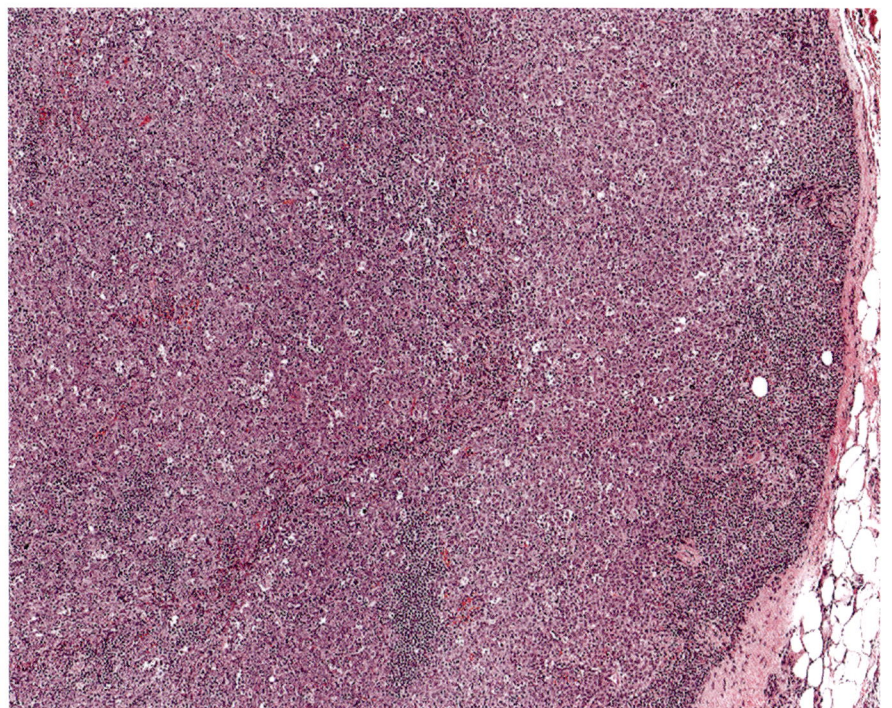

Figure 30-2

PERIPHERAL T-CELL LYMPHOMA-NOS, INVOLVING LYMPH NODE

The neoplasm has a vaguely nodular and diffuse pattern (hematoxylin and eosin [H&E] stain).

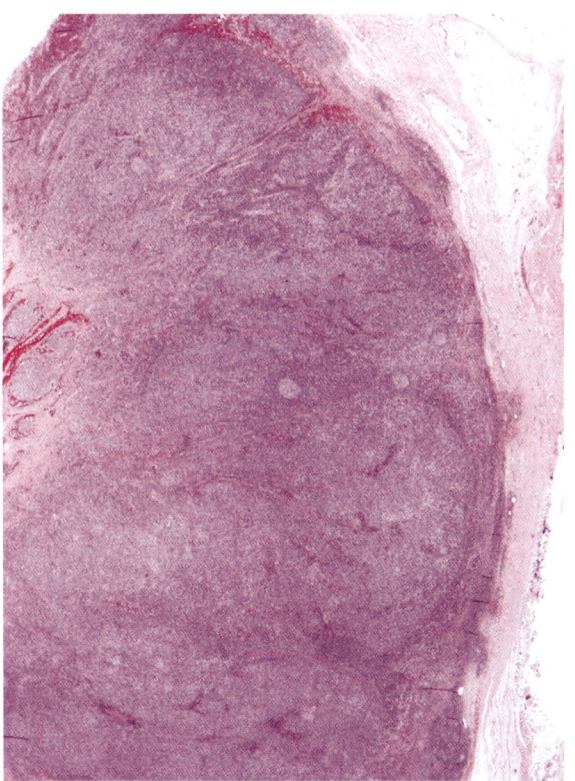
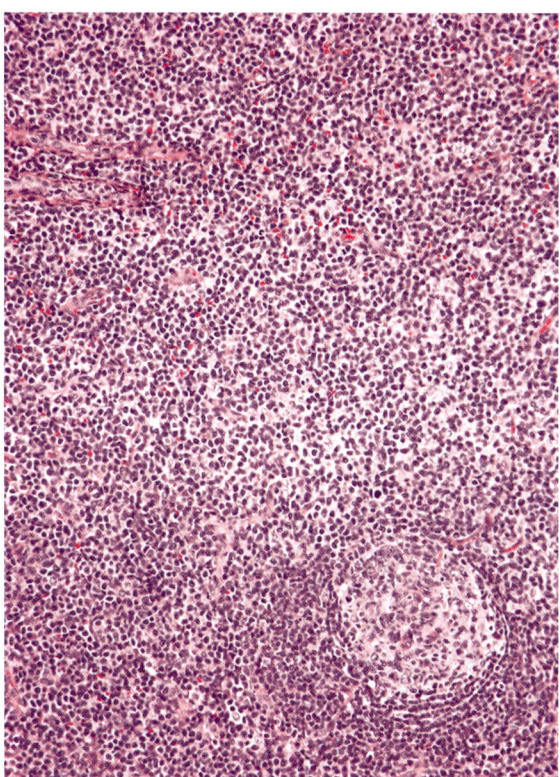

Figure 30-3

PERIPHERAL T-CELL LYMPHOMA-NOS INCOMPLETELY REPLACING LYMPH NODE
Some lymphoid follicles are spared (left, right: H&E stain).

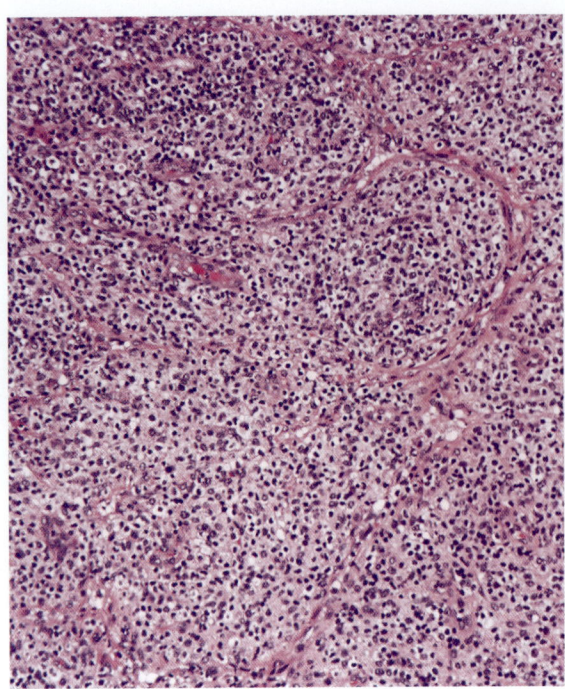
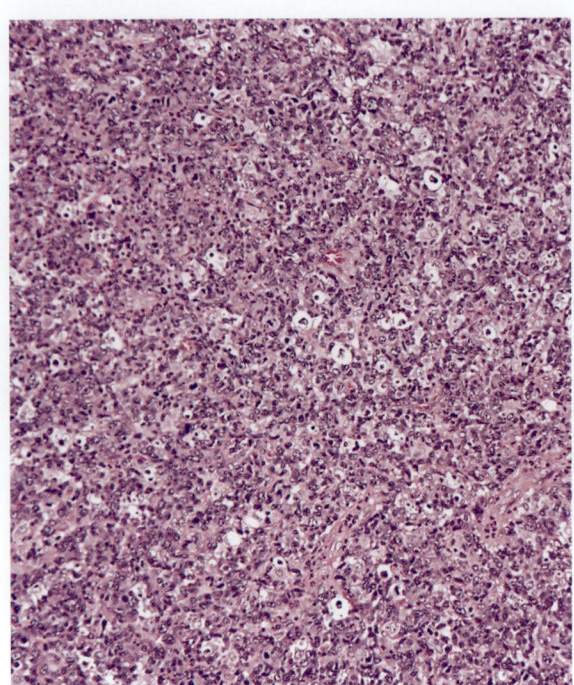

Figure 30-4

PERIPHERAL T-CELL LYMPHOMA-NOS: MORPHOLOGIC SPECTRUM

Left: In this case the neoplasm is associated with prominent vascularity.
Right: In another case, the tumor has a starry sky pattern (left, right: H&E stain).

clusters. Reed-Sternberg–like or Hodgkin-like cells may be present, usually scattered, but these cells may be more numerous (4). A variable number of eosinophils, plasma cells, small reactive lymphocytes, and epithelioid histiocytes can be observed in the background of PTCL-NOS.

MORPHOLOGIC VARIANTS

Currently, three morphologic variants of PTCL-NOS are recognized, but their morphologic, immunophenotypic, and molecular features are not considered sufficiently distinctive to justify their own category in the WHO classification (21,28a).

Lymphoepithelioid Variant

The *lymphoepithelioid variant*, also known as *Lennert lymphoma*, is characterized by an interfollicular or diffuse infiltrate of atypical small to medium-sized neoplastic T cells (fig. 30-6). Scattered, admixed large cells that may exhibit Reed-Sternberg and Hodgkin (RS+H)-like features also may be present. The microenvironment of these neoplasms is their most distinctive feature. Numerous reactive epithelioid histiocytes that form irregular and confluent clusters or rows are admixed with the lymphoma cells (6,13a). Eosinophils and plasma cells also may be present; usually, reactive cells greatly outnumber the neoplastic cells in the specimen. The proliferation of high endothelial venules is not usually prominent in the lympho-epithelioid variant of PTCL-NOS.

Based on the heterogeneous immunophenotypic features it seems likely that the lympho-epithelioid variant is heterogeneous, with one subset having a T follicular helper cell immunophenotype, likely related to angioimmunoblastic T-cell lymphoma (13a).

T-Zone Variant

T-zone lymphoma is characterized by a distinctive paracortical and perifollicular growth pattern, with partial distortion of the lymph node architecture (21). The neoplastic cells are numerous and usually small to medium in size with mild cytologic atypia. The tumor cell cytoplasm is often pale or clear. Occasional large

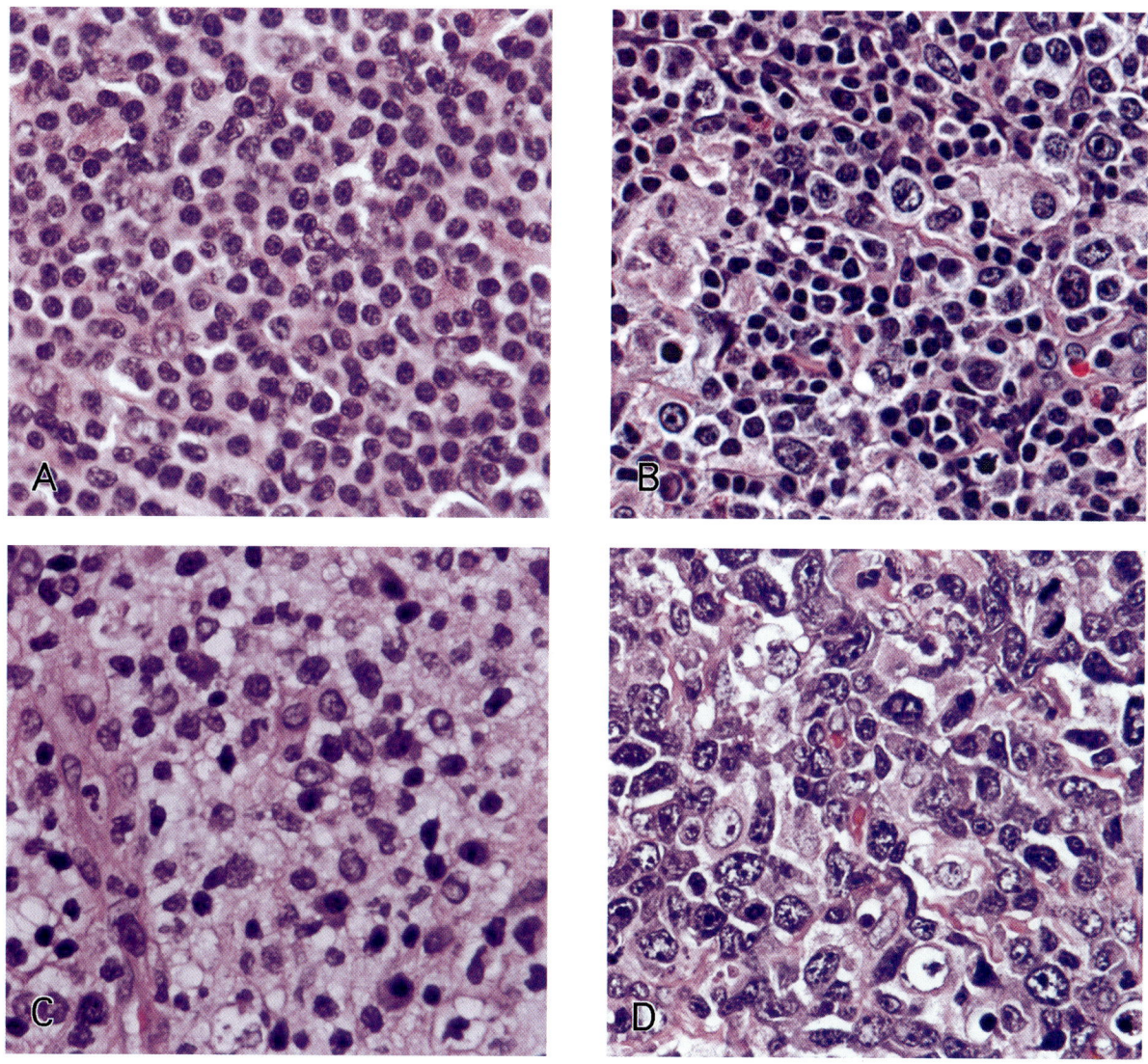

Figure 30-5

PERIPHERAL T-CELL LYMPHOMA-NOS: CYTOLOGIC SPECTRUM

A: The neoplastic cells are predominantly small cells. Occasional eosinophils are present in the background.
B: Mixed small and large cells are seen in this case.
C: Small and large cells have pale cytoplasm; plasma cells are in the background.
D: A monotonous population of large cells is present in this neoplasm (A–D: H&E stain).

neoplastic cells are present. Capsular fibrosis, polytypic plasmacytosis, and proliferation of high endothelial venules also may be present in these neoplasms.

Follicular Variant

Follicular T-cell lymphoma is a rare variant that represents 1 percent or less of all cases of PTCL-NOS (fig. 30-7) (12,16). These neoplasms likely arise from follicular helper T cells (T_{FH}) in the normal germinal center and, therefore, the growth pattern may be confined to follicles and mimic follicular lymphoma or progressive transformation of germinal centers. The neoplastic T cells also may spill over to the perifollicular area, mimicking a marginal zone lymphoma (25). The neoplastic cells are small to medium sized, with irregular or round nuclei and clear cytoplasm.

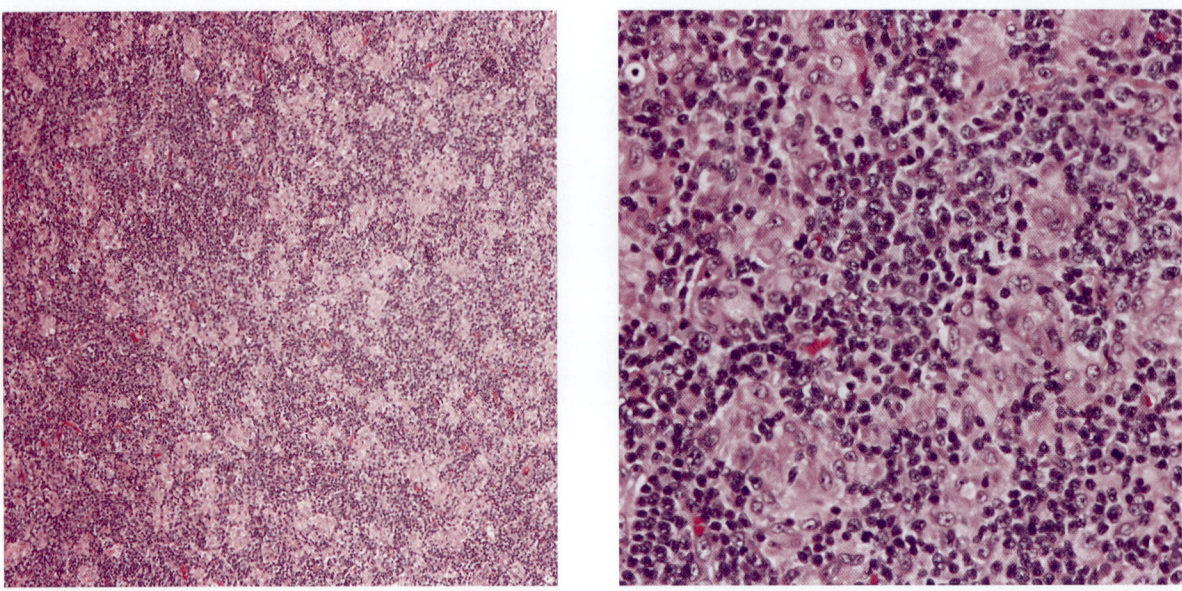

Figure 30-6

**LYMPHOEPITHELIOID VARIANT OF PERIPHERAL
T-CELL LYMPHOMA-NOS (LENNERT LYMPHOMA)**

Left: The neoplasm diffusely replaces the lymph node architecture (left, right: H&E stain).
Right: The neoplastic lymphoid cells are associated with numerous epithelioid histiocytes in clusters and rows.

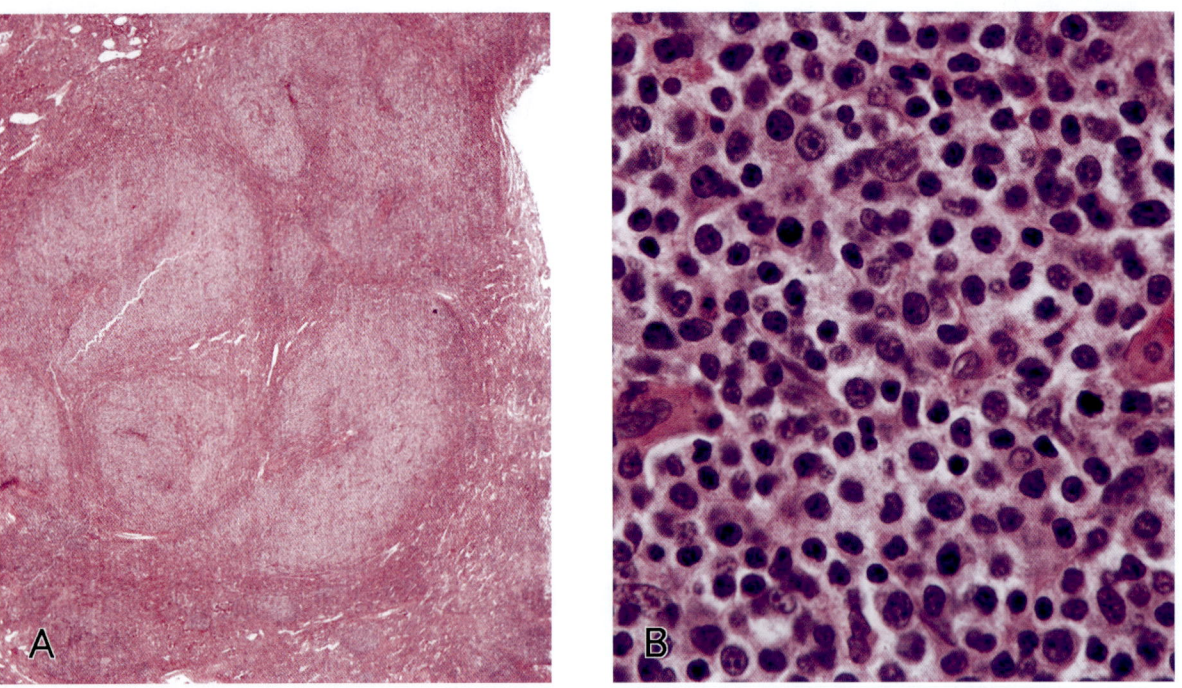

Figure 30-7

FOLLICULAR VARIANT OF PERIPHERAL T-CELL LYMPHOMA-NOS

A: The neoplasm is composed of large, expansile nodules (A,B: H&E stain).
B: High magnification shows mostly small neoplastic cells with abundant pale cytoplasm.

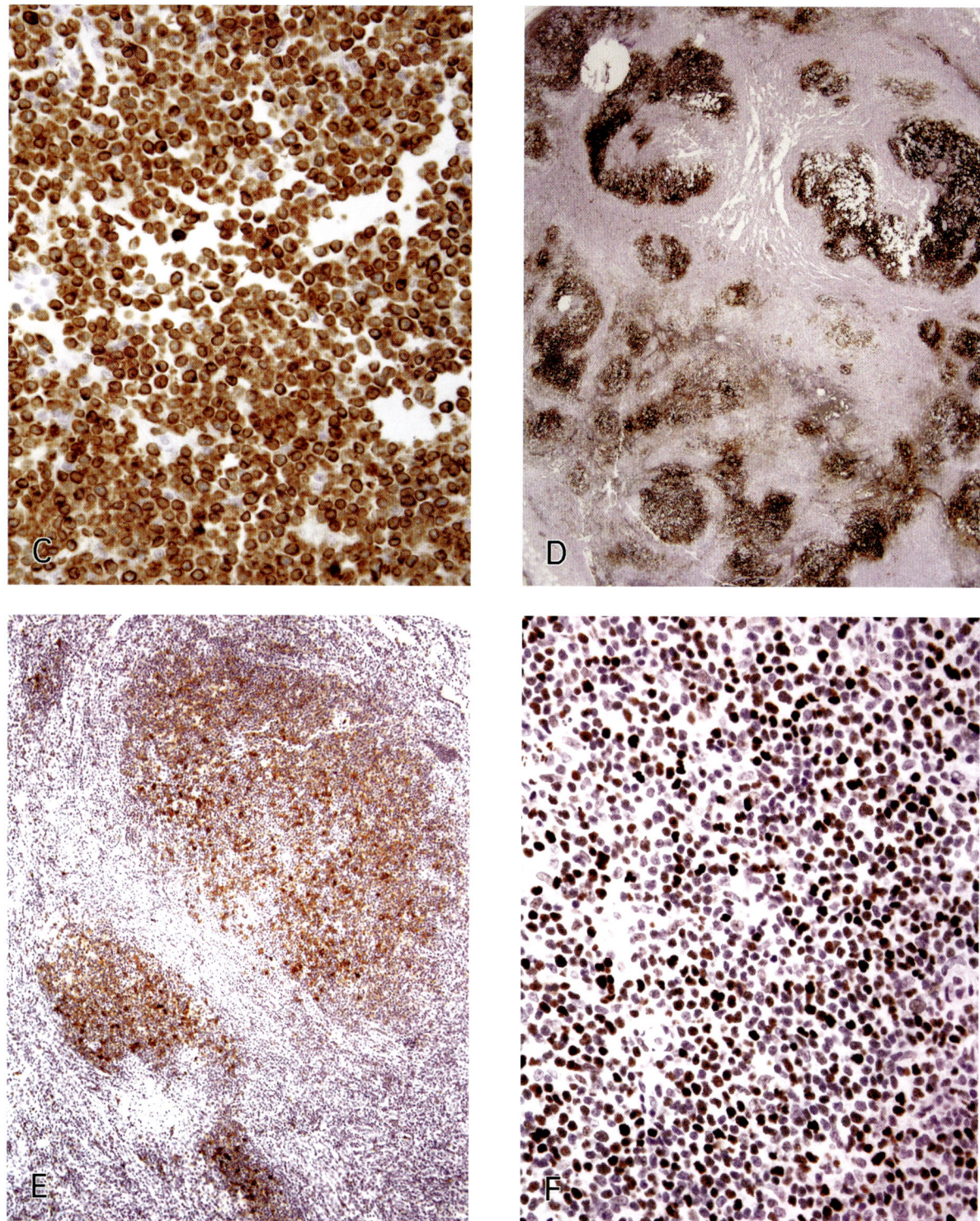

Figure 30-7, continued

C: The nodules are composed mostly of CD3-positive neoplastic T cells.

D: CD21 is expressed by many follicular dendritic cells within the tumor nodules.

E,F: The cells in the nodules are positive for PD-1/CD279 (E) and BCL6 (F), two markers expressed by follicular T-helper cells (C–F: immunohistochemistry with hematoxylin counterstain).

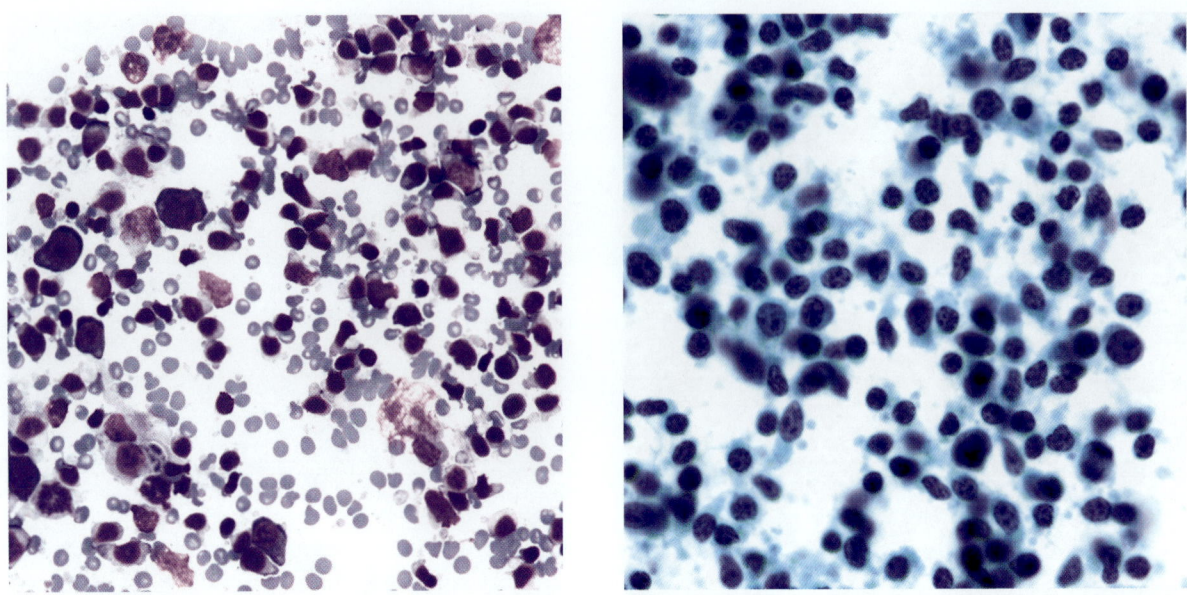

Figure 30-8

PERIPHERAL T-CELL LYMPHOMA-NOS

A polymorphic mixture of angulated lymphoma cells of small to medium size, large transformed cells, and scattered plasmacytoid cells is seen. This polymorphous mixture of cells can be misinterpreted as a reactive process without clinical correlation and immunophenotypic analysis (left: Diff-Quik stain; right: Papanicolaou stains).

Genetic data obtained on a few of these tumors suggest that follicular T-cell lymphoma may represent a distinctive subset of PTCL-NOS. In addition, some patients with follicular T-cell lymphoma at one biopsy site have had other biopsy specimens involved by angioimmunoblastic T-cell lymphoma (9,12), suggesting a close relationship. The update of the WHO classification also recognizes a subset of PTCL-NOS, diffuse pattern with a T_{FH} immunophenotype that may be related to the follicular variant of PTCL-NOS (28a).

CYTOLOGIC FINDINGS

Aspirate smears of PTCL-NOS can be quite variable, ranging from a polymorphic to a monomorphic lymphoid population. Smears may show atypical lymphocytes of variable size (small, medium, and large) with angulated or convoluted nuclei (fig. 30-8). These cells are often admixed with mature lymphocytes, plasma cells, neutrophils, and epithelioid histiocytes. Monomorphic populations may contain atypical small or large lymphocytes, also with convoluted nuclei (fig. 30-9). RS+H-like cells may also be seen.

The several morphologic variants of PTCL-NOS are usually difficult to distinguish on cytologic preparations alone. Aspirates of the lymphoepithelioid variant contain numerous epithelioid histiocytes, eosinophils, and plasma cells, in addition to lymphoma cells (fig. 30-10). Epithelioid histiocytes have oval nuclei and abundant cytoplasm, and when numerous, a lesion may mimic chronic granulomatous inflammation (29).

Aspirated material can be triaged for flow cytometry immunophenotypic analysis or molecular studies. It is important to correlate the flow cytometry results with the cytomorphologic features because T cells in smears may represent peripheral blood contamination.

IMMUNOPHENOTYPIC FINDINGS

PTCL-NOS expresses a variety of antigens or patterns of antigens. Both flow cytometry immunophenotypic and immunohistochemical analysis are helpful to establish immunophenotype (21,33). Unlike B-cell lymphomas in which monotypic light chain is used for the determination of clonality, no similar reliable and analogous marker is available to assess clonality

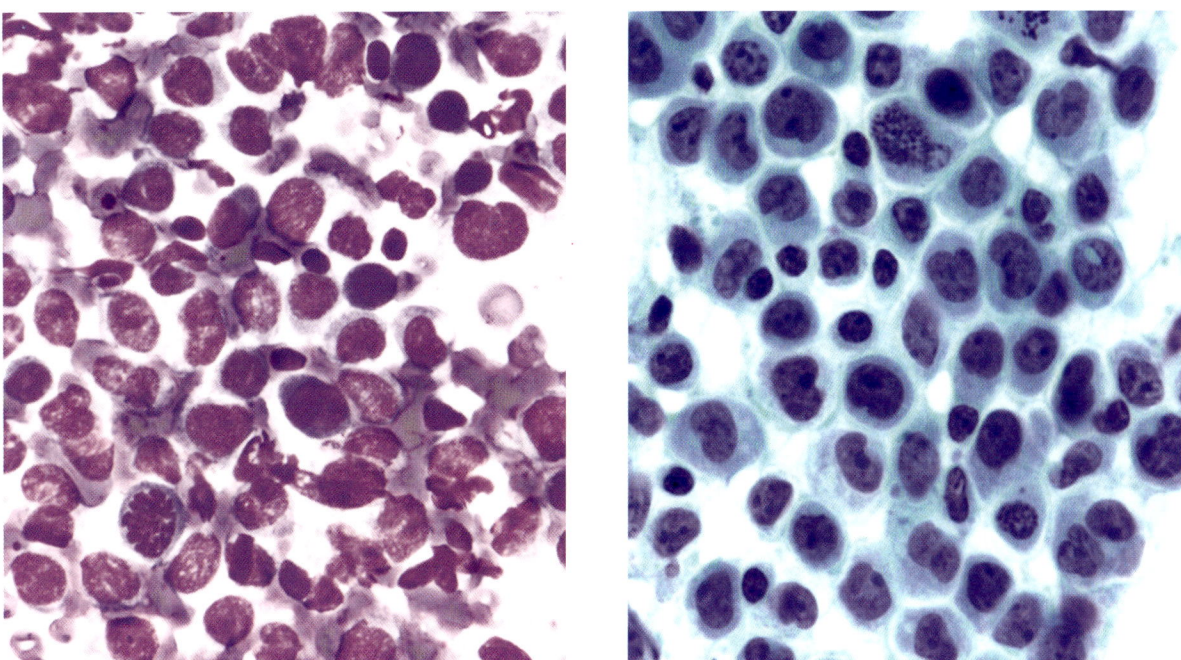

Figure 30-9

PERIPHERAL T-CELL LYMPHOMA-NOS

Medium to large lymphoma cells, many with convoluted nuclei, are present in an aspirate smear (left: Diff-Quik stain; right: Papanicolaou stain).

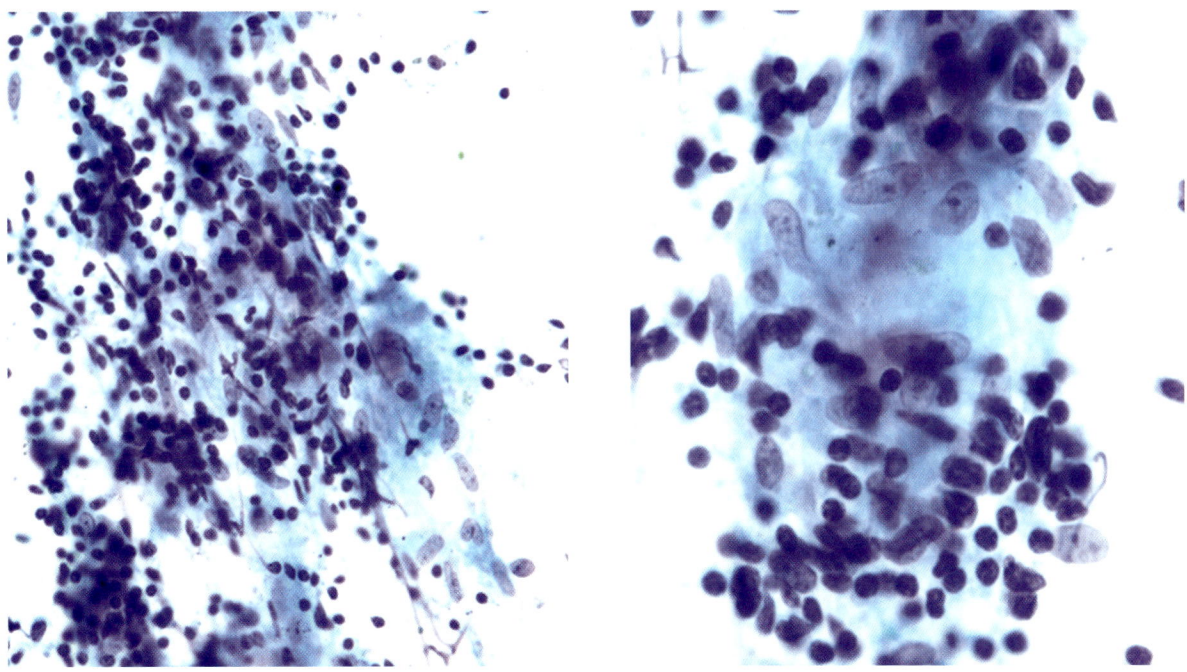

Figure 30-10

LYMPHOEPITHELIOID VARIANT OF PERIPHERAL T-CELL LYMPHOMA-NOS (LENNERT LYMPHOMA)

Small lymphocytes and epithelioid histiocytes mimic granulomatous inflammation (left, right: Papanicolaou stain).

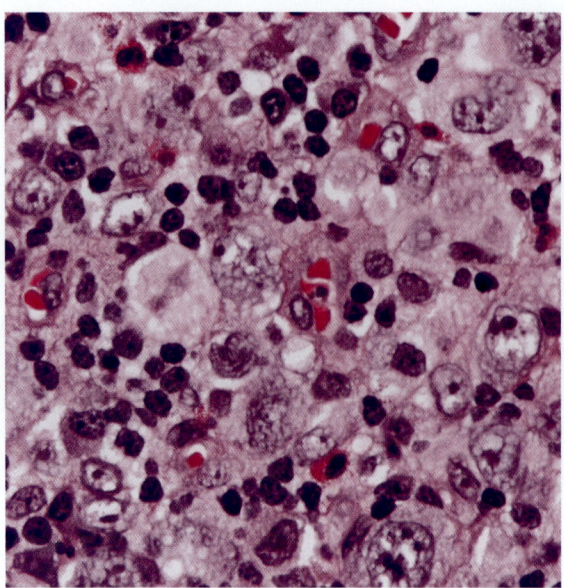
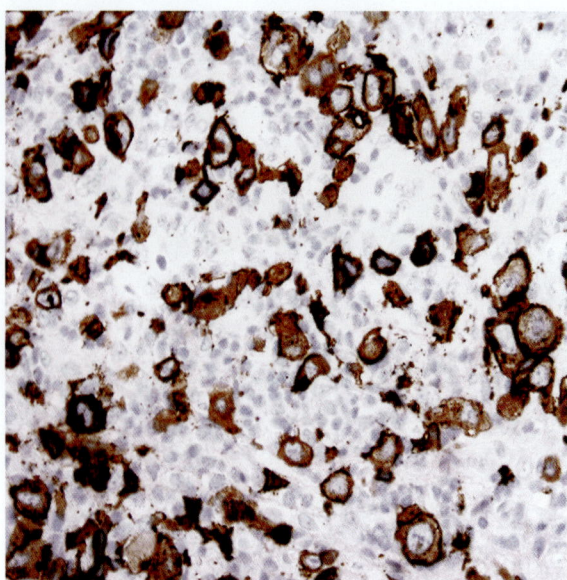

Figure 30-11

PERIPHERAL T-CELL LYMPHOMA-NOS WITH CD30-POSITIVE CELLS

Left: The neoplastic cells are large and many cells have prominent nucleoli. Eosinophils are present in the background (H&E stain).

Right: The neoplastic cells express cytoplasmic CD3 (not shown) and a subset of cells were CD30 positive (immunohistochemistry with hematoxylin counterstain).

in T-cell lymphomas. Therefore, the detection of aberrant immunophenotypes, either loss or gain of antigen(s), and detection of unusual levels of expression (high or low), are helpful findings that imply malignancy.

All cases of PTCL-NOS express at least one pan-T-cell–associated antigen, including CD2, CD3, CD5, CD7, and T-cell receptor (TCR) (αβ or γδ). About two thirds of cases of PTCL-NOS are CD4 positive and are likely derived from activated mature CD4-positive memory T cells. CD8 is expressed in 15 to 20 percent of cases and small subsets of tumors are CD4/CD8 positive or double negative for CD4 and CD8. Most cases of PTCL-NOS express TCRαβ, in accord with the normal distribution of TCRαβ and TCRγδ T cells. In our experience, however, TCRβ, as detected by the βF1 antibody, is not expressed in a subset of PTCL-NOS cases; this finding does not imply necessarily a γδ T-cell immunophenotype. Also, occasional cases of PTCL-NOS are positive for both βF1 and TCR γδ.

Ki-67 expression in PTCL-NOS is highly variable, being lower in tumors composed mostly of small cells, but usually ranges from 40 to 90 percent (33,34). MYC is overexpressed in 10 to 15 percent of PTCL-NOS and correlates with high proliferation (14a). CD30 is expressed by at least a few cells in most cases of PTCL-NOS (18a) and by an appreciable subset of tumor cells in about 33 percent of PTCL-NOS. CD30 can be strongly expressed by many lymphoma cells in a smaller subset of cases (fig. 30-11). Cytotoxic markers, including perforin, granzyme B, and TIA1, are expressed in 15 to 20 percent of PTCL-NOS cases, usually tumors that are CD8 positive and frequently associated with EBV infection (fig. 30-12) (13).

FOXP3 is expressed in a small subset of cases of PTCL-NOS and this subset may be distinctive. As has been reported by Satou et al. (27), patients with FOXP3-positive PTCL-NOS are usually older men (median age, 65 years) with advanced-stage disease and a high IPI score. These tumors usually express TCRαβ, may be positive for EBV infection, and are negative for cytotoxic markers. FOXP3 may have a role in altering the host immune response, which may explain, at least in part, the poorer prognosis associated with these tumors (27).

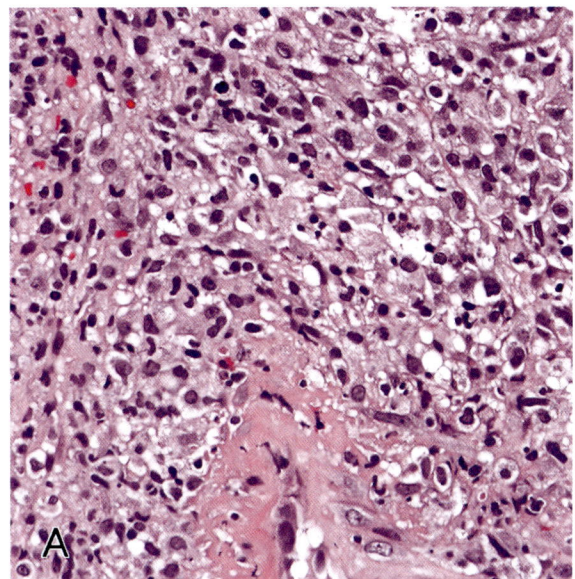

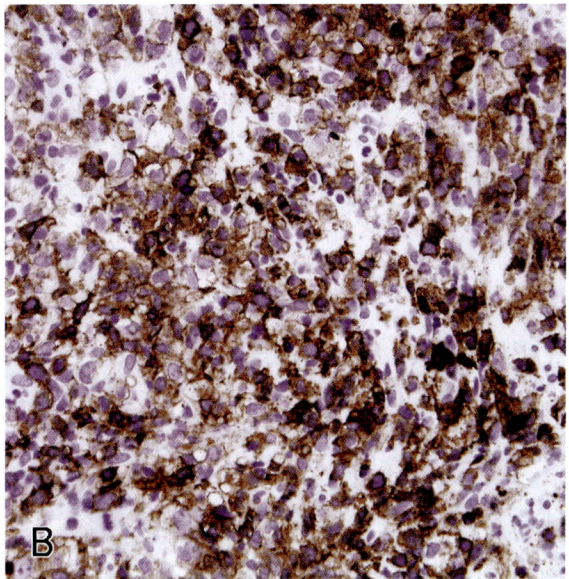

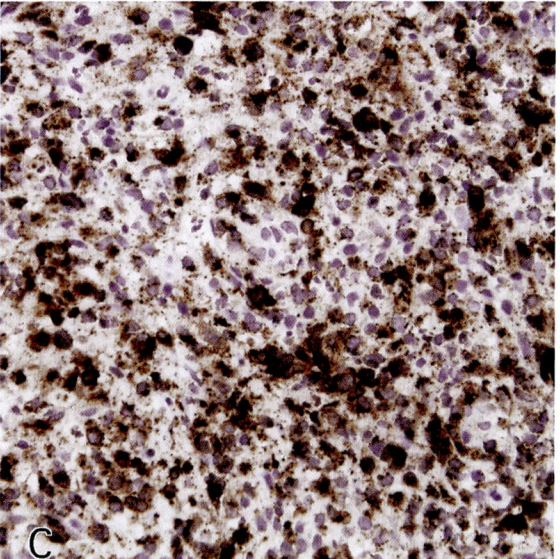

Figure 30-12

CYTOTOXIC PERIPHERAL T-CELL LYMPHOMA-NOS

A: The neoplastic cells are a mixture of small and large cells with abundant cytoplasm (H&E stain).

B,C: The neoplastic cells are positive for CD8 (B), granzyme B (C), and TIA-1 (not shown) (B,C: immunohistochemistry with hematoxylin counterstain).

CD56 is positive in 5 to 10 percent of PTCL-NOS cases and CD15 in about 5 percent, usually in tumors with large cells that can resemble RS+H cells (fig. 30-13). PTCL-NOS cases are almost always negative for pan-B-cell antigens, but rare cases express CD19, CD20 (most common), or CD79A, usually as a single aberrant marker (fig. 30-14) (22,23). Cyclin D1 is expressed usually weakly in rare cases. Myeloid-associated and NK-specific markers are negative.

Flow cytometry immunophenotyping is helpful for detecting an aberrant T-cell immunophenotype, which is present in approximately 75 percent of cases. Surface antigens most frequently lost (or showing decreased expression) include CD5, CD7, and CD3. An aberrant immunophenotype is also shown by immunohistochemistry, but generally this approach is less quantitative and less sensitive (fig. 30-15). Assessment of TCRβ receptor expression is also helpful, as expression of a single receptor implies malignancy; however, this method is successful in only about 75 percent of PTCL-NOS cases.

The morphologic variants of PTCL-NOS have some unusual features, particularly the follicular variant of PTCL. The neoplastic T$_{FH}$ cells reside

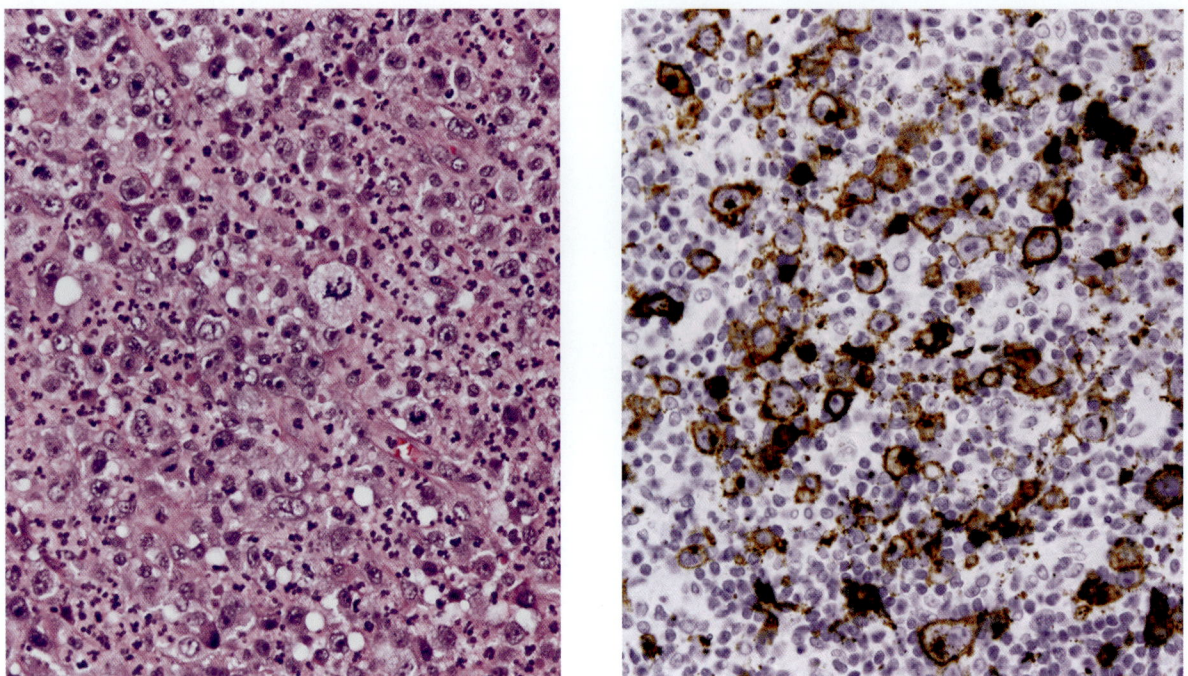

Figure 30-13

PERIPHERAL T-CELL LYMPHOMA-NOS

Left: The neoplastic cells are large and anaplastic and are associated with many background neutrophils (H&E stain).

Right: Many of the neoplastic cells are CD15 positive in this case (immunohistochemistry with hematoxylin counterstain).

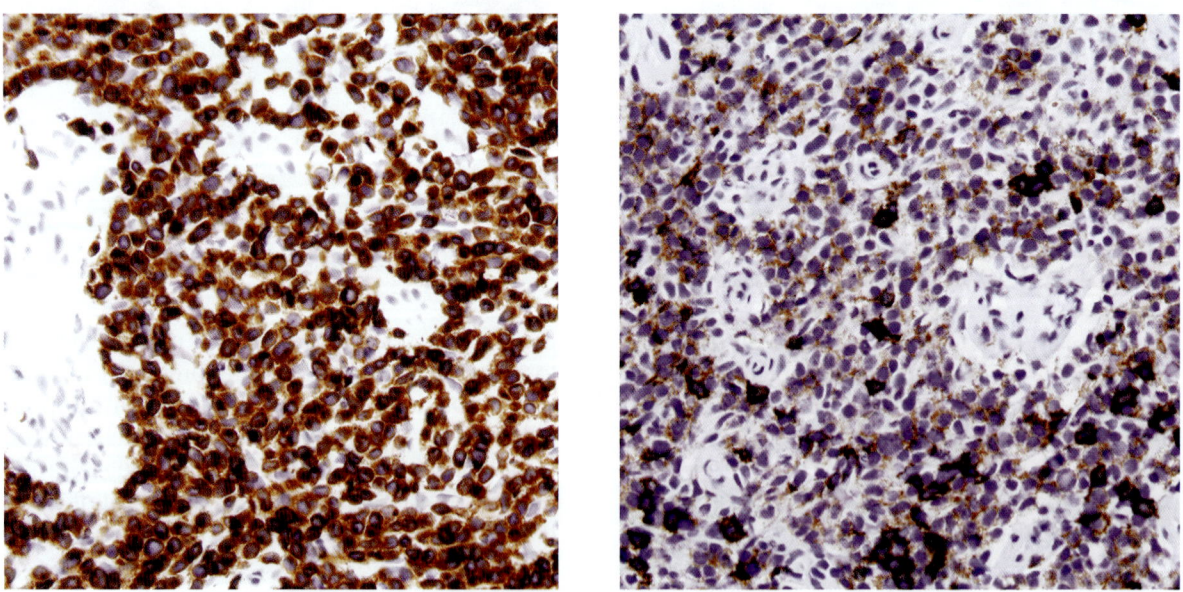

Figure 30-14

PERIPHERAL T-CELL LYMPHOMA-NOS WITH CD20 EXPRESSION

Left: The lymphoma cells are positive for CD3 and other T-cell markers (not shown).

Right: The neoplasm cells are also aberrantly positive for CD20 (immunohistochemistry with hematoxylin counterstain).

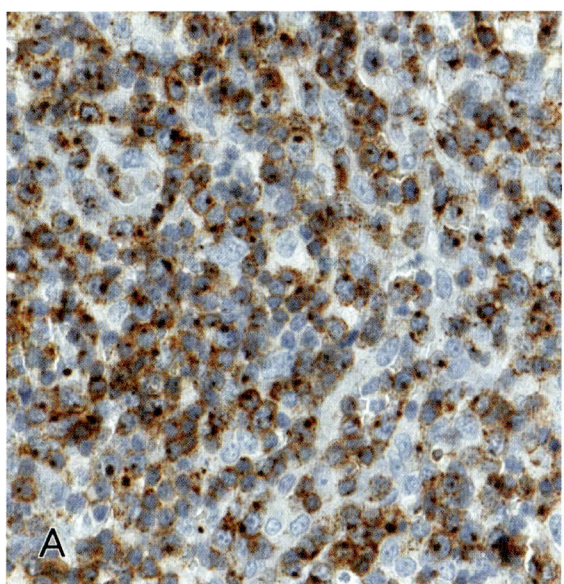

Figure 30-15

PERIPHERAL T-CELL LYMPHOMA-NOS WITH AN ABERRANT T-CELL IMMUNOPHENOTYPE

CD2 is positive (A), CD3 is positive (B), and CD5 shows dim and partial positivity (C). Reactive T cells are positive for all three antigens (immunohistochemistry with hematoxylin counterstain).

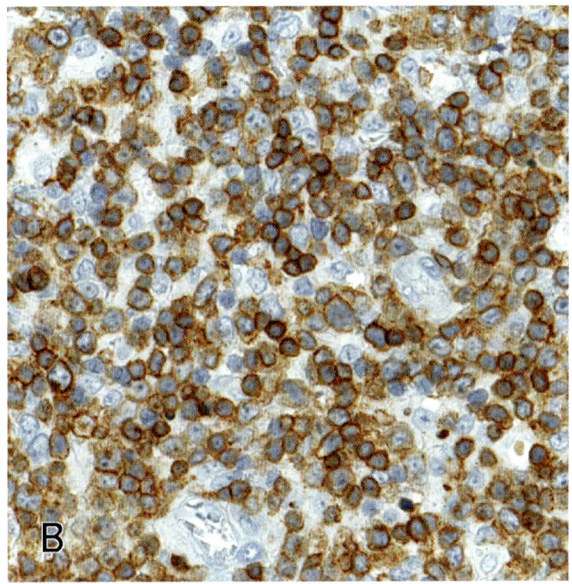

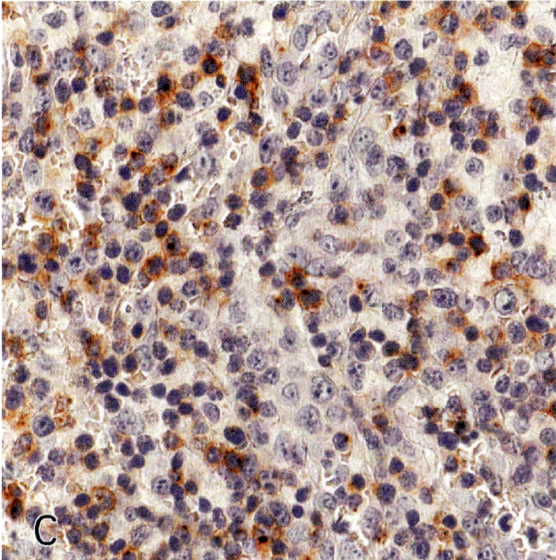

in follicles that contain abundant follicular dendritic cells and express CD10, BCL6 (see fig. 30-7), PD-1/CD279, CXCL13, and ICOS (8). These tumors are usually negative for cytotoxic markers. T-zone lymphomas are usually CD4 positive, do not express cytotoxic markers, and have generally lower Ki-67 (proliferation) rates (5,33). The lymphoepithelioid variant is heterogeneous with a CD4-positive, T$_{FH}$-positive subset and a CD8-positive, often cytotoxic, subset (13a).

Newly developed markers enable better segregation of PTCL cases into more meaning-ful biologic and prognostic subtypes (11,32). Two markers reported recently as useful for identifying subgroups with prognostic importance in PTCL-NOS are: *TBX21* (*T-bet*) and *GATA-3*, correlating with better and worse outcome, respectively.

MOLECULAR GENETIC FINDINGS

Most cases of PTCL-NOS show monoclonal rearrangement of the T-cell receptor genes (fig. 30-16). The immunoglobulin genes are in the germline configuration. Conventional cytogenetic analysis has shown that PTCL-NOS cases

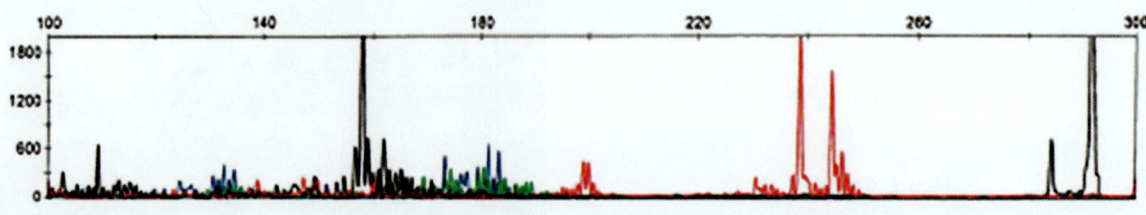

Figure 30-16

PERIPHERAL T-CELL LYMPHOMA-NOS ANALYZED FOR *TRG* REARRANGEMENTS

Rearrangements involve the V gamma I (two red peaks) and the V gamma III family (one black peak). A smear pattern of polyclonal T cells is present in the background (low level peaks of all colors). (The methods used for this analysis have been described in reference 30.)

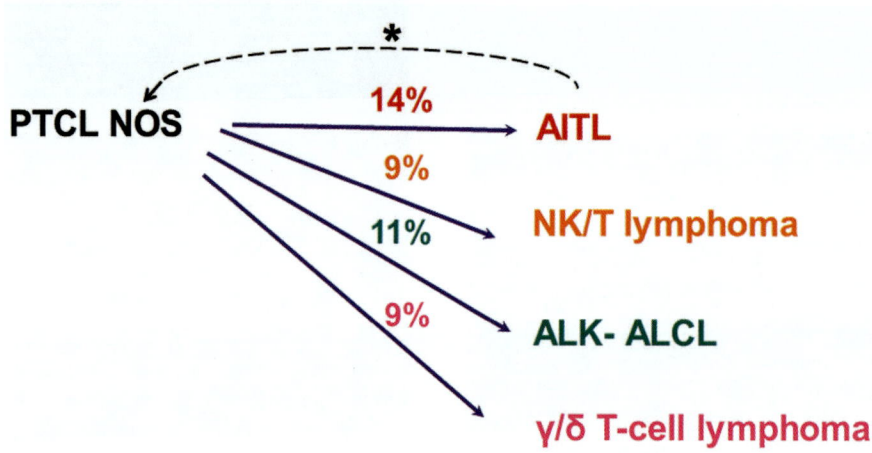

Figure 30-17

GENE EXPRESSION PROFILING ANALYSIS OF PERIPHERAL T-CELL LYMPHOMA-NOS

As shown in this schematic, some cases of PTCL-NOS have a signature more in keeping with other types of peripheral T-cell lymphoma. The arrows pointing to the right are the category suggested by the signature. The dashed line and asterisk indicate that a subset (13 percent) of cases that had been classified as AITL had signatures that were atypical for AITL and might be better classified in the PTCL-NOS category. These data highlight the fluidity of the T-cell lymphoma classification as new data emerge. (These data are based on the work of reference 11.)

commonly have highly complex karyotypes (18), data supported by the results of conventional and array-based comparative genomic hybridization studies (7). Commonly, there are gains in chromosome loci 7q, 8q, 17q, and 22q, and losses in chromosome loci 4q, 5q, 6q, 9p, 10q, 12q, and 13q (7,37). A subset of tumors shows abnormalities that involve the *REL* locus at 2p13-12 (7). The t(5;9)(q33;q22)/*TYK-SYK* is a recurrent translocation, but this abnormality occurs in only a few cases of PTCL-NOS, and appears to be most common in the follicular variant (28).

Gene expression profiling studies of PTCL-NOS have shown that these are a heterogeneous group of neoplasms (10,11). Iqbal et al. (11) have shown that about one third of cases currently classified as PTCL-NOS using traditional criteria have profiles supporting classification as more specific types of T-cell lymphoma, such as angioimmunoblastic T-cell lymphoma and anaplastic large cell lymphoma (fig. 30-17). A much smaller subset of cases, mostly classified as angioimmunoblastic T-cell lymphoma, had a profile more akin to PTCL-NOS. This study also showed that the cases with the molecular

Table 30-1

GENETIC ABNORMALITIES IDENTIFIED IN PERIPHERAL T-CELL LYMPHOMA, NOT OTHERWISE SPECIFIED (PTCL-NOS)

Molecular Abnormalities	Frequency
TBX21 signature	~50%
GATA3 signature	~30%
REL (gains/rearrangements)	~20%
CDK6 amplification	~20%
t(5;9)(q33; q22); *ITK-SYK* fusion	Follicular T-cell lymphoma (subset)
t(14;19)(q11;q13)/*BCL3* rearrangements	<5%
Gene mutations	
DNMT3A	~25%[a]
RHOA G17V	~20%[a]
TET2	~20%[a]
IDH2 mutation	≤5%
PLCG1 mutation	≤5%
CD28 mutation	≤5%

[a]Present in subset of PTCL-NOS with T_{FH} immunophenotype.

signature of PTCL-NOS can be further classified into at least two novel subgroups with distinct clinical outcomes, one with high expression of *GATA3* and its known target genes (*CCR4, IL18RA, CXCR7*) and the other with high expression of *TBX21* and its target genes including *CXCR3, IL2RB, CCL3,* and *IFN-γδ* (10,11).

These are different molecular subgroups of PTCL-NOS, with activation of different oncogenetic pathways and prognostic significance (10,11). The *GATA3* high expression subgroup is associated with poor survival and enrichment of gene signatures related to proliferation, *mTOR* and *Wnt/β-catenin*. *GATA3* also is thought to promote macrophage polarization and therefore highlights the prognostic importance of the tumor microenvironment (32). The *TBX21* high subgroup shows enrichment of IFN-γ- and NF-κB-induced gene signatures and a more favorable clinical outcome (except for a subset of cases with a cytotoxic phenotype).

A number of gene mutations have been reported in PTCL-NOS, although none are completely specific (Table 30-1) (14,15,19,26). Approximately 20 percent of cases have mutations of *RHOA* (one of the Rho GTPases), leading to alteration of this

pathway involved in cytoskeleton regulation. Almost all of these mutations target the same amino acid (glycine 17) in the GTD/GDP-binding domain of *RHOA* (15,19,26).

Other mutations in PTCL-NOS involve epigenetic regulation and T-cell activation. PTCL-NOS cases, particularly tumors that express T_{FH} markers, carry *TET2* and *DNMT3A* mutations. *IDH2^{R172}, PLCG1, CTNNB1, GTF21,* and *CD28* mutations occur infrequently (5 percent of cases or less) (19,24,29a). Yoo et al. (35) reported a *CTLA4-CD28* fusions in 9 of 39 (23 percent) cases of PTCL-NOS. *CTLA4-CD28* fusions and mutations of *RHOA, TET2, DNMT3A,* and *IDH2* are also seen in angioimmunoblastic T-cell lymphoma cases at a higher frequency (19,26,35). *CCR4* frameshift mutations were reported in 9 percent of PTCL-NOS cases in one study (36).

DIFFERENTIAL DIAGNOSIS

The diagnosis of PTCL-NOS is one of exclusion and therefore all other types of mature T-cell lymphoma should be considered in the differential diagnosis.

Angioimmunoblastic T-Cell Lymphoma (AITL). PTCL-NOS may have overlapping features with AITL. The morphologic, immunophenotypic, and genetic characteristics of AITL include vascular proliferation, clear cell cytology, follicular dendritic cell expansion encircling high endothelial venules, EBV-positive large B cells, and expression of markers of T_{FH} cells. Some cases of PTCL-NOS express markers of T_{FH} cells, and these cases overlap with and may be morphologically underdeveloped cases of AITL.

ALK-Negative Anaplastic Large Cell Lymphoma (ALCL). ALK-negative ALCL can be difficult to distinguish from cases of PTCL-NOS that express CD30. ALK-negative ALCLs have uniform and strong expression of CD30 and expression of cytotoxic markers, in addition to the characteristic morphologic and cytologic findings ("hallmark" cells) of ALCL. The presence of *DUSP22-IRF4* or *TP63* rearrangements also supports the diagnosis of ALK-negative ALCL over PTCL-NOS (3,20).

Small T-Cell Lymphomas. When a lymph node is involved by a proliferation of small to medium-sized T cells, the possibilities of adult T-cell lymphoma/leukemia, T-cell prolymphocytic leukemia, and mycosis fungoides need to be considered. Evidence of HTLV-1 infection supports adult T-cell lymphoma/leukemia. A high leukocyte and prolymphocyte count or characteristic skin lesions, help in the recognition of T-cell prolymphocytic leukemia and mycosis fungoides, respectively.

Classic Hodgkin Lymphoma. Cases of PTCL-NOS, including all variants, may have large lymphoid cells resembling RS+H cells, mimicking Hodgkin lymphoma (4,16). These large cells are commonly positive for CD30 and rarely positive for CD15, further complicating the differential diagnosis. In these cases an extended panel of B- and T-cell markers as well as analysis of the T-cell receptor genes is helpful for establishing the diagnosis of PTCL-NOS.

Nodal Marginal Zone Lymphoma. Cases of PTCL-NOS that partially involve the lymph node, sparing lymphoid follicles, and composed of clear cells can resemble nodal marginal zone lymphoma. Cases of the follicular variant of PTCL-NOS also resemble nodal marginal zone lymphoma. Immunophenotypic analysis resolves this issue because nodal marginal zone B-cell lymphomas are of B-cell lineage, express monotypic Ig, and carry monoclonal immunoglobulin rearrangements.

Follicular Lymphoma. The growth pattern of the follicular variant of PTCL-NOS closely mimics follicular lymphoma. Immunophenotypic analysis resolves this issue because follicular lymphomas are of B-cell lineage, positive for CD10 and BCL6, and carry monoclonal immunoglobulin rearrangements and t(14;18)(q32;q21)/*IGH-BCL2*.

Reactive Conditions. There are a number of benign conditions involving lymph nodes that histologically may resemble PTCL-NOS, including paracortical lymph node hyperplasia induced by viral infections or drug reactions; infectious mononucleosis; and Kikuchi-Fujimoto lymphadenitis. In particular, needle core biopsies of lymph nodes with the early/proliferative phase of Kikuchi-Fujimoto lymphadenitis can be problematic as there may be numerous immunoblasts of T-cell lineage positive for CD8 and CD30. The clinical history, the absence of architectural effacement, and no evidence of an aberrant immunophenotype or monoclonal T-cell receptor gene rearrangements support a benign disease.

TREATMENT AND PROGNOSIS

There is no consensus on the best frontline therapy for patients with PTCL-NOS. Most patients are treated with combination chemotherapy containing an anthracycline. Traditionally, cyclophosphamide, doxorubicin, vincristine, and prednisone (CHOP) have been used with overall response rates of 70 to 80 percent, but 25 percent of patients have primary refractory disease, remissions are not durable, and relapses are frequent (1,17,31). Patients with PTCL-NOS have a poor 5-year overall survival and failure-free survival rate, 20 to 30 percent (17,33). Patients with localized disease appear to have better survival rates.

A number of therapeutic approaches have been advocated for patients with PTCL-NOS. Some of these approaches build on the CHOP regimen, as reviewed by Moskowitz et al. (17). The addition of etoposide (CHOEP regimen) appears to be promising although there are concerns about toxicity. Others have advocated autologous stem cell transplantation in the first complete remission for patients who are fit and eligible. There appears to be no benefit to using allogeneic stem cell transplantation. For patients who fail these approaches, more recently developed agents that may be beneficial include brentuximab vedotin, histone deacetylase inhibitors, and SYK inhibitors among other agents (17).

In recent years a number of pathologic features have been suggested as poor prognostic indicators in patients with PTCL-NOS. These features include: proliferation (Ki-67) rate over 25 percent, number of large and transformed tumor cells over 70 percent, large numbers of EBV-positive B cells, CD56 expression, and CD30 expression by more than 20 percent of the tumor cells (5,33). The follicular variant of PTCL-NOS is usually clinically aggressive and refractory to standard chemotherapy regimens (8,9). Some data available, mostly from Asia, support the concept that PTCL-NOS patients with a cytotoxic immunophenotype and EBV infection have a poorer prognosis (13). As already mentioned, high *GATA3* or *TBX21* groups with poorer or better prognosis have been proposed (11,32).

REFERENCES

1. Abramson JS, Feldman T, Kroll-Desrosiers AR, et al. Peripheral T-cell lymphomas in a large US multicenter cohort: prognostication in the modern era including impact of frontline therapy. Ann Oncol 2014;25:2211-2217.
2. Adams SV, Newcomb PA, Shustov AR. Racial patterns of peripheral T-cell lymphoma incidence and survival in the United States. J Clin Oncol 2016;34:963-971.
3. Feldman AL, Dogan A, Smith DI, et al. Discovery of recurrent t(6;7)(p25.3;q32.3) translocations in ALK-negative anaplastic large cell lymphomas by massively parallel genomic sequencing. Blood 2011;117:915-919.
4. Eladl AE, Satou A, Elsayed AA, et al. Clinicopathological study of 30 cases of peripheral T-cell lymphoma with Hodgkin and Reed-Sternberg-like B-cells from Japan. Am J Surg Pathol 2017;41:506-516.
5. Gallamini A, Stelitano C, Calvi R, et al. Peripheral T-cell lymphoma unspecified (PTCL-U): a new prognostic model from a retrospective multicentric clinical study. Blood 2004;103:2474-2479.
6. Geissinger E, Odenwald T, Lee SS, et al. Nodal peripheral T-cell lymphomas and, in particular, their lymphoepithelioid (Lennert's) variant are often derived from CD8(+) cytotoxic T-cells. Virchows Arch 2004;445:334-343.
7. Hartmann S, Gesk S, Scholtysik R, et al. High resolution SNP array genomic profiling of peripheral T cell lymphomas, not otherwise specified, identifies a subgroup with chromosomal aberrations affecting the REL locus. Br J Haematol 2010;148:402-412.
8. Hu S, Young KH, Konoplev SN, Medeiros LJ. Follicular T-cell lymphoma: a member of an emerging family of follicular helper T-cell derived T-cell lymphomas. Hum Pathol 2012;43:1789-1798.
9. Huang Y, Moreau A, Dupuis J, et al. Peripheral T-cell lymphomas with a follicular growth pattern are derived from follicular helper T cells (TFH) and may show overlapping features with angioimmunoblastic T-cell lymphomas. Am J Surg Pathol 2009;33:682-690.
10. Iqbal J, Weisenburger DD, Greiner TC, et al. Molecular signatures to improve diagnosis in peripheral T-cell lymphoma and prognostication in angioimmunoblastic T-cell lymphoma. Blood 2010;115:1026-1036.
11. Iqbal J, Wright G, Wang C, et al. Gene expression signatures delineate biological and prognostic subgroups in peripheral T-cell lymphoma. Blood 2014;123:2915-2923.
12. Jiang L, Jones D, Medeiros LJ, Orduz YR, Bueso-Ramos CE. Peripheral T-cell lymphoma with a "follicular" pattern and the perifollicular sinus phenotype. Am J Clin Pathol 2005;123:448-455.
13. Kato S, Takahashi E, Asano N, et al. Nodal cytotoxic molecule (CM)-positive Epstein-Barr virus (EBV)-associated peripheral T cell lymphoma (PTCL): a clinicopathologic study of 26 cases. Histopathology 2012;61:186-199.
13a. Kurita D, Miyoshi H, Yoshida N, et al. A clinicopathologic study of Lennert lymphoma and possible prognostic factors: the importance of follicular helper T-cell markers and the association with angioimmunoblastic T-cell lymphoma. Am J Surg Pathol 2016;40:1249-1260.
14. Lemonnier F, Couronné L, Parrens M, et al. Recurrent TET2 mutations in peripheral T-cell lymphomas correlate with TFH-like features and adverse clinical parameters. Blood 2012;120:1466-1469.
14a. Manso R, Bellas C, Martín-Acosta P, et al. C-MYC is related to GATA3 expression and associated with poor prognosis in nodal peripheral T-cell lymphomas. Haematologica 2016;101:e336-338.
15. Manso R, Sanchez-Beato M, Monsalvo S, et al., The RHOA G17V gene mutation occurs frequently in peripheral T-cell lymphoma and is associated with a characteristic molecular signature. Blood 2014;123:2893-2894.
16. Moroch J, Copie-Bergman C, de Leval L, et al. Follicular peripheral T-cell lymphoma expands the spectrum of classical Hodgkin lymphoma mimics. Am J Surg Pathol 2012;36:1636-1646.
17. Moskowitz AJ, Lunning MA, Horwitz SM. How I treat peripheral T-cell lymphomas. Blood 2014;123:2636-2644.
18. Nelson M, Horsman DE, Weisenburger DD, et al. Cytogenetic abnormalities and clinical correlations in peripheral T-cell lymphoma. Br J Haematol 2008;141:461-469.
18a. Onaindia A, Martínez N, Montes-Moreno S, et al. CD30 expression by B and T cells: a frequent finding in angioimmunoblastic T-cell lymphoma and peripheral T-cell lymphoma-not otherwise specified. Am J Surg Pathol 2016;40:378-385.
19. Palomero T, Couronne L, Khiabanian H, et al., Recurrent mutations in epigenetic regulators, RHOA and FYN kinase in peripheral T cell lymphomas. Nat Genet 2014;46:166-170.
20. Pedersen MB, Hamilton-Dutoit SJ, Bendix K, et al. DUSP22 and TP63 rearrangements predict outcome of ALK-negative anaplastic large cell lymphoma: a Danish cohort study. Blood 2017. [Epub ahead of print]

21. Pileri S, Weisenburger D, Sng I, Jaffe ES, Ralfkiaer E, Nakamura S. Peripheral T-cell lymphoma not otherwise specified. In: Swerdlow SH, Campo E, Harris NL, et al., eds. WHO classification of tumours of haematopoietic and lymphoid tissues, 4th ed. Lyon: IARC Press; 2008:306-308.

22. Rahemtullah A, Longtine JA, Harris NL, et al. CD20+ T-cell lymphoma: clinicopathologic analysis of 9 cases and a review of the literature. Am J Surg Pathol 2008;32:1593-1607.

23. Rizzo K, Stetler-Stevenson M, Wilson W, Yuan CM. Novel CD19 expression in a peripheral T cell lymphoma: A flow cytometry case report with morphologic correlation. Cytometry B Clin Cytom 2009;76:142-149.

24. Rohr J, Guo S, Huo J, et al. Recurrent activating mutations of CD28 in peripheral T-cell lymphomas. Leukemia 2016;30:1062-1070.

25. Rudiger T, Ichinohasama R, Ott MM, et al. Peripheral T-cell lymphoma with distinct perifollicular growth pattern: a distinct subtype of T-cell lymphoma? Am J Surg Pathol 2000;24:117-122.

26. Sakata-Yanagimoto M, Enami T, Yoshida K, et al. Somatic RHOA mutation in angioimmunoblastic T cell lymphoma. Nat Genet 2014;46:171-175.

27. Satou A, Asano N, Kato S, et al. FoxP3-positive T-cell lymphoma arising in non-HTLV1 carrier: clinicopathological analysis of 11 cases of PTCL-NOS and 2 cases of mycosis fungoides. Histopathology 2016;68:1099-1108.

28. Streubel B, Vinatzer U, Willheim M, et al. Novel t(5;9)(q33;q22) fuses ITK to SYK in unspecified peripheral T-cell lymphoma. Leukemia 2006;20:313-318.

28a. Swerdlow SH, Campo E, Pileri SA, et al. The 2016 revision of the World Health Organization classification of lymphoid neoplasms. Blood 2016;127:2375-2390.

29. Vaillo Vinagre A, Gutierrez Martin A, Perez Barrios A, Alberti Masgrau N, Ruiz Liso JM. Lymphoepithelioid cell lymphoma (Lennert's lymphoma). Report of a case with fine needle aspiration cytology. Acta Cytol 2004;48:234-238.

29a. Vallois D, Dobay MP, Morin RD, et al. Activating mutations in genes related to TCR signaling in angioimmunoblastic and other follicular helper T-cell-derived lymphomas. Blood 2016;128:1490-1502.

30. Vega F1, Medeiros LJ, Jones D, et al. A novel four-color PCR assay to assess T-cell receptor gamma gene rearrangements in lymphoproliferative lesions. Am J Clin Pathol 2001;116:17-24.

31. Vose J, Armitage J, Weisenburger D, International T-Cell Lymphoma Project. International peripheral T-cell and natural killer/T-cell lymphoma study: pathology findings and clinical outcomes. J Clin Oncol 2008;26:4124-4130.

32. Wang T, Feldman AL, Wada DA, et al. GATA-3 expression identifies a high-risk subset of PTCL, NOS with distinct molecular and clinical features. Blood 2014;123:3007-3015.

33. Weisenburger DD, Savage KJ, Harris NL, et al. Peripheral T-cell lymphoma, not otherwise specified: a report of 340 cases from the International Peripheral T-cell Lymphoma Project. Blood 2011;117:3402-3408.

34. Xu P, Yu D, Wang L, Shen Y, Shen Z, Zhao W. Analysis of prognostic factors and comparison of prognostic scores in peripheral T cell lymphoma, not otherwise specified: a single-institution study of 105 Chinese patients. Ann Hematol 2015;94:239-247.

35. Yoo HY, Kim P, Kim WS, et al. Frequent CTLA4-CD28 gene fusion in diverse types of T-cell lymphoma. Haematologica 2016;101:757-763.

36. Yoshida N, Miyoshi H, Kato T. CCR4 frameshift mutation identified a distinct group of adult T-cell leukemia/lymphoma with poor prognosis. J Pathol 2016;238:621-626.

37. Zettl A, Rudiger T, Konrad MA, et al. Genomic profiling of peripheral T-cell lymphoma, unspecified, and anaplastic large T-cell lymphoma delineates novel recurrent chromosomal alterations. Am J Pathol 2004;164:1837-1848.

31 ANGIOIMMUNOBLASTIC T-CELL LYMPHOMA

GENERAL FEATURES

Angioimmunoblastic T-cell lymphoma (AITL) is a type of peripheral T-cell lymphoma (PTCL) characterized by generalized lymphadenopathy, frequent extranodal involvement, and immune dysregulation resulting in a variety of autoimmune manifestations and laboratory abnormalities. The lymph nodes are involved by a polymorphous population of T cells associated with a prominent proliferation of high endothelial venules (HEV) and expansion of follicular dendritic cells (12).

AITL was described initially in the German literature (16), but was not widely recognized until 1974 when Frizzera et al. (17) more fully described and designated the disease as *angioimmunoblastic lymphadenopathy with dysproteinemia* (AILD). Almost simultaneously, others also described this disease using terms such as *immunoblastic lymphadenopathy* and *lymphogranulomatosis X*, but the designation of AILD was used most widely for the next two decades.

Initially, AILD was considered to be an abnormal immune reaction or premalignant condition and affected patients were thought to have an increased risk of progression to lymphoma. Subsequently, immunophenotypic and molecular analyses showed evidence of T-cell monoclonality in many cases of AILD (so-called AILD-like lymphoma), resulting in the inclusion of AILD as a specific type of T-cell lymphoma in the updated Kiel classification (see chapter 4). In the Revised European-American classification, AILD and AILD-like T-cell lymphoma were redesignated as angioimmunoblastic T-cell lymphoma and this name was adopted in the third and fourth editions and the 2016 revision of the World Health Organization (WHO) classification (12,45).

AITL is a lymphoma that is derived from follicular T-helper cells (T_{FH}) (11,38). This concept is supported by the fact that normal T_{FH} cells and neoplastic AITL cells show similar upregulation or expression of a number of T_{FH} markers including CXCL13, a chemokine essential for the recruitment of B cells into lymph nodes and their activation in germinal centers (11,19). The functional properties of neoplastic T_{FH} cells may explain several of the peculiar biological and clinical features inherent to this lymphoma, including the laboratory abnormalities, the heterogeneous morphologic findings in lymph nodes including expansion of B cells and follicular dendritic cell networks, and the associated host immunodeficiency.

With the recognition of a distinctive immunophenotype, there has been some shift in the criteria used for the diagnosis of AITL. Traditionally, the diagnosis was based on distinctive histologic features combined with a characteristic clinical context and laboratory abnormalities. Currently, the combination of histologic findings and a T_{FH} immunophenotype may be used to support the diagnosis of AITL, even when typical clinical and laboratory findings are only partially present or even absent. In addition, some patients have typical clinical and laboratory findings, but their lymph node biopsy findings are not typical or are less well-developed; a T_{FH} immunophenotype can be used to support classification as AITL in this circumstance. In these two scenarios, the distinctive immunophenotype probably facilitates recognition of AITL at an earlier stage in its evolution, before the clinical and laboratory findings develop, or before characteristic morphologic features are formed. The use of the distinctive immunophenotype likely has some impact on inter-pathologist reproducibility and perhaps may have an effect on the length of patient survival following the initial diagnosis of AITL.

AITL is the second most common type of PTCL in Western countries, representing approximately 20 percent of all cases of PTCL and 1 to 2 percent of all non-Hodgkin lymphomas (1,28,50). AITL is more common in western

Table 31-1	
CLINICAL FINDINGS IN PATIENTS WITH ANGIOIMMUNOBLASTIC T-CELL LYMPHOMA	
Finding	**Frequency**
Generalized lymphadenopathy	>90%
Bone marrow involvement	60-70%
Hepatosplenomegaly	50-60%
B symptoms	40-50%
Poor performance status	40-50%
Effusions (all body cavities)	40-50%
Skin manifestations	30-40%
High IPI[a] score (4-5)	30-40%
Bulky mass	10-20%
Arthralgias/arthritis	10-15%
Neurologic manifestations (various)	10%
Lung involvement	10%

[a]IPI = International Prognostic Index.

Table 31-2	
LABORATORY FINDINGS IN PATIENTS WITH ANGIOIMMUNOBLASTIC T-CELL LYMPHOMA	
Finding	**Frequency**
Anemia (often Coombs positive)	60-70%
Serum hypergammaglobulinemia	60-70%
Elevated serum LDH[a]	50-60%
Hypereosinophilia	30-40%
Lymphopenia	30-40%
Thrombocytopenia	15-25%

[a]LDH = lactate dehydrogenase.

Europe than in the United States or Asia, and is also more common in Caucasians than African-Americans. No etiologic agents or risk factors have been identified. In older reports, antecedent antibiotic therapy was suggested as a potential cause of AITL in some patients. In retrospect, most likely these patients had an early phase of AITL associated with infection for which the antibiotics were prescribed.

CLINICAL FEATURES

Most patients with AITL are elderly adults with a median age range of 59 to 65 years. Various studies report a slightly greater predominance in men or an equal sex ratio (12,28,50). Patients with AITL usually present with generalized lymphadenopathy (Table 31-1). B-type symptoms (fever, night sweats, weight loss) are seen in up to 50 percent of patients. Hepatosplenomegaly and serous effusions of the pleural or peritoneal cavities are common. The bone marrow is involved in 60 to 70 percent of cases and skin involvement occurs in about 30 to 40 percent. A maculopapular eruption is the most common skin manifestation (27). Approximately 80 percent of patients with AITL have advanced clinical stage disease (Ann Arbor stage III or IV) (1,15,28,29,50).

Most patients with AITL have an aggressive clinical course, but some, presumably at an early point in the evolution of disease, have a more indolent course. This subset of patients responds well to steroid therapy; occasionally spontaneous regression, usually temporary, occurs. Most of these patients, however, eventually progress to more aggressive disease associated with greater host immune compromise and opportunistic infections.

Laboratory abnormalities are common in AITL patients (Table 31-2). Hematologic abnormalities include hemolytic anemia (often Coombs positive), eosinophilia, and lymphopenia; lymphocytosis is uncommon (12,15,29). The absolute monocyte count is increased in a subset of patients (56). Serum chemistry studies often show polyclonal hypergammaglobulinemia and a number of autoantibodies, including rheumatoid factor, antinuclear antibody, and antismooth muscle antibody.

HISTOLOGIC FINDINGS

Lymph Node

The lymph node architecture is effaced by a polymorphous cellular infiltrate that often extends beyond the capsule. In cases with subtotal effacement, the neoplasm has a paracortical distribution. The subcapsular and trabecular sinuses are often patent. A characteristic feature is the proliferation of HEVs arranged in a branching pattern.

Three overlapping architectural patterns that correspond, in part, to morphologic stages of disease, have been described in AITL (3,46). These patterns reflect the presence of residual reactive hyperplastic B-cell follicles and the degree of nodal architectural effacement. In

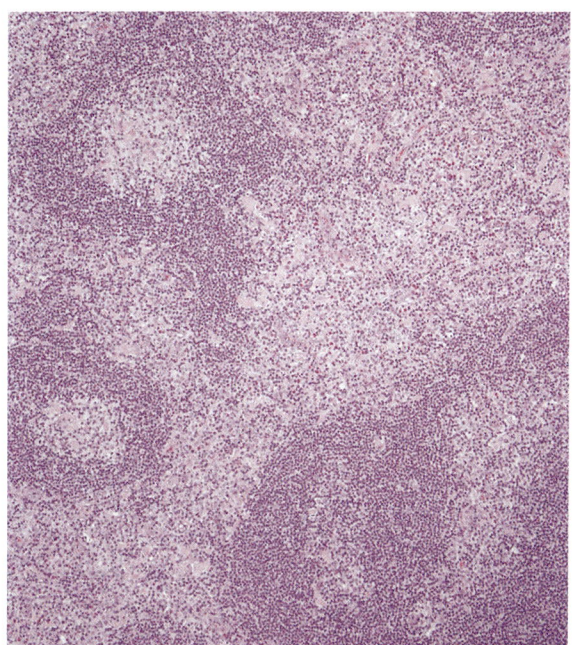 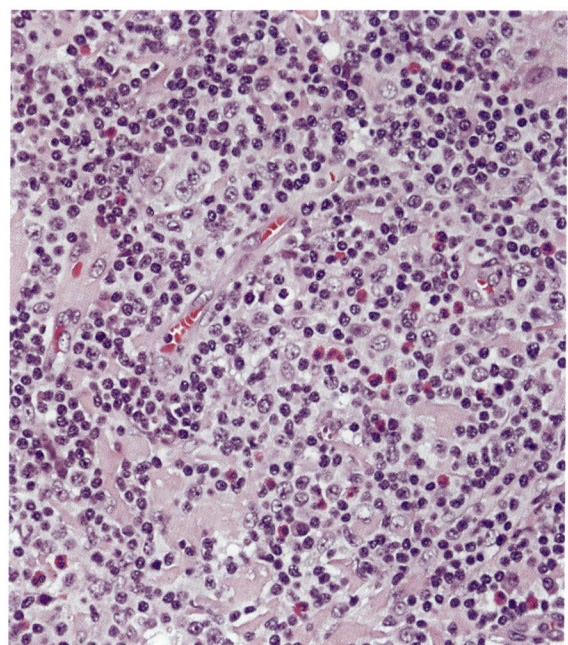

Figure 31-1

ANGIOIMMUNOBLASTIC T-CELL LYMPHOMA, PATTERN I, INVOLVING LYMPH NODE

Left: Low-power view shows intact and reactive follicles scattered throughout the lymph node.

Right: High-power view shows a proliferation of high endothelial venules (HEVs) and neoplastic cells with pale cytoplasm (left, right: hematoxylin and eosin [H&E] stain).

pattern I (about 15 percent of cases), the lymph node architecture is partially preserved and hyperplastic, or normal lymphoid follicles are present (fig. 31-1). There is little proliferation of follicular dendritic cells at this stage. In pattern II (about 25 percent of cases), the architecture is mostly effaced, with only some residual, often regressed ("burned out") follicles present. In some cases, the regressed follicles resemble hyaline-vascular follicles as observed in Castleman disease (fig. 31-2). The most common pattern in AITL is pattern III (about 60 percent of cases), in which the architecture is almost completely replaced without residual follicles or only a few regressed follicles (fig. 31-3) (3,17). Follicular dendritic cell proliferation is usually marked. Commonly, more than one pattern is present in an individual lymph node biopsy specimen. Some patients who initially have findings of pattern I, subsequently show patterns II or III, suggesting morphologic progression and that pattern III represents more advanced disease (3).

The number of neoplastic lymphoid cells and the cell composition of the microenvironment

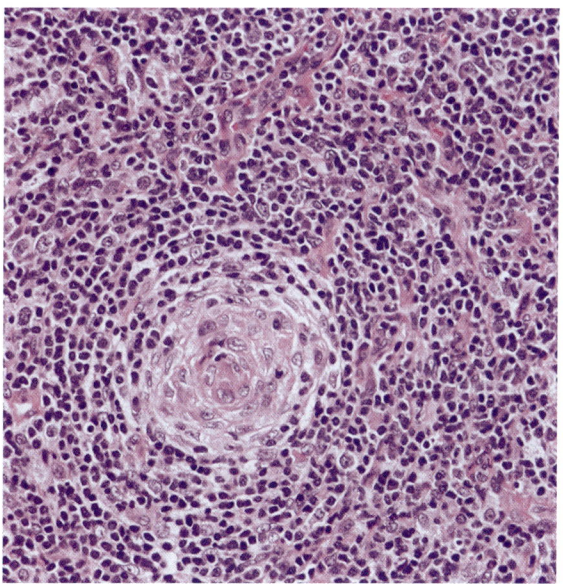

Figure 31-2

ANGIOIMMUNOBLASTIC T-CELL LYMPHOMA INVOLVING LYMPH NODE

High-power magnification shows a highly regressed residual lymphoid follicle that resembles, in part, a follicle in hyaline-vascular Castleman disease (H&E stain).

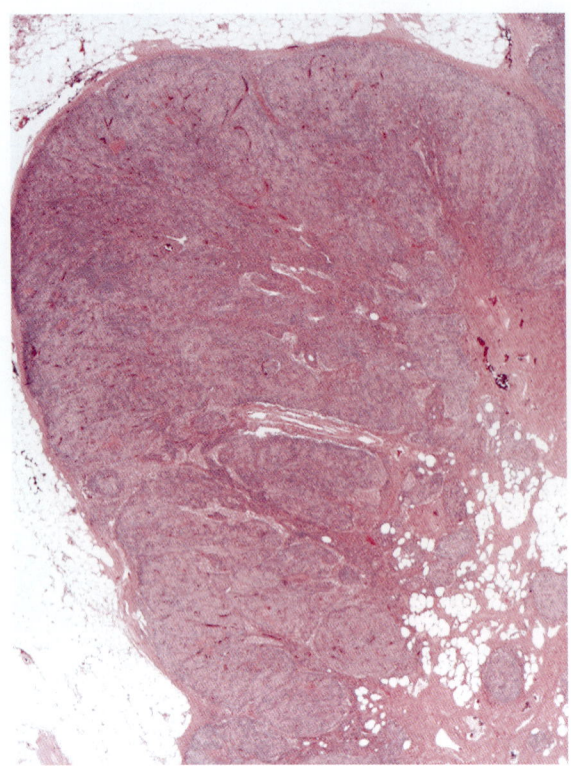
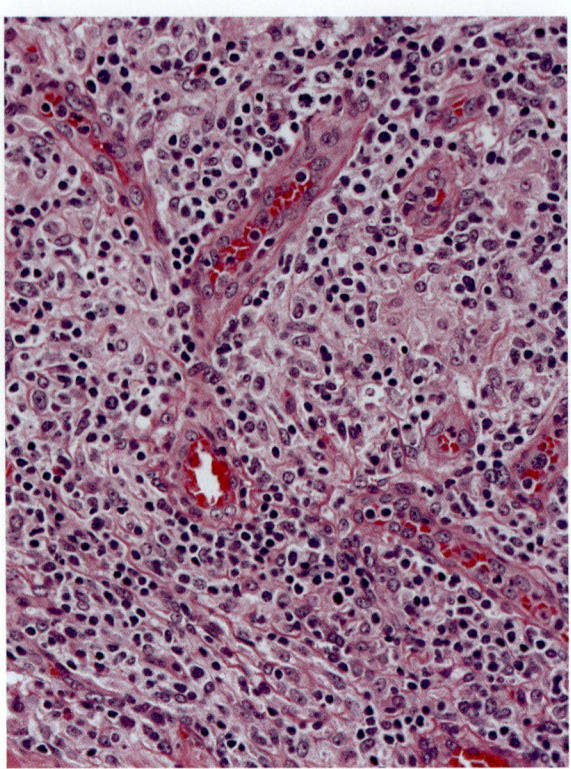

Figure 31-3

ANGIOIMMUNOBLASTIC T-CELL LYMPHOMA, PATTERN III, INVOLVING LYMPH NODE

Left: Low-power view shows diffuse effacement of the lymph node architecture. Some sinuses are patent and others distended in this field.

Right: Prominent, branching HEVs and a polymorphous cell population are present (left, right: H&E stain).

are highly variable in AITL. Although morphologic grading has no established prognostic significance, the concept is used here to describe the range of morphologic findings. In lower grade (often early) lesions (fig. 31-4), the neoplastic cells are few and are small to medium in size with clear or pale cytoplasm and minimal to moderate cytologic atypia. Mitotic figures are infrequent. The neoplastic cells often form clusters around follicles, HEVs, or both. The neoplastic cells are admixed with reactive small lymphocytes (T and B cells), immunoblasts, histiocytes (which can have an epithelioid appearance), eosinophils, plasma cells, and other cell types. By contrast, in higher-grade (probably advanced) lesions (fig. 31-5), the neoplastic cells are numerous, arranged in large nodules or sheets, and exhibit obvious cytologic atypia and an appreciable mitotic rate. In these cases the inflammatory cells are less numerous. These cases also have been referred to as the *clear cell-rich variant*.

Histologic Variants of Angioimmunoblastic T-Cell Lymphoma

Lennert-Like AITL. Epithelioid histiocytes are a common finding in AITL, but in rare cases these cells are numerous and form clusters or small granulomas that can mimic the lymphoepithelioid variant of PTCL, not otherwise specified (NOS), so-called Lennert lymphoma (fig. 31-6). Usually, these tumors have at least some areas of typical AITL associated with the Lennert-like areas.

Plasma Cell-Rich AITL. Plasma cells are a common component of AITL, but usually they are scattered and represent less than 5 percent of all cells. Rare cases, however, contain numerous plasma cells that form large aggregates or sheets (fig. 31-7). As a result, a plasma cell neoplasm may be considered, but areas of unequivocal AITL are also present and allow the correct diagnosis.

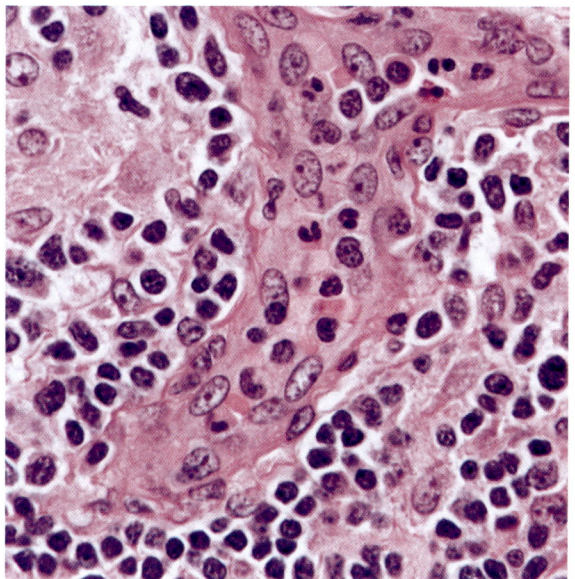

Figure 31-4

ANGIOIMMUNOBLASTIC T-CELL LYMPHOMA INVOLVING LYMPH NODE

The neoplastic lymphocytes are small, have clear cytoplasm, and surround HEVs (H&E stain).

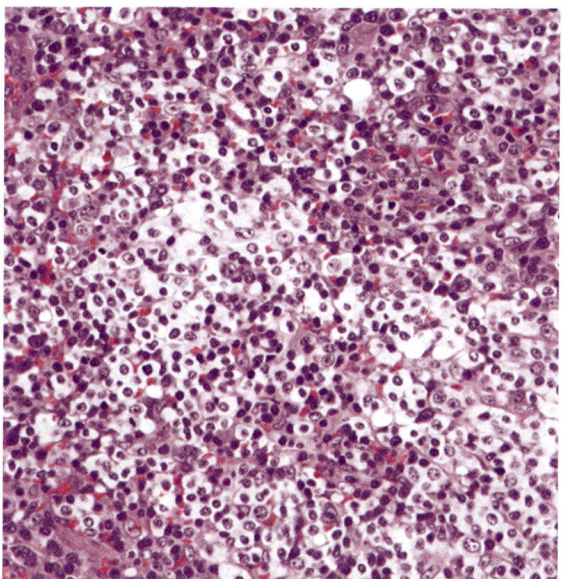

Figure 31-5

ANGIOIMMUNOBLASTIC T-CELL LYMPHOMA, CLEAR CELL-RICH VARIANT, INVOLVING LYMPH NODE

The lymphoma is composed of numerous neoplastic lymphocytes with abundant clear cytoplasm (H&E stain).

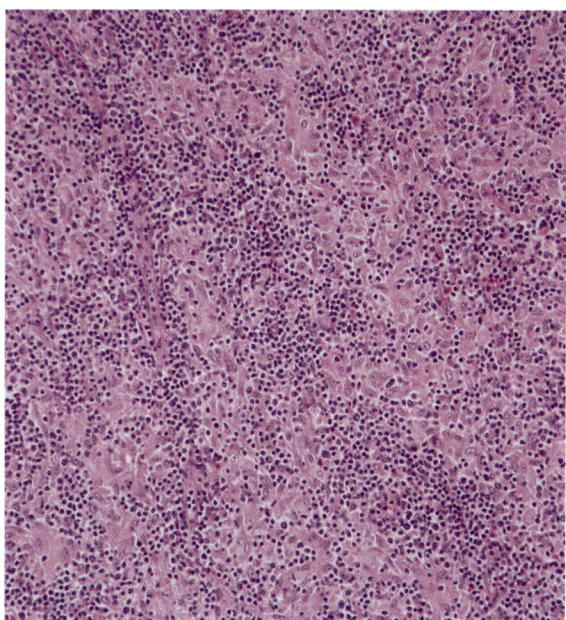

Figure 31-6

ANGIOIMMUNOBLASTIC T-CELL LYMPHOMA, LENNERT-LIKE VARIANT, INVOLVING LYMPH NODE

Numerous epithelioid histiocytes are seen. Other fields in this specimen had findings typical of AITL and the lymphoma cells had an appropriate immunophenotype (H&E stain).

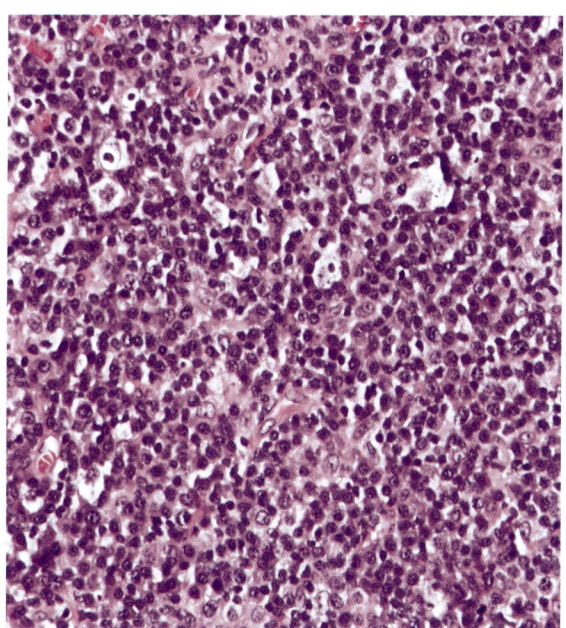

Figure 31-7

ANGIOIMMUNOBLASTIC T-CELL LYMPHOMA, PLASMA CELL-RICH, INVOLVING LYMPH NODE

There are numerous plasma cells without cytologic atypia. Other areas in this biopsy specimen had features of AITL and the neoplastic cells had an appropriate immunophenotype (H&E stain).

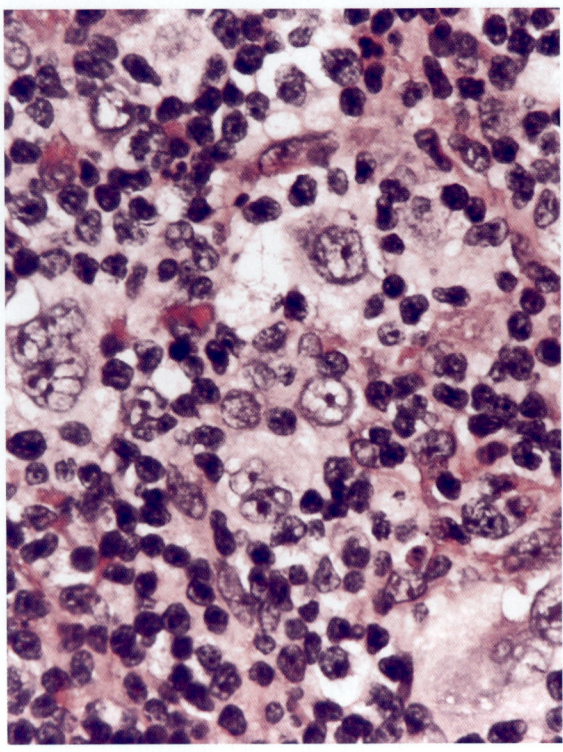

Figure 31-8

**ANGIOIMMUNOBLASTIC T-CELL LYMPHOMA
WITH REED-STERNBERG AND HODGKIN CELLS
INVOLVING LYMPH NODE**

Oil immersion magnification shows RS+H cells in AITL. These cells were shown to be positive for CD15, CD30, and PAX5 (not shown) (H&E stain).

AITL with Reed-Sternberg and Hodgkin Cells. In a small subset of cases of AITL, scattered large cells that resemble Reed-Sternberg and Hodgkin (RS+H) cells are present (fig. 31-8). These cells have a RS+H cell immunophenotype (positive for CD15, CD30, PAX5) and are usually Epstein-Barr virus (EBV) positive (32). In another subset of AITL cases, large cells that resemble RS+H cells are present that are often CD15(-), CD20(+), CD30(+), and CD45(+); these cells are often designated as RS+H-like cells. Despite these large cells, these cases usually resemble AITL, with the characteristic HEV and follicular dendritic cell proliferations.

Bone Marrow

AITL is challenging to recognize in aspirate smears due to the heterogeneous mixture of inflammatory cells and the rarity of neoplastic cells in some cases. Therefore, evaluation for AITL is best performed by analysis of the bone marrow biopsy specimen. The neoplasm is frequently multifocal and often vaguely nodular, although interstitial, paratrabecular, and diffuse patterns are observed (8,24).

The neoplastic lymphoid aggregates are commonly associated with many reactive inflammatory cells, and it may be difficult to specifically identify the neoplastic cells within these aggregates in hematoxylin and eosin (H&E)-stained slides (fig. 31-9). Nevertheless, the lymphoma cells are identified by a combination of immunohistochemical markers supporting a T_{FH} immunophenotype (24). In situ hybridization for EBV-encoded RNA1 (EBER1) is also helpful for establishing the presence of bone marrow involvement by AITL.

The reactive cells associated with AITL in bone marrow are usually small lymphocytes and histiocytes, with scattered eosinophils and plasma cells (8,24). In some patients, however, eosinophils are numerous and may be associated with peripheral eosinophilia, raising the possibility of hypereosinophilic syndrome. Polytypic plasma cells in bone marrow also may be numerous, up to about 20 percent, and may suggest plasma cell myeloma. These plasma cells, however, are usually small and lack nucleoli or evidence of cytologic atypia. Rarely, fibrosis or hemophagocytosis is found in the bone marrow

Peripheral Blood

In blood smears, normochromic normocytic anemia is common and rouleaux, although usually not prominent, may be observed. Absolute lymphocytosis is unusual and a leukemic phase occurs only rarely in patients with AITL. By morphologic examination of a peripheral blood smear, the small neoplastic T cells of AITL are not easily recognized in many patients. Instead, a low number of intermediate to large cells with basophilic cytoplasm, referred to in the literature as "immunocytes," may be observed (fig. 31-10). These cells are usually of B-cell lineage and occur more often in AITL cases with numerous B cells.

Although morphologic review of the blood smear may be negative for AITL cells, analysis of blood specimens by more sensitive methods of detection, such as flow cytometry, commonly shows the presence of lymphoma cells with an

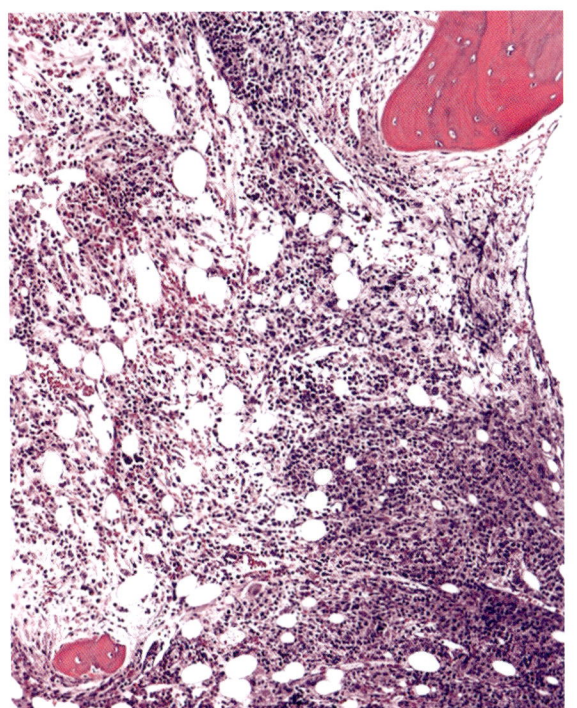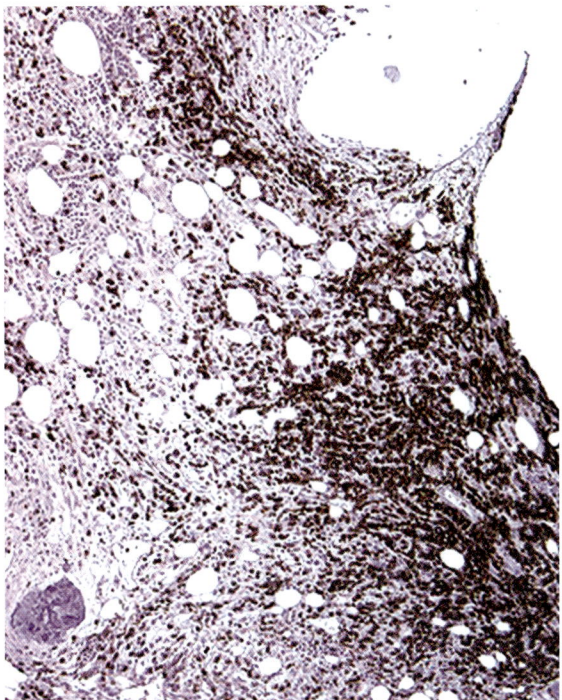

Figure 31-9

ANGIOIMMUNOBLASTIC T-CELL LYMPHOMA INVOLVING BONE MARROW

Left: The bone marrow is partially replaced by lymphoma (H&E stain).
Right: The anti-CD3 antibody highlights the neoplastic cells (immunohistochemistry with hematoxylin counterstain).

aberrant CD4-positive T_{FH} immunophenotype, albeit in low numbers.

Other Sites of Involvement

In liver biopsy specimens, AITL tends to preferentially involve the portal tracts but can more extensively replace the hepatic parenchyma. In the spleen, AITL involves the white or red pulp. In the skin, histologic findings may be subtle and mimic an infectious process; less often, the histologic changes are extensive (fig. 31-11). In most cases, the AITL cells infiltrate the dermis, either as a mildly atypical perivascular infiltrate or more extensively. Epidermotropism is not a feature of AITL involving the skin. Patients with AITL can develop tonsillar enlargement; histologic examination often shows paracortical involvement similar to pattern I in lymph nodes. Immunohistochemical studies, by showing that the cells in an extranodal lesion have a T_{FH} immunophenotype, help distinguish AITL from reactive lesions or other types of lymphoma (2,3).

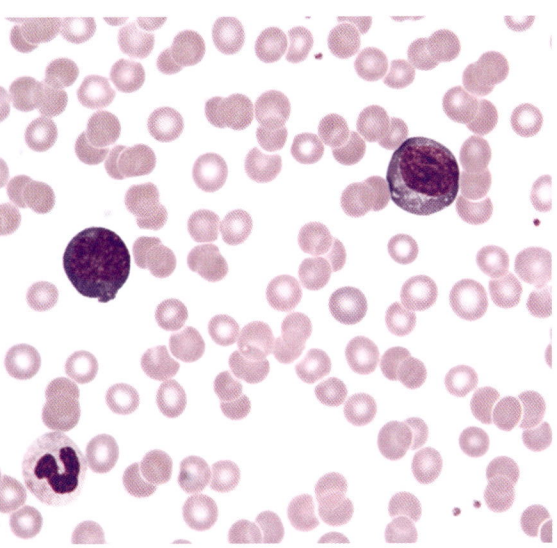

Figure 31-10

ANGIOIMMUNOBLASTIC T-CELL LYMPHOMA INVOLVING BLOOD

A peripheral blood smear shows lymphocytes with abundant basophilic cytoplasm (so-called "immunocytes") (Wright-Giemsa stain).

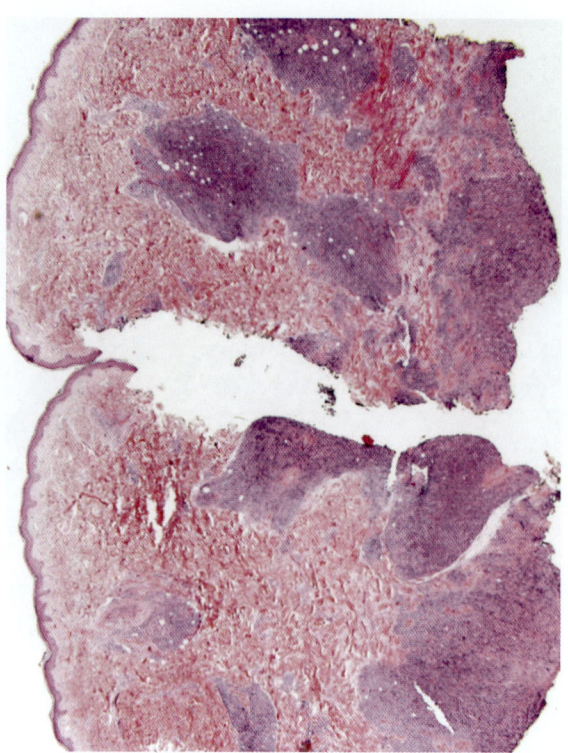 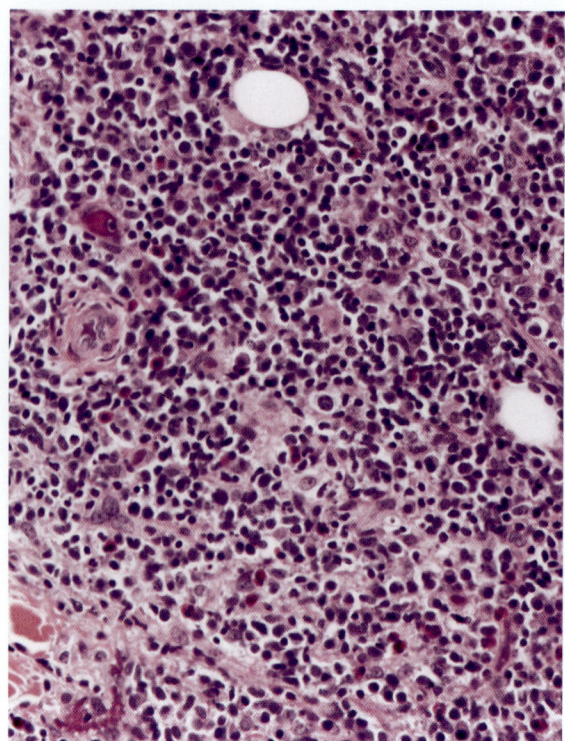

Figure 31-11

ANGIOIMMUNOBLASTIC T-CELL LYMPHOMA INVOLVING SKIN

Left: The neoplasm has a perivascular and periadnexal pattern in the dermis. The epidermis is spared.

Right: A polymorphous infiltrate consists of medium-sized atypical lymphocytes admixed with histiocytes and scattered eosinophils (left, right: H&E stain).

CYTOLOGIC FINDINGS

Aspirate smears show a heterogeneous population of cells including a variable number of small to medium-sized neoplastic lymphoid cells, reactive lymphocytes and immunoblasts, histiocytes, plasma cells, and eosinophils (fig. 31-12) (31). In some cases, small fragments of lymphoid tissue have a prominent HEV network. In high-grade cases, the neoplastic cells are much more numerous. Reed-Sternberg-like cells are present in some cases.

In cytologic preparations of AITL, particularly the low-grade lesions, the findings can mimic a reactive or inflammatory process. Ancillary studies may be essential for establishing the diagnosis (see below). Detection of an aberrant T-cell or T_{FH} immunophenotype or monoclonal T-cell receptor gene rearrangements may be essential for establishing the diagnosis of AITL. In some cases, monoclonal *IGH* rearrangements are also detected. Ancillary methods may fail to detect an aberrant immunophenotype or monoclonal gene rearrangements, especially in tumors with few neoplastic cells.

IMMUNOHISTOCHEMICAL FINDINGS

Immunohistochemical analysis shows characteristic immunoarchitectural features in cases of AITL involving lymph nodes, which evolve with disease progression. In pattern I, lymphoid follicles, as observed by pan-B-cell antibodies, are common and small B cells are often compressed toward the lymph node capsule (seemingly pushed by the lymphoma) (fig. 31-13). At this stage, there may be few large B immunoblasts scattered throughout the tumor. Follicular dendritic cells (CD21 positive) are often focal and not well-developed. Neoplastic T cells are present in the paracortical region, but they are often small, do not form clusters, and are intermixed with many reactive cells. It therefore can be difficult to identify the neoplastic cells morphologically.

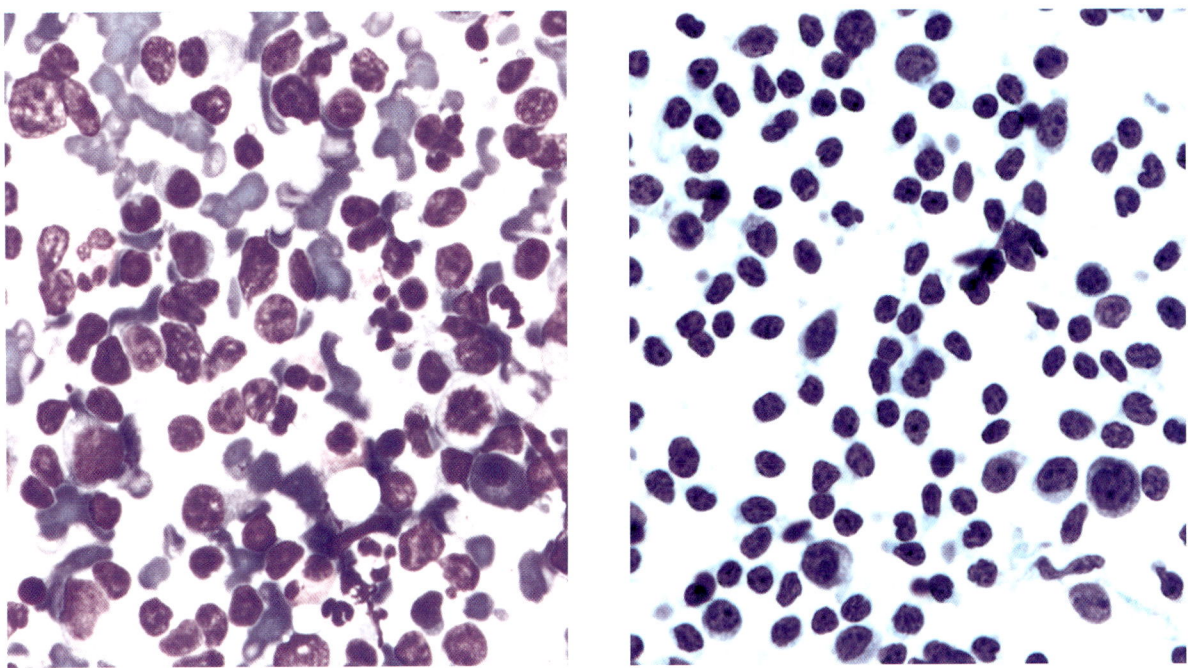

Figure 31-12

ANGIOIMMUNOBLASTIC T-CELL LYMPHOMA INVOLVING LYMPH NODE

Cytologic smears obtained by fine-needle aspiration from a lymph node show a highly polymorphous cellular infiltrate (Left: Diff-Quik stain; right: Papanicolaou stain).

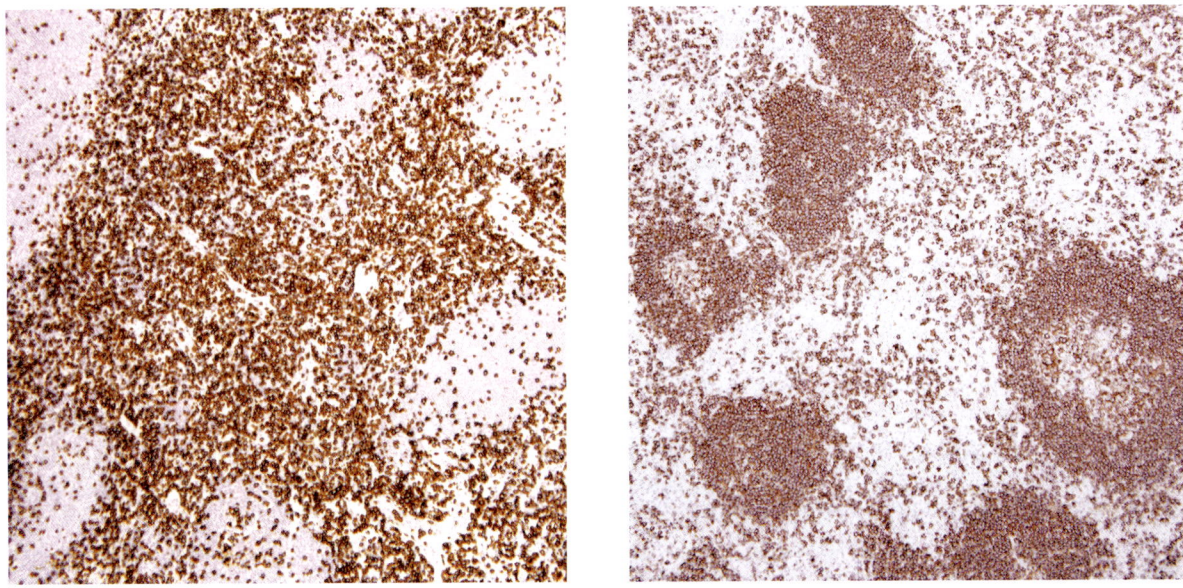

Figure 31-13

ANGIOIMMUNOBLASTIC T-CELL LYMPHOMA, PATTERN I, INVOLVING LYMPH NODE

Left: The neoplastic cells are CD3 positive and are located primarily in the paracortical regions. Lymphoid follicles are negative for CD3.

Right: Scattered CD20-positive B cells are also present in the paracortical areas, intermixed within the lymphoma cell population. Follicles are also positive for CD20 (left, right: immunohistochemistry with hematoxylin counterstain).

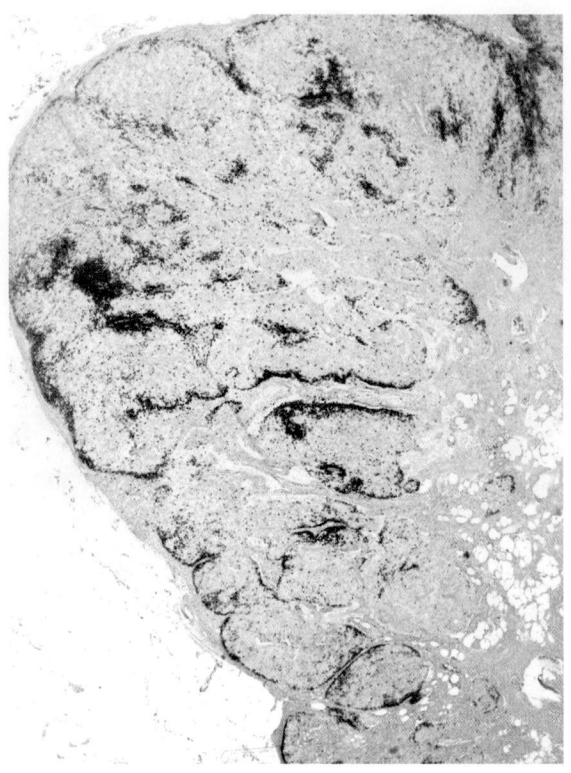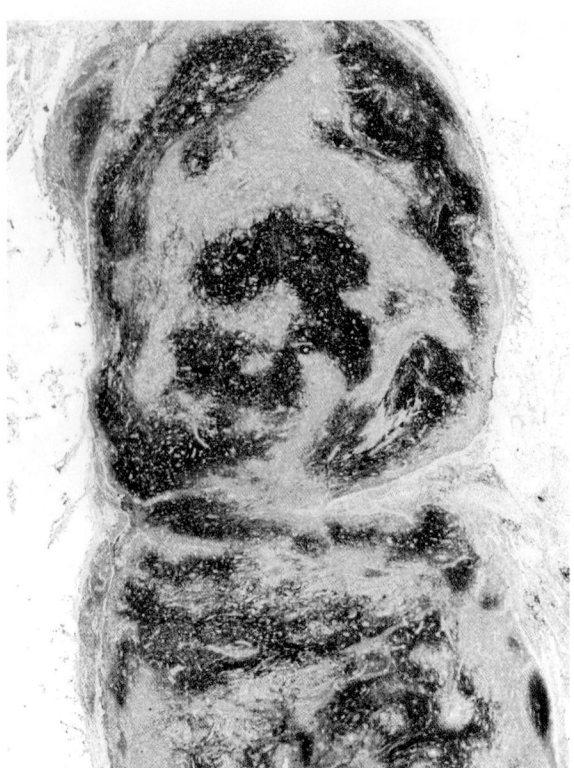

Figure 31-14

ANGIOIMMUNOBLASTIC T-CELL LYMPHOMA, PATTERN III, INVOLVING LYMPH NODE

Left: Few CD20-positive B cells remain and are pushed underneath the capsule.

Right: Marked proliferation of CD21-positive follicular dendritic cells (left, right: immunohistochemistry with hematoxylin counterstain).

As AITL progresses through pattern II to pattern III, the lymphoid follicles become disrupted and depleted of B cells. Small B cells are compressed up against the lymph node capsule and their overall number is decreased, while large B immunoblasts scattered throughout the paracortical regions become increased (fig. 31-14). These B cells are usually polytypic, commonly express CD30 (fig. 31-15), and are commonly positive for EBER1 (fig. 31-16) (12,35,53). In a small subset of cases, the B cells are monotypic (see below). Neoplastic T cells are more numerous in this phase and may exhibit an aberrant immunophenotype. Follicular dendritic cells progressively increase near the follicles and form disorganized networks around HEVs. Antibodies that highlight follicular dendritic cells are reactive with CD21, CD23, CD35, CXCL13, clusterin, and others; CD21 is the most sensitive (49).

In patterns II and III, the paracortical T-cell regions expand and the number of morpho-logically abnormal T cells increases. These neoplastic T cells often form clusters and have abundant pale cytoplasm, facilitating their recognition by immunohistochemistry stains (fig. 31-17). The neoplastic T cells are derived from CD4-positive T_{FH} cells (11) and typically express pan-T-cell markers including CD2, CD3, CD5, and T-cell receptor α/β and are negative for CD1a, CD8, and TdT. The neoplastic T cells (as well as reactive cells) also commonly express CD30 with variable intensity (35). The tumor cells, however, may show aberrant loss or reduced expression of surface CD3, CD7, or other T-cell antigens.

A defining feature of AITL is that the lymphoma cells express one or more of several markers of T_{FH} cells (fig. 31-18). The T_{FH} markers include: CD10, BCL6, CXCL13, PD1/CD279 (programmed death-1, a member of the CD28 costimulatory membrane receptor family), ICOS (inducible T-cell co-stimulator molecule),

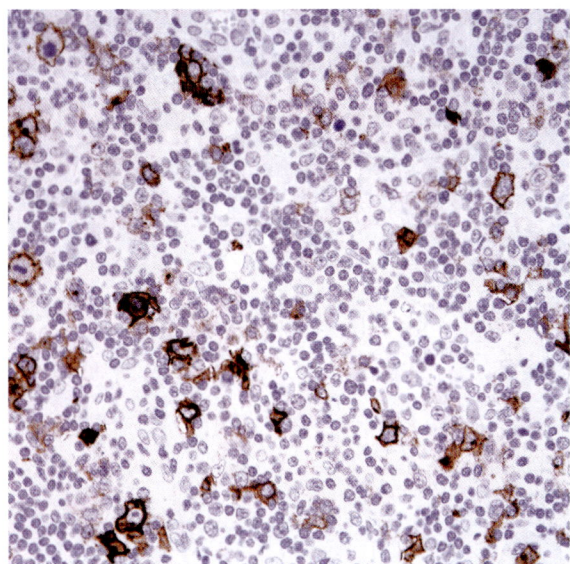

Figure 31-15

CD30-POSITIVE CELLS IN ANGIOIMMUNOBLASTIC T-CELL LYMPHOMA

Scattered large cells consistent with B immunoblasts are positive for CD30 (immunohistochemistry with hematoxylin counterstain).

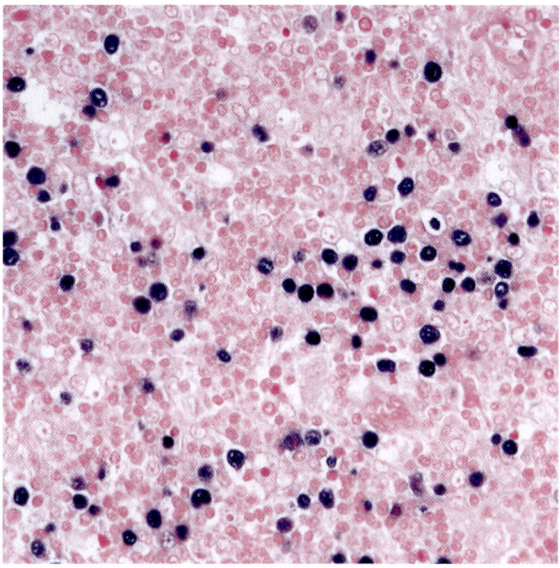

Figure 31-16

EBER1-POSITIVE CELLS IN ANGIOIMMUNOBLASTIC T-CELL LYMPHOMA

Scattered small lymphocytes and larger immunoblasts (of B-cell lineage) are positive for Epstein-Barr virus (EBV)-encoded RNA1 (in situ hybridization with eosin counterstain).

CD200, CXCR5, CD154, and cytoplasmic SAP (signaling lymphocyte activation molecule [SLAM]-associated protein) (5,11,13,14,59). CD10 expression by T cells may be the most specific finding supporting the diagnosis of AITL, but the sensitivity is low and the use of a combination of T_{FH} markers is recommended to establish a T_{FH} immunophenotype (59).

Commonly, numerous histiocytes and macrophages are admixed within AITL. The prognostic importance of tumor-associated macrophages has been assessed in AITL in a few studies, with no correlation with prognosis in most reports; one study, however, showed that the ratio of CD163/CD68 macrophages correlated with an M2 state of polarization and outcome (33). The results of this study need to be validated in a larger group of patients.

Flow cytometry immunophenotypic analysis is also useful for establishing the diagnosis of AILT in tissues and is ideally suited to the analysis of peripheral blood and bone marrow specimens (fig. 31-19). The total number of aberrant T cells in AITL ranges from less than 5 percent up to 90 percent (4,5). The lymphoma cells express CD2, CD4, and CD5 (dim in about

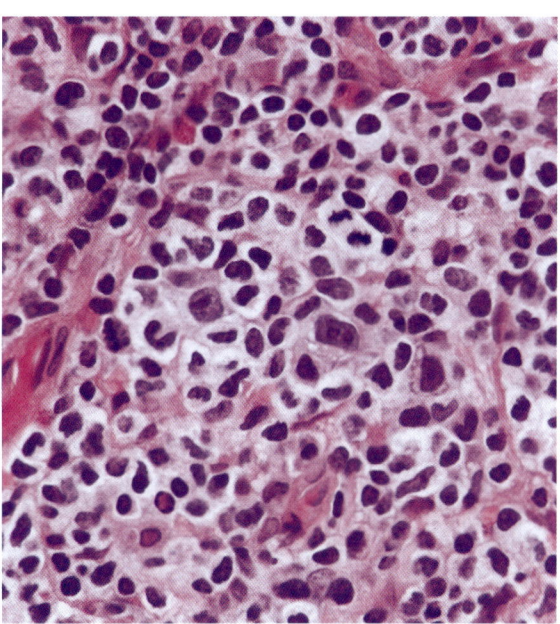

Figure 31-17

ANGIOIMMUNOBLASTIC T-CELL LYMPHOMA INVOLVING LYMPH NODE

Oil immersion magnification shows that the lymphoma cells have abundant clear (pale) cytoplasm and form clusters, helpful features when assessing T_{FH} markers by immunohistochemistry (H&E stain).

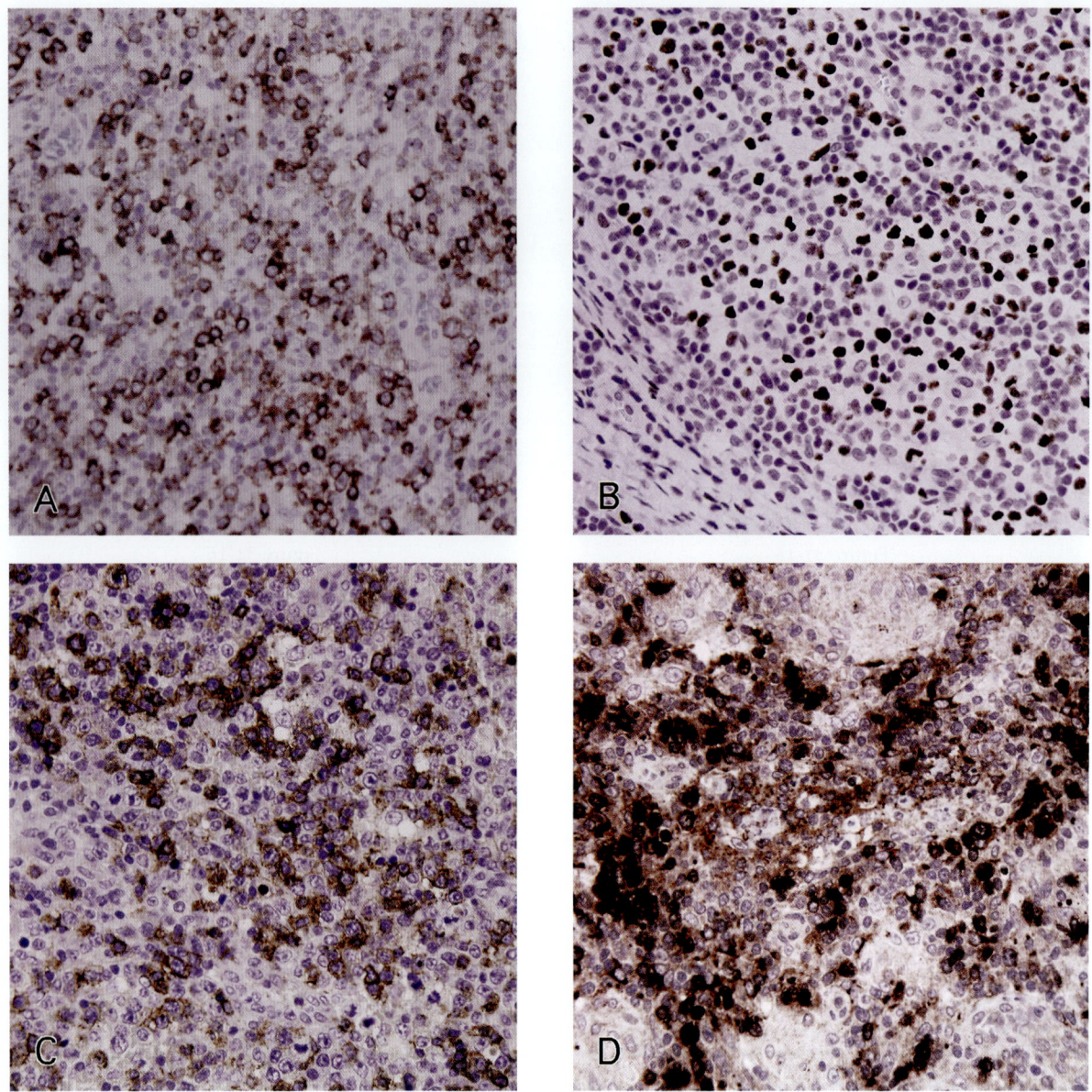

Figure 31-18

T$_{FH}$ MARKER EXPRESSION BY ANGIOIMMUNOBLASTIC T-CELL LYMPHOMA

Expression of CD10 (A), BCL6 (B), PD1/CD279 (C), and CXCL13 (D) (immunohistochemistry with hematoxylin counterstain).

10 percent of cases). Surface CD3 is commonly absent, CD7 is absent in about one third of cases, and surface T-cell receptors are absent in one third of cases. CD26 is absent in about 20 percent of cases. CD56 and CD57 are rarely positive and CD16 and CD94 are absent.

In biopsy specimens analyzed by flow cytometry, polytypic B cells are usually present and can be numerous. Although a T$_{FH}$ immunophenotype is characteristic of AITL, it can be difficult to demonstrate in some cases and overall, fewer (compared with immunohistochemistry) T$_{FH}$ markers have been applied to flow cytometry detection. CD10 is positive in 60 to 70 percent of all cases of AITL; levels of expression may be variable (4,5,26a).

Prominent B-Cell or Plasma Cell Populations in AITL

Using flow cytometry immunophenotyping or immunohistochemical analysis, a monotypic B-cell or plasma cell population may be identified in some AITL cases. In biopsy specimens of AITL, prominent proliferations of B cells are detected in about 20 percent of cases (52). The B cells are often large and positive for EBER1 (about 75 percent of cases) and may be polytypic or monotypic (about 40 percent of cases) (52). In a subset of cases these large B-cell proliferations meet the criteria for diffuse large B-cell lymphoma (see below) (54,58).

Proliferations of small B cells or plasma cells also occur in AITL but are less common and often EBER1 negative. In general, the diagnosis of coexistent small B-cell lymphoma or plasmacytoma requires morphologic evidence of architectural replacement as well as monotypic Ig expression (52).

MOLECULAR GENETIC FINDINGS

Conventional cytogenetic analysis of cases of AITL has shown that the most common abnormalities are trisomies of chromosome 3, 5, or 21; gain of chromosome X; and loss of 6q (30,43,47). The t(5;9)(q33;q22)/*ITK-SYK* has been reported in a small subset of cases (20), but gains of *ITK* and *SYK* (without translocation) are much more common, in 38 and 14 percent of cases, respectively, in one study (26).

Analysis of the antigen receptor genes by either Southern blot analysis or polymerase chain reaction (PCR)-based methods has shown that most cases of AITL carry rearrangements of T-cell receptor genes, usually monoclonal but sometimes oligoclonal (44). In about 10 percent of cases, however, no T-cell receptor gene rearrangements are identified. *IGH* also is rearranged, in a monoclonal/oligoclonal pattern, in about 25 percent of cases (2,12).

The B cells of AITL are commonly infected by EBV (53) and the virus is commonly present in monoclonal or oligoclonal form. The EBV-positive B cells carry mutated *IGH* variable region genes, suggesting that they traversed the germinal center (6). The mutational load is often high and because mutations are destructive these cells would be expected to undergo apoptosis; as these cells do not, the microenvironment

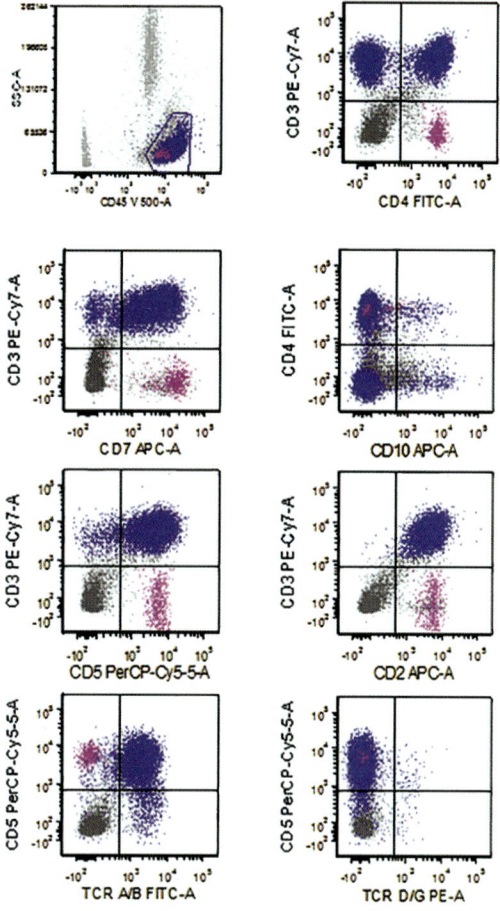

Figure 31-19

ANGIOIMMUNOBLASTIC T-CELL LYMPHOMA INVOLVING BONE MARROW

Flow cytometry immunophenotypic analysis shows lymphoma cells that are positive for CD2, CD3, CD4, CD5, CD7, CD10 (subset), and T-cell receptor α/β. (Courtesy of Dr. S. Loghavi, Houston, Texas.)

or EBV itself likely is involved in maintaining B-cell proliferation (6).

Array comparative genomic hybridization or single nucleotide polymorphism microarrays have shown common areas of copy number gain that include chromosomes 8, 9, and 19, and loci 11p11-q14 and 22q. Chromosome locus 13q is a frequent area of loss (18,47). One microRNA study of AITL showed upregulation of miR-34a, miR-146a, and miR-193b and downregulation of miR-140-3p, let-7g, miR-30b, and miR-664 (40).

Gene expression profiling studies have shown a distinctive T_{FH} signature in most cases of AITL

(11,21,22,38). The gene expression signature is characterized by the expression of genes involved in B-cell biology, angiogenesis, endothelial biology and cell migration, reflecting the contribution of the heterogeneous microenvironment (11,38). Wang et al. (51) reported that AITL cases with an *IDH2^{R172}* mutation have a unique profile characterized by an interleukin 12-induced gene expression signature.

Gene mutations have been identified in many AITL cases (reviewed by Cortes and Palomero in reference 8a). Mutations of *RHOA* (one of the Rho GTPases) are common (in about 70 percent of cases) (42). *RHOA* mutations correlate with an increased frequency of B symptoms and splenomegaly as well as increased microvessel density and expression of T_{FH} markers (36). *RHOA*-mutated AITL cases may represent a distinctive subset. Mutations of *TET2* are also common (about 70 percent of cases) (34,37). Many AITL cases harbor two or three *TET2* mutations, indicating a strong selective pressure to inactivate *TET2* early during lymphomagenesis (9). *DNMT3A* mutations occur in up to one third of cases and *IDH2^{R172}* in 20 to 30 percent (7,9,34,51). *TET2* mutations are strongly associated with coexistent *RHOA*, *DNMT3A*, and *IDH2^{R172}* mutations, suggesting cooperation between these oncogenic events (9,34). *TET2* mutations also have been identified in polyclonal B cells within AITL (43a). Overall, these mutations indicate that epigenetic transcriptional regulation is often abnormal in AITL, resulting in increased methylation of various gene promoters (51).

Mutations in the T-cell receptor pathway also occur in AITL (8a). Mutations of *CD28* and *CTLA4-CD28* fusions have been reported in 11 percent and 58 percent of AITL cases, respectively (41,57). Mutations in *FYN* and *PLCG1* also have been identified in a subset of AITL (37,49a). *TP53* mutations are rare in AITL.

Is AITL Related to T_{FH} Cell Lymphomas

In some patients with follicular T-cell lymphoma (discussed in chapter 30), follow-up biopsy specimens have shown features of AITL. The t(5;9)(q33;q22), found in about 20 percent of follicular T-cell lymphomas, also has been reported uncommonly in AITL (20). This suggests that a small subset of cases of follicular T-cell lymphoma represents an early manifestation of AITL. It also seems likely that cases of PTCL-NOS with a T_{FH} immunophenotype are also biologically related to AITL.

RISK OF OTHER LYMPHOMAS

Patients with AITL are at increased risk of developing B-cell non-Hodgkin lymphomas. In a study from Kiel, about 12 percent of AITL patients developed B-cell non-Hodgkin lymphomas, of which diffuse large B-cell lymphoma was, by far, the most common (54). Diffuse large B-cell lymphoma can involve the same or different anatomic sites and at least half of these cases are EBV positive (54,58). Diffuse large B-cell lymphoma usually follows the diagnosis of AITL, but rarely, EBV-positive diffuse large B-cell lymphoma can precede the diagnosis of AITL, usually by 1 year or less.

Patients with AITL also develop classic Hodgkin lymphoma or plasma cell neoplasms, but these tumors are much less common. About 1 percent of AITL patients develop classic Hodgkin lymphoma (54), which is usually EBV positive. Plasma cell neoplasms arising in AITL patients are rare and are commonly EBV negative (52).

DIFFERENTIAL DIAGNOSIS

Reactive Paracortical Hyperplasia. There is significant morphologic overlap between early AITL (pattern I) and reactive paracortical hyperplasia, which is also associated commonly with reactive follicles. Prominent and often atypical T-cell hyperplasia can be associated with non-specific viral infections, drug reactions, and autoimmune diseases. Morphologic findings that suggest AITL are the presence of lymphocytes with clear cytoplasm that often form aggregates surrounding follicles or HEVs, as well as follicular dendritic cells encircling HEVs. The demonstration that the clusters or sheets of cells with clear cytoplasm are T cells with a T_{FH} immunophenotype supports the diagnosis of AITL. Clonality and mutational studies also help in establishing a diagnosis of AITL.

Castleman Disease. In AITL it is common for residual lymphoid follicles to show regressive changes and, in some cases, these follicles mimic the follicles of hyaline vascular Castleman disease. Unlike AITL, the follicles of Castleman disease are usually larger. In addition, the prominent branching HEVs or neoplastic clear cells of AITL are absent in Castleman disease. Ancillary studies do not show evidence of an aberrant T-cell immunophenotype or T-cell receptor gene rearrangements in Castleman disease.

Angiolymphoid Hyperplasia with Eosinophilia. Angiolymphoid hyperplasia with eosinophilia (ALHE), also known as epithelioid hemangioma, may be associated with a marked polymorphous infiltrate that mimics AITL. However, ALHE is typically extranodal and lacks evidence of an aberrant T-cell immunophenotype or a monoclonal T-cell population.

Peripheral T-Cell Lymphoma, Not Otherwise Specified (PTCL-NOS). A constellation of clinical and laboratory findings favor AITL over PTCL-NOS, including rash, body cavity effusions, serum hypergammaglobulinemia, and hemolytic anemia. Helpful pathologic features that support AITL are: prominent HEVs, lymphocytes with clear cytoplasm, cytologic atypia of lymphocytes, numerous plasma cells, and a patent or distended subcapsular sinus combined with involvement of perinodal tissues (59). Immunophenotypic features, however, are usually essential to distinguish AITL from PTCL-NOS. Cases of AITL are characterized by a proliferation of CD21-positive follicular dendritic cell networks, numerous B cells that are often EBV-positive, and expression of T_{FH} markers by the neoplastic cells. Expression of CD10, BCL6, CXCL13, and PD-1/CD279 by the tumor cells, particularly if only a single marker, is not entirely specific for AITL and is seen in other PTCL types (59). A combination of T_{FH} markers is most helpful to support AITL.

A small subset of cases that morphologically resembles AITL is composed of neoplastic cells that express CD8. Traditionally, these cases were classified as AITL, but with recognition of the T_{FH} immunophenotype as a characteristic feature, these cases may be better classified as PTCL-NOS (22).

T-Cell/Histiocyte-Rich Large B-Cell Lymphoma. T-cell/histiocyte-rich large B-cell lymphoma can simulate AITL, but usually these tumors are not associated with EBV-positive B cells and lack branching HEVs, follicular dendritic cell proliferations, or T cells with clear cytoplasm or cytologic atypia.

EBV-Positive Diffuse Large B-Cell Lymphoma. EBV-positive diffuse large B-cell lymphoma, particularly the polymorphous variant, may morphologically mimic AITL. However, the lack of neoplastic T cells with an aberrant T_{FH} immunophenotype excludes the diagnosis of AILT. As mentioned above, AITL patients have an increased risk of developing secondary lymphomas, most frequently diffuse large B-cell lymphoma that is usually EBV positive (54,58). Diffuse large B-cell lymphoma arising in the setting of AITL is supported by the presence of sheets of large atypical EBV-positive B cells, with a dominant B-cell clone identified by gene rearrangement studies.

Classic Hodgkin Lymphoma. Analogies can be drawn between AITL and classic Hodgkin lymphoma. In both diseases, the neoplastic cells may be few, representing less than 10 percent of all cells in a lymph node. In both tumors the neoplastic cells are associated with numerous inflammatory cells, including reactive lymphocytes, histiocytes, eosinophils, plasma cells, and mast cells, in other words, a prominent inflammatory microenvironment. The microenvironment in both diseases is sustained by various cytokines and other factors released or expressed by neoplastic or inflammatory cells. In AITL the microenvironment is sustained by interleukin-17–producing T cells and mast cells, as well as other inflammatory cells (48).

In typical examples of classic Hodgkin lymphoma and AITL, the diagnosis is straightforward. Patients with classic Hodgkin lymphoma are younger and usually lack extranodal sites of disease or widespread laboratory abnormalities, unlike patients with AITL who are often elderly and commonly have extranodal disease. Morphologically, classic Hodgkin lymphoma is characterized by large RS+H cells that are of B-cell lineage [CD15(+/-), CD30(+), PAX5(dim)] (32). In contrast, in most cases of AITL, RS+H cells are absent, the neoplastic cells have clear cytoplasm, and a T_{FH} immunophenotype and monoclonal T-cell receptor gene rearrangements are present.

Complicating the differential diagnosis, some AITL cases have large cells that closely mimic RS+H cells, including expression of CD15, CD30, PAX5, and usually EBV. In these cases, however, the background cell population is not reactive, as in classic Hodgkin lymphoma. Instead, there are atypical lymphocytes with clear cytoplasm, HEV proliferation, and expanded FDC networks. In addition, monoclonal T-cell receptor gene rearrangements are present.

TREATMENT AND PROGNOSIS

Currently, anthracycline-based treatment is considered the first line of therapy for patients with AITL (1,15,29). Rituximab is added to the regimen by some oncologists since AITL is known to contain many B cells. Clinical trials are currently evaluating antibody-based therapies that target CD4 (zanolimumab) or CD52 (alemtuzumab), and bortezomib to target the NF-κB pathway (10,23,25). Other potentially valuable agents used in small numbers of patients include thalidomide, lenalidomide, pralatrexate, brentuximab vedotin (anti-CD30), cyclosporine, and anti-vascular endothelial growth factor (VEGF), as well as others (28,39). There is no clear benefit to using intensive chemotherapy regimens or stem cell transplantation (1,28).

The median survival period of patients with AITL is about 3 years or less, and many patients die of infectious complications (15,29); 20 to 30 percent of patients, however, respond well to steroids and have a longer survival time (15,17). There has been little improvement in overall prognosis during the past two decades (55). Early-stage disease and initial response to therapy correlate with a better prognosis (1,15). An elevated absolute monocyte count in the peripheral blood correlates with a poorer prognosis (56).

The International Prognostic Index (IPI) and the prognostic index for PTCL (PIT) have limited value in the prognostication of AITL patients. Federico et al. (15) have suggested an alternative prognostic index for AITL that subdivides patients into low- and high-risk groups. This index is composed of age over 60 years, performance status of 2 or greater, more than one extranodal site, B symptoms, and platelet count of less than 150×10^9/L.

Traditionally, no pathologic findings have correlated with prognosis. However, in a small study, Tan et al. (46) suggested that patients with pattern I AITL have better survival and a lower risk of developing diffuse large B-cell lymphoma. This study needs further validation.

REFERENCES

1. Abramson JS, Feldman T, Kroll-Desrosiers AR, et al. Peripheral T-cell lymphomas in a large US multicenter cohort: prognostication in the modern era including impact of frontline therapy. Ann Oncol 2014;25:2211-2217.

2. Attygalle AD, Chuang SS, Diss TC, Du MQ, Isaacson PG, Dogan A. Distinguishing angioimmunoblastic T-cell lymphoma from peripheral T-cell lymphoma, unspecified, using morphology, immunophenotype and molecular genetics. Histopathology 2007;50:498-508.

3. Attygalle AD, Kyriakou C, Dupuis J, et al. Histologic evolution of angioimmunoblastic T-cell lymphoma in consecutive biopsies: clinical correlation and insights into natural history and disease progression. Am J Surg Pathol 2007;31: 1077-1088.

4. Baseggio L, Berger F, Morel D, et al. Identification of circulating CD10 positive T cells in angioimmunoblastic T-cell lymphoma. Leukemia 2006;20:296-303.

5. Baseggio L, Traverse-Glehen A, Berger F, et al. CD10 and ICOS expression by multiparametric flow cytometry in angioimmunoblastic T-cell lymphoma. Mod Pathol 2011;24:993-1003.

6. Brauninger A, Spieker T, Willenbrock K, et al. Survival and clonal expansion of mutating "forbidden" (immunoglobulin receptor-deficient) Epstein-Barr virus-infected B cells in angioimmunoblastic T cell lymphoma. J Exp Med 2001;194:927-940.

7. Cairns RA, Iqbal J, Lemonnier F, et al. IDH2 mutations are frequent in angioimmunoblastic T-cell lymphoma. Blood 2012;119:1901-1903.

8. Cho YU, Chi HS, Park CJ, Jang S, Seo EJ, Huh J. Distinct features of angioimmunoblastic T-cell lymphoma with bone marrow involvement. Am J Clin Pathol 2009;131:640-646.

8a. Cortés JR, Palomero T. The curious origin of angioimmunoblastic T-cell lymphoma. Curr Opin Hematol 2016;23:434-443.

9. Couronne L, Bastard C, Bernard OA. TET2 and DNMT3A mutations in human T-cell lymphoma. N Engl J Med 2012;366:95-96.

10. d'Amore F, Radford J, Relander T, et al. Phase II trial of zanolimumab (HuMax-CD4) in relapsed or refractory non-cutaneous peripheral T cell lymphoma. Br J Haematol 2010;150:565-573.

11. de Leval L, Rickman DS, Thielen C, et al. The gene expression profile of nodal peripheral T-cell lymphoma demonstrates a molecular link between angioimmunoblastic T-cell lymphoma (AITL) and follicular helper T (TFH) cells. Blood 2007;109:4952-4963.

12. Dogan A, Gaulard P, Sng I, Jaffe ES, Ralfkiaer E, Muller-Hermelink HK. Angioimmunoblastic T-cell lymphoma. In: Swerdlow SH, Campo E, Harris NL, et al., eds. WHO Classification of tumours of haematopoietic and lymphoid tissues. Lyon: IARC Press; 2008:309-311.

13. Dorfman DM, Brown JA, Shahsafaei A, Freeman GJ. Programmed death-1 (PD-1) is a marker of germinal center-associated T cells and angioimmunoblastic T-cell lymphoma. Am J Surg Pathol 2006;30:802-810.

14. Dorfman DM, Shahsafaei A. CD200 (OX-2 membrane glycoprotein) is expressed by follicular T helper cells and in angioimmunoblastic T-cell lymphoma. Am J Surg Pathol 2011;35:76-83.

15. Federico M, Rudiger T, Bellei M, et al. Clinicopathologic characteristics of angioimmunoblastic T-cell lymphoma: analysis of the international peripheral T-cell lymphoma project. J Clin Oncol 2013;31:240-246.

16. Forster G, Moeschlin S. [Extramedullary, leukemic plasmacytoma with dysproteinemia and acquired hemolytic anemia.] Schweiz Med Wochenschr 1954;84:1106-1110. [German]

17. Frizzera G, Moran EM, Rappaport H. Angio-immunoblastic lymphadenopathy with dysproteinaemia. Lancet 1974;1:1070-1073.

18. Fujiwara SI, Yamashita Y, Nakamura N, et al. High-resolution analysis of chromosome copy number alterations in angioimmunoblastic T-cell lymphoma and peripheral T-cell lymphoma, unspecified, with single nucleotide polymorphism-typing microarrays. Leukemia 2008;22:1891-1898.

19. Grogg KL, Attygalle AD, Macon WR, Remstein ED, Kurtin PJ, Dogan A. Expression of CXCL13, a chemokine highly upregulated in germinal center T-helper cells, distinguishes angioimmunoblastic T-cell lymphoma from peripheral T-cell lymphoma, unspecified. Mod Pathol 2006;19:1101-1107.

20. Huang Y, Moreau A, Dupuis J, et al. Peripheral T-cell lymphomas with a follicular growth pattern are derived from follicular helper T cells (TFH) and may show overlapping features with angioimmunoblastic T-cell lymphomas. Am J Surg Pathol 2009;33:682-690.

21. Iqbal J, Weisenburger DD, Greiner TC, et al. Molecular signatures to improve diagnosis in peripheral T-cell lymphoma and prognostication in angioimmunoblastic T-cell lymphoma. Blood 2010;115:1026-1036.

22. Iqbal J, Wright G, Wang C, et al. Gene expression signatures delineate biological and prognostic subgroups in peripheral T-cell lymphoma. Blood 2014;123:2915-2923.

23. Jiang L, Yuan CM, Hubacheck J, et al. Variable CD52 expression in mature T cell and NK cell malignancies: implications for alemtuzumab therapy. Br J Haematol 2009;145:173-179.

24. Khokhar FA, Payne WD, Talwalkar SS, et al. Angioimmunoblastic T-cell lymphoma in bone marrow: a morphologic and immunophenotypic study. Hum Pathol 2010;41:79-87.

25. Kim SJ, Yoon DH, Kang HJ, et al. Bortezomib in combination with CHOP as first-line treatment for patients with stage III/IV peripheral T-cell lymphomas: a multicentre, single-arm, phase 2 trial. Eur J Cancer 2012;48:3223-3231.

26. Liang PI, Chang ST, Lin MY, et al. Angioimmunoblastic T-cell lymphoma in Taiwan shows a frequent gain of ITK gene. Int J Clin Exp Pathol 2014;7:6097-6107.

26a. Loghavi S, Wang SA, Medeiros JL, et al. Immunophenotypic and diagnostic characterization of angioimmunoblastic T-cell lymphoma by advanced flow cytometric technology. Leuk Lymphoma 2016;57:2804-2812.

27. Martel P, Laroche L, Courville P, et al. Cutaneous involvement in patients with angioimmunoblastic lymphadenopathy with dysproteinemia: a clinical, immunohistological, and molecular analysis. Arch Dermatol 2000;136:881-886.

28. Mosalpuria K, Bociek RG, Vose JM. Angioimmunoblastic T-cell lymphoma management. Semin Hematol 2014;51:52-58.

29. Mourad N, Mounier N, Briere J, et al. Clinical, biologic, and pathologic features in 157 patients with angioimmunoblastic T-cell lymphoma treated within the Groupe d'Etude des Lymphomes de l'Adulte (GELA) trials. Blood 2008;111:4463-4470.

30. Nelson M, Horsman DE, Weisenburger DD, et al. Cytogenetic abnormalities and clinical correlations in peripheral T-cell lymphoma. Br J Haematol 2008;141:461-469.

31. Ng WK, Ip P, Choy C, Collins RJ. Cytologic findings of angioimmunoblastic T-cell lymphoma: analysis of 16 fine needle aspirates over 9-year period. Cancer 2002;96:166-173.

32. Nicolae A, Pittaluga S, Venkataraman G, et al. Peripheral T-cell lymphomas of follicular T-helper cell derivation with Hodgkin/Reed-Sternberg cells of B-cell lineage: both EBV-positive and EBV-negative variants exist. Am J Surg Pathol 2013;37:816-826.

33. Niino D, Komohara Y, Murayama T, et al. Ratio of M2 macrophage expression is closely associated with poor prognosis for angioimmunoblastic T-cell lymphoma (AITL). Pathol Int 2010;60:278-83.

34. Odejide O, Weigert O, Lane AA, et al. A targeted mutational landscape of angioimmunoblastic T-cell lymphoma. Blood 2014;123:1293-1296.

35. Onaindia A, Martinez N, Montes-Moreno S, et al. CD30 expression by B and T cells: a frequent finding in angioimmunoblastic T-cell lymphoma and peripheral T-cell lymphoma-not otherwise specified. Am J Surg Pathol 2016; 40:378-385.

36. Ondrejka SL, Grzywacz B, Bodo J, et al. Angioimmunoblastic T-cell lymphomas with the RHOA p.Gly17Val mutation have classic clinical and pathologic features. Am J Surg Pathol 2016;40:335-341.

37. Palomero T, Couronne L, Khiabanian H, et al. Recurrent mutations in epigenetic regulators, RHOA and FYN kinase in peripheral T cell lymphomas. Nat Genet 2014;46:166-170.

38. Piccaluga PP, Agostinelli C, Califano A, et al. Gene expression analysis of angioimmunoblastic lymphoma indicates derivation from T follicular helper cells and vascular endothelial growth factor deregulation. Cancer Res 2007;67:10703-10710.

39. Ramasamy K, Lim Z, Pagliuca A, Salisbury JR, Mufti GJ, Devereux S. Successful treatment of refractory angioimmunoblastic T-cell lymphoma with thalidomide and dexamethasone. Haematologica 2006;91(Suppl):ECR44.

40. Reddemann K, Gola D, Schillert A, et al. Dysregulation of microRNAs in angioimmunoblastic T-cell lymphoma. Anticancer Res 2015;35:2055-2061.

41. Rohr J, Guo S, Huo J, et al. Recurrent activating mutations of CD28 in peripheral T-cell lymphomas. Leukemia 2016;30:1062-1070.

42. Sakata-Yanagimoto M, Enami T, Yoshida K, et al. Somatic RHOA mutation in angioimmunoblastic T cell lymphoma. Nat Genet 2014;46:171-175.

43. Schlegelberger B, Zhang Y, Weber-Matthiesen K, Grote W. Detection of aberrant clones in nearly all cases of angioimmunoblastic lymphoadenopathy with dysproteinemia-type T-cell lymphoma by combined interphase and metaphase cytogenetics. Blood 1994;84:2640-2648.

43a. Schwartz FH, Cai Q, Fellmann E, et al. TET2 mutations in B cells of patients affected by angioimmunoblastic T cell lymphoma. J Pathol 2017;242:129-133.

44. Shah ZH, Harris S, Smith JL, Hodges E. Monoclonality and oligoclonality of T cell receptor beta gene in angioimmunoblastic T cell lymphoma. J Clin Pathol 2009;62:177-181.

45. Swerdlow SH, Campo E, Pileri SA, et al. The 2016 revision of the World Health Organization classification of lymphoid neoplasms. Blood 2016;127:2375-2390.

46. Tan LH, Tan SY, Tang T, et al. Angioimmunoblastic T-cell lymphoma with hyperplastic germinal centres (pattern 1) shows superior survival to patterns 2 and 3: a meta-analysis of 56 cases. Histopathology 2012;60:570-585.

47. Thorns C, Bastian B, Pinkel D, et al. Chromosomal alterations in angioimmunoblastic T-cell lymphoma and peripheral T-cell lymphoma unspecified: a matrix-based approach. Genes Chromosomes Cancer 2007;46:37-44.

48. Tripodo C, Gri G, Piccaluga PP, et al. Mast cells and Th17 cells contribute to the lymphoma-associated pro-inflammatory microenvironment of angioimmunoblastic T-cell lymphoma. Am J Pathol 2010;177:792-802.

49. Troxell ML, Schwartz EJ, van de Rijn M, et al. Follicular dendritic cell immunohistochemical markers in angioimmunoblastic T-cell lymphoma. Appl Immunohistochem Mol Morphol 2005;13: 297-303.

49a. Vallois D, Dobay MP, Morin RD, et al. Activating mutations in genes related to TCR signaling in angioimmunoblastic and other follicular helper T-cell-derived lymphomas. Blood 2016;128:1490-1502.

50. Vose J, Armitage J, Weisenburger D, International T-Cell Lymphoma Project. International peripheral T-cell and natural killer/T-cell lymphoma study: pathology findings and clinical outcomes. J Clin Oncol 2008;26:4124-4130.

51. Wang C, McKeithan TW, Gong Q, et al. IDH2R172 mutations define a unique subgroup of patients with angioimmunoblastic T-cell lymphoma. Blood 2015;126:1741-1752.

52. Warnke RA, Jones D, Hsi ED. Morphologic and immunophenotypic variants of nodal T-cell lymphomas and T-cell lymphoma mimics. Am J Clin Pathol 2007;127:511-527.

53. Weiss LM, Jaffe ES, Liu XF, Chen YY, Shibata D, Medeiros LJ. Detection and localization of Epstein-Barr viral genomes in angioimmunoblastic lymphadenopathy and angioimmunoblastic lymphadenopathy-like lymphoma. Blood 1992;79:1789-1795.

54. Willenbrock K, Brauninger A, Hansmann ML. Frequent occurrence of B-cell lymphomas in angioimmunoblastic T-cell lymphoma and proliferation of Epstein-Barr virus-infected cells in early cases. Br J Haematol 2007;138:733-739.

55. Xu B, Liu P. No survival improvement for patients with angioimmunoblastic T-cell lymphoma over the past two decades: a population-based study of 1207 cases. PLoS One 2014;9:e92585.

56. Yang YQ, Liang JH, Wu JZ, et al. Elevated absolute monocyte count predicts unfavorable outcomes in patients with angioimmunoblastic T-cell lymphoma. Leuk Res 2015;42:88-92.

57. Yoo HY, Kim P, Kim WS, et al. Frequent CTLA4-CD28 gene fusion in diverse types of T cell lymphoma. Haematologica 2016;101:757-763.

58. Zettl A, Lee SS, Rudiger T, et al. Epstein-Barr virus-associated B-cell lymphoproliferative disorders in angioimmunoblastic T-cell lymphoma and peripheral T-cell lymphoma, unspecified. Am J Clin Pathol 2002;117:368-379.

59. Zhan HQ, Li XQ, Zhu XZ, Lu HF, Zhou XY, Chen Y. Expression of follicular helper T cell markers in nodal peripheral T cell lymphomas: a tissue microarray analysis of 162 cases. J Clin Pathol 2011;64:319-324.

32 ADULT T-CELL LEUKEMIA/LYMPHOMA

GENERAL FEATURES

Adult T-cell leukemia/lymphoma (ATLL) is a mature T-cell neoplasm, often with a T-regulatory immunophenotype. It is caused by infection by human T-cell lymphotropic virus 1 (HTLV-1).

HTLV-1 Virus

HTLV-1 was the first retrovirus proven to cause a malignant neoplasm, ATLL. The virus is 80 to 100 nm and is composed of a single-stranded RNA surrounded by an envelope (16). The virus spreads via cell to cell contact using a cell surface HTLV-1 receptor (a complex of molecules including glucose transporter-1, neuropilin, and heparin sulfate proteoglycan).

HTLV-1 infects a number of cell types, including various T-cell subsets, B cells, histiocytes, dendritic cells, and hematopoietic stem cells (16). Infection most often occurs by transmission of HTLV-1–positive CD4-positive T cells and dendritic cells. Infection of CD4-positive mature T cells, hematopoietic stem cells, or both, is most important in the pathogenesis of ATLL. After HTLV-1 is transmitted to another cell, the viral RNA is converted to proviral (double-stranded) DNA; provirus then integrates into the host cell DNA via the enzyme viral integrase.

The HTLV-1 genome is flanked by long terminal repeats (LTRs) and has a limited number of genes, including *GAG, POL,* and *ENV*; there is also a pX region near the 3′ LTR that encodes via differential mRNA splicing for TAX, REX, and other viral proteins (see chapter 9, fig. 9-13) (16,35). Two viral genes are essential for HTLV-1 infection: HTLV-1 transactivator X (*TAX*) and HTLV-1 basic leucine zipper factor (*HBZ*).

TAX is a promiscuous transcriptional activator that induces the expression of viral genes and cellular genes through the interaction with pleiotropic transcription factors involved in the NF-κB, PI3K/AKT, AP-1 pathways, and others (16). TAX drives cell proliferation, inhibits apoptosis, and increases genetic instability. TAX is essential for initial infection and early proliferation. However, in a substantial subset of ATLL cases, TAX expression is absent; apparently the TAX-positive cells in these patients have been eliminated by the host cytotoxic T-cell response (16,35). Once HTLV-1 is integrated into the host genome, a host cytotoxic T-cell response can eliminate most virally infected (TAX positive) cells. It seems that TAX is important early, but not later, in pathogenesis. TAX-negative virally infected cells escape detection and survive. TAX-negative cells express HBZ, and HBZ appears to be important for the maintenance of infection. HBZ also plays an important role in cell proliferation and clonal expansion.

Other HTLV viruses share many genes with HTLV-1, but their role in human disease is not well established. HTLV-2 is the best known. In the United States, HTLV-2 infection is endemic in intravenous drug users in some urban areas (5); HTLV-2 is not a cause of ATLL. HTLV-3 and HLTV-4 occur in Central Africa and do not appear to be associated with ATLL (14).

Primates are infected by similar viruses (STLV), of which there are multiple types. Interspecies transmission of HTLV-1, from primates to humans, is a low frequency event that can occur, particularly in central Africa and southeast Asia, likely related to hunting and bites by an infected animal, exposure to the carcass, or ingestion of infected meat (14).

Epidemiology of HTLV-1 Infection

HTLV-1 infection is distributed around the world and the estimated number of infected persons (carriers) ranges from 5 to 20 million (6,35). The distribution of carriers, however, is not homogeneous (fig. 32-1). Geographic clusters of high infection frequency (endemic regions) are often located near areas where viral infection is rare or absent. The most highly endemic regions are southwestern Japan (Kyushu and Okinawa islands), sub-Saharan Africa (especially western

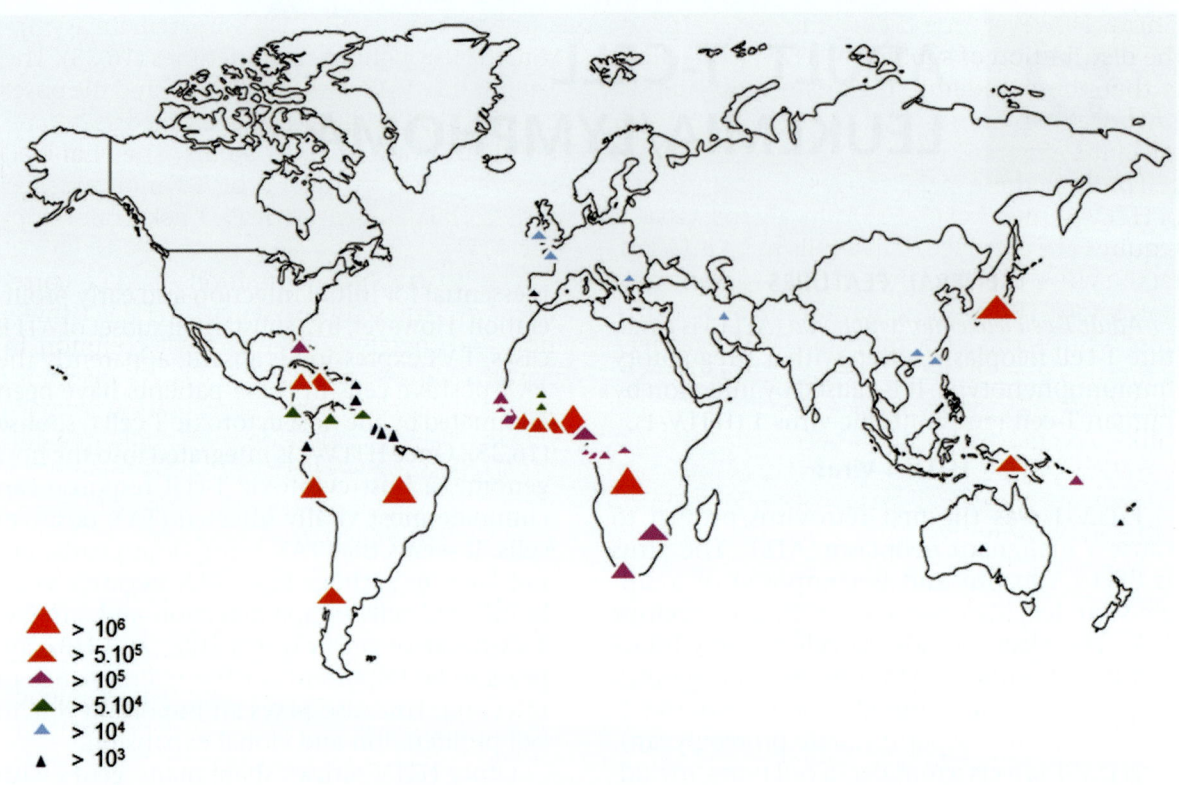

Figure 32-1

HTLV-1 CARRIERS AROUND THE WORLD

Brazil, Central Africa, and Japan have the highest seroprevalence, each with greater than 1 x 10^6 carriers.

and central nations), the Caribbean islands, South America (Brazil, Chile, and Peru), Iran (in particular, the northeast Mashhad region), Romania, and the Melanesian Islands (6,35). The prevalence of HTLV-1 infection is low in western Europe and the United States, and most often HTLV-1 carriers in these nations are immigrants from endemic regions or their descendents (40). HTLV-1 infections cluster in families, related to its most common mode of transmission (see below); about 10 percent of ATLL patients have a positive family history. Coastal regions have a higher prevalence of HTLV-1 infection (6).

The HTLV-1 virus is fairly stable from the genetic point of view, likely related to its integration into DNA and clonal expansion in infected cells. As a result, there is little sequence variation; nevertheless, variation has resulted in seven viral strains, designated A to G, corresponding with the geographic distribution of HTLV-1 infection (6). The most common

and widely distributed viral strain is subtype A (or Cosmopolitan subtype). Subtype A predominates in southwestern Japan, the Caribbean islands, South America, countries in West and North Africa, and Iran. There are also four subgroups of viral strain A that correspond to geographic regions, likely related to divergent evolution (designated as transcontinental, Japanese, West African, and North African). There are three other major subtypes of HTLV-1 designated as B, C, and D and three minor subtypes designated as E to G. Subtype B occurs in Central Africa; subtype C in Australia and nearby Pacific islands; and subtype D in Central African pygmies. Subtypes E, F, and G are minor viral strains in Central Africa, possibly related to interspecies transmission (6).

The reason for the geographic distribution of HTLV-1 infection is unknown, and few studies are available on the prevalence of HTLV-1 infection in large countries such as India and

China. However, one theory that may explain the distribution of subtype A HTLV-1 infection is that these endemic regions correspond to historical exploration and travel routes of the ancient slave trade (36).

There are three major modes of transmission of HTLV-1 infection (5,6,16). Since transmission requires the presence of live cells to be infected by the virus, the efficiency of HTLV-1 transmission is low. The most important mode of transmission in terms of number of HTLV-1 carriers is mother to child transmission, which occurs via breast milk (by lymphocytes present in the milk). The risk of an infant becoming infected correlates with the HTLV-1 proviral load of the mother and the length of time of breast feeding. With maximum exposure, about 20 percent of infants of carrier mothers become HTLV-1 carriers themselves (6,40). In addition, about 3 percent of non-breastfed babies born to HTLV-1 carrier mothers become infected (2). Exposure of a baby to infected blood during delivery is a possible means of such transmission.

A second mode of transmission is by unprotected sexual contact, mostly male to female via infected lymphocytes in semen. As a result of this mode, the frequency of the HTLV-1 carrier status in women increases with age (40).

Exposure to blood and blood products is a third mode of HTLV-1 transmission, and is divided into two major types: intravenous drug use and therapeutic administration of blood products, of which packed red blood cell transfusion carries the greatest risk. For the past 20 years, in most industrialized nations, the blood supply has been screened routinely for HTLV-1 infection, reducing the transmission of HTLV-1 infection as a result of blood transfusion (6). A few cases of donor-derived infection following stem cell transplantation also have been reported (19).

HTLV-1–Associated Diseases

Due to the long latency interval between exposure to HTLV-1 infection and the development of ATLL, exposure usually occurs early in life, usually acquired by breast feeding. Nevertheless, the lifetime risk of developing ATLL in HTLV-1 carriers is low, estimated to be between 2 and 4 percent, and slightly higher for men (about 5 percent) than women. Most HTLV-1 carriers never develop ATLL and remain asymptomatic throughout their lifetimes (16,35). The latency interval between infection and the onset of ATLL is 20 to 40 years, and the disease predominantly affects older adults. The viral load in circulating peripheral blood mononuclear cells correlates with increased risk of developing ATLL.

The geographic distribution of ATLL correlates with the seroprevalence of HTLV-1 infection and therefore ATLL is most common in nations highly endemic for HTLV-1 infection. Japan has the highest known seroprevalence rate for HTLV-1 worldwide, with about one million HTLV-1 carriers (35). Not surprisingly, ATLL is the most common type of T-cell lymphoma in Japan, where 800 to 1,000 new cases occur each year, and ATLL represents up to 25 percent of all T-cell lymphomas (35,37). ATLL is also common in other highly endemic nations, such as Brazil and West and Central Africa and is rare in Europe and North America (6,37). The frequency of HTLV-1 carriers is increasing in nonendemic regions, however, possibly related to migration from endemic to nonendemic regions (40).

Several other diseases are associated with HTLV-1. HTLV-1–associated myelopathy/tropical spastic paraparesis is a demyelinating disease of the spinal cord, particularly the lateral and anterior columns, that commonly affects the lower extremities, bladder, and erectile function in men. Other HTLV-1–associated diseases, although less well established, include a rheumatoid-like arthropathy, uveitis in Japan, dermatitis in children in the Caribbean islands, and a form of interstitial pneumonia known as HTLV-1–associated bronchioloalveolar disorder (6,21). These diseases are not the focus of this chapter.

CLINICAL FEATURES

The median age of onset in patients with ATLL is most often the seventh decade, but there is a broad age range, from 20 to 80 years (11,21,25,35). Children rarely develop ATLL, but the rare cases that do occur are most often the acute variant (13). The male to female ratio is 1.5 to 1.0.

Patients with ATLL commonly present with widely disseminated disease and involvement of multiple sites including lymph nodes, spleen, skin, peripheral blood, bone

Table 32-1

CLINICOPATHOLOGIC FEATURES OF ADULT T-CELL LEUKEMIA/LYMPHOMA VARIANTS

Feature	Acute	Lymphomatous	Chronic	Smoldering
Lymphocytosis	present, often marked elevation	absent	present, usually mild elevation	absent
Flower cells in blood smear	numerous	present, but no leukemic phase	~5%	3-5% atypical small lymphocytes
Serum lactate dehydrogenase	increased	increased	minimally increased	normal
Serum calcium	high	variable levels	present in subset of patients (unfavorable group)	normal
Lymphadenopathy	present	present	can be present, but mild	absent
Hepatosplenomegaly	usually present	often present	can be present, but mild	absent
Skin lesions	frequent, sometimes erythroderma	frequent	frequent, often exfoliative rash	frequent, often patch lesions
BM infiltration	may be present	may be present	absent	absent
Lytic bone lesions	present	present	absent	absent
Median survival	6-12 months	10-12 months	~2 years	2-4 years

marrow, lungs, liver, central nervous system, and gastrointestinal tract (21,29,35). Over 50 percent of ATLL patients exhibit skin manifestations (33). High levels of soluble CD25 may be detected in the serum and correlate with disease activity. About 90 percent of patients present with stage III to IV disease, and the bone marrow is involved in almost one third of patients. Approximately two thirds of patients present with a high International Prognostic Index (37).

Patients with ATLL, particularly those with the acute and lymphomatous variants, frequently become severely immunocompromised and are prone to opportunistic organisms including *Pneumocystis jirovecii* (previously known as *Pneumocystis carinii*), *Aspergillus fumigatus*, *Cryptococcus neoformans*, and *Strongyloides stercolaris*; the latter may be particularly virulent in ATLL patients (21,29,30). Malignant tumors associated with immunodeficiency, such as Kaposi sarcoma and Epstein-Barr virus (EBV)-associated lymphomas, also occur in patients with ATLL.

Clinical Variants

The Shimoyama classification (Table 32-1) recognizes four clinical variants of ATLL: acute, lymphomatous, chronic, and smoldering (29). This classification has been adopted by the World Health Organization (WHO) classifica-

tion (21). The *acute variant* of ATLL represents approximately 60 percent of all cases. Patients present with leukemia and often an extremely high peripheral leukocyte count, commonly accompanied by eosinophilia, B-type symptoms, hypercalcemia (serum calcium over 20 mg/mL), a high serum lactate dehydrogenase (LDH) level, generalized lymphadenopathy, hepatosplenomegaly, lytic bone lesions, and cutaneous lesions including rashes, papules, and nodules/tumors (28,29,33). The central nervous system is involved in about 10 percent of patients. The prognosis is poor, with a median survival period of 6 to 12 months. The acute variant is the most common variant of ATLL in Japan.

The *lymphomatous variant* represents approximately 20 percent of all cases (11,29). This variant clinically overlaps with the acute variant, except that patients usually do not have a leukemic phase. Patients present with prominent lymphadenopathy and cutaneous manifestations. Hypercalcemia and lytic bone lesions occur, but less often than in the acute variant. Lymphoma cells are identified in the blood smear. The prognosis of patients with the lymphomatous variant is also poor, with a median survival period of about 10 to 12 months. The lymphomatous variant is less common than the acute variant in Japan, but is the predominant presentation for patients with ATLL in the Caribbean islands (21).

The *chronic variant* of ATLL represents approximately 15 percent of all cases (11,29). Patients with the chronic variant characteristically have an exfoliative rash and the peripheral leukocyte count is often mildly elevated; atypical lymphocytes represent about 5 percent of blood lymphocytes. This variant is subdivided into unfavorable and favorable subsets. Patients with the *unfavorable chronic variant* may have mild lymphadenopathy or hepatosplenomegaly, an elevated serum LDH or blood urea nitrogen level, and low serum albumin. Hypercalcemia occurs in some patients. Patients with the unfavorable chronic variant have a poor prognosis and are considered to have aggressive disease. Patients lacking these features have the favorable chronic variant.

The *smoldering variant* of ATLL represents approximately 5 percent of all cases (11,29). This variant is characterized by a normal leukocyte count, but 3 to 5 percent of the circulating ATLL cells exhibit slight atypia. Patients with the smoldering variant often have skin and pulmonary manifestations, but do not have a leukemic phase, widespread lymphadenopathy, organomegaly, or hypercalcemia. The smoldering variant and the favorable chronic variant are usually lumped together as clinically indolent ATLL.

Transition from the smoldering or chronic variant to the aggressive acute variant of ATLL occurs in 25 to 50 percent of cases and the long-term outlook for these patients is generally unfavorable (11). In one study, the median time for this transition to occur was 18.8 months (range, 0.3 months to 17.6 years) (31).

HISTOLOGIC FINDINGS

Lymph Node

The morphologic features of ATLL involving lymph nodes are diverse (20,21,25). The pattern of involvement can be paracortical, leaving the B-cell compartment relatively unaffected, or the neoplasm can diffusely replace the lymph node architecture (fig. 32-2). A starry sky pattern is common. In some cases, a leukemic pattern of spread is observed, with prominent intrasinusoidal involvement (fig. 32-3). The wide cytologic spectrum seen in ATLL may be subdivided, in part arbitrarily, into five subgroups: pleomorphic small cell, pleomorphic medium and large cell, anaplastic large cell-like, angioimmunoblastic T-cell lymphoma-like, and Hodgkin-like (9,22,24,25).

The pleomorphic small cell and pleomorphic medium and large cell subgroups are the most common. In the pleomorphic small cell subgroup, the tumor cells are monotonous, small lymphoid cells with irregular nuclear contours. In the pleomorphic medium and large cell subgroup, the tumor cells range from small to intermediate to large, with highly irregular nuclear contours in varying proportions (fig. 32-4). Giant cells with convoluted or cerebriform nuclei are sometimes present (24). Small lymphocytes, histiocytes, and, in some cases, many eosinophils are present in the background.

The anaplastic large cell-like variant is composed of large neoplastic cells with anaplastic features (38). In general, the cells are more pleomorphic than observed in anaplastic lymphoma kinase (ALK)-positive ALCL, and more similar to ALK-negative ALCL. The angioimmunoblastic T-cell lymphoma-like variant of ATLL is uncommon, representing less than 10 percent of all cases (9). These tumors are characterized by a proliferation of high endothelial venules, neoplastic cells with abundant clear cytoplasm, associated plasma cells and eosinophils, and EBV-positive large B cells; however, there is no expansion of CD21-positive follicular dendritic cell networks. In addition, the lymphoma cells do not express follicular T-helper cell markers, such as PD1/CD279, CD10, BCL6, or CXCL13 (9).

In cases of ATLL with a Hodgkin-like morphologic appearance, the tumor often partially involves lymph nodes, and large tumor cells that closely resemble Reed-Sternberg or Hodgkin cells are present (fig. 32-5) (22). These cases are associated with a less aggressive clinical course (22). The Hodgkin-like cells are often of B-cell lineage; positive for CD15, CD30, PAX5, and EBV; and are present in a background of neoplastic T cells that may show minimal or more obviously irregular nuclear contours (21,24). The Hodgkin-like cells lack integration of HTLV-1 and likely arise secondary to superimposed EBV infection due to the underlying immunodeficiency observed in ATLL patients (21,24).

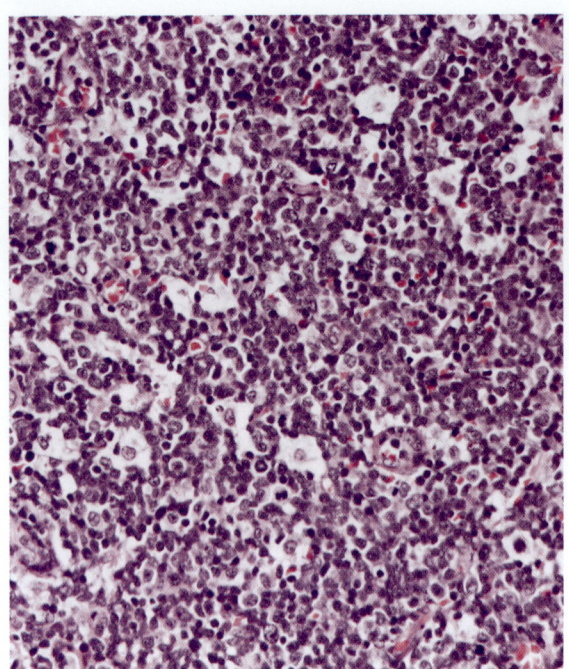 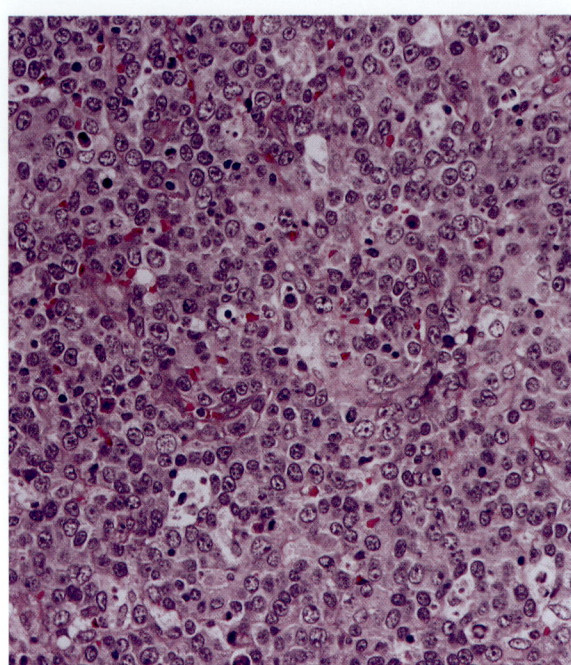

Figure 32-2

ADULT T-CELL LEUKEMIA/LYMPHOMA EFFACING LYMPH NODE

Left: In this case the lymphoma cells are mostly small to medium-sized with occasional large cells.

Right: In another case the lymphoma cells are predominantly large and, in part, resemble centroblasts. In the left and right images a starry sky pattern is present (left, right: hematoxylin and eosin [H&E] stain).

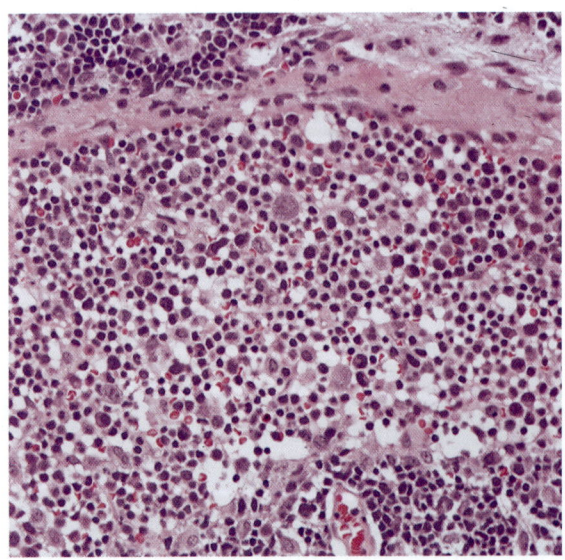 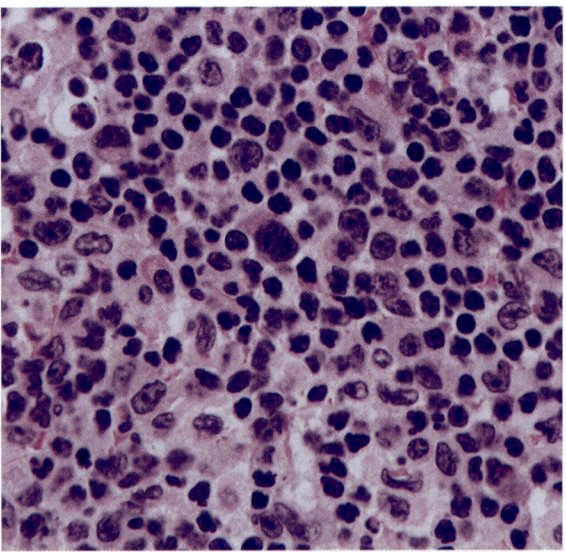

Figure 32-3

ADULT T-CELL LEUKEMIA/LYMPHOMA INVOLVING LYMPH NODE SINUS

A dilated subcapsular sinus is filled with many small and scattered large lymphoma cells (H&E stain).

Figure 32-4

ADULT T-CELL LEUKEMIA/LYMPHOMA, PLEOMORPHIC MIXED SMALL AND LARGE CELL, INVOLVING LYMPH NODE

High-power magnification shows a neoplasm composed of many small lymphoid cells and scattered large cells with highly irregular nuclear contours (H&E stain).

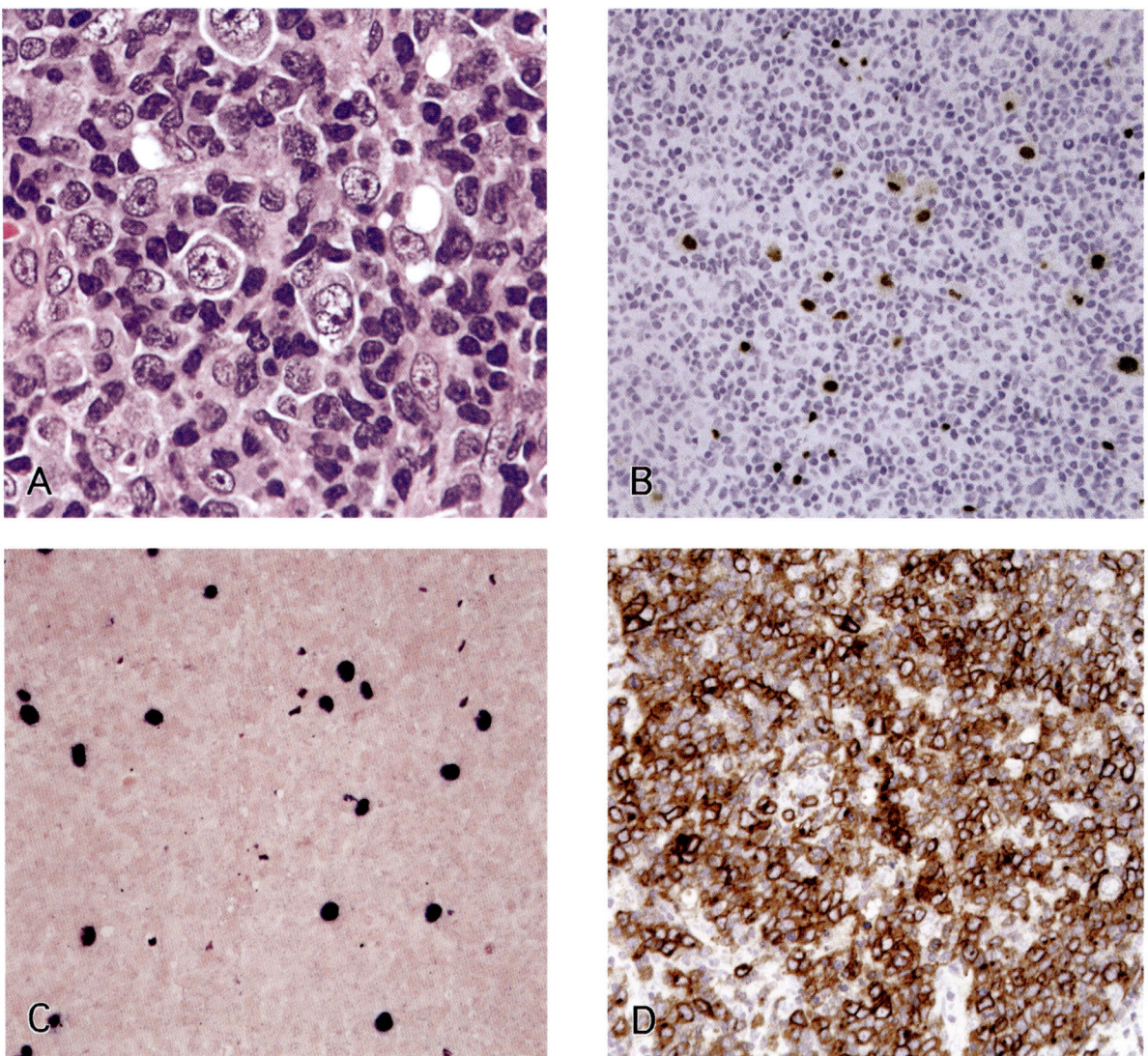

Figure 32-5

ADULT T-CELL LEUKEMIA/LYMPHOMA WITH LARGE HODGKIN-LIKE CELLS INVOLVING LYMPH NODE

A: Oil immersion magnification shows large Hodgkin-like cells in a background of smaller atypical lymphoid cells (H&E stain).

B,C: The Hodgkin-like cells are positive for PAX5 (B) and Epstein-Barr virus-encoded RNA1 (EBER1) (C).

D: The background atypical cells are T cells positive for CD25 (D), FOXP3 (not shown), and CD3 (not shown) (B,D: immunohistochemistry with hematoxylin counterstain; C: in situ hybridization with eosin counterstain).

Peripheral Blood and Bone Marrow

Patients with ATLL, particularly those with the acute variant, commonly have a leukemic phase; leukocyte and absolute lymphocyte counts can be very high. In blood smears, the lymphoma cells commonly have characteristic morphologic features and are known as flower cells. Flower cells are medium-sized or large and have lobulated nuclei, with the lobules resembling the petals of a flower (fig. 32-6) (20,21). Nucleoli are often prominent and the cytoplasm is deeply basophilic. Patients with unfavorable chronic variant disease may have prominent leukocytosis (up to 50×10^9/L), lower degrees of leukocytosis, or a normal leukocyte count. In patients with the chronic or smoldering variant, the circulating lymphoma cells are

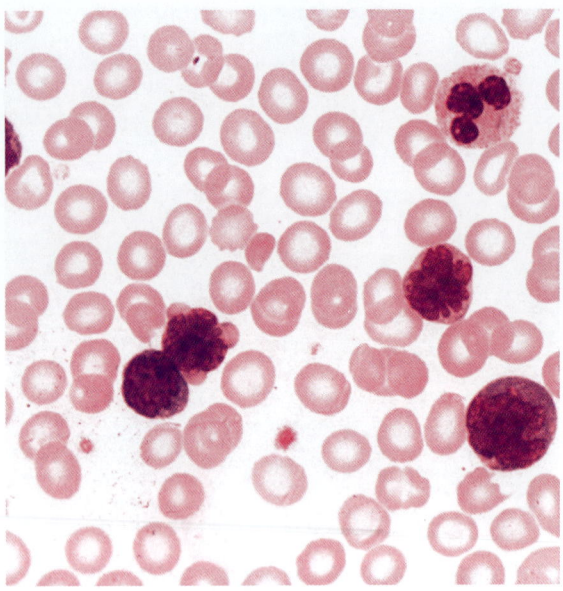

Figure 32-6

**ADULT T-CELL LEUKEMIA/LYMPHOMA
INVOLVING PERIPHERAL BLOOD**

Many leukemia cells are present in a patient with the acute variant of ATLL. The cells have lobulated nuclei that resemble petals of a flower, hence the nickname "flower cells" (Wright-Giemsa stain).

small to medium-sized, with more convoluted (rather than lobulated) nuclei, resembling, in part, Sezary cells and smaller variants (Lutzner cells) or, less often, the lymphocytes of chronic lymphocytic leukemia.

About one third of patients with ATLL have bone marrow involvement, which can be interstitial and subtle or extensive and diffuse (fig. 32-7). Osteoclastic activity may be prominent in bone marrow or bone (fig. 32-8) biopsy specimens, likely explaining the hypercalcemia in affected patients. Osteoclastic activity, however, is not linked with morphologic evidence of bone marrow involvement by ATLL (21).

Skin

At least half of ATLL patients have skin involvement (15,28,33). Skin lesions occur with all four clinical variants of disease. The skin lesions manifest as patches, plaques, papules, nodules/tumors, erythroderma, or a purpuric rash. Nodules and tumors are the most frequent (about 40 percent of patients) followed by plaques (25 to 30 percent) (33). Erythroderma occurs in 3 to 5 percent of patients, most often in those with

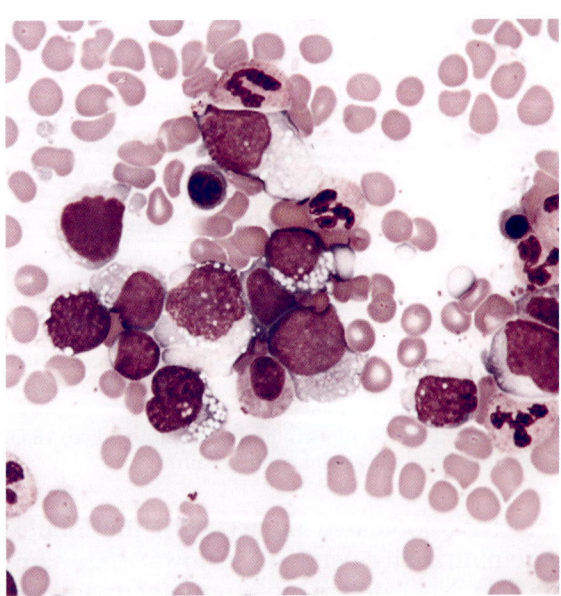
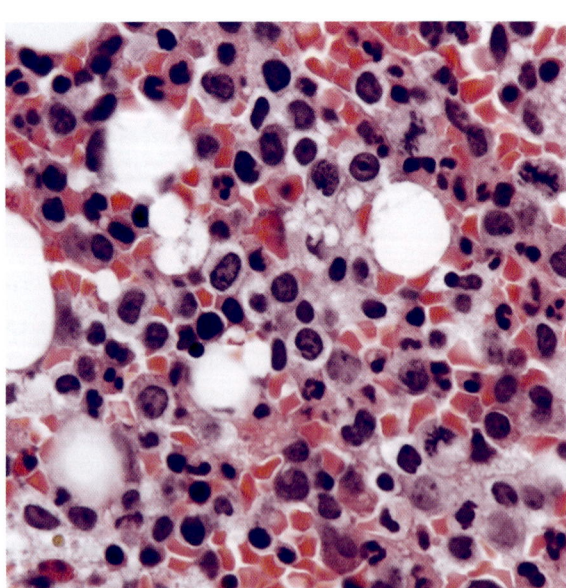

Figure 32-7

ADULT T-CELL LEUKEMIA/LYMPHOMA INVOLVING BONE MARROW

Left: A bone marrow aspirate smear shows many leukemic cells with abundant basophilic cytoplasm and cytoplasmic vacuoles (Wright-Giemsa stain).

Right: The aspirate clot specimen shows lymphoma cells intermingled with hematopoietic cells. Many mitotic figures are seen (H&E stain).

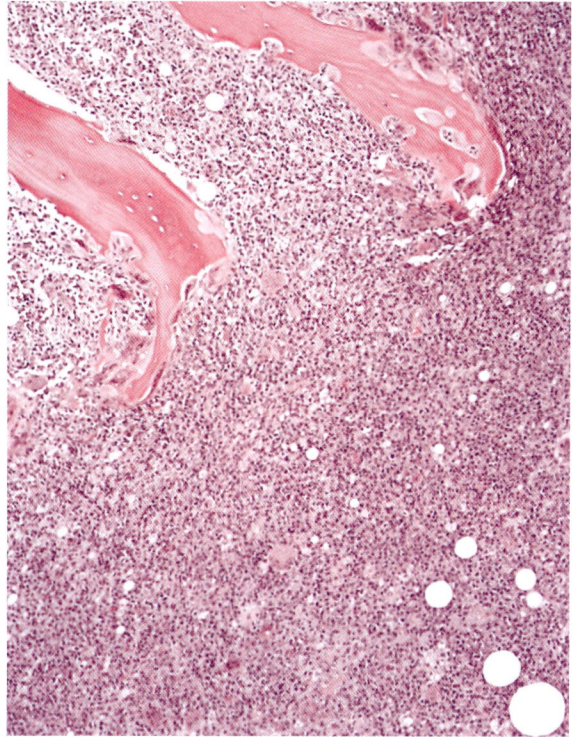

Figure 32-8

**ADULT T-CELL LEUKEMIA/
LYMPHOMA INVOLVING BONE**

A lytic bone lesion shows extensive involvement by ATLL. The osteoclastic activity is marked (H&E stain).

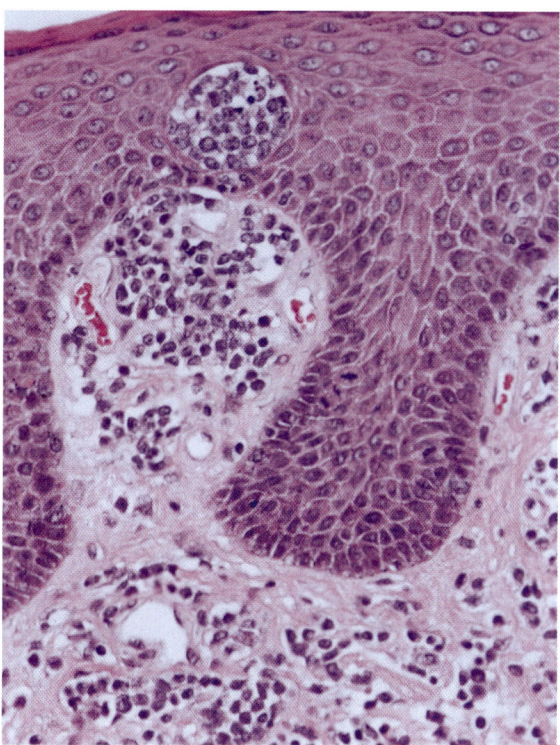

Figure 32-9

**ADULT T-CELL LEUKEMIA/
LYMPHOMA INVOLVING SKIN**

The lymphoma cells involve the dermis and infiltrate the epidermis, forming a Pautrier-type microabscess (H&E stain).

the acute variant of ATLL (33). An exfoliative rash or patch lesion is more common in patients with the smoldering variant (28). Skin disease is often the first manifestation of ATLL in patients from the Caribbean basin (15).

Histologic examination of skin biopsy specimens show a perivascular, nodular, or diffuse pattern of involvement. Larger nodules may extend into the deep dermis and subcutaneous adipose tissue. An angiocentric pattern is common. Follicotropism and epidermotropism occur in up to two thirds of cases (15); Pautrier-like microabscesses occur in approximately half of skin biopsy specimens (fig. 32-9). Follicular mucinosis, which also occurs in ATLL, can mimic mycosis fungoides (15,28).

Other Organ Systems

Since ATLL is a systemic disease, theoretically any organ in the body can be involved. Particularly in patients with the acute or lymphomatous variant, other organs are often involved and a biopsy specimen may show diffuse infiltration or a leukemic pattern. The lungs, liver, gastrointestinal tract, and central nervous system are the most frequent sites (21). Lung lesions are often detected as interstitial infiltrates. The cerebrospinal fluid is often involved in patients with central nervous system disease (lymphomatous meningitis). In the gastrointestinal tract, ATLL may cause ulcers or develop as tumor masses.

CYTOLOGIC FINDINGS

The spectrum of cytologic features of ATLL cells is broad, ranging from small to medium-sized atypical cells with coarse chromatin and irregular nuclear contours, to large lymphoid cells with more open chromatin, to giant cells with polylobated nuclear contours and prominent nucleoli (4,20). Most frequently, the tumor cells have the features of flower cells, with coarse nuclear chromatin, sometimes small or

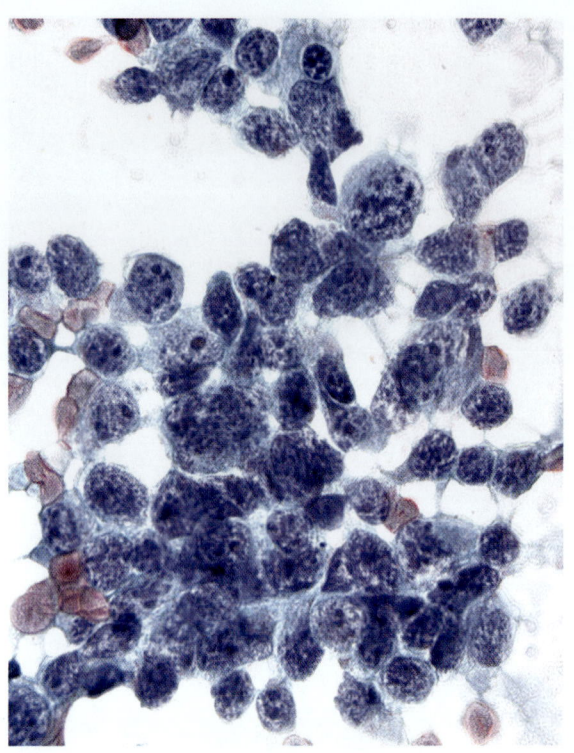 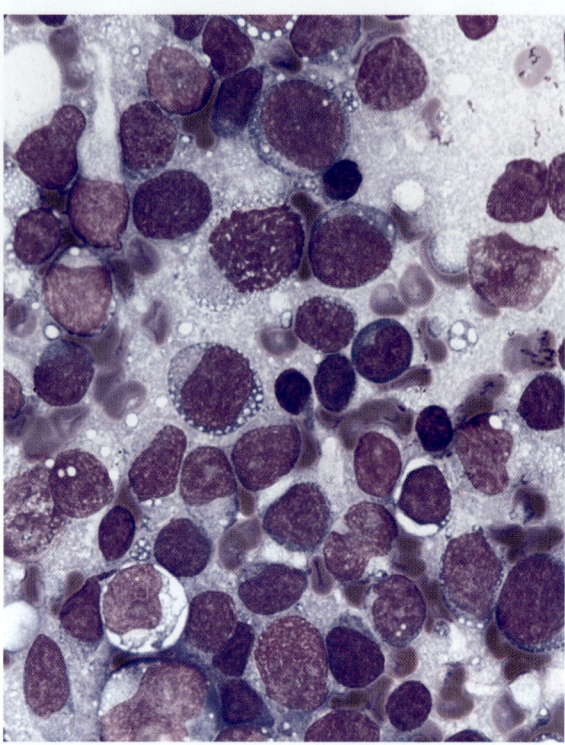

Figure 32-10

FINE-NEEDLE ASPIRATE SMEARS OF ADULT T-CELL LEUKEMIA/LYMPHOMA

Left: A fixed smear shows medium to large lymphoma cells with irregular nuclei, coarse chromatin, and prominent nucleoli (Papanicolaou stain).

Right: An air-dried smear highlights the deeply basophilic cytoplasm, which contains fine vacuoles (Diff-Quik stain). (Courtesy of Dr. W. Geddie, Toronto, Canada.)

prominent nucleoli (fig. 32-10, left), and deeply basophilic cytoplasm, occasionally with fine vacuoles (fig. 32-10, right). The cells in Diff-Quik smears resemble those observed in Wright-Giemsa–stained blood smears.

IMMUNOPHENOTYPIC FINDINGS

The cells of ATLL express a mature, often aberrant T-cell immunophenotype, being positive for CD2, CD3 (fig. 32-11A), CD5, CD43, CD45RO, and usually T-cell receptor α/β (BF-1), and negative for CD7 (4,39). CD3 expression is often dim and this feature can be used as part of gating strategies (39). Approximately 90 percent of ATLL cases are positive for CD4 and negative for CD8, but 5 to 10 percent are CD4(+)/CD8(+) or CD4(-)/CD8(+) (4,39). The tumor cells also usually express CD25 (fig. 32-5D), the chemokine receptor CCR4, and about 70 percent are positive for FOXP3, supporting a T-regulatory cell immunophenotype (8). CD30 can be expressed in ATLL

cases, usually in a subset, and often in the largest lymphoma cells (fig. 32-11B).

FOXP3 expression correlates with the pleomorphic small and medium-sized cell morphologic subgroup of ATLL, and may be lost with large cell transformation and CD30 expression (38). CD52 is usually positive in ATLL and the cytotoxic markers TIA-1, granzyme B, and perforin are usually negative. IRF4/MUM1 is expressed commonly by ATLL cells (fig. 32-11C); expression of IRF4/MUM1, and nuclear c-REL is associated with resistance to antiviral agents (27). The proliferation rate shown by Ki-67 expression may be very high (fig. 32-11D).

In cases of Hodgkin-like ATLL, the large Reed-Sternberg-like and Hodgkin-like cells express CD15, CD30, and PAX5 (fig. 32-5B) in a background of CD4-positive T cells (21). In situ hybridization for EBV-encoded RNA1 (EBER1) shows positive cells in some ATLL cases, particularly in Hodgkin-like cells (fig.

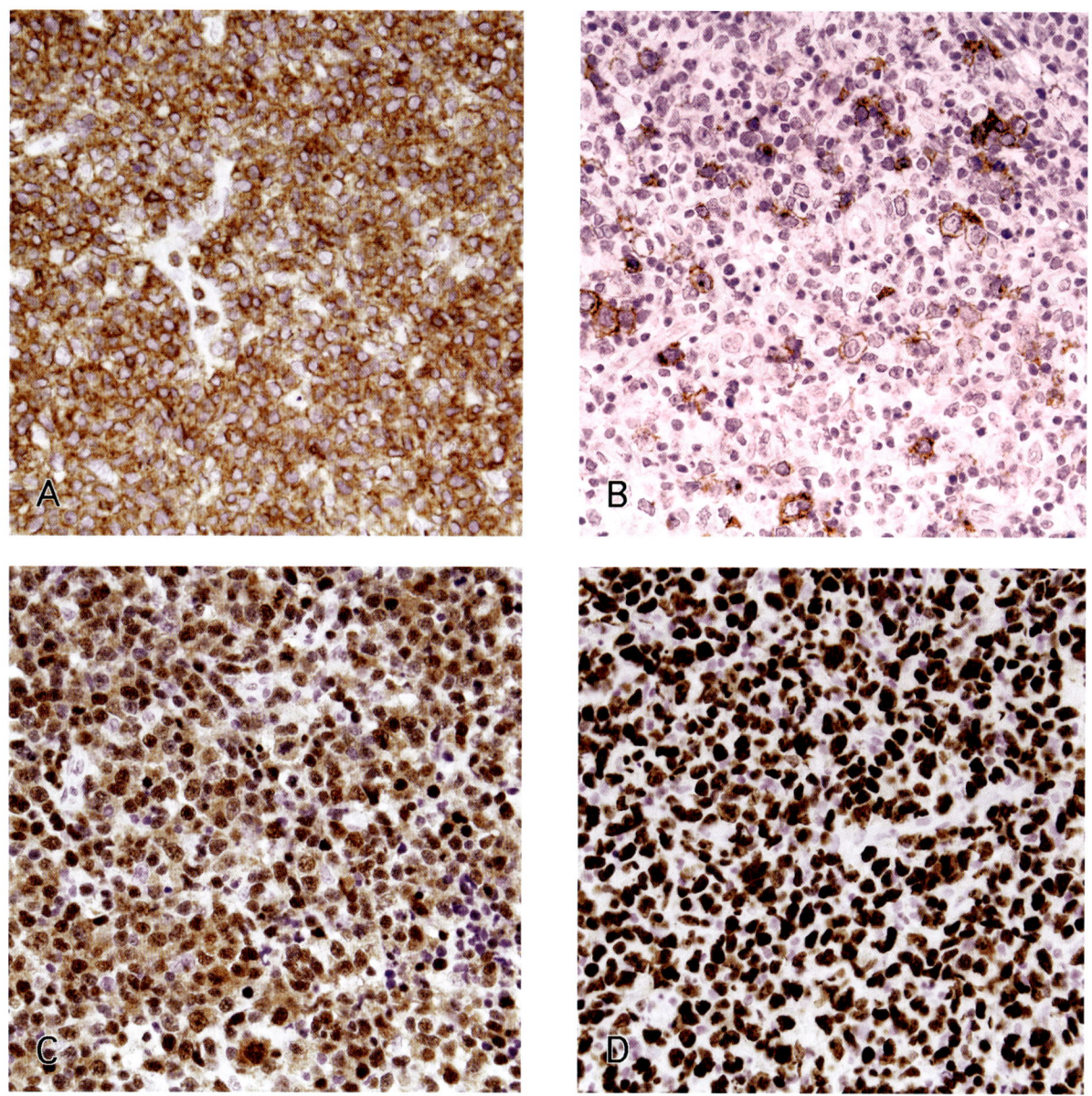

Figure 32-11

ADULT T-CELL LEUKEMIA/LYMPHOMA: IMMUNOHISTOCHEMISTRY

A–D: The lymphoma cells are positive for CD3 (A), CD30 (subset of large cells) (B), MUM1/IRF4 (C), and are highly proliferative as shown by expression of Ki-67 (D) (immunohistochemistry with hematoxylin counterstain).

32-5C), usually associated with more severe host immunosuppression.

MOLECULAR GENETIC FINDINGS

The cytogenetic, gene mutation, and methylation profiles of ATLL have been reviewed by Watanabe (37a). Conventional cytogenetic analysis of ATLL cases commonly shows a complex karyotype, but no recurrent or characteristic chromosomal aberrations (7). Approximately 80 percent of ATLL cases are aneuploid (7). The acute variant usually has a more complex karyotype than the chronic variant. The chromosomal loci most often involved are 1p, 2q, 3q, 6q, 9q, 12q, and 14q (7). Structural abnormalities in chromosome 6 are the most frequent chromosomal alteration and loss of heterozygosity on chromosome 6q has been noted in about half of ATLL cases, suggesting that a tumor suppressor gene may be located in this region. Comparative genomic hybridization analysis similarly has shown numerous chromosomal gains and losses in ATLL (34,41). Gains of chromosome loci 1q and 4q and loss of 13q are more common in aggressive variants of ATLL (34). The acute variant usually has the greatest number of chromosomal abnormalities (41).

Application of next-generation sequencing methods to the study of ATLL has shown many abnormalities, up to 90 per tumor involving approximately 50 different genes (10). The most common activating mutations involved *PLCG1* (64 percent), *PRKCB* (33 percent), *CCR4* (29 percent), *CARD11* (24 percent), *VAV1* (18 percent), *IRF4* (14 percent), and *CCR7* (11 percent) (10). A number of other genes were mutated at lower frequencies including *GATA3, FYN, TBL1XR1,* and *TP53* (10). *RHOA* mutations have been identified in about 15 percent of cases of ATLL, which are heterogeneous and can be activating or inactivating (10,17).

Gene mutations correlate, in part, with the variants of ATLL. Mutations of *CD58, IRF4,* and *TBL1XR1* and loss of *CDKN2A/p16* are more common in the acute variant, suggesting that cell dysregulation and escape from immunosurveillance are involved in the evolution to the acute variant (10). P53 is commonly inactivated in ATLL, via interaction with TAX or HBZ. *TP53* mutations are less common and correlate with progression of ATLL from an indolent to an aggressive variant (32). *STAT3* is more commonly mutated in the chronic and smoldering variants (10). A number of genes in ATLL are also inactivated via methylation (37a). The great number of molecular abnormalities and the long latency interval suggest a multi-hit pathogenesis, with HTLV-1 infection being the likely first event in the sequence.

CCR4 (CC chemokine 4) mutations are reported in about 25 percent of cases of ATLL (10,18,42). These mutations may be of frameshift or nonsense type, resulting in truncation of the carboxy terminus of CCR4; frameshift mutations are associated with a poorer prognosis (42). Gain of function *CCR4* mutations are also reported (18).

Gene expression profiling analysis has shown upregulation of a number of genes in ATLL, including *CDC2/cyclin B1, SYK/LYN,* and the antiapoptotic gene *BIRC5/survivin* (26). The gene expression profiles of different clinical variants of ATLL are similar.

The acute and lymphomatous variants demonstrate monoclonal rearrangements of the T-cell receptor genes (21,23). Clonal integration of HTLV-1 provirus is invariably present in all cases of ATLL. The virus integrates into host DNA randomly and there are no hotspots for integration (1,3,23). Integration, however, is biased toward areas of euchromatin (allowing viral access to DNA) as well as short, palindromic DNA motifs (facilitating the action of viral integrase) (1). In a small percentage of cases, the viral insertion site is in proximity to a cellular gene that has been linked to leukemogenesis (3). Alternatively, viral insertion can dysregulate or otherwise modulate host cellular pathways, likely playing a role in lymphomagenesis. The virus is often partially deleted or mutated in ATLL cases (10).

By analyzing the integration site, the random nature of HTLV-1 proviral insertion into host DNA can be exploited to understand the pathogenesis of ATLL. Virtually all patients with the acute and lymphomatous variants of ATLL have a single dominant clone attributable to HTLV-1 infection of a T cell prior to clonal expansion (1,3,23). This implicates the virus as having a role in clonal expansion. In some patients with the acute or lymphomatous variant, a dominant clone and a second or third prominent, but smaller, clone is present, and usually there is a background of minor clones of HTLV-1–infected cells (1,3). Patients with the smoldering and chronic variants of ATLL generally have clones of smaller size and may carry one (monoclonal) or multiple (oligoclonal) small T-cell populations with the clonally integrated HTLV-1 provirus.

The risk of progression of an indolent variant to an aggressive variant of ATLL may correlate with the total number of HTLV-1–infected T-cell clones, presumably increasing the chance that one dominant clone will emerge (1). HTLV-1 carriers have innumerable minute T-cell clones (20,000 to 50,000) corresponding to different T cells infected by HTLV-1 (1).

DIFFERENTIAL DIAGNOSIS

ATLL closely resembles a number of other T-cell neoplasms as well as Hodgkin lymphoma. In nonendemic regions where ATLL is rare, it is common to misdiagnose these tumors as other types of T-cell lymphoma, particularly if routine screening for HTLV-1 is not performed.

Testing for HTLV-1 infection is essential for establishing the diagnosis of ATLL. In nonendemic areas, serologic testing for HTLV-1 is often performed using an enzyme-linked immunoassay (ELISA) and confirmed by Western blot analysis. Analysis for HTLV-1 integration is not usually required. Molecular assessment of HTLV-1 may be needed in rare seronegative patients with clinical features suspicious for ATLL.

In endemic regions, where serology is commonly positive for HTLV-1, the chance that a T-cell lymphoma unrelated to HTLV-1 infection may occur in a seropositive patient is increased, compromising the specificity of serologic testing. HTLV-1 molecular analysis by either Southern blot or polymerase chain reaction (PCR) to assess integration into tumor DNA, in situ hybridization to detect virus in tumor cells, or PCR to detect provirus in serum plays a more prominent role in diagnosis. Identification of HTLV-1 within lymphoma cells or clonal integration of HTLV-1 into the neoplastic cells is diagnostic of ATLL. A high serum HTLV-1 provirus load is highly suspicious for ATLL.

The main entities in the differential diagnosis of patients with leukemic involvement by ATLL include T-cell prolymphocytic leukemia, Sézary syndrome, and mycosis fungoides with a leukemic phase. Sézary syndrome, mycosis fungoides, and reactive skin infiltrates are included in the differential diagnosis of patients with the smoldering and chronic variants of ATLL. For patients who present with lymphadenopathy, the major entities in the differential diagnosis are peripheral T-cell lymphoma not otherwise specified, anaplastic large cell lymphoma (ALCL), angioimmunoblastic T-cell lymphoma, and classic Hodgkin lymphoma.

Clinical clues to the correct diagnosis of ATLL include patient origin from an endemic area, history of or simultaneous opportunistic infections, and hypercalcemia. The morphologic identification of characteristic lymphoma (flower) cells in the peripheral blood smear and immunophenotypic evidence that the lymphoma cells have a T-regulatory cell immunophenotype [CD3dim(+), CD4(+), CD25(+), FOXP3(+)] are also helpful clues. In addition to features that support the diagnosis of ATLL, there are also findings that occur in other types of T-cell leukemia or lymphoma that make the diagnosis of ATLL unlikely.

T-Cell Prolymphocytic Leukemia. T-cell prolymphocytic leukemia is usually positive for TCL1 and shows one of the following chromosomal abnormalities: inv(14)(q11q32), t(14;14)(q11;q32), or t(X;14)(q28;q11) involving the *TCL1* or *MTCP1* genes.

Anaplastic Large Cell Lymphoma. There is some overlap between anaplastic lymphoma kinase (ALK)-negative ALCL and ATLL. Some cases of ALK-negative ALCL brightly express CD25, like ATLL, and in some cases of ATLL, the lymphoma cells are anaplastic, express CD30, and are negative for FOXP3. Uniform and strong expression of CD30 by all lymphoma cells and expression of cytotoxic markers support the diagnosis of ALK-negative ALCL. ALK-positive ALCL is easier to distinguish from ATLL because ATLL does not express ALK.

Angioimmunoblastic T-Cell Lymphoma. Immunophenotypic features that support AITL over ATLL include the presence of sheets or clusters of tumor cells positive for PD1/CD279, CD10, and CXCL13, supporting a follicular T-helper cell immunophenotype, and expansion of follicular dendritic cell networks entrapping high endothelial venules (9). Infection by EBV can be detected in both AITL and ATLL.

TREATMENT AND PROGNOSIS

Patients with the acute and lymphomatous variants, as well as the unfavorable chronic variant, are grouped together as having aggressive ATLL (29,35). Overall, the morphologic features of these neoplasms have no or minimal impact on overall survival (21,29). In general, treatment for patients with ATLL is inadequate (reviewed in reference 35). Most patients with the aggressive variants of ATLL are treated with combination chemotherapy regimens. Prophylaxis for the central nervous system is also recommended. There is some evidence to support the use of antiviral agents, such as zidovudine (AZT) or interferon-α, combined with chemotherapy. Promising data are emerging using a humanized monoclonal antibody directed against CCR4, mogamulizumab (35). As ATLL cells express CD25 and a subset expresses CD30, some patients may be suitable candidates for treatment with monoclonal anti-CD25 or anti-CD30 antibodies. Allogeneic hematopoietic stem cell transplantation is the only curative option although only a subset of patients is eligible for this approach: about 25 percent survive long-term, but treatment-related mortality is high (35).

The overall prognosis for patients with the aggressive variants of ATLL has been poor historically, with a median overall survival time of 1 year or less due to chemotherapy resistance and profound immunosuppression (11,21). Those with the more favorable chronic and smoldering variants have a longer disease evolution and overall survival, and are often grouped together as having indolent ATLL (21,31). The combination of AZT, interferon-α, and arsenic trioxide has induced a high response rate in clinical trials. If patients are completely asymptomatic, watchful waiting may be used. As shown by Katsuya et al. (11), however, the long-term outlook for patients with chronic and smoldering ATLL is also poor, with 4-year overall survival rates of 36 percent and 52 percent, respectively.

A number of findings have been reported to be associated with a poorer prognosis in ATLL patients (12): markedly elevated serum calcium or LDH dehydrogenase levels, advanced performance status, high serum soluble IL-2α receptor, more than three extranodal lesions, hepatosplenomegaly, and high-stage disease. Patients die due to widespread tumor or opportunistic infections as a result of severe immunodeficiency.

REFERENCES

1. Bangham CR, Cook LB, Melamed A. HTLV-1 clonality in adult T-cell leukaemia and non-malignant HTLV-1 infection. Semin Cancer Biol 2014;26: 89-98.
2. Carneiro-Proietti AB, Amaranto-Damasio MS, Leal-Horiguchi CF, et al. Mother-to-child transmission of human T-cell lymphotropic viruses-1/2: what we know, and what are the gaps in understanding and preventing this route of infection. J Pediatric Infect Dis Soc 2014;3(suppl 1):S24-S29.
3. Cook LB, Melamed A, Niederer H, et al. The role of HTLV-1 clonality, proviral structure, and genomic integration site in adult T-cell leukemia/lymphoma. Blood 2014;123:3925-3931.
4. Dahmoush L, Hijazi Y, Barnes E, Stetler-Stevenson M, Abati A. Adult T-cell leukemia/lymphoma: a cytopathologic, immunocytochemical, and flow cytometric study. Cancer 2002;96:110-116.
5. Freeman RC, Rodriguez GM, French JF. Seroprevalence and risk factors associated with HTLV-I/II infection in injection drug users in northern New Jersey. J Addict Dis 1995;14:51-66.
6. Gessain A, Cassar O. Epidemiological aspects and world distribution of HTLV-1 infection. Front Microbiol 2012;3:388.
7. Itoyama T, Chaganti RS, Yamada Y, et al. Cytogenetic analysis and clinical significance in adult T-cell leukemia/lymphoma: a study of 50 cases from the human T-cell leukemia virus type-1 endemic area, Nagasaki. Blood 2001;97:3612-3620.
8. Karube K, Ohshima K, Tsuchiya T. Expression of FoxP3, a key molecule in CD4+CD25+ regulatory T cells, in adult T-cell leukaemia/lymphoma cells. Br J Haematol 2004;126:81-84.
9. Karube K, Suzumiya J, Okamoto M, et al. Adult T-cell lymphoma/leukemia with angioimmunoblastic T-cell lymphomalike features: Report of 11 cases. Am J Surg Pathol 2007;31:216-223.
10. Kataoka K, Nagata Y, Kitanaka A, et al. Integrated molecular analysis of adult T cell leukemia/lymphoma. Nat Genet 2015;47:1304-1315.
11. Katsuya H, Ishitsuka K, Utsunomiya A, et al. Treatment and survival among 1594 patients with ATL. Blood 2015;126:2570-2577.
12. Katsuya H, Yamanaka T, Ishitsuka K, et al. Prognostic index for acute- and lymphoma-type adult T-cell leukemia/lymphoma. J Clin Oncol 2012;30:1635-1640.
13. Lin B, Musset M, Szekely AM, et al. Human T-cell lymphotropic virus-1-positive T-cell leukemia/lymphoma in a child. Report of a case and review of the literature. Arch Pathol Lab Med 1997;121:1282-1286.
14. Mahieux R, Gessain A. The human HTLV-3 and HTLV-4 retroviruses: new members of the HTLV family. Pathol Biol 2009;57:161-166.
15. Marchetti MA, Pulitzer MP, Myskowski PL, et al. Cutaneous manifestations of human T-cell lymphotropic virus type-1-associated adult T-cell leukemia/lymphoma: a single-center, retrospective study. J Am Acad Dermatol 2015;72:293-301.
16. Matsuoka M, Jeang KT. Human T-cell leukaemia virus type 1 (HTLV-1) infectivity and cellular transformation. Nat Rev Cancer 2007;7:270-280.

17. Nagata Y, Kontani K, Enami T, et al. Variegated RHOA mutations in adult T-cell leukemia/lymphoma. Blood 2016;127:596-604.
18. Nakagawa M, Schmitz R, Xiao W, et al. Gain-of-function CCR4 mutations in adult T cell leukemia/lymphoma. J Exp Med 2014;211:2497-2505.
19. Nakamizo A, Akagi Y, Amano T, et al. Donor-derived adult T-cell leukaemia. Lancet 2011;377:1124.
20. Ohshima K. Pathological features of diseases associated with human T-cell leukemia virus type I. Cancer Sci 2007;98:772-778.
21. Ohshima K, Jaffe ES, Kikuchi M. Adult T-cell leukaemia/lymphoma. In: Swerdlow SH, Campo E, Harris NL, et al., eds. WHO classification of tumours of haematopoietic and lymphoid tissues. Lyon: IARC Press; 2008:281-284.
22. Ohshima K, Kikuchi M, Yoshida T, Masuda Y, Kimura N. Lymph nodes in incipient adult T-cell leukemia-lymphoma with Hodgkin's disease-like histologic features. Cancer 1991;67:1622-1628.
23. Ohshima K, Mukai Y, Shiraki H, Suzumiya J, Tashiro K, Kikuchi M. Clonal integration and expression of human T-cell lymphotropic virus type I in carriers detected by polymerase chain reaction and inverse PCR. Am J Hematol 1997;54:306-312.
24. Ohshima K, Suzumiya J, Kato A, Tashiro K, Kikuchi M. Clonal HTLV-I-infected CD4+ T-lymphocytes and non-clonal non-HTLV-I-infected giant cells in incipient ATLL with Hodgkin-like histologic features. Int J Cancer 1997;72:592-598.
25. Ohshima K, Suzumiya J, Sato K, et al. Nodal T-cell lymphoma in an HTLV-I-endemic area: proviral HTLV-I DNA, histological classification and clinical evaluation. Br J Haematol 1998;101:703-711.
26. Pise-Masison CA, Radonovich M, Dohoney K, et al. Gene expression profiling of ATL patients: compilation of disease-related genes and evidence for TCF4 involvement in BIRC5 gene expression and cell viability. Blood 2009;113:4016-4026.
27. Ramos JC, Ruiz P Jr, Ratner L, et al. IRF-4 and c-Rel expression in antiviral-resistant adult T-cell leukemia/lymphoma. Blood 2007;109:3060-3068.
28. Sawada Y, Hino R, Hama K, et al. Type of skin eruption is an independent prognostic indicator for adult T-cell leukemia/lymphoma. Blood 2011;117:3961-3967.
29. Shimoyama M. Diagnostic criteria and classification of clinical subtypes of adult T-cell leukaemia-lymphoma. A report from the Lymphoma Study Group (1984-87). Br J Haematol 1991;79:428-437.
30. Sugata K, Satou Y, Yasunaga J, et al. HTLV-1 bZIP factor impairs cell-mediated immunity by suppressing production of Th1 cytokines. Blood 2012;119:434-444.
31. Takasaki Y, Iwanaga M, Imaizumi Y, et al. Long-term study of indolent adult T-cell leukemia-lymphoma. Blood 2010;115:4337-4343.
32. Tawara M, Hogerzeil SJ, Yamada Y, et al. Impact of p53 aberration on the progression of adult T-cell leukemia/lymphoma. Cancer Lett 2006;234:249-255.
33. Tokura Y, Sawada Y, Shimauchi T. Skin manifestations of adult T-cell leukemia/lymphoma: clinical, cytological and immunological features. J Dermatol 2014;41:19-25.
34. Tsukasaki K, Krebs J, Nagai K,et al. Comparative genomic hybridization analysis in adult T-cell leukemia/lymphoma: correlation with clinical course. Blood 2001;97:3875-3881.
35. Tsukasaki K, Tobinai K. Human T-cell lymphotropic virus type 1-associated adult T-cell leukemia-lymphoma: new directions in clinical research. Clin Cancer Res 2014;20:5217-5225.
36. Van Dooren S, Salemi M, Vandamme AM. Dating the origin of the African human T-cell lymphotrophic virus type 1 (HTLV-1) subtypes. Mol Biol Evol 2001;18:661-671.
37. Vose J, Armitage J, Weisenburger D, International T-Cell Lymphoma Project. International peripheral T-cell and natural killer/T-cell lymphoma study: pathology findings and clinical outcomes. J Clin Oncol 2008;26:4124-4130.
37a. Watanabe T. Adult T-cell leukemia: molecular basis for clonal expansion and transformation of HTLV-1-infected T cells. Blood 2017;129:1071-1081.
38. Yao J, Gottesman SR, Ayalew G, Braverman AS, Axiotis CA. Loss of Foxp3 is associated with CD30 expression in the anaplastic large cell subtype of adult T-cell leukemia/lymphoma (ATLL) in US/Caribbean patients: potential therapeutic implications for CD30 antibody-mediated therapy. Am J Surg Pathol 2013;37:1407-1412.
39. Yokote T, Akioka T, Oka S, et al. Flow cytometric immunophenotyping of adult T-cell leukemia/lymphoma using CD3 gating. Am J Clin Pathol 2005;124:199-204.
40. Yoshida N, Chihara D. Incidence of adult T-cell leukemia/lymphoma in nonendemic areas. Curr Treat Options Oncol 2015;16:7.
41. Yoshida N, Karube K, Utsunomiya A, et al. Molecular characterization of chronic-type adult T-cell leukemia/lymphoma. Cancer Res 2014;74:6129-6138.
42. Yoshida N, Miyoshi H, Kato T, et al. CCR4 frameshift mutation identifies a distinct group of adult T-cell leukemia/lymphoma with poor prognosis. J Pathol 2016;268:621-626.

33 ALK-POSITIVE ANAPLASTIC LARGE CELL LYMPHOMA

GENERAL FEATURES

Anaplastic lymphoma kinase (ALK)-positive anaplastic large cell lymphoma (ALCL) is a systemic lymphoma of T/null-cell lineage. It is characterized by strong and uniform CD30 expression and chromosome 2p23.2/*ALK* rearrangements that result in ALK expression (11,48a). Although cases of ALK-positive ALCL have been recognized for many years, the understanding of this neoplasm and the designation as ALK-positive anaplastic large cell lymphoma is relatively recent.

These tumors were designated by a variety of terms in the past, reflecting their poorly differentiated, often cohesive appearance and the common location of the lymphoma cells within lymph node sinuses. One commonly used older term was malignant histiocytosis. Alfred Stansfeld in London recognized the distinctive features of a case of the lymphohistiocytic variant of ALCL in a woman named Linda Brown and the informal designation "Linda Brown's disease" was often used with his colleagues in the Kiel Classification Group including Karl Lennert (Dr. Peter Banks, personal communication, 2015).

The more modern history of ALK-positive ALCL begins with the description of Ki-1 lymphoma in 1985 by Harald Stein et al. (47). This group of lymphomas showed strong immunoreactivity with the Ki-1 antibody, subsequently shown to react with CD30 and to be encoded by tumor necrosis factor superfamily member 8 (*TNFSF8*). The category of ALCL has evolved substantially since its description as Ki-1 lymphoma (fig. 33-1) and, in retrospect, the study by Stein et al. likely included cases of ALK-positive ALCL, ALK-negative ALCL, primary cutaneous ALCL, and CD30-positive B-cell lymphomas.

A major advance was the discovery and subsequent recognition that t(2;5)(p23.2;q35) is highly associated with a subset of cases of ALCL (21). Subsequently, the breakpoints of t(2;5) were cloned and the translocation was shown to create a *NPM-ALK* fusion gene that results in overexpression of ALK (27). Antibodies specific for ALK were developed, with the ALK-1 monoclonal antibody becoming most popular (35). It was recognized that localized skin tumors and B-cell lymphomas were sufficiently different, and should be excluded, from the ALCL

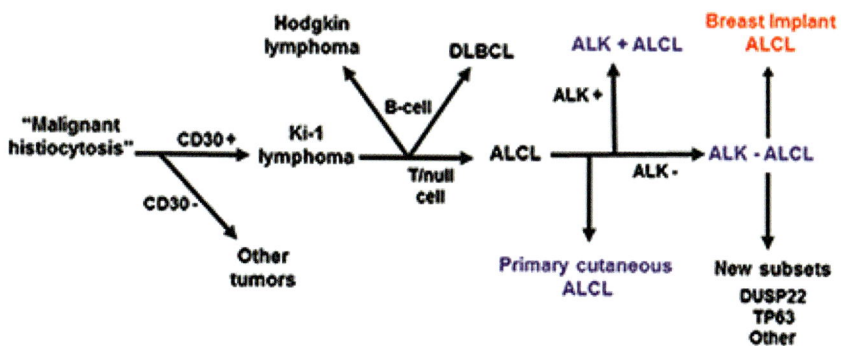

Figure 33-1

EVOLUTION OF THE CATEGORY OF ANAPLASTIC LARGE CELL LYMPHOMA (ALCL)

In the revised Health Organization (WHO) classification, three types of ALCL are formally recognized (in blue). Breast implant-associated ALCL (in red) is a provisional entity and new subsets of ALK-negative ALCL are likely to be delineated in the future.

Table 33-1

FREQUENCY OF ANAPLASTIC LARGE CELL LYMPHOMA RELATIVE TO
OTHER TYPES OF T-CELL LYMPHOMA IN THREE GEOGRAPHIC REGIONS[a]

Lymphoma Type	North America	Europe	Asia
Peripheral T-cell lymphoma, NOS[b]	34.4%	34.3%	22.4%
Angioimmunoblastic T-cell lymphoma	16%	28.7%	17.9%
ALK[b]-positive anaplastic large cell lymphoma	16%	6.4%	3.2%
ALK-negative anaplastic large cell lymphoma	7.8%	9.4%	2.6%

[a]Data from table 1 in reference 50.
[b]NOS = not otherwise specified; ALK = anaplastic lymphoma kinase.

category. Skin lesions are almost always ALK negative and patients usually have an excellent prognosis. These tumors are currently designated as *primary cutaneous anaplastic large cell lymphomas*. CD30-positive B-cell lymphomas are biologically distinct from ALCL and genetically heterogeneous, and are therefore reassigned to the category of diffuse large B-cell lymphoma.

Currently, ALCL is separated into two major categories in the World Health Organization (WHO) classification: ALK-positive ALCL, the subject of this chapter, and ALK-negative ALCL (48a). ALK-positive ALCL represents 2 to 3 percent of adult non-Hodgkin lymphomas and up to 30 percent of all childhood lymphomas (11,50); it also represents 16 percent of T-cell lymphomas in North America, second only to peripheral T-cell lymphoma not otherwise specified. ALK-positive ALCL is less common in Europe and Asia, representing 6.4 percent and 3.2 percent of all T-cell lymphomas, respectively (Table 33-1) (50).

CLINICAL FEATURES

Patients with ALK-positive ALCL are most commonly children or young adults in the second and third decades of life (6,26,46). Patients of all ages are affected, however, with the exception of infants, in whom ALK-positive ALCL is rare (6). There is a slight male predominance, more pronounced in adolescents and young adults. B-type symptoms are present in 50 to 75 percent of patients. Lymphadenopathy occurs in 80 to 90 percent and mediastinal lymph nodes are enlarged in one third of patients (6,46). Extranodal sites of involvement are present in about 60 percent of patients and include bone marrow (10 to 30 percent), gastrointestinal tract, soft tissue, skin, and bone (26,46). Fifty to 60 percent of patients present

with stage III or IV disease and about 50 percent have a high-risk International Prognostic Index score (46,50). Patients with the lymphohistiocytic and small cell variants of ALK-positive ALCL have a higher frequency of enlarged mediastinal lymph nodes and skin lesions (6).

Rarely, patients with ALK-positive ALCL, most often the lymphohistiocytic or small cell variant, develop leukemic involvement and the leukocyte count may be very high (2,30). Patients may present initially with fever, leukocytosis, and peripheral blood neutrophilia with left-shifted granulopoiesis and toxic granulation, all of which may suggest an infectious/inflammatory process. The leukemic presentation of ALK-positive ALCL is associated with an aggressive clinical course and poor outcome (2).

HISTOLOGIC FINDINGS

Lymph Node

In most cases, ALK-positive ALCL preferentially involves the paracortical regions, sparing lymphoid follicles, or diffusely effaces the lymph node architecture (fig. 33-2) (3,11,26,46). A starry sky pattern is prominent in 10 to 20 percent of cases (fig. 33-3). Areas of coagulative necrosis are common and may sometimes be prominent (fig. 33-4). Sinusoidal involvement is common, and in a small subset of biopsy specimens, the lymphoma cells are mostly confined to the lymph node sinuses (figs. 33-5, 33-6). The lymphoma cells often exhibit a cohesive growth pattern, and within sinuses may resemble a metastatic tumor. Cytologically, the lymphoma cells are usually large with a pleomorphic, often horseshoe-shaped nucleus, prominent central perinuclear clearing (Golgi zone), and abundant cytoplasm; these are known as hallmark cells (fig. 33-6B) (3,11,26,46).

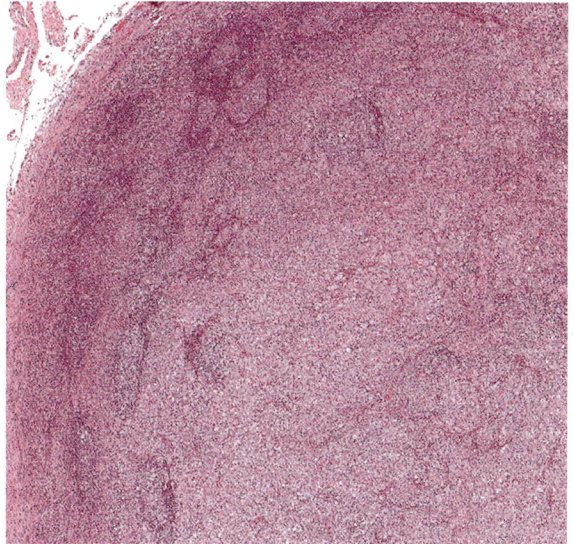

Figure 33-2

**ANAPLASTIC LYMPHOMA KINASE (ALK)-POSITIVE
ANAPLASTIC LARGE CELL LYMPHOMA
INVOLVING LYMPH NODE**

Overall, the neoplasm has a diffuse pattern, but in some areas the tumor has a paracortical distribution and spares lymphoid follicles (hematoxylin and eosin [H&E] stain).

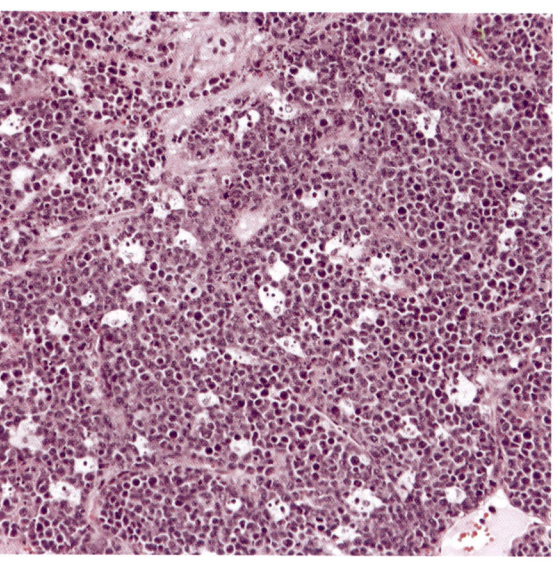

Figure 33-3

**ALK-POSITIVE ANAPLASTIC LARGE CELL
LYMPHOMA INVOLVING LYMPH NODE**

The lymphoma has a prominent starry sky pattern (H&E stain).

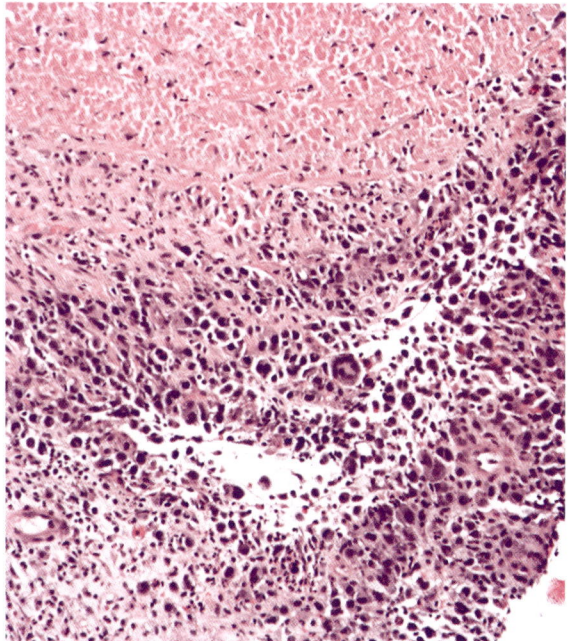

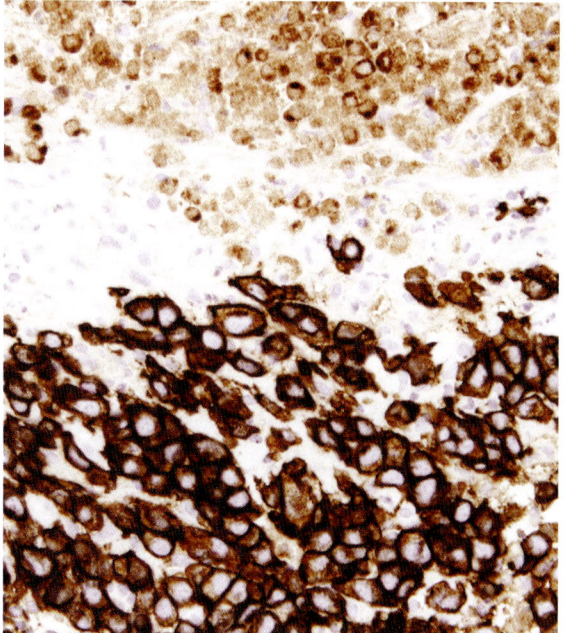

Figure 33-4

ALK-POSITIVE ANAPLASTIC LARGE CELL LYMPHOMA INVOLVING LYMPH NODE

Left: A needle biopsy specimen of a lymph node shows large areas of coagulative necrosis (upper part of field) (H&E stain).
Right: The anti-CD30 antibody highlights both viable (bright) and necrotic (dim, upper part of field) lymphoma cells (immunohistochemistry with hematoxylin counterstain).

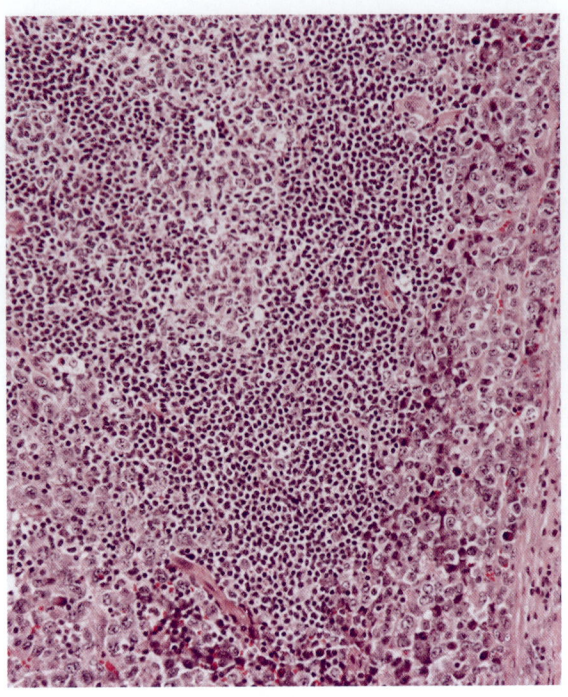

Figure 33-5

ALK-POSITIVE ANAPLASTIC LARGE CELL LYMPHOMA INVOLVING LYMPH NODE

The lymphoma cells preferentially involve the subcapsular sinus (right of field) and spare a lymphoid follicle (H&E stain).

The morphologic spectrum of ALK-positive ALCL is broad and includes a number of variants (3,26,46). Four main variants are recognized in the current WHO classification listed in Table 33-2 (11). In up to 20 percent of cases, more than one morphologic pattern is observed in a single lymph node biopsy specimen. Relapses may reveal morphologic features different from those seen initially. These observations suggest that morphologic variants represent variations of the same entity. There is no correlation between the type of ALK translocation and the morphologic variant (11).

In the *common* (or *classic*) *variant* of ALK-positive ALCL, the neoplastic cells exhibit a spectrum of morphologic atypia. They are large and pleomorphic, frequently with horseshoe-shaped or wreath-like nuclei, and some resemble hallmark cells (figs. 33-2–33-6) (3,11,26,46).

The *lymphohistiocytic variant* is characterized by few tumor cells admixed with numerous reactive lymphocytes and histiocytes (fig. 33-7). The histiocytes are usually not epithelioid and some have eccentric nuclei, a prominent golgi region, and abundant cytoplasm that appears purple on Giemsa stain (19). The lymphoma cells can represent less than 10 percent of all

Table 33-2

MORPHOLOGIC PATTERNS IN ALK-POSITIVE ANAPLASTIC LARGE CELL LYMPHOMA

Morphologic Pattern	Frequency	Key Features
Common	~70%	Sinusoidal involvement is common Pleomorphic large cells and many hallmark cells
Lymphohistiocytic	~10%	Numerous histiocytes can obscure lymphoma cells Hallmark cells aggregate around blood vessels
Small cell	5-10%	Many small cells that are ALK+ and CD30- Few large cells that are ALK+ and CD30+ Hallmark cells aggregate around blood vessels
Hodgkin-like	1-3%	Can mimic nodular sclerosis Hodgkin lymphoma (low power magnification) Usually lymphoma cell rich
Composite	10-20%	More than one pattern in biopsy specimen Lymphohistiocytic and small cell most common mixture

Other patterns
  Sarcomatoid
  Monomorphic
  Giant cell rich
  Neutrophil rich
  Eosinophil rich
  Edematous/myxoid
  Signet ring cell-like
	Rare	Not formally recognized as distinctive morphologic patterns in the WHO classification

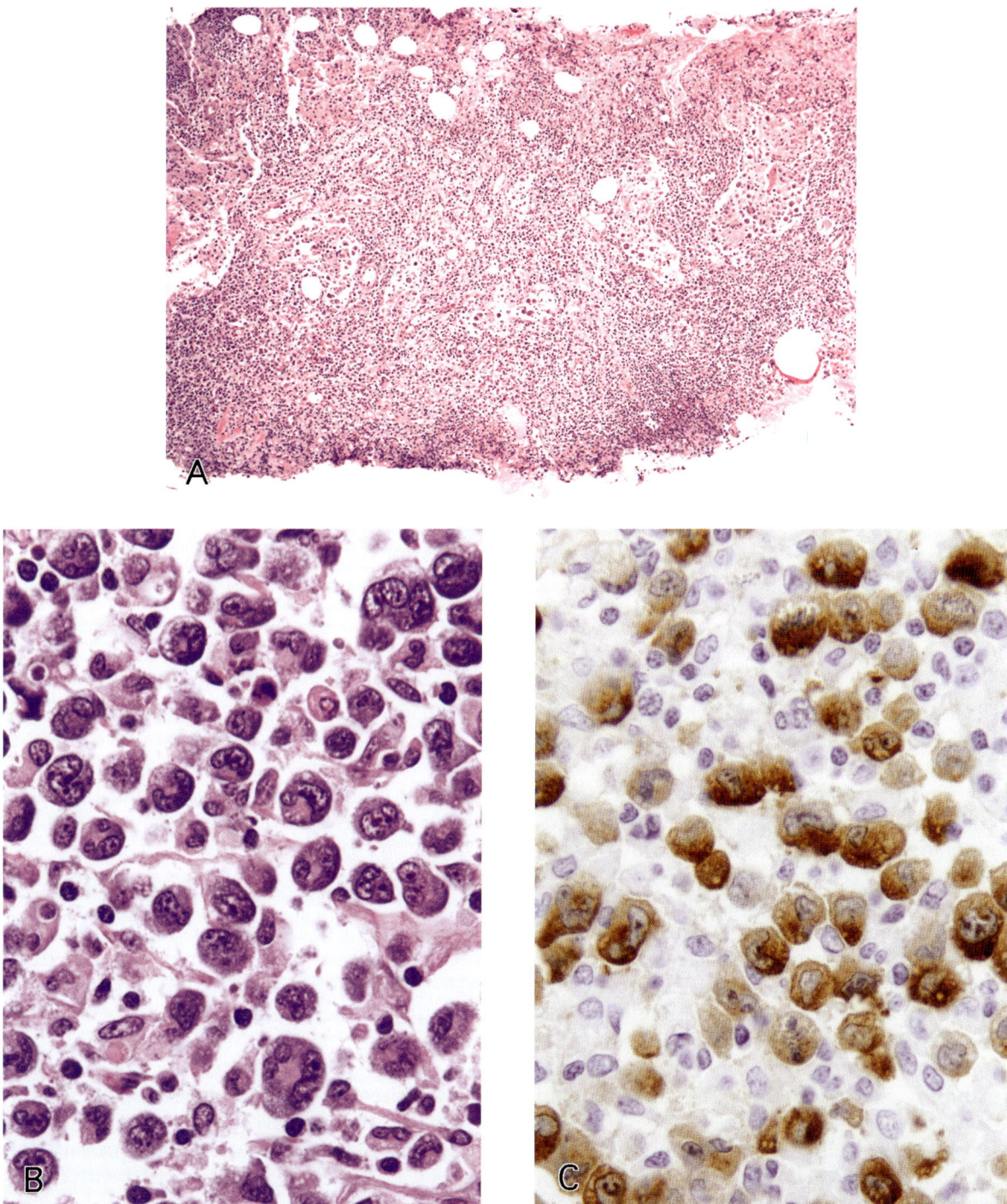

Figure 33-6

ALK-POSITIVE ANAPLASTIC LARGE CELL LYMPHOMA INVOLVING LYMPH NODE

A: A needle biopsy specimen of a lymph node shows patent sinuses and large atypical cells within the sinuses. The remainder of the lymph node parenchyma is not or only minimally involved (A,B: H&E stain).

B: Oil immersion magnification shows many hallmark cells within a lymph node sinus.

C: The lymphoma cells are positive for ALK in a cytoplasmic pattern, suggesting a non-t(2;5) *ALK* translocation (immunohistochemistry with hematoxylin counterstain).

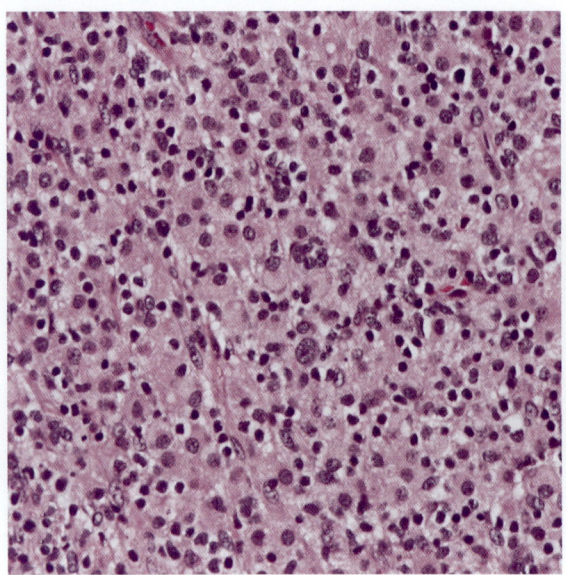 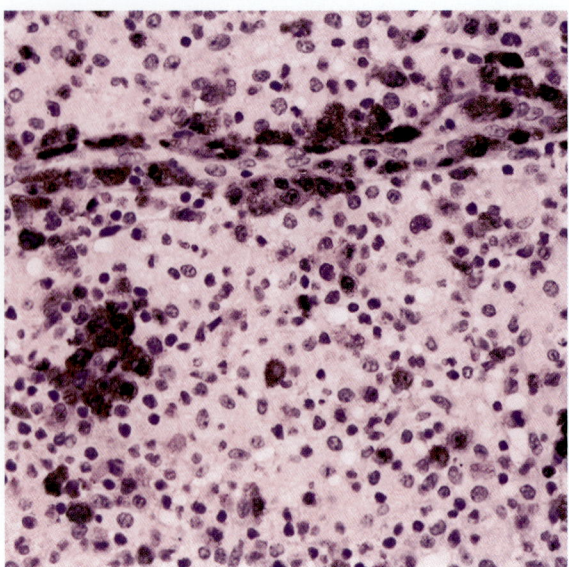

Figure 33-7

ALK-POSITIVE ANAPLASTIC LARGE CELL LYMPHOMA, LYMPHOHISTIOCYTIC VARIANT, INVOLVING LYMPH NODE

Left: Most of the cells in this field are reactive lymphocytes and histiocytes. However, some larger lymphoma cells are seen (H&E stain).

Right: The ALK-positive lymphoma cells tend to line up along blood vessels (immunohistochemistry with hematoxylin counterstain).

cells in a biopsy specimen and therefore may be difficult to appreciate in hematoxylin and eosin (H&E)-stained tissue sections. The lymphoma cells tend to cluster around the blood vessels and are much easier to appreciate when highlighted by antibodies specific for CD30 or ALK.

In the *small cell variant* (fig. 33-8), the tumor cells are predominantly small to intermediate in size and often have pale cytoplasm. Hallmark cells are infrequent but may aggregate around blood vessels. Often the lymphohistiocytic and small cell variants coexist in a single biopsy specimen (11). The *"Hodgkin-like" variant* (fig. 33-9) is an uncommon morphologic variant that resembles, in part, nodular sclerosis Hodgkin lymphoma (see Differential Diagnosis) (11,49).

Other morphologic patterns of ALK-positive ALCL have been reported, although they are not formally recognized in the WHO classification. The importance of these patterns lies primarily in being aware that they exist to avoid misdiagnosis. In the *sarcomatoid variant*, the neoplastic cells are spindle-shaped and resemble, more or less, sarcoma cells (fig. 33-10). Some cases of ALK-positive ALCL are monomorphic and resemble diffuse large B-cell lymphoma,

plasmacytoma, or plasmablastic lymphoma (fig. 33-11) (24,26). Rare examples of ALK-positive ALCL are associated with numerous eosinophils, neutrophils (fig. 33-12), or giant cells (3,26,46). Other rare cases have a prominent myxoid or edematous background (fig. 33-13).

Peripheral Blood and Bone Marrow

Leukemia can occur in patients with either the lymphohistiocytic or small cell variant of ALK-positive ALCL. The leukocyte count in these patients can be higher than 100 x 10^9/L and, rarely, much higher (30). The lymphoma cells are usually small and therefore the diagnosis ALK-positive ALCL may not be considered initially (fig. 33-14). Less often, the circulating cells are large and anaplastic. A leukemic presentation of ALK-positive ALCL is associated with an aggressive clinical course and poor outcome (2).

ALK-positive ALCL in the bone marrow can be morphologically obvious or subtle, the latter best appreciated by immunohistochemistry (fig. 33-15). The tumor cells may be widely scattered and blend in with normal hematopoietic cells. Erythrohemophagocytosis by lymphoma cells may be observed.

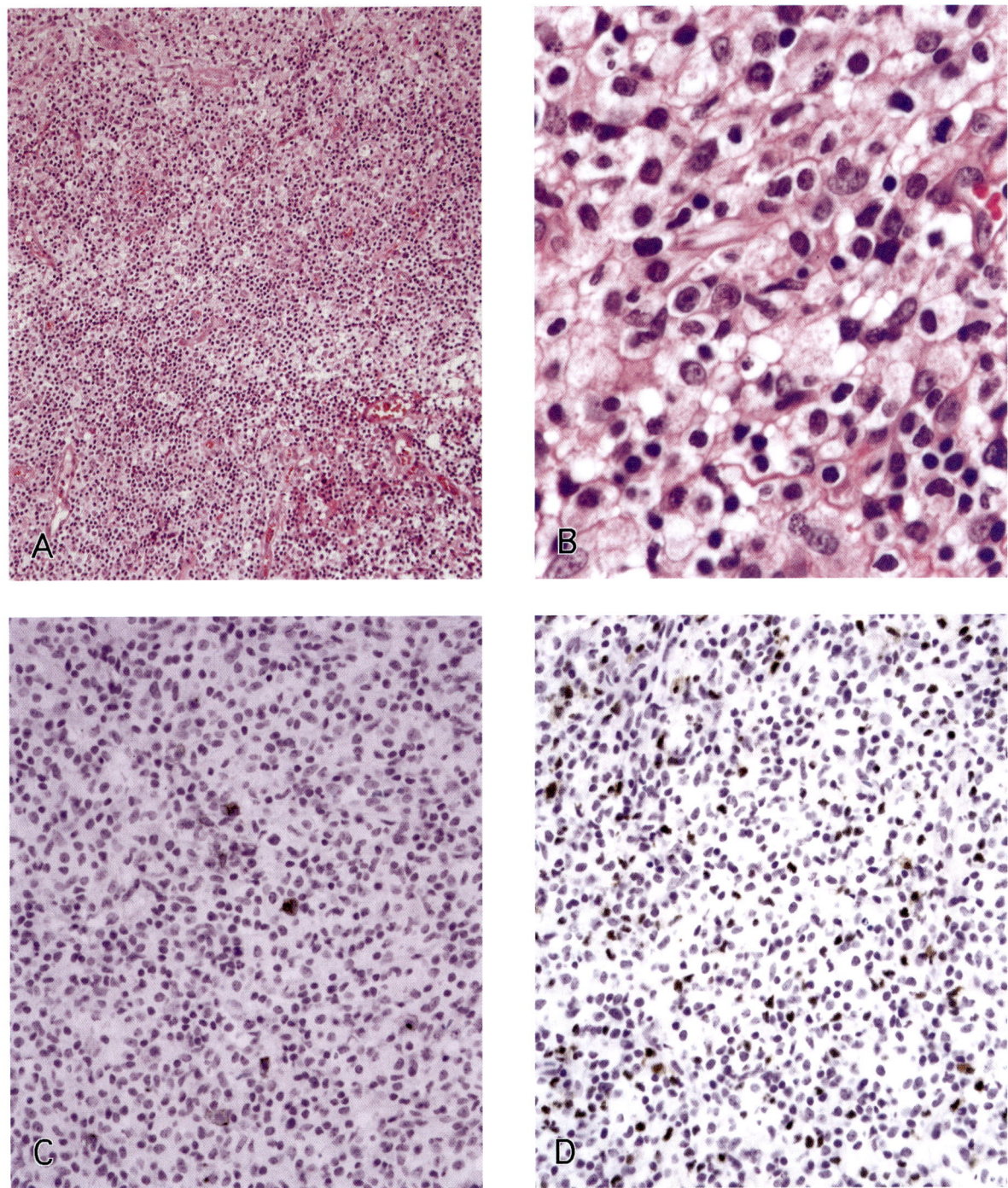

Figure 33-8

ALK-POSITIVE ANAPLASTIC LARGE CELL LYMPHOMA, SMALL CELL VARIANT, INVOLVING LYMPH NODE

A: The lymph node architecture is diffusely replaced by lymphoma (A,B: H&E stain).

B: Numerous small lymphoma cells with pale or clear cytoplasm are associated with reactive lymphocytes and histiocytes; only a few large, more obvious lymphoma cells are observed in this field.

C,D: Only the large lymphoma cells are positive for CD30 (C), but all of the lymphoma cells (small and large) are positive for ALK (D) in a nuclear pattern. The few large lymphoma cells exhibit both nuclear and cytoplasmic ALK reactivity (C,D: immunohistochemistry with hematoxylin counterstain).

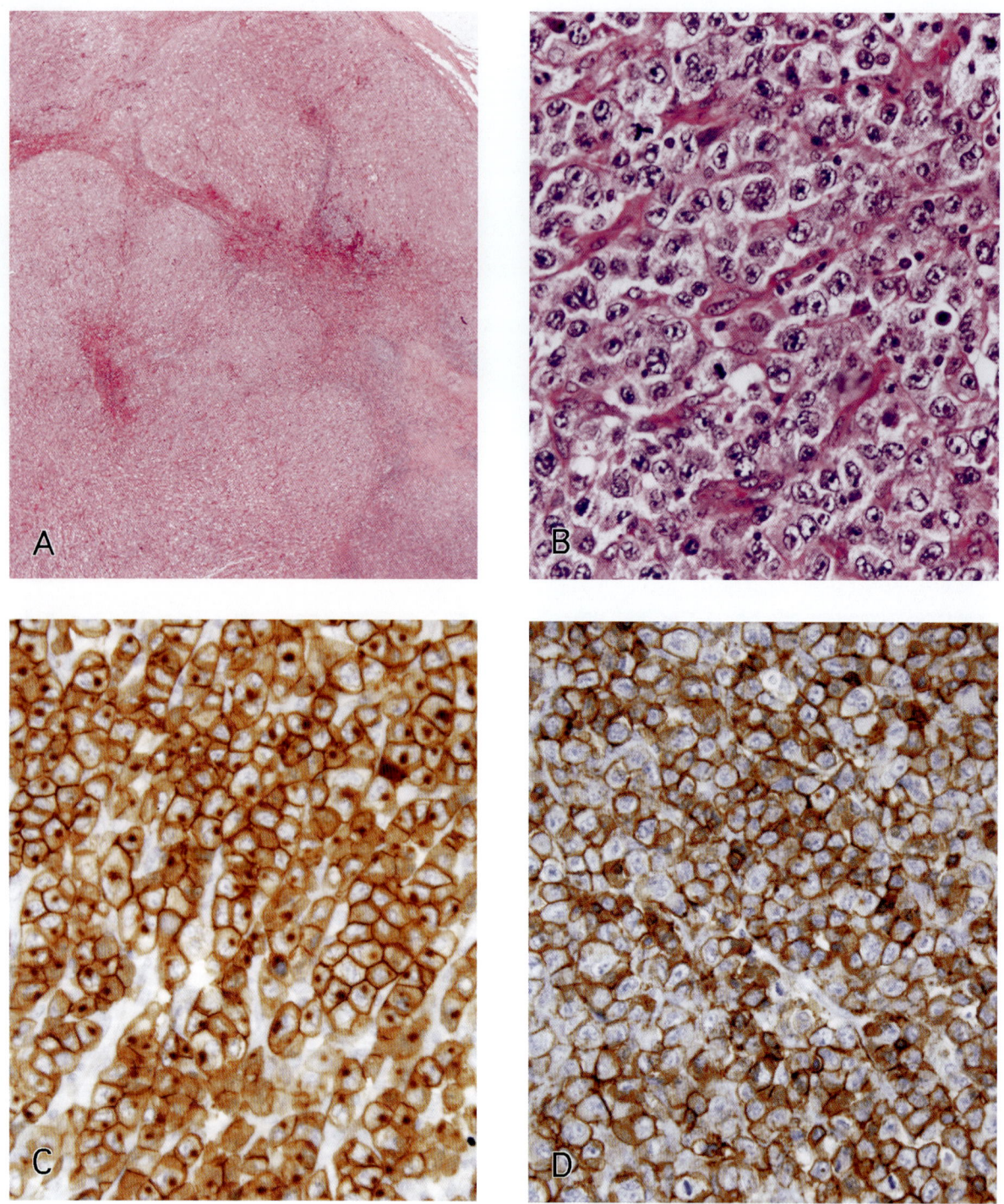

Figure 33-9

ALK-POSITIVE ANAPLASTIC LARGE CELL LYMPHOMA, HODGKIN-LIKE VARIANT, INVOLVING LYMPH NODE

A: The lymph node is replaced by tumor with a vaguely nodular pattern. Fibrous bands are present between some of the nodules (A,B: H&E stain).

B: The nodules are composed of sheets of lymphoma cells.

C,D: The neoplastic cells are positive for CD30 (C) and CD43 (D) (C,D: immunohistochemistry with hematoxylin counterstain).

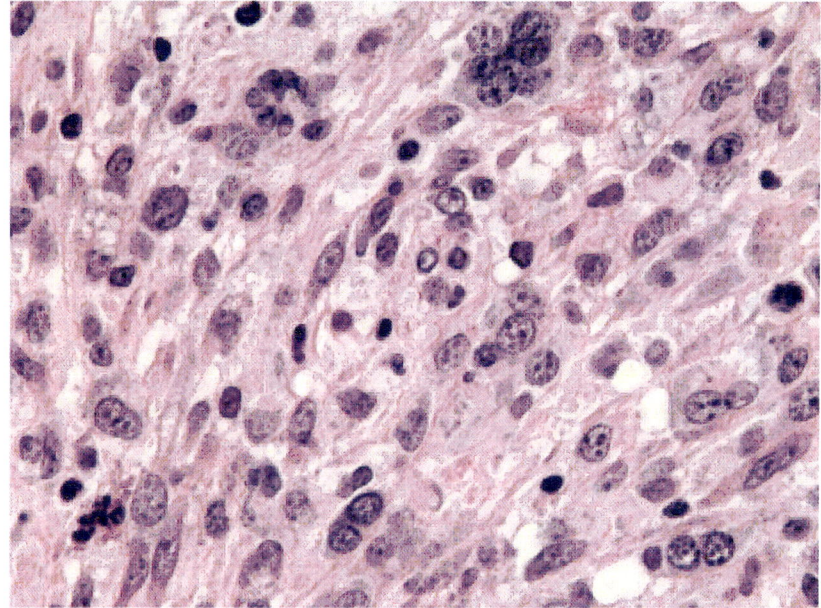

Figure 33-10

ALK-POSITIVE ANAPLASTIC LARGE CELL LYMPHOMA, SARCOMATOID VARIANT

Many of the lymphoma cells are spindled and some large and atypical nuclei are seen (H&E stain).

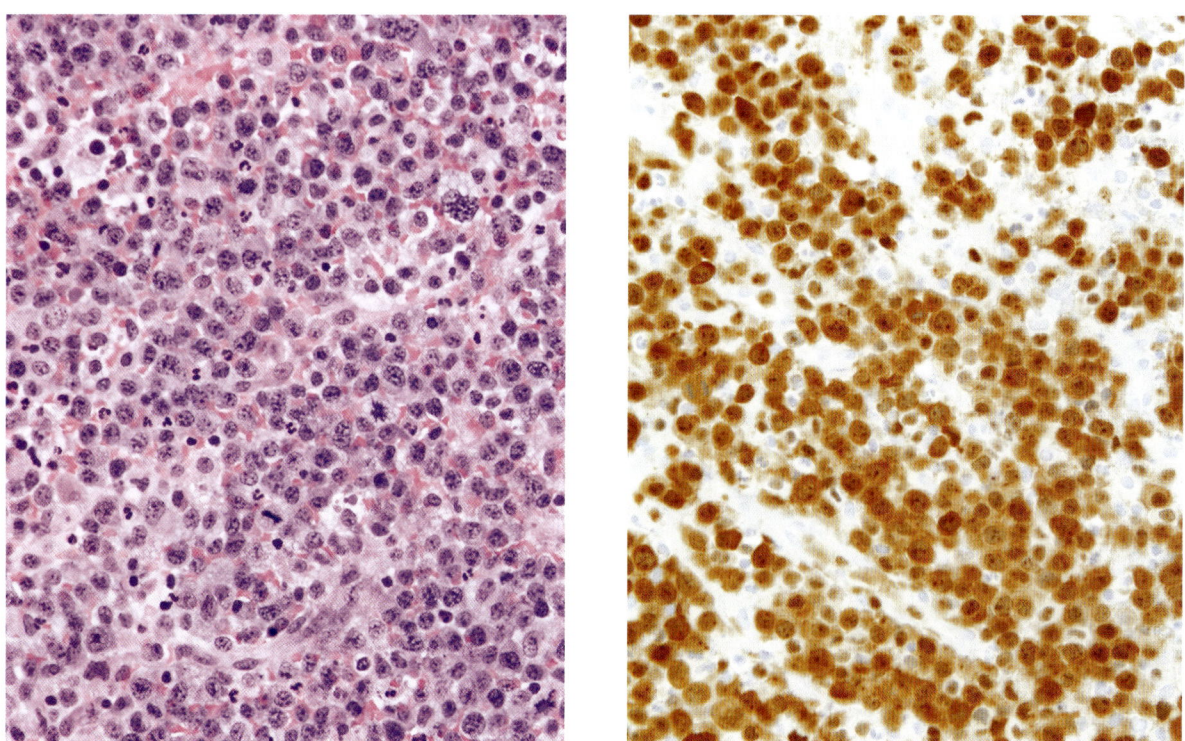

Figure 33-11

ALK-POSITIVE ANAPLASTIC LARGE CELL LYMPHOMA, MONOMORPHIC VARIANT, INVOLVING SOFT TISSUE OF THE NECK

Left: The lymphoma cells are arranged in a diffuse pattern, with abundant cytoplasm and some eccentrically located nuclei, suggestive of plasmacytoid differentiation (H&E stain).

Right: The lymphoma cells are brightly positive for ALK in a nuclear and cytoplasmic pattern. These cells were also strongly and uniformly positive for CD30, positive for CD4 and CD43, and negative for CD20 (not shown) (immunohistochemistry with hematoxylin counterstain).

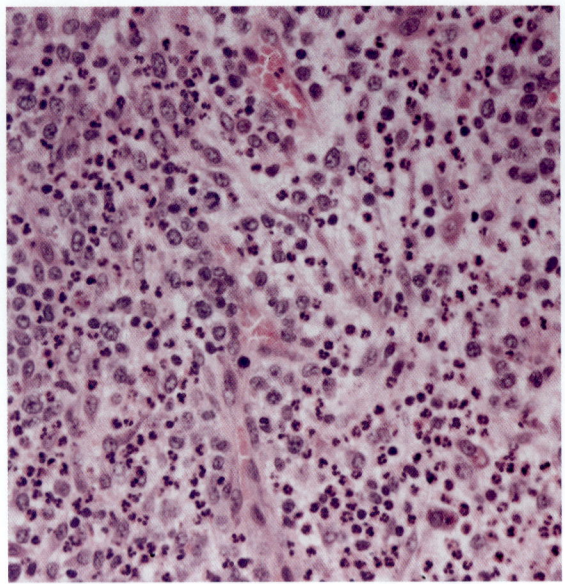

Figure 33-12

ALK-POSITIVE ANAPLASTIC LARGE CELL LYMPHOMA WITH A NEUTROPHIL-RICH BACKGROUND

The tumor was detected as a lytic lesion. Some of the lymphoma cells have a spindled shape and are associated with numerous neutrophils (H&E stain).

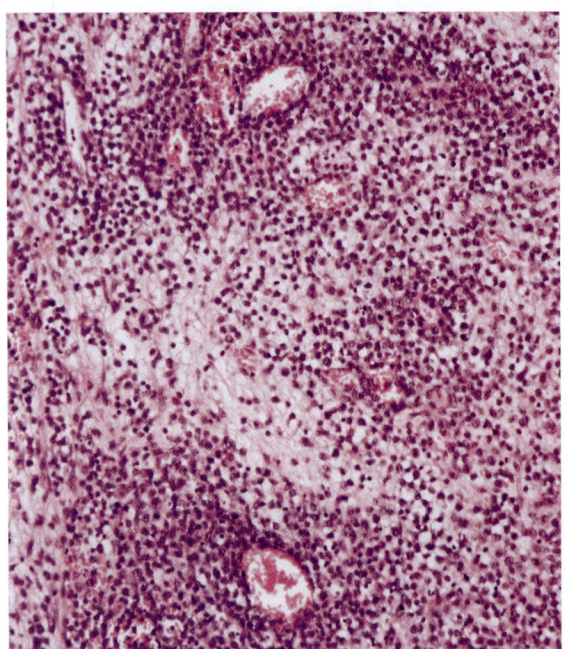

Figure 33-13

ALK-POSITIVE ANAPLASTIC LARGE CELL LYMPHOMA INVOLVING LYMPH NODE

Many areas have a prominent edematous or myxoid background (H&E stain).

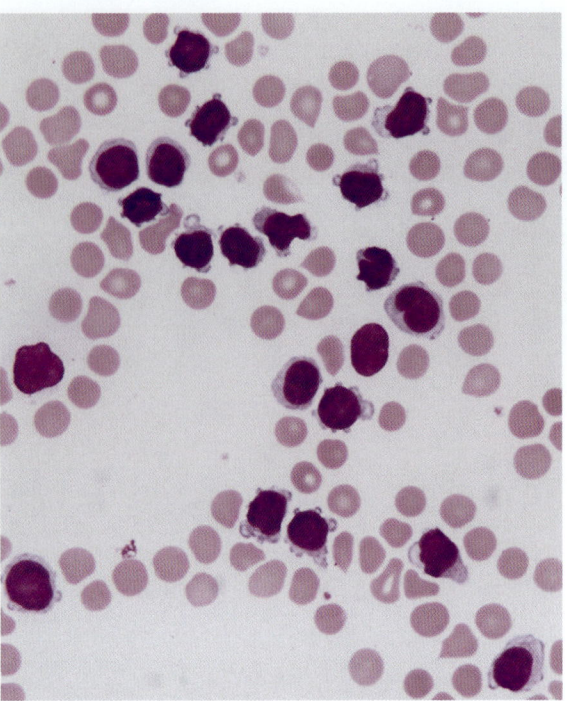

Figure 33-14

ALK-POSITIVE ANAPLASTIC LARGE CELL LYMPHOMA IN PERIPHERAL BLOOD

Numerous lymphoma cells are present in the peripheral blood smear (Wright-Giemsa stain).

Using morphology alone, bone marrow involvement is detected in about 10 percent of patients. In contrast, using immunohistochemistry with antibodies specific for CD30 and ALK, up to 30 percent of patients are seen to have bone marrow involvement (11,28). Using molecular methods, the detection rate is higher (50 to 60 percent of patients) (10).

CYTOLOGIC FINDINGS

Aspirate specimens vary considerably in cell size and composition, depending on the morphologic variant described above, but typically contain large pleomorphic cells with hyperchromatic nuclei and varying amounts of cytoplasm (figs. 33-16–33-18). The cells may be dispersed or loosely cohesive, mimicking an epithelial neoplasm. The nuclei are C-shaped, wreath-shaped, doughnut-shaped, multinucleated, or binucleated with one or more nucleoli; the latter can mimic Reed-Sternberg cells. The cytoplasm can be vacuolated or have a prominent Golgi region. Classic hallmark cells are present variably and

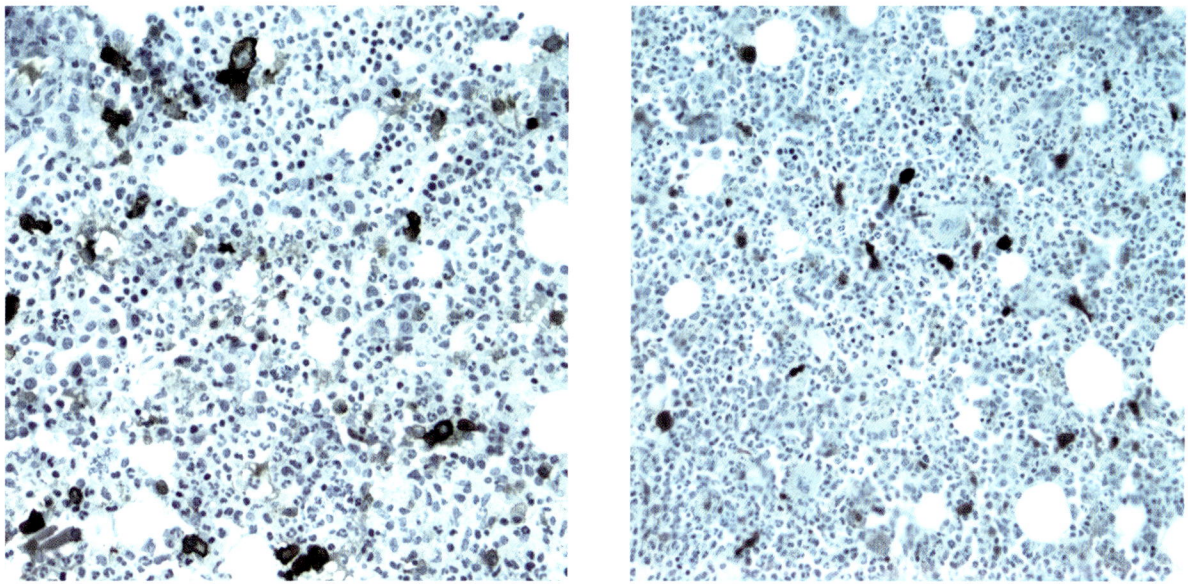

Figure 33-15

ALK-POSITIVE ANAPLASTIC LARGE CELL LYMPHOMA INVOLVING BONE MARROW

The bone marrow can be involved by ALCL in a subtle fashion but immunohistochemical analysis using antibodies specific for CD30 and ALK-1 can facilitate the detection of single cells or small aggregates of lymphoma cells. The lymphoma cells shown are positive for CD30 (left) and ALK (right) (immunohistochemistry with hematoxylin counterstain).

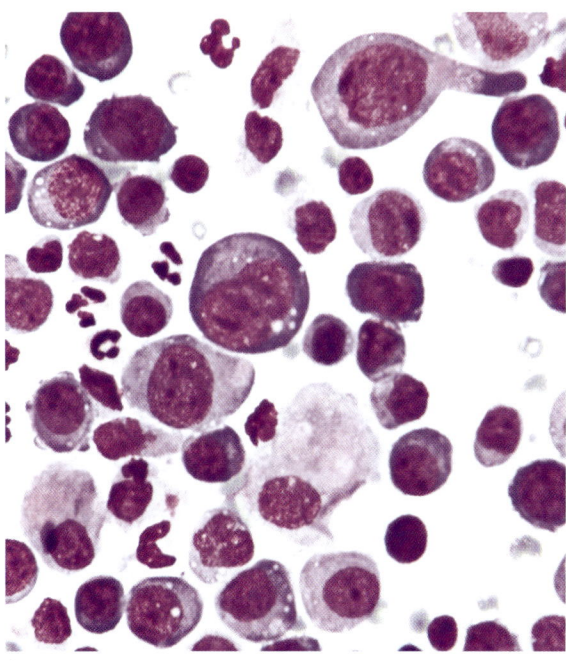

Figure 33-16

ALK-POSITIVE ANAPLASTIC LARGE CELL LYMPHOMA INVOLVING LYMPH NODE

A touch imprint of a biopsy specimen shows tumor cells with abundant cytoplasm and vacuoles. The cells can show variation in size and shape (Wright-Giemsa stain).

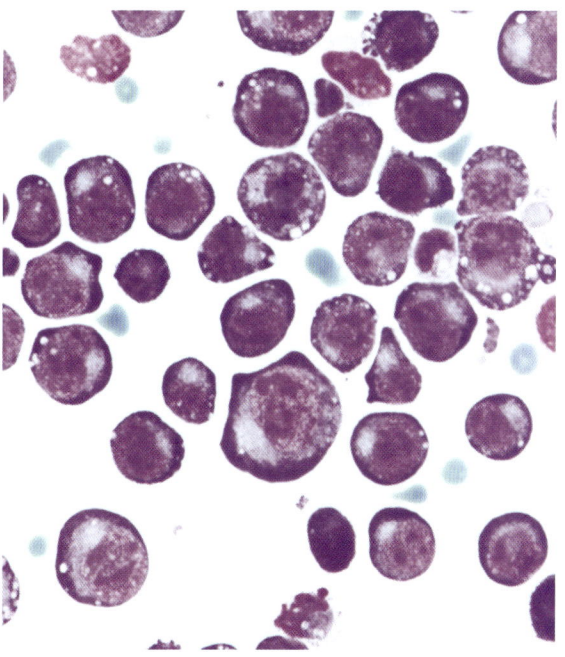

Figure 33-17

ALK-POSITIVE ANAPLASTIC LARGE CELL LYMPHOMA INVOLVING LYMPH NODE

A fine-needle aspiration shows tumor cells with abundant cytoplasm. Some cells have eccentrically located nuclei, imparting a plasmacytoid appearance (Diff-Quik stain).

527

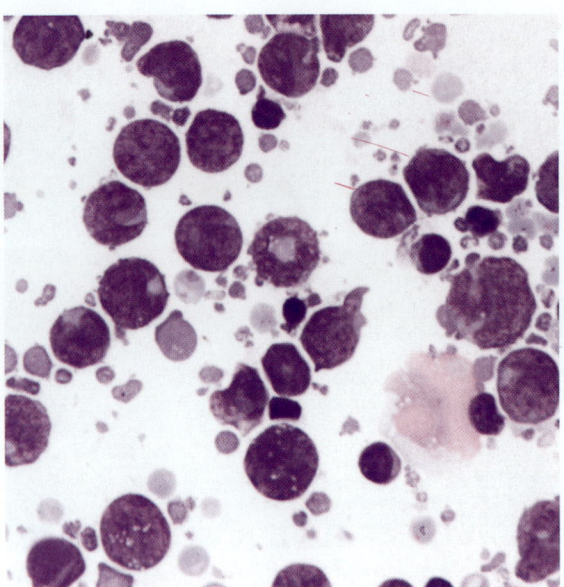 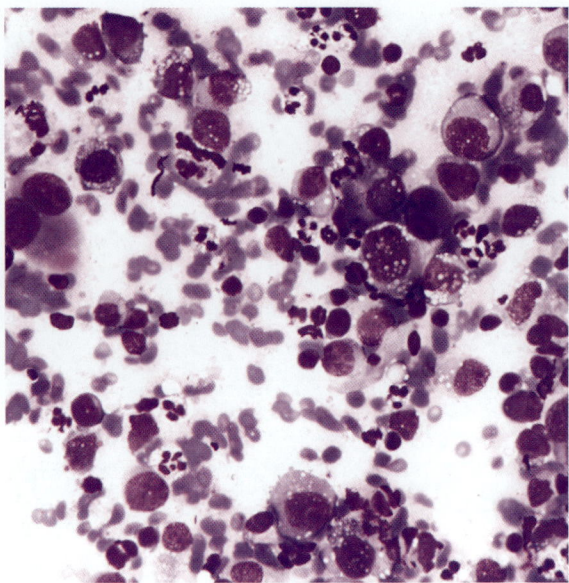

Figure 33-18

ALK-POSITIVE ANAPLASTIC LARGE CELL LYMPHOMA INVOLVING LYMPH NODE

Left: Fine-needle aspiration smear shows large cells with C-shaped or circular nuclei and scant cytoplasm.
Right: An atypical binucleated cell and some mononuclear variants in a background of inflammatory cells can mimic Hodgkin lymphoma (left, right: Diff-Quick stain).

can be readily identified on Romanowsky preparations. In other cases, the neoplastic cells are more monotonous, with oval nuclei, prominent nucleoli, and scant pale cytoplasm.

The lymphoma cells are often present in a mixed inflammatory background containing small lymphocytes, neutrophils, or eosinophils. Lymphoglandular bodies are generally seen in aspirate smears prepared from involved lymph nodes (37). ALK-positive ALCL cannot be reliably distinguished from ALK-negative ALCL by cytomorphologic features alone. Cell block preparations are helpful for diagnosis as they allow for immunohistochemical analysis.

IMMUNOPHENOTYPIC FINDINGS

By definition, ALK-positive ALCL expresses CD30 (figs. 33-4, right; 33-9C) and ALK (fig. 33-6C, 33-8D; Table 33-3). CD30 is expressed strongly by the neoplastic cells in a characteristic membranous and paranuclear (Golgi) pattern (26,46). ALK (CD246) is a tyrosine kinase that belongs to the insulin receptor superfamily. It is normally expressed by a small subset of cells in the central and peripheral nervous systems and is not expressed normally in lymphocytes

(35). As a result, immunohistochemical analysis for ALK expression is a helpful and commonly used test to support the diagnosis of ALK-positive ALCL. Molecular analysis to show specific ALK fusions or ALK rearrangements is usually not required for diagnosis.

The pattern of ALK expression in ALK-positive ALCL is determined by the partner of ALK in the fusion protein and therefore pattern can suggest the specific fusion gene present in the tumor (Table 33-4). ALK is overexpressed in four patterns (3,26,46). In cases where the partner is nucleophosmin (*NPM1*), ALK expression is cytoplasmic and nuclear (fig. 33-11, right). This is because NPM-ALK forms heterodimers with normal NPM and is carried into the nucleus. In most cases with variant translocations, ALK expression is usually confined to the cytoplasm with a diffuse, homogeneous pattern (fig. 33-6C). In cases where the ALK partner is the clathrin heavy polypeptide-like gene (*CLTC*), ALK expression is cytoplasmic and coarsely granular, correlating with the location of clathrin in cytoplasmic vesicles. Rarely, ALK expression is membranous in cases where the partner is moesin (*MSN*) which encodes a membrane-bound protein.

Table 33-3

IMMUNOPHENOTYPIC FINDINGS IN ALK-POSITIVE AND ALK-NEGATIVE ANAPLASTIC LARGE CELL LYMPHOMA

Antigen	ALK-positive ALCL	ALK-negative ALCL	Pattern or Comment
CD30	Positive	Positive	Strong and uniform membranous and para-nuclear/Golgi pattern
ALK-1	Positive	Negative	See Table 33-4 for patterns in ALK-positive ALCL
CD2	Can be negative or positive	Can be negative but more often positive	
CD3	Often negative	Often negative	Defective T-cell signaling pathway; also applies to TCRβ and ZAP-70
CD4	Commonly positive	Commonly positive	Membrane and cytoplasm
CD5	Often negative	Often negative	
CD8	Usually negative	Usually negative	Small subset positive; more often in ALK-negative ALCL
CD43	Usually positive	Usually positive	Membrane and cytoplasm
TCRβ	Often negative	Often negative	
CD13	~40% positive	Usually negative	CD13 often detected by flow cytometry in ALK-positive ALCL
CD15	Usually negative	Minority subset of cases can be positive	Membrane and paranuclear
CD45	Positive or negative	Positive or negative	CD45 can be negative by immunohistochemistry (usually positive by flow cytometry)
CD56	Positive in subset of cases	Positive in subset of cases	
Cytotoxic proteins	Often positive	Less often positive; cases with *DUSP22* rearrangement often negative	TIA-1, granzyme B, and perforin are commonly tested
Clusterin	Usually positive, ~90% of cases	Positive less often	Paranuclear/Golgi pattern
B-cell antigens	Negative	Rare cases are PAX5+	
BCL2	Negative	Positive in 40-50% of cases	Rare cases of ALK-positive ALCL are weakly BCL2 positive by immunohistochemistry
ZAP-70	Often negative	Often negative	
TdT	Negative	Negative	
Cyclin D1	~25% positive	<10% negative	
EBV	Negative	Negative	Rare ALK-negative tumors can be positive

Both flow cytometry immunophenotyping and immunohistochemistry are used to assess ALK-positive ALCL. Flow cytometry is more sensitive and therefore can detect dimly expressed markers that may appear to be negative by immunohistochemistry (29). When using flow cytometry, the number of lymphoma cells is often lower than expected by morphologic assessment of the tumor, suggesting that there is some loss of tumor cells during preparation of the specimen for analysis.

ALK-positive ALCL is of T-cell or null-cell lineage (fig. 33-19). In cases of T-cell lineage, aberrant T-cell immunophenotypes are common and many tumors do not express CD3 (fig. 33-19A), ZAP-70, or T-cell receptors, indicating defective T-cell signaling by the lymphoma cells (13). Epigenetic modification of T-cell gene promoters and upregulation of suppressor molecules are possible explanations for the loss of T-cell antigen expression (17,44).

CD4 (fig. 33-19B) and CD43 (fig. 33-9D) are the most frequently expressed T-cell markers in ALK-positive ALCL. CD8 is positive in a small subset of neoplasms and is more commonly expressed in the lymphohistiocytic and small cell

Table 33-4

ALK TRANSLOCATIONS AND GENE PARTNERS IN ALK-POSITIVE ANAPLASTIC LARGE CELL LYMPHOMA

Translocation	Gene Partner	Frequency	ALK Pattern
t(2;5)(p23.2;q35)	*NPM1*	80-85%	Nucleus and cytoplasm
t(1;2)(q21.2;p23.2)	*TPM3*	~10%	Cytoplasm
t(2;3)(p23.2;q21)	*TFG*	1-2%	Cytoplasm
inv(2)(p23.2q35)	*ATIC*	1-2%	Cytoplasm
t(2;17)(p23.2;q23)	*CLTC*	Rare	Granular cytoplasmic
t(2;X)(p23.2;q11-12)	*MSN*	Rare	Membranous
t(2;17)(p23.2;q25)	*RNF213 (ALO17)*	Rare	Cytoplasm
t(2;22)(p23.2;q13.1)	*MYH9*	Rare	Cytoplasm
t(2;19)(p23.2;p13.1)	*TPM4*	Rare	Cytoplasm
t(2;9)(p23.2;q33)	*TRAF1*	Rare	Cytoplasm
t(2;11;2)(p23.2;p15;q31)	*CARS*	Rare	Cytoplasm
t(2;11)(2p23.2;11q12.3)	EEFIG	Rare	Cytoplasm

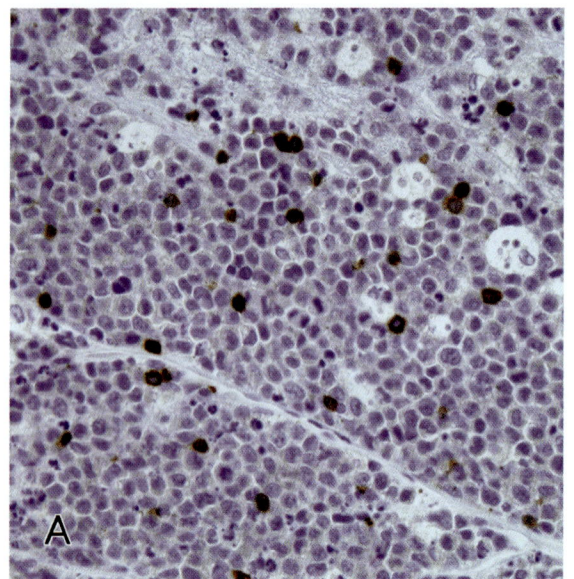
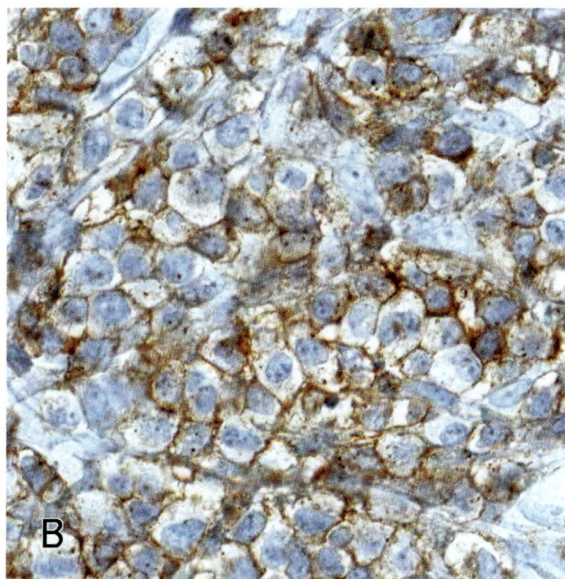

Figure 33-19

ALK-POSITIVE ANAPLASTIC LARGE CELL LYMPHOMA: IMMUNOHISTOCHEMISTRY

A,B: In this case the lymphoma cells are CD3 negative (A) and CD4 positive (B).

variants (1). Some cases of ALK-positive ALCL are negative for both CD4 and CD8 but these molecules are rarely (if ever) both expressed by the lymphoma cells (1,46). Null-cell tumors do not express cell-specific antigens but usually carry monoclonal T-cell receptor gene rearrangements.

In most cases of ALK-positive ALCL, the lymphoma cells have a cytotoxic immuno-phenotype and express TIA-1 (fig. 33-19C), granzyme B, and perforin (11,26,46). The proliferation rate is often very high, shown by Ki-67 expression (fig. 33-19D). EMA/MUC1 (fig. 33-19E) and clusterin (fig. 33-19F) are commonly positive (26,42,46). CD45/LCA may be negative by immunohistochemistry (46). Approximately 70 to 80 percent of ALK-positive ALCL cases are

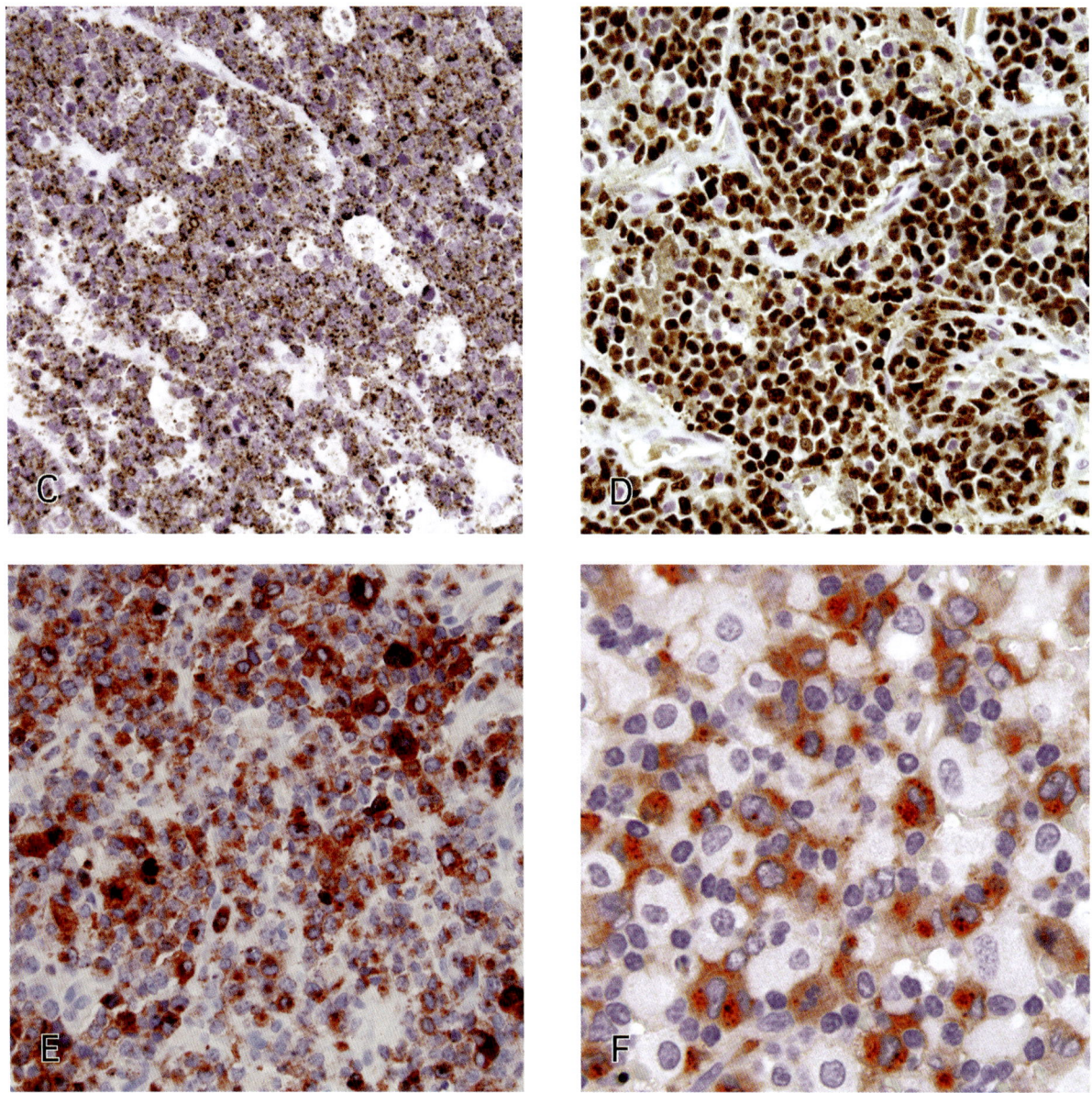

Figure 33-19, continued

C: The lymphoma cells express cytotoxic proteins such as TIA-1 (C) and granzyme B (not shown).

D,E: Ki-67 is often very high (D) and EMA/MUC1 is often positive (E).

F: Clusterin is often positive with a paranuclear pattern of staining (A–F: immunohistochemistry with hematoxylin counterstain).

positive for CD99. The myeloid-associated markers CD11b, CD13, and CD33 are positive in 30 to 40 percent of cases (26). CD56 is positive in about 20 percent of tumors. ALK-positive ALCL has a high apoptotic rate compared with other types of T-cell lymphoma (38). ALK-positive ALCL is negative for pan-B-cell antigens and

is not associated with Epstein-Barr virus (EBV) infection in developed nations (15).

A number of other molecules are expressed in ALK-positive ALCL. Although the diagnostic utility of these markers is currently limited, many are downstream targets of cell pathways activated by NPM-ALK. NPM-ALK activates the

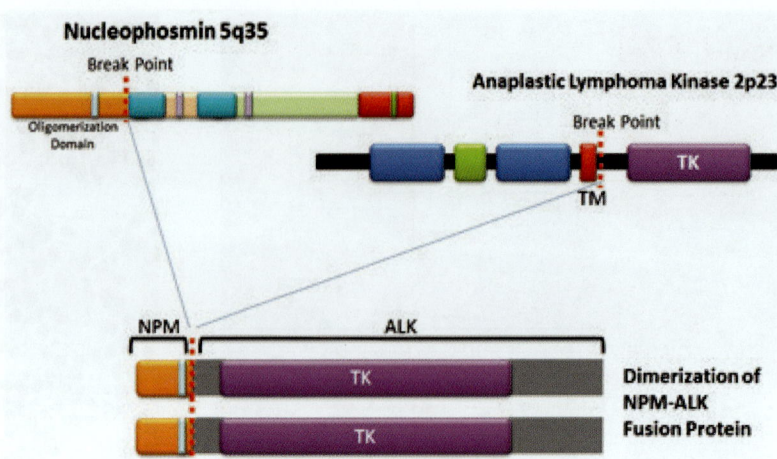

Figure 33-20

NPM-ALK t(2;5)(p23;q35)

A schematic diagram of the t(2;5) (p23.2;q35), resulting in oncogenic chimeric fusion (and overexpression of ALK).

JAK/STAT pathway, and as a result, STAT3 is expressed at high levels (7,18). STAT3 is phosphorylated (activated) and translocated into the nucleus. In accord with JAK/STAT activation, downstream targets of STAT3, such as suppressor of cytokine signaling 3 (SOCS3), are overexpressed (8). NPM-ALK activates members of the AP1 transcription family that are expressed highly in most cases of ALK-positive ALCL (22). P53 is commonly overexpressed in ALK-positive ALCL although corresponding genetic alterations are uncommon (41,43). MUM1/IRF4 and MYC are overexpressed in a subset of ALK-positive ALCL cases; MYC is a downstream target of MUM1/IRF4 (51). Apoptotic molecules are downstream of NPM-ALK and JAK/STAT. The profile of apoptotic molecule expression is distinctive in ALK-positive ALCL: positive for MCL1 and negative or uncommonly dimly positive for BCL2 by immunohistochemistry (38,40). About 25 percent of cases of ALK-positive ALCL express cyclin D1 (44a). A small number of cases of ALK-positive ALCL express keratins.

MOLECULAR GENETIC FINDINGS

Conventional cytogenetic analysis facilitates the detection of all chromosomal translocations involving 2p23.2/*ALK*, with t(2;5)(p23.2;q35) being the most common recurrent abnormality (32,43). This method also allows for the detection of additional chromosomal abnormalities likely to be involved in pathogenesis or tumor progression. Translocations involving ALK are detected in 80 to 90 percent of children and 50 to 60 percent of adults with ALCL (43,46). In general, karyotypes in ALK-positive ALCL are less complex than in ALK-negative ALCL (see chapter 34).

Comparative genomic hybridization studies have shown that cases of ALK-positive ALCL, whether carrying t(2;5)/*NPM-ALK* or other variant *ALK* abnormalities, have a similar profile of secondary abnormalities. In 43 cases of ALK-positive ALCL studied by Salaverria et al. (43), a mean of four chromosomal imbalances per case were found, and the most common abnormalities were gains of 2q, 7p, 17p, and 17q and losses of 4q, 11q, and 13q. This study also showed common abnormalities in ALK-positive and ALK-negative ALCL, but ALK-positive ALCL more often had gains of 17p and 17q24-qter and losses of 4q13-q21 and 11q14.

At the molecular level, all cases of ALK-positive ALCL carry a fusion gene involving ALK at chromosome 2p23.2. The most common fusion gene is *NPM-ALK* in about 80 to 85 percent of cases (fig. 33-20) (11,26,46) which encodes for NPM-ALK. Dimerization of NPM-ALK via the oligomerization domain contributed by NPM simulates physiologic ligand binding and induces autophosphorylation, leading to the activation of the kinase domain of ALK in a deregulated manner (fig. 33-21) (7,35). Using mass spectrophotometry, NPM-ALK has been shown to bind with numerous molecules, including JAK2, JAK3, STAT3, PI3K, PLCG1, adaptor molecules (e.g., SOCS), kinases, phosphatases, and heat shock proteins (9). In accord with these data, ALK activation begins a cascade of events by activating several signaling pathways, such

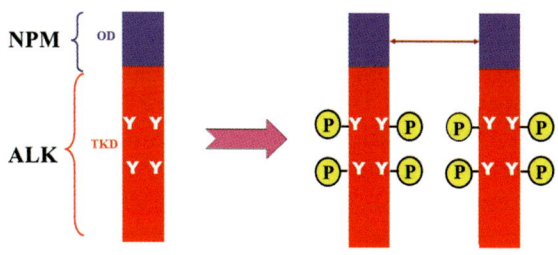

Figure 33-21

**DIMERIZATION OF NPM-ALK MIMICS
LIGAND BINDING AND RESULTS
IN CONSTITUTIVE ACTIVATION OF ALK**

Schematic illustrative of constitutive activation of ALK. Dimerization of NPM-ALK molecules via the oligomerization domain (OD) of NPM mimics normal ligand binding thereby facilitating autophosphorylation of the tyrosine kinase domain (TKD) of ALK. NPM, nucleophosmin; ALK, anaplastic lymphoma kinase; Y, tyrosine; P, phosphate.

as the JAK-STAT, RAS-ERK, PI3K/AKT and NF-κB pathways involved in cell survival, cell proliferation, and cell cycle progression (7,36). Of these pathways, STAT3 activation appears to be particularly important in lymphomagenesis and is an attractive research area for targeted therapy (45).

The remaining 15 percent of cases of ALK-positive ALCL harbor variant fusion partners that also result in *ALK* activation (Table 33-4). The partner genes identified include *CLTC*, *MSN*, nonmuscle tropomyosin 3 gene (*TPM3*), nonmuscle tropomyosin 4 (*TPM4*), Trk fused gene (*TFG*), eukaryotic translation elongation factor 1 gamma (*EEFIG*), myosin heavy chain (*MYH9*), 5-aminoimidazole-4-carboxamide ribonucleotide formyltransferase/IMP cyclohydrolase gene (*ATIC*), and TNF receptor associated factor 1 (*TRAF1*) (6,7,26,32a). For most of the fusion genes, the *ALK* partner gene contributes a domain that facilitates the formation of dimers similar to the role performed by NPM, and results in autophosphorylation and activation of cellular pathways that eventually lead to lymphomagenesis. Due to their rarity, however, few studies have focused specifically on the pathways activated by the variant fusion proteins. Presumably much is shared with the actions of NPM-ALK, but it seems likely there may be some differences.

ALK rearrangements are detected by fluorescence in situ hybridization (FISH) studies using *ALK* breakapart probes. This approach documents the presence of *ALK* rearrangements, but does not provide information about the specific gene partner and is less convenient than immunohistochemistry for ALK assessment. One advantage of FISH is that this method facilitates the detection of *ALK* amplification, which has been observed in a small subset of ALK-positive ALCLs (and more commonly in solid tumors).

Gene expression profiling studies have shown that ALK-positive and ALK-negative ALCLs share aspects of their signatures, suggesting that they have shared mechanisms in lymphomagenesis (16,20,34). Nevertheless, the expression profile of ALK-positive ALCL is distinctive from ALK-negative ALCL. ALK-positive ALCL cases are enriched for expression of HIF1-α target genes and *IL10-* and *HRAS/KRAS*-induced genes (16,25). MicroRNA profiling studies have shown commonly altered microRNAs as well as different profiles for ALK-positive ALCL versus ALK-negative ALCL (23,45,48). Liu et al. (23) reported a 7-microRNA signature characteristic of ALK-positive ALCLs. Other microRNA combinations also distinguish ALK-positive from ALK-negative ALCL (48). The miR-17~92 cluster is highly expressed in ALK-positive ALCL and thought to be involved in STAT3 activation (45). Downregulation of miR-146a and miR-155 also seems to be characteristic of ALK-positive ALCL (23,48).

Most cases of ALK-positive ALCL carry monoclonal rearrangements of the T-cell receptor (TCR) genes, but in 10 percent of cases no monoclonal TCR gene rearrangements are detected, suggesting origin from a T cell at a stage before initiation of physiologic gene rearrangement (26,46). Immunoglobulin gene rearrangements are uncommon.

A number of other genetic abnormalities have been identified in ALK-positive ALCL and are likely involved in oncogenesis or tumor progression. AP1 family members are involved in cell-cycle progression in ALK-positive ALCL (22). As a result, most cases of ALK-positive ALCL are positive for cyclins A, D2, and D3. Expression of AP1 family members also has been linked to CD30 expression, and C-JUN and JUNB can bind the AKT promoter, possibly explaining PI3K/AKT pathway activation. NPM-ALK binds with MSH2, a key protein involved in DNA mismatch repair (5).

PRDM1/BLIMP1 and *RB* are often deleted or otherwise inactivated in ALK-positive ALCL (and ALK-negative ALCL) (4,39). Although MYC is commonly expressed, rearrangements or other genetic lesions are reported rarely. *TP53* mutations or amplification are uncommon in ALK-positive ALCL (less than 10 percent of cases) (41). ALK-positive ALCL is not associated with chromosomal translocations that involve *DUSP22/6p25.3* or *TP63/3q28*, as occurs in a subset of ALK-negative ALCL cases (33).

DIFFERENTIAL DIAGNOSIS

ALK-Negative ALCL. ALK-negative ALCL is more common in older adults than ALK-positive ALCL, and ALK-negative ALCL tumors are often more anaplastic with numerous "doughnut"-like or "wreath"-like cells. However, both tumors are often indistinguishable, and immunophenotypically both frequently share an aberrant T-cell immunophenotype and strong and uniform CD30 immunoreactivity. In contrast with ALK-positive ALCL, ALK-negative ALCL is negative for ALK expression or *ALK* translocations. In addition, ALK-negative ALCL is frequently positive for BCL2 and has a lower frequency of positivity for cytotoxic molecules, EMA/MUC1 or clusterin (6,26). At the molecular level, about 30 percent and 10 percent of cases of ALK-negative ALCL have rearrangements involving *DUSP22/6p25.3* and *TP63/3q28*, respectively, abnormalities that do not occur in ALK-positive ALCLs (33). ALK-negative ALCL is the focus of chapter 34.

Primary Cutaneous ALCL. ALK-positive ALCL secondarily involving skin and primary cutaneous ALCL can be morphologically identical, and both neoplasms express CD30 in a uniform and bright fashion. The clinical history of localized skin disease supports primary cutaneous ALCL and therefore this differential diagnosis is often resolved by clinical staging. Immunohistochemical demonstration of ALK expression and genetic studies for *ALK* translocations support ALK-positive ALCL, with the caveat that rare cases of primary cutaneous ALCL that express ALK have been described (31). Rearrangements of *DUSP22/6p25.3* are detected in a subset of cases of primary cutaneous ALCL but are not present in ALK-positive ALCL (33).

Peripheral T-Cell Lymphoma, Not Otherwise Specified. Because of the broad morphologic spectrum of ALK-positive ALCL, all cases of peripheral T-cell lymphoma, not otherwise specified (PTCL-NOS), should be evaluated for the expression of CD30. Most cases of PTCL-NOS are CD30 negative; however, in some cases a subset of lymphoma cells variably and weakly expresses CD30. There are rare cases of PTCL, however, in which CD30 is expressed moderately or strongly by most of the tumor cells. These cases do not exhibit anaplastic cytologic features (otherwise they would be designated as ALK-negative ALCL). Immunohistochemical analysis for ALK expression or molecular evidence of *ALK* translocation resolves this differential diagnosis.

The small cell variant of ALK-positive ALCL does not have the typical, uniform CD30 expression pattern observed in other variants; only a minority of the lymphoma cells are positive for CD30, often located around blood vessels. These cases can be mistaken for PTCL-NOS if ALK expression is not assessed.

Hodgkin Lymphoma. Rare cases of ALK-positive ALCL morphologically simulate nodular sclerosis Hodgkin lymphoma (49). These tumors show capsular thickening and vague or well-developed fibrous bands that can subdivide the tumor into nodules. Some of the neoplastic cells resemble classic Reed-Sternberg cells, but hallmark cells are also present. Unlike nodular sclerosis Hodgkin lymphoma, the tumor cells are positive for ALK; variably positive for T-cell antigens, epithelial membrane antigen (EMA), and CD45/LCA; and are negative for CD15 and PAX5.

CD30-Positive Diffuse Large B-Cell Lymphoma. Approximately 2 to 3 percent of diffuse large B-cell lymphomas have anaplastic cytologic features, express CD30, and resemble ALK-positive ALCL. These tumors tend to occur in older adults and immunohistochemical analysis shows expression of pan-B-cell antigens including CD20. In addition, the pattern of CD30 expression is often cytoplasmic, although it can be membranous and cytoplasmic, similar to ALCL.

Other CD30-Positive B-Cell Lymphomas. Other rare B-cell lymphomas also express CD30. The solid (extracavitary) variant of primary effusion lymphoma may exhibit marked sinusoidal involvement and anaplastic morphologic features resembling ALCL. These tumors, however, occur in human immunodeficiency virus (HIV)-

infected patients with severe immunodeficiency and are positive for human herpesvirus (HHV) 8.

ALK-positive large B-cell lymphoma also may resemble ALCL morphologically. These lymphomas express ALK in a pattern that most often is coarsely granular and cytoplasmic, but rarely, nuclear and cytoplasmic, corresponding to the t(2;17) and t(2;5), respectively. ALK-positive large B-cell lymphoma is usually positive for CD138, MUM1/IRF4, and intracytoplasmic immunoglobulins (often IgA) and is negative for CD30.

Other Hematopoietic Tumors. Other hematopoietic tumors that may express CD30 include myeloid sarcoma and mast cell neoplasms. Myeloid sarcoma with monocytic differentiation may be positive for CD4 in addition to CD30, mimicking ALCL. Some ALK-positive ALCLs express the myeloid-associated antigens, CD13 and less often CD33, further complicating the differential diagnosis. ALK, however, is not expressed by myeloid sarcoma or mast cell neoplasms.

In the blood, the diagnosis of acute myeloid leukemia may be considered because the circulating ALK-positive ALCL cells may be weakly positive or negative for CD30 and express myeloid-associated markers such as CD11b, CD13, or lysozyme (26,30). The lymphoma cells, however, express ALK and ALK translocations are present.

Nonhematopoietic Tumors. In lymph nodes involved by ALK-positive ALCL in a predominantly sinusoidal pattern, the possibility of metastatic tumor is likely to be considered, particularly metastatic carcinoma or melanoma. The lymphoma cells also appear cohesive and can be associated with sclerosis, further misleading the observer (fig. 33-22). Once the possibility of ALCL is considered, immunohistochemical studies resolve the issue if antibodies specific for CD30 and ALK are used. It is important to remember that ALK-positive ALCL commonly expresses EMA/MUC1 and can be CD45/LCA negative.

A number of nonhematopoietic neoplasms express CD30. A well known example is embryonal cell carcinomas of the testis and ovary, which can express CD30 brightly and uniformly, much like ALCL. A subset of nasopharyngeal carcinomas, other carcinomas, and mesotheliomas also may express CD30, more often in a cytoplasmic pattern. The clinical context of these tumors is unlike that of patients with ALK-positive ALCL and these tumors are negative for ALK.

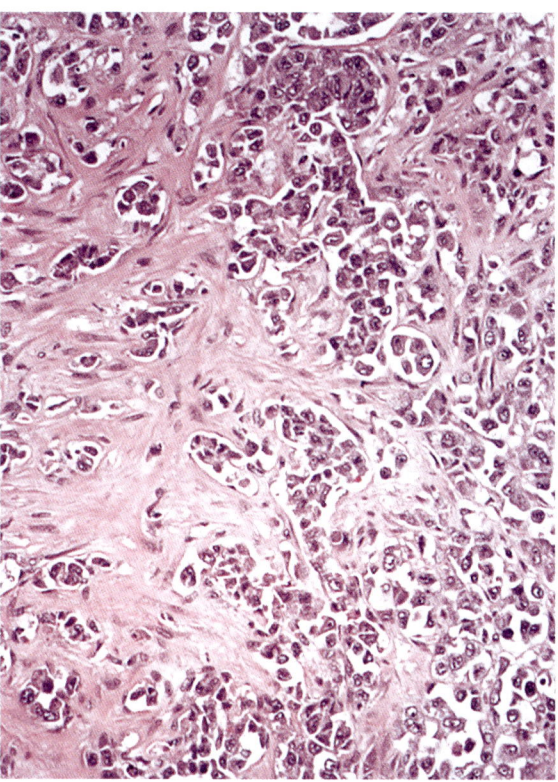

Figure 33-22

ALK-POSITIVE ANAPLASTIC LARGE CELL LYMPHOMA ASSOCIATED WITH SCLEROSIS

The cohesive appearance of the nests of tumor cells resembles, in part, carcinoma (H&E stain).

A distinctive form of lung adenocarcinoma is positive for ALK and carries an *ALK* translocation, usually with *EML4* as the partner. These tumors are usually well differentiated, show the obvious features of adenocarcinoma, express keratin, and are CD30 negative. Some inflammatory myofibroblastic tumors (IMTs) express ALK and carry *ALK* translocations and a subset of these tumors is also positive for CD30 (21a). A number of partners of ALK have been identified in IMTs, but not NPM. These tumors are also usually soft tissue based and have histologic features unlike most cases of ALK-positive ALCL.

Other solid tumors express full length ALK receptor, including neuroblastoma, glioblastoma, and melanoma, or show immunoreactivity (usually weak) for ALK, such as breast carcinoma and liposarcoma. Importantly, the clinical context for these solid tumors differs greatly from that of ALK-positive ALCL. In addition, these tumors are negative for CD30 and have immunophenotypic profiles appropriate for their cell lineage.

TREATMENT AND PROGNOSIS

Most adults with ALK-positive ALCL are treated with anthracycline-based multiagent chemotherapy, typically the CHOP (cyclophosphamide, doxorubicin, vincristine, and prednisone) regimen (14,48b). In children, the ALCL99 (doxorubicin, dexamethasone, cyclophosphamide, ifosfamide, methotrexate, cytarabine, and etoposide) regimen is commonly used. Patients with relapsed disease have been traditionally offered stem cell transplantation. The CD30-targeted antibody drug conjugate, brentuximab vedotin, has clinical efficacy in patients with relapsed/refractory ALCL and may be used as a bridge to or combined with stem cell transplantation (14,48b). Brentuximab vedotin combined with CHOP chemotherapy in the front-line setting is being evaluated in clinical trials. The ALK inhibitor, crizotinib, also has shown encouraging responses in patients with relapsed ALK-positive ALCL (12). *ALK* mutations have been described following crizotinib therapy in a subset of ALK-positive ALCL patients and explain the resistance to crizotinib in some patients; however, not all mutations interfere with sensitivity to crizotinib (52). Second generation ALK inhibitors have been developed (e.g., ceritinib).

The 5-year overall survival rate for patients with ALK-positive ALCL treated with current chemotherapeutic regimens is 70 to 80 percent (11,14,46). Approximately 30 percent of patients develop late relapses and about half of these patients completely respond to additional therapies. Aggressive assessment for minimal residual disease using polymerase chain reaction (PCR) methods to detect *NPM-ALK* in blood or bone marrow has prognostic value (10,28,48b). Many patients with ALK-positive ALCL also develop serum antibodies to ALK which can be monitored after therapy (10).

Patients with ALK-positive ALCL have a better prognosis than patients with other types of peripheral T-cell lymphoma, including ALK-negative ALCL (14,50). Overall, pediatric patients have a better prognosis. For patients less than 40 years of age, there are minimal differences in overall survival between patients with ALK-positive versus ALK-negative ALCL (14). In the pediatric age group, patients with the small cell and lymphohistiocytic variants have a worse prognosis than patients with the common variant. Leukemic involvement and CD8 expression, seen more often in the uncommon variants, also correlate with poorer prognosis (1).

REFERENCES

1. Abramov D, Oschlies I, Zimmermann M, et al. Expression of CD8 is associated with non-common type morphology and outcome in pediatric anaplastic lymphoma kinase-positive anaplastic large cell lymphoma. Haematologica 2013;98:1547-1553.
2. Bayle C, Charpentier A, Duchayne E, et al. Leukaemic presentation of small cell variant anaplastic large cell lymphoma: report of four cases. Br J Haematol 1999;104:680-688.
3. Benharroch D, Meguerian-Bedoyan Z, Lamant L, et al. ALK-positive lymphoma: a single disease with a broad spectrum of morphology. Blood 1998;91:2076-2084.
4. Boi M, Rinaldi A, Kwee I, et al. PRDM1/BLIMP1 is commonly inactivated in anaplastic large T-cell lymphoma. Blood 2013;122:2683-2693.
5. Bone KM, Wang P, Wu F, et al. NPM-ALK mediates phosphorylation of MSH2 at tyrosine 238, creating a functional deficiency in MSH2 and the loss of mismatch repair. Blood Cancer J 2015;5:e311.
6. Bonzheim I, Steinhilber J, Fend F, Lamant L, Quintanilla-Martinez L. ALK-positive anaplastic large cell lymphoma: an evolving story. Front Biosci (Schol Ed) 2015;7:248-259.
7. Chiarle R, Voena C, Ambrogio C, Piva R, Inghirami G. The anaplastic lymphoma kinase in the pathogenesis of cancer. Nat Rev Cancer 2008;8:11-23.
8. Cho-Vega JH, Rassidakis GZ, Amin HM, et al. Suppressor of cytokine signaling 3 expression in anaplastic large cell lymphoma. Leukemia 2004;18:1872-1878.

9. Crockett DK, Lin Z, Elenitoba-Johnson KS, Lim MS. Identification of NPM-ALK interacting proteins by tandem mass spectrophotometry. Oncogene 2004;23:2617-2629.

10. Damm-Welk C, Mussolin L, Zimmermann M, et al. Early assessment of minimal residual disease identifies patients at very high relapse risk in NPM-ALK-positive anaplastic large-cell lymphoma. Blood 2014;123:334-337.

11. Delsol G, Fallini B, Muller-Hermelink HK, et al. Anaplastic large cell lymphoma (ALCL) ALK-positive. WHO classification of tumours of haematopoietic and lymphoid tissues. Swerdlow SH, Campo E, Harris NL, et al., eds. Lyon: IARC Press: 2008;312-316.

12. Gambacorti-Passerini C, Farina F, Stasia A, et al. Crizotinib in advanced, chemoresistant anaplastic lymphoma kinase-positive lymphoma patients. J Natl Cancer Inst 2014;106:djt378.

13. Geissinger E, Sadler P, Roth S, et al. Disturbed expression of the T-cell receptor/CD3 complex and associated signaling molecules in CD30+ T-cell lymphoproliferations. Haematologica 2010;95:1697-1704.

14. Hapgood G, Savage KJ. The biology and management of systemic anaplastic large cell lymphoma. Blood 2015;126:15-25.

15. Herling M, Rassidakis GZ, Jones D, Schmitt-Graeff A, Sarris AH, Medeiros LJ. Absence of Epstein-Barr virus in anaplastic large cell lymphoma: a study of 64 cases classified according to World Health Organization criteria. Hum Pathol 2004;35:455-459.

16. Iqbal J, Wright G, Wang C, et al. Gene expression signatures delineate biological and prognostic subgroups in peripheral T-cell lymphoma. Blood 2014;123:2915-2923.

17. Joosten M, Seitz V, Zimmermann K, et al. Histone acetylation and DNA demethlyation of T cells result in an anaplastic large cell lymphoma-like phenotype. Haematologica 2013;98:247-254.

18. Khoury JD, Medeiros LJ, Rassidakis GZ, et al. Differential expression and clinical significance of tyrosine-phosphorylated STAT3 in ALK+ and ALK- anaplastic large cell lymphoma. Clin Cancer Res 2003;9(Pt 1):3692-3699.

19. Klapper W1, Böhm M, Siebert R, Lennert K. Morphological variability of lymphohistiocytic variant of anaplastic large cell lymphoma (former lymphohistiocytic lymphoma according to the Kiel classification). Virchows Arch 2008;452:599-605.

20. Lamant L, de Reyniès A, Duplantier MM, et al. Gene-expression profiling of systemic anaplastic large-cell lymphoma reveals differences based on ALK status and two distinct morphologic ALK+ subtypes. Blood 2007;109:2156-2164.

21. Le Beau MM, Bitter MA, Larson RA, et al. The t(2;5)(p23;q35): a recurring chromosomal abnormality in Ki-1-positive anaplastic large cell lymphoma. Leukemia 1989;3:866-870.

21a. Lee JC, Li CF, Huang HY, et al. ALK oncoproteins in atypical inflammatory myofibroblastic tumours: novel RRBP1-ALK fusions in epithelioid inflammatory myofibroblastic sarcoma. J Pathol 2017;241:316-323.

22. Leventaki V, Drakos E, Medeiros LJ, et al. NPM-ALK oncogenic kinase promotes cell-cycle progression through activation of JNK/cJun signaling in anaplastic large-cell lymphoma. Blood 2007;110:1621-1630.

23. Liu C, Iqbal J, Teruya-Feldstein J, et al. MicroRNA expression profiling identified molecular signatures associated with anaplastic large cell lymphoma. Blood 2013;122:2083-2092.

24. Lones MA, Sanger W, Perkins SL, Medeiros LJ. Anaplastic large cell lymphoma arising in bone: report of a case of the monomorphic variant with the t(2;5)(p23;q35) translocation. Arch Pathol Lab Med 2000;124:1339-1343.

25. Martinengo C, Poggio T, Menotti M, et al. ALK-dependent control of hypoxia-inducible factors mediates growth and metastasis. Cancer Res 2014;74:6094-6106.

26. Medeiros LJ, Elenitoba-Johnson KS. Anaplastic large cell lymphoma. Am J Clin Pathol 2007;127:707-722.

27. Morris SW, Kirstein MN, Valentine MB, et al. Fusion of a kinase gene, ALK, to a nucleolar protein gene, NPM, in non-Hodgkin's lymphoma. Science 1994;263:1281-1284.

28. Mussolin L, Pillon M, d'Amore ES, et al. Prevalence and clinical implications of bone marrow involvement in pediatric anaplastic large cell lymphoma. Leukemia 2005;19:1643-1647.

29. Muzzafar T, Wei EX, Lin P, Medeiros LJ, Jorgensen JL. Flow cytometric immunophenotyping of anaplastic large cell lymphoma. Arch Pathol Lab Med 2009;133:49-56.

30. Nguyen JT, Condron MR, Nguyen ND, De J, Medeiros LJ, Padula A. Anaplastic large cell lymphoma in leukemic phase: extraordinarily high white blood cell count. Pathol Int 2009;59:345-353.

31. Oschlies I, Lisfeld J, Lamant L, et al. ALK-positive anaplastic large cell lymphoma limited to the skin: clinical, histopathological and molecular analysis of 6 pediatric cases. A report from the ALCL99 study. Haematologica 2013;98:50-56.

32. Ott G, Katzenberger T, Siebert R, et al. Chromosomal abnormalities in nodal and extranodal CD30+ anaplastic large cell lymphomas: infrequent detection of the t(2;5) in extranodal lymphomas. Genes Chromosomes Cancer 1998;22:114-121.

32a. Palacios G, Shaw TI, Li Y, et al. Novel ALK fusion in anaplastic large cell lymphoma involving EEF1G, a subunit of the eukaryotic elongation factor-1 complex. Leukemia 2017;31:743-747.

33. Parilla Castellar ER, Jaffe ES, Said JW, et al. ALK-negative anaplastic large cell lymphoma is a genetically heterogeneous disease with widely disparate clinical outcomes. Blood 2014;124: 1473-1480.

34. Piva R, Agnelli L, Pellegrino E, et al. Gene expression profiling uncovers molecular classifiers for the recognition of anaplastic large-cell lymphoma within peripheral T-cell neoplasms. J Clin Oncol 2010;28:1583-1590.

35. Pulford K, Lamant L, Morris SW, et al. Detection of anaplastic lymphoma kinase (ALK) and nucleolar protein nucleophosmin (NPM)-ALK proteins in normal and neoplastic cells with the monoclonal antibody ALK1. Blood 1997;89:1394-1404.

36. Pulford K, Morris SW and Turturro F. Anaplastic lymphoma kinase proteins in growth control and cancer. J Cell Physiol 2004;199:330-358.

37. Rapkiewicz A, Wen H, Sen F, Das K. Cytomorphologic examination of anaplastic large cell lymphoma by fine-needle aspiration cytology. Cancer 2007;111:499-507.

38. Rassidakis GZ, Jones D, Lai R, et al. BCL-2 family proteins in peripheral T-cell lymphomas: correlation with tumour apoptosis and proliferation. J Pathol 2003;200:240-248.

39. Rassidakis GZ, Lai R, Herling M, Cromwell C, Schmitt-Graeff A, Medeiros LJ. Retinoblastoma protein is frequently absent or phosphorylated in anaplastic large-cell lymphoma. Am J Pathjol 2004;164:2259-2267.

40. Rassidakis GZ, Lai R, McDonnell TJ, Cabanillas F, Sarris AH, Medeiros LJ. Overexpression of Mcl-1 in anaplastic large cell lymphoma cell lines and tumors. Am J Pathol 2002;160:2309-2310.

41. Rassidakis GZ, Thomaides A, Wang S, et al. p53 gene mutations are uncommon but p53 is commonly expressed in anaplastic large-cell lymphoma. Leukemia 2005;19:1663-1669.

42. Saffer H, Wahed A, Rassidakis GZ, Medeiros LJ. Clusterin expression in malignant lymphomas: a survey of 266 cases. Mod Pathol 2002;15:1221-1226.

43. Salaverria I, Bea S, Lopez-Guillermo A, et al. Genomic profiling reveals different genetic aberrations in systemic ALK-positive and ALK-negative anaplastic large cell lymphomas. Br J Haematol 2008;140:516-526.

44. Schiefer AI, Vesely P, Hassler MR, Egger G, Kenner L. The role of AP-1 and epigenetics in ALCL. Front Biosci (Schol Ed) 2015;7:226-235.

44a. Song JY, Song L, Herrera AF, et al. Cyclin D1 expression in peripheral T-cell lymphomas. Mod Pathol 2016;29:1306-1312.

45. Spaccarotella E, Pellegrino E, Ferracin M, et al. STAT3-mediated activation of microRNA cluster 17~92 promotes proliferation and survival of ALK-positive anaplastic large cell lymphoma. Haematologica 2014;99:116-124.

46. Stein H, Foss HD, Durkop H, et al. CD30(+) anaplastic large cell lymphoma: a review of its histopathologic, genetic, and clinical features. Blood 2000;96:3681-3695.

47. Stein H, Mason DY, Gerdes J, et al. The expression of the Hodgkin's disease associated antigen Ki-1 in reactive and neoplastic lymphoid tissue: evidence that Reed-Sternberg cells and histiocytic malignancies are derived from activated lymphoid cells. Blood 1985;66:848-858.

48. Steinhilber J, Bonin M, Walter M, Fend F, Bonzheim I, Quintanilla-Martinez L. Next-generation sequencing identifies deregulation of microRNAs involved in both innate and adaptive immune response in ALK+ ALCL. PLoS One 2015;10:e0117780.

48a. Swerdlow SH, Campo E, Pileri SA, et al. The 2016 revision of the World Health Organization classification of lymphoid neoplasms. Blood 2016;127:2375-2390.

48b. Turner SD, Lamant L, Kenner L, Brugières L. Anaplastic large cell lymphoma in paediatric and young adult patients. Br J Haematol 2016;173:560-572.

49. Vassallo J, Lamant L, Brugieres L, et al. ALK-positive anaplastic large cell lymphoma mimicking nodular sclerosis Hodgkin's lymphoma: report of 10 cases. Am J Surg Pathol 2006;30:223-229.

50. Vose J, Armitage J, Weisenburger D; International T-Cell Lymphoma Project. International peripheral T-cell and natural killer/T-cell lymphoma study: pathology findings and clinical outcomes. J Clin Oncol 2008;26:4124-4130.

51. Weilemann A, Grau M, Erdmann T, et al. Essential role of IRF4 and MYC signaling for survival of anaplastic large cell lymphoma. Blood 2015;125:124-132.

52. Zdzalik D, Dymek B, Grygielewicz P, et al. Activating mutations in ALK kinase domain confer resistance to structurally unrelated ALK inhibitors in NPM-ALK-positive anaplastic large cell lymphoma. J Cancer Res Clin Oncol 2014;140:589-598.

34 ALK-NEGATIVE ANAPLASTIC LARGE CELL LYMPHOMA

GENERAL FEATURES

Anaplastic lymphoma kinase (ALK)-negative anaplastic large cell lymphoma (ALCL) was included in the 2008 World Health Organization (WHO) classification as a provisional category (18). The provisional designation is dropped in the 2016 revision (33a). This tumor is morphologically indistinguishable from ALK-positive ALCL, but lacks *ALK* gene rearrangement and ALK expression (18).

The evolution of our current understanding of ALCL began in 1985 with the first description of Ki-1 lymphoma, as was reviewed in the previous chapter (see fig. 33-1). Recent studies have shown that ALK-negative ALCL, as currently defined, is genetically heterogeneous, with molecular subtypes conferring markedly different prognoses, and this category will likely evolve further (26). An argument can be made to split the category of ALK-negative ALCL into two or three different diseases, and this seems to be inevitable if additional studies further confirm initial reports.

Observations also suggest that ALK-negative ALCL, as currently defined, is clinically heterogeneous. A subset of patients with a history of peripheral T-cell lymphoma (PTCL), not otherwise specified, can relapse with an anaplastic, uniformly CD30-positive tumor that closely resembles ALK-negative ALCL. This suggests that some cases of ALK-negative ALCL may have originated as PTCL. Similarly, in a subset of patients with either lymphomatoid papulosis or primary cutaneous ALCL, the lesion may eventually disseminate, initially to regional lymph nodes and less often widely; these tumors also can resemble ALK-negative ALCL. Although a history of skin disease may not be reported by the patient, skin lesions may be remote.

ALK-negative ALCL represents 2 to 3 percent of all non-Hodgkin lymphomas and up to about 10 percent of all T-cell lymphomas in adults

(4,18,33). In one study, ALK-negative ALCL represented 9.4 percent, 7.8 percent, and 2.6 percent of T-cell lymphomas in Europe, North America, and Asia, respectively (see Table 33-1) (37).

CLINICAL FEATURES

Most patients with ALK-negative ALCL are adults with a median age in the sixth decade (4,19,31). ALK-negative ALCL, however, also occurs in children. There is a slight male predominance. B-type symptoms are present in at least half of all patients. Approximately 50 percent of patients present initially with lymphadenopathy (4,18,31). Extranodal involvement occurs in about 25 percent. Common extranodal sites of disease include skin, lung, gastrointestinal tract, and liver. Bone marrow involvement is detected in 5 to 10 percent of patients (4,18,31).

Rare patients develop a leukemic phase. Serum lactate dehydrogenase (LDH) and beta-2-microglobulin levels are commonly elevated and approximately 60 percent of patients have widespread disease, Ann Arbor stage III or IV (18,31). Most patients have an International Prognostic Index (IPI) score that is moderate or high risk. The relapse rate is higher and overall survival is inferior in patients with ALK-negative ALCL compared with patients with ALK-positive ALCL (26,31).

HISTOLOGIC FINDINGS

ALK-negative ALCL commonly effaces the lymph node architecture in a diffuse pattern (fig. 34-1). In a subset of cases, the tumor is present in a paracortical distribution, sparing and often surrounding residual lymphoid follicles (fig. 34-2). Sinusoidal involvement is common (fig. 34-3) and coagulative necrosis can be prominent (19,33).

Most cases of ALK-negative ALCL closely resemble the common (or classic) variant of ALK-positive ALCL (figs. 34-1–34-3). The lymphoma cells may show a spectrum of cell sizes, from intermediate-size to large, or entirely large

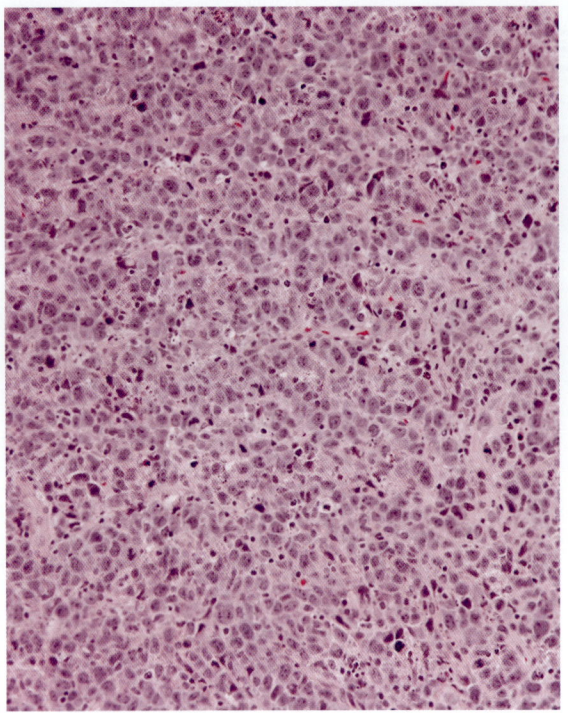

Figure 34-1

ANAPLASTIC LYMPHOMA KINASE (ALK)-NEGATIVE
ANAPLASTIC LARGE CELL
LYMPHOMA, COMMON VARIANT

The tumor diffusely replaces lymph node (hematoxylin and eosin (H&E) stain).

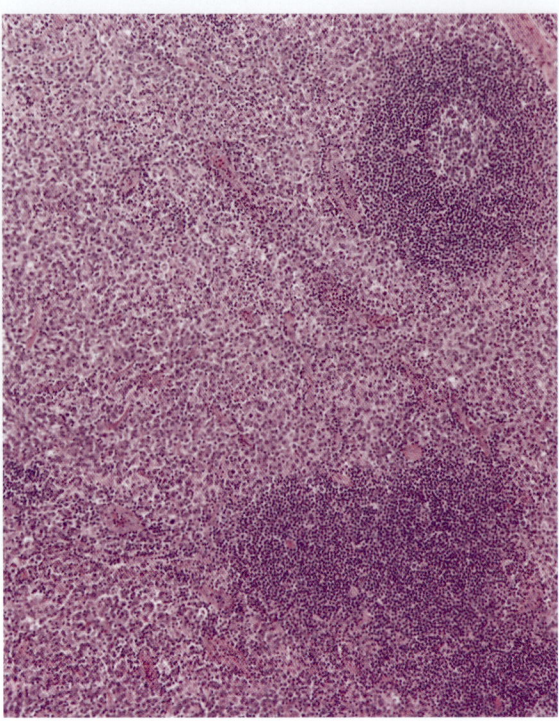

Figure 34-2

ALK-NEGATIVE ANAPLASTIC LARGE CELL LYMPHOMA, COMMON VARIANT, INVOLVING LYMPH NODE

A paracortical pattern is present, sparing some lymphoid follicles (H&E stain).

(figs. 34-4, 34-5). Hallmark cells are present although often less frequent than observed in ALK-positive ALCL (18,19,33). Some lymphoma cells are pleomorphic, often more pleomorphic than the cells in ALK-positive ALCL. The cells can be multinucleated, wreath-like or spindled (fig. 34-6). These tumors may be associated with numerous neutrophils or eosinophils (fig. 34-7). Rare tumors have neoplastic cells with a signet ring-like morphology (fig. 34-8).

Of the four morphologic variants recognized by the WHO classification for ALK-positive ALCL, the Hodgkin-like variant of ALK-negative ALCL can be recognized. In these tumors, fibrous bands may subdivide the lymphoma cells into vague nodules resembling, at low magnification, Hodgkin lymphoma (fig. 34-9). The lymphohistiocytic variant of ALK-negative ALCL can be difficult to recognize and the small cell variant (if it exists) cannot be recognized using morphologic and immunophenotypic criteria.

CYTOLOGIC FINDINGS

Cytologic preparations typically contain large pleomorphic cells with hyperchromatic nuclei and a variable amount of cytoplasm. The cytomorphologic features are similar to those of ALK-positive ALCL (see previous chapter), including hallmark cells, mononuclear cells with "doughnut"-like or "wreath"-like cells, and binucleated cells with prominent nucleoli (Reed-Sternberg–like cells) (fig. 34-10). Likewise, the cells can be dispersed or loosely cohesive, mimicking an epithelial malignancy. Varying numbers of inflammatory cells may be present in the background, including small lymphocytes, histiocytes, plasma cells, and eosinophils. Cell block preparations are optimal to perform immunohistochemical analysis because the differential diagnosis is broad (see below).

IMMUNOPHENOTYPIC FINDINGS

ALK-negative ALCL shares many immunophenotypic features with ALK-positive ALCL (see

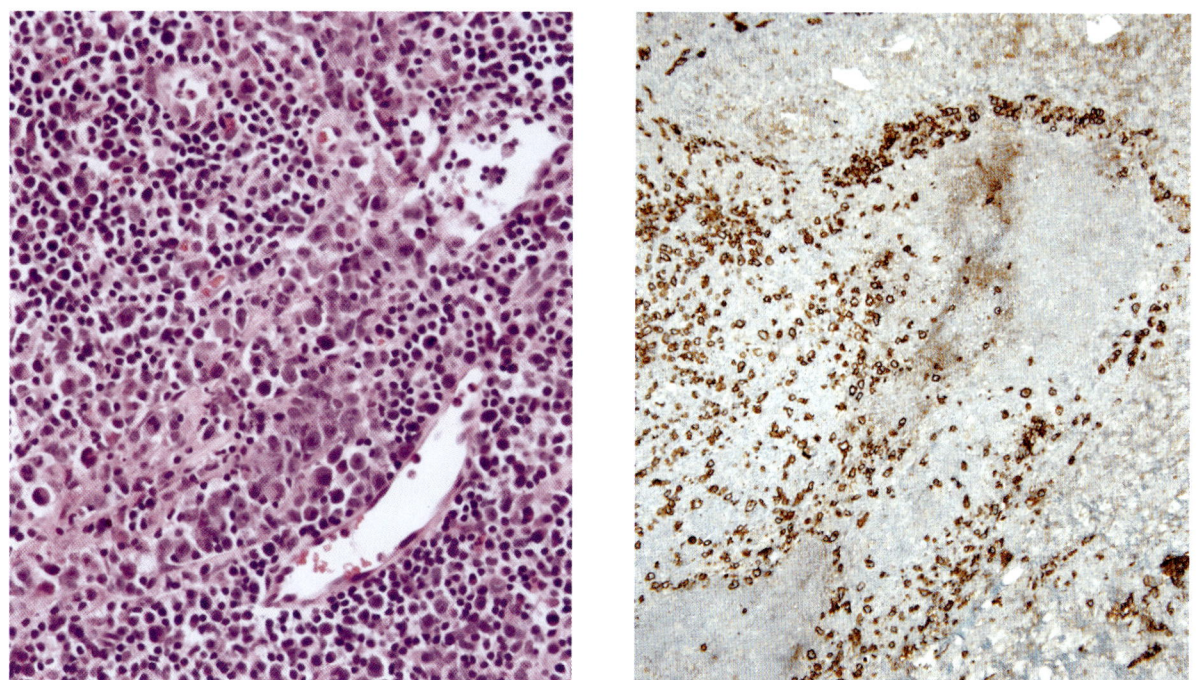

Figure 34-3

ALK-NEGATIVE ANAPLASTIC LARGE CELL LYMPHOMA INVOLVING LYMPH NODE SINUSES

Left: The lymphoma cells fill a sinus in the center of the field, parallel to a blood vessel (H&E stain).

Right: In another case, the CD30 antibody highlights involvement of the subcapsular sinus (immunohistochemistry with hematoxylin counterstain).

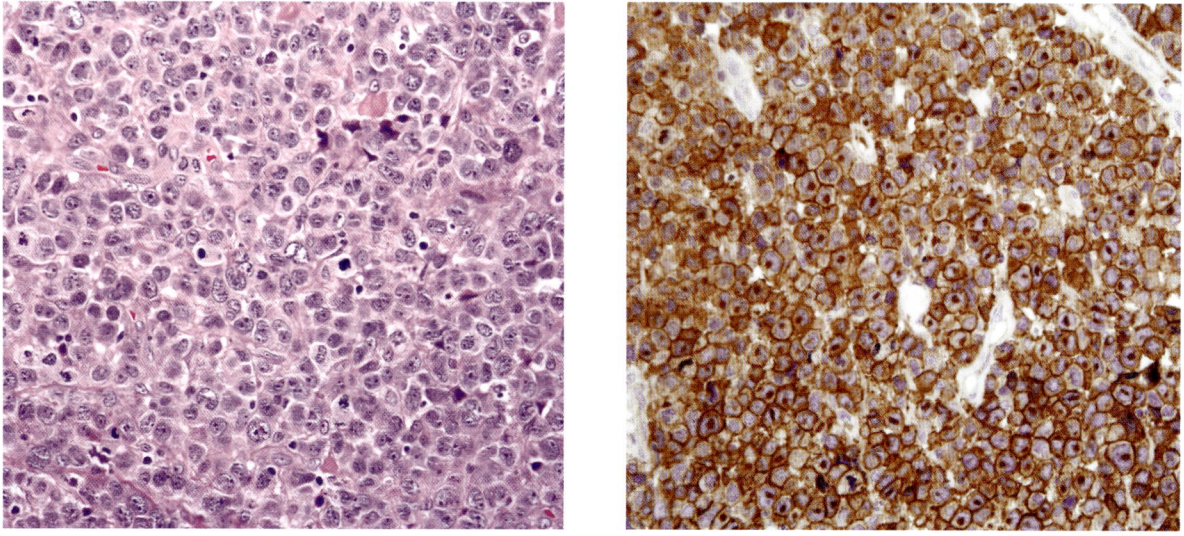

Figure 34-4

ALK-NEGATIVE ANAPLASTIC LARGE CELL LYMPHOMA, COMMON VARIANT

Left: The lymphoma cells are large, with abundant cytoplasm. Some cells meet the criteria for hallmark cells with horseshoe-shaped nuclei (H&E stain).

Right: The lymphoma cells are uniformly and strongly positive for CD30 (immunohistochemistry with hematoxylin counterstain).

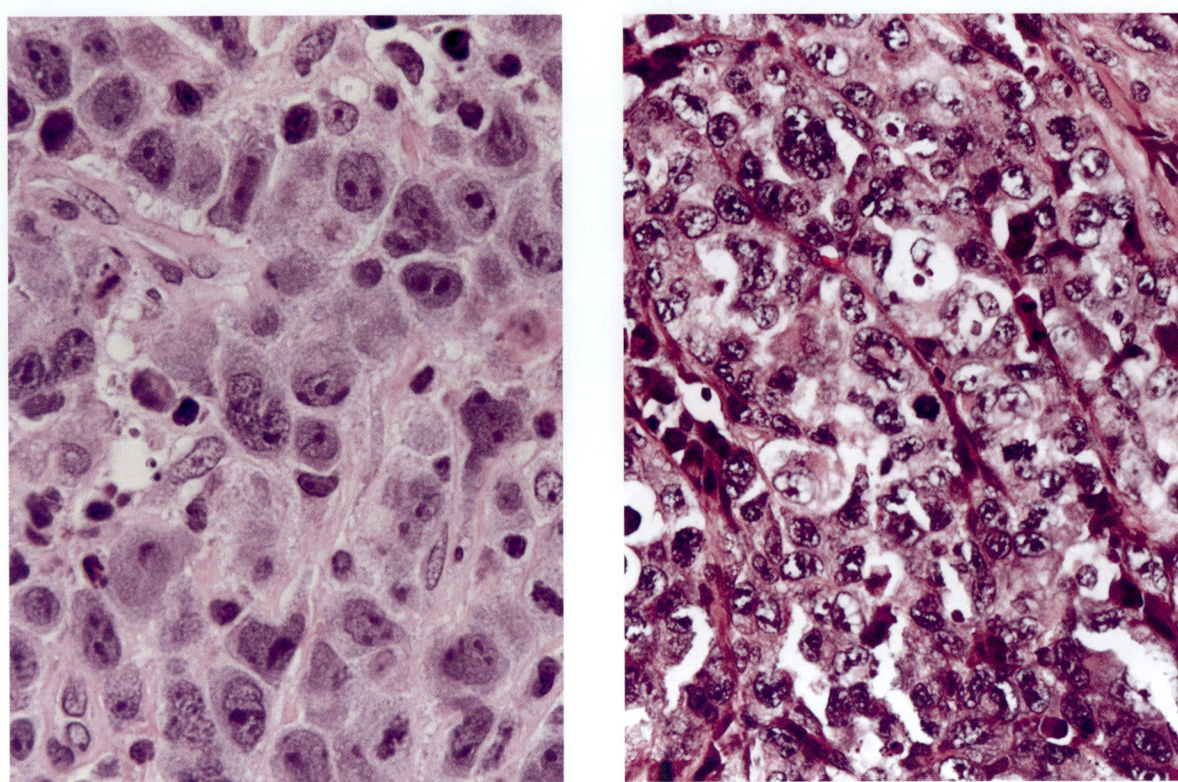

Figure 34-5

ALK-NEGATIVE ANAPLASTIC LARGE CELL LYMPHOMA, COMMON VARIANT

Left: This neoplasm is fairly monomorphous, but a hallmark cell is present in the center of the field (same case as fig. 34-1). Right: In this case, the lymphoma cells are more pleomorphic, with a brisk apoptotic rate (left, right: H&E stain).

Figure 34-6

ALK-NEGATIVE ANAPLASTIC LARGE CELL LYMPHOMA, SARCOMATOID VARIANT

The lymphoma cells are spindled, and initially a sarcoma was suspected. However, the neoplastic cells were shown to be positive for CD30 and T-cell antigens (not shown) (H&E stain)

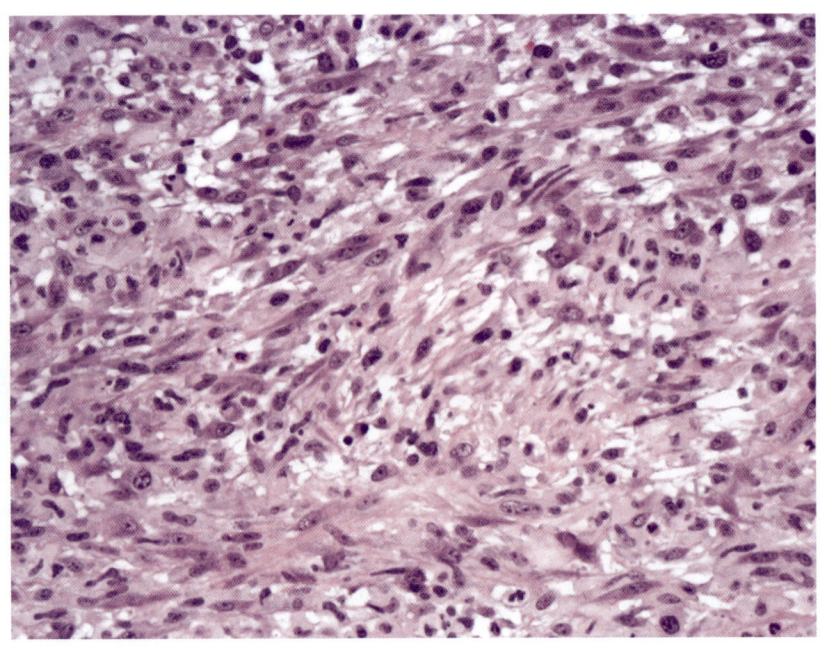

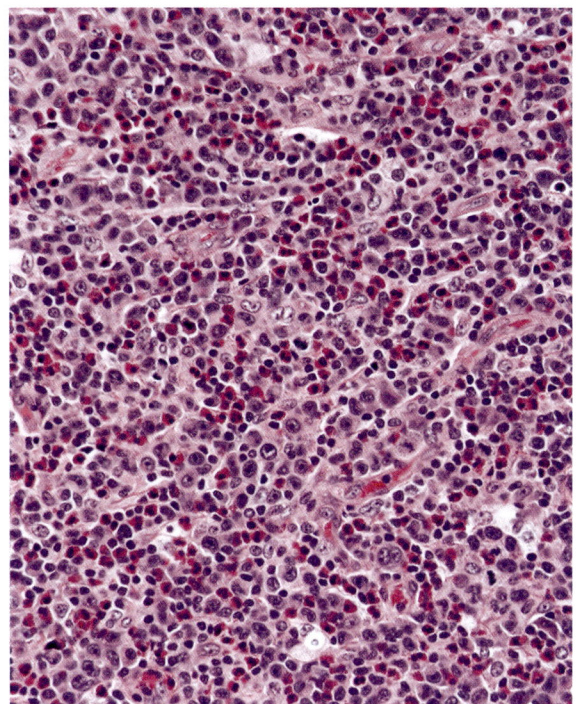

Figure 34-7

ALK-NEGATIVE ANAPLASTIC LARGE CELL LYMPHOMA ASSOCIATED WITH EOSINOPHILS

The lymphoma cells are associated with numerous eosinophils (H&E stain).

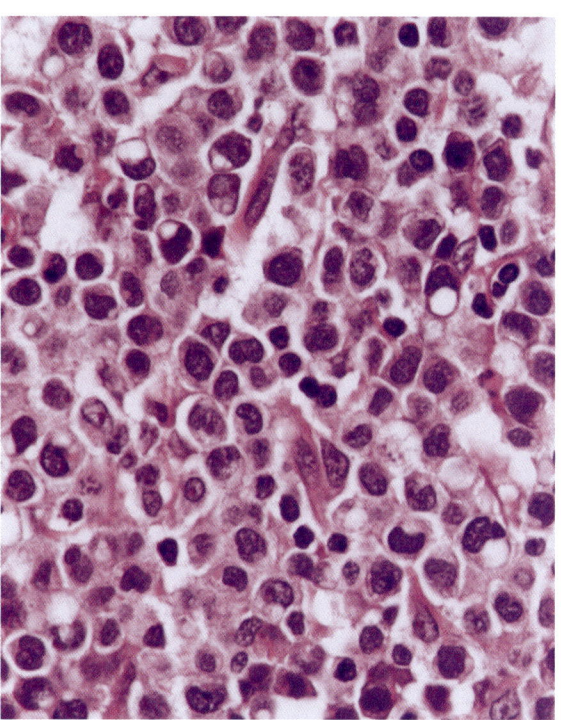

Figure 34-8

ALK-NEGATIVE ANAPLASTIC LARGE CELL WITH SIGNET RING CELLS

Some of the lymphoma cells have vacuolated cytoplasm, imparting a signet ring-like appearance. The lymphoma cells were of T-cell lineage and uniformly positive for CD30 (not shown) (H&E stain).

Table 33-3). By definition, ALK-negative ALCL uniformly and strongly expresses CD30 (fig. 34-3, right; 34-4, right) and is negative for ALK (18,19). Cases that morphologically resemble, more or less, ALK-negative ALCL but weakly, partially, or do not express CD30 are classified as PTCL.

An aberrant T-cell immunophenotype with loss of CD3 (fig. 34-11), CD5, or molecules of the T-cell receptor signaling pathway (e.g., TCRβ and ZAP-70) is common (11,18,33). CD2, CD4, and CD43 are the most frequently expressed T-cell antigens. CD8 is rarely expressed by ALK-negative ALCL (18). Cytotoxic proteins such as TIA-1, granzyme B (fig. 34-12) and perforin are detected commonly in ALK-negative ALCL, but at a lower frequency than observed in ALK-positive ALCL (18,19). One subset of ALK-negative ALCL cases associated with *DUSP22* rearrangement is often negative for cytotoxic proteins (26).

PD-L1 is positive in about two thirds of ALK-negative ALCL (3a). LEMA/MUC1 and clusterin may be expressed, but less commonly

than observed in ALK-positive ALCL (18). BCL2 is expressed in 40 to 50 percent of cases of ALK-negative ALCL, unlike in ALK-positive ALCL, which is usually negative (29). The apoptotic rate in cases of ALK-negative ALCL is usually moderate to high (29). CD45/LCA is often positive but can be negative (fig. 34-13, left) and CD15 (fig. 34-13, right) can be brightly positive in a small subset of cases (18). ALK-negative ALCL is negative for B-cell antigens including CD10, CD19, CD20, CD22, and CD79A. Almost all cases are also negative for PAX5, but rare cases of ALK-negative ALCL with PAX5 immunoreactivity (usually dim) are reported (fig. 34-14) (10). Most cases of ALK-negative ALCL in developed nations are negative for Epstein-Barr virus (EBV) infection (13).

MOLECULAR GENETIC FINDINGS

Conventional cytogenetic analysis of ALK-negative ALCL often shows a complex karyotype, commonly more complex than ALK-positive

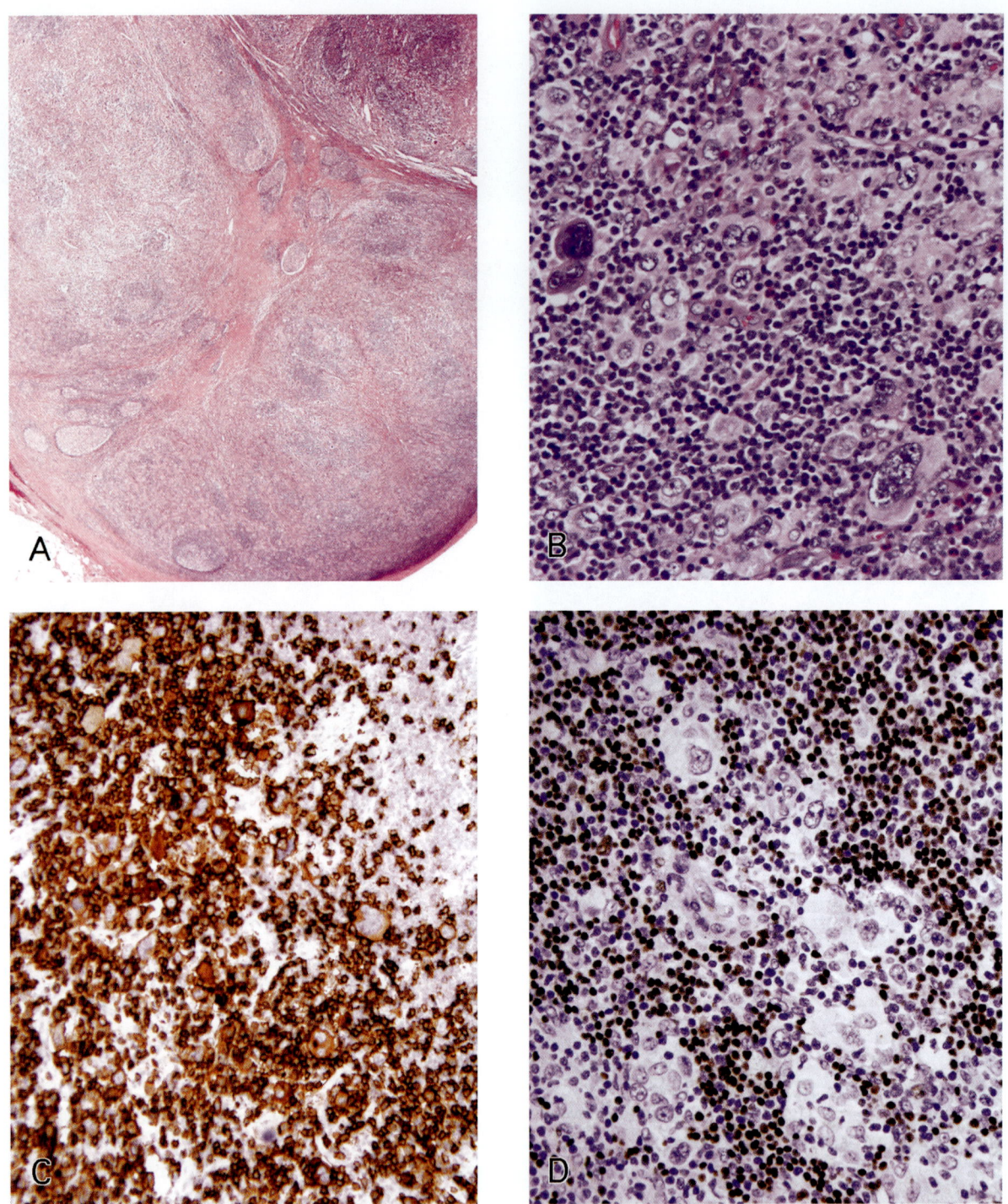

Figure 34-9

ALK-NEGATIVE ANAPLASTIC LARGE CELL LYMPHOMA, HODGKIN-LIKE VARIANT, INVOLVING LYMPH NODE

A: The lymphoma has a nodular appearance at low magnification (A,B: H&E stain).

B: The neoplasm is composed of large pleomorphic lymphoma cells in a background of reactive small lymphocytes, histiocytes, and a few eosinophils.

C,D: The lymphoma cells were positive for CD4 (not shown), CD5 (C), CD30 (not shown), and CD45/LCA (not shown) and were negative for PAX5 (D) and CD20 (not shown) (C,D: immunohistochemistry with hematoxylin counterstain).

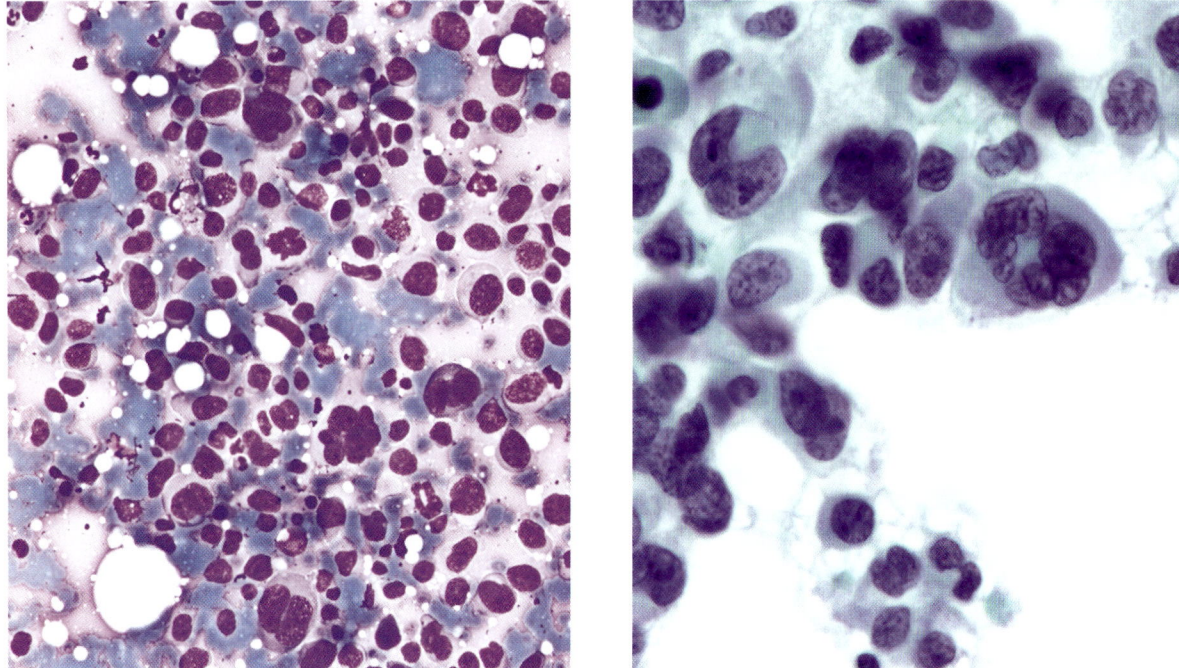

Figure 34-10

ALK-NEGATIVE ANAPLASTIC LARGE CELL LYMPHOMA

Aspirate smears contain pleomorphic mononuclear, binucleated, and multinucleated cells (left: Diff-Quik stain; right: Papanicolaou stain).

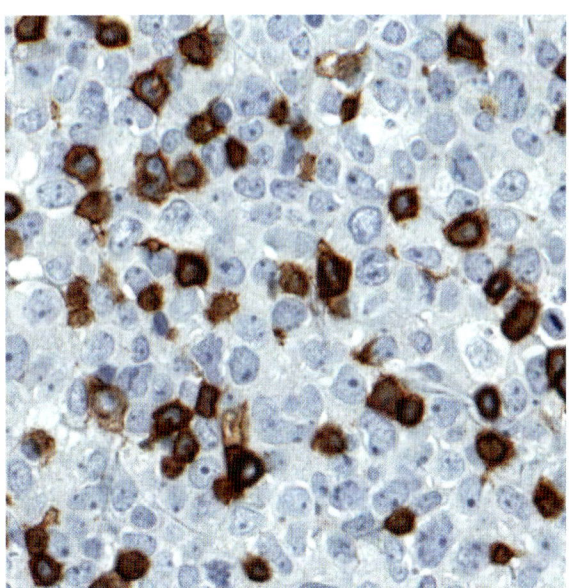

Figure 34-11

ALK-NEGATIVE ANAPLASTIC LARGE CELL LYMPHOMA

The lymphoma cells are negative for CD3. Reactive lymphocytes in the field are positive (immunohisto-chemistry with hematoxylin counterstain).

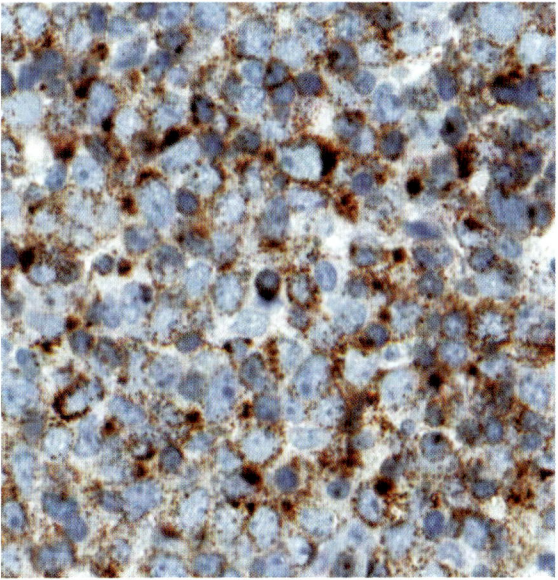

Figure 34-12

ALK-NEGATIVE ANAPLASTIC LARGE CELL LYMPHOMA

The lymphoma cells are positive for granzyme B, supporting a cytotoxic immunophenotype (immuno-histochemistry with hematoxylin counterstain).

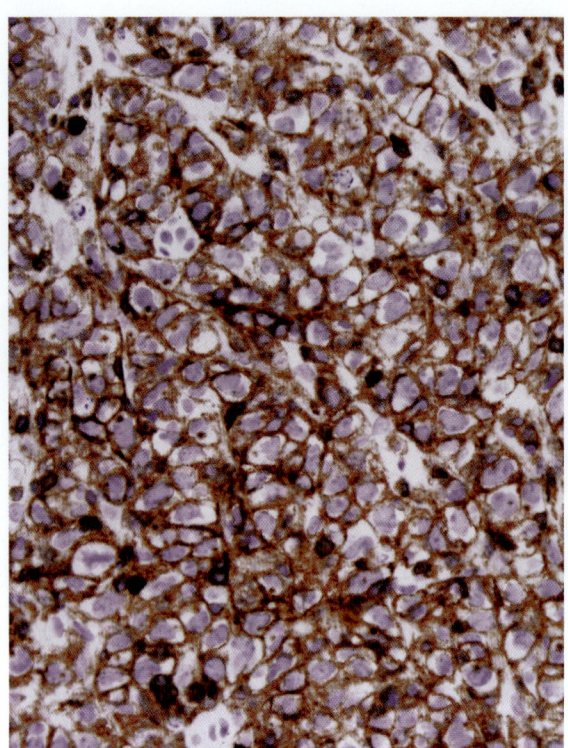 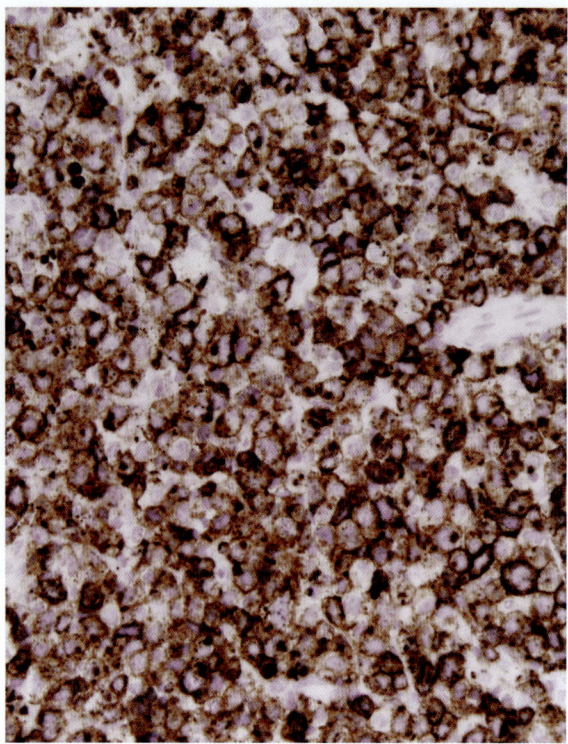

Figure 34-13

ALK-NEGATIVE ANAPLASTIC LARGE CELL LYMPHOMA: IMMUNOHISTOCHEMICAL FEATURES

The cells are positive for CD45/LCA (left) and CD15 (right) (left, right: immunohistochemistry with hematoxylin counterstain). (Same case as shown in figs. 34-1 and 34-5, left.)

ALCL (25). There is no evidence of transloca-tions or other abnormalities involving the chro-mosomal 2p23 locus. The t(6;7)(p25.3;q32.3) has been detected in approximately 20 percent of ALK-negative ALCLs (as well as in primary cutaneous ALCL and lymphomatoid papulosis) (8,26). Some ALK-negative ALCLs have abnor-malities involving chromosome 3q28 (26).

Comparative genomic hybridization reveals chromosomal imbalances in 60 to 70 percent of cases of ALK-negative ALCL. In a study by Salaverria et al. (30), the mean number of genetic abnormalities was 5.4. The most fre-quent alterations included gains of 1q, 5q, 6p, 7p, 7q, 8q, 12q, and 17q and losses of 4q, 6q, 11q, and 13q. There were shared abnormalities with ALK-positive ALCL, but gains of 1q41-qter and 6p21 were significantly more common in ALK-negative cases (30).

Gene expression profiling analysis has shown that ALK-negative ALCLs are enriched for ex-pression of *MYC* and *IRF4* target genes, and have overexpression of signatures for proliferation and the mTOR pathway as compared with PTCL (14,27). A three-gene model of *CD30/TNFRSF8*, *BATF3*, and *TMOD1* distinguishes ALK-nega-tive ALCL from PTCL in most of the cases (1). MicroRNA analysis has shown different profiles of ALK-negative versus ALK-positive ALCL (17,20,21). ALK-negative ALCL has high expres-sion of miR-155, miR-29a, miR-29b-1-5p, and miR-720 (20,21).

Parillar et al. (26) recently divided cases of ALK-negative ALCL (fig. 34-15) into three sub-sets with clinical meaning. About 30 percent of cases (the first subset) harbor recurrent balanced translocations disrupting the *DUSP22* locus on 6p25.3 and adjoining the FRA7H fragile site on 7q32.3 (8,26). *DUSP22* is located within 40 kb of *MUM1/IRF4* and is a dual-specificity phospha-tase that physiologically has a role in inhibiting T-cell receptor signaling and may be a tumor suppressor gene (3). Translocations involving *DUSP22* result in reduced DUSP22 expression;

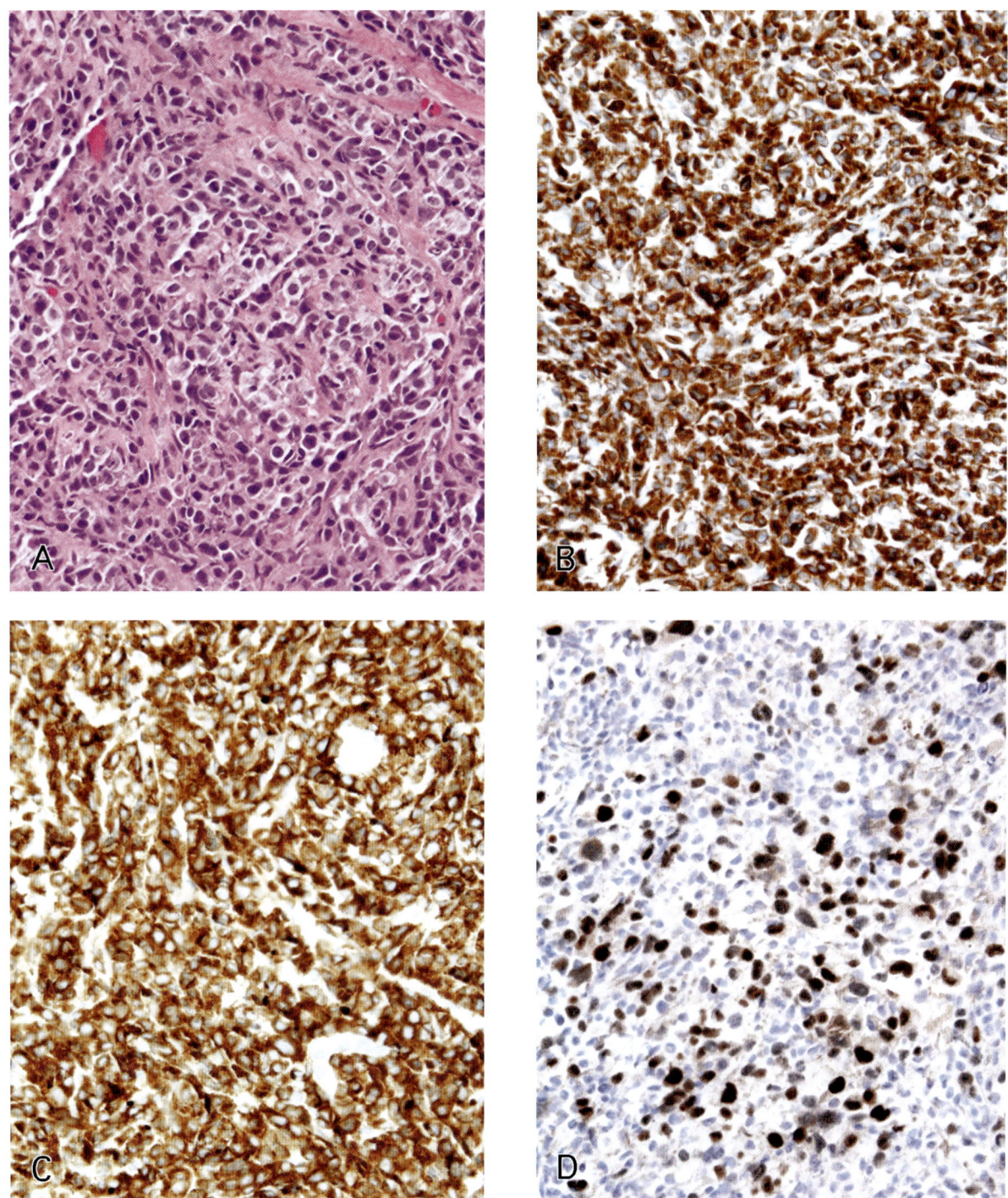

Figure 34-14

ALK-NEGATIVE ANAPLASTIC LARGE CELL LYMPHOMA WITH PAX5 EXPRESSION

This case was unusual because a subset of the lymphoma cells were positive for PAX5.

A: This biopsy specimen was not well prepared or fixed, but the lymphoma cells are large and some cells are consistent with hallmark cells (H&E stain).

B–D: The lymphoma cells are positive for CD3 (B), CD30 (C), and some cells are positive for PAX5 (D). Not shown: CD2 was positive and CD20 was negative (B–D: immunohistochemistry with hematoxylin counterstain).

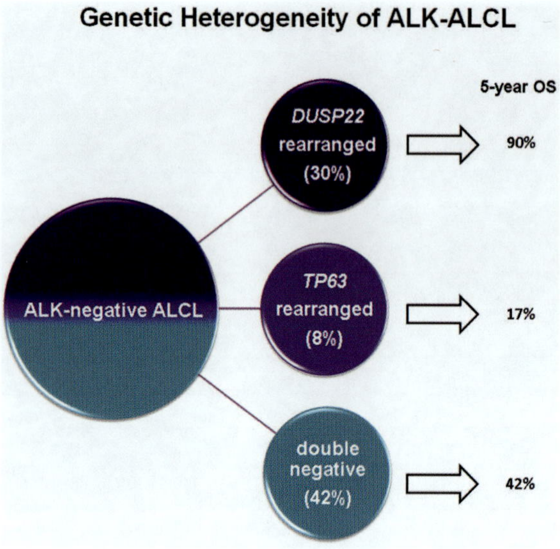

Genetic Heterogeneity of ALK-ALCL

Figure 34-15

GENETIC FINDINGS IN ALK-NEGATIVE ANAPLASTIC LARGE CELL LYMPHOMA

The genetic findings and their reported impact on overall survival are shown. (Data are derived from reference 26; courtesy of Dr. S. Loghavi, Houston, TX.)

these data suggest translocations disrupt the regulatory functions of *DUSP22* (26). Others have suggested that *DUSP22*-rearranged tumors have distinctive morphologic features (see below).

A second subset of ALK-negative ALCL, about 8 percent of cases, is associated with rearrangements of *TP63*, a homologue of *TP53*, located at chromosome on 3q28 (26). Fluorescence in situ hybridization (FISH) studies can be used to identify these chromosomal translocations. The remaining cases of ALK-negative ALCL have neither *DUSP22* or *TP63* translocations.

Scarfo et al. (32) have identified another subset, representing 24 percent of cases of ALK-negative ALCL, associated with aberrant expression of *ERBB4* transcripts. Immunohistochemistry also identifies overexpression of ERBB4 in these tumors, which more often have Hodgkin-like morphologic features (32).

Most cases of ALK-negative ALCL carry monoclonal rearrangements of the T-cell receptor genes and the immunoglobulin genes are in the germline configuration (18,19,33). Next-generation sequencing and other high-throughput molecular methods have shown a high frequency (about 20 percent) of *JAK1* and *STAT3* muta-

tions in ALK-negative ALCLs. These mutations occur singly, but also often occur together to synergistically activate the JAK/STAT pathway (6). Whole transcriptome sequencing identified gene fusions between the transcription factors *NF-κB2* or *NCOR2* with the tyrosine kinases *ROS1* or *TYK2* in another 20 percent of ALK-negative ALCL cases that also activate the JAK/STAT pathway (6,36).

DIFFERENTIAL DIAGNOSIS

ALK-Positive ALCL. Histologically, ALK-positive and ALK-negative ALCL cannot be reliably distinguished. ALK-negative ALCL tends to be more anaplastic, with numerous doughnut-like or wreath-like cells; hallmark cells, although present, are usually less numerous than in ALK-positive ALCL (18,19,33). Both neoplasms frequently have an aberrant T-cell immunophenotype and express CD30 uniformly and strongly in a membranous and paranuclear (target-like) pattern. There are some other, more "soft" differences in immunophenotype. Compared with ALK-positive ALCL, cases of ALK-negative ALCL are less frequently positive for EMA/MUC1 or clusterin and more frequently positive for BCL2, which can be strongly expressed (18,19). CD15 can be uniformly positive in some ALK-negative cases. Although uncommon, PAX5 positivity has been shown in a small subset of ALK-negative ALCLs (10).

The most important and reliable way to distinguish ALK-negative ALCL from ALK-positive ALCL is to assess for ALK by immunohistochemistry, FISH, or other genetic methods. As is self-evident, there is no evidence of ALK expression or ALK translocations in ALK-negative ALCL.

Primary Cutaneous ALCL. Primary cutaneous ALCL presents as localized skin disease, disseminates infrequently, and patients have an excellent prognosis, often treated with only local therapy. Secondary skin involvement by ALK-negative ALCL can be morphologically identical to primary cutaneous ALCL and both neoplasms express CD30 in a uniform and bright fashion. At this time, there are no other immunophenotypic markers that substantially assist in this differential diagnosis.

The clinical history of localized skin disease supports primary cutaneous ALCL and the history of systemic disease makes ALK-negative ALCL more likely. Although rare, ALK expression has been described in primary cutaneous ALCL and this finding would exclude ALK-negative ALCL (24).

Rare primary cutaneous ALCLs are associated with t(6;7)(p25.3;q32.3) involving *DUSP22* at chromosome 6p25.3 (23). These tumors are described as having unusual features in the skin. There is a diffuse dermal component composed of sheets of medium-sized to large cells, often with doughnut-shaped cells. In addition, there is marked epidermotropism with intraepidermal small cells (16,23). The history and staging information are essential to separate primary cutaneous ALCL from ALK-negative ALCL.

Lymphomatoid Papulosis. Some cases of lymphomatoid papulosis (LyP), mostly the so-called type C, closely resemble primary cutaneous ALCL and can mimic ALK-negative ALCL involving the skin. Some of these cases also have *DUSP22*/6p25.3 rearrangements (15). The clinical history is helpful. Patients with LyP tend to have waxing and waning crops of skin lesions that are usually small, with no evidence of systemic disease.

Breast Implant-Associated ALCL. Rarely, patients with breast implants develop anaplastic, CD30-positive and ALK-negative lymphomas in the seroma fluid and capsule around the implant (fig. 34-16). The implants may be placed for either cosmetic or breast reconstruction purposes and the time interval between implant and lymphoma can be many years (fig. 34-17). Although these neoplasms were designated as ALK-negative ALCL in the past, recent studies indicate that they are a distinct entity better designated as breast implant-associated ALCL (22,34).

Overall, most patients with breast implant-associated ALCL have disease confined to seroma fluid or superficial involvement of the capsule, and at this stage patients can be treated by surgical excision alone, resulting in an excellent prognosis (2,22). A few patients have a tumor mass that invades through the capsule and, rarely, spreads to regional lymph nodes. Dissemination is most likely to occur in patients in whom the original tumor is incompletely excised and is allowed to fester for a prolonged time. Usually, the location of the neoplasm and the presence or history of a breast implant is sufficient to alert the pathologist to the correct diagnosis.

CD30-Positive Transformation of Mycosis Fungoides. A small subset of patients with mycosis fungoides develops CD30-positive transformation. In some instances, the transformed cells uniformly and strongly express CD30 and arise in the skin, thereby mimicking primary cutaneous ALCL or ALK-negative ALCL secondarily involving the skin.

Patients with mycosis fungoides usually have a long history of disease as well as multiple skin lesions (7). In some biopsy specimens, there may be foci of epidermotropism or other features of mycosis fungoides at the edge of the transformed tumor that help resolve this differential diagnosis.

Peripheral T-Cell Lymphoma, Not Otherwise Specified. Most cases of PTCL are composed of a mixture of small and large cells. CD30 is negative or a subset of cells variably and weakly express CD30 (fig. 34-18). It is unusual for PTCL to be composed entirely of large anaplastic cells. Even in cases of PTCL that morphologically approximate ALCL, CD30 expression may be weak or partial inconsistent with the diagnosis of ALCL.

However, in cases in which all of the lymphoma cells are strongly CD30 positive, the relative contribution of morphology and immunophenotype toward diagnosis has not been established and the boundaries between ALK-negative ALCL and CD30-positive PTCL are not well defined. For pathologists who believe the morphologic findings are most important, most of the tumor cells need to be anaplastic and include hallmark cells to establish the diagnosis of ALK-negative ALCL. For other pathologists, the presence of strong and uniform CD30 expression allows for the morphologic features to be less perfect. The detection of *DUSP22* rearrangements supports ALK-negative ALCL over PTCL. *TP63* rearrangements have been reported in both ALK-negative ALCL and PTCL (26,35).

Hodgkin Lymphoma. Rare cases of ALK-negative ALCL morphologically simulate nodular sclerosis Hodgkin lymphoma. These tumors show capsular thickening and poorly or well-developed fibrous bands that subdivide the tumor into nodules. Some of the lymphoma cells resemble classic Reed-Sternberg cells and express of CD30 and CD15, also resembling nodular sclerosis Hodgkin lymphoma.

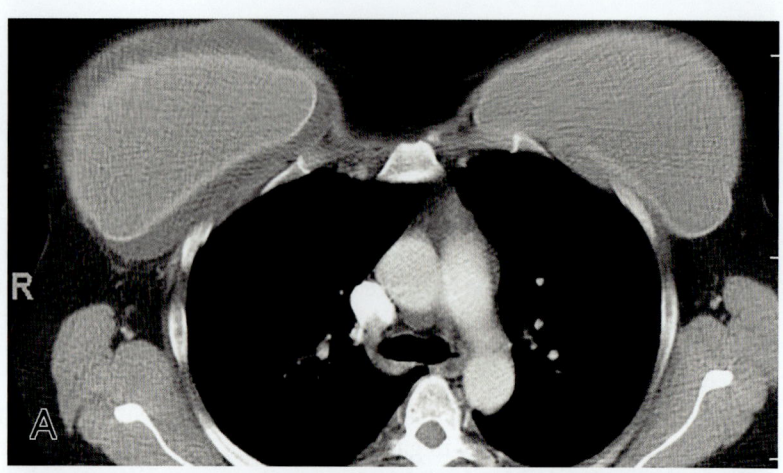

Figure 34-16

BREAST-IMPLANT ASSOCIATED ANAPLASTIC LARGE CELL LYMPHOMA

A: A computerized tomography (CT) scan shows breast implants and seroma fluid surrounding the right (R) implant.

B: Gross image of the fibrous capsule that surrounded the right breast implant.

C: The lymphoma cells line the capsule and are large and anaplastic (H&E stain).

D: The lymphoma cells are uniformly positive for CD30 (immunohistochemistry with hematoxylin counterstain). (A and B courtesy of Dr. R. Miranda, Houston, TX.)

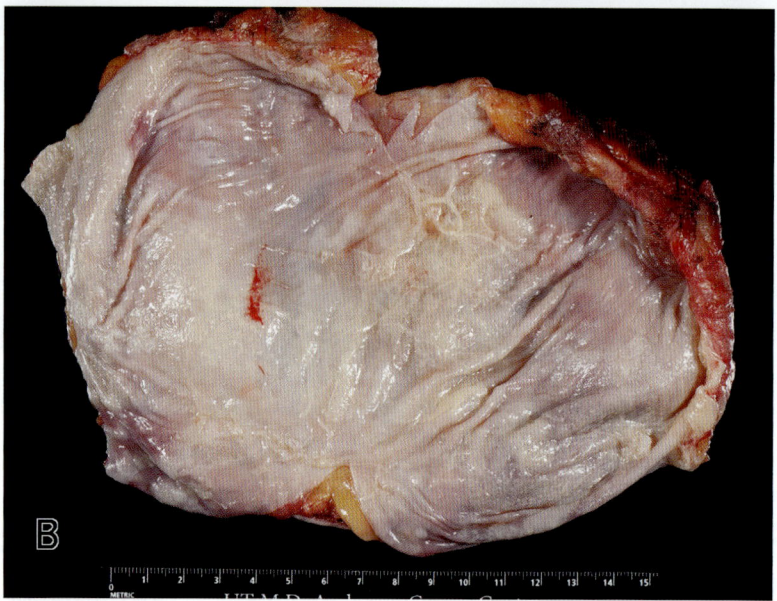

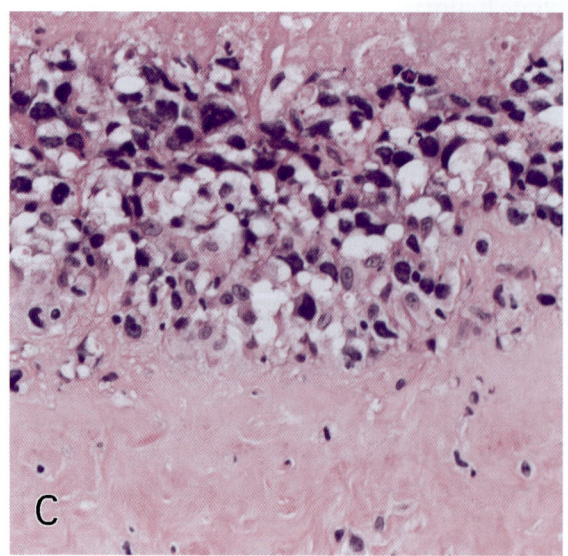

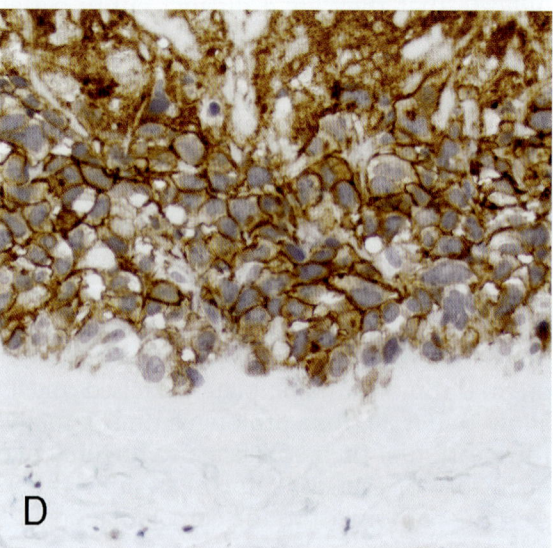

Years Since Diagnosis

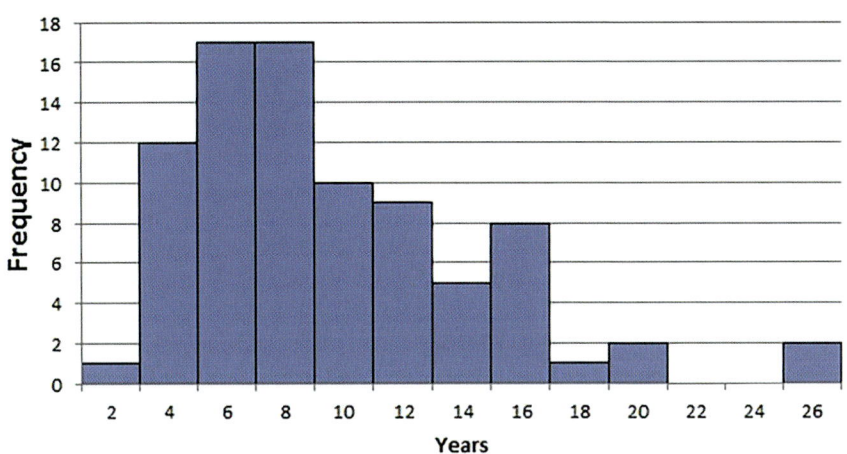

Figure 34-17

BREAST-IMPLANT ASSOCIATED ANAPLASTIC LARGE CELL LYMPHOMA

Histogram showing the time interval from the insertion of the breast implant to the diagnosis of breast implant-associated ALCL. (Courtesy of Dr. R. Miranda, Houston, TX.)

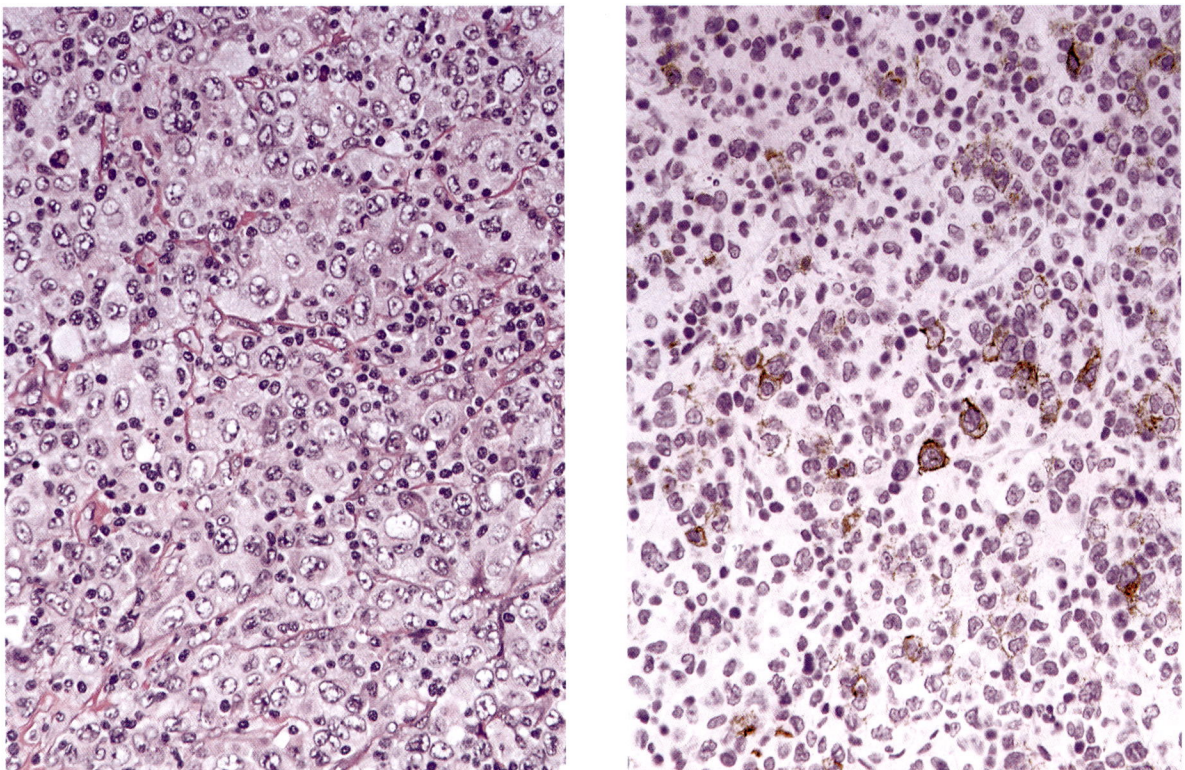

Figure 34-18

PERIPHERAL T-CELL LYMPHOMA, NOT OTHERWISE SPECIFIED

Left: The lymphoma is composed of a spectrum of cell sizes including some large and pleomorphic forms (H&E stain).
Right: CD30 is expressed by a subset of lymphoma cells with low intensity, unlike ALK-negative ALCL (immunohistochemistry with hematoxylin counterstain).

Importantly, in ALK-negative ALCL the lymphoma cells show a spectrum of sizes, from intermediate-size to large, and hallmark cells are present. Immunohistochemical analysis shows that the lymphoma cells are positive for a combination of T-cell antigens (most often CD4 and CD43), CD45/LCA, CD56, clusterin, and EMA/MUC1, and are negative for B-cell antigens. PAX5 is absent in ALK-negative ALCL, with very rare exceptions. The presence of PAX5 and Epstein-Barr virus favors the diagnosis of classic Hodgkin lymphoma. The presence of monoclonal T-cell receptor gene rearrangements supports the diagnosis of ALK-negative ALCL.

Other Hematopoietic Neoplasms. B-cell non-Hodgkin lymphomas may express CD30 and resemble ALK-negative ALCLs, including a subset of diffuse large B-cell lymphomas and the solid variant of primary effusion lymphoma. Both of these tumors may exhibit anaplastic morphologic features and sinusoidal involvement. Detection of B-cell lineage and human herpesvirus 8 (HHV8) in primary effusion lymphoma allows resolution of this differential diagnosis.

Other hematopoietic tumors that may express CD30 include myeloid sarcoma and mast cell neoplasms. Immunophenotypic studies that show expression of myeloid-associated and mast cell-associated markers, respectively, will resolve this issue.

Nonhematopoietic Tumors. Embryonal carcinoma of the testis or in the mediastinum is commonly positive for CD30. Other tumors, such as melanoma and carcinomas, also rarely express CD30. The clinical context and immunohistochemical analysis determine the diagnosis.

TREATMENT AND PROGNOSIS

Most patients with ALK-negative ALCL are treated with anthracycline-based multiagent chemotherapy, most often the regimen of cyclophosphamide, doxorubicin, vincristine, and prednisone (CHOP) (4,12). Brentuximab vedotin, an anti-CD30 drug conjugate, has clinical efficacy in patients with relapsed/refractory ALCL (28) and may be a bridge to stem cell transplant (34a). Brentutimab vedotin when combined with CHOP in the frontline setting is being evaluated in ongoing clinical trials (12). Bortezomib may have value in the treatment of ALK-negative ALCL (5).

Patients with ALK-negative ALCL have a worse prognosis than patients with ALK-positive ALCL, but an outcome superior to that of PTCL patients (31). The 5-year overall survival rate for all patients with ALK-negative ALCL is 40 to 50 percent. The genetic heterogeneity recognized in ALK-negative ALCL also has prognostic relevance. Patients with ALK-negative ALCL associated with a *DUSP22*/6p25.3 rearrangement have a 5-year overall survival rate of 90 percent, similar to or better than patients with ALK-positive ALCL (26). By contrast, patients with *TP63*-rearranged ALK-negative ALCL have a 5-year overall survival rate of 17 percent and patients without either abnormality have an intermediate 5-year overall survival rate of 42 percent (26). These data were confirmed in a larger study by Pedersen et al. (26a).

REFERENCES

1. Agnelli L, Mereu E, Pellegrino E, et al., Identification of a 3-gene model as a powerful diagnostic tool for the recognition of ALK-negative anaplastic large-cell lymphoma. Blood 2012;120:1274-1281.
2. Aladily TN, Medeiros LJ, Amin MB, et al. Anaplastic large cell lymphoma associated with breast implants: a report of 13 cases. Am J Surg Pathol 2012;36:1000-1008.
3. Alonso A, Merlo JJ, Na S, et al. Inhibition of T cell antigen receptor signaling by VHR-related MKPX (VHX), a new dual specificity phosphatase related to VH1 related (VHR). J Biol Chem 2002;277:5524-5528.
3a. Atsaves V, Tsesmetzis N, Chioureas D, et al. PD-L1 is commonly expressed and transcriptionally regulated by STAT3 and MYC in ALK-negative anaplastic large-cell lymphoma. Leukemia 2017;31:1633-1637.
4. Boi M, Zucca E, Inghirami G, Bertoni F. Advances in understanding the pathogenesis of systemic anaplastic large cell lymphoma. Br J Haematol 2015;168:771-783.
5. Cillessen SA, Hijmering NJ, Moesbergen LM, et al. ALK-negative anaplastic large cell lymphoma is sensitive to bortezomib through Noxa upregulation and release of Bax from Bcl-2. Haematologica 2015;100:e365-368.
6. Crescenzo R, Abate F, Lasorsa E, et al. Convergent mutations and kinase fusions lead to oncogenic STAT3 activation in anaplastic large cell lymphoma. Cancer Cell 2015;27:516-532.
7. Fauconneau A, Pham-Ledard A, Cappellen D, et al. Assessment of diagnostic criteria between primary cutaneous anaplastic large-cell lymphoma and CD30-rich transformed mycosis fungoides; a study of 66 cases. Br J Dermatol 2015;172:1547-1554.
8. Feldman AL, Dogan A, Smith DI, et al. Discovery of recurrent t(6;7)(p25.3;q32.3) translocations in ALK-negative anaplastic large cell lymphomas by massively parallel genomic sequencing. Blood 2011;117:915-919.
9. Feldman AL, Grogg KL, Knudson RA, Inwards DJ. Secondary cutaneous involvement by systemic ALK-negative anaplastic large cell lymphoma with 6p25.3 rearrangement. Histopathology 2015;67:932-935.
10. Feldman AL, Law ME, Inwards DJ, Dogan A, McClure RF, Macon WR. PAX5-positive T-cell anaplastic large cell lymphomas associated with extra copies of the PAX5 gene locus. Mod Pathol 2010;23:593-602.
11. Geissinger E, Sadler P, Roth S, et al. Disturbed expression of the T-cell receptor/CD3 complex and associated signaling molecules in CD30+ lymphoproliferations. Haematologica 2010;95:1697-1704.
12. Hapgood G, Savage KJ. The biology and management of systemic anaplastic large cell lymphoma. Blood 2015;126:17-25.
13. Herling M, Rassidakis GZ, Jones D, Schmitt-Graeff A, Sarris AH, Medeiros LJ. Absence of Epstein-Barr virus in anaplastic large cell lymphoma: a study of 64 cases classified according to World Health Organization criteria. Hum Pathol 2004;35:455-459.
14. Iqbal J, Wright G, Wang C, et al. Gene expression signatures delineate biological and prognostic subgroups in peripheral T-cell lymphoma. Blood 2014;123:2915-2923.
15. Karai LJ, Kadin ME, Hsi ED, et al. Chromosomal rearrangements of 6p25.3 define a new subtype of lymphomatoid papulosis. Am J Surg Pathol 2013;37:1173-1181.
16. King RL, Dao LN, McPhail ED, et al. Morphologic features of ALK-negative anaplastic large cell lymphomas with DUSP22 rearrangements. Am J Surg Pathol 2016;40:36-43.
17. Liu C, Iqbal J, Teruya-Feldstein J, et al. MicroRNA expression profiling identifies molecular signatures associated with anaplastic large cell lymphoma. Blood 2013;122:2083-2092.
18. Mason DY, Harris N, Delsol G, et al. Anaplastic large cell lymphoma, ALK-negative. In: Swerdlow SH, Campo E, Harris NL, et al., eds. WHO classification of tumours of haematopoietic and lymphoid tissues. Lyon: IARC Press; 2008;317-319.
19. Medeiros LJ, Elenitoba-Johnson KS. Anaplastic large cell lymphoma. Am J Clin Pathol 2007;127:707-722.
20. Mehrotra M, Medeiros LJ, Luthra R, et al. Identification of putative pathogenic microRNA and its downstream targets in anaplastic lymphoma kinase-negative anaplastic large cell lymphoma. Hum Pathol 2014;45:1995-2005.
21. Merkel O, Hamacher F, Griessl R, et al. Oncogenic role of miR-155 in anaplastic large cell lymphoma lacking the t(2;5) translocation. J Pathol 2015;236:445-456.
22. Miranda RN, Aladily TN, Prince HM, et al. Breast implant-associated anaplastic large-cell lymphoma: long-term follow-up of 60 patients. J Clin Oncol 2014;32:114-120.
23. Onaindia A, Montes-Moreno S, Rodriguez-Pinilla SM, et al. Primary cutaneous anaplastic large cell lymphomas with 6p25.3 rearrangement exhibit particular histological features. Histopathology 2015;66:846-855.

24. Oschlies I, Lisfeld J, Lamant L, et al. ALK-positive anaplastic large cell lymphoma limited to the skin: clinical, histopathological and molecular analysis of 6 pediatric cases. A report from the ALCL99 study. Haematologica 2013;98:50-56.

25. Ott G, Katzenberger T, Siebert R, et al. Chromosomal abnormalities in nodal and extranodal CD30+ anaplastic large cell lymphomas: infrequent detection of the t(2;5) in extranodal lymphomas. Genes Chromosomes Cancer 1998;22:114-121.

26. Parrilla Castellar ER, Jaffe ES, Said JW, et al. ALK-negative anaplastic large cell lymphoma is a genetically heterogeneous disease with widely disparate clinical outcomes. Blood 2014;124:1473-1480.

26a. Pedersen MB, Hamilton-Dutoit SJ, Bendix K, et al. DUSP22 and TP63 rearrangements predict outcome of ALK-negative anaplastic large cell lymphoma: a Danish cohort study. Blood 2017. [Epub ahead of print]

27. Piva R, Agnelli L, Pellegrino E, et al. Gene expression profiling uncovers molecular classifiers for the recognition of anaplastic large-cell lymphoma within peripheral T-cell neoplasms. J Clin Oncol 2010;28:1583-1590.

28. Pro B, Advani R, Brice P, et al. Brentuximab vedotin (SGN-35) in patiens with relpased or refractory systemic anaplastic large-cell lymphoma: results of a phase II study. J Clin Oncol 2012;30:2190-2196

29. Rassidakis GZ, Jones D, Lai R, et al. BCL-2 family proteins in peripheral T-cell lymphomas: correlation with tumour apoptosis and proliferation. J Pathol 2003;200:240-248.

30. Salaverria I, Beà S, Lopez-Guillermo A, et al. Genomic profiling reveals different genetic aberrations in systemic ALK-positive and ALK-negative anaplastic large cell lymphomas. Br J Haematol 2008;140:516-526.

31. Savage KJ, Harris NL, Vose JM, et al. ALK- anaplastic large-cell lymphoma is clinically and immunophenotypically different from both ALK+ ALCL and peripheral T-cell lymphoma, not otherwise specified: report from the International Peripheral T-Cell Lymphoma Project. Blood 2008;111:5496-5504.

32. Scarfo I, Pellegrino E, Mereu E, et al. Identification of a new subclass of ALK-negative ALCL expressing aberrant levels of ERBB4 transcripts. Blood 2016;127:221-232.

33. Stein H, Foss HD, Durkop H, et al. CD30(+) anaplastic large cell lymphoma: a review of its histopathologic, genetic, and clinical features. Blood 2000;96:3681-3695.

33a. Swerdlow SH, Campo E, Pileri SA, et al. The 2016 revision of the World Health Organization classification of lymphoid neoplasms. Blood 2016;127:2375-2390.

34. Thompson PA, Lade S, Webster H, Ryan G, Prince HM. Effusion-associated anaplastic large cell lymphoma of the breast: time for it to be defined as a distinct clinico-pathological entity. Haematologica 2010;95;1977-1979.

34a. Turner SD, Lamant L, Kenner L, Brugières L. Anaplastic large cell lymphoma in paediatric and young adult patients. Br J Haematol 2016;173:560-572.

35. Vasmatzis G, Johnson SH, Knudson RA, et al. Genome-wide analysis reveals recurrent structural abnormalities of TP63 and other p53-related genes in peripheral T-cell lymphomas. Blood 2012;120:2280-2289.

36. Velusamy T, Kiel MJ, Sahasrabuddhe AA, et al. A novel recurrent NPM1-TYK2 gene fusion in cutaneous CD30-positive lymphoproliferative disorders. Blood 2014;124:3768-3771.

37. Vose J, Armitage J, Weisenburger D, International T-Cell Lymphoma Project. International peripheral T-cell and natural killer/T-cell lymphoma study: pathology findings and clinical outcomes. J Clin Oncol 2008;26:4124-4130.

35 EXTRANODAL NK/T-CELL LYMPHOMA, NASAL TYPE

GENERAL FEATURES

Extranodal NK/T-cell lymphoma of nasal type is a lymphoma of natural killer (NK) or, less often, T-cell lineage with a cytotoxic phenotype associated consistently with Epstein-Barr virus (EBV) infection. The nasal cavity is the most common site of involvement but other so-called extranasal anatomic sites can be involved. Therefore the qualifier "nasal type" is applied to this neoplasm in the current World Health Organization (WHO) classification (3,34).

NK cells exhibit non-major histocompatibility complex (MHC)-restricted antibody-independent cytotoxicity. Cytotoxicity is mediated by the FAS-FAS ligand system and cytoplasmic cytotoxic molecules include perforin, T-cell-restricted intracellular antigen1 (TIA-1), and granzyme B. NK cells express killer immunoglobulin-like receptors and CD94/NKG2, which are important in distinguishing non-host (e.g., infectious organisms) from host (self) antigens. NK cells do not express a functional surface T-cell receptor or rearrange their T-cell receptor genes, but otherwise share some immunophenotypic features with cytotoxic T cells. This is likely explained by origin from a common precursor cell with the potential to differentiate into NK or T cells (20).

Extranodal NK/T-cell lymphoma, nasal type, is a disease that has been known by a number of other terms over the years including lethal midline granuloma, polymorphic reticulosis, malignant midline reticulosis, and angiocentric lymphoma (3). The term lethal midline granuloma still has value and is best considered a clinical term for a midline destructive lesion attributable to a number of etiologies including infections and tumors. The other terms, direct synonyms for extranodal NK/T-cell lymphoma of nasal type, are obsolete.

Extranodal NK/T-cell lymphoma, nasal type, shows pronounced ethnic and geographic predilections (3,24,38). The tumor is most common in Asians and Central and South Americans of Native American heritage. It represents 5 to 6 percent of all cases of non-Hodgkin lymphoma in these patient populations (3,24). By comparison, these tumors represent about 1 percent of all non-Hodgkin lymphomas in North America and Western Europe (3,24,38). Restricting this comparison to NK- and T-cell lymphomas, extranodal NK/T-cell lymphoma, nasal type represents approximately 22 percent of all tumors in Asia compared with about 5 percent in North America and Europe (3). In certain parts of Southeastern Asia, such as Hong Kong, extranodal NK/T-cell lymphoma, nasal type represents almost half of all NK- or T-cell lymphomas.

EBV infection likely plays an important role in the etiology/pathogenesis of extranodal NK/T-cell lymphoma of nasal type. Originally described by Harabuchi et al. (7) in 1990, viral infection occurs in virtually 100 percent of cases. The virus is present within the lymphoma cells in monoclonal episomal form, implying the presence of virus before neoplastic transformation (3,28,29). Host genetic predisposition, environmental exposure (e.g., diet), and tumor-associated genetic abnormalities are also involved in etiology/pathogenesis. Rare cases also have been reported in organ transplant recipients, suggesting that immunosuppression may play a role in pathogenesis (3).

CLINICAL FEATURES

Extranodal NK/T-cell lymphoma of nasal type occurs most often in adults with a median age in the sixth decade (3,24). The male to female ratio is about 2 to 1. In 70 to 75 percent of all patients, the tumor arises in midline upper aerodigestive tract structures, usually the nasal cavity and nasopharynx. The tumor often locally invades contiguous structures, such as the orbit, paranasal sinuses, palate, oropharynx, and oral cavity. Invasion of bone, best observed by radiologic imaging studies, is common (3,17,24). Based on the extent of local invasion, patients can present with nasal obstruction, epistaxis, palatal destruction, orbital swelling, and edema. Systemic symptoms, including fever and weight loss, are present in some patients. About 75 percent present with localized disease, stage I or II. Regional lymphadenopathy, most often in the cervical region, occurs in about 20 percent of patients (23,24).

Staging bone marrow specimens show involvement in 5 to 10 percent of patients. Rarely, patients present initially with bone marrow disease. Serum lactate dehydrogenase (LDH) levels can be high. More than half of patients present with a low-risk International Prognostic Index (IPI) score and less than 5 percent present with a high IPI score (24,38). Patients with extranodal NK/T-cell lymphoma, nasal type, can develop a hemophagocytic syndrome (36).

Extranasal (non-nasal) sites are involved in 25 to 30 percent of patients. The most common extranasal sites include skin, soft tissue, gastrointestinal tract, kidneys, and testis. There are some epidemiologic and clinical differences between nasal and primary extranasal cases. Extranasal NK/T-cell lymphoma occurs in younger adults with a median age of 44 years, and a male predominance (3,23,24,38). About two thirds of patients with extranasal NK/T-cell lymphoma have stage III or IV disease and bone marrow involvement is more common (about 20 percent of patients). Approximately 20 percent of patients have a high IPI score. Some patients who present initially with an extranasal site of disease are subsequently shown to have nasal involvement. A small subset of patients develops a leukemic phase of disease.

Aggressive NK-Cell Leukemia/Lymphoma. Rare patients present with a disease involving the peripheral blood and bone marrow that is morphologically and immunophenotypically similar to extranodal NK/T-cell lymphoma of nasal type, although the epidemiologic features differ. *Aggressive NK/T-cell leukemia/lymphoma* occurs much more frequently in Asia (3,13,24). The median age is 39 years and the male to female ratio is approximately equal. Patients present with B-type symptoms, lymphadenopathy, hepatosplenomegaly, and leukemic involvement, and have a clinically aggressive

course that is usually fatal. Some patients respond to stem cell transplantation (13).

The peripheral blood smear shows few to numerous atypical leukemic cells that usually contain cytoplasmic azurophilic granules (4). Tissue sites involved by leukemic cells mimic extranodal NK/T-cell lymphoma at nasal or extranasal sites. The lymphoma cells have an NK-cell immunophenotype [cytoplasmic CD(3+), surface CD3(-), CD56(+), cytotoxic molecules(+)] and may share a common cell of origin (22,25). Cases of aggressive NK-cell leukemia/lymphoma lack monoclonal T-cell receptor gene rearrangements and are usually positive for EBV infection (25).

The relationship between extranodal NK/T-cell lymphoma of nasal type and aggressive NK-cell leukemia/lymphoma is not clear. There is much overlap between these two diseases and they are likely closely related, but the differences in epidemiologic features suggest these diseases are not one entity. Some patients with aggressive NK-cell leukemia/lymphoma have been shown by staging workup to have nasal disease, suggesting that this subset of patients has a nasal-type NK-cell lymphoma in leukemic phase (25).

HISTOLOGIC FINDINGS

Lymph Node

In regional lymph nodes the architecture is usually diffusely replaced or partially effaced by lymphoma in a predominantly paracortical distribution. Areas of coagulative necrosis within the lymph node (fig. 35-1), which can be extensive, are common. The perinodal adipose tissue may be involved by lymphoma and the tumor may show an angiocentric growth pattern. Mitotic figures and apoptotic cells are usually present and may be numerous.

The cellular composition of NK/T-cell lymphoma, nasal type in lymph nodes is highly variable and usually correlates with the primary neoplasm. The tumor can be composed mostly of small, intermediate/medium-sized, or large cells, or a mixture of cell sizes (figs. 35-2, 35-3). Binucleated and multinucleated large cells are frequently seen. Occasionally, the large cells are anaplastic, with horseshoe-shaped nuclei (simulating anaplastic large cell lymphoma). The background cellular infiltrate is usually composed of small lymphocytes, histiocytes, and occasional plasma cells. Granulocytes and particularly eosinophils are uncommon.

Nasal Region/Upper Aerodigestive Tract

Extranodal NK/T-cell lymphoma of nasal type involving the nasal and other regions in the upper aerodigestive tract has a diffuse pattern and is almost always associated with coagulative necrosis, ranging from focal to extensive (fig. 35-4) (3,6,23). An angiocentric and angiodestructive growth pattern is seen in about two thirds of cases (fig. 35-5) (23). Even in cases in which blood vessels lack infiltration by lymphoma cells, the blood vessels often show fibrinoid necrosis, fragmentation of the elastic lamina, and thrombosis possibly related to damage by cytotoxic molecules (3). When the tumor cells infiltrate minor salivary glands, the glandular epithelium can show partially cleared out cytoplasm (fig. 35-6).

Extranodal NK/T-cell lymphomas of nasal type have a wide cytologic spectrum (fig. 35-7) (3,6,23). Most cases are composed of a mixture of intermediate-sized and large atypical cells in variable percentages. Nevertheless, 5 to 10 percent of tumors are composed predominantly of small cells with a deceptively low-grade appearance (fig. 35-7A). These small cell tumors, referred to as the small cell variant in some reports, infrequently show angiodestruction or extensive necrosis and the mitotic rate can be low. Other cases are composed predominantly of large cells and rarely, anaplastic cells (so-called anaplastic variant). The lymphoma cells can be elongated with folded or angulated nuclei, and the nickname "cucumber cells" has been used in the literature (fig. 35-7B). A correlation between the number of large cells and poorer prognosis has been reported (38). In touch imprints of these lesions, the lymphoma cells may exhibit azurophilic cytoplasmic granules (fig. 35-8).

Extranodal NK/T-cell lymphoma of nasal type may be difficult to recognize as a lymphoma, particularly in tumors composed of small or intermediate-sized cells. As these tumors in the nasal region are commonly associated with ulcer, superficial areas may have many granulocytes and plasma cells, making the diagnosis challenging, particularly in small biopsy specimens. When extranodal NK/T-cell lymphoma of nasal type involves the overlying mucosa, it can

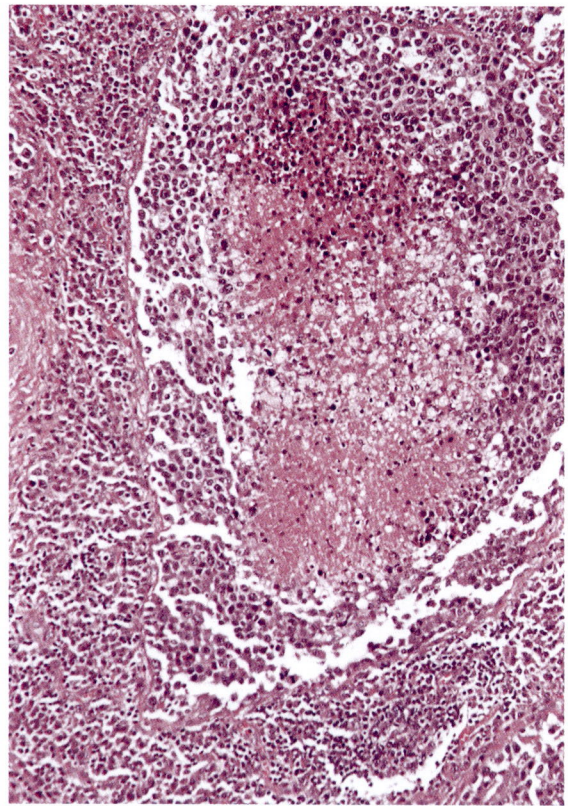

Figure 35-1

EXTRANODAL NK/T-CELL LYMPHOMA, NASAL TYPE, INVOLVING LYMPH NODE

The lymph node shows prominent areas of coagulative necrosis (hematoxylin and eosin [H&E] stain).

induce hyperplasia of epithelial cells (so-called pseudoepitheliomatous hyperplasia), which may be misinterpreted as squamous cell carcinoma.

Extranasal Sites

The morphologic findings of nasal-type NK/T-cell lymphoma at extranasal sites resemble those of tumors in the nasal region (figs. 35-9–35-11). There are some site-specific findings. In the skin, the infiltrate surrounds blood vessels in the dermis and may be associated with hemorrhage, mimicking vasculitis (3,23). The infiltrate in the subcutaneous tissue can surround adipocytes, mimicking panniculitis. In the gastrointestinal tract, the lymphoma infiltrate can be associated with transmural necrosis and perforation may occur. In soft tissues, extranodal NK/T-cell lymphoma can be associated with marked destruction of skeletal muscle.

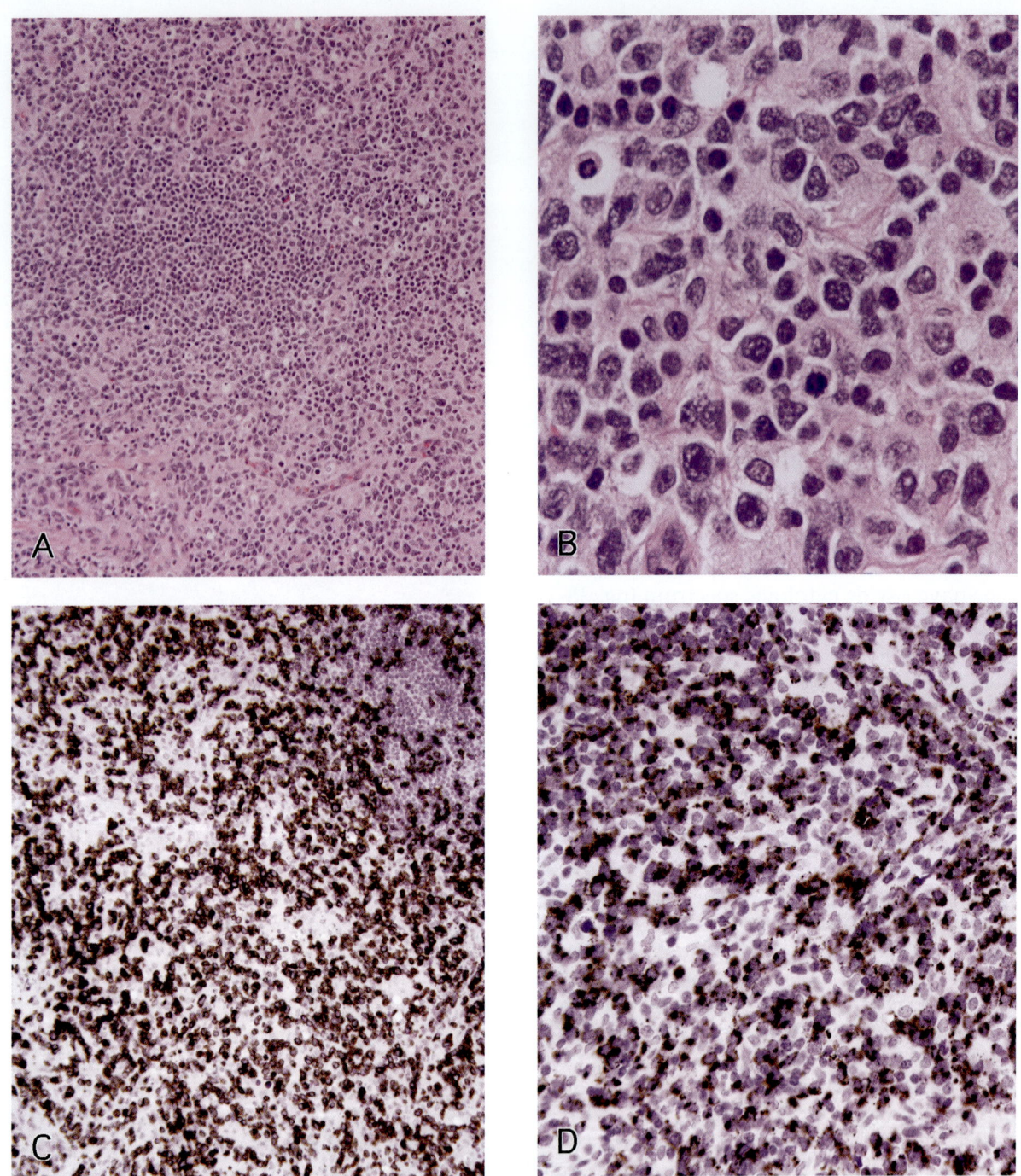

Figure 35-2

EXTRANODAL NK/T-CELL LYMPHOMA, NASAL TYPE, INVOLVING LYMPH NODE

This patient presented initially with lymphadenopathy and the biopsy specimen showed involvement by NK/T-cell lymphoma, nasal type. Nasopharyngeal disease was identified subsequently.

A: The lymphoma replaces most of the lymph node parenchyma, but small residual benign areas (center) are present.

B: There is a mixture of small and large lymphoma cells.

C,D: The lymphoma cells have a cytotoxic NK-cell immunophenotype positive for cytoplasmic CD3 (C), and granzyme B (D). This tumor was also positive for CD56 (not shown) and Epstein-Barr virus (EBV) encoded RNA1 (EBER1) and negative for surface CD3 and CD8 (not shown) (A,B: H&E stain; C,D: immunohistochemistry with hematoxylin counterstain).

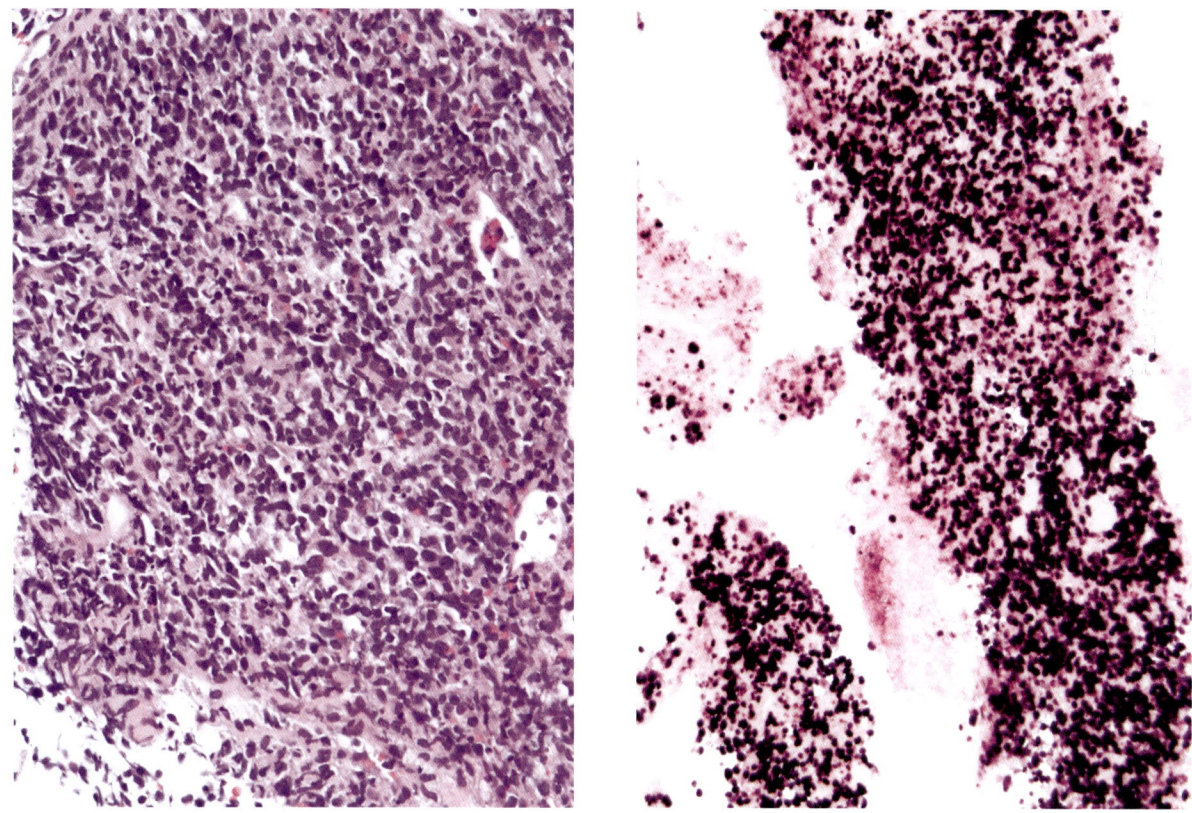

Figure 35-3

EXTRANODAL NK/T-CELL LYMPHOMA, NASAL TYPE, INVOLVING LYMPH NODE

Needle core biopsy specimen of a cervical lymph node in a patient who had known nasal disease.

Left: The lymphoma cells are mostly small but there is distortion and crush of the cytologic features, most likely attributable to artifact associated with using a small gauge needle. Apoptotic cells are seen (H&E stain).

Right: In situ hybridization for EBER1 shows that virtually all cells are positive (in situ hybridization with eosin counterstain).

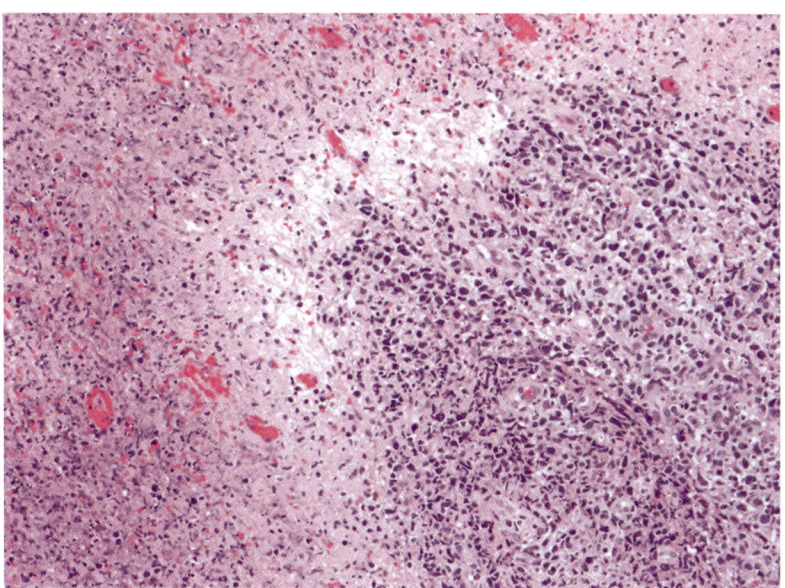

Figure 35-4

EXTRANODAL NK/T-CELL LYMPHOMA, NASAL TYPE, INVOLVING NASOPHARYNX

The patient presented with a mass involving the nasopharynx. Large areas of coagulative necrosis are present in this biopsy specimen. Necrosis is very common in these tumors and may be attributable to vascular occlusion or release of cytotoxic proteins from the lymphoma cells (H&E stain).

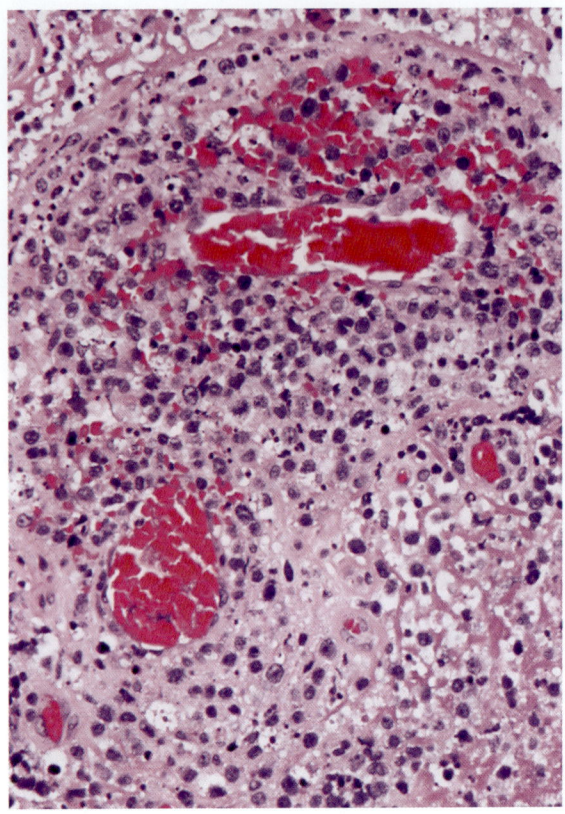

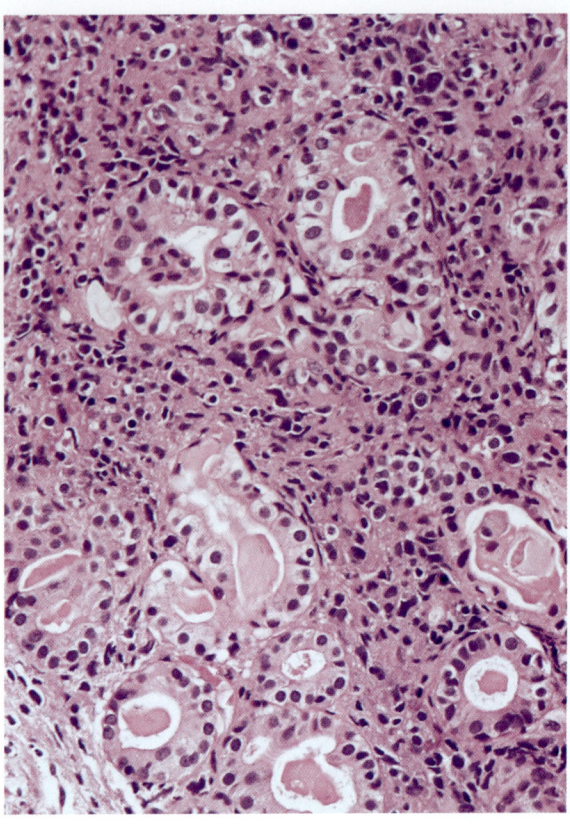

Figure 35-5

EXTRANODAL NK/T-CELL LYMPHOMA, NASAL TYPE

An angiocentric growth pattern, which is often angiodestructive, is present. Highly atypical lymphoma cells surround blood vessels; abundant coagulative necrosis is also present (H&E stain).

Figure 35-6

EXTRANODAL NK/T-CELL LYMPHOMA, NASAL TYPE, INVOLVING PARANASAL SINUS

The neoplastic cells infiltrate between benign glands that show epithelial cells with clear cytoplasmic changes. These changes are common in biopsy specimens of mucosal tissues involved by these tumors (H&E stain).

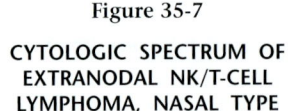

Figure 35-7

CYTOLOGIC SPECTRUM OF EXTRANODAL NK/T-CELL LYMPHOMA, NASAL TYPE

A: The neoplasm is composed of small cells with pale or clear cytoplasm.

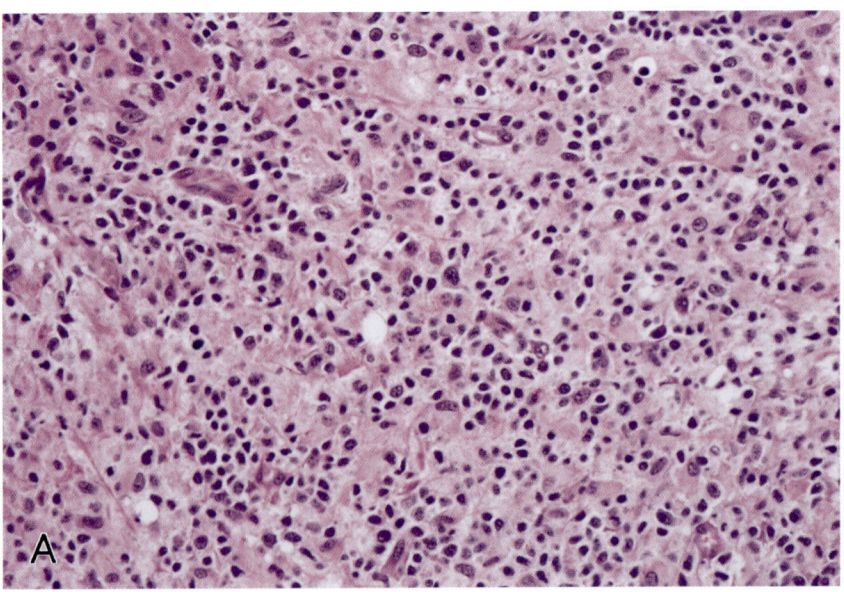

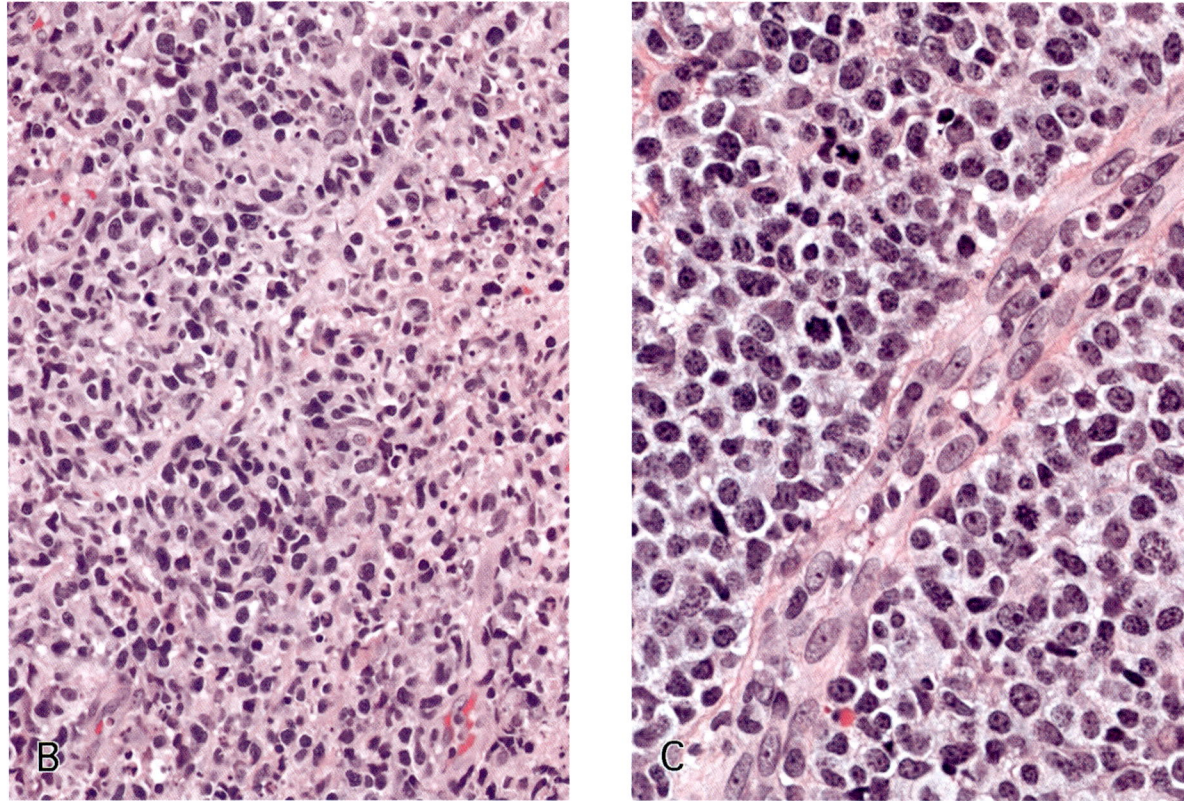

Figure 35-7, continued

B: There is a mixture of small and large cells. Some of the cells have elongated nuclei and have been designated as "cucumber cells."

C: This tumor is composed mostly of large cells. Mitotic figures are easily identified (A–C: H&E stain).

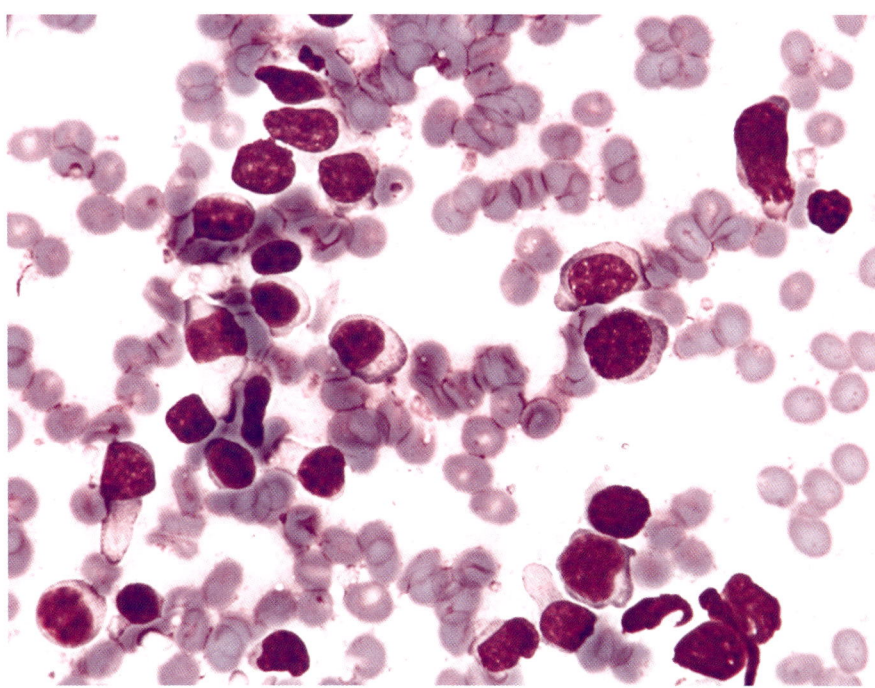

Figure 35-8

TOUCH IMPRINT OF EXTRANODAL NK/T-CELL LYMPHOMA, NASAL TYPE

The lymphoma cells have moderate amounts of cytoplasm. Some cells have cytoplasm with fine azurophilic granules (Wright-Giemsa stain).

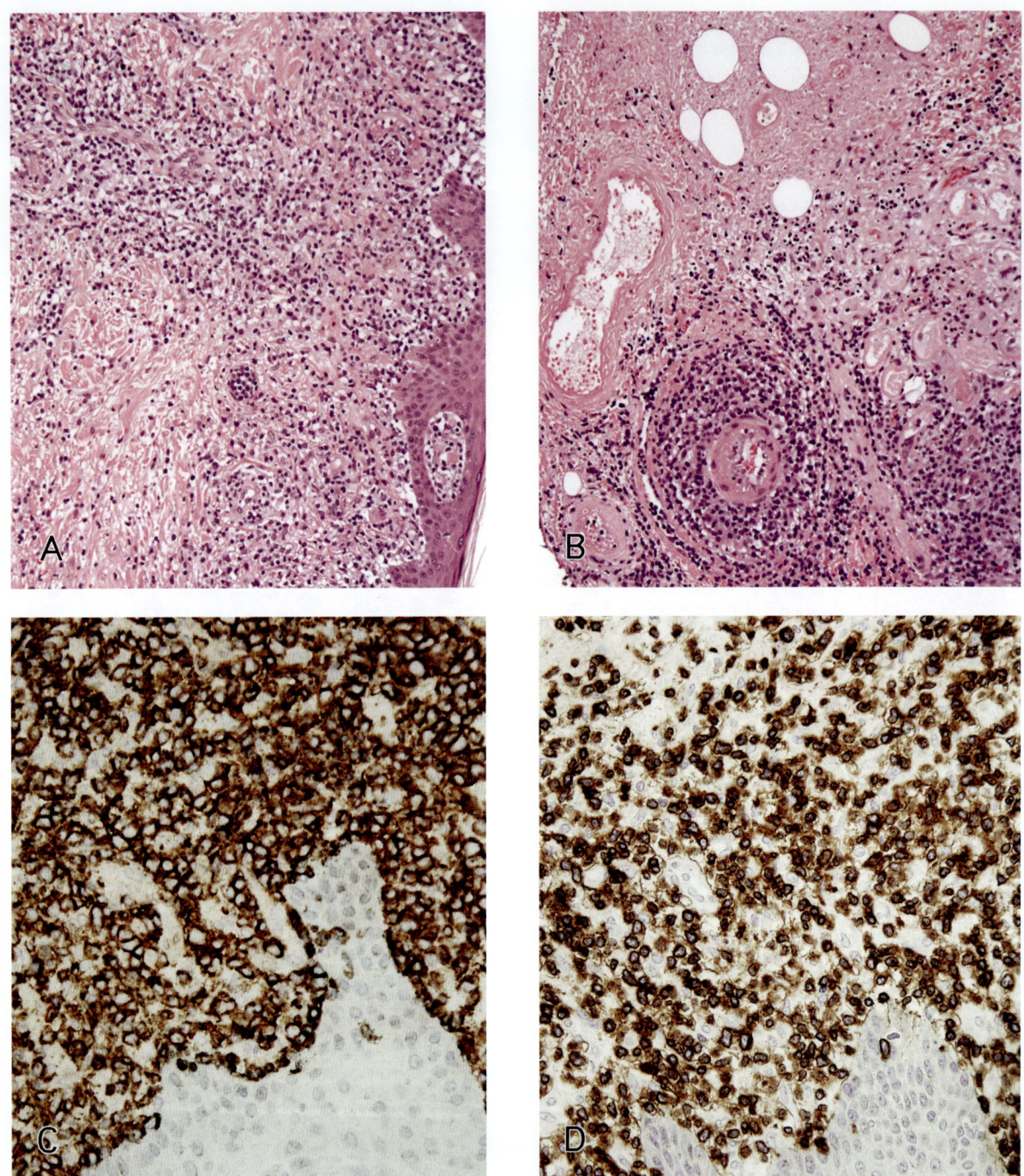

Figure 35-9

EXTRANODAL NK/T-CELL LYMPHOMA, NASAL TYPE, INVOLVING SKIN

This patient initially presented with skin lesions. The lymphoma cells had a T-cell immunophenotype as is common in extranasal lesions.

A: The lymphoma cells are mostly small and located in the superficial and deep dermis (A,B: H&E stain).

B: In the deeper dermis and subcutaneous tissue, the tumor has an angiocentric growth pattern and is associated with coagulative necrosis.

C,D: The lymphoma cells are positive for CD8 (C) and βF1 (D). The lymphoma cells were also positive for cytotoxic markers and EBER1 and were negative for CD56 (not shown) (C,D: immunohistochemistry with hematoxylin counterstain).

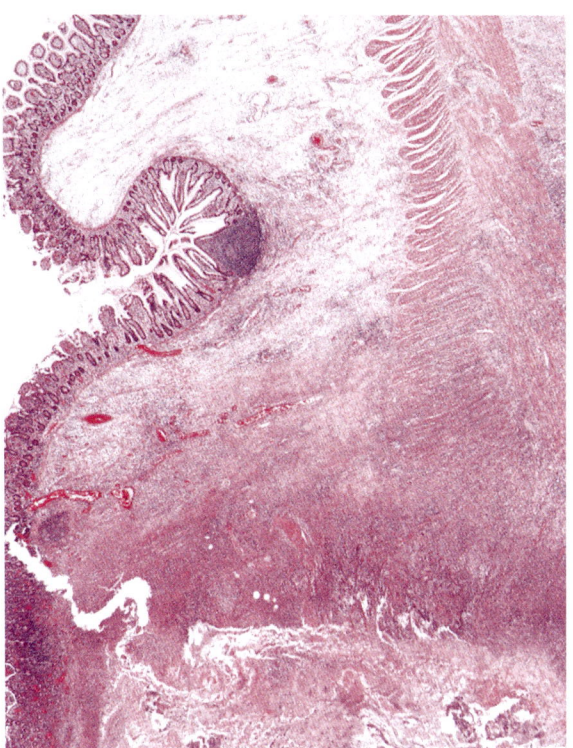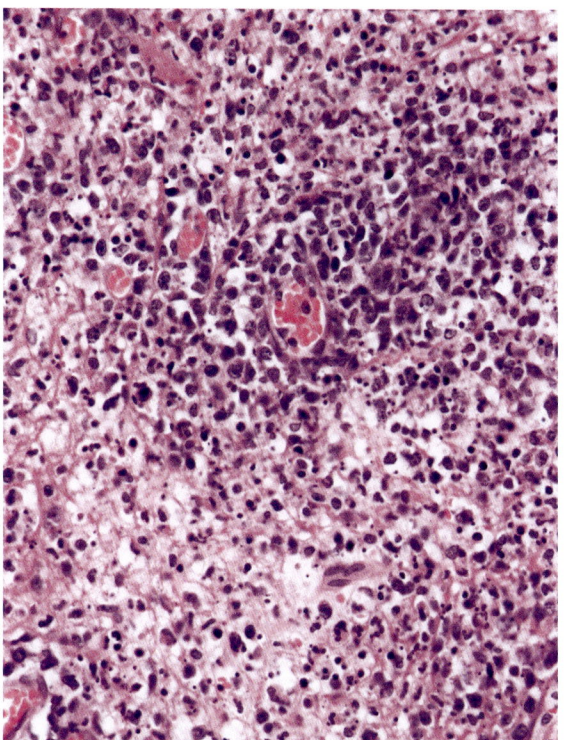

Figure 35-10

EXTRANODAL NK/T-CELL LYMPHOMA, NASAL TYPE, INVOLVING SMALL INTESTINE

This patient presented with small intestinal obstruction and excision showed extranodal NK/T-cell lymphoma of nasal type. The tumor had an NK-cell immunophenotype.

Left: The transition from normal small intestine to a large tumor (bottom of field) is shown, with necrosis replacing much of the intestinal wall.

Right: High magnification of the tumor shows an angiocentric pattern, tumor cell apoptosis, and coagulative necrosis (left, right: H&E stain).

Staging bone marrow specimens may be extensively involved by extranodal NK/T-cell lymphoma of nasal type, but more often the findings are subtle. The infiltrate can be composed of mostly small cells in an interstitial pattern, without the formation of aggregates or focal replacement of the medullary space (fig. 35-12). In aspirate smears, the lymphoma cells may have cytoplasmic azurophilic granules.

CYTOLOGIC FINDINGS

Tumors involving the nasal region rarely undergo fine-needle aspiration and therefore the cytologic findings are biased toward extranasal tumors (fig. 35-13). The cytologic spectrum of extranasal tumors is broad. The neoplastic cells show a spectrum of cell sizes: small, medium-sized, or large. The cells show irregular nuclei with mature to vesicular chromatin. The cytoplasm is scant to moderate and may contain small granules. The nucleoli are typically inconspicuous or small. Mitotic figures, karyorrhectic debris, fibrinoid exudate, and blood are commonly observed. In Giemsa-stained touch preparations, azurophilic cytoplasmic granules are often present. Two reports in the literature have described highly unusual cytologic features in nasal type NK/T-cell lymphoma. These include lymphoma cells in cellular aggregates with occasional spindled tumor cells and absence of lymphoglandular bodies (16,39).

IMMUNOPHENOTYPIC FINDINGS

Flow cytometry immunophenotypic analysis can be performed on NK/T-cell lymphomas, nasal type, but due to the small size of the biopsy specimens and extensive necrosis immunohistochemistry is more often used for

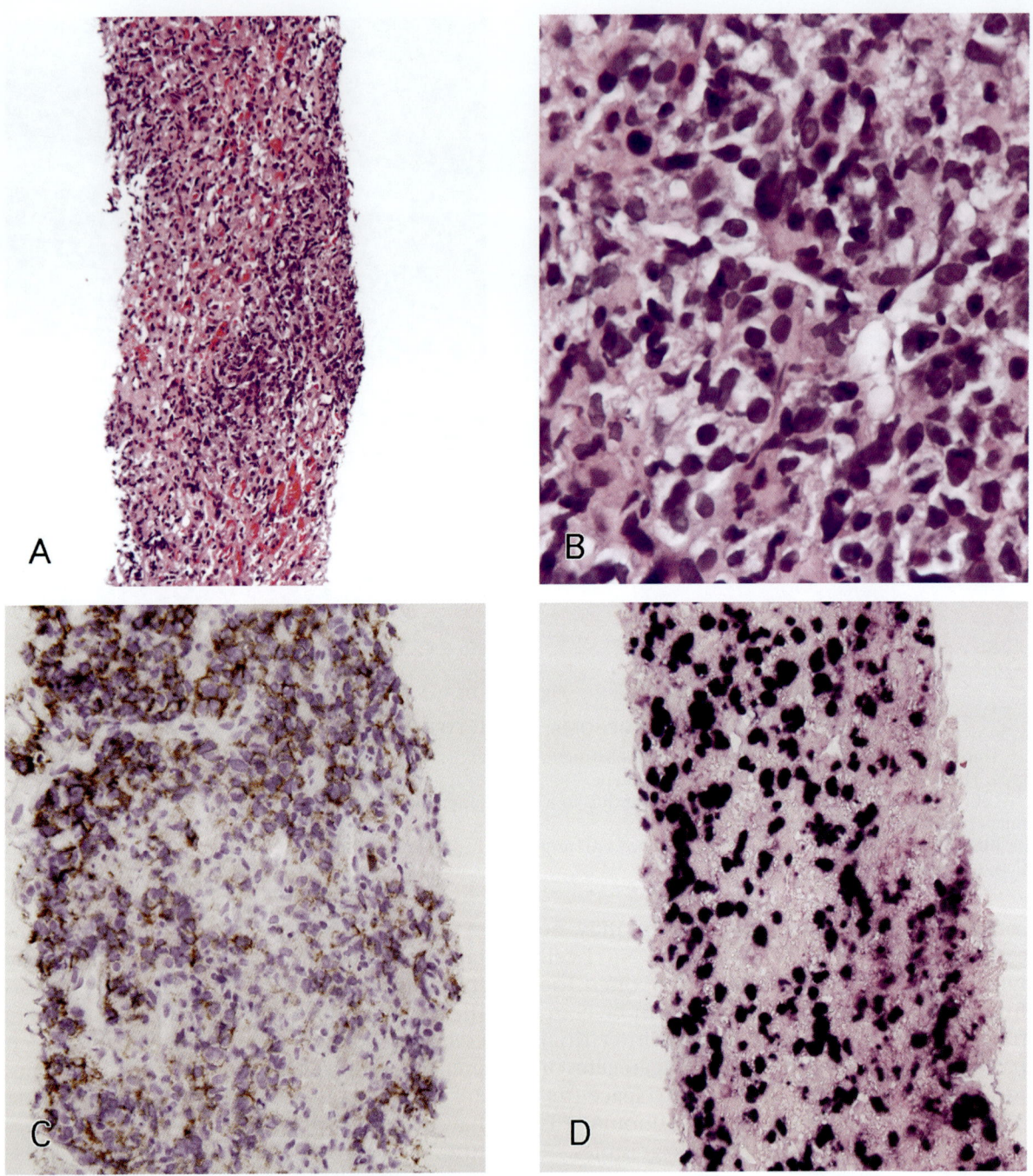

Figure 35-11

EXTRANODAL NK/T-CELL LYMPHOMA, NASAL TYPE, INVOLVING LIVER

This patient had widely disseminated extranodal NK/T-cell lymphoma of nasal type and underwent liver biopsy to evaluate a liver nodule.

A: Low-power image of needle biopsy specimen shows replacement of the parenchyma by tumor.

B: The lymphoma cells are not well-preserved but appear to be of intermediate and large size; some cells have elongated and angulated nuclei (A,B: H&E stain).

C: The lymphoma cells have a NK-cell immunophenotype positive for CD56 and cytoplasmic CD3 (not shown) (immunohistochemistry with hematoxylin counterstain).

D: The lymphoma cells are brightly positive for EBER1 (in situ hybridization with eosin counterstain).

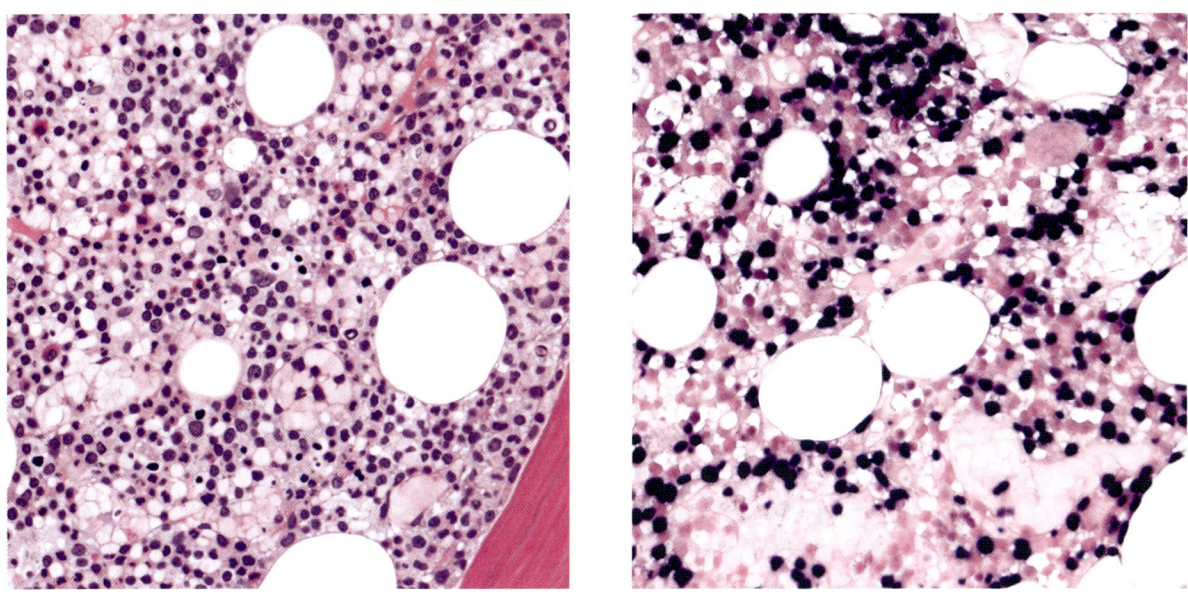

Figure 35-12

EXTRANODAL NK/T-CELL LYMPHOMA, NASAL TYPE, INVOLVING BONE MARROW

Left: The bone marrow biopsy specimen shows an interstitial infiltrate of small to intermediate-sized cells that blend in with hematopoietic elements (H&E stain).

Right: In situ hybridization for EBER1 helps highlight the lymphoma cells (in situ hybridization with eosin counterstain).

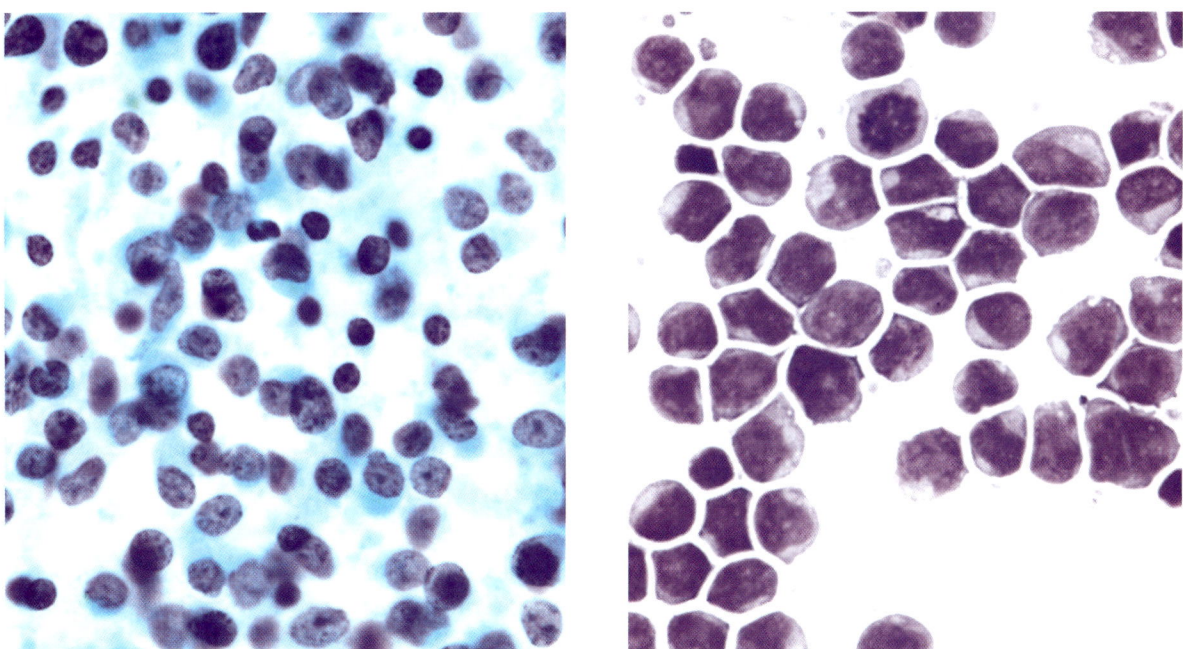

Figure 35-13

EXTRANODAL NK/T-CELL LYMPHOMA, NASAL TYPE: CYTOLOGIC FEATURES

Left: Fine needle aspirate smear (Papanicolaou stain). The lymphoma cells are intermediate-sized cells with oval nuclei and fine chromatin.

Right: In the air-dried cytospin preparation the lymphoma cells have pale cytoplasm (Diff-Quik stain).

immunophenotyping. Extranodal NK/T-cell lymphoma of nasal type shares features with non-neoplastic NK or T cells. About 75 percent of cases have an NK-cell immunophenotype overall, but extranasal tumors are more frequently of T-cell lineage (23,38).

Tumors of NK-cell lineage are positive for CD2, cytoplasmic CD3 (epsilon chain), CD43, CD45RO, CD56, CD94, FAS (CD95), FAS ligand (CD178), and the cytotoxic molecules TIA-1, perforin, and granzyme B (3,6,23,26,32). Granzyme H has been proposed as a new diagnostic marker that is brightly expressed in extranodal NK/T-cell lymphoma of nasal type (9). CD7 (about 15 percent of patients) and CD25 (about 25 percent) are also expressed (3,32). About 40 percent of tumors show CD30 expression, usually by a subset of tumor cells; this expression correlates with large cell size. MYC and Ki-67 are high in some cases and have been reported to predict poorer prognosis in Chinese patients (11).

Extranodal NK/T-cell lymphoma of nasal type is negative for CD1A, surface CD3, CD4, CD5, CD7 (usually), CD8, CD15, CD16, CD57, ALK, T-cell receptors (α/β) and (γ/δ), TdT, and B-cell and myeloid-associated antigens. In contrast, nasal-type lymphomas of true T-cell lineage express surface CD3, CD8 (uncommonly CD4), and T-cell receptors (3,23,31).

Immunohistochemical results are in keeping with the flow cytometry data. All extranodal NK/T-cell lymphomas of nasal type (NK and T cell) are positive for cytoplasmic CD3 (figs. 35-2C, 35-14A) and about 85 percent of cases are CD56 positive (fig. 35-11C); negative cases may be attributable, in part, to the lower sensitivity of paraffin section immunohistochemistry. In support of this statement, cases assessed by both flow cytometry and immunohistochemistry may be positive only by flow cytometry (23). CD56 is also expressed less often by tumors of T-cell lineage. MUM1/IRF4 is positive in approximately half of nasal-type NK/T-cell lymphomas (more often in NK-lineage tumors) (31). The combination of CD3(+) and CD5(-) by immunohistochemistry favors the possibility of an NK-cell neoplasm (fig. 35-14).

In virtually all cases of extranodal NK/T-cell lymphoma of nasal type, the lymphoma cells are positive for one or more cytotoxic proteins including TIA-1, granzyme B, and perforin

(22,31). The percentage of cells expressing Ki-67 is usually over 50 percent, including tumors composed of small cells, and the proliferation rate can be much higher. T-bet, a transcription factor required for Th1 T-cell development and differentiation of lymphocytes and NK cells, is often positive (23). P-glycoprotein is commonly positive (3). p53 is positive in about half (or more) of cases and is more frequent in tumors of large cell size (4,22).

Nasal-type NK/T-cell lymphoma is always associated with EBV infection, independent of patient ethnicity or geographic region, and EBV infection is included in the definition of the disease (3). Although rare EBV-negative cases are reported in the literature, there are questions about the classification of these cases. In situ hybridization for EBV-encoded RNA1 (EBER1) is an excellent method for the detection of the virus (figs. 35-3, right; 35-12B) (28). Most cases of nasal-type NK/T-cell lymphoma have a type I or, less often, a type II latency program. As EBV latent membrane protein 1 (LMP1) is not expressed in type I latent infection. Therefore, in situ hybridization for EBER1 is superior to immunohistochemistry for LMP1 for establishing the presence of viral infection.

MOLECULAR GENETIC FINDINGS

NK cells do not rearrange their T-cell receptor (TCR) genes. Not surprisingly, cases of nasal-type NK/T-cell lymphoma of NK cell lineage also do not carry monoclonal TCR gene rearrangements. In contrast, cases of true T-cell derivation carry monoclonal rearrangements of *TRB* or *TRG*, or both. The immunoglobulin genes are in the germline configuration.

As mentioned above, EBV is present in monoclonal, episomal form, proving the monoclonal nature of nasal-type NK/T-cell lymphoma. There are a number of viral subtypes that can occur in these tumors, with type A being the most common (3). A 30 base pair deletion in the *EBV LMP1* gene occurs in a subset of tumors. Viral microRNA molecules suppress *TP53* transcription and inhibit the interferon γ-STAT1 pathway, and therefore may be involved in tumor progression (8).

Few studies using conventional cytogenetic analysis have been performed on extranodal NK/T-cell lymphoma of nasal type, likely attributable to the small and necrotic nature of many biopsy specimens. Comparative genomic hybridization

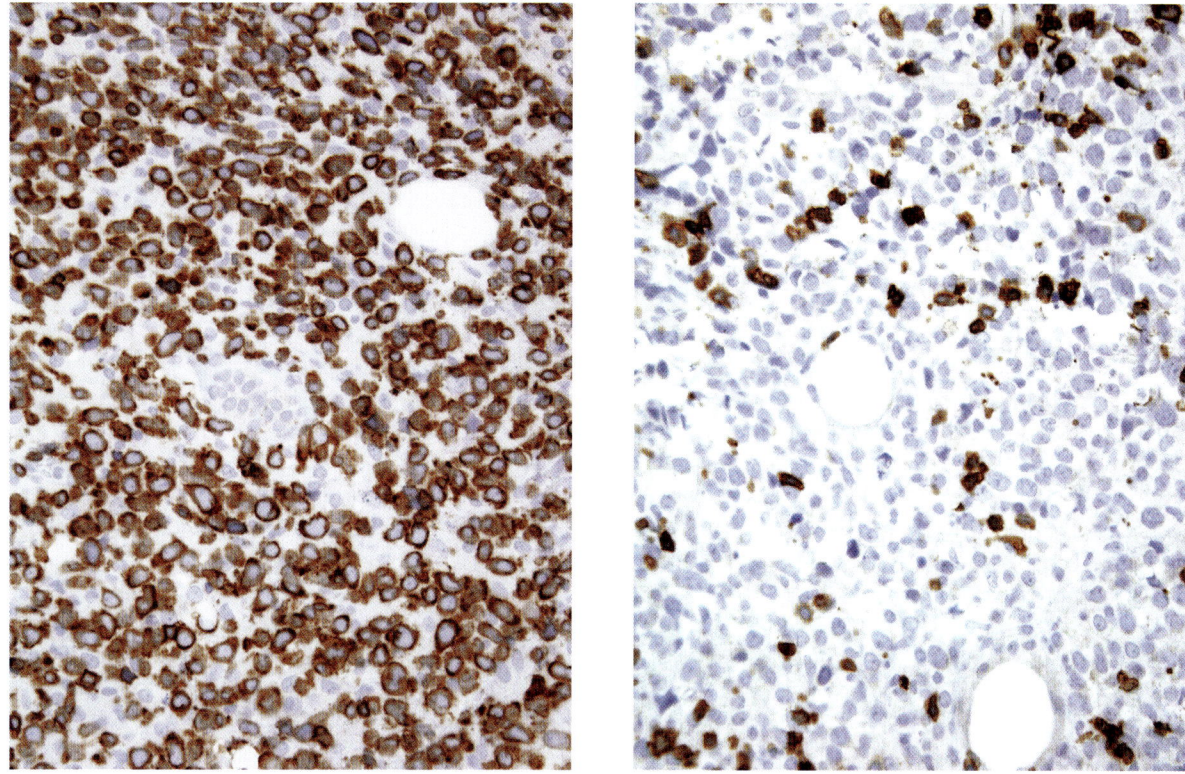

Figure 35-14

EXTRANODAL NK/T-CELL LYMPHOMA, NASAL TYPE: IMMUNOHISTOCHEMICAL FEATURES

The neoplastic cells are positive for CD3 (left) and negative for CD5 (right), consistent with a NK-cell lineage (left, right: immunohistochemistry with hematoxylin counterstain).

has shown numerous chromosomal abnormalities. Common abnormalities include gains of 1q, 2q, 3q26.1, 7q34, and 8q24.3, and losses of 1p, 1q21.1, 5p13.2, 6q, 8p11.23 (possibly *ADAM3A*), 11q, 13q, 14q11.1-11.2, 15q11.2, 15q24.2, 17p (likely *TP53*), 19p13.32, and 22q11.23 (possibly *GSTT1*) (33). Partial deletion of chromosome 6q21-25 is one of the most common recurrent aberrations present in up to 50 percent of cases (3,33). Several candidate tumor-suppressor genes map to this locus, for example, *PRDM1* and *HACE1* (10).

A number of gene mutations have been reported in extranodal NK/T-cell lymphoma of nasal type. The JAK-STAT pathway is commonly activated in these tumors and activating *JAK3* mutations have been detected in 20 to 35 percent of cases, resulting in constitutive STAT3 activation (2,18,19,21). Receptor-type tyrosine-protein phosphatase κ, encoded by a gene on chromosome 6q, is thought to be a tumor suppressor that regulates STAT3; del(6q)

is thought to result in underexpression of receptor-type tyrosine-protein phosphatase κ and STAT3 activation (5). *TP53* mutations have been reported in 15 to 60 percent of cases in different studies. The *BCL6* corepressor (*BCOR*) gene, located at chromosome Xp11.4, is mutated in 20 to 30 percent of cases (5a,21). Mutations of *CTNNB1* (β-catenin), *KRAS, TP53, DDX3S, FAT4, NRAS, KMT2C*, and *KIT* have been reported in about 5 to 15 percent of cases (3,5a).

The gene expression signature of extranodal NK/T-cell lymphoma, nasal type, of either NK- or T-cell immunophenotype is similar to that of activated NK cells, and these tumors are distinct from other types of T-cell lymphoma (10). In one study, 80 unique genes were identified in extranodal NK/T-cell lymphoma including *FAS* ligand, *CD244*, killer immunoglobulin-like receptors, and other genes associated with NK-cell activation or survival (12). These tumors also overexpress genes involved in angiogenesis, genotoxic stress, proliferation, and the TGFβ, Notch, Wnt, PDGFRα, AKT, and NF-κB pathways (10,12).

MicroRNA profiling has been performed in a limited number of nasal-type extranodal NK/T-cell lymphomas. The data are currently too preliminary to fully understand the pathogenesis of many of the reported abnormalities. miR-155 and miR-21 are overexpressed and a number of microRNAs are downregulated in these neoplasms (9,15,30).

DIFFERENTIAL DIAGNOSIS

The differential diagnosis of extranodal NK/T-cell lymphoma, nasal type, is greatly influenced by the anatomic site of disease.

Cytotoxic Peripheral T-Cell Lymphoma. There is overlap between extranodal NK/T-cell lymphoma of nasal type and cytotoxic peripheral T-cell lymphoma. Both tumors share expression of T-cell-associated antigens and a cytotoxic immunophenotype. Location in the nasal region and evidence of EBV infection support nasal-type NK/T-cell lymphoma, as does expression of CD56 and other NK-cell–associated antigens.

In non-nasal extranodal sites, a typical NK-cell immunophenotype and EBV positivity help establish a diagnosis of NK-cell lymphoma, nasal type (3,4). Distinguishing extranasal NK/T-cell lymphoma, nasal type of true T-cell lineage, from cytotoxic peripheral T-cell lymphoma is problematic: both tumors are of T-cell lineage and express cytotoxic molecules, and cytotoxic peripheral T-cell lymphoma is commonly positive for EBV infection. Necrosis and vascular invasion are more common in nasal type NK/T-cell lymphoma but these findings are not completely reliable for the differential diagnosis.

For lesions involving the skin, if the lymphoma is EBV positive and otherwise resembles extranodal T-cell lymphoma, nasal type, but is positive for T-cell receptor gamma or delta by immunohistochemistry, the possible diagnosis of primary cutaneous γ/δ T-cell lymphoma is raised since both tumors share a cytotoxic T-cell immunophenotype. In our opinion, the presence of EBV supports nasal-type T-cell lymphoma over the primary cutaneous γ/δ T-cell lymphoma. Furthermore, the latter tumor is often negative for CD4 and CD8, unlike nasal-type T-cell lymphoma, which is often CD8 positive. There is

no consensus currently for distinguishing these two tumors in the literature.

Cases reported as extranodal NK/T-cell lympoma of nasal type have been described to arise in lymph nodes, usually cervical, in patients without evidence of nasal disease (14,35), but this designation is controversial. This diagnosis may be appropriate for tumors of NK-cell lineage. For tumors of T-cell lineage, the WHO classification recommends the designation node-based EBV-positive peripheral T-cell lymphoma, not otherwise specified, with a cytotoxic immunophenotype (34).

Diffuse Large B-Cell Lymphoma. In the nasopharynx, diffuse large B-cell lymphoma (DLBCL) is far more common than extranodal NK/T-cell lymphoma of nasal type. Cases of DLBCL are characterized by sheets of large lymphoma cells of B-cell lineage and lack an angiocentric growth pattern.

Lymphomatoid Granulomatosis. The lung is involved in 5 to 10 percent of patients with extranodal NK/T-cell lymphoma of nasal type, usually as a part of disseminated disease, suggesting a diagnosis of lymphomatoid granulomatosis (LYG). Unlike nasal-type NK/T-cell lymphoma, patients with LYG almost always present initially with bilateral lung lesions and respiratory tract symptoms such as cough and shortness of breath. In some patients, the lesions disseminate to other extranodal sites, most often the brain, kidney, and skin, where the diagnosis can be highly challenging without knowledge of the lung lesions.

Histologically, LYG is characterized by an angiocentric and angiodestructive, EBV-positive polymorphous lymphoid infiltrate that can resemble extranodal NK/T-cell lymphoma of nasal type. The EBV-positive lymphoma cells, however, are of B-cell lineage and carry monoclonal immunoglobulin rearrangements.

Lymphomas Involving Skin. Extranodal NK/T-cell lymphoma of nasal type involving the skin may be confused with a number of cutaneous tumors. NK-cell–derived lymphomas have an NK-cell immunophenotype but lack evidence of EBV infection. Blastic plasmacytoid dendritic cell neoplasms (BPDCN) express CD56 and therefore extranodal NK/T-cell lymphoma of nasal type may be considered. There is often less necrosis, no evidence of an angiocentric growth pattern, and the neoplastic cells are positive for CD4, CD123 and TCL1, and negative for cytoplasmic CD3 and EBV in BPDCN. Primary cutaneous γ/δ T-cell lymphomas express T-cell receptor γ and are usually negative for EBV.

Nasal-type NK/T-cell lymphomas can involve subcutaneous adipose tissue and the lymphoma cells can rim adipocytes, similar to subcutaneous panniculitis-like T-cell lymphoma (SPTCL). However, SPTCL is negative for EBV. Some cases of nasal-type NK/T-cell lymphoma are composed of large cells that express CD30 and may be mistaken for cutaneous anaplastic large cell lymphoma. However, most cases of NK/T-cell lymphoma of nasal type, even tumors with many large cells, show a range of cell sizes and CD30 expression is variable. In contrast, cutaneous ALCL is composed predominantly of large cells that uniformly and brightly express CD30 and are negative for EBV.

Lymphomas Involving Gastrointestinal Tract. Extranodal NK/T-cell lymphoma, nasal type, involving the gastrointestinal tract may be confused with enteropathy-associated T-cell lymphoma (ETL). Unlike nasal-type NK/T-cell lymphoma, ETL is often associated with a history of celiac disease, the tumors occur most often in the jejunum, and most tumors are negative for EBV. The differential diagnosis with monomorphic epitheliotropic intestinal T-cell lymphoma (previously known as ETL type II) is more challenging because the lymphoma cells have a cytotoxic immunophenotype (34). These tumors, however, are usually negative for EBV.

A clinically indolent NK-cell lymphoproliferative disease of the gastrointestinal tract has been reported, designated as NK-cell enteropathy (27). Patients with NK-cell enteropathy have multiple superficial ulcers of the gastrointestinal mucosa, characterized by a dense mucosal lymphoid infiltrate of intermediate-sized to large atypical lymphoid cells without necrosis or angiodestruction. The lymphoid cells have a cytotoxic NK-cell immunophenotype (positive for CD56, negative for T-cell antigens and EBV), and they lack monoclonal T-cell receptor gene rearrangements (27,37). These lesions persist without progression and follow an indolent clinical course even without therapy.

Wegener Granulomatosis. Wegener granulomatosis (also known as granulomatosis with polyangiitis) is an important entity in the differential diagnosis of extranodal NK/T-cell lymphoma of nasal type. Clinically, patients with Wegener granulomatosis present with disease involving the upper respiratory tract, lungs, and kidneys, and they have characteristic serologic abnormalities (e.g., antineutrophil cytoplasmic antibody). Histologically, a triad of vasculitis, granulomatous inflammation, and geographic necrosis is described in Wegener granulomatosis, but the frequency of this triad is low.

Wegener granulomatosis often shows necrosis and mucosal ulceration that can mimic nasal-type NK/T-cell lymphoma. In Wegener granulomatosis, however, there is no bone destruction, mitotic activity is low, and the infiltrate can be rich in eosinophils and granulocytes. There is no evidence of EBV infection in Wegener granulomatosis.

Other Reactive Conditions in the Nasal Region. Mucosal-associated lymphoid tissue (MALT) in the nasopharynx can be prominent and mimic a mass lesion, suggesting the possibility of lymphoma. Unlike lymphoma, MALT does not destroy normal tissues and is a mixed infiltrate of lymphocytes, histiocytes, and plasma cells. Immunohistochemical analysis shows well-defined B- and T-cell compartments and polytypic plasma cells; EBV infection is either absent or rare (less than 1 percent of EBV cells are positive).

Herpes simplex infection of the nasopharynx can form a mass lesion and be associated with extensive necrosis that may simulate extranodal NK/T-cell lymphoma of nasal type. Unlike lymphoma, the T cells in the infiltrate are mostly CD4 positive and do not express cytotoxic molecules. There is also no evidence of EBV infection. Detection of herpesvirus Cowdry type A nuclear inclusions and multinucleated giant cells in the epithelial cell layer support the diagnosis of herpes simplex infection.

TREATMENT AND PROGNOSIS

The overall prognosis of patients with extranodal NK/T-cell lymphoma of nasal type is poor. Patients with localized nasal disease have a 5-year overall survival rate ranging from 42 to 64 percent in most recent series (1,17,24,40). In contrast, patients with high-stage disease and those with extranasal disease have an abysmal prognosis. Extranasal disease, high IPI score, and a high proliferation rate correlate with poorer prognosis (23,38). Recent studies have correlated vascular invasion and overexpression of both MYC and BCL2 with poorer prognosis (38a,38b). CD94 expression correlates with a better prognosis (26).

Radiotherapy was used traditionally for patients with localized disease, but relapses were common and currently radiation and chemotherapy are used for these patients (24,40). Commonly used regimens for aggressive lymphoma, such as the CHOP (cyclophosphamide, doxorubicin, vincristine, and prednisone) regimen, are not effective. A regimen composed of steroid (dexamethasone), methotrexate, ifosfamide, L-asparaginase, and etoposide (SMILE) has been developed and is associated with improved rates of complete response (24,40). There may be a role for high-dose chemotherapy with hematopoietic stem cell transplantation (41). A pre-clinical investigation suggests a potential benefit for drugs that target the JAK-STAT pathway (2).

REFERENCES

1. Bossard C, Belhadj K, Reyes F, et al. Expression of the granzyme B inhibitor PI9 predicts outcome in nasal NK/T-cell lymphoma: results of a Western series of 48 patients treated with first-line polychemotherapy within the Groupe d'Etude des Lymphomes de l'Adulte (GELA) trials. Blood 2007;109:2183-2189.

2. Bouchekioua A, Scourzic L, de Wever O, et al. JAK3 deregulation by activating mutations confers invasive growth advantage in extranodal nasal-type natural killer cell lymphoma. Leukemia 2014;28:338-348.

3. Chan JK, Quintanilla-Martinez L, Ferry JA, Peh SC. Extranodal NK/T-cell lymphoma, nasal type. In: Swerdlow SH, Campo E, Harris NL, et al., eds. WHO classification of tumours of haematopoietic and lymphoid tissues Lyon: IARC Press; 2008:285-288.

4. Chan JK, Sin VC, Wong KF, et al. Nonnasal lymphoma expressing the natural killer cell marker CD56: a clinicopathologic study of 49 cases of an uncommon aggressive neoplasm. Blood 1997;89:4501-4513.

5. Chen YW, Guo T, Shen L, et al. Receptor-type tyrosine-protein phosphatase κ directly targets STAT3 activation for tumor suppression in nasal NK/T-cell lymphoma. Blood 2015;125:1589-1600.

5a. Dobashi A, Tsuyama N, Asaka R, et al. Frequent BCOR aberrations in extranodal NK/T-cell lymphoma, nasal type. Genes Chromosomes Cancer 2016;55:460-471.

6. Gualco G, Domeny-Duarte P, Chioato L, Barber G, Natkunam Y, Bacchi CE. Clinicopathologic and molecular features of 122 Brazilian cases of nodal and extranodal NK/T-cell lymphoma, nasal type, with EBV subtyping analysis. Am J Surg Pathol 2011;35:1195-1203.

7. Harabuchi Y, Yamanaka N, Kataura A, et al. Epstein-Barr virus in nasal T-cell lymphomas in patients with lethal midline granuloma. Lancet 1990;335:128-130.

8. Huang WT, Lin CW. EBV-encoded miR-BART20-5p and miR-BART8 inhibit the IFN-γ-STAT1 pathway associated with disease progression in nasal NK-cell lymphoma. Am J Pathol 2014; 184:1185-1197.

9. Huang Y, de Leval L, Gaulard P. Molecular underpinning of extranodal NK/T-cell lymphoma. Best Pract Res Clin Haematol 2013;26:57-74.

10. Huang Y, de Reynies A, de Leval L, et al. Gene expression profiling identifies emerging oncogenic pathways operating in extranodal NK/T-cell lymphoma, nasal type. Blood 2010;115:1226-1237.

11. Huang X, Sun Q, Fu H, Zhou X, Guan X, Wang J. Both c-Myc and Ki-67 expression are predictive markers in patients with extranodal NK/T-cell lymphoma, nasal type: a retrospective study in China. Pathol Res Pract 2014;210:351-356.

12. Iqbal J, Wright G, Wang C, et al. Gene expression signatures delineate biological and prognostic subgroups in peripheral T-cell lymphoma. Blood 2014;123:2915-2923.

13. Ishida F, Ko YH, Kim WS, et al. Aggressive natural killer cell leukemia: therapeutic potential of L-asparaginase and allogeneic hematopoietic stem cell transplantation. Cancer Sci 2012;103:1079-1083.

14. Jeon YK, Kim JH, Sung JY, Han JH, Ko YH; Hematopathology Study Group of the Korean Society of Pathologists. Epstein-Barr virus-positive nodal T/NK-cell lymphoma: an analysis of 15 cases with distinct clinicopathological features. Hum Pathol 2015;46:981-990.

15. Ji WG, Zhang XD, Sun XD, Wang XQ, Chang BP, Zhang MZ. miRNA-155 modulates the malignant biological characteristics of NK/T-cell lymphoma cells by targeting FOXO3a gene. J Huazhong Univ Sci Technolog Med Sci 2014;34:882-888.

16. Jimenez-Heffernan JA, Gonzalez-Peramato P, Perna C, Alvarez-Ferreira J, López-Ferrer P, Viguer JM. Fine-needle aspiration cytology of extranodal natural killer/T-cell lymphoma. Diagn Cytopathol 2002;27:371-374.

17. Kim TM, Park YH, Lee SY, et al. Local tumor invasiveness is more predictive of survival than International Prognostic Index in stage I(E)/II(E) extranodal NK/T-cell lymphoma, nasal type. Blood 2005;106:3785-3790.

18. Koo GC, Tan SY, Tang T, et al. Janus kinase 3-activating mutations identified in natural killer/T-cell lymphoma. Cancer Discov 2012;2:591-597.

19. Küçük C, Jiang B, Hu X, et al. Activating mutations of STAT5B and STAT3 in lymphomas derived from γδ-T or NK cells. Nat Commun 2015;6:6025.

20. Lanier LL, Chang C, Spits H, Phillips JH. Expression of cytoplasmic CD3 epsilon proteins in activated human adult natural killer (NK) cells and CD3 gamma, delta, epsilon complexes in fetal NK cells. Implications for a relationship of NK and T lymphocytes. J Immunol 1992;149:1876-1880.

21. Lee S, Park HY, Kang SY, et al. Genetic alterations of JAK/STAT cascade and histone modification in extranodal NK/T-cell lymphoma nasal type. Oncotarget 2015;6:17764-17776.

22. Li C, Tian Y, Wang J, et al. Abnormal immunophenotype provides a key diagnostic marker: a report of 29 cases of de novo aggressive natural killer cell leukemia. Transl Res 2014;163:565-577.

23. Li S, Feng X, Li T, et al. Extranodal NK/T-cell lymphoma, nasal type: a report of 73 cases at MD Anderson Cancer Center. Am J Surg Pathol 2013;37:14-23.

24. Liang R. Advances in the management and monitoring of extranodal NK/T-cell lymphoma, nasal type. Br J Haematol 2009;147:13-21.

25. Lima M. Extranodal NK/T cell lymphoma and aggressive NK cell leukaemia: evidence for their origin on CD56+bright CD16-/+dim NK cells. Pathology 2015;47:503-514.

26. Lin CW, Chen YH, Chuang YC, Liu TY, Hsu SM. CD94 transcripts imply a better prognosis in nasal-type extranodal NK/T-cell lymphoma. Blood 2003;102:2623-2631.

27. Mansoor A, Pittaluga S, Beck PL, Wilson WH, Ferry JA, Jaffe ES. NK-cell enteropathy: a benign NK-cell lymphoproliferative disease mimicking intestinal lymphoma: clinicopathologic features and follow-up in a unique case series. Blood 2011;117:1447-1452.

28. Medeiros LJ, Jaffe ES, Chen YY, Weiss LM. Localization of Epstein-Barr viral genomes in angiocentric immunoproliferative lesions. Am J Surg Pathol 1992;16:439-447.

29. Medeiros LJ, Peiper SC, Elwood L, Yano T, Raffeld M, Jaffe ES. Angiocentric immunoproliferative lesions: a molecular analysis of eight cases. Hum Pathol 1991;22:1150-1157.

30. Ng SB, Yan J, Huang G, et al. Dysregulated microRNAs affect pathways and targets of biologic relevance in nasal-type natural killer/T-cell lymphoma. Blood. 2011;118: 4919-4929.

31. Pongpruttipan T, Sukpanichnant S, Assanasen T, et al. Extranodal NK/T-cell lymphoma, nasal type, includes cases of natural killer cell and αβ, γδ, and αβ/γδ T-cell origin: a comprehensive clinicopathologic and phenotypic study. Am J Surg Pathol 2012;36:481-499.

32. Schwartz EJ, Molina-Kirsch H, Zhao S, Marinelli RJ, Warnke RA, Natkunam Y. Immunohistochemical characterization of nasal-type extranodal NK/T-cell lymphoma using a tissue microarray: an analysis of 84 cases. Am J Clin Pathol 2008;130:343-351.

33. Sun L, Li M, Huang X, Xu J, Gao Z, Liu C. High-resolution genome-wide analysis identified recurrent genetic alterations in NK/T-cell lymphoma, nasal type, which are associated with disease progression. Med Oncol 2014;31:71.

34. Swerdlow SH, Campo E, Pileri SA, et al. The 2016 revision of the World Health Organization classification of lymphoid neoplasms. Blood 2016;127:2375-2390.

35. Takahashi E, Asano N, Li C, et al. Nodal T/NK-cell lymphoma of nasal type: a clinicopathological study of six cases. Histopathology 2008;52:585-596.

36. Takahashi N, Miura I, Chubachi A, Miura AB, Nakamura S. A clinicopathological study of 20 patients with T/natural killer (NK)-cell lymphoma-associated hemophagocytic syndrome with special reference to nasal and nasal-type NK/T-cell lymphoma. Int J Hematol 2001;74:303-308.

37. Vega F, Chang CC, Schwartz MR, et al. Atypical NK-cell proliferation of the gastrointestinal tract in a patient with antigliadin antibodies but not celiac disease. Am J Surg Pathol 2006;30:539-544.

38. Vose J, Armitage J, Weisenburger D; International T-Cell Lymphoma Project. International peripheral T-cell and natural killer/T-cell lymphoma study: pathology findings and clinical outcomes. J Clin Oncol 2008;26:4124-4130.

38a. Wang H, Li P, Zhang X, Xia Z, Lu Y, Huang H. Histological vascular invasion is a novel prognostic indicator in extranodal natural killer/T-cell lymphoma, nasal type. Oncol Lett 2016;12:825-836.

38b. Wang JH, Bi XW, Li PF, et al. Overexpression of MYC and BCL2 predicts poor prognosis in patients with extranodal NK/T-cell lymphoma, nasal type. J Cancer 2017;8:793-800.

39. Wright CA, Cooper K, Leiman G, Davidge-Pitts M. Natural killer cell lymphoma in cytology: breaking all the rules—a case report. Diagn Cytopathol 1998;19:9-11.

40. Yang Y, Zhu Y, Cao JZ, et al. Risk-adapted therapy for early-stage extranodal nasal-type NK/T-cell lymphoma: a comprehensive analysis from a multicenter study. Blood 2015;126:1424-1432.

41. Yhim HY, Kim JS, Mun YC, et al. Clinical outcomes and prognostic factors of up-front autologous stem cell transplantation in patients with extranodal natural killer/T cell lymphoma. Biol Blood Marrow Transplant 2015;21:1597-1604.

36 MYCOSIS FUNGOIDES

GENERAL FEATURES

Mycosis fungoides (MF) is a mature T-cell lymphoma arising in skin and characterized by a protracted clinical course with a stepwise evolution from patches to plaques and ultimately tumors. The lymphoma cells in MF have a pronounced tendency to infiltrate the epidermis (epidermotropism). Although some patients with advanced disease develop leukemic involvement and erythroderma resembling Sézary syndrome (SS), de novo SS is considered to be a separate disease (28,29,36a).

Mycosis fungoides is the most common type of primary cutaneous lymphoma, representing about half of all primary lymphomas involving the skin and about 70 percent of cutaneous T-cell lymphomas (6). The annual incidence is 6 to 7 cases per 1 million persons per year (6,19), and is 1.5 times higher in African-Americans than in Caucasians. From the 1970s until 2009, there was a substantial rise in the incidence of MF, likely due, at least in part, to increased efficiency of detection and improvement of diagnostic methods; the incidence has held steady since 2009 (6,19).

The cell of origin of MF is thought to be a CD45RO-positive effector memory T cell that expresses cutaneous lymphocyte-associated antigen (CLA) and normally resides in the skin. These T cells express molecules that facilitate their ability to migrate into the skin, such as the chemokine receptors CCR4, CCR6, and CCR10. Cutaneous effector memory T cells have a number of subsets, such as TH1, TH2, and TH17 cells, and therefore the cell of origin of MF is somewhat heterogeneous, although currently, derivation from these subsets is not thought to be clinically important.

The etiology of MF is unknown. Rare families with MF have been described, and there are associations with human leukocyte antigen (HLA) alleles, suggesting that genetic inheritance plays a role, at least in some patients. Chronic antigen stimulation is likely involved in pathogenesis, but no infectious organisms or chemical exposures have been identified (28). Although almost all cases of MF in the plaque and tumor stages carry monoclonal T-cell receptor gene rearrangements, some patch stage MF cases are polyclonal (27). This finding is consistent with the hypothesis that chronic antigenic stimulation leads to polyclonal T-cell expansion and prolonged T-cell survival, increasing the opportunity for the genetic hits that lead to a monoclonal T-cell population.

The genetic abnormalities in MF are numerous and complex, and the overall profile is suggestive of ultraviolet light-induced genetic damage (reviewed in reference 9a). This finding is surprising as there is no obvious epidemiologic connection between MF and heavy sun exposure. The tumor microenvironment of MF is also important in tumorigenesis as well as disease progression. There is an interplay between MF cells and host reactive T cells, macrophages, dendritic cells, and keratinocytes, in part related to the secretion of various chemokines and cytokines, such as interleukin (IL)-10. Many of these molecules have growth promoting properties whereas others (e.g., IL-10) induce an immunosuppressive microenvironment. Cells within the tumor microenvironment also have prognostic implications. Studies have shown that patients with MF lesions characterized by a high number of CD8-positive reactive T-cells have a better prognosis, suggesting that the host CD8-positive cytotoxic T cells can keep MF in check (12). In contrast, high numbers of CD163-positive macrophages (TH2 polarization) correlate with progressive disease and a poorer prognosis (36).

CLINICAL FEATURES

MF is mostly a disease of adults, usually in the sixth decade of life (28,48). In one large study from the United States, the mean age at time of diagnosis was 53.6 years (7). Males are more commonly

Table 36-1

TNMB SYSTEM FOR PATIENTS WITH MYCOSIS FUNGOIDES

Skin

T1 Limited patches (any size) and/or plaques covering <10% of skin surface

T2 Patches, papules, or plaques covering ≥10% of skin surface

T3 One of more tumors (≥1 cm in diameter)

T4 Confluence of erythema covering ≥80% of body surface area

Lymph Node (see Table 36-2)

N0 No clinically abnormal peripheral lymph nodes

N1 Clinically abnormal peripheral lymph nodes (Dutch grade 1 or NCI[a] LN0-2)
　　N1a: T-cell clonal population absent
　　N1b: T-cell clonal population present

N2 Clinically abnormal peripheral lymph nodes (Dutch grade 2 or NCI LN3)
　　N2a: T-cell clonal population absent
　　N2b: T-cell clonal population present

N3 Clinically abnormal peripheral lymph nodes (Dutch grade 3-4 or NCI LN4)

NX Clinically abnormal peripheral lymph nodes; no histologic examination

Viscera

M0 No visceral organ involvement

M1 Visceral involvement (must be histologically confirmed); specify organ

Blood

B0 No substantial involvement: ≤5% atypical lymphocytes (Sézary cells); not B2
　　B0a: T-cell clonal population absent
　　B0b: T-cell clonal population present

B1 Low tumor burden: >5% atypical lymphocytes (Sézary cells); not B2
　　B1a: T-cell clonal population absent
　　B1b: T-cell clonal population present

B2 High tumor burden: >1 x 10^6 Sézary cells with T-cell clone present

[a]NCI = National Cancer Institute.

TABLE 36-2

INTERNATIONAL SOCIETY FOR CUTANEOUS LYMPHOMAS/EUROPEAN ORGANIZATION OF RESEARCH AND TREATMENT OF CANCER STAGING SYSTEM FOR PATIENTS WITH MYCOSIS FUNGOIDES[a]

Stage	T	N	M	B
IA	1	0	0	0, 1
IB	2	0	0	0, 1
IIA	1, 2	1	0	0, 1
IIB	3	0-2	0	0, 1
IIIA	4	0-2	0	0
IIIB	4	0-2	0	1
IVA1	1-4	0-2	0	2
IVA2	1-4	3	0	0-2
IVB	1-4	0-3	1	0-2

[a]Criteria for T, N, M, and B are outlined in Table 36-1.

with MF (and SS) may have a compromised immunosurveillance system, due to dysfunctional T cells and associated with an increased frequency of infections and second tumors (44).

Extracutaneous dissemination is observed in a subset of MF patients: most frequently in patients with advanced stage disease with skin tumors or erythroderma (about 40 percent of patients), uncommonly in patients with plaques (about 10 percent), and rarely in patients with patches (28,48). The lymph nodes draining areas of skin involvement are usually the first and most common extracutaneous sites involved. Following the criteria of the International Society for Cutaneous Lymphomas (ISCL) and the European Organization of Research and Treatment of Cancer (EORTC), a clinically abnormal lymph node is defined as at least 1.5 cm in diameter or larger or any palpable lymph node, regardless of size, that is firm, irregular, or fixed (24).

Rarely, patients with MF develop widespread dissemination to visceral sites and the blood (28,47,48). Usually this occurs in patients who have a long history of clinically indolent MF who then develop a more clinically aggressive phase of disease. Dissemination is more common in patients with skin tumors, lymphadenopathy, or following large cell transformation. Virtually any visceral site can be involved, with the lungs, liver, spleen, blood, and gastrointestinal tract the most common (28,30).

affected with reported male to female ratios ranging from 1.1 to 1.0 up to 2.0 to 1.0 (7,28,48).

Classic MF usually begins as patches with scale that are often confined to sun-protected areas ("bathing suit" distribution), although any skin site may be affected (28,48). Over time the disease evolves to plaques and then skin tumors. In many patients, patches, plaques, and tumors coexist. Plaques, and particularly tumors, may ulcerate and cause secondary infection.

MF is characterized by an indolent clinical course, with disease persistence or gradual progression over years or decades (28,47,48). Patients

Table 36-3

HISTOPATHOLOGIC STAGING OF LYMPH NODES IN MYCOSIS FUNGOIDES

Updated ISCL/EORTC[a]	Dutch System[b]	NCI Classification[c]
N1	Grade 1, dermatopathic lymphadenopathy	LN0, no atypical lymphocytes LN1, occasional and isolated atypical lymphocytes (not arranged in clusters) LN2, many atypical lymphocytes in clusters of 3-6
N2	Grade 2, dermatopathic lymphadenopathy; early involvement by MF (presence of cerebriform nuclei >7.5 μm)	LN3, aggregates of atypical lymphocytes; nodal architecture preserved
N3	Grade 3, partial effacement of LN architecture; many atypical cerebriform mononuclear cells Grade 4, complete effacement	LN4, partial/complete effacement of nodal architecture by atypical lymphocytes or frankly neoplastic cells

[a]ISCL = International Society for Cutaneous Lymphomas; EORTC = European Organization of Research and Treatment of Cancer.
[b]Data from reference 34.
[c]NCI = National Cancer Institute; data from reference 32.

A clinical staging system developed by the ISCL and EORTC is used to determine the extent of disease, which has therapeutic and prognostic implications (Tables 36-1, 36-2). This is a TNMB type system based on the extent of skin surface involved by tumor (T), nodal status (N), presence or absence of metastasis (M), and blood status (B). In estimating skin surface involvement, a convenient rule of thumb is that the hand (palm and digits) represents about 1 percent of the total skin surface area.

The clinical and pathologic findings of MF are highly heterogeneous. Approximately 15 "variant" forms have been described including: palmoplantar, isolated alopecia, unilesional MF, pagetoid reticulosis, hypopigmented MF, bullous MF, folliculotropic MF, syringotropic MF, and granulomatous slack skin among other rare variants (5,28,48).

Rarely, MF occurs in young children and adolescents. In a large study at MD Anderson Cancer Center, 34 of 1,902 (1.8 percent) patients with MF were under 20 years of age (2). The median age at time of onset of MF was 9 years and diagnosis was often delayed due, in part, to the unusually young age of the patients. Patients presented with patches or plaques and over 95 percent had stage I disease. MF in young patients can closely resemble typical adult-onset disease, however, about 50 percent of lesions are hypopigmented; a subset of these lesions has a CD8-positive immunophenotype (2,28,48).

HISTOLOGIC FINDINGS

Lymph Node

Lymph nodes in patients with MF show a range of histologic findings, from dermatopathic lymphadenopathy with no evidence of MF to extensive replacement by lymphoma that can mimic other types of peripheral T-cell lymphoma (28,32,43). This spectrum is encompassed in the two main histopathologic grading systems for lymph nodes involved by MF in the past: the National Cancer Institute system and a system from The Netherlands (32,34). These systems have been integrated by the ISCL and EORTC classification (Table 36-3).

Dermatopathic lymphadenopathy or less well-developed dermatopathic changes are frequent in regional lymph nodes draining the skin lesions of MF. Dermatopathic lymphadenopathy consists of expanded pale areas within the paracortex due to clusters of interdigitating reticulum cells, Langerhans cells, macrophages with phagocytized melanin, and small T lymphocytes (fig. 36-1). Dermatopathic changes are usually associated with follicular hyperplasia. The presence of dermatopathic lymphadenopathy does not exclude the presence of MF in the same lymph node.

In early lymph node involvement, the overall architecture is well preserved and the neoplastic lymphocytes are located in the paracortical regions, but MF lymphocytes may be few and difficult to identify or present as small clusters

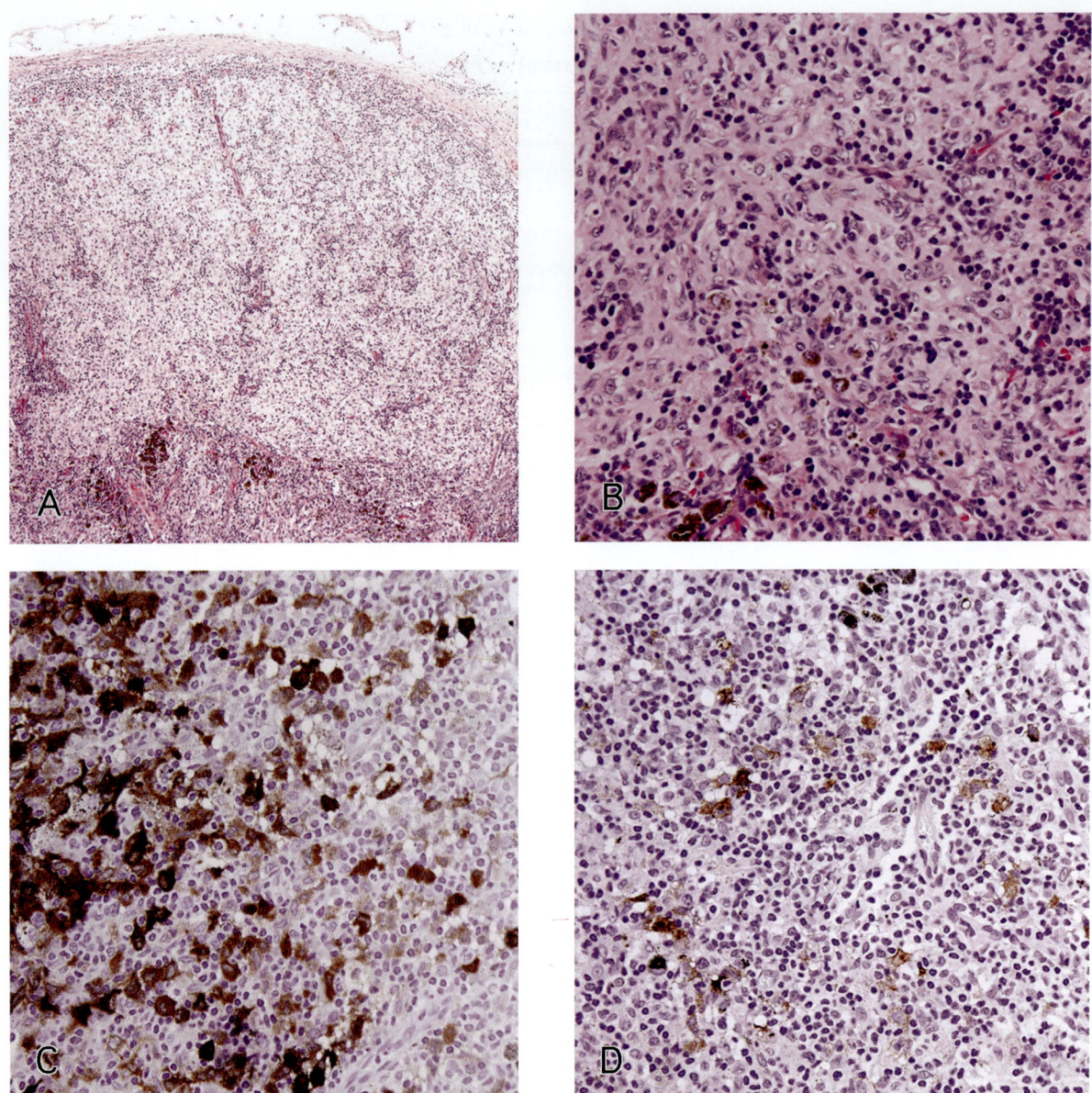

Figure 36-1

DERMATOPATHIC LYMPHADENOPATHY IN PATIENT WITH MYCOSIS FUNGOIDES

A palpable lymph node from a patient with mycosis fungoides (MF) showed dermatopathic lymphadenopathy and molecular studies performed to assess *TRG* showed a polyclonal pattern.

A,B: Histologic sections show many interdigitating dendritic cells with scattered small lymphocytes. Few and small lymphocyte clusters are present (hematoxylin and eosin [H&E] stain).

C,D: Immunohistochemical studies highlight many S-100 protein-positive interdigitating dendritic cells (C) and fewer CD1a-positive Langerhans cells (D) (C,D: immunohistochemistry with hematoxylin counterstain).

more easily recognized by morphologic examination (fig. 36-2) (32,34). The recognition of low numbers of small MF lymphocytes in lymph nodes is challenging. These small cells are cytologically atypical, but assessment of atypia is somewhat subjective. In general, atypical lymphocytes are usually medium-sized, with irregular (cerebriform) nuclear contours; in contrast, reactive lymphocytes are smaller, with less irregular nuclear contours. Examination

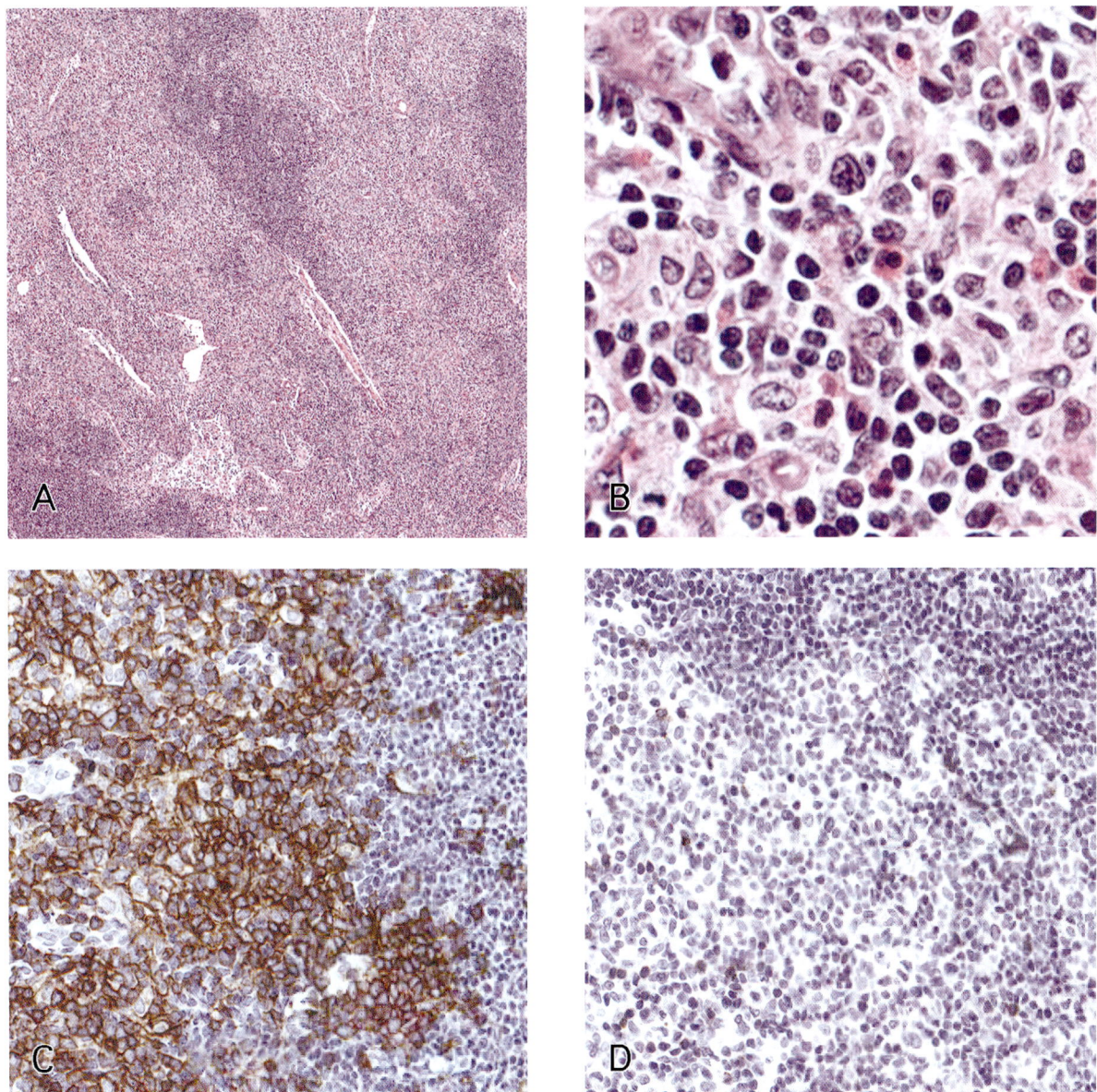

Figure 36-2

MYCOSIS FUNGOIDES INVOLVING LYMPH NODE

A: In a lymph node partially involved by lymphoma, there is paracortical expansion by aggregates of atypical lymphocytes, which in some areas form diffuse sheets (A,B: H&E stain).

B: The lymphocytes of MF in this case show mild to moderate cytologic atypia with a moderate amount of pale cytoplasm. The nuclei are highly convoluted and have cerebriform nuclear contours. Eosinophils are present in background.

C,D: The MF cells are of mature T-cell lineage and are positive for CD4 (C) with aberrant downregulation of CD7 (D); CD3 was also positive (not shown) (C,D: immunohistochemistry with hematoxylin counterstain).

using oil magnification helps delineate the cerebriform nuclear features of MF lymphocytes. Immunophenotypic analysis and molecular studies help support early/partial involvement of lymph nodes by MF (24).

In lymph nodes with more extensive involvement by MF, the nodal architecture is partially or totally effaced by a diffuse infiltrate of medium-sized lymphoma cells (figs. 36-3, 36-4). In some patients, large cell transformation occurs and lymph nodes show a mixture of medium-sized and large cells or sheets of large cells that can resemble centroblasts and immunoblasts or may be pleomorphic or anaplastic. Although usually some large cells have cerebriform nuclear contours, in some cases MF in lymph nodes cannot be distinguished from other types of peripheral T-cell lymphoma (fig. 36-4C). Large cell transformation in lymph nodes is associated with disease progression and poorer prognosis (28,48). LeBlanc et al. (20) described a small series of MF patients in whom the lymph nodes had features similar to angioimmunoblastic T-cell lymphoma, including proliferation of high endothelial venules, cells with clear cytoplasm, and expression of some follicular T-helper cell markers.

Excisional biopsy is the preferred method to evaluate abnormal lymph nodes in patients with MF, but core needle biopsy or fine-needle aspiration specimens can be used if combined with immunophenotypic analysis (11,42). It is best to biopsy lymph nodes with the highest standardized uptake value as assessed by fludeoxyglucose positron emission tomography (FDG-PET) scan. In patients with multiple lymph nodes, biopsy of inguinal lymph nodes is discouraged because cervical or axillary lymph nodes are more likely to be involved by lymphoma (24,43). Central enlarged lymph nodes are excluded from the determination of "N" status except in patients where an excisional biopsy of a central lymph node has proven involvement by MF (N3 stage).

Skin

The diagnosis of MF, particularly in patch stage, can be difficult because at this stage MF can mimic a variety of benign skin diseases (5,22,28). The "gold standard" for diagnosis is a combination of clinical and pathologic findings. In patients with a classic clinical presentation of MF, unimpressive histologic findings may be adequate to support the diagnosis. In contrast, for patients with classic histologic findings in a biopsy specimen, the clinical presentation still must be appropriate to support the diagnosis of MF.

In *patch stage MF* (fig. 36-5), classic morphologic criteria include a band-like (lichenoid) lymphoid infiltrate in the papillary dermis and infiltration of lymphocytes into the overlying epidermis (epidermotropism), with little spongiosis (compared with benign diseases) (22). Infiltration of the epidermis

can be marked or minimal, with lymphocytes lined up at the dermal-epidermal junction ("toy soldier" or "string of pearls" pattern). The MF cells are often surrounded by clear spaces or "halos." Epidermal changes, such as parakeratosis and wiry collagen in the papillary dermis (indicating that the process is chronic), also support a diagnosis of MF. The neoplastic lymphocytes of MF usually are slightly larger, with more irregular nuclear contours than reactive lymphocytes, but this degree of cytologic atypia may be difficult to appreciate because the lymphoma cells may represent only a minor subset of the lymphocytes in the specimen. In general, Pautrier (also known as Pautrier-Darier) microabscesses, are uncommon or not well-developed in patch stage disease. A Pautrier microabscess consists of round clusters of T cells that often surround central Langerhans cells located within the epidermis. Eosinophils are less common in patch stage MF than in many reactive skin diseases, and are particularly uncommon within the epidermis of MF lesions.

In *plaque stage MF*, the histologic findings are similar to those in patch stage disease, but more pronounced (fig. 36-6). The epidermal layer is raised above the surrounding uninvolved skin and the papillary dermis is partially or more extensively filled by lymphoma cells. The MF cells in the plaques are often more obviously atypical and have cerebriform nuclear contours that are best appreciated by examination using oil magnification. The lymphoma cells also represent a greater percentage of the total lymphocytes in the biopsy specimen. Pautrier microabscesses are well-developed in over half of biopsy specimens derived from plaque lesions. Eosinophils and plasma cells are also common within the dermis of plaque (and tumor) stage MF.

Tumor stage MF is characterized by extensive involvement of the papillary and reticular dermis by lymphoma cells (fig. 36-7). These cells are obviously atypical and are intermediate-sized or large (3,28,48). Tumor stage is often (but not invariably) associated with large cell transformation of MF, defined by the presence of large tumor cells representing more than the 25 percent of the infiltrate (3,8,33,41). Epidermotropism can be absent in this stage. Superficial ulceration of skin tumors may occur, with secondary bacterial or fungal infection, resulting in abundant superficial acute inflammation.

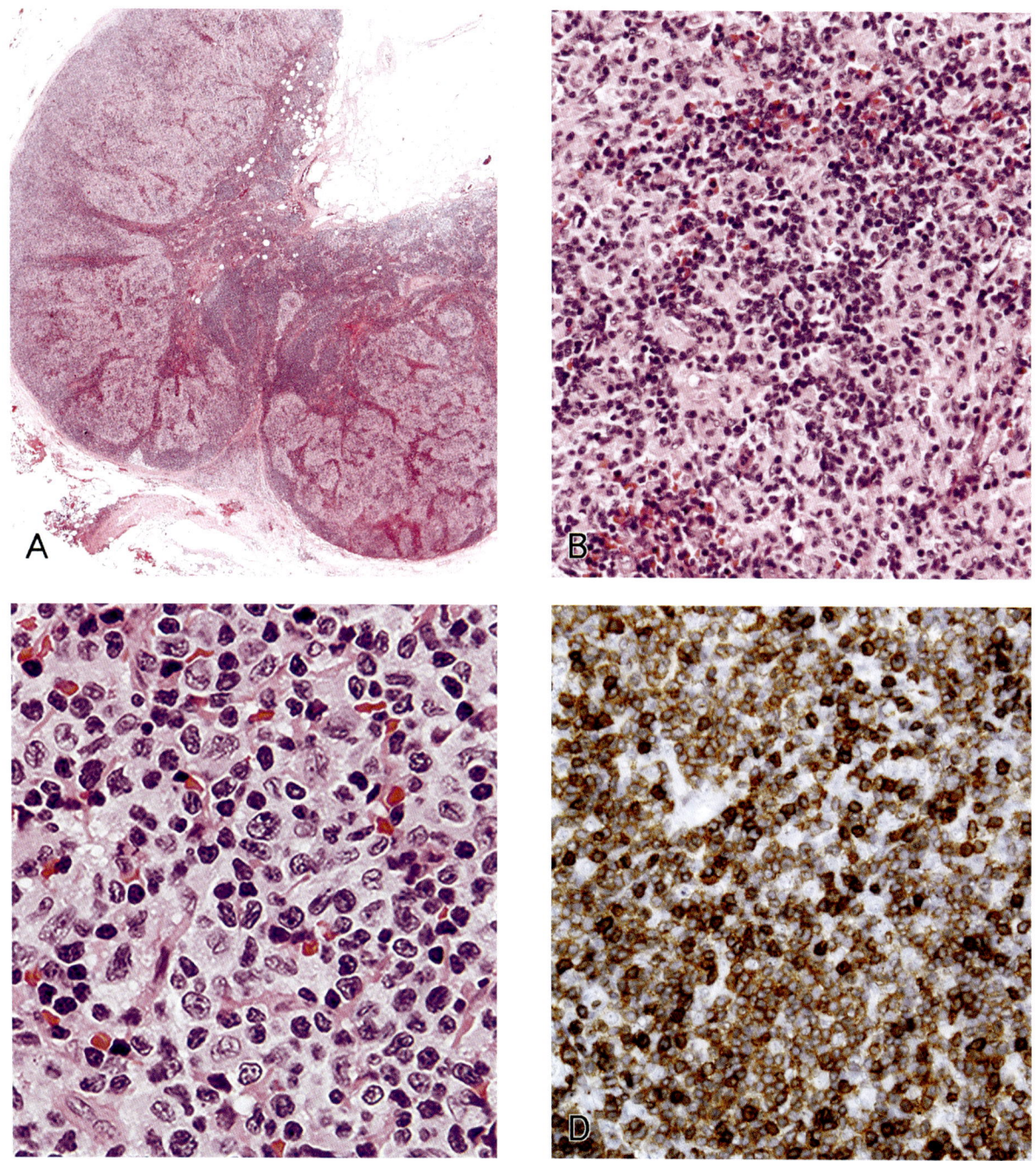

Figure 36-3

MYCOSIS FUNGOIDES INVOLVING LYMPH NODE

This patient with MF had prominent axillary lymphadenopathy that prompted lymph node biopsy.

A: This low magnification image shows that the paracortical regions are expanded by dermatopathic lymphadenopathy and MF (A–C: H&E stain).

B: Clusters of MF lymphocytes are intermixed with dendritic cells and histiocytes in this field.

C: In other areas of the lymph node, the clusters are more prominent, with some large cells, and under oil magnification cerebriform nuclear contours can be appreciated.

D: Immunohistochemistry for CD3 highlights the lymphocytes. The MF cells express CD3 more dimly than scattered reactive T cells in the field (D: Immunohistochemistry with hematoxylin counterstain)

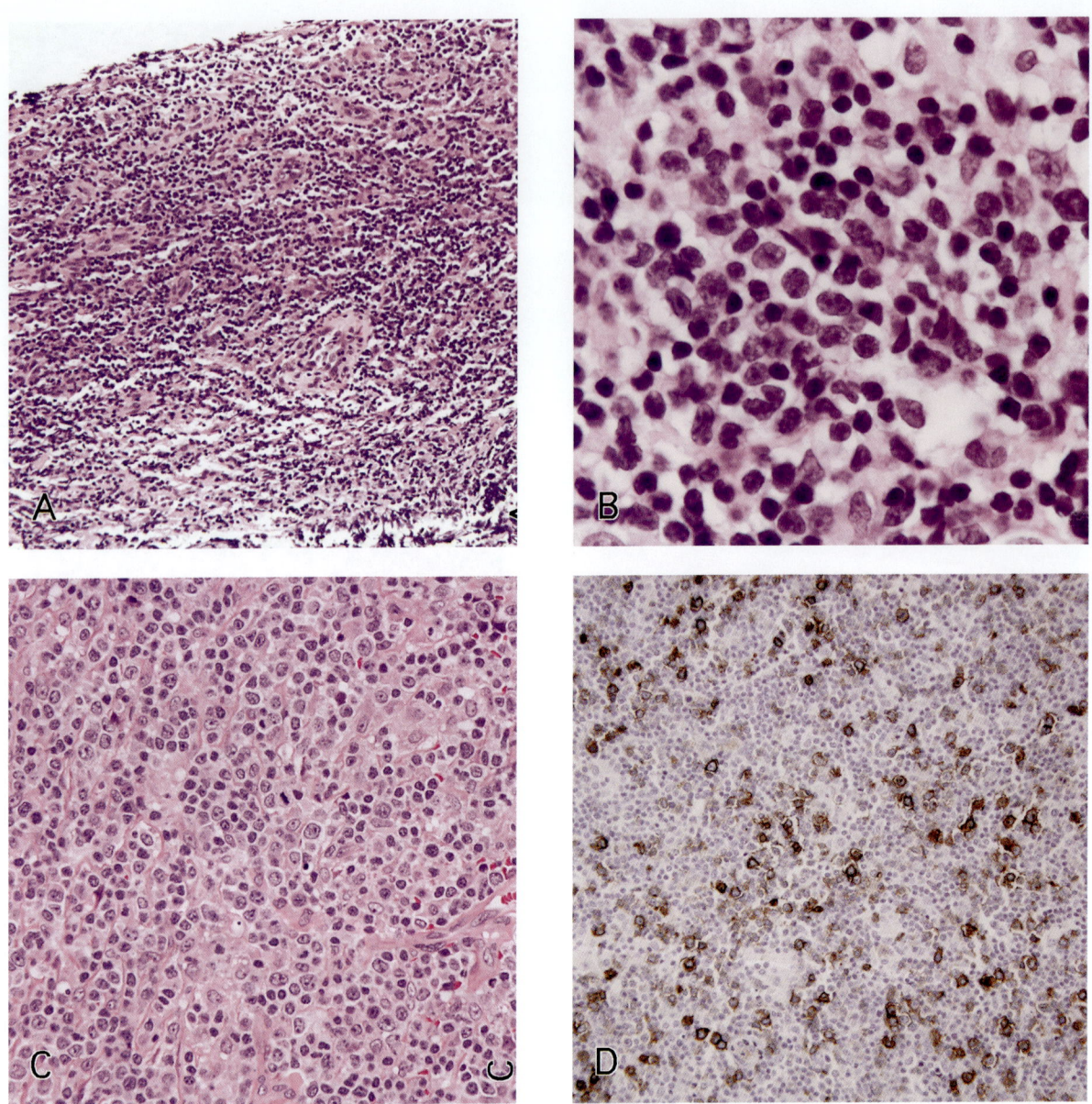

Figure 36-4

MYCOSIS FUNGOIDES WITH SUBSEQUENT LARGE CELL TRANSFORMATION INVOLVING LYMPH NODE

This patient with MF had bilateral inguinal lymphadenopathy and both sides were biopsied 14 months apart.

A,B: Needle biopsy of the left side shows that the lymph node architecture is extensively replaced by mostly small cerebriform cells, with some medium-sized to large cells (A,B: H&E stain).

C,D: Excisional biopsy of the right side shows obvious large cell transformation that is indistinguishable from other forms of peripheral T-cell lymphoma. Some of these large cells (D) are positive for CD30 (D: immunohistochemistry with hematoxylin counterstain).

Peripheral Blood and Bone Marrow

The blood may be involved by MF, most often in patients with advanced-stage disease. The term *Sézary cell* has been used to designate circulating intermediate-sized to large lymphoma cells with irregular contours that resemble the outlines of a closed fist (fig. 36-8). Smaller MF cells in the blood have been designated as *Lutzner cells*; these cells have irregular nuclear

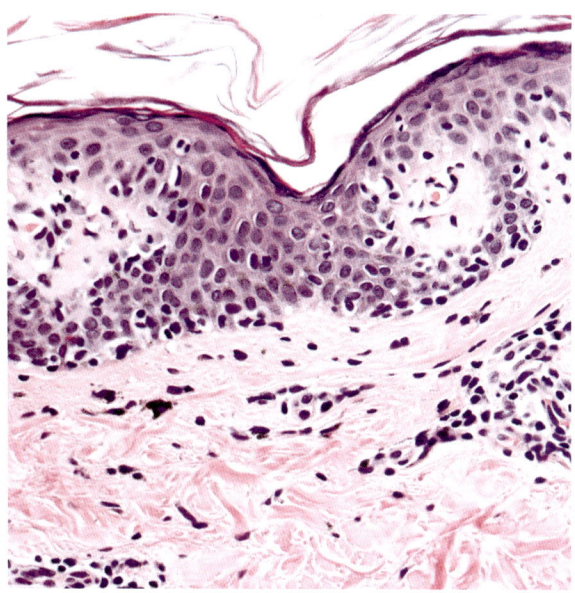

Figure 36-5

PATCH STAGE MYCOSIS FUNGOIDES INVOLVING SKIN

The lesion is flat and epidermotropism is present, best appreciated as a linear arrangement ("string of pearls") in the basal epithelial layer of the dermis. There is also some subepidermal fibrosis and a scant perivascular lymphoid infiltrate in the superficial dermis (H&E stain).

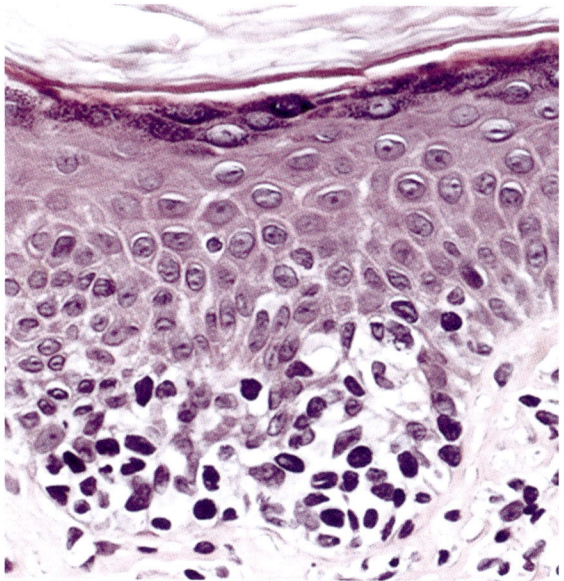

Figure 36-6

PLAQUE STAGE MYCOSIS FUNGOIDES INVOLVING SKIN

Although difficult to appreciate in this image, the lesion formed a plaque that was raised relative to the surrounding skin surface. In this field, a Pautrier microabscess is present at the epidermal-dermal junction. In addition, prominent ("wiry") subepidermal fibrosis is present indicating that the lesion is chronic (H&E stain).

contours but may be difficult to distinguish from reactive lymphocytes morphologically (fig. 36-9). Flow cytometry immunophenotypic analysis is helpful for identifying neoplastic lymphocytes in the blood of MF patients.

The blood involvement may be minimal or prominent (leukemic phase). In MF patients with lesser blood involvement and no erythroderma, the tumor is designated as *mycosis fungoides with leukemic involvement*. In MF patients with a prominent leukemic phase with erythroderma, the tumor is designated as *Sézary syndrome preceded by mycosis fungoides*. These terms are useful for distinguishing these tumors from de novo Sézary syndrome (28,48).

The bone marrow can be involved in patients with MF. Commonly, the degree of involvement is minimal and therefore often requires immunophenotypic analysis for its reliable identification. For this reason, the bone marrow is often described as being relatively spared in patients with MF. The cells of MF may be difficult to identify in aspirate smears, but resemble MF cells in blood smears. In some patients, usually those with advanced disease, the bone marrow

is extensively involved (fig. 36-10). The authors also have observed large cell transformation in the bone marrow (fig. 36-11).

Viscera

MF can involve almost any visceral organ. Patients develop tumor masses that replace the normal architecture. The tumors are usually composed of a mixture of small and large lymphoma cells, or mostly large cells, some of which are pleomorphic or anaplastic (28,30). In many cases, MF involving viscera cannot be reliably distinguished from other types of peripheral T-cell lymphoma without a clinical history. In some cases, transformed MF can mimic anaplastic large cell lymphoma.

CYTOLOGIC FINDINGS

Cytologic diagnosis by fine-needle aspiration (FNA) is most often used to evaluate potential involvement of lymph nodes or visceral sites by MF (fig. 36-12). In lymph nodes with partial

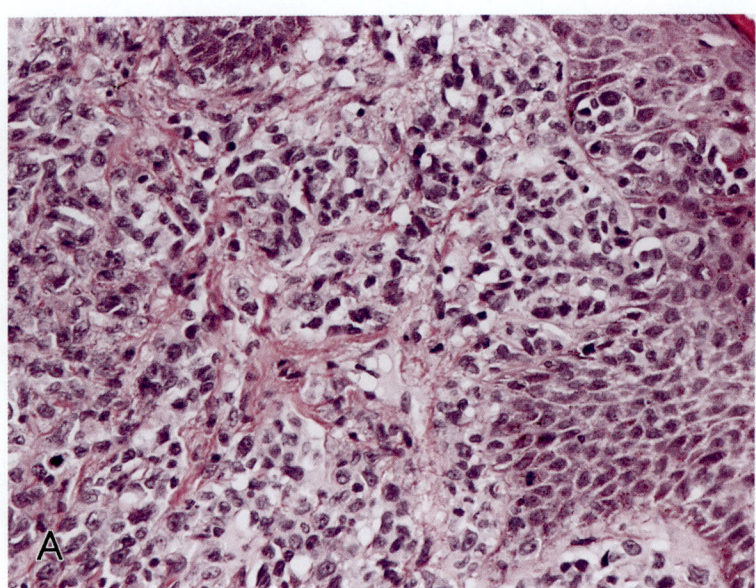

Figure 36-7

TUMOR STAGE MYCOSIS FUNGOIDES WITH LARGE CELL TRANSFORMATION

A: Large and atypical lymphoid cells diffusely replace the dermis. Epidermotropism is also present, including a Pautrier microabscess (far right of field) (H&E stain).

B,C: The lymphoma cells are uniformly and brightly positive for CD3 (B) and some aberrantly express CD20 (C). CD79a (not shown) and PAX5 (not shown) were negative in the lymphoma cells (B,C: Immunohistochemistry with hematoxylin counterstain).

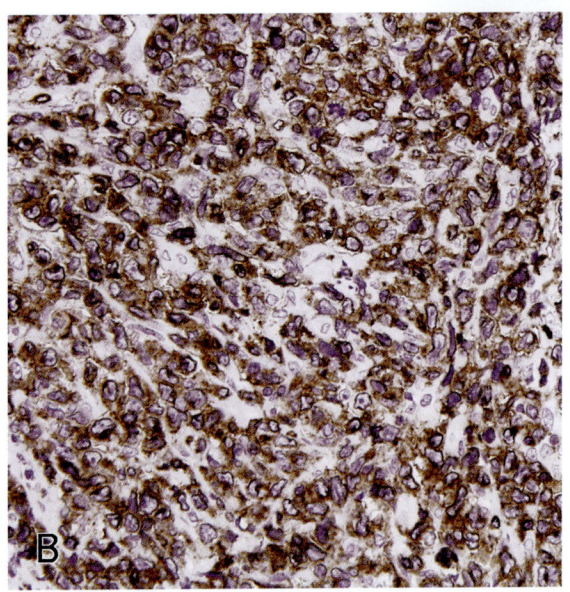

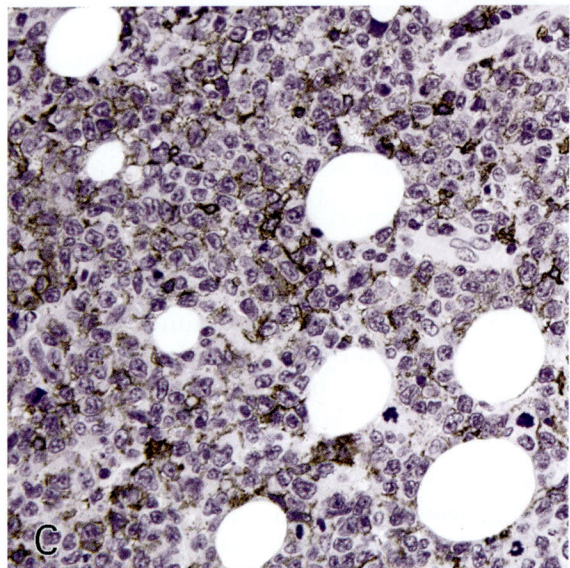

involvement by MF, establishing the diagnosis may be difficult (11). Aspirate smears may show very few neoplastic cells. The lymph nodes of MF patients commonly show dermatopathic changes that may obscure the presence of the lymphoma cells. When combined with ancillary techniques, however, such as flow cytometry immunophenotyping and molecular studies, FNA is an effective tool for evaluating lymph node status in patients with MF.

The reliability of FNA is further enhanced when the immunophenotype or molecular signature of the neoplastic clone is known. In cases with extensive lymph node or visceral involvement, smears may show a large number of atypical, medium-sized lymphoid cells with dense nuclear chromatin and irregular nuclear contours (42). Larger neoplastic cells with prominent nucleoli are observed in cases with large cell transformation.

IMMUNOPHENOTYPIC FINDINGS

The neoplastic cells of MF likely arise from skin resident effector memory T-cells and exhibit a mature T-cell immunophenotype. In most cases, the tumor cells are CD4 positive (figs. 36-2C, 36-11C).

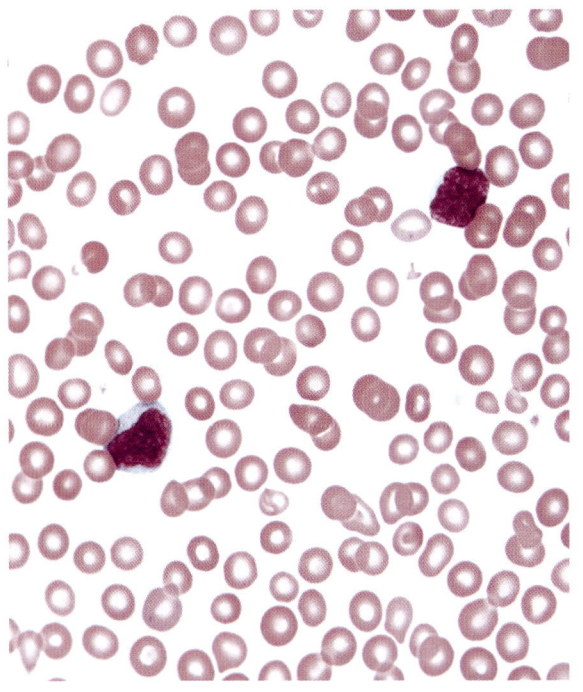

Figure 36-8

MYCOSIS FUNGOIDES INVOLVING BLOOD

Two Sézary cells, which have nuclear contours that resemble the outlines of a closed fist, are present (Wright-Giemsa stain).

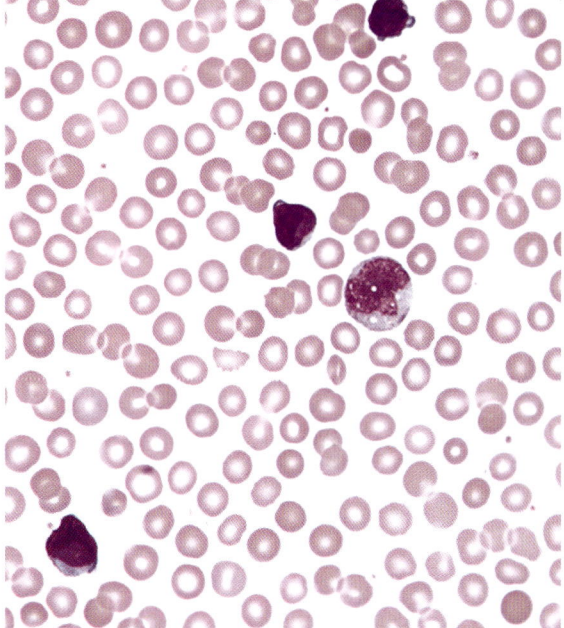

Figure 36-9

MYCOSIS FUNGOIDES WITH LEUKEMIC INVOLVEMENT

The lymphoma cells are small (Lutzner cells) and morphologically overlap with other leukemic T-cell neoplasms (Wright-Giemsa stain).

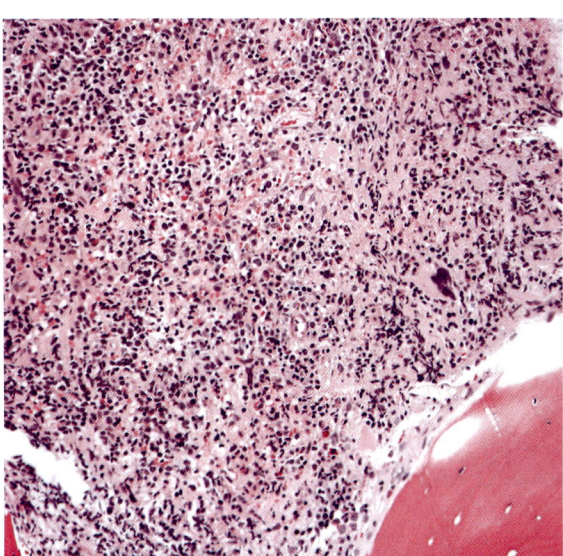

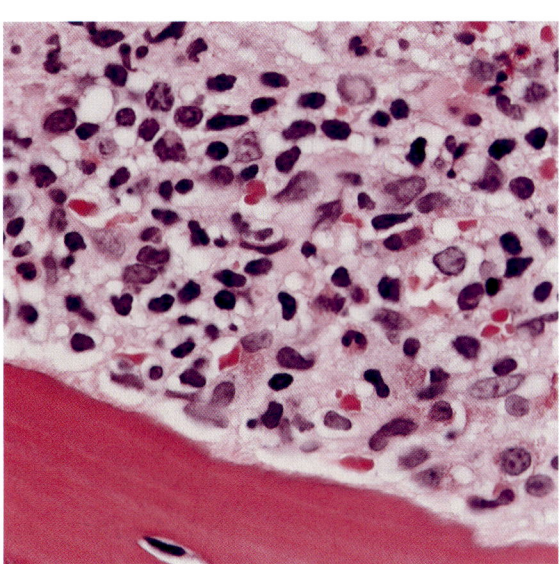

Figure 36-10

MYCOSIS FUNGOIDES INVOLVING BONE MARROW

Left, right: This patient had advanced skin disease, lymphadenopathy, and blood involvement. The bone marrow medullary space is replaced by a mixture of small and large lymphoma cells that were positive for T-cell markers including CD3 and CD4 (not shown) (H&E stain).

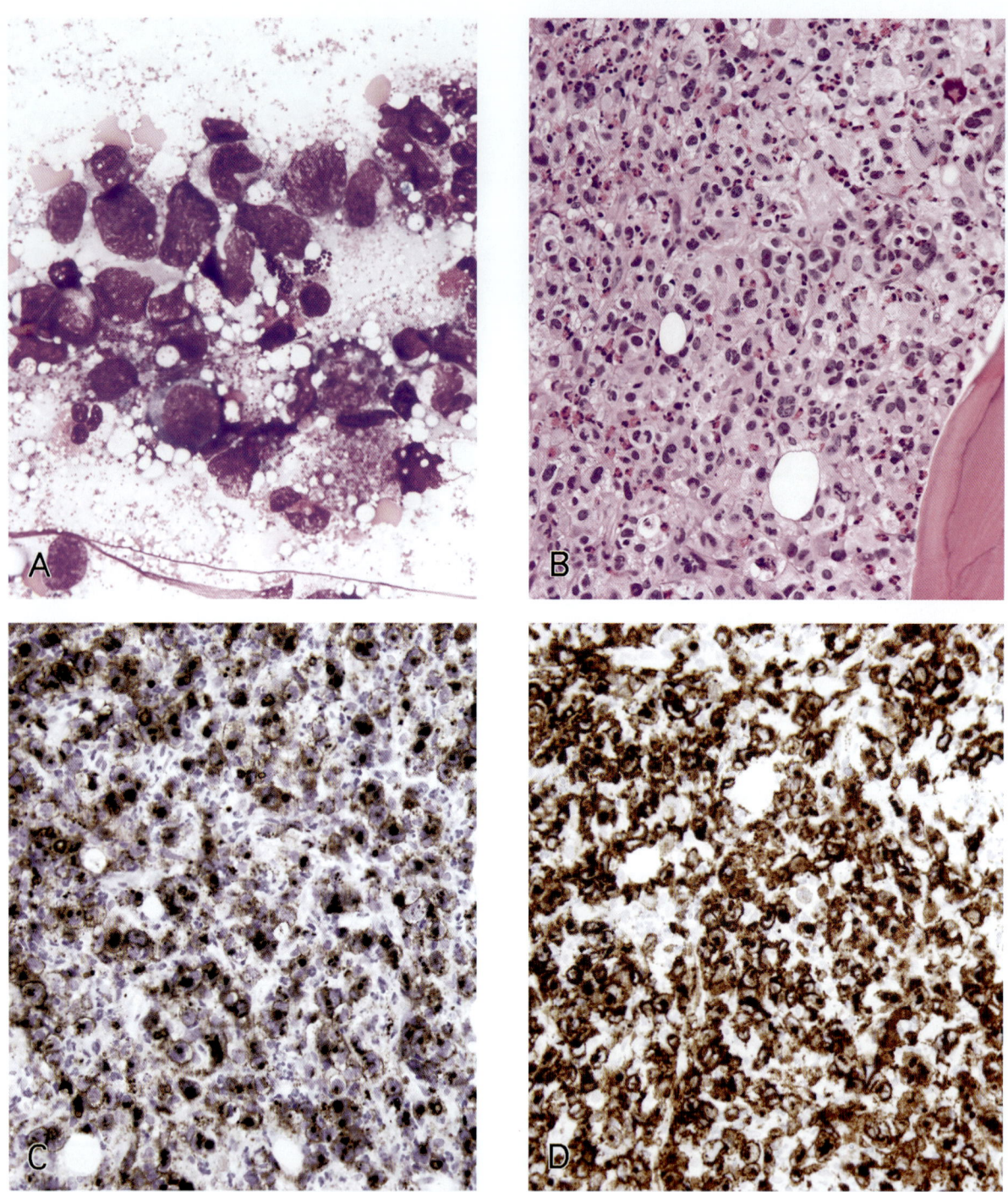

Figure 36-11

MYCOSIS FUNGOIDES WITH ANAPLASTIC LARGE CELL TRANSFORMATION INVOLVING BONE MARROW

A: The touch imprint shows many large cells (Wright-Giemsa stain).

B: The bone marrow medullary space is replaced by large cells with prominent nucleoli including some cells with horseshoe-shaped nuclei resembling hallmark cells (H&E stain).

C,D. Immunohistochemical analysis shows that the lymphoma cells were T cells dimly positive for CD4 (C) and brightly and uniformly positive for CD30 (D). The lymphoma cells were negative for ALK (not shown) (C,D: immunohistochemistry with hematoxylin counterstain).

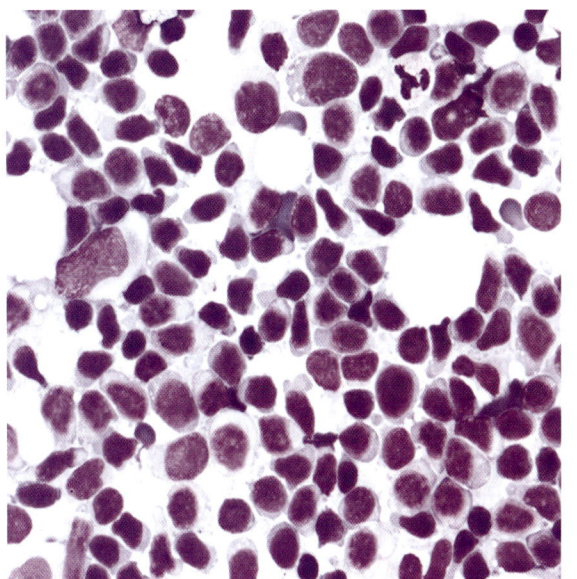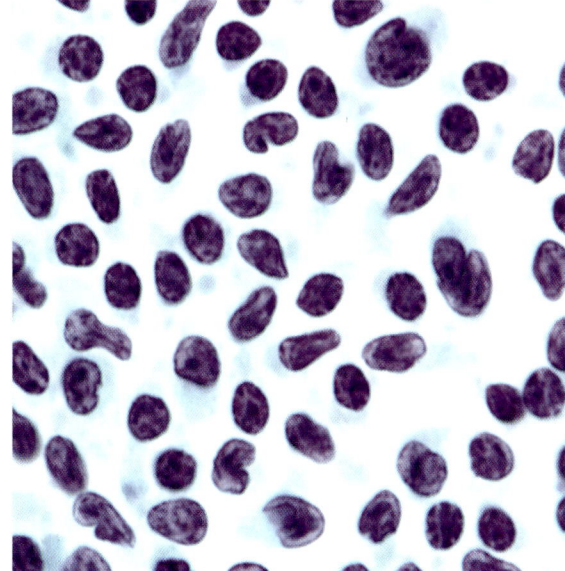

Figure 36-12

MYCOSIS FUNGOIDES INVOLVING LYMPH NODE: CYTOLOGIC FEATURES

Left, right: The fine-needle aspirate shows small to medium-sized cells with convoluted nuclei. The cerebriform nuclei are best observed on fixed smears (left: Diff-Quik stain; right: Papanicolaou stain).

The lymphoma cells are usually positive for CD2, CD3 (figs. 36-3D, 36-7B), CD5, and cytotoxic T-lymphocyte antigen 4 (CTLA-4), and are negative for CD8 (T-helper cell immunophenotype). Rare cases are CD8 positive (and CD4 negative) and very rare cases are CD4/CD8 positive or CD4/CD8 negative. CD8-positive cases of MF are more common in children and in hypopigmented lesions, but CD8 expression in otherwise typical cases of MF seems to have no importance.

Cases of MF can express CD30, usually variably in a subset of cells (fig. 36-4D). CCR4 and BCL2 are positive in many cases of MF. The proliferation rate in MF, assessed by anti-Ki67, is low in patch stage disease but can be high in tumor stage lesions. Some cells express PD1/CD279. In a small subset of MF cases, the lymphoma cells express CD56. Rare cases of MF have been reported to express TCRγ (but primary cutaneous γ/δ T-cell lymphoma needs to be excluded). The cells of MF are negative for CD1a, CD7 (usually), CD10, B-cell antigens, myeloid-associated antigens, cyclin D1, TCL1, TdT, ALK (very rare positive cases have been reported), and Epstein-Barr virus (EBV).

During the course of the disease, partial or complete loss of T-cell antigens can be observed including CD3, CD4, and βF1. Reactive B cells can be present in the background of MF and may be positive for EBV, presumably related to host immunosuppression. Rare cases of MF expressing CD20 (fig. 36-7C) have been reported; these tumors often show increased large cells and are negative for other B-cell antigens.

Large cell transformation is often accompanied by an altered immunophenotype. The large cells often express CD30 and in some cases, CD30 is expressed uniformly (similar to anaplastic large cell lymphoma) (fig. 36-11D). CD25, clusterin, and cytotoxic molecules can be expressed in MF, more often in tumor stage disease or large cell transformation (3,4). Rare cases of MF in large cell transformation are characterized by Hodgkin-like cells that may express CD15 and CD30 and resemble classic Hodgkin lymphoma (9,31). In most of these cases the large cells express one or more T-cell antigens, but T-cell antigens also may be absent (31).

Abnormalities detected by flow cytometry include the presence of a T-cell population with an increased CD4/CD8 ratio, absence of CD26, decreased intensity or complete absence of expression of CD7, and dim expression of CD2, CD3, CD4 or CD5 (10,14). CD26 expression is useful in samples collected from peripheral blood, but less so in lymph node or skin biopsy specimens because decreased expression of CD26 has been reported in reactive T cells in these tissue sites (26). Approximately 75 percent of cases of MF express a single TCR-Vβ region, supporting the presence of a monoclonal T-cell population (10). Flow cytometry analysis assessing TCR-Vβ region expression also allows for quantification of the T-cell clone and helps assess for minimal residual disease (10).

MOLECULAR GENETIC FINDINGS

Conventional cytogenetic analysis of MF cases characteristically reveals complex karyotypes, particularly in advanced stage disease. Comparative genomic hybridization methods have identified several alterations or copy number changes involving a variety of loci (21,39). Lin et al. (21), for example, reported 17 areas of copy number amplification and 40 areas of deletion. Some of the most common alterations include deletions of chromosomes 1p36, 10q, 17p, and 19, and gains on 4q, 8q,18, and 17q (21,39).

As has been reviewed (9a), genome wide studies of MF have shown great complexity, with 21 to 27 copy number variations per case, with deletions and amplifications more common than gene mutations. Pathways involved include T-cell receptor signaling, NF-κB, epigenetic modifiers, histone remodelers, regulators of the cell cycle, and apoptosis (9a). Molecular studies of MF also have shown that the number of genetic alterations is lowest in patch stage and highest in tumor stage disease. Inactivation of TP53 and the cyclin-dependent kinase inhibitors *CDKN2A*/p16^{INK4A}, *CDKN2B*/p15^{INK4A}, and *PTEN* are associated with disease progression (28,47).

Whole genome sequencing of MF cases shows mutations in genes important in chromatin remodeling and histone modification, specifically *NCOR1*, *FAT3*, *CLUAP1*, *BAI3*, and *ZEB1* (23). Mutations involving genes in the JAK-STAT pathway are reported in 10 to 20 percent of cases and the JAK-STAT pathway is activated in MF (25,35). Mutations in the JAK-STAT pathway repress miR-22, a tumor suppressor gene (35). Copy number gains of *NOTCH1* and less often *NOTCH2* mutations correlate with overexpression and advanced disease stage (15,23).

Monoclonal rearrangements of the T-cell receptor (TCR) genes are detected in most cases of MF (27,40). A polyclonal or oligoclonal pattern is seen in 15 percent of cases, particularly in early patch stage. Multicolor capillary electrophoresis (Genescan) methods to assess the TCR genes provide a molecular signature of the neoplastic clone (size and variable segment utilized) (40). Several studies have shown that detection of the same T-cell clone in more than one lesion or in a given patient over time is associated with an increased risk of disease progression (27,40).

SÉZARY SYNDROME

Sézary syndrome (SS) is related to MF and some authors have suggested that SS is the leukemic counterpart of MF. Some patients with advanced MF develop a leukemic phase of disease, with circulating Sézary cells, that resembles SS. Unlike MF (see above), the cell of origin of SS is thought to be a central memory T cell, and there are some differences in the epidemiologic features, clinical presentation, and morphologic features of the two (24,29,47,48). The genetic profiles of MF and SS also are distinctive although there is some overlap (9a). MF and SS are considered as separate diseases in the WHO classification (29,36a). SS is rare and represents only 2 to 3 percent of all T-cell lymphomas in the skin.

SS is defined as a de novo disease characterized by a triad of erythroderma, generalized lymphadenopathy, and the presence of monoclonal T cells with cerebriform nuclei in skin, lymph nodes, and peripheral blood (29). In addition, at least one of the following three criteria must be fulfilled: absolute Sézary cell count of more than 1,000 cells/mm^3, expanded CD4 cells with a CD4/CD8 ratio of greater than 10 to 1, and an aberrant T-cell immunophenotype with absence of one or more T-cell antigens (29).

Most patients are middle-aged or elderly and there is a male predominance (24,29,48). Patients often present with pruritus, which may be nearly intolerable, alopecia, palmar and plantar hyperkeratosis, and changes of the nails of the fingers and toes. As stated in the definition, patients have erythroderma, defined as diffusely red and often scaly skin (fig. 36-13), and not simply multiple, disconnected red skin lesions.

Morphologically, the lymph nodes in SS patients show involvement by a small cell infiltrate that can partially or extensively replace the parenchyma (29). Dermatopathic changes

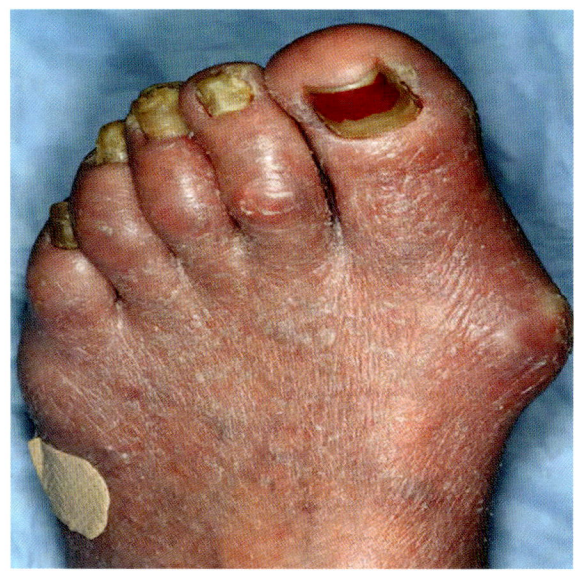

Figure 36-13

SÉZARY SYNDROME: ERYTHRODERMA

The foot of a patient with Sézary syndrome shows diffusely red skin (erythroderma).

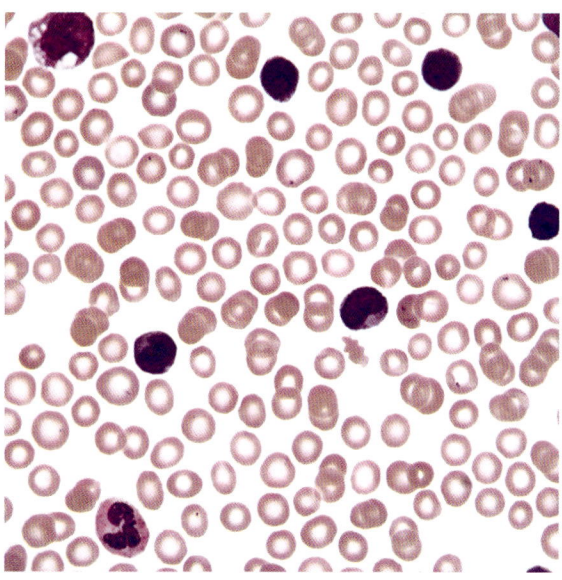

Figure 36-14

SÉZARY SYNDROME

Numerous leukemic lymphocytes are seen in a blood smear of a patient with Sézary syndrome (Wright-Giemsa stain).

may be present in lymph nodes with partial involvement. Skin biopsy specimens involved by SS may closely resemble patch stage MF, but Pautrier microabcesses are identified in only about 25 percent of cases and, in some SS biopsy specimens, there is minimal or no epidermotropism (18,29,48). Peripheral blood smears show many leukemic cells including classic Sézary cells and small cell variants that have cerebriform or rounder nuclear contours (fig. 36-14). The bone marrow is often involved, but is relatively spared considering the extent of the leukemic disease.

The cells of SS are mature T cells, usually with a T-helper cell immunophenotype, positive for CD4 and negative for CD8. Sezary cells usually express CD2, CD5, and TCRα/β and are often positive for CD25 (fig. 36-15). In some cases the lymphoma cells also express MUM1/IRF4, PD1/CD279, and CD158k (a natural killer immunoglobulin-like receptor) (18,47,48). The lymphoma cells commonly express a single TCR-Vβ region, supporting T-cell monoclonality (10). Ki-67 expression is variable, but can be high. The cells of SS often have an aberrant immunophenotype, with the absence of T-cell antigens: most often CD7 (about 67 percent) and CD26, but less often other T-cell antigens. The cells of

SS are negative for CD1a, TdT, TCL1, ALK, and B-cell– and myeloid-associated antigens (18,29).

Molecular studies have shown that the cells of SS carry monoclonal T-cell receptor gene rearrangements (27) and share molecular abnormalities with MF, but SS also has unique molecular findings (9a,37,39). TOX is highly expressed in SS cells and appears to be important in oncogenesis (13). Sequencing studies have shown that the genomic landscape of SS is complex. Loss of function mutations in chromatin remodeling and trithorax family genes (e.g., *ARID1A*) occur in most SS cases (16). Other loss of function mutations occur commonly in histone methyltransferases (e.g., *KMT2D* [*MLL2*], *KMT2C* [*MLL3*]), histone deacetylase (e.g., *NCOR1*), DNA methyltransferase (e.g., *DNMT3A*), and other genes including *CDKN1B*, *RB1*, *ZEB1*, *CARD11*, *CCR4*, *PLCG1*, and *RPS6KA1* (16,45). In some cases, gain of function mutations occur in T-cell receptor signaling and *JAK-STAT* pathway genes (16,25) as do a variety of low-level gene fusions including *TPR-MET, MYBL1-TOX, EZH2-FOXP1*, and *DNAJC15-ZMYM2* (16).

In skin biopsy specimens, SS can be difficult to distinguish from reactive skin diseases that cause erythroderma. The features more common in SS and helpful for diagnosis include cerebriform

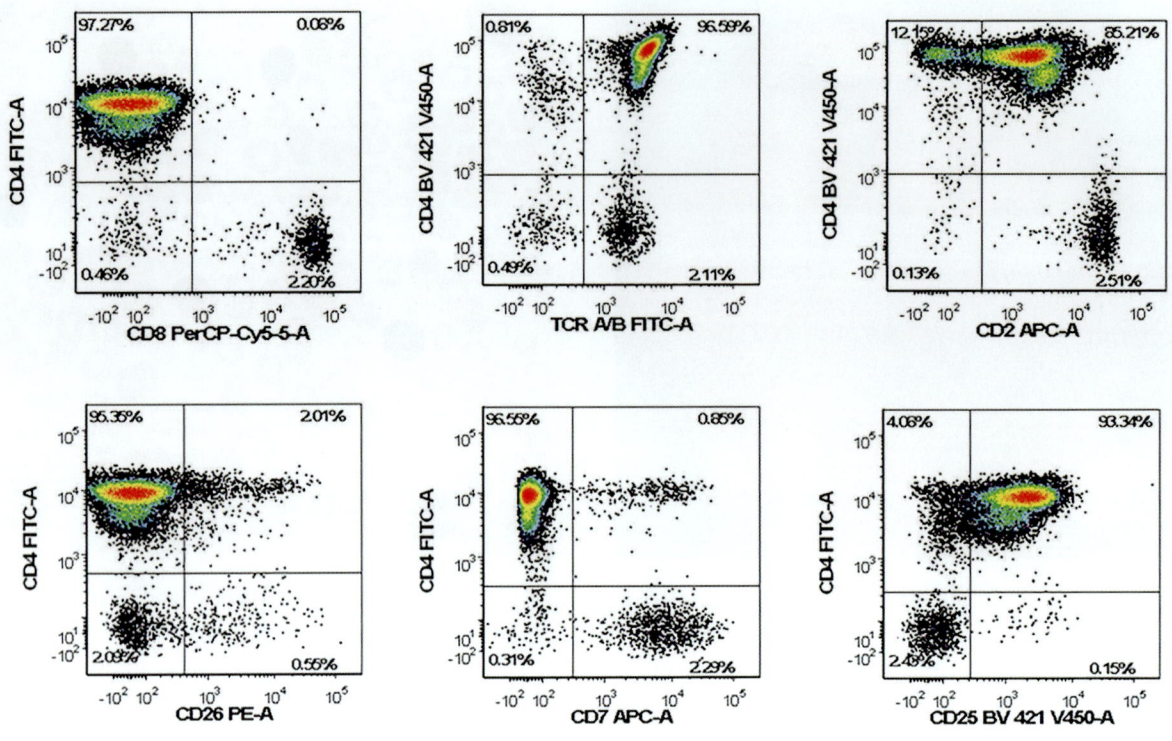

Figure 36-15

IMMUNOPHENOTYPE OF SÉZARY SYNDROME

Flow cytometry immunophenotypic results show that the neoplastic cells are positive for CD2, CD4, CD25, and TCRα/β (A/B) and are negative for CD7, CD8, and CD26. (Courtesy of Dr. S. Wang, Houston, TX.)

tumor cells, a high percentage of Ki-67-positive cells, and less reactive CD8-positive lymphocytes admixed within the tumor infiltrate (18).

The prognosis of patients with SS is generally poor. The 5-year overall survival rate is less than 20 percent. Due to either symptoms or advanced stage disease, SS patients need to be treated. Extracorporeal ultraviolet phototherapy, single agent chemotherapy (e.g., methotrexate), or combination chemotherapy has been used, but response rates are poor and recurrences in patients who do respond to therapy are common.

DIFFERENTIAL DIAGNOSIS

A clinical history, physical examination, and biopsy evaluation are fundamental to establishing the diagnosis of MF, since the gold standard for diagnosis is clinical and pathologic correlation. The differential diagnosis is broad and includes a number of inflammatory and neoplastic diseases. In general, the differential diagnosis of patch stage MF is mostly composed of reactive and inflammatory skin diseases whereas the differential diagnosis of plaque or tumor stage disease includes several other types of cutaneous lymphoma as well as systemic lymphomas involving skin.

Benign Diseases of Skin. There are a large number of benign skin diseases that present as macules or papules of inflamed and scaling skin and thus clinically mimic patch stage MF, including forms of spongiotic dermatitis and interface dermatitis. The differential diagnosis for variants of MF is broader. For example, the differential diagnosis of atrophic (poikilodermatous) MF includes other benign diseases that destroy rete ridges such as the atrophic variant of lichen planus and poikilodermatomyositis. The differential diagnosis of hypopigmented MF includes vitiligo and other diseases that cause loss of skin pigmentation. Other sources are recommended for an in depth discussion of these differential diagnoses.

Spongiotic Dermatitis. In spongiotic dermatitis, eosinophils may be common in both the epidermis and dermis; in patch stage MF, eosinophils are rare in the epidermis and usually present in low numbers in the dermis. In addition, histiocytes and Langerhans cells can collect in the epidermis of spongiotic dermatitis and mimic Pautrier microabscesses. Unlike the Pautrier microabscesses in MF, these collections of cells have a flask-like shape rather than being round or oval. Immunohistochemical analysis helps in diagnosis by determining the immunophenotype of the histiocytes (CD11c/CD68 positive) and Langerhans cells (CD1a/CD207 positive) in spongiotic dermatitis.

Interface Dermatitis. In interface dermatitis, there are numerous lymphocytes at the dermal-epidermal junction, often associated with vacuolar change or cytotoxic damage to keratinocytes and eradication of rete ridges. These changes can occur in MF, but are not a dominant feature.

Primary Cutaneous γ/δ T-Cell Lymphoma. Primary cutaneous γ/δ T-cell lymphoma is an aggressive type of lymphoma that most often involves the subcutaneous tissue and dermis, but can be epidermotropic and simulate MF. In primary cutaneous γ/δ T-cell lymphoma, the lymphoma cells are often obviously atypical and necrosis is common. The lymphoma cells express TCRγ and usually have a cytotoxic immunophenotype. Lymph nodes are usually not involved by primary cutaneous γ/δ T-cell lymphoma. Uncommon cases classified as MF that express TCRγ have been reported in the literature. There also may be an epidermotropic variant of primary cutaneous γ/δ T-cell lymphoma and criteria to distinguish diseases are not well defined (23a). Clinicopathologic correlation may be helpful in this circumstance.

CD8-Positive Aggressive Epidermotropic Cytotoxic T-Cell Lymphoma. This is a rare and very aggressive cutaneous form of CD8-positive T-cell lymphoma, also known as Berti lymphoma. Patients with these tumors usually present with widespread erosive/necrotic skin lesions and often experience a fulminant clinical course with dissemination to extracutaneous sites. Skin biopsy specimens of this lymphoma show prominent epidermotropism with extensive epidermal necrosis, and the tumors cells have a cytotoxic immunophenotype with positivity for CD8, TIA-1, and TCRβ (BF1). CD30 is typically negative.

Primary Cutaneous Anaplastic Large Cell Lymphoma. Rare cases of MF exhibit large cell transformation and uniform CD30 expression, mimicking cutaneous anaplastic large cell lymphoma (ALCL). The clinical history and presentation are more in keeping with MF: patients tend to be middle-aged or elderly and have multiple skin lesions without evidence of spontaneous regression. Other skin biopsy specimens may show typical MF or there may be evidence of MF at the edges of a CD30-positive skin lesion. In contrast, patients with cutaneous ALCL are often young adults who present with a solitary skin lesion and may show spontaneous regression.

In lymph nodes, distinguishing MF in CD30-positive large cell transformation from cutaneous ALCL or systemic anaplastic lymphoma kinase (ALK)-negative ALCL is challenging. Correlation with the clinical history, earlier or current skin biopsy specimens, and staging studies are often needed to work through this differential diagnosis. Immunophenotypic and molecular analyses are helpful. Unlike MF, the lymphoma cells of ALCL more commonly have an aberrant T-cell immunophenotype and commonly express cytotoxic markers. If present, the *DUSP22* or *TP63* rearrangement supports cutaneous or systemic ALK-negative ALCL.

Adult T-Cell Leukemia/Lymphoma. Adult T-cell leukemia/lymphoma (ATLL) can involve skin with well-formed Pautrier-like microabscesses that can mimic MF. Lymph nodes involved by ATLL may be composed predominantly of highly convoluted, small to medium-sized T cells that resemble MF involving lymph nodes. A rapid clinical course, high leukocyte count, hypercalcemia, and evidence of human T-cell lymphotropic virus (HTLV)-1 infection support the diagnosis of ATLL. Strong CD25 expression, typical of ATLL, also can occur uncommonly in MF (44).

Classic Hodgkin Lymphoma. Rare cases of MF undergo large cell transformation with Hodgkin-like cells. In the skin, differentiation from Hodgkin lymphoma is usually not problematic, but in lymph nodes distinguishing MF with Hodgkin-like cells from classic Hodgkin lymphoma can be challenging. The Hodgkin-like cells in MF may express CD15 and CD30, as occurs in classic Hodgkin lymphoma (9,31). A previous history of MF is helpful to establish the correct diagnosis. Additional features that support the diagnosis of large cell transformation of MF include: a lymph node located in a region draining cutaneous lesions, Hodgkin-like cells that are variably sized, frequent sinusoidal infiltration, expression of T-cell antigens, PAX5 negativity in Hodgkin-like cells, and the presence of monoclonal T-cell receptor gene rearrangement (9).

Angioimmunoblastic T-Cell Lymphoma. Patients with angioimmunoblastic T-cell lymphoma (AITL) have systemic disease. Almost all have lymphadenopathy and some have skin lesions. Most patients have serum hypergammaglobulinemia or other laboratory abnormalities. Gene expression profiling and other methods have shown that most cases of AITL have an immunophenotype consistent with follicular T-helper cells.

Lymph nodes in patients with AITL are usually distinguishable from those involving MF. AITL shows prominent high endothelial venules, lymphoma cells with clear cytoplasm, a highly polymorphous mixed inflammatory cell background, and proliferation of CD21-positive follicular dendritic cells. Nevertheless, LeBlanc et al. (20) have reported four patients with MF in which lymph node biopsy specimens showed features similar to those of AITL, including a proliferation of high endothelial venules and CD21-positive follicular dendritic cells. All four patients had a history of well-established MF or SS.

T-Cell Prolymphocytic Leukemia. Patients with T-cell prolymphocytic leukemia (T-PLL) may have skin lesions that might raise the possibility of MF. The lymphocytes in these skin lesions usually have prominent nucleoli, but in some cases the lymphocytes are convoluted and cytologically mimic MF cells (38). Unlike MF, patients have a high leukocyte count with numerous prolymphocytes and extensive bone marrow involvement. In addition, the lymphocytes of T-PLL are usually positive for TCL1 and show one of the following chromosomal abnormalities: inv(14)(q11q32), t(14;14)(q11;q32), or t(X;14)(q28;q11) involving the *TCL1* or *MTCP1* gene.

TREATMENT AND PROGNOSIS

Most patients with MF have limited patch stage disease, with or without plaques, and have an excellent survival rate. The goal of therapy for these patients is to provide relief from symptoms and maintain life quality. Watchful waiting or skin directed therapies are employed. Topical therapies (e.g., steroids), phototherapy, and external beam radiation therapy are also used.

For patients with advanced stage MF, the goal is to tailor therapy to each patient based on their age, performance status, extent of disease (stage), presence or absence of large cell transformation, and pace and progression (if present) of disease (33). Previous therapies used for a given patient also factor into treatment decisions. The therapeutic options for patients with advanced MF include retinoids, histone deacetylase inhibitors, interferon-α, extracorporeal photophoresis, and monoclonal antibodies (reviewed in references 46 and 47). Anti-CD25 antibody, as part of an antibody drug conjugate (e.g., denileukin diftitox), has induced good responses. Antibodies specific for CD2, CD4, CCR4 (mogamulizumab), PD-1, and other molecules are being evaluated. A phase II study has shown that many patients respond to brentuximab vedotin (anti-CD30 drug conjugate), especially in lesions that contain many CD30-positive cells (17).

The therapeutic options for patients with progressive or disseminated disease also include single and multiagent systemic chemotherapy, but most regimens result in temporary palliative control, with a short (1 year or less) median duration of response. Investigational therapies for these unfortunate patients include: lenalidomide, toll-like receptor agonists, phosphoinositide 3-kinase inhibitors, and protein kinase C inhibitors (46,47). High-dose chemotherapy supported by autologous bone marrow transplantation is another experimental treatment strategy.

Adverse prognostic factors in patients with low-stage MF include male gender, age over 60 years, folliculotropic disease, elevated serum lactate dehydrogenase (LDH) level, large cell transformation, and extensive (high-stage) disease involving blood, lymph nodes, or viscera (1,7,33,47). Lymph node evaluation is an important step in the staging of patients with MF. Patients with only dermatopathic changes (N1) or minimal (early) lymph node involvement (N2) have an 80 percent 5-year survival rate. In contrast, patients with more extensive lymph node involvement have a 5-year survival rate of less than 30 percent. Large cell transformation of MF, defined as 25 percent or more large cells in skin biopsy specimens, has a negative prognostic impact in some studies (8).

REFERENCES

1. Alberti-Violetti S, Talpur R, Schlichte M, Sui D, Duvic M. Advanced-stage mycosis fungoides and Sezary syndrome: survival and response to treatment. Clin Lymhoma Myeloma Leuk 2015;15:e105-112.
2. Boulos S, Vaid R, Aladily TN, Ivan DS, Talpur R, Duvic M. Clinical presentation, immunopathology, and treatment of juvenile-onset mycosis fungoides: a case series of 34 patients. J Am Acad Dermatol 2014;71:1117-1126.
3. Cerroni L, Rieger E, Hodl S, Kerl H. Clinicopathologic and immunologic features associated with transformation of mycosis fungoides to large-cell lymphoma. Am J Surg Pathol 1992;16:543-552.
4. Chandra P, Plaza JA, Zuo Z, et al. Clusterin expression correlates with stage and presence of large cells in mycosis fungoides. Am J Clin Pathol 2009;131:511-515.
5. Cho-Vega JH, Tschen JA, Duvic M, Vega F. Early-stage mycosis fungoides variants: case-based review. Ann Diagn Pathol 2010;14:369-385.
6. Criscione VD, Weinstock MA. Incidence of cutaneous T-cell lymphoma in the United States, 1973-2002. Arch Dermatol 2007;143:854-859.
7. Desai M, Liu S, Parker S. Clinical characteristics, prognostic factors, and survival of 393 patients with mycosis fungoides and Sezary syndrome in the southeastern United States: a single-institution cohort. J Am Acad Dermatol 2015;72:276-285.
8. Diamandidou E, Colome-Grimmer M, Fayad L, Duvic M, Kurzrock R. Transformation of mycosis fungoides/Sezary syndrome: clinical characteristics and prognosis. Blood 1998;92:1150-1159.
9. Eberle FC, Song JY, Xi L, et al. Nodal involvement by cutaneous CD30-positive T-cell lymphoma mimicking classical Hodgkin lymphoma. Am J Surg Pathol 2012;36:716-725.
9a. Elenitoba-Johnson KS, Wilcox R. A new molecular paradigm in mycosis fungoides and Sézary syndrome. Semin Diagn Pathol 2017;34:15-21.
10. Feng B, Jorgensen JL, Jones D, et al. Flow cytometric detection of peripheral blood involvement by mycosis fungoides and Sezary syndrome using T-cell receptor Vbeta chain antibodies and its application in blood staging. Mod Pathol 2010;23:284-295.
11. Galindo LM, Garcia FU, Hanau CA, et al. Fine-needle aspiration biopsy in the evaluation of lymphadenopathy associated with cutaneous T-cell lymphoma (mycosis fungoides/Sézary syndrome). Am J Clin Pathol 2000;113:865-871.
12. Hoppe RT, Medeiros LJ, Warnke RA, Wood GS. CD8-positive tumor-infiltrating lymphocytes influence the long-term survival of patients with mycosis fungoides. J Am Acad Dermatol 1995;32:448-453.
13. Huang Y, Su MW, Jiang X, Zhou Y. Evidence of an oncogenic role of aberrant TOX activation in cutaneous T-cell lymphoma. Blood 2015;125:1435-1443.
14. Jokinen CH, Fromm JR, Argenyi ZB, Olerud J, Wood BL, Greisman HA. Flow cytometric evaluation of skin biopsies for mycosis fungoides. Am J Dermatopathol 2011;33:483-491.
15. Kamstrup MR, Gjerdrum LM, Biskup E, et al. Notch1 as a potential therapeutic target in cutaneous T-cell lymphoma. Blood 2010;116:2504-2512.
16. Kiel MJ, Sahasrabuddhe AA, Rolland DC, et al. Genomic analyses reveal recurrent mutations in epigenetic modifiers and the JAK-STAT pathway in Sézary syndrome. Nat Comm 2015;6:8470.
17. Kim YH, Tavallaee M, Sundram U, et al. Phase II investigator-initiated study of brentuximab vedotin in mycosis fungoides and Sézary syndrome with variable CD30 expression level: A multi-institution collaborative project. J Clin Oncol 2015;33:3750-3758.
18. Klemke CD, Booken N, Weiss C, et al. Histopathologic and immunophenotypical criteria for the diagnosis of Sézary syndrome in differentiation from other erythrodermic skin diseases: an EORTC Cutaneous Lymphoma Task Force Study of 97 cases. Br J Dermatol 2015;173:93-105.
19. Korgavkar K, Xiong M, Weinstock M. Changing incidence trends of cutaneous T-cell lymphoma. JAMA Dermatol 2013;149:1295-1299.
20. LeBlanc RE, Lefterova MI, Suarez CJ, et al. Lymph node involvement by mycosis fungoides and Sézary syndrome mimicking angioimmunoblastic T-cell lymphoma. Hum Pathol 2015;46:1382-1389.
21. Lin WM, Lewis JM, Filler RB, et al. Characterization of the DNA copy-number genome in the blood of cutaneous T-cell lymphoma patients. J Invest Dermatol 2012;132:188-197.
22. Massone C, Kodama K, Kerl H, Cerroni L. Histopathologic features of early (patch) lesions of mycosis fungoides: a morphologic study on 745 biopsy specimens from 427 patients. Am J Surg Pathol 2005;29:550-560.
23. McGirt LY, Jia P, Baerenwald DA, et al. Whole-genome sequencing reveals oncogenic mutations in mycosis fungoides. Blood 2015;126:508-519.
23a. Merrill ED, Agbay R, Miranda RN, et al. Primary cutaneous T-cell lymphomas showing gamma-delta (γδ) phenotype and predominantly epidermotropic pattern are clinicopathologically distinct from classic primary cutaneous γδ T-cell lymphomas. Am J Surg Pathol 2017;41:204-215.

591

24. Olsen E, Vonderheid E, Pimpinelli N, et al. Revisions to the staging and classification of mycosis fungoides and Sézary syndrome: a proposal of the International Society for Cutaneous Lymphomas (ISCL) and the cutaneous lymphoma task force of the European Organization of Research and Treatment of Cancer (EORTC). Blood 2007;110:1713-1722.

25. Pérez C, González-Rincón J, Onaindia A, et al. Mutated JAK kinases and deregulated STAT activity are potential therapeutic targets in cutaneous T cell lymphoma. Haematologica 2015;100:e450-453.

26. Pierson DM, Jones D, Muzzafar T, et al. Utility of CD26 in flow cytometric immunophenotyping of T-cell lymphomas in tissue and body fluid specimens. Cytometry B Clin Cytom 2008;74:341-348.

27. Ponti R, Quaglino P, Novelli M, et al. T-cell receptor gamma gene rearrangement by multiplex polymerase chain reaction/heteroduplex analysis in patients with cutaneous T-cell lymphoma (mycosis fungoides/Sezary syndrome) and benign inflammatory disease: correlation with clinical, histological and immunophenotypical findings. Br J Dermatol 2005;153:565-573.

28. Ralfkiaer E, Cerroni L, Sander CA, Smoller BK, Willemze R. Mycosis fungoides. In: Swerdlow SH, Campo E, Harris NL, et al., eds. WHO classification of tumours of haematopoietic and lymphoid tissues. Lyon: IARC Press; 2008:296-298.

29. Ralfkiaer E, Willemze R, Whittaker SJ. Sezary syndrome. Swerdlow SH, Campo E, Harris NL, Jaffe ES, Pileri SA, Stein H, Thiele J, Vardiman JW (Eds). 2008, Lyon IARC; 299.

30. Rappaport H, Thomas LB. Mycosis fungoides: the pathology of extracutaneous involvement. Cancer 1974;34:1198-1229.

31. Reddi DM, Sebastian S, Wang E. Acquisition of CD30 and CD15 accompanied with simultaneous loss of all pan-T-cell antigens in a case of histological transformation of mycosis fungoides with involvement of regional lymph node: an immunophenotypic alteration resembling classical Hodgkin lymphoma. Am J Dermatopathol 2015;37:249-253.

32. Sausville EA, Worsham GF, Matthews MJ, et al. Histologic assessment of lymph nodes in mycosis fungoides/Sezary syndrome (cutaneous T-cell lymphoma): clinical correlations and prognostic import of a new classification system. Hum Pathol 1985;16:1098-1109.

33. Scarisbrick JJ, Prince HM, Vermeer MH, et al. Cutaneous Lymphoma International Consortium Study of outcome in advanced stages of mycosis fungoides and Sezary syndrome: effect of specific prognostic markers on survival and development of a prognostic model. J Clin Oncol 2015;33:3766-3773

34. Scheffer E, Meijer CJ, Van Vloten WA, Dermatopathic lymphadenopathy and lymph node involvement in mycosis fungoides. Cancer 1980;45:137-148.

35. Sibbesen NA, Kopp KL, Litvinov IV, et al. JAK3, STAT3, and STAT5 inhibit expression of miR-22, a novel tumor suppressor microRNA, in cutaneous T-cell lymphoma. Oncotarget 2015;6:20555-20569.

36. Sugaya M, Miyagaki T, Ohmatsu H, et al. Association of the numbers of CD163(+) cells in lesional skin and serum levels of soluble CD163 with disease progression of cutaneous T cell lymphoma. J Dermatol Sci 2012;68:45-51.

36a. Swerdlow SH, Campo E, Pileri SA, et al. The 2016 revision of the World Health Organization classification of lymphoid neoplasms. Blood 2016;127:2375-2390.

37. Ungewickell A, Bhaduri A, Rios E, et al. Genomic analysis of mycosis fungoides and Sézary syndrome identifies recurrent alterations in TNFR2. Nat Genet 2015;47:1056-1060.

38. Valbuena JR, Herling M, Admirand JH, Padula A, Jones D, Medeiros LJ. T-cell prolymphocytic leukemia involving extramedullary sites. Am J Clin Pathol 2005;123:456-464.

39. van Doorn R, van Kester MS, Djikman R, et al. Oncogenomic analysis of mycosis fungoides reveals major differences with Sézary syndrome. Blood 2009;113:127-136.

40. Vega F, Luthra R, Medeiros LJ, et al. Clonal heterogeneity in mycosis fungoides and its relationship to clinical course. Blood 2002;100:3369-3373.

41. Vergier B, de Muret A, Beylot-Barry M, et al. Transformation of mycosis fungoides: clinicopathological and prognostic features of 45 cases. French Study Group of Cutaneous Lymphomas. Blood 2000;95:2212-2218.

42. Vigliar E, Cozzolino I, Picardi M, et al. Lymph node fine needle cytology in the staging and follow-up of cutaneous lymphomas. BMC Cancer 2014;14:8.

43. Vonderheid EC, Diamond LW, Lai SM, Au F, Dellavecchia MA. Lymph node histopathologic findings in cutaneous T-cell lymphoma. A prognostic classification system based on morphologic assessment. Am J Clin Pathol 1992;97:121-129.

44. Wada DA, Pittelkow MR, Comfere NI, et al. CD4(+) CD25(+)FOXP3(+) malignant T cells in Sézary syndrome are not necessarily functional regulatory T cells. J Am Acad Dermatol 2013;69: 485-489.

45. Wang L, Ni X, Covington KR, et al. Genomic profiling of Sézary syndrome identifies alterations of key T cell signaling and differentiation genes. Nat Genet 2015;47:1426-1434.

46. Whittaker S, Hoppe R, Prince HM. How I treat mycosis fungoides and Sézary syndrome. Blood 2016;127:3142-3153.

47. Wilcox RA. Cutaneous T-cell lymphoma: 2016 update on diagnosis, risk-stratification, and management. Am J Hematol 2016;91:151-165.

48. Willemze R, Jaffe ES, Burg G. WHO-EORTC classification for cutaneous lymphomas. Blood 2005;105:3768-3785.

OVERVIEW OF HODGKIN LYMPHOMAS

GENERAL FEATURES

Hodgkin lymphomas (HL) affect approximately 9,000 new patients per year and represent about 11 percent of all lymphomas in the United States (70). The incidence of HL is similar in the United States and other resource-rich countries; it has increased over the past few decades, particularly the nodular sclerosis type in adolescents and younger adults (50). Incidence statistics for HL in resource-poor nations are less known, but overall, the nodular sclerosis type is less common, resulting in an overall lower incidence of HL.

The current classification system of HL is derived from the system developed initially by Lukes and Butler in the 1960s (45) and the terminology has undergone little change over the past 50 years. Nevertheless, although the names of current disease categories are similar to those proposed originally, the criteria for diagnosis of HL and practice patterns have changed substantially. The World Health Organization (WHO) classification system recognizes five categories: nodular sclerosis, mixed cellularity, lymphocyte-rich classic, lymphocyte depleted, and nodular lymphocyte predominant (73,75a).

Traditionally, the histologic diagnosis and classification of HL was based purely on morphologic criteria. In particular, HL was defined by the presence of Reed-Sternberg (RS) and Hodgkin (H) cells in an inflammatory cell background. The classic RS cell is a large, binucleated lymphoid cell with eosinophilic inclusion-like nucleoli, paranucleolar chromatin clearing, and thick nuclear membranes imparting an "owl's eye" appearance (fig. 37-1). H cells are large, mononucleated lymphoid cells that can have a prominent nucleolus or are multilobated and resemble, in part, RS cells (fig. 37-2). In most cases of HL, RS+H cells represent less than 5 percent and often less than 1 percent of all cells in the biopsy specimen, the remainder of the cells being benign inflammatory and lymph node stromal cells.

A major change in the approach to HL diagnosis came with the development of routine immunohistochemical analysis which facilitated direct observation of the immunophenotype of the neoplastic cells. Previously, using other methods, it had been difficult to directly assess the neoplastic cells because they were so few. Immunohistochemical studies showed that the

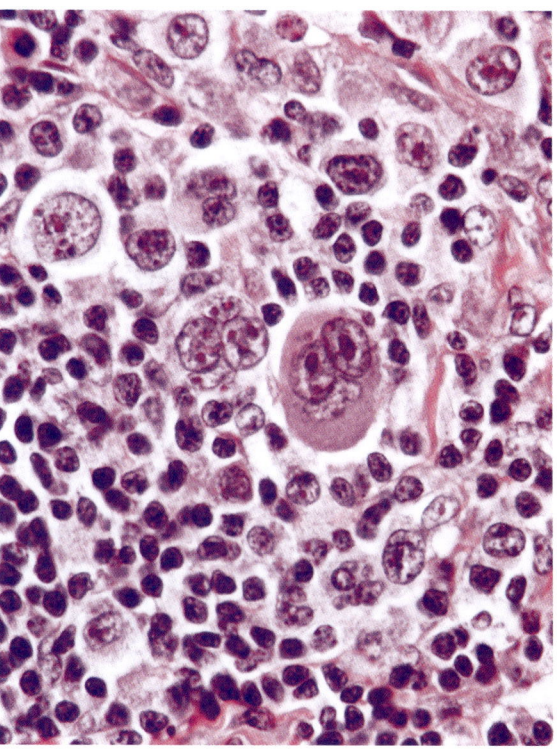

Figure 37-1

MIXED CELLULARITY HODGKIN LYMPHOMA

A classic Reed-Sternberg cell is in the center of the field. This cell is bilobed, with two prominent nucleoli surrounded by perinucleolar halos, thick nuclear membranes, and abundant cytoplasm. A few mononuclear variant (Hodgkin) cells are also present in this field (hematoxylin and eosin [H&E] stain).

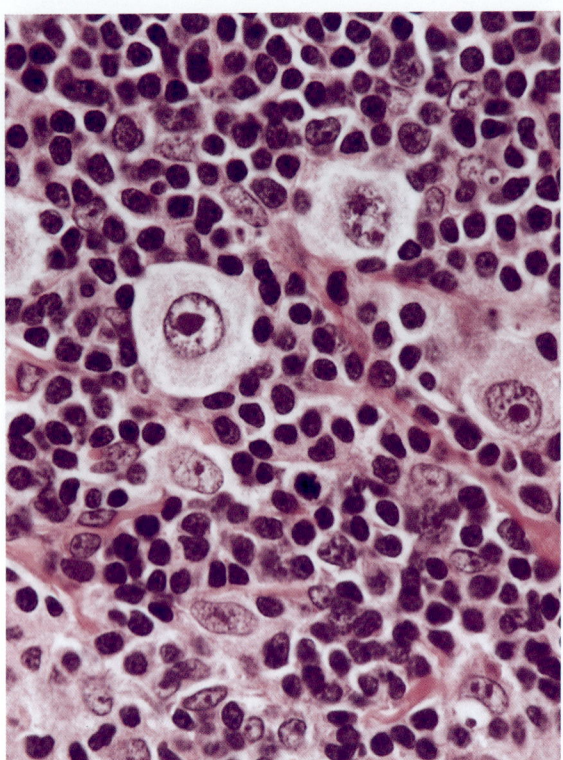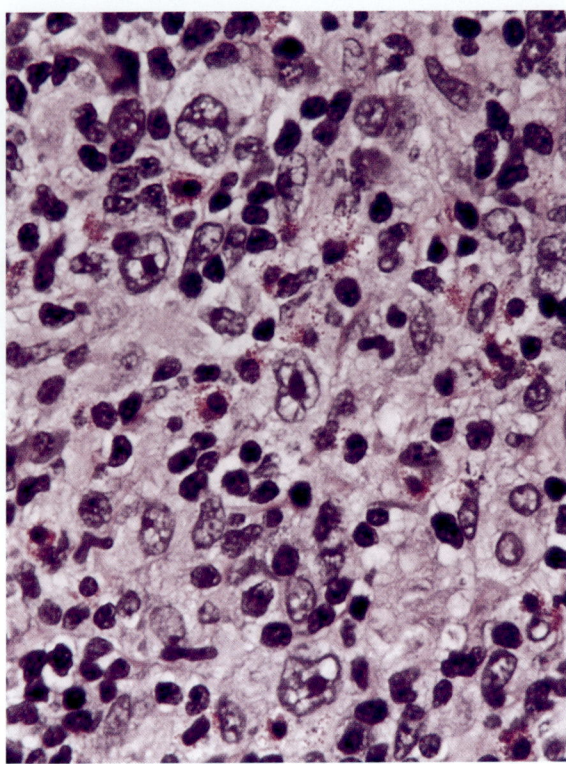

Figure 37-2

MONONUCLEAR VARIANT (HODGKIN) CELLS IN CLASSIC HODGKIN LYMPHOMA

Left: Nodular sclerosis HL with Hodgkin cells in lacunar spaces, also known as lacunar cells.
Right: Mixed cellularity HL with many Hodgkin cells in a background of small lymphocytes, histiocytes, and eosinophils (left, right: H&E stain).

lymphocyte-predominant (LP) cells of nodular lymphocyte-predominant HL have a well-developed germinal center B-cell immunophenotype and are positive for CD20 and BCL6. In contrast, the RS+H cells of all other types of HL are also of B-cell lineage, but their B-cell differentiation program is highly abnormal: usually PAX5 (dim) and CD20 and BCL6 negative (73). Molecular analysis of RS+H cells (see below) has confirmed that these cells are of germinal center B-cell origin.

Although morphologic features remain extremely important for diagnosis, the availability of routine immunohistochemical analysis has resulted in a shift in the criteria for diagnosis from those based purely on morphologic features to a combination of morphologic and immunophenotypic features. This combined approach for diagnosis has resulted in the following: 1) cases once designated as HL are reclassified as other tumor types based on immunophenotypic data; 2) refinement of the criteria for the diagnosis of

classic HL types has resulted in changes in the absolute incidence and relative frequency of diseases; 3) availability of routine immunohistochemical analysis confirms morphologic experience that classic RS cells may be rare, although distinctive mononuclear cells are easily identified in certain types of HL (e.g., nodular sclerosis); and 4) immunohistochemical studies facilitate the recognition of classic HL in small needle biopsy specimens in which RS+H cells may be difficult to appreciate morphologically due to small sample size or crush artifact. In summary, immunohistochemical analysis has become an essential part of the workup of HL cases, and the overall impact of combined morphologic and immunohistochemical analysis has improved our understanding of HL, refined classification, and changed practice patterns.

Using current diagnostic criteria for HL, in resource-rich countries, nodular sclerosis is the most common type. In the United States, nodular sclerosis represents 60 to 70 percent of all cases of HL, with a frequency up to 80 percent in certain subpopulations (50,73). Mixed cellularity is the second most common type of HL, representing 20 to 25 percent of all cases, followed by nodular lymphocyte predominant, 5 to 6 percent; lymphocyte-rich classic, 4 to 5 percent; and lymphocyte depletion, less than 1 percent of all HL cases. In resource-poor nations, mixed cellularity HL is much more common.

Nodular lymphocyte-predominant HL is different from the other types of HL in terms of clinical behavior, morphologic features, immunophenotype, and treatment approach, and therefore is discussed separately in chapter 42. The other four types of HL share immunophenotypic and molecular abnormalities, and are treated similarly. This had led to the use of the umbrella term *classic HL* for these diseases (73). Although this term is convenient and useful for highlighting the similarities between these four types of HL, this term underemphasizes the fact that the different types of classic HL have distinctive epidemiologic features, patterns of disease distribution, and morphologic features. The results of molecular studies, such as gene expression profiling, also suggest some differences between different histologic types of classic HL (9).

Bimodal Incidence of HL

When the incidence of HL is plotted against age, a bimodal distribution is observed, with incidence peaks from 15 to 25 years of age and after 45 to 50 years of age (15,47). This pattern is explained by the differences in the incidence of the two major types of classic HL. Patients with nodular sclerosis HL tend to be adolescents or younger adults, with a disease peak in the third decade. In contrast, patients with mixed cellularity HL are most often adults past the age of 30 years, with a disease peak after 45 to 50 years of age. These data led MacMahon to propose the "two disease" hypothesis for HL (47). Nodular lymphocyte predominant is a third group of HL and pediatric HL may be another group (83).

As other types of HL are uncommon relative to nodular sclerosis and mixed cellularity, their incidence patterns are difficult to appreciate when all cases of HL are plotted in this manner. Patients with lymphocyte-depleted HL are almost always adults over the age of 40 years, with their incidence contributing to the latter part of the bimodal incidence (47,50). This type of classic HL may be an end-stage of other types. Patients with nodular lymphocyte-predominant HL tend to have a low, but continuous incidence over young and older patient ages. The peak age for patients with lymphocyte-rich classic HL is the tail end of the fourth decade (73).

Epstein-Barr Virus in HL

Worldwide, Epstein-Barr virus (EBV) infection occurs in 40 to 50 percent of cases of classic HL (39,83). When present, the virus is detected in virtually all RS+H cells. Southern blot analysis using EBV terminal repeat region probes of classic HL tissues has shown that the virus is present in monoclonal form, indicating that EBV is present prior to monoclonal expansion, and therefore implicating EBV as an early event in pathogenesis (2). At least three EBV proteins expressed by RS+H cells likely provide antiapoptotic signals, thereby rescuing RS+H cells from apoptosis.

EBV nuclear antigen 1 (EBNA1), in addition to being essential for viral episome replication, helps to maintain the HL microenvironment by upregulating chemokines that attract reactive cells to the involved tumor site (e.g., CCL20 attracts T regulatory cells). Viral latent membrane protein 1 (LMP-1) aggregates on the cell membrane of RS+H cells and mimics activated CD40 receptor, thereby activating the NF-κB pathway. LMP-1 has been shown to activate other cellular pathways, including the JAK/STAT, PI3K, and AP1 pathways. Viral LMP-2a has a cytoplasmic motif that resembles the B-cell receptor (83).

The frequency of EBV in HL correlates greatly with type. In developed nations, EBV infection is most frequent in the mixed cellularity type (up to 75 percent of cases) (50,73). The lymphocyte-depleted type also is commonly positive for EBV. The frequency of EBV infection is lower in lymphocyte-rich classic HL (30 to 40 percent), and nodular sclerosis HL (about 20 percent). EBV is present rarely (less than 1 percent) in nodular lymphocyte-predominant HL (85).

EBV-infected cells in HL show a type 2 pattern of latent infection (83). Therefore, the virus is detected by immunohistochemistry for LMP1 and EBNA1 or by in situ hybridization for EBV encoded RNA1 (EBER1) (fig. 37-3).

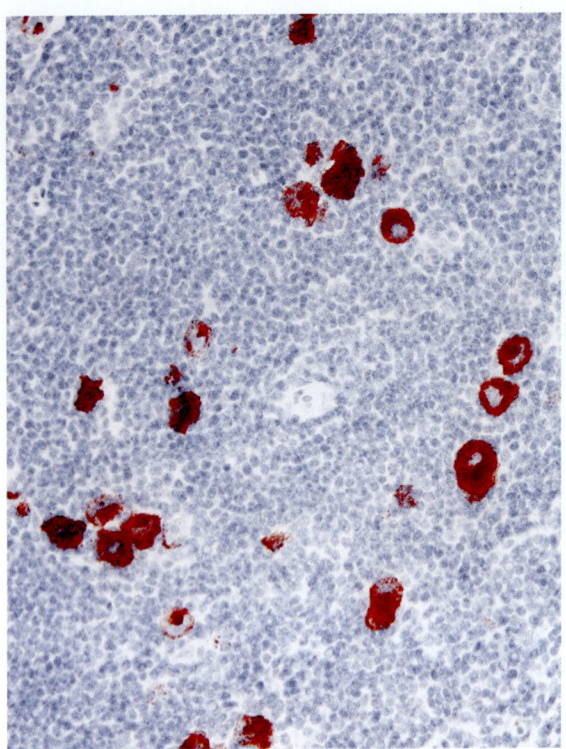 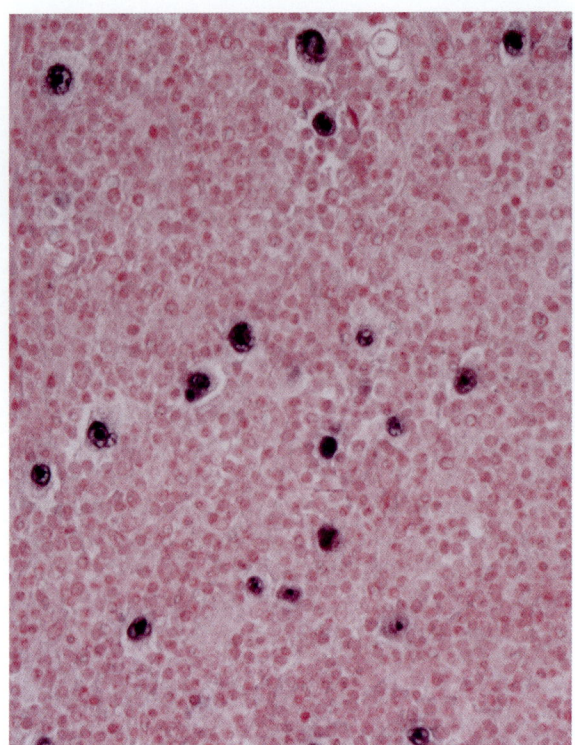

Figure 37-3

EBV-POSITIVE CLASSIC HODGKIN LYMPHOMA

Left, right: The Reed-Sternberg and Hodgkin (RS+H) cells are positive for Epstein-Barr virus (EBV) latent membrane protein 1 (left) and EBV encoded RNA1 (right) (left: immunohistochemistry with hematoxylin counterstain; right: in situ hybridization with eosin counterstain).

Risk Factors for Classic HL

Although the cause of HL is unknown, there are known risk factors that provide clues to the pathogenesis. It seems likely that there is an inherited predisposition to developing HL. This genetic risk may be specific for the onset of HL itself, or it may convey susceptibility to certain infections that may increase the risk of disease. Monozygotic twins are known to share an increased risk of classic HL (46). Patients who have first-degree relatives with HL are at greater risk of developing HL and same sex siblings, particularly sisters, are also at increased risk (19,32). Persons with multiple older (but not younger) siblings seem to be protected from developing classical HL (7).

It is known that viral infection plays a role in the risk of HL. Patients who develop infectious mononucleosis are at increased risk of developing classic HL (22,51) and EBV has been shown to be present within the RS+H cells of many classic HL cases (83). Patients with human immunodeficiency virus (HIV) have a higher risk for lymphomas including classic HL (79). There are also data suggesting that inherited human leukocyte antigen (HLA) alleles correlate with EBV status and better or worse host cytotoxic T-cell responses to classic HL (22,26). Other viral infections may be protective. For example, individuals who have developed chickenpox, pertussis, measles, rubella or mumps have a lower frequency of classic HL and therefore these infections may have a protective effect (1). Perhaps loss of this protection is a casualty of highly successful vaccine programs and may explain the increasing incidence of some types of HL.

CLINICAL FEATURES

Patients with all types of HL often present with lymphadenopathy involving the central or axial lymph node groups. The enlarged lymph nodes are firm, but not hard, and are usually painless. In most patients, the lymphadenopathy presents above the diaphragm (8).

Symptoms in patients with HL can be localized and related to the site of disease or constitutional such as fever, drenching night sweats, weight loss, and fatigue. Uncommon symptoms include intractable pruritus and painful lymph nodes after ingestion of alcohol (8). A number of uncommon autoimmune and paraneoplastic manifestations occur rarely in HL patients (Table 37-1).

Patterns of Spread and Relapse in Patients with Classic HL

As was shown by detailed staging studies, including staging laparotomy in the 1970s, classic HL is known to spread in a predictable manner. The disease begins in one lymph node, spreads to multiple lymph nodes within a group, and then to other contiguous lymph node groups (42,73). Extranodal sites of disease are uncommon and occur as a result of either localized spread or distant dissemination. Localized extranodal spread is most common and is explained by direct invasion or trafficking through lymphatics from an involved, usually large lymph node. Distant spread of HL occurs less often and usually to only four sites: spleen, liver, bone marrow, and lungs. Usually the spleen is involved first, although splenic disease may not be appreciated (8). The pattern of spread makes classic HL well suited for disease staging and, in fact, the Ann Arbor staging system was designed for HL patients.

HISTOLOGIC FINDINGS

The morphologic findings in the various types of HL are discussed individually in chapters 38 through 42.

IMMUNOPHENOTYPIC FINDINGS

In general, there has been a limited role for flow cytometry in the analysis of HL, in large part due the low number of RS+H cells; however, it has been used in some laboratories with success (61) and is likely to be more widely used in the future. To date, immunohistochemical analysis is used by most investigators. It is now recognized that nodular lymphocyte predominant and the other types of HL are fundamentally different (Table 37-2). The LP cells of nodular lymphocyte-predominant HL

Table 37-1
CLINICAL MANIFESTATIONS OF HODGKIN LYMPHOMA

Manifestations	Frequency
Lymphadenopathy	~95%
Above diaphragm	~85%
Below diaphragm	~10%
Extranodal sites	
None	~70%
Local extension from contiguous LNs[a]	~10%
Disseminated	~20%
	(Classic HL >NLPHL)
Symptoms	Common
Localized	>50%
B-type symptoms	~33%
Intractable pruritus	2-3%
Alcohol-induced pain at disease sites	1-2%
Autoimmune cytopenia	Rare
Hemolytic anemia	
Thrombocytopenia	
Kidney abnormalities	Rare
Glomerulonephritis (various types)	
Nephrotic syndrome	
Various neurologic manifestations	Rare
Cerebellar degeneration	
Guillain-Barre syndrome	
Limbic encephalitis	
Others	

[a]LN = lymph node; HL = Hodgkin lymphoma; NLPHL = nodular lymphocyte-predominant HL.

have a well-developed, albeit abnormal, B-cell differentiation program (see chapter 42). In contrast, the RS+H cells of all types of classic HL have a markedly abnormal, poorly developed B-cell differentiation program (73). Here the focus is on the immunophenotype of RS+H cells in classic HL.

The RS+H cells of classic HL are positive for CD15 (70 to 80 percent) and CD30 (virtually 100 percent) (fig. 37-4) (56,73). Both antigens are expressed characteristically in a membranous and paranuclear (Golgi) pattern. Cytoplasmic expression also occurs, but cytoplasmic expression alone is less specific, particularly for CD15. In general, CD30-positive cells outnumber CD15-positive cells in classic HL tissues. In large part, this is explained by the anti-CD30 antibody, which also highlights reactive immunoblasts, and may be more sensitive than CD15. Analysis of CD15, however, is influenced by tissue

Table 37-2
IMMUNOHISTOCHEMICAL RESULTS IN HODGKIN LYMPHOMA

Antibody	RS+H[a] Cells of Classic HL	LP Cells of NLPHL
CD3	−[b]	−
CD5	−[b]	−
CD15	+ (~70-80%)	− (rare cases +)
CD19	−/+ (5-10%+)	+
CD20	−/+ (~15%); variable and dim	LP cells +; small B cells +
CD22	−/+ (5-10%)	+
CD30	+	−/+ (5-10% dim +)
CD45/LCA	−	+ (~90%)
CD79A	−/+ (5-10%)	+
J chain	−	+
PU.1	−	+
PAX5	+ (~95%, dim)	+
EMA	− /+ (5-10%)	+/− (50-60%)
OCT2	−/+ (5-10%, dim)	+
BOB.1	−/+ (5-10%, dim)	+
BCL2	−/+ (~50%)	−
BCL6	−	+
MUM1/IRF4	+ (~90%)	−/+ (25%, dim/moderate)
Cytotoxic markers	−/+ (10-20%)	−
AP1 transcription family proteins	+	−
Galectin-1	+	−
Fascin	+/−	−/+ (10-15%, dim)
EBV	+ 75% MC; lower frequency in other types	− (very rare cases +)

[a]RS+H = Reed-Sternberg and Hodgkin cells; HL = Hodgkin lymphoma; LP = lymphocyte predominant; NLP = nodular lymphocyte predominant; EBV = Epstein-Barr virus; MC = mixed cellularity.
[b]About 5% of classic HL is positive for CD3 or CD5, usually nodular sclerosis (NS).

fixation; the frequency of expression stated above is for formalin-fixed tissue specimens. CD15 is more often (and more sharply) positive and CD30 expression can be compromised in B5-fixed tissue specimens (fig. 37-5).

The RS+H cells of classic HL are positive for the B-cell–associated transcription factor PAX5 in 90 to 95 percent of cases (fig. 37-6, left) (56,73). Typically, PAX5 intensity of expression is dim compared with reactive B lymphocytes. RS+H cells are usually negative for B-cell antigens such as CD19, CD20, CD22, and CD79A (fig. 37-6, right) (66). One or more of these antigens may be expressed in about 20 percent of cases of classic HL; usually only a subset of cells are positive with variable, but usually dim, intensity of expression (58). OCT2 and BOB.1

are uncommonly expressed by RS+H cells, and when present, usually only one marker is present and dim (44,74). The transcription factor PU.1 is consistently negative in RS+H cells (44,77). It is highly unusual for the RS+H cells of classic HL to uniformly and brightly express one or more B-cell antigens or both OCT2 and BOB.1, and other possible diagnoses need to be considered in this circumstance. Nevertheless, moderate or bright CD20 expression can occur in rare cases of classic HL that lack expression of other B-cell antigens except PAX5.

The RS+H cells are positive for MUM1/IRF4 in about 90 percent of cases (fig. 37-7) and virtually always positive for Ki-67 (73,80). Fascin is commonly positive (fig. 37-8). BCL2 is expressed by RS+H in 50 to 60 percent of cases (57). RS+H cells

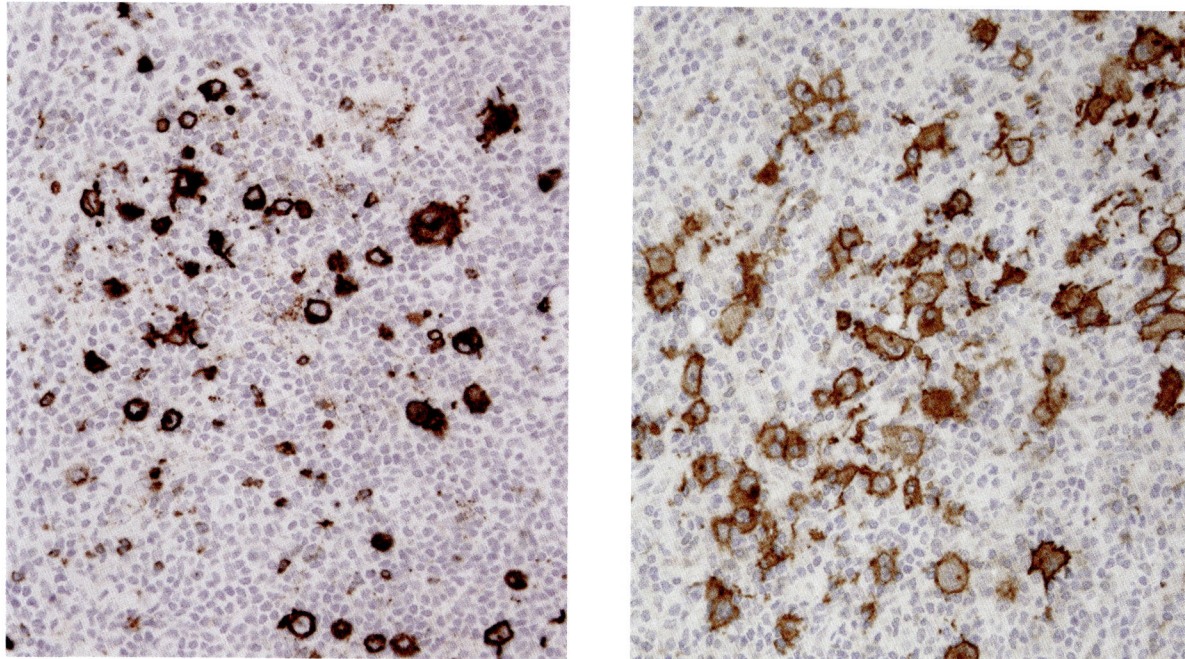

Figure 37-4

NODULAR SCLEROSIS HODGKIN LYMPHOMA: FORMALIN FIXATION

The RS+H cells are positive for CD15 (left) and CD30 (right) in a membranous and paranuclear pattern. The anti-CD15 antibody (left) also highlights granulocytes in the background. The anti-CD30 antibody (right) highlights reactive immunoblasts in the background. The biopsy specimen was fixed in neutral buffered formalin (immunohistochemistry with hematoxylin counterstain).

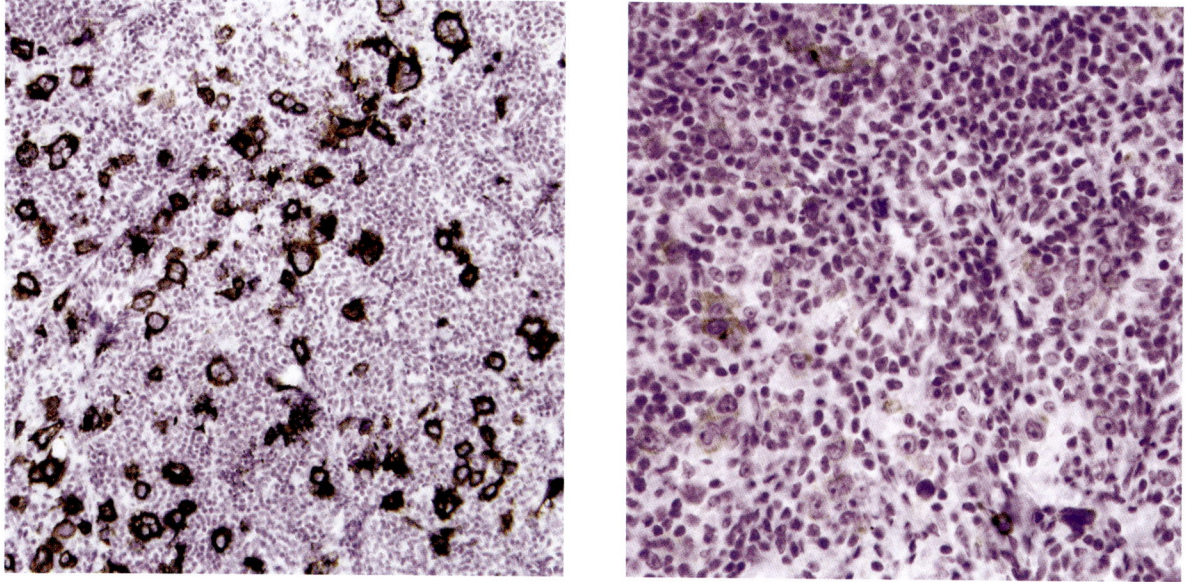

Figure 37-5

NODULAR SCLEROSIS HODGKIN LYMPHOMA: B5 FIXATION

The RS+H cells are brightly positive for CD15 (left) but the CD30 reactivity (right) is suboptimal. This biopsy specimen was fixed in B5 (immunohistochemistry with hematoxylin counterstain).

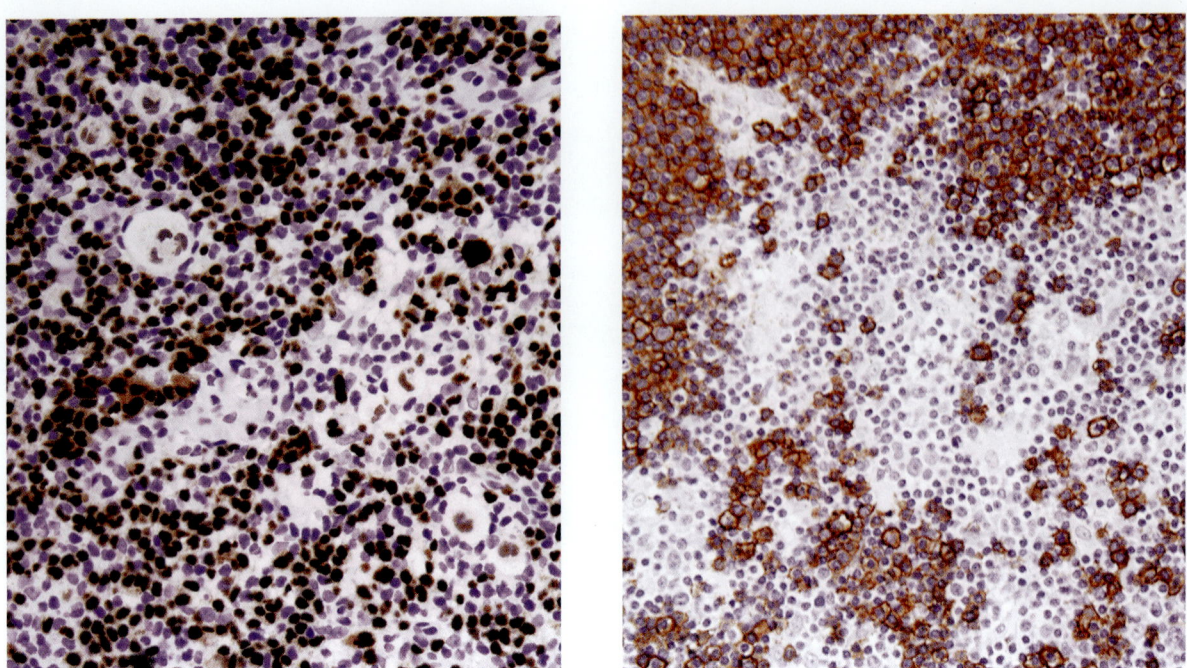

Figure 37-6

CLASSIC HODGKIN LYMPHOMA: ABERRANT B-CELL IMMUNOPHENOTYPE

The RS+H cells have an aberrant B-cell immunophenotype: dimly positive for PAX5 (left) and negative for CD20 (right). Many small reactive B cells (PAX5 and CD20 positive) are present (immunohistochemistry with hematoxylin counterstain).

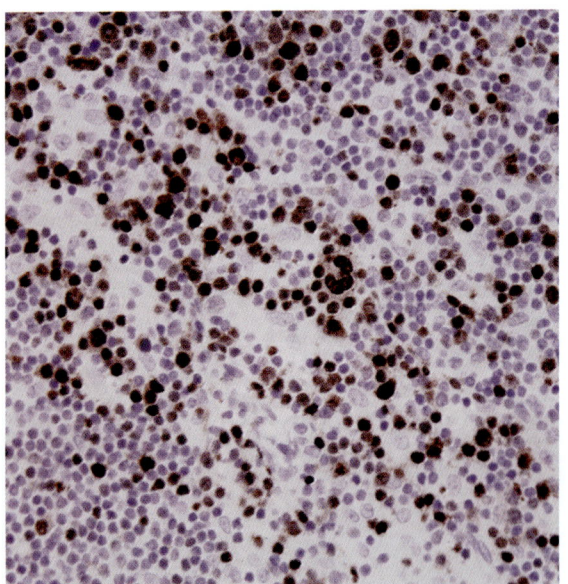

Figure 37-7

CLASSIC HODGKIN LYMPHOMA: MUM1/IRF4

The RS+H cells are positive for MUM1/IRF4 (immuno-histochemistry with hematoxylin counterstain) (same case as shown in fig. 37-4).

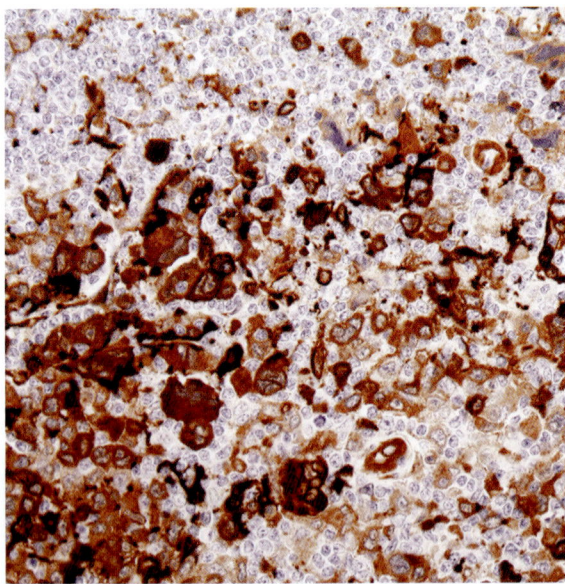

Fig. 37-8

CLASSIC HODGKIN LYMPHOMA: FASCIN

The RS+H cells are positive for fascin (immunohisto-chemistry with hematoxylin counterstain).

are usually negative for follicular dendritic cell markers, but CD21 is expressed in 5 to 10 percent of cases (33). RS+H cells express cytotoxic markers including TIA-1, granzyme B, and perforin, in 10 to 20 percent of cases (6). Epithelial membrane antigen (EMA) and BCL6 are uncommonly expressed and clusterin is usually negative (62). The neoplastic cells are negative for CD45/LCA, CD117/KIT, and podoplanin (33,73).

RS+H cells express one or more T-cell antigens in 10 to 15 percent of cases of classic HL, most often in nodular sclerosis type (69). In almost all of these cases, the RS+H cells are also positive for PAX5 and carry *IGH* rearrangements, supporting the interpretation that the RS+H cells are B cells that aberrantly express T-cell antigens. A few cases that express T-cell antigens may be truly of T-cell lineage (69). This issue is discussed in detail in chapter 38.

A number of other markers are expressed by the RS+H cells although antibodies specific for these markers rarely are used for routine diagnosis or prognostic assessment. A few markers that may become more relevant are mentioned here. RS+H cells commonly express molecules of the AP1 transcription factor family, such as JunB, c-JUN, and c-JUN N-terminal kinase (JNK), supporting activation of this pathway (40). IRF5 expression by RS+H cells may drive activation of the AP1 pathway (36). p53 is commonly expressed by RS+H cells although *TP53* is mutated rarely (12). PD-L1/CD274 and PD-L2/CD273 are strongly and uniformly expressed by RS+H cells in a subset of cases (18). RS+H cells also commonly express glioma-associated homologue 3 (GLI3) of the hedgehog pathway (16). Bruton tyrosine kinase is positive in about 25 percent of cases and is a potential target for therapy (14). Based upon their review of gene expression profiling data, Doring et al. (10) proposed four additional markers useful to support the diagnosis of classic HL: macrophage-derived chemokine/CCL22, CD83, STAT3, and tubulin beta 2 (TUBB2B); these markers are positive in over 80 percent of RS+H cells.

The background population in most cases of classic HL is composed of numerous T cells, and usually CD4-positive cells outnumber CD8-positive cells (73). T cells may form rosettes around RS+H cells; these cells are usually positive for CD4 and also often positive for follicular

T-helper cell–associated antigens such as PD1/CD279. B-cells also occur in the background of classic HL, show a range in differentiation, and in some cases, can be numerous, especially in the nodular variant of lymphocyte-rich classic type HL (78).

Other cells in the background include histiocytes, plasma cells, eosinophils, granulocytes, mast cells, fibroblasts, and endothelial cells in variable proportions. These cells express markers appropriate for their lineage and it is important to not mistake antigen expression by background cells for expression by RS+H cells.

MOLECULAR GENETIC FINDINGS

The molecular findings in all types of classic HL are thought to be similar and are discussed here as a group. To date, however, most molecular studies of classic HL have focused on nodular sclerosis HL because it is most common. There are likely some molecular differences between nodular sclerosis and other types of classic HL, as has been suggested by others (discussed in chapter 38).

Conventional cytogenetic analysis of classic HL cases has shown a variety of cytogenetic abnormalities including complex karyotypes in a subset of cases, but no consistent recurrent changes have been identified. Standard fluorescence in situ hybridization (FISH) is problematic because of the low percentage of RS+H cells. The technique of fluorescence immunophenotyping and interphase cytogenetic analysis (FICTION), which allows FISH analysis on CD30-positive RS+H cells, has shown many numerical chromosome abnormalities in classic HL (86).

Comparative genomic hybridization using whole tissue sections or microdissected CD30-positive RS+H cells has shown amplification of chromosomes 2p/*REL* and 9p24/*JAK2* (18,28). In one study, a large number of recurrent gains and losses identified subsets of classic HL more responsive or resistant to therapy (71). Many of the gains involved loci with genes associated with growth and proliferation, NF-κB activation, cell cycle control, and immune development. The losses were associated with loci of known tumor suppressor genes.

A major advance in our understanding of HL came as a result of single cell polymerase chain reaction (PCR) analysis. The results showed that all cases of nodular lymphocyte-predominant HL and virtually all cases of classic HL carry *IGH* rearrangements (reviewed in reference 38). Molecular analysis of the *IGH* variable region genes in HL also has shown a high load of somatic mutations (41). This finding suggests that the cell of origin of HL is a germinal center B cell. Rare cases of classic HL, however, are reported to carry T-cell receptor gene rearrangements, suggesting a T-cell origin (see chapter 38).

The molecular events of classic HL can be divided into two general groups: genetic changes that involve the RS+H cells themselves and changes that alter the tumor microenvironment including host immunosurveillance (reviewed in reference 49). Many cellular pathways are constitutively activated in RS+H cells and function to promote RS+H cell survival and proliferation. The NF-κB and JAK-STAT pathways have particularly prominent roles. Pathway activation is the result of a number of gene mutations and amplifications that affect the components that either activate or inhibit these pathways. In the NF-κB pathway, mutations in *NFKN1A*, *NFKB1B*, and *TNFAIP3* (encoding A20, a suppressor of NF-κB) and *REL* amplification result in NF-κB activation. HAP3K14, TRAF3, and BCL3 also can be mutated, at lower frequency, and as mentioned above, EBV can play a role in NK-κB activation, bypassing the need for genetic changes. Protein tyrosine phosphatase nonreceptor 1 (*PTPN1*), located at chromosome 20q13.13, is an inhibitor of the JAK-STAT pathway and is mutated in about 20 percent of cases of classic HL (20). Suppressor of cytokine signaling 1 (*SOCS1*) is another inhibitor of the JAK-STAT pathway that is commonly mutated. Mutations of these genes appear to be oncogenic and have a role in activating the JAK-STAT pathway. Genomic amplification of JAK2 at chromosome 9p24.1 also activates this pathway (18).

The B-cell differentiation program in RS+H cells is highly defective or suppressed and this observation has been supported by single gene experiments and gene expression profiling analysis (60,65). These results explain the highly unusual immunophenotype of RS+H cells, in particular, the common absence of expression of CD20 and other B-cell antigens. There are a number of potential explanations for the abnormal B-cell program in RS+H cells. Immunoglobulin gene

rearrangements in RS+H cells are abnormal, with crippling mutations occurring in about 25 percent of cases, usually in EBV-positive tumors (38,83). In cases with functional gene rearrangements, defects in transcription occur. RS+H cells overexpress molecules that suppress B-cell differentiation, such as NOTCH1, ABF-1, and ID2 (49). Epigenetic modification of promoters of genes that encode for IG and B-cell transcription factors (e.g., PU1, BOB.1) also has been shown (11). All of these mechanisms likely apply in different subsets of classic HL cases.

The tumor microenvironment plays a role in HL pathogenesis (reviewed in references 43, 49, and 68). One in vivo example highlighting the importance of the microenvironment is classic HL in HIV-positive patients. With the advent of highly effective retroviral therapy, the frequency of nodular sclerosis HL has increased, suggesting that the partially restored microenvironment is essential to pathogenesis (79). It seems likely that secretion of chemokines, antiapoptotic molecules, and growth factors by RS+H cells and various inflammatory and stromal cells in the microenvironment provide abundant opportunity for crosstalk, thereby promoting survival and growth of RS+H cells. Genomic amplification of 9p24.1 also leads to PD-L1 and PD-L2 being expressed by RS+H cells which can negate the host T-cell–mediated immune response (5,59a).

CIITA, located at chromosome 16p13.13, is a non-DNA binding coactivator of the major histocompatibility complex (MHC) class II promoter. Translocations/gene fusions involving *CIITA* have been described in about 15 percent of cases of classic HL (72). *CIITA* can partner with a number of other genes, creating in-frame gene fusions that result in downregulation of surface HLA class II expression by RS+H cells. Mutations in *CD58* and *B2M* also can result in decreased MHC class I expression (59b). These events make it more difficult for the host immune system to recognize and attack RS+H cells.

DIFFERENTIAL DIAGNOSIS

The differential diagnosis of HL is extensive and dependent on the type of HL. It is discussed in subsequent chapters on each type of HL. A summary of the differential diagnosis of classic HL is provided in Table 37-3.

TREATMENT AND PROGNOSIS

The treatment of patients with HL has been one of the great success stories of oncology. Currently, the overall survival of patients with all types and stages of classic HL is about 80 percent (4,25,81). Risk stratification and tailoring of therapy for patients in different risk groups has been an important part of this success. Patients with classic HL are typically divided into three prognostic groups: early stage favorable, early stage unfavorable, and advanced stage disease.

Patients with early stage favorable disease have stage I/II disease and lack all risk factors. Standard therapy for this group is 2 to 4 cycles of combination chemotherapy, most often a regimen of doxorubicin, bleomycin, vinblastine, and dacarbazine (ABVD) in the United Sates, combined with 30 Gray (Gy) of involved-field radiotherapy. Patients with early stage unfavorable disease have at least one risk factor; this factor differs somewhat between different systems employed worldwide but includes: older patient age (over 40 or 50 years), a large mediastinal mass, an elevated erythrocyte sedimentation rate (ESR), extranodal disease, 3 to 4 or more lymph node sites of disease, and histology other than nodular sclerosis type. These patients receive 4 to 6 cycles of ABVD (or alternative regimen) associated with involved-field radiotherapy (30 Gy).

Patients with advanced stage HL typically receive 6 to 8 cycles of chemotherapy and radiotherapy for residual masses. Use of fludeoxyglucose-positron emission tomography (FDG-PET) imaging after two courses of therapy helps determine the presence of residual active disease versus inflammation and scar, and a positive PET scan will likely lead to a biopsy to exclude persistent disease; if disease is present, additional therapy is indicated.

With a cure rate of about 80 percent for all patients with classic HL, there is great interest in reducing toxicity while maintaining the current outcome (4,25). It is a major challenge to design regimens that will improve the cure rate above the current level of success without increasing toxicity. Of the four drugs that comprise ABVD, bleomycin is known for its lung toxicity. In older patients, therefore, some oncologists omit bleomycin from the regimen. Brentuximab vedotin (see below) has been combined with AVD in clinical trials in the frontline setting, with the goal of increasing cure rate and reducing pulmonary toxicity and this approach appears to be promising (37).

Other therapeutic regimens have been designed to replace ABVD for the treatment of patients with classic HL. Bleomycin, etoposide, doxorubicin, cyclophosphamide, vincristine, procarbazine, and prednisone (BEACOPP) is a regimen designed by the German Hodgkin Lymphoma Study Group and is commonly used in Europe. Although BEACOPP therapy results in a higher short-term complete response and progression-free survival, this regimen is associated with more toxicity and a higher frequency of long-term complications (e.g., secondary solid tumors) and therefore long-term progression-free survival is similar to ABVD (4). Other therapeutic regimens for HL patients have been designed but, in general, they have been used less frequently than BEACOPP and appear to be associated with greater toxicity than ABVD. These data illustrate that a balance must be achieved between using more aggressive regimens that may bump up initial response rates but are associated with toxicity versus the excellent results that are achieved using salvage regimens for patients who relapse after therapy.

Novel therapies for classic HL have been developed recently and have shown promising results. As mentioned above, the anti-CD30 monoclonal antibody drug conjugate, brentuximab vedotin, has resulted in a good response in some patients who have failed standard therapies; a subset of patients has completely responded to brentuximab vedotin (4,25). This agent is becoming essential to the care of patients with refractory disease and its role in the frontline setting is being evaluated. More recently, anti-PD1 antibodies that inhibit the PD1-PD-L1 axis have been shown to be highly active in patients with refractory or relapsed classic HL (5).

Prognostic Factors

For patients with advanced classic HL, Hasenclever and Diehl (21) developed a score (known as the International Prognostic Score [IPS]) using seven factors, each representing 1 point: serum albumin less than 4 g/d dL, hemoglobin less than 10.5 g/dL, male sex, age 45 or more years, stage IV disease, leukocyte count over 15,000/mm^3, and lymphopenia of less than 600/mm^3

Table 37-3

DIFFERENTIAL DIAGNOSIS OF HODGKIN LYMPHOMA

Type of HL[a]	Tumor in Differential Diagnosis	Useful Findings for Distinguishing the Entities
NSHL	Other HL types in lymph node with fibrosis	Fibrosis is not dense and does not polarize Rare cases of NLPHL can have polarizing fibrous bands and resemble NSHL, but are CD20+, CD45/LCA+, CD15-
	Primary mediastinal large B-cell lymphoma	Sheets of neoplastic cells Minimal inflammatory cell background CD20+ CD45/LCA+ CD23+/- CD30+/- CD15-
	T-cell/histiocyte-rich large B-cell lymphoma	Large cells are CD20+ CD30+/- CD45/LCA+ CD15-
	Gray zone lymphoma	CD20+, CD30+, CD45/LCA+, CD79A+, PAX5 (bright +) CD15+/-
	ALK+ anaplastic large cell lymphoma	Hallmark cells are present Sinusoidal pattern often prominent Rarely fibrous bands surrounding nodules are present CD30+, ALK+, cytotoxic molecules+; CD15-, PAX5-, CD3-, CD5-
	ALK- anaplastic large cell lymphoma	Hallmark cells present, but less numerous Sinusoidal pattern often prominent Rarely fibrous bands surrounding nodules are present CD30+ cytotoxic molecules+/-, CD3-/+, CD5-/+ ALK-, PAX5- (rare cases +)
	Metastatic nasopharyngeal carcinoma	Posterior cervical lymph nodes Neoplastic cells are cohesive Keratin+, EMA+
	Mediastinal germ cell tumors	Oct 3/4+, PLAP+, CD117+, CD15-, PAX5- Embryonal carcinoma is CD30+
	Thymoma	Keratin+; T-cells are TdT+
	Sclerosing mediastinitis	No RS+H cells IgG4+ plasma cells
LRCHL	Nodular LPHL	Can closely resemble nodular variant of LRCHL LP cells resemble "popped corn" Nodules centered on follicles without expansion of mantle zones CD20+, CD15-, CD30-
	Nodular sclerosis HL	Collagenous bands and capsular fibrosis Lacunar cells
	Mixed cellularity HL	Background cells are heterogeneous with many histiocytes, plasma cells and/or eosinophils
MCHL	Chronic granulomatous inflammation	No RS+H cells
	T-cell/histiocyte-rich large B-cell lymphoma	Less mixed inflammatory cell background (no eosinophils) CD20+, CD45/LCA+, CD15-, CD30-/+
	Nodular sclerosis HL	Collagenous bands and lacunar cells
	Peripheral T-cell lymphoma	Lymphocytes usually show atypia and a range of cell sizes T-cell immunophenotype CD45/LCA+, CD15-, CD30-/+
LDHL	Anaplastic large cell lymphoma	Hallmark cells and extensive sinusoidal pattern T-cell or null-cell immunophenotype ALK+, CD15-, EBV-
	Syncytial variant of NSHL	Often some residual evidence of typical NSHL Mediastinum involved often (rare in LDHL)
	Diffuse large B-cell lymphoma	Sheets of neoplastic B-cells Few granulocytes or plasma cells CD30+, CD45/LCA+, CD15-
	Peripheral T-cell lymphoma	ALK- ALCL included here T-cell immunophenotype CD30-/+, CD15- Mediastinum is unusual location for PTCL
	Nonhematopoietic tumors	Clinical history often helpful Immunohistochemistry often needed CD15-, CD30-, CD45/LCA-, EBV- Solid tumor markers +

Table 37-3, continued

Type of HL[a]	Tumor in Differential Diagnosis	Useful Findings for Distinguishing the Entities
NLPHL	Progressive transformation of germinal centers	No effacement of nodal architecture No LP cells
	Follicular lymphoma	Numerous well-formed follicles Follicles in perinodal adipose tissue CD10+ monotypic Ig *IGH-BCL2*/t(14;18)(q32;q21)+
	Lymphocyte-rich classic HL, nodular variant	Expanded mantle zones Residual germinal centers+/- CD15+, CD30+, CD45/LCA-, EBV+/-
	T-cell/histiocyte-rich large B-cell lymphoma	Diffuse pattern CD20+, CD45/LCA+, CD15-, CD30-

[a]HL = Hodgkin lymphoma; NSHL = nodular sclerosis HL; NLPHL = nodular lymphocyte-predominant HL; ALK = anaplastic lymphoma kinase; EMA = epithelial membrane antigen; LRCHL = lymphocyte-rich classic HL; RS+H = Reed-Sternberg and Hodgkin cells; MCHL = mixed cellularity HL; LDHL = lymphocyte-depleted HL; LP = lymphocyte-predominant; EBV = Epstein-Barr virus; ALCL = anaplastic large cell lymphoma.

or 8 percent of total leukocytes. A higher score predicts lower freedom from progression of disease (FFP). In their study, patients had an FFP of 84 percent for score 0; 77 percent for score 1; 67 percent for score 2; 60 percent for score 3; 51 percent for score 4; and 42 percent for score 5 or more (21).

As a result of the great success of current therapy for patients with classic HL, it has been challenging to identify markers that can predict the small subset of patients who will fail standard therapy. Proposed prognostic markers include serum/plasma markers, single molecule expression by RS+H cells or cells in the microenvironment usually assessed by immunohistochemistry, and whole tissue assessment achieved by using gene expression profiling or other high-throughput methods (reviewed in reference 81). To date, many markers have correlated with prognosis, although few have been incorporated into standard patient care. Prognostication in classic HL is an area of active research and a list (although incomplete) of some of the markers reported in the literature is provided in Table 37-4.

Table 37-4

PROGNOSTIC MARKERS IN CLASSIC HODGKIN LYMPHOMA

Marker	Prognostic Impact	Reference
Nodular sclerosis (NS) type	Favorable	Many studies
Grade 2 (NS type only)	Unfavorable	Many studies
Syncytial variant (NS type only)	Unfavorable	69a
High number of eosinophils	Unfavorable in NS	84
High number of macrophages	Unfavorable	59
High number of mast cells	Unfavorable in MC	3
Macrophage gene expression profile and high number CD68 cells	Unfavorable	68
High absolute monocytes and low lymphocyte/monocyte ratio in blood	Unfavorable	76
High neutrophil/lymphocyte ratio	Unfavorable in NS	47a
High TARC (CCL17) in plasma	Unfavorable	55
High EBV[a] DNA in plasma	Unfavorable	24, 30
High interleukin (IL) 6 and IL-2R in serum	Unfavorable	48
High IL-10 in serum	Unfavorable	23, 82
High beta-2-microglobulin in serum	Unfavorable	52
High galectin-1 in serum	Unfavorable	54
Increased T-regulatory cells in tumor microenvironment	Favorable	31
Galectin-1 expression by cells in tumor microenvironment	Unfavorable	29
CSF-1R expression by cells in tumor microenvironment	Unfavorable	35
HGAL expression by RS+H cells	Favorable	53
COX2 expression by RS+H cells	Unfavorable	34
Cytotoxic markers by RS+H cells	Unfavorable	6
T-cell antigens by RS+H cells	Unfavorable	6
EBV infection of RS+H cells	Unfavorable	13, 27
BCL2 expression by RS+H cells	Unfavorable	57, 75
ABCC1 expression by RS+H	Unfavorable	17
KDM4B or KDM4D expression by RS+H cells	Unfavorable	6a
Decreased expression of MHC class I by RS+H cells	Unfavorable	59b
Gene expression profile (11 genes)	Unfavorable	64
Gene expression profile (23 genes)	Unfavorable	67
MicroRNA profile (overexpression of MIR21, MIR92B*,MIR30D, MIR30E)	Unfavorable	63
Genetic alteration of PD-L1 and PD-L2 by RS&H cells	Unfavorable	59a

[a]EBV = Epstein Barr virus; RS+H cells = Reed-Sternberg and Hodgkin cells; NS = nodular sclerosis; MC = mixed cellularity.

REFERENCES

1. Alexander FE, Jarrett RF, Lawrence D, et al. Risk factors for Hodgkin's disease by Epstein-Barr virus (EBV) status: prior infection by EBV and other agents. Br J Cancer 2000;82:1117-1121.
2. Anagnostopoulos I, Herbst H, Niedobitek G, Stein H. Demonstration of monoclonal EBV genomes in Hodgkin's disease and Ki-1-positive anaplastic large cell lymphoma by combined Southern blot and in situ hybridization. Blood 1989;74:810-816.
3. Andersen MD, Kamper P, Nielsen PS, et al. Tumour-associated mast cells in classical Hodgkin's lymphoma: correlation with histological subtype, other tumour-infiltrating inflammatory cell subsets and outcome. Eur J Haematol 2016;96:252-259.
4. Ansell SM. Hodgkin lymphoma: 2016 update on diagnosis, risk-stratification, and management. Am J Hematol 2016;91:434-442.
5. Ansell SM, Lesokhin AM, Borrello I, et al. PD-1 blockade with nivolumab in relapsed and refractory Hodgkin's lymphoma. N Engl J Med 2015;372:311-319.
6. Asano N, Oshiro A, Matsuo K, et al. Prognostic significance of T-cell or cytotoxic molecules phenotype in classical Hodgkin's lymphoma: a clinicopathologic study. J Clin Oncol 2006;24:4626-4633.
6a. Bur H, Haapasaari KM, Turpeenniemi-Hujanen T, et al. Strong KDM4B and KDM4D expression associates with radioresistance and aggressive phenotype in classical hodgkin lymphoma. Anticancer Res 2016;36:4677-4683.
7. Chang ET, Montgomerey SM, Richiardi L, Ehlin A, Ekbom A, Lambe M. Number of siblings and risk of Hodgkin's lymphoma. Cancer Epidemiol Biomarkers Prev 2004;13:1236-1243.
8. Connors JM. Clinical manifestations and natural history of Hodgkin's lymphoma. Cancer J 2009;15:124-128.
9. Devilard E, Bertucci F, Trempat P, et al. Gene expression profiling defines molecular subtypes of classical Hodgkin's disease. Oncogene 2002;21:3095-3102.
10. Döring C, Hansmann ML, Agostinelli C, et al. A novel immunohistochemical classifier to distinguish Hodgkin lymphoma from ALK anaplastic large cell lymphoma. Mod Pathol 2014;27:1345-1354.
11. Ehlers A, Oker E, Bentink S, Lenze D, Stein H, Hummel M. Histone acetylation and DNA demethylation of B cells result in a Hodgkin-like phenotype. Leukemia 2008;22:835-841.
12. Elenitoba-Johnson KS, Medeiros LJ, Khorsand J, King TC. P53 expression in Reed-Sternberg cells does not correlate with gene mutations in Hodgkin's disease. Am J Clin Pathol 1996;106:728-738.
13. Elsayed AA. Asano N, Ohshima K, Izutsu K, Kinoshita T, Nakamura S. Prognostic significance of CD20 expression and Epstein-Barr virus (EBV) association in classical Hodgkin lymphoma in Japan: a clinicopathologic study. Pathol Int 2014;64:336-345.
14. Fernández-Vega I, Quirós LM, Santos-Juanes J, Pane-Foix M, Marafioti T. Bruton's tyrosine kinase (Btk) is a useful marker for Hodgkin and B cell non-Hodgkin lymphoma. Virchows Arch 2015;466:229-235.
15. Glaser SL, Jarrett RF. The epidemiology of Hodgkin's disease. Bailleres Clin Haematol 1996;9:401-416.
16. Greaves WO, Kim JE, Singh RR, et al. Glioma-associated oncogene homologue 3, a hedgehog transcription factor, is highly expressed in Hodgkin and Reed-Sternberg cells of classical Hodgkin lymphoma. Hum Pathol 2011;42:1643-1652.
17. Greaves W, Xiao L, Sanchez-Espiridion B, et al. Detection of ABCC1 expression in classical Hodgkin lymphoma is associated with increased risk of treatment failure using standard chemotherapy protocols. J Hematol Oncol 2012;5:47.
18. Green MR, Monti S, Rodig SJ, et al. Integrative analysis reveals selective 9p24.1 amplification, increased PD-1 ligand expression, and further induction via JAK2 in nodular sclerosis Hodgkin lymphoma and primary medistinal large B-cell lymphoma. Blood 2010;116:3268-3277.
19. Grufferman S, Cole P, Smith PG, Lukes RJ. Hodgkin's disease in siblings. N Engl J Med 1977;296:248-250.
20. Gunawardana J, Chan FC, Telenius A, et al. Recurrent somatic mutations of PTPN1 in primary mediastinal B cell lymphoma and Hodgkin lymphoma. Nat Genet 2014;46:329-335.
21. Hasenclever D, Diehl V. A prognostic score for advanced Hodgkin's disease. International Prognostic Factors Project for Advanced Hodgkin's disease. N Engl J Med 1998;339:1506-1514.
22. Hjalgrim H, Rostgaard K, Johnson PC, et al. HLA-A alleles and infectious mononucleosis suggest a critical role for cytotoxic response in EBV-related Hodgkin lymphoma. Proc Natl Acad Sci USA 2010;107:6400-6405.
23. Hohaus S, Giachelia M, Massini G, et al. Clinical significance of interleukin-10 gene polymorphisms and plasma levels in Hodgkin lymphoma. Leuk Res 2009;33:1352-1356.

607

24. Hohaus S, Santangfelo R, Giachelia M, et al. The viral load of Epstein-Barr virus (EBV) DNA in peripheral blood predicts for biological and clinical characteristics in Hodgkin lymphoma. Clin Cancer Res 2011; 17:2885-2892.

25. Hoppe RT, Advani RH, Ai WZ, et al. Hodgkin lymphoma, version 2.2015. J Natl Compr Canc Netw 2015;13:554-586.

26. Huang X, Kushekhar K, Nolte I, et al. Multiple HLA class I and II associations in classical Hodgkin lymphoma and EBV status defined subgroups. Blood 2011;118:5211-5217.

27. Jarrett RF, Stark GL, White J, et al. Impact of tumor Epstein-Barr virus status on presenting features and outcome in age-defined subgroups of patients with classic Hodgkin lymphoma. Blood 2005;106:2444-2451.

28. Joos S, Menz CK, Wrobel G, et al. Classical Hodgkin lymphoma is characterized by recurrent copy number gains of the short arm of chromosome 2. Blood 2002;99:1381-1387.

29. Kamper P, Ludvigsen M, Bendix K, et al. Proteomic analysis identifies galectin-1 as a predictive biomarker for relapsed/refractory disease in classical Hodgkin lymphoma. Blood 2011;117:6638-6649.

30. Kanakry JA, Li H, Gellert LL, et al. Plasma Epstein-Barr virus DNA predicts outcome in advanced Hodgkin lymphoma: correlative analysis from a large North American cooperative group trial. Blood 2013;121:3547-3553.

31. Kelley TW, Pohlman B, Elson P, Hsi ED. The ratio of FOXP3+ regulatory T cells to granzyme B+ cytotoxic T/NK cells predicts prognosis in classical Hodgkin lymphoma and is independent of bcl-2 and MAL expression. Am J Clin Pathol 2007;128:958-965.

32. Kharazmi E, Fallah M, Pukkala E, et al. Risk of familial classical Hodgkin lymphoma by relationship, histology, age, and sex: a joint study from five Nordic countries. Blood 2015;126:1990-1995.

33. Kim SH, Choe JY, Jeon Y, et al. Frequent expression of follicular dendritic cell markers in Hodgkin lymphoma and anaplastic large cell lymphoma. J Clin Pathol 2013;66:589-596.

34. Koh YW, Park C, Yoon DH, Suh C, Huh J. Prognostic significance of COX-2 expression and correlation with Bcl-2 and VEGF expression, microvessel density, and clinical variables in classical Hodgkin lymphoma. Am J Surg Pathol 2013;37:1242-1251.

35. Koh YW, Park C, Yoon DH, Suh C, Huh J. CSF-1R expression in tumor-associated macrophages is associated with worse prognosis in classical Hodgkin lymphoma. Am J Clin Pathol 2014;141:573-583.

36. Kreher S, Bouhlel MA, Cauchy P, et al. Mapping of transcription factor motifs in active chromatin identifies IRF5 as key regulator in classical Hodgkin lymphoma. Proc Natl Acad Sci USA 2014;111:E4513-4522.

37. Kumar A, Casulo C, Yahalom J, et al. Brentuximab vedotin and AVD followed by involved-site radiotherapy in early stage, unfavorable risk Hodgkin lymphoma. Blood 2016;128:1458-1464.

38. Küppers R, Rajewsky K. The origin of Hodgkin and Reed/Sternberg cells in Hodgkin's disease. Annu Rev Immunol 1998;16:471-493.

39. Lee JH, Kim Y, Choi JW, Kim YS. Prevalence and prognostic significance of Epstein-Barr virus infection in classical Hodgkin's lymphoma: a meta-analysis. Arch Med Res 2014;45:417-431.

40. Leventaki V, Drakos E, Karanikou M, et al. c-JUN N-terminal kinase (JNK) is activated and contributes to tumor cell proliferation in classical Hodgkin lymphoma. Hum Pathol 2014;45:565-572.

41. Liso A, Capello D, Marafioti T, et al. Aberrant somatic hypermutation in tumor cells of nodular-lymphocyte-predominant and classic Hodgkin lymphoma. Blood 2006;108:1013-1020.

42. Lister TA, Crowther D, Sutcliffe SB, et al. Report of a committee convened to discuss the evaluation and staging of patients with Hodgkin's disease: Cotswolds meeting. J Clin Oncol 1989;7:1630-1636.

43. Liu Y, Sattarzadeh A, Diepstra A, Visser L, van den Berg A. The microenvironment in classical Hodgkin lymphoma: an actively shaped and essential tumor component. Semin Cancer Biol 2014;24:15-22.

44. Loddenkemper C, Anagnostopoulos I, Hummel M, et al. Differential Emu enhancer activity and expression of BOB.1/OBF.1, Oct2, PU.1, and immunoglobulin in reactive B-cell populations, B-cell non-Hodgkin lymphomas, and Hodgkin lymphomas. J Pathol 2004;202:60-69.

45. Lukes RJ, Butler JJ. The pathology and nomenclature of Hodgkin's disease. Cancer Res 1966;26:1063-1083.

46. Mack TM, Cozen W, Shibata DK, et al. Concordance for Hodgkin's disease in identical twins suggesting genetic susceptibilty to the young-adult form of the disease. N Engl J Med 1995;332:413-418.

47. MacMahon B. Epidemiology of Hodgkin's disease. Cancer Res 1966;26:1189-1200.

47a. Marcheselli R, Bari A, Tadmor T, et al. Neutrophil-lymphocyte ratio at diagnosis is an independent prognostic factor in patients with nodular sclerosis Hodgkin lymphoma: results of a large multicenter study involving 990 patients. Hematol Oncol 2016. [Epub ahead of print]

608

48. Marri PR, Hodge LS, Maurer MJ, et al. Prognostic significance of pretreatment serum cytokines in classical Hodgkin lymphoma. Clin Cancer Res 2013;19:6812-6819.

49. Mathas S, Hartmann S, Küppers R. Hodgkin lymphoma: pathology and biology. Semin Hematol 2016;53:139-147.

50. Medeiros LJ, Greiner TC. Hodgkin's disease. Cancer 1995;75(Suppl):357-369.

51. Mueller N, Evans A, Harris NL, et al. Hodgkin's disease and Epstein-Barr virus. Altered antibody pattern before diagnosis. N Engl J Med 1989;320:689-695.

52. Nakajima Y, Tomita N, Watanabe R, et al. Prognostic significance of serum beta-2 microglobulin level in Hodgkin lymphoma treated with ABVD-based therapy. Med Oncol 2014;31:185.

53. Natkunam Y, Hsi ED, Aoun P, et al. Expression of the human germinal center-associated lymphoma (HGAL) protein identifies a subset of classic Hodgkin lymphoma of germinal center derivation and improved survival. Blood 2007;109:298-305.

54. Ouyang J, Plütschow A, Pogge von Strandmann E, et al. Galectin-1 serum levels reflect tumor burden and adverse clinical features in classical Hodgkin lymphoma. Blood 2013;121:3431-3433.

55. Plattel WJ, van den Berg A, Visser L, et al. Plasma thymus and activation-regulated chemokine as an early response marker in classical Hodgkin's lymphoma. Haematologica 2012;97:410-415.

56. Poppema S. Immunobiology and pathophysiology of Hodgkin lymphomas. Hematology Am Soc Hematol Educ Program 2005;231-238.

57. Rassidakis GZ, Medeiros LJ, Vassilakopoulos TP, et al. BCL-2 expression in Hodgkin and Reed-Sternberg cells of classical Hodgkin disease predicts a poorer prognosis in patients treated with ABVD or equivalent regimens. Blood 2002; 100:3935-3941.

58. Rassidakis GZ, Medeiros LJ, Viviani S, et al. CD20 expression in Hodgkin and Reed-Sternberg cells of classical Hodgkin's disease: associations with presenting features and clinical outcome. J Clin Oncol 2002;20:1278-1287.

59. Ree HJ, Kadin ME. Macrophage-histiocytes in Hodgkin's disease. The relation of peanut-agglutinin-binding macrophage-histiocytes to clinicopathologic presentation and course of disease. Cancer 1985;56:333-338.

59a. Roemer MG, Advani RH, Ligon AH, et al. PD-L1 and PD-L2 genetic alterations define classical Hodgkin lymphoma and predict outcome. J Clin Oncol 2016;34:2690-2697.

59b. Roemer MG, Advani RH, Redd RA, et al, Classical Hodgkin lymphoma with reduced β2M/MHC class I expression is associated with inferior outcome independent of 9p24.1 status. Cancer Immunol Res 2016;4:910-916.

60. Rosenwald A, Wright G, Leroy K, et al. Molecular diagnosis of primary mediastinal B cell lymphoma identifies a clinically favorable subgroup of diffuse large B cell lymphoma related to Hodgkin lymphoma. J Exp Med 2003;198:851-862.

61. Roshal M, Wood BL, Fromm JR. Flow cytometric detection of the classical Hodgkin lymphoma: clinical and research applications. Adv Hematol 2011;2011:387034.

62. Saffer H, Wahed A, Rassidakis GZ, Medeiros LJ. Clusterin expression in malignant lymphomas: a survey of 266 cases. Mod Pathol 2002;15:1221-1226.

63. Sánchez-Espiridión B, Martín-Moreno AM, Montalbán C, et al. MicroRNA signatures and treatment response in patients with advanced classical Hodgkin lymphoma. Br J Haematol 2013;162:336-347.

64. Sánchez-Espiridión B, Montalbán C, López A, et al. A molecular risk score based on 4 functional pathways for advanced classical Hodgkin lymphoma. Blood 2010;116:e12-17.

65. Savage KJ, Monti S, Kutok KL, et al. The molecular signature of mediastinal large B-cell lymphoma differs from that of other diffuse large B-cell lymphomas and shares features with classical Hodgkin lymphoma. Blood 2003;102:3871-3879.

66. Schwering I, Brauninger A, Klein U, et al. Loss of the B-lineage-specific gene expression program in Hodgkin and Reed-Sternberg cells of Hodgkin lymphoma. Blood 2003;101:1505-1512.

67. Scott DW, Chan FC, Hong F, et al. Gene expression-based model using formalin-fixed paraffin-embedded biopsies predicts overall survival in advanced-stage classical Hodgkin lymphoma. J Clin Oncol 2013;31:692-700.

68. Scott DW, Steidl C. The classical Hodgkin lymphoma tumor microenvironment: macrophages and gene expression-based modeling. Hematology Am Soc Hematol Educ Program 2014;2014:144-150.

69. Seitz V, Hummel M, Marafioti T, Anagnostopoulos I, Assaf C, Stein H. Detection of clonal T-cell receptor gamma-chain gene rearrangements in Reed-Sternberg cells of classic Hodgkin disease. Blood 2000;95:3020-3024.

69a. Sethi T, Nguyen V, Li S, Morgan D, Greer J, Reddy N. Differences in outcome of patients with syncytial variant Hodgkin lymphoma compared with typical nodular sclerosis Hodgkin lymphoma. Ther Adv Hematol 2017;8:13-20.

70. Siegel RL, Miller KD, Jemal A. Cancer statistics, 2015. CA Cancer J Clin 2015;65:5-29.

71. Slovak ML, Bedell V, Hsu YH, et al. Molecular karyotypes of Hodgkin and Reed-Sternberg cells at disease onset reveal distinct copy number alterations in chemosensitive versus refractory Hodgkin lymphoma. Clin Cancer Res 2011;17:3443-3454.

72. Steidl C, Shah SP, Woolcock BW, et al. MHC class II transactivator CIITA is a recurrent gene fusion partner in lymphoid cancers. Nature 2011;471:377-381.

73. Stein H, Delsol G, Pileri SA, Weiss LM, Poppema S, Jaffe ES. Classical Hodgkin lymphoma, introduction. In: Swerdlow SH, Campo E, Harris NL, et al., eds. WHO classification of tumours of haematopoietic and lymphoid tissues. Lyon: IARC Press; 2008;326-329.

74. Stein H, Marafioti T, Foss HD, et al. Down-regulation of BOB.1/OBF.1 and Oct2 in classical Hodgkin disease but not in lymphocyte predominant Hodgkin disease correlates with immunoglobulin transcription. Blood 2001;97:496-501.

75. Sup SJ, Alemañy CA, Pohlman B, et al. Expression of bcl-2 in classical Hodgkin's lymphoma: an independent predictor of poor outcome. J Clin Oncol 2005;23:3773-3779.

75a. Swerdlow SH, Campo E, Pileri SA, et al. The 2016 revision of the World Health Organization classification of lymphoid neoplasms. Blood 2016;127:2375-2390.

76. Tadmor T, Bari A, Marcheselli L, et al. Absolute monocyte count and lymphocyte-monocyte ratio predict outcome in nodular sclerosis Hodgkin lymphoma: evaluation based on data from 1450 patients. Mayo Clin Proc 2015;90:756-764.

77. Torlakovic E, Tierens A, Dang HD, Delabie J. The transcription factor PU.1, necessary for B-cell development is expressed in lymphocyte predominance, but not classical Hodgkin's disease. Am J Pathol 2001;159:1807-1814.

78. Tudor CS, Distel LV, Eckhardt J, Hartmann A, Niedobitek G, Buettner M. B cells in classical Hodgkin lymphoma are important actors rather than bystanders in the local immune reaction. Hum Pathol 2013;44:2475-2486.

79. Uldrick TS, Little RF. How I treat classical Hodgkin lymphoma in patients infected with human immunodeficiency virus. Blood 2015;125:1226-1235.

80. Valsami S, Pappa V, Rontogianni G, et al. A clinicopathological study of B-cell differentiation markers and transcription factors in classical Hodgkin's lymphoma: a potential prognostic role of MUM1/IRF4. Haematologica 2007;92:1343-1350.

81. Venkataraman G, Mirza MK, Eichenauer DA, Diehl V. Current status of prognostication in classical Hodgkin lymphoma. Br J Haematol 2014;165:287-299.

82. Visco C, Vassilakopoulos TP, Kliche KO, et al. Elevated serum levels of IL-10 are associated with inferior progression-free survival in patients with Hodgkin's disease treated with radiotherapy. Leuk Lymphoma 2004;45:2085-2092.

83. Vockerodt M, Cader FZ, Shannon-Lowe C, Murray P. Epstein-Barr virus and the origin of Hodgkin lymphoma. Chin J Cancer 2014;33:591-597.

84. von Wasielewski R, Seth S, Franklin J, et al. Tissue eosinophilia correlates strongly with poor prognosis in nodular sclerosis Hodgkin's disease, allowing for known prognostic factors. Blood 2000;95:1207-1213.

85. Wang S, Medeiros LJ, Xu-Monette ZY, et al. Epstein-Barr virus-positive nodular lymphocyte predominant Hodgkin lymphoma. Ann Diagn Pathol 2014;18:203-209.

86. Weber-Matthiesen K, Deerberg J, Poetsch M, Grote W. Numerical chromosome aberrations are present within the CD30+ Hodgkin and Reed-Sternberg cells in 100% of analyzed cases of Hodgkin's disease. Blood 1995;86:1464-1468.

38 NODULAR SCLEROSIS HODGKIN LYMPHOMA

GENERAL FEATURES

Nodular sclerosis (NS) Hodgkin lymphoma (NSHL) is characterized by capsular fibrosis and dense collagenous bands that compartmentalize the tumor into nodules. The nodules contain an infiltrate composed of neoplastic cells, often comprising about 1 percent of all cells, scattered within a reactive inflammatory environment composed of small reactive lymphocytes, histiocytes, plasma cells, and granulocytes. In NSHL, Reed-Sternberg (RS) cells are often rare and most of the neoplastic cells are Hodgkin (H) cells but more specifically designated as lacunar cells. A triad of findings, therefore, supports the classification of NS type: nodules, collagen-dense fibrous bands surrounding tumor nodules, and lacunar cells.

The epidemiologic features associated with NSHL differ from those associated with mixed cellularity HL. Patients tend to be from families of higher socioeconomic status and have fewer siblings (8,13). Patients with NSHL have some features analogous to the paralytic polio model in that first exposure at a later age to a possible infectious agent, such as a virus, can be associated with a catastrophic event, i.e., development of HL. However, to date there is no proof of a viral etiology for NSHL. By contrast, patients with mixed cellularity HL are commonly from families of lower socioeconomic status and have a greater number of siblings, suggesting the possibility of infection early in life; Epstein-Barr virus (EBV) is a likely candidate (8,13,14).

CLINICAL FEATURES

The peak age incidence for patients with NSHL is 15 to 34 years of age (9,25). The male to female ratio is about 1 to 1, unlike other types of HL in which males predominate (25). Most often, patients present with disease involving cervical, supraclavicular, or axillary lymph nodes. About 75 percent of patients have a mediastinal mass (fig. 38-1) attributable to involvement of the thymus gland, mediastinal lymph nodes, or both (9,20a,25).

In about half of all patients, the mass is bulky and may invade locally into the lungs. Patients with a bulky mediastinal mass may present with cough, dyspnea, or rarely, superior vena cava syndrome. Most patients present with localized (stage I or II) disease. In some patients, NSHL spreads to the spleen (8 to 10 percent), bones (about 5 percent), bone marrow (3 to 5 percent), and liver (2 to 3 percent) (25). Extranodal sites are rarely involved unless adjacent to an involved lymph node.

HISTOLOGIC FINDINGS

Lymph Nodes

Histologic sections of involved lymph nodes show capsular fibrosis and dense collagenous bands projecting into the nodal parenchyma, surrounding variably sized tumor nodules (fig. 38-2) (1,25). Lukes and Butler (16) emphasized that the use of polarized light is helpful for diagnosis because the collagenous bands exhibit yellow birefringence. In most cases, numerous tumor nodules are surrounded by dense collagenous bands; uncommonly, these bands are underdeveloped compared with the nodularity and the number of neoplastic cells.

In the World Health Organization (WHO) classification, a minimum of one tumor nodule surrounded by a collagenous band is required for diagnosis (25). This is a reasonable position, but perhaps too restrictive. In a small subset of cases of NSHL, the nodules are incompletely surrounded by fibrous bands or only marked perivascular sclerosis is present. The absence of at least one collagenous band surrounding a tumor nodule occurs more often in small needle biopsy specimens. Coagulative necrosis is common in NSHL, usually located in the center of the tumor nodules (fig. 38-3).

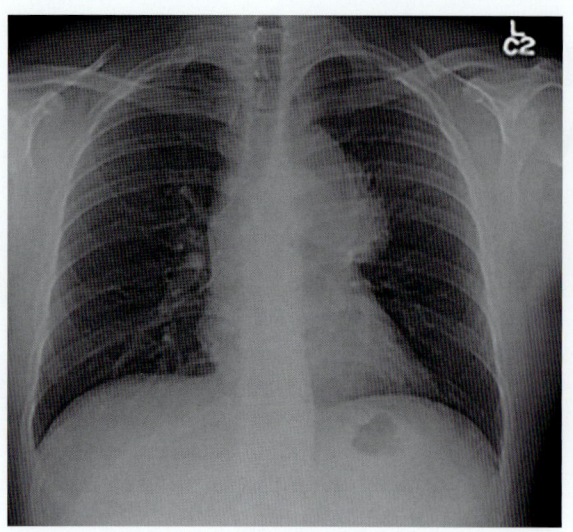
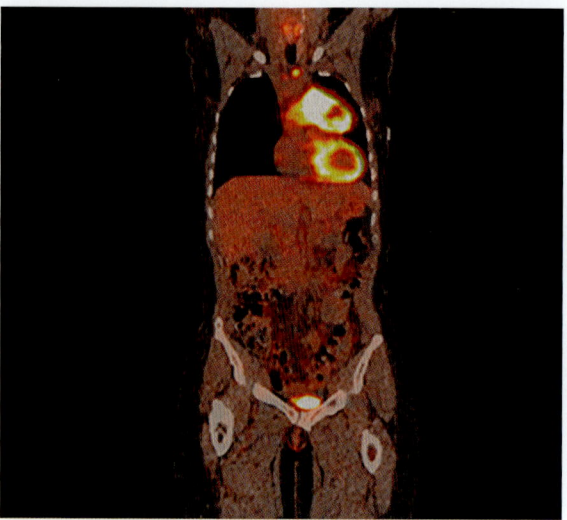

Figure 38-1

NODULAR SCLEROSIS HODGKIN LYMPHOMA (NSHL): RADIOLOGIC FEATURES

The patient presented with a mediastinal mass (left: chest radiograph; right: positron emission tomography [PET]/ computerized tomography [CT] scan).

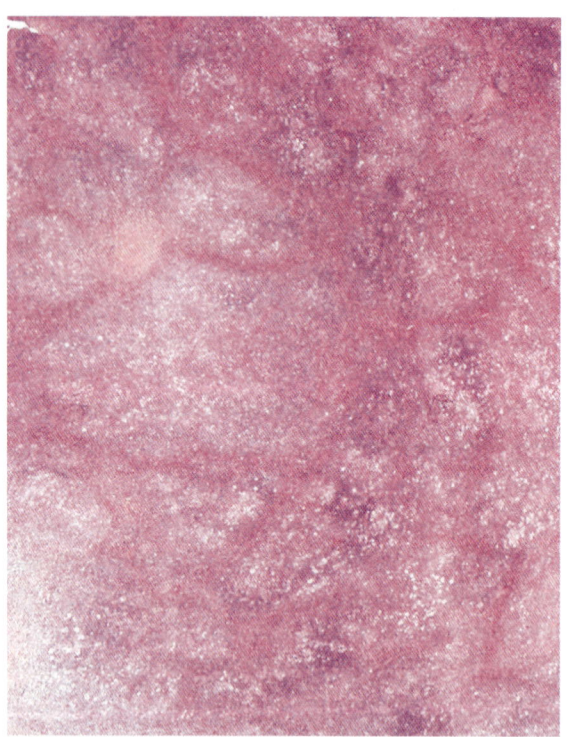
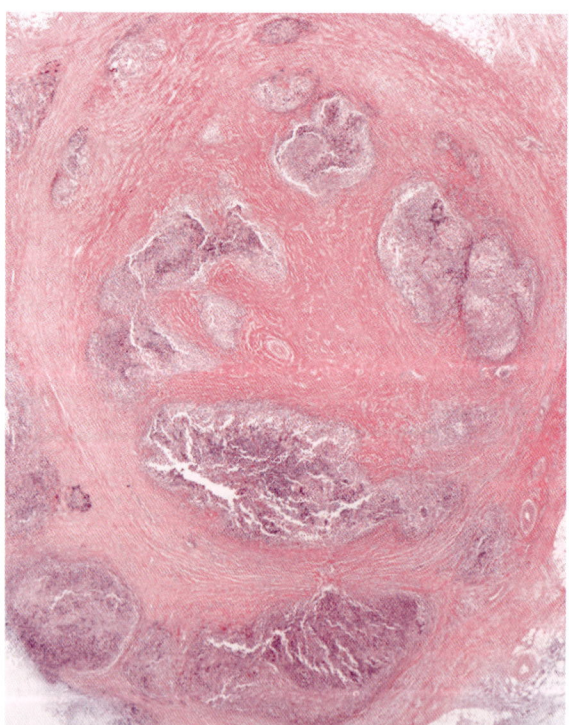

Figure 38-2

NODULAR SCLEROSIS HODGKIN LYMPHOMA INVOLVING LYMPH NODE

Left: In this case, there were areas of capsular fibrosis (not shown) but most of the tumor nodules are not surrounded by fibrous bands, similar to the so-called cellular phase of NSHL.

Right: In this case, the lymph node capsule is thickened, and dense collagenous bands course through the lymph node, surrounding tumor nodules (left, right: hematoxylin and eosin [H&E] stain).

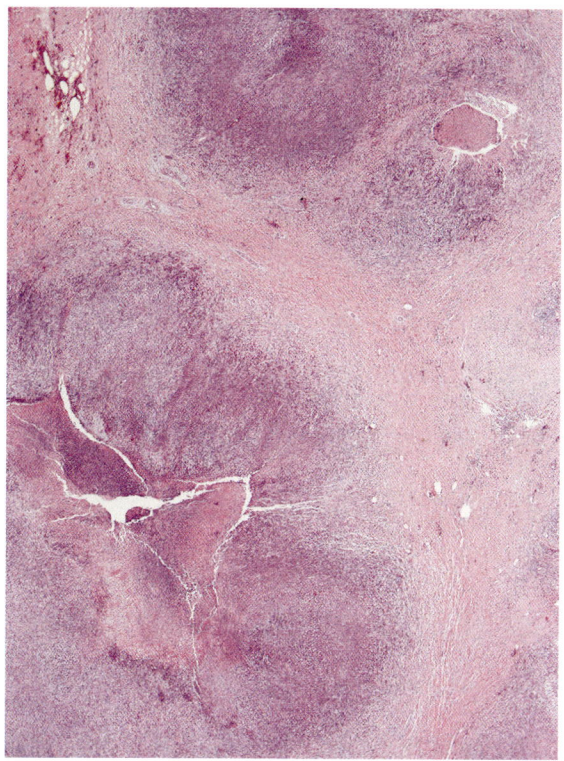

Figure 38-3

NODULAR SCLEROSIS HODGKIN LYMPHOMA: NECROSIS IN TUMOR NODULES

Necrosis is present in the center of tumor nodules (H&E stain).

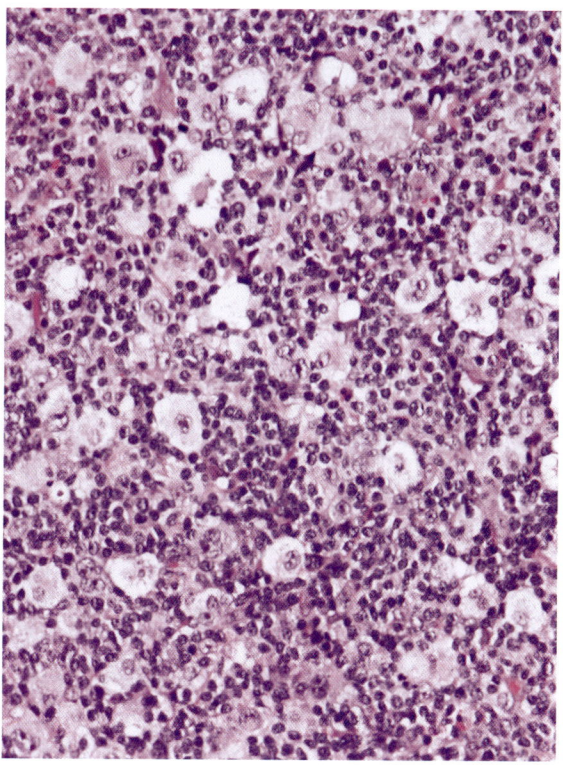

Figure 38-4

NODULAR SCLEROSIS HODGKIN LYMPHOMA: LACUNAR CELLS

High magnification shows many lacunar cells in a background of small lymphocytes and fewer histiocytes. The lacunar cells have retracted cytoplasm, an artifact of formalin fixation, and therefore the cells appear to lie within lacunar spaces (H&E stain).

RS cells are often few or rare in NSHL, but Hodgkin cells are readily identified, more specifically designated as lacunar cells (fig. 38-4). Lacunar cells are so-named because their cytoplasm is artifactually retracted in formalin-fixed paraffin-embedded sections and these cells appear to lie within lacunar spaces (fig. 38-4). Compared with RS cells, lacunar cells have smaller nuclei and nucleoli, and more abundant cytoplasm. Lacunar cells can be few or numerous, and form sheets. Mummified cells, in which there are early signs of cellular necrosis with blurring of cellular details, are also present in NSHL (as well as other types of HL).

The background cells in NSHL vary from case to case and include small lymphocytes, histiocytes, eosinophils, neutrophils, plasma cells, and mast cells in varying proportions (1,20a,25). Histiocytes are often epithelioid in appearance and may be numerous; sarcoid-like granulomas also may be present (fig. 38-5) (23). Eosinophils can form clusters. Neutrophilic granulocytes can be numerous and are often associated with necrosis forming microabscesses. Mast cells may be subtle in the background cell population, but are usually more common in NSHL than other types of classic HL; they can be highlighted with Giemsa or other metachromatic cytochemical stains or by immunohistochemistry (3).

For patients who completely respond to therapy, lesions that were once NSHL can persist for some time as areas of dense fibrosis devoid of neoplastic lacunar cells or an inflammatory infiltrate (fig. 38-6). In patients who are treated and then develop relapsed NSHL, the lesions tend to have a greater number of neoplastic cells; these cells can form sheets (fig. 38-7). In relapsed disease, lacunar cells are often atypical and can be anaplastic. Sinusoidal invasion by

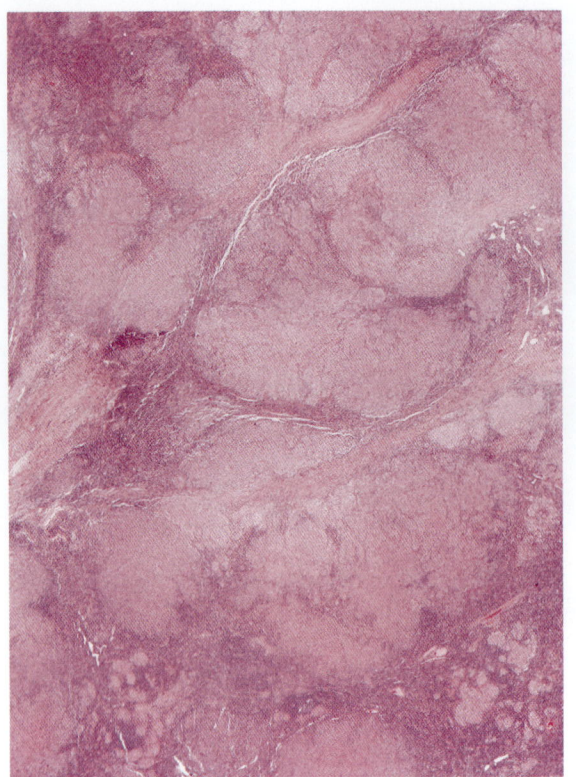 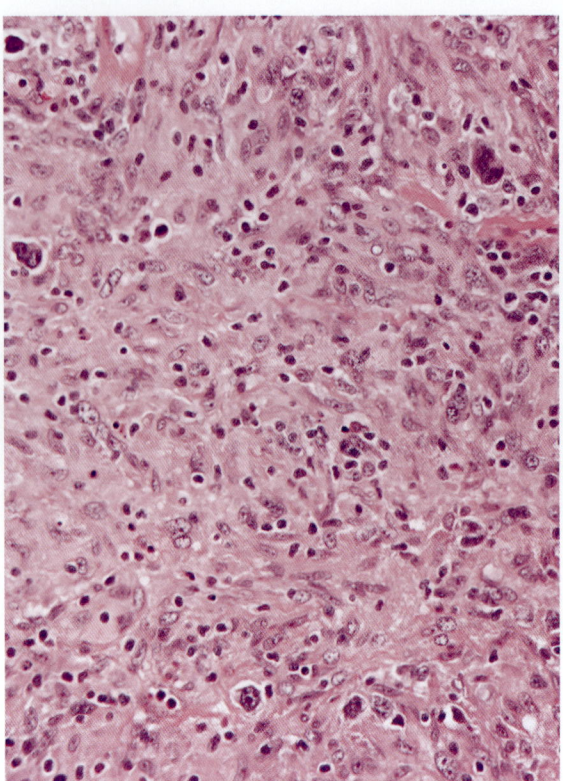

Figure 38-5

**NODULAR SCLEROSIS HODGKIN LYMPHOMA WITH EXTENSIVE
EPITHELIOID GRANULOMAS INVOLVING LYMPH NODE**

Left: The large nodules observed at low power are epithelioid granulomas. Fibrous bands were present in this case but are not well shown here.

Right: Scattered large neoplastic cells are appreciated in a background of numerous histiocytes (left, right: H&E stain).

Figure 38-6

SCLEROSIS FOLLOWING THERAPY FOR NODULAR SCLEROSIS HODGKIN LYMPHOMA

This patient with NSHL was treated with chemotherapy. A persistent small cervical lymph node was excised. The biopsy specimen showed extensive replacement of lymph node by dense sclerosis with no foci of residual disease (H&E stain).

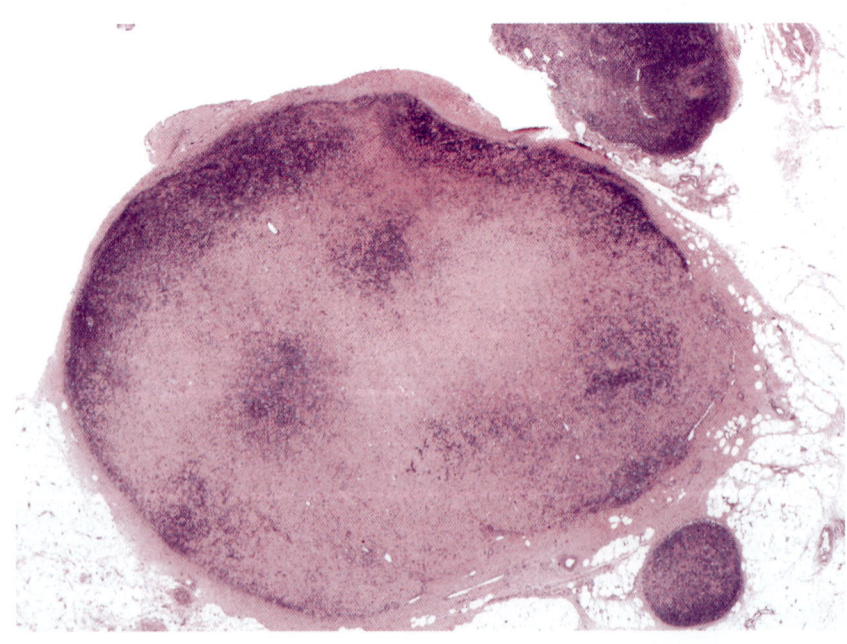

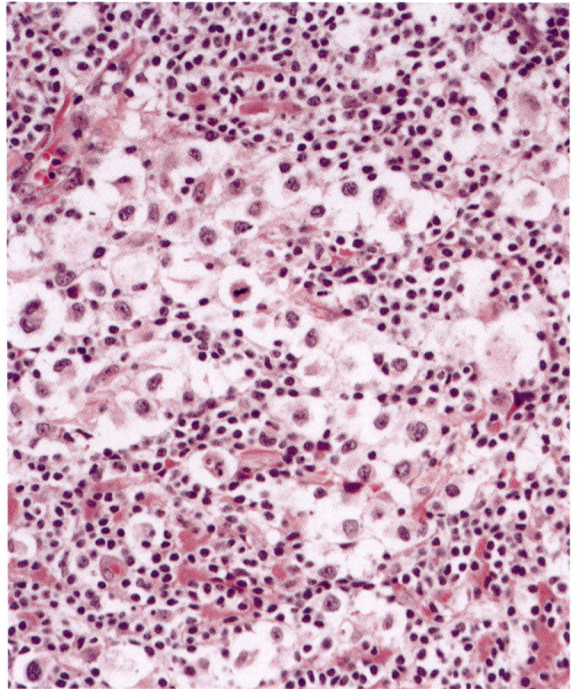

Figure 38-7

**RELAPSED NODULAR SCLEROSIS HODGKIN
LYMPHOMA INVOLVING LYMPH NODE**

The lacunar cells are numerous and present in sheets (H&E stain).

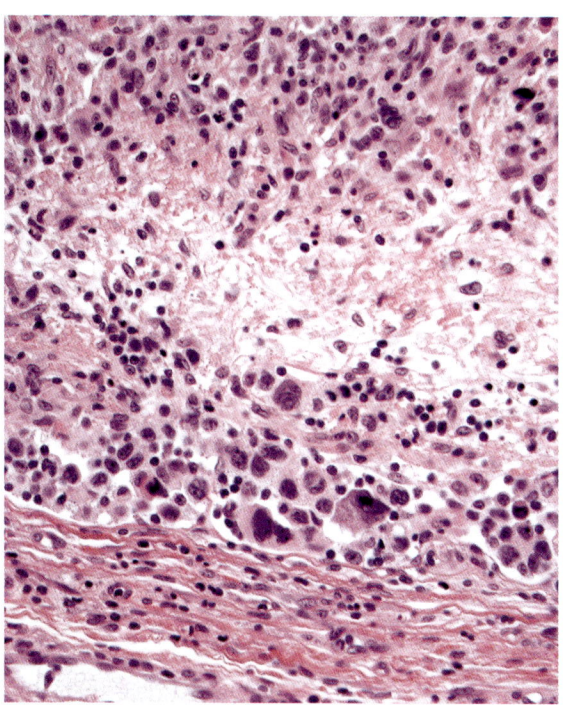

Figure 38-8

**RELAPSED NODULAR SCLEROSIS HODGKIN
LYMPHOMA INVOLVING LYMPH NODE SINUS**

Large neoplastic cells fill the subcapsular sinus (right) (H&E stain).

lacunar cells is an unusual finding in NSHL pretherapy, but can be prominent at time of relapse (fig. 38-8). Necrosis may be more prominent. The cellular background of NSHL after therapy is commonly depleted of small, reactive lymphocytes, with an increased proportion of histiocytes (9). After therapy and relapse, NSHL can resemble the syncytial variant of NSHL (see below) or lymphocyte-depleted HL.

Grading. In many (but not all) studies, grading NSHL has been shown to have prognostic value (12,17,31,32). Typically, grading is restricted to pretherapy lymph node biopsy specimens because relapse after therapy is often associated with a higher-grade tumor; in one study, however, grading NSHL also had prognostic value after relapse (12).

There are two well-known grading systems, developed by the British National Lymphoma Investigation (BNLI) group and the German Hodgkin Lymphoma Study Group (GHLSG) (17,31). These systems divide cases into grades 1 and 2, with grade 2 associated with a worse prognosis. The BNLI system (17) has three criteria, with the presence of one criterion adequate to support grade 2. The criteria are: 1) over 25 percent reticular or pleomorphic lymphocytic depletion of tumor nodules; 2) over 80 percent fibrohistiocytic depletion of tumor nodules; and 3) over 25 percent bizarre and anaplastic neoplastic cells (17). In the GHLSG system (31), three criteria are used in grading: lymphocyte depletion (over 33 percent of entire tumor), atypia of lacunar cells (over 25 percent), and eosinophilia (fig. 38-9). Eosinophilia is defined as more than 5 percent of all cells in the tumor or clusters of eosinophils in at least 5 high-power microscopic fields. Substantial necrosis also correlates with survival but is not included in the GHLSG grading system.

Morphologic Variants. *Syncytial Variant.* The term syncytial variant is used to designate a subset of cases of NSHL in which the lacunar cells are present in sheets (5,26). Other terms used in the past to designate this variant include sarcomatous lacunar cell Hodgkin disease and lymphocyte-

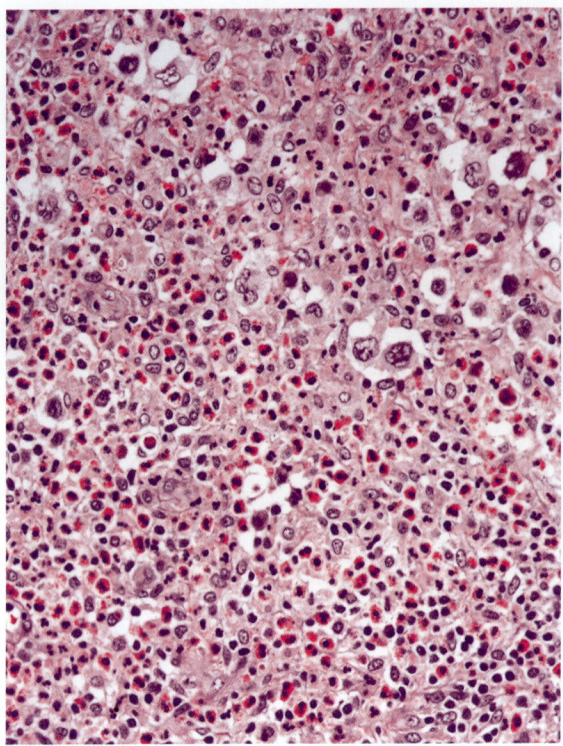

Figure 38-9

NODULAR SCLEROSIS HODGKIN LYMPHOMA GRADE 2

The numerous eosinophils support the designation of grade 2, using the German Hodgkin Lymphoma Study Group system (31) (H&E stain).

depleted variant of NS. The syncytial variant of NS represents 5 to 15 percent of all cases of NSHL in different studies. Patients commonly present with B-type symptoms, a large mediastinal mass, or advanced stage disease (1). Patients treated with standard HL therapy had a lower complete response rate and progression-free survival rate in one large study (24a).

Histologically, in addition to sheets of lacunar cells, large foci of coagulative necrosis and atypia of the lacunar cells are common in the syncytial variant of NSHL (fig. 38-10) (5,26). Sinusoidal invasion may be observed (21). The findings resemble, in part, non-Hodgkin lymphomas such as diffuse large B-cell lymphoma or anaplastic large cell lymphoma. Regarding grade, all cases of syncytial variant NSHL are grade 2, but not all grade 2 cases of NSHL qualify as the syncytial variant. In most biopsy specimens of syncytial variant NSHL, if large enough, there are also areas of more typical NSHL, facilitating the correct diagnosis.

Fibroblastic Variant. This term is used for an uncommon morphologic variant of NSHL in which lacunar cells are present in a background composed of histiocytes and fibroblasts, with or without granulocytes, with marked depletion of small reactive lymphocytes (9). The neoplastic cells may have a partially spindled low-power appearance (fig. 38-11). These tumors are recognized because capsular fibrosis and collagenous bands are present in at least some areas of the biopsy specimen (or in concurrent specimens). These tumors, based on the extensive lymphocyte depletion, are grade 2.

Cellular Phase. Rare cases of HL are nodular at low power and have neoplastic cells suggestive of lacunar cells, yet dense collagenous bands are absent and capsular fibrosis is minimal or absent (figs. 38-2, left; 38-12). The designation cellular phase of NSHL has been used for these cases, with the presumption that they are an early phase of NSHL.

HL cases with cellular phase morphology can be subdivided into two groups. In one, the presence of a mediastinal mass or a subsequent biopsy specimen at relapse may show the typical features of NS, supporting a close relationship to NSHL. Another, probably larger subset of cases, is more likely related to either the nodular variant of lymphocyte-rich classic HL or mixed cellularity HL (7,9). The presence of EBV in the neoplastic cells, uncommon in NSHL and more common in other types of classic HL, is a clue that the tumor may not be related to NSHL (7).

Thymus

NSHL may involve the thymus gland. As in the lymph nodes, the thymic parenchyma is subdivided by collagenous bands that surround tumor nodules. There are two distinctive features that occur in the thymus when involved by NSHL. One feature is the tendency to develop epithelial-lined cysts, which may be small or large (fig. 38-13). In large cysts, it may be difficult to identify foci of HL, particularly in needle biopsy specimens. A second feature is that thymic epithelial cells may become hyperplastic and spindled (and can resemble, more or less, spindle cell thymoma).

Spleen and Liver

NSHL involves the spleen, preferentially the white pulp (fig. 38-14) (9,25). In cases with

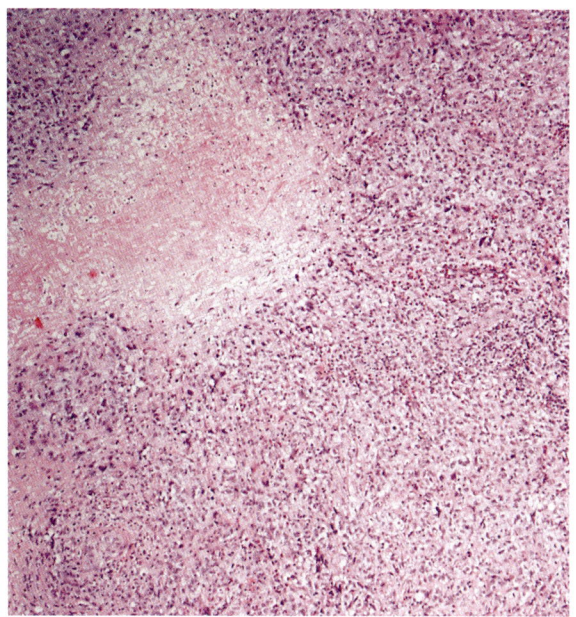
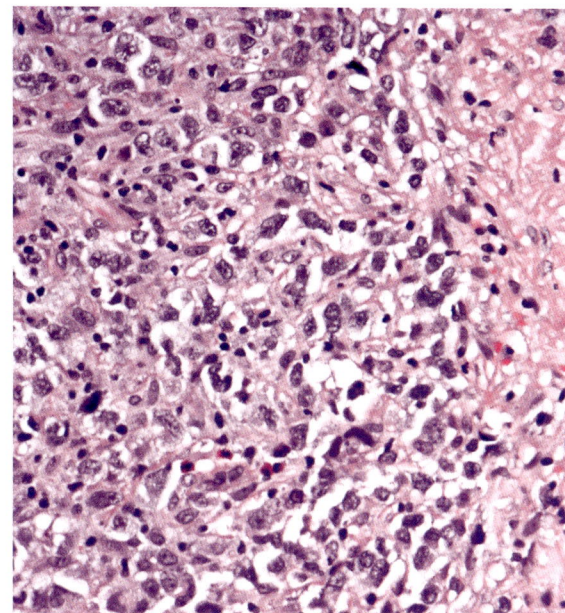

Figure 38-10

NODULAR SCLEROSIS HODGKIN LYMPHOMA, SYNCYTIAL VARIANT

Left: Sheets of lacunar cells and areas of coagulative necrosis (upper left) are present.
Right: High magnification of the sheets of lacunar cells, with eosinophils in the background (left, right: H&E stain).

extensive involvement, the tumor forms nodules surrounded by collagenous bands, but in cases with lesser involvement, not all of the features of NSHL may be present and lacunar cells may be surrounded by loose aggregates of reactive lymphoid cells and less well-developed fibrosis. Liver involvement by NSHL is almost always preceded by splenic disease and preferentially involves and expands the portal tracts (fig. 38-15) (9,25).

Bone Marrow

Patients with bone marrow disease commonly show peripheral cytopenia(s). Due to the presence of fibrosis, it is unusual to detect NSHL in aspirate smears. Even in patients with extensive replacement of the medullary space by NSHL, aspirate smears can be negative (fig. 38-16).

CYTOLOGIC FINDINGS

Cytologic preparations of NSHL show variable numbers of RS+H cells in a background of small lymphocytes, plasma cells, eosinophils, histiocytes, and occasional neutrophils (figs. 38-17, 38-18). Some fine-needle aspirate specimens are hypocellular due to fibrosis, or they contain primarily inflammatory cells with rare classic

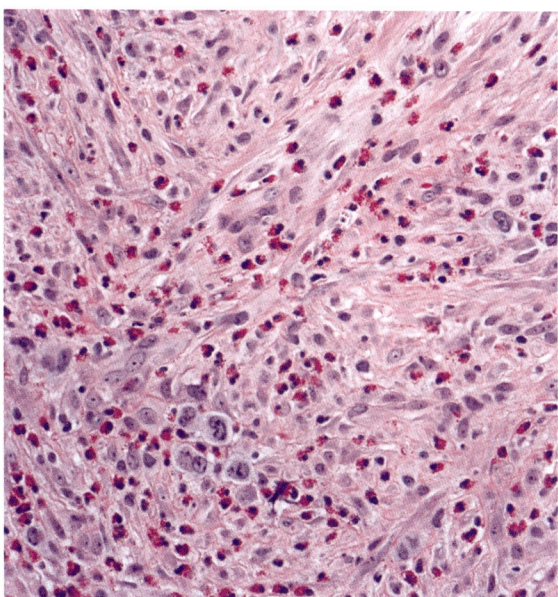

Figure 38-11

NODULAR SCLEROSIS HODGKIN LYMPHOMA, FIBROBLASTIC VARIANT

Numerous spindle-shaped fibroblasts and eosinophils are present with a few neoplastic cells (cluster in lower left). This patient had morphologically more typical NSHL in another lymph node (H&E stain).

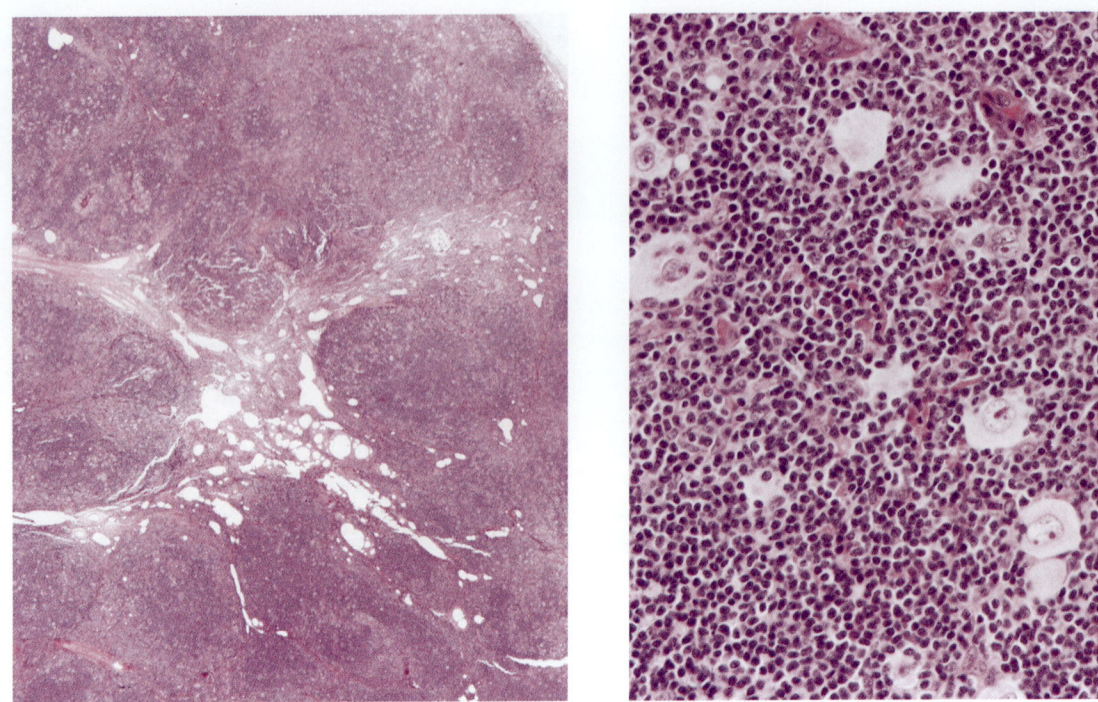

Figure 38-12

CELLULAR PHASE OF NODULAR SCLEROSIS HODGKIN LYMPHOMA

Left: The neoplasm is obviously nodular but there was no capsular fibrosis or fibrous bands around the nodules.

Right: The neoplastic cells have features suggestive of lacunar cells. This patient had a mediastinal mass and the tumor cells were negative for Epstein-Barr virus (EBV)-encoded RNA1, evidence thought suggestive of NSHL (left, right: H&E stain).

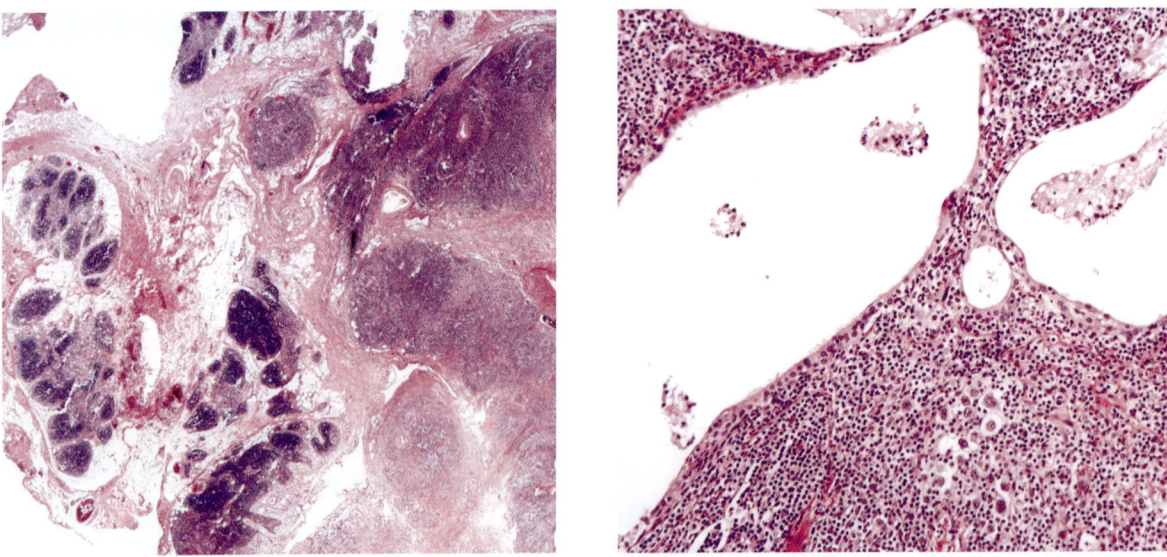

Figure 38-13

NODULAR SCLEROSIS HODGKIN LYMPHOMA INVOLVING THYMUS GLAND

Left: At low-power magnification, NSHL (right of field) partially replaces thymic parenchyma (left of field).

Right: High magnification shows cysts lined by ciliated epithelium. Lacunar cell are present at the bottom center of the field (left, right: H&E stain).

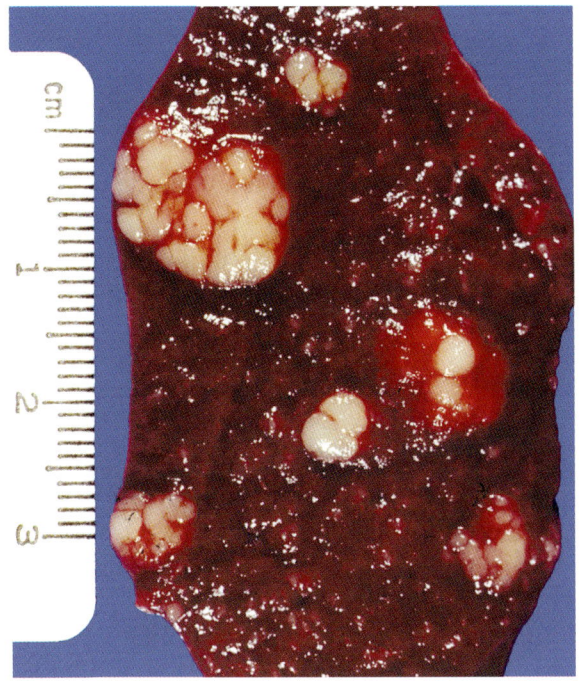
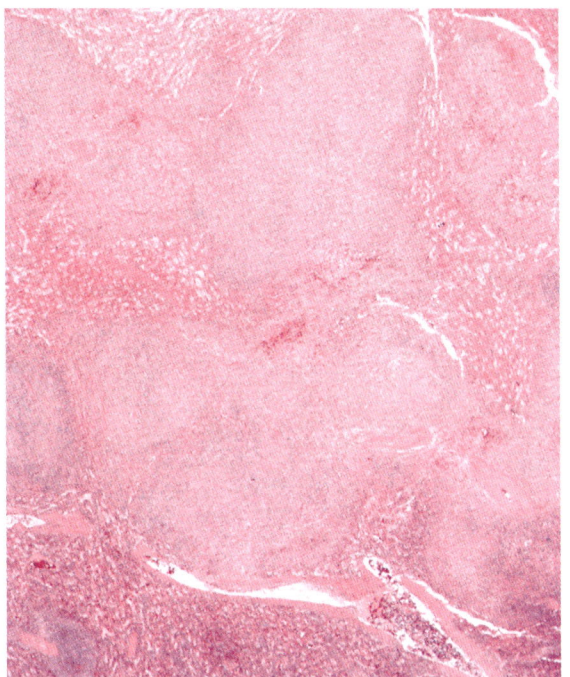

Figure 38-14

NODULAR SCLEROSIS HODGKIN LYMPHOMA INVOLVING SPLEEN

Left: Gross image of large tumor nodules.
Right: Histologic section shows extensive replacement and expansion of white pulp (H&E stain).

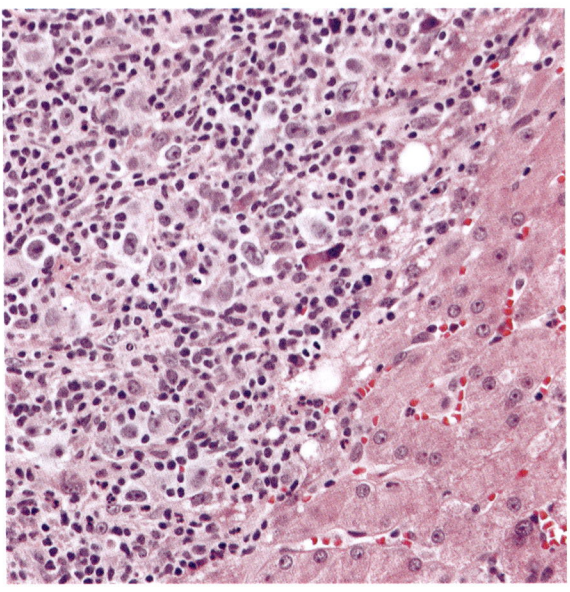

Figure 38-15

NODULAR SCLEROSIS HODGKIN LYMPHOMA INVOLVING LIVER

The neoplasm preferentially involves the portal tracts (H&E stain).

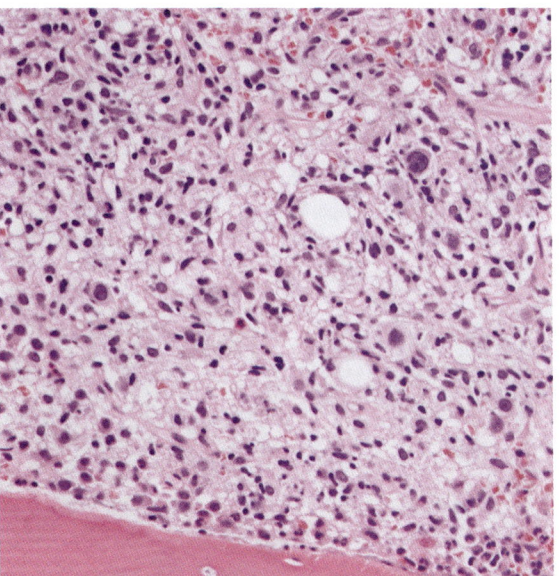

Figure 38-16

NODULAR SCLEROSIS HODGKIN LYMPHOMA INVOLVING BONE MARROW

The medullary space is replaced by lymphoma, with scattered large neoplastic cells in a background of reactive cells and fibrosis (H&E stain).

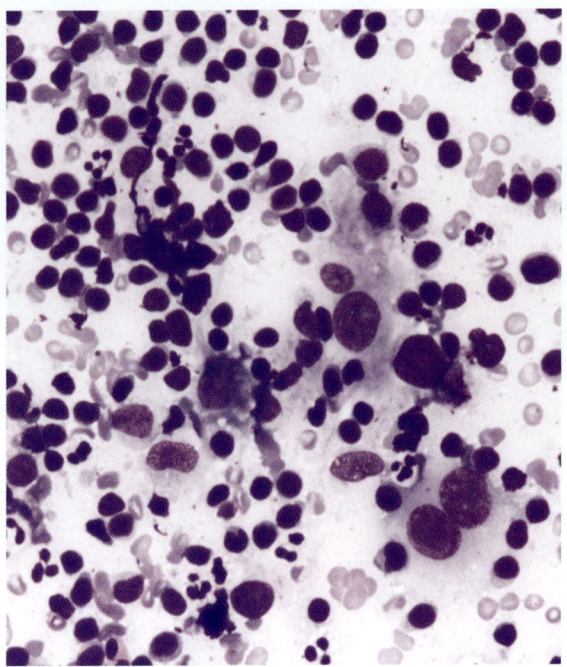
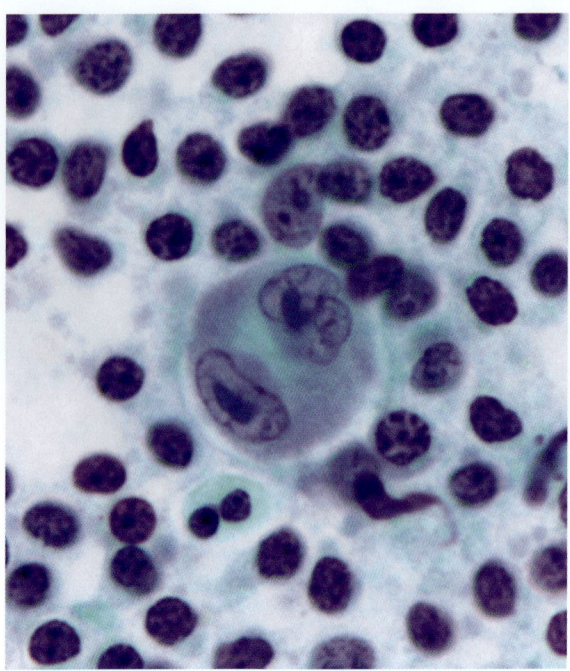

Figure 38-17

NODULAR SCLEROSIS HODGKIN LYMPHOMA: ASPIRATE SMEARS

Left: Large tumor cells in a background of lymphocytes, histiocytes, plasmacytoid cells, and eosinophils are shown. A Reed-Sternberg (RS) cell is present (lower right) (Diff-Quik stain).

Right: A classic RS cell with prominent nucleoli is shown (Papanicolaou stain).

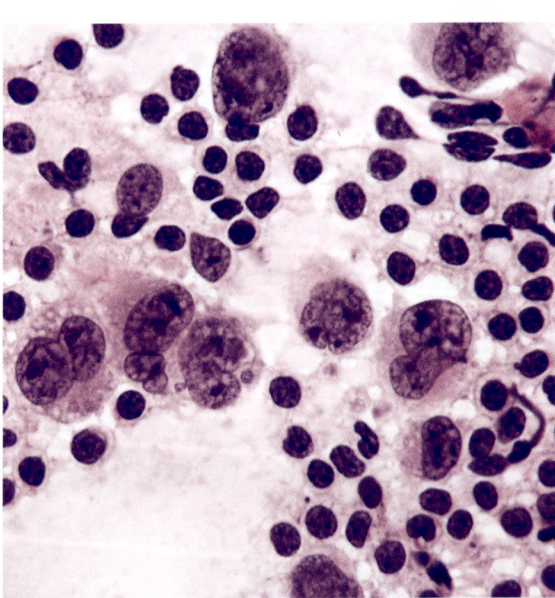

Figure 38-18

NODULAR SCLEROSIS HODGKIN LYMPHOMA: TOUCH IMPRINT

Image taken using oil magnification shows lacunar cells in a reactive cell background (H&E stain).

RS or lacunar cells. Cases of grade 2 or syncytial variant NSHL can be highly challenging because of the large number of RS+H cells, leading to misdiagnosis as non-Hodgkin lymphoma or a solid tumor (24b).

IMMUNOHISTOCHEMICAL FINDINGS

The lacunar (and rare RS) cells of NSHL express CD15 (70 to 80 percent) (fig. 38-19), CD30 (virtually 100 percent), MUM1/IRF4 (over 90 percent), and PAX5 (dim, 90 to 95 percent) and are negative for CD45/LCA. B-cell antigens are usually negative, but scattered and variable reactivity for CD20 may be observed in some RS+H cells in up to 20 percent of cases. In about 20 percent of cases the neoplastic cells are positive for EBV.

Cytotoxic molecules are expressed by the lacunar cells in 10 to 20 percent of cases of classic HL (25). Cytotoxic molecule expression has been described most often in NSHL. In a study by Asano et al. (4), about 70 percent of cases of classic HL with neoplastic cells positive for cytotoxic molecules were of NS type. Whether the frequency of cytotoxic molecule expression reflects the overall frequency of the different types of classic HL or is a property inherent to NSHL is unclear.

Does T-Cell Classic HL Exist?

Expression of T-cell antigens has been reported in 10 to 15 percent of cases of classic HL (24). In a study by Venkataraman et al. (30), 80 percent of cases of HL with T-cell antigen expression by the neoplastic cells were of NS type (30). CD2, CD4, and CD7 are positive most often in the neoplastic cells. In most cases, expression of T-cell antigens is aberrant because the neoplastic cells are positive for PAX5 and carry monoclonal *IGH* rearrangements, supporting B-cell lineage (fig. 38-20) (24,30).

Rare cases classified as classic HL, usually NS type, have neoplastic cells that express T-cell antigens, lack PAX5 expression, and carry monoclonal T-cell receptor gene rearrangements without monoclonal *IGH* rearrangements, supporting T-cell lineage (18,24). In these cases the neoplastic cells express CD15, CD30, and MUM1/IRF4, similar to RS+H cells in classic HL. Are these neoplasms truly classic HL or cases of peripheral T-cell lymphoma that mimic classic HL?

Currently, there is no clear answer to this question and the approach taken by various observers seems more philosophical than scientific. For those pathologists who favor the diagnosis of classic HL, it seems that traditional morphologic criteria and CD15 and CD30 immunoreactivity are most important. For those pathologists who believe these tumors should be classified as peripheral T-cell lymphoma, the goal is to identify pure and homogeneous diagnostic categories, and these investigators view HL as a purely B-cell neoplasm. There is some follow-up data showing that patients with classic HL with T-cell antigen expression (some cases also carrying monoclonal T-cell receptor gene rearrangements) have a poorer prognosis (30). These data seem to provide some support for at least distinguishing so-called T-cell classic HL from other cases of classic HL.

Some patients with mycosis fungoides or lymphomatoid papulosis develop a tumor that meets the morphologic criteria for classic HL, most often of NS type. Eberle et al. (11) studied 10 such cases and showed a T-cell immunophenotype and monoclonal T-cell receptor gene rearrangements in many. The authors

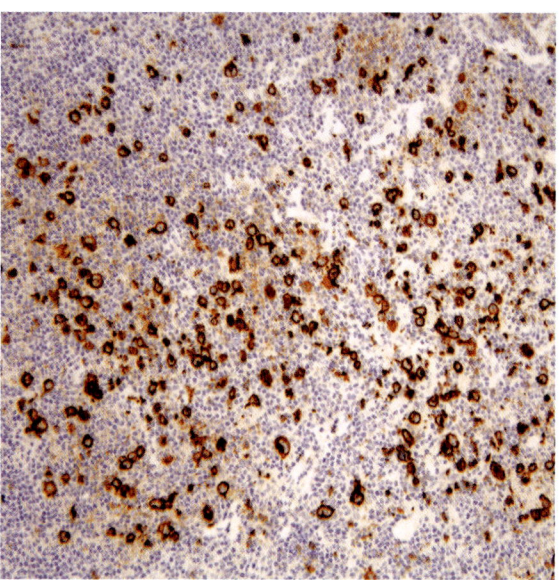

Figure 38-19

NODULAR SCLEROSIS HODGKIN LYMPHOMA: CD15

The lacunar cells are positive for CD15, and at this magnification tumor nodules can be appreciated (immunohistochemistry with hematoxylin counterstain).

concluded that the NSHL-like tumors in which T-cell clonality could be established were better classified as T-cell lymphoma. In the clinical context of mycosis fungoides or lymphomatoid papulosis, the approach advocated by Eberle et al. seems reasonable.

MOLECULAR GENETIC FINDINGS

The molecular findings in NSHL are thought to be similar to those of other types of classic HL and are reviewed in chapter 37.

At the gene expression level, there are some differences between the NS and mixed cellularity types of HL (6,10,28). Early work using gene expression profiling of whole tissues showed similarities between classic HL and primary mediastinal B-cell lymphoma (PMBL), with an overlap of 33 percent of genes in one study (22). Tiacci et al. (28) used gene expression profiling methods on microdissected tumor cells to show this overlap is in genes specifically between NSHL and PBML. In contrast, mixed cellularity HL overlapped much more with nodular lymphocyte-predominant HL. The work also showed possible roles for MYC, IRF4, and NOTCH1 activation in classic HL that

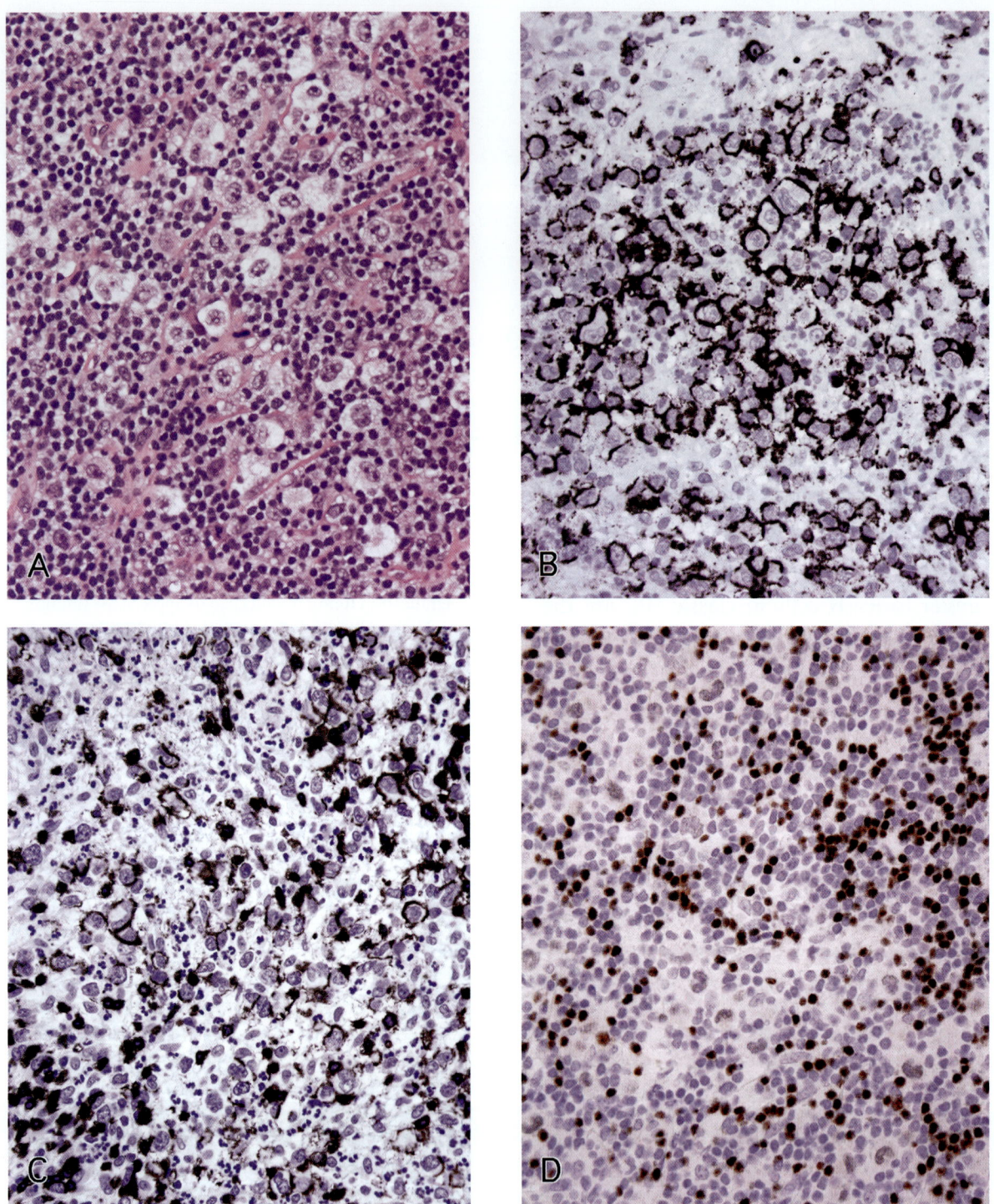

Figure 38-20

NODULAR SCLEROSIS HODGKIN LYMPHOMA WITH ABERRANT T-CELL ANTIGEN EXPRESSION

A: Lacunar cells are present in a reactive cellular background (H&E stain).

B–D: The lacunar cells are positive for CD2 (B), betaF1 (C), and PAX5 (D). PAX5 expression is weak compared to reactive lymphocytes. Not shown, the lacunar cells were also positive for CD15 and CD30 (B–D: immunohistochemistry with hematoxylin counterstain).

did not correlate with histologic type of HL or EBV infection.

The collagenous fibrosis of NSHL is a distinctive feature that is absent in other types of HL. In earlier studies, the interleukin 13 and transforming growth factor beta (TGFβ) by the tumor cells of NSHL were implicated in inducing fibrosis (19,20). Gene expression profiling has shown that NSHL is characterized by upregulation of genes involved in extracellular matrix deposition and remodeling, including *SPARC* and connective tissue growth factor (6,10,28). In contrast, cases of mixed cellularity HL had overexpression of many genes involved in inflammation (6,28). Devilard et al. (10) showed that upregulation of genes involved fibroblast activation, extracellular matrix remodeling, angiogenesis, and cell proliferation correlated with poorer prognosis in patients with NSHL.

DIFFERENTIAL DIAGNOSIS

Other Types of Hodgkin Lymphoma. As described above, NSHL is characterized by a triad of findings: sclerosis (which can be capsular or perivascular but usually surrounds tumor nodules), nodules surrounded by sclerotic bands, and lacunar cells. This combination of features is absent in other types of HL. The features of NSHL take precedence in cases of HL, even in cases in which NS features are minimal. Lymphocyte-rich classic HL and nodular lymphocyte-predominant HL may have prominent nodular patterns, but the former lacks sclerosis and classic-appearing lacunar cells and the latter is composed of LP cells with a different immunophenotype [CD20(+), CD45/LCA(+), CD15(-), CD30(-)]. Importantly, other types of HL can involve a fibrotic lymph node (attributable to other causes) and should not be mistaken for NSHL.

Primary Mediastinal Large B-Cell Lymphoma (PMBL). These tumors are composed of sheets of large cells that are often associated with sclerosis. In addition, the neoplastic cells can resemble lacunar cells or, rarely, RS cells, and therefore, the diagnosis of the syncytial variant NSHL may be considered. Unlike NSHL, however, the sclerosis is usually finer in PMBL and the tumor cells have a B-cell immunophenotype positive for CD19, CD20 (bright), CD79a, and PAX5 (bright) as well as CD45/LCA and CD23 (about 70 percent of cases). CD30 is positive

in about 75 percent of PMBL cases, but usually weakly or in a cytoplasmic pattern, and CD15 is negative. Hoeller et al. (15) suggested that assessing for expression of BOB.1, CD79a, and cyclin E is particularly helpful for distinguishing classic HL from PMBL: these markers are usually positive in PMBL.

T-Cell/Histiocyte-Rich Large B-Cell Lymphoma (THRLBCL). Cases of THRLBCL are composed of scattered large neoplastic B cells in a background of reactive small T cells and histiocytes, and can be associated with sclerosis. The large cells may resemble lacunar or RS cells in some cases, and may express CD30. NSHL is considered in the differential diagnosis. However, the neoplastic cells are B cells that express CD19, CD20 (bright), CD79a, and PAX5 (bright) as well as CD45/LCA and are negative for CD15.

B-Cell Lymphoma, Unclassifiable, with Features Intermediate Between Classic HL and Diffuse Large B-Cell Lymphoma (Gray Zone Lymphoma). These rare tumors occur in the mediastinum or at other sites and can closely mimic NSHL morphologically; they also express CD30. Unlike NSHL, gray zone lymphomas have large neoplastic cells that strongly and uniformly express CD20, express other B-cell antigens (e.g., CD79a, PAX5 [bright], OCT2, and BOB.1), and are often positive for CD45/LCA.

Anaplastic Lymphoma Kinase (ALK)-Positive Anaplastic Large Cell Lymphoma (ALCL). Rare cases of ALK-positive ALCL present as a mediastinal mass, have a nodular pattern, and can be associated with sclerosis, mimicking NSHL (29). The large neoplastic cells also can resemble lacunar cells and are positive for CD30. By definition, however, the neoplastic cells in ALK-positive ALCL express ALK, usually also express T-cell antigens, and usually lack CD15 or evidence of EBV infection.

ALK-Negative Anaplastic Large Cell Lymphoma. The large lymphoma cells of this tumor can resemble RS+H cells but are usually present in a sinusoidal pattern or in diffuse sheets, unlike NSHL. The neoplastic cells are of T-cell lineage, often express cytotoxic markers, and usually carry monoclonal T-cell receptor gene rearrangements. ALK-negative ALCL cases infrequently express CD15 and very rarely are PAX5 positive. In general, PAX5 expression supports classic HL or B-cell lymphoma over ALCL.

623

Peripheral T-Cell Lymphoma (PTCL), Not Otherwise Specified. Some cases of PTCL can have large RS-like cells in a prominent inflammatory background and resemble classic HL. The RS-like cells also express CD30. A useful distinguishing feature is the spectrum of neoplastic cells, from small to large and RS-like, present in PTCL. In contrast, in classic HL, there is a "gap" between the large neoplastic cells and the background inflammatory cells. Immunohistochemical studies show that the RS-like cells of PTCL may express CD30 and rarely CD15, but are positive for CD45/LCA and one or more pan-T-cell antigens and are negative for PAX5.

Mediastinal Germ Cell Tumors. Seminoma is often associated with numerous small lymphocytes, plasma cells, and histiocytes, and sclerosis may be present. The neoplastic cells in seminoma also commonly have prominent nucleoli. In the mediastinum, particularly in small needle biopsy specimens, seminoma can resemble NSHL at the histologic level. Immunohistochemical studies help because the cells of seminoma are positive for CD117, PLAP, SOX17, OCT3/4, and keratin (in a subset), and are negative for CD15, CD30 and PAX5.

Embryonal carcinoma cells express CD30 and in the mediastinum these tumors are associated with necrosis or sclerosis, and therefore may resemble the syncytial variant NSHL. Embryonal carcinoma cells, however, are positive for keratins and lack CD15 and PAX5.

Thymoma. At low power, thymoma can have a nodular pattern and is commonly associated with bands of sclerosis. However, thymoma lacks RS or lacunar cells that express CD15 and CD30. Instead, thymoma cells express keratins and are associated with immature T lymphocytes [CD1a(+), TdT(+)].

Sarcoidosis. As mentioned above, sarcoid-like granulomas can be present in the background of NSHL (23). Rarely, these granulomas are very prominent, leading one to consider the possibility of sarcoidosis, particularly in biopsy specimens from the mediastinum. A search for RS+H cells is required to distinguish sarcoidosis from classic HL. The presence of many eosinophils is also suggestive of classic HL.

Sclerosing Mediastinitis. Some of these rare lesions are now thought to be part of the spectrum of IgG4-related disease. Biopsy specimens show reactive lymphocytes, plasma cells, histiocytes, and rarely, granulocytes, and are often associated with sclerosis. However, no RS+H cells are identified.

TREATMENT AND PROGNOSIS

The standard therapy for patients with NSHL is usually similar to that of other types of classic HL and is based on risk stratification (see chapter 37). There are three general prognostic groups of patients: early stage favorable, early stage unfavorable, and advanced stage disease. Patients are treated with combination chemotherapy; radiation therapy is also used for patient subsets.

For patients with NSHL, bulky disease in the mediastinum is an adverse prognostic factor. In general, the histologic type is not a powerful predictor of prognosis in HL patients. Nevertheless, in some studies, patients with NSHL have a more favorable prognosis when compared to patients with other types of classic HL (2). The grade of NSHL also correlates with prognosis. An absolute monocyte count of over 750 cells/mm^3 and an absolute monocyte to lymphocyte ratio 2.1 or less have been correlated with poorer prognosis in patients with classic HL and particularly for patients with NSHL (27). A large number of other markers in serum/plasma and tissue have been suggested as having prognostic value in classic HL (see Table 37-4).

REFERENCES

1. Agostinelli C, Pileri S. Pathobiology of Hodgkin lymphoma. Med J Hematol Infect Dis 2014;6: e2014040.
2. Allemani C, Sant M, De Angelis R, Marcos-Gragera R, Coebergh JW; EUROCARE Working Group. Hodgkin disease survival in Europe and the U.S.: prognostic significance of morphologic groups. Cancer 2006;107:352-360.
3. Andersen MD, Kamper P, Nielsen PS, et al. Tumour-associated mast cells in classical Hodgkin lymphoma: correlation with histological subtype, other tumour-infiltrating inflammatory cell subsets, and outcome. Eur J Haematol 2016;96;252-259.
4. Asano N, Kinoshita T, Tamaru J, et al. Cytotoxic molecule-positive classical Hodgkin lymphoma: a clinicopathological comparison with cytotoxic molecule-positive peripheral T-cell lymphoma of not otherwise specified type. Haematologica 2011;96:1636-1643.
5. Ben-Yehuda-Salz D, Ben-Yehuda A, Polliack A, Ron N, Okon E. Syncytial variant of nodular sclerosing Hodgkin's disease. A new clinicopathologic entity. Cancer 1990;65:1167-1172.
6. Birgersdotter A, Baumforth KR, Porwit A, et al. Inflammation and tissue repair markers distinguish the nodular sclerosis and mixed cellularity subtypes of classical Hodgkin's lymphoma. Br J Cancer 2009;101:1393-1401.
7. Boiocchi M, De Re V, Dolcetti R, Carbone A, Scarpa A, Menestrina F. Association of Epstein-Barr virus genome with mixed cellularity and cellular phase nodular sclerosis Hodgkin's disease subtypes. Ann Oncol 1992;3:307-310.
8. Clarke CA, Glaser SL, Keegan TH, Stroup A. Neighborhood socioeconomic status and Hodgkin's lymphoma incidence in California. Cancer Epidemiol Biomarkers Prev 2005;14:1441-1447.
9. Colby TV, Hoppe RT, Warnke RA. Hodgkin's disease: a clinicopathologic study of 659 cases. Cancer 1982;49:1848-1858.
10. Devilard E, Bertucci F, Trempat P, et al. Gene expression profiling defines molecular subtypes of classical Hodgkin's disease. Oncogene 2002;21:3095-3102.
11. Eberle FC, Song JY, Xi L, et al. Nodal involvement by cutaneous CD30-positive T-cell lymphoma mimicking classical Hodgkin lymphoma. Am J Surg Pathol 2012;36:716-725.
12. Ferry JA, Linggood RM, Convery KM, Efird JT, Eliseo R, Harris NL. Hodgkin's disease, nodular sclerosis type. Implications of histologic subclassification. Cancer 1993;71:457-463.
13. Grufferman S, Cole P, Smith PG, Lukes RJ. Hodgkin's disease in siblings. N Engl J Med 1977;296:248-250.
14. Gutensohn N, Cole P. Childhood social environment and Hodgkin's disease. N Engl J Med 1981;304:135-140.
15. Hoeller S, Zihler D, Zlobec I, et al. BOB.1, CD79a and cyclin E are the most appropriate markers to discriminate classical Hodgkin's lymphoma from primary mediastinal large B-cell lymphoma. Histopathology 2010;56:217-228.
16. Lukes RJ, Butler JJ. The pathology and nomenclature of Hodgkin's disease. Cancer Res 1966;26:1063-1083.
17. MacLennan KA, Bennett MH, Tu A, et al. Relationship of histopathologic features to survival and relapse in nodular sclerosing Hodgkin's disease. A study of 1659 patients. Cancer 1989;64:1686-1693.
18. Müschen M, Rajewsky K, Bräuninger A, et al. Rare occurrence of classical Hodgkin's disease as a T cell lymphoma. J Exp Med 2000;191:387-394.
19. Newcom SR, Kadin ME, Ansari AA. Production of transforming growth factor-beta activity by Ki-1 positive lymphoma cells and analysis of its role in in the regulation of Ki-1 positive lymphoma growth. Am J Pathol 1988;131:569-577.
20. Ohshima K, Akaiwa M, Umeshita R, Suzumiya J, Izuhara K, Kikuchi M. Interleukin-13 and interleukin-13 receptor in Hodgkin's disease: possible autocrine mechanism and involvement in fibrosis. Histopathology 2001;38:368-375.
20a. Piña-Oviedo S, Moran CA. Primary mediastinal classical Hodgkin lymphoma. Adv Anat Pathol 2016;23:285-309.
21. Rodriguez-Justo M, Fisher T, Wotherspoon AC. Hodgkin's disease with an intrasinusoidal pattern of infiltration. A report of two cases. Virchows Arch 2001;439:691-696.
22. Rosenwald A, Wright G, Leroy K, et al. Molecular diagnosis of primary mediastinal B cell lymphoma identifies a clinically favorable subgroup of diffuse large B cell lymphoma related to Hodgkin lymphoma. J Exp Med 2003;198:851-862.
23. Sacks EL, Donaldson SS, Gordon J, Dorfman RF. Epithelioid granulomas associated with Hodgkin's disease: clinical correlations in 55 previously untreated patients. Cancer 1978;41:562-567.
24. Seitz V, Hummel M, Marafioti T, Anagnostopoulos I, Assaf C, Stein H. Detection of clonal T-cell receptor gamma-chain gene rearrangements in Reed-Sternberg cells of classic Hodgkin disease. Blood 2000;95:3020-3024.

24a. Sethi T, Nguyen V, Li S, Morgan D, Greer J, Reddy N. Differences in outcome of patients with syncytial variant Hodgkin lymphoma compared with typical nodular sclerosis Hodgkin lymphoma. Ther Adv Hematol 2017;8:13-20.

24b. Sharma S, Dey P, Mitra S, et al. Nodular sclerosis Hodgkin lymphoma grade 2: a diagnostic challenge to the cytopathologists. Cancer 2017; 125:104-113.

25. Stein H, Von Wasielewski R, Poppema S, Mac Lennan KA, Guenova M. Nodular sclerosis classical Hodgkin lymphoma. In: Swerdlow SH, Campo E, Harris NL, et al., eds. WHO classification of tumours of haematopoietic and lymphoid tissues. Lyon: IARC Press; 2008;330.

26. Strickler JG, Michie SA, Warnke RA, Dorfman RF. The "syncytial variant" of nodular sclerosing Hodgkin's disease. Am J Surg Pathol 1986;10:470-477.

27. Tadmor T, Bari A, Marcheselli L, et al. Absolute monocyte count and lymphocyte-monocyte ratio predict outcome in nodular sclerosis Hodgkin lymphoma: evaluation based on data from 1450 patients. Mayo Clin Proc 2015;90:756-964.

28. Tiacci E, Döring C, Brune V, et al. Analyzing primary Hodgkin and Reed-Sternberg cells to capture the molecular and cellular pathogenesis of classical Hodgkin lymphoma. Blood 2012;120:4609-4620.

29. Vassallo J, Lamant L, Brugieres L, et al. ALK-positive anaplastic large cell lymphoma mimicking nodular sclerosis Hodgkin's lymphoma: report of 10 cases. Am J Surg Pathol 2006;30:223-229.

30. Venkataraman G, Song JY, Tzankov A, et al. Aberrant T-cell antigen expression in classical Hodgkin lymphoma is associated with decreased event-free survival and overall survival. Blood 2013;121:1795-1804.

31. von Wasielewski S, Franklin J, Fischer R, et al. Nodular sclerosing Hodgkin disease: new grading predicts prognosis in intermediate and advanced stages. Blood 2003;101:4063-4069.

32. Wijhuizen TJ, Vrints LW, Jairam R, et al. Grades of nodular sclerosis (NSI-II) in Hodgkin's disease. Are they of independent prognostic value? Cancer 1989;63:1150-1153.

39 LYMPHOCYTE-RICH CLASSIC HODGKIN LYMPHOMA

GENERAL FEATURES

Lymphocyte-rich classic Hodgkin lymphoma (LRCHL) is characterized by Reed-Sternberg and Hodgkin (RS+H) cells in a reactive background of predominantly small lymphocytes and fewer histiocytes; granulocytes are absent or rare (1,10). Nodular and diffuse variants of LRCHL are well described, but the former is much more common, representing over 75 percent of all cases.

LRCHL is a relatively recently described type of HL that was included initially as a provisional entity in the Revised European American Lymphoma Classification in 1994. Overall, LRCHL is uncommon, representing 4 percent of HL cases in the large database of the German Hodgkin Lymphoma Study Group (9). However, there may be variation in incidence by geographic region. A study from the European Organization for Research and Treatment of Cancer found that 0.8 percent of all cases of HL were LRCHL (4). In contrast, a small study from Armenia reported a 25 percent frequency of LRCHL (3). LRCHL can closely mimic other types of HL, in particular, nodular lymphocyte-predominant HL (see below), and immunohistochemical analysis is essential for establishing the diagnosis.

CLINICAL FEATURES

The median patient age at the time of diagnosis of LRCHL is 38 to 40 years (5,9). Men are affected more often than women, with a male to female ratio of at least 2 to 1 (5,9). Patients most often present with painless peripheral lymphadenopathy, commonly involving the cervical region (2,9). A large mediastinal mass or involvement of multiple lymph node sites is uncommon. Fever, weight loss, and night sweats (B symptoms) occur in about 15 percent of patients. In the German Hodgkin Lymphoma Study Group database, 80 percent of patients with LRCHL had either stage I or II disease (5,9). In many ways, the clinical presentation of patients with LRCHL is similar to that of patients with nodular lymphocyte-predominant HL and, before the advent of immunophenotyping, the nodular variant of LRCHL was likely grouped with the latter (2).

HISTOLOGIC FINDINGS

Lymph Nodes

In the *nodular variant of LRCHL*, the lymph node is extensively replaced by lymphoma composed of large expansile nodules (figs. 39-1, 39-2) (1,8,9). These nodules correspond to the mantle zones of follicles expanded by small reactive lymphocytes. Reactive germinal centers are common in these nodules and are often eccentrically located (fig. 39-1B). The RS+H cells are predominantly distributed within the expanded mantle zones and are not identified within the germinal centers (fig. 39-1C). Importantly, the tumor nodules are not surrounded or compartmentalized by broad, fibrous bands and capsular fibrosis is absent or minimal. T-cell zones between the tumor nodules are attenuated and, particularly at the border between nodules and T zones, small numbers of granulocytes may be identified (fig. 39-1D). Necrosis is absent in almost all cases of nodular variant LRCHL.

The *diffuse variant of LRCHL* (fig. 39-3) is characterized by scattered RS+H cells in a background of small lymphocytes and fewer histiocytes, distributed in a diffuse pattern throughout the lymph node parenchyma (1,2). In some cases, aggregates of histiocytes, often with an epithelioid appearance, are present. Granulocytes or areas of necrosis are rare.

The neoplastic RS+H cells in LRCHL may be numerous or sparse and they show a spectrum of cytologic features. They often resemble classic RS+H cells (fig. 39-4), but also may resemble lymphocyte-predominant (LP) cells as are observed in nodular lymphocyte-predominant HL (fig. 39-2, right).

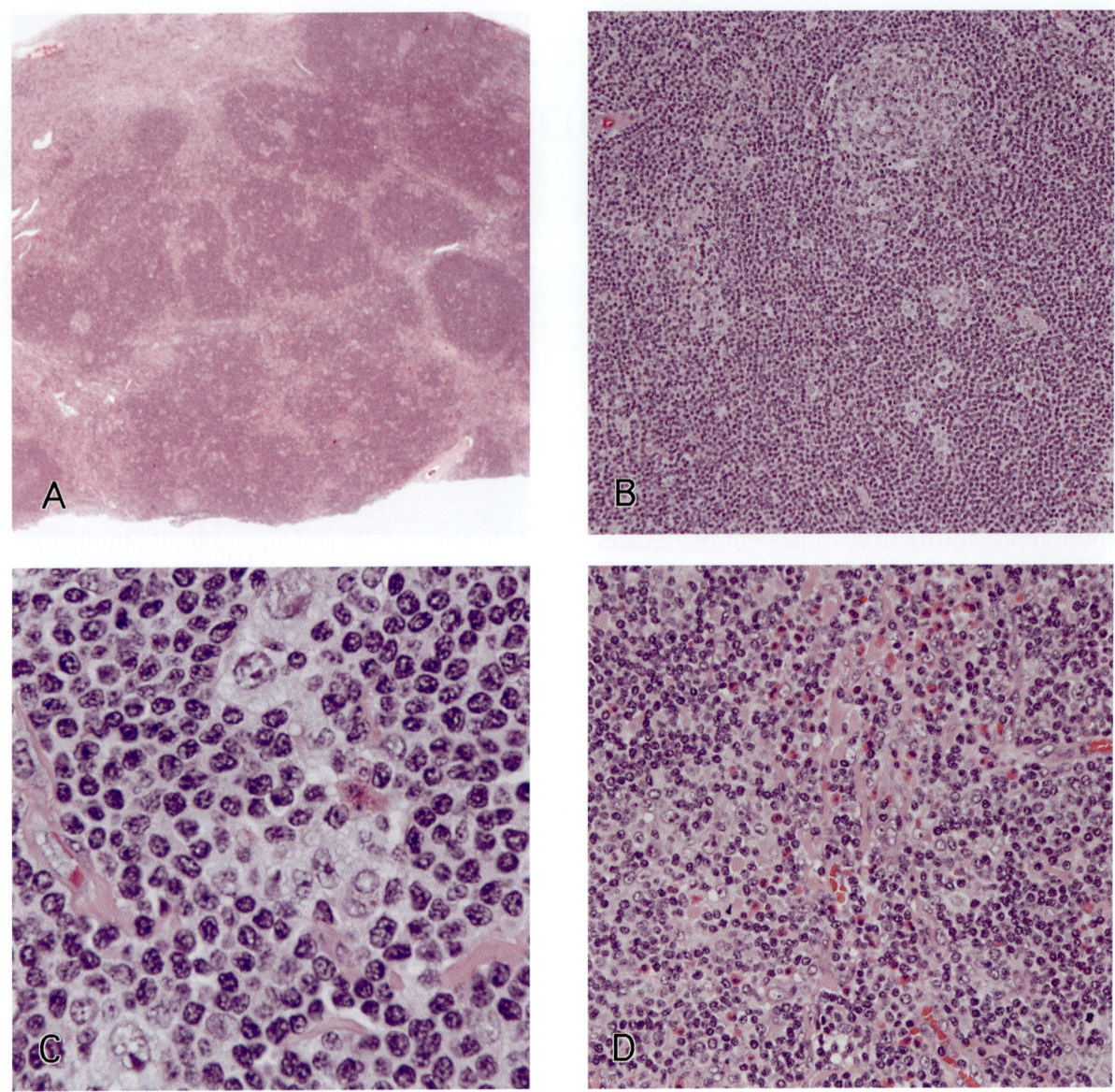

Figure 39-1

LYMPHOCYTE-RICH CLASSIC HODGKIN LYMPHOMA, NODULAR VARIANT, INVOLVING LYMPH NODE

A: The lymph node parenchyma is extensively replaced by lymphoma with a vaguely nodular pattern.

B: Higher-power magnification of one nodule shows many small reactive lymphocytes, scattered Reed-Sternberg and Hodgkin cells, and a small reactive germinal center (upper portion of field).

C: Large Hodgkin cells are present in a background of numerous small reactive lymphocytes and one eosinophil.

D: At the border between a tumor nodule and the T-cell compartments, many eosinophils are present, a useful clue for distinguishing LRCHL from nodular lymphocyte-predominant HL (A–D: hematoxylin and eosin [H&E] stain).

Other Sites

As stated above, most patients with LRCHL have stage I or II disease (9). Uncommonly, the organs of Waldeyer ring, spleen, liver, and bone marrow are involved. Cases of nodular variant LRCHL can retain the nodular pattern or become diffuse. The lymphocyte-rich background may be retained, but some cases recur with a more histiocyte-rich or mixed inflammatory background.

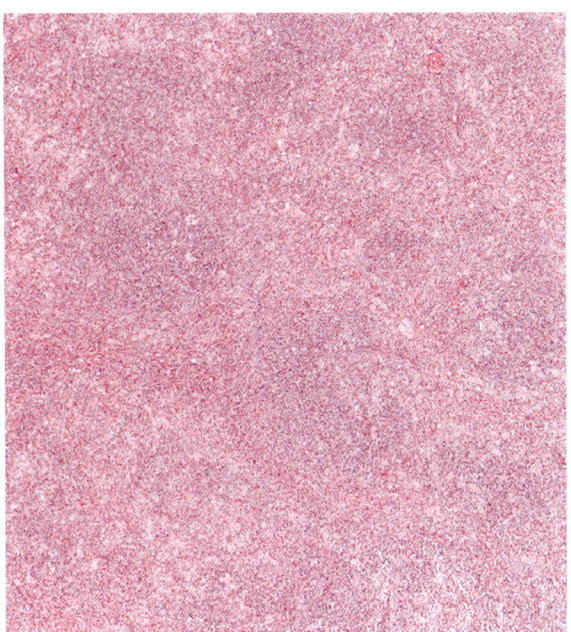 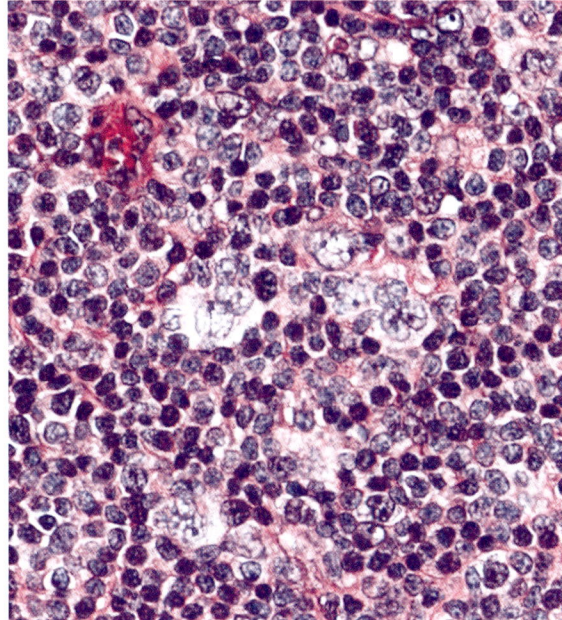

Figure 39-2

LYMPHOCYTE-RICH CLASSIC HODGKIN LYMPHOMA, NODULAR VARIANT

Left: The lymph node is subtotally replaced by a vaguely nodular neoplasm. At low power, small lymphocytes and scattered histiocytes are appreciated.

Right: The neoplastic cells are multilobulated and resemble lymphocyte-predominant (LP) cells as typically occur in nodular lymphocyte-predominant HL. The background cells are almost entirely small lymphocytes without eosinophils, neutrophils, or plasma cells (left, right: H&E stain).

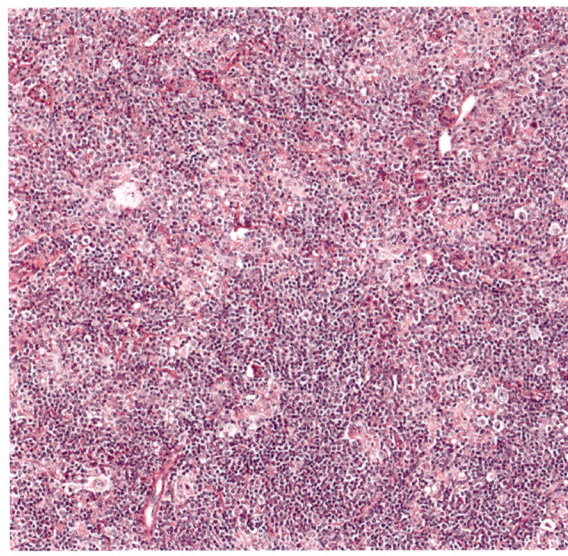 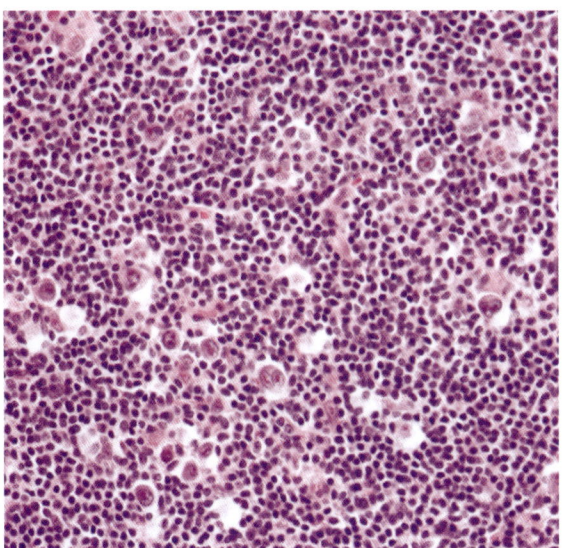

Figure 39-3

LYMPHOCYTE-RICH CLASSIC HODGKIN LYMPHOMA, DIFFUSE VARIANT

This lymphoma had a diffuse pattern but the cellular composition otherwise resembles the nodular variant cases shown previously (H&E stain).

Figure 39-4

LYMPHOCYTE-RICH CLASSIC HODGKIN LYMPHOMA

The neoplastic cells have features of typical RS+H cells (H&E stain).

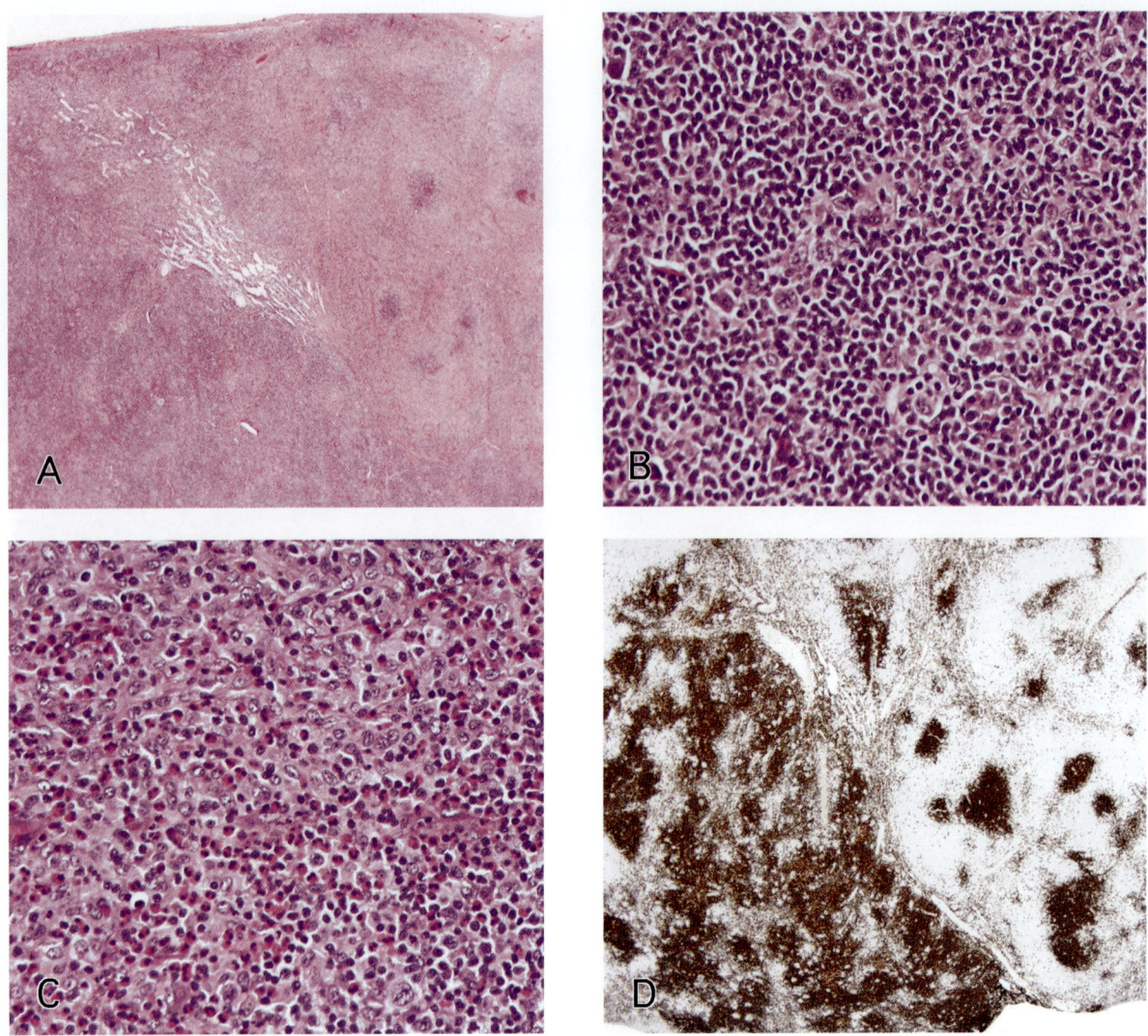

Figure 39-5

CLASSIC HODGKIN LYMPHOMA WITH LYMPHOCYTE-RICH AND NODULAR SCLEROSIS AREAS

A cervical lymph node biopsy specimen shows some areas that resemble LRCHL and other areas that resemble typical nodular sclerosis HL.

A: At low power, an area of LRCHL (left) and an area of nodular sclerosis HL (right) are appreciated (A–C: H&E stain).

B,C: High-magnification images of LRCHL (B) and nodular sclerosis HL areas (C).

D: Anti-CD20 antibody highlights the small B lymphocytes in the background, which are much more numerous in the LRCHL area (left) than in the nodular sclerosis HL area (right) (immunohistochemistry with hematoxylin counterstain).

The Relationship of LRCHL to Nodular Sclerosis HL

After therapy, some patients with LRCHL relapse with a tumor that has the features of nodular sclerosis HL, including well-formed fibrous bands surrounding nodules, neoplastic cells that resemble lacunar cells, and a mixed inflammatory background. In some cases of nodular sclerosis HL, the involved lymph node has areas that closely resemble the nodular variant LRCHL in addition to areas of typical nodular sclerosis HL (fig. 39-5). These observations suggest that a subset of cases currently designated as LRCHL may be an early phase of nodular sclerosis HL and the criteria for LRCHL may need to be further refined. The presence of a mediastinal mass may be a clue suggesting early phase nodular sclerosis.

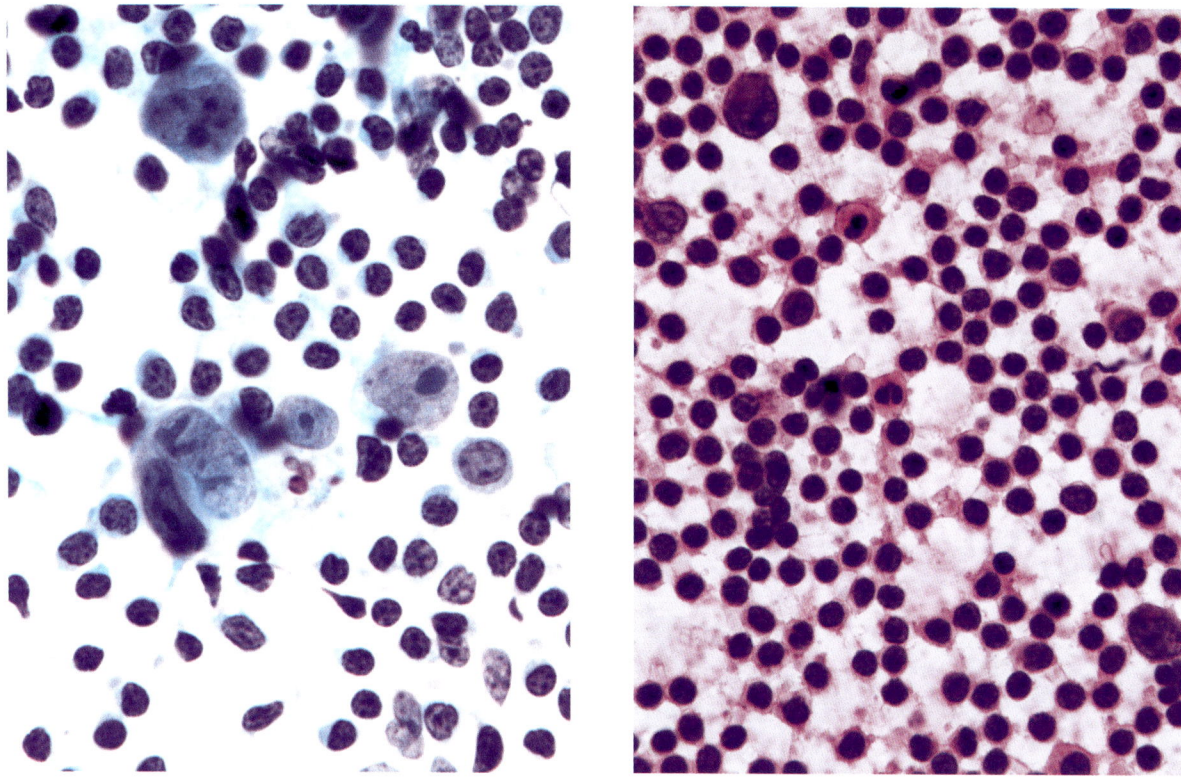

Figure 39-6

LYMPHOCYTE-RICH CLASSIC HODGKIN LYMPHOMA: CYTOLOGIC FINDINGS

Left: A fine-needle aspirate of lymph node shows RS+H cells and variants admixed with small lymphocytes (Papanicolaou stain).

Right: A lymph node scrape preparation shows scattered large Hodgkin cells with numerous small lymphocytes in the background (H&E stain).

CYTOLOGIC FINDINGS

Cytologic preparations of LRCHL show numerous small reactive lymphocytes with a variable number of histiocytes that can have epithelioid features. Large neoplastic cells that resemble RS+H cells, LP cells, or both may be present (fig. 39-6). In some cases, the neoplastic cells are sparse in number and the cell population mimics a reactive process. Granulocytes and plasma cells are rare to absent in the background.

IMMUNOHISTOCHEMICAL FINDINGS

The RS+H cells of LRCHL express CD30 (fig. 39-7A), CD15 (70 to 80 percent) (fig. 39-7B), IRF4/MUM1 (over 90 percent), and PAX5 (dim, 90 to 95 percent); they are negative for CD3, CD43, CD45/LCA (fig. 39-7C), and J chain (1,2,8). CD20 is usually negative (fig. 39-7D), but some cases have weak and variable expression.

In the nodular variant of LRCHL, the background small lymphocytes are mostly B cells. Scattered small reactive T cells commonly form rosettes around the neoplastic cells (fig. 39-8). CD57-positive T cells are also scattered throughout the nodules, as are many CD21-positive follicular dendritic cells, supporting a relationship to normal follicles (fig. 39-9).

In a study by Nam-Cha et al. (8), LRCHL cases were assessed with a large panel of antibodies. The authors concluded that cases of LRCHL have a B-cell transcription profile intermediate between nodular lymphocyte-predominant HL and other types of classic HL. The RS+H cells have an intermediate frequency of expression of B-cell transcription factors, such as OCT.2, BOB.1, BCL6, GCET1, and more often brightly express PAX5 than other types of classic HL, although less than in cases of nodular

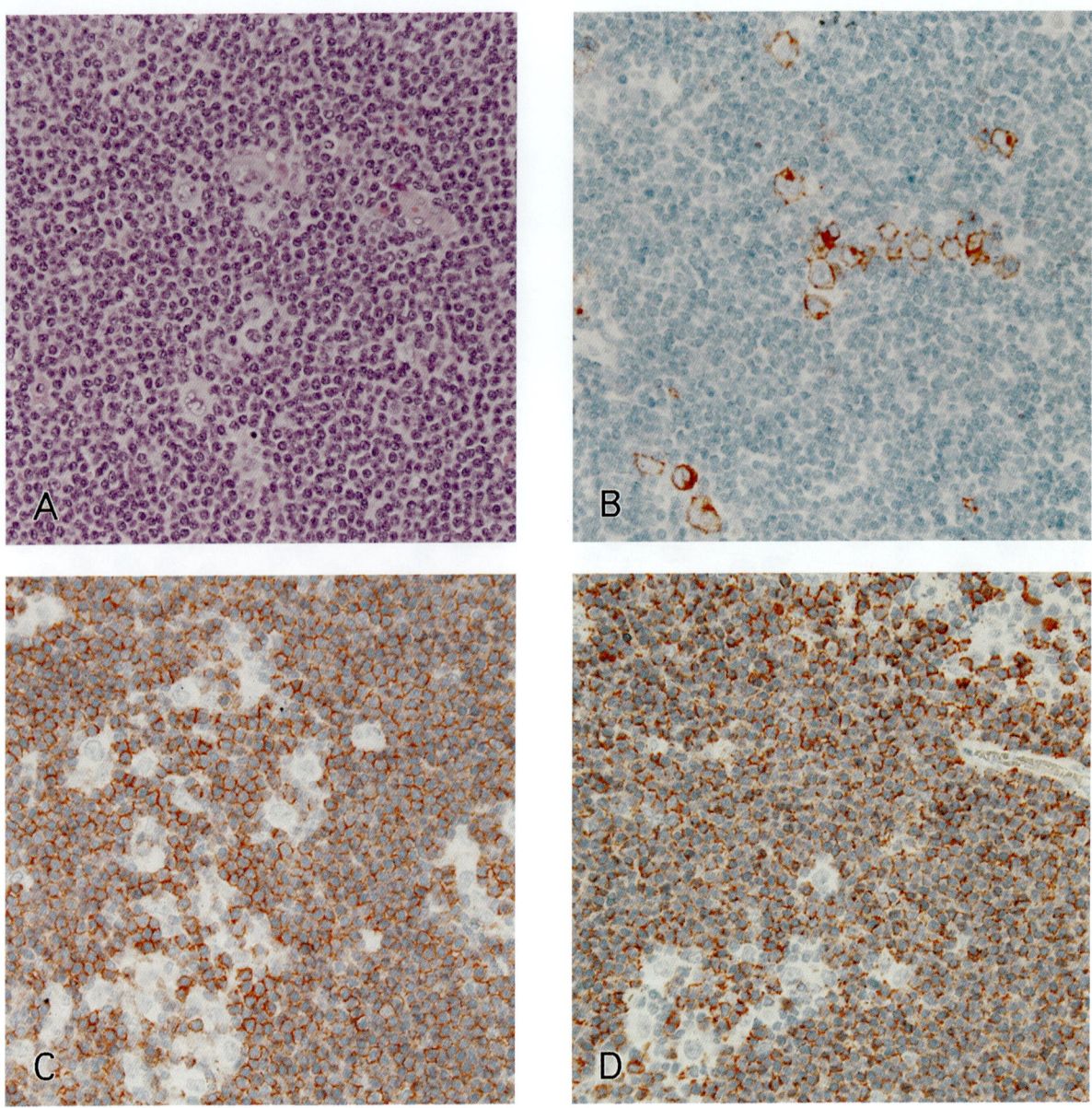

Figure 39-7

IMMUNOPHENOTYPE OF LYMPHOCYTE-RICH CLASSIC HODGKIN LYMPHOMA, NODULAR VARIANT

A: High magnification of RS+H cells (H&E stain).

B–D: The neoplastic cells are positive for CD30 (B) and negative for CD45/LCA (C) and CD20 (D). Many small reactive B cells are seen in the tumor nodules (A–C: immunohistochemistry with hematoxylin counterstain) (same case as shown in figure 39-1).

lymphocyte-predominant HL. Markers of the NF-κB pathway, however, are expressed commonly, similar to other types of classic HL. They further concluded that the microenvironment in cases of nodular variant LRCHL mimics the outer zone of the germinal center.

Evidence of Epstein-Barr virus (EBV) infection is present in about 40 percent of LRCHL cases. The RS+H cells have a type II latency pattern: positive for EBV latent membrane protein type 1 (LMP1) and EBV nuclear antigen 1 (EBNA1) but negative for EBNA2. The RS+H

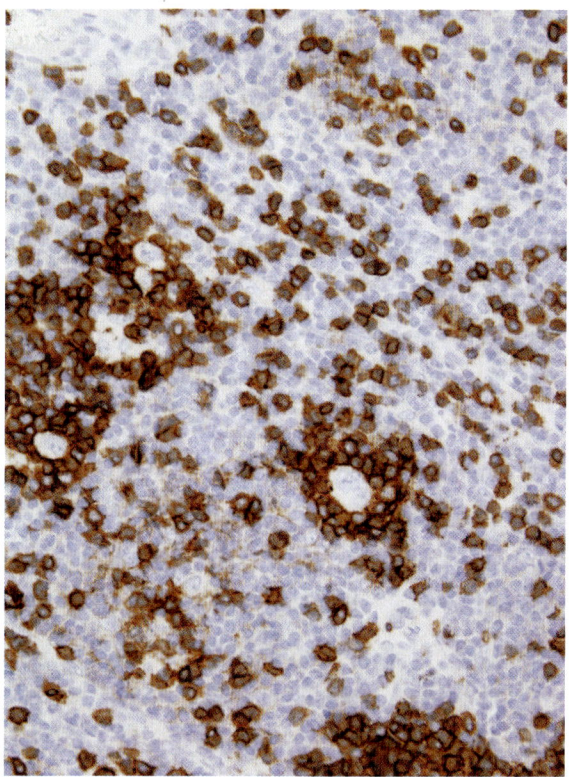

Figure 39-8

T-CELL ROSETTES IN LYMPHOCYTE-RICH CLASSIC HODGKIN LYMPHOMA, NODULAR VARIANT

The anti-CD3 antibody highlights small T cells that form rosettes around the neoplastic cells (immunohistochemistry with hematoxylin counterstain).

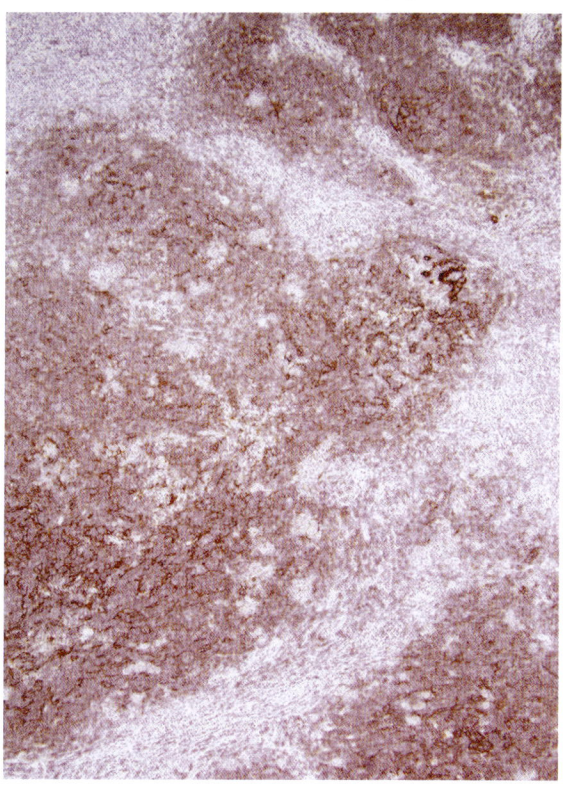

Figure 39-9

LYMPHOCYTE-RICH CLASSIC HODGKIN LYMPHOMA, NODULAR VARIANT: CD21

The anti-CD21 antibody highlights large networks of follicular dendritic cells within the tumor nodules (immunohistochemistry with hematoxylin counterstain).

cells are also positive for EBV encoded RNA1 (EBER1) (fig. 39-10).

MOLECULAR GENETIC FINDINGS

The molecular findings in cases of LRCHL are similar to those in other types of classic HL, as is discussed in chapter 37.

DIFFERENTIAL DIAGNOSIS

Nodular Lymphocyte-Predominant HL. The nodular variant of LRCHL can closely mimic nodular lymphocyte-predominant HL (2,5). The nodular variant of LRCHL and nodular lymphocyte-predominant HL are composed of expansile nodules composed of many small reactive B lymphocytes, fewer histiocytes, and rare or absent granulocytes.

Histologic clues to the diagnosis of LRCHL include: reactive germinal centers within the

tumor nodules, neoplastic cells that appear to be located in the periphery of the nodules, and granulocytes that are present at the margins of the tumor nodules. In contrast, in nodular lymphocyte-predominant HL reactive germinal centers are uncommon in tumor nodules (about 15 percent of cases), the tumor cells are distributed throughout the tumor nodules, and eosinophils are usually not present or are rare (6). Although the neoplastic cells often resemble typical RS+H cells in LRCHL, this feature is not reliable as the neoplastic cells can resemble LP cells as well. Immunohistochemical studies are essential for this differential diagnosis because the histologic features alone are often misleading.

Nodular Sclerosis HL. Unlike the nodular variant of LRCHL, nodular sclerosis HL is characterized by capsular fibrosis, perivascular fibrosis, and collagenous fibrous bands that

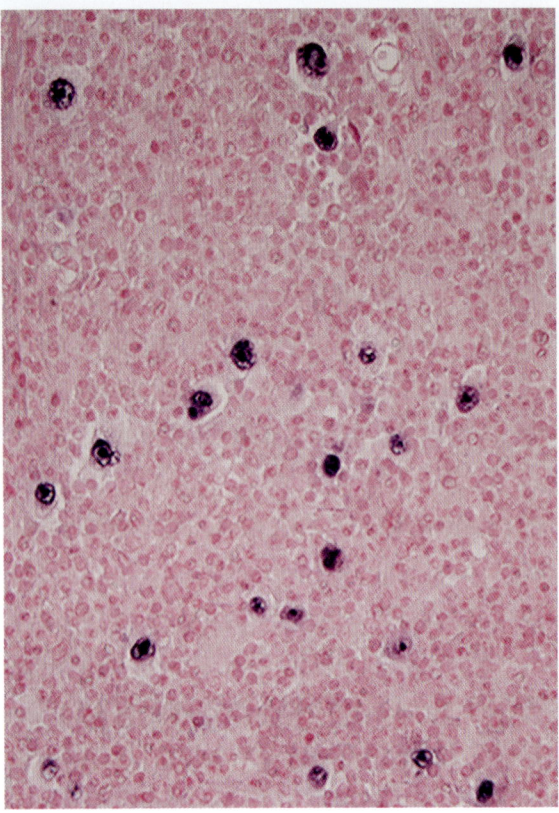

Figure 39-10

**LYMPHOCYTE-RICH CLASSIC HODGKIN
LYMPHOMA, NODULAR VARIANT**

The neoplastic cells are positive for Epstein-Barr virus encoded RNA1 (EBER1) (in situ hybridization with eosin counterstain).

surround tumor nodules. In addition, the neoplastic cells are lacunar cells. As stated above, in some patients who initially have a lymph node involved by LRCHL, the relapse can have features of nodular sclerosis HL.

Mixed Cellularity HL. The diffuse variant of LRCHL can resemble mixed cellularity HL. The quality of the background cells helps distinguish these neoplasms. Mixed cellularity HL is characterized by a mixture of small lymphocytes, histiocytes, eosinophils, or plasma cells whereas LRCHL is characterized by mostly small lymphocytes with fewer histiocytes. Mixed cellularity HL also often has a greater number of classic RS cells.

T-Cell/Histiocyte-Rich Large B-Cell Lymphoma. The diffuse variant of LRCHL shares features with T-cell/histiocyte-rich large B-cell lymphoma. Scattered large neoplastic cells are present in a sea of small lymphocytes and histiocytes. Unlike LRCHL, the large lymphoma cells in T-cell/histiocyte-rich large B-cell lymphoma are B cells positive for CD20, PAX5 (bright), and CD45/LCA and negative for CD15. CD30 can be expressed by the tumor cells of T-cell/histiocyte-rich large B-cell lymphoma.

Follicular T-Helper Cell Lymphoma. Follicular T-helper cell lymphoma is a rare subtype of peripheral T-cell lymphoma recognized in the 2016 WHO classification revision (10) that usually mimics follicular lymphoma or, less often, marginal zone lymphoma. However, Moroch et al. (7) described four cases that were nodular and mimicked LRCHL. In all cases, the lymphoma cells (including RS+H-like cells), had a T-helper cell immunophenotype positive for CD10, BCL6, CXCL13, or ICOS and carried monoclonal T-cell receptor gene rearrangements, unlike HL (7).

B-Cell Non-Hodgkin Lymphomas with a Nodular Pattern. The nodular variant of LRCHL may resemble, in part, follicular lymphoma, nodular pattern of mantle cell lymphoma, or marginal zone lymphoma with follicular colonization. RS+H cells are not observed in non-Hodgkin lymphomas. In follicular lymphoma, the mixture of centrocytes and centroblasts is unlike the background cells of LRCHL. In mantle cell lymphoma, the neoplastic cells typically show greater nuclear irregularity, unlike LRCHL. In marginal zone lymphoma, the cell population is more heterogeneous than LRCHL, with monocytoid B cells, plasmacytoid cells, and scattered intermixed large cells. Immunophenotypic and molecular studies make the recognition of B-cell non-Hodgkin lymphomas easier since these neoplasms express monotypic surface immunoglobulin and carry monoclonal immunoglobulin gene rearrangements. The t(14;18)(q32;q21)/*IGH-BCL2* and t(11;14)(q13;q32)/*CCND1-IGH* support follicular lymphoma and mantle cell lymphoma, respectively.

TREATMENT AND PROGNOSIS

The standard therapy for patients with LRCHL is similar to that for other types of classic Hodgkin lymphoma. Combination chemotherapy and radiation therapy are used for most patients (see chapter 37).

The progression-free and overall survival rates of patients with LRCHL are slightly more favorable than for other subtypes of classic HL and are comparable to patients with nodular lymphocyte-predominant HL, with the exception of the pattern of relapse. Patients with LRCHL may relapse in the first 2 to 3 years after therapy, but subsequently relapse-free survival curves show a plateau correlating with cure. In contrast, patients with nodular lymphocyte-predominant HL relapse over time in a continuous manner, without a plateau (2,5,9).

REFERENCES

1. Agnastopoulos I, Isaacson PG, Stein H, et al. Lymphocyte-rich classical Hodgkin lymphoma. In: Swerdlow SH, Campo E, Harris NL, et al., eds. WHO classification of tumours of haematopoietic and lymphoid tissues. Lyon: IARC Press; 2008;323-333.
2. Anagnostopoulos I, Hansmann ML, Franssila K, et al. European Task Force on Lymphoma project on lymphocyte predominance Hodgkin disease: histologic and immunohistologic analysis of submitted cases reveals 2 types of Hodgkin disease with a nodular growth pattern and abundant lymphocytes. Blood 2000;96:1889-1899
3. Avagyan A, Danielyan S, Voskanyan A, et al. Treating adults with Hodgkin lymphoma in the developing world: a hospital-based cohort study from Armenia. Asian Pac J Cancer Prev 2016;17:101-104.
4. de Jong D, Bosq J, MacLennan KA, et al. Lymphocyte-rich classical Hodgkin lymphoma (LRCHL): clinico-pathological characteristics and outcome of a rare entity. Ann Oncol 2006;17:141-145.
5. Diehl V, Sextro M, Franklin J, et al. Clinical presentation, course, and prognostic factors in lymphocyte-predominant Hodgkin's disease and lymphocyte-rich classical Hodgkin's disease: report from the European Task Force on Lymphoma Project on Lymphocyte-Predominant Hodgkin's Disease. J Clin Oncol 1999;17:776-783.
6. Fan Z, Natkunam Y, Bair E, Tibshirani R, Warnke RA. Characterization of variant patterns of nodular lymphocyte predominant Hodgkin lymphoma with immunohistologic and clinical correlation. Am J Surg Pathol 2003;27:1346-1356.
7. Moroch J, Copie-Bergman C, de Leval L, et al. Follicular peripheral T-cell lymphoma expands the spectrum of classical Hodgkin lymphoma mimics. Am J Surg Pathol 2012;36:1636-1646.
8. Nam-Cha SH, Montes-Moreno S, Salcedo MT, Sanjuan J, Garcia JF, Piris MA. Lymphocyte-rich classical Hodgkin's lymphoma: distinctive tumor and microenvironment markers. Mod Pathol 2009;22:1006-1015.
9. Shimabukuro-Vornhagen A, Haverkamp H, Engert A, et al. Lymphocyte-rich classical Hodgkin's lymphoma: clinical presentation and treatment outcome in 100 patients treated within German Hodgkin's Study Group trials. J Clin Oncol 2005;23:5739-5745.
10. Swerdlow SH, Campo E, Pileri SA, et al. The 2016 revision of the World Health Organization classification of lymphoid neoplasms. Blood 2016;127:2375-2390.

40

MIXED CELLULARITY HODGKIN LYMPHOMA

GENERAL FEATURES

Mixed cellularity Hodgkin lymphoma (MCHL) is characterized histologically by numerous classic Reed-Sternberg and Hodgkin (RS+H) cells in a mixed inflammatory background. There is no evidence of tumor-associated nodularity or sclerosis. The World Health Organization (WHO) classification also allows the use of the mixed cellularity category as a "wastebasket" for cases of classic HL that do not readily fit into other well-defined types (15).

MCHL is the second most common type of HL. In well-developed nations, such as the United States and those of Europe, MCHL represents 20 to 25 percent of all cases of HL (9,15). In developing countries, MCHL is more frequent and the most common type of HL in some nations (7a). In Asia, the frequency of MCHL may be changing as a western type lifestyle or diet has become more common. In a study from Japan, almost 50 percent of HL cases were MCHL (4). Patients with immunodeficiency, such as human immunodeficiency virus (HIV) infection, also have a higher frequency of MCHL (11). Young children (peak age of 5 to 10 years) have a higher frequency as well (12).

Among all types of HL, the frequency of Epstein-Barr virus (EBV) infection is highest in MCHL: up to 75 percent of all cases are positive (9,15). Poorer economic status, social factors such as lower parent education level (often associated with lower economic status), and a larger number of siblings are associated with a higher frequency of MCHL. These factors suggest exposure to an infectious agent in early life, likely EBV. Primary EBV infection could play a role in the small peak of incidence of MCHL in young children (12). Reactivation of viral infection may be involved in adult cases of MCHL.

CLINICAL FEATURES

MCHL is most frequently seen in adults with a median age of 38 years or older in various studies. The male to female ratio is 2.3 to 1.0 (5,9,15). B symptoms are present in 30 to 40 percent of patients. Patients commonly present with lymphadenopathy involving cervical or other peripheral lymph nodes. As compared with patients who have nodular sclerosis HL, patients with MCHL have a higher frequency of advanced stage disease (9,12,13,15). Common sites of dissemination include: spleen, about 30 percent of patients; abdominal lymph nodes, 25 percent; bone marrow, about 10 percent; bones, 5 percent; and liver, 3 percent (5,15).

HISTOLOGIC FINDINGS

Lymph Nodes

The lymph node architecture may be subtotally effaced by the neoplasm, with a preferential interfollicular and paracortical pattern of involvement (fig. 40-1) or completely and diffusely effaced (fig. 40-2) (15). The RS+H cells are usually easily identified and have classic features (discussed in chapter 37). The RS cells are large, with moderate to abundant cytoplasm and two nuclear lobes (fig. 40-3, left). These lobes have a thick and irregular nuclear membrane; a prominent, round, eosinophilic inclusion-like nucleolus ("owl's eye"); pale chromatin; and a perinucleolar clear zone (or "halo"). The Hodgkin cells are mononuclear, but otherwise have similar cytologic features (fig. 40-2, right; 40-3, right). Variable numbers of large transformed cells with pyknotic nuclei, "mummified cells," also may be seen (fig. 40-3, right). In some cases Hodgkin cells have abundant, retracted cytoplasm and resemble lacunar cells, however, these cells are usually not numerous and the designation lacunar cell is not useful in this context.

The background cells in MCHL are highly variable: a mixture of small lymphocytes, histiocytes, plasma cells, and eosinophils. In most cases of MCHL, the small lymphocytes and histiocytes are the most numerous and eosinophils,

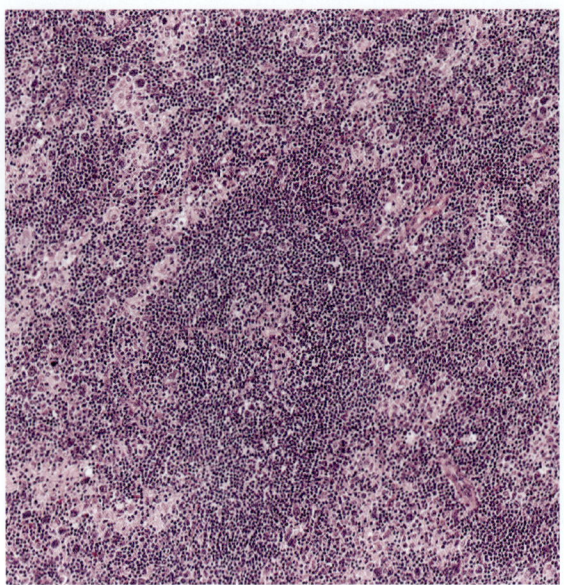

Figure 40-1

**MIXED CELLULARITY HODGKIN LYMPHOMA
SUBTOTALLY REPLACING LYMPH NODE**

The neoplasm has a paracortical pattern, sparing a central lymphoid follicle (hematoxylin and eosin [H&E] stain).

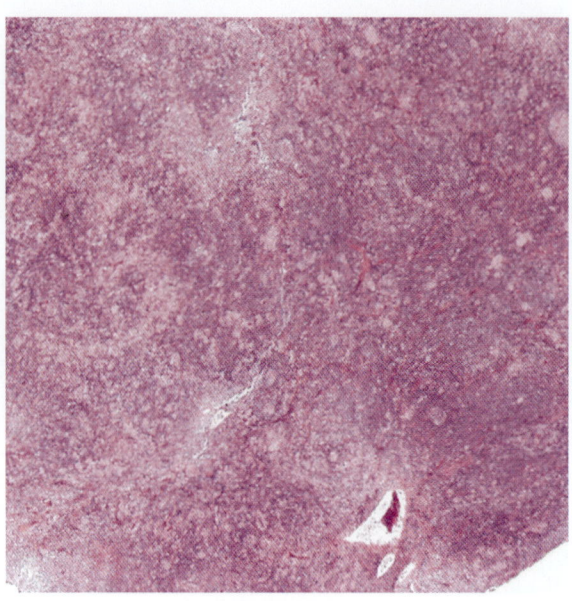

Figure 40-2

**MIXED CELLULARITY HODGKIN LYMPHOMA
INVOLVING LYMPH NODE**

The neoplasm almost completely replaces the lymph node in a diffuse pattern. A few reactive follicles and sinuses are spared (H&E stain).

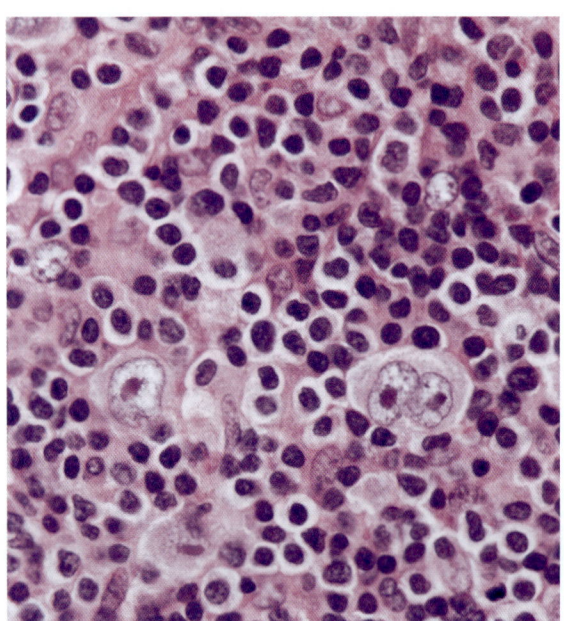

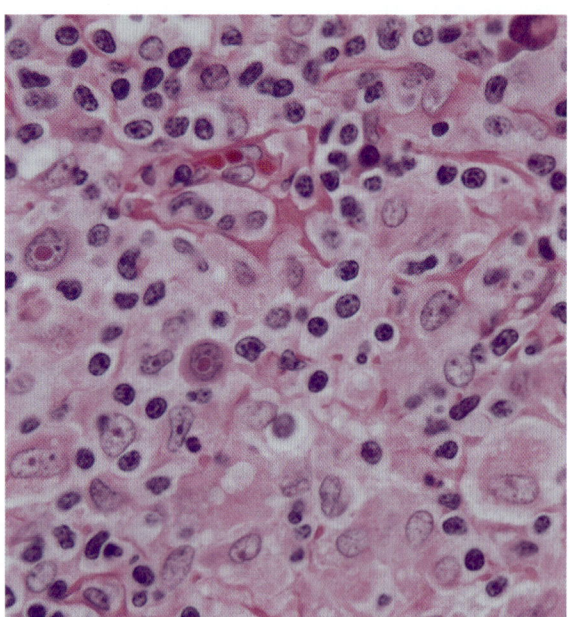

Figure 40-3

REED-STERNBERG AND HODGKIN CELLS

Left: At high magnification, one bilobed Reed-Sternberg (RS) cell (middle right) and mononuclear Hodgkin cells are seen.
Right: Two Hodgkin cells (left) have a prominent eosinophilic nucleolus and a well-developed perinucleolar halo. In addition, one mummified cell (far upper right) is appreciated. The background cell population in this tumor is histiocyte-rich (left, right: H&E stain) (same case as from fig. 40-2).

although often present, are less numerous. Some cases of MCHL have many plasma cells in the background (fig. 40-4). Neutrophilic granulocytes occur in some cases but are usually not numerous. Foci of necrosis are unusual.

Interfollicular Variant. In this variant, RS+H cells and associated background cells exclusively involve the interfollicular areas of the lymph node. The RS+H cells may be few, replacing only a small percentage of the lymph node (fig. 40-5) (6). This variant is often associated with reactive plasmacytosis and follicular hyperplasia that can be prominent, superficially mimicking a reactive lymph node process. Although rare cases of the interfollicular variant have been of nodular sclerosis type, most are best classified as MCHL (6).

Histiocyte-Rich or Granulomatous Variant. In this variant, numerous histiocytes, often with epithelioid features, are present in the background throughout the lymph node. The histiocytes may be scattered singly or form epithelioid or, less often, sarcoid-like granulomas (fig. 40-6) (2,14). In some cases, the histiocytes are so numerous that

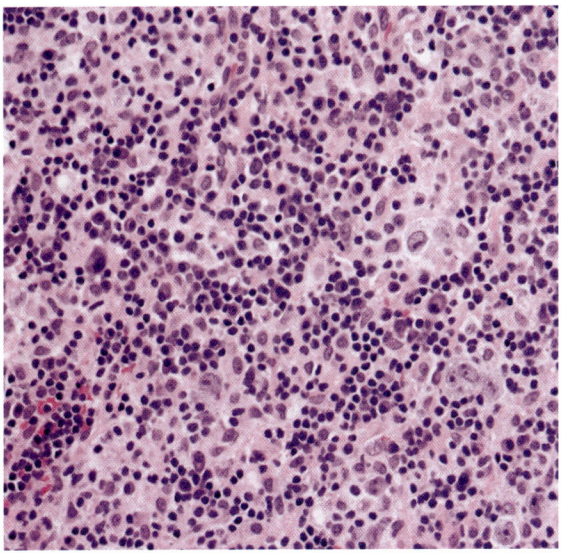

Figure 40-4

MIXED CELLULARITY HODGKIN LYMPHOMA INVOLVING LYMPH NODE

The background is composed of many lymphocytes and plasma cells and fewer histiocytes. Hodgkin cells also are seen (H&E stain).

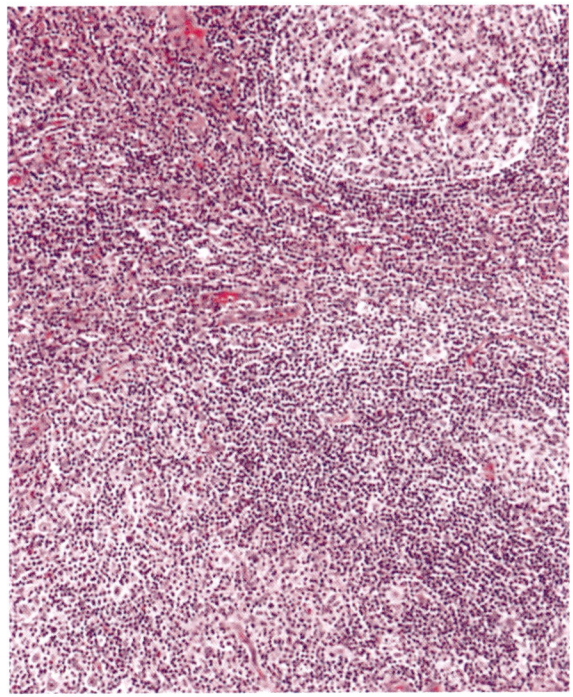 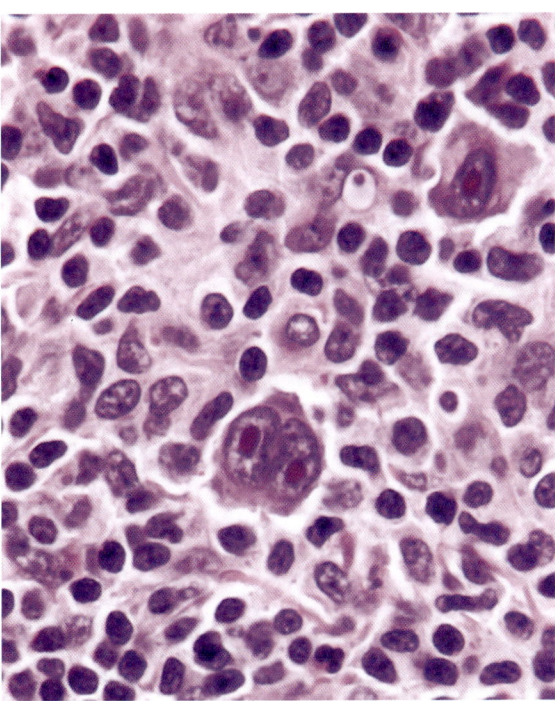

Figure 40-5

MIXED CELLULARITY HODGKIN LYMPHOMA, INTERFOLLICULAR VARIANT

Left: The neoplasm focally involves the lymph node (lower left). Reactive follicles are present.
Right: High-power magnification shows a classic RS cell (center) and a mononuclear Hodgkin cell (top right) (left, right: H&E stain).

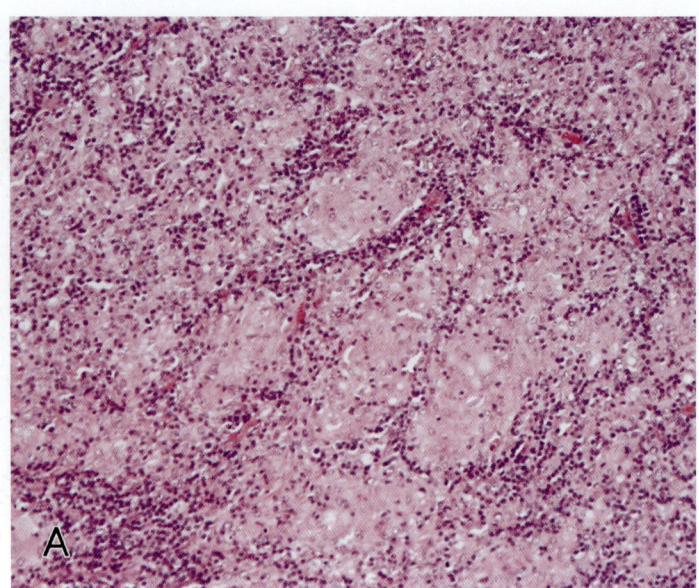

Figure 40-6

MIXED CELLULARITY HODGKIN LYMPHOMA WITH EXUBERANT HISTIOCYTE-RICH BACKGROUND

A: Many sarcoid-like granulomas are seen.

B: A Langerhans-type giant cell and numerous epithelioid histiocytes are present. The histiocytes partially obscure the neoplastic cells but a Hodgkin cell can be seen in this field (arrow).

C: High magnification shows a RS cell and a mononuclear Hodgkin cell (A–C: H&E stain).

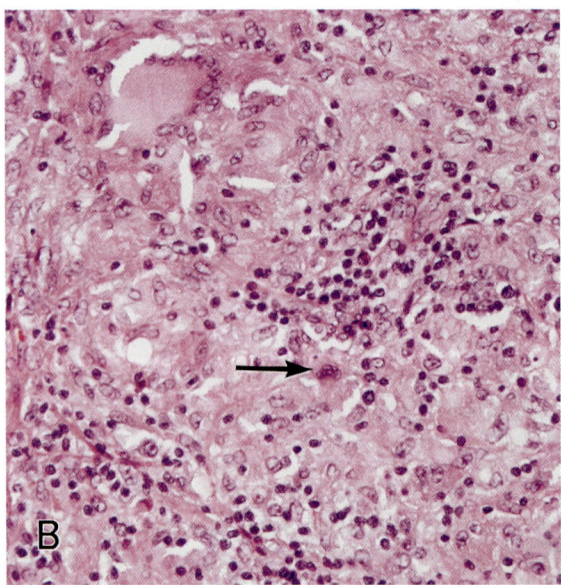

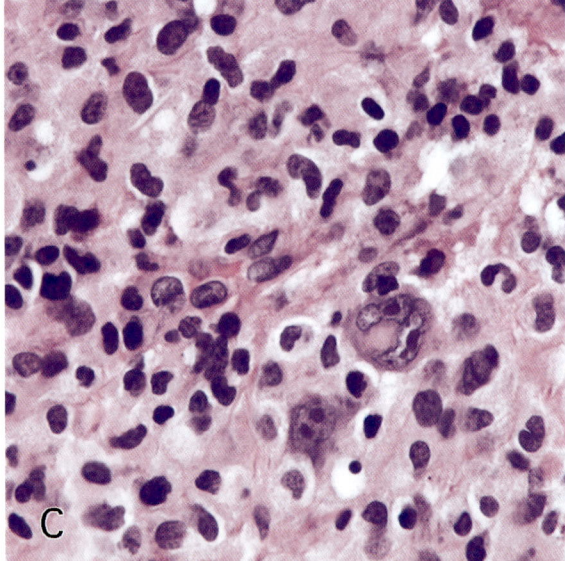

they obscure recognition of the RS+H cells. The histiocyte-rich variant of MCHL also may have plasma cells in the background, but eosinophils and neutrophils are infrequent. Areas of necrosis are present in some cases.

Sinusoidal Involvement Associated with Marginal Zone B-Cell Clusters/Hyperplasia. In this variant, the RS+H cells are located within the lymph node sinuses, which are often expanded by monocytoid B cells; these B cells can form prominent clusters (fig. 40-7) (10). The sinusoidal monocytoid B cells are often associated with neutrophils in the background. The lymph node is usually partially involved in this variant, and the uninvolved lymph node often shows reactive follicular and paracortical hyperplasia.

Castleman-Like Changes. In some cases of MCHL, the neoplasm is associated with prominent interfollicular plasmacytosis, and germinal centers in reactive follicles show regressive changes, mostly depletion of germinal center lymphocytes. Less often, surrounding "onion skin" change in the mantle zones and hyaline-vascular lesions can be present. These changes resemble, in part, the plasma cell variant of Castleman disease (8,16). Rare cases of

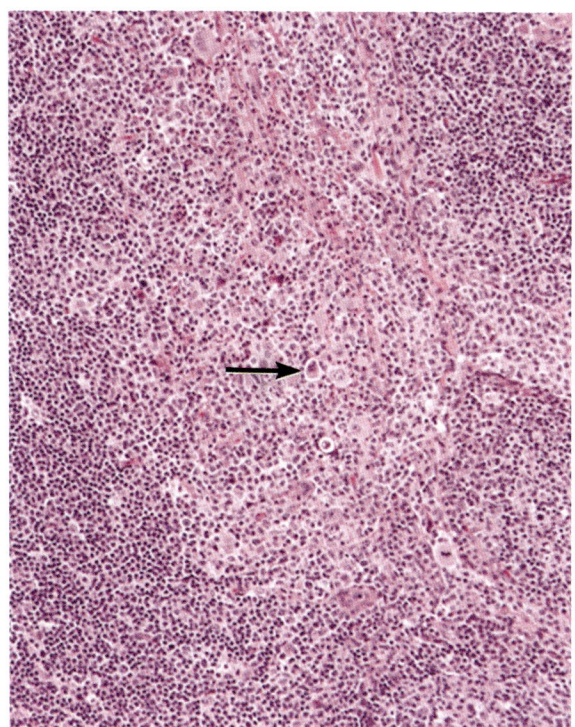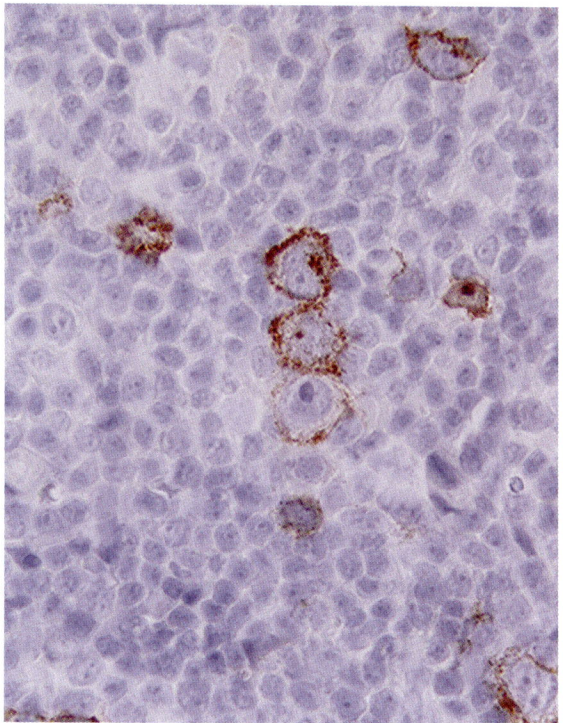

Figure 40-7

MIXED CELLULARITY HODGKIN LYMPHOMA INVOLVING AN EXPANDED LYMPH NODE SINUS

Left: In this field, Hodgkin cells (arrow) are associated with monocytoid B cells and neutrophils (H&E stain).
Right: The neoplastic cells are positive for CD30 and were negative for CD20 (not shown) (immunohistochemistry with hematoxylin counterstain).

HL, often the interfollicular variant, have been reported to be associated with Castleman disease, usually the plasma cell variant and negative for human herpesvirus 8 (HHV-8) infection (7).

Spleen, Liver, and Bone Marrow

MCHL lymphoma can involve the spleen, preferentially involving the white pulp (fig. 40-8). In cases with splenic disease, nodules are often visible grossly and the white pulp is expanded by RS+H cells in a mixed inflammatory background. In the liver, MCHL preferentially involves the portal tracts but can extensively replace the parenchyma (fig. 40-9). In bone marrow, MCHL is usually associated with fibrosis and therefore is best detected in a bone marrow biopsy specimen.

CYTOLOGIC FINDINGS

In aspirate smears, MCHL is characterized by a high proportion of RS+H cells with classic features, mummified cells, and background inflammatory cells in variable proportions (fig. 40-10). The reactive inflammatory background includes small lymphocytes, eosinophils, neutrophils, plasma cells, and histiocytes. The histiocytes may exhibit epithelioid features and form aggregates or microgranulomas (17).

IMMUNOPHENOTYPIC FINDINGS

The RS+H cells of MCHL express CD30 (fig. 40-7B), CD15 (65 to 75 percent) (fig. 40-11), IRF4/MUM1 (over 90 percent) and PAX5 (dim, 90 to 95 percent) and are negative for CD45/LCA. EBV infection of RS+H cells is present in up to 75 percent of cases. RS+H cells show a type II latency pattern: positive for EBV latent membrane protein type 1 (LMP1) and EBV nuclear antigen 1 (EBNA1) but negative for EBNA2. The RS+H cells are also positive for EBV-encoded RNA1 (EBER1).

MOLECULAR GENETIC FINDINGS

The molecular findings in cases of MCHL are similar to those in other types of classic HL, as is discussed in chapter 37.

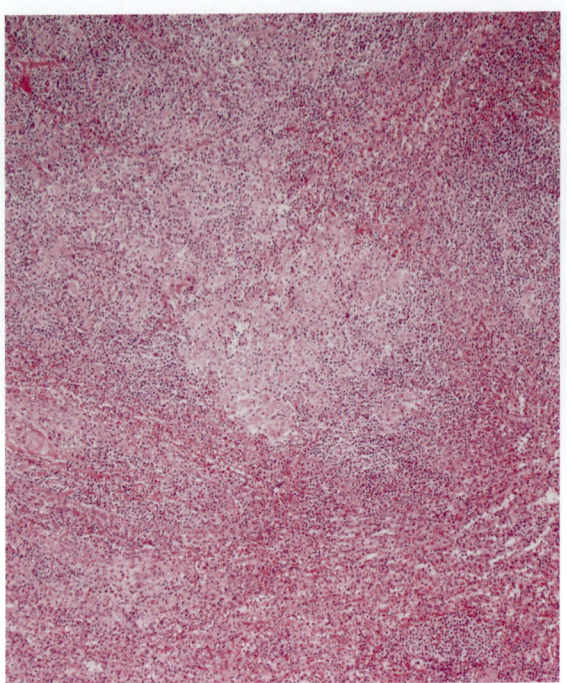
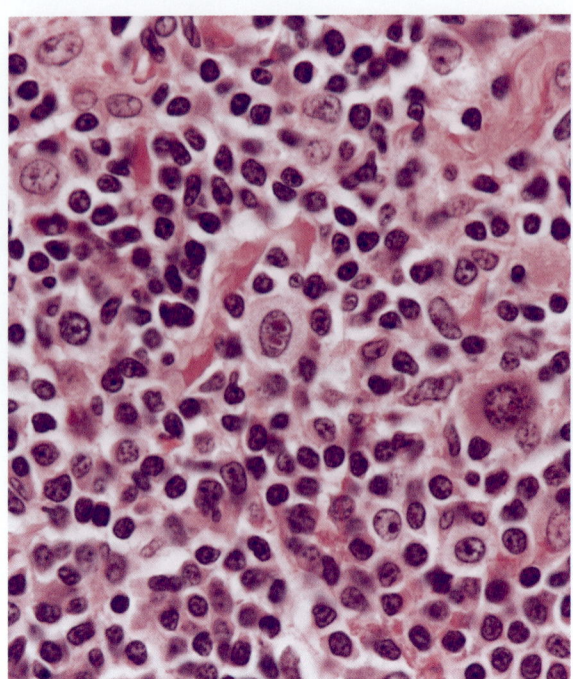

Figure 40-8

MIXED CELLULARITY HODGKIN LYMPHOMA INVOLVING SPLEEN

Left: A splenectomy specimen shows MCHL predominantly located in the white pulp.
Right: Hodgkin cells are present in a reactive background (left, right: H&E stain).

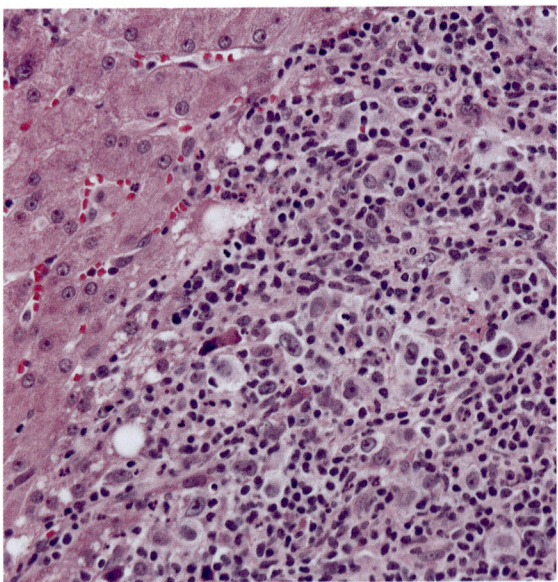
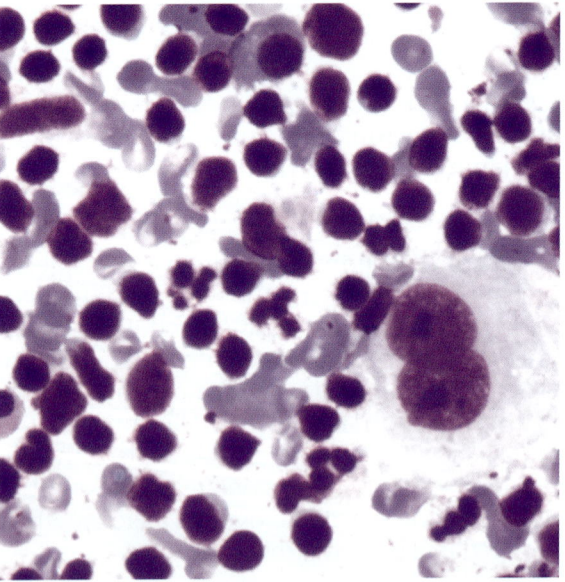

Figure 40-9

**MIXED CELLULARITY HODGKIN
LYMPHOMA INVOLVING LIVER**

A wedge biopsy specimen of the liver shows extensive involvement by MCHL (H&E stain).

Figure 40-10

MIXED CELLULARITY HODGKIN LYMPHOMA

The fine-needle aspirate smear shows a RS cell in a background of lymphocytes and eosinophils (Diff-Quik stain).

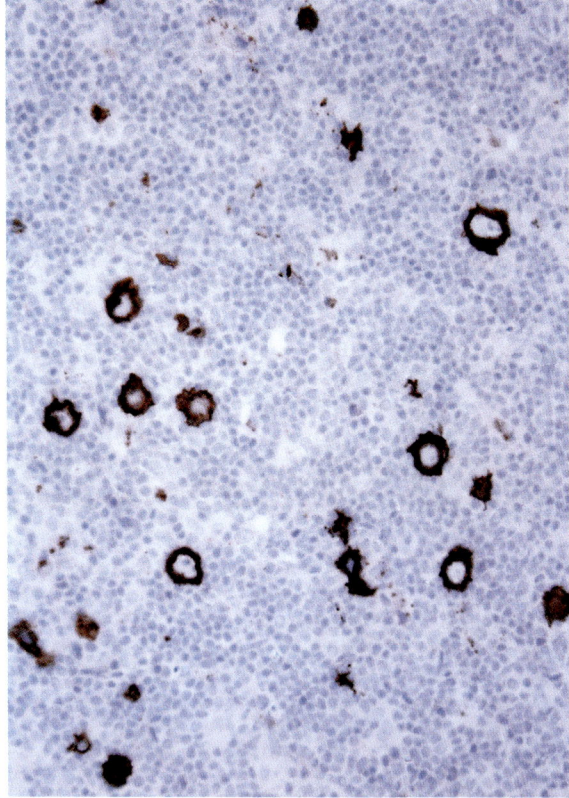

Figure 40-11

MIXED CELLULARITY HODGKIN LYMPHOMA: CD15

The neoplastic cells are positive for CD15 (immunohisto-chemistry with hematoxylin counterstain).

DIFFERENTIAL DIAGNOSIS

Chronic Granulomatous Inflammation. Cases of MCHL with a histiocyte-rich background can obscure RS+H cells, and particularly if necrosis is present, can be confused with infectious causes of chronic granulomatous inflammation (14,17). If a case of MCHL has numerous epithelioid or sarcoid-like granulomas, the possibility of sarcoidosis also may be considered. The key features in distinguishing HL from benign causes is the presence of RS+H cells. Immunohistochemical studies are very helpful by highlighting the neoplastic cells.

Nodular Sclerosis HL. Distinguishing nodular sclerosis HL from MCHL is usually straightforward as the former has a nodular pattern, the nodules are surrounded by dense collagenous fibrous bands, and the neoplastic cells have features of lacunar cells. However, areas of nodular sclerosis can have a highly mixed background, with numerous eosinophils, often more exuberant than observed in MCHL. Particularly in a needle biopsy specimen or small biopsy specimens of nodular sclerosis HL, fibrous bands and nodules can be under-represented or underdeveloped and these cases can mimic MCHL. A search for perivascular or capsular fibrosis and assessment of the quality of the lacunar cells in nodular sclerosis HL are helpful for establishing the diagnosis, but in some small needle biopsy specimens, the distinction is not possible, forcing the diagnosis of classic HL, not otherwise specified.

Lymphocyte-Rich Classic Hodgkin Lymphoma, Diffuse Pattern. The quality of the background reactive cell population is helpful in this differential diagnosis. In lymphocyte-rich classic HL, the background cells are small lymphocytes and histiocytes. Granulocytes are absent or rare. In MCHL, the background cell population is highly mixed, with granulocytes and plasma cells in variable proportions.

T-Cell/Histiocyte-Rich Large B-Cell Lymphoma (TCRLBCL). Most cases of MCHL have a more mixed population of cells in the background, unlike cases of TCRLBCL in which the background infiltrate is composed of small lymphocytes and histiocytes. Immunohistochemical studies are essential for distinguishing these neoplasms. The neoplastic cells of TCRLBCL are strongly and uniformly positive for CD20 and other B-cell markers as well as CD45/LCA, and are negative for CD15 and usually negative for CD30. Cases of TCRLBCL are also usually negative for EBV.

Peripheral T-Cell Lymphoma, Not Otherwise Specified (PTCL-NOS). Cases of PTCL-NOS and MCHL may closely resemble each other. Clues that support MCHL are the dichotomy between the large RS+H cells and small lymphocytes in the background population as well as the presence of classic RS+H cells. Cases of PTCL-NOS, however, can exhibit RS+H-like cells and have a mixed inflammatory background. Immunophenotypic studies are very helpful. Flow cytometry immunophenotyping of PTCL-NOS often shows an aberrant T-cell immunophenotype. Immunohistochemical analysis shows that the large neoplastic cells in PTCL-NOS express T-cell antigens and CD45/LCA, usually are negative for CD15 and CD30, and are negative for PAX5.

TREATMENT AND PROGNOSIS

The standard therapy for patients with MCHL is similar to that of other types of classic HL (3). Combination chemotherapy and radiation therapy are used for most patients (see chapter 37).

About 80 percent of patients with MCHL completely respond to therapy, and most of those patients are cured of disease. The progno-sis of patients with MCHL correlates with the stage of the disease. Stage for stage, the prognosis of patients with MCHL is slightly worse than that of patients with nodular sclerosis HL, but better that of patients with lymphocyte-depleted HL (1).

REFERENCES

1. Allemani C, Sant M, De Angelis R, Marcos-Gragera R, Coebergh JW; EUROCARE Working Group. Hodgkin disease survival in Europe and the U.S.: prognostic significance of morphologic groups. Cancer 2006;107:352-360.

2. Al-Maghrabi JA, Sawan AS, Kanaan HD. Hodgkin's lymphoma with exuberant granulomatous reaction. Saudi Med J 2006;27:1905-1907.

3. Ansell SM. Hodgkin lymphoma: 2016 update on diagnosis, risk-stratification, and management. Am J Hematol 2016;91:434-442.

4. Asano N, Oshiro A, Matsuo K, et al. Prognostic significance of T-cell or cytotoxic molecules phenotype in classical Hodgkin's lymphoma: a clinicopathologic study. J Clin Oncol 2006;24:4626-4633.

5. Colby TV, Hoppe RT, Warnke RA. Hodgkin's disease: a clinicopathologic study of 659 cases. Cancer 1982;49:1848-1858.

6. Doggett RS, Colby TV, Dorfman RF. Interfollicular Hodgkin's disease. Am J Surg Pathol 1983;7:145-149.

7. Haque S, van Kirk R. Three patients with both Hodgkin's lymphoma and Castleman's disease: Clinicopathologic correlations and lack of association with HHV-8. Indian J Med Paediatr Oncol 2009;30:76-79.

7a. Konkay K, Paul TR, Uppin SG, Rao DR. Hodgkin lymphoma: a clinicopathological and immunophenotypic study. Indian J Med Paediatr Oncol 2016;37:59-65.

8. Maheswaran PR, Ramsay AD, Norton AJ, Roche WR. Hodgkin's disease presenting with the histological features of Castleman's disease. Histopathology 1991;18:249-253.

9. Medeiros LJ, Greiner TC. Hodgkin's disease. Cancer 1995;75(Suppl):357-369.

10. Mohrmann RL, Nathwani BN, Brynes RK, Sheibani K. Hodgkin's disease occurring in monocytoid B-cell clusters. Am J Clin Pathol 1991;95:802-808.

11. Serraino D, Carbone A, Franceschi S, Tirelli U. Increased frequency of lymphocyte depletion and mixed cellularity subtypes of Hodgkin's disease in HIV-infected patients. Italian Cooperative Group on AIDS and Tumours. Eur J Cancer 1993;29A:1948-1950.

12. Sherief LM, Elsafy UR, Abdelkhalek ER, et al. Hodgkin lymphoma in childhood: clinicopathological features and therapy outcome at 2 centers from a developing country. Medicine (Baltimore) 2015;94:e670.

13. Shimabukuro-Vornhagen A, Haverkamp H, Engert A, et al. Lymphocyte-rich classical Hodgkin's lymphoma: clinical presentation and treatment outcome in 100 patients treated within German Hodgkin's Study Group trials. J Clin Oncol 2005;23:5739-5745.

14. Szumera-Cieckiewic A, Prochorec-Sobieszek M, Lech-Maranda E. Hodgkin's lymphoma mimicking tuberculosis in cervical lymph nodes. Pol J Pathol 2014;65:83-88.

15. Weiss LM, von Wasielewski R, Delsol G, Poppena S, Stein H. Mixed cellularity classical Hodgkin lymphoma. In: Swerdlow SH, Campo E, Harris NL, et al., eds. Who classification of tumours of haematopoietic and lymphoid tissues. Lyon: IARC Press; 2008;331.

16. Zarate-Osorno A, Medeiros LJ, Danon AD, Neiman RS. Hodgkin's disease with coexistent Castleman-like histologic features. A report of three cases. Arch Pathol Lab Med 1994;118:270-274.

17. Zardawi IM, Barker BJ, Simons DP. Hodgkin's disease masquerading as granulomatous lymphadenitis on fine needle aspiration cytology. Acta Cytol 2005;49:224-226.

41

LYMPHOCYTE-DEPLETED HODGKIN LYMPHOMA

GENERAL FEATURES

Lymphocyte-depleted Hodgkin lymphoma (LDHL) is the least common form of HL. It is characterized by Reed-Sternberg and Hodgkin (RS+H) cells in a background enriched with histiocytes and fibroblasts, with depletion of small reactive lymphocytes.

LDHL has been known by a number of names over the years. These tumors were designated as sarcoma in the Jackson-Parker classification (6) and were subdivided into two disease categories in the Lukes and Butler classification system (10): diffuse fibrosis and reticular. These two categories were combined in the Rye classification as lymphocyte depletion (see chapter 4), and are now known as *lymphocyte-depleted classic HL* in the World Health Organization (WHO) classification (4,12a).

With the advent of immunophenotypic and molecular studies, it became clear that many neoplasms once classified as LDHL were, in fact, examples of other types of HL, non-Hodgkin lymphomas, or nonhematolymphoid tumors. This realization has resulted in a progressive decrease in the frequency of LDHL. The reticular variant, as described by Lukes and Butler, has been particularly reduced in frequency. Currently, the relative frequency of LDHL in the United States and Europe is 1 to 2 percent (8). The frequency appears to be higher in developing nations, particularly in Africa, South America, and Asia. In one large study from Brazil, almost 5 percent of all HL cases were LDHL (13). The frequency of LDHL also appears to be higher in Israel and Japan, 5.9 percent and 9.0 percent, respectively (3,7). As pointed out by the authors of the study from Japan, however, not all cases were assessed rigorously by immunophenotypic and molecular methods and therefore the reported frequency may be misleadingly high. LDHL is also more common in patients with human immunodeficiency virus (HIV) infection (5).

CLINICAL FEATURES

The male to female ratio is at least 2 to 1 with a ratio closer to 3 to 1 in some studies. Patients with LDHL are usually older than those with other HL types, with a median age of approximately 34 years (2). Compared with other types of HL, B-type symptoms and advanced stage are more common (5,8,11). Extranodal, abdominal, and retroperitoneal disease is also more common in this type of HL (8,9,11).

Bone marrow involvement is more common in patients with LDHL than in those with other types of classic HL. Bone marrow involvement by most types of classic HL is often associated with dense fibrosis and the tumor cannot be aspirated. In contrast, in patients with LDHL, associated fibrosis is less well developed and the tumor is more often aspirated, and therefore detectable in aspirate smears as well as in biopsy sections. Rarely, LDHL is better represented in aspirate smears than in the biopsy specimen.

HISTOLOGIC FINDINGS

Lymph Nodes

LDHL diffusely replaces lymph nodes (fig. 41-1) or extranodal sites, and is histologically characterized by relatively numerous RS+H cells and relatively few small lymphocytes, compared with other HL types. The RS+H cells are more often pleomorphic or multinucleated in LDHL (fig. 41-1B). In some cases, the neoplastic cells prominently invade the lymph node sinuses (fig. 41-1C). Eosinophils and plasma cells are infrequent.

Foci of coagulative necrosis with acute inflammation may be present. The stroma appears hyalinized, with varying levels of reticular (fig. 41-2) or diffuse fibrosis. The fibrosis is usually not birefringent when viewed with polarized light. In some cases both neoplastic and stromal cells are spindled, imparting a sarcomatoid appearance (figs. 41-3, 41-4).

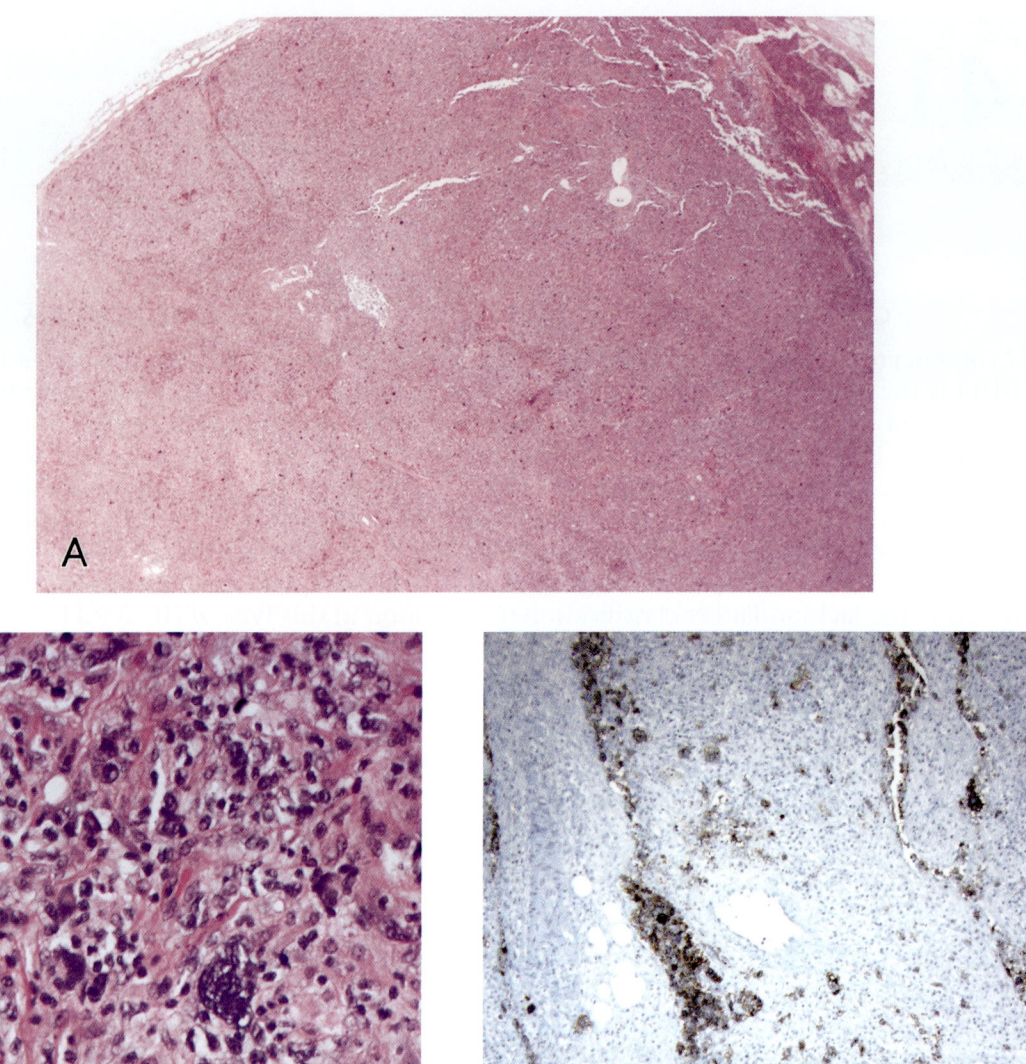

Figure 41-1

LYMPHOCYTE-DELETED HODGKIN LYMPHOMA, INVOLVING LYMPH NODE

A: The neoplasm diffusely replaces the lymph node architecture. Large pleomorphic Reed-Sternberg and Hodgkin (RS+H) cells are seen even at low magnification (A,B: hematoxylin and eosin [H&E] stain).

B: Large and pleomorphic neoplastic cells are present in a background of numerous histiocytes and few small lymphocytes or granulocytes.

C: The anti-CD30 antibody highlights prominent invasion of lymph node sinuses by the RS+H cells (immunohistochemistry with hematoxylin counterstain).

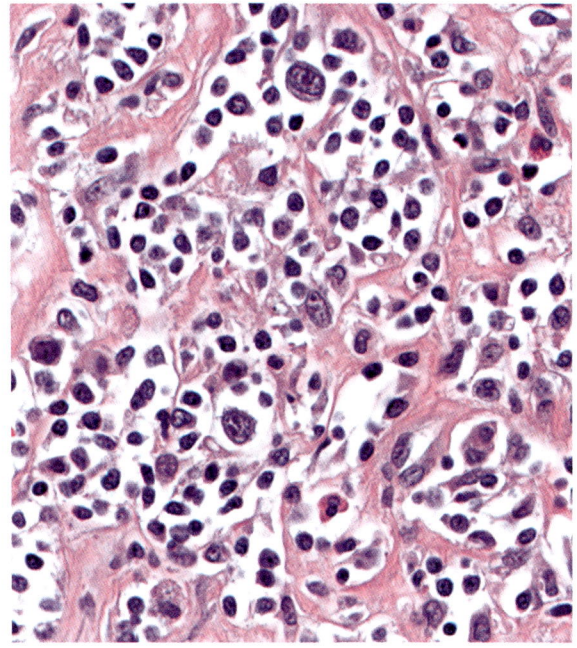

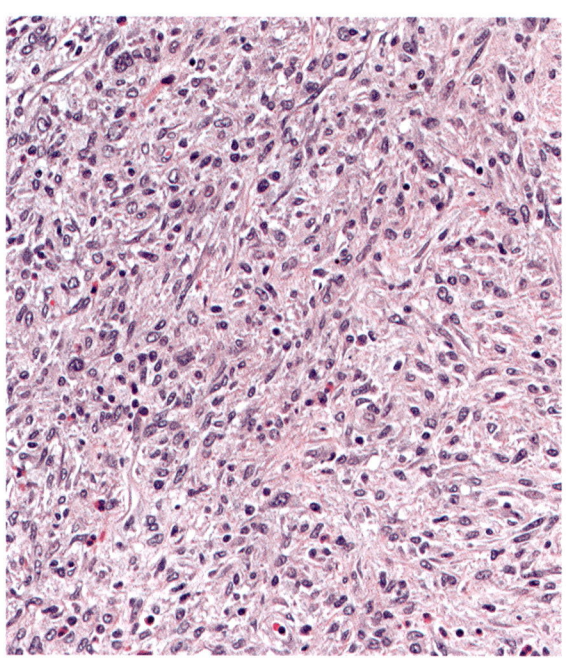

Figure 41-2

LYMPHOCYTE-DELETED HODGKIN LYMPHOMA ASSOCIATED WITH FIBROSIS

The lymph node architecture is effaced by large RS+H cells in a background of fine reticular and nonpolarizable fibrosis. Histiocytes, small lymphocytes, and eosinophils are also seen (H&E stain).

Figure 41-3

LYMPHOCYTE-DELETED HODGKIN LYMPHOMA WITH A SPINDLED APPEARANCE

The neoplastic cells and background histiocytes and fibroblasts appear spindled in this field (H&E stain).

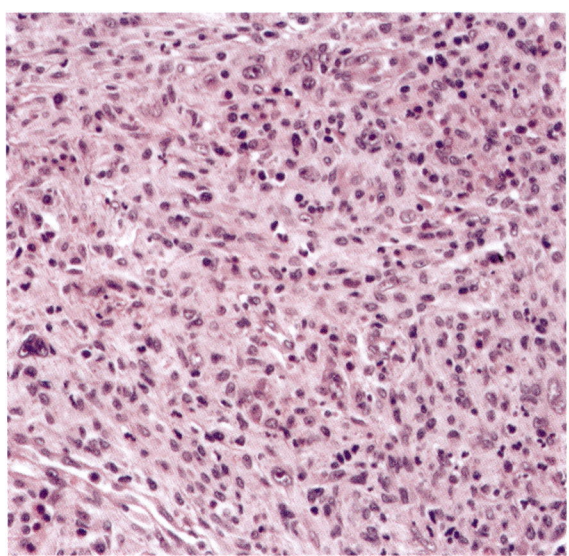

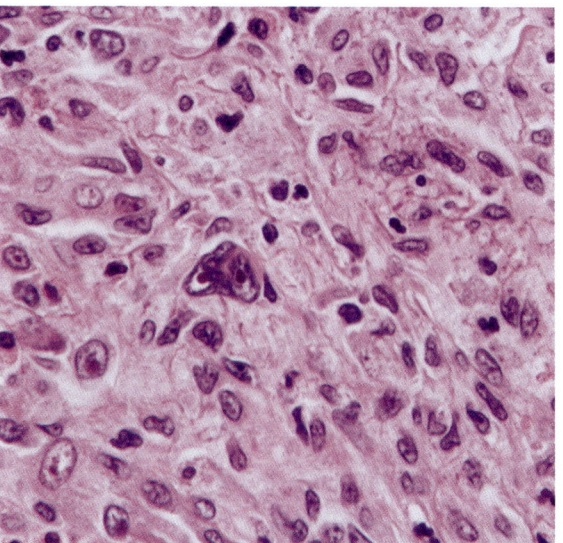

Figure 41-4

LYMPHOCYTE-DELETED HODGKIN LYMPHOMA INVOLVING ABDOMINAL LYMPH NODE

Left: An atypical RS cell and mononuclear variant cells are present in a background of numerous histiocytes with a partial spindled appearance.

Right: Oil-immersion magnification of a RS cell (left, right: H&E stain).

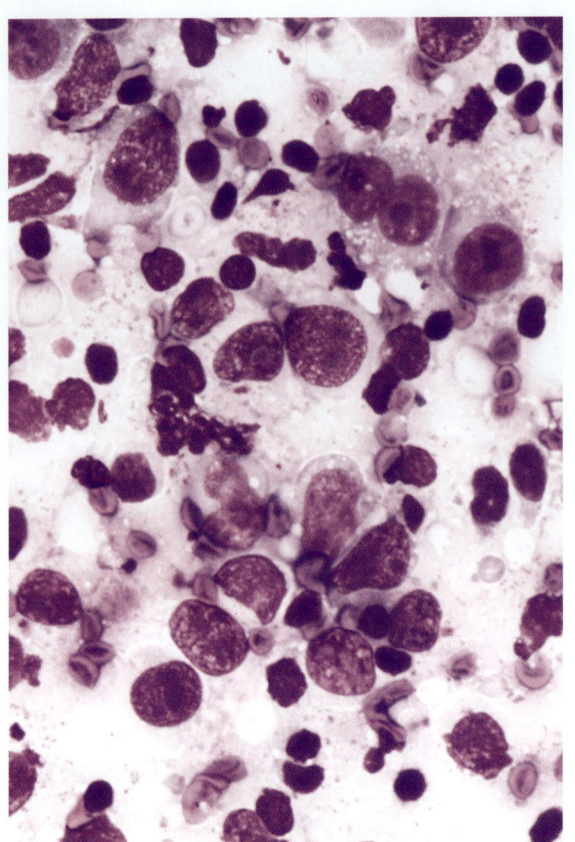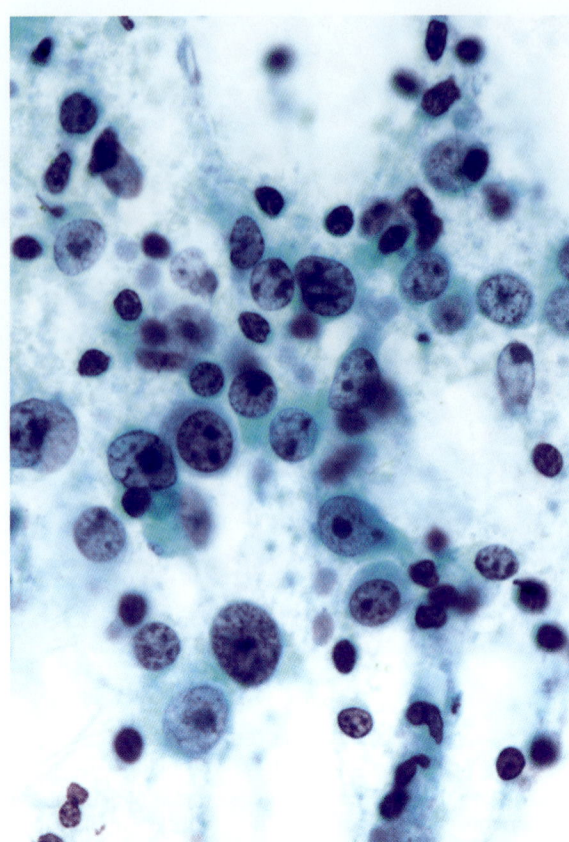

Figure 41-5

LYMPHOCYTE-DELETED HODGKIN LYMPHOMA IN ASPIRATE SMEARS

Numerous RS+H cells and sparse small lymphocytes are seen in the aspirate smear (left: Diff-Quik stain; right: Papanicolaou stain).

CYTOLOGIC FINDINGS

A prominent aspect of LDHL in cytologic preparations is the abundance of the RS+H cells, including highly pleomorphic cells (fig. 41-5). The pleomorphic cells are large and multinucleated, with prominent nucleoli that are round, oval, or polygonal. The cytoplasm is abundant and eosinophilic in most cases. In some cases, bizarre pleomorphic variant neoplastic cells have a spindled shape.

IMMUNOPHENOTYPIC FINDINGS

As is true for other types of classic HL, the RS+H cells are virtually always positive for CD30 (fig. 41-1C) and PAX5 is dimly expressed in 90 to 95 percent of cases. IRF4/MUM1 is positive in about 90 percent of cases and CD15 is expressed in about two thirds (fig. 41-6). CD20 is usually negative on RS+H cells, but dim and variable CD20 expression is observed in about 20 percent of cases. Cytotoxic antigens, such as TIA-1, are expressed in 10 to 20 percent of cases (12). RS+H cells are negative for CD3, CD10, CD19, CD45/LCA, and CD68. Epstein-Barr virus (EBV) LMP1 (fig. 41-7) and EBV- encoded RNA1 (EBER1) are detectable in over 50 percent of cases (12).

MOLECULAR GENETIC FINDINGS

The molecular findings in cases of LDHL are similar to those in other types of classic HL, as discussed in chapter 37.

DIFFERENTIAL DIAGNOSIS

The differential diagnosis of LDHL is very broad (see Table 37-3). Immunophenotypic analysis and, in some cases, molecular studies, are needed to exclude lacunar cell-rich nodular sclerosis HL, diffuse large B-cell lymphoma not

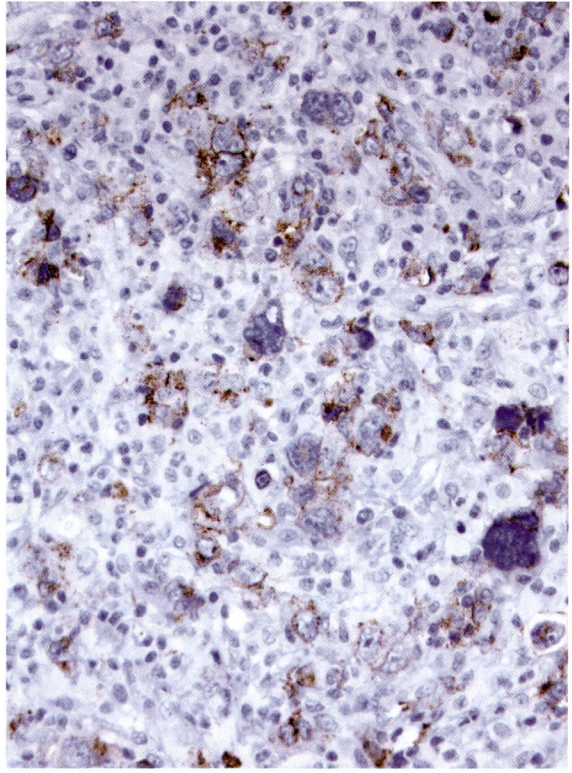

Figure 41-6

LYMPHOCYTE-DELETED HODGKIN LYMPHOMA: CD15

The neoplastic cells are positive for CD15 (immuno-histochemistry with hematoxylin counterstain) (same case as shown in fig. 41-1).

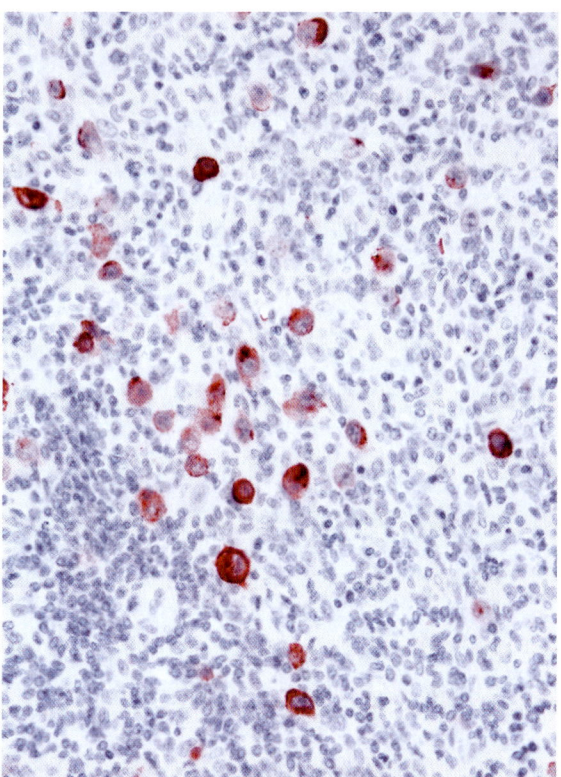

Figure 41-7

LYMPHOCYTE-DELETED HODGKIN LYMPHOMA: EBV INFECTION

The neoplastic cells are positive for Epstein-Barr virus (EBV) latent membrane protein type 1 (immunohistochemistry with hematoxylin counterstain) (same case as shown in fig. 41-4).

otherwise specified, EBV-positive diffuse large B-cell lymphoma of the elderly, B-cell lymphoma unclassifiable with features intermediate between diffuse large B-cell lymphoma and classic HL, anaplastic large cell lymphoma, sarcomas, and sarcomatoid or pleomorphic carcinomas.

TREATMENT AND PROGNOSIS

The standard therapy for patients with LDHL is similar to that for patients with other types of classic HL. Combination chemotherapy and radiation therapy are used for most patients (see chapter 37).

Compared with other types of classic HL, patients with LDHL have a statistically higher frequency of advanced stage disease, B-type symptoms, greater than 3 or more sites of lymph node disease, liver or bone marrow involvement, a higher International Prognostic Score, and worse overall and progression-free survival rates. In a large study from Germany, the overall and progression-free survival rates for patients with LDHL were 83 percent and 71 percent, respectively (8).

The prognosis of patients with LDHL is somewhat controversial. As patients are older and present with advanced disease and other poor risk factors, as a group, patients with LDHL exhibit lower progression-free and overall survival rates compared with patients with other types of HL. When adjustments are made for age, stage, and other factors, however, investigators disagree about the prognostic importance of the lymphocyte-depleted (LD) morphology. In a German study, LD morphology was not an independent poor risk factor (8). In other studies, LD morphology was proposed as a poor risk factor (1,7).

REFERENCES

1. Ali S, Olszewski AJ. Disparate survival and risk of secondary non-Hodgkin lymphoma in histologic subtypes of Hodgkin lymphoma: a population-based study. Leuk Lymphoma 2014;55:1570-1577.

2. Allemani C, Sant M, De Angelis R, Marcos-Gragera R, Coebergh JW; EUROCARE Working Group. Hodgkin disease survival in Europe and the U.S.: prognostic significance of morphologic groups. Cancer 2006;107:352-360.

3. Benharroch D, Levy A, Gopas J, Sacks M. Lymphocyte-depleted classic Hodgkin lymphoma—a neglected entity? Virchows Arch 2008;453:611-616.

4. Benharroch D, Stein H, Peh SC. Lymphocyte-depleted classical Hodgkin lymphoma. In: Swerdlow SH, Campo E, Harris NL, et al., eds. WHO classification of tumours of haematopoietic and lymphoid tissues. Lyon: IARC Press; 2008:334.

5. Glaser SL, Clarke CA, Gulley ML, et al. Population-based patterns of human immunodeficiency virus-related Hodgkin lymphoma in the Greater San Francisco Bay Area, 1988-1998. Cancer 2003; 98:300-309.

6. Jackson HJ Jr, Parker F Jr. Hodgkin's disease and allied disorders. New York: Oxford University Press; 1947.

7. Karube K, Niino D, Kimura Y, Ohshima K. Classical Hodgkin lymphoma, lymphocyte depleted type: clinicopathological analysis and prognostic comparison with other types of classical Hodgkin lymphoma. Pathol Res Pract 2013;209:201-207.

8. Klimm B, Franklin J, Stein H, et al. Lymphocyte-depleted classical Hodgkin's lymphoma: a comprehensive analysis from the German Hodgkin study group. J Clin Oncol 2011;29:3914-3920.

9. Laurent C, Do C, Gourraud PA, de Paiva GR, Valmary S, Brousset P. Prevalence of common non-Hodgkin lymphomas and subtypes of Hodgkin lymphoma by nodal site of involvement: a systematic retrospective review of 938 cases. Medicine (Baltimore) 2015;94:e987.

10. Lukes RJ, Butler JJ. The pathology and nomenclature of Hodgkin's disease. Cancer Res 1966; 26:1063-1081.

11. Neiman RS, Rosen PJ, Lukes RJ. Lymphocyte-depletion Hodgkin's disease. A clinicopathological entity. N Engl J Med 1973;288:751-755.

12. Slack GW, Ferry JA, Hasserjian RP, et al. Lymphocyte depleted Hodgkin lymphoma: an evaluation with immunophenotyping and genetic analysis. Leuk Lymphoma 2009;50: 937-943.

12a. Swerdlow SH, Campo E, Pileri SA, et al. The 2016 revision of the World Health Organization classification of lymphoid neoplasms. Blood 2016;127:2375-2390.

13. Vassallo J, Paes RP, Soares FA, et al. Histological classification of 1,025 cases of Hodgkin's lymphoma from the State of São Paulo, Brazil. Sao Paulo Med J 2005;123:134-136.

42 NODULAR LYMPHOCYTE-PREDOMINANT HODGKIN LYMPHOMA

GENERAL FEATURES

Nodular lymphocyte-predominant Hodgkin lymphoma (NLPHL) is a neoplasm of germinal center B-cell origin with a characteristic nodular pattern. It is composed of scattered large neoplastic cells, known as lymphocyte-predominant (LP) cells, in a background of numerous reactive small lymphocytes, histiocytes, and follicular dendritic cell (FDC) networks (33,43a). Some cases exhibit variant patterns, including tumors with a nodular and diffuse pattern and rare tumors that have a diffuse pattern (10,16).

The nodular pattern included in the definition is not simply based on morphologic evidence. A nodule in the context of NLPHL is defined by morphologic features, but also by appropriate cellular composition, including FDCs, small reactive B lymphocytes, and follicular helper T lymphocytes. Immunohistochemical studies are essential for recognizing these cell types and are needed to unequivocally recognize a nodular pattern in NLPHL.

Other designations for NLPHL used in the past have included paragranuloma (Jackson and Parker classification), lymphocytic and histiocytic (Lukes and Butler classification), and lymphocytic predominance (Rye conference) (see fig. 4-1). In large part, these terms are obsolete, with the possible exception of paragranuloma, which was incorporated into the designation *nodular paragranuloma* by Poppema et al. (34). The term nodular paragranuloma is still occasionally used as a synonym for NLPHL, particularly in Europe.

NLPHL is a rare disease. The overall incidence rate in the United States is 0.08 per 10^6 person per year (27). NLPHL represents about 5 percent of all HLs and approximately 0.5 percent of all lymphomas (33).

The etiology of NLPHL is poorly understood, but there is evidence that genetic predisposition has a role. First-degree relatives of patients with NLPHL have an increased risk of developing NLPHL and rare families have a high frequency of disease, supporting familial NLPHL (38). In one NLPHL family, whole exome sequencing identified a germline mutation in the nuclear protein ataxia-telangiectasia *(NPAT)* gene at chromosome 11q22.3 (37). The mutation is a 2 base pair deletion that causes a frameshift and truncation of NPAT protein, compromising function. This mutation, however, shows low penetrance, suggesting that other genetic or environmental factors are required for lymphomagenesis. *NPAT* mutations also have been identified in a few cases of sporadic NLPHL; the mutation in these cases was a 3-base pair deletion resulting in loss of a serine at codon 724 (37). Wild-type NPAT is involved in cell cycle control as well as other functions.

Although NLPHL has been traditionally classified as a type of HL, it has become clear that it is distinct from the other types of HL, commonly designated using the umbrella term classic HL, which includes nodular sclerosis, mixed cellularity, lymphocyte-rich classic, and lymphocyte-depleted HL.

NLPHL and classic HL (all types) differ at the morphologic, immunophenotypic, and genetic level (3,14,21,22). In NLPHL, the neoplastic LP cells have a functional (although abnormal) B-cell differentiation program. The LP cells express pan-B-cell antigens (e.g., CD19, CD20) and CD45/LCA and are negative for CD15 and CD30 (14,33). The tumor microenvironment is rich in reactive small B lymphocytes and FDCs. At the molecular level, LP cells carry functional immunoglobulin gene rearrangements and somatic mutations of the immunoglobulin variable region genes that are ongoing (26).

The neoplastic Reed-Sternberg and Hodgkin (RS+H) cells of classic HL are also of B-cell lineage, but these cells have a markedly dysfunctional B-cell differentiation program (reviewed in reference 21). The RS+H cells usually do not express pan-B-cell antigens, are positive for CD15 (often) and CD30, and are negative for CD45/LCA. The tumor microenvironment is usually poor in reactive small B lymphocytes and FDCs and rich in T cells, granulocytes, and other inflammatory cells. At the molecular level, RS+H cells carry nonfunctional immunoglobulin gene rearrangements or the expression of the B-cell genes is stunted, either by epigenetic mechanisms (methylation) or expression of molecules (e.g., NOTCH1, ID2) that suppress B-cell differentiation.

These differences in biology likely explain, at least in part, differences in behavior between NLPHL and classic HL as summarized in Table 37-1. The natural history of NLPHL is similar to various types of indolent B-cell non-Hodgkin lymphomas: a clinically indolent disease that commonly relapses over time, including late relapses, and has no cure (i.e., a staircase-shaped relapse-free survival curve) (14,22,28). The pattern of spread in NLPHL is often discontiguous and patients have an increased risk of developing diffuse large B-cell lymphoma (DLBCL) (2,5,9).

These features are in contrast with classic HL (Table 42-1). If there is a relapse in classic HL patients it occurs early, within the first 3 years of therapy, after which time relapse is rare and cure can be attained (plateau-shaped relapse-free survival curve). Classic HL usually spreads in a contiguous manner and patients rarely develop DLBCL (21).

CLINICAL FEATURES

The median age of patients with NLPHL is 35 to 40 years at the time of initial diagnosis and the male to female ratio is about 3 to 1 (14,22). B-type symptoms are uncommon (about 10 percent of patients). Most patients present with localized disease (Ann Arbor stage I or II) involving peripheral lymph nodes in the cervical, axillary, or inguinal regions. Mediastinal lymph nodes are involved in 10 to 20 percent of patients. About 25 percent of NLPHL patients present with advanced stage disease and involvement of the spleen is one of the most common sites supporting stage III disease (47). Some patients with splenic disease also have liver involvement, but other visceral organs and bone marrow are rarely involved.

Table 42-1

CLINICAL FEATURES OF PATIENTS WITH NODULAR LYMPHOCYTE-PREDOMINANT HODGKIN LYMPHOMA (NLPHL) AND CLASSIC HL[a]

Clinical Feature	NLPHL	Classic HL (all types)
Median age (years)	35-40	30-35
Male to female ratio	3 to 1	1.5 to 1
Low stage (I + II) disease	~80%	50-60%
B symptoms	~10%	~40%
Elevated serum LDH[b]	10-20%	~35%
Mediastinal disease[c]	10-20%	50-60%
≥3 lymph node sites	25-30%	50-60%
Extranodal sites of disease	~5%	10-20%
Pattern of spread	Not contiguous	Contiguous
Late relapses	Common	Rare
Complete response to therapy	~90%	~80%
10-year overall survival	~90%	80%
Risk of DLBCL	5-15%	Rare

[a]Based mostly on the experience of the German Hodgkin Lymphoma Study Group, but other sources were also consulted.
[b]LDH = lactate dehydrogenase; DLBCL = diffuse large B-cell lymphoma.
[c]Usually lymph nodes are involved in NLPHL patients.

Radiologic imaging studies are essential for staging patients with NLPHL. Usually computerized tomography (CT) scans of the neck, chest, and abdomen are performed. NLPHL is fluorodeoxyglucose (FDG) avid and therefore FDG-position emission tomography (PET) is useful for staging and assessing response to therapy.

Patients with NLPHL are at risk of developing DLBCL, often a manifestation of histologic transformation. Al-Mansour et al. (2) reported that 13 (14 percent) of 95 patients followed for a median of 6.5 years developed DLBCL. These authors emphasized the need for long follow-up and reported an actuarial risk of DLBCL of 7 percent at 10 years, 15 percent at 15 years, and 31 percent at 20 years. In three other studies of NLPHL patients with long follow-up, Biasoli et al. (5) reported a cumulative risk of DLBCL at 10 years of 12 percent; Eyre et al. (9) reported that 17 percent of patients developed DLBCL; and Kenderian et al. (19a) reported that 7.6 percent of patients developed DLBCL. Currently, it is difficult

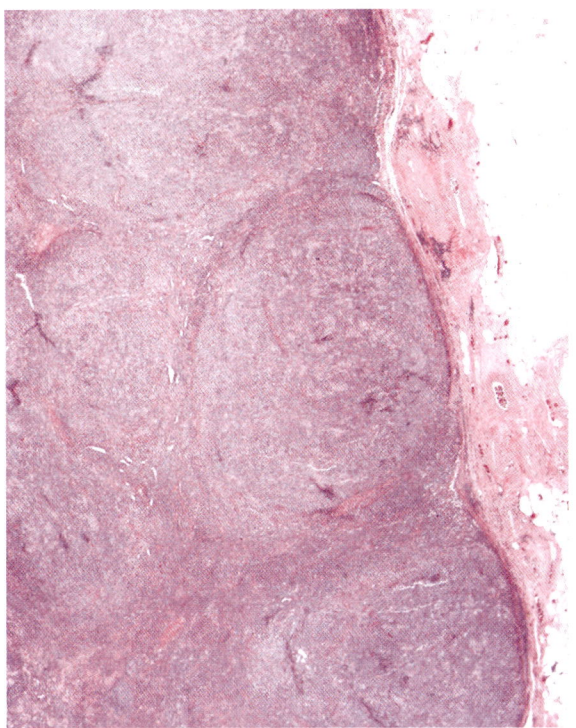

Figure 42-1

NODULAR LYMPHOCYTE-PREDOMINANT HODGKIN LYMPHOMA INVOLVING LYMPH NODE

The neoplastic nodules are large and back-to-back, replacing the lymph node architecture (hematoxylin and eosin [H&E] stain).

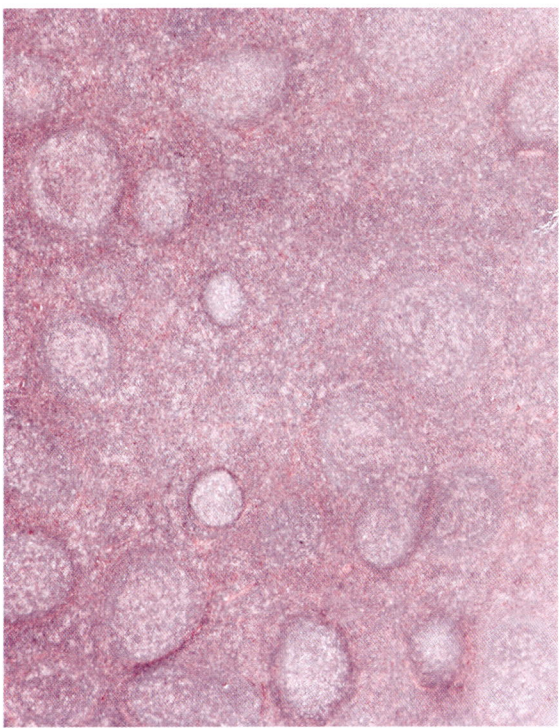

Figure 42-2

NODULAR LYMPHOCYTE -PREDOMINANT HODGKIN LYMPHOMA INVOLVING LYMPH NODE

The neoplastic nodules are small and widely spaced. A few small reactive germinal centers (two in center) are present (H&E stain).

to identify which NLPHL patients are most likely to develop DLBCL. Splenic involvement by NLPHL has been reported to be an independent risk factor for subsequent DLBCL (2). Variant histologic patterns (described below) also correlate with an increased risk of DLBCL (16).

The development of DLBCL usually follows the diagnosis of NLPHL: Al-Mansour et al. (2) reported a median time interval of 8.1 years, with some DLBCLs occurring less than 1 year and others up to 20 years after an NLPHL diagnosis. Rarely, the diagnosis of DLBCL is established initially and a subsequent biopsy, often within a year, shows NLPHL. The anatomic site of DLBCL usually differs from the site of the initial biopsy, but rarely, the same lymph node is involved by both NLPHL and DLBCL (i.e., composite lymphoma). At time of onset of DLBCL, patients usually show the findings expected with an aggressive lymphoma including B symptoms, poor performance status, elevated serum lactate dehydrogenase (LDH) level, high International Prognostic Index (IPI), and advanced stage disease (2,5,9,19a).

HISTOLOGIC FINDINGS

Lymph Nodes

NLPHL is characterized by expansive, vague nodules that are usually larger than the size of reactive follicles (3,10,16,33). The nodules are composed of large neoplastic LP cells in a benign background of small round lymphocytes and fewer epithelioid histiocytes. In many cases, the tumor nodules are arranged back-to-back, but in other cases, the interfollicular regions are expanded and the tumor nodules are widely separated (figs. 42-1, 42-2). In most cases, numerous small round lymphocytes predominate in the interfollicular regions, but in a small subset (less than 5 percent) of cases, the interfollicular lymphocytes are activated and have more irregular

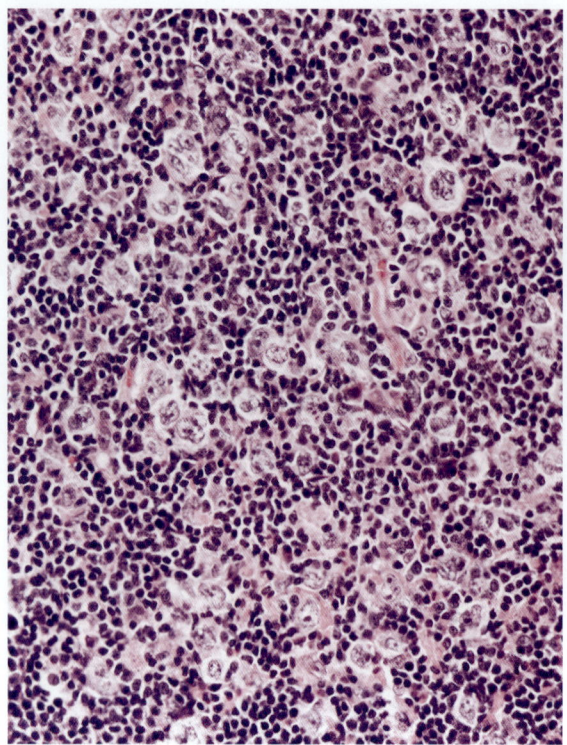

Figure 42-3

NODULAR LYMPHOCYTE PREDOMINANT HODGKIN LYMPHOMA INVOLVING LYMPH NODE

The tumor is rich in lymphocyte-predominant (LP) cells. The background cells are mostly small lymphocytes and scattered histiocytes (H&E stain).

nuclear contours or are medium-sized; this occurs more commonly in children (40).

Although the LP cells in NLPHL usually represent 1 to 2 percent of all cells in the tumor, this percentage is variable, ranging from difficult to identify to numerous (tumor cell rich) (fig. 42-3). These LP cells, known previously as lymphocytic and histiocytic (L&H) cells, commonly resemble popped kernels of corn and hence the nickname "popcorn cell" (fig. 42-4A). The LP cells of NLPHL are large, with folded or multilobated nuclei that contain clear or vesicular nucleoplasm and small or inconspicuous nucleoli. LP cells, however, do not always resemble popcorn: in some cases the cell nuclei are round, resembling, in part, centroblasts (fig. 42-4B); in other cases the LP cells have prominent nucleoli and can reside in lacunar-like spaces resembling lacunar cells of nodular sclerosis HL (fig. 42-4C). Classic Reed-Sternberg cells are usually absent

in NLPHL, but can coexist with LP cells in some cases (fig. 42-4D) (3).

The reactive cells within the tumor nodules include small B lymphocytes with a mantle zone immunophenotype, small T lymphocytes, epithelioid histiocytes, and follicular dendritic cells. Granulocytes and plasma cells are absent within the nodules (figs. 42-1–42-3). Reactive germinal centers are observed within tumor nodules in 10 to 20 percent of cases (fig. 42-5) (10). In some cases, small epithelioid granulomas are numerous and can form a wreath around the tumor nodules (fig. 42-6). Larger, sarcoid-like granulomas also may be present. Uncommonly, plasma cells and rarely, eosinophils in small numbers, are observed at the periphery of the tumor nodules. In uninvolved lymph node at the margins of NLPHL, reactive follicular hyperplasia (fig. 42-7) or progressive transformation of germinal centers, the latter invariably associated with reactive follicular hyperplasia, is common (15).

Variant Patterns in NLPHL. A variety of patterns in NLPHL have been described by Fan et al. (10), designated A through F (fig. 42-8), and more recently these patterns were shown to have prognostic impact by the German Hodgkin Study Group (16). These patterns are best recognized by using both routinely stained histologic sections and the results of immunohistochemistry analysis, particularly anti-CD20 and antibodies specific for FDCs. Pattern A is the typical nodular pattern described above (figs. 42-1, 42-9). Pattern B (serpiginous/interconnected) is characterized by tumor nodules that partially fuse together forming a "chain-like" or serpiginous pattern (fig. 42-9). Pattern C (extranodular LP cells) is characterized by B-cell–rich tumor nodules, but many of the LP cells are situated at the periphery and outside the B-cell regions (fig. 42-10). Pattern D (T-cell–rich nodular) is composed of tumor nodules in which small B cells are few and LP cells represent most of the B cells in the nodules (fig. 42-11). These nodules are T-cell–rich. Pattern E (diffuse T-cell/histiocyte-rich B-cell lymphoma) has a diffuse pattern and is composed of scattered LP cells in a background of numerous reactive T cells (often CD8 positive) and histiocytes, with few small B cells (fig. 42-12). Pattern F (diffuse moth-eaten pattern) has a diffuse pattern and is composed of many small B cells and scattered LP

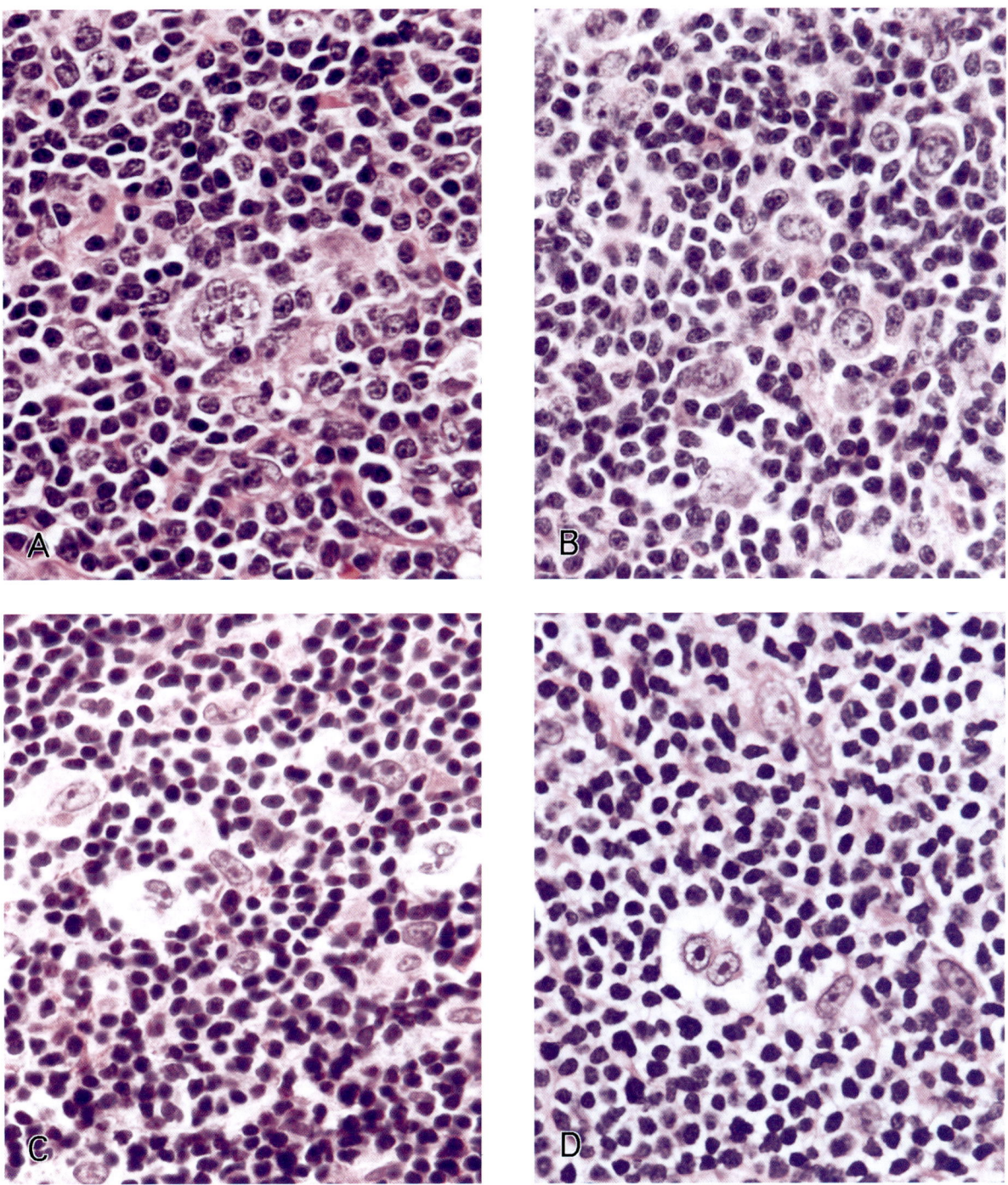

Figure 42-4

NODULAR LYMPHOCYTE-PREDOMINANT HODGKIN LYMPHOMA: SPECTRUM OF NEOPLASTIC CELLS

A: A LP cell with multilobated nuclear contours (popcorn-shaped) is present in the center of the field. (Some popcorn-shaped LP cells are also present in figure 42-3).

B: The LP cells are mostly round and resemble, in part, centroblasts.

C: Here the LP cells have eosinophilic nucleoli and reside in lacunar-like spaces, resembling Hodgkin cells of classic HL.

D: A Reed-Sternberg cell (center of field) is seen. Reed-Sternberg cells are uncommon in NLPHL and are not required for diagnosis (A–D: H&E stain).

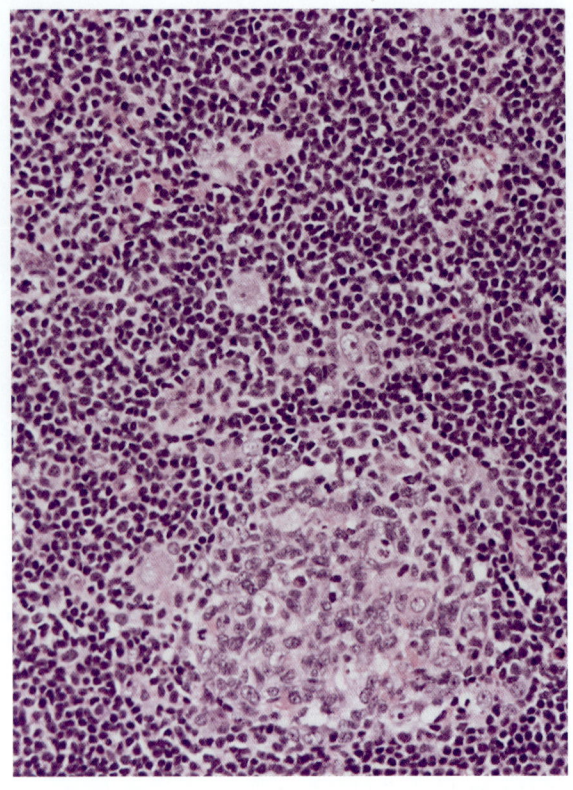

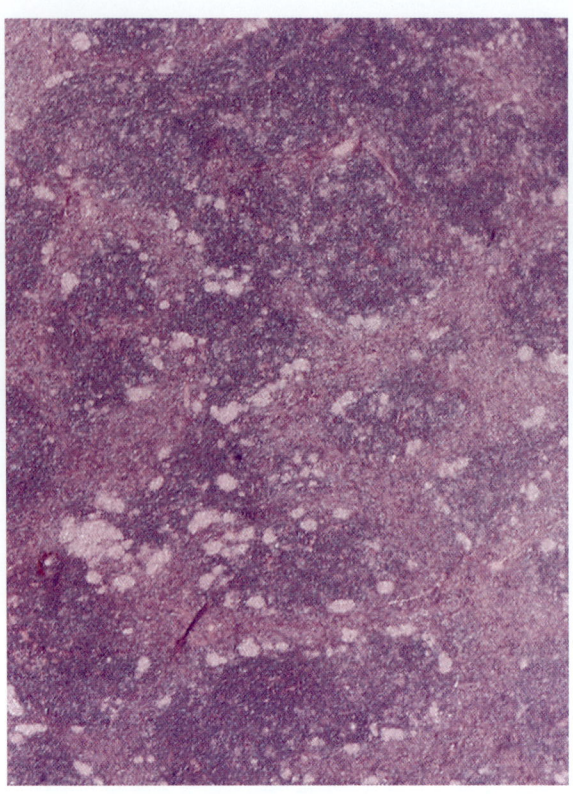

Figure 42-5

NODULAR LYMPHOCYTE-PREDOMINANT HODGKIN LYMPHOMA INVOLVING LYMPH NODE

The tumor nodule contains a reactive germinal center, which can occur in 10 to 20 percent of cases of NLPHL (H&E stain).

Figure 42-6

NODULAR LYMPHOCYTE-PREDOMINANT HODGKIN LYMPHOMA ASSOCIATED WITH EPITHELIOID GRANULOMAS

Many epithelioid histiocytes and granulomas are present, some of which surround tumor nodules in a wreath-like configuration (H&E stain).

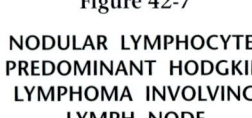

Figure 42-7

NODULAR LYMPHOCYTE-PREDOMINANT HODGKIN LYMPHOMA INVOLVING LYMPH NODE

Large tumor nodules replace over 95 percent of the parenchyma. However, in the upper portion of the field at the margin of the tumor, small hyperplastic lymphoid follicles are present (H&E stain).

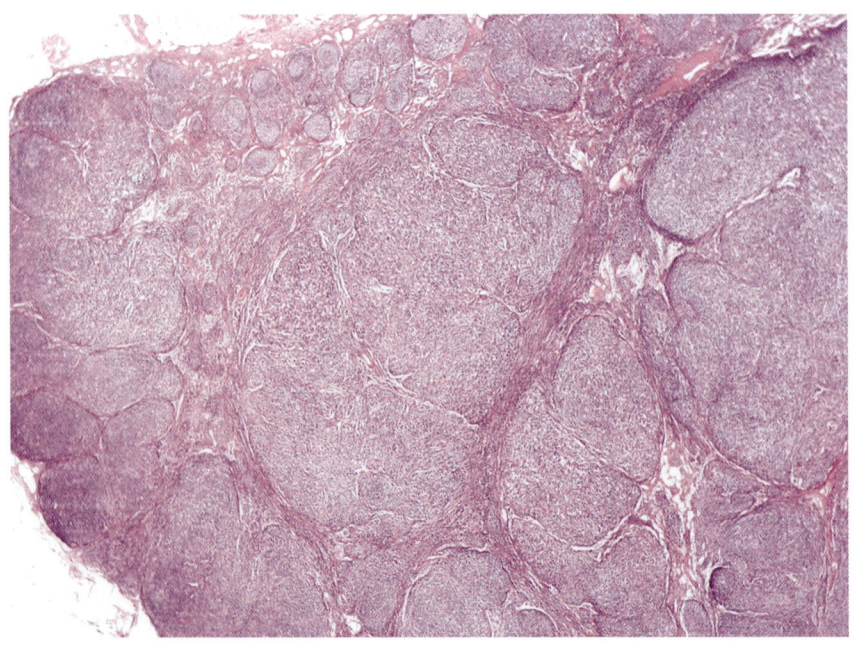

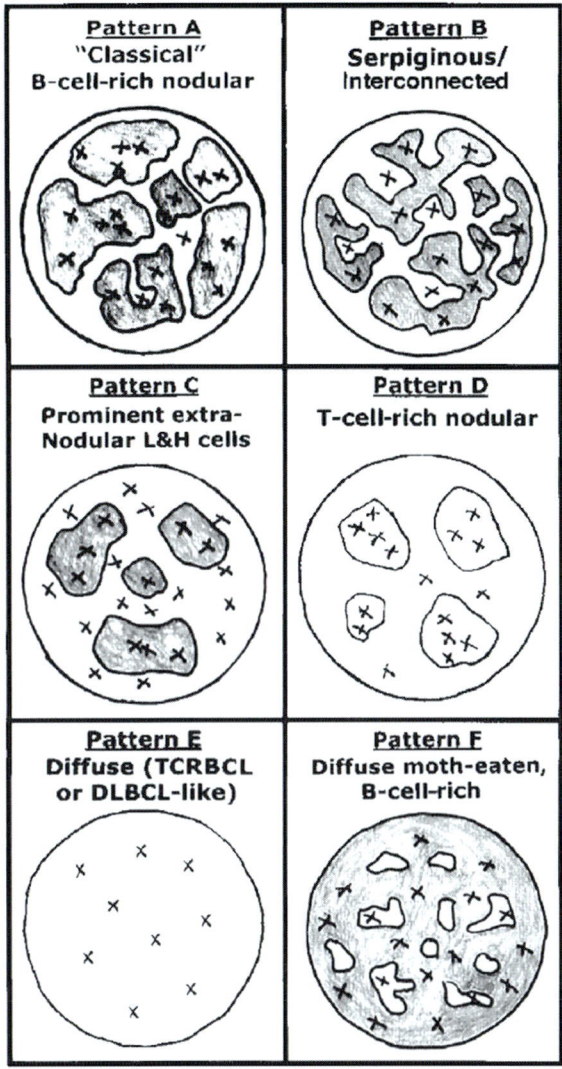

Figure 42-8

PATTERNS OF NODULAR LYMPHOCYTE-
PREDOMINANT HODGKIN LYMPHOMA

Patterns A to F are shown. Patterns C–F are considered variants associated with a poorer prognosis. The X indicates LP cells. (Fig. 3 from Fan Z, Natkunam Y, Bair E, Tibshirani R, Warnke RA. Characterization of variant patterns of nodular lymphocyte predominant Hodgkin lymphoma with immunohistologic and clinical correlation. Am J Surg Pathol 2003;27:1351.)

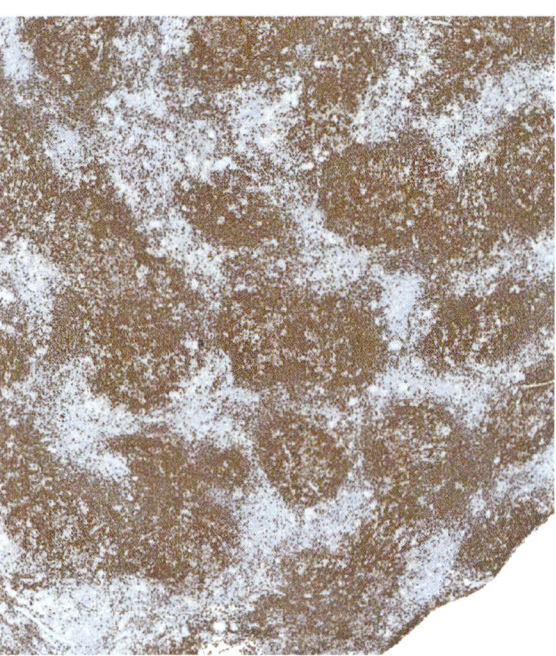

Figure 42-9

PATTERNS A AND B OF NODULAR LYMPHOCYTE-
PREDOMINANT HODGKIN LYMPHOMA

CD20 showing areas of patterns A and B. These two patterns are not associated with a poorer prognosis (immunohistochemistry with hematoxylin counterstain).

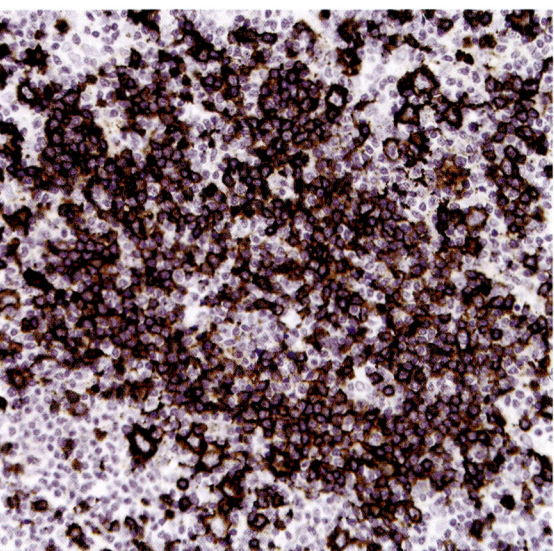

Figure 42-10

PATTERN C OF NODULAR LYMPHOCYTE-
PREDOMINANT HODGKIN LYMPHOMA

CD20 showing pattern C, which is characterized by LP cells outside the confines of tumor nodules (immunohistochemistry with hematoxylin counterstain).

cells (fig. 42-13). Patterns A and B are associated with a better prognosis and patterns C through F, also known as variant patterns, are associated with a poorer prognosis (16). Variant patterns occur in about 25 percent of cases of NLPHL.

Two additional rare variant patterns are worthy of mention. We have observed cases of

Figure 42-11

PATTERN D OF NODULAR LYMPHOCYTE-PREDOMINANT HODGKIN LYMPHOMA

CD20 showing pattern D, which is characterized by T-cell-rich nodules with LP cells and a few small, reactive B cells. Two tumor nodules are seen (immunohistochemistry with hematoxylin counterstain).

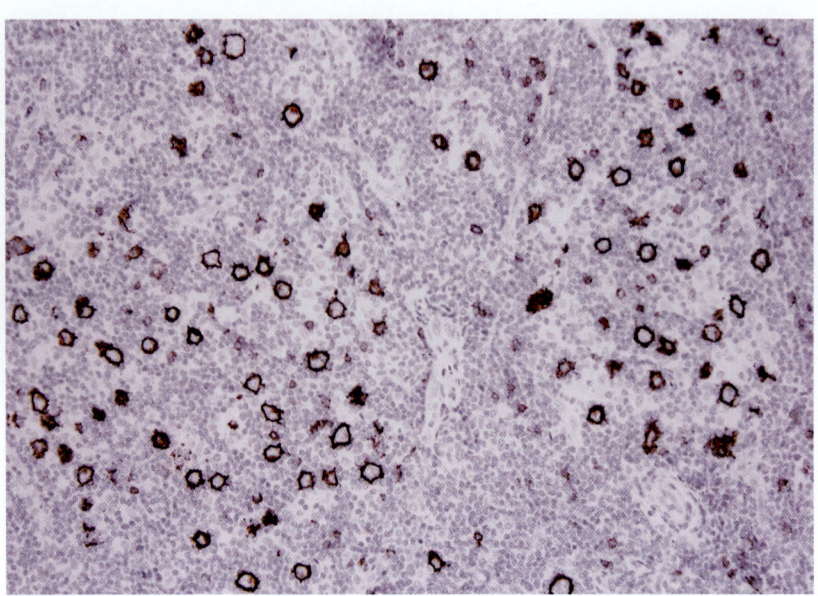

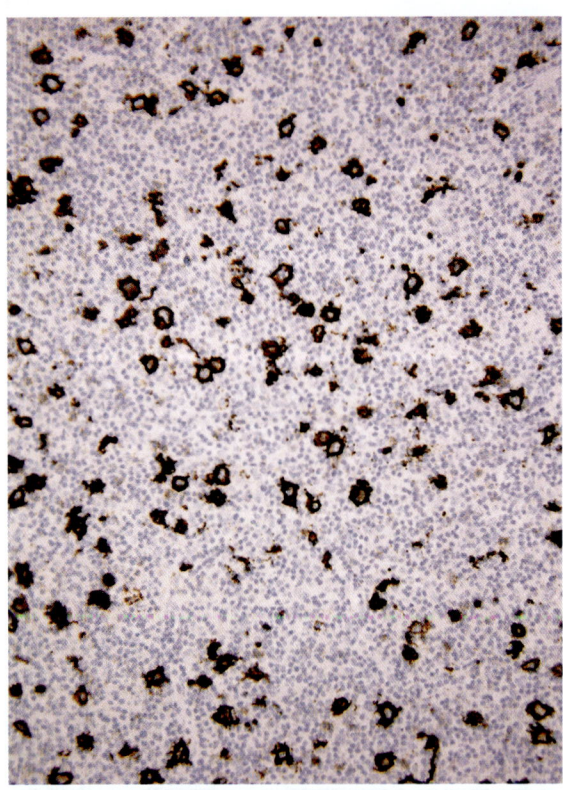

Figure 42-12

PATTERN E OF NODULAR LYMPHOCYTE-PREDOMINANT HODGKIN LYMPHOMA

The lymph node had about 25 percent pattern A (not shown) and about 75 percent pattern E. CD20 highlights scattered LP cells in a background of lymphocytes and histiocytes (immunohistochemistry with hematoxylin counterstain).

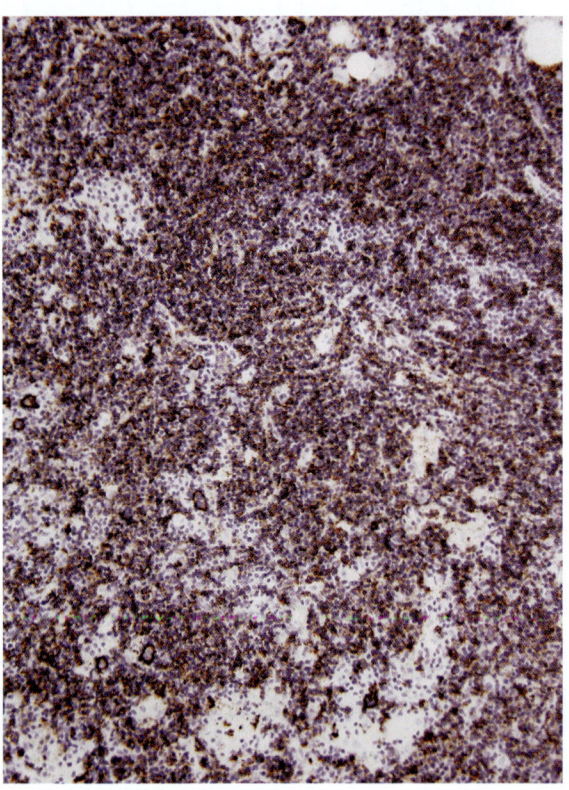

Figure 42-13

PATTERN F OF NODULAR LYMPHOCYTE-PREDOMINANT HODGKIN LYMPHOMA

CD20 immunostaining of pattern F, which is characterized by diffuse areas with LP cells, small reactive B cells, and T cells (not shown) (immunohistochemistry with hematoxylin counterstain).

NLPHL in which nodules are surrounded by collagenous bands that polarize light and the neoplastic cells resemble, more or less, lacunar cells (fig. 42-14). Occasional eosinophils or small foci of necrosis with granulocytes also may be present. Nevertheless, the neoplastic cells have an appropriate immunophenotype, being CD20(+), CD45/LCA(+), BCL6(+), and CD15(-). For lack of a better term, we designate these tumors as a nodular sclerosis-like variant. A second rare variant pattern has been described by Treetipsatit et al. (44) who reported a few neoplasms in which the pattern was nodular or nodular and diffuse. The tumor nodules contained CD4(+), PD1(+) T cells, some of which formed rosettes around large B cells, but the nodules had few small B cells and completely lacked FDCs as assessed by immunohistochemical analysis for CD21 or CD23. The authors concluded that these neoplasms were best classified as large B-cell lymphoma, but likely represented a "gray zone" or an early stage of transformation between NLPHL and T-cell/histiocyte-rich large B-cell lymphoma (44).

Histologic Changes Associated with Recurrent Disease. When NLPHL recurs in lymph nodes, the pattern and cell composition of the tumor often changes. Variant histologic patterns are more common at disease recurrence, particularly patterns D and E. Areas of fibrosis or sclerosis that replace the lymph node parenchyma also may be present, perhaps related to prior therapy (fig. 42-15). The LP cells may be more numerous or acquire more prominent nucleoli, and the number of small B cells within the tumor nodules is commonly decreased and may be few. The immunophenotype of the LP cells also can change over time; in particular, LP cells may acquire CD15 (fig. 42-16, left) and CD30 (fig. 42-16, right), the latter often dimly expressed.

Foci of Rosai-Dorfman Disease Associated with NLPHL. Rarely, foci of Rosai-Dorfman disease (sinus histiocytosis with massive lymphadenopathy) are associated with lymphomas, almost always of B-cell lineage, and commonly NLPHL (24). Typically, Rosai-Dorfman disease associated with NLPHL is microscopic and composed of typical S-100 protein-positive histiocytes, some of which show emperipolesis (fig. 42-17). These patients have no evidence of Rosai-Dorfman disease elsewhere, suggesting that this finding is of no clinical importance (24).

The etiology of focal Rosai-Dorfman disease is unknown; a viral infection or a hyperplastic process seems possible.

Spleen, Liver, and Bone Marrow

The spleen is the most commonly involved anatomic site in patients with advanced stage NLPHL (2,47). The tumor usually involves and expands the splenic white pulp and, if disease is extensive, a nodular pattern may be appreciated. In the liver, NLPHL tends to involve the portal tracts (fig. 42-18). The bone marrow is rarely involved by NLPHL, but when involved, the neoplasm often diffusely replaces the medullary space (fig. 42-19), is T-cell rich, and there is usually clinical evidence to support transformation to a T-cell/histiocyte-rich large B-cell lymphoma (20).

CYTOLOGIC FINDINGS

Fine-needle aspirate smears typically show predominantly small lymphocytes with variable numbers of LP cells (fig. 42-20A,B). Smears also may contain large nuclei with prominent nucleoli, often stripped of cytoplasm. In some cases, the LP cells are sparse and obscured by a background of lymphocytes, mimicking a reactive process. As noted above, there are variable numbers of histiocytes, but eosinophils are not observed (43).

IMMUNOPHENOTYPIC FINDINGS

Flow cytometry immunophenotypic analysis of NLPHL cases shows a mixture of polytypic B cells and T cells (33,35). The T cells do not show evidence of an aberrant immunophenotype and CD4-positive cells usually outnumber CD8-positive cells. In up to 50 percent of cases, a population of T cells is present that is positive for both CD4 and CD8 (dim). These cells range from 10 to 40 percent of all events (35). LP cells are difficult to assess by flow cytometry because they are present in low numbers.

Immunohistochemical analysis is more helpful for assessing cases of NLPHL since this approach directly assesses the neoplastic cells. The LP cells in NLPHL have an immunophenotype of germinal center B cells (fig. 42-21). They are positive for pan-B-cell antigens (CD19, CD20, CD22, CD79a), B-cell transcription factors (BCL6, PAX5, OCT2, and BOB.1) (fig. 42-21A,B), and CD45/LCA (fig. 42-21D) (33,42). PAX5 expression

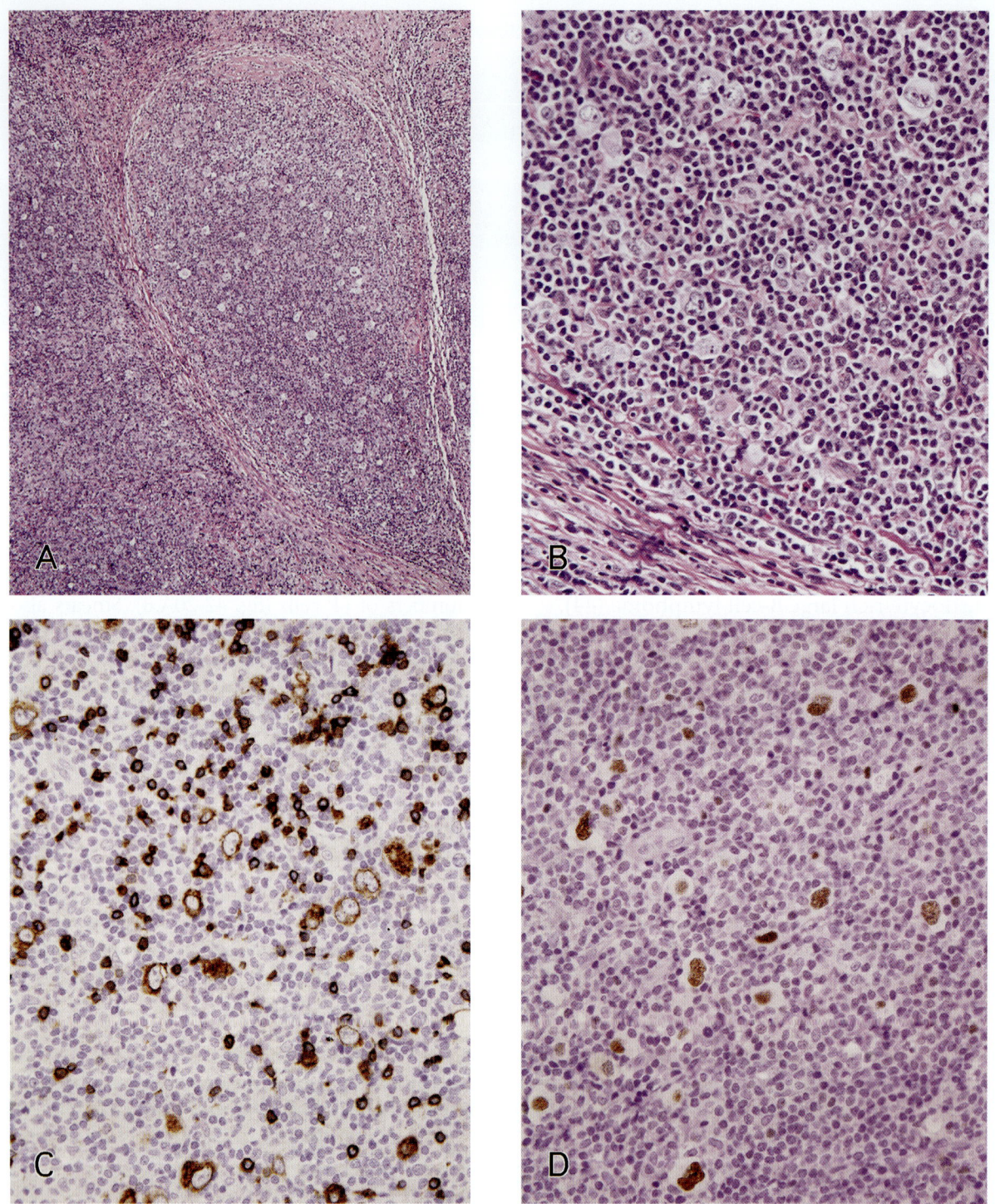

Figure 42-14

NODULAR LYMPHOCYTE-PREDOMINANT HODGKIN LYMPHOMA WITH NODULAR SCLEROSIS-LIKE FEATURES

A: A fibrous band surrounds a tumor nodule (A,B: H&E stain).

B: The tumor cells have mixed features, with some cells resembling LP cells and others resembling lacunar cells.

C,D: The LP cells are positive for CD79A (C) and BCL6 (D). Not shown: the LP cells were also positive for CD20 and IgD and were negative for CD15 and CD30 (C,D: immunohistochemistry with hematoxylin counterstain).

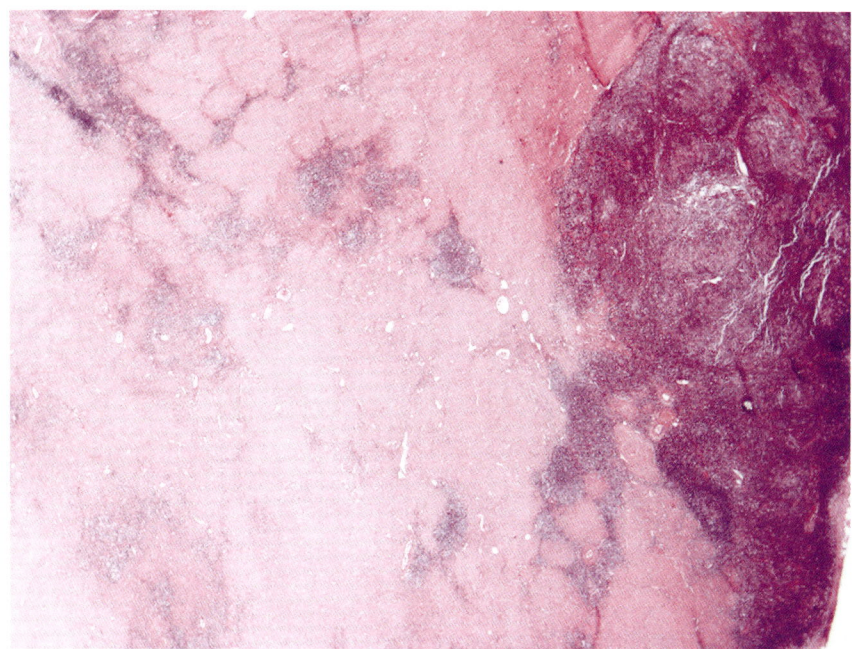

Figure 42-15

RECURRENT NODULAR LYMPHOCYTE-PREDOMINANT HODGKIN LYMPHOMA: FIBROSIS

Wide areas of fibrosis replace the lymph node parenchyma. Recurrent tumor is present at the right of the field (H&E stain).

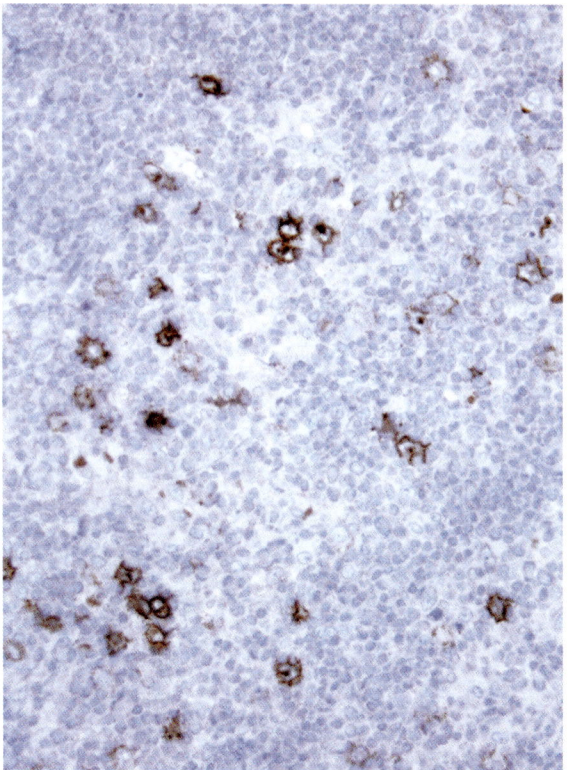 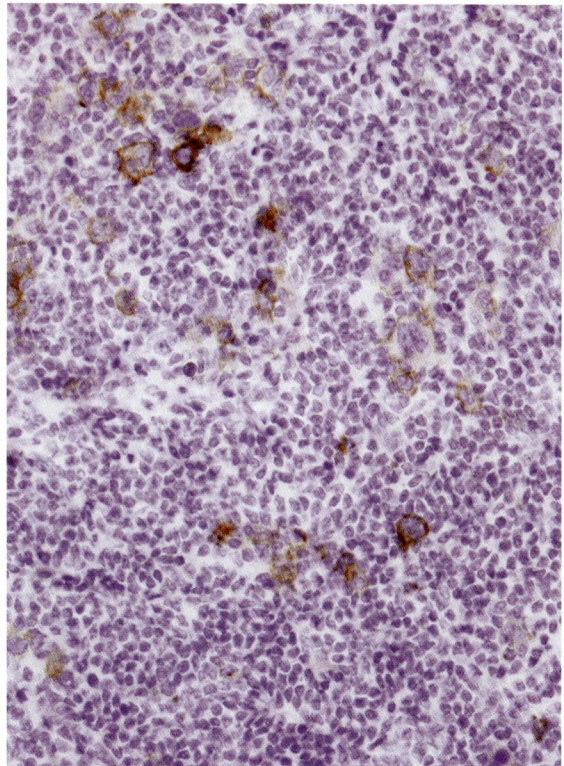

Figure 42-16

RECURRENT NODULAR LYMPHOCYTE-PREDOMINANT HODGKIN LYMPHOMA: CD15 AND CD30 POSITIVE

Left, right: The LP cells in this specimen were positive for CD15 (left) and dimly positive for CD30 (right), unlike the initial biopsy specimen. The LP cells retained bright expression of CD20 (not shown) (immunohistochemistry with hematoxylin counterstain).

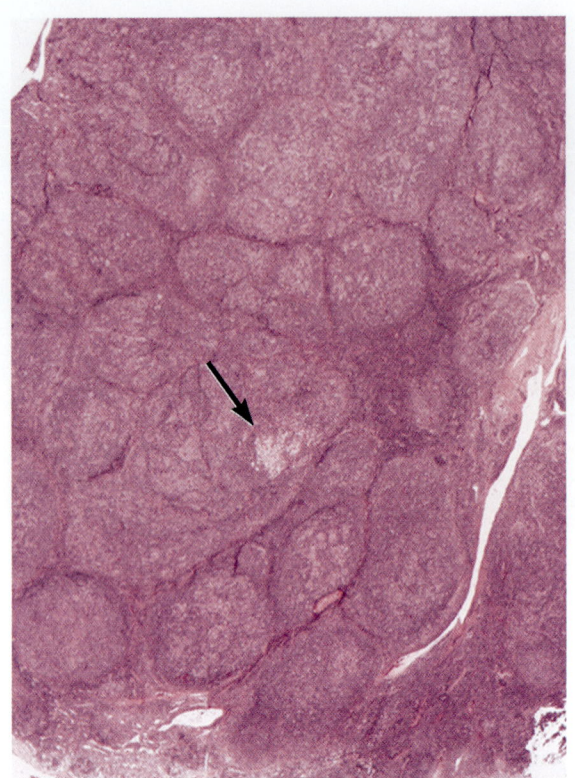
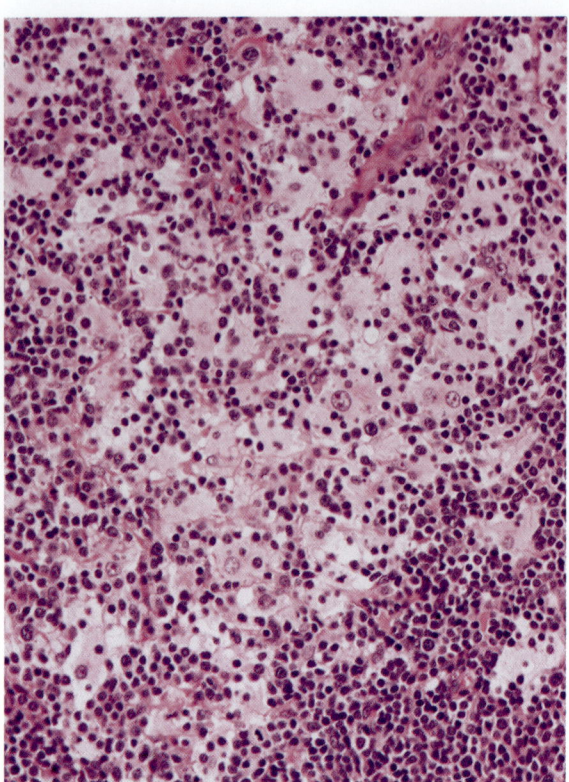

Figure 42-17

**NODULAR LYMPHOCYTE-PREDOMINANT HODGKIN LYMPHOMA
ASSOCIATED WITH A FOCUS OF ROSAI-DORFMAN DISEASE**

Left: The lymph node is replaced by back-to-back nodules of NLPHL. In the center of the field, a small focus (arrow) of Rosai-Dorfman disease is present.

Right: High magnification of Rosai-Dorfman disease shows histiocytes with abundant pale and plate-like cytoplasm. Emperipolesis (lymphocytes within histiocyte cytoplasm) is also present in this field (left, right: H&E stain).

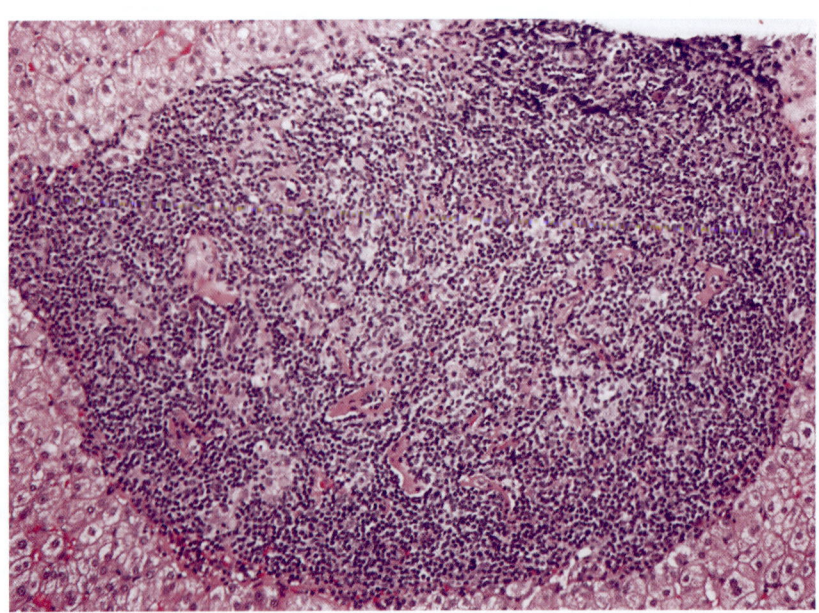

Figure 42-18

NODULAR LYMPHOCYTE-PREDOMINANT HODGKIN LYMPHOMA INVOLVING LIVER

NLPHL expands a portal tract in the liver (H&E stain).

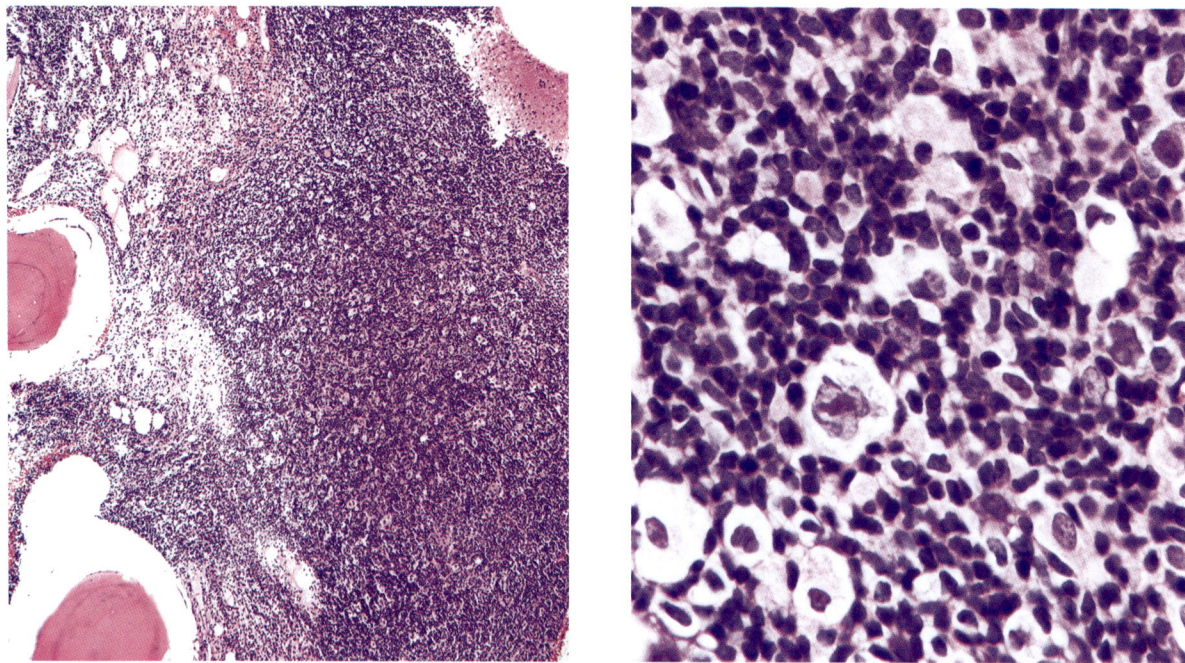

Figure 42-19

**T-CELL/HISTIOCYTE-RICH LARGE B-CELL LYMPHOMA INVOLVING BONE MARROW IN A PATIENT WITH
NODULAR LYMPHOCYTE-PREDOMINANT HODGKIN LYMPHOMA INVOLVING LYMPH NODE**

Left: The medullary space is substantially and diffusely replaced by lymphoma.
Right: Large neoplastic cells with prominent nucleoli are present in a background of small lymphocytes and histiocytes.
The neoplastic cells were CD20(+) (not shown) (left, right: H&E stain).

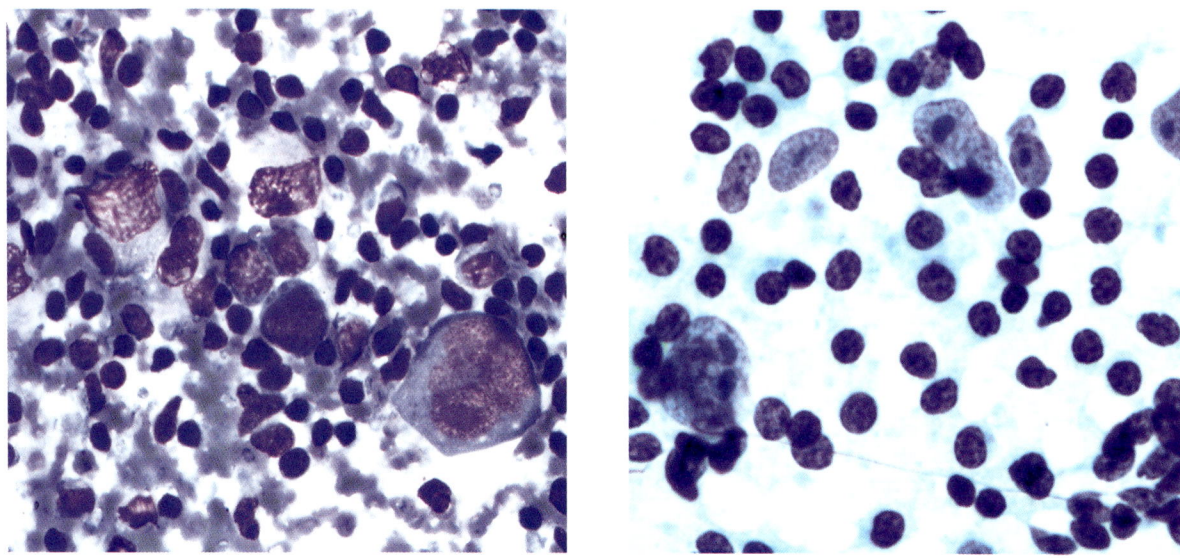

Figure 42-20

NODULAR LYMPHOCYTE-PREDOMINANT HODGKIN LYMPHOMA: CYTOLOGIC FEATURES

Left: In this fine-needle aspirate smear a large LP cell with a multilobated nucleus is seen in a background of small
lymphocytes (Diff-Quik stain). (Courtesy of Dr. J. Stewart, Houston, TX.)
Right: LP cells with convoluted bare nuclei and nucleoli admixed with small lymphocytes (Papanicolaou stain).

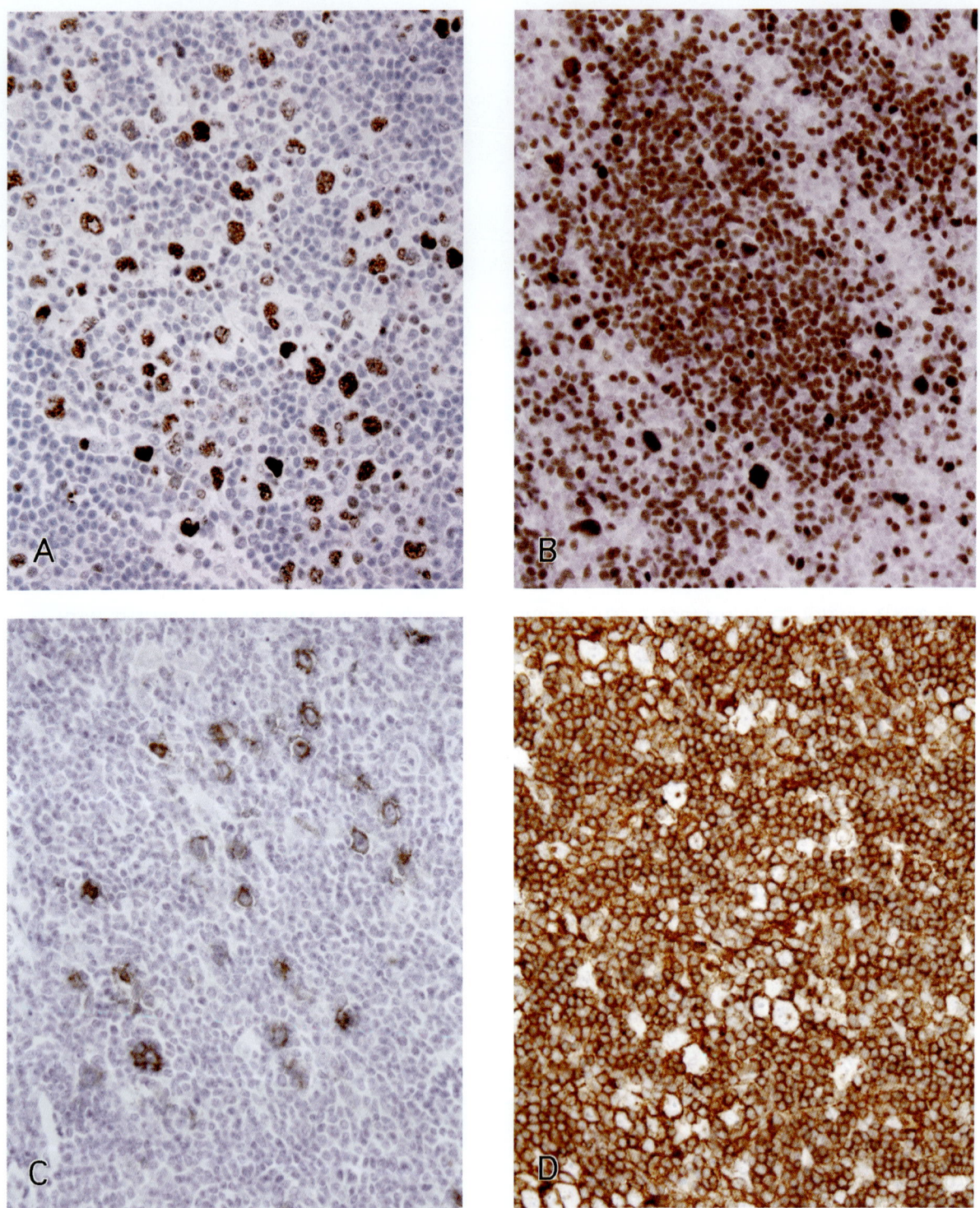

Figure 42-21

NODULAR LYMPHOCYTE-PREDOMINANT HODGKIN LYMPHOMA: IMMUNOHISTOCHEMISTRY

A–D: The LP cells in this case of NLPHL are positive for BCL6 (A), OCT2 (B), epithelial membrane antigen (EMA) (C), and CD45/LCA (D). BCL6 expression by LP cells supports a germinal center B-cell origin. In image B, many LP cells are outside the B-cell nodule (pattern C) (A–D, immunohistochemistry with hematoxylin counterstain).

Table 42-2

CAVEATS AND POTENTIAL PITFALLS IN INTERPRETING IMMUNOHISTOCHEMICAL RESULTS IN NODULAR LYMPHOCYTE-PREDOMINANT HODGKIN LYMPHOMA (NLPHL)

Antibody	Caveat/Pitfall
CD15	In rare (<1%) cases of NLPHL the LP[a] cells are CD15(+). This is more common in cases with a variant pattern or at time of relapse.
CD30	In ~10% of cases of NLPHL, LP cells express CD30, usually variably and with dim to moderate intensity. More often, CD30+ reactive immunoblasts are present.
CD45/LCA	CD45/LCA can be difficult to interpret in NLPHL because the LP cells are surrounded by CD45(+) small lymphocytes. In addition, CD45/LCA appears to be negative in 10 to 20 percent of NLPHL cases.
Epstein-Barr virus	Rare (~1%) cases of NLPHL can be EBV(+). EBV(+) cases often have a variant pattern, may be associated with fibrosis, or the LP cells have atypical features (e.g., prominent nucleoli) suggesting that the neoplasm may be undergoing histologic progression.
T-cell rosettes	LP cells in NLPHL are commonly surrounded by rosettes of T cells that are often follicular T-helper cells. The anti-CD3 antibody is more sensitive, compared with CD57, BCL6, and PD1, for showing the rosettes, but CD3(+) rosettes are less specific for NLPHL.

[a]LP = lymphocyte predominant; EBV = Epstein-Barr virus.

by LP cells is of moderate to bright intensity (equivalent to reactive small B cells). LP cells also express LRF/pokemon (6) and J chain, and are variably positive for Bruton tyrosine kinase (about 85 percent), epithelial membrane antigen (EMA) (about 50 percent) (fig. 42-21C), cyclin D1 (very dim, about 25 percent) and IgD (about 25 percent) (6,12,33,42). LP cells are usually in cycle and therefore positive for Ki-67 and are negative for pan-T-cell antigens, CD1a, CD4, CD8, CD10, CD15, CD21, CD23, CD30, CD43, CD57, CD68, BCL2, PD1, TdT, and NOTCH1 (6,16,33). There are some pitfalls and caveats regarding the interpretation of these immunohistochemical results (Table 42-2).

The reactive background in NLPHL cases is distinctive and helpful in establishing the diagnosis (fig. 42-22). The nodules of NLPHL are composed predominantly of small B cells with an immunophenotype of mantle zone B cells (10,33). These cells express pan-B-cell antigens, B-cell transcription factors, IgD (fig. 42-22A), CD23, and BCL2 and are negative for pan-T-cell antigens, CD10, and BCL6. Reactive T cells are also present in the tumor nodules and are numerous in some cases (fig. 42-22B). Many of these T cells are of follicular T-helper cell lineage, positive for CD4 (fig. 42-22C), CD57 (fig. 42-22D), BCL6, and PD1/CD273 (fig. 42-22E), and these cells tend to surround LP cells forming rosettes (10,33). T cells within the nodules of NLPHL are CD134(+) and CD38(-), consistent with an early or transient activation profile; by contrast, in diffuse areas of NLPHL, the T cells are CD134(-) and CD38(+), supporting persistent T-cell activation (23).

Networks of FDCs are also present within the tumor nodules; usually these cells are positive for CD21 (fig. 42-22F), CD23, CD35, and other markers associated with FDCs. However, there is incomplete concordance in expression of FDC markers in the nodules of NLPHL, suggesting that different stages of FDC differentiation or other factors play a role in their expression.

The above immunophenotypic findings apply to cases with a nodular pattern. In variant patterns of NLPHL, particularly cases with patterns D and E, the LP cells retain their B-cell immunophenotype, but the background cell population is markedly different. Small B lymphocytes are infrequent or entirely absent, and FDCs are also absent in pattern E. The background is composed of numerous small T cells and histiocytes. The T cells are commonly positive for CD8 and often express cytotoxic markers.

Evidence of Epstein-Barr virus (EBV) is also negative in typical cases of NLPHL. However, EBV can be present in rare (less than 1 percent) of cases of NLPHL, shown by either immunohistochemistry for latent membrane protein type 1 (LMP1) or in situ hybridization for EBV-encoded RNA1 (EBER1) (18,45). Usually cases of EBV-positive NLPHL have atypical morphologic features, such as fibrosis, a diffuse pattern, or LP cells with prominent nucleoli (Hodgkin cell-like) (45).

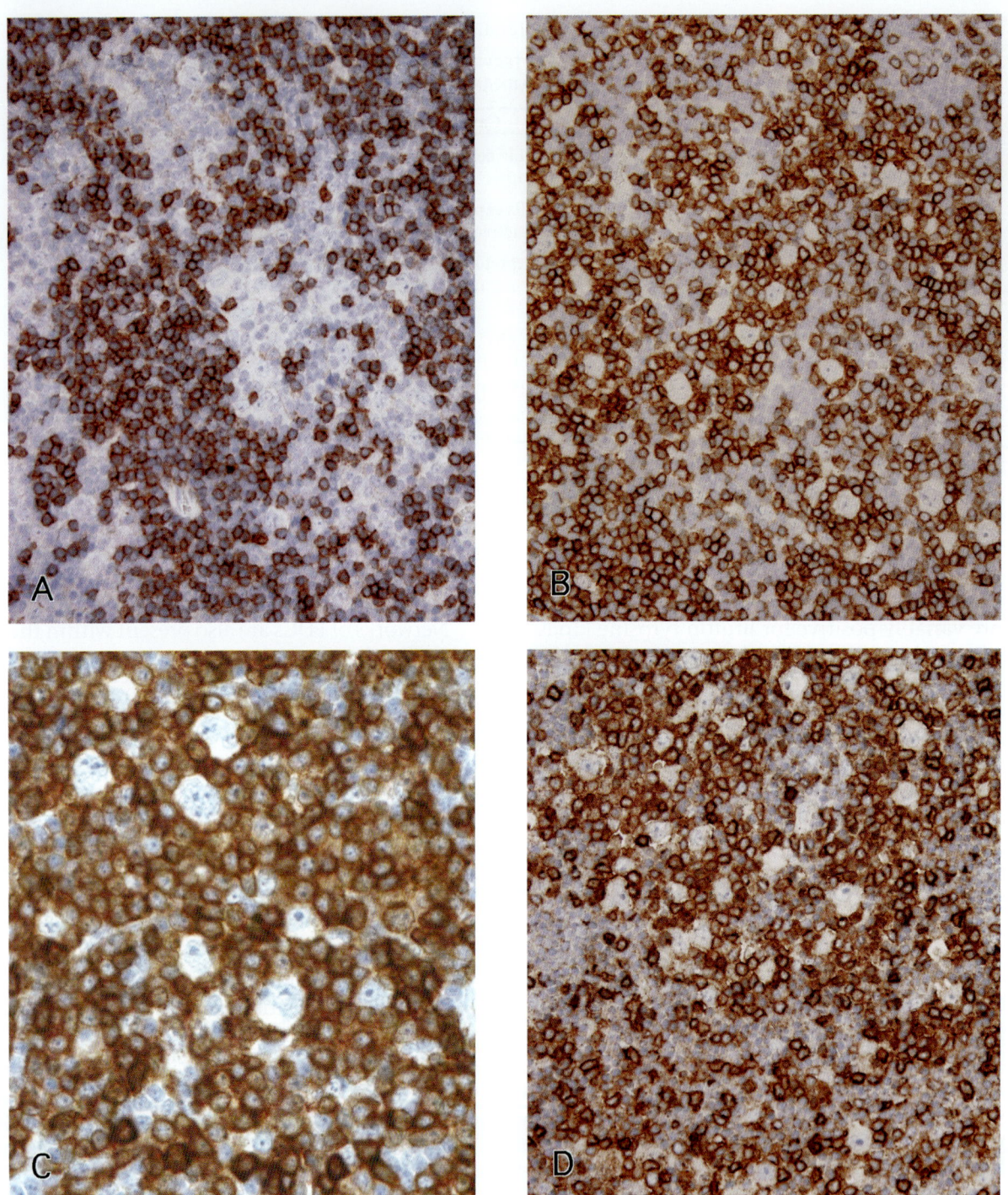

Figure 42-22

NODULAR LYMPHOCYTE PREDOMINANT HODGKIN LYMPHOMA: IMMUNOHISTOCHEMISTRY

The reactive cell population in the nodules of NLPHL is characteristic of the follicular microenvironment and is helpful for diagnosis.

A: IgD is expressed by small B cells consistent with a mantle zone immunophenotype. The LP cells are negative in this case.

B–E: The T-cells in the nodules often have a follicular T-helper cell immunophenotype positive for CD3 (B), CD4 (C), CD57 (D) and PD-1 (E). The T cells often form rosettes around the LP cells.

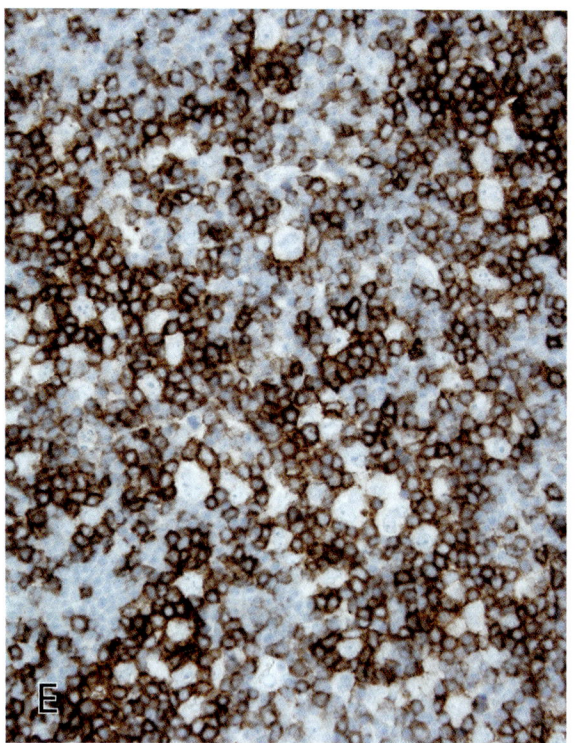
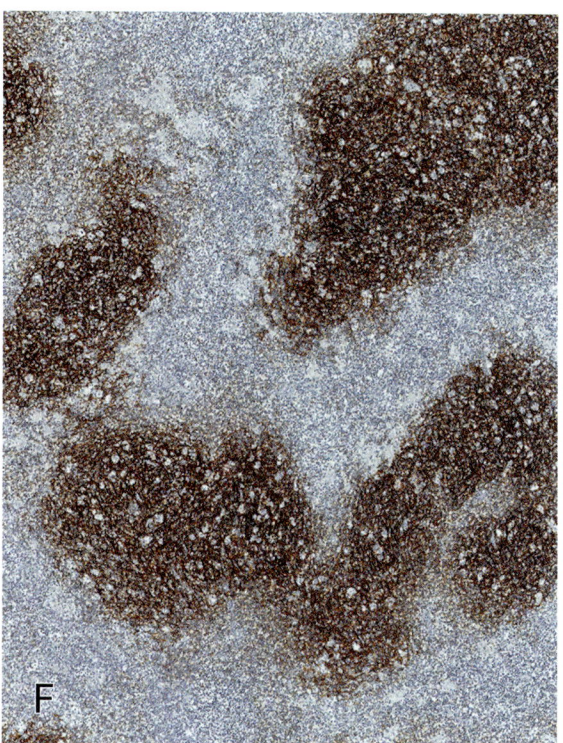

Figure 42-22, continued

F: The anti-CD21 antibody (reactive with C3d receptor) highlights networks of follicular dendritic cells within the tumor nodules (A–F: immunohistochemistry with hematoxylin counterstain).

MOLECULAR GENETIC FINDINGS

Conventional cytogenetic analysis has been performed on a small number of cases. The results, using standard methods, are often diploid because LP cells are few in the specimen. However, in a study by Stamatoullas et al (41), 12 of 13 cases of NLPHL showed clonal karyotypes that were complex in 11 cases. Rearrangements of the chromosome 3q27 locus were the most common (two thirds of cases), with multiple partner loci. Other cytogenetic abnormalities included chromosome 9 (58 percent), 14q32 (50 percent), del(4q28-q32) (50 percent), del(7) or del(7q23-q33) (42 percent), and del(13) (25 percent) (41).

Comparative genomic hybridization analysis of microdissected LP cells supports the results of conventional cytogenetic analysis, since LP cells have been shown to carry numerous abnormalities, with a median of 10.8 in one study (13). These chromosomal aberrations include gains of chromosomes 1, 2q, 3, 4q, 5q, 6, 8q, 11q, 12q, and X, and loss of 17, with a frequency ranging from 35 to 70 percent (13). A number of studies have shown a high frequency of *BCL6* alterations in NLPHL, the result of translocations and less often gene amplification (4,36,46). *BCL6* often partners with *IGH*, but a number of other partner chromosomal loci have been reported (41).

Gene expression profiling analysis of microdissected LP cells was performed by Brune et al. (8). They reported that LP cells show increased expression of molecules in the NF-κB and ERK pathways, dysregulation of many regulators of apoptosis, and partial loss of B-cell differentiation molecules.

Clonality, using routine polymerase chain reaction (PCR)-based methods, is often not identified in NLPHL because of the low percentage of LP cells in these specimens. However, single-cell PCR of LP cells has shown that these carry monoclonally rearranged immunoglobulin genes with evidence of somatic hypermutation of the variable regions (25,30). These mutations show intraclonal diversity, evidence that

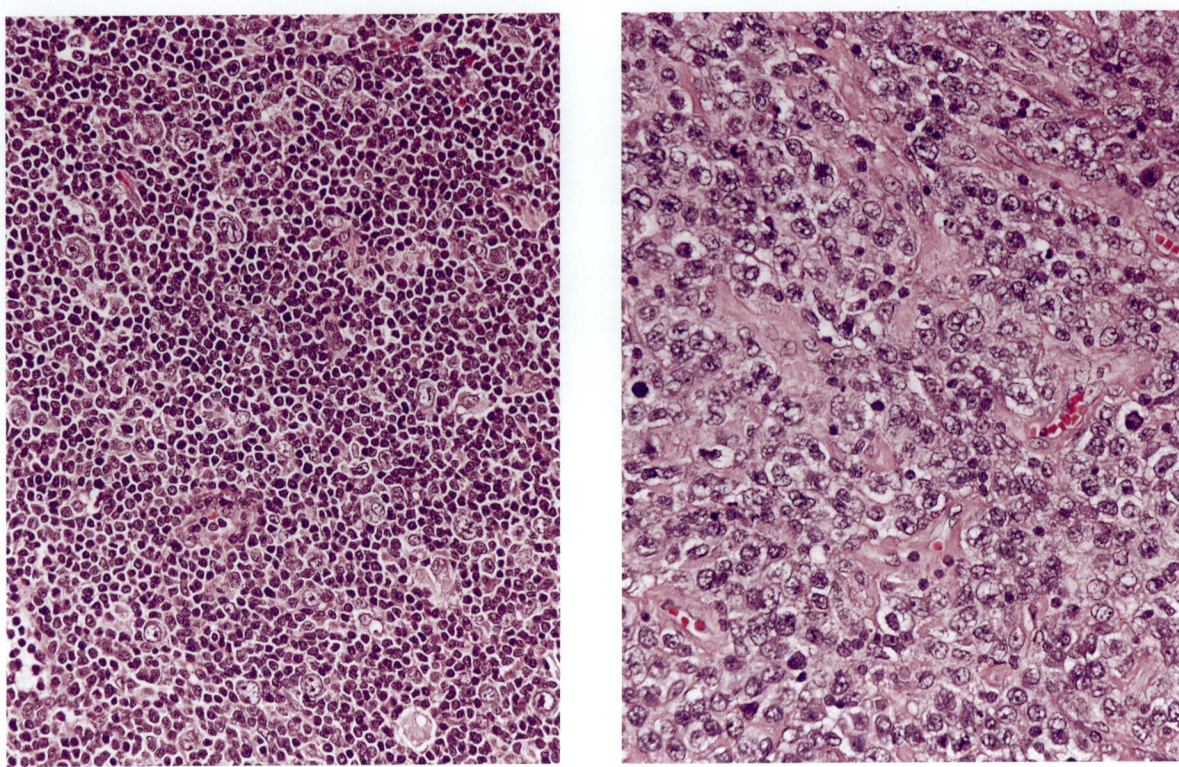

Figure 42-23

NODULAR LYMPHOCYTE-PREDOMINANT HODGKIN LYMPHOMA AND
DIFFUSE LARGE B-CELL LYMPHOMA (DLBCL) INVOLVING DIFFERENT LYMPH NODES

Left: A tumor nodule and scattered LP cells of NLPHL can be appreciated in this field.
Right: In DLBCL, sheets of large cells, some with multilobated nuclei resembling LP cells, are associated with sclerosis. The neoplastic cells were strongly positive for CD20 and had a brisk proliferation (Ki-67) rate (not shown) (left, right: H&E stain).

mutations are ongoing as would be expected of a tumor arising in the germinal center (25,30). In one study by Marafioti et al. (25), the immunoglobulin variable regions showed a mutational load ranging from 7.5 to 27.2 percent. The T-cell receptor genes are in the germline configuration. LP cells do not carry t(11;14)(q13;q32/ *CCND1-IGH*, *MYC* rearrangements, or any of the other known oncogene translocations except *BCL6* alterations (described above).

One study of NLPHL using next generation sequencing showed a high frequency of mutations involving *DUSP2*, *SGK1*, and *JUNB* (17a).

DIFFUSE LARGE B-CELL LYMPHOMA IN PATIENTS WITH NLPHL

As stated previously, patients with NLPHL have an increased risk of transformation to DLBCL. DLBCLs that arise in patients with NLPHL are not easily distinguished from de novo DLBCL,

although there are some morphologic clues. The lymphoma cells may have multilobated nuclei with abundant pale cytoplasm, resembling LP cells (fig. 42-23). NLPHL can also transform to T-cell/histiocyte-rich large B-cell lymphoma (THRLBCL) although distinguishing these lesions from pattern E of NLPHL is problematic using only pathologic findings (fig. 42-24). Criteria to distinguish NLPHL pattern E from THRLBCL are poorly defined, although aggressive clinical findings support THRLBCL (see section in differential diagnosis). In the WHO classification update these cases are designated as THRLBCL-like transformation of NLPHL (43a).

The immunophenotype of DLBCL arising in patients with NLPHL often shares many features with NLPHL, including expression of BCL6, J chain, EMA, and MUM1/IRF4, but there are also some differences (17). Unlike NLPHL, in DLBCL, J chain and EMA may be more dimly positive,

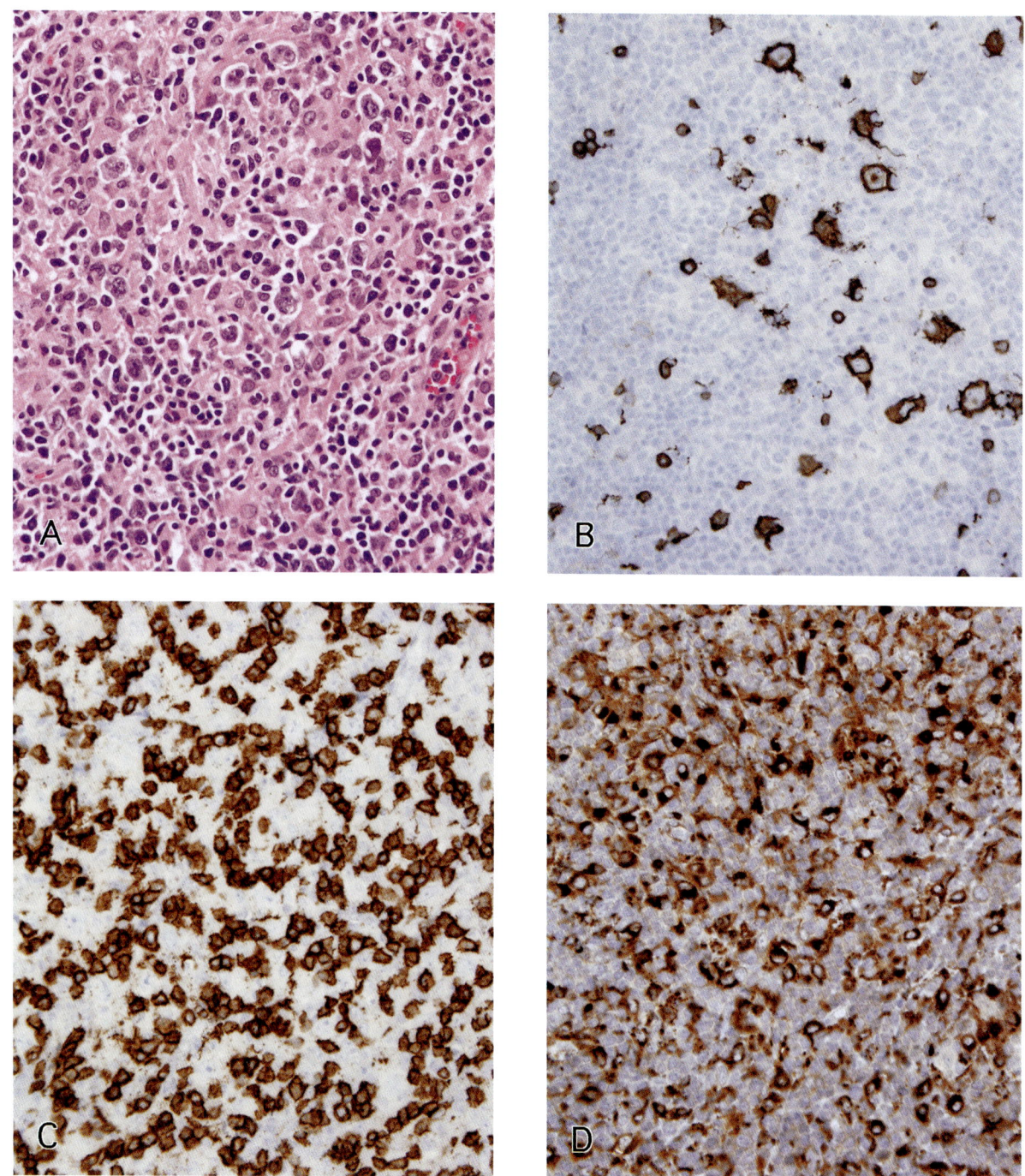

Figure 42-24

**T-CELL/HISTIOCYTE-RICH LARGE B-CELL LYMPHOMA IN A PATIENT
WHO HAD NODULAR LYMPHOCYTE-PREDOMINANT HODGKIN LYMPHOMA**

This patient with a history of NLPHL subsequently developed B symptoms and bone marrow involvement. The lymph node biopsy showed T-cell/histiocyte-rich large B-cell lymphoma.

A: Scattered large neoplastic cells are present in a background of small lymphocytes and histiocytes (H&E stain).

B: The neoplastic cells are positive for CD20, with few small reactive B cells present.

C,D: Most of the background cells are CD8(+) T cells (C) and CD68(+) histiocytes (D) (B–D: immunohistochemistry with hematoxylin counterstain).

CD19 and CD79a may be more brightly positive, and BCL2, often negative in LP cells of NLPHL, may be positive (17).

A small number of patients with paired samples of NLPHL and DLBCL have been studied by molecular methods. These tumor pairs are commonly clonally related, supporting histologic transformation (29,32). The molecular events involved in transformation are poorly understood.

DIFFUSE LYMPHOCYTE-PREDOMINANT HODGKIN LYMPHOMA

The category of diffuse lymphocyte-predominant Hodgkin lymphoma (LPHL) is a rare and controversial entity that is not recognized as such in the WHO classification. With the advent of immunohistochemical and molecular studies, almost all cases once designated as diffuse lymphocyte-predominant Hodgkin disease (Rye classification) have been reclassified as classic HL or non-Hodgkin lymphoma, in particular, THRLBCL. For the few cases that remain as diffuse LPHL, some of these cases may fit into variant pattern F of NLPHL.

DIFFERENTIAL DIAGNOSIS

Progressive Transformation of Germinal Centers. Progressive transformation of germinal centers (PTGC) is a lesion that occurs in 3 to 5 percent of benign lymph nodes, most often in young adults and more often in males (15). Patients usually present with painless lymphadenopathy, most often involving the cervical, axillary, or inguinal regions. Rarely, patients with PTGC present with systemic lymphadenopathy and a viral-like illness after initial diagnosis. Twenty-five to 33 percent of patients with PTGC have persistent lymphadenopathy or develop recurrent lymphadenopathy. Usually, no therapy is required for PTGC, but in some patients rituximab may be beneficial (31).

Histologically, PTGC is characterized by large nodules that are usually 4 to 5 times the size of reactive follicles (fig. 42-25). The PTGC nodules do not fuse or replace the lymph node architecture (15). Mantle zone B cells infiltrate into and disrupt the germinal centers. Over time, the germinal center cells disappear and PTGC nodules are composed almost entirely of small lymphocytes, before the nodules shrink

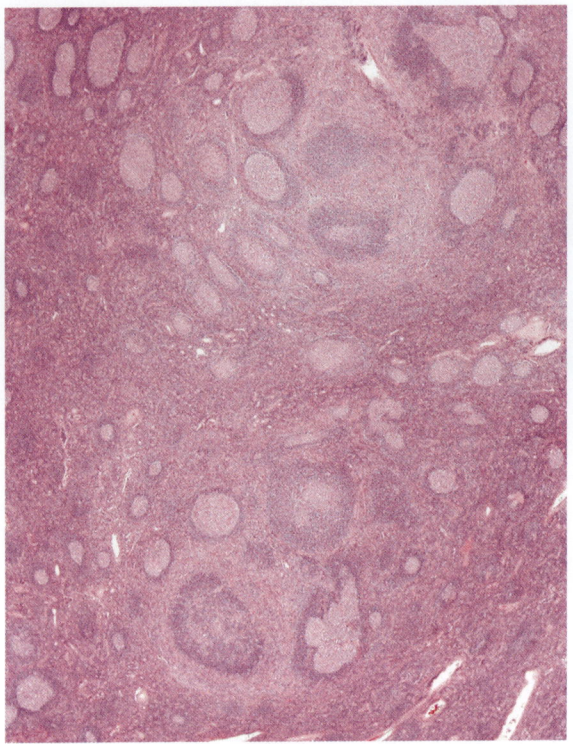

Figure 42-25

PROGRESSIVE TRANSFORMATION OF GERMINAL CENTERS (PTGC) INVOLVING LYMPH NODE

The lymph node shows numerous reactive follicles and some very large nodules of PTGC. At low magnification, the pattern of PTGC is reminiscent of NLPHL (H&E stain).

and resolve. No LP cells are present in PTGC. Immunophenotypic and molecular analyses of PTGC do not yield any evidence of an aberrant immunophenotype or monoclonality.

There is a well-known association between PTGC and NLPHL (and a much weaker association with classic HL). As was shown by others, some patients with NLPHL have simultaneous evidence of PTGC in the same lymph nodes or subsequently develop lymphadenopathy attributable to PTGC. There are also patients who have lymph nodes involved by PTGC before NLPHL. About 10 percent of patients with HL (all types) have evidence of PTGC in another lymph node at some point in time; however, the frequency of PTGC in NLPHL patients is higher. These observations have led to the hypothesis that PTGC is a precursor lesion or possibly a predisposing factor for the development of NLPHL. Prospective follow-up studies of patients with

PTGC, however, have not shown that these patients have an increased risk of NLPHL. Therefore, the evidence supports a linkage between PTGC and NLPHL, but the relationship between these two lesions is otherwise unclear.

One hypothesis is that PTGC is a nonspecific reaction pattern that can be explained by a number of etiologies. In support of this idea, PTGC can be subdivided into general groups: focal PTGC in otherwise reactive lymph nodes, tumor-associated PTGC, and rarely, systemic lymphadenopathy attributable to PTGC (15). Although the exact etiologies are unknown, it seems likely that advances in understanding of PTGC may further stratify these cases. It also seems possible that one specific etiology of PTGC may result in an increased risk of NLPHL. One case of PTGC associated with a t(3;22)(q27;q11), likely involving *BCL6*, but not proven, has been reported (7). This finding lends some credence to the hypothesis that some PTGC cases may be precursors of NLPHL.

Nodular Variant of Lymphocyte-Rich Classic Hodgkin Lymphoma. The differential diagnosis of the nodular variant of lymphocyte-rich classic Hodgkin lymphoma (LRCHL) is discussed in more detail in chapter 39. Briefly, LRCHL and NLPHL may be morphologically indistinguishable in some cases. Histologic clues to LRCHL include reactive germinal centers within tumor nodules, Hodgkin cells with prominent eosinophilic nucleoli, classic Reed-Sternberg cells, and granulocytes or plasma cells surrounding tumor nodules. Most of these features, however, can occur in NLPHL, although granulocytes are rare. Immunohistochemical analysis is essential as the neoplastic cells in LRCHL have the typical immunophenotype for classic HL [CD15(+), CD30(+), PAX5 (dim), CD45/LCA(-)].

Follicular Lymphoma. Follicular lymphoma and NLPHL share a nodular pattern. Although the nodules are usually vague in NLPHL and are often well-formed in follicular lymphoma, in some cases the nodular pattern of both diseases overlaps. Unlike NLPHL, the nodules of follicular lymphoma are composed of a monotonous population of centrocytes and centroblasts. In the few cases where ancillary studies are needed, the cells of follicular lymphoma express CD10 and monotypic Ig, unlike NLPHL. Follicular lymphoma also carries monoclonal immunoglobulin

gene rearrangements and t(14;18)(q32;q21)/ *IGH-BCL2*.

T-Cell/Histiocyte-Rich Large B-Cell Lymphoma. Distinguishing NLPHL with a variant pattern from THRLBCL can be highly challenging. As stated in the World Health Organization (WHO) classification, any degree of tumor nodularity supports the diagnosis NLPHL over de novo THRLBCL (33). Patients with NLPHL, however, can undergo transformation to an aggressive large cell lymphoma that has features of so-called THRLBCL-like transformation of NLPHL (43a). Using morphologic criteria alone, it is difficult (if not impossible) to distinguish NLPHL with large diffuse areas (variant pattern E) from NLPHL with true transformation to THRLBCL. Currently, there are no consensus criteria available for separating these two possible diagnoses. When faced with this differential diagnosis, additional clinical information should be sought as the clinical context is useful. Evidence of B symptoms, elevated serum LDH, bone marrow involvement, and radiologic images showing lytic bone lesions or widespread disease correlate with a poorer prognosis and can be used to support transformation to THRLBCL (2).

TREATMENT AND PROGNOSIS

Patients with NLPHL are traditionally subdivided into those with early stage versus advanced stage disease (1,11,22,26,28,39). A number of prognostic factors have been developed for NLPHL patients that allow their disease designation as favorable or unfavorable. The following findings are poor prognostic factors in different studies: age 45 years or older, advanced stage, three or more nodal sites of disease, extranodal sites of disease, and abnormal laboratory findings including elevated erythrocyte sedimentation rate or serum LDH and low (less than 10.5 g/dL) hemoglobin level.

Regardless of the prognostic factors, the current standard treatment for patients with early stage NLPHL is involved field radiotherapy at 30 to 36 Gy (1,22). The response to radiation therapy is excellent in patients with early stage disease, with complete remission rates of over 90 percent; overall survival is similarly high. Relapses occur in 10 to 20 percent of patients, and in this patient subset the relapses can be multiple (1,11,22). As radiation therapy is associated with toxicity, there are efforts to reduce the dose of radiation by treating only involved sites (effectively reducing the margins of the radiation field). There are some data, mostly in children in whom radiation treatment is avoided, that complete excision of involved lymph nodes can be followed by observation alone (1,39). The important feature using this strategy is complete excision of disease.

For patients with advanced stage disease, the traditional regimen of chemotherapy (doxorubicin [Adriamycin®], bleomycin, vinblastine, and dacarbazine [ABVD]), which is used for patients with classic HL, is recommended (1,11,22,26). Rituximab adds value to traditional therapy (1,26,26a). Overall survival is good, but late relapses occur in a subset of patients. Some data suggest that relapse or poor response is more common in patients with variant histology (39a). There are also some data suggesting that rituximab, cyclophosphamide, doxorubin, vincristine, and prednisolone (R-CHOP) is a better regimen for NLPHL; these data are better developed for patients at the time of relapse than as initial therapy, but some patients who received R-CHOP upfront have done well (1,10a,47). When patients experience multiple relapses, autologous stem cell transplantation is an option (19). For patients who develop DLBCL or THRLBCL, therapy with R-CHOP is usually recommended.

REFERENCES

1. Advani RH, Hoppe RT. How I treat nodular lymphocyte predominant Hodgkin lymphoma. Blood 2013;122:4182-4188.
2. Al-Mansour M, Connors JM, Gascoyne RD, Skinnider B, Savage KJ. Transformation to aggressive lymphoma in nodular lymphocyte-predominant Hodgkin's lymphoma. J Clin Oncol 2010;28:793-799.
3. Anagnostopoulos I, Hansmann ML, Franssila K, et al. European Task Force on Lymphoma project on lymphocyte predominance Hodgkin disease: histologic and immunohistologic analysis of submitted cases reveals 2 types of Hodgkin disease with a nodular growth pattern and abundant lymphocytes. Blood 2000;96:1889-1899.
4. Bakhirev AG, Vasel MA, Zhang QY, Reichard KK, Czuchlewski DR. Fluorescence immunophenotyping and interphase cytogenetics (FICTION) detects BCL6 abnormalities, including gene amplification, in most cases of nodular lymphocyte-predominant Hodgkin lymphoma. Arch Pathol Lab Med 2014;138:538-542.
5. Biasoli I, Stamatoullas A, Meignin V, et al. Nodular, lymphocyte-predominant Hodgkin lymphoma: a long-term study and analysis of transformation to diffuse large B-cell lymphoma in a cohort of 164 patients from the Adult Lymphoma Study Group. Cancer 2010;116:631-639.
6. Bohn O, Maeda T, Filatov A, Lunardi A, Pandolfi PP, Teruya-Feldstein J. Utility of LRF/pokemon and NOTCH1 protein in expression in the distinction between nodular lymphocyte-predominant Hodgkin lymphoma and classical Hodgkin lymphoma. Int J Surg Pathol 2014;22:6-11.
7. Bouron-Dal Soglio D, Truong F, Fetni R, et al. A B-cell lymphoma-associated chromosomal translocation in a progression transformation of germinal center. Hum Pathol 2008;39:292-297.
8. Brune V, Tiacci E, Pfeil I, et al. Origin and pathogenesis of nodular lymphocyte-predominant Hodgkin lymphoma as revealed by global gene expression analysis. J Exp Med 2008;205:2251-2268.
9. Eyre TA, Gatter K, Collins GP, Hall GW, Watson C, Hatton CS. Incidence, management and outcome of high grade transformation of nodular lymphocyte predominant Hodgkin lymphoma: long-term outcomes from a 30-year experience. Am J Hematol 2015;90:E103-110.
10. Fan Z, Natkunam Y, Bair E, Tibshirani R, Warnke RA. Characterization of variant patterns of nodular lymphocyte predominant Hodgkin lymphoma with immunohistologic and clinical correlation. Am J Surg Pathol 2003;27:1346-1356.
10a. Fanale MA, Cheah CY, Rich A, et al. Encouraging activity for R-CHOP in advanced stage nodular lymphocyte predominant Hodgkin lymphoma. Blood 2017. [Epub ahead of print]
11. Farrell K, McKay P, Leach M, et al. Nodular lymphocyte predominant Hodgkin lymphoma behaves as a distinct clinical entity with good outcome: evidence from 14-year follow-up in the West of Scotland Cancer Network. Leuk Lymphoma 2011;52:1920-1928.

12. Fernandez-Vega I, Quiros LM, Santos-Juanes J, Pane-Foix M, Marafioti T. Bruton's tyrosine kinase (Btk) is a useful marker for Hodgkin and B cell non-Hodgkin lymphoma. Virchow Archiv 2015;466:229-235.

13. Franke S, Wlodarska I, Maes B, et al. Lymphocyte predominance Hodgkin disease is characterized by recurrent genomic imbalances. Blood 2001;97:1845-1853.

14. Goel A, Fan W, Patel AA, Devabhaktuni M, Grossbard ML. Nodular lymphocyte predominant Hodgkin lymphoma: biology, diagnosis and treatment. Clin Lymphoma Myeloma Leuk 2014;14:261-270.

15. Hansmann ML, Fellbaum C, Hui PK, Moubayed P. Progressive transformation of germinal centers with and without association to Hodgkin's disease. Am J Clin Pathol 1990;93:219-226.

16. Hartmann S, Eichenauer DA, Plütschow A, et al. The prognostic impact of variant histology in nodular lymphocyte-predominant Hodgkin lymphoma: a report from the German Hodgkin Study Group (GHSG). Blood 2013;122:4246-4252.

17. Hartmann S, Eray M, Doring C, et al. Diffuse large B cell lymphoma derived from nodular lymphocyte predominant Hodgkin lymphoma presents with variable histopathology. BMC Cancer 2014;14:332.

17a. Hartmann S, Schuhmacher B, Rausch T, et al. Highly recurrent mutations of SGK1, DUSP2 and JUNB in nodular lymphocyte predominant Hodgkin lymphoma. Leukemia 2016;30:844-853.

18. Huppmann AR, Nicolae A, Slack GW, et al. EBV may be expressed in the LP cells of nodular lymphocyte-predominant Hodgkin lymphoma (NLPHL) in both children and adults. Am J Surg Pathol 2014;38:316-324.

19. Karuturi M, Hosing C, Fanale M, et al. High-dose chemotherapy and autologous stem cell transplantation for nodular lymphocyte-predominant Hodgkin lymphoma. Biol Blood Marrow Transplant 2013;19:991-994.

19a. Kenderian SS, Habermann TM, Macon WR, et al. Large B-cell transformation in nodular lymphocyte-predominant Hodgkin lymphoma: 40-year experience from a single institution. Blood 2016;127:1960-1966.

20. Khoury JD, Jones D, Yared MA, et al. Bone marrow involvement in patients with nodular lymphocyte predominant Hodgkin lymphoma. Am J Surg Pathol 2004;28:489-495.

21. King RL, Howard MT, Bagg A. Hodgkin lymphoma: pathology, pathogenesis, and a plethora of potential prognostic markers. Adv Anat Pathol 2014;21:12-25.

22. Lee AI, LaCasce AS. Nodular lymphocyte predominant Hodgkin lymphoma. Oncologist 2009;14:739-751.

23. Lin P, Medeiros LJ, Wilder RB, Abruzzo LV, Manning JT, Jones D. The activation profile of tumour-associated reactive T-cells differs in the nodular and diffuse patterns of lymphocyte predominant Hodgkin's disease. Histopathology 2004;44:561-569.

24. Lu D, Estalilla OC, Manning JT Jr, Medeiros LJ. Sinus histiocytosis with massive lymphadenopathy and malignant lymphoma involving the same lymph node: a report of four cases and review of the literature. Mod Pathol 2000;13:414-419.

25. Marafioti T, Hummel M, Anagnostopoulos I, et al. Origin of nodular lymphocyte-predominant Hodgkin's disease from a clonal expansion of highly mutated germinal-center B cells. N Engl J Med 1997;337:453-458.

26. McKay P, Fielding P, Gallop-Evans E, et al. Guidelines for the investigation and management of nodular lymphocyte predominant Hodgkin lymphoma. Br J Haematol 2016;172:32-43.

26a. Molin D, Linderoth J, Wahlin BE. Nodular lymphocyte predominant Hodgkin lymphoma in Sweden between 2000 and 2014: an analysis of the Swedish Lymphoma Registry. Br J Haematol 2017;177:449-456.

27. Morton LM, Wang SS, Devesa SS, Hartge P, Weisenburger DD, Linet MS. Lymphoma incidence patterns by WHO subtype in the United States, 1991-2001. Blood 2006;107:265-276.

28. Nogova L, Reineke T, Brillant C, et al. Lymphocyte-predominant and classical Hodgkin's lymphoma: a comprehensive analysis from the German Hodgkin Study Group. J Clin Oncol 2008;26:434-439.

29. Ohno T, Huang JZ, Wu G, Park KH, Weisenburger DD, Chan WC. The tumor cells in nodular lymphocyte-predominant Hodgkin disease are clonally related to the large cell lymphoma occurring in the same individual. Direct demonstration by single cell analysis. Am J Clin Pathol 2001;116:506-511.

30. Ohno T, Stribley JA, Wu G, Hinrichs SH, Weisenburger DD, Chan WC. Clonality in nodular lymphocyte-predominant Hodgkin's disease. N Engl J Med 1997;337:459-465.

31. Picardi M, Zeppa P, Ciancia G, et al. Efficacy and safety of rituximab treatment in patients with progressive transformation of germinal centers after Hodgkin lymphoma in complete remission post-induction chemotherapy and radiotherapy. Leuk Lymphoma 2011;52:2082-2089.

32. Pijuan L, Vicioso L, Bellosillo B, et al. CD20-negative T-cell-rich B-cell lymphoma as a progression of a nodular lymphocyte-predominant Hodgkin's lymphoma treated with rituximab: a molecular analysis using laser capture microdissection. Am J Surg Pathol 2005;29:1399-1403.

33. Poppema S, Delsol G, Pileri SA, et al. Nodular lymphocyte predominant Hodgkin lymphoma. In: Swerdlow SH, Campo E, Harris NL, et al., eds. WHO classification of tumours of haematopoietic and lymphoid tissues. Lyon: IARC Press; 2008:323-325.

34. Poppema S, Kaiserling E, Lennert K. Hodgkin's disease with lymphocytic predominance, nodular type (nodular paragranuloma) and progressively transformed germinal centres—a cytohistological study. Histopathology 1979;3:295-308.

35. Rahemtullah A, Reichard KK, Preffer FI, Harris NL, Hasserjian RP. A double-positive CD4+CD8+ T-cell population is commonly found in nodular lymphocyte predominant Hodgkin lymphoma. Am J Clin Pathol 2006;126:805-814.

36. Renné C, Martin-Subero JI, Hansmann ML, Siebert R. Molecular cytogenetic analyses of immunoglobulin loci in nodular lymphocyte predominant Hodgkin's lymphoma reveal a recurrent IGH-BCL6 juxtaposition. J Mol Diagn 2005;7:352-356.

37. Saarinen S, Aavikko M, Aittomaki K, et al. Exome sequencing reveals germline NPAT mutation as a candidate risk factor for Hodgkin lymphoma. Blood 2011;118:493-498.

38. Saarinen S, Pukkala E, Vahteristo P, Mäkinen MJ, Franssila K, Aaltonen LA. High familial risk in nodular lymphocyte-predominant Hodgkin lymphoma. J Clin Oncol 2013;31:938-943,

39. Shankar A, Daw S. Nodular lymphocyte predominant Hodgkin lymphoma in children and adolescents—a comprehensive review of biology, clinical course and treatment options. Br J Haematol 2012;159:288-298.

39a. Shankar AG, Kirkwood AA, Depani S, et al. Relapsed or poorly responsive nodular lymphocyte predominant Hodgkin lymphoma in children and adolescents—a report from the United Kingdom's Children's Cancer and Leukaemia Study Group. Br J Haematol 2016;173:421-431.

40. Sohani AR, Jaffe ES, Harris NL, Ferry JA, Pittaluga S, Hasserjian RP. Nodular lymphocyte-predominant Hodgkin lymphoma with atypical T cells: a morphologic variant mimicking peripheral T-cell lymphoma. Am J Surg Pathol 2011;35:1666-1678.

41. Stamatoullas A, Picquenot JM, Dumesnil C, et al. Conventional cytogenetics of nodular lymphocyte-predominant Hodgkin's lymphoma. Leukemia 2007;21:2064-2067.

42. Stein H, Hansmann ML, Lennert K, Brandtzaeg P, Gatter KC, Mason DY. Reed-Sternberg and Hodgkin cells in lymphocyte-predominant Hodgkin's disease of nodular subtype contain J chain. Am J Clin Pathol 1986;86:292-297.

43. Subhawong AP, Ali SZ, Tatsas AD. Nodular lymphocyte-predominant Hodgkin lymphoma: cytopathologic correlates on fine-needle aspiration. Cancer Cytopathol 2012;25:254-260.

43a. Swerdlow SH, Campo E, Pileri SA, et al. The 2016 revision of the World Health Organization classification of lymphoid neoplasms. Blood 2016;127:2375-2390.

44. Treetipsatit J, Metcalf RA, Warnke RA, Natkunam Y. Large B-cell lymphoma with T-cell-rich background and nodules lacking follicular dendritic cell meshworks: description of an insufficiently recognized variant. Hum Pathol 2015;46:74-83.

45. Wang S, Medeiros LJ, Xu-Monette ZY, et al. Epstein-Barr virus-positive nodular lymphocyte predominant Hodgkin lymphoma. Ann Diagn Pathol 2014;18:203-209.

46. Wlodarska I, Stul M, De Wolf-Peters C, Hagemeijer A. Heterogeneity of BCL6 rearrangements in nodular lymphocyte predominant Hodgkin's lymphoma. Haematologica 2004;89:965-972.

47. Xing KH, Connors JM, Lai A, et al. Advanced-stage nodular lymphocyte predominant Hodgkin lymphoma compared with classical Hodgkin lymphoma: a matched pair analysis. Blood 2014;123:3567-3573.

43 HUMAN IMMUNODEFICIENCY VIRUS-ASSOCIATED LYMPHOPROLIFERATIVE DISORDERS

GENERAL FEATURES

In the World Health Organization (WHO) classification, immunodeficiency-associated lymphoproliferative disorders are grouped according to the clinical setting or background in which they arise and there are four major categories: human immunodeficiency virus infection, iatrogenic (chapter 44), primary immunodeficiency (chapter 46), and following organ transplantation (chapter 47). In this chapter, we focus on lymphoproliferative disorders that develop in the context of human immunodeficiency virus (HIV) infection and often, acquired immunodeficiency syndrome (AIDS) (47). *HIV-associated lymphoproliferative disorders* are heterogeneous and include lymphomas that are virtually unique to patients with HIV infection as well as lymphomas that arise in immunocompetent patients (47).

HIV is a retrovirus that belongs to the genus *Lentivirus* (48,57). There are two major types of virus, HIV-1 and HIV-2, based on organizational differences in their genomes; both viruses cause AIDS. HIV-2 infection appears to be more indolent than HIV-1; in other words, it takes longer for infected patients to develop AIDS (58).

HIV is highly variable at a genetic and structural level. This variability allows the virus to overcome host immune defenses and maintain survival (at low levels) in the face of antiretroviral therapy, and therefore presents a major challenge in developing an effective vaccine (30,38). The genetic variation of HIV is attributable to two features of the virus. First, reverse transcriptase is error prone. As viral replication occurs rapidly and generates innumerable virions per day, many mutations are introduced into the viral genome. Secondly, two or more HIV viruses can recombine in an infected individual.

As a result of HIV variability, there are three major groups of HIV-1: Major (M), Outlier (O), and non-M, non-O (N). Group M includes many subtypes, A to K. Each subtype also has sub-subtypes, designated by a number, for example, subtype A has four sub-subtypes (A1-A4). In large part, group M of HIV-1 is responsible for the worldwide AIDS pandemic, involving most countries including Africa. Groups O and N of HIV-1 are confined to Africa. HIV-2 is mostly confined to sub-Saharan, central, and western Africa (57). HIV-2 also exhibits variability and multiple strains occur, but this topic is much less studied.

Viral Structure and Replication

HIV is a sphere of about 120 nm and contains a central capsid (or core) surrounded by an outer envelope or membrane (24,30,48). The capsid contains a RNA molecule that has long terminal repeat (LTR) regions at each end. Similar to other retroviruses, the RNA has *GAG*, *POL*, and *ENV* genes that encode a structural core (e.g., p24), viral enzymes (i.e., reverse transcriptase and integrase), and viral envelope glycoproteins. The virus also has a number of unique genes, including *TAT, REV, VPR, VPU, VIF*, and *NEF* (fig. 43-1). Each of the genes is essential for HIV survival, replication, or spread of infection. For example, *TAT* encodes for a protein that is expressed early in HIV infection and promotes expression of other HIV genes; *VPR* is involved in the arrest of the cell cycle and allows reverse transcribed DNA to enter the nucleus in macrophages. In HIV-2, *VPR* is replaced by *VPX* (24).

The envelope of HIV is rich in protein and lipids. The two major components of the envelope are glycoprotein (gp) 41 and gp120, which bind to each other. During the process of budding, the envelope also incorporates proteins from host cells, for example, human leukocyte antigen (HLA) or adhesion molecules (38).

The HIV replication cycle can be subdivided into six general steps: 1) binding of the virus and cell entry; 2) viral shedding of its surrounding

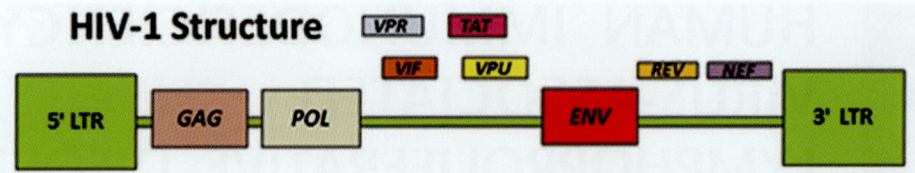

Figure 43-1

HUMAN IMMUNODEFICIENCY VIRUS (HIV) TYPE 1

The genes in the small boxes in this schematic representation are unique to HIV, and *VPU* is unique to type 1.

membrane (i.e., uncoating); 3) reverse transcription of RNA into proviral DNA; 4) integration of provirus into DNA of infected cell; 5) synthesis of viral proteins; and 6) budding, which allows viral transfer to another cell (30). During the initial step in this process, gp120 of the viral envelope binds to CD4 expressed predominantly by T cells and macrophages (24,30,38). The process of binding also involves chemokine receptors on the cell membrane that function as co-receptors. Although a number of chemokines may be involved, when HIV binds to T cells and macrophages, the major co-receptors are CXCL4 and CCR5, respectively. Different strains of HIV have a preference for binding to T cells versus macrophages, in part related to co-receptor use. Dendritic cells also are infected by HIV, perhaps via phagocytosis of immune complexes.

Natural History of HIV Infection

HIV thrives in human lymphoid tissues and the bloodstream, but cannot survive outside the human body for any length of time (11,48,57). Also, the virus is easily inactivated by commonly used disinfectants. Therefore, a person acquires HIV infection only by exposure to infected blood or body secretions. Sexual intercourse is the most common means of transmission, and the risk of infection is greatly increased in the context of skin or mucosal cuts or abrasions. Other means of transmission include the use of infected needles, usually related to illicit drug use, or blood transfusions. The use of sharp instruments, including medical or dental tools, also has been connected to HIV transmission. Fortunately, HIV transmission via blood products or medical instruments is currently low in developed countries, due to effective screening and instrument sterilization.

Once a person is infected by HIV, the virus quickly spreads to regional lymph nodes and the bloodstream (7,48). In lymph nodes, HIV is identified in CD4-positive T cells, macrophages, and follicular dendritic cells in germinal centers. Within 2 weeks, infected patients have viremia and are capable of spreading the infection. Around this time, infected patients often develop a flu-like illness with malaise, fever, pharyngitis, mouth ulcers, rash, arthralgias and myalgias, and lymphadenopathy, which usually lasts for 7 to 10 days (7). Subsequently, the initial phase of viremia and the acute illness resolve as the host immune system seemingly brings the virus under control over the next few weeks.

Antibodies to HIV in serum first appear 3 to 5 weeks after infection. An apparent asymptomatic phase then follows that can last years. During the asymptomatic interval, however, HIV continues to replicate, destroying CD4-positive T cells and the architecture of lymphoid tissues (22,25,58).

Although progressive impairment of the immune system occurs in virtually all patients, the rate of impairment is variable and depends, in part, on host factors. CD4-positive T cells have varying capability to resist destruction, and different patients have differences in their CD8-positive cytotoxic T-cell response as well as other factors (22,49). Eventually, the impairment of the immune system becomes extreme, with very low CD4-positive T-cell counts, and patients become symptomatic. The combination of B symptoms, low CD4-positive T-cell count, and hypergammaglobulinemia is known as AIDS-related complex (ARC). The onset of severe opportunistic infections, non-Hodgkin lymphomas (NHL), Kaposi sarcoma, and invasive cervical carcinoma are defining features of AIDS.

Patients with AIDS commonly develop opportunistic infections by organisms such as *Pneumocystis jiroveci*, *Mycobacteria avium-intracellulare* or *tuberculosis*, various fungi, *Toxoplasma gondii*, gastrointestinal tract parasites, and viruses (e.g., cytomegalovirus, herpes viruses) (48,49). The combination of HIV infection and opportunistic infections results in fever, low body weight, and symptoms related to respiratory and gastrointestinal tract diseases (48,57). Patients with AIDS also have a greatly increased risk of developing viral-driven tumors, particularly viral-driven lymphomas, Kaposi sarcoma, and viral-induced carcinomas (15). If a patient is not treated, the median time interval from initial HIV infection to death with AIDS is about 11 years (48).

HIV-Associated Benign Lymphadenopathy

Patients with HIV infection usually develop lymphadenopathy, which is commonly benign in the early stages of disease (11,31,40). The most commonly involved lymph node groups are those around the salivary gland and the cervical, supraclavicular, axillary, and inguinal regions. Lymphadenopathy attributable to benign causes commonly precedes the onset of lymphoma, but a clear relationship showing that benign lymph nodes are precursors to lymphoma is not established (31,40). Nevertheless, this sequence implies a multistep pathogenesis for lymphomas arising in HIV-positive patients.

Initially, lymph nodes in HIV-positive patients exhibit florid follicular hyperplasia (also known as type A) (20,31). In these lymph nodes, lymphoid follicles are large and irregular (map-like shape) and composed predominantly of germinal centers with a starry-sky pattern (due to admixed histiocytes) and numerous centroblasts. The mantle zones are underdeveloped and can be nearly absent (fig. 43-2).

Using immunohistochemistry, HIV can be shown in lymph nodes with reactive follicular hyperplasia, particularly in follicular dendritic cells within follicles (20). In addition, at this stage, monocytoid B cells are increased and expand sinuses, and plasma cells may be increased between follicles. With time and as the patient's immune system is further compromised, lymph nodes begin to undergo follicular involution, with hemorrhage into germinal centers (also known as follicle lysis) (fig. 43-3). As this process progresses there is disruption and collapse of the follicular dendritic cell networks within germinal centers (type B) and then near total depletion of lympho-

cytes (type C). In this last stage, opportunistic infections, such as *Mycobacterium avium-intracellulare*, are commonly present (fig. 43-4) (31).

Cystic Lymphoepithelial Lesion. These lesions occur in salivary gland lymph nodes of HIV-positive patients. Patients present with tenderness, pain, or progressive swelling that can result in a cystic mass(es) that may be unilateral or bilateral. In some patients, these lesions are prominent, up to 6 or 7 cm in diameter. The etiology is thought to be the result of HIV infection attributable to either an autoimmune reaction or duct blockage as a result of marked lymphoid hyperplasia (or both).

Histologically, cystic lymphoepithelial lesions are characterized by marked follicular hyperplasia (type A as described above) associated with proliferation and squamous metaplasia of intranodal salivary gland duct inclusions that can closely mimic myoepithelial sialadenitis (or benign lymphoepithelial lesion) as occurs in patients with Sjogren syndrome. The intranodal ducts become microscopically or grossly cystic and filled with keratin (fig. 43-5). Cyst contents leak into the surrounding tissues, inducing chronic inflammation and a foreign body giant cell reaction.

Risk of Lymphoma

Compared with the general population, lymphomas occur with a markedly increased frequency in patients with HIV infection (6,47). Prior to the era of highly active antiretroviral therapy (HAART), also referred to in the literature as anti-retroviral therapy (ART) or combination ART (cART), the overall risk of lymphoma was 60 times greater than the general population and up to 3 percent of all patients with AIDS developed NHL (4). The risk of NHL is currently much lower in the HAART era, most substantially for primary diffuse large B-cell lymphoma (DLBCL) arising in the central nervous system, and to a lesser degree, Burkitt lymphoma (5,6).

Factors other than HAART also are involved in lymphoma risk, such as genetic susceptibility. Patients with HIV infection who have inherited *CCR5-delta32* mutations have a reduced risk of lymphoma (17,46). Conversely, *SDF-1* polymorphisms, more common in the white population, have been reported to increase the risk of NHL up to 4-fold in those with HIV infection (46).

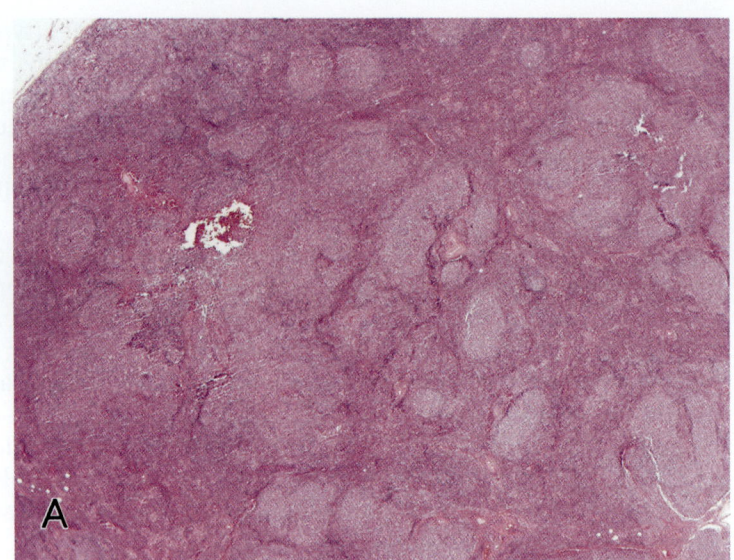

Figure 43-2

FLORID REACTIVE FOLLICULAR HYPERPLASIA IN LYMPH NODE OF HIV-POSITIVE PATIENT

A: At low-power magnification, numerous reactive follicles of different shapes are present (A,B: hematoxylin and eosin [H&E] stain).

B: At high-power magnification, the follicles lack well-defined mantle zones.

C: Immunohistochemical study for HIV p24 shows reactivity within the germinal centers and is usually abundant in follicle dendritic cells (immunohistochemistry with hematoxylin counterstain).

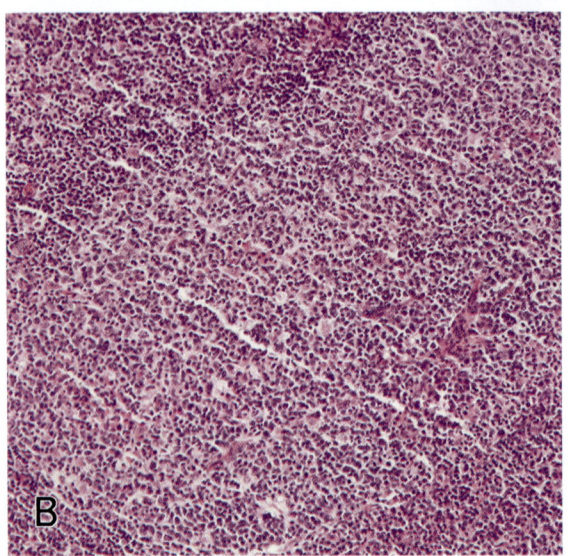

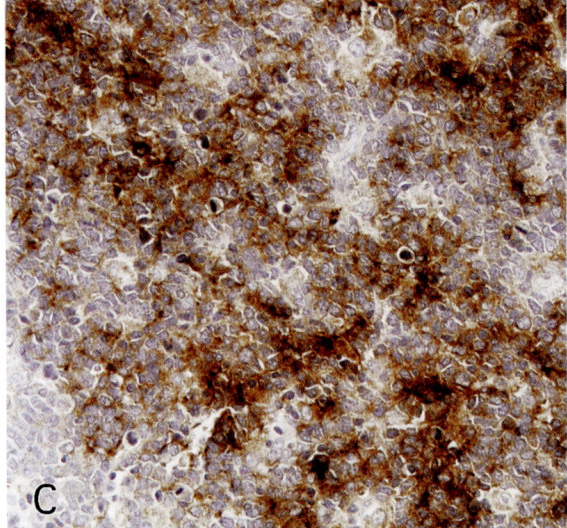

Despite the progress that has accompanied the advent of HAART, HIV-positive patients remain at a substantial risk for lymphoma. In the HAART era, about 50 percent of HIV-positive patients present with lymph node-based disease, an increase from the pre-HAART era. There is also a higher prevalence in women and often a longer time interval between first diagnosis of HIV infection and onset of lymphoma (5,6,29). In different studies, HIV-positive patients remain 25 to 100 times more likely to develop NHL than the general population and 1 to 5 percent of these patients develop NHL each year (5,6,29,34,44). The risk of Hodgkin lymphoma is also increased, approximately 10 to 20 times. Unlike NHLs, the frequency of Hodgkin lymphoma, in particular nodular sclerosis type, has increased in the era of HAART (39,47). This increase is thought to be related to the improved immune status of HIV-positive patients as a result of antiretroviral therapy, implicating the microenvironment in facilitating the development of Hodgkin lymphoma.

The role of HIV in the pathogenesis of lymphomas is thought most likely to be indirect (11). HIV is usually not integrated into the lymphoma cell genome (although rare exceptions are described in the literature) and therefore is not directly involved in neoplastic cell transformation. There are at least five factors

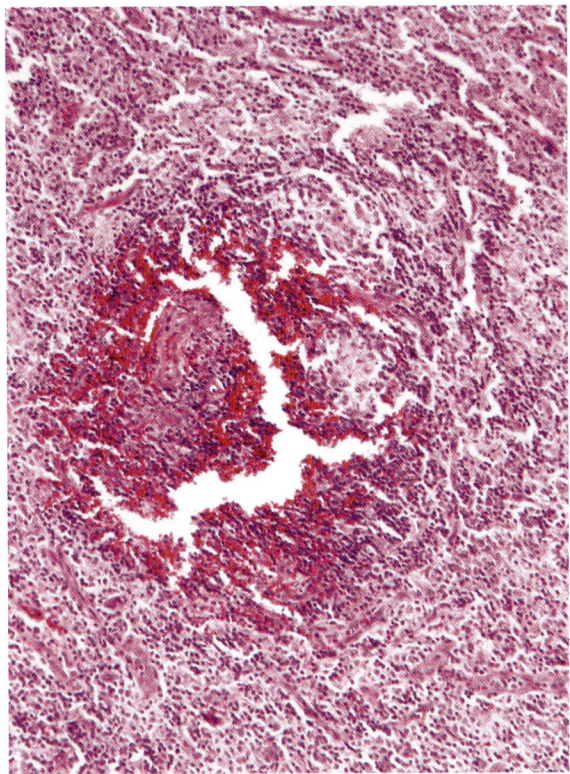

Figure 43-3

**FOLLICLE LYSIS IN LYMPH NODE
OF HIV-POSITIVE PATIENT**

Lysis and hemorrhage are seen within the reactive follicle. Hemorrhage into follicles is characteristic although not specific of HIV infection in lymph nodes (H&E stain).

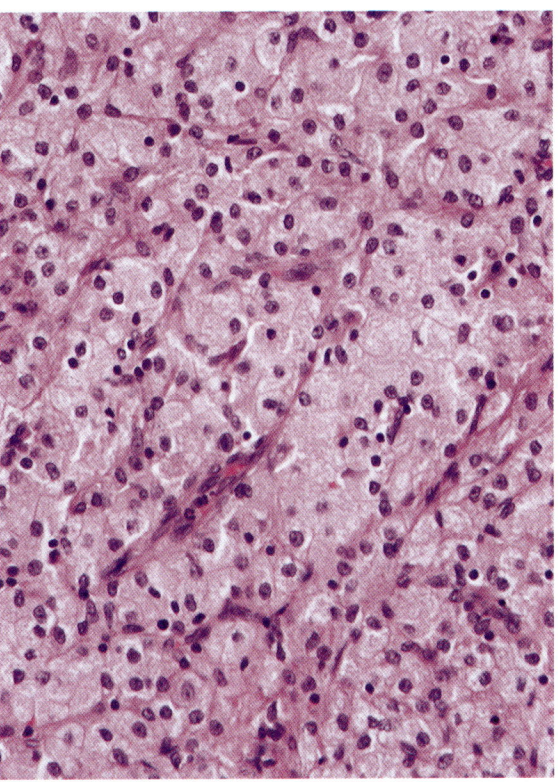

Figure 43-4

**OPPORTUNISTIC INFECTION INVOLVING
LYMPH NODE IN HIV-POSITIVE PATIENT**

The lymph node is replaced by sheets of histiocytes with foamy cytoplasm. An acid-fast stain showed numerous bacilli of *Mycobacterium avium-intracellulare* (H&E stain). (Courtesy of Dr. M. Garcia, Zaragoza, Spain.)

involved in lymphomagenesis: 1) chronic antigenic stimulation leading to B-cell proliferation and prolonged lifespan, thereby increasing the chance that molecular alterations arise that promote lymphomagenesis; 2) dysregulation of various cytokines (e.g., interleukins 6 and 10); 3) impaired T-cell immunosurveillance as a result of the destruction of T cells by HIV; 4) genetic aberrations; and 5) infection by other oncogenic viruses, in particular, Epstein-Barr virus (EBV) and human herpesvirus 8 (HHV8) (19,27,34). These factors are not mutually exclusive.

Nevertheless, it is possible that HIV also has some direct effects, perhaps via the secretion of viral proteins that may act more directly on the host cells. As has been reviewed by Dolcetti et al. (21), HIV p17 protein variants may enhance B-clonogenic activity. The virus also may foster a tumor-promoting role of the microenvironment.

CLINICAL FEATURES

The demographic features of patients with HIV-associated lymphoma reflect those of HIV-infected patients in general (34,41). The onset of NHL in an HIV-positive patient is an AIDS-defining illness. HIV-associated NHLs arise in extranodal locations in up to 60 percent of patients. The digestive tract and central nervous system are the most common extranodal sites (34,41). Most patients have high-stage disease and an aggressive clinical course. Unlike NHLs, Hodgkin lymphoma in an HIV-positive patient is not considered an AIDS-defining illness, is clinically more aggressive, and patients more often present with advanced-stage disease compared with immunocompetent patients (39,54).

Almost all cases of NHL in HIV-positive patients are of B-cell lineage. It is useful to divide

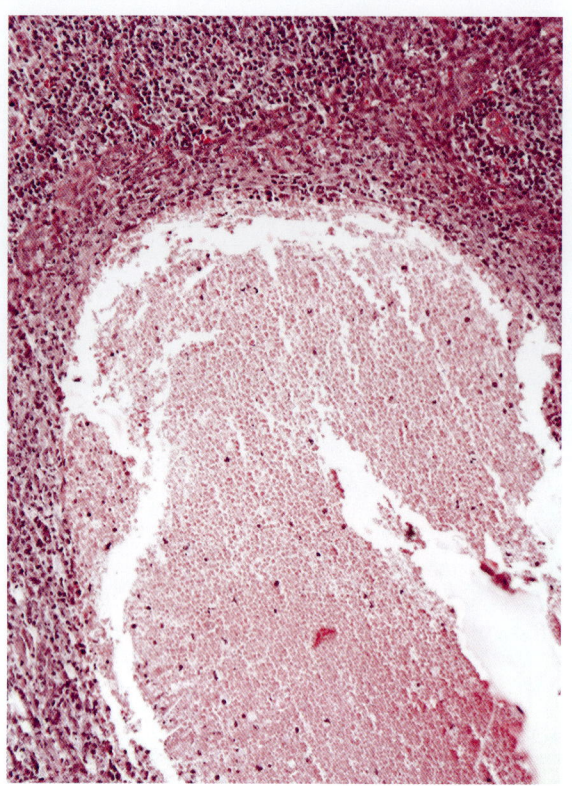
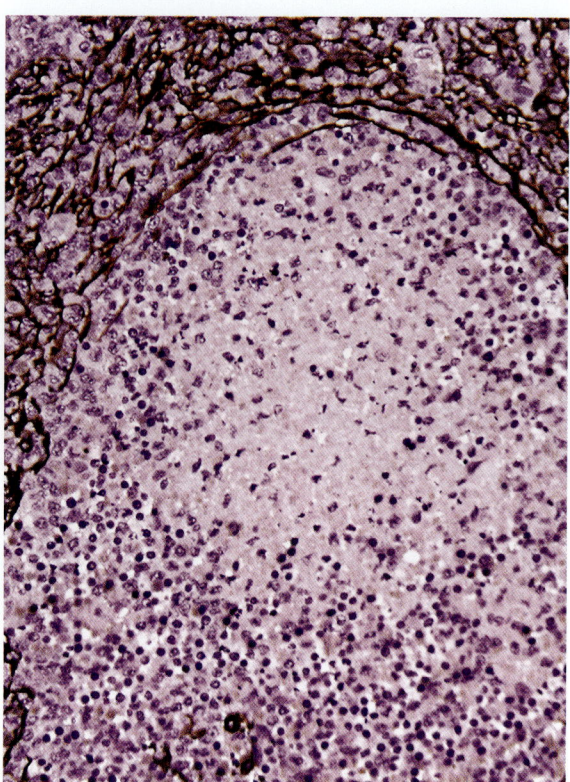

Figure 43-5

CYSTIC LYMPHOEPITHELIAL LESION IN HIV-POSITIVE PATIENT

Left: A dilated salivary gland duct is filled with keratin and debris. The duct is lined by hyperplastic epithelium with squamous metaplasia and lymphoepithelial lesions (H&E stain).

Right: Keratin negatively outlines lymphoepithelial lesions in the lining of the cyst (immunohistochemistry with hematoxylin counterstain).

these lymphomas into two groups: 1) lesions that are highly characteristic and, in some cases, almost unique to patients with HIV infection; and 2) lymphomas that also occur in the immunocompetent patient population (47).

LYMPHOMAS CHARACTERISTIC OF HIV INFECTION

HIV-Positive Multicentric Castleman Disease and Associated Large B-Cell Lymphoma

HIV-related multicentric Castleman disease is usually positive for HHV8 infection. Rarely, large B-cell lymphoma with plasmablastic or immunoblastic features arises in patients with HHV8-positive multicentric Castleman disease, usually associated with severe immune compromise. These two diseases are discussed in detail in chapter 22.

Primary Effusion Lymphoma

Definition. *Primary effusion lymphoma* (PEL) is a neoplasm of HHV8-infected large B cells that occurs usually in the clinical context of immunodeficiency and most often presents as a serous effusion in body cavities without a tumor mass. Less often, PEL presents as a mass involving extranodal sites or lymph nodes; this is designated as the *extracavitary variant* (50).

General Features. The causative agent of PEL is HHV8, which is a gamma herpes virus that is transmitted via body fluids (see chapter 9 and fig. 9-10) (12). Once infection occurs, host cytotoxic T cells are able to bring the infection under control, but HHV8 evades T cells by establishing lifelong latent infection in B cells (12). HHV8 viral infection is reactivated and becomes lytic in the context of impaired host immunosurveillance.

The seroprevalence of HHV8 is geographically restricted (12,50). The frequency of HHV8 infection is high in Africa and the Amazon region of South America, where up to 50 percent of persons are seropositive. In nations that border the Mediterranean Sea, the seropositive rate ranges from 5 to 20 percent and in Asia, Europe, and North America it is less than 5 percent (often less than 1 percent).

In developed nations, HHV8 seroprevalence is increased in immunocompromised patients (up to 30 percent in patients with HIV infection). As a result, in developed nations almost all cases of PEL occur in patients with HIV infection and PEL is an AIDS-defining illness. Patients with PEL who are not HIV positive are often also immunocompromised, for example, organ transplant recipients (13,37). Rarely in North America, and more often in nations endemic for HHV8 infection, patients with PEL are HIV negative and are usually elderly at the time of diagnosis (50). PEL is a rare lymphoma, even in patients with AIDS, representing less than 5 percent of all lymphomas in this patient group.

Clinical Features. The clinical features of patients with PEL in developed nations are essentially those of AIDS patients. These patients are usually 30 to 40 years old, with a male predominance, and are severely immunosuppressed with very low CD4-positive counts (less than 100 cells/mm^3) (34,45). Patients commonly have B-type symptoms and up to one third have Kaposi sarcoma in addition to PEL (50).

There are two forms of PEL: classic and extracavitary (or solid). The classic form is the most common. Patients present with an effusion involving the pleural, pericardial, or abdominal body cavity (usually only one cavity) without a discrete tumor mass (50). Rare cases involving cerebrospinal fluid or the space around breast implants are also described. Severe dyspnea or symptoms related to marked ascites may be present. The extracavitary variant of PEL is less common. Patients present with a tumor mass involving lymph nodes (over half the cases) or extranodal sites (gastrointestinal tract, spleen, skin, and liver), without a body cavity effusion (28,35,45).

In some patients, an initial extracavitary variant of PEL relapses as the classic form with body cavity effusion. Conversely, about 25 percent of patients with classic PEL have a tumor mass, usually contiguous with the effusion and attributable to direct invasion of adjacent organs by tumor cells. In addition, the classic form of PEL can disseminate to extracavitary sites, including lymph nodes, extranodal sites, and bone marrow (28,50).

Histologic Findings. The classic form of PEL is usually diagnosed in cytologic smears and cytospin preparations. The lymphoma cells are large, with multilobated nuclear contours, large nucleoli, and abundant cytoplasm (fig. 43-6) (33,50). The cytoplasm is often basophilic and can be vacuolated. Reed-Sternberg-like cells may be observed.

The extracavitary form of PEL is usually diagnosed by a tissue biopsy. In lymph nodes, the neoplasm may preferentially involve sinuses or diffusely replace the lymph node architecture (fig. 43-7) (28,35,45). At extranodal sites, the neoplasm usually diffusely replaces the architecture. A starry sky pattern is common, and apoptotic cells and mitotic figures may be numerous (fig. 43-8). The lymphoma cells may exhibit plasmablastic, immunoblastic, or anaplastic cytologic features.

Immunophenotypic Findings. The cells of PEL are always positive for HHV8, as is shown by in situ hybridization or immunohistochemistry using an antibody specific for latency-associated nuclear antigen 1 (LANA1) (fig. 43-7, right; 43-8, right) (12). The anti-LANA1 antibody typically yields a speckled nuclear pattern of reactivity.

The cells of the classic form of PEL are usually positive for CD38, CD45/LCA, CD71, CD138, EMA, HLA-DR, MUM1/IRF4, and often CD30, and are negative for pan-B-cell antigens such as CD19, CD20, CD22, and PAX5 as well as CD10 and BCL6 (50). Surface immunoglobulin is negative and cytoplasmic immunoglobulin is usually negative, but a small subset of cases expresses monotypic immunoglobulin. Aberrant expression of pan-T-cell antigens, particularly CD45RO, CD7, and CD4, is best appreciated by flow cytometry (33,50). The proliferation rate is usually high, 80 to 90 percent, as shown by Ki-67 expression. Rare cases of HHV8-positive lymphoma with a T-cell immunophenotype have been reported (16). Whether these cases reflect lineage infidelity at the protein and DNA level or are true T-cell mimics of PEL is not clear.

The immunophenotype of extracavitary PEL is similar to that of the classic form, but these

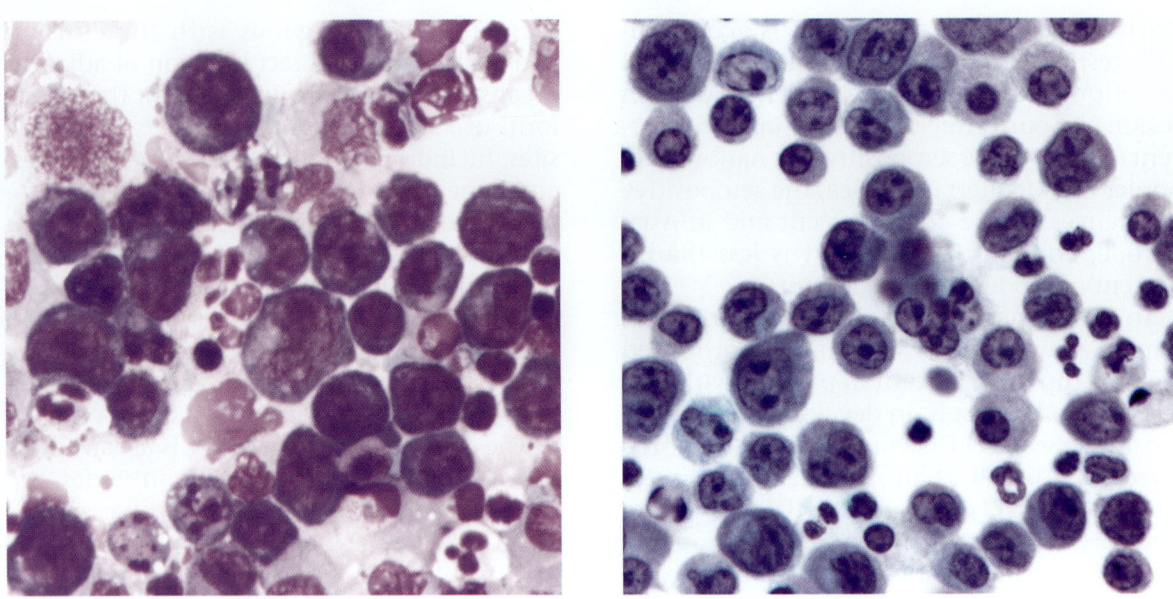

Figure 43-6

PRIMARY EFFUSION LYMPHOMA, CLASSIC VARIANT: CYTOLOGIC FINDINGS

Effusion in which lymphoma cells are large and pleomorphic, with eccentrically located nuclei, irregular nuclear membranes, several nucleoli, and abundant basophilic cytoplasm (left: Diff-Quik stain; right: Papanicolaou stain).

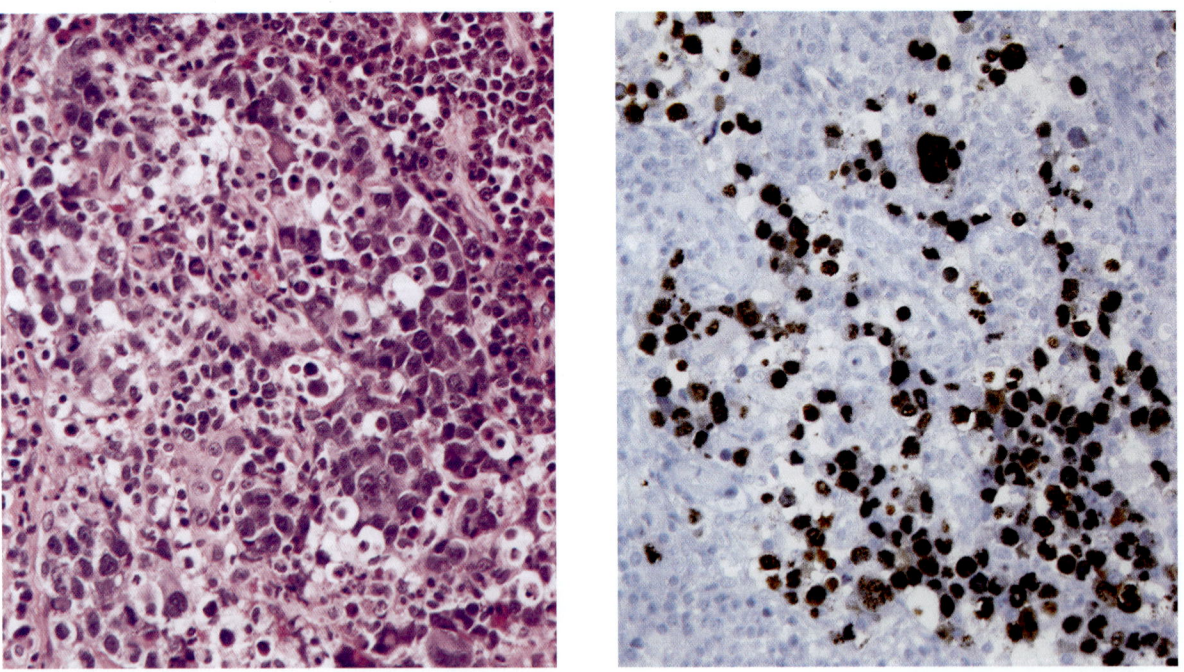

Figure 43-7

PRIMARY EFFUSION LYMPHOMA, EXTRACAVITARY VARIANT, INVOLVING LYMPH NODE

Left: The neoplastic cells preferentially involve the sinuses and are large with abundant cytoplasm. Many apoptotic cells and some mitotic figures are observed in this field (H&E stain).

Right: The nuclei of the lymphoma cells are positive for HHV8 (immunohistochemistry with hematoxylin counterstain).

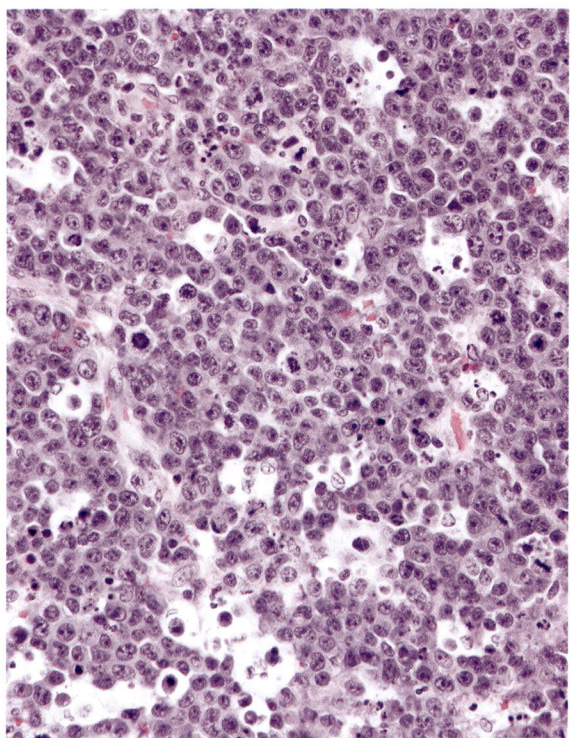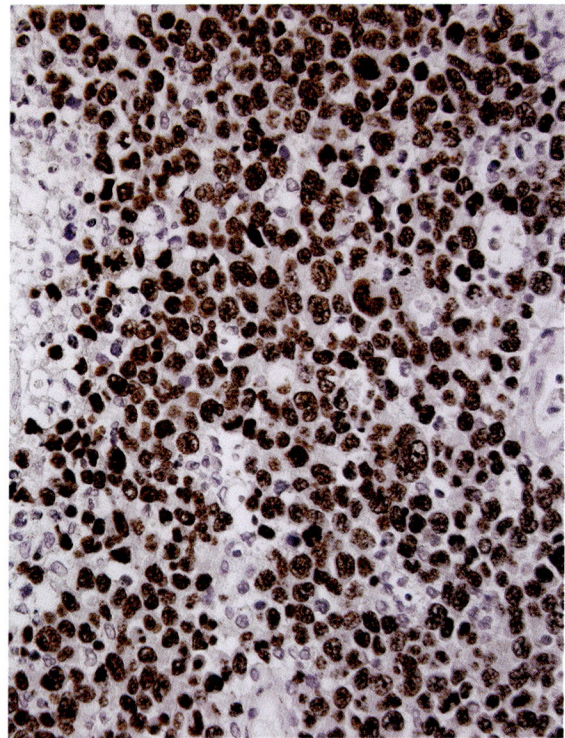

Figure 43-8

PRIMARY EFFUSION LYMPHOMA, EXTRACAVITARY VARIANT, INVOLVING THE GASTROINTESTINAL TRACT

Left: Sheets of lymphoma cells are arranged in a starry sky pattern. The lymphoma cells have abundant cytoplasm and plasmablastic morphologic features (H&E stain).

Right: The nuclei of the lymphoma cells are positive for HHV8 (immunohistochemistry with hematoxylin counterstain).

tumors less often express CD45/LCA and more often express CD20 and CD79a (20 percent of cases). Extracavitary/solid PEL also less frequently expresses CD138 (30 to 50 percent of tumors) (13,35,45).

EBV is present in virtually all cases of PEL that arise in AIDS patients. The virus usually is present in a type I latency pattern. EBV-encoded RNA1 (EBER1) is detected by in situ hybridization, and EBV nuclear antigen 1 (EBNA1) is detected by immunohistochemistry, but EBV latent membrane protein is not expressed (12,50).

Molecular Genetic Findings. Conventional cytogenetic studies of PEL, mostly the classic form, commonly show complex karyotypes. No recurrent translocations have been identified and there are no rearrangements of *MYC*, *BCL2*, *BCL6*, or *CCND1* (50). *TP53* and *RAS* are rarely mutated. Molecular analysis of the antigen receptor genes usually shows monoclonal *IGH* rearrangements, with monoclonal T-cell receptor gene rearrangements also present in some cases (35,45,50). Gene expression profiling studies have shown that the neoplastic cells have features similar to both plasma cells and immunoblasts (32,36). The cells of PEL show downregulation of B-cell differentiation antigens and upregulation of plasma cell markers such as MUM1/IRF4 as well as interleukin 10 and vascular endothelial growth factor.

Differential Diagnosis. A number of entities that exhibit the morphologic features of immunoblasts or plasmablasts are included in the differential diagnosis of PEL. The classic form of PEL should be distinguished from HHV8-negative body cavity lymphoma (1,13) and pyothorax-associated lymphoma (also known as DLBCL associated with chronic inflammation) (Table 43-1) (14). The extracavitary variant of PEL should be distinguished from the

Table 43-1

DIFFERENTIAL DIAGNOSIS OF CLASSIC VARIANT PRIMARY EFFUSION LYMPHOMA

Feature	Primary Effusion Lymphoma, Classic Variant	HHV8[a]-Negative Effusion-Based Lymphoma[b]	Pyothroax-Associated Lymphoma[c]
Median age (yrs)	35-45	65-75	65-70
Male to female ratio	8-9 to 1	~2 to 1	~4 to 1
HIV+	Almost 100%	<10%	<5%
Immunosuppression	Marked	Absent or mild	Absent or mild
Tuberculosis	Simultaneous infection may be present as part of AIDS	Absent	Remote history of active infection in almost all patients
Hepatitis C infection	Uncommon	~25%	Uncommon
Other relevant medical history	Absent	Fluid overload states (e.g., congestive heart failure, cirrhosis)	Therapeutically induced pyothorax for tuberculosis
Effusion(s)	Typical/some patients have mass (extracavitary variant)	Typical/no mass	Uncommon/usually a serosa-based mass
Body cavities	All	All	Pleural cavities
Pan-B-cell antigens+	Often negative	Positive in ~85% of cases	Common
HHV8	Present	Absent	Absent
EBV	Present	~30%	Very common
IGH	Monoclonal	Monoclonal	Monoclonal
TP53 mutation	Minimal data available	Minimal data available	~75%
Survival	Median, 4-6 months	Median, ~ 1 year	~25% 5-year survival

[a]HHV8 = human herpesvirus 8; HIV = human immunodeficiency virus; EBV = Epstein-Barr virus.
[b]From reference 1.
[c]From reference 14.

immunoblastic variant of DLBCL, not otherwise specified (see chapter 17), anaplastic lymphoma kinase (ALK)-positive large B-cell lymphoma (see chapter 21), HHV8-positive germinotropic B-cell lymphoproliferative disorder (see chapter 22), large B-cell lymphoma associated with HHV8-positive multicentric Castleman disease (see chapter 22), plasmablastic lymphoma (see chapter 23), and anaplastic large cell lymphoma (see chapters 33 and 34).

Treatment and Prognosis. There is no consensus therapy for patients with PEL (34,45,50). Standard therapeutic approaches used for DLBCL patients have not been successful, in part attributable to tumor resistance, but also related to the poor immune status of AIDS patients, with the coexistence of opportunistic infections or Kaposi sarcoma. Treatment with HAART is recommended. The median survival period of HIV-positive patients with PEL is less than 6 months and few patients survive longer than 1 year after diagnosis (43,45,50).

AIDS-Related Polymorphic Lymphoproliferative Disorder

These lesions represent approximately 5 percent or less of lymphoproliferative disorders in HIV-positive patients (8). There is no correlation between the means of HIV infection and the frequency of these lesions. Males and females are affected equally. Extranodal sites and lymph nodes are involved. In many patients the disease is localized. These lesions appear to be analogous to post-transplant polymorphic lymphoproliferative disorders, but their clinical behavior in HIV-positive patients is poorly understood. In rare cases, they resolve after initiation of HAART therapy (8).

Morphologically, these lesions have a diffuse pattern and can exhibit necrosis (42). They are composed of a mixture of small and larger lymphocytes, immunoblasts, plasma cells, and histiocytes. A subset of cases exhibits plasmacytoid differentiation. The lymphoid cells are B cells

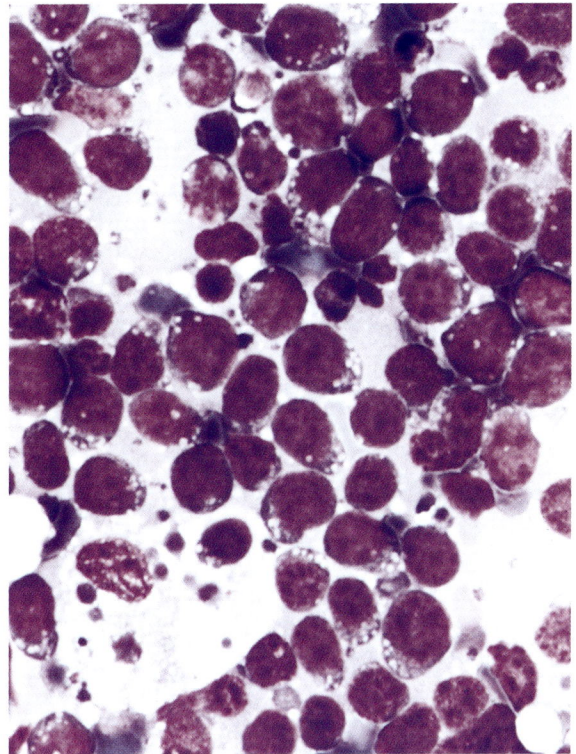 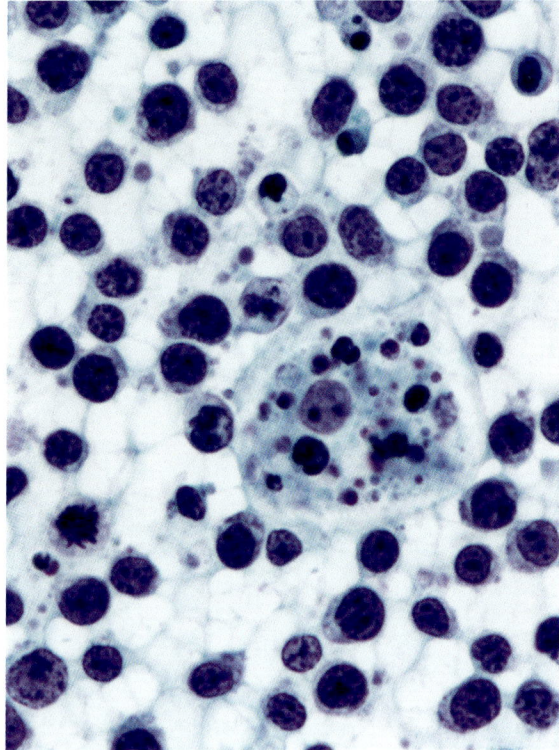

Figure 43-9

BURKITT LYMPHOMA IN A HIV-POSITIVE MAN: CYTOLOGIC FINDINGS

Left, right: The lymphoma cells are of intermediate size, with round nuclei, multiple small nucleoli, and small cytoplasmic vacuoles best observed in Romanowsky stained slides. Histiocytes and mitotic figures are also noted (left: Diff-Quik stain; right: Papanicolaou stain).

that are CD20 positive and they often express monotypic surface immunoglobulin. Approximately 75 percent of cases carry monoclonal *IGH* rearrangements, but the monoclonal B-cell populations often represent only a small minority of the total cells. EBV was present in 4 of 10 cases in one study (42). A small subset of cases has shown evidence of HHV8 infection or mutations involving *RAS, MYC, BCL6,* or *TP53* (42).

LYMPHOMAS THAT ALSO OCCUR IN IMMUNOCOMPETENT PATIENTS

Most lymphoma types that occur in immunocompetent patients also can arise in HIV-positive patients. Overwhelmingly, these tumors are of B-cell lineage; T-cell lymphomas are rare (44,47). Although the context of HIV infection increases the risk of these tumors, and also complicates the therapeutic approach, these lymphomas are presumably similar to their counterparts in immunocompetent patients.

Burkitt Lymphoma

Burkitt lymphomas account for 30 to 40 percent of HIV-associated lymphomas (47,52). Affected patients tend be younger and immunosuppression is less severe than in patients with DLBCL (52). The CD4-positive T-cell count is usually over 200 cells/mm³. Most HIV-positive patients with Burkitt lymphoma present with advanced-stage disease including bone marrow involvement. B-type symptoms are common.

The morphologic features of HIV-associated Burkitt lymphoma resemble their counterparts in immunocompetent patients: sheets of intermediately sized tumor cells and a prominent starry sky pattern (see chapter 25, figs. 25-2 and 25-4). There are, however, some differences. The neoplastic cells can show more variability in size and shape, with more prominent nucleoli (fig. 43-9). Some cases have eccentrically located nuclei and more abundant cytoplasm suggestive

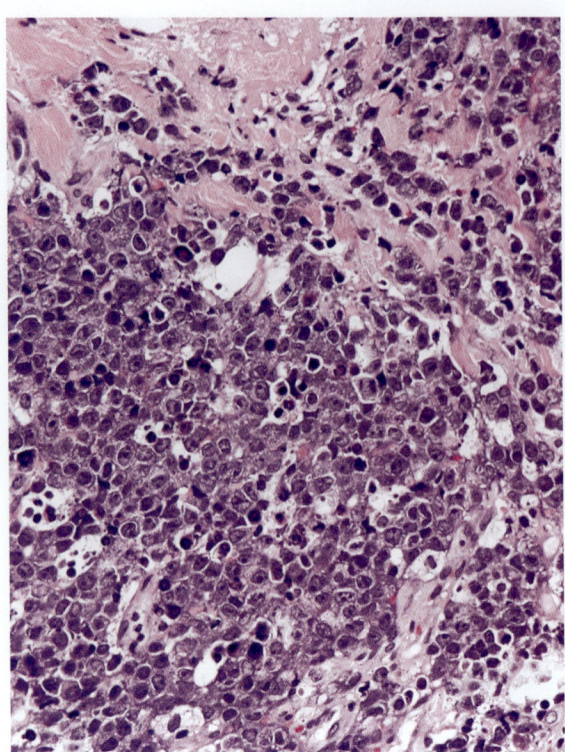
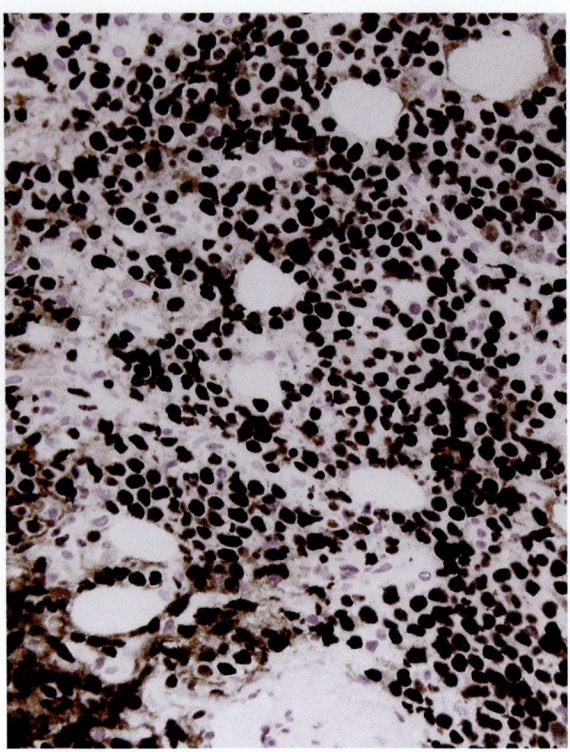

Figure 43-10

DIFFUSE LARGE B-CELL LYMPHOMA ARISING IN A HIV-POSITIVE MAN

Left: The lymphoma cells are arranged in a diffuse pattern and have centroblastic features (H&E stain).
Right: The neoplastic cells have a high proliferation rate as shown with the anti-Ki-67 antibody and were also positive for Epstein-Barr virus infection (not shown) (immunohistochemistry with hematoxylin counterstain).

of plasmacytoid differentiation (11). Plasmacytoid differentiation is rare in Burkitt lymphoma arising in non-HIV-positive patients.

Burkitt lymphoma cells express monotypic surface Ig, pan-B-cell antigens, CD10, BCL6, and MYC and are negative for T-cell antigens and BCL2. The proliferation rate as shown by Ki-67 expression is very high, usually over 95 percent. EBV is present in 30 to 40 percent of all Burkitt lymphomas, but is more common in the tumors with plasmacytoid features (about 75 percent). Conventional karyotyping and molecular studies have shown chromosomal translocations and rearrangements involving *MYC* at chromosome 8q24. Point mutations in the *MYC* regulatory regions and *TP53* point mutations are found in up to 50 percent of cases (26,47).

Diffuse Large B-Cell Lymphoma

DLBCL accounts for almost one third of lymphomas in HIV-positive patients (26,47).

DLBCLs may involve lymph nodes but commonly involve extranodal sites including the central nervous system (CNS). HIV-positive patients with DLBCL arising at non-CNS sites are usually much less immunosuppressed than patients with CNS disease (discussed below).

Histologically, biopsy specimens are replaced by sheets of large lymphoma cells that most often have centroblastic features, with oval nuclei, vesicular chromatin, and 2 to 3 small nucleoli (fig. 43-10) (47). These tumors have a B-cell immunophenotype. Approximately 60 percent of DLBCLs have a germinal center B-cell immunophenotype and 40 percent have an activated B-cell-like immunophenotype; classification does not correlate with prognosis in HIV-positive patients. PD-L1 is expressed in a subset of tumors. The proliferation rate, as assessed by Ki-67 (fig. 43-10, right), can be very high. The frequency of EBV infection in these tumors is about 30 percent (11,26).

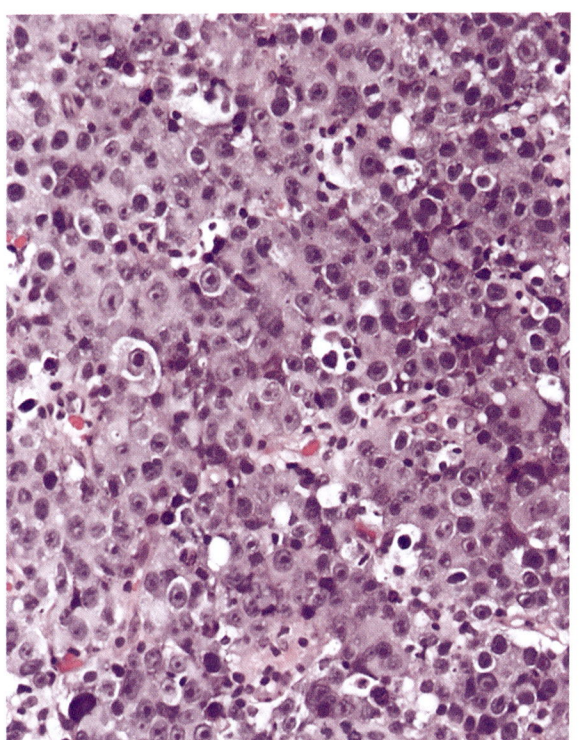 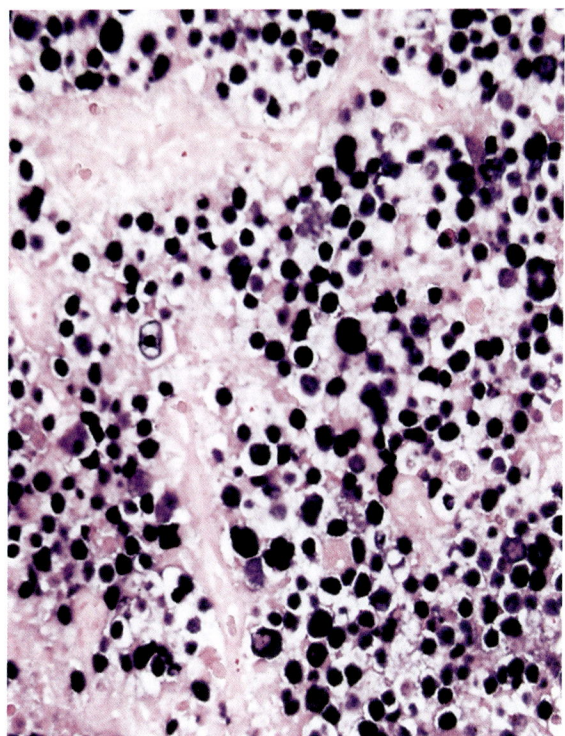

Figure 43-11

PRIMARY DIFFUSE LARGE B-CELL LYMPHOMA OF THE CENTRAL NERVOUS SYSTEM IN A HIV-POSITIVE MAN

Left: The lymphoma cells are arranged in a diffuse pattern and have central nuclei with prominent nucleoli and abundant cytoplasm (immunoblastic features) (H&E stain).

Right: Virtually all of the lymphoma cells are positive for EBER1 (in situ hybridization with eosin counterstain).

Molecular studies of HIV-positive DLBCL have shown monoclonal immunoglobulin gene rearrangements. *RAS* or *TP53* point mutations have been reported in up to 40 percent of DLBCL cases and some tumors have *BCL6* rearrangements (26).

Primary DLBCL of the Central Nervous System

Primary DLBCL of the central nervous system (DLBCL-CNS) occurs in immunocompetent and HIV-positive patients. DLBCL-CNS in HIV-positive patients is an AIDS-defining illness and is associated with marked immunodeficiency, manifested by extremely low CD4-positive counts (less than 50 cells/mm^3) in the blood and often simultaneous opportunistic infections (47). In the pre-HAART era, DLBCL-CNS was approximately 1,000-fold more frequent in AIDS patients than in immunocompetent patients and about 2 to 9 percent of AIDS patients in different studies developed DLB-

CL-CNS (3). The frequency of these tumors has dropped dramatically in the HAART era (2,6).

HIV-positive patients with DLBCL-CNS are younger, have a lower performance status, and have a higher serum lactate dehydrogenase (LDH) level than their immunocompetent counterparts (3). HIV-positive patients also have a worse survival rate. Patients with DLBCL-CNS present with headaches, confusion, personality changes, memory loss, focal neurologic deficits, and seizures. These tumors are often multifocal and seem to preferentially involve the periventricular areas. The brainstem and cerebellum also may be involved.

Histologically, DLBCL-CNS in HIV-positive patients commonly surrounds blood vessels, at least initially, and is composed of sheets of immunoblasts with prominent central nucleoli and abundant cytoplasm (fig. 43-11) (9,10). These tumors often show plasmacytoid differentiation. Multilobated cells and Reed-Sternberg-like cells can be present.

These neoplasms have a B-cell immunophenotype: positive for CD20, CD22, CD79a, and PAX5; CD45/LCA is usually positive (11,47). In cases with plasmacytoid differentiation, CD20 and CD45/LCA may be dim or absent but CD38, CD138, or MUM1/IRF4, or all of these antigens may be present. These tumors usually have an activated B-cell or nongerminal center B-cell immunophenotype (9,11). Evidence of EBV infection is present in virtually all cases of DLBCL-CNS in HIV-positive patients (fig. 43-11, right) (11). *MYC* rearrangements do not occur (or are rare).

The prognosis of HIV-positive patients is worse than that of immunocompetent patients who develop DLBCL-CNS. The median survival period for HIV-positive patients is usually less than 1 year, in part because of their severely compromised immune status (3,10). The prognosis, however, has improved in the era of HAART therapy.

Patients with HIV-associated DLBCL-CNS are treated with whole brain radiation therapy or high-dose methotrexate and/or cytarabine (3). Antiviral agents are also used as the tumors are EBV positive. For patients who are not on HAART treatment when DLBCL-CNS develops, HAART is administered with other therapies.

Plasmablastic Lymphoma

Plasmablastic lymphoma (PBL) is an aggressive NHL with an immunophenotype of plasma cells (53). PBL was described initially in HIV-positive patients, but was reported subsequently in patients with other types of immunodeficiency (18,59), elderly patients presumably as a result of immunosenescence, and immunocompetent patients (discussed in detail in chapter 23).

PBL in the context of HIV infection occurs mostly in men, with a male to female ratio of at least 5 to 1 (18,53). The interval from diagnosis of HIV infection to PBL is prolonged, with a mean interval of about 5 years. Most cases arise at extranodal sites, such as the nasopharynx, skin, soft tissues, and the gastrointestinal tract (53). Lymph nodes are uncommonly involved. Most patients have advanced-stage disease, B-type symptoms, and a high International Prognostic Index (IPI) (53).

Histologically, cases of PBL have a diffuse pattern and are composed of sheets of large neoplastic cells that may resemble immunoblasts or plasmablasts (18,53,56): the nuclei are large and blastic in appearance, nucleoli may be prominent, and cytoplasm is amphophilic. Some cases have more cytoplasm and more obvious evidence of plasmacytic differentiation. The immunophenotype is that of plasmablasts: CD38(+), CVD138(+), MUM1/IRF4(+), cytoplasmic light chain (+), CD20(-), CD79a(-), PAX5(-) (rarely these B-cell antigens can be dim+), CD45/LCA(-) and HHV8(-) (18,53). A minority of cases expresses CD30, usually focally. The neoplastic cells are often positive for EBER (52). Molecular analysis has shown monoclonal rearrangements of the immunoglobulin genes. *MYC* translocations have been reported in up to 50 percent of cases of PBL (56).

Hodgkin Lymphoma

Patients with HIV infection are at increased risk of developing classic *Hodgkin lymphoma* (HL) (15,39). The mean interval from HIV infection to classic HL is about 5 years. Most patients present with advanced-stage disease with abdominal and bone marrow involvement. Mediastinal disease is uncommon. Most cases of classic HL in HIV-positive patients are positive for EBV (39,54).

In HIV-positive patients, classic HL often exhibits some degree of small lymphocyte depletion, and the mixed cellularity and lymphocyte depletion types are more common (fig. 43-12) (54). The number of Reed-Sternberg and Hodgkin cells is often high. The neoplastic cells express CD15 (about 70 percent), CD30, MUM1/IRF4, and PAX5 (dim), and are negative for CD45/LCA. The neoplastic cells also express EBER1 and EBV latent membrane protein type 1. The background lymphocytes are mostly CD8-positive cells, unlike classic HL in immunocompetent patients in which CD4-positive cells usually predominate (47,54). The nodular sclerosis type of classic HL is uncommon (about 10 percent of patients), however, the incidence of nodular sclerosis has increased in the HAART era (5,39).

Other Lymphomas

Patients with HIV infection are at increased risk for *plasma cell myeloma*, although quantifying this risk in the literature is somewhat muddled by the overlap between plasma cell myeloma and PBL (47). In general, most patients

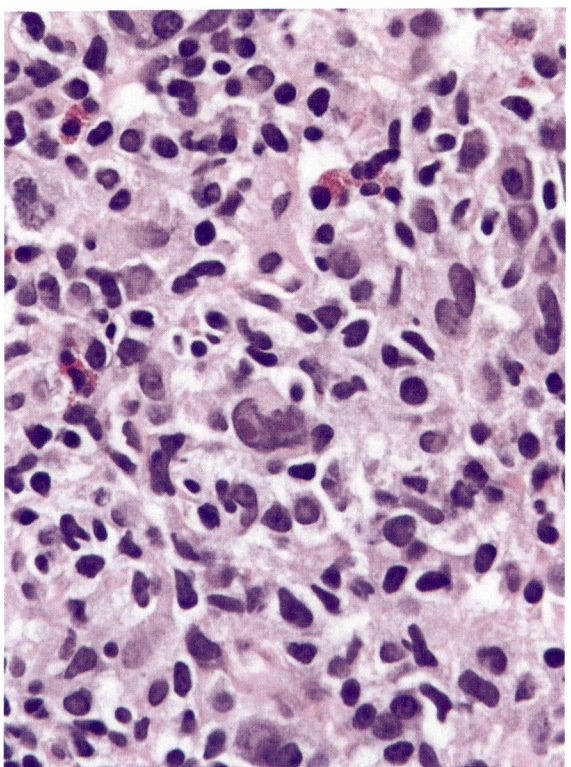 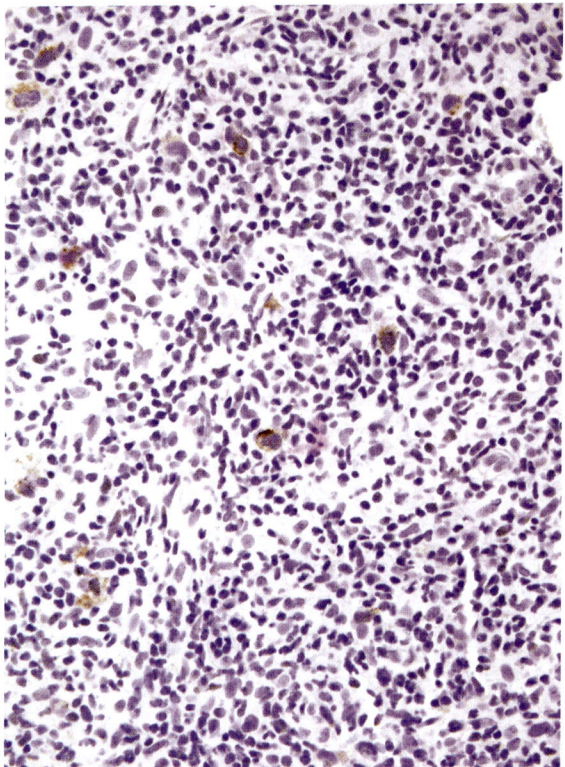

Figure 43-12

MIXED CELLULARITY HODGKIN LYMPHOMA IN A HIV-POSITIVE MAN

Left: This oil immersion image shows a large neoplastic cell in an inflammatory cell background of many histiocytes, moderately depleted small lymphocytes, and scattered eosinophils (H&E stain).

Right: At lower magnification, multiple Hodgkin cells are positive for EBV latent membrane protein type 1 (immunohistochemistry with hematoxylin counterstain).

who present initially with extramedullary or nonosseous disease are best classified as having PBL. Evidence of EBV infection also supports PBL, since EBV is rare in plasma cell myeloma. HIV-positive patients with plasma cell myeloma often present with a serum paraprotein, hypercalcemia, and/or bone lesions. Bone marrow aspiration and biopsy specimens show plasma cells that are well to poorly differentiated.

The frequency of *extranodal marginal zone lymphoma of mucosa-associated lymphoid tissue (MALT lymphoma)* may be increased in HIV-positive patients. *Peripheral T-cell lymphomas* also have been reported rarely in HIV-positive patients. Morphologically, these tumors resemble their counterparts arising in immunocompetent patients. In a small subset of T-cell lymphomas in HIV-positive patients, the HIV virus has been shown to be integrated into the host genome.

TREATMENT AND PROGNOSIS

The advent of HAART therapy has resulted in improved prognosis for HIV-positive patients with lymphoma, in large part, by controlling, but not totally eradicating, HIV; therefore, immune function is partially preserved. Patients are in overall better condition and can tolerate chemotherapy regimens that are administered to immunocompetent patients with the same lymphoma types. It is therefore recommended that patients be treated with intent to cure (assuming no other contraindications) using chemotherapy regimens appropriate for these tumors in immunocompetent patients (23,34,41,55). Nevertheless, although the prognosis of HIV-positive patients with lymphoma has improved in the HAART era, it is not equivalent to that of immunocompetent patients (28a).

For patients that require only a short course of chemotherapy, HAART is temporarily suspended as the potential interactions between HAART and chemotherapy are not well understood. For patients who require chemotherapy over longer time intervals, HAART is administered simultaneously with chemotherapy. Occasional patients have undergone regression of lymphoma after HAART therapy, suggesting that HAART therapy alone is beneficial. Control of viral infection most likely allows for improved immunosurveillance, but simultaneous direct effects on the lymphoma cells cannot be completely excluded.

In general, the prognosis of HIV-positive patients with lymphomas that are not unique to HIV, such as DLBCL, Burkitt lymphoma, and Hodgkin lymphoma, has improved (23,34,41,54). In these patients, the best indicators of prognosis are use of HAART therapy and overall immune status. The IPI also has value and Barta et al. (2) have proposed an AIDS-related lymphoma IPI that may be of more prognostic value. The AIDS-related IPI includes the age-adjusted traditional IPI, the number of extranodal sites, and an HIV score, the latter composed of CD4-positive T-cell count, HIV load, and history of AIDS (2). In contrast, the prognosis of patients with lymphomas unique to HIV infection, such as primary effusion lymphoma and plasmablastic lymphoma, remains poor (23,34,43,53).

REFERENCES

1. Alexanian S, Said J, Lones M, Pullarkat ST. KSHV/HHV8-negative effusion-based lymphoma, a distinct entity associated with fluid overload states. Am J Surg Pathol 2013;37:241-249.
2. Barta SK, Xue X, Wang D, et al. A new prognostic score for AIDS-related lymphomas in the rituximab era. Haematologica 2014;99:1731-1737.
3. Bayraktar S, Bayraktar UD, Ramos JC, Stefanovic A, Lossos IS. Primary CNS lymphoma in HIV positive and negative patients: comparison of clinical characteristics, outcome and prognostic factors. J Neurooncol 2011;101:257-265.
4. Beral V, Peterman T, Berkelman R, Jaffe H. AIDS associated non-Hodgkin lymphoma. Lancet 1991;337:805-809.
5. Bernstein WB, Little RF, Wilson WH, Yarchoan R. Acquired immunodeficiency syndrome-related malignancies in the era of highly active antiretroviral therapy. Int J Hematol 2006;84:3-11.
6. Bonnet F, Balestre E, Thiebaut R, et al. Factors associated with the occurrence of AIDS-related non-Hodgkin lymphoma in the era of highly active antiretroviral therapy: Aquitane Cohort, France. Clin Infect Dis 2006;42:411-417.
7. Busch MP, Satten GA. Time course of viremia and antibody seroconversion following human immunodeficiency virus exposure. Am J Med 1997;102:117-124.
8. Buxton J, Leen C, Goodlad JR. Polymorphic lymphoid proliferations occurring in HIV-positive patients: report of a case responding to HAART. Virchows Arch 2012;461:93-98.
9. Camilleri-Broet S, Criniere E, Broet P, et al. A uniform activated B-cell-like immunophenotype might explain the poor prognosis of primary central nervous system lymphomas: Analysis of 83 cases. Blood 2006;107:190-196.
10. Camilleri-Broët S, Davi F, Feuillard J, et al. AIDS-related primary brain lymphomas: histopathologic and immunohistochemical study of 51 cases. The French Study Group for HIV-Associated Tumors. Hum Pathol 1997; 28:367-374.
11. Carbone A, Gloghini A. AIDS-related lymphomas: from pathogenesis to pathology. Br J Haematol 2005;130:662-670.
12. Cesarman E. Gammaherpesvirus and lymphoproliferative disorders in immunocompromised patients. Cancer Lett 2011;305:163-174.
13. Chadburn A, Said J, Chan JK, et al. HHV8/KSHV-positive lymphoproliferative disorders and the spectrum of plasmablastic and plasma cell neoplasms: 2015 SH/EAHP Workshop Report–Part 3. Am J Clin Pathol 2017;147:171-187.
14. Chan JK, Aozasa K, Gaulard P. DLBCL associated with chronic inflammation. In: Swerdlow SH, Campo E, Harris NL, et al., eds. WHO classification of tumours of haematopoietic and lymphoid tissues. Lyon: IARC Press; 2008:245-246.
15. Clifford GM, Franceschi S. Cancer risk in HIV-infected persons: influence of CD4(+) count. Future Oncol 2009;5:669-678.

16. Coupland SE, Charlotte F, Mansour G, Maloum K, Hummel M, Stein H. HHV-8-associated T-cell lymphoma in a lymph node with concurrent peritoneal effusion in an HIV-positive man. Am J Surg Pathol 2005;29:647-652.

17. Dean M, Jacobson LP, McFarlane G, et al. Reduced risk of AIDS lymphoma in individuals heterozygous for the CCR5-delta32 mutation. Cancer Res 1999;59:3561-3564.

18. Delecluse HJ, Anagnostopoulos I, Dallenbach F, et al. Plasmablastic lymphomas of the oral cavity: a new entity associated with the human immunodeficiency virus infection. Blood 1997;89:1413-1420.

19. Delecluse HJ, Hummel M, Marafioti T, Anagnostopoulos I, Stein H. Common and HIV-related diffuse large B-cell lymphoma differ in their immunoglobulin gene mutation pattern. J Pathol 1999;188:133-138.

20. De Paiva GR, Laurent C, Godel A, et al. Discovery of human immunodeficiency virus infection by immunohistochemistry on lymph node biopsies from patients with unexplained follicular hyperplasia. Am J Surg Pathol 2007;31:1534-1538.

21. Dolcetti R, Gloghini A, Caruso A, Carbone A. A lymphomagenic role for HIV beyond immunosuppression? Blood 2016;127:1403-1409.

22. Douek DC. Disrupting T-cell homeostasis: how HIV-1 infection causes disease. AIDS Rev 2003;5:172-177.

23. Dunleavy K, Wilson WH. How I treat HIV-associated lymphoma. Blood 2012;119:3245-3255.

24. Emerman M, Malim MH. HIV-1 regulatory/accessory genes: keys to unraveling viral and host biology. Science 1998;280:1880-1884.

25. Ford ES, Puronen CE, Sereti I. Immunopathogenesis of asymptomatic chronic HIV infection: the calm before the storm. Curr Opin HIV AIDS 2009;4:206-214.

26. Gaidano G, Carbone A, Dalla-Favera R. Pathogenesis of AIDS-related lymphomas. Molecular and histogenetic heterogeneity. Am J Pathol 1998;152:623-630.

27. Grulich AE, Wan X, Law MG, et al. B-cell stimulation and prolonged immune deficiency are risk factors for non-Hodgkin's lymphoma in people with AIDS. AIDS 2000;14:133-140.

28. Guillet S, Gerard L, Meignin V, et al. Classical and extracavitary primary effusion lymphoma in 51 HIV-infected patients from a single institution. Am J Hematol 2016;91:233-237.

28a. Han X, Jemal A, Hulland E, et al. HIV infection and survival of lymphoma patients in the era of highly active antiretroviral therapy. Cancer Epidemiol Biomarkers Prev 2017;26:303-311.

29. Herida M, Mary-Krause M, Kaphan R, et al. Incidence of non-AIDS-defining cancers before and during the highly active antiretroviral era in a cohort of human immunodeficiency virus-infected patients. J Clin Oncol 2003;21:3447-3453.

30. Ho DD. Perspective series: host/pathogen interactions. Dynamics of HIV-1 replication in vivo. J Clin Invest 1997;99:2565-2567.

31. Ioachim HL, Cronin W, Roy M, Maya M. Persistent lymphadenopathies in people at high risk for HIV infection. Clinicopathologic correlations and long-term follow-up in 79 cases. Am J Clin Pathol 1990;93:208-218.

32. Jenner RG, Maillard K, Cattini N, et al. Kaposi's sarcoma-associated herpesvirus-infected primary effusion lymphoma has a plasma cell gene expression profile. Proc Natl Acad Sci USA 2003;100:10399-10404.

33. Kalogeraki A, Haniotis V, Karvelas-Kalogerakis M, Karvela-Kalogeraki I, Psyllaki M, Tamiolakis D. Primary effusion lymphoma with aberrant T-cell phenotype in an iatrogenically immunosuppressed renal transplant male: cytologic diagnosis in peritoneal fluid. Diagn Cytopathol 2015;43:144-148.

34. Kaplan LD. HIV-associated lymphoma. Best Pract Res Clin Haematol 2012;25:101-117.

35. Kim Y, Leventaki V, Bhaijee F, Jackson CC, Medeiros LJ, Vega F. Extracavitary/solid variant of primary effusion lymphoma. Ann Diagn Pathol 2012;16:441-446.

36. Klein U, Gloghini A, Gaidano G, et al. Gene expression profile analysis of AIDS-related primary effusion lymphoma (PEL) suggests a plasmablastic derivation and identifies PEL-specific transcripts. Blood 2003;101:4115-4121.

37. Lebbe C, Porcher R, Marcelin AG, et al. Human herpesvirus 8 (HHV8) transmission and related morbidity in organ recipients. Am J Transplant 2013;13:207-213.

38. Martin N, Sattentau Q. Cell-to-cell HIV-1 spread and its implications for immune evasion. Curr Opin HIV AIDS 2009;4:143-149.

39. Martis N, Mounier N. Hodgkin lymphoma in patients with HIV infection. Curr Hematol Rep 2012;7:228-234.

40. Mathur-Wagh U, Enlow RW, Spigland I, et al. Longitudinal study of persistent generalised lymphadenopathy in homosexual men: relation to acquired immunodeficiency syndrome. Lancet 1984;1:1033-1038.

41. Mounier N, Spina M, Gisselbrecht C. Modern management of non-Hodgkin lymphoma in HIV-infected patients. Br J Haematol 2007;136:685-698.

42. Nador RG, Chadburn A, Gundappa G, Cesarman E, Said JW, Knowles DM. Human immunodeficiency virus (HIV)-associated polymorphic lymphoproliferative disorders. Am J Surg Pathol 2003;27:293-302.

43. Okada S, Goto H, Yotsumoto M, Current status of treatment for primary effusion lymphoma. Intractable & Rare Diseases Research 2014;3:65-74.

44. Ota Y, Hishima T, Mochizuki M, et al. Classification of AIDS-related lymphoma cases between 1987 and 2012 in Japan based on the WHO classification of lymphomas, fourth edition. Cancer Med 2014;3:143-153.

45. Pan ZG, Zhang QY, Lu ZB, et al. Extracavitary KSHV-associated large B-cell lymphoma. A distinct entity or a subtype of primary effusion lymphoma? Study of 9 cases and review of an additional 43 cases. Am J Surg Pathol 2012;36:1129-1140.

46. Rabkin CS, Yang Q, Goedert JJ, Nguyen G, Mitsuya H, Sei S. Chemokine and chemokine receptor gene variants and risk of non-Hodgkin's lymphoma in human immunodeficiency virus-1-infected individuals. Blood 1999;93:1838-1842.

47. Raphael M, Said J, Borisch B, Cesarman E, Harris NL. Lymphomas associated with HIV infection. In: Swerdlow SH, Campo E, Harris NL, et al, eds. WHO classification of tumours of haematopoietic and lymphoid tissues. Lyon: IARC Press; 2008:340-342.

48. Sabin CA, Lundgren JD. The natural history of HIV infection. Curr Opin HIV AIDS 2013;8:11-317.

49. Saharia KK, Koup RA. T cell susceptibility to HIV influences outcome of opportunistic infections. Cell 2013;155:505-514.

50. Said J, Cesarman E. Primary effusion lymphoma. In: Swerdlow SH, Campo E, Harris NL, et al. eds. WHO classification of tumours of haematopoietic and lymphoid tissues. Lyon: IARC Press; 2008:260-261.

51. Shiramizu B, Herndier BG, McGrath MS. Identification of a common clonal human immunodeficiency virus integration site in human immunodeficiency virus-associated lymphomas. Cancer Res 1994;54:2069-2072.

52. Spina M, Tirelli U, Zagonel V, et al. Burkitt's lymphoma in adults with and without human immunodeficiency virus infection: a single-institution clinicopathologic study of 75 patients. Cancer 1998;82:766-774.

53. Stein H, Harris NL, Campo E. Plasmablastic lymphoma. In: Swerdlow SH, Campo E, Harris NL, et al., eds. WHO classification of tumours of haematopoioetic and lymphoid tissues. Lyon: IARC Press; 2008:256-257.

54. Tirelli U, Errante D, Dolcetti R, et al. Hodgkin's disease and human immunodeficiency virus infection: clinicopathologic and virologic-features of 114 patients from the Italian Cooperative Group on AIDS and tumors. J Clin Oncol 1995;13:1758-1767.

55. Uldrick TS, Little RF. How I treat classical Hodgkin lymphoma in patients infected with human immunodeficiency virus. Blood 2015;125:1226-1235.

56. Valera A, Balagué O, Colomo L, et al. IG/MYC rearrangements are the main cytogenetic alteration in plasmablastic lymphomas. Am J Surg Pathol 2010;34:1686-1694.

57. Vergis EN, Mellors JW. Natural history of HIV-1 infection. Infect Dis Clin North Am 2000;14:809-825, v-vi.

58. Whittle H, Morris J, Todd J, et al. HIV2-infected patients survive longer than HIV-1 infected patients. AIDS 1994;8:1617-1620.

59. Zeng M, Haase AT, Schacker TW. Lymphoid tissue structure and HIV-1 infection: life or death for T cells. Trends Immunol 2012;33:306-314.

60. Zimmermann H, Oschlies I, Fink S, et al. Plasmablastic posttransplant lymphoma: cytogenetic aberrations and lack of Epstein-Barr virus association linked with poor outcome in the prospective German Posttransplant Lymphoproliferative Disorder Registry. Transplantation 2012;93:543-550.

44 IATROGENIC LYMPHOPROLIFERATIVE DISORDERS

GENERAL FEATURES

Iatrogenic lymphoproliferative disorders (LPDs) occur in patients who have compromised or dysregulated immune function as a result of being treated with immunosuppressive or immune-modulating drugs (6). Patients who have LPDs associated with other causes of immunodeficiency, such as organ transplantation, human immunodeficiency virus infection, or anticancer therapies are excluded from this chapter.

In terms of absolute number, the most common autoimmune disease in which patients have an increased risk of an iatrogenic LPD is rheumatoid arthritis (1,8,10). Other autoimmune diseases, however, have been linked to an increased incidence of lymphoproliferative diseases including: systemic lupus erythematosus, dermatomyositis, Sjögren syndrome, ankylosing spondylitis, and inflammatory bowel disease, among others.

The drug most tightly linked to iatrogenic LPDs is methotrexate (8–10,17,20). Other immune-modulating agents linked to LPD include azathioprine, 6-mercaptopurine, and monoclonal antibodies or agonists that inhibit tumor necrosis factor alpha (TNFα), CD11a, CD25, CD52, CD121, and interleukin-12/interleukin-23 (also known as ustekinumab) (7,12,14,21). The data linking TNFα inhibitors and other biologic agents to LPDs are less persuasive than the data for methotrexate. One factor complicating the assessment of risk of TNFα inhibitors is that patients who receive these drugs also commonly receive other immunomodulator agents, most often methotrexate (7,14,21).

The cause of LPDs in patients with autoimmune disease is most likely multifactorial. As affected patients may develop lymphoma without being treated with immunosuppressive or immune modulator drugs, it seems likely that the immunodysregulatory state may facilitate a form of chronic antigen stimulation, a known risk factor for lymphoma in other clinical contexts (1). It is possible that some patients have a genetic predisposition for developing lymphoma. Immunosuppression also has been implicated in the pathogenesis, including the degree (or dose) of drug therapy, the duration of therapy, and the drug(s) used to induce immunosuppression. Perhaps the most persuasive evidence implicating these therapeutic agents is that some patients with LPDs undergo spontaneous and rapid resolution of disease after the drug is discontinued, commonly within 4 weeks (1,8,20). Spontaneous regression of LPDs occurs in about 25 percent of patients who have been treated with methotrexate (fig. 44-1) but is uncommon in patients who have received TNFα inhibitors.

The mechanisms by which methotrexate and other immunosuppressive or immuno-modulator agents contribute to the genesis of LPDs are largely unknown. Typically, the dose of methotrexate administered to patients with rheumatoid arthritis or other autoimmune diseases is substantially lower than doses used to treat cancers as part of traditional chemotherapy regimens. The known anti-cancer mechanism of methotrexate, inhibition of the enzyme dihydro-folate reductase, leading to decreased production of thymidine and impaired DNA synthesis, is not thought to be involved in the pathogenesis of iatrogenic LPDs (6). Instead, methotrexate is thought to impair T-cell function via a number of mechanisms including: decreased activation, decreased expression of adhesion molecules, increased number of T-regulatory cells, and shifting of the T-cell phenotype from TH1 to TH2. The anticancer mechanism of azathioprine, inhibition of nucleotide synthesis, is also not likely to be involved in the pathogenesis of iatrogenic LPDs. Instead, azathioprine has been reported to directly inhibit natural killer cell and

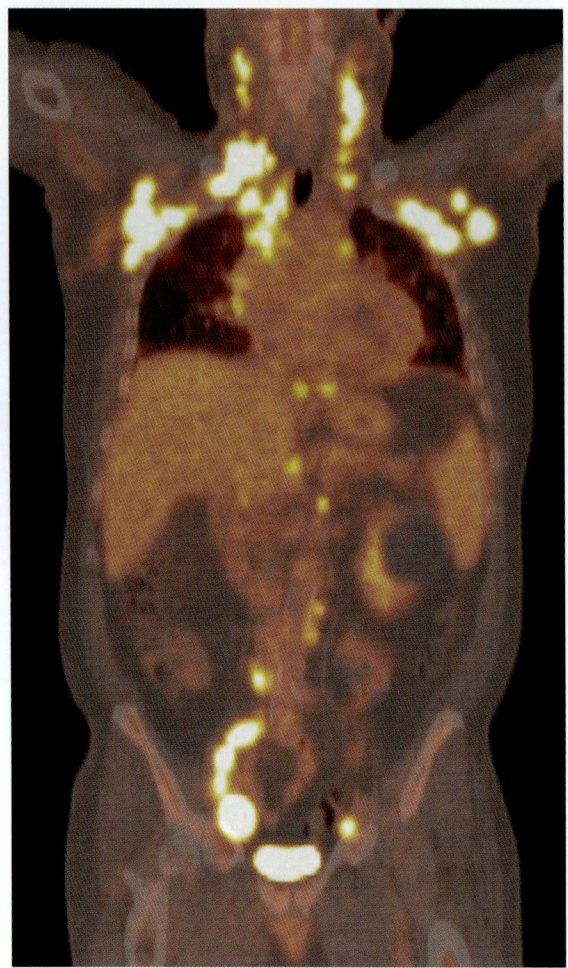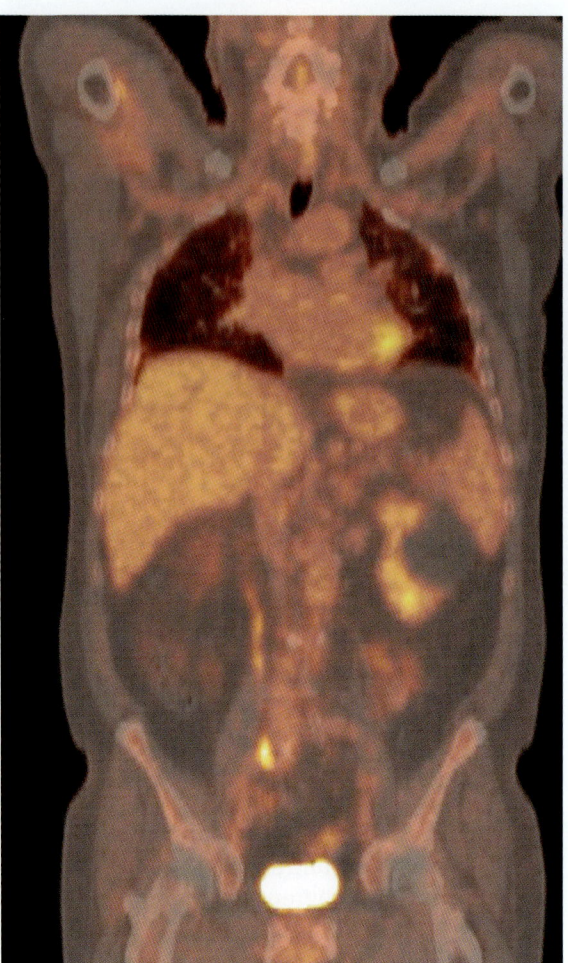

Figure 44-1

EPSTEIN-BARR VIRUS (EBV)-POSITIVE DIFFUSE LARGE B-CELL LYMPHOMA

Left: A 69-year-old man with rheumatoid arthritis was treated with methotrexate. A positron emission tomography-computed tomography (PET-CT) scan shows numerous hypermetabolic lymph nodes and a pericardial effusion.

Right: Methotrexate therapy was discontinued and 6 weeks later the PET-CT shows complete resolution of disease. (Modified from images 1 and 2 from reference 16. Courtesy of Dr. K. Nader, Camden, NJ.)

cytotoxic T-cell function. The role that recently developed immunomodulator agents may play in the pathogenesis of iatrogenic LPDs is poorly understood.

Infection by Epstein-Barr virus (EBV) appears to play an important role in the pathogenesis of a subset of iatrogenic LPDs. EBV is present in approximately 40 percent of these lesions overall, and varies according to the histologic type of LPD (8,10,20). Reactivation of primary EBV infection by therapeutic agents seems to be a likely explanation for the presence of EBV in iatrogenic LPDs.

CLINICAL FEATURES

Patients with iatrogenic LPDs clinically resemble patients with other immunodeficiency-associated lymphoproliferative disorders (e.g., following organ transplantation) or immunocompetent patients. Patients present with localized or generalized disease, B-type symptoms, and large masses (1,6,10,12,20). Approximately 50 percent of patients present with lymphadenopathy. Extranodal sites of disease are seen in approximately 50 percent of patients, and patients may present initially with extranodal disease. The histologic type of iatrogenic LPD

Table 44-1

RELATIVE FREQUENCY OF IATROGENIC LYMPHOPROLIFERATIVE DISORDERS

Histologic Type of LPD[a]	Relative Frequency
Diffuse large B-cell lymphoma	~50%
Classic Hodgkin lymphoma	~20%
Polymorphic LPD	7-10%
Follicular lymphoma	~5%
Hodgkin-like lesion	~4%
Peripheral T-cell lymphoma, NOS	~4%
Burkitt lymphoma	~2%
Marginal zone lymphoma	~2%
Lymphoplasmacytic lymphoma	1-2%
Hepatosplenic T-cell lymphoma	~1%
Chronic lymphocytic leukemia/small lymphocytic lymphoma	<1%
Plasma cell tumors	<1%
Extranodal NK/T-cell lymphoma, nasal type	<1%

[a]LPD = lymphoproliferative disorder; NOS = not otherwise specified; NK = natural killer.

correlates, in part, with the anatomic distribution of disease.

The relative frequency of various iatrogenic LPDs is shown in Table 44-1. Diffuse large B-cell lymphoma (DLBCL) is the most common type (1,6,8,11,12,20), followed by classic Hodgkin lymphoma and polymorphous LPDs. A number of other lymphoma types occur at a lower frequency, about 5 percent or less.

HISTOLOGIC AND IMMUNOPHENOTYPIC FINDINGS

Diffuse Large B-Cell Lymphoma

DLBCLs account for about 50 percent of all cases of iatrogenic LPD (1,6,8,10,20). Extranodal involvement occurs in 50 to 60 percent of patients and the most common extranodal sites of involvement are skin, soft tissue, and gastrointestinal tract. The lymphoma cells of iatrogenic DLBCL are arranged in diffuse sheets and are monomorphous, large cells with either centroblastic or immunoblastic cytologic features (fig. 44-2). Reed-Sternberg- and Hodgkin (RS+H)-like cells may be present. Plasmacytic differentiation or geographic necrosis is common (6,8,10,11).

Mitotic figures are usually easily identified. A small subset of iatrogenic DLBCL cases has features of lymphomatoid granulomatosis (6).

At the immunophenotypic and molecular level, these tumors resemble DLBCLs that occur in immunocompetent patients. The lymphoma cells express CD20 and other pan-B-cell antigens and are negative for pan-T-cell antigens (1,6,11,12,20). The neoplastic cells are also usually CD45/LCA(+) and CD15(-). CD30 is often positive in some of the large neoplastic cells. Monotypic cytoplasmic immunoglobin is present in some cases. Some DLBCLs have a germinal center B-cell immunophenotype, but a nongerminal center B-cell immunophenotype is more common. PD-L1 is expressed by a subset of cases. The proliferation (Ki-67) rate is high, often 60 to 80 percent. EBV is positive in 20 to 30 percent of DLBCL cases, including cases with features of lymphomatoid granulomatosis (8,10). Molecular analysis shows monoclonal immunoglobulin rearrangements in 40 percent of cases (8).

Classic Hodgkin Lymphoma and Hodgkin-Like Lesions

Classic Hodgkin lymphoma accounts for about 20 percent of iatrogenic LPDs (5,13,15). Miranda et al. (15) reviewed the literature and identified 54 reported cases. The median age of the patients was 51 years (range, 8 to 82) and the male to female ratio was 1.0 to 1.4. In this review, over half of all patients had rheumatoid arthritis, and Crohn's disease was the second most common autoimmune disease. In a study of Swedish patients, however, a greater number of autoimmune diseases predisposed to an increased risk of Hodgkin lymphoma, including systemic lupus erythematosus, dermatomyositis, Sjogren syndrome, ankylosing spondylitis, inflammatory bowel disease (particularly Crohn's disease), autoimmune hematolytic anemia or thrombocytopenic purpura, sarcoidosis, polyarteritis nodosa, polymyalgia rheumatica, Behcet disease, and psoriasis (5). Classic Hodgkin lymphoma occurs in patients treated with methotrexate, azathioprine, or TNFα inhibitors, but most often patients have been treated with both methotrexate and a TNFα inhibitor.

Patients with iatrogenic classic Hodgkin lymphoma most often present with lymphadenopathy (75 percent of patients). The most

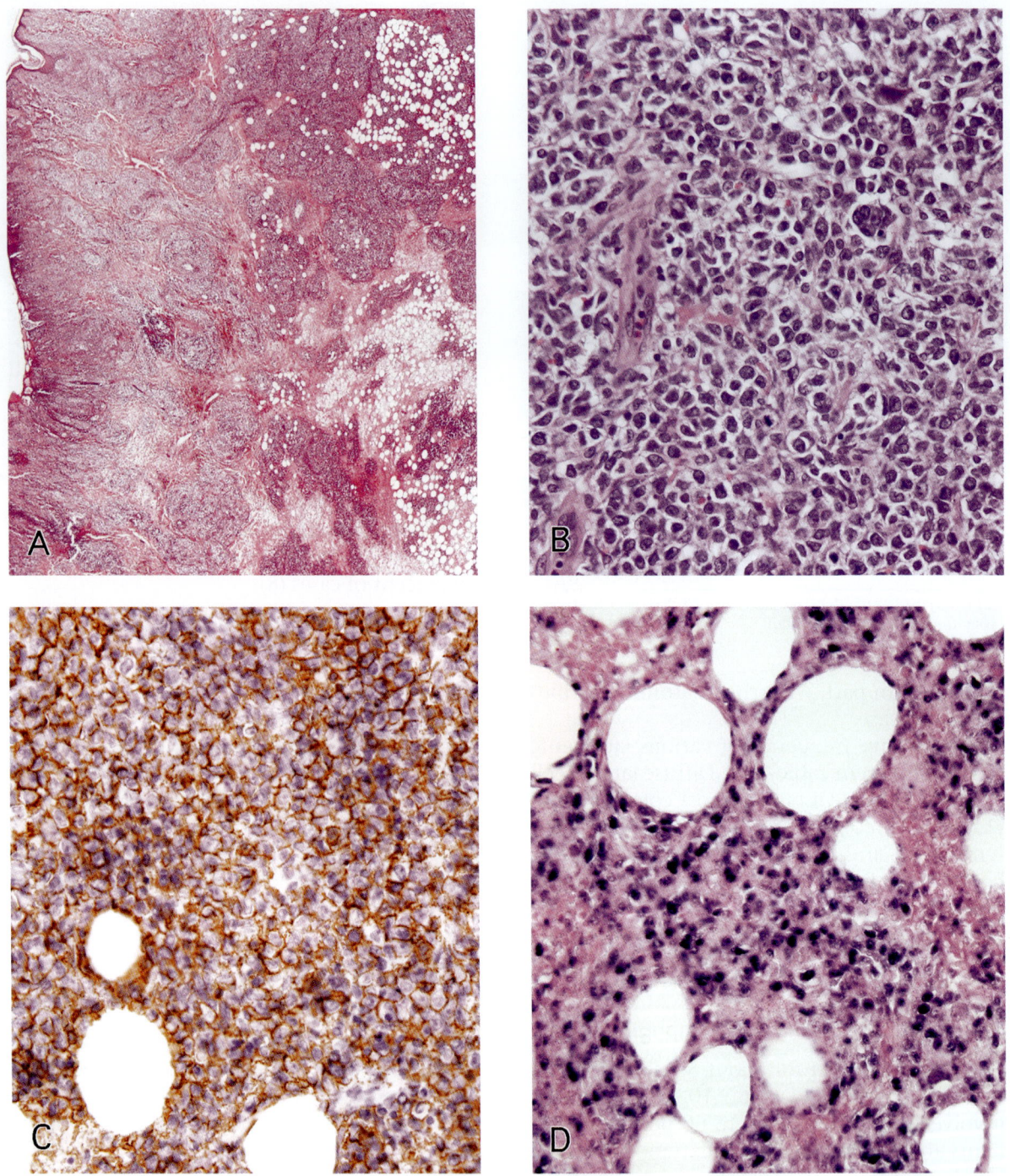

Figure 44-2

EBV-POSITIVE DIFFUSE LARGE B-CELL LYMPHOMA ARISING IN SKIN

This man was being treated with methotrexate for rheumatoid arthritis.

A: The lymphoma subtotally and diffusely replaces the dermis and subcutaneous tissue.

B: The lymphoma cells are a mixture of intermediate size and large cells (A,B: hematoxylin and eosin [H&R] stain).

C: CD20 highlights virtually all of the lymphoma cells, supporting B-cell lineage (immunohistochemistry with hematoxylin counterstain).

D: Many lymphoma cells are positive for EBV-encoded RNA1 (EBER1) (in situ hybridization with eosin counterstain).

commonly reported extranodal site is the gastrointestinal tract. (Some cases in the gastrointestinal tract overlap histologically with EBV-positive mucocutaneous ulcer [see below].) Skin and bone marrow involvement also are reported and there are other rare extranodal sites.

Classic Hodgkin lymphoma arising in the context of drug therapy morphologically resembles classic Hodgkin lymphoma in immunocompetent patients (fig. 44-3) (6,8,13). RS+H cells are present in an inflammatory cell background of reactive T cells, histiocytes, plasma cells, and granulocytes in varying proportions. Mixed cellularity is the most common histologic type and nodular sclerosis represents 10 to 20 percent of cases (13). Nevertheless, all histologic types can occur (5).

The RS+H cells of classic Hodgkin lymphoma are positive for CD15 (about 70 percent), CD30, PAX5 (dim), and MUM1/IRF4 and are negative for CD45/LCA. Dim and variable expression of CD20 occurs in 10 to 20 percent of cases. In approximately 75 percent of cases, the RS+H cells have a type II latency pattern [EBER1(+), LMP1(+)] of EBV infection (13). Preliminary analysis of the background cells in classic Hodgkin lymphoma has shown increased numbers of FOXP3-positive lymphocytes, presumably T-regulatory cells, and increased CD163-positive histiocytes, suggesting an M2 phenotype (13).

Approximately 4 percent of iatrogenic LPDs are Hodgkin-like lesions (6). These lesions may be included in the polymorphic LPD category, but are morphologically distinctive based on the presence of RS+H-like cells. (At mucosal sites, these lesions also overlap histologically with EBV-positive mucocutaneous ulcer.) Hodgkin-like lesions more commonly present at extranodal than nodal sites.

Histologically, Hodgkin-like lesions may closely resemble classic Hodgkin lymphoma (fig. 44-4). In some cases, however, the large neoplastic cells are poor mimics of true RS+H cells, one clue pointing to the correct diagnosis. Hodgkin-like lesions also tend to have few or no eosinophils in the background. The small lymphocytes in the background of Hodgkin-like lesions have a spectrum of cell sizes, and include immunoblasts, which is unusual in classic Hodgkin lymphoma.

The distinction between classic Hodgkin lymphoma and Hodgkin-like lesion is based primarily

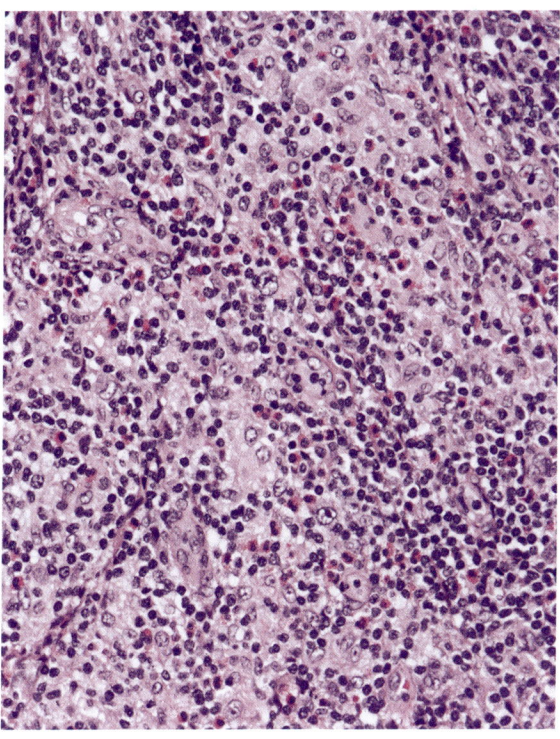

Figure 44-3

EBV-POSITIVE CLASSIC HODGKIN LYMPHOMA INVOLVING LYMPH NODE

This woman was treated with methotrexate for rheumatoid arthritis. The immunophenotype of the Reed-Sternberg and Hodgkin (RS+H) cells in this case was: CD15(+), CD30(+), and CD20(-), and cells were positive for EBER1 (not shown) (H&E stain).

on immunophenotypic data. Molecular studies are also helpful. In Hodgkin-like lesions, the large neoplastic cells are CD20(bright +), CD30(+), CD45/LCA (+/-), and CD15(-). In the background, small B cells are more common in Hodgkin-like lesion than classic Hodgkin lymphoma. In situ hybridization for EBER1 in Hodgkin-like lesions highlights both RS+H-like cells and many small lymphocytes, in contrast with classic Hodgkin lymphoma in which EBER1 is present primarily in the RS+H cells. Monoclonal *IGH* rearrangements are commonly detected in Hodgkin-like lesions, unlike classic Hodgkin lymphoma.

Polymorphic Lymphoproliferative Disorders

Polymorphic LPDs represent 7 to 10 percent of all iatrogenic cases (6,8). These lesions involve nodal or extranodal sites. Histologically, polymorphic LPDs share many features in

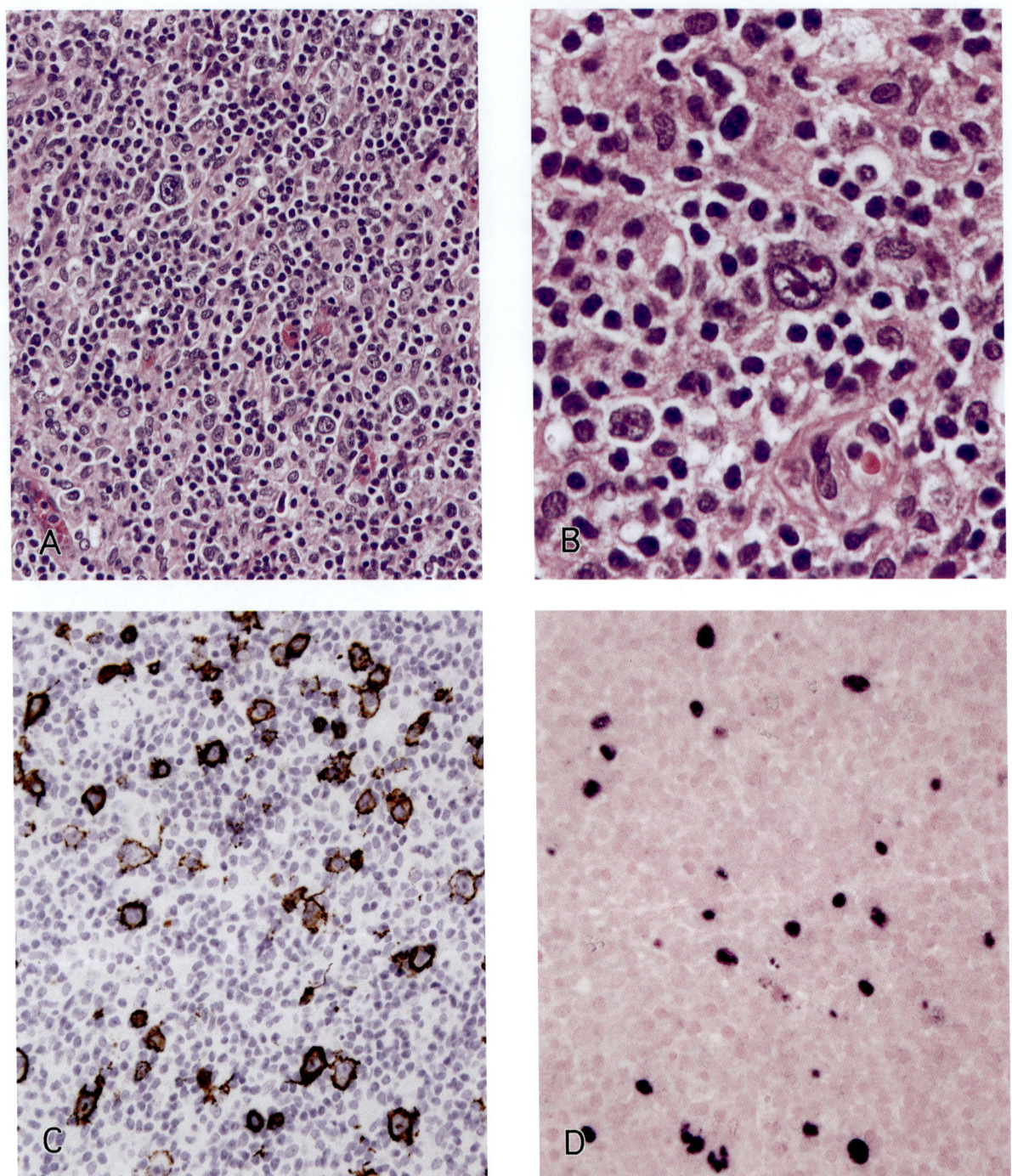

Figure 44-4

EBV-POSITIVE HODGKIN-LIKE LESION INVOLVING LYMPH NODE

A: This woman was treated with azathioprine for systemic lupus erythematosus. The lymph node architecture is replaced by the lesion (A,B: H&E stain).

B: Oil magnification shows a large RS-like cell.

C: The RS+H-like cells are strongly positive for CD20. These cells were also positive for CD45/LCA and negative for CD15 (not shown) (immunohistochemistry with hematoxylin counterstain).

D: The RS+H-like cells (and a few small lymphocytes) are positive for EBER1 (in situ hybridization with eosin counterstain).

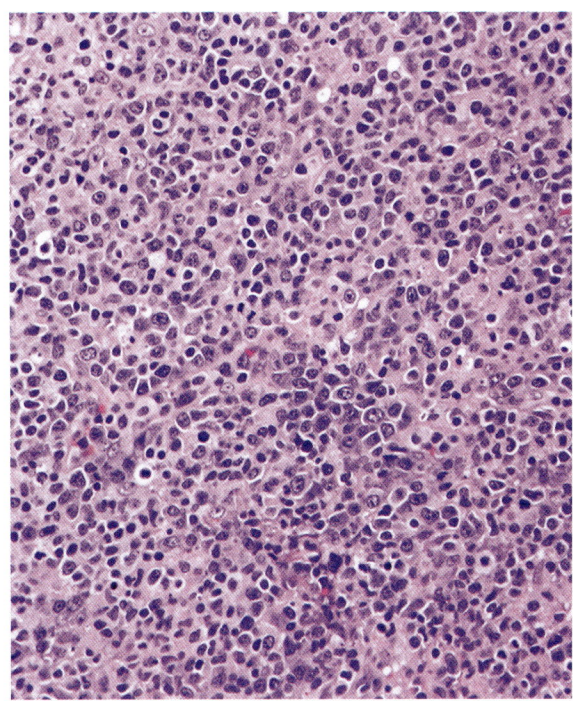 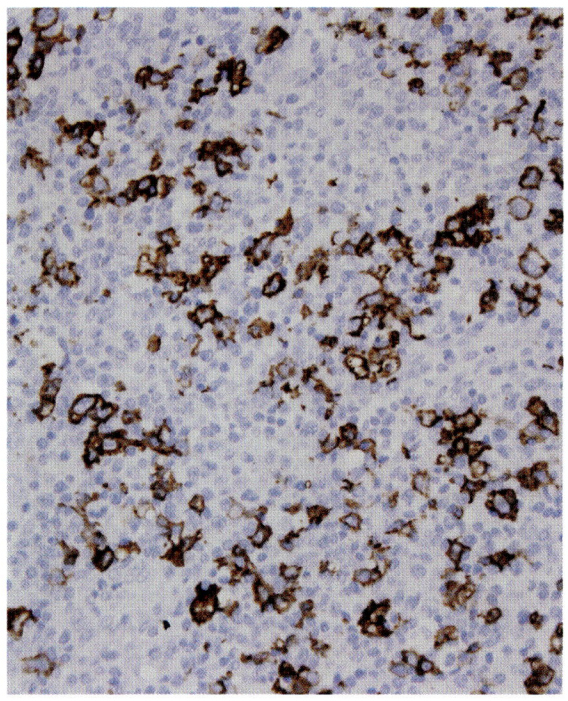

Figure 44-5

EBV-POSITIVE POLYMORPHIC LYMPHOPROLIFERATIVE DISORDER

Left: The patient was being treated with methotrexate for rheumatoid arthritis. The lesion is composed of a heterogeneous mixture of cells including small lymphocytes, larger lymphocytes, immunoblasts, and plasma cells (H&E stain).

Right: CD20 highlights a subset of cells, mostly large lymphocytes and immunoblasts that were also positive for EBER1 (not shown) (immunohistochemistry with hematoxylin counterstain).

common with polymorphic post-transplant LPDs. The lesions are diffuse and composed of small and intermediate sized lymphocytes, scattered large centroblasts or immunoblasts, plasma cells, and histiocytes (fig. 44-5). The large lymphoid cells may exhibit plasmacytoid features. The number of large centroblasts may be overestimated in routinely stained sections because the histiocytes can be numerous and form sheets. Some pathologists have included cases of atypical follicular or paracortical hyperplasia in this category as well.

Immunohistochemical studies show that the large lymphoid cells express pan-B-cell antigens and are negative for T-cell markers. Flow cytometry analysis detects a monotypic B-cell population in up to 50 percent of cases, although the number of monotypic B cells may be low. Monotypic cytoplasmic Ig light chain may be detected if the large lymphoid cells show plasmacytoid differentiation or in cases with numerous plasma cells. The proliferation

(Ki-67) rate is variable but often brisk. Evidence of EBV infection is common.

EBV-Positive Mucocutaneous Ulcer

This lesion is a recently described clinicopathologic entity that occurs in the setting of immunosuppression (4). *EBV-positive mucocutaneous ulcer* fits within the polymorphic LPD category, albeit with distinctive features, and is included as a provisional entity in the 2016 update of the World Health Organization (WHO) classification (19a).

EBV-positive mucocutaneous ulcer is reported most often in elderly patients with presumed age-associated immunodeficiency (4). These lesions also occur in patients with autoimmune diseases who have received methotrexate, azathioprine, or less often, other immunosuppressive agents (4) but few (if any) cases have been reported in patients who received anti-TNFα agents or other monoclonal antibodies. Rarely, EBV-positive mucocutaneous ulcer can occur in the post-transplant setting and in patients with a history of malignancy treated with chemotherapy (17a).

Patients with EBV-positive mucocutaneous ulcer are usually adults and more often women, particularly patients with autoimmune diseases (4). Patients present with well-circumscribed, superficial ulcers that most often involve the oral mucosa, but also have been reported at various sites in the gastrointestinal tract or skin. Regional lymph nodes may be enlarged but patients invariably have localized disease (stage I or II).

Morphologically, EBV-positive mucocutaneous ulcer has a circumscribed appearance, and often a band of small lymphocytes and histiocytes forms a rim around the base of the lesion (fig. 44-6) (4). Necrosis and angioinvasion occur in about 25 percent of cases. Cytologically, lesions are polymorphous and composed of scattered RS+H-like cells in a background rich in small T cells and histiocytes. In a subset of cases, plasma cells and eosinophils are prominent.

Immunohistochemical analysis has shown that the large cells are always CD30 positive and express a variety of B-cell antigens including CD20 (about 90 percent of cases), CD79A, PAX5, OCT2, and IRF4/MUM1. In approximately half of cases, the RS+H-like cells are positive for CD45/LCA, CD15, and BCL6 (4). Some cases are CD10 positive. The presence of EBV is required for diagnosis; the virus is positive for EBER1 and usually also for LMP1 (4). Molecular analysis has shown monoclonal *IGH* or, less often, T-cell receptor gene rearrangements in about 40 percent of cases. Little cytogenetic or molecular data are available for these lesions.

Patients with EBV-positive mucocutaneous ulcer often regress following the discontinuation of methotrexate or other immunosuppressive therapeutic agents employed (4). These lesions can recur, however, usually locally, and at that point patients may require chemotherapy. Rarely, patients with recurrences fail therapy and Saton et al. (17a) reported a patient who died.

Other Iatrogenic LPDs

A number of other histologic types of iatrogenic LPD occur at a much lower frequency (Table 44-1). These lesions resemble their counterparts in immunocompetent patients. The etiologic relationship between drug therapy and these lymphoma types is not well established. Coincidental occurrence cannot be excluded, particularly for unusual histologic types of disease that are EBV negative.

Low-grade B-cell lymphomas represent 6 to 7 percent of iatrogenic LPDs and include *follicular lymphoma, extranodal marginal zone B-cell lymphoma of mucosa-associated lymphoid tissue, chronic lymphocytic leukemia/small lymphocytic lymphoma,* and *lymphoplasmacytic lymphoma/Waldenstrom macroglobulinemia* (fig. 44-7) (7,12). Follicular lymphoma is the most common. Most low-grade B-cell lymphomas are EBV negative and may be coincidental, but EBV-positive low-grade B-cell lymphomas, particularly those with plasmacytic differentiation, may be related to immunodeficiency. In addition, rare low-grade B-cell lymphomas regress after discontinuing drug therapy, suggesting an etiologic relationship (2).

Burkitt lymphoma represents about 2 percent of iatrogenic LPDs (6). These neoplasms generally resemble sporadic Burkitt lymphomas. EBV is positive in 20 to 30 percent of cases. *Plasma cell lesions* represent less than 1 percent of iatrogenic LPDs. These lesions can involve the bone marrow or extramedullary sites (fig. 44-8). The plasma cells are well or poorly differentiated.

Overall, about 5 percent of iatrogenic LPDs are T-cell lymphomas of which *peripheral T-cell lymphoma not otherwise specified* is the most common (6). Other T-cell lymphomas reported include *hepatosplenic T-cell lymphoma, extranodal NK/T-cell lymphoma of nasal type, cutaneous anaplastic large cell lymphoma,* and *angioimmunoblastic T-cell lymphoma* (6). T-cell lymphomas express pan-T-cell antigens and are negative for B-cell antigens. T-cell lymphomas are infrequently EBV positive, with the exception of extranodal NK/T-cell lymphoma of nasal type.

Hepatosplenic T-cell lymphoma (HSTCL) is unique in the context of iatrogenic LPDs. These tumors have been reported most often in young men who are being treated with anti-TNFα therapy, particularly infliximab, for Crohn's disease. In a recent review by Yabe et al. (22), a total of 67 cases have been reported. The true risk of anti-TNFα therapy remains controversial (18,19,22). Patients with Crohn's disease treated with azathioprine (without an anti-TNFα inhibitor) also may develop HSTCL as do some patients who have not received any immunomodulating

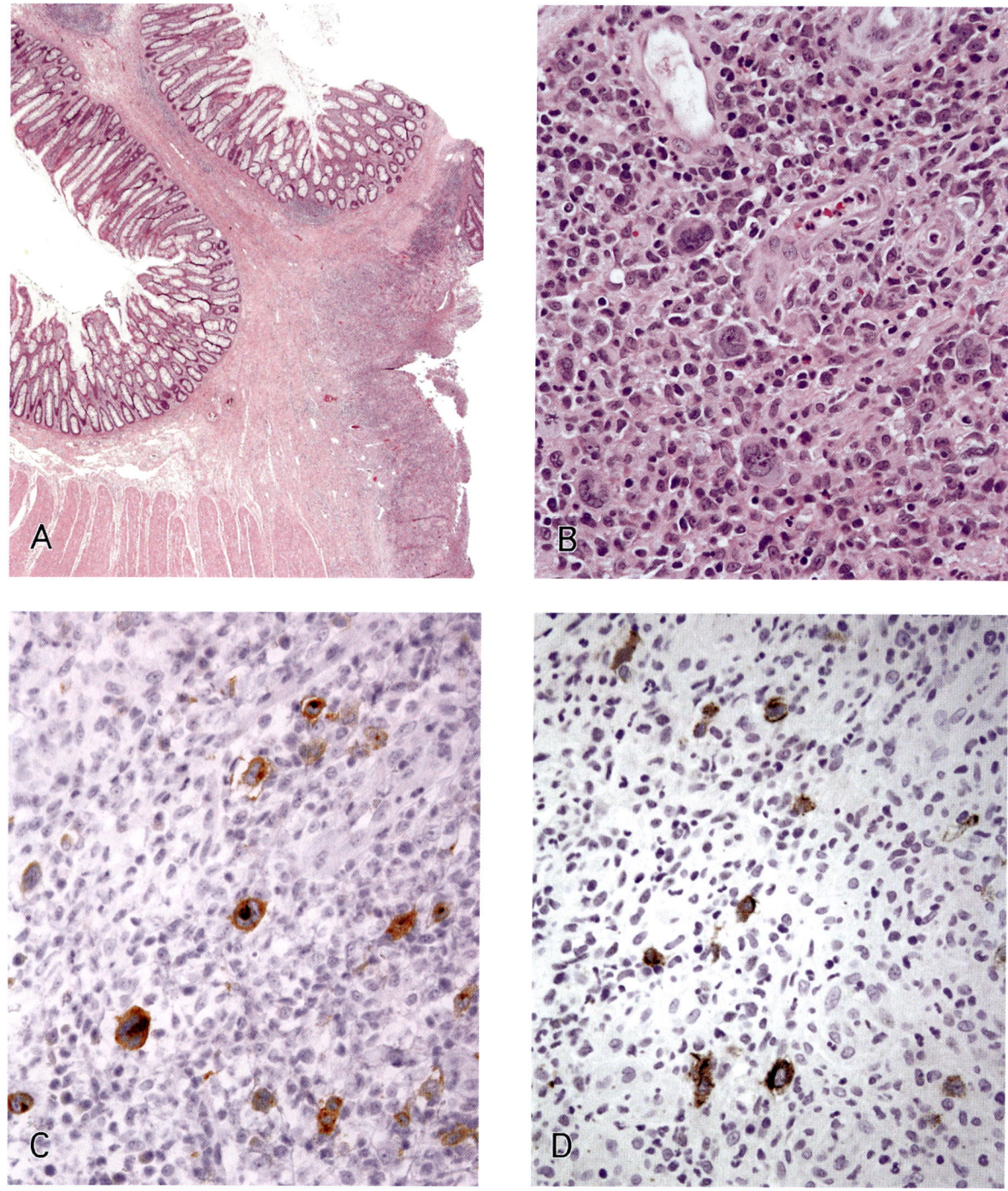

Figure 44-6

EBV-POSITIVE MUCOCUTANEOUS ULCER IN SIGMOID COLON

A: This woman with a history of systemic lupus erythematosus was treated with methotrexate and mycophenolate. A circumscribed ulcer is present (right side of field) (A,B: H&E stain).

B. High magnification shows large cells with RS+H-like features in an inflammatory background.

C,D: The large cells are positive for CD30 (C) and EBV latent membrane protein 1 (LMP1) (D). These cells were also positive for PAX5 and negative for CD15, CD20, and CD45/LCA (not shown). The histologic findings and immunophenotype are consistent with EBV-positive mucocutaneous ulcer (C,D: immunohistochemistry with hematoxylin counterstain).

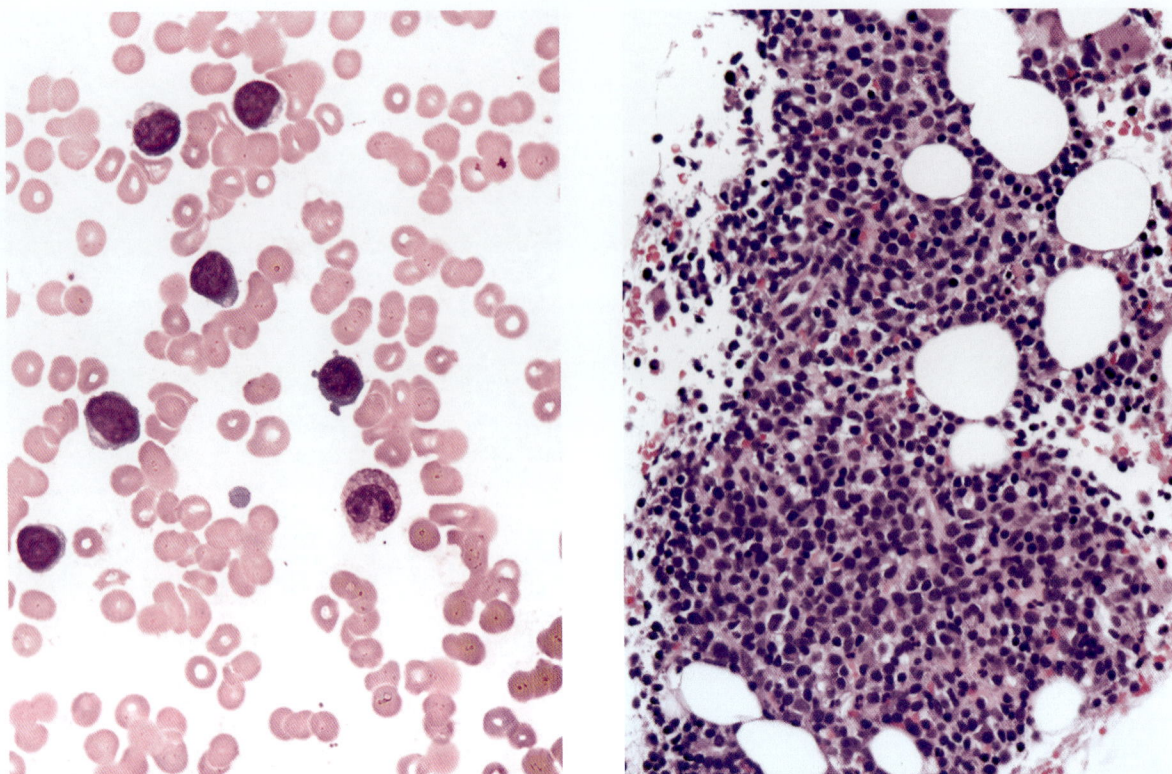

Figure 44-7

LYMPHOPLASMACYTIC LYMPHOMA/WALDENSTROM MACROGLOBULINEMIA

Left: An elderly woman who had a history of rheumatoid arthritis was treated with methotrexate and the tumor necrosis factor alpha (TNFα) inhibitor, adalimumab (Humira™). This bone marrow aspirate smear shows increased small lymphocytes, including plasmacytoid cells (Wright-Giemsa stain).

Right: The bone marrow aspirate clot specimen shows many small lymphocytes and fewer plasma cells (H&E stain).

Figure 44-8

EBV-NEGATIVE PLASMACYTOMA

This patient with rheumatoid arthritis was treated with adalimumab. The patient had received methotrexate in the past. The lesion is composed of sheets of mature-appearing plasma cells that were CD138 positive (not shown) (H&E stain).

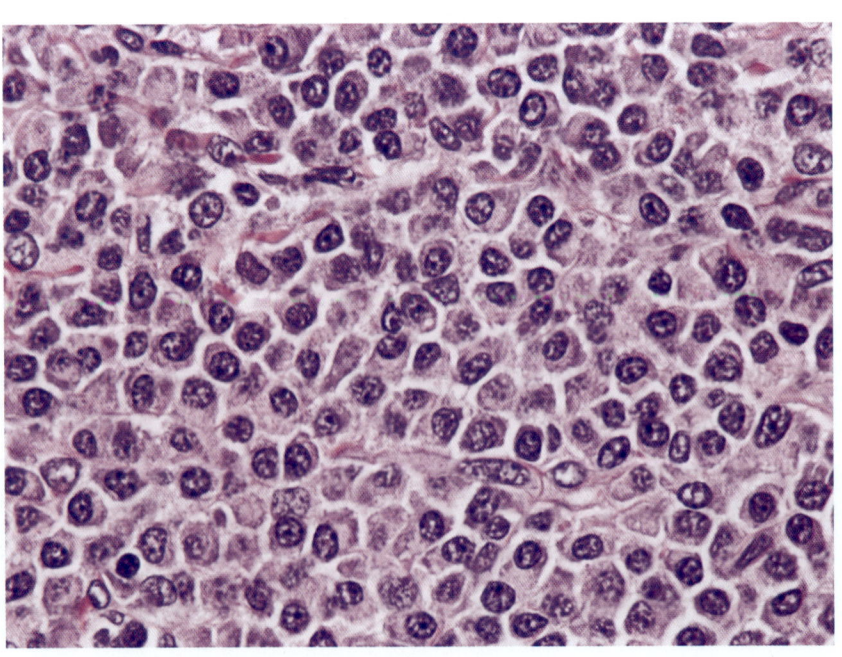

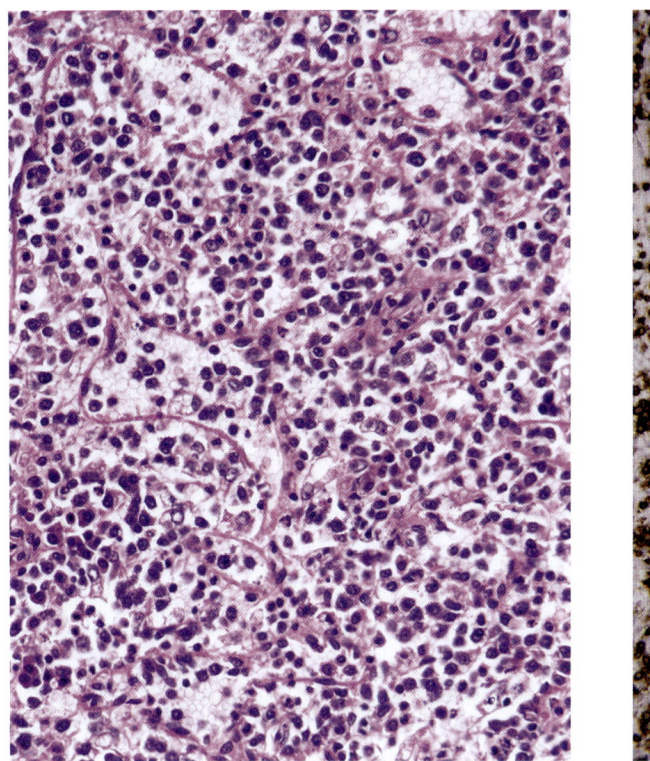 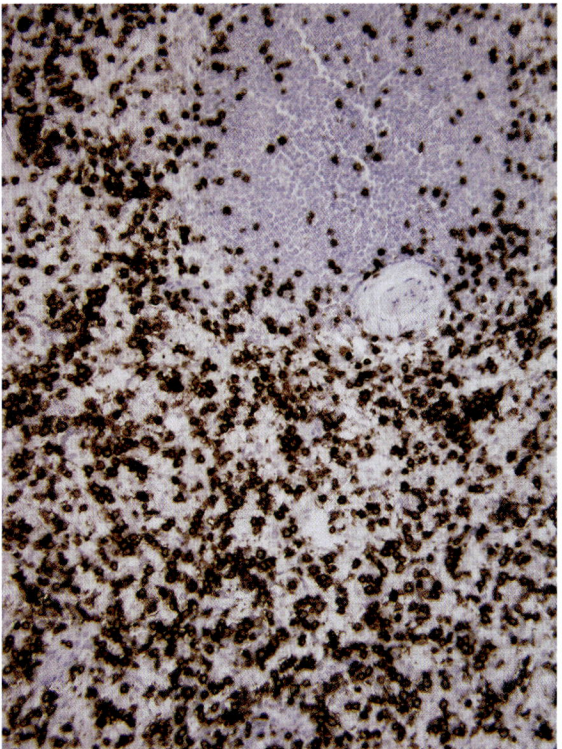

Figure 44-9

HEPATOSPLENIC T-CELL LYMPHOMA

Left: A young man with Crohn's disease was being treated with infliximab (Remicade™). The red pulp of the spleen is extensively infiltrated by small to intermediate sized lymphoid cells (H&E stain).

Right: The neoplastic cells are positive for CD3 and were negative for CD4 and CD8 (not shown). Flow cytometry immunophenotypic analysis of bone marrow confirmed these results and showed that the tumor cells were positive for TCR γ/δ (not shown) (immunohistochemistry with hematoxylin counterstain).

agents. HSTCL has not yet been reported in patients treated with methotrexate for Crohn's disease. Patients with ulcerative colitis do not appear to be at increased risk of HSTCL.

Histologically, HSTCL in patients with Crohn's disease closely resembles the disease in other clinical settings (fig. 44-9). HSTCLs are virtually always EBV negative. In the iatrogenic context, most patients with HSTCL have a very aggressive course and a poor prognosis unless treated by stem cell transplantation (19,22).

CYTOLOGIC FINDINGS

Fine-needle aspirate smears of iatrogenic LPDs show morphologic findings that are often indistinguishable from those of lymphomas arising in immunocompetent patients. The reader is referred to other chapters that describe these cytologic findings. In cases of DLBCL, the most common

iatrogenic LPD, the neoplastic cells are large with vesicular chromatin and contain 2 to 3 distinct nucleoli to a single, central prominent nucleolus. Necrosis and apoptotic cells are common.

MOLECULAR GENETIC FINDINGS

Little is known about the genetics of iatrogenic LPDs and the limited data available are heavily biased toward cases of DLBCL. Conventional cytogenetic analysis has not shown specific findings. In a study of 14 cases, 9 had an abnormal karyotype (20). Cases of follicular lymphoma and a proportion of DLBCL cases carry t(14;18)(q32;q21)/*IGH-BCL2*. Cases of peripheral T-cell lymphoma often have a complex karyotype. Some cases of HSTCL carry isochromosome 7 and/or trisomy 8.

Data are available on the analysis of antigen receptor genes in iatrogenic LPDs, usually by polymerase chain reaction methods. Most cases of DLBCL and Burkitt lymphoma carry monoclonal immunoglobulin rearrangements. *MYC* rearrangements are characteristic of Burkitt lymphoma and are uncommon in iatrogenic DLBCL. T-cell lymphomas usually carry monoclonal T-cell receptor gene rearrangements. In iatrogenic LPDs positive for EBV, the virus is usually present in monoclonal episomal form. Data regarding other genes in iatrogenic LPD are sparse. In a brief correspondence, two cases of methotrexate-associated DLBCL did not have mutations in the *CD79A*, *CD79B*, or *EZH2* genes (3).

DIFFERENTIAL DIAGNOSIS

The essential information required for the diagnosis of iatrogenic LPD is the knowledge that the patient is receiving immunosuppressive or immunomodulator therapeutic agents. If the history is unknown, clues to suspect the possibility include: unusual clinical findings or anatomic sites of disease for the histologic type and the presence of a polymorphous infiltrate composed of a spectrum of lymphocytes from small to large immunoblasts, histiocytes, and plasma cells. Lesions that resemble Hodgkin lymphoma at extranodal sites are often associated with some form of immunosuppression, including iatrogenic causes (13). In some patients with iatrogenic LPD, however, the clinical presentation and morphologic findings are not unusual. For individual iatrogenic LPDs, the differential diagnosis is similar to their morphologic counterparts in immunocompetent patients.

TREATMENT AND PROGNOSIS

The prognosis of patients with iatrogenic LPD is variable, and correlates in part with the drugs used prior to the onset of the LPD, morphologic findings, immunophenotype, and EBV and *IGH* status (1,6,7,8-10,20). Patients treated with methotrexate or azathioprine before onset are more likely to regress after discontinuation than patients who received anti-TNFα agents. Low-grade B-cell and T-cell iatrogenic LPDs rarely regress. Iatrogenic LPDs that are EBV positive are most likely to regress after the offending drug is discontinued; EBV-negative iatrogenic LPDs regress uncommonly. The presence of monoclonal *IGH* rearrangement also may cor-

relate with a lower frequency of regression and more aggressive disease course (8). For patients who do not experience regression after discontinuing drug therapy, cytotoxic chemotherapy is usually required and a substantial number of patients experience an aggressive disease course and poor response to therapy.

Diffuse Large B-Cell Lymphoma

About 20 percent of patients treated with methotrexate who develop DLBCL regress after the methotrexate is discontinued (1,6,6a,9,10,20). Regression can be complete or partial. Regression is most likely for patients with EBV-positive DLBCL. In some patients, a prolonged interval of "watchful waiting" is needed following discontinuation for regression to occur (9). Some patients with complete regression will never require additional therapy, but in others, disease will recur and chemotherapy will be required. Nevertheless, the prognosis for these patients is good and in one study, the 5-year overall survival rate was 100 percent for the subgroup of patients who underwent regression (20).

The most commonly used chemotherapy regimen for patients with iatrogenic DLBCL is cyclophosphamide, doxorubicin, vincristine, and prednisone (CHOP), often combined with rituximab. The overall survival rate for patients with DLBCL arising in the context of iatrogenic LPD, including all patients who required therapy, and therefore not patients who completely regressed, is approximately 50 percent (1,8).

Classic Hodgkin Lymphoma and Hodgkin-Like Lesion

Although classic Hodgkin lymphoma is commonly EBV positive, these lesions rarely regress after discontinuing methotrexate (6,6a,13). In contrast, Hodgkin-like lesions are more likely to regress than classic Hodgkin lymphoma.

Most patients with classic Hodgkin lymphoma are treated with combination chemotherapy with an overall good outcome. In a literature review by Miranda et al. (15), about 80 percent of patients with classic Hodgkin lymphoma responded well to therapy and were alive at last follow-up. Much less information is available for patients with Hodgkin-like lesions who did not undergo regression.

Polymorphic LPD and
EBV-Positive Mucocutaneous Ulcer

Many polymorphic LPDs are EBV positive, as is EBV-positive mucocutaneous ulcer. Patients with these lesions often regress once drug therapy is stopped (4,6). The prognosis of patients with EBV-positive mucocutaneous ulcer is particularly good, which may be related to the low disease stage and superficial location of these lesions. In one study, all patients with EBV-positive mucocutaneous ulcer underwent regression after the offending agent was discontinued (4). Nevertheless, some patients with either polymorphic LPD or EBV-positive mucocutaneous ulcer may progress or the lesion may recur after regression and chemotherapy is then required.

REFERENCES

1. Baecklund E, Backlin C, Iliadou A, et al. Characteristics of diffuse large B cell lymphomas in rheumatoid arthritis. Arthritis Rheum 2006;54: 3774-3781.
2. Baird RD, van Zyl-Smit RN, Dilke T, Scott SE, Rassam SM. Spontaneous remission of low- grade B-cell non-Hodgkin's lymphoma following withdrawal of methotrexate in a patient with rheumatoid arthritis: case report and review of the literature. Br J Haematol 2002;118:567-568.
3. Capello D, Gloghini A, Martini M, et al. Mutations of CD79A, CD79B, and EZH2 genes in immunodeficiency-related non-Hodgkin lymphomas. Br J Haematol 2011;152:777-786.
4. Dojcinov SD, Venkataraman G, Raffeld M, Pittaluga S, Jaffe ES. EBV positive mucocutaneous ulcer – a study of 26 cases associated with various sources of immunosuppression. Am J Surg Pathol 2010;34:405-417.
5. Fallah M, Liu X, Ji J, Försti A, Sundquist K, Hemminki K. Hodgkin lymphoma after autoimmune disease by age at diagnosis and histologic type. Ann Oncol 2014;25:1397-1404.
6. Gaulard P, Swerdlow SH, Harris NL, Jaffe ES, Sundström C. Other iatrogenic immunodeficiency-associated lymphoproliferative disorders. In: Swerdlow SH, Campo E, Harris NL, et al., eds. WHO classification of tumours of haematopoietic and lymphoid tissues. Lyon: IARC Press; 2008;350-351.
6a. Gion Y, Iwaki N, Takata K, et al. Clinicopathological analysis of methotrexate-associated lymphoproliferative disorders: comparison of diffuse large B-cell lymphoma and classical Hodgkin lymphoma types. Cancer Sci 2017;108:1271-1280.
7. Hasserjian RP, Chen S, Perkins SL, et al. Immunomodulator agent-related lymphoproliferative disorders. Mod Pathol 2009;22:1532-1540.
8. Ichikawa A, Arakawa F, Kiyasu J, et al. Methotrexate/iatrogenic lymphoproliferative disorders in rheumatoid arthritis: histology, Epstein-Barr virus, and clonality are important predictors of disease progression and regression. Eur J Haematol 2013;91:20-28; Erratum in: Eur J Haematol 2013;91:565.
9. Inui Y, Matsuoka H, Yakushijin K, et al. Methotrexate-associated lymphoproliferative disorders: management by watchful waiting and observation of early lymphocyte recovery after methotrexate withdrawal. Leuk Lymphoma 2015;56:3045-3051.
10. Kamel OW. Iatrogenic lymphoproliferative disorders in non-transplantation settings. Recent Results Cancer Res 2002;159:19-26.
11. Kojima M, Itoh H, Hirabayashi K, et al. Methotrexate-associated lymphoproliferative diseases. A clinicopathological study of 13 Japanese cases. Pathol Res Pract 2006;202:679-685.
12. Larvol L, Soule JC, Le Tourneau A. Reversible lymphoma in the setting of azathioprine therapy for Crohn's disease. N Engl J Med 1994;331:883-884.
13. Loo EY, Medeiros LJ, Aladily TN, et al. Classical Hodgkin lymphoma arising in the setting of iatrogenic immunodeficiency: a clinicopathologic study of 10 cases. Am J Surg Pathol 2013;37:1290-1297.
14. Mariette X, Tubach F, Bagheri H, et al. Lymphoma in patients treated with anti-TNF: results of the 3-year prospective French RATIO registry. Ann Rheum Dis 2010;69:400-408.
15. Miranda RN, Loo E, Medeiros LJ. Iatrogenic immunodeficiency-associated classical Hodgkin lymphoma. Am J Surg Pathol 2013;37:1895-1897.
16. Nader K, Behrens DS, Leon CA, Schwarting R, Ferber A. Iatrogenic lymphoproliferative disorder. Am J Hematol 2014;89:787-788.

17. Rizzi R, Curci P, Delia M, et al. Spontaneous remission of "methotrexate-associated lymphoproliferative disorders" after discontinuation of immunosuppressive treatment for autoimmune disease. Review of the literature. Med Oncol 2009;26:1-9.

17a. Satou A, Kohno A, Fukuyama R, Elsayed AA, Nakamura S. EBV-positive mucocutaneous ulcer arising in a post-hematopoietic cell transplant patient followed by polymorphic post-transplant lymphoproliferative disorder and cytomegalovirus colitis. Hum Pathol 2017;59:147-151.

18. Selvaraj SA, Chairez E, Wilson LM, Lazarev M, Bass EB, Hutfless S. Use of case reports and the Adverse Event Reporting System in systematic reviews: overcoming barriers to assess the link between Crohn's disease medications and hepatosplenic T-cell lymphoma. Syst Rev 2013;2:53.

19. Subramaniam K, Yeung D, Grimpen F, et al. Hepatosplenic T-cell lymphoma, immunosuppressive agents and biologicals: what are the risks? Int Med J 2014;44:287-290.

19a. Swerdlow SH, Campo E, Pileri SA, et al. The 2016 revision of the World Health Organization classification of lymphoid neoplasms. Blood 2016; 127:2375-2390.

20. Tokuhira M, Watanabe R, Nemoto T, et al. Clinicopathological analyses in patients with other iatrogenic immunodeficiency-associated lymphoproliferative diseases and rheumatoid arthritis. Leuk Lymphoma 2012;53:616-623.

21. Wong AK, Kerkoutian S, Said J, Rashidi H, Pullarkat ST. Risk of lymphoma in patients receiving antitumor necrosis factor therapy: a meta-analysis of published randomized controlled studies. Clin Rheumatol 2012;31:631-636.

22. Yabe M, Medeiros LJ, Daneshbod Y, et al. Hepatosplenic T-cell lymphoma arising in patients with immunodysregulatory disorders: a study of 7 patients who did not receive tumor necrosis factor-a inhibitor therapy and literature review. Ann Diagn Pathol 2017;26:16-22.

45 CANCER THERAPY-ASSOCIATED LYMPHOPROLIFERATIVE DISORDERS

GENERAL FEATURES

As has been described, the World Health Organization (WHO) classification segregates immunodeficiency-associated lymphoproliferative disorders (LPDs) into four categories based on the clinical setting in which they arise. Nevertheless, as has been reported by others, LPDs in each WHO category show a similar range of morphologic features and a high frequency of Epstein-Barr virus (EBV) infection, suggesting common pathogenic mechanisms (20a). In this chapter, we describe another group of lesions that we believe may fit within the overall framework of immunodeficiency-associated LPDs. These lesions are alluded to, but not formerly covered, in the WHO classification (9).

Patients with cancer of various types and who were treated with a variety of chemotherapeutic agents, with or without radiation therapy, can subsequently develop lymphoproliferative disorders designated here as *cancer therapy-associated lymphoproliferative disorders* (CT-LPD). Patients who develop LPDs associated with other WHO classification recognized causes of immunodeficiency, such as allogeneic solid organ or stem cell transplantation, human immunodeficiency virus infection, or immunomodulator agent therapy for nonmalignant diseases, are excluded from this category.

In this patient subset, the essential requirement is a history of a cancer that has been treated prior to the onset of LPD. Therefore, in a larger sense, CT-LPD is a form of iatrogenic LPD, although not as this category is strictly defined in the WHO classification (see chapter 44). We believe the category of CT-LPD is justified because these lesions share morphologic features and likely pathogenetic mechanisms with other types of immunodeficiency-associated LPDs. However, unlike patients with other types of immunodeficiency-associated LPDs, patients with CT-LPD uncommonly undergo partial or rarely complete regression.

Patients treated for a wide variety of hematologic neoplasms as well as solid tumors have gone on to develop CT-LPDs. The many hematologic malignancies include both myeloid and lymphoid neoplasms as well as leukemias and lymphomas, and are summarized in Table 45-1. There is an increased risk of non-Hodgkin lymphomas in patients who have been treated for breast, testicular, or ovarian cancer (12,15). Children with neuroblastoma or less often retinoblastoma who have been treated with high-dose therapy and often autologous stem cell transplantation have gone on to develop CT-LPD (24).

The etiology of CT-LPD is poorly understood and is likely multifactorial (Table 45-2). Immunodeficiency in this patient group is probably an important factor and is attributable to a number of causes, as has been reviewed by Friman et al.

Table 45-1

HEMATOLOGIC MALIGNANCIES THAT PRECEDE CANCER THERAPY-ASSOCIATED LYMPHOPROLIFERATIVE DISORDERS

Acute myeloid leukemia

Acute mixed lineage leukemia

Acute lymphoblastic leukemia (B and T cell)

Chronic myeloid leukemia

Chronic myelomonocytic leukemia

Lymphoplasmacytic lymphoma/Waldenstrom macroglobulinemia

Marginal zone lymphomas (extranodal and splenic)

Follicular lymphoma

Diffuse large B-cell lymphoma

Plasma cell myeloma

T-cell prolymphocytic leukemia

Mycosis fungoides

Angioimmunoblastic T-cell lymphoma

Peripheral T-cell lymphoma, not otherwise specified

Classic Hodgkin lymphoma

Table 45-2

FACTORS THAT MAY BE INVOLVED IN THE PATHOGENESIS OF CANCER THERAPY-ASSOCIATED LYMPHOPROLIFERATIVE DISORDERS

Immune defects associated with cancer

Age-associated immunosenescence

Therapy-associated immunosuppression

Virus infection (most often Epstein-Barr virus)

Chemotherapy-induced DNA damage

Host genetic susceptibility

(8a). One possible etiology may be the qualitative and quantitative defects in host immunity known to be associated with cancers. A good example among lymphoid tumors is chronic lymphocytic leukemia/small lymphocytic lymphoma (CLL/SLL); patients are known to have many immune defects independent of therapy that contribute to the overall degree of immunosuppression (5,6,8a). A second possible cause is physiologic immunosenescence, which is known to be associated with age. Many patients with CT-LPD are older and may have immunocompromise as a result of immunosenescence of both the innate and adaptive immune systems (reviewed in reference 19). Another more hypothetical possibility is that patients who develop CT-LPD have an underlying genetic predisposition, although, at this time, there is little literature addressing this issue. Lastly, immunosuppression related to the class(es) of chemotherapeutic agents used to treat the initial cancer are likely to be important in pathogenesis (1,15,24). Here we expand on therapy-related immunocompromise since the literature suggests that this etiology is very important.

Purine and pyrimidine analogs that inhibit DNA synthesis have immunosuppressive effects. Fludarabine is the most frequently used drug in this class, but others include cladribine, clofarabine, and azacytidine (1,2,7,8,11,16,18,27). Patients treated with fludarabine may have suppressed CD4-positive T-cell counts that can persist for prolonged intervals after therapy is completed. Fludarabine also causes neutropenia. In patients with CLL/SLL, fludarabine is often combined with cyclophosphamide and rituximab (the FCR regimen), further adding to

overall immunosuppression and likely increasing the risk of CT-LPD (1).

Alemtuzamab (anti-CD52) is a highly immunosuppressive agent that has been implicated in patients with CT-LPD (14,26). The combination of fludarabine and alemtuzumab appears to be particularly immunosuppressive (1). Cytotoxic chemotherapy drugs also appear to predispose to CT-LPD, particularly in patients who have undergone multiple relapses requiring many salvage regimens (22). Patients with chronic myeloid leukemia treated with imatinib may develop CT-LPD that may or may not resolve after discontinuation of the drug (17). Imatinib inhibits T-cell proliferation and activation, which may play a role in pathogenesis (25).

Autologous stem cell transplantation also has been implicated in the pathogenesis of CT-LPD (3,10,23,24). Reports suggest that cumulative high-dose chemotherapy presumably induces a greater degree of immunosuppression that is involved in pathogenesis (3,10,24). Procedures that have been used as part of the process of autologous stem cell transplantation, such as T-cell depletion or CD34 selection, or the use of tandem transplant strategies, are associated with greater immunosuppression and a greater risk of CT-LPD (23,24).

Most reported cases of CT-LPD are positive for Epstein-Barr virus (EBV) (1,14,17,21,22,26). These cases support a role for compromised immunosurveillance and also point to a role for EBV or other viral infections in pathogenesis (1,21,22,26).

Chemotherapeutic agents themselves also have a role in oncogenesis. The mechanisms involved in the pathogenesis of therapy-related myeloid neoplasms, as reviewed by Leone et al. (18), may be involved in the pathogenesis of CT-LPD. Cytotoxic agents such as cyclophosphamide and etoposide are known to damage DNA via distinct pathways. Induction of double-stranded DNA breaks provides an opportunity for chromosomal translocations or somatic mutations to occur during the process of DNA repair (15,18).

CLINICAL FEATURES

There is a latency interval from the treatment of the initial cancer to the development of CT-LPD. In the literature, this interval ranges from a few weeks to many years. In general, the interval is longer for patients who develop classic Hodgkin lymphomas than for patients who develop non-Hodgkin lymphomas (1,4).

Patients with CT-LPD have clinical features similar to those of patients with other types of immunodeficiency-associated LPD (1,4). Many patients have localized disease, but some have multiple lesions. B-type symptoms may be present. Patients present with lymphadenopathy, extranodal sites of disease, or both. The distribution of disease in patients with CT-LPD correlates, in part, with histologic findings. Polymorphic lesions and lesions that resemble diffuse large B-cell lymphoma (DLBCL) are commonly extranodal. Patients with classic Hodgkin lymphoma more often present with lymphadenopathy (4,7,8).

HISTOLOGIC FINDINGS

The most common histologic form of CT-LPD is a polymorphic lesion that can resemble a post-transplant LPD or classic Hodgkin lymphoma. The most common monomorphic CT-LPD resembles DLBCL, but cases of plasmablastic lymphoma and T-cell lesions that resemble peripheral T-cell lymphoma have been reported rarely (8,13,27).

Areas of coagulative necrosis are common and mitotic figures and apoptotic cells are often numerous in CT-LPD (1). Polymorphic lesions are composed of a spectrum of lymphoid cells including small lymphocytes, larger cells, immunoblasts, and, in some cases, Reed-Sternberg–like cells associated with plasma cells and histiocytes (figs. 45-1, 45-2) (1,14). Cases of classic Hodgkin lymphoma are similar to lesions that arise in immunocompetent patients. Most cases reported have been nodular sclerosis or mixed cellularity type (fig. 45-3) (4,7,8). In monomorphic cases that resemble DLBCL, the lymphoma cells have centroblastic or immunoblastic features.

CYTOLOGIC FINDINGS

Little in the literature is available regarding the cytologic features of CT-LPD. In our experience, fine-needle aspirate smears of these lesions usually are associated with necrosis and a polymorphic or monomorphic infiltrate of cells indistinguishable from those of LPDs that arise in patients with various other types of immunodeficiency or immunodysregulation.

IMMUNOPHENOTYPIC FINDINGS

Most cases of CT-LPD reported have been of B-cell lineage (1,10,14,17,20,26). The large cells express pan-B-cell antigens (figs. 45-1, 45-2) and are negative for CD5 and other T-cell antigens. Large B cells usually express CD45/LCA and commonly express CD30 (fig. 45-2C). Plasma cells may express polytypic or monotypic cytoplasmic immunoglobulin. CD15 is negative. In cases of classic Hodgkin lymphoma, the Reed-Sternberg and Hodgkin (RS+H) cells have an appropriate immunophenotype: CD15(+), CD30(+), MUM1/IRF4(+), PAX5 (dim+), and CD45/LCA(-) (4,7). Cases of CT-LPD of T-cell lineage are rare; these tumors express pan-T-cell markers.

Most cases of CT-LPD reported have been positive for EBV, shown either by in situ hybridization for EBV-encoded RNA1 (EBER1) (figs. 45-1D, 45-2D) or less often immunohistochemical evaluation for EBV latent membrane protein type 1. EBV nuclear antigens are variably positive.

MOLECULAR GENETIC FINDINGS

Little is known about the genetics of CT-LPD. Immunoglobulin gene rearrangements are common. In a small group of patients with CLL/SLL who developed CT-LPD, Abruzzo et al. (1) compared the antigen receptor genes and showed that 3 of 4 cases were not clonally related to the CLL/SLL (1). In a study by Fong et al. (7), 2 of 4 CT-LPD cases with features of Hodgkin lymphoma were not clonally related to the CLL/SLL. For clonally related cases, the pathogenesis of the CT-LPD is unknown. Histologic transformation of CLL/SLL to CT-LPD is possible. A common stem cell origin for the CLL/SLL and CT-LPD is also a possibility although the presence of contaminating CLL/SLL cells in the CT-LPD specimen is difficult to completely exclude.

DIFFERENTIAL DIAGNOSIS

The information essential for the diagnosis of CT-LPD is the knowledge that the patient has a history of a cancer that was treated with chemotherapy, with or without radiation therapy or autologous stem cell transplantation. If the history is unknown, presentation of disease at extranodal sites, a polymorphous infiltrate, and EBV positivity are clues to the diagnosis of CT-LPD.

In patients with CLL/SLL, the presence of CT-LPD can be viewed as a form of Richter

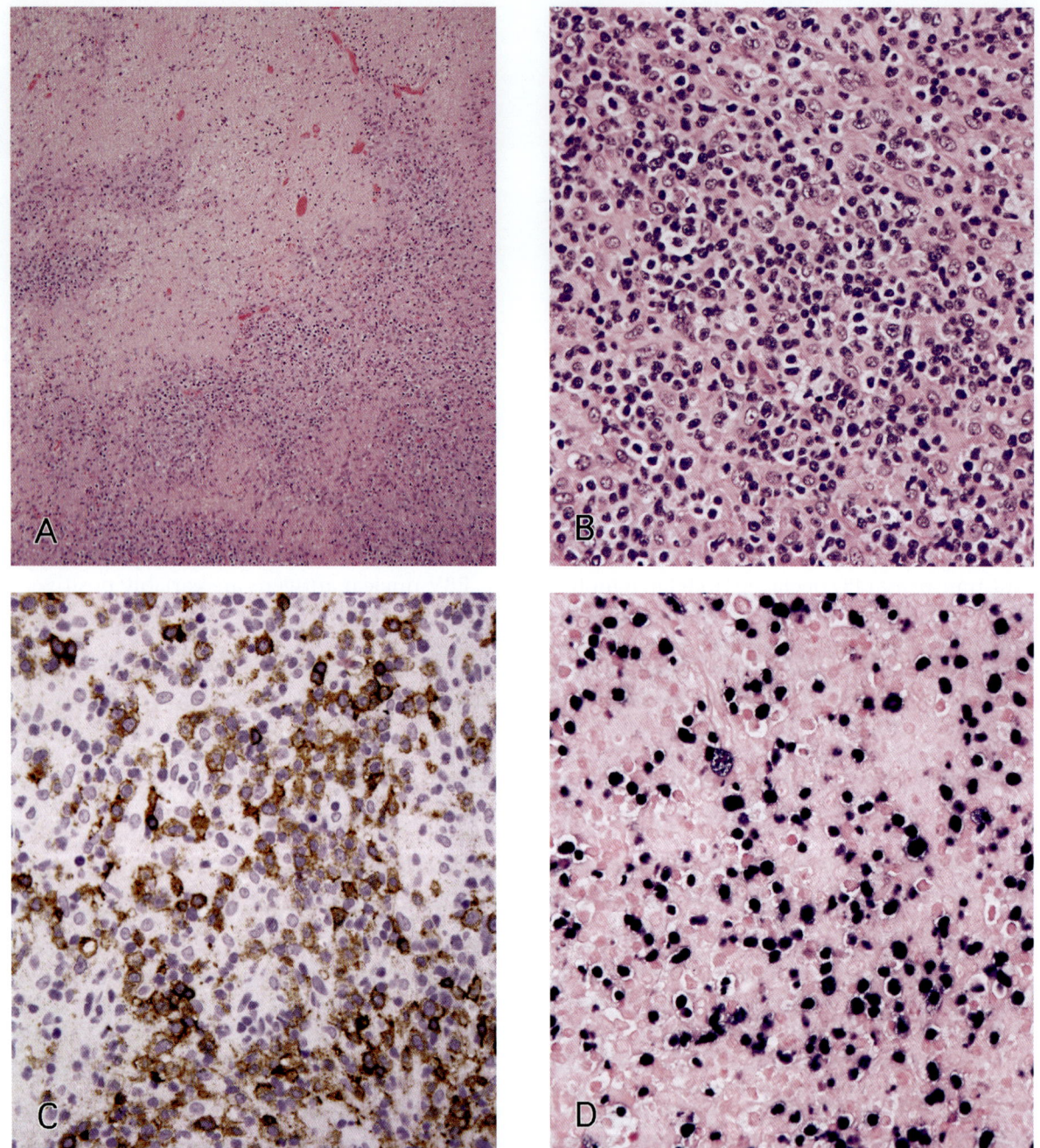

Figure 45-1

EPSTEIN-BARR VIRUS (EBV)-POSITIVE POLYMORPHIC LYMPHOPROLIFERATIVE DISORDER INVOLVING LYMPH NODE

This lesion occurred 7 years after initial the diagnosis of chronic lymphocytic leukemia and 5 years after treatment with the fludarabine, cyclophosphamide, and rituximab (FCR) chemotherapy regimen.

A: At low magnification extensive coagulative necrosis is seen (A,B: hematoxylin and eosin [H&E] stain).

B: High-power magnification shows a polymorphic population of cells including mainly small and large lymphocytes and histiocytes.

C: Many large lymphocytes are CD19-positive B cells. The cells were negative for CD20 (not shown), common after rituximab therapy (immunohistochemistry with hematoxylin counterstain).

D: In situ hybridization shows many cells positive for EBV-encoded RNA1 (EBER1) (In situ hybridization with eosin counterstain).

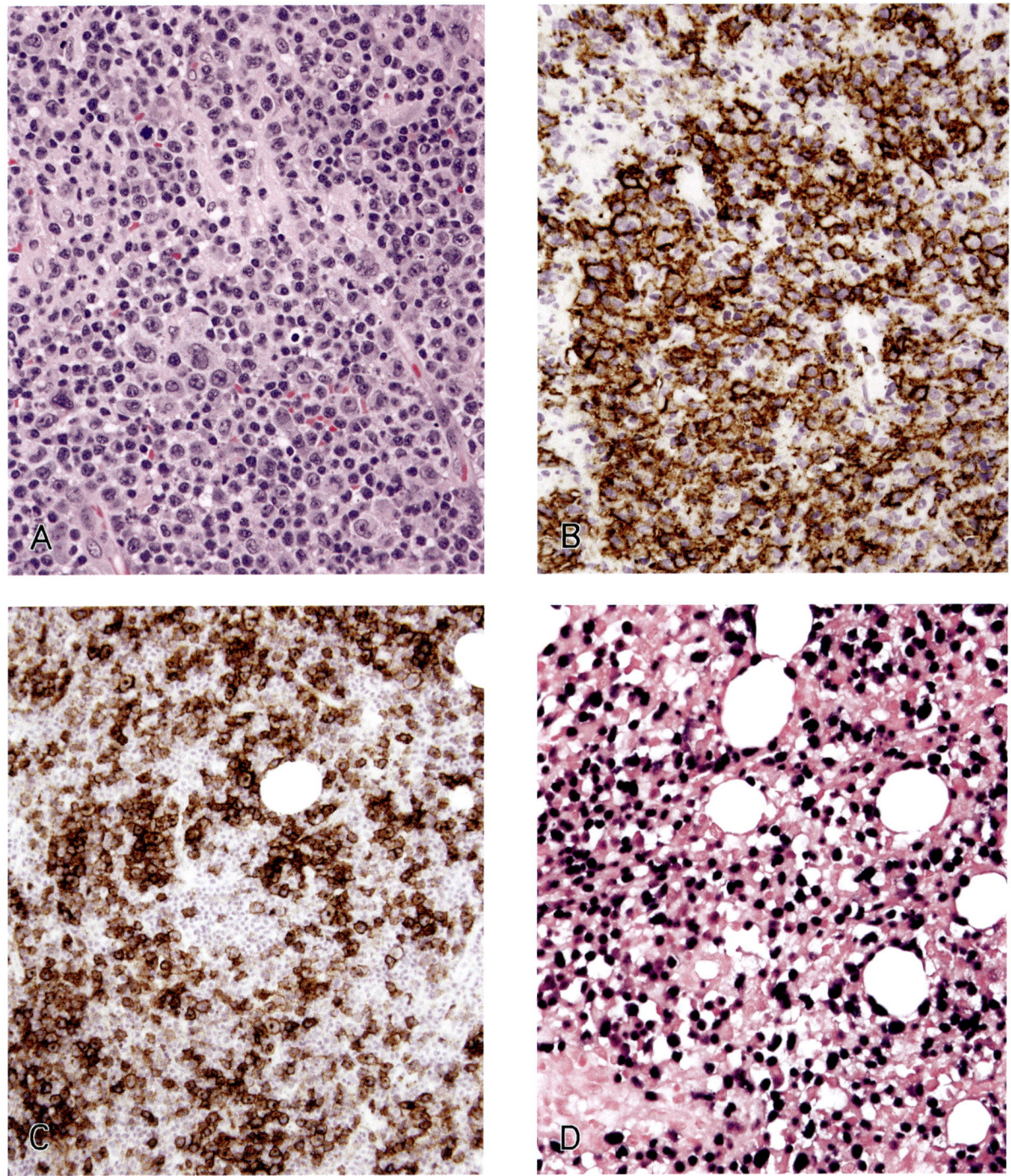

Figure 45-2

EBV-POSITIVE POLYMORPHIC LYMPHOPROLIFERATIVE DISORDER INVOLVING SOFT TISSUE

This lesion occurred 3 months after the diagnosis of acute monocytic leukemia with FLT3 mutation and treatment with the clofarabine, idarubicin, and cytarabine (CIA) chemotherapy regimen.

A: There is a mixture of small lymphocytes, plasma cells, immunoblasts, and multilobated large cells. Mitotic figures are seen (H&E stain).

B,C: Most cells are positive for CD20 (B) and CD30 (C) (immunohistochemistry with H&E counterstain).

D: In situ hybridization shows that many cells are positive for EBER1 (in situ hybridization with eosin counterstain).

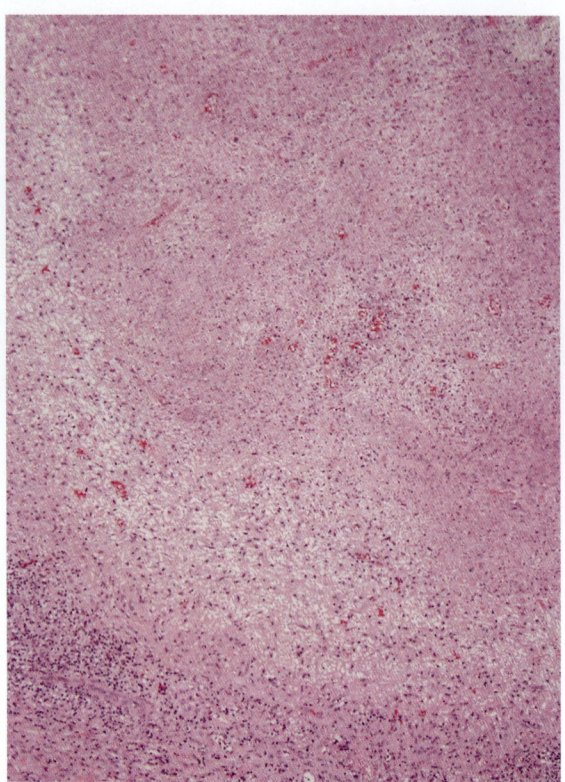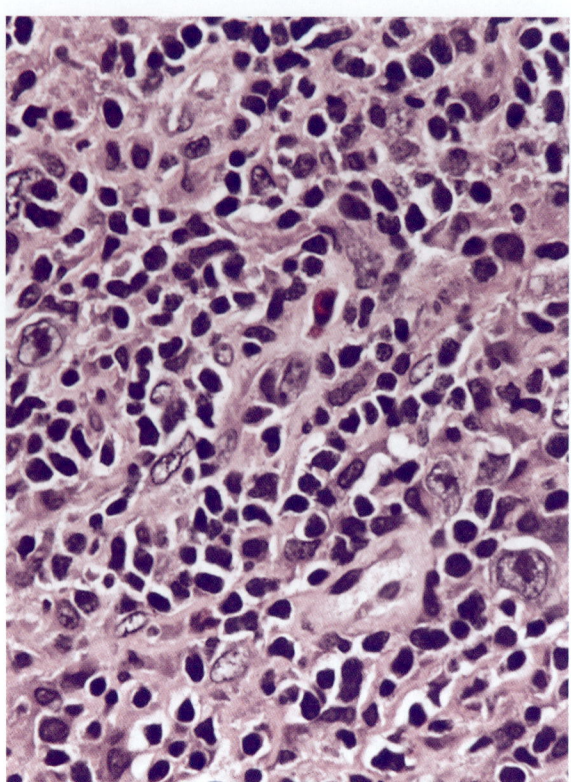

Figure 45-3

EBV-POSITIVE CLASSIC HODGKIN LYMPHOMA

This lesion occurred 13 years after the diagnosis of splenic marginal zone lymphoma and following cytotoxic chemotherapy with rituximab.

Left: Large areas of necrosis are present in this tumor.

Right: High magnification shows large Hodgkin cells in an inflammatory background of lymphocytes, histiocytes, and occasional plasma cells and eosinophils. The Hodgkin cells and rare Reed-Sternberg cells (not shown) had an appropriate immunophenotype and were EBV positive (not shown) (left, right: H&E stain).

syndrome. However, we suggest that CT-LPD should be distinguished from Richter syndrome. In CLL/SLL patients with Richter syndrome, transformation to DLBCL occurs and the neoplasm is typically EBV negative, unlike many cases of CT-LPD. Molecular studies showing clonal identity between the CLL/SLL and the DLBCL also supports Richter syndrome. However, there is overlap between CT-LPD and Richter syndrome and more studies are needed.

TREATMENT AND PROGNOSIS

The prognosis of patients with CT-LPD is variable, and correlates with the morphologic findings and immunophenotype. Rarely, EBV-positive lesions, particular those with polymorphic features, regress spontaneously (1,2). Some of these cases recur, however, and patients then require chemotherapy (1). Monomorphic lesions that resemble DLBCL usually require chemotherapy. Patients with classic Hodgkin lymphoma, even if disseminated, often respond well to chemotherapy (4,7). The most commonly used chemotherapy regimen for patients with CT-LPD is rituximab, cyclophosphamide, doxorubicin, vincristine, and prednisone (R-CHOP) or CHOP. The overall survival for patients with CT-LPD is generally poor, but more studies are needed to understand the natural history of these lesions.

REFERENCES

1. Abruzzo LV, Rosales CM, Medeiros LJ, et al. Epstein-Barr virus-positive B-cell lymphoproliferative disorders arising in immunodeficient patients previously treated with fludarabine for low-grade B-cell neoplasms. Am J Surg Pathol 2002;26:630-636.

2. Bhamidipati PK, Jabbour E, Konoplev S, Estrov Z, Cortes J, Daver N. Epstein-Barr virus-induced CD30-positive diffuse large B-cell lymphoma in a patient with mixed-phenotypic leukemia treated with clofarabine. Clin Lymphoma Myeloma Leuk 2013;13:342-346.

3. Briz M, Forés R, Regidor C, et al. Epstein-Barr virus associated B-cell lymphoma after autologous bone marrow transplantation for T-cell acute lymphoblastic leukaemia. Br J Haematol 1997;98:485-487.

4. Cheminant M, Galicier L, Briere J, et al. Therapy-related classical Hodgkin lymphoma after a primary haematological malignancy: a report on 13 cases. Br J Haematol 2012;158:644-648.

5. Cutucache CE. Tumor-induced host immunosuppression: special focus on CLL. Int Immunopharmacol 2013;17:35-41.

6. Dhalla F, Lucas M, Schuh A, et al. Antibody deficiency secondary to chronic lymphocytic leukemia: Should patients be treated with prophylactic replacement immunoglobulin? J Clin Immunol 2014;34:277-282.

7. Fong D, Kaiser A, Spizzo G, Gastl G, Tzankov A. Hodgkin's disease variant of Richter's syndrome in chronic lymphocytic leukaemia patients previously treated with fludarabine. Br J Haematol 2005;129:199-205.

8. Foo WC, Huang Q, Sebastian S, Hutchinson CB, Burchette J, Wang E. Concurrent classical Hodgkin lymphoma and plasmablastic lymphoma in a patient with chronic lymphocytic leukemia/small lymphocytic lymphoma treated with fludarabine: a dimorphic presentation of iatrogenic immunodeficiency-associated lymphoproliferative disorder with evidence suggestive of mutliclonal transformability of B cells by Epstein-Barr virus. Human Pathol 2010;41:1802-1808.

8a. Friman V, Winqvist O, Blimark C, Langerbeins P, Chapel H, Dhalla F. Secondary immunodeficiency in lymphoproliferative malignancies. Hematol Oncol 2016;34:121-132.

9. Gaulard P, Swerdlow SH, Harris NL, et al. Other iatrogenic immunodeficiency-associated lymphoproliferative diorders. In Swerdlow SH, Campo E, Harris NL, et al., eds. WHO classification of tumours of haematopoietic and lymphoid tissues. Lyon: IARC Press; 2008:350-351.

10. Izumiya S, Ishida M, Hodohara K, Yoshida T, Okabe H Epstein-Barr virus-associated lymphoproliferative disorder developed following autologous peripheral blood stem cell transplantation for relapsing Hodgkin's lymphoma. Oncol Lett 2012;6:1203-1206.

11. Jain P, Benjamini O, Konoplev S, Mohamed MS, Romo CG, Estrov Z. Spontaneous remission of chemo-immunotherapy related, non-transplant Epstein-Barr virus-associated lymphoproliferative disorder in a patient with chronic lymphocytic leukemia. Leuk Lymphoma 2013;54:2540-2542.

12. Kaldor JM, Day NE, Band P, et al. Second malignancies following testicular cancer, ovarian cancer and Hodgkin's disease: an international collaborative study among cancer registries. Int J Cancer 1987;39:571-585.

13. Kilner MF, Merante S, Svec A. The development of peripheral T-cell lymphoma after successful treatment for diffuse large B-cell lymphoma in a patient with suspected adult onset immunodeficiency: more questions than answers? BMJ Case Rep 2013; doi:10.1136/bcr-2013-200079.

14. Kluin-Nelemans HC, Coeneb JL, Boers JE, van Imhoff GW, Rosati S. EBV-positive immunodeficiency lymphoma after alemtuzamab-CHOP therapy for peripheral T-cell lymphoma. Blood 2008;112:1036-1041.

15. Krishnan B, Morgan GJ. Non-Hodgkin lymphoma secondary to cancer chemotherapy. Cancer Epidemiol Biomarkers Prev 2007;16:377-380.

16. Lazzarino M, Orlandi E, Baldanti F, et al. The immunosuppression and potential for EBV reactivation of fludarabine combined with cyclophosphamide and dexamethasone in patients with lymphoproliferative disorders. Br J Haematol 1999;107:877-882.

17. Leguay T, Foucaud C, Parrens M, et al. EBV-positive lymphoproliferative disease with medullary, splenic and hepatic infiltration after imatinib therapy for chronic myeloid leukemia. Leukemia 2007;21:2208-2210.

18. Leone G, Fianchi L, Voso MT. Therapy-related myeloid neoplasms. Curr Opin Oncol 2011;23:672-680.

19. Malaguarnera L, Cristaldi E, Malaguarnera M. The role of immunity in elderly cancer. Crit Rev Oncol Hematol 2010;74:40-60.

20. Menter T, Schlageter M, Bastian L, Haberthür R, Rätz Bravo AE, Tzankov A. Development of an Epstein-Barr virus-associated lymphoproliferative disorder in a patient treated with azacitidine for chronic myelomonocytic leukaemia. Hematol Oncol 2014;32:47-51.

20a. Natkunam Y, Gratzinger D, de Jong D, et al. Immunodeficiency and dysregulation: report of the 2015 Workshop of the Society for Hematopathology/European Association for Haematopathology. Am J Clin Pathol 2017;147:124-128.

21. Niesvizky R, Zhu AX, Louie D, Michaeli J. Epstein-Barr virus-positive lymphoma after treatment of macroglobulinemia with cladribine. N Engl J Med 1999;341:55.

22. Orlandi E, Paulli M, Viglio A, et al. Epstein-Barr virus positive aggressive lymphoma as a consequence of immunosuppression after multiple salvage treatments for follicular lymphoma. Br J Haematol 2001;112:373-376.

23. Peniket AJ, Perry AR, Williams CD, et al. A case of EBV-associated lymphoproliferative disease following high-dose therapy and CD34-purified autologous peripheral blood progenitor cell transplantation. Bone Marrow Transplant 1998;22:307-309.

24. Powell JL, Bunin NJ, Callahan, Aplenc R, Griffin G, Grupp SA. Post-transplant lymphoproliferative disorder. An unexpectedly high incidence of Epstein-Barr virus lymphoproliferative disease after CD34+ selected autologous peripheral blood stem cell transplant in neuroblastoma. Bone Marrow Transplantation 2004;33:651-657.

25. Seggewiss R, Lore K, Greiner E, et al. Imatinib inhibits T-cell receptor-mediated T-cell proliferation and activation in a dose-dependent manner. Blood 2005;105:2473-2479.

26. Sohani AR, Ferry JA, Chang PS, Abramson JS. Epstein-Barr virus-positive diffuse large B-cell lymphoma during therapy with alemtuzumab for T-cell prolymphocytic leukemia. J Clin Oncol 2010;28:e69-72.

27. Wu JZ, Min K, Fan L, et al. Plasmablastic lymphoma following combination treatment with fludarabine and rituximab for nongastric mucosa-associated lymphoid tissue lymphoma: a case report and review of literature. Int J Clin Exp Pathol 2014;7:4400-4407.

46 PRIMARY IMMUNODEFICIENCY-ASSOCIATED LYMPHOPROLIFERATIVE DISORDERS

GENERAL FEATURES

Primary immunodeficiency-associated lymphoproliferative diseases arise in patients who have an immunodeficiency that is a result of a primary (inherited) immunodeficiency or immunodysregulatory disorder (38). They encompass a wide spectrum of lesions attributable, in part, to the variability of *primary immunodeficiency disorders* (PIDs) and the marked differences in their pathogenesis (5).

The first well-described PID in the English literature was reported by Ogden Bruton in 1952 (8); currently over 200 PIDs are described in the literature (6). Because the field is vast, the International Union of Immunological Societies (IUIS) has formed an expert committee that meets regularly to summarize novel developments; the proceedings of the last meeting were published in 2015 (6). PIDs are divided into nine general categories (Table 46-1) and a number of subgroups are included within each general category.

Traditionally, PIDs are defined as diseases that compromise the development or function of the humoral or cellular immune system, leading to increased susceptibility to infection by microbes as well as dysfunctional immune phenomena. Essentially, this is a definition based on a clinical and immunologic phenotype. However, with the great progress in our understanding of molecular abnormalities, should PIDs now be classified on the basis of their molecular defects? Although such a classification seems likely in the future, this approach is complicated by the fact that different mutations in the same gene can lead to distinctive phenotypes. Also, a similar phenotype can result from more than one gene mutation. Phenocopies of PID also occur; in these conditions patients present with an immunodeficiency syndrome that closely mimics a PID that occurs as a result of a germline mutation, but instead, in these patients the phenotype is a result of a somatic gene mutation or an autoantibody. Until there is a clear consensus, the criteria used for the diagnosis of PIDs will continue to evolve.

The known incidence of PIDs is based heavily on registry data, but it seems likely that these registries under-capture cases of PID and also under-represent adults with PID. With improved methods of detection and increased awareness of PIDs, it is becoming apparent that milder forms of PID occur in many adults. As a result of improved screening in asymptomatic patients, the prevalence of PIDs has been increasing. The current frequency of clinically evident PIDs in the United States, based on registry data, is 1 child in 10,000, or about 400 newly diagnosed cases per year. Bousfiha et al. (5), however, have suggested that up to 6 million persons worldwide have some form of PID. This incidence is based on the results of two surveys performed in the United States, the combined results of which suggest a much higher prevalence of PIDs than is currently assumed (7,19).

Primary immunodeficiency diseases are inherited in an X-linked or autosomal fashion, and autosomal diseases show recessive or dominant inheritance. The molecular defects associated with PIDs affect the development, function, and regulation of T cells, B cells, natural killer (NK) cells, and other components of the immune system (6). The frequency of PIDs is variable in different geographic regions, between different continents, and on the same continent, implying that some patients variably inherit a genetic susceptibility for the development of PIDs (1). Consanguineous marriage increases the risk of PIDs in children (1). In some geographic regions, such as the Middle East, there is a higher frequency of autosomal recessive forms of PID compared with the United States or Europe; this may be attributable to a higher frequency of consanguineous marriage in the Middle East (1).

Table 46-1

GROUPING OF PRIMARY IMMUNODEFICIENCY DISEASES[a]

IUIS Group	No. of Subgroups[b]	No. Subgroups with Lymphoma	Subgroups[c]
Combined immunodeficiencies	29	8	Severe combined immunodeficiency (SCID) Hyper-IgM syndrome Cartilage hair hypoplasia ITK[d] deficiency Coronin-1A deficiency XLP type 1 (*SH2D1A*) Activated PI3K-δ CD27 deficiency
Combined immunodeficiencies with associated or syndromic features	16	3	Wiskott-Aldrich syndrome Ataxia-telangiectasia Nijmegen breakage syndrome
Predominantly antibody deficiencies	6	3	X-linked agammaglobulinemia Common variable immunodeficiency disorders Hyper-IgM syndrome
Diseases of immune dysregulation	7	5	XLP type 1 (*SH2D1A*) XLP type 2 (*XIAP/BIRC*) ALPS ITK deficiency CD27 deficiency
Congenital defects of phagocyte number and/or function	5	0	
Defects in innate immunity	11	0	
Autoinflammatory disorders	18	0	
Complement deficiencies	25	0	
Phenocopies	2	1	ALPS

[a]Recommended by the Expert Committee of the International Immunological Societies (IUIS).
[b]Many major subgroups contain multiple additional entities.
[c]Some subgroups are listed more than once because there are disease variants. See also Table 46-2.
[d]ITK = interleukin-2-inducible T-cell kinase; XLP = X-linked lymphoproliferative syndrome; ALPS = autoimmune lymphoproliferative syndrome.

A specific PID diagnosis commonly requires a careful clinical history, particularly a family history, as well as routine and highly specialized immunologic and molecular testing for the specific gene mutation, at least for those diseases in which the defect(s) are known. The workup should include a complete blood cell count; enumeration of T, NK, and B cells; immunophenotypic expression of various activation markers such as CD25, CD80, and CD154; and quantification of serum immunoglobulins and complement components. A functional evaluation of B cells, T cells, and macrophages is also often needed and includes: natural or acquired antibodies and responses to protein or carbohydrate antigens (B cells); delayed hypersensitivity skin tests, proliferative response to mitogens, and cytokine levels (T cells); and chemotaxis, bactericidal activity, and reduction of nitroblue tetrazolium (macrophages) (10).

It was appreciated 40 years ago that patients with PIDs have an increased risk of lymphoma and, to a lesser extent, solid tumors (14). In a large study from Italy, Arico et al. (3) reported that 34 (2.4 percent) children out of 1,430 with lymphoma had an associated inherited genetic disease. Lymphomas represent approximately 60 percent of all cancers in PID patients and the overall risk of lymphoma ranges from 10 to 200 times above similarly aged patents without PID. The greatest risk is associated with non-Hodgkin lymphomas (30,38), although Hodgkin lymphomas and leukemias are also increased in PID patients. Increased awareness and earlier diagnosis of PID, better control of infections, and longer patient survival also explain, at least in part, the increased risk of

Table 46-2

PRIMARY IMMUNODEFICIENCY DISEASES (PIDs) ASSOCIATED WITH LYMPHOPROLIFERATIVE DISORDERS (LPDs)[a]

PID	Frequency[b]	Genetic Mutation	Inheritance Pattern	Clinical Manifestations	Most Common LPDs
Common variable immunodeficiency syndrome	21-31%	many defects resulting in low serum IgG and IgA levels	variable	bacterial infections; hypogamma-globulinemia; recurrent herpes infections; autoimmune diseases; diarrhea secondary to *Giardia lamblia*	DLBCL[c]; CHL, EMZL, atypical lymphoproliferative lesions (not clonal)
Ataxia telangiec-tasia	2-8%	*ATM*	AR	combined immunodeficiency; ataxia from progressive neu-ronal degeneration; occular telangiectasia; radiosensitivity	DLBCL, CHL, T-ALL, T-PLL
Severe combined immunodeficiency	1-5%	many defects; in-adequate humoral and cell-mediated immunity	AR or XL	infections in first few months; short survival without therapy; patients often die before LPDs can develop	EBV+LPDs
Wiskott-Aldrich syndrome	1-3%	*WAS*	XL	bacterial infections, eczema; microthrombocytopenia; autoimmune diseases	EBV+ DLBCL, CHL, LYG
Hyper-IgM syn-drome (Ig class switch recombin-ation deficiency)	1-2%	*CD40* ligand, *CD40*, and other defects	XL or AR	bacterial infections; lymphoid hyperplasia; normal or elevated IgM in serum with low IgA, IgG, and IgE	EBV+ LPDs, DLBCL, CHL, T-cell large granular lymphocytic leukemia
Nijmegen break-age syndrome	1-2%	*NBS1*	AR	combined immunodeficiency; microcephaly, mental retarda-tion, radiosensitivity	DLBCL, CHL
Cartilage hair hypoplasia	<1%	*RMRP*	AR	combined immunodeficiency; metaphyseal chondroplasia; sparse hair; anemia	EBV+ NHL, cutan-eous CD30+ T-cell LPD
X-linked agam-maglobulinemia	<1%	*BTK*; many other ab-normalities	XL	bacterial infections; low or absent pre-B cells or mature B cells; low serum Ig levels	DLBCL
X-linked lympho-proliferative syndrome type 1		*SH2D1A*	XL	EBV-triggered infectious mono-nucleosis (often fatal), hepatitis, aplastic anemia	Burkitt; CHL; DLBCL
Autoimmune lymphoprolif-erative syndrome	<1%	*FAS, FAS* ligand,	AD	recurrent infections; lympha-denopathy; splenomegaly; autoimmune cytopenias	DLBCL, Burkitt lymphoma; CHL NLPHL
Interleukin-2-in-ducible T-cell kinase deficiency	<1%	*ITK*	AR	infections; inability to control EBV infection (can mimic XLP)	CHL, DLBCL, polymorphic B-cell LPD
Activated phospho-inositide 3-kinase δ syndrome	<1%	*PIK3CD*	AD (gain-of-function)	recurrent respiratory infections; defective antibody production; progressive lymphopenia	DLBCL, CHL, marginal zone lymphoma
CD27 deficiency	<1%	*CD27*	AR	symptoms associated with hemophagocytosis or lymphoma	B-cell NHL, can be EBV+

[a]This table is incomplete as there are other PIDs in which LPDs have been reported rarely. In addition, cancer predisposition syndromes in which lymphomas may occur (e.g., Lynch syndrome or congenital mismatch repair deficiency) are not included.
[b]Frequency among all PIDs.
[c]LPD = lymphoproliferative disorder; DLBCL = diffuse large B-cell lymphoma; CHL = classic Hodgkin lymphoma; EMZL = extranodal marginal zone lymphoma; T-ALL = T-acute lymphoblastic leukemia; T-PLL = T-prolymphocytic leukemia; LYG = lymphomatoid granulomatosis; AR = autosomal recessive; AD = autosomal dominant; XL= X-linked; EBV = Epstein-Barr Virus.

lymphoproliferative disorders in PID patients. The frequency of some types of malignant tumor in patients with PID ranges from 4 to 25 percent (30).

Nevertheless, only a subset of the over 200 PIDs known currently is associated with an increased risk of lymphoma (Table 46-2) (1).

The median age at which PID patients develop lymphoma is around 7 years (38). It is probable that a latency interval is required before the lymphoma can develop. The specific type of PID and the age of onset play a role in the determination of this interval.

The etiology of lymphomas in patients with PID is not fully understood. Because patients with PID who undergo stem cell transplantation may be cured and do not have an increased risk of lymphoma, this implies that at least some types of PID predispose to lymphoma and some do not. Mechanisms that are thought to contribute to the pathogenesis of lymphomas in patients with PID, similar to those in patients with other types of immunodeficiency who develop lymphomas, include: 1) impaired host immunosurveillance; 2) chronic antigenic stimulation resulting in a polyclonal proliferation of lymphoid cells; 3) defective responses to DNA damage thereby causing genomic instability and predisposing to the genesis of molecular abnormalities (e.g., chromosomal translocations); 4) systemic dysregulation of the immune system; and 5) possibly, unknown oncogenic viruses (9,13).

CLINICAL FEATURES

Most patients who have a PID are diagnosed in the first year of life and recurrent infections are a frequent clinical manifestation of these diseases (10,39). Infections commonly involve the ears, sinuses, or lungs, with less common bouts of diarrhea, conjunctivitis, cellulitis, or meningitis/encephalitis. Patients with common variable immunodeficiency (CVID) syndrome present later in life, often between 20 to 30 years of age, also with various infections (13). Symptoms of PID include fever, fatigue, lethargy, or an infectious mononucleosis-like syndrome. Physical examination may show lymphadenopathy or hepatosplenomegaly. Laboratory findings show defects in humoral, cell-mediated immunity, or phagocytic function. Low serum immunoglobulin levels are a feature of patients with humoral defects. Lymphopenia is a characteristic finding in patients with severe combined immunodeficiency; the absolute lymphocyte count is a useful screening tool for infants. Because of an increased awareness and better detection methods, PID is often detected early in patients without or with fewer symptoms.

Lymphoproliferative disorders usually follow the diagnosis of PID, but occasionally, the lymphoproliferative disorder is the first manifestation of PID. As mentioned, patients with PID develop lymphoma or leukemia at around 7 years of age (38). There is often a mass at an extranodal site, most commonly the gastrointestinal tract, skin, and less often, other viscera including the brain. Lymphadenopathy and hepatosplenomegaly, more common in certain types of PID, are associated with the onset of lymphoma or leukemia. Some types of PID show a spectrum of severity or exhibit more than one phenotype based on different genetic abnormalities or dosage effects, and the risk of lymphoma is not identical with each variant.

TYPES OF PID

A complete discussion of the different types of PID and their lymphoma risk is a vast subject and the reader is referred to other textbooks for a more thorough discussion. Here some of the best known types of PID, as well as a few more recently described PIDs in which patients appear to have an increased risk of lymphoma, are discussed.

Common Variable Immunodeficiency Syndrome

Common variable immunodeficiency (CVID) is the most common form of PID associated with an increased risk of lymphoma (9,13). The incidence of CVID ranges from 1 in 10,000 to 1 in 50,000 persons and seems to be more common in Caucasians (13). Although patients with most types of PID present with symptoms as infants or young children, this is not the case for those with CVID who typically develop symptoms attributable to recurrent infections in the second or third decade of life.

CVID results from defects in antibody production (1,13). Patients have a low number of B cells in the blood, which respond to antigen but are unable to differentiate into plasma cells and produce antibody. The genetic defects that result in a failure to produce antibody are known for only a subset of patients with CVID, but include defects in inducible costimulator (ICOS), CD19, B-cell activating factor receptor (BAFFR), and transmembrane activator and calcium-modulating cyclophilin-ligand interactor (TACI) (6). T-cell defects also occur in CVID patients and

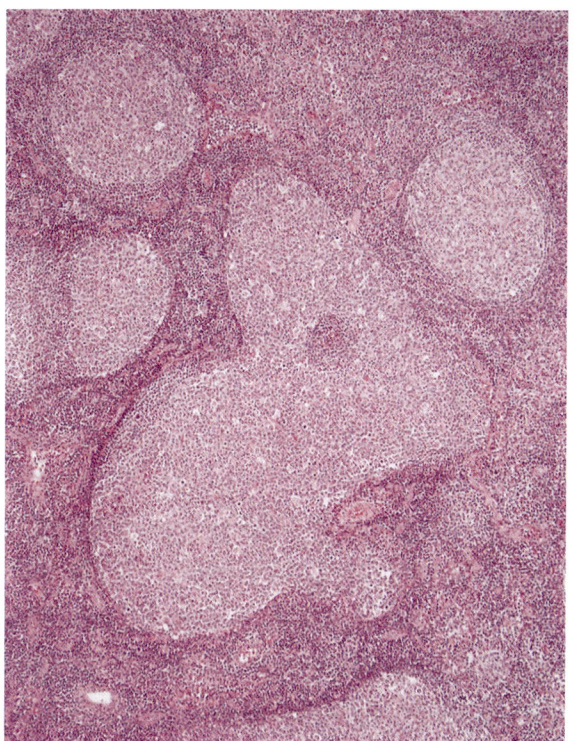 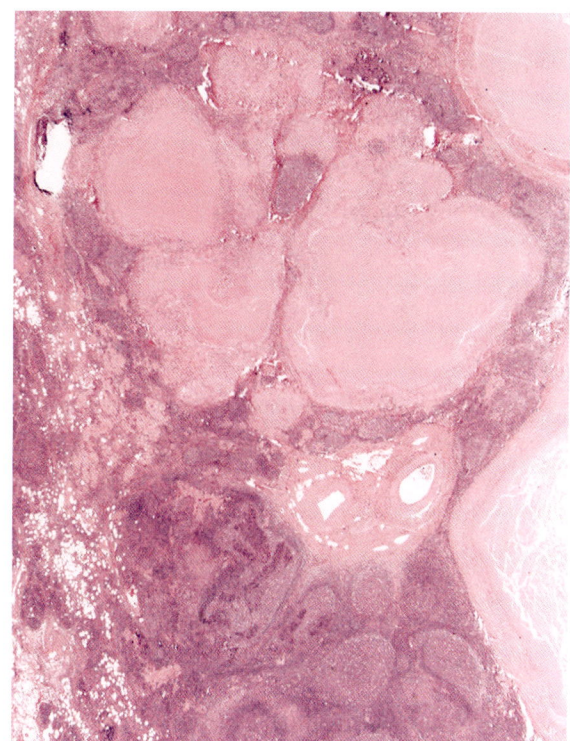

Figure 46-1

LYMPH NODE FINDINGS IN PATIENTS WITH COMMON VARIABLE IMMUNODEFICIENCY

Left: Reactive follicular hyperplasia.
Right: Chronic granulomatous inflammation with necrosis (left, right: hematoxylin and eosin [H&E] stain).

the different defects or combination of defects are likely to be associated with the different risks for developing lymphoma (13).

Patients with CVID manifest a number of phenotypes that are not mutually exclusive. Most patients present with infections and their complications. Some manifest autoimmune manifestations or gastrointestinal tract symptoms as a result of prominent nodular lymphoid hyperplasia (13). A small subset develops lymphoma.

The clinical phenotypes are reflected, in part, in the spectrum of findings in biopsy and splenectomy specimens of CVID patients (12a,32). Sander et al. (32) reviewed 30 biopsy specimens from 17 CVID patients and divided the lesions into four groups: reactive lymphoid hyperplasia (about 27 percent), chronic granulomatous inflammation (about 20 percent), atypical lymphoid hyperplasia (about 46 percent), and lymphoma (about 7 percent) (figs. 46-1, 46-2). In this study, most lymph node biopsy specimens showed benign findings, attributable to either infection or autoimmune polyclonal lymphocytic infiltration. In contrast, most lymphomas in patients with CVID are extranodal and of B-cell lineage. Epstein-Barr virus (EBV) is positive in some benign/reactive lymph nodes and lymphomas in CVID patients (32).

In the study by Sander et al. (32), the cases of atypical lymphoid hyperplasia were clinically suspicious for lymphoma, either because the involved area was a large mass or the patients had widespread disease. The biopsy specimens, however, showed florid expansion of the B- and T-cell compartments with ill-defined germinal centers (fig. 46-2C), often best appreciated by immunohistochemical assessment, and there was no evidence of clonality. Unger et al. (37) reported similar findings in CVID patients. In their study, they reported that germinal centers had high numbers of infiltrating CD8-positive T cells and reduced class-switched plasma cells. The authors suggested that these germinal centers probably develop normally, but there is a failure of germinal center output (37).

719

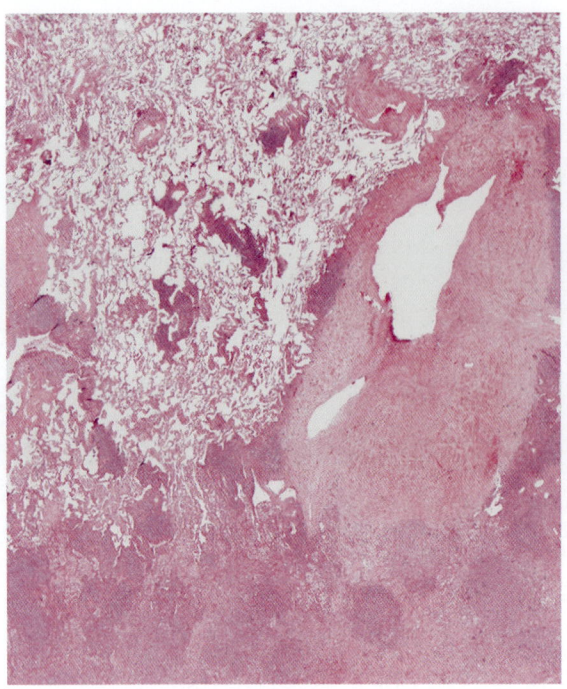
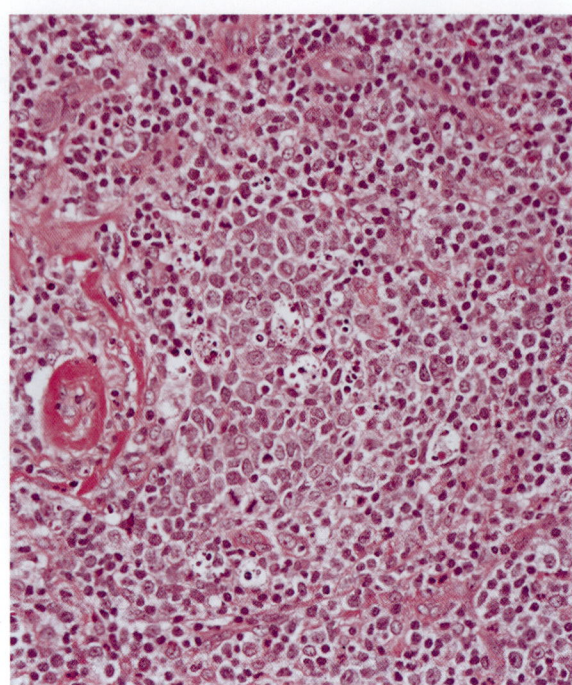

Figure 46-2

ATYPICAL LYMPHOID HYPERPLASIA IN COMMON VARIABLE IMMUNODEFICIENCY

Wedge biopsy specimen from the lung of a patient with CVID showed a vaguely nodular, florid lymphoid infiltrate diagnosed as atypical lymphoid hyperplasia. Immunohistochemical studies (not shown) showed B- and T-cell compartments and molecular studies showed no evidence of monoclonality.

Left: Low-power magnification shows alveolar lung parenchyma and infiltrate (right) (left, right: H&E stain).

Right: Hyperplastic germinal centers without mantle zones were observed in many of the nodules.

The most common type of lymphoma in patients with CVID is diffuse large B-cell lymphoma (DLBCL), which can be EBV positive. Patients also are reported with classic Hodgkin lymphoma and extranodal marginal zone lymphoma of mucosa-associated lymphoid tissue (MALT lymphoma) (9,13).

Ataxia-Telangiectasia

Ataxia-telangiectasia (AT) is a rare disorder occurring in approximately 1 in 80,000 births (23). Patients inherit heterozygous or homozygous mutations in the ataxia-telangiectasia mutated (*ATM*) gene in an autosomal recessive fashion. *ATM* is located on chromosome 11q22.3-23.1 and encodes a serine-threonine kinase that is normally involved in activation of cell cycle checkpoints, apoptosis, and repair of double-stranded DNA breaks (34,38). Patients with AT develop progressive neuronal degeneration, radiosensitivity, and combined immunodeficiency. These patients also have an increased risk of cancers, greater

in patients with homozygous *ATM* mutations. The cumulative incidence of cancer is estimated to be 1 percent per year for up to 40 years (34). The estimated risk of hematopoietic tumors in patients with AT is 70 to 250 times greater than the normal population (23,38).

Both solid tumors and hematopoietic malignancies can occur in AT patients. Most patients who develop hematopoietic tumors do so in the second decade of life. In a study from the French National Registry of Primary Immune Deficiencies, Suarez et al. (34) reported that 69 of 279 (24.5 percent) patients with AT developed cancers and 61 of these were hematopoietic, including 38 cases of non-Hodgkin lymphoma of different types, 12 cases of classic Hodgkin lymphoma, 8 acute leukemia, and 3 T-cell prolymphocytic leukemia. Approximately 75 percent of the non-Hodgkin lymphomas arose at extranodal sites and about 85 percent were of B-cell lineage. Half of non-Hodgkin lymphomas and all cases of classic Hodgkin lymphoma were positive for EBV. The cases of acute leukemia included four T-cell acute lymphoblastic leukemias, one case of acute myeloid leukemia, and three that were not further specified.

Severe Combined Immunodeficiency

Severe combined immunodeficiency (SCID) is the most severe form of all inherited immunodeficiency syndromes in its fully developed phenotype (6,38). Patients present within the first few months of life with failure to thrive and recurrent bacterial or opportunistic infections. Up to 10 genetic defects have been recognized as a cause of SCID, with a number of distinctive phenotypes, although various authors recognize four main phenotypes (9). In each phenotype, T cells are deficient, but B and NK cells also may be singly deficient [i.e., B(+) NK(-) or B(-) NK(+)] or both deficient [B(-) NK(-)]. Adenosine deaminase deficiency results in deficiency of T, B, and NK cells (9).

If not successfully treated and cured by stem cell transplantation or replacement therapy, most patients with SCID have a short survival period and die as very young children. For patients who survive a number of years there is an increased risk of EBV-associated LPDs, most often of polymorphic type (9).

Wiskott-Aldrich Syndrome

Wiskott-Aldrich syndrome (WAS) is named after two pediatricians who described it, Alfred Wiskott from Germany and Robert Aldrich from the United States. The incidence of Wiskott-Aldrich syndrome is 1 in 250,000 and the disease is the result of mutations in the Wiskott-Aldrich syndrome (*WAS*) gene located on chromosome Xp11.4-11.21 (6). Over 300 mutations in *WAS* are known. This gene encodes a protein that is expressed by hematopoietic cells and is involved in the actin cytoskeleton. Patients with *WAS* mutations have decreased numbers of T cells, defects in T- and NK-cell function, impaired antibody production, defects in phagocytes and dendritic cells, and abnormalities in apoptosis (6,38).

Patients who present with fully developed clinical manifestations of WAS exhibit a triad of eczema, microthrombocytopenia, and recurrent infections as a result of immunodeficiency (38). Patients have an increased risk of autoimmune diseases and lymphoma. There are milder forms of WAS, known as X-linked thrombocytopenia or X-linked neutropenia, with a lower risk of developing lymphoma.

Patients with WAS can develop benign lesions involving lymph nodes and spleen; about 10 percent develop lymphomas. These tumors are commonly extranodal, of B-cell lineage, and EBV positive and include DLBCL, classic Hodgkin lymphoma, and lymphomatoid granulomatosis (33,38).

Hyper-IgM Syndrome

Hyper-IgM syndrome, also known as *immunoglobulin class switch recombination deficiency*, is a family of genetic disorders in which patients have normal or elevated serum levels of IgM and IgD antibodies, but IgG, IgA, or IgE are low or absent as a result of defects in Ig class switch recombination and somatic hypermutation (11,38).

At least five genetic defects have been reported (6,11). The most common defect, in about 75 percent of patients, is a mutation in the gene encoding for CD40 ligand (CD40L) which is located on chromosome Xq26-27 and therefore inheritance is X-linked. CD40L is expressed normally on activated CD4-positive T cells and the interaction between T cells and CD40-positive B cells is essential for Ig class switching. Other mutations known to result in hyper-IgM syndrome, with an autosomal recessive pattern of inheritance, involve the genes that encode for CD40 (about 10 percent of cases), NF-κB essential modulator (NEMO, less than 2 percent), and activation-induced cytidine deaminase (AID, less than 1 percent).

All patients with hyper-IgM syndrome are susceptible to bacterial infection. Patients with the most common form of the disease also have defects in cell-mediated immunity and are predisposed to opportunistic infections as well as an increased risk of lymphoid hyperplasia and lymphomas (11). DLBCL, classic Hodgkin lymphoma, and T-cell large granular lymphocytic leukemia have been reported (38).

Nijmegen Breakage Syndrome

Patients with *Nijmegen breakage syndrome* inherit a mutation in *NBS1*, located at chromosome 8p21.3, which encodes the nibrin protein normally involved in DNA damage repair (6,38). This disease is rare, occurring in 1 of 100,000 births (15). Patients with Nijmegen breakage syndrome develop short stature, microcephaly, dysmorphic facial features, and intellectual impairment (6,15). These features are usually evident by 3 years of age. Patients also have recurrent infections as a result of cellular and humoral immune defects, gonadal failure, chromosomal instability, sensitivity to ionizing radiation, and an increased risk of hematopoietic tumors and to a lesser degree solid tumors; these patients have a 1,000-fold increased risk of developing lymphoma (15,41).

Gladkowska-Dura et al. (15) described the features of 14 non-Hodgkin lymphomas that arose in patients with Nijmegen breakage syndrome. The median age at the time of diagnosis of lymphoma was 9.5 years (range, 4 to 24 years). Eight patients developed DLBCL, 3 T-acute lymphoblastic leukemia, 1 Burkitt-like lymphoma, 1 mixed cellularity Hodgkin lymphoma, and 1 was designated as AITL-like B-cell lymphoma. The cases of DLBCL showed an activated B-cell immunophenotype and 25 percent were EBV positive (15).

X-Linked Agammaglobulinemia

The PID described by Bruton (8) is now designated as *X-linked agammaglobulinemia.* The patient was an 8-year-old boy who had at least 19 episodes of pneumococcal infection of the lungs. Analysis of this boy's serum showed virtually no IgG. The patient is typical of most patients with fully developed X-linked agammaglobulinemia. The disease results from mutations in the Bruton tyrosine kinase (*BTK*) gene which is critical to normal B-lymphocyte development. As a result of *BTK* mutations, B-cell maturation is blocked at a very early (pro-B) stage and patients cannot make antibodies (21,40).

X-linked agammaglobulinemia is rare, with a birthrate of 1 in 100,000. There is no ethnic preference. Patients have an increased risk of non-Hodgkin lymphomas, in particular, DLBCL.

Cartilage Hair Hypoplasia Syndrome

Patients with this disease have mutations in *RMRP*, a gene that encodes for the RNA component of the mitochondrial RNA processing endoribonuclease (6). *Cartilage hair hypoplasia syndrome* is rare and autosomal recessive. Patients have a wide variety of abnormalities including sparse hair, metaphyseal chondrodysplasia, anemia, combined immunodeficiency, and an increased risk of basal cell carcinoma and

non-Hodgkin lymphomas. In one study, 10 of 123 (8 percent) patients with cartilage hair hypoplasia syndrome developed lymphomas (35). The lymphomas in these patients are usually of B-cell lineage and can be positive for EBV; one patient developed a cutaneous CD30-positive lymphoproliferative disorder (35,36).

X-Linked Lymphoproliferative Syndrome

The classic form of *X-linked lymphoproliferative syndrome* (XLP), also known as XLP1, was first described by David Purtilo in 1975 (27). Purtilo's initial designation for this entity was Duncan disease, after the affected family he described. XLP affects young boys who are highly susceptible to EBV infection (28). After viral exposure, the boys develop lymphoma, hemophagocytic lymphohistiocytosis, or both. There is a second form of this disease, known as XLP2. These patients develop hemophagocytic lymphohistiocytosis, but have a much lower risk (if any) of developing lymphomas (12).

The molecular defects in XLP patients result from mutations involving either the *SH2D1A* (*XLP1*) or *XIAP* (*BIRC*) genes (6,28). The *SH2D1A* gene, located on chromosome Xq25, encodes the cytoplasmic signaling lymphocytic activation molecule-associated protein, also known as SLAM-associated protein (SAP). T cells require SAP to interact with antigen-presenting B cells, and since EBV infects B cells, XLP patients have no effective T-cell defense against EBV-infected B cells. Defects downstream of SAP that impair the interaction between T cells and B cells also can result in a similar syndrome, explaining the second type of X-linked lymphoproliferative syndrome, or XLP2.

Patients with XLP are boys who often present with lymphadenopathy and hepatosplenomegaly (28,38). In the classic form of XLP, the disease presents initially or the patient subsequently develops fatal infectious mononucleosis due to an inability to handle EBV infection. However, about 20 percent of patients have no evidence of EBV infection. In biopsy or autopsy specimens that show fatal infectious mononucleosis, there is a florid proliferation of small and large lymphocytes, immunoblasts, and plasma cells that expands and replaces the parenchyma of the lymph nodes and extranodal sites, particularly the liver, spleen (fig. 46-3), and gastrointestinal tract.

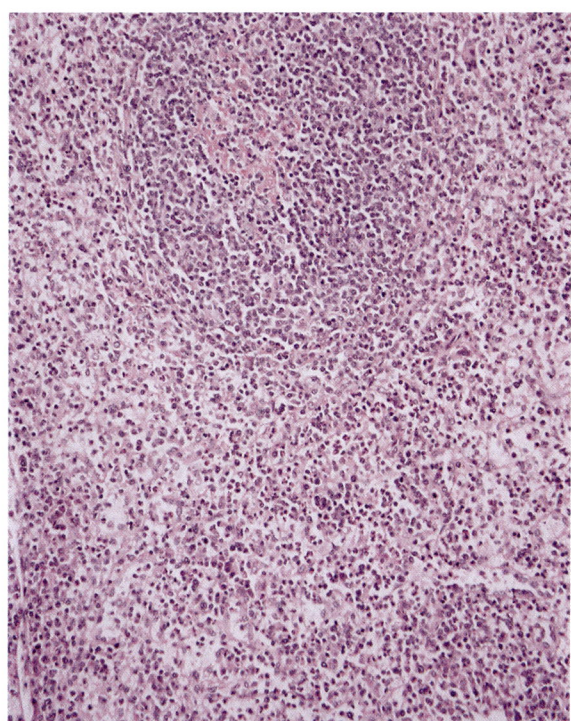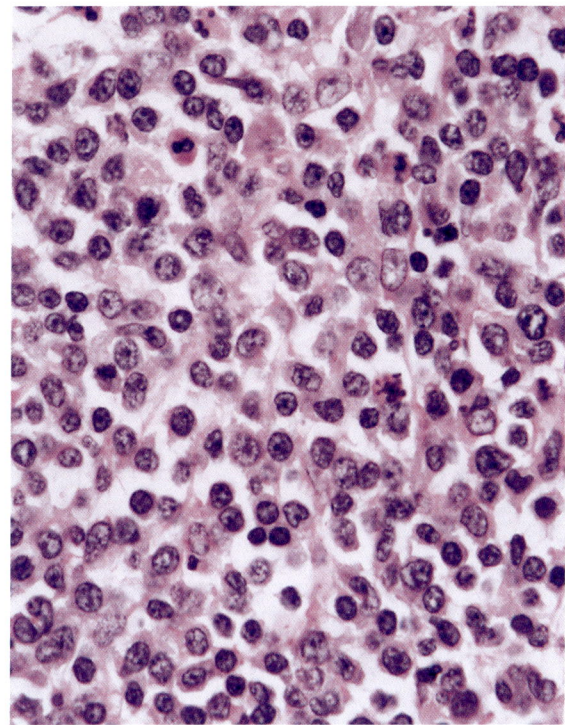

Figure 46-3

INFECTIOUS MONONUCLEOSIS INVOLVING SPLEEN IN X-LINKED LYMPHOPROLIFERATIVE SYNDROME

A teenage boy with X-linked lymphoproliferative syndrome subsequently died from infectious mononucleosis.
Left: At low magnification, the red pulp is expanded and infiltrated by lymphocytes of various sizes.
Right: High magnification of red pulp shows many lymphocytes of varying sizes (left, right: periodic acid–Schiff [PAS] stain).

Most lymphomas in patients with XLP are extranodal. The gastrointestinal tract and particularly the ileocecal region is a common site (28,38). Almost all lymphomas are of B-cell lineage and the most common histologic types include Burkitt lymphoma, DLBCL, and classic Hodgkin lymphoma. About two thirds of these lymphomas are positive for EBV (28,38).

Autoimmune Lymphoproliferative Syndrome

Autoimmune lymphoproliferative syndrome (ALPS) is a rare disease characterized by defective lymphocyte apoptosis that results from mutations involving genes encoding for components of the extrinsic apoptotic pathway. The most common mutation involves *FAS* (also known as *TNFRSF6*), but mutations also occur in FAS ligand or caspases 8 or 10 (26,38). The mutations may be germline (most often) or somatic (phenocopies), and either heterozygous or homozygous (26). The mTOR pathway is hyperactive in ALPS and may be a therapeutic target (39).

Patients tend to present as children or young adults with recurrent infections, lymphadenopathy or splenomegaly, and often autoimmune cytopenias (26). Patients have a characteristic expansion of mature α/β T cells that are negative for CD4 and CD8 (double negative). Double-negative T cells are increased in blood, bone marrow, lymph nodes (fig. 46-4), and spleen (26). Patients also have mild defects in marginal zone B-cell function, possible related to infiltration or replacement of splenic marginal zones by double-negative T cells (25).

Patients with ALPS have an increased risk of both non-Hodgkin lymphomas and Hodgkin lymphomas, including classic and nodular lymphocyte-predominant Hodgkin lymphoma (26,30,38). Price et al. (26) reported 18 patients with ALPS who developed lymphoma. Their median age was 18 years (range, 5 to 60 years) and 14 were male. All patients had *FAS* mutations and the lymphomas included Hodgkin lymphomas and non-Hodgkin lymphomas. Mixed

723

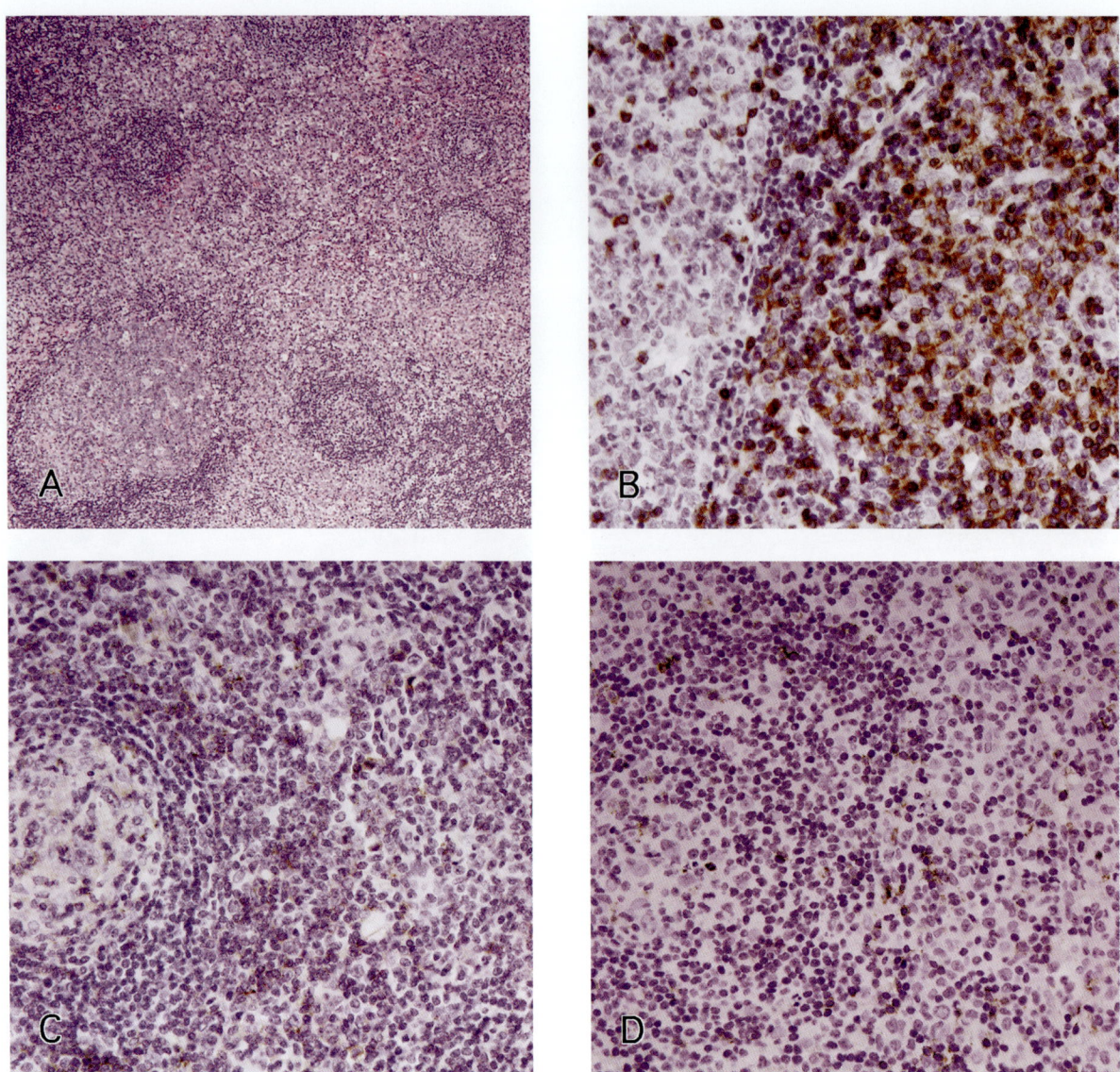

Figure 46-4

AUTOIMMUNE LYMPHOPROLIFERATIVE DISORDER INVOLVING LYMPH NODE

A: Follicular and paracortical hyperplasia are present (H&E stain).

B: The anti-CD3 antibody highlights many T cells in the paracortical compartment (reactive follicle is at left).

C,D: The T cells in the paracortex are negative for CD4 (C) and CD8 (D) (B–D: immunohistochemistry with hematoxylin counterstain).

cellularity was the most common type of Hodgkin lymphoma, followed by the nodular lymphocyte-predominant and lymphocyte-rich classic types. The non-Hodgkin lymphomas were mostly of B-cell lineage and included T-cell/histiocyte-rich large B-cell lymphoma, Burkitt lymphoma, follicular lymphoma, and mantle cell lymphoma. There was also one case of peripheral T-cell lymphoma and a case of histiocytic sarcoma.

Activated Phosphoinositide 3-Kinase δ Syndrome

Patients with activated phosphoinositide 3-kinase δ syndrome (APDS) have heterozygous gain-of-function mutations in the *PIK3Cδ* gene that encodes for p110δ protein, the catalytic component of phosphoinositide 3-kinase δ (2). Patients with this form of PID present with recurrent respiratory infections, progressive lymphopenia, and defective antibody production. Patients also have an increase of lymphoma, particularly B-cell lymphomas of various types (2,10a,20).

Interleukin-2-Inducible T-Cell Kinase Deficiency

Patients with *interleukin-2-inducible T-cell kinase (ITK) deficiency* have an autosomal recessive disease associated with lymphadenopathy, lung involvement, and a poor prognosis. These patients have homozygous mutations of *ITK*, located at 5q31-32, that result in ITK deficiency, impaired T-cell receptor signaling, and abnormal effector function of CD4-positive and CD8-positive T cells (17). Patients are unable to control EBV infection and develop signs and symptoms that overlap with patients who have XLP.

Patients with ITK deficiency have an increased risk of EBV-positive lymphoproliferative disorders. EBV infection with a type 2 latency pattern is present in most cases. The most common lymphoma is classic Hodgkin lymphoma, most often mixed cellularity type. Other patients develop polymorphic B-cell lymphoproliferative disorders, monomorphic B-cell lesions that resemble DLBCL, and rarely, Hodgkin-like lesions (4).

Other Immunodeficiency Disorders Likely Associated with an Increased Risk of Lymphoma

In recent years, other PIDs have been reported that are likely to be associated with an increased risk of lymphoma.

Coronin-1A Deficiency. A family of three children was reported with an inability to control EBV infection (24). The patients were young, about 1 year of age or less, and all three had a missense mutation in the *CORO1A* that encodes for coronin-1A. These patients had severe CD4-positive T-cell lymphopenia, impaired T-cell development, and low numbers of T and NK cells. The patients developed extranodal, B-lineage and EBV-positive lymphoproliferative disorders that were associated with oligoclonal or monoclonal *IGH* and T-cell receptor gene rearrangements (24).

CD27 Deficiency. Three families have been reported with CD27 deficiency as a result of a homozygous mutation in the gene encoding for the transmembrane receptor of CD27 (31). Patients with this defect show a spectrum of abnormalities including asymptomatic deficiency of memory B cells, hypogammaglobulinemia, EBV-associated hemophagocytic lymphohistiocytosis, and EBV-positive lymphoproliferative disorders and lymphomas.

HISTOLOGIC FINDINGS

The full range of LPDs that occur in patients with secondary immunodeficiency of various types also occurs in patients with PIDs. In general, patients with DNA repair defects have a higher frequency of monomorphic LPDs or overt lymphomas. In contrast, patients with other types of PID more often develop polymorphic B-cell LPDs as well as monomorphic LPDs. Here we focus on monomorphic lesions that occur in patients with PID.

In PID patients, 75 percent of all lymphoid neoplasms are non-Hodgkin lymphomas, with DLBCL being the most common type (figs. 46-5, 46-6) (38). Some DLBCLs show polymorphous features or exhibit plasmacytoid differentiation similar to DLBCL arising in other immunodeficiency settings. Other non-Hodgkin lymphomas that occur in PID patients include Burkitt lymphoma, follicular lymphoma, lymphomatoid granulomatosis, extranodal marginal zone B-cell lymphoma, and rarely, peripheral T-cell lymphoma (30).

Hodgkin lymphomas represent up to 15 percent of lymphomas in PID patients (fig. 46-7) (16,29,38). Classic Hodgkin lymphoma is the most common and the mixed cellularity and lymphocyte depleted types are over-represented compared with immunocompetent patients (16). Nodular lymphocyte-predominant Hodgkin lymphoma is rare in PID patients, with the exception of patients with ALPS. EBV is commonly positive in the Reed-Sternberg and Hodgkin (RS+H) cells of classic Hodgkin lymphoma cases; the virus can be present in small lymphocytes in addition to the neoplastic cells, similar to Hodgkin lymphoma in other immunodeficiency disorders.

Approximately 10 percent of lymphoid neoplasms in patients with PID are leukemias.

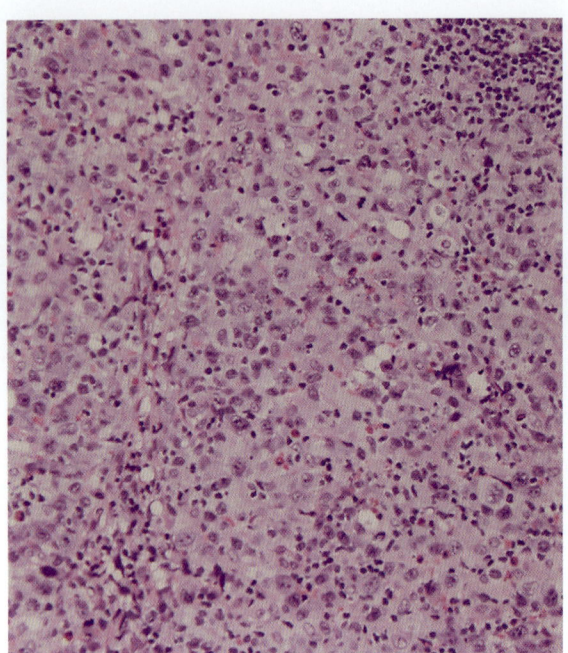
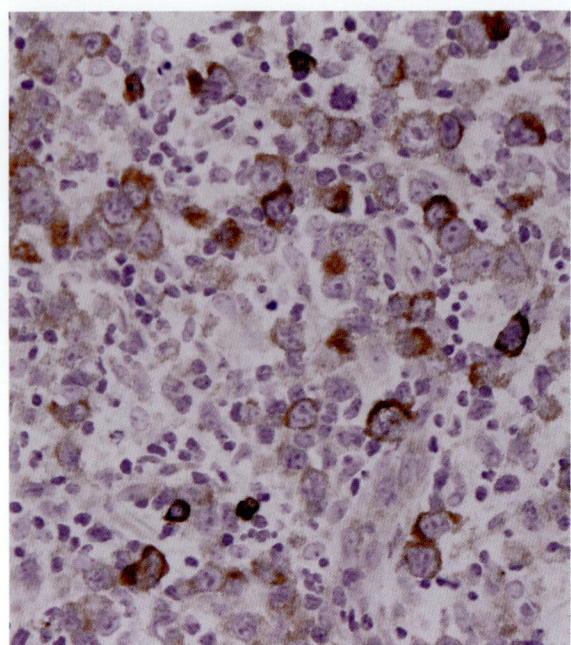

Figure 46-5

DIFFUSE LARGE B-CELL LYMPHOMA IN PATIENT WITH WISKOTT-ALDRICH SYNDROME

Left: The lymphoma is composed of large cells, some of which have plasmacytoid differentiation (H&E stain).
Right: Immunohistochemical analysis shows that a subset of large cells expresses cytoplasmic monotypic lambda light chain (immunohistochemistry with hematoxylin counterstain).

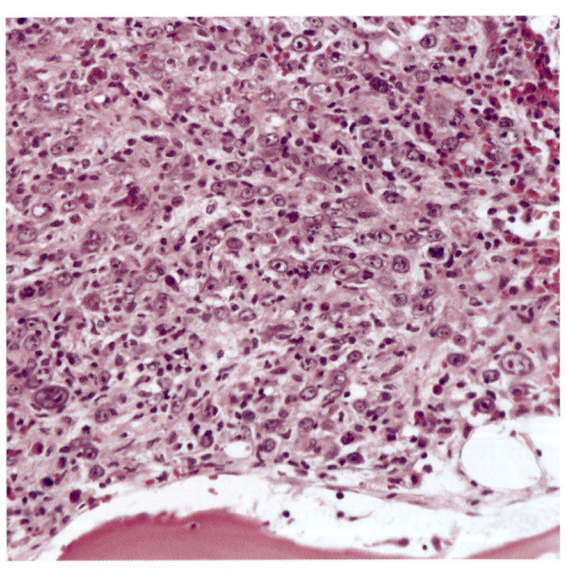

Figure 46-6

DIFFUSE LARGE B-CELL LYMPHOMA IN A PATIENT WITH COMMON VARIABLE IMMUNODEFICIENCY

The bone marrow medullary space is extensively replaced by lymphoma. The lymphoma cells had Hodgkin-like features but were CD20(+) and CD15(-) (not shown) (H&E stain).

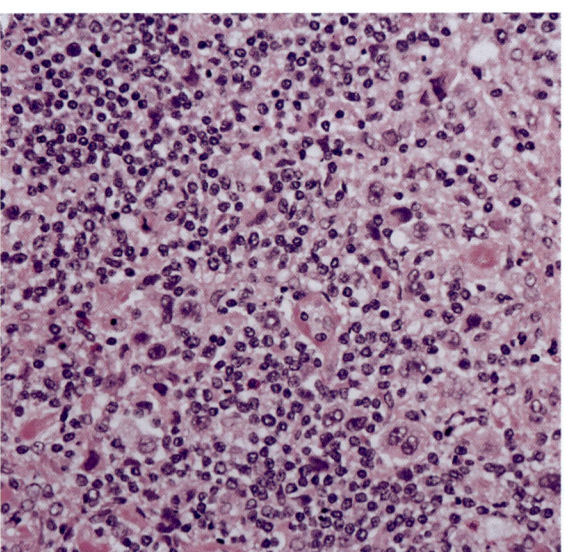

Figure 46-7

CLASSIC HODGKIN LYMPHOMA INVOLVING CERVICAL LYMPH NODE

A teenage boy had a poorly characterized primary immunodeficiency disorder. Many Hodgkin cells are present in a reactive cellular background (H&E stain).

These include T-acute lymphoblastic leukemia and T-cell prolymphocytic leukemia (38).

CYTOLOGIC FINDINGS

Few cases of PID assessed by fine-needle aspiration are reported in the literature. In our experience, smears of lymphomas associated with PID resemble their counterparts in immunocompetent patients.

IMMUNOPHENOTYPIC FINDINGS

Most lymphomas that arise in PID patients are of B-cell lineage (38). Cases of DLBCL are similar to those arising in other immunodeficiency diseases. The lymphoma cells express pan-B-cell antigens. In cases with plasmacytoid differentiation, monotypic cytoplasmic immunoglobulin may be expressed and B-cell antigens such as CD20 can be downregulated. EBV is present in a subset of cases of DLBCL and Burkitt lymphoma. In EBV-positive DLBCLs, CD30 is often expressed by some cells. In the few cases assessed, most DLBCLs have an activated B-cell immunophenotype and are negative for CD10 (15). T-cell antigens, including CD5, are negative. The proliferation (Ki-67) rate is usually high in DLBCL and over 95 percent in Burkitt lymphoma. EBV infection can show various patterns of viral latency, depending on the degree of host immune compromise and histologic type. Many EBV-positive cases of DLBCL exhibit a type 2 (or less often type 3) latency pattern and are positive for EBV-encoded RNA1 (EBER1) by in situ hybridization and latent membrane protein-1 (LMP1).

Cases of classic Hodgkin lymphoma have an immunophenotype similar to cases in immunocompetent patients. The RS+H cells are CD15(+/-), CD30(+), PAX5(+) (dim), and CD45/LCA(-). EBV can be present in the neoplastic cells, particularly in mixed cellularity type. Peripheral T-cell lymphomas may have aberrant patterns of expression. Cases of T-cell prolymphocytic leukemia are often positive for TCL1. T-cell acute lymphoblastic leukemia has an immature T-cell immunophenotype (TdT positive).

MOLECULAR GENETIC FINDINGS

A number of specific molecular defects have been identified in PIDs (4,22). Although this topic is beyond the scope of this chapter, some of the common defects in PIDs associated with an increased risk of lymphoma are listed in Table 46-2.

Most B-cell lymphomas carry monoclonal immunoglobulin gene rearrangements. Monoclonal T-cell receptor gene rearrangements occur in T-cell lymphomas. In addition, T-cell clones of small size have been reported in a subset of B-cell lymphomas. The presence of a monoclonal B- or rarely T-cell population supports lymphoma, but integration with clinical and pathologic findings is required because small monoclonal populations and oligoclonal populations may occur in reactive lesions (38). In EBV-positive lymphomas, analysis of the EBV terminal repeat regions can be used to establish monoclonality. *MYC* translocations are associated with Burkitt lymphoma arising in PID patients.

In ataxia-telangiectasia, inversions or translocations of the T-cell receptor gene loci at 14q11, 7q32-35, and 7p15 are identified in approximately 10 percent of patients without lymphoma (22). These chromosomal abnormalities include inv(7)(p13q35), t(7;7)(p13;q35), t(7;14)(p13;q11), and t(14;14)(q11;q32). *TCL1* gene abnormalities have been reported in T-cell prolymphocytic leukemia.

DIFFERENTIAL DIAGNOSIS

Patients with PID may have highly atypical lymphoproliferative lesions that morphologically mimic lymphoma, but which lack immunophenotypic or molecular evidence of monoclonality and pursue a nonmalignant clinical course (32). It is also true that patients with PID die from aggressive lymphoproliferative disorders that fail to meet the criteria for lymphoma, but which cannot be controlled because of the immune defect; X-linked lymphoproliferative syndrome is such an example (28). The differential diagnosis of lymphoproliferative disorders in PID patients is otherwise similar to the differential diagnosis of similar lymphomas that occur in the context of other types of immunodeficiency as well as in immunocompetent patients.

TREATMENT AND PROGNOSIS

For severe immune defects, such as SCID, patients are treated and cured by stem cell transplantation if the disease is recognized early (9). For some defects, replacement therapy is effective. Gene therapy has been used for disorders where the molecular defect can be partially or completely repaired, such as X-linked hyper-IgM syndrome or adenosine deaminase deficiency (9,18). Patients with less severe immunodeficiency are managed conservatively by aggressive treatment of their infections, using prophylactic antibiotics. Intravenous immunoglobulin can be helpful for patients with antibody deficiency, such as those with CVID. Rituximab or prednisone may be helpful for manifestations of autoimmunity.

Prognosis needs to be assessed on an individual patient basis and depends on the underlying PID, the type of LPD, and the overall immunologic status of the patient. Patients with defects in cell-mediated (T-cell) immunity tend to do worse than patients with B-cell immune defects. Patients with PID have a substantially shorter survival period than immunocompetent patients when they develop lymphoma or leukemia (3,13). The shorter survival period is attributable to compromised host immunodeficiency as well as the challenges in administering the therapy as a result of the immunologic defect. Therefore, chemotherapy doses are often adjusted. Patients with ataxia-telangiectasia are highly sensitive to radiation therapy and therefore this modality is avoided, when possible.

REFERENCES

1. Al-Herz Aldhekri H, Barbouche MR, Rezaei N. Consanguinity and primary immunodeficiencies. Hum Hered 2014;77:138-143.

2. Angulo I, Vadas O, Garçon F, et al. Phosphoinositide 3-kinase γ gene mutation predisposes to respiratory infection and airway damage. Science 2013;342(6160):866-871.

3. Arico M, Mussolin L, Carraro E, et al. Non-Hodgkin lymphoma in children with an associated inherited condition: a retrospective analysis of the Associazione Italiana Ematologic Oncologia Pediatrica (AIEOP). Pediatr Blood Cancer 2015;62:1782-1789.

4. Bienemann K, Borkhardt A, Klapper W, Oschlies I. High incidence of Epstein-Barr virus (EBV)-positive Hodgkin lymphoma and Hodgkin lymphoma-like B-cell lymphoproliferations with EBV latency profile 2 in children with interleukin-2-inducible T-cell kinase deficiency. Histopathology 2015;67:607-616.

5. Bousfiha AA, Jeddane L, Ailal F, et al. Primary immunodeficiency diseases worldwide: more common than generally thought. J Clin Immunol 2013;33:1-7.

6. Bousfiha A, Jeddane L, Al-Herz W, et al. The 2015 IUIS phenotypic classification for primary immunodeficiencies. J Clin Immunol 2015;35:727-738.

7. Boyle JM, Buckley RH. Population prevalence of diagnosed primary immunodeficiency diseases in the United States. J Clin Immunol 2007;27:497-502.

8. Bruton OC. Agammaglobulinemia. Pediatrics 1952;9:722-728.

9. Cunningham-Rundles C, Ponda PP. Molecular defects in T- and B-cell primary immunodeficiency diseases. Nat Rev Immunol 2005;5:880-892.

10. de Vries E, Clinical Working Party of the European Society for Immunodeficiencies (ESID). Patient-centered screening for primary immunodeficiency: a multi-stage diagnostic for non-immunologists. Clin Exp Immunol 2006;145:204-214.

10a. Elkaim E, Neven B, Bruneau J, et al. Clinical and immunologic phenotype associated with activated phosphoinositide 3-kinase δ syndrome 2: a cohort study. J Allergy Clin Immunol 2016;138:210-218.

11. Etzioni A, Ochs HD. The Hyper IgM syndrome—an evolving story. Pediatr Res 2004;56:519-525.

12. Filipovich AH, Zhang K, Snow AL, Marsh RA. X-linked lymphoproliferative syndromes: brothers or distinct cousins? Blood 2010;116:3398-3408.

12a. Furudoï A, Gros A, Stanislas S, et al. Spleen histologic appearance in common variable immunodeficiency: analysis of 17 cases. Am J Surg Pathol 2016;40:958-967.

13. Gangemi S, Allegra A, Musolino C. Lymphoproliferative disease and cancer among patients with common variable immunodeficiency. Leuk Res 2015;39:389-396.

14. Gatti RA, Good RA. Occurrence of malignancy in immunodeficiency diseases. A literature review. Cancer 1971;28:89-98.

15. Gladkowska-Dura M, Dzierzanowska-Fangrat K, Dura WT et al. Unique morphological spectrum of lymphomas in Nijmegen breakage syndrome (NBS) patients with high frequency of consecutive lymphoma formation. J Pathol 2008;216:337-344.

16. Hummel JM, Thorland EC, Lim MS. Hodgkin lymphoma in a young child contributing to the diagnosis of ataxia telangiectasia: review of the literature. J Hematop 2010; 3:69-76.

17. Huck K, Feyen O, Niehues T, et al. Girls homozygous for an IL-2-inducible T cell kinase mutation that leads to protein deficiency develop fatal EBV-associated lymphoproliferation. J Clin Invest 2009;119:1350-1358.

18. Jain A. Kovacs JA, Nelson DL, et al. Partial immune reconstitution of X-linked hyper IgM syndrome with recombinant CD40 ligand. Blood 2011;118:3811-3817.

19. Joshi AY, Iyer VN, Hagan JB, St Sauver JL, Boyce TG. Incidence and temporal trends of primary immunodeficiency: a population-based cohort study. Mayo Clin Proc 2009;84:16-22.

20. Kracker S, Curtis J, Ibrahim MAA, et al. Occurrence of B-cell lymphoma in patients with activated phosphoinositide 3-kinase γ syndrome. J Allergy Clin Immunol 2014;134:233-236.

21. Lee PP, Chen TX. Jiang LP, et al. Clinical characteristics and genotype-phenotype correlation in 62 patients with X-linked agammaglobulinemia. J Clin Immunol 2010;30:121-131.

22. Lim MS, Elenitoba-Johnson KS. The molecular pathology of primary immunodeficiencies. J Mol Diagn 2004;6:59-83.

23. Morrell D, Cromartie E, Swift M. Mortality and cancer incidence in 263 patients with ataxia-telangiectasia. J Natl Cancer Inst 1986;77:89-92.

24. Moshous D, Martin E, Carpentier W, et al. Whole-exome sequencing identifies coronin-1A deficiency in 3 siblings with immunodeficiency and EBV-associated lymphoproliferation. J Allergy Clin Immunol 2013;131:1594-1603.

25. Neven B, Magerus-Chatiner A, Florkin B, et al. A survey of 90 patients with autoimmune lymphoproliferative syndrome related to TNFRSF6 mutation. Blood 2011;118:4798-4807.

26. Price S, Shaw PA, Seitz A, et al. Natural history of autoimmune lymphoproliferative syndrome associated with FAS gene mutations. Blood 2014;123:1989-1999.

27. Purtilo DT, Cassel CK, Yang JP, Harper R. X-linked recessive progressive combined variable immunodeficicency (Duncan's disease). Lancet 1975;1:935-940.

28. Rezaei N, Mahmoudi E, Aghamohammadi A, Das R, Nichols KE. X-linked lymphoproliferative syndrome: a genetic condition typified by the triad of infection, immunodeficiency and lymphoma. Br J Haematol 2011;152:13-30.

29. Robison LL, Stoker V, Frizzera G, Heinitz K, Meadows AT, Filipovich AH. Hodgkin's disease in pediatric patients with naturally-occurring immunodeficiency. Am J Pediatr Hematol Oncol 1987;9:189-192.

30. Salavoura K, Kolialexi A, Tsangaris G, Mavrou A. Development of cancer in patients with primary immunodeficiencies. Anticancer Res 2008;28:1263-1269.

31. Salzer E, Daschkey S, Choo S, et al. Combined immunodeficiency with life-threatening EBV-associated lymphoproliferative disorder in patients lacking functional CD27. Haematologica 2013;98:473-478.

32. Sander CA, Medeiros LJ, Weiss LM, Yano T, Sneller MC, Jaffe ES. Lymphoproliferative lesions in patients with common variable immunodeficiency syndrome. Am J Surg Pathol 1992;16:1170-1182.

33. Snover DC, Frizzera G, Spector BD, Perry GS 3rd, Kersey JH. Wiskott-Aldrich syndrome: histopathologic findings in the lymph nodes and spleens of 15 patients. Hum Pathol 1981;12:821-831.

34. Suarez F, Mahlaoui N, Canioni D, et al. Incidence, presentation, and prognosis of malignancies in ataxia-telangiectasia: a report from the French National Registry of Primary Immune Deficiencies. J Clin Oncol 2015;33:202-208.

35. Taskinen M, Jeskanen L, Karjalainen-Lindsberg ML, Mäkitie A, Mäkitie O, Ranki A. Combating cancer predisposition in association with idiopathic immune deficiency: a recurrent nodal and cutaneous T-cell lymphoproliferative disease in a patient with cartilage-hair hypoplasia. Clin Lymphoma Myeloma Leuk 2013;13:73-76.

36. Taskinen M, Ranki A, Pukkala E, Jeskanen L, Kaitila I, Mäkitie O. Extended follow-up of the Finnish cartilage-hair hypoplasia cohort confirms high incidence of non-Hodgkin lymphoma and basal cell carcinoma. Am J Med Genet A 2008;146A:2370-2375.

37. Unger S, Seidl M, Schmitt-Graeff A, et al. Ill-defined germinal centers and severely reduced plasma cells are histological hallmarks of lymphadenopathy in patients with common variable immunodeficiency. J Clin Immunol 2014;34:615-626.

38. Van Krieken JH, Onciu M, Elenitoba-Johnson KS, Jaffe ES. Lymphoproliferative diseases associated with primary immune disorders. In: Swerdlow SH, Campo E, Harris NL, et al., eds. WHO classification of tumours of haematopoietic and lymphoid tissues. Lyon: IARC Press; 2008:336-339.

39. Völkl S, Rensing-Ehl A, Allgäuer A, et al. Hyperactive mTOR pathway promotes lymphoproliferation and abnormal differentiation in autoimmune lymphoproliferative syndrome. Blood 2016;128:227-238.

40. Winkelstein JA, Marino MC, Lederman HM, et al. X-linked agammaglobulinemia: report on a United States registry of 201 patients. Medicine 2006;85:193-202.

41. Wolska-Kusnierz B, Gregorek H, Chrzanowska K, et al. Nijmegen breakage syndrome: clinical and immunological features, long-term outcome and treatment options—a retrospective analysis. J Clin Immunol 2015;35:538-549.

47 POST-TRANSPLANT LYMPHOPROLIFERATIVE DISORDERS

GENERAL FEATURES

Post-transplant lymphoproliferative disorders (PTLDs) are a highly heterogeneous group of diseases that arise following solid organ or hematopoietic stem cell transplantation. In the World Health Organization (WHO) classification (43a,44) PTLDs are subdivided into four broad groups based, in part, on their resemblance to lymphoid lesions arising in immunocompetent patients as follows: 1) nondestructive/early lesions that are clearly reactive; 2) polymorphic lesions that are composed of a highly heterogeneous population of cells not readily classified as one of the known types of lymphoma; 3) monomorphic lesions that meet the criteria for known types of lymphoma; and 4) classic Hodgkin lymphoma.

Although the PTLD classification system adopted by the WHO system has been in wide use for a number of years, this system has some limitations. As discussed by others and in the following chapter, the four major categories of PTLD are heterogeneous at the clinicopathologic and molecular levels, and likely reflect different etiologies. In particular, Epstein-Barr virus (EBV) infection is very important because EBV-positive B-cell nondestructive/early and polymorphic PTLDs are more likely to respond to reduced immunosuppression. These lesions can be polyclonal or oligoclonal, or in the case of polymorphic lesions, often monoclonal. In contrast, monomorphic PTLD lesions, even those lesions that can be EBV-positive (e.g., Burkitt lymphoma), are virtually always monoclonal and infrequently respond to reduced immunosuppression. Weisenburger and Gross (49a) have suggested a new schema for the classification of PTLDs that emphasizes EBV and clonality status. In the remainder of this chapter, we follow the WHO classification system, but we acknowledge the merit of developing a newer approach to the classification of PTLDs.

There are approximately 115,000 transplants performed worldwide each year (34). Kidney transplants, by far, are the most frequent. The overall frequency of PTLD in patients who undergo allogeneic transplantation is 1 to 3 percent (33), a frequency that is 20 to 120 percent higher than that in the general population (31). The risk of developing PTLD correlates with the type of transplant: highest in patients who have undergone more than one organ transplant (near 10 percent of all patients), lower in patients who have heart (5 to 6 percent) or lung (about 3 percent) transplants, lower still in patients who have undergone liver (1 to 3 percent) or kidney (0.5 to 1.0 percent) transplants, and the lowest risk in patients who undergo hematopoietic stem cell transplant (less than 1 percent) (5,18,22,34,44).

The major risk factor for developing PTLD is the extent of immunosuppression patients must experience to undergo the organ transplantation and subsequently maintain host tolerance for the transplant (18,20,44). The immunosuppression is thought to impair host T-cell function, particularly cytolytic T cells, which are responsible for attacking viruses, in particular, Epstein-Barr virus (EBV).

EBV plays a major role in the pathogenesis of PTLDs. Most of the adult population has been exposed to infection by EBV, present in a quiescent state in memory B cells once a host recovers from infection. EBV is kept under control in a healthy person by host immunosurveillance, particularly by cytolytic CD8-positive T cells. As a result of the immunosuppression needed to facilitate allograft transplantation, EBV infection can be reactivated. In addition, primary infection of an EBV-negative host via the allograft can occur (18,34).

From 60 to 80 percent of all cases of PTLD, depending on the study, are positive for EBV infection (24,34,44). EBV is commonly present in PTLDs in monoclonal form. EBV infection has two phases: lytic and latent. Since lytic infection by EBV results in cell death, EBV-infected tumors, such as PTLD, exhibit latent infection by the virus, usually a type III latency pattern with expression of EBV-small encoded RNA1 (EBER1), latent membrane protein type 1 (LMP1), and all EBV nuclear antigens (EBNA) by the infected cells. EBV LMP1, via its CD40-like functions, can activate the NF-κB pathway, resulting in induction of telomerase. High telomerase activity inhibits the viral protein BZLF-1 which is a regulator of viral lytic phase infection, driving infected cells to a latent pattern of EBV infection (34). EBV also co-opts the host B-cell microRNA program. By viral suppression of host miR-194, the B cells in PTLD secrete interleukin 10, which stimulates B-cell growth in an autocrine manner (15).

Based on the important role of EBV and impaired host T-cell function in pathogenesis, it is not surprising that major risk factors for PTLD include: 1) the EBV status of the host prior to transplant (EBV-negative patients are at greater risk); 2) the dose of immunosuppression; and 3) the length of time the patient is immunosuppressed. Patient age of under 10 or over 60 years is a risk factor because these patients are at higher risk of primary infection or reactivation, respectively. Higher EBV viral load in the serum or whole blood after transplant also correlates with increased risk of PTLD, as does the use of certain immunosuppressive drugs including antithymocyte globulin, anti-CD3 antibody, tacrolimus, cyclosporine, and calcineurin inhibitors (20,22–24,26).

Before transplant, certain infections are also thought to be risk factors for PTLD, including infection by hepatitis C, cytomegalovirus, and human herpesvirus 8 (HHV-8) (18,47). These infections are probably a manifestation of the compromised host immune status, although other mechanisms may be involved. Similarly, patients with certain types of cancer pretransplant also may be at increased risk for PTLDs (18).

Host genetic makeup also plays a role in predisposing patients to PTLD. Caucasians appear to be at a higher risk than African Americans (28). Certain HLA alleles associated with the development of PTLDs include: HLA-A2, HLA-A11, HLA-A26, HLA-B5, HLA-B18, HLA-B21, HLA-B35, and HLA-B38, Others have suggested that inherited cytokine polymorphisms (e.g., interferon-γ, TGF-β, TNFα) are involved in increased risk of PTLD (18,39,42).

For patients who undergo hematopoietic stem cell transplant, additional risk factors for PTLD include T-cell depletion of the allograft, HLA-mismatched graft, umbilical cord blood transplant, matched unrelated donor (MUD) graft, severity of graft-versus-host disease, use of total body irradiation, and hosts who have immunodeficiency diseases prior to receiving a graft (2,18,23,36).

The risk factors for patients with EBV-negative PTLDs are poorly understood. It seems likely that a subset of these cases, perhaps a large subset, are de novo lymphomas with their pathogenesis being unrelated to the history of transplantation. For cases related to transplant, there is speculation that these cases may be infected by EBV initially, but the virus is somehow lost, the so-called hit and run theory. Infection by unknown viruses, in the host or the allograft, may be a source of chronic antigenic stimulation (34). Genetic predisposition, as discussed above for EBV-positive cases, is likely relevant.

Some cases of PTLD are associated with either HHV-6 or HHV-8 infection. The cases associated with HHV-6 are so few that if the virus has any role in etiology it must be minor. It seems likely that most PTLDs associated with HHV-8 are better classified as primary effusion lymphoma involving body cavities or, rarely, tissue sites (so-called solid or extracavitary variant) because these lymphomas are likely driven primarily by HHV-8 and are clearly different from most cases of PTLD. Patients with HHV-8 infection also have an increased frequency of Kaposi sarcoma and other HHV-8-associated diseases following transplant (14).

CLINICAL FEATURES

PTLDs can arise "early" or "late" after transplantation (18,24,29,34,44). Early lesions are more often EBV-positive and arise within 1 to 2 years. Late lesions are more often EBV negative and occur 4 or more years after transplant. In general, patients who undergo hematopoietic stem cell transplantation develop PTLDs earlier, often within the first year. Most cases of PTLD following hematopoietic stem cell transplant are EBV positive (2,23,33,36).

Patients with PTLD present with systemic symptoms including weight loss, fever, anorexia, and fatigue (12,18,29,44). Sepsis can be an initial manifestation. In patients with B-cell PTLD,

Table 47-1

FEATURES OF NONDESTRUCTIVE (EARLY) LESIONS ARISING IN THE POST-TRANSPLANT SETTING

Category	Morphology	Immunophenotype	EBV[a]	Clonality Studies
Plasmacytic hyperplasia	Intact architecture; small lymphocytes, plasma cells, and few immunoblasts	Polytypic B cells and plasma cells; T cells not aberrant	Usually +	Typically polyclonal; small *IGH* clones identified by PCR-based methods in subset; no oncogene abnormalities
Infectious mononucleosis-like	Intact architecture; numerous immunoblasts; plasma cells and small lymphocytes present	Polytypic B cells and plasma cells; T cells not aberrant	Usually +	Typically polyclonal; small *IGH* clones identified by PCR-based methods in subset; no oncogene abnormalities
Florid follicular hyperplasia	Intact architecture	Polytypic B cells; germinal centers are CD10(+), BCL6(+), and BCL2(-)	+ / -	Polyclonal

[a]EBV = Epstein-Barr virus; PCR = polymerase chain reaction.

extranodal sites of disease are common (70 to 80 percent of patients) (12,22,26). The most common extranodal site of PTLD is the gastrointestinal tract (25 percent of patients) followed by bone marrow (10 percent of patients) (22). Other extranodal sites include the lung, liver, skin, and central nervous system. The allograft is involved in about a quarter of patients (12,18). Lymphadenopathy, with or without extranodal disease, occurs in 30 to 40 percent of patients.

In 2007, Swerdlow (43) reviewed the literature and identified 130 cases of NK/T-cell PTLD. This subset of PTLD is highly heterogeneous. In patients with NK/T-cell PTLD, extranodal sites of disease are most common, including bone marrow, blood, spleen, liver, skin, gastrointestinal tract, and the central nervous system. Lymphadenopathy occurs in approximately 25 percent of patients (43).

HISTOLOGIC AND IMMUNOPHENOTYPIC FINDINGS

The morphologic features of PTLD are highly variable (12,21,43,44,47). There are four major categories specified in the WHO classification. In the following discussion, we separate monomorphic B-cell from T-cell PTLDs based on their many differences and to better organize the information presented.

Nondestructive Lesions

Most nondestructive (formerly known as early) lesions are EBV positive and occur early after transplantation (Table 47-1). Nondestruc-

tive lesions are subdivided into three types: *plasmacytic hyperplasia* (fig. 47-1), *infectious mononucleosis-like,* and *florid follicular hyperplasia*. These lesions occur commonly in lymph nodes, but can involve extranodal sites. The lymphoid tissue of Waldeyer ring is a common extranodal site; another is the bone marrow.

In plasmacytic hyperplasia, tissues show architectural preservation and expanded interfollicular regions with many plasma cells and immunoblasts. In infectious mononucleosis-like lesions, the paracortical regions are expanded by many immunoblasts and fewer plasma cells. These two types of nondestructive/early lesions are composed of a mixture of small lymphocytes, mature-appearing plasma cells, and immunoblasts.

The small lymphocytes of plasmacytic hyperplasia and infectious mononucleosis-like lesions are a mixture of B cells and T cells. Immunoblasts are of B- or T-cell lineage and are CD30(+), CD45/LCA(+), and CD15(-). Plasma cells express CD138 and other plasma cell-associated markers and are polytypic (fig. 47-1). Plasmacytoid dendritic cells are increased in all types of PTLDs, but particularly so in these lesions (17).

Follicular Hyperplasia. Although follicular hyperplasia was not included in the 2008 WHO classification of PTLDs, lymph nodes and extranodal sites (fig. 47-2) showing prominent reactive follicular hyperplasia often are present early after transplantation. These lesions include cases in which EBV-positive cells are preferentially located in germinal centers, as well as EBV-negative cases. Monoclonal karyotypes also

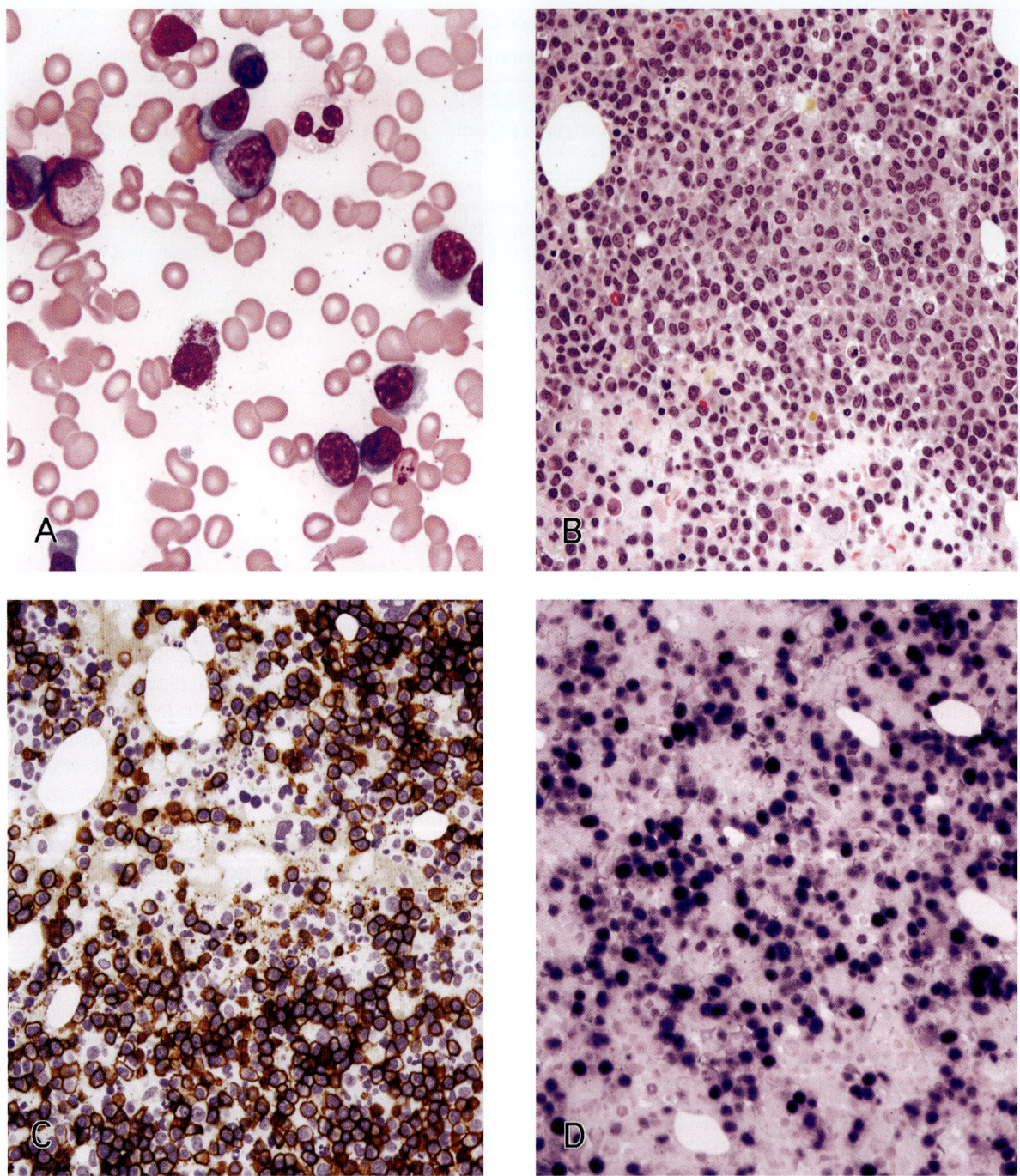

Figure 47-1

NONDESTRUCTIVE EPSTEIN-BARR VIRUS (EBV)-POSITIVE POST-TRANSPLANT LYMPHOPROLIFERATIVE DISORDER (PTLD)

This case of plasmacytic hyperplasia type involved the bone marrow. The patient was a 57-year-old man with a history of aplastic anemia who underwent allogeneic bone marrow transplantation.

A: The bone marrow aspirate smear shows many, mostly mature, plasma cells (Wright-Giemsa stain).

B: The aspirate clot specimen also shows many plasma cells (hematoxylin and eosin [H&E] stain).

C: The plasma cells are positive for CD138 (Immunohistochemistry with hematoxylin counterstain).

D: In situ hybridization for EBV-encoded RNA1 (EBER1) shows many positive cells (in situ hybridization with eosin counterstain).

Table 47-2

FEATURES OF POLYMORPHIC AND MONOMORPHIC B-CELL PTLDs

Category	Morphology	Immunophenotype	EBV [a]	Clonality Studies
Polymorphic	Partially or completely effaced architecture	Full spectrum of lymphoid maturation (small to immunoblasts), plasma cells, and histiocytes	Usually +	Monoclonal *IGH* rearrangements common; cytogenetic abnormalities in up to 30%; no rearrangements of *MYC, BCL6, BCL2*
Diffuse large B-cell lymphoma	Effaced architecture	Pan-B-cell antigens + (CD19, CD20, CD22, PAX5), CD45+, CD5-, CD30+/- (often partial+), sIg +/-, BCL2+/-, CD10-/+, Ki-67 high but variable	50-75% +	Monoclonal *IGH* rearrangements cytogenetic abnormalities in up to 75%; *MYC* rearrangements -/+ *BCL6* mutations common
Burkitt lymphoma	Effaced architecture	Pan-B-cell antigens+, CD10+, BCL6+, PAX5+, sIg+, CD5-, CD30-, BCL2, Ki-67 very high	~50% +	Monoclonal *IGH* rearrangements; *MYC* rearrangements with immunoglobulin partner
Plasma cell myeloma	Effaced architecture	cIg+, CD38+, CD138+, CD20-, Ki-67 intermediate but variable	Usually -	Monoclonal *IGH* rearrangements
Plasmacytoma-like	Effaced architecture	cIg+, CD38+, CD138+, CD20-, Ki-67 intermediate but variable	Variable	Monoclonal *IGH* rearrangements
Plasmablastic lymphoma	Effaced architecture	CD38+, CD138+, cIg +/-, CD30+/-, CD20-, CD45-, Ki-67 high but variable	60-90% +	Monoclonal *IGH* rearrangements
Small B-cell lymphoma	Marginal zone lymphomas most common; often plasmacytic	Pan B-cell antigens+, CD5-, CD10-, CD23-/+; EBER+ cIg+/-	Usually +	Monoclonal *IGH* rearrangements

[a]EBV = Epstein-Barr virus; s = surface; c = cytoplasmic.

have been identified in about 10 percent of cases (48). For these reasons florid follicular hyperplasia has been included in the 2016 revision of the WHO classification (43a). In follicular hyperplasia, the germinal center B cells are polytypic, CD10(+) and BCL6(+), and BCL2(-).

Polymorphic Lesions

Polymorphic PTLDs represent 15 to 20 percent of all cases of B-cell PTLD and are the most common type of PTLD in the pediatric age group (Table 47-2) (18,44). These lesions involve lymph nodes or extranodal sites, and are usually EBV positive.

The architecture of affected organs is effaced by a highly heterogeneous infiltrate that includes small lymphocytes, immunoblasts, histiocytes, and plasma cells (figs. 47-3, 47-4). Reed-Sternberg-like cells are found in some cases. Granulocytes are rare. Areas of geographic necrosis are common and the mitotic rate is often high. These lesions do not resemble any known types of de novo lymphoma. The lymphoid cells are a mixture of B cells, T cells,

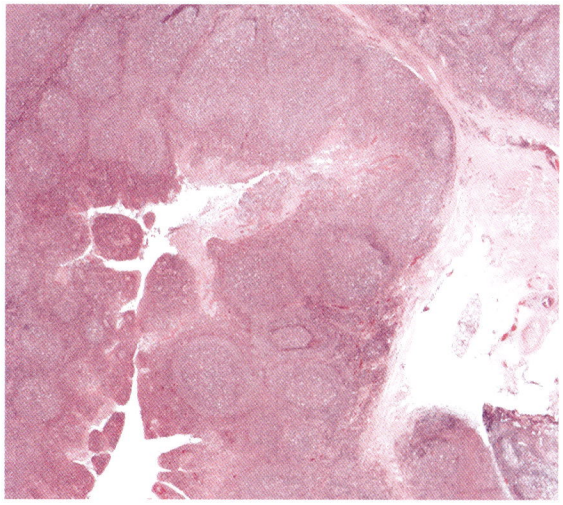

Figure 47-2

FLORID FOLLICULAR HYPERPLASIA

This lesion occurred in the tonsil of an adolescent boy a few months following allogeneic hematopoietic stem cell transplantation and is consistent with a nondestructive lesion. EBV-positive cells were present in moderate number in this specimen (not shown). Cases of follicular hyperplasia that arise after transplant have been included in the 2016 revision of the WHO classification (H&E stain).

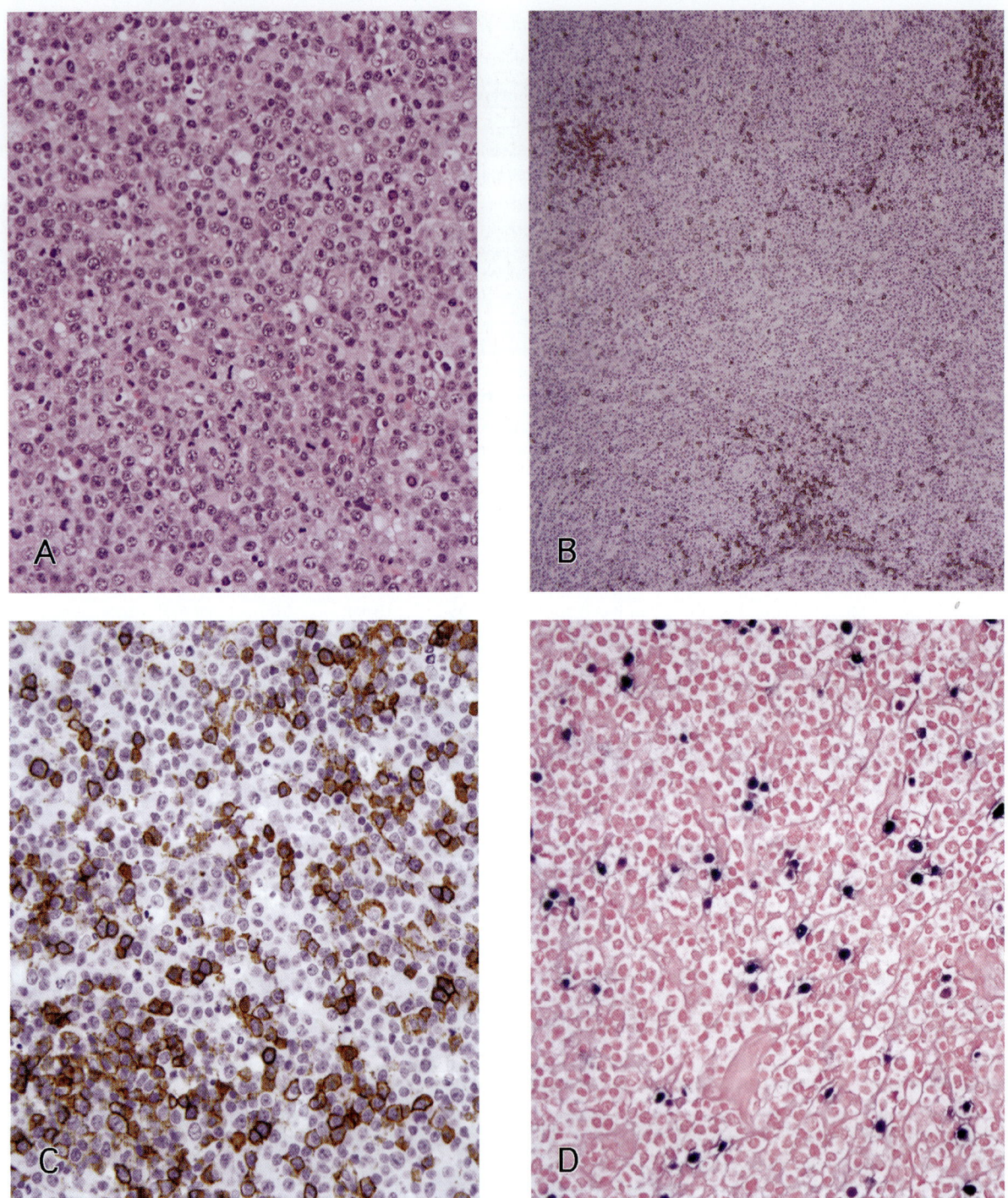

Figure 47-3

EBV-POSITIVE POLYMORPHIC POST-TRANSPLANT LYMPHOPROLIFERATIVE DISORDER INVOLVING LYMPH NODE

A 55-year-old woman previously underwent allogeneic hematopoietic stem cell transplant for acute myeloid leukemia.
A: The lesion has a diffuse pattern and is composed of plasma cells, lymphocytes, and histiocytes (H&E stain).
B,C: The lesion is composed of few CD20-positive B cells (B) and many CD138-positive plasma cells (C) (immuno-histochemistry with hematoxylin counterstain).
D: Scattered cells are positive for EBER1 (in situ hybridization with eosin counterstain).

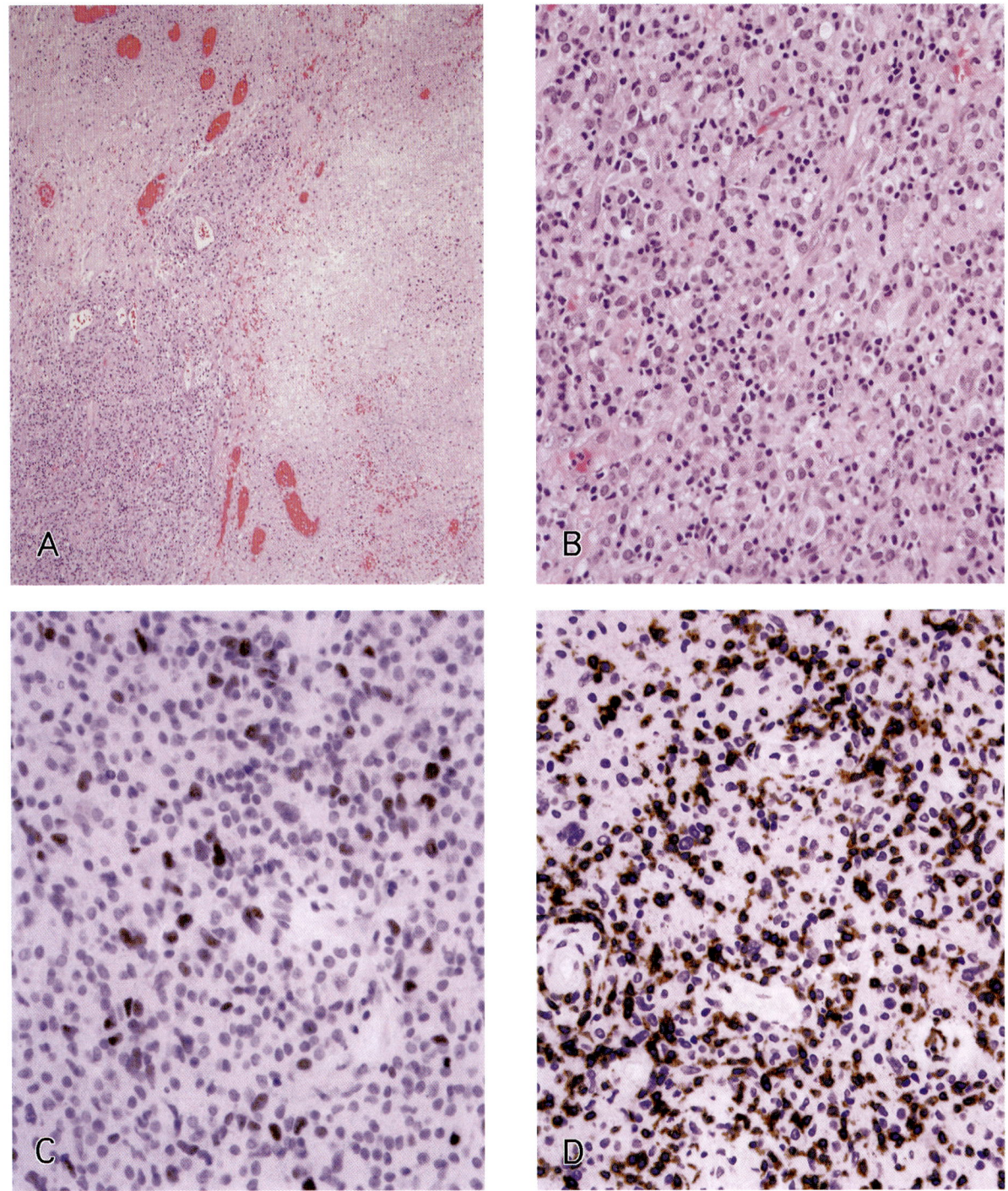

Figure 47-4

EBV-POSITIVE POLYMORPHIC POST-TRANSPLANT LYMPHOPROLIFERATIVE DISORDER INVOLVING BRAIN

A 47-year-old man previously underwent kidney transplantation.

A: There is extensive necrosis in the biopsy specimen (A,B: H&E stain).

B: The lesion is diffuse and composed of many lymphocytes and histiocytes.

C,D: Immunohistochemical studies showed scattered PAX5-positive B cells (C) and many CD3-positive T cells (D). This lesion was also positive for EBER1 (not shown) (immunohistochemistry with hematoxylin counterstain).

and histiocytes; T cells and histiocytes often predominate. The large immunoblasts are frequently CD30 positive. Plasmacytoid lymphocytes or plasma cells express CD138 and either polytypic or monotypic immunoglobulin light chains. The proliferation rate, as assessed by Ki-67, is usually 50 to 80 percent.

Monomorphic Lesions: B Cell

About 90 to 95 percent of monomorphic PTLDs are of B-cell lineage and most of these lesions (about 75 percent), are EBV positive (Table 47-2) (12,44). Monomorphic lesions are composed of a uniform population of cells that appear transformed and usually large. Although most monomorphic PTLDs are composed of a monotonous population of cells, some are composed of transformed lymphoid cells, including plasmacytoid lymphocytes, centroblasts, and immunoblasts, and do not appear monotonous. Therefore, a predominance of transformed cells and not monotony (although these two features are often present together) is required for the diagnosis of monomorphic PTLD.

Diffuse Large B-Cell Lymphoma. The most common type of monomorphic PTLD is diffuse large B-cell lymphoma (DLBCL) (12,18,21,44). These lesions have a diffuse pattern; a starry sky appearance is present in a minority of cases (figs. 47-5–47-7). Geographic areas of necrosis are common, as are mitotic figures and apoptotic cells. The lymphoid cells most often have centroblastic features, but immunoblastic or anaplastic features also occur.

The lymphoid cells are predominantly B cells positive for pan-B-cell antigens (fig. 47-5B) and negative for CD3 and CD5. Some large lymphoid cells are often CD30 positive (fig. 47-5C). MUM1/IRF4 is often positive and CD138 highlights the plasmacytoid lymphocytes and plasma cells that may be present. Most cases have a high proliferation rate, ranging from 50 to 90 percent (fig. 47-6, right).

These lesions most often have an activated B-cell immunophenotype, but some have a germinal B-cell immunophenotype [CD10(+) and BCL6(+)]. Cell of origin classification does not appear to have prognostic value in the post-transplant setting (49). EBV is present in 50 to 75 percent of DLBCL cases (fig. 47-5D); cases with a germinal center B-cell immunophe-

notype are less often EBV positive compared with cases that have an activated B-cell immunophenotype. (It seems possible that some EBV-negative germinal center B-cell DLBCLs are unrelated to the transplant.)

Burkitt Lymphoma. This tumor is an uncommon form of monomorphic PTLD. Burkitt lymphoma arises more often in children than adults (25,35,51), and males are affected more often than females in both children and adults. Burkitt lymphoma tends to arise late after transplant: in children, the median interval was 52 months (range, 6 to 107 months) in one study of 12 cases (35) and in adults, it was 5.7 years (51).

Histologically, Burkitt lymphoma arising in the post-transplant setting closely resembles Burkitt lymphoma in immunocompetent patients (35,44). The neoplasms have a diffuse and starry sky pattern, with high mitotic and apoptotic activity. Cytologically, the lymphoma cells are intermediate in size, with multiple small nucleoli. The neoplastic cells express pan-B-cell antigens, CD10, and BCL6, and are BCL2 negative. Over 95 percent of the cells are proliferating, as shown by the Ki-67 immunostain. The frequency of EBV infection is higher in Burkitt lymphoma arising in the post-transplant setting than in immunocompetent patients. Approximately half of cases in adults are EBV positive, with a higher frequency in children (35,51).

Plasma Cell Myeloma. Less than 1 percent of PTLDs closely resemble plasma cell myeloma (3,8). Older patient age, infection by hepatitis C, and therapy with antithymocyte globulin (ATG) appears to correlate with an increased risk of plasma cell myeloma. Patients commonly present with lytic bone lesions, serum and/or urine paraprotein, and sheets of plasma cells in the bone marrow (3,8). The plasma cells express monotypic cytoplasmic immunoglobulin and plasma cell-associated antigens.

Plasmacytoma-Like Lesion. These tumors represent about 4 percent of all PTLDs (46). They can arise early or late after transplant, but most arise late, with a median interval of approximately 8 years after transplant. Patients commonly present with an extranodal mass, and either localized or disseminated disease. A serum paraprotein is common, osteolytic bone lesions are uncommon, and the bone marrow

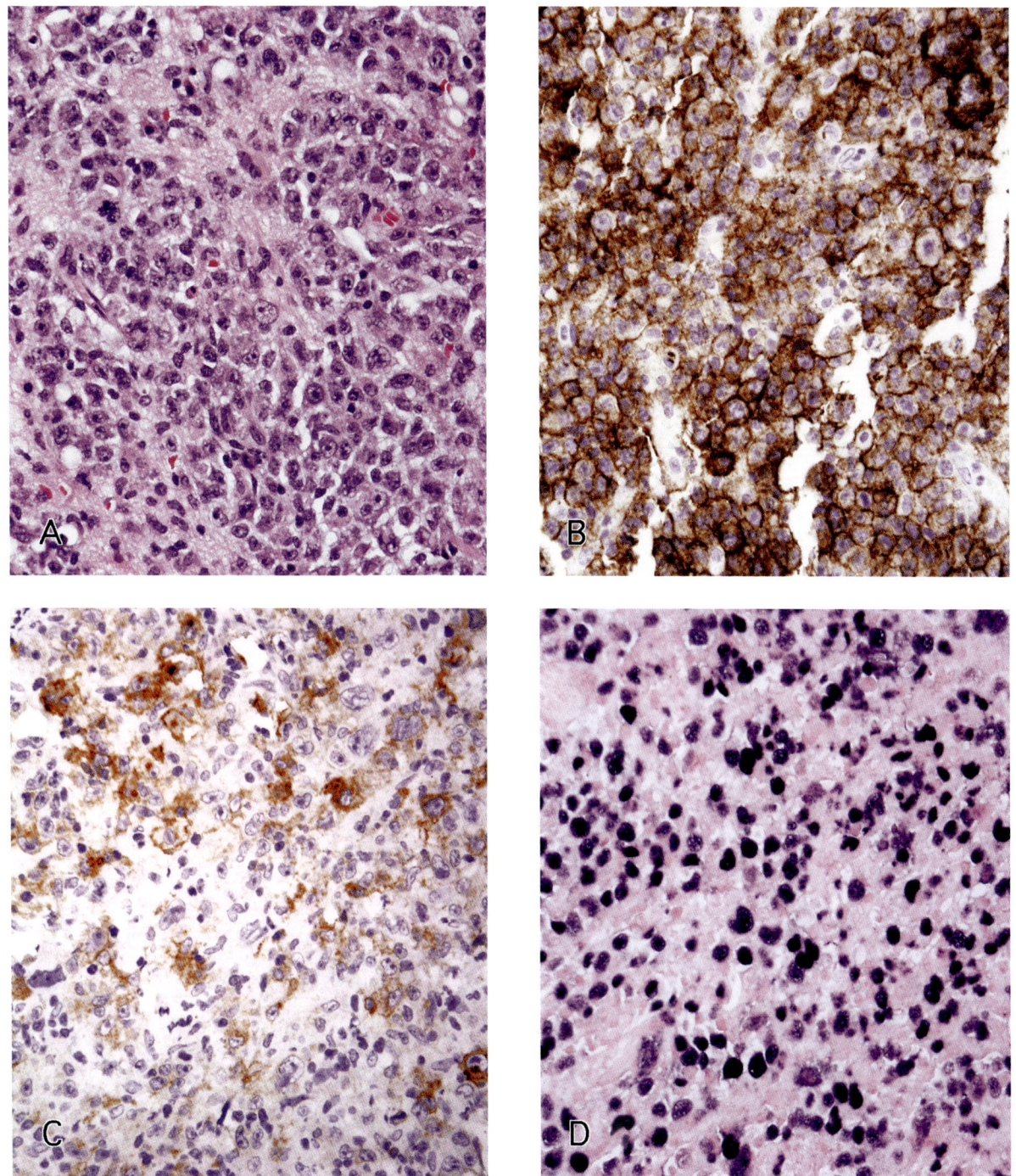

Figure 47-5

**EBV-POSITIVE MONOMORPHIC POST-TRANSPLANT LYMPHOPROLIFERATIVE
DISORDER CONSISTENT WITH DIFFUSE LARGE B-CELL LYMPHOMA INVOLVING BRAIN**

A 14-year-old boy had undergone umbilical cord transplantation for B-acute lymphoblastic leukemia.

A: Sheets of large lymphoid cells are present in a diffuse pattern (H&E stain).

B,C: The cells are diffusely positive for CD19 (B) and some express CD30 (C) (immunohistochemistry with hematoxylin counterstain).

D: Many EBER1-positive cells are present (in situ hybridization with eosin counterstain).

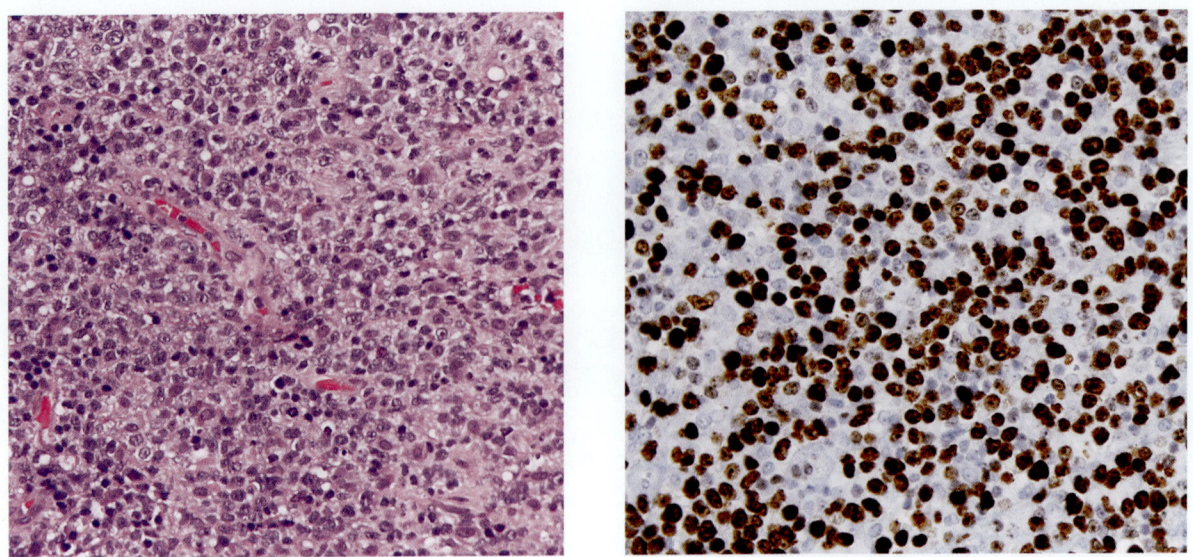

Figure 47-6

EBV-POSITIVE MONOMORPHIC POST-TRANSPLANT LYMPHOPROLIFERATIVE DISORDER CONSISTENT WITH DIFFUSE LARGE B-CELL LYMPHOMA INVOLVING NECK LYMPH NODE

Left: In a patient who had earlier undergone a kidney transplant, the lymph node is replaced by a monomorphic population of large lymphoid cells (H&E stain).

Right: This lesion was positive for CD20 (not shown) and EBER1 (not shown) and has a brisk proliferation (Ki-67) rate (immunohistochemistry with hematoxylin counterstain).

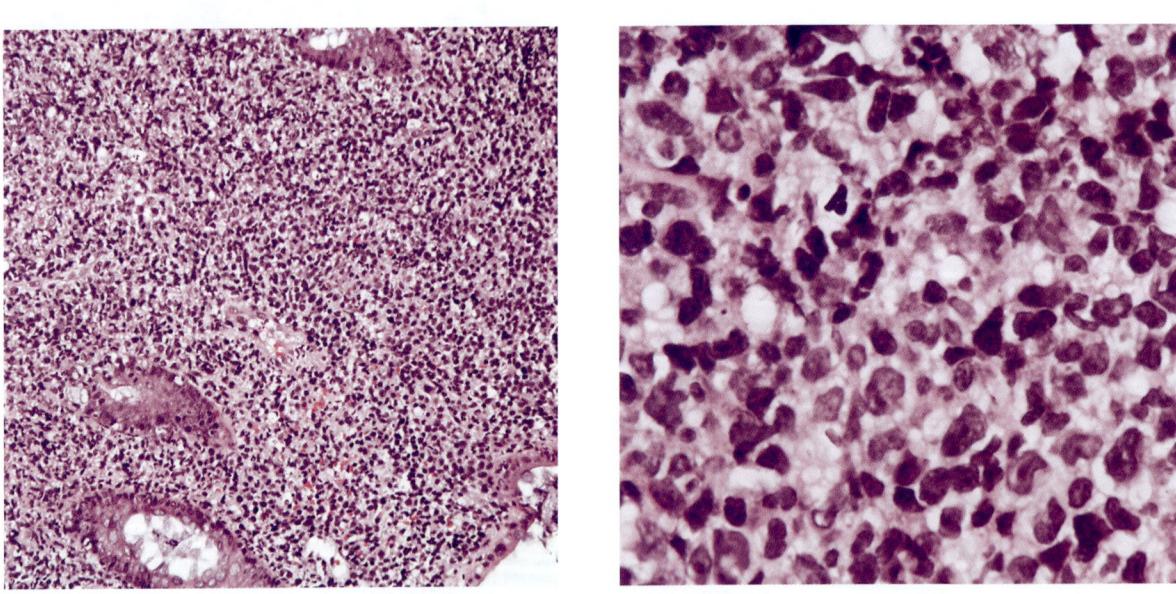

Figure 47-7

EBV-NEGATIVE MONOMORPHIC POST-TRANSPLANT LYMPHOPROLIFERATIVE DISORDER CONSISTENT WITH DIFFUSE LARGE B-CELL LYMPHOMA INVOLVING GASTROINTESTINAL TRACT

A 68-year-old woman who was treated for breast carcinoma subsequently developed therapy-related acute myeloid leukemia for which she underwent hematopoietic stem cell transplant. Subsequently the patient developed this lesion. The relationship of this lesion to the prior transplant is uncertain.

Left, Right: Low- and high-power magnification show a diffuse proliferation of large lymphoid cells. These cells were positive for CD20 (not shown) and negative for EBER1 (not shown) (H&E stain).

Table 47-3

FEATURES OF CLASSIC HODGKIN LYMPHOMA AND HODGKIN-LIKE PTLD

Category	Morphology	Immunophenotype	EBV [a]	Clonality Studies
Classic Hodgkin lymphoma	Effaced architecture resembles HL in immunocompetent patients	RS+H cells are CD15+, CD30+, MUM1+, PAX5 dim+, CD20-/+, CD45-	RS+H cells usually EBV+; background cells -	Usually not monoclonal using standard PCR methods
Hodgkin lymphoma-like lesions	Effaced architecture; often resembles HL in immunocompetent patients	RS+H-like cells are CD15-, CD30+ MUM+/-, PAX5+ CD20+, CD45+	RS+H-like cells usually EBV+; background cells often +	Often monoclonal

[a]EBV = Epstein-Barr virus; RS+H = Reed-Sternberg and Hodgkin cells.

is not involved. Cytologically, the plasma cells are most often well differentiated (Marschalko type), with a low mitotic rate (19,46). The plasma cells have the expected immunophenotype. EBV infection occurred in 3 of 8 cases in a German study (46).

Plasmablastic Lymphoma. These tumors are another uncommon type of PTLD that usually arises at extranodal sites and can be localized or disseminated (44,50). In one study, this type of PTLD arose most often in men who had undergone heart transplantation (50). Histologically, there is a diffuse pattern, often with a starry sky appearance, and a composition of plasmablasts and immunoblasts. The mitotic rate is usually high and apoptosis is brisk. The lymphoma cells are CD138(+), MUM1/IRF4(+), and CD20(-). Five of 8 (63 percent) cases of plasmablastic lymphoma arising in the post-transplant setting were EBV positive in one study (50).

Small B-Cell Lymphomas. Mucosa-associated lymphoid tissue (MALT) lymphoma is the most common small B-cell lymphoma that can arise in the post-transplant setting. Gibson et al. (13) described four cases of MALT lymphoma that arose late (about 10 years) after solid organ transplantation. These tumors were nongastric, involved subcutaneous tissue or the periorbital region, and were uniformly positive for EBER1. In all four patients, reduction of immunosuppression (often associated with other treatments) led to complete regression. Subsequent studies have shown that other small B-cell lymphomas, usually with extensive plasmacytic differentiation, can arise in the post-transplant setting including nodal marginal zone lymphoma and, rarely, lymphoplasmacytic lymphoma (6a). These tumors are usually EBV positive.

Classic Hodgkin Lymphoma

Classic Hodgkin lymphoma is a rare type of PTLD, occurring in less than 1 percent of patients (44). These lesions morphologically resemble their counterparts in immunocompetent patients (Table 47-3). The architecture is effaced by a neoplasm composed of Reed-Sternberg and Hodgkin (RS+H) cells within an inflammatory background. Mixed cellularity is the most common type of classic Hodgkin lymphoma arising in the post-transplant setting, but nodular sclerosis and lymphocyte depletion also occur.

Similar to classic Hodgkin lymphoma in immunocompetent patients, the RS+H cells are CD15+, CD30(+), PAX5 (dim+), and CD45/LCA(-). Unlike de novo cases, in the post-transplant setting RS+H cells are almost always EBV positive and more commonly express a number of B-cell antigens including BOB.1, OCT2, CD79a, and CD20 (1).

Hodgkin Lymphoma-Like Lesions. These tumors are a rarely reported form of PTLD that morphologically resemble classic Hodgkin lymphoma (fig. 47-8), most often of mixed cellularity type (37,38). It is uncommon for Hodgkin lymphoma-like lesions to have sclerotic bands or other features of nodular sclerosis, although cases are reported. The immunophenotype of the RS+H-like cells is distinctive. These large cells are CD20(+) (fig. 47-8B), CD79a(+), CD45/LCA(+), PAX5 (bright+), CD30 (variably +) (fig. 47-8C), and CD15(-). The RS+H-like cells may be positive for EBER1; small background lymphocytes are often EBER1 positive as well (fig. 47-8D). Unlike most cases of classic Hodgkin lymphoma, Hodgkin lymphoma-like lesions commonly carry monoclonal immunoglobulin

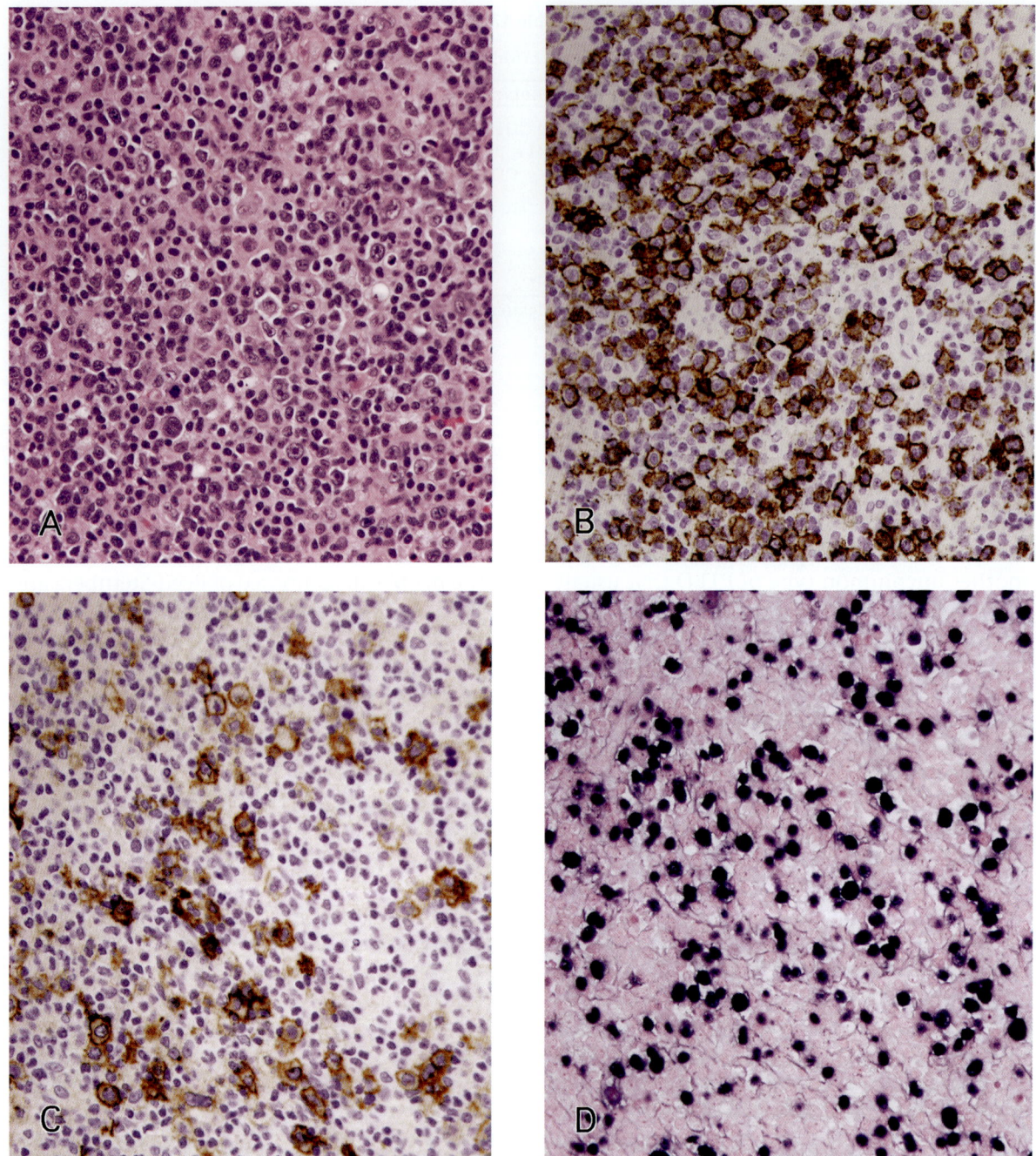

Figure 47-8

HODGKIN-LIKE POST-TRANSPLANT LYMPHOPROLIFERATIVE DISORDER

A 38-year-old man underwent umbilical stem cell transplantation for relapsed classic Hodgkin lymphoma and developed this lesion involving the tonsils 4 months after transplant.

A: Scattered large Reed-Sternberg and Hodgkin (RS+H)-like cells are present in a background of smaller lymphocytes and histiocytes (H&E stain).

B,C: The RS+H-like cells are positive for CD20 (B) and CD30 (C), but were negative for CD15 (not shown) (immunohistochemistry with hematoxylin counterstain).

D. The RS+H-like cells and many background small lymphocytes are positive for EBER1 (in situ hybridization with eosin counterstain).

Table 47-4

FEATURES OF T-CELL POST-TRANSPLANT LYMPHOPROLIFERATIVE DISORDERS

Category	Morphology	Immunophenotype	EBV[a]	Clonality Studies
Peripheral T-cell lymphoma, NOS	Effaced architecture	Pan-T-cell-antigens+ CD30-/+, Ki-67 variable	~50% +	Monoclonal *TRB* and/or *TRG* rearrangements; cytogenetic abnormalities common
Hepatosplenic T-cell lymphoma	Expansion of splenic red pulp; infiltration of liver sinusoids	CD56+, TCR γ/δ often+, CD4-, CD8-/+	-	Monoclonal *TRB* and/or *TRG* rearrangements; iso(7q),+8
ALK+ ALCL	Sinusoidal infiltration, paracortical pattern, or complete effacement	CD30+, ALK+, T cell or null cell, cytotoxic+ often CD3- or CD5-, Ki-67 high	-	Monoclonal *TRB* and/or *TRG* rearrangements; *ALK* rearrangements
ALK- ALCL	Sinusoidal infiltration paracortical pattern, or complete effacement	CD30+, ALK-, T cell or null cell, cytotoxic+, often CD3- or CD5-, Ki-67 high	-/+	Monoclonal *TRB* and/or *TRG* rearrangements
Large granular lymphocytic leukemia	Lymphocytosis in blood; subtle sinusoidal involvement in bone marrow	CD3+, CD16+/-, CD57+, CD56-	-	Monoclonal *TRB* and/or *TRG* rearrangements
Extranodal NK/T-cell lymphoma	Effaced architecture	cCD3+, sCD3-/+, CD56+, CD5-, Ki-67 variable	+	NK cells lack rearrangements; T-cell cases with monoclonal *TRB* and/or *TRG* rearrangements
Adult T-cell leukemia/ lymphoma	Effaced architecture; wide cytologic spectrum	Pan-T-cell antigens+	-	Monoclonal *TRB* and/or *TRG* rearrangements; HTLV-1+
Cutaneous ALCL	Dermal involvement of skin; large anaplastic cells; often associated eosinophilia	CD30+, CD4+/-, pan-T-cell antigen +, ALK-	-	Monoclonal *TRB* and/or *TRG* rearrangements
Mycosis fungoides	Patch, plaque, or tumor stage; cerebriform cells	Pan-T-cell antigen +, CD4+	-	Monoclonal *TRB* and/or *TRG* rearrangements

[a]EBV = Epstein-Barr virus; *TRB* = T-cell receptor beta gene; *TRG* = T-cell receptor gamma gene; NOS = not otherwise specified; ALK = anaplastic lymphoma kinase; ALCL = anaplastic large cell lymphoma; c = cytoplasmic; s = surface; HTLV-1 = human T-cell leukemia virus-1.

rearrangements (37). The prognosis of patients appears to be poorer than that of patients with classic Hodgkin lymphoma, and more in keeping with patients who have polymorphic B-cell PTLD.

Monomorphic Lesions: T Cell

All *NK/T-cell PTLDs* are included in the monomorphic category in the current WHO classification system and represent 5 to 10 percent of monomorphic cases (43,44). In our opinion, however, NK/T-cell PTLDs are sufficiently heterogeneous and distinctive to merit classification in a separate category in future classification schemes for PTLDs (Table 47-4) and their relationship to transplantation and immunosuppression is unclear.

Approximately one third of NK/T-cell PTLDs are EBV positive. T-cell PTLDs develop following any type of organ transplant, but most often

occur in patients who have received a kidney allograft. T-cell PTLDs tend to arise late after transplant, with a median interval of 66 months, but some arise within 6 months of transplant (43). EBV-positive T-cell PTLDs tend to develop earlier than EBV-negative cases; the median time from transplant to T-cell PTLD is approximately 4 years for EBV-positive lesions. Morphologically, T-cell PTLDs closely resemble their counterparts arising in immunocompetent patients.

As is the case in immunocompetent patients, *PTCL, NOS,* is the most common type of T-cell PTLD, representing approximately one third of cases. These lesions diffusely replace tissue architecture and exhibit a wide cytologic spectrum (fig. 47-9). Geographic necrosis is less common than in B-cell PTLDs, and the mitotic rate may be variable. These tumors express pan-T-cell antigens, CD30 is commonly expressed by some

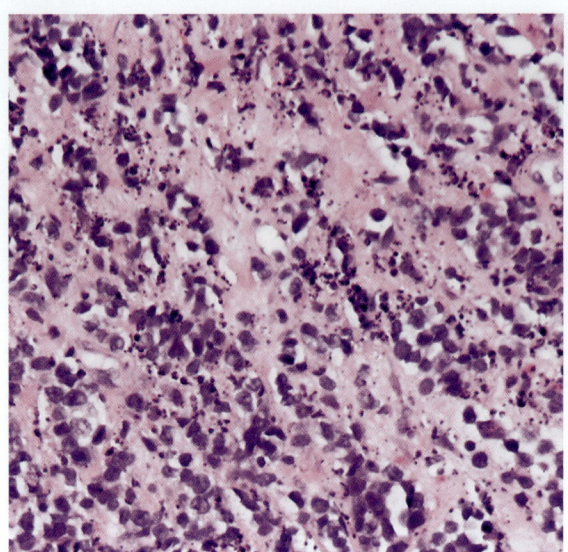
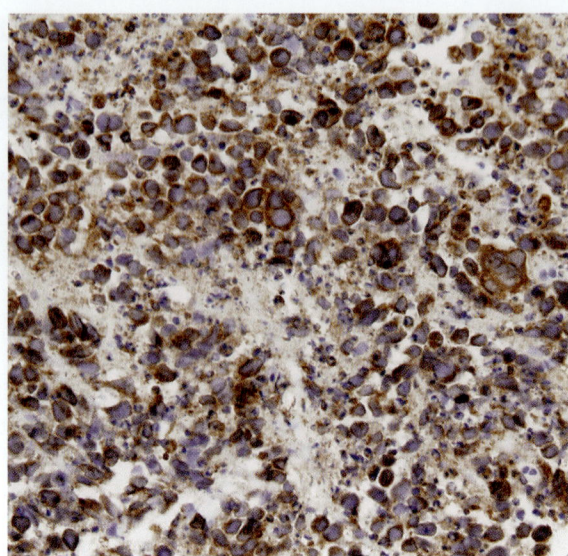

Figure 47-9

EBV-NEGATIVE T-CELL POST-TRANSPLANT LYMPHOPROLIFERATIVE DISORDER CONSISTENT WITH PERIPHERAL T-CELL LYMPHOMA

The patient had a remote history of a kidney transplant.

Left: The lesion has a diffuse pattern and is composed of large cells with abundant apoptosis (H&E stain).

Right: The cells were positive for CD3 and other T-cell antigens (not shown) (immunohistochemistry with hematoxylin counterstain).

cells, and the proliferation rate as assessed by Ki-67 is variable. Approximately half of these cases are EBV positive.

As reviewed by Swerdlow (43), *hepatosplenic T-cell lymphoma* (13.8 percent) is the second most frequent type of T-cell PTLD, followed by *anaplastic large cell lymphoma* (7.7 percent), *T-cell large granular lymphocytic leukemia* (6.9 percent), and other types with a frequency of 5 percent or less (*extranodal NK/T-cell lymphoma of nasal type, adult T-cell leukemia/lymphoma, mycosis fungoides,* and *cutaneous anaplastic large cell lymphoma*).

There are rare polyclonal T-cell lesions that arise after solid organ transplant. In one case at MD Anderson Cancer Center, the lesion involved a cervical lymph node and was composed primarily of small T cells, histiocytes, and scattered immunoblasts and polytypic plasma cells. This lesion arose approximately 5 years after a kidney transplant, was EBV negative, and showed no evidence of monoclonal T-cell receptor gene rearrangements.

CYTOLOGIC FINDINGS

Fine-needle aspiration specimens of PTLD reflect their wide morphologic spectrum (11).

In nondestructive lesions, a mixture of plasma cells, lymphocytes, and immunoblasts is present. Typically, necrosis is not present and mitotic activity is low to moderate. In polymorphic PTLDs, fine needle aspirates show a mixed population of small and large lymphocytes with a variable number of mitotic figures and necrosis. Histiocytes and scattered plasma cells are present in the background (fig. 47-10). In monomorphic PTLDs, the cytologic findings are similar to their de novo lymphoma counterparts. There is a predominance of large transformed lymphoid cells and mitotic figures are usually easily appreciated (fig. 47-11).

MOLECULAR GENETIC FINDINGS

PTLDs can be of donor or host/recipient origin. Most often the origin is assessed by fluorescence in situ hybridization (FISH) or microsatellite polymorphism analysis. Following solid organ transplantation, PTLDs are more commonly of host origin. In a study of 43 PTLDs, 27 (63 percent) were of host and 16 (37 percent) were of donor origin; the latter group included most cases that involved the allograft (30). In contrast, PTLDs that arise following hematopoietic stem cell

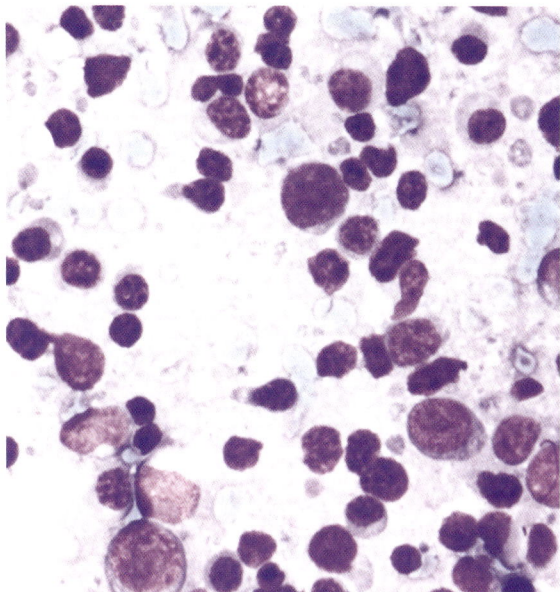

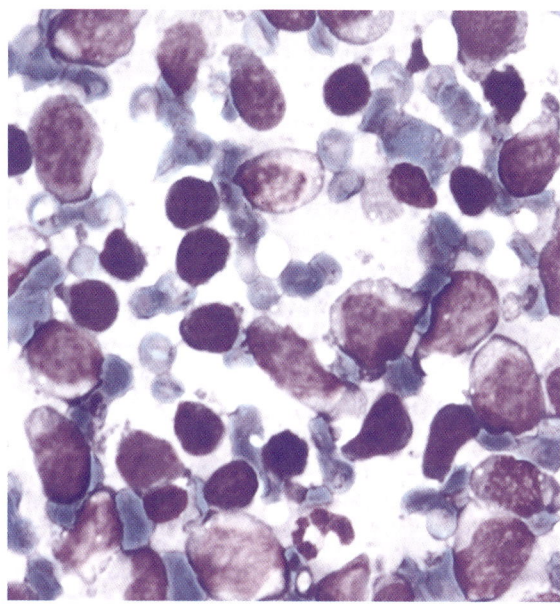

Figure 47-10

POLYMORPHIC POST-TRANSPLANT LYMPHOPROLIFERATIVE DISORDER

Fine-needle aspirate smear from a patient who had undergone bone marrow and cord blood transplants for acute myeloid leukemia. This smear shows a polymorphous population of small and larger lymphocytes as well as plasma cells consistent with a polymorphic PTLD (Diff-Quik stain).

Figure 47-11

MONOMORPHIC POST-TRANSPLANT LYMPHOPROLIFERATIVE DISORDER

In this fine-needle aspiration smear, there are many large transformed cells, consistent with a monomorphic PTLD (Diff-Quik stain).

transplantation have been reported to be more commonly of donor origin. Our experience with hematopoietic stem cell transplantation at MD Anderson Cancer Center, however, is somewhat at variance with the literature: PTLDs following hematopoietic stem cell transplantation are equally of host or donor origin.

In nondestructive lesions, cytogenetic abnormalities are rare and the analysis of antigen receptor genes is usually polyclonal (21,32,44). In some cases, small B-cell or T-cell clones are detected. EBV terminal repeat region analysis shows that EBV is usually present in a polyclonal or oligoclonal pattern.

Up to one third of polymorphic PTLDs show cytogenetic abnormalities, although consistent and recurrent abnormalities are usually not present (21,32,44). Most polymorphic PTLDs carry monoclonal immunoglobulin gene rearrangements and EBV terminal repeat region analysis shows that the virus is usually present in monoclonal form. The T-cell receptor genes are polyclonal or, in some cells, have low-level

monoclonal gene rearrangements. Approximately 40 percent of cases show *BCL6* mutations (29). Rearrangements or translocations of known oncogenes such as *MYC*, *BCL2*, *BCL6*, and *RAS*, and *TP53* mutation or deletion are uncommon (21).

Monomorphic B-cell PTLDs are the best studied PTLD category, particularly cases that fulfill the criteria for DLBCL. Up to 75 percent of cases have abnormalities detected by conventional cytogenetics; these include trisomy of chromosomes X, 2, 7, 9, and 11, and monosomy of chromosome 22 (7). *8q24/MYC* translocations occur in some cases of DLBCL and plasmablastic lymphoma (21,50). *MYC* translocation also occurs in Burkitt lymphoma. A recent study of seven Burkitt-like cases arising in the post-transplant setting, however, showed that the three cases that arose after solid organ transplant did not carry *MYC* rearrangements and had a distinctive pattern of 11q23.3 gain and 11q24.1qter loss involving *PAFAH1B2* and *FLI1/ETS1*, respectively (9).

Analysis of the antigen receptor genes in DLBCL arising after transplant shows monoclonal immunoglobulin gene rearrangements, with the T-cell receptor genes usually in the germline configuration (21,32,44). EBV is typically present in a monoclonal pattern. *BCL6* is mutated in most cases, *RAS* and *TP53* genes are commonly mutated, and *MYC* and *PAX5* are mutated in a subset of cases. Mentor et al. (25b) performed next generation sequencing on 50 cases of PTLD. Compared with immunocompetent patients with DCLCL, post-transplant DLBCL cases more often had *TP53* mutations and rarely *ATM* or *B2M* mutations. Overall, *KMT2D* was most frequently mutated and EBV-positive PTLD had a lower frequency of mutations. *NF-kB* mutations are also infrequent in EBV-positive PTLDs (4,25b).

Comparative genomic hybridization of post-transplant DLBCL has shown gains of chromosomal loci 5p and 11p, and deletions of 4p, 4q, 12p, 12q, 17p, and 18q (41). There are also differences between EBV-positive and -negative cases. EBV-negative PTLD cases share many molecular abnormalities with cases of DLBCL arising in immunocompetent patients, and some have suggested that EBV-negative cases of PTLD are de novo tumors (i.e., unrelated to transplant) (10). However, in a study in which monomorphic PTLD was compared with immunocompetent DLBCL using high-density single nucleotide polymorphism (SNP) arrays, there was a higher frequency of deletions involving fragile sites, in particular, del(2p16.1)/*FRA2E* in monomorphic PTLD of DLBCL type. Monomorphic PTLD of DLBCL type also had a lower frequency of del(13q14.3)/*MIR15* and *MIR16*, gains at 18q21/*BCL2*, or abnormalities of 6p/MHC complex compared with de novo DLBCL (40).

Gene expression profiling comparing EBV-positive and EBV-negative monomorphic B-cell PTLD resembling DLBCL found that EBV-positive cases had high expression of EBV genes and other genes consistent with a viral-induced immune response (6,27). By contrast, EBV-negative cases showed no overexpression of EBV genes, but there was overexpression of a number of pathways that are often abnormal in immunocompetent DLBCLs, including genes involved in B-cell receptor signaling, cell cycle control, DNA synthesis and replication, and cell proliferation. These data suggest that EBV-positive and -negative monomorphic PTLDs of DLBCL type have a distinct pathogenesis. The data also suggest that the "hit and run" theory

of PTLD pathogenesis, i.e., EBV is present when the lesion initially develops, but is subsequently lost, is unlikely.

Little is known regarding PTLD of classic Hodgkin lymphoma type. Antigen receptor gene rearrangement and oncogene abnormalities are typically absent. By contrast, in Hodgkin lymphoma-like lesions, monoclonal immunoglobulin rearrangements were common in over half of cases analyzed in one study (37).

In T-cell PTLDs, conventional cytogenetic abnormalities are common as are monoclonal T-cell receptor gene rearrangements (43,44). One study has shown mutations in epigenetic modifier genes (e.g., *TET2*, *KMT2C/MLL3*, *KMT2D/MLL2*), *TP53*, and *JAK/STAT* pathway genes in T-cell PTLDs, similar to de novo T-cell lymphomas (24a). EBV is present in monoclonal form in extranodal NK/T-cell lymphoma of nasal type, but uncommonly in most other types of T-cell PTLD. Chromosomal 2p23/*ALK* rearrangements are present in rare cases of anaplastic lymphoma kinase (ALK)-positive anaplastic large cell lymphoma (ALCL) arising post-transplant.

DIFFERENTIAL DIAGNOSIS

The clinical history of transplantation is essential for the diagnosis of PTLD. Lesions involving extranodal sites, geographic necrosis, and a polymorphous cell population are features that suggest the possibility of immunodeficiency of various types including tumors arising in the post-transplant setting. The differential diagnoses of the various types of monomorphic PTLD are similar to their counterparts in immunocompetent patients.

TREATMENT AND PROGNOSIS

The treatment of PTLD is complicated by the presence of the allograft and the need to preserve its function. The first step in therapy is usually reduction of immunosuppression (12,18,20). Typically, the dose of immunosuppression is reduced by approximately half, and in approximately half of patients the PTLD regresses. It often takes 3 to 5 weeks for regression to occur. Complete regression of PTLD occurs in 20 to 25 percent of patients (12). EBV-positive PTLDs are most likely to regress. Reduced immunosuppression, however, brings a risk of graft rejection.

Rituximab (anti-CD20) therapy has been an important advance and is standard in treating PTLDs (12,18,45). Rituximab therapy may follow reduced immunosuppression but a recent trend is to combine reduced immunosuppression and rituximab therapy, with overall response rates of up to 70 percent. Data also suggest that rituximab is best administered early in patients with PTLDs (18). If patients do not respond to rituximab alone, chemotherapy is often required. Traditionally, the CHOP (cyclophosphamide, doxorubicin, vincristine, and prednisone) regimen has been used, but currently rituximab-CHOP is favored (12,45,51).

There is a limited role for surgery or radiation therapy in the treatment of patients with PTLDs, except for those with localized lesions (12,18). Antiviral agents may have a role in the prevention of EBV-positive PTLDs, but there are few data that support their use once a PTLD has developed. This is true, in part, because antiviral agents such as ganciclovir are active in cells in the lytic phase of EBV infection. A potential therapy being explored is inducing reactivation of lytic phase of EBV in PTLD combined with antiviral agents. Similarly, donor-derived EBV-specific cytotoxic T-cell therapy has been used to treat patients with EBV-positive tumors. This approach, however, requires substantial time to grow the cells ex vivo and may not be available in real time; it may be better suited for use in prevention rather than as a treatment once a PTLD has developed (18).

The prognosis of patients with nondestructive (early) lesions is excellent. Virtually all respond to reduced immunosuppression, although rituximab may be required in some patients (18,21,44). The prognosis of patients with other types of PTLD is highly variable. Most patients with polymorphic PTLDs respond to reduced immunosuppression, but a subset of patients relapse. In patients who initially do not respond or who relapse, rituximab or rituximab with chemotherapy is needed (12,20,45).

The overall prognosis of patients with monomorphic PTLD is poorer, but the prognosis largely depends on the type of PTLD. Monomorphic PTLD of DLBCL, Burkitt, or plasmablastic lymphoma types are rarely successfully treated by reduced immunosuppression alone (44,45,50,51). Rituximab plus chemotherapy is usually used for CD20-positive lymphomas. The median survival period of patients with B-cell PTLD in a Mayo Clinic study, based on 33 years experience, was 31.5 months (12). Nevertheless, the addition and earlier use of rituximab in treatment regimens has improved overall survival somewhat in recent years (18). Patients with most T-cell monomorphic PTLDs usually require chemotherapy and have a poor prognosis. CD30-positive cells are common in most cases of PTLD and are associated with a better prognosis. This finding also suggests a possible role for brentuximab vedotin in patients who fail standard therapy (49).

The following prognostic factors are associated with a poorer prognosis in patients with PTLD: older age, B-type symptoms, poor performance status, more than one extranodal site of disease, involvement of the brain or bone marrow, advanced stage, involvement of the allograft, high serum lactate dehydrogenase level, monomorphic type, and EBV-negative lesions (12,18,20,26,45). Montanari et al. (26) suggested a prognostic score based on Eastern Cooperative Oncology Group performance score (0-1 versus 2-4), age (less than 16 years, 16 to 60 years, and over 60 years), and CD20 positivity. This system divides patients with PTLD into four prognostic groups. Patients with classic Hodgkin lymphoma post transplant have a poorer prognosis than their immunocompetent counterparts (41a).

Patients with plasmacytoma-like B-cell PTLD and those with T-cell large granular lymphocytic leukemia arising after transplant have an indolent clinical course. Patients with MALT lymphomas also tend to do well (13,16). The above prognostic factors do not seem to apply to these tumors.

REFERENCES

1. Adams H, Campidelli C, Dirnhofer S, Pileri SA, Tzankov A. Clinical, phenotypic and genetic similarities and disparities between post-transplant and classical Hodgkin lymphomas with respect to therapeutic targets. Expert Opin Ther Targets 2009;13:1137-1145.

2. Bhatia S, Ramsay NK, Steinbuch M, et al. Malignant neoplasms following bone marrow transplantation. Blood 1996;87:3633-3639.

3. Caillard S, Agodoa LY, Bohen EM, Abbott KC. Myeloma, Hodgkin's disease, and lymphoid leukemia after renal transplantation: characteristics, risk factors, and prognosis. Transplantation 2006;81:888-895.

4. Capello D, Gloghini A, Martini M, et al. Mutations of CD79A, CD79B and EZH2 genes in immunodeficiency-related non-Hodgkin lymphomas. Br J Haematol 2011;152:777-780.

5. Clarke CA, Morton LM, Lynch C, et al. Risk of lymphoma subtypes after solid organ transplantation in the United States. Br J Cancer 2013;109:280-288.

6. Craig FE, Johnson LR, Harvey SA, et al. Gene expression profiling of Epstein-Barr virus-positive and -negative monomorphic posttransplant lymphoproliferative disorders. Diagn Mol Pathol 2007;16:158-168.

6a. de Jong D, Roemer MG, Chan JK, et al. B-cell and classical Hodgkin lymphomas associated with immunodeficiency: 2015 SH/EAHP Workshop Report-Part 2. Am J Clin Pathol 2017;147:153-170.

7. Djokic M, Le Beau MM, Swinnen LJ, et al. Post-transplant lymphoproliferative disorder subtypes correlate with different recurring chromosomal abnormalities. Genes Chromosome Cancer 2006;45:313-318.

8. Engels EA, Clarke CA, Pfeiffer RM, et al. Plasma cell neoplasms in US solid organ transplant recipients. Am J Transplant 2013;13:1523-1532.

9. Ferreiro JF, Morscio J, Dierickx D, et al. Post-transplant molecularly defined Burkitt lymphomas are frequently MYC-negative and characterized by the 11q-gain/loss pattern. Haematologica 2015;100:e275.

10. Ferreiro JF, Morscio J, Dierickx D, et al. EBV-positive and EBV-negative posttransplant diffuse large B-cell lymphomas have distinct genomic and transcriptomic features. Am J Transplant 2016; 16:414-425.

11. Gattuso P, Manosca F. Fine-needle aspiration of posttransplant lymphoproliferative disorders: a review. Diagn Cytopathol 2005;33:273-278.

12. Ghobrial IM, Habermann TM, Maurer MJ, et al. Prognostic analysis for survival in adult solid organ transplant recipients with post-transplantation lymphoproliferative disorders. J Clin Oncol 2005;23:7574-7582.

13. Gibson SE, Swerdlow SH, Craig FE, et al. EBV-positive extranodal marginal zone lymphoma of mucosa-associated lymphoid tissue in the posttransplant setting: a distinct type of post-transplant lymphoproliferative disorder? Am J Surg Pathol 2011;35:807-815.

14. Grulich AE, Vajdic CM. The epidemiology of cancers in human immunodeficiency virus infection and after organ transplantation. Sem Oncol 2015;42:247-257.

15. Harris-Arnold A, Arnold CP, Schaffert S, et al. Epstein-Barr virus modulates host cell microRNA-194 to promote IL-10 production and B lymphoma cell survival. Am J Transplant 2015;15:2814-2824.

16. Hsi ED, Singleton TP, Swinnen L, Dunphy CH, Alkan S. Mucosa-associated lymphoid tissue-type lymphomas occurring in post-transplantation patients. Am J Surg Pathol 2000;24:100-106.

17. Ibrahim HA, Menasce L, Pomplun S, Burke M, Bower M, Naresh KN. Tumour infiltrating plasmacytoid dendritic cells in B cell post-transplant lymphoproliferative disorders, human immunodeficiency virus-associated B cell lymphomas and immune competent diffuse large B cell lymphomas. Histopathology 2011;59:152-156.

18. Jagadeesh D, Woda BA, Draper J, Evens AM. Post transplant lymphoproliferative disorders: risk, classification, and therapeutic recommendations. Curr Treat Options Oncol 2012;13:122-136.

19. Joseph G, Barker RL, Yuan B, Martin A, Medeiros LJ, Peiper SC. Posttransplantation plasma cell dyscrasias. Cancer 1994;74:1959-1964.

20. Knight JS, Tsodikov A, Cibrik DM, Ross CW, Kaminski MS, Blayney DW. Lymphoma after solid organ transplantation: risk, response to therapy and survival at a transplantation center. J Clin Oncol 2009;27:3354-3362.

21. Knowles DM, Cesarman E, Chadburn A, et al. Correlative morphologic and molecular genetic analysis demonstrates three distinct categories of posttranplantation lymphoproliferative disorders. Blood 1995;85:552-565.

22. Kumarasinghe G, Lavee O, Parker A, et al. Post-transplant lymphoproliferative disease in heart and lung transplantation: defining risk and prognostic factors. J Heart Lung Transplant 2015;34:1406-1414.

23. Landgren O, Gilbert ES, Rizzo JD, et al. Risk factors for lymphoproliferative disorders after allogeneic hematopoietic cell transplantation. Blood 2009;113:4992-5001.

24. Luskin MR, Heil DS, Tan KS, et al. The impact of EBV status on characteristics and outcomes of posttransplantation lymphoproliferative disorder. Am J Transplant 2015;15:2665-2673.

24a. Margolskee E, Jobanputra V, Jain P, et al. Genetic landscape of T- and NK-cell post-transplant lymphoproliferative disorders. Oncotarget 2016;7:37636-37648.

25. Mbulaiteye SM, Clarke CA, Morton LM, et al. Burkitt lymphoma risk in U.S. solid organ transplant recipients. Am J Hematol 2013;88:245-250.

25b. Menter T, Juskevicius D, Alikian M, et al. Mutational landscape of B-cell post-transplant lymphoproliferative disorders. Br J Haematol 2017;178:48-56.

26. Montanari F, Radeski D, Seshan V, Alobeid B, Bhagat G, O'Connor OA. Recursive partitioning analysis of prognostic factors in post-transplant lymphoproliferative disorders (PTLD): a 120 case single institution series. Br J Haematol 2015;171:491-500.

27. Morscio J, Dierickx D, Ferreiro JF, et al. Gene expression profiling reveals clear differences between EBV-positive and EBV-negative post-transplant lymphoproliferative disorders. Am J Transplant 2013;13:1305-1316.

28. Nee R, Hurst FP, Dharnidharka VR, Jindal RM, Agodoa LY, Abbott KC. Racial variation in the development of post-transplantation lymphoproliferative disorders after renal transplantation. Transplantation 2011;92:190-195.

29. Nourse JP, Jones K, Gandhi MK. Epstein-Barr Virus-related post-transplant lymphoproliferative disorders: pathogenetic insights for targeted therapy. Am J Transplant 2011;11:888-895.

30. Olagne J, Caillard S, Gaub MP, Chenard MP, Moulin B. Post-transplant lymphoproliferative disorders: determination of donor/recipient origin in a large cohort of kidney recipients. Am J Transplant 2011;11:1260-1269.

31. Opelz G, Henderson R. Incidence of non-Hodgkin lymphoma in kidney and heart transplant recipients. Lancet 1993;342:746-748.

32. Parker A, Bowles K, Bradley JA, et al. Diagnosis of post-transplantation lymphoproliferative disorders in solid organ recipients-BCHS and BTS guidelines. Br J Haematol 2010;149:675-692.

33. Paya CV, Fung JJ, Nalesnik MA, et al. Epstein-Barr virus-induced posttransplant lymphoproliferative disorders. ASTS/ASTP EBV-PTLD Task Force and The Mayo Clinic Organized International Consensus Development Meeting. Transplantation 1999;68:1517-1525.

34. Petrara MR, Giunco S, Serraino D, Dolcetti R, De Rossi A. Post-transplant lymphoproliferative disorders: from epidemiology to pathogenesis-driven treatment. Cancer Lett 2015;369:37-44.

35. Picarsic J, Jaffe R, Mazariegos G, et al. Post-transplant Burkitt lymphoma is a more aggressive and distinct form of post-transplant lymphoproliferative disorder. Cancer 2011;117:4540-4550.

36. Piñana JL, Sanz J, Esquirol A, et al; GETH GITMO groups. Umbilical cord blood transplantation in adults with advanced Hodgkin's disease: high incidence of post-transplant lymphoproliferative disease. Eur J Haematol 2016;96:128-135.

37. Pitman SD, Huang Q, Zuppan CW, et al. Hodgkin lymphoma-like posttransplant lymphoproliferative disorder (HL-like PTLD) simulates monomorphic PTLD both clinically and pathologically. Am J Surg Pathol 2006;30:470-476.

38. Ranganathan S, Webber S, Ahuja S, Jaffe R. Hodgkin-like post-transplant lymphoproliferative disorder in children: does it differ from posttranplant Hodgkin lymphoma? Pediatr Dev Pathol 2004;7:348-360.

39. Reshef R, Luskin MR, Kamoun M, et al. Association of HLA polymorphisms with post-transplant lymphoproliferative disorder in solid-organ transplant recipients. Am J Transplant 2011;11:817-825.

40. Rinaldi A, Capello D, Scandurra M, et al. Single nucleotide polymorphism-arrays provide new insights in the pathogenesis of post-transplant diffuse large B-cell lymphoma. Br J Haematol 2010;149:569-577.

41. Rinaldi A, Kwee I, Poretti G, et al. Comparative genome-wide profiling of post-transplant lymphoproliferative disorders and diffuse large B-cell lymphomas. Br J Haematol 2006;134:27-36.

41a. Rosenberg AS, Klein AK, Ruthazer R, Evens AM. Hodgkin lymphoma post-transplant lymphoproliferative disorder: a comparative analysis of clinical characteristics, prognosis, and survival. Am J Hematol 2016;91:560-565.

42. Stern M, Opelz G, Dohler B, Hess C. Natural killer-cell receptor polymorphisms in post-transplantation non-Hodgkin lymphoma. Blood 2010;115:3960-3965.

43. Swerdlow SH. T-cell and NK-cell posttransplantation lymphoproliferative disorders. Am J Clin Pathol 2007;127:887-895.

43a. Swerdlow SH, Campo E, Pileri SA, et al. The 2016 revision of the World Health Organization classification of lymphoid neoplasms. Blood 2016;127:2375-2390.

44. Swerdlow SH, Webber SA, Chadburn A, Ferry JA. Post-transplant lymphoproliferative disorders. In: Swerdlow SH, Campo E, Harris NL, et al., eds. WHO classification of tumours of haemato-poietic and lymphoid tissues. Lyon: IARC Press; 2008:343-349.

45. Trappe R, Oertel S, Leblond V, et al. Sequential treatment with rituximab followed by CHOP chemotherapy in adult B cell post-transplant lymphoproliferative disorder (PTLD): the prospective international multicentre phase 2 PTLD-1 trial. Lancet Oncol 2012;13:196-206.

46. Trappe R, Zimmerman H, Fink S, et al. Plasma-cytoma-like post-transplant lymphoproliferative disorder, a rare subtype of monomorphic B-cell post-transplant lymphoproliferation, is associated with a favorable outcome in localized as well as in advanced disease: a prospective analysis of 8 cases. Haematologica 2011;96:1067-1074.

47. Tsao L, Hsi ED. The clinicopathologic spectrum of posttransplantation lymphoproliferative disorders. Arch Pathol Lab Med 2007;131:1209-1218.

48. Vakiani E, Nandula SV, Subramaniyam S, et al. Cytogenetic analysis of B-cell posttransplant lymphoproliferations validates the World Health Organization classification and suggests inclusion of florid follicular hyperplasia as a precursor lesion. Hum Pathol 2007;38:315-325.

49. Vase MØ, Maksten EF, Bendix K, et al. Occurrence and prognostic relevance of CD30 expression in post-transplant lymphoproliferative disorders. Leuk Lymphoma 2015;56:1677-1685.

49a. Weisenburger DD, Gross TG. Post-transplant lymphoproliferative disorder: a heterogeneous conundrum. Br J Haematol 2016. [Epub ahead of print]

50. Zimmermann H, Oschlies I, Fink S, et al. Plasmab-lastic posttransplant lymphoma: cytogenetic ab-errations and lack of Epstein-Barr virus association linked with poor outcome in the prospective German Posttransplant Lymphoproliferative Disorder Registry. Transplantation 2012;93:543-550.

51. Zimmermann H, Reinke P, Neuhaus R, et al. Burkitt post-transplantation lymphoma in adult solid organ transplant recipients: sequential im-munochemotherapy with rituximab (R) followed by cyclophosphamide, doxorubicin, vincristine, and prednisone (CHOP) or R-CHOP is safe and effective in an analysis of 8 patients. Cancer 2012;118:4515-4724.

48 BLASTIC PLASMACYTOID DENDRITIC CELL NEOPLASM

GENERAL FEATURES

Blastic plasmacytoid dendritic cell neoplasm (BPDCN) is an aggressive neoplasm likely derived from a bone marrow–based cell that normally gives rise to plasmacytoid dendritic cells. In the World Health Organization (WHO) classification, BPDCN is thought to be more closely related to myeloid diseases than to lymphoid neoplasms and is therefore grouped with acute myeloid leukemias (2,5). BPDCNs commonly involve skin, bone marrow, blood, and lymph nodes.

These neoplasms are rare and represent less than 1 percent of all hematologic malignancies. Due in part to their rarity, BPDCN was not a well-characterized entity until the past decade. Nevertheless, these tumors were described over 30 years ago (or perhaps earlier). Older names used for BPDCN in the literature include *agranular CD4-positive natural killer cell leukemia* (3) and *CD4/CD56-positive hematodermic neoplasm* (23). Two additional designations that were once used for this disease, blastic natural killer (NK)-cell lymphoma/leukemia and plasmacytoid T-cell lymphoma (21), are scientifically inaccurate and extinct.

CLINICAL FEATURES

BPDCNs occur predominantly in the elderly, with a median age at time of diagnosis of approximately 65 years, but they can occur at any age including children (5,7,13). There is a male predilection of up to 3 to 1 in some studies (7,13).

Patients with BPDCN most frequently present with skin lesions (80 to 85 percent of patients) (4,13,23). The skin lesions are solitary or multiple, appearing as plaques, nodules, or foci resembling bruises. In about two thirds of patients with skin lesions, the skin is the only site of disease at the time of initial diagnosis, but the disease often disseminates rapidly (13). Peripheral lymphadenopathy is observed in 40 to 50 percent of patients and splenomegaly also

occurs (5,7,15). A small subset of patients has symptoms or signs of the central nervous system being involved, but occult disease is more common (17a).

Blood and bone marrow involvement are common at the time of initial diagnosis (5,7,22,26). Patients present with either mild or severe peripheral cytopenias; the latter portend bone marrow failure. Some patients present with a leukemic blood picture with a moderately high, or rarely, very high leukocyte count (22,26). Patients who present with cytopenias also may develop leukemia during the clinical course of the disease, often heralding a fulminant, rapidly progressive phase of disease (7). Approximately 10 percent of patients develop secondary myeloid leukemia, either within a preexisting background of myelodysplasia or abruptly during disease progression or relapse (7,10,15).

HISTOLOGIC FINDINGS

Lymph Node

In lymph nodes, the neoplastic cells exhibit an interfollicular, medullary, or "leukemic" distribution or may totally efface the lymph node architecture (5,15). The neoplasm has a diffuse pattern and in many cases, tingible body macrophages in a starry sky pattern are observed (figs. 48-1, 48-2A). The neoplastic cells are monotonous, intermediately sized cells with slightly or more markedly irregular nuclear contours, delicate chromatin, and scant cytoplasm, and often have a blastic appearance. Mitotic figures and apoptotic cells can be numerous.

Skin

Skin lesions are characterized by a "bottom-heavy" distribution of BPDCN cells forming aggregates and sheets in the dermis (figs. 48-2B, 48-3, 48-4) (4,13,23,24). The tumor cells often displace, but do not destroy, dermal collagen bundles. The cells also may involve the dermis

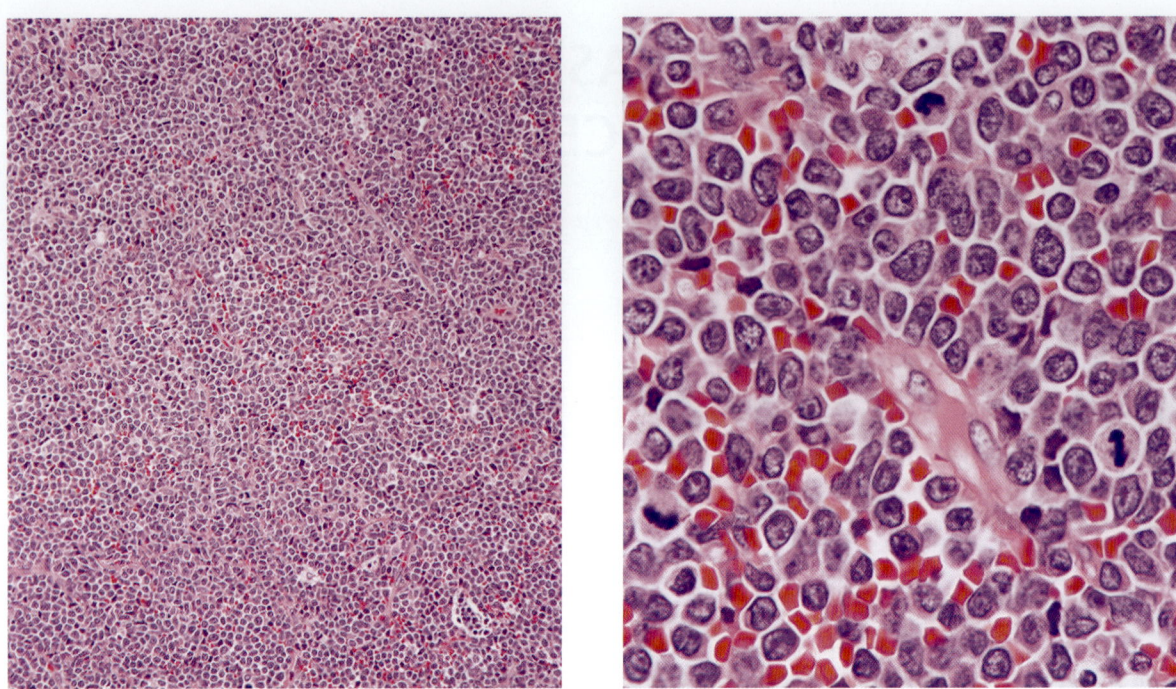

Figure 48-1

BLASTIC PLASMACYTOID DENDRITIC CELL NEOPLASM INVOLVING LYMPH NODE

Left: The architecture is diffusely replaced. A hint of a starry sky pattern can be appreciated in this field.
Right: The neoplastic cells are intermediate in size with immature chromatin. Mitotic figures are numerous (hematoxylin and eosin [H&E] stain).

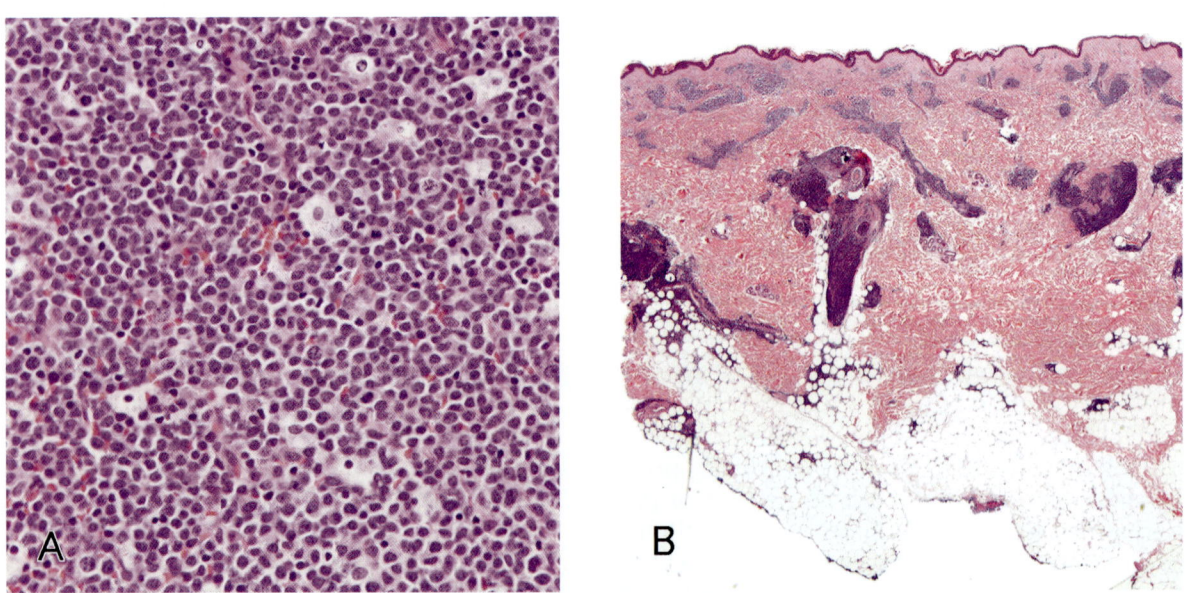

Figure 48-2

MULTIPLE ANATOMIC SITES INVOLVED BY BLASTIC PLASMACYTOID DENDRITIC CELL NEOPLASM IN A SINGLE PATIENT

A: The neoplasm diffusely replaces the lymph node architecture and has a prominent starry sky pattern.
B: A skin biopsy specimen shows a dermal perivascular and periadnexal infiltrate of neoplastic cells.

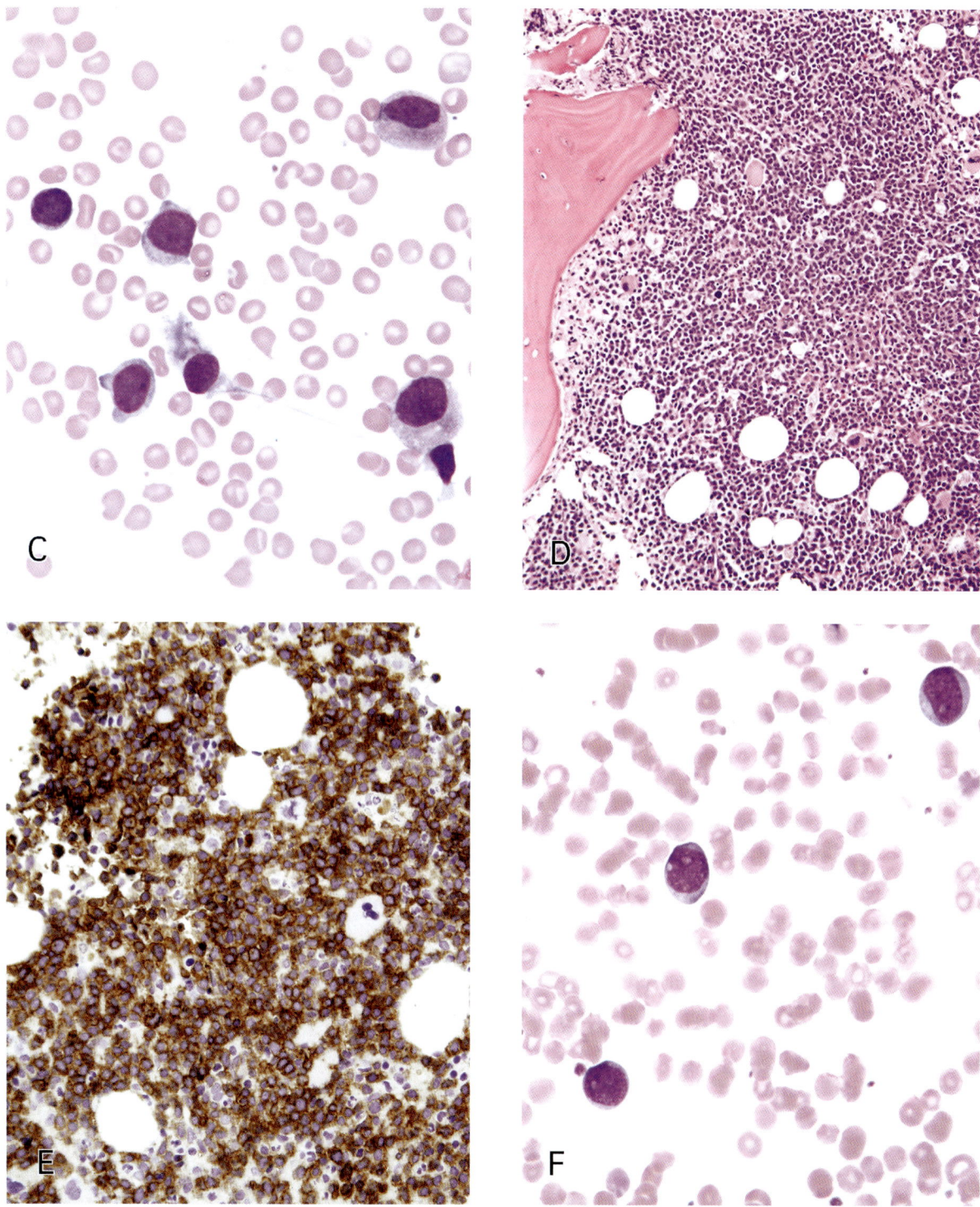

Figure 48-2, continued

C: The neoplastic cells in the bone marrow aspirate smear show moderate agranular cytoplasm with pseudopodia.

D: The bone marrow medullary space is extensively replaced in an interstitial and diffuse pattern.

E: The neoplastic cells in the bone marrow are positive for CD123.

F: Neoplastic cells in the blood smear are not distinctive and resemble blasts (A,B,D: H&E stain; C,F: Wright-Giemsa stain; E: immunohistochemistry with hematoxylin counterstain).

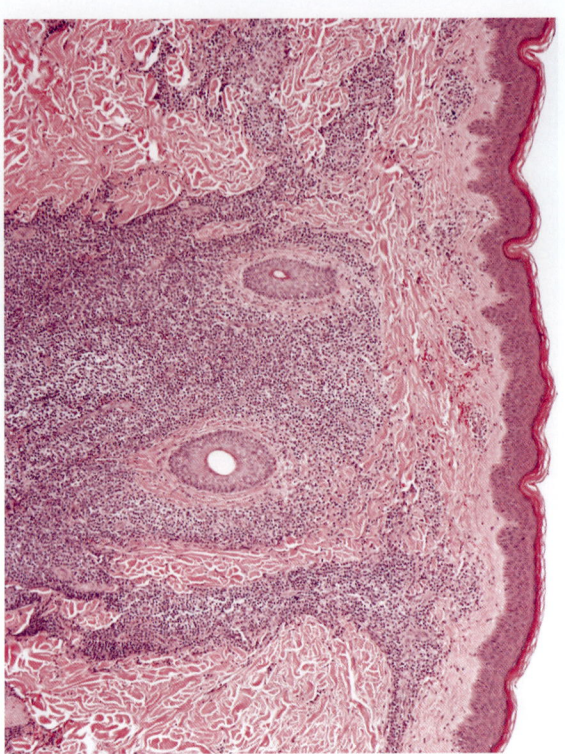 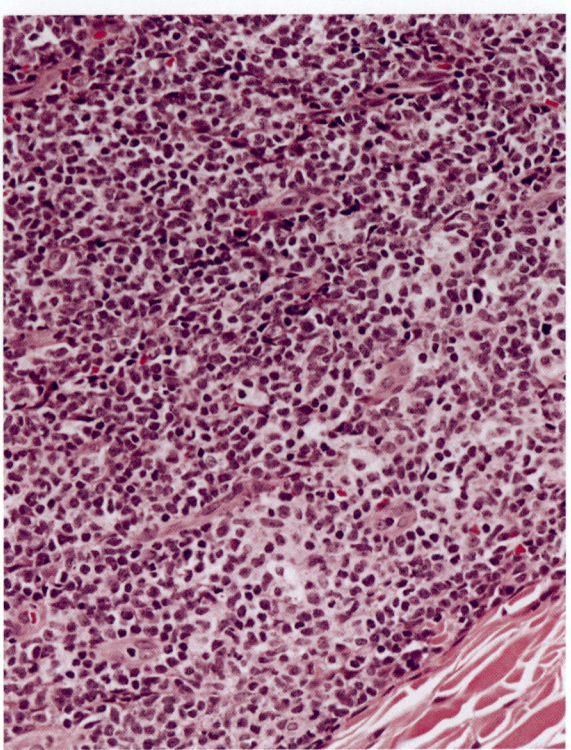

Figure 48-3

BLASTIC PLASMACYTOID DENDRITIC CELL NEOPLASM INVOLVING SKIN

Left: The neoplasm involves the dermis and surrounds hair follicles.
Right: The neoplastic cells are small to intermediate in size, and do not appear blastic (H&E stain).

in a perivascular or periadnexal distribution. Neoplastic cells may extend into subcutaneous adipose tissue (fig. 48-4), but usually spare the epidermis. Angioinvasion is not a feature of BPDCN.

Bone Marrow

In bone marrow aspirate smears, the cells of BPDCN show unipolar cytoplasmic processes (pseudopodia) or resemble poorly differentiated myeloblasts or lymphoblasts (1,26). The cytoplasm of BPDCN cells is agranular and nucleoli are clearly recognizable and can be conspicuous. Cytoplasmic microvacuoles oriented toward the cell membrane ("pearl necklace-like" appearance) may be observed (fig. 48-5).

In bone marrow biopsy sections, BPDCN may be present as nonparatrabecular clusters scattered among normal bone marrow cellular elements; more often, however, the disease is more extensive, with an interstitial or diffuse pattern and minimal or almost imperceptible residual hematopoiesis (fig. 48-2D).

Peripheral Blood

In blood smears, the cells are of intermediate size, with round or slightly indented nuclei containing finely reticulated chromatin, conspicuous nucleoli, and scant amounts of lightly basophilic cytoplasm (fig. 48-2F). Unlike the situation in bone marrow smears, in our experience, the neoplastic cells less often exhibit cytoplasmic pseudopodia or cytoplasmic microvacuoles and can closely resemble leukemic blasts (myeloid or lymphoid).

CYTOLOGIC FINDINGS

The cytologic findings resemble those observed in bone marrow and peripheral blood smears. Fine-needle aspirate smears are commonly hypercellular. The tumor cells are monotonous and intermediate sized, and are arranged in loose aggregates or as single cells. These cells have round to oval nuclei, finely stippled chromatin, one or multiple nucleoli that

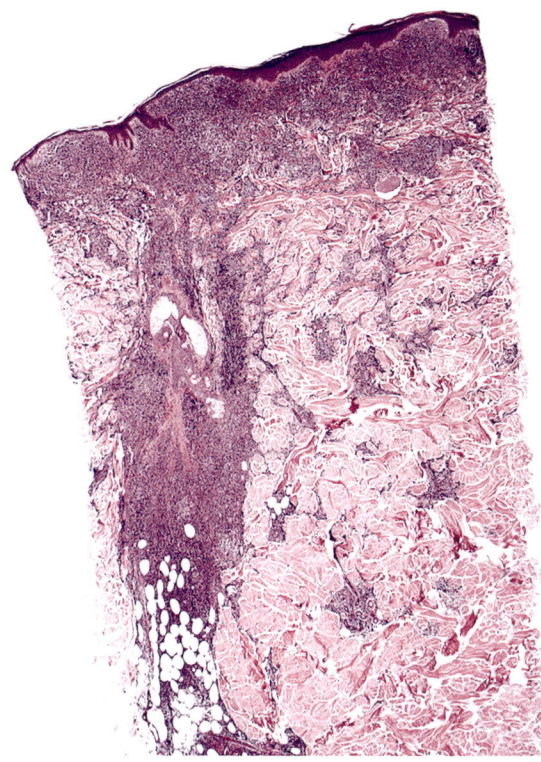

Figure 48-4

BLASTIC PLASMACYTOID DENDRITIC CELL NEOPLASM INVOLVING SKIN

In this case, the neoplastic cells are located primarily in the dermis, but also invade more deeply into adipose tissue (H&E stain).

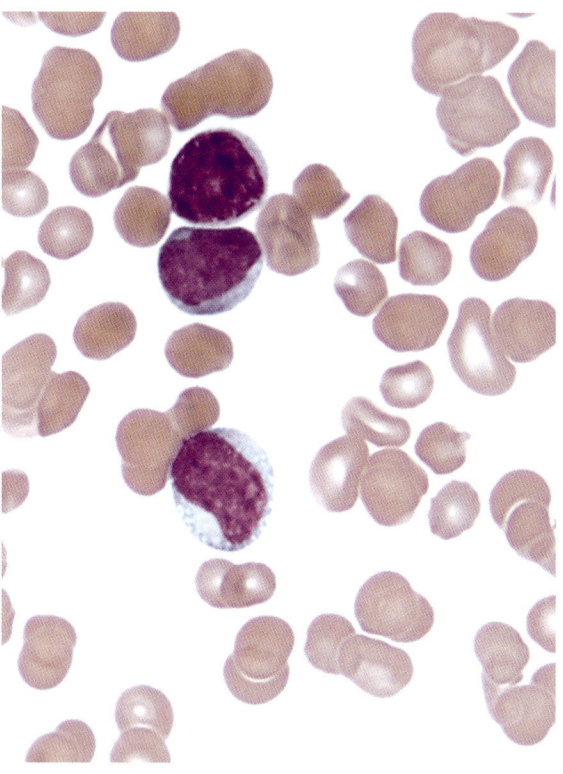

Figure 48-5

BLASTIC PLASMACYTOID DENDRITIC CELL NEOPLASM INVOLVING BONE MARROW

Two neoplastic cells and a lymphocyte are shown. The lower cell has multiple cytoplasmic vacuoles, resembling a pearl necklace (Wright-Giemsa stain).

can be prominent, and scant lightly basophilic and agranular cytoplasm that often contains small vacuoles (fig. 48-6) (6).

CYTOCHEMICAL FINDINGS

Cytochemical assessment using the periodic acid–Schiff (PAS) reaction is positive in less than half of BPDCNs and is not conspicuous (3). Uncommonly, PAS-positive cytoplasmic vacuoles are more prominent. Cytochemical stains for myeloperoxidase (MPO) and esterases are negative in BPDCN cells.

IMMUNOPHENOTYPIC FINDINGS

Using flow cytometry immunophenotypic analysis, the cells of BPDCN are virtually always positive for CD4, CD43, CD45RA, CD56, CD123, and HLA-DR (5,9,18). Other markers positive in many cases of BPDCN include CD36, CD38 (heterogeneous), CD45, CD71 (often dim or mod-

erate), and CD99. Some cases express the T-cell–associated antigens CD7 (about 75 percent), CD2 (about 25 percent), CD5 (about 15 percent), and cytoplasmic CD3 (rare), but are negative for surface CD3 and CD8. The myeloid-associated antigens CD13 (about 20 percent), CD33 (60 to 70 percent), and CD117 (10 to 20 percent) also may be positive. The tumor cells are characteristically negative for CD1a, CD10, CD15, CD16, CD19, CD20, CD22, CD25, CD34, CD45RO, CD79a, CD79b, CD117, MPO, and LAT (linker for activation of T cells).

Martin-Martin et al. (18) suggested that BPDCN can be subdivided into three groups that have prognostic relevance: immature, intermediate, and mature. The immature group is bone marrow–based and shares immunophenotypic features with acute myeloid leukemia (AML). In this subtype, the BPDCN cells are partially positive for CD34, may be dimly positive for CD117, and are often negative for CD56 and

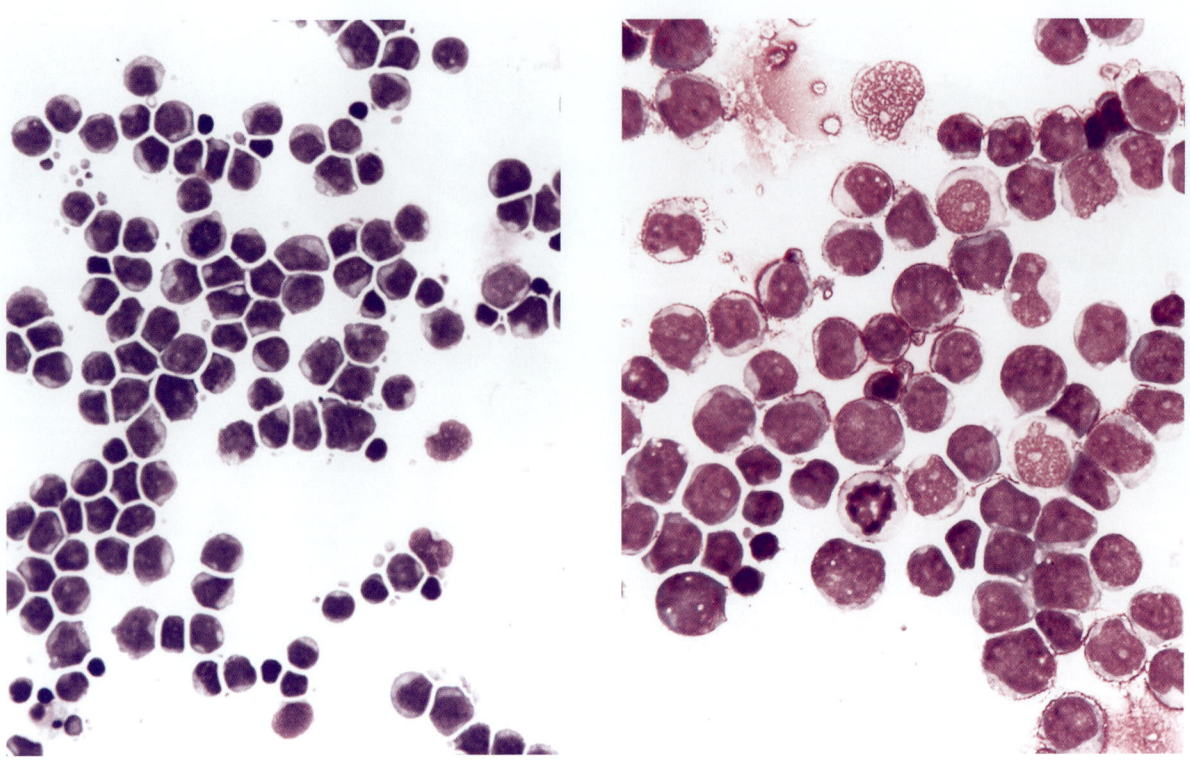

Figure 48-6

BLASTIC PLASMACYTOID DENDRITIC CELL NEOPLASM: CYTOLOGIC FEATURES

Left: In this cytospin smear the neoplastic cells have a high nucleus to cytoplasmic ratio, fine chromatin, and pale cytoplasm (Diff-Quik stain). (Courtesy of Dr. J. Stewart, Houston, TX.)

Right: In this imprint, the neoplastic cells also have a high nucleus to cytoplasm ratio and prominent nucleoli, and resemble blasts as might be observed in myeloid sarcoma (Wright-Giemsa stain).

more mature markers. Commonly, this immature plasmacytoid dendritic cell population coexists with the blasts of AML [CD34(+), CD117(+)] or less often, acute lymphoblastic leukemia. Patients in the immature group infrequently have extramedullary disease. Using the WHO criteria, these cases most likely would be classified as acute leukemia of ambiguous lineage or minimally differentiated AML (18). The intermediate group of BPDCN cases is CD34(-), CD117(+) and the mature group has a characteristic plasmacytoid dendritic cell immunophenotype that is CD34(-), CD117(-). In large part, the mature group fits the definition of BPDCN in the WHO classification and patients have a typical presentation with extramedullary disease involving skin, lymph nodes, and viscera. The prognosis is poor in all three groups, but the disease is more aggressive in the intermediate and mature groups (18). The approach of Martin-Martin et

al. needs validation, but the attempt to further characterize the immunophenotypic spectrum of BPDCN cases seems to be worthy.

Using immunohistochemical methods and routinely processed tissue sections, the cells of BPDCN are positive for CD4, CD45RA, CD45/LCA, CD123, CD303/blood dendritic cell antigen-2 (BDCA-2), TCL1, and BCL2 (figs. 48-2, 48-7) (10,15,23,27,29). Additional recently developed markers of BPDCN of value include: SPIB, CD162/cutaneous lymphocyte-associated antigen (CLA), BDCA-4, myxovirus A (MxA), CD2AP, IRF8, TCF4, and brain and dendritic cell-associated membrane protein (BAD-LAMP) (3a,20,25,29).

CD56 is usually positive, but can be negative or very dim in 10 to 20 percent of cases. Some tumors are positive for CD68 (about 50 percent), MUM1/IRF4, CD99, and TdT (about 33 percent). TdT is usually expressed by only a subset of cells with variable intensity. Blastic plasmacytoid

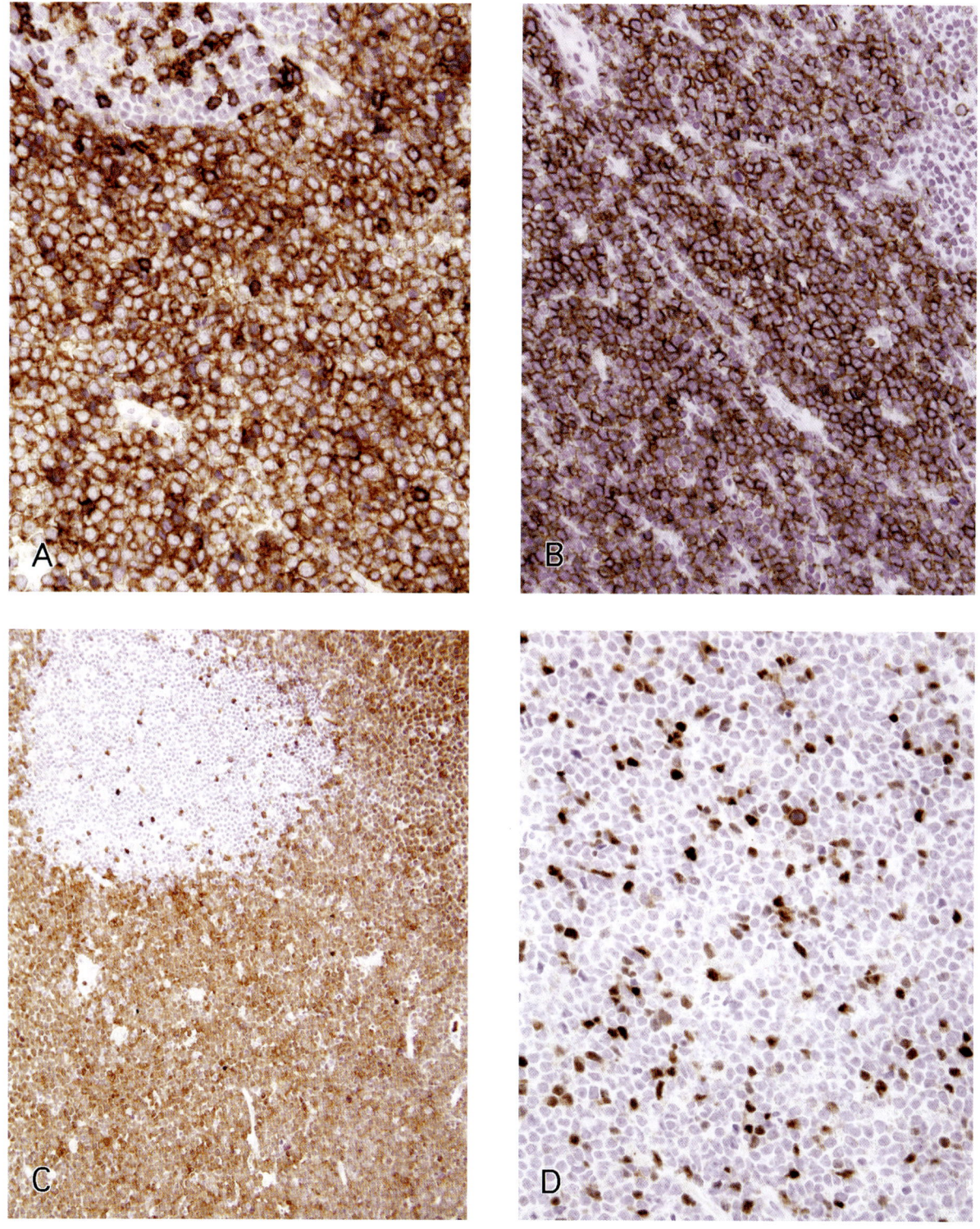

Figure 48-7

IMMUNOHISTOCHEMICAL FINDINGS OF BLASTIC PLASMACYTOID DENDRITIC CELL NEOPLASM IN LYMPH NODE

A–C: The neoplastic cells are strongly positive for CD4 (A), CD56 (B), and TCL1 (C).

D: Some cells are positive for TdT, a common result in BPDCN (immunohistochemistry with hematoxylin counterstain).

dendritic cell neoplasms are negative for B-cell antigens including PAX5 and BCL6, CD1a, CD3 (almost all cases), CD34, CD207/langerin, S-100 protein, lysozyme, MPO, cyclin D1, Epstein-Barr virus (EBV) latent membrane protein, and cytotoxic markers (TIA1, perforin, and granzyme B). In situ hybridization for EBV-encoded RNA (EBER1) is negative.

MOLECULAR GENETIC FINDINGS

Conventional cytogenetic analysis of BPDCN has shown that about 75 percent of cases have a complex (often highly complex) karyotype. Leroux et al. (16) reported a mean number of 6.8 alterations (range, 1 to 16) per clone. The six chromosomes altered most frequently in cases of BPDCN are chromosomes 5, 6, 9, 12, 13, and 15; each chromosome is altered in 30 to 40 percent of cases. Numerical aberrations are more frequent for chromosomes 9, 13, and 15 and structural aberrations are more common in chromosomes 5, 6, and 12.

Comparative genomic hybridization analysis has further confirmed the complexity of chromosomal changes in BPDCN (11,17). The most common sites of abnormality include: deletions or losses at 5q21 or 5q34 in about 75 percent of cases, 12p13 and 13q13-21 in about 65 percent, 6q in about 50 percent, as well as 15q, 7p12.2, and monosomy 9 (about 30 percent). Overall, the pattern of these chromosomal changes is similar to those observed in cases of AML and myelodysplastic syndrome (MDS) (13,19,20).

At the gene level, a number of mutations have been reported in BPDCN using targeted and small whole exome sequencing studies. In one study by Menezes et al. (19), the most common mutated genes were: *TET2*, 36 percent; *ASXL1*, 32 percent; *NRAS*, 20 percent; *NPM1*, 20 percent; *IKAROS* family genes, 20 percent; and *ZEB2*, 16 percent. Approximately half of all cases of BPDCN have gene mutations involved in DNA methylation and chromatin remodeling (19). Other investigators have shown a similar or higher frequency of *TET2* mutations as well as mutations in *TP53, PHF6, EZH2, SHOC2, RB1,* and *BCOR* (1,12,30a). Suzuki et al. (30a) also have reported *MYB* rearrangements, mostly gene fusions partnered with *ZFAT, PLEHO1, DCPS,* or *MIR3134* in approximately two thirds of cases including 100 percent of childhood BPDCNs.

The *IGH* and T-cell receptor genes are typically in the germline configuration in BPDCN, although rare cases with monoclonal *TRG* or *TRB* rearrangements, detected by polymerase chain reaction methods, have been reported. A gene expression profiling study of BPDCN cases showed a signature similar to resting precursors of plasmacytoid dendritic cells (30). In addition, the profile showed overexpression of genes in the NF-κB pathway, suggesting a potential therapeutic target.

DIFFERENTIAL DIAGNOSIS

Benign Proliferations of Plasmacytoid Dendritic Cells. In lymph nodes, a number of reactive conditions can result in hyperplasia of plasmacytoid dendritic cells. In our experience, some adjuvant therapies for solid tumors result in prominent plasmacytoid dendritic cell hyperplasia in regional lymph nodes. Typically, plasmacytoid dendritic cells are present as well-defined nodules, but rarely, the plasmacytoid dendritic cell hyperplasia is more diffuse, although some nodules are also present. Reactive plasmacytoid dendritic cells do not replace architecture or exhibit cytologic atypia.

Kikuchi-Fujimoto disease is a benign disease that tends to occur in cervical lymph nodes of younger patients and spontaneously resolves. The cause of Kikuchi-Fujimoto disease is unknown. Histologically, the paracortical regions are expanded by numerous plasmacytoid dendritic cells [CD43(+), CD68(+), CD123(+), TCL1(+)], immunoblasts, and T cells associated with abundant apoptosis. The lymph node architecture is not completely replaced.

Myeloid Sarcoma/Acute Myeloid Leukemia. In lymph nodes and skin, particularly in patients without evidence of leukemia, BPDCN may closely resemble myeloid sarcoma, and in bone marrow, AML. Expression of CD68 in about 50 percent of cases of BPDCN and CD123 in both BPDCN and a subset of AML cases can result in misdiagnosis. In addition, rare problematic cases classified as BPDCN but reported to show focal MPO expression (usually shown by immunohistochemistry) further complicate the diagnosis. Markers helpful for distinguishing BPDCN from myeloid sarcoma/AML include: TCL1, CD303, SPIB, and CD162, which are positive and CD34, lysozyme, and MPO, which are negative in BPDCN (29). A summary of markers useful for distinguishing BPDCN from myeloid sarcoma/AML is provided in Table 48-1.

Extramedullary Chronic Myelomonocytic Leukemia (CMML). Patients with CMML can develop extramedullary disease involving skin, lymph nodes, and other sites. In extramedullary biopsy specimens of CMML, aggregates of plasmacytoid dendritic cells with a mature immunophenotype [CD123(+), CD303(+), TCL1(+), CD1A(-), S-100 protein(-)] can be present, likely clonally related to the CMML. Unlike BPDCN, aggregates of mature plasmacytoid dendritic cells represent only a small component of the CMML, do not show cytologic atypia, and are typically CD56 negative (fig. 48-8). Importantly, true BPDCN, often involving the skin, can also occur in patients with CMML (31).

Lymphoblastic Lymphoma/Leukemia. The blastic appearance of the cells in many cases of BPDCN can resemble lymphoblastic lymphoma (LBL) of either T- or B-cell lineage. Expression of TdT as well as T-cell–associated antigens in

Table 48-1

MARKERS USEFUL FOR DISTINGUISHING BLASTIC PLASMACYTOID DENDRITIC CELL NEOPLASM (BPDCN) FROM ACUTE MYELOID LEUKEMIA/MYELOID SARCOMA (AML/MS)

Stain	BPDCN	AML/MS
CD4	+	–/+ (~20%)
CD123	+	–/+ (30-40%)
SPIB	+	–
TCL1	+ (~95%)	–
TCF4	+ (80-90%)	–/+ (10-20%)
CD56	+ (~85%)	–/+ (5-10%)
Myxovirus A	+/– (60-70%)	–/+ (~33%)
CD303/BDCA2	+/– (50-60%)	–
CD162/CLA	+/– (~50%)	–
Lysozyme	–	+/– (~90%)
Myeloperoxidase	–	+ (60-70%)
CD163	–	+ (~33%)
TdT	+/– (40-50%)	–/+ (10-20%)
CD34	–	+/– (~50%)

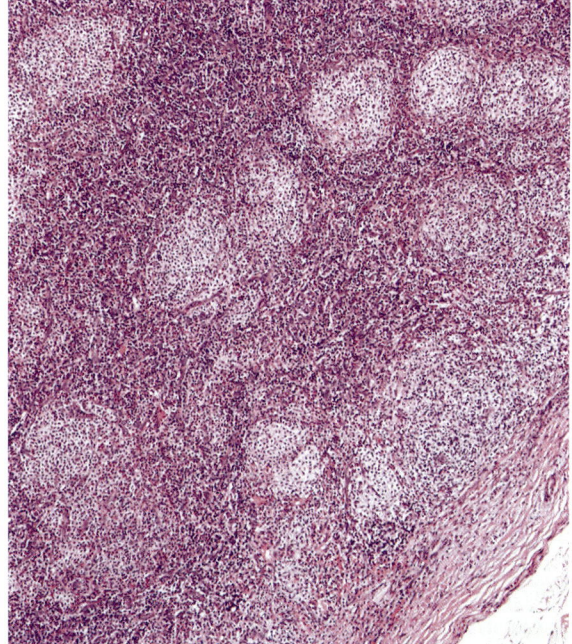 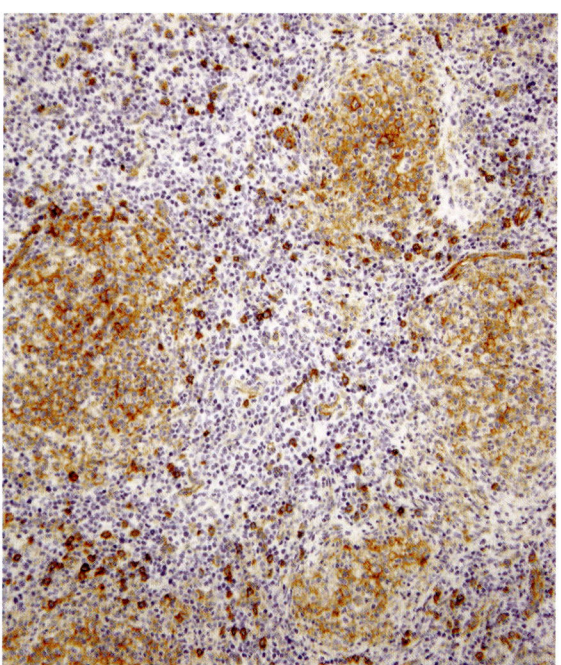

Figure 48-8

LYMPH NODE FROM A PATIENT WITH CHRONIC MYELOMONOCYTIC LEUKEMIA (CMML) SHOWING AGGREGATES OF PLASMACYTOID DENDRITIC CELLS

Left: Plasmacytoid dendritic cells form pale nodules throughout the lymph node otherwise involved by CMML in transformation (H&E stain).

Right: The plasmacytoid dendritic cells are positive for CD123 (immunohistochemistry with hematoxylin counterstain).

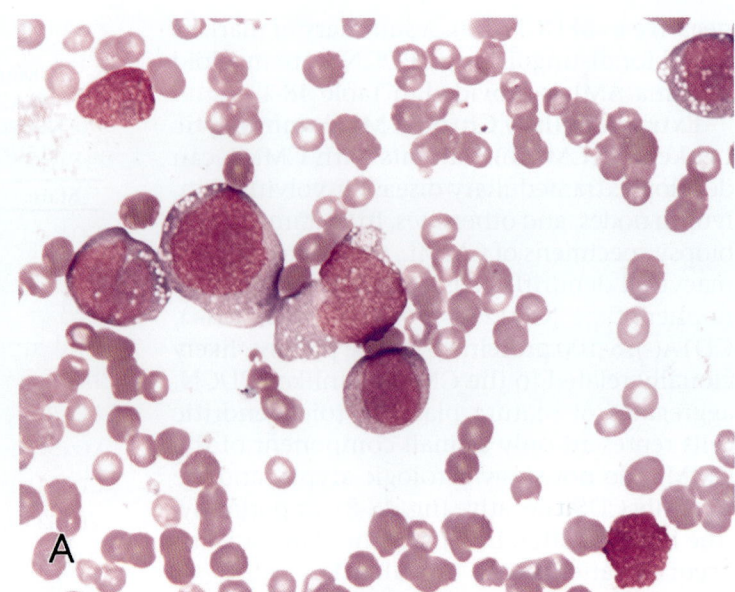

Figure 48-9

ACUTE MYELOID LEUKEMIA ARISING IN A PATIENT WHO INITIALLY HAD BLASTIC PLASMACYTOID DENDRITIC CELL NEOPLASM INVOLVING SKIN AND LYMPH NODES

A: The bone marrow aspirate smear shows many blasts with agranular cytoplasm and vacuoles (Wright-Giemsa stain).

B: The blasts are positive for myeloperoxidase (MPO) by cytochemistry (cytochemistry with Wright-Giemsa counterstain).

C: The bone marrow biopsy specimen shows replacement by myeloblasts (H&E stain).

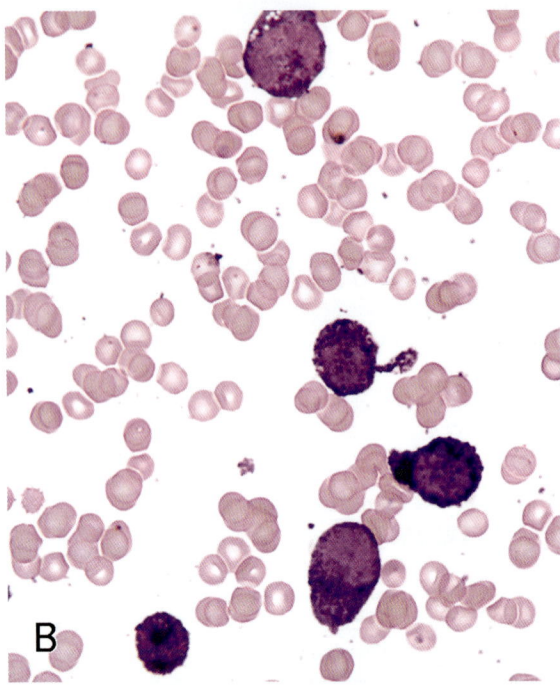

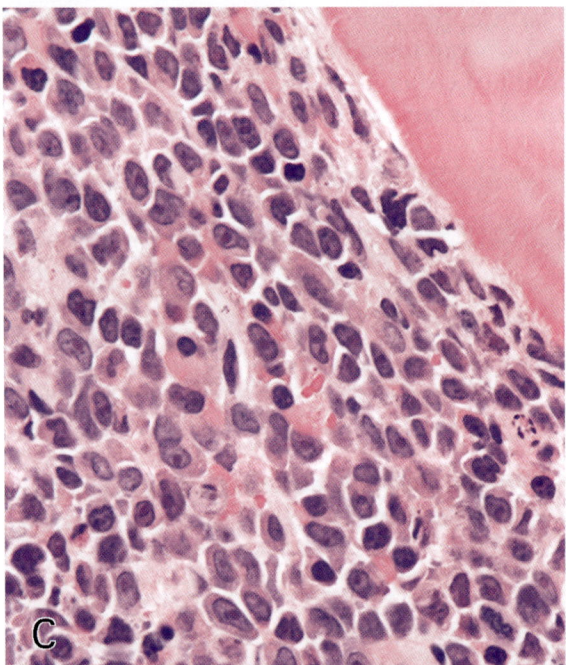

BPDCN complicates the differential diagnosis with T-LBL. The cells of T-LBL, unlike BPDCN, usually express TdT uniformly, often express CD1a or CD10, are positive for T- or B-cell–specific antigens, and carry monoclonal T-cell receptor or *IGH* gene rearrangements.

Mycosis Fungoides. Skin lesions of BPDCN need to be distinguished from mycosis fungoides and both lesions express CD4, which may complicate distinguishing these diseases. Unlike BPDCN, mycosis fungoides usually shows epidermal involvement by neoplastic cells (epidermotropism), parakeratosis, and dermal fibrosis, indicating a chronic disease process. Mycosis fungoides is CD3(+), CD123(-), CD303(-), and TCL1(-). Most cases carry monoclonal T-cell receptor gene rearrangements (except a subset of cases of early patch stage disease).

Extranodal NK/T-Cell Lymphoma, Nasal Type. Particularly in skin, BPDCN can resemble nasal type extranodal NK/T-cell lymphoma and both diseases express CD56. Unlike BPDCN, extranodal NK/T-cell lymphomas often show angioinvasion, express cytotoxic markers and EBER1, and are negative for CD123 and TCL1.

Mantle Cell Lymphoma, Blastoid Variant. In lymph nodes and bone marrow, in particular, BPDCN and the blastoid variant of mantle cell lymphoma can closely resemble each other. Unlike BPDCN, mantle cell lymphoma expresses pan-B-cell antigens and cyclin D1, and carries t(11;14)(q13;q32)/*CCND1-IGH*.

TREATMENT AND PROGNOSIS

Patients with BPDCN have a rapidly progressive disease that requires aggressive combination chemotherapy. Therapies developed for AML and acute lymphoblastic leukemia have been used for BPDCN patients; the latter appears to be better in terms of inducing clinical remission and extending survival (22,28,32). Allogeneic hematopoietic stem cell transplantation has resulted in prolonged clinical remission in a small number of patients (7,14,22,28). Overexpression of CD123 (interleukin-3 receptor) by the cells of BPDCN is the target of a recently developed agent, SL-401, which is composed of diphtheria toxin linked with an anti-CD123 antibody. In vitro and in vivo studies using SL-401 appear to be promising (8). A recent study has identified TCF4 as a marker of BPDCN suggesting a potential target for novel therapy (3a).

The overall survival of patients with BPDCN is poor, with a median survival period of 12 to 18 months (5,15). About 10 percent of patients progress to myeloid leukemia, either acute myeloid leukemia (fig. 48-9) or acute or chronic myelomonocytic leukemia (7,10,15,27).

REFERENCES

1. Alayed K, Patel KP, Konoplev S, et al. TET2 mutations, myelodysplastic features, and a distinct immunoprofile characterize blastic plasmacytoid dendritic cell neoplasm in the bone marrow. Am J Hematol 2013;88:1055-1061.
2. Arber DA, Orazi A, Hasserjian R, et al. The 2016 revision to the World Health Organization classification of myeloid neoplasms and acute leukemia. Blood 2016;127:2391-2405.
3. Brody JP, Allen S, Schulman P, et al. Acute agranular CD4-positive natural killer cell leukemia. Comprehensive clinicopathologic studies including virologic and in vitro culture with inducing agents. Cancer 1995;75:2474-2483.
3a. Ceribelli M, Hou ZE, Kelly PN, et al. A druggable TCF4- and BRD4-dependent transcriptional network sustains malignancy in blastic plasmacytoid dendritic cell neoplasm. Cancer Cell 2016;30:764-778.
4. Cota C, Vale E, Viana I, et al. Cutaneous manifestations of blastic plasmacytoid dendritic cell neoplasm-morphologic and phenotypic variability in a series of 33 patients. Am J Surg Pathol 2010;34:75-87.
5. Facchetti F, Jones DM, Petrella T. Blastic plasmacytoid dendritic cell neoplasm. In: Swerdlow SH, Campo E, Harris NL, Jaffe ES, Pileria SA, Thiele J, Vardiman JW, eds. WHO classification of tumours of haematopoietic and lymphoid tissues, 4th ed. Lyon: IARC Press; 2008;145-147.
6. Ferreira J, Gasparinho MG, Fonseca R. Cytomorphological features of blastic plasmacytoid dendritic cell neoplasm on FNA and cerebrospinal fluid cytology: a review of 6 cases. Cancer Cytopathol 2016;124:196-202.
7. Feuillard J, Jacob MC, Valensi F, et al. Clinical and biologic features of CD4(+)CD56(+) malignancies. Blood 2002;99:1556-1563.
8. Frankel AE, Woo JH, Ahn C, et al. Activity of SL-401, a targeted therapy directed to interleukin-3 receptor, in blastic plasmacytoid dendritic cell neoplasm patients. Blood 2014;124:385-392.
9. Garnache-Ottou F, Feuillard J, Ferrand C, et al. Extended diagnostic criteria for plasmacytoid dendritic cell leukaemia. Br J Haematol 2009;145:624-636.
10. Herling M, Teitell MA, Shen RR, Medeiros LJ, Jones D. TCL1 expression in plasmacytoid dendritic cells (DC2s) and the related CD4+ CD56+ blastic tumors of skin. Blood 2003;101:5007-5009.
11. Jardin F, Callanan M, Penther D, et al. Recurrent genomic aberrations combined with deletions of various tumour suppressor genes may deregulate the G1/S transition in CD4+ CD56+ hematodermic neoplasms and contribute to the aggressiveness of disease. Leukemia 2009;23:698-707.

12. Jardin F, Ruminy P, Parmentier F, et al. TET2 and TP53 mutations are frequently observed in blastic plasmacytoid dendritic cell neoplasm. Br J Haematol 2011;153:413-416.

13. Julia F, Dalle S, Duru G, et al. Blastic plasmacytoid dendritic cell neoplasms. clinico-immunohisto-chemical correlations in a series of 91 patients. Am J Surg Pathol 2014;38:673-680.

14. Kharfan-Dabaja MA, Lazarus HM, Nishihori T, Mahfouz RA, Hamadani M. Diagnostic and therapeutic advances in blastic plasmacytoid dendritic cell neoplasm: a focus on hematopoietic cell transplantation. Biol Blood Marrow Transplant 2013;19:1006-1012.

15. Khoury JD, Medeiros LJ, Manning JT, Sulak LE, Bueso-Ramos C, Jones D. CD56(+) TdT(+) blastic natural killer cell tumor of the skin: a primitive systemic malignancy related to myelomonocytic leukemia. Cancer 2002;94:2401-2408.

16. Leroux D, Mugneret F, Callanan M, et al. CD4(+), CD56(+) DC2 acute leukemia is characterized by recurrent clonal chromosomal changes affecting 6 major targets: a study of 21 cases by the Groupe Francais de Cytogenetique Hematologique. Blood 2002;99:4154-4159.

17. Lucioni M, Novara F, Fiandrino G, et al. Twenty-one cases of blastic plasmacytoid dendritic cell neoplasm: focus on biallelic locus 9p21.3 deletion. Blood 2011;118:4591-4594.

17a. Martín-Martín L, Almeida J, Pomares H, et al. Blastic plasmacytoid dendritic cell neoplasm frequently shows occult central nervous system involvement at diagnosis and benefits from intrathecal therapy. Oncotarget 2016;7:10174-10181.

18. Martin-Martin L, Lopez A, Vidriales B, et al. Classification and clinical behavior of blastic plasmacytoid dendritic cell neoplasms according to their maturation-associated immunophenotypic profile. Oncotarget 2015;6:19204-10216.

19. Menezes J, Acquadro F, Wiseman M, et al. Exome sequencing reveals novel and recurrent mutations with clinical impact in blastic plasmacytoid dendritic cell neoplasm. Leukemia 2014;28:823-829.

20. Montes-Moreno S, Ramos-Medina R, Martinez-Lopez A, et al. SPIB, a novel immunohisto-chemical marker for human blastic plasmacytoid dendritic cell neoplasms: characterization of its expression in major hematolymphoid neoplasms. Blood 2013;121:643-647.

21. Muller-Hermelink HK, Stein H, Steinmann G, Lennert K. Malignant lymphoma of plasma-cytoid T-cells. Morphologic and immunologic studies characterizing a special type of T-cell. Am J Surg Pathol 1983;7:849-862.

22. Pagano L, Valentini CG, Grammatico S, Pulsoni A. Blastic plasmacytoid dendritic cell neoplasm: diagnostic criteria and therapeutical approaches. Br J Haematol 2016;174:188-202.

23. Petrella T, Comeau MR, Maynadié M, et al. Agranular CD4+ CD56+ hematodermic neoplasm' (blastic NK-cell lymphoma) originates from a population of CD56+ precursor cells related to plasmacytoid monocytes. Am J Surg Pathol 2002;26:852-862.

24. Petrella T, Dalac S, Maynadié M, et al. CD4+ CD56+ cutaneous neoplasms: a distinct hematological entity? Groupe Francais d'Etude des Lymphomes Cutanes (GFELC). Am J Surg Pathol 1999;23:137-146.

25. Pilichowska ME, Fleming MD, Pinkus JL, Pinkus GS. CD4+/CD56+ hematodermic neoplasm ("blastic natural killer cell lymphoma"): neoplastic cells express the immature dendritic cell marker BDCA-2 and produce interferon. Am J Clin Pathol 2007;128:445-453.

26. Rauh MJ, Rahman F, Good D, et al. Blastic plasmacytoid dendritic cell neoplasm with leukemic presentation, lacking cutaneous involvement: Case series and literature review. Leuk Res 2012;36:81-86.

27. Reichard KK, Burks EJ, Foucar MK, et al. CD4(+) CD56(+) lineage-negative malignancies are rare tumors of plasmacytoid dendritic cells. Am J Surg Pathol 2005;29:1274-1283.

28. Roos-Weil D, Dietrich S, Boumendil A, et al. Stem cell transplantation can provide durable disease control in blastic plasmacytoid dendritic cell neoplasm: a retrospective study from the European Group for Blood and Marrow Transplantation. Blood 2013;121:440-446.

29. Sangle NA, Schmidt RL, Patel JL, et al. Optimized immunohistochemical panel to differentiate myeloid sarcoma from blastic plasmacytoid dendritic cell neoplasm. Mod Pathol 2014;27:1137-1143.

30. Sapienza MR, Fuligni F, Agostinelli C, et al. Molecular profiling of blastic plasmacytoid dendritic cell neoplasm reveals a unique pattern and suggests selective sensitivity to NF-kB pathway inhibition. Leukemia 2014;28:1606-1616.

30a. Suzuki K, Suzuki Y, Hama A, et al. Recurrent MYB rearrangement in blastic plasmacytoid dendritic cell neoplasm. Leukemia 2017;31:1629-1633.

31. Vitte F, Fabiani B, Bénet C, et al. Specific skin lesions in chronic myelomonocytic leukemia: a spectrum of myelomonocytic and dendritic cell proliferations: a study of 42 cases. Am J Surg Pathol 2012;36:1302-1316.

32. Wright KD, Onciu MM, Coustan-Smith E, et al. Successful treatment of pediatric plasmacytoid dendrtitic cell tumors with a contemporary regimen for acute lymphoblastic leukemia. Pediatr Blood Cancer 2013;60:E38-E41.

MASTOCYTOSIS

GENERAL FEATURES

Mastocytosis, also known as *mast cell disease*, is a monoclonal expansion of abnormal mast cells in various tissues, most often skin and bone marrow. The cells commonly carry activating mutations of *KIT*.

Mast cells were first described by Paul Ehrlich in 1878 because of their large cytoplasmic granules with unique staining characteristics: the granules were metachromatic in tissue sections. These granules led Ehrlich to conclude incorrectly that mast cells nourish the surrounding tissues, and he named them *mastzellen* (from German meaning "fattening"). Mast cells are now known to be the major effectors of allergic reactions and their cytoplasmic granules contain many substances, such as heparin, histamine, serotonin, proteases (e.g., tryptase and chymase), and tumor necrosis factor alpha.

Normal or reactive mast cells are usually 5 to 15 μm in size and are round with a single eccentric nucleus and moderate amounts of granulated cytoplasm. In most organs, small numbers of mast cells, either singly or in small groups (1 to 3 cells), are present within interstitial spaces. In bone marrow aspirate smears, mast cells are found within or in close proximity to bone marrow particles and differ from basophils in their nuclear shape. Unlike mast cells, basophils have segmented nuclei.

Mastocytosis is a rare disease in all of its forms and the etiology is poorly understood. Cutaneous mastocytosis is the most frequent type, but data on its incidence are not clear. The incidence of systemic mastocytosis is lower, approximately 0.9 cases per 100,000 persons per year in a study from Denmark (10). Environmental factors are known to trigger exacerbations of disease (see below), but are not implicated in the etiology. Inheritance plays a role as a small subset of cases runs in families.

The presence of activating point mutations of *KIT* (located at chromosome 4q12) is the molec-ular hallmark of mastocytosis. The most frequent mutation is D816V (Asp816Val) in exon 17 located within the activation loop, which causes a conformational change in the juxtamembrane region of the protein, resulting in constitutive receptor dimerization and signaling activation in the absence of stem cell factor (KIT ligand) (3,25). KIT (CD117) is a type III transmembrane tyrosine kinase receptor expressed widely by hematopoietic stem cells and multipotential progenitor cells, and is necessary for the differentiation of the myeloid and lymphoid lineages, but it is downregulated in all mature myeloid lineage cells except mast cells.

Mastocytosis, as currently defined, is a markedly heterogeneous disease ranging from asymptomatic skin lesions that usually regress to aggressive neoplasms. For this reason, mastocytosis is subdivided into two broad categories: cutaneous and systemic (16,48). *Cutaneous mastocytosis* is defined as mast cell disease confined to the skin (Table 49-1). Patients do not have evidence of organomegaly and serum tryptase levels are normal. The most common variant of cutaneous mastocytosis is *urticaria pigmentosa* (UP), also known more recently as *maculopapular cutaneous mastocytosis*. The justification for this newer term is that the lesions of UP are stable, whereas urticaria lesions as currently defined are usually transient wheals (8). For historical reasons, however, UP is a term that is well entrenched in the literature and it seems unlikely to be completely replaced by the term maculopapular cutaneous mastocytosis.

Systemic mastocytosis (SM) is defined as mast cell disease involving at least one extracutaneous organ, with or without coexistent skin infiltration. A consensus group (50) developed a system for the diagnosis of mastocytosis based on the one major and four minor criteria and this system is used in the World Health Organization (WHO) classification (Table 49-2) (2a,16). The major criterion is the presence of

Table 49-1

CLASSIFICATION OF CUTANEOUS MASTOCYTOSIS[a]

Category	Clinical Features	Pathologic Features
Urticaria pigmentosa	Red or brown-red macules or maculopapular lesions; larger papules more common in children; dissemination more common in adults; a rare variant in children presents as a nonpigmented plaque	Aggregates of spindle-shaped mast cells in dermis; often perivascular
Diffuse cutaneous mastocytosis	Diffusely thickened skin with peau d'orange appearance	Band-like infiltration by mast cells in superficial dermis
Solitary mastocytoma of skin	Infants with single lesion	Single lesion of mast cells filling dermis

[a]Patients with cutaneous mastocytosis lack evidence of systemic involvement. There is no organomegaly and the serum tryptase level is normal.

Table 49-2

WORLD HEALTH ORGANIZATION (WHO) CRITERIA FOR DIAGNOSIS OF SYSTEMIC MASTOCYTOSIS

Major Criterion
Biopsy sections (bone marrow [BM] or extracutaneous organs) show dense infiltrates or aggregates of mast cells (>15 mast cells per aggregate)

Minor Criteria
1. Biopsy sections (BM or extracutaneous organs) show >25% mast cells with spindle shape or atypical morphologic features; or in BM aspirate smear >25% masts cells are immature or atypical
2. Detection of activating point mutation of *KIT* at codon 816
3. Mast cells are positive for CD2 and/or CD25 in addition to normal mast cell markers
4. Serum tryptase level >20 ng/mL (unless an associated monoclonal myeloid disorder is present which precludes the use of this criterion)

resulting in compromised organ function. B findings include increased mast cell burden, dysplasia or myeloproliferation without criteria to diagnose a hematopoietic neoplasm, and organomegaly. C findings include cytopenias (indicating bone marrow dysfunction), palpable hepatomegaly with evidence of functional compromise, bone lesions, palpable splenomegaly with hypersplenism, and malabsorption with weight loss as a result of involvement of the gastrointestinal tract (2a,16).

CLINICAL FEATURES

Cutaneous Mastocytosis

Cutaneous mastocytosis is the most common form of mast cell disease and it occurs most frequently in children. There are three variants of cutaneous mastocytosis: urticaria pigmentosa (or maculopapular cutaneous mastocytosis), diffuse cutaneous mastocytosis, and mastocytoma of skin (8,15,28). Urticaria pigmentosa is characterized by multiple skin lesions that show variably sized, hyperpigmented (red-brown) macular or maculopapular lesions that become urticarial when rubbed or scratched, known as Darier sign (8). A recent proposal divides urticaria pigmentosa into polymorphic and monomorphic variants (15). The polymorphic variant is composed of larger lesions of variable size and shape (fig. 49-1, left). These most often occur in children and commonly resolve around the time of puberty. The monomorphic variant is composed of smaller maculopapular lesions that occur in children or adults, and are more often disseminated (fig. 49-1, right). The

extracutaneous organ involvement with multifocal dense infiltrates of over 15 mast cells per aggregate. The four minor criteria are: 1) over 25 percent of mast cells in infiltrates that are spindle shaped or atypical; 2) *KIT*-activating mutation in codon 816 in blood, bone marrow, or extracutaneous organ; 3) mast cells that aberrantly express CD2 and/or CD25; and 4) serum total tryptase level consistently greater than 20 ng/mL. The diagnosis of SM requires 1 major and 1 minor or at least 3 minor criteria.

SM is further subclassified into six subcategories based on the integration of "B" and "C" findings (Table 49-3). B findings generally correlate with the degree of infiltration whereas C findings are related to more severe infiltration

Table 49-3

WHO CLASSIFICATION OF MASTOCYTOSIS

Category	Criteria	Prognosis
Cutaneous mastoctosis	See Table 49-1	Good
Indolent systemic mastocytosis	Meets criteria for SM (Table 49-2), but no "C" findings[a]; mast cell burden is low and skin lesions are very common; A subset of patients has disease only in BM[b]	Good
Smoldering systemic masto-cytosis	Similar to indolent SM with two or more "B" findings[c]	Good
Systemic mastocytosis with an associated hematologic neo-plasm (SM-AHN)	Meets criteria for SM (Table 49-2) and associated with MDS, MPN, MDS/MPN, and rarely AML, lymphoma, or myeloma	Determined by the type of AHNMD
Aggressive systemic masto-cytosis	Meets criteria for SM (Table 49-2) with one or more "C" findings; no evidence of mast cell leukemia; usually no skin lesions	Variably aggressive clinical course
Mast cell leukemia	Meets criteria for SM (Table 49-2) with atypical or imma-ture mast cells diffusely infiltrating BM medullary space; BM aspirate smears with $\geq$20% mast cells; in peripheral blood smear $\geq$10% mast cells	Very poor
Mast cell sarcoma	Unifocal mast cell tumor with a destructive growth pattern and obvious, high-grade cytologic atypia; no evidence of systemic mastocytosis	Very poor; the tumor often disseminates or converts into mast cell leukemia

[a]"C" findings: 1) BM dysfunction manifested by one or more cytopenias, but no obvious nonmast cell hematopoietic malignancy; 2) palpable hepatomegaly with impairment of liver function, ascites, and/or portal hypertension; 3) skeletal involvement with large osteolytic lesions and/or pathologic fractures; 4) palpable splenomegaly with hypersplenism; and 5) malabsorption with weight loss due to mast cell infiltrates in gastrointestinal tract.
[b]BM = bone marrow; MDS = myelodysplastic syndrome; MPN = myeloproliferative neoplasm; AML = acute myeloid leukemia.
[c]"B" findings: 1) BM biopsy shows >30% infiltration by mast cells (focal, dense aggregates) and/or serum total tryptase level >20 ng/mL; 2) signs of dysplasia or myeloproliferation in nonmast cell lineage but insufficient criteria for definitive diagnosis of AHNMD, with normal or only slightly abnormal blood counts; and 3) hepatomegaly without impairment of liver function, and/or splenomegaly without hypersplenism, and/or lymphadenopathy on palpation or imaging.

monomorphic variant in children often persists into adulthood (15).

The other two variants of cutaneous masto-cytosis are uncommon. Diffuse cutaneous mas-tocytosis occurs almost exclusively in children who present with thickened skin with a peau d'orange (orange peel) appearance, without any individual skin lesions. Mastocytoma of skin is usually a single lesion, but can be multiple, and occurs almost exclusively in infants (8,16).

Systemic Mastocytosis

SM is most common in adults with a mean age of 60 years, and is rare in patients under 30 years of age (16,26,33). Men are more commonly affected in a ratio of about 1.5 to 1. Symptoms can be subgrouped into two categories: those related to the activation of neoplastic mast cells, with the release of granule contents, and those related to tissue infiltration by mast cells and, if severe, compromised organ function. This second group also includes organ compromise as a result of in-filtration by an associated hematologic neoplasm (AHN) (16,26,55).

The release of mast cell mediators and/or cyto-kines (e.g., interleukin-1B, interleukin-6) results in a myriad of symptoms (22,52). Generalized symptoms include weight loss, night sweats, fever, fatigue, and anorexia. The skin may show flushing, pruritus, and urticaria. Cardiovascular symptoms include palpitations, syncope, or dizziness, and central nervous system/psychiatric symptoms include anxiety, depression, and cognitive impair-ment. Abdominal pain is the most common symptom of the gastrointestinal tract, followed by diarrhea, anorexia, and nausea. Osteoporosis or fibromyalgia also occurs in a subset of patients. The acute release of mediators renders patients

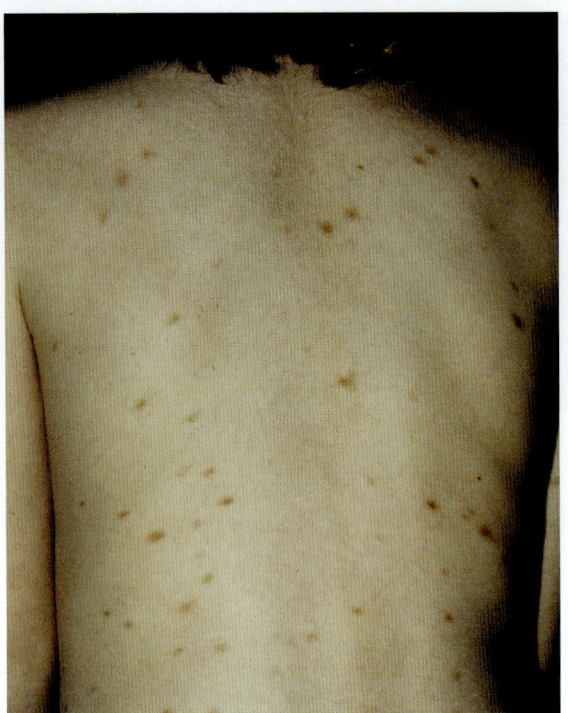
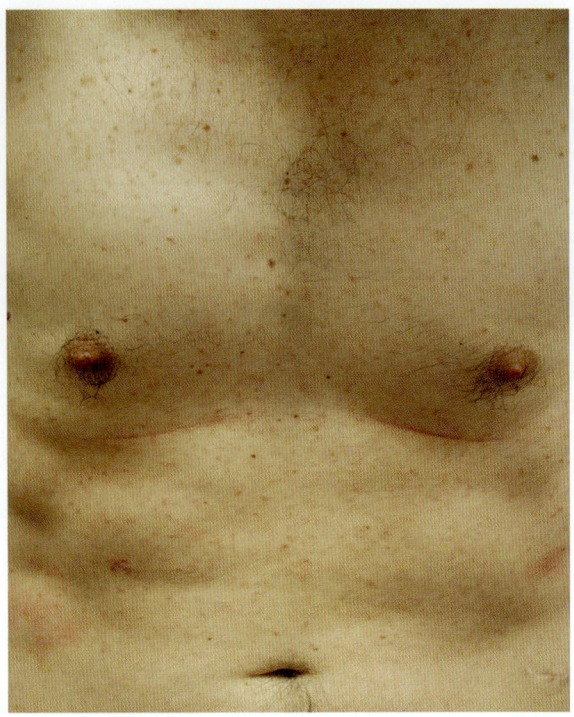

Figure 49-1

URTICARIA PIGMENTOSA (CUTANEOUS MASTOCYTOSIS)

Left: The back of a young girl with the polymorphous variant is seen. The lesions are variably sized and pigmented.
Right: The abdomen of an adult man with multiple small lesions on the chest and abdomen that are more monomorphic compared with the lesions of the young girl. (Courtesy of Dr. A. Ciurea, Houston, TX.)

with SM at increased risk of anaphylaxis. Patients must avoid potential triggers of mast cell release, often unique for each patient, a few of which include ingestion of alcohol (especially red wine) and drugs (e.g., aspirin, codeine, morphine, and others), insect bites or stings, and emotional stress (22). Patients have an increased risk of duodenal ulcer as a consequence of increased acid production induced by elevated histamine levels. Bleeding can occur, thought to be attributable to the release of heparin-like substances from mast cell granules. Tissue infiltration by mast cells also results in a number of symptoms or physical findings, depending on the anatomic site and extent of infiltration and accounted for, at least in part, by the subdivision of SM into categories (Table 49-3).

The most useful laboratory study in the workup of patients with SM is serum tryptase. As stated in the WHO classification, a serum tryptase level greater than 20 ng/mL in a patient clinically suspected of having SM supports the diagnosis. The serum tryptase level correlates with overall mast cell burden, however, it is not specific and can be increased in patients with anaphylactic reactions or hematologic malignancies as well as other causes (7,38). For this reason, a high serum tryptase level cannot be used as a criterion to support the diagnosis of SM in patients with SM-AHN (24). Urine testing for N-methylhistamine and methylimidazole acetic acid, markers of elevated histamine levels, are surrogates for mast cell activity and SM. Patients with aggressive SM may have an elevated serum lactate dehydrogenase or beta-2-microglobulin level. Hematologic abnormalities are common in patients with SM. Anemia occurs in about half of patients, most often in patients with SM-AHN, aggressive SM, and mast cell leukemia. Thrombocytopenia and leukocytosis also occur. About 15 percent of patients have eosinophilia and, uncommonly, eosinophilia may be an isolated finding (30). *KIT* mutation testing is very helpful, but using standard assays is less sensitive when performed using a blood specimen compared with bone marrow. Recently developed highly sensitive assays can be used to assess blood specimens and therefore are an advantage for monitoring disease (3).

Indolent Systemic Mastocytosis. Patients with indolent SM have involvement of the bone marrow, often with skin lesions. They tend to have a low disease burden and do not have C findings or evidence of AHN (26).

Smoldering Systemic Mastocytosis. Patients with smoldering SM have two or more B findings but no C findings (49). Some patients with smoldering SM (1 to 5 percent) progress to aggressive SM.

Well-Differentiated Systemic Mastocytosis. This is a rare variant of SM involving primarily skin and bone marrow, with organomegaly in less than 25 percent of patients (2). Most patients are children, with a girl-to-boy ratio of 4 to 1 and about 40 percent of cases run in families. The skin lesions are most often maculopapular, but other variants are described. The bone marrow shows infiltrates of mature mast cells otherwise similar to other cases of SM in bone marrow. However, the mast cells are positive for CD30 and negative for CD2 and CD25 in about 80 percent of cases. In addition, *KIT* mutations are detected in only about one third of cases and *D816V* mutations are less common (2).

Systemic Mastocytosis with an Associated Hematologic Neoplasm. Patients with SM-AHN have evidence of a myeloproliferative neoplasm (MPN), myelodysplastic syndrome (MDS), or MDS/MPN, or uncommonly, acute myeloid leukemia, lymphomas of various types, or plasma cell myeloma (36,55). Patients with SM-AHN are usually older, more frequently have constitutional symptoms and hematologic abnormalities, and less often have skin lesions. They also have a lower overall survival rate compared to patients with pure SM (36,55). Eosinophilia is observed in approximately 15 percent of patients with SM-AHN, possibly related to the chemotaxis attributable to cytokine release from mast cells or related to the coexistent nonmast cell hematologic neoplasm.

Aggressive Systemic Mastocytosis. Patients with aggressive SM have one or more C findings that include bone marrow dysfunction (as shown by the presence of cytopenias), palpable hepatomegaly with impaired liver function, palpable splenomegaly with hypersplenism, bone lesions, and malabsorption or weight loss as a result of mast cells infiltrating the gastrointestinal tract (16,26). Most patients with hepatomegaly, splenomegaly, or lymphadenopathy fall within this category. Patients with aggressive SM usually do not have skin lesions at the time of initial presentation. Skin involvement can be marked and plaque-like, however, in the terminal stages of disease.

Mast Cell Leukemia. Mast cell leukemia is rare; about 100 cases have been reported in the literature, representing less than 1 percent of all cases of SM (16,20,33,41,51). There is a marked male predominance, with about 80 percent of all cases in men. In these patients the bone marrow is extensively involved. Mast cells represent 20 percent or more of all cells in aspirate smears and they diffusely replace the medullary space in the biopsy specimen. Mast cells usually represent 10 percent or more of all cells in the peripheral blood smear. If the blood smear shows less than 10 percent mast cells, the term *aleukemic mast cell leukemia* is used. Valent et al. (51) suggested subdividing mast cell leukemia cases into acute and chronic types based on the presence or absence of C findings, respectively.

Mast Cell Sarcoma and Extracutaneous Mastocytoma. Patients with these lesions do not have other evidence of SM (16,50). Mast cell sarcoma is rare and presents as a unifocal tumor that exhibits a destructive growth pattern and marked or high-grade cytologic atypia. Some patients with mast cell sarcoma subsequently develop widespread disease or mast cell leukemia.

Patients with an extracutaneous mastocytoma present with a solitary mast cell tumor involving a non-skin site. In general, these lesions do not have a destructive growth pattern and have minimal or no cytologic atypia. The clinical course is usually indolent.

HISTOLOGIC FINDINGS

Cutaneous Mastocytosis

The skin lesions of cutaneous mastocytosis show an increased number of mast cells in the dermis. Normal skin from healthy persons contains about 40 mast cells/mm^2 whereas mast cells in cutaneous mastocytosis are 4 to 8 times

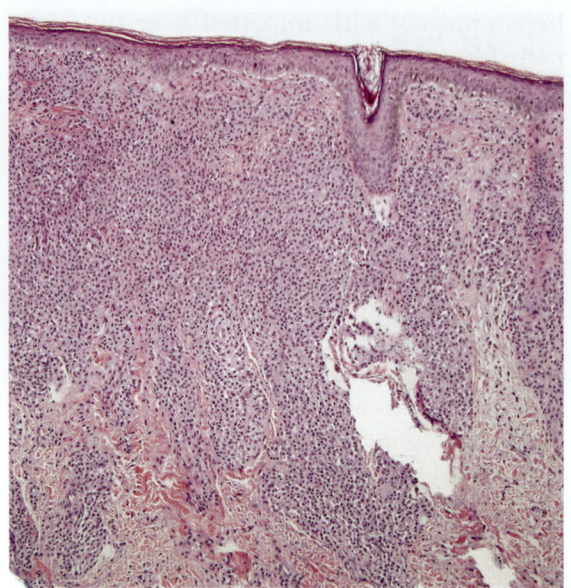
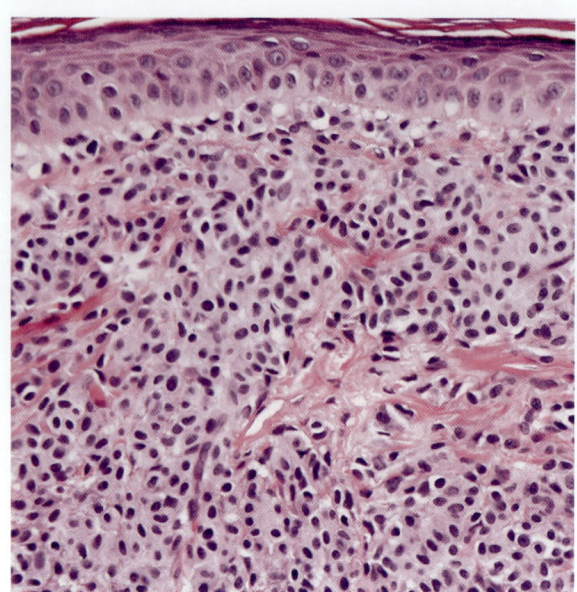

Figure 49-2

CUTANEOUS MASTOCYTOSIS

Left: Mast cells fill the papillary dermis and extend into the deep dermis.
Right: High-magnification image shows mast cells with oval or mildly spindled nuclei and abundant pale cytoplasm (left, right: hematoxylin and eosin [H&E] stain).

more numerous; mast cells are increased to a lesser extent, 2 to 3 times normal, in inflammatory cutaneous diseases (15). The number of mast cells in the dermis of patients with cutaneous mastocytosis varies, however, and can overlap with that of normal healthy skin.

In urticaria pigmentosa, mast cells are either loosely scattered, with a tendency to aggregate around blood vessels and adnexa in the upper dermis, or form small compact infiltrates (fig. 49-2) (8,15,28). They usually have a spindle-shaped appearance. In contrast, in patients with mastocytoma of skin, the mast cells are often round and can fill and expand the dermis. Mast cells usually contain many metachromatic granules and are easily detectable with cytochemical stains (e.g., Giemsa).

Systemic Mastocytosis

Lymph Node. Approximately half of patients with SM have lymph node involvement, but the degree of involvement is highly variable, ranging from subtle disease that may require immunohistochemical analysis for recognition, to obvious replacement of lymph node parenchyma (11,17,46). In a study from the Mayo Clinic, 21 percent of patients with mastocytosis had clinical evidence of lymphadenopathy (46).

Single scattered mast cells may be increased in non-neoplastic conditions but the presence of compact clusters of mast cells is required to establish the diagnosis of SM in lymph node. Mast cell clusters can involve any lymph node compartment (17,46). The paracortex is involved most often, but mast cell clusters are observed within lymphoid follicles, medullary cords, and sinuses (fig. 49-3). Mast cells also commonly surround arterioles or involve lymph node trabeculae, and these may have a round, ovoid, or spindle shape (fig. 49-4). Infiltrates of mast cells are often associated with eosinophils (which may be numerous) and fibrosis. Involved lymph nodes also may show plasmacytosis and follicular or paracortical hyperplasia (17).

Spleen. Splenomegaly occurs in up to 40 percent of patients with SM (11,18,46). However, the true prevalence of splenic involvement is uncertain because splenectomy is rarely performed in these patients. Mast cell aggregates involve the red or white pulp, and may have a granulomatous appearance at low magnification (fig. 49-5). Similar to lymph nodes, mast

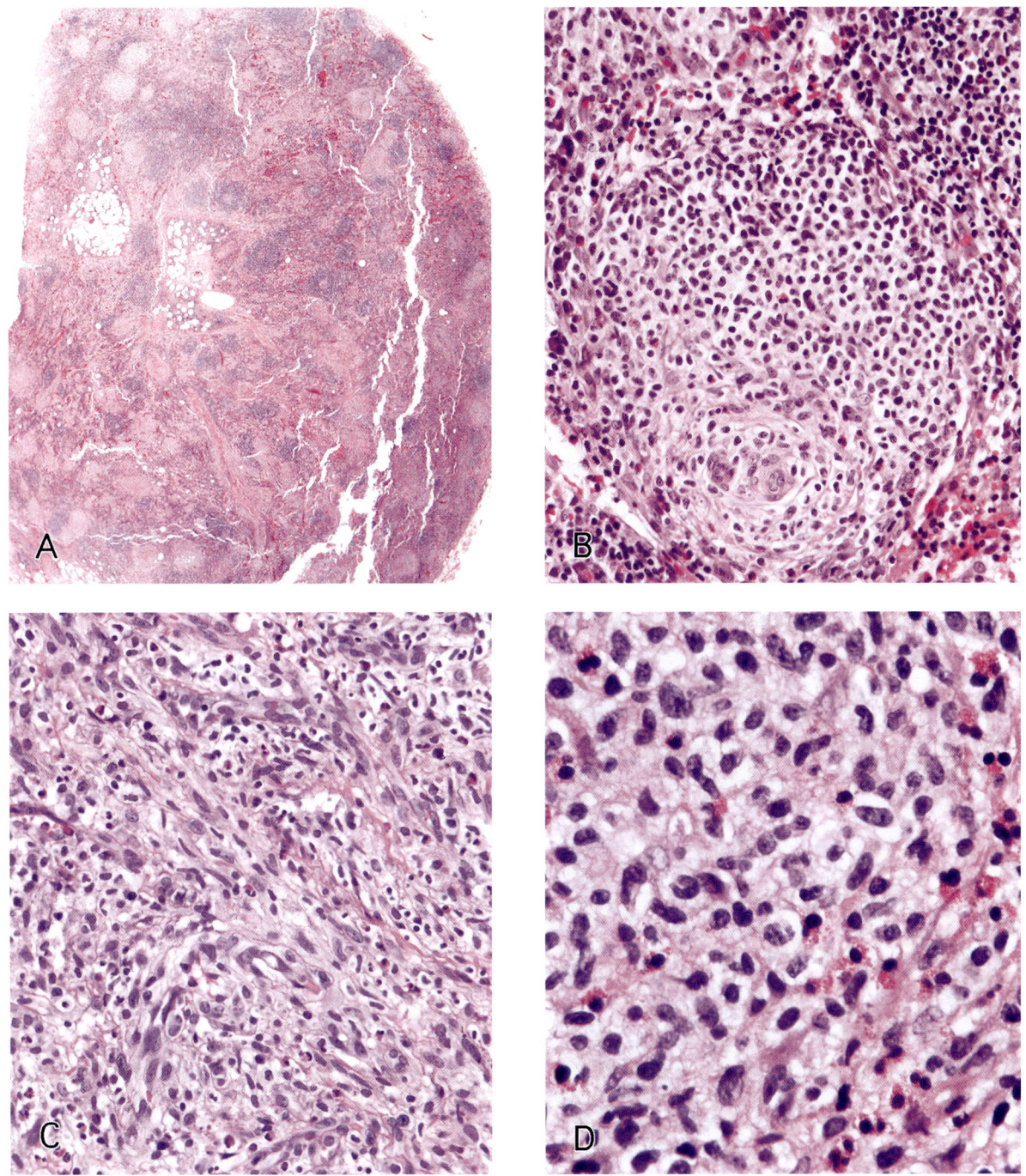

Figure 49-3

SYSTEMIC MASTOCYTOSIS INVOLVING LYMPH NODE

A: Low-magnification view shows a lymph node partially involved by pale nodules of mast cells located predominantly in the paracortical region (A–D: H&E stain).

B: A mast cell nodule surrounds a blood vessel. The mast cells have pale cytoplasm, and a few eosinophils are present in the background.

C: In this field the mast cells have a spindle shape and are associated with fibrosis and scattered eosinophils.

D: In another field the mast cells have an oval or mildly spindled appearance, with more numerous eosinophils and no fibrosis.

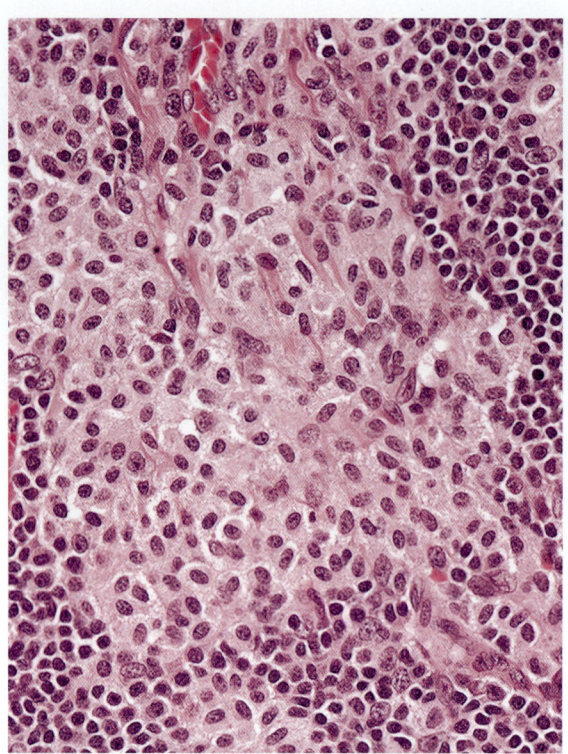 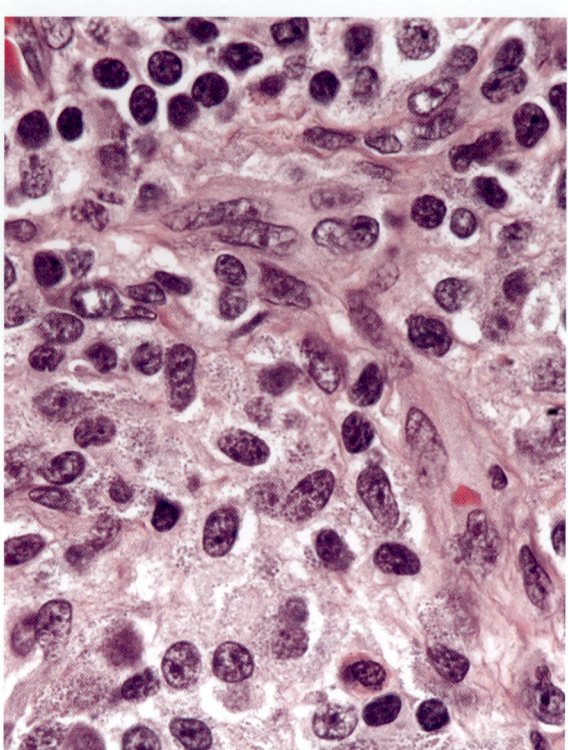

Figure 49-4

SYSTEMIC MASTOCYTOSIS INVOLVING LYMPH NODE

Left: Mast cells are present within a lymph node sinus.
Right: Mast cells surround a blood vessel in the lymph node paracortex. In both images the mast cells have round or oval nuclei and abundant, pale, finely granulated cytoplasm (H&E stain).

cells in the spleen may show the same range of cytologic appearances and are commonly associated with fibrosis, eosinophils, or both. Less frequently, mastocytosis diffusely infiltrates the splenic parenchyma with minimal fibrosis/sclerosis (see also chapter 62) (18).

Liver. Hepatomegaly occurs in about 20 percent of patients with SM who also may exhibit ascites and other signs of portal hypertension (29,57). Mast cell infiltration is associated with elevated liver function tests, but it seems likely that liver involvement is underestimated because small mast cell aggregates have been detected in the liver of patients without hepatomegaly or abnormal liver enzyme levels.

Mast cell infiltrates are usually observed in portal triads and within sinusoids (fig. 49-6). Portal spaces can be enlarged and contain mast cells associated with numerous small lymphocytes and eosinophils. Portal tract fibrosis is common, but cirrhosis does not occur as a result of mast cell infiltration. Mast cells in the liver commonly have a spindle shape. The gallbladder also may be involved by mast cells (fig. 49-7).

Gastrointestinal Tract. Occasionally, the first diagnosis of SM is made on the basis of an endoscopic biopsy of the gastrointestinal tract (12,23). The most common sites involved by SM in the gastrointestinal tract are: colon, 95 percent; ileum, 86 percent; duodenum, 80 percent; and stomach, 54 percent (12). Biopsy specimens commonly show infiltrates of ovoid to spindle-shaped mast cells within the lamina propria, sometimes forming a confluent band underneath the surface epithelium (fig. 49-8). Focal involvement of the gastrointestinal tract is common (about 25 percent of patients). Mast cell infiltration is often associated with eosinophils, which can be prominent, particularly in lesions involving the colon or ileum, but are uncommon in the stomach (12).

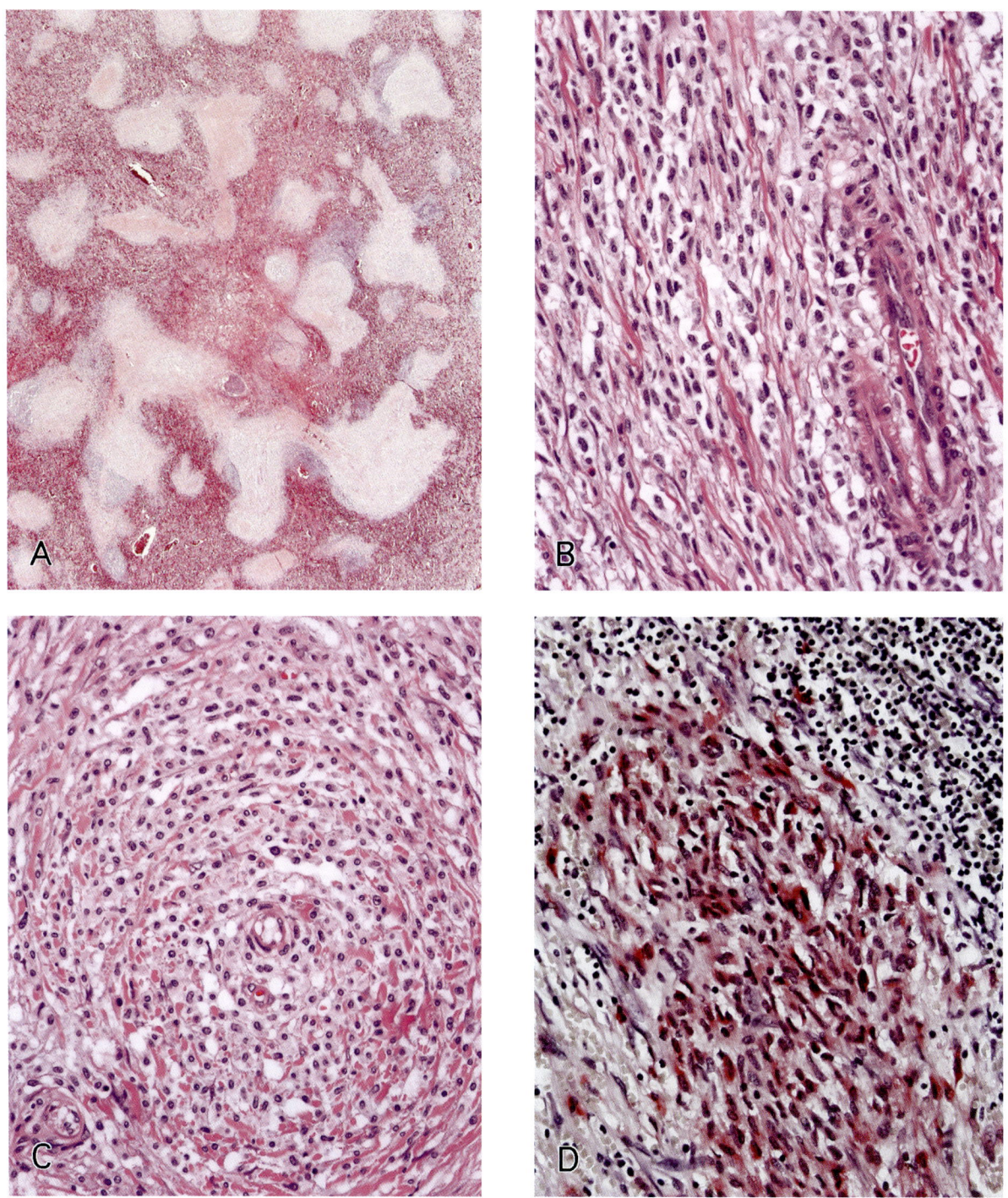

Figure 49-5

SYSTEMIC MASTOCYTOSIS INVOLVING SPLEEN

A: Low-power magnification shows numerous aggregates of mast cells involving the spleen, many of which surround blood vessels. The aggregates are pale because the mast cells have abundant pale cytoplasm (A–C: H&E stain).

B: Higher magnification shows the spindle shape of the mast cells.

C: A different field where the mast cells are mostly oval.

D: A chloroacetate esterase (Leder) stain highlights mast cells with a spindle shape (Napthol AS-D chloroacetate esterase).

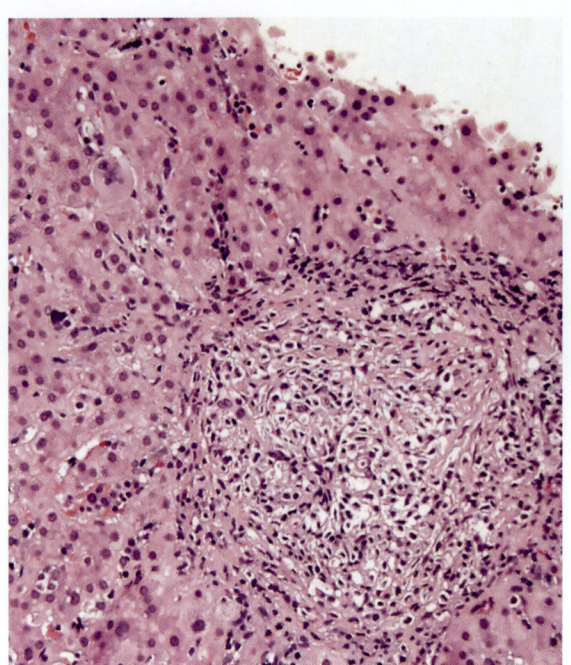
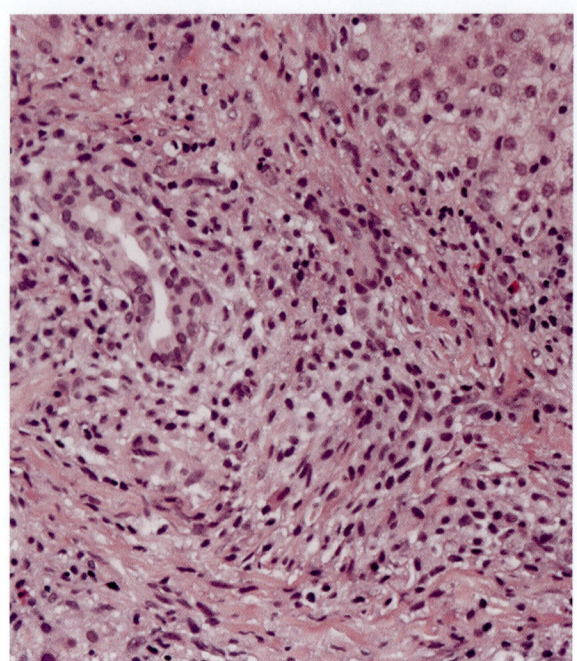

Figure 49-6

SYSTEMIC MASTOCYTOSIS INVOLVING LIVER

Left: Mast cells expand a portal tract.

Right: High magnification shows that the mast cells are mildly to moderately spindled and have abundant pale cytoplasm.

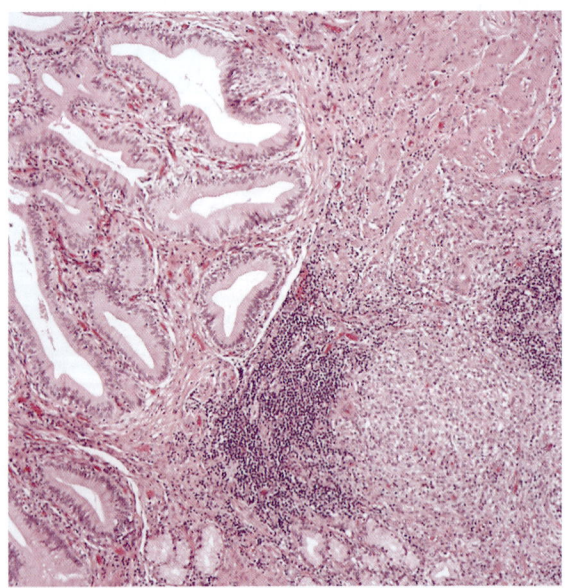
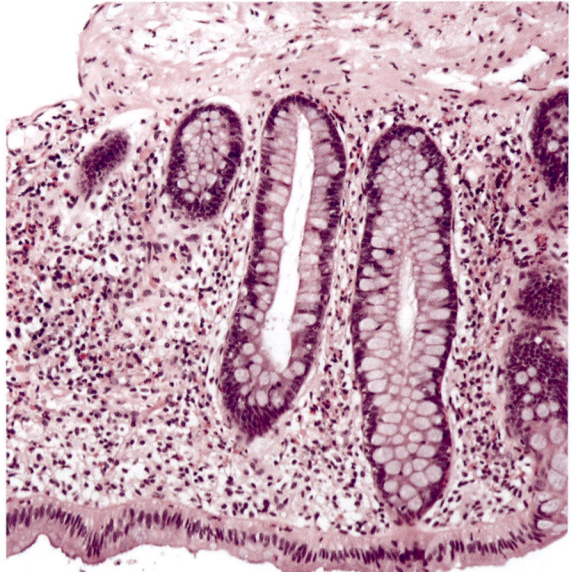

Figure 49-7

SYSTEMIC MASTOCYTOSIS INVOLVING GALLBLADDER

The mast cell aggregates involve the gallbladder wall (lower right) and surround blood vessels.

Figure 49-8

SYSTEMIC MASTOCYTOSIS INVOLVING COLON

An endoscopic biopsy specimen from the left colon shows systemic mastocytosis involving the lamina propria. The mast cells are associated with eosinophils (H&E stain).

Bone Marrow. The bone marrow is the most common (over 95 percent) site of involvement by SM and therefore bone marrow aspiration and biopsy should be performed on all adult patients with a clinical suspicion of SM. In addition, bone marrow examination allows assessment for a potential associated hematologic neoplasm.

Involvement of the bone marrow medullary space by mastocytosis is usually manifested as multifocal, compact mast cell aggregates (7,16,24,49). Mast cells are commonly located in a paratrabecular or perivascular distribution, or both (figs. 49-9, 49-10). Mast cells also can be present as nonparatrabecular nodules. The morphology of the mast cells is variable; they can be spindle shaped, oval, or round. Mast cells have abundant pale or pink cytoplasm.

Mast cells are commonly accompanied by eosinophils, small lymphocytes, and to a lesser extent, plasma cells. Small lymphocytes are of B- or T-cell lineage, and often both lineages are present. Reactive cells may be at the center or the periphery of mast cell aggregates, and may be few or numerous. These lesions are also often associated with fibrosis and angiogenesis (capillaries) (fig. 49-9C). The term eosinophilic fibrohistiocytic lesion, proposed by Arkadi Rywlin over 40 years ago, descriptively captures the features of these bone lesions although this term is currently considered obsolete. Rarely, mast cells are associated with histiocytes with cytoplasm filled with Charcot-Leyden crystals, a form of crystal-storing histiocytosis (fig. 49-10B). In advanced mast cell lesions, trabecular bone may show osteosclerosis or evidence of increased osteoclastic activity.

In general, mast cells are less numerous in aspirate smears than in biopsy sections (16,24). In cases of indolent SM, the mast cells may represent less than 5 percent or even 1 percent of all cells in the smear. They are most easily found in crushed bone marrow particles.

Cytologically, mast cells often have a spindle shape (fig. 49-9A). Neoplastic mast cells show a range in cytoplasmic granulation, correlating with differentiation, but are often less well granulated than normal mast cells.

Mast Cell Leukemia. Mast cell leukemia is rare. It is characterized by the presence of mast cells equal to or greater than 20 percent of all nucleated cells in bone marrow aspirate smears (16,51). Unlike normal mast cells, leukemic mast cells are commonly hypogranular and may have an immature blast-like morphology with monocytoid or lobulated nuclei (promastocytes).

In patients with mast cell leukemia the bone marrow is hypercellular and diffusely infiltrated or completely replaced by mast cells (fig. 49-11). Mast cells are infrequently identified in the peripheral blood of patients with SM, with the exception of those with mast cell leukemia

Systemic Mastocytosis with an Associated Hematologic Neoplasm. Examination of bone marrow or other biopsied sites not affected by SM is important because some patients have concurrent hematologic neoplasms. The uninvolved bone marrow may be hypercellular and reveal the presence of a coexisting myeloid neoplasm, such as a myeloproliferative neoplasm (MPN), myelodysplastic syndrome (MDS), or MDS/MPN (36,54). Uncommonly, SM is associated with chronic lymphocytic leukemia (fig. 49-12), other types of lymphoma, or plasma cell myeloma. In a large study of 123 patients with SM-AHN, almost 90 percent of the patients had an associated myeloid neoplasm, including 45 percent with MPN, 29 percent with chronic myelomonocytic leukemia, and 23 percent with MDS (36). Less often, a nonmast cell hematologic neoplasm can be detected in a lymph node biopsy specimen or FNA smears (fig. 49-13).

Limitations of Current Criteria for Diagnosis of Systemic Mastocytosis. The current criteria are not entirely sensitive for establishing a diagnosis of SM. As the bone marrow is almost invariably involved in patients with SM and is relatively easy to biopsy, bone marrow examination in usually an early step in the workup of patients with suspected SM. Nevertheless, the major criterion, compact clusters of more than 15 mast cells, is not present in a subset of patients with SM. In studies from the Mayo Clinic and MD Anderson Cancer Center, the major criterion was present in 80 percent and 68 percent of patients, respectively (24,38). In some bone marrow biopsy specimens, mast cells may be present in loose clusters (admittedly compact versus loose is somewhat subjective) of less than 15 cells, or single scattered mast cells that are not appreciable in routinely stained sections, therefore requiring immunohistochemical analysis for recognition.

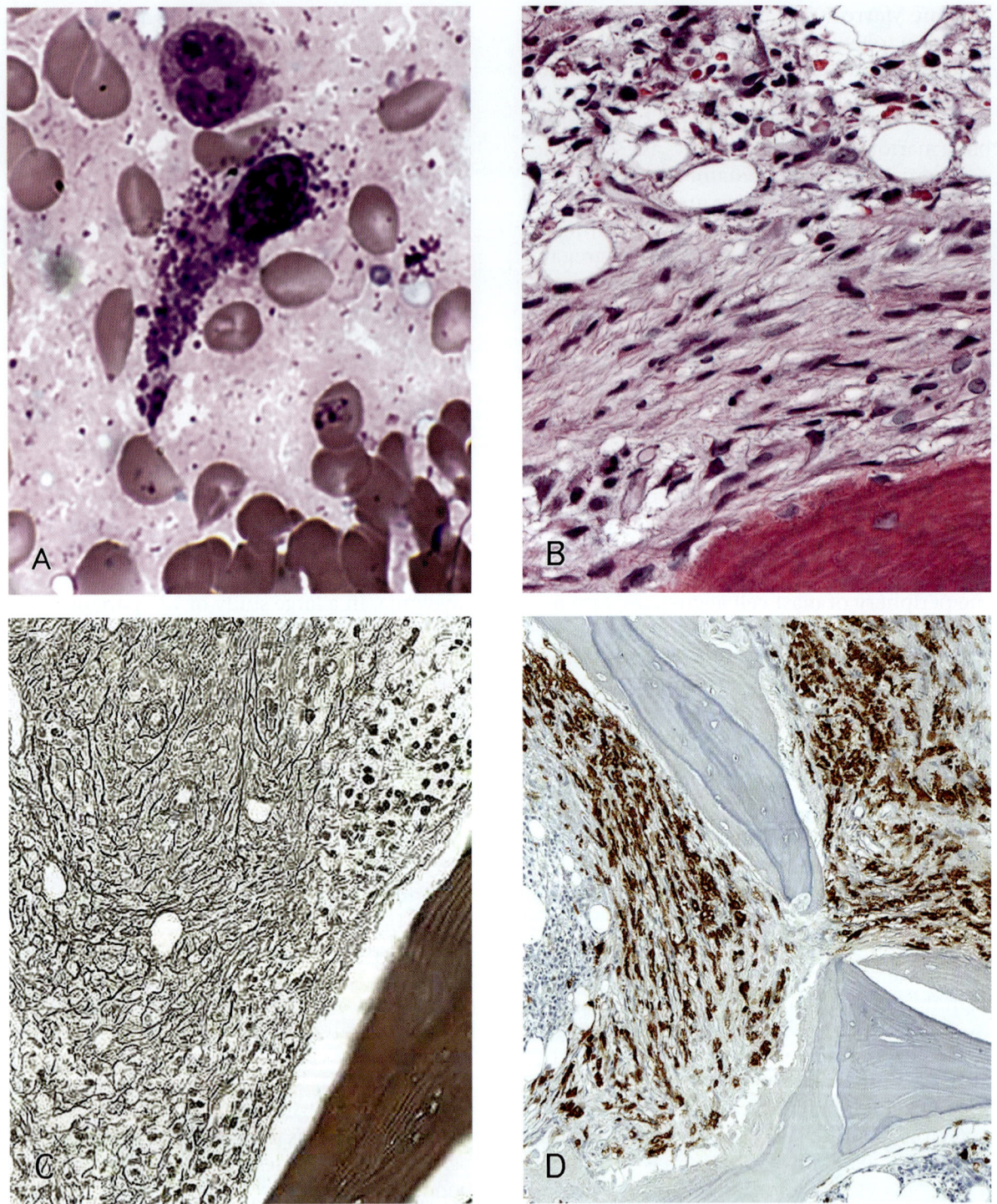

Figure 49-9

SYSTEMIC MASTOCYTOSIS INVOLVING BONE MARROW

A: A spindle-shaped mast cell in an aspirate smear (Wright-Giemsa stain).
B: Spindle shaped mast cells are located in a paratrabecular distribution in the biopsy specimen (H&E stain).
C: A reticulin stain shows increased reticulin fibrosis associated with mast cell aggregates (Gomori reticulin stain).
D: The mast cells are positive for tryptase (immunohistochemistry with hematoxylin counterstain).

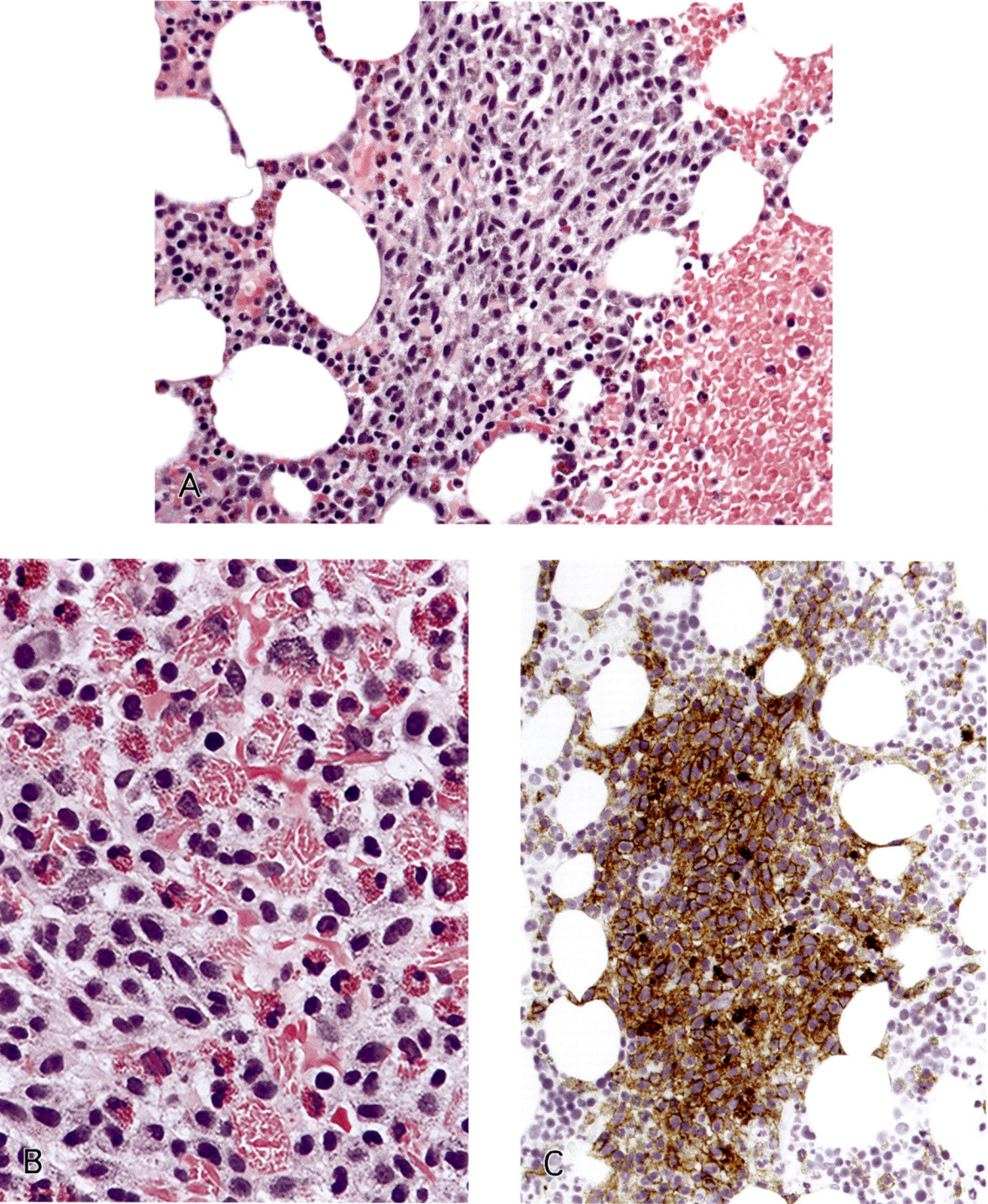

Figure 49-10

SYSTEMIC MASTOCYTOSIS INVOLVING BONE MARROW

A: An aggregate of mast cells is identified in the aspirate clot specimen. Iron pigment is also present in this field as a result of earlier transfusion (A,B: H&E stain).

B: High magnification shows many Charcot-Leyden–type crystals within histiocytes associated with neoplastic mast cells.

C: The mast cells are aberrantly positive for CD25 (immunohistochemistry with hematoxylin counterstain).

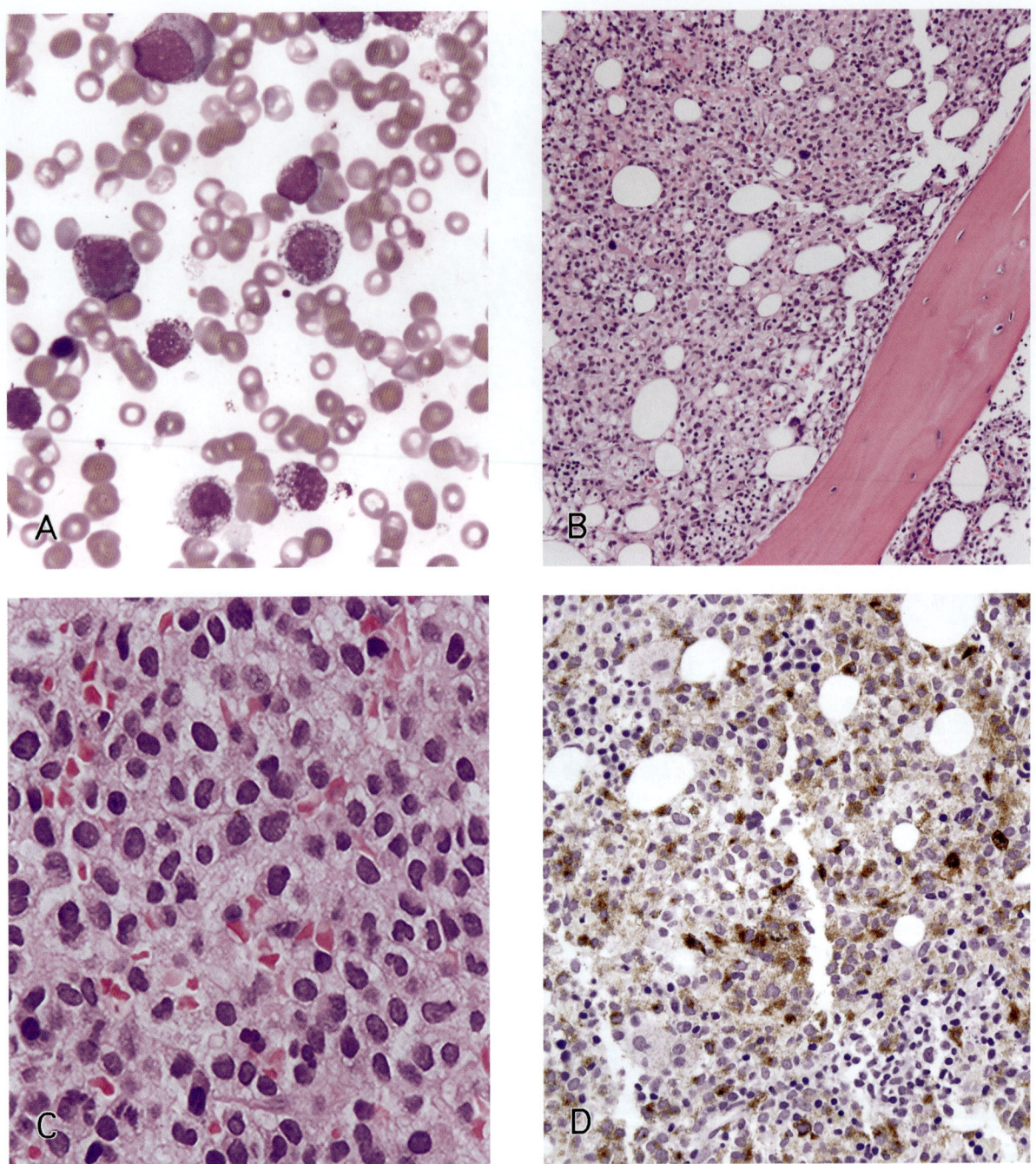

Figure 49-11

MAST CELL LEUKEMIA, ALEUKEMIC VARIANT, INVOLVING BONE MARROW

This 68-year-old woman had no history of mastocytosis. The leukocytic count was low (2×10^9/L) and the peripheral blood smear had only a few mast cells.

A: Numerous mast cells with variable cytoplasmic granularity are present in the bone marrow aspirate smear (Wright-Giemsa stain).

B: Mast cells replace the bone marrow medullary space in an interstitial and diffuse pattern (B,C: H&E stain).

C: High magnification of the bone marrow medullary space shows a sheet of mast cells.

D: Tryptase is expressed variably in the mast cells because the cells are poorly granulated (immunohistochemistry with hematoxylin counterstain).

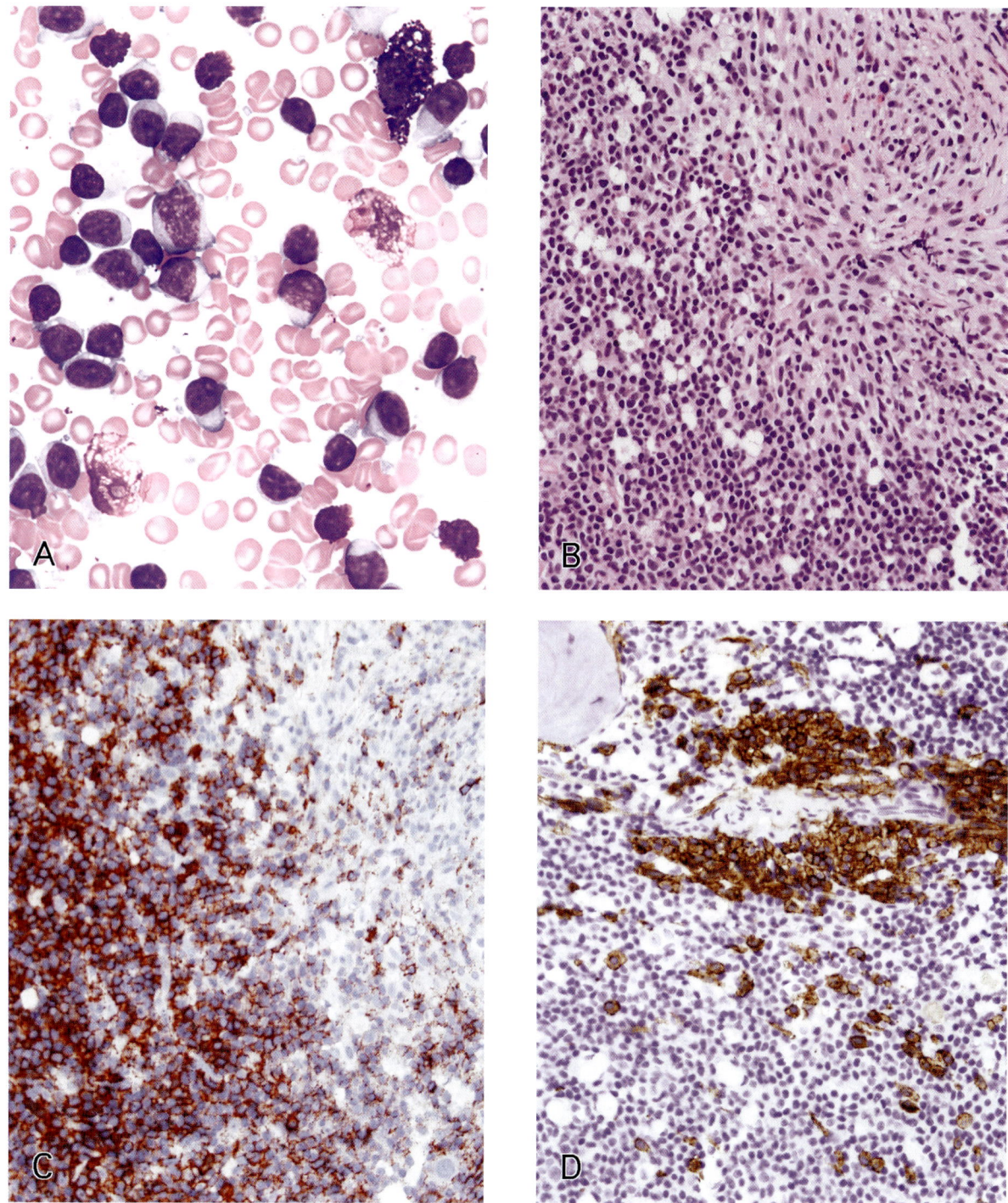

Figure 49-12

SYSTEMIC MASTOCYTOSIS ASSOCIATED WITH CHRONIC LYMPHOCYTIC LEUKEMIA (CLL) INVOLVING BONE MARROW

A: Numerous lymphocytes and a spindle-shaped mast cell (upper right) are present (Wright-Giemsa stain).

B: This field shows an aggregate of mast cells (upper right) and CLL cells (lower left) (H&E stain).

C: The same field as B assessed for CD20 shows that the mast cells are negative and CLL cells are positive (C,D: immunohistochemistry with hematoxylin counterstain)

D: The mast cells are positive for KIT.

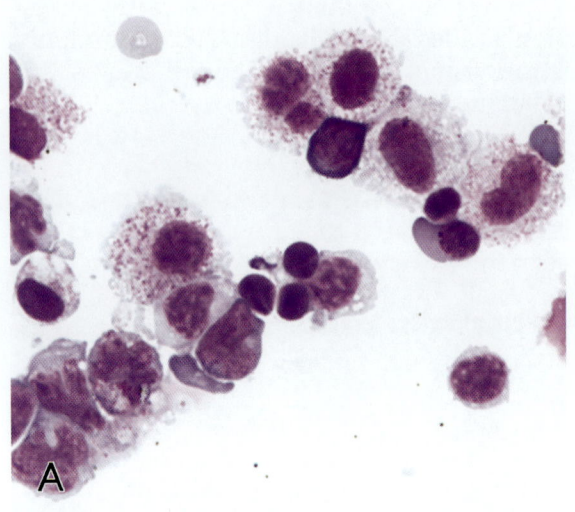

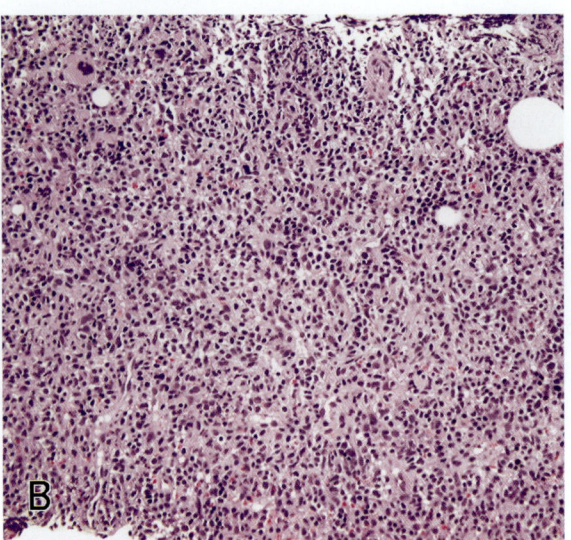

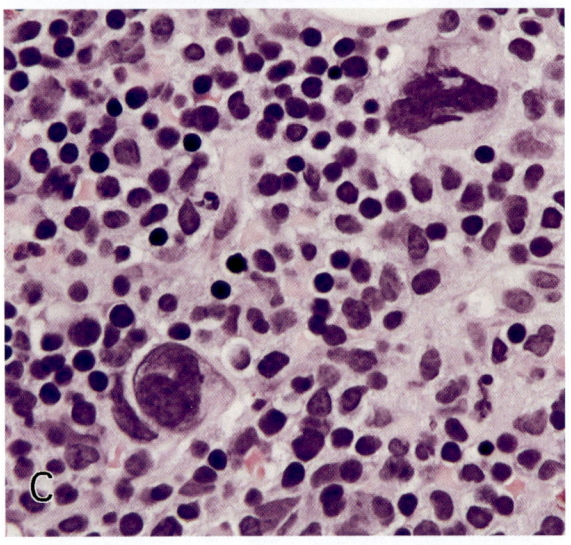

Figure 49-13

SYSTEMIC MASTOCYTOSIS AND CHRONIC MYELOMONOCYTIC LEUKEMIA INVOLVING LYMPH NODE

A: The fine-needle aspirate smear shows mast cells with cytoplasmic granules admixed with blasts, maturing myelomonocytic cells, and erythroid cells (Diff-Quik stain). (Courtesy of Dr. J. Stewart, Houston, TX.)

B: At this power the biopsy specimen shows that the lymph node architecture is replaced by a mixture of cells including atypical megakaryocytes (B,C: H&E stain).

C: High magnification shows a mixed population of myelomonocytic cells, mast cells, and megakaryocytes.

D: Immunohistochemical analysis for tryptase highlights mast cells (D,E: immunohistochemistry with hematoxylin counterstain).

E: Immunohistochemical analysis for KIT highlights mast cells and myelomonocytic cells.

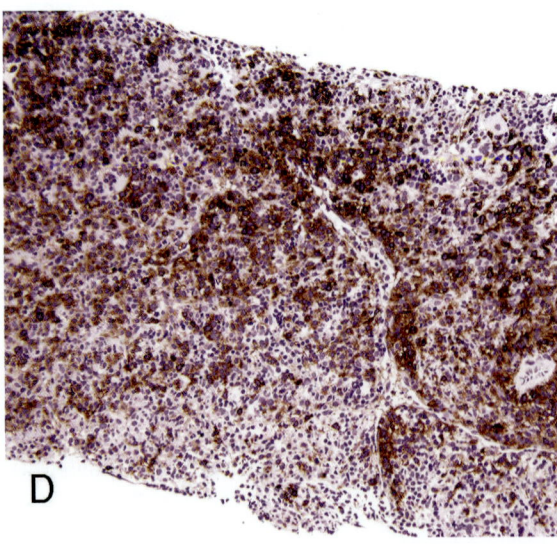

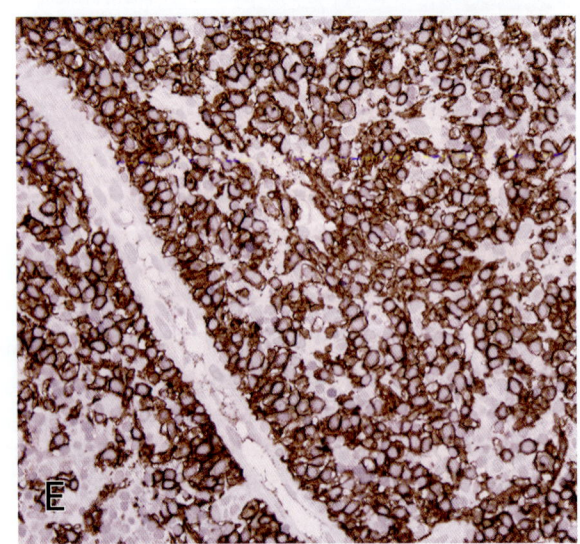

There are also challenges associated with using the current minor criteria. Two of the minor criteria, *KIT* mutations and an elevated serum tryptase level, have suboptimal sensitivity, being present in 33 of 44 (75 percent) and 44 of 52 (85 percent) of specimens in one study (24). These criteria are particularly ill suited for cases of well-differentiated SM in which aberrant expression of CD2 or CD25 and *KIT* mutations occur in a minority of cases (2). Furthermore, an elevated serum tryptase level is not specific and was considered impractical in one study (38). In contrast, atypical mast cell morphology and an aberrant immunophenotype are very sensitive, each present in over 95 percent of all cases of SM (24,38).

CYTOLOGIC FINDINGS

In fine-needle aspirate smears, the neoplastic mast cells are frequently oval or spindle shaped, with a central round nucleus with variable degrees of cytoplasmic granularity (fig. 49-13) (59). The granules may be sparse and clustered around a bare nucleus since mast cell cytoplasm is fragile. Neoplastic mast cells also may degranulate completely, making their identification more challenging.

CYTOCHEMICAL FINDINGS

Mast cells are identified by conventional metachromatic stains such as Giemsa or toluidine blue (pH dependent) and by using enzymatic cytochemical stains such as naphthol-ASD-chloroacetate esterase (fig. 49-5D), elastase, and tartrate-resistant acid phosphatase (50). They are not reactive with myeloperoxidase and alpha-naphthyl acetate and butyrate esterases.

IMMUNOPHENOTYPIC FINDINGS

Flow cytometry immunophenotypic and immunohistochemical analyses are the two methods used most frequently to support the diagnosis of mastocytosis. Flow cytometry immunophenotyping is well suited to the analysis of liquid specimens, such as bone marrow aspirate and fine-needle aspiration specimens. Mast cells, however, are often under-represented in bone marrow aspirate specimens compared with bone marrow biopsy specimens. Immunohistochemical analysis is more often used to assess tissue biopsy specimens.

Using flow cytometry, normal mast cells express a wide variety of antigens used commonly in the diagnostic workup of bone marrow specimens including CD9, CD11b, CD11c, CD13, CD18, CD22, CD33, CD35, CD44, CD45, CD61, CD71, and CD117, and are negative for CD2 and CD25 (19,44). Neoplastic mast cells have higher side scatter than normal mast cells and aberrantly express CD2 and CD25. Neoplastic mast cells also abnormally express high levels of CD35, CD45/LCA, CD59, CD63, CD69, CD123, and CD203c (fig. 49-14) (19,34,44,53).

Because expression of CD2 and CD25 supports the diagnosis of mastocytosis, it is important that assessment of these antigens be sensitive. To improve the sensitivity of detection it has been recommended that the anti-CD2 and anti-CD25 antibodies be conjugated with a bright fluorochrome such as phycoerythrin (PE) (fig. 49-15) (19,24). In general, CD2 expression is less frequent and often less intense than CD25 by neoplastic mast cells. CD2 is also less specific as it is expressed by nearly all T cells and a subset of NK cells. Therefore, CD25 assessment is the more reliable test for neoplastic mast cells. There are two potential pitfalls in using CD2 and CD25 for the diagnosis of SM. First, although these markers are sensitive, mast cells positive for CD2 or CD25 have been observed uncommonly in patients without evidence of SM (9). Secondly, in the analysis of skin lesions in SM patients, the mast cells can be negative for CD2 or CD25 even though bone marrow mast cells are positive for these antigens (15).

Using immunohistochemistry, antibodies specific for tryptase and KIT (CD117) are widely used for highlighting and quantifying mast cells. Tryptase is a cytoplasmic serine protease that is expressed in a granular and cytoplasmic staining pattern almost exclusively by mast cells. For this reason, tryptase is the standard marker recommended for quantifying mast cells in skin or other tissue sites (15). CD117 exhibits a membranous pattern of staining and is a sensitive marker for mast cells, but is less specific than tryptase as it is also expressed in other neoplasms including melanoma, seminoma, acute leukemias, plasma cell neoplasms, and gastrointestinal stromal tumors. Chymase is another marker of normal mast cells, but chymase is negative in some cases of mastocytosis and is therefore less sensitive. Mast cells are also positive for other, less specific antibodies

Figure 49-14

FLOW CYTOMETRY OF SYSTEMIC MASTOCYTOSIS

Flow cytometry immuno-phenotypic analysis of neo-plastic mast cells (systemic mastocytosis) and normal mast cells, gated as shown in figure 49-15. The mast cells in systemic mastocytosis show aberrant expression or brighter intensity of expression of many antigens including CD2 (A,B), CD59 (C,D), CD25 (E,F), CD63 (G,H), CD35 (I,J), and CD69 (K,L). (Fig. 2 from KJ Jabbar, LJ Medeiros, SA Wang, et al. Flow cytometric immunophenotypic analysis of systemic mastocytosis involving bone marrow. Arch Pathol Lab Med 2014;138:1212.)

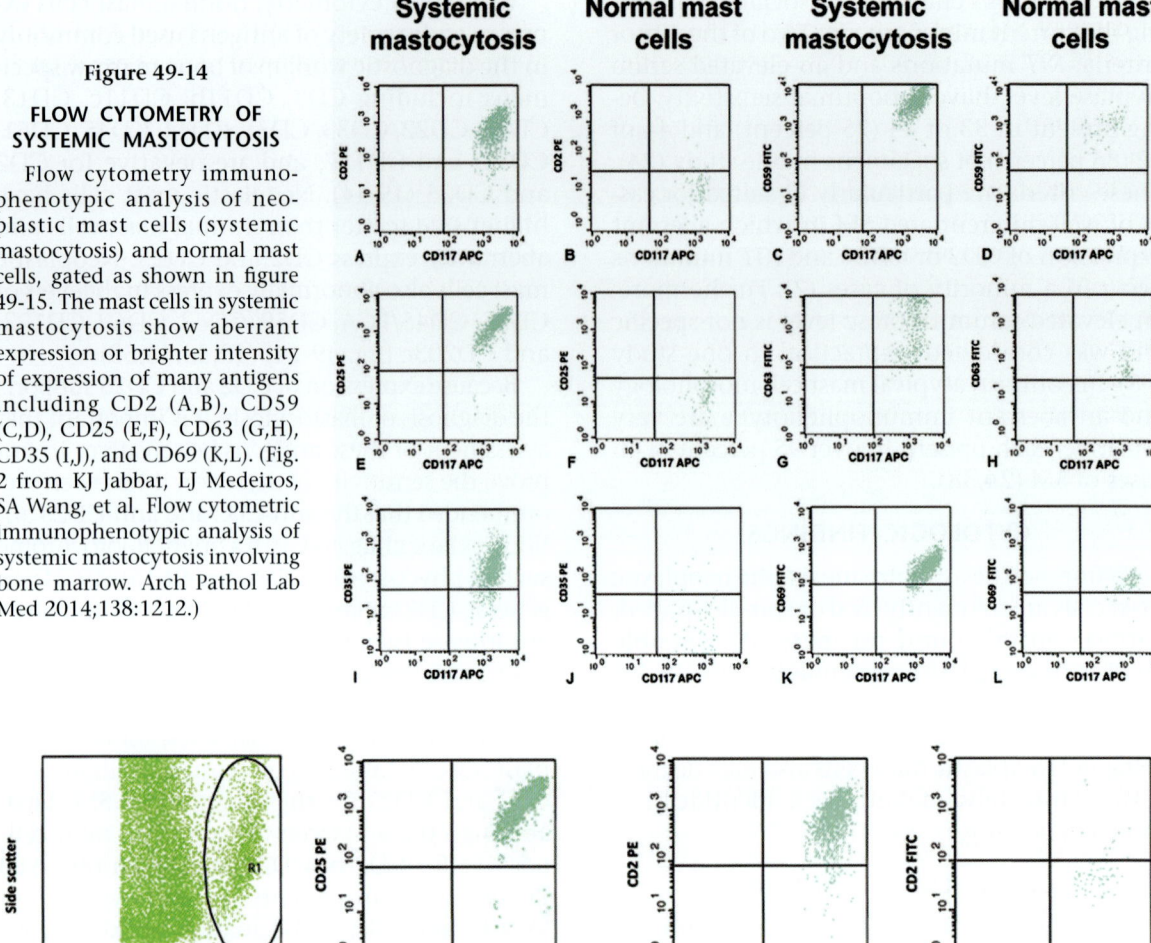

Figure 49-15

FLOW CYTOMETRY OF SYSTEMIC MASTOCYTOSIS

Flow cytometry immunophenotypic analysis of systemic mastocytosis illustrating the need to use bright fluorochromes to assess for CD25 and particularly for CD2 expression by neoplastic mast cells.

A: Total CD117-positive mast cells are collected and gated for analysis.

B,C: The neoplastic mast cells express CD25 (B) and CD2 (C) using antibodies conjugated with a bright fluorochrome, phycoerythrin (PE).

D: The mast cells were also assessed using an anti-CD2 antibody conjugated with fluorescein isothiocyanate (FITC) which showed a false negative result. (Fig. 1 from KJ Jabbar, LJ Medeiros, SA Wang, et al. Flow cytometric immunophenotypic analysis of systemic mastocytosis involving bone marrow. Arch Pathol Lab Med 2014;138:1211.)

used diagnostically, such as (but not restricted to) CD11c, CD30 (subset), CD43, CD45/LCA, CD68, CD123, and microphthalmia transcription factor (MITF) (16,42).

MOLECULAR GENETIC FINDINGS

Conventional cytogenetic analysis of bone marrow specimens involved by SM almost always shows a diploid karyotype (55). These results may be explained by the small number of mast cells in aspirate specimens, poor growth of mast cells in culture, or possibly both. The exception is SM-AHN in which approximately one third of cases have an abnormal karyotype, most likely attributable to the AHN component (55). In a study that used single nucleotide polymorphism arrays to assess a small number of cases of SM and AHN, about two thirds of cases of SM had chromosomal abnormalities involving chromosomes 2, 7, 12, 13, 14, and X although a breakdown between SM versus SM-AHN was not provided in this study (45).

The most important molecular finding in mastocytosis is the common presence of *KIT* mutations, which are almost always somatic and thought to be a later event in the pathogenesis of the disease. Germline *KIT* mutations have been described in rare cases of familial mastocytosis. The most common *KIT* mutation, in over 90 percent of mutated cases, is D816V in which aspartic acid (D) is replaced by valine (V). This point mutation results in a gain-of-function in the catalytic domain of *KIT* (3,5,6,14,27). *KIT* D816V has been found in 30 to 40 percent of patients with cutaneous mastocytosis and most cases of childhood-onset mastocytosis as well as familial cases (5). Most of patients with adult-onset SM, irrespective of WHO subtype, also carry *KIT* mutations (3).

Other somatic *KIT* mutations have been identified in SM, but much less often (less than 5 percent of cases). These variant mutations are more common in adults than children and include: V560G, D815K, D816Y, insVI815-816, D816F, D816H, and D820G (3,6,27,40). Most of these *KIT* mutations cluster in exons 8-11 and 17 and are confined to mast cells and their precursors. *KIT* mutations, however, can involve multiple hematopoietic lineages, and when this occurs, patients most often have more aggressive disease. Importantly, somatic *KIT* mutations are not specific for SM and are found in other neoplasms, such as gastrointestinal stromal tumor and seminoma.

The pathogenetic role of *KIT* mutations is incompletely understood. Both childhood and adult-onset mastocytosis are clonal diseases and associated with the same activating *KIT* mutations. However, the clinical behavior in these age groups is often different (see above). Transgenic mice carrying *KIT* D816V mutations show incomplete disease penetrance, suggesting that additional somatic mutations are necessary for full malignant transformation (58).

Other oncogenic mutations have been identified in cases of SM (39,43,55,56). Jawhar et al. (21) found the following mutations: *TET2*, 47 percent; *SRSF2*, 43 percent; *ASXL1*, 29 per-cent; *RUNX1*, 23 percent, *JAK2*, 16 percent; *N/KRAS*, 14 percent; *CBL*, 13 percent; and *EZH2*, 10 percent. Other mutated genes (less than 10 percent of cases) include *IDH2, KMT2A, NPM1, DNMT3A,* and *TP53* (21). In different studies, one or combinations of these genes, when mutated, correlate with a poorer prognosis (20,21, 35). Importantly, patients with SM do not have other disease-defining molecular abnormalities such as *BCR-ABL1, FIP1L1-PDGFRA,* or breaks involving *PDGFRB* or *FGFR1*.

DIFFERENTIAL DIAGNOSIS

The differential diagnosis of SM is broad and includes inflammatory and neoplastic diseases in which the number of mast cells is increased.

Mast Cell Syndromes. Two mast cell–associated syndromes have been proposed: monoclonal mast cell activation syndrome and idiopathic mast cell activation syndrome (1,37). These syndromes are increasingly recognized in patients with symptoms attributable to mast cell activation, such as hymenoptera sting-induced or idiopathic anaphylaxis. In both of these syndromes, the criteria for mastocytosis are not fulfilled.

In monoclonal mast cell activation syndrome, the bone marrow shows monoclonal mast cells with a *KIT* D816V mutation or mast cells with an aberrant immunophenotype (e.g., CD25 positive). Classification of these cases as monoclonal mast cell activation syndrome rather than occult SM is controversial at this time (1,38). Patients with idiopathic mast cell activation syndrome lack evidence of monoclonal mast cells, but otherwise present with symptoms of mast cell activation comparable to those of monoclonal mast cell activation syndrome.

Mast Cell Hyperplasia. In mast cell hyperplasia, by definition, mast cells are loosely scattered without forming compact infiltrates and the three minor criteria for mastocytosis are not met. Mast cells may be increased in the bone marrow and other organs in patients with reactive processes. Increased mast cells are also associated with certain types of neoplasms including lymphoplasmacytic lymphoma/Waldenstrom macroglobulinemia, chronic lymphocytic leukemia, and neural tumors.

Nodal Marginal Zone Lymphoma. In lymph nodes, SM cells with moderate or abundant pale cytoplasm may resemble, in part, monocytoid B cells or nodal marginal zone lymphoma (MZL) cells. SM in lymph nodes may spare lymphoid follicles, which can be hyperplastic, as is common in nodal MZL. Unlike nodal MZL, SM in lymph nodes is often associated with fibrosis or eosinophilia and can exhibit a prominent perivascular pattern of infiltration. In nodal MZL, large lymphoid cells are present in variable number and plasmacytoid differentiation is common. Immunophenotypic and molecular analysis resolves this differential diagnosis because nodal MZL cells are B cells that express monotypic immunoglobulin (Ig) and carry monoclonal immunoglobulin gene rearrangements.

Peripheral T-Cell Lymphoma. In peripheral T-cell lymphoma, the neoplastic cells may be small and have abundant pale cytoplasm that can resemble mast cells. Peripheral T-cell lymphomas also may have increased mast cells or many eosinophils and therefore mimic, in part, SM. Both mast cells and neoplastic T cells can express CD2 or CD25 as well. However, neoplastic T cells express a variety of other T-cell antigens (e.g., CD3, CD5) and carry monoclonal T-cell gene rearrangements.

Hairy Cell Leukemia. Sheets of mast cells with pale cytoplasm can resemble hairy cell leukemia cells. In SM, mast cell infiltrates are commonly associated with eosinophils, a feature not present in hairy cell leukemia. Mastocytosis is also commonly associated with collagenous fibrosis, which is uncommon in hairy cell leukemia. Cytochemical and immunophenotypic studies resolve this issue: hairy cell leukemia cells are positive for pan-B-cell antigens, CD103, and annexin A1. Both SM and hairy cell leukemia, however, can be positive for CD11c, CD25, and tartrate-resistant acid phosphatase (TRAP).

Langerhans Cell Histiocytosis. Langerhans cell histiocytosis, particularly bone lesions, can have numerous eosinophils and fibrosis, and therefore a diagnosis of SM might be considered. Unlike SM, Langerhans cells have delicate, folded (grooved) nuclei and are positive for S-100 protein, CD1a, and langerin/CD207. Although unlikely to be needed for diagnosis, molecular studies are helpful: *BRAF*V600E and *MAP2K1* mutations are common and *KIT*D816V mutations do not occur in Langerhans cell histiocytosis.

Acute Myeloid Leukemia with Tryptase-Positive Blasts. In the setting of aggressive myeloid neoplasms, usually AML, MDS with excess blasts, or MDS/MPN, myeloblasts may show evidence of mast cell differentiation (51). The blasts may have metachromatic cytoplasmic granules (Giemsa stain) or be positive for tryptase. These findings do not fulfill the criteria for SM, although serum tryptase levels are often elevated. If the number of blasts with mast cell differentiation is more than 10 percent the designation myelomastocytic leukemia has been suggested (51). In contrast to SM, myelomastocytic leukemia does not show *KIT* D816V point mutations or aberrant expression of CD25.

Acute Basophilic Leukemia. Normal basophils have segmented nuclei, unlike mast cells. In acute basophilic leukemia, however, the blasts may be morphologically indistinguishable from the metachromatic blasts of mast cell leukemia. Unlike mast cells, basophilic blasts are negative for CD117, have low tryptase expression, and are positive for myeloid markers.

Hematolymphoid neoplasms with fusions involving *PDGFRA*, *PDGFRB*, and *FGFR1*. These neoplasms, defined by the presence of gene fusions involving *PDGFRA*, *PDGFRB*, or *FGFR1* (see chapter 50), show diverse pathologic findings including leukocytosis and eosinophilia, myeloid neoplasms involving bone marrow, and, in patients with *FGFR1* fusions, lymphadenopathy (reviewed by Vega et al. [54]). Although these three gene fusions are disease defining, thereby excluding SM, loose aggregates of spindle-shaped mast cells that express CD2 and/or CD25 may be present in a small subset of cases. There is, however, usually no evidence of *KIT* mutation in these cases (33,54).

TREATMENT AND PROGNOSIS

Cutaneous mastocytosis in children, particularly the polymorphic type, often resolves spontaneously, usually around the time of puberty (15,16). Indolent SM is a chronic disease that may cause symptoms of mast cell activation but rarely compromises the patient's lifespan. A small number of patients (approximately 15 percent or less) develop aggressive SM. These patients may have florid symptoms related to mast cell activation and organ infiltration. The prognosis of patients with SM-AHN is linked to the underlying myeloid disorder (55). Mast cell leukemia/sarcoma is an aggressive and invariably fatal disease with a survival period of 6 to 18 months (20,33,41).

Avoidance of factors that trigger mast cell activation (variation in temperature, excess exercise, certain drugs, and alcohol) and use of histamine antagonists and H1 and H2 receptor blockers are important therapeutic cornerstones. In patients with aggressive SM, cytoreductive therapy with interferon-alpha, corticosteroids, and 2-chlorodeoxyadenosine have been used. Importantly, the *KIT* D816V mutation results in resistance to imatinib, precluding the use of this tyrosine kinase inhibitor. Alternative tyrosine kinase inhibitors that target *KIT* mutated mast cells are potential candidates for future therapies (32,47).

Midostaurin, an inhibitor of KIT D816V, appears to be particularly promising as 60 percent of patients with advanced stage SM responded in one trial (14a). Patients with SM-AHN are treated in a dichotomous fashion, with the AHN treated independently of the SM and vice versa.

CD30 is expressed by neoplastic mast cells in a number of patients with SM, particularly those with aggressive or advanced disease (4,31). Preliminary experimental studies have suggested that brentuximab vedotin, an anti-CD30 drug conjugate, is effective for the treatment of patients with CD30-positive SM (4). Newer, highly sensitive methods to detect *KIT* mutations in blood specimens are helpful for monitoring response to therapy and minimal residual disease (3,13).

REFERENCES

1. Akin C, Valent P, Metcalfe DD. Mast cell activation syndrome: proposed diagnostic criteria. J Allergy Clin Immunol 2010;126:1099-1104.
2. Alvarez-Twose I, Jara-Acevedo M, Morgado JM, et al. Clinical, immunophenotypic, and molecular characteristics of well-differentiated systemic mastocytosis. J Allergy Clin Immunol 2016;137:168-178.
2a. Arber DA, Orazi A, Hasserjian R, et al. The 2016 revision to the World Health Organization classification of myeloid neoplasms and acute leukemia. Blood 2016;127:2391-2405.
3. Arock M, Sotlar K, Akin C, et al. KIT mutation analysis in mast cell neoplasms: recommendations of the European Competence Network on Mastocytosis. Leukemia 2015;29:1223-1232.
4. Blatt K, Cerny-Reiterer S, Schwaab J, et al. Identification of the Ki-1 antigen (CD30) as a novel therapeutic target in systemic mastocytosis. Blood 2015;126:2832-2841.
5. Bodemer C, Hermine O, Palmerini F, et al. Pediatric mastocytosis is a clonal disease associated with D816V and other activating c-KIT mutations. J Invest Dermatol 2010;130:804-815.
6. Buttner C, Henz BM, Welker P, Sepp NT, Grabbe J. Identification of activating c-kit mutations in adult-, but not in childhood-onset indolent mastocytosis: a possible explanation for divergent clinical behavior. J Invest Dermatol 1998;111:1227-1231.
7. Carter MC, Clayton ST, Komarov HD, et al. Assessment of clinical findings, tryptase levels, and bone marrow histopathology in the management of pediatric mastocytosis. J Allergy Clin Immunol 2015;136:1673-1679.
8. Castells M, Metcalfe DD, Escribano L. Diagnosis and treatment of cutaneous mastocytosis in children: practical recommendations. Am J Clin Dermatol 2011;12:259-270.
9. Cherian S, McCullouch V, Miller V, Dougherty K, Fromm JR, Wood BL. Expression of CD2 and CD25 on mast cell populations can be seen outside the setting of systemic mastocytosis. Cytometry B Clin Cytom 2016;90:387-392.
10. Cohen SS, Skovbo S, Vestergaard H, et al. Epidemiology of systemic mastocytosis in Denmark. Br J Haematol 2014;166:521-528.
11. Doyle LA, Hornick JL. Pathology of extramedullary mastocytosis. Immunol Allergy Clin North Am 2014;34:323-339.
12. Doyle LA, Sepehr GJ, Hamilton MJ, Akin C, Castells MC, Hornick JL. A clinicopathologic study of 24 cases of systemic mastocytosis involving the gastrointestinal tract and assessment of mucosal mast cell density in irritable bowel syndrome and asymptomatic patients. Am J Surg Pathol 2014;38:832-843.

13. Erben P, Schwaab J, Metzgeroth G, et al. The KIT D816V expressed allele burden for diagnosis and disease monitoring of systemic mastocytosis. Ann Hematol 2014;93:81-88.

14. Garcia-Montero AC, Jara-Acevedo M, Teodosio C, et al. KIT mutation in mast cells and other bone marrow hematopoietic cell lineages in systemic mast cell disorders: a prospective study of the Spanish Network on Mastocytosis (REMA) in a series of 113 patients. Blood 2006;108:2366-2372.

14a. Gotlib J, Kluin-Nelemans HC, George TI, et al. Efficacy and safety of midostaurin in advanced systemic mastocytosis. N Engl J Med 2016;374:2530-2541.

15. Hartmann K, Escribano L, Grattan C, et al., Cutaneous manifestations in patients with mastocytosis: Consensus report of the European Competence Network on Mastocytosis; the American Academy of Allergy, Asthma & Immunology; and the European Academy of Allergology and Clinical Immunology. J Allergy Clin Immunol 2016;137:35-45.

16. Horny HP, Metcalfe DD, Bennett JM, et al. Mastocytosis. In: Swerdlow SH, Campo E, Harris NL, et al., eds. WHO classification of tumours of haematopoietic and lymphoid tissues. Lyon: IARC Press; 2008:54-63.

17. Horny HP, Kaiserling E, Parwaresch MR, Lennert K. Lymph node findings in generalized mastocytosis. Histopathology 1992;21:439-446.

18. Horny HP, Ruck MT and Kaiserling E, Spleen findings in generalized mastocytosis. A clinicopathologic study. Cancer 1992;70:459-468.

19. Jabbar KJ, Medeiros LJ, Wang SA, et al. Flow cytometric immunophenotypic analysis of systemic mastocytosis involving bone marrow. Arch Pathol Lab Med 2014;138:1210-1214.

20. Jawhar M, Schwaab J, Meggendorfer M, et al. The clinical and molecular diversity of mast cell leukemia with or without associated hematologic neoplasm. Haematologica 2017;102:1035-1043.

21. Jawhar M, Schwaab J, Schnittger S, et al. Additional mutations in SRSF2, ASXL1, and/or RUNX1 identify a high-risk group of patients with KIT D816V+ advanced systemic mastocytosis. Leukemia 2016;30:136-143.

22. Jennings S, Russell N, Jennings B, et al. The Mastocytosis Society survey on mast cell disorders: patient experiences and perceptions. J Allergy Clin Immunol Pract 2014;2:70-76.

23. Jensen RT. Gastrointestinal abnormalities and involvement in systemic mastocytosis. Hematol Oncol Clin North Am 2000;14:579-623.

24. Johnson MR, Verstovsek S, Jorgensen JL, et al. Utility of the World Health Organization classification criteria for the diagnosis of systemic mastocytosis in bone marrow. Mod Pathol 2009; 22:50-57.

25. Laine E, Chauvot de Beauchene I, Perahia D, Auclair C, Tchertanov L. Mutation D816V alters the internal structure and dynamics of c-KIT receptor cytoplasmic region: implications for dimerization and activation mechanisms. PLoS Comput Biol 2011;7:e1002068.

26. Lim KH, Tefferi A, Lasho TL, et al. Systemic mastocytosis in 342 consecutive adults: survival studies and prognostic factors. Blood 2009;113:5727-5736.

27. Longley BJ Jr, Metcalfe DD, Tharp M, et al. Activating and dominant inactivating c-KIT catalytic domain mutations in distinct clinical forms of human mastocytosis. Proc Natl Acad Sci USA 1999;96:1609-1614.

28. Meni C, Bruneau J, Georgin-Lavialle S, et al. Paediatric mastocytosis: a systematic review of 1747 cases. Br J Dermatol 2015;172:642-651.

29. Mican JM, Di Bisceglie AM, Fong TL, et al. Hepatic involvement in mastocytosis: clinicopathologic correlations in 41 cases. Hepatology 1995;22(4 Pt 1):1163-1170.

30. Miranda RN, Esparza AR, Sambandam S, Medeiros LJ. Systemic mast cell disease presenting with peripheral blood eosinophilia. Hum Pathol 1994;25:727-730.

31. Morgado JM, Perbellini O, Johnson RC, et al. CD30 expression by bone marrow mast cells from different diagnostic variants of systemic mastocytosis. Histopathology 2013;63:780-787.

32. Pan J, Quintas-Cardama A, Kantarjian HM, et al. EXEL-0862, a novel tyrosine kinase inhibitor, induces apoptosis in vitro and ex vivo in human mast cells expressing the KIT D816V mutation. Blood 2007;109:315-322.

33. Pardanani A. Systemic mastocytosis in adults: 2017 update on diagnosis, risk stratification, and management. Am J Hematol 2016;91:1146-1159.

34. Pardanani A, Lasho T, Chen D, et al. Aberrant expression of CD123 (interleukin-3 receptor-α) on neoplastic mast cells. Leukemia 2015;29:1605-1608.

35. Pardanani AD, Lasho TL, Finke C, et al. ASXL1 and CBL mutations are independently predictive of inferior survival in advanced systemic mastocytosis. Br J Haematol 2016;175:534-536.

36. Pardanani A, Lim KH, Lasho TL, et al. Prognostically relevant breakdown of 123 patients with systemic mastocytosis associated with other myeloid malignancies. Blood 2009;114:3769-3772.

37. Picard M, Giavina-Bianchi P, Mezzano V, Castells M. Expanding spectrum of mast cell activation disorders: monoclonal and idiopathic mast cell activation syndromes. Clin Ther 2013;35:548-562.

38. Reichard KK, Chen D, Pardanani A, et al. Morphologically occult systemic mastocytosis in bone marrow: clinicopathologic features and an algorithmic approach to diagnosis. Am J Clin Pathol 2015;144:493-502.

39. Schwaab J, Schnittger S, Sotlar K, et al. Comprehensive mutational profiling in advanced systemic mastocytosis. Blood 2013;122:2460-2466.

40. Sotlar K, Escribano L, Landt O, et al. One-step detection of c-kit point mutations using peptide nucleic acid-mediated polymerase chain reaction clamping and hybridization probes. Am J Pathol 2003;162:737-746.

41. Sperr WR, Valent P. Diagnosis, progression patterns and prognostication in mastocytosis. Expert Rev Hematol 2012;5:261-274.

42. Sundram UN, Natkunam Y. Mast cell tryptase and microphthalmia transcription factor effectively discriminate cutaneous mast cell disease from myeloid leukemia cutis. J Cutan Pathol 2007;34:289-295.

43. Tefferi A, Levine RL, Lim KH, et al. Frequent TET2 mutations in systemic mastocytosis: clinical, KITD816V and FIP1L1-PDGFRA correlates. Leukemia 2009;23:900-904.

44. Teodosio C, Mayado A, Sánchez-Muñoz L, et al. The immunophenotype of mast cells and its utility in the diagnostic work-up of systemic mastocytosis. J Leukoc Biol 2015;97:49-59.

45. Traina F, Visconte V, Janlowska AM, et al. Single nucleotide polymorphism array lesions, TET2, DNMT3A, ASXL1, and CBL mutations are present in systemic mastocytosis. PLOS One 2012;7:e43090.

46. Travis WD, Li CY. Pathology of the lymph node and spleen in systemic mast cell disease. Mod Pathol 1988;1:4-14.

47. Ustun C, DeRemer DL, Akin C. Tyrosine kinase inhibitors in the treatment of systemic mastocytosis. Leuk Res 2011;35:1143-1152.

48. Valent P, Akin C, Escribano L, et al. Standards and standardization in mastocytosis: consensus statements on diagnostics, treatment recommendations and response criteria. Eur J Clin Invest 2007;37:435-453.

49. Valent P, Akin C, Sperr WR, Horny HP, Metcalfe DD. Smouldering mastocytosis: a novel subtype of systemic mastocytosis with slow progression. Int Arch Allergy Immunol 2002;127:137-139.

50. Valent P, Horny HP, Escribano L, et al. Diagnostic criteria and classification of mastocytosis: a consensus proposal. Leuk Res 2001;25:603-625.

51. Valent P, Sotlar K, Sperr WR, et al. Refined diagnostic criteria and classification of mast cell leukemia (MCL) and myelomastocytic leukemia (MML): a consensus proposal. Ann Oncol 2014;25:1691-1700.

52. Valent P, Sperr WR, Samorapoompichit P, et al. Myelomastocytic overlap syndromes: biology, criteria, and relationship to mastocytosis. Leuk Res 2001;25:595-602.

53. Valent P, Sperr WR, Schwartz LB, Horny HP. Diagnosis and classification of mast cell proliferative disorders: delineation from immunologic diseases and non-mast cell hematopoietic neoplasms. J Allergy Clin Immunol 2004;114:3-11; quiz 12.

54. Vega F, Medeiros LJ, Bueso-Ramos CE, Arboleda P, Miranda RN. Hematolymphoid neoplasms associated with rearrangements of PDGFRA, PDGFRB, and FGFR1. Am J Clin Pathol 2015;144:377-392.

55. Wang SA, Hutchinson L, Tang G, et al. Systemic mastocytosis with associated clonal hematological non-mast cell lineage disease: clinical significance and comparison of chomosomal abnormalities in SM and AHNMD components. Am J Hematol 2013;88:219-224.

56. Wilson TM, Maric I, Simakova O, et al. Clonal analysis of NRAS activating mutations in KIT-D816V systemic mastocytosis. Haematologica 2011;96:459-463.

57. Yam LT, Chan CH, Li CY. Hepatic involvement in systemic mast cell disease. Am J Med 1986;80:819-826.

58. Zappulla JP, Dubreuil P, Desbois S, et al. Mastocytosis in mice expressing human Kit receptor with the activating Asp816Val mutation. J Exp Med 2005;202:1635-1641.

59. Zardawi IM. Fine needle aspiration appearances of mastocytosis. Acta Cytol 2010;54(5 Suppl):1066-1069.

50 BLASTIC HEMATOPOIETIC NEOPLASMS ASSOCIATED WITH t(8;13)(p11;q12)/*ZMYM2-FGFR1*

GENERAL FEATURES

Blastic hematopoietic neoplasms associated with t(8;13)(p11;q12)/ZMYM2-FGFR1 are tumors that exhibit the clinical and morphologic features of a lymphoid and myeloid neoplasm. Affected patients present with or develop lymphadenopathy. The bone marrow often has features similar to a myeloproliferative neoplasm and there is a propensity for developing acute myeloid leukemia (1,9,14). In the literature the tumor in lymph nodes most often has been classified as a T-cell lymphoblastic lymphoma.

Blastic hematopoietic neoplasms associated with t(8;13)(p11;q12)/*ZMYM2-FGFR1* are part of a larger group of neoplasms for which the designation *8p11 myeloproliferative syndrome* has been used most commonly in the literature (14). The 8p11 locus is the site of *FGFR1*. Other names for the tumors discussed in this chapter include *stem cell leukemia/lymphoma syndrome, T-lymphoblastic lymphoma associated with eosinophilia*, and *t(8;13)-positive bilineal lymphoma* (1,9,26). In the 2016 revised World Health Organization (WHO) classification (3), these tumors are included in a broader category under the umbrella term *myeloid/lymphoid neoplasms with eosinophilia and rearrangement of PDGRFA, PDGFRB, or FGFR1, or with PCM1-JAK2*, and more specifically as *myeloid/lymphoid neoplasms with FGFR1 rearrangement*. In this chapter we focus on this entity because patients often present with a lymphoma-like picture, unlike the other entities without *FGFR1* rearrangements.

Tumors included in the category of 8p11 myeloproliferative syndrome are clinically and morphologically heterogeneous. A number of partner genes of *FGFR1* have been reported (see Table 50-1). t(8;13)(p11;q12)/*ZMYM2-FGFR1* is the most common molecular abnormality in this group, occurring in about 50 percent of cases (10,14).

Fibroblast growth factor receptor (FGFR) 1 is a member of a family of receptor tyrosine kinas-es that play a role in embryonic development and wound repair by controlling cell growth, differentiation, and migration. The FGFR family is composed of 18 ligands that exert their actions through four highly conserved transmembrane tyrosine kinase receptors (FGFR1-4) (11). FGFR1 activation leads to downstream signaling via the PI3K/AKT, PLC-gamma, and RAS/MAPK pathways, which are central to growth, survival, migration, and angiogenesis in many cancers (7,15,24). Dysregulation of FGFR signaling has been reported in many cancers, with amplifications, translocations, and point mutations described in a broad range of tumor types including carcinomas of the breast, prostate gland, bladder, lung, and endometrium; plasma cell myeloma (FGFR3); and sarcomas, among others (7,15,24).

The partner genes involved in *FGFR1* translocations seem to contribute to the clinical and morphologic phenotype. Patients with tumors associated with t(8;13)(p11;q12) and *ZMYM2* as the partner of *FGFR1* are almost unique in that they present commonly with lymphadenopathy in addition to having features of a myeloproliferative neoplasm (10,14). In patients with neoplasms in which *FGFR1* is partnered with other genes, blood and bone marrow manifestations predominate and lymphadenopathy is uncommon (10,14,25). Patients with a hematopoietic neoplasm associated with t(8;22)(p11;q11)/*BCR-FGFR1* often present with basophilia, which may lead to confusion with chronic myeloid leukemia. Monocytosis seems to be more frequent in patients with hematopoietic neoplasms associated with t(8;9)(p11;q34)/*CNTRL-FGFR1* and t(1;8)(q25;p11.2) (10,12). Patients who have tumors associated with t(6;8)(q27;p11)/*FGFP10-FGFR1* may present with erythrocytosis and a polycythemia vera-like picture (27).

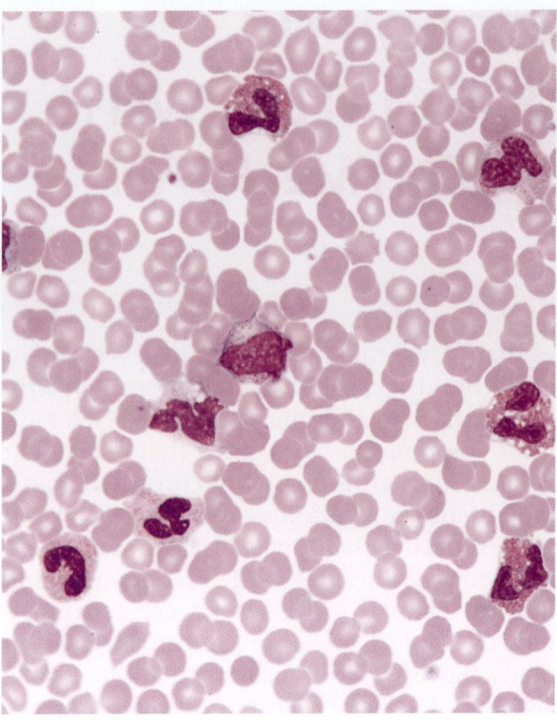

Figure 50-1

BLASTIC HEMATOPOIETIC NEOPLASM ASSOCIATED WITH t(8;13)(p11;q12)/*ZMYM2-FGFR1*

The total leukocyte count in the peripheral blood smear was 75.9 x 10⁹/L with 13 percent eosinophils (absolute count 9.9 x 10⁹/L) (Wright-Giemsa stain).

In t(8;13)/*ZMYM2-FGFR1*-positive blastic hematopoietic neoplasms, the molecular lesion is present in both myeloblasts and lymphoblasts (10). This finding supports the hypothesis that the tumor arises from a common progenitor or stem cell. In the mouse, *ZMYM2-FGFR1* induces tumors that resemble those in humans, including an immature T-cell lymphoma involving lymph nodes and a myeloproliferative-like neoplasm in the bone marrow, indicating that the *ZMYM2-FGFR1* fusion gene is oncogenic (21). Other fusion genes also have been shown to be oncogenic in mouse models (2,21).

CLINICAL FEATURES

The median age of patients with these neoplasms is 44 years, but there is a wide age range, from 3 years to the ninth decade (10,25). There is a slight predominance of males, with a reported male to female ratio of 1.2 to 1.0. Patients present with systemic symptoms in-cluding fatigue, night sweats, weight loss, and fever; about 20 percent are asymptomatic at the time of initial diagnosis. Lymphadenopathy (about 65 percent) and splenomegaly (about 60 percent) are common (10). Laboratory studies invariably show hematologic abnormalities. Eosinophilia is very common (about 85 percent of patients) (fig. 50-1). Neutrophilia, monocytosis, or both are also common, in up to 70 percent of patients. In about 60 percent of patients, the leukocyte count is greater than 20 x 10⁹/L, with absolute neutrophilia and increased bands, metamyelocytes, and myelocytes. Circulating blasts are detected in more than half of patients; in about 15 percent these blasts are greater than 20 percent of the cells, in the range of acute leukemia. The blasts are of myeloid, lymphoid, or mixed lineage. Serum tryptase levels may be elevated in some patients.

HISTOLOGIC FINDINGS

Lymph Nodes

Blastic hematopoietic neoplasms associated with t(8;13)(p11;q12)/*ZMYM2-FGFR1* can partially or completely replace lymph nodes (26). The pattern is diffuse. In cases with partial lymph node involvement, the tumor is located in the paracortex and spares lymphoid follicles. At low to intermediate magnification, a two-tone appearance is often observed, with darker and paler areas (figs. 50-2, 50-3). At high-power magnification, these dark and pale areas correspond to two cellular components, both with blastic features (26). One component (darker areas) is composed of lymphoblasts of small to medium size with scant cytoplasm. The other component (paler areas) is composed of imma-ture myeloid cells including many myeloblasts; these cells are larger with more abundant, pale or eosinophilic cytoplasm. The myeloblastic component tends to surround blood vessels or residual lymphoid follicles. Mitotic figures are usually easy to identify and a starry sky pattern may observed (fig. 50-4). Numerous mature eosinophils are often sprinkled throughout the tumor and prominent high endothelial venules are common, two clues suggesting the diagnosis. Eosinophils are often more numerous in the myeloblastic areas (26); eosinophils, however, are sometimes inconspicuous.

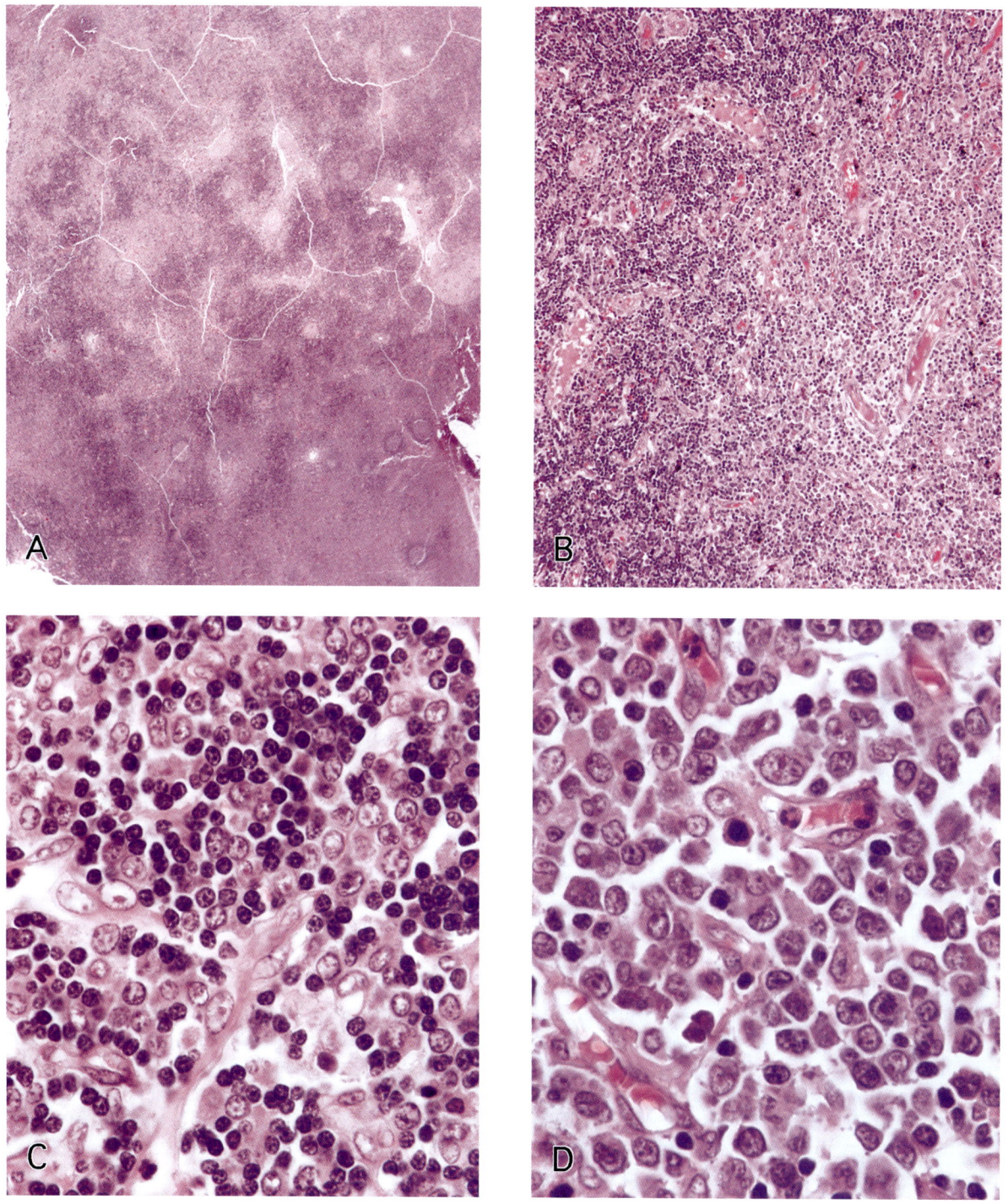

Figure 50-2

BLASTIC HEMATOPOIETIC NEOPLASM ASSOCIATED WITH t(8;13)/*ZMYM2-FGFR1*

A: At low magnification the lymph node is replaced by a neoplasm with darker and paler areas.

B: At intermediate magnification, a pale area surrounds a blood vessel.

C,D: Oil immersion magnification of the lymphoblastic (C) and myeloblastic (D) components (hematoxylin and eosin [H&E] stain; this case was fixed in B5 and some mercuric chloride crystals incompletely removed during processing can be seen in the B image).

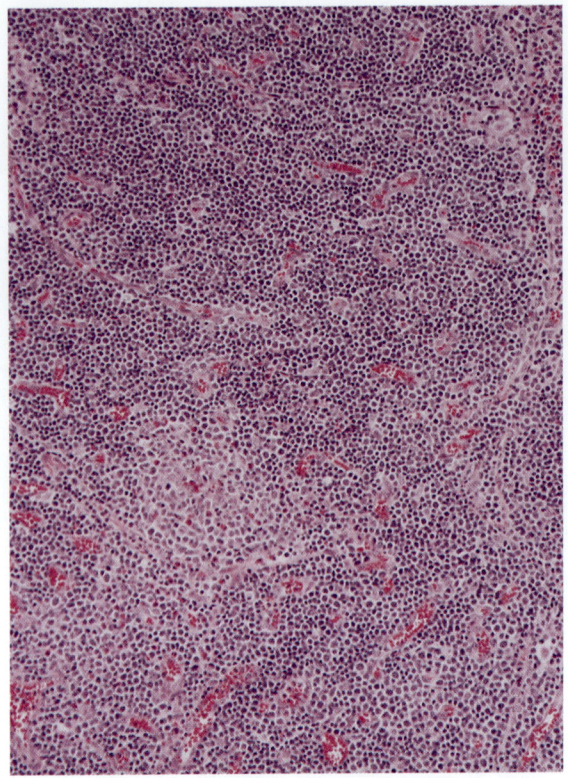

Figure 50-3

BLASTIC HEMATOPOIETIC NEOPLASM ASSOCIATED WITH t(8;13)/*ZMYM2-FGFR1* INVOLVING LYMPH NODE

The lymphoblastic component is predominant and a small myeloid (pale) area surrounds a blood vessel (H&E stain).

The relative proportions of the lymphoblastic and myeloblastic components in t(8;13)-positive blastic hematopoietic neoplasms are highly variable (figs. 50-2, 50-3). The lymphoblastic or myeloblastic component can predominate or be subtle, and immunohistochemical studies are often needed to appreciate their presence. The variable presence of these components may explain the apparent discordant classification of the tumors that have been reported. In the literature, about 80 percent of these tumors are classified as lymphoblastic lymphoma, with the other 20 percent classified as myeloid sarcoma (9,14,22).

Bone Marrow

In most patients, the bone marrow aspirate smears are cellular or hypercellular (fig. 50-5) (8,10,14). Neutrophilic precursors are increased and may be left-shifted in maturation, and eosinophilia is common. Spindled or hypo-

granular mast cells are observed in some cases. The bone marrow core biopsy usually shows a hypercellular bone marrow with myeloid predominance, with or without left-shifted maturation, and eosinophilia in about 70 percent of patients (fig. 50-6). The bone marrow biopsy specimen is normocellular in about 10 percent of patients and hypocellular in less than 5 percent. Mast cells may be increased; plasma cells and lymphoid aggregates are rare.

On the basis of these findings, a myeloproliferative neoplasm is often the initial impression, particularly without knowledge that a *FGFR1* translocation is present. In some patients, dysplastic changes are observed that lead to consideration of a myelodysplastic/myeloproliferative neoplasm. In other patients, myeloblasts are increased and if 20 percent or more, the diagnosis of acute leukemia can be established. The blasts may be purely of myeloid, lymphoid, or bilineal (myeloid and lymphoid) lineage (10).

CYTOLOGIC FINDINGS

There are few reports that describe the cytologic findings of blastic hematopoietic neoplasms associated with (t(8;13)/*ZMYM2-FGFR1*. Smears of involved lymph nodes show mature neutrophils and neutrophilic precursors in varying proportions, as well as eosinophils, lymphoblasts, and small lymphocytes (fig. 50-7). Lymphoblasts or myeloblasts are numerous in some cases. Eosinophils may show cytologic abnormalities including nuclear hyposegmentation and sparse granulation with clear cytoplasmic areas (17).

IMMUNOPHENOTYPIC FINDINGS

The lymphoblastic component is almost always of immature T-cell lineage. The lymphoblasts are commonly positive for TdT, CD1a, CD2, CD3 (usually cytoplasmic), CD5, CD7, CD45, and CD99, and are negative for myeloid markers (fig. 50-4B,C) (26,28). A subset of T-cell tumors express CD4, CD7, and CD8. In rare patients the lymphoblastic component is of immature B-cell lineage (23).

In the myeloblastic component, the cells usually express at least one marker of myeloid differentiation including lysozyme, CD43 (moderate or bright), CD68, CD117, myeloperoxidase, and PU.1 (fig. 50-4D) (26). CD15 may

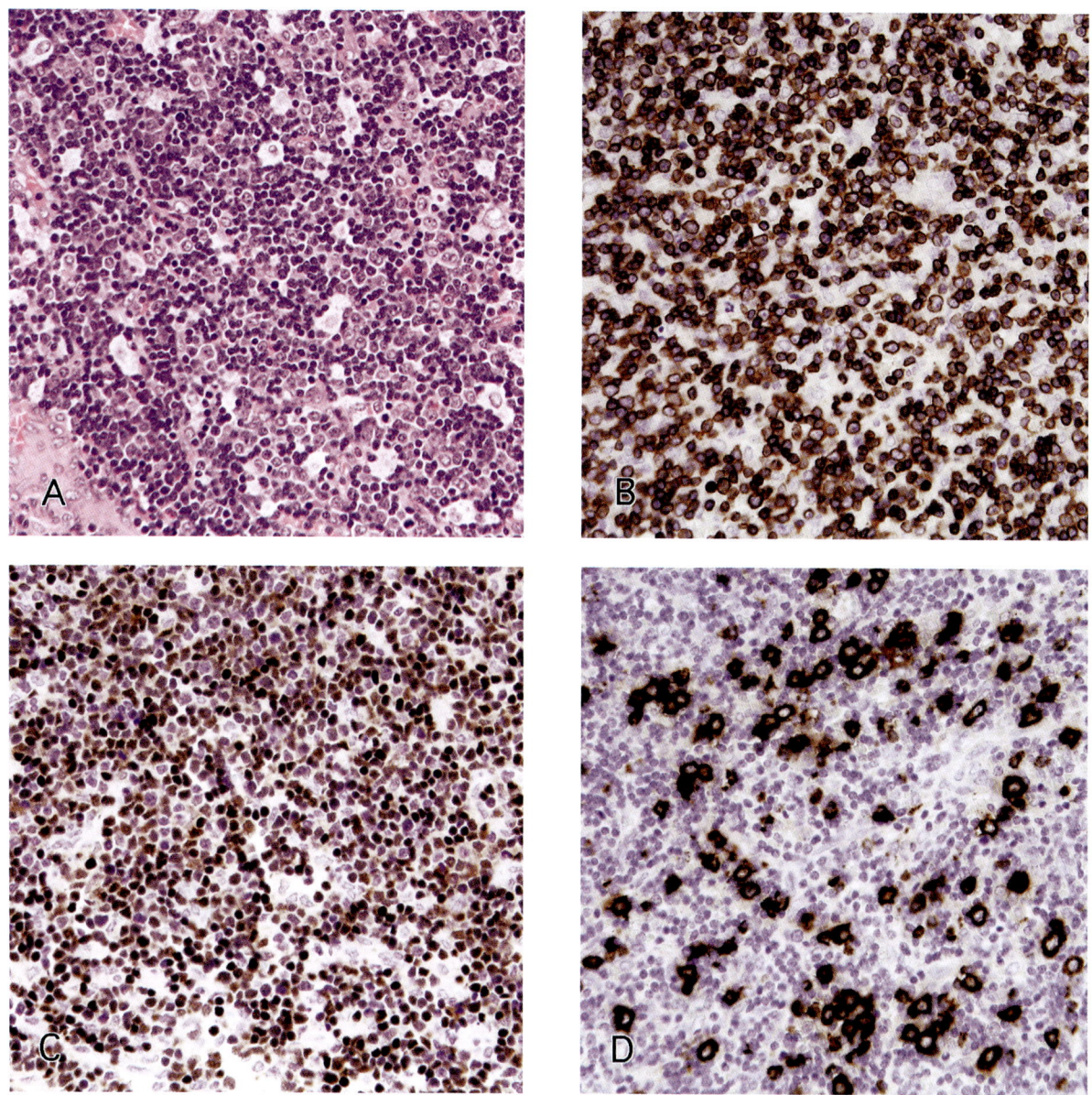

Figure 50-4

BLASTIC HEMATOPOIETIC NEOPLASM ASSOCIATED WITH t(8;13)/*ZMYM2-FGFR1*

A. A starry sky pattern is appreciated in this lymph node specimen (H&E stain).

B–D. Most of the neoplastic cells in this case were positive for CD3 (B) and TdT (C) with a small subset positive for myeloperoxidase (D) and lysozyme (not shown) (B–D: immunohistochemistry with hematoxylin counterstain).

be expressed by a subset of cases. The myeloblasts can be positive for CD3 (as detected by immunohistochemistry and likely cytoplasmic), but negative for surface CD3 (as detected by flow cytometry immunophenotyping) (26). The myeloid component is negative for most T-cell antigens.

MOLECULAR GENETIC FINDINGS

Currently, at least 15 genes can partner with *FGFR1* via 14 translocations and 1 insertion (Table 50-1). These translocations result in fusion genes. The partner genes that are fused to *FGFR1* encode proteins that foster dimerization and activation of FGFR1, thereby mimicking normal

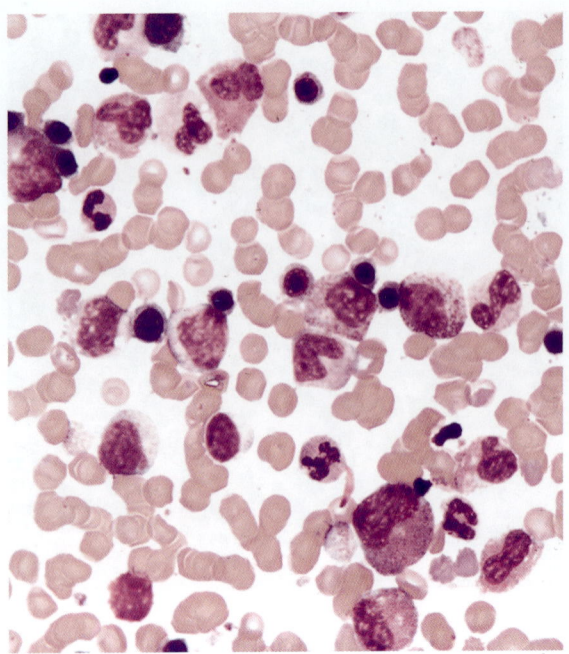
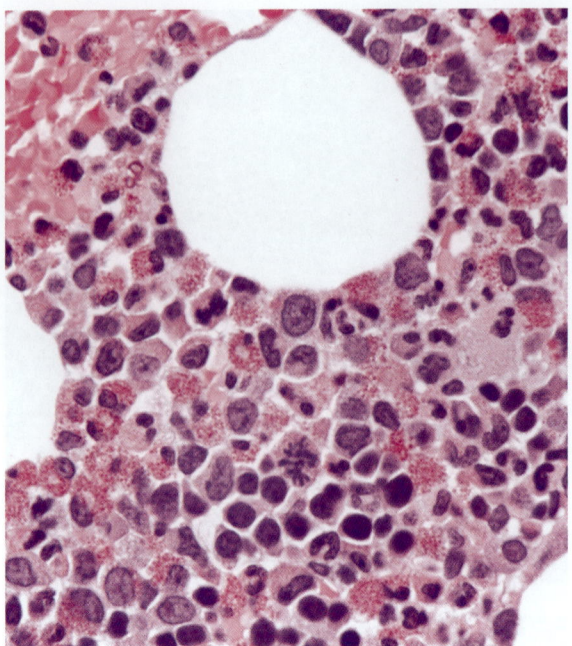

Figure 50-5

BLASTIC HEMATOPOIETIC NEOPLASM ASSOCIATED WITH t(8;13)/*ZMYM2-FGFR1*

In the bone marrow, the tumor had features of a myeloproliferative neoplasm with eosinophilia.
Left: Neutrophilic precursors and eosinophils are present in an aspirate smear (Wright-Giemsa stain).
Right: Aspirate clot specimen shows a hypercellular particle with numerous eosinophils. The core biopsy specimen was of suboptimal size and poorly preserved in this patient and therefore is not shown (H&E stain).

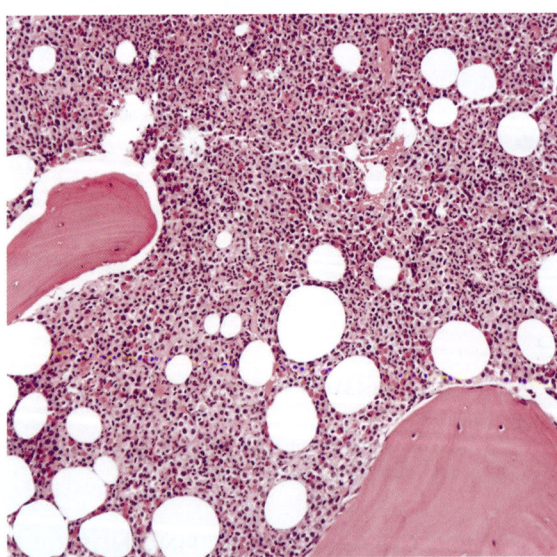

Figure 50-6

BLASTIC HEMATOPOIETIC NEOPLASM ASSOCIATED WITH t(8;13)/*ZMYM2-FGFR1*

The bone marrow is hypercellular and eosinophilia is present (H&E stain).

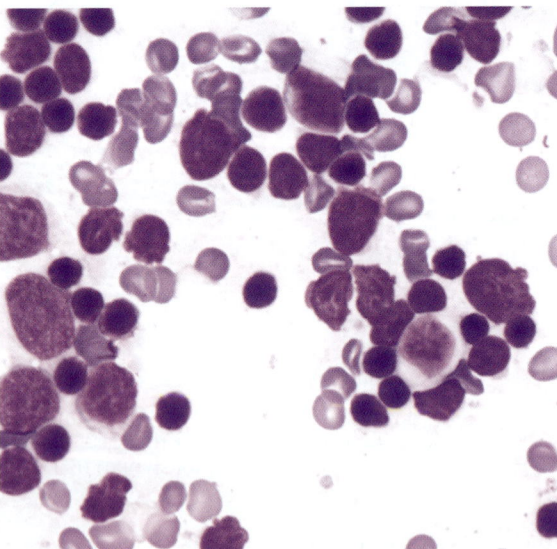

Figure 50-7

BLASTIC HEMATOPOIETIC NEOPLASM ASSOCIATED WITH t(8;13)/*ZMYM2-FGFR1*

The fine-needle aspirate smear of a lymph node shows large neoplastic cells with fine chromatin admixed with small lymphocytes (Diff-Quik stain).

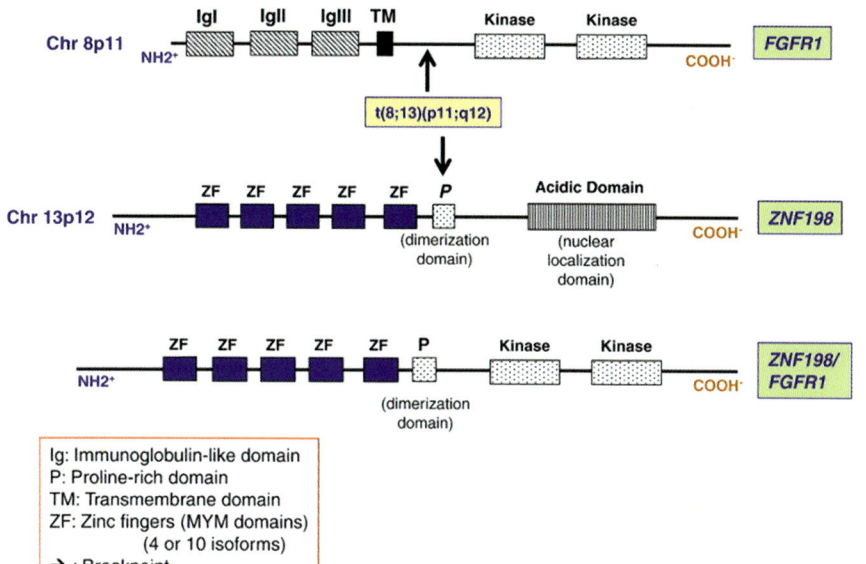

Figure 50-8

WILD TYPE *FGFR1* AND *ZMYM2* (FORMERLY KNOWN AS *ZNF198*) GENES AND THE *ZMYM2-FGFR1* FUSION GENE

In this schematic representation, the fusion gene (bottom) retains the zinc finger and proline-rich domains of ZMYM2/ZNF198 and the kinase domain of FGFR1 (Fig. 3 from Jackson CC, Medeiros LJ, Miranda RN. 8p11 myeloproliferative syndrome: a review. Hum Pathol 2010;41:461-476.)

ligand binding and promoting activation of the downstream pathways involved in oncogenesis. t(8;13)(p11;q12)/*ZMYM2-FGFR1* (fig. 50-8) is the most frequent of the translocations that occur in the 8p11 myeloproliferative syndrome. There are three other common translocations, t(8;9)(p11;q33)/*CEP110-FGFR1*, t(6;8)(q27;p11-12)/*FGFR1OP1-FGFR1,* and t(8;22)(p11;q11)/*BCR-FGFR1;* all others reported are rare.

ZMYM2, formerly known as *ZNF198*, encodes a zinc finger protein that functions as a transcription factor. The ZMYM2-FGFR1 fusion protein contains a number of zinc finger motifs, a proline-rich region contributed by ZMYM2, and an intracellular FGFR1 that contains a tyrosine kinase domain. The proline-rich domain of ZMYM2 promotes self-oligomerization, forming dimers that mimic normal ligand binding (fig. 50-9). Dimerization results in constitutive activation of FGFR1 and downstream cellular pathways including the phospholipase C gamma, PI3K/AKT, and RAS/MAPK pathways.

Trisomy 21 is the most common secondary chromosomal abnormality in blastic hematopoietic neoplasms associated with t(8;13) (10). *RUNX1* mutations have been reported in a few cases, including t(8;13)-positive tumors and tumors with other partners of *FGFR1* (4,13,20). The *RUNX1* mutations may be of nonsense or truncated type, are thought to be secondary events, and have been correlated with disease progression. In a mouse model, the NOTCH pathway is activated in T-cell tumors associated with t(8;13)/*ZMYM2-FGFR1* (18).

Conventional cytogenetics is the best technique for identifying translocations or insertions involving *FGFR1* at 8p11. Conventional

Table 50-1

KARYOTYPES AND PARTNER GENES REPORTED IN PATIENTS WITH 8P11 MYELOPROLIFERATIVE SYNDROME

Karyotype	Partner of *FGFR1*
t(8;13)(p11;q12)	*ZMYM2 (ZNF198)*
t(8;9)(p11;q33)	*CNTRL (CEL110)*
t(6;8)(q27;p11-12)	*FGFR1OP*
t(8;22)(p11;q11)	*BCR*
t(8;19)(p12;q13.3)	*HERVK*
t(7;8)(q34;p11)	*TIF1 (TRIM24)*
t(2;8)(q37;p11)	*LRRFIP1*
t(8;17)(p11;q23)	*MYO18A*
t(8;12)(p11;q15/dic(8;12)(p11;p11)	*CPSF6*
t(8;11)(p11;p15)	*NUP98*
t(7;8)(q22;p11)	*CUX1*
t(2;8)(q12;p11)	*RANBP2/NUP358*
t(3;8;9)(p25;p21;q34)	Unknown
ins(12;8)(p11;p11p22)	*FGFR1OP2*
t(1;8)(q25;p11.2)	*TPR*

Figure 50-9

WILD TYPE FGFR1 AND ZMYM2 (ZNF198) PROTEINS AT THE CELL SURFACE

A: The schematic representation shows the resting state where FGFR1 is a monomer.

B: Physiologic binding and dimerization of FGFR1 results in autophosphorylation of intracellular tyrosine kinase domains and activation of intracellular pathways including the PLC-gamma and RAS/MAPK pathways.

C. Chimeric ZMYM2-FGFR1 proteins form dimers that mimic normal ligand binding and result in constitutive activation of FGFR1. (Fig. 4 from Jackson CC, Medeiros LJ, Miranda RN. 8p11 myeloproliferative syndrome: a review. Hum Pathol 2010;41:461-476.)

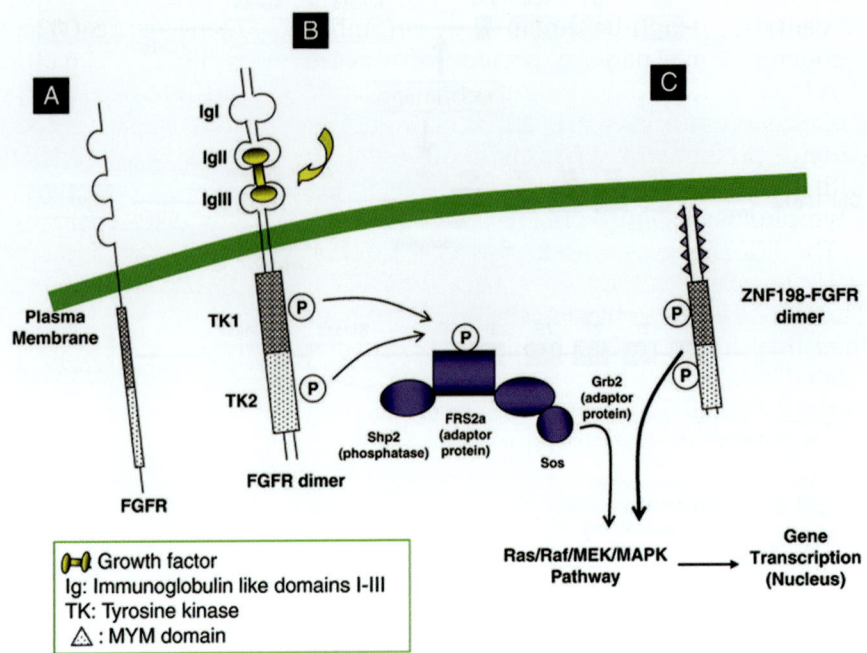

cytogenetics can identify all loci (and presumed partner genes) involved in the *FGFR1* translocation, however, viable cells are required. The diagnosis also can be established by using fluorescence in situ hybridization (FISH) with a *FGFR1* breakapart probe. This approach can be applied to the study of fixed, paraffin-embedded tissue sections. Commercial probes for *ZMYM2* are available to establish the presence of *ZMYM2-FGFR1*. FISH probes are not available to allow identification of all gene partners (25). Reverse transcriptase-polymerase chain reaction (RT-PCR) assays can be designed to detect *FGFR1* fusion genes when the partner is known. This approach may be most applicable for monitoring minimal residual disease.

DIFFERENTIAL DIAGNOSIS

T-Cell Lymphoblastic Lymphoma/Leukemia, Not Otherwise Specified. A high index of suspicion is required to distinguish a blastic hematopoietic neoplasm associated with t(8;13) (p11;q12)/*ZMYM2-FGFR1* from other types of T-lymphoblastic lymphoma/leukemia. The presence of eosinophilia (greater than 1.5×10^9/L) and particularly the combination of eosinophilia, a myeloid neoplasm (either a myeloproliferative neoplasm or acute myeloid leukemia), and lymphoblastic lymphoma, should suggest the possibility of a t(8;13)/*ZMYM2-FGFR1* blastic hematopoietic neoplasm (10). Morphologically, cases of t(8;13) blastic hematopoietic neoplasm usually have a myeloid component, usually best observed surrounding blood vessels, that can be subtle or more obvious (26). Eosinophilia also may be intermixed with the lymphoma cells (1,26).

Hematopoietic Neoplasms Associated with *PDFGRA* or *PDGFRB* Fusions. Hematolymphoid neoplasms associated with *PDFGRA* or *PDFGRB* abnormalities exhibit some of the clinicopathologic features of the *FGFR1*-associated hematolymphoid neoplasms in general, although these patients rarely present with lymphoblastic leukemia/lymphoma, unlike patients with tumors associated with t(8;13)(p11;q12)/*ZMYM2-FGFR1*.

Hematopoietic Neoplasms Associated with PDFGRA Fusions. The median patient age of patients with *PDFGRA* fusions is the fifth decade with a wide age range (7 to 77 years) and the male to female ratio is over 10 to 1 (3,16,25). Many patients present with features of chronic eosinophilic leukemia, with symptoms related to the release of eosinophilic granules, most often rash and erythema, and less frequently, pulmonary, gastrointestinal tract, or cardiac manifestations. Splenomegaly is present in about 60 percent of patients. The complete blood count may show eosinophilia (about 70 percent), neutrophilia, anemia, or thrombocytopenia. Some patients present with acute myeloid leukemia or acute lymphoblastic leukemia/lymphoma (16) and uncommonly patients present with a lymphoma-like picture with lymphadenopathy and a tumor resembling T-lymphoblastic lymphoma (8).

The *PDGFRA* gene is located at chromosome 4q12; its most common gene partner is *FIP1L1*. The *FIP1L1-PDGFRA* fusion gene results from an interstitial deletion of 800kb (6). This abnormality is often undetectable by conventional cytogenetic analysis because of its small size and therefore the best test to detect this abnormality in clinical practice is FISH. Other uncommon gene partners of *PDGFRA* include *BCR, ETV6, KIF5B, STRN,* and *CDK5RAP2* (8). These rare gene partners occur via translocations that are detected by conventional karyotyping. The clinicopathologic features of cases with *PDFGRA* deletions or translocations, regardless of the gene partner, are indistinguishable and almost all patients with these tumors are sensitive to tyrosine kinase inhibitors.

Hematopoietic Neoplasms Associated with PDFGRB Fusions. The median patient age is 42 years and the male to female ratio is 2 to 1 (3,8,25). These neoplasms are often classified as chronic myelomonocytic leukemia, atypical chronic myelogenous leukemia *BCR-ABL1* negative, juvenile myelomonocytic leukemia, myelodysplastic syndrome, acute myeloid leukemia, or T-cell acute lymphoblastic leukemia. Patients commonly present with anemia, leukocytosis, monocytosis, and eosinophilia. Lymphadenopathy and splenomegaly are less prominent and a lymphoma-like presentation is rare in these patients.

More than 20 gene partners of *PDGFRB* have been identified. The most frequent translocation is t(5;12)(q33;p13)/*ETV6-PDGFRB* (8,25). Conventional cytogenetic analysis and FISH using a breakapart probe are the best techniques to identify abnormalities of *PDGFRB*. Almost all patients with tumors associated with *PDGFRB* fusion are sensitive to tyrosine kinase inhibitors.

Myeloid Sarcoma Associated with Eosinophilia. Patients with acute myeloid leukemia (AML) with inv(16)(p13.1q22) or t(16;16)(p13.1;q22) resulting in *CBFB-MYH11* or AML with t(8;21)(q22;q22)/*RUNX1-RUNX1T1* can have prominent eosinophilia. The eosinophils in this context are usually derived from the leukemic clone. In a subset of patients, these neoplasms involve lymph nodes or other extramedullary sites, leading to the diagnosis of myeloid sarcoma. In patients who present with myeloid sarcoma and lack bone marrow disease, it is important to procure viable cells for conventional cytogenetic analysis. FISH and molecular studies are also helpful for establishing the presence of the *CBFB-MYH11* or *RUNX1-RUNX1T1* fusion genes in myeloid sarcoma.

TREATMENT AND PROGNOSIS

Patients with blastic hematopoietic neoplasms associated with *FGFR1* translocations usually have a clinically aggressive disease that responds poorly to conventional chemotherapy as well as first generation tyrosine kinase inhibitors such as imatinib. There are some pre-clinical data suggesting that ponatinib may have activity against this disease (19). Aggressive chemotherapy and hematopoietic stem cell transplantation have shown some success, but overall the prognosis of these patients is poor (5).

REFERENCES

1. Abruzzo LV, Jaffe ES, Cotelingam JD, Whang-Peng J, Del Duca V Jr, Medeiros LJ. T-cell lymphoblastic lymphoma with eosinophilia associated with subsequent myeloid malignancy. Am J Surg Pathol 1992;16:236-245.
2. Agerstam H, Järås M, Andersson A, et al. Modeling the human 8p11-myeloproliferative syndrome in immunodeficient mice. Blood 2010;116:2103-2111.
3. Arber DA, Orazi A, Hasserjian R, et al. The 2016 revision to the World Health Organization classification of myeloid neoplasms and acute leukemia. Blood 2016;127:2391-2405.
4. Buijs A, van Wijnen M, van den Blink D, van Gijn M, Klein SK. A ZMYM2-FGFR1 8p11 myeloproliferative neoplasm with a novel nonsense RUNX1 mutation and tumor lysis upon imatinib treatment. Cancer Genet 2013;206:140-144.

5. Dolan M, Cioc A, Cross NC, Neglia JP, Tolar J. Favorable outcome of allogeneic hematopoietic cell transplantation for 8p11 myeloproliferative syndrome associated with BCR-FGFR1 gene fusion. Pediatr Blood Cancer 2012;59:194-196.

6. Gotlib J, Cools J. Five years since the discovery of FIP1L1-PDGFRA: what we have learned about the fusion and other molecularly defined eosinophilias. Leukemia 2008;22:1999-2010.

7. Haugsten EM, Wiedlocha A, Olsnes S, Wesche J. Roles of fibroblast growth factor receptors in carcinogenesis. Mol Cancer Res 2010;8:1439-1452.

8. Holroyd A, Cross NC, Macdonald DH. The two faces of myeloproliferative neoplasms: molecular events underlying lymphoid transformation. Leuk Res 2011;35: 1279-1285.

9. Inhorn RC, Aster JC, Roach SA, et al. A syndrome of lymphoblastic lymphoma, eosinophilia, and myeloid hyperplasia/malignancy associated with t(8;13)(p11;q11): description of a distinctive clinicopathologic entity. Blood 1995;85:1881-1887.

10. Jackson CC, Medeiros LJ, Miranda RN. 8p11 myeloproliferative syndrome: a review. Hum Pathol 2010;41:461-476.

11. Katoh M, Nakagama H. FGF receptors: cancer biology and therapeutics. Med Res Rev 2014;34:280-300.

12. Kim WS, Park SG, Park G, Jang SJ, Moon DS, Kang SH. 8p11 myeloproliferative syndrome with t(1;8)(q25;p11.2): a case report and review of the literature. Acta Haematol 2015;133:101-105.

13. Kumar KR, Chen W, Koduru PR, Luu HS. Myeloid and lymphoid neoplasm with abnormalities of FGFR1 presenting with trilineage blasts and RUNX1 rearrangement: a case report and review of literature. Am J Clin Pathol 2015;143:738-748.

14. Macdonald D, Aguiar RC, Mason PJ, Goldman JM, Cross NC. A new myeloproliferative disorder associated with chromosomal translocations involving 8p11: a review. Leukemia 1995;9:1628-1630.

15. Mason I. Initiation to end point: the multiple roles of fibroblast growth factors in neural development. Nat Rev Neurosci 2007;8:583-596.

16. Metzgeroth G, Walz C, Score J, et al. Recurrent finding of the FIP1L1-PDGFRA fusion gene in eosinophilia-associated acute myeloid leukemia and lymphoblastic T-cell lymphoma. Leukemia 2007;21:1183-1188.

17. Patel RA, Sheehan AM, Finch CJ, Lopez-Terrada D, Hernandez VS, Curry CV. Fine-needle aspiration cytology of T-lymphoblastic lymphoma associated FGFR1 rearrangement myeloproliferative neoplasm. Diagn Cytopathol 2014;42:45-48.

18. Ren M, Cowell JK. Constitutive Notch pathway activation in murine ZMYM2-FGFR1-induced T-cell lymphomas associated with atypical myeloproliferative disease. Blood 2011;117:6837-6847.

19. Ren M, Quin H, Ren R, Cowell JK. Ponatinib suppresses the development of myeloid and lymphoid malignancies associated with FGFR1 abnormaities. Leukemia 2013;27:32-40.

20. Richebourg S, Theisen O, Plantier I, et al. Chronic myeloproliferative disorder with t(8;22)(p11;q11) can mime clonal cytogenetic evolution of authentic chronic myelogeneous leukemia. Genes, Chromosomes Cancer 2008;47:915-918.

21. Roumiantsev S, Krause DS, Neumann CA, et al. Distinct stem cell myeloproliferative/T lymphoma syndromes induced by ZNF198-FGFR1 and BCR-FGFR1 fusion genes from 8p11 translocations. Cancer Cell 2004;5:287-298.

22. Somers GR, Slater H, Rockman S, et al. Coexistent T-cell lymphoblastic lymphoma and an atypical myeloproliferative disorder associated with t(8;13)(p21;q14). Pediatr Pathology Lab Med 1997;17:141-158.

23. Trimaldi J, Carballido EM, Bowers JW, et al. B-lymphoblastic leukemia/lymphoma associated with t(8;13)(p11;q12)/ZMYM2 (ZNF198)-FGFR1: rare case and review of the literature. Acta Haematol 2013;130:127-134.

24. Turner N, Grose R. Fibroblast growth factor signalling: from development to cancer. Nat Rev Cancer 2010;10:116-129.

25. Vega F, Medeiros LJ, Bueso-Ramos CE, Arboleda P, Miranda RN. Hematolymphoid neoplasms associated with rearrangements of PDGFRA, PDGFRB, and FGFR1. Am J Clin Pathol 2015;144:377-392.

26. Vega F, Medeiros LJ, Davuluri R, Cromwell CC, Alkan S, Abruzzo LV. t(8;13)-positive bilineal lymphomas: report of 6 cases. Am J Surg Pathol 2008;32:14-20.

27. Vizmanos JL, Hernandez R, Vidal MJ, et al. Clinical variability of patients with the t(6;8)(q27;p12) and FGFR1OP-FGFR1 fusion: two further cases. Hematol J 2004;5:534-537.

28. Wong WS, Cheng KC, Lau KM, et al. Clonal evolution of 8p11 stem cell syndrome in a 14-year-old Chinese boy: a review of literature of t(8;13) associated myeloproliferative diseases. Leuk Res 2007;31:235-238.

51 MYELOID SARCOMA

GENERAL FEATURES

Myeloid sarcoma is a tumor mass composed of blasts of myeloid lineage occurring at an anatomic site other than the bone marrow (2a,16). The term does not include tissue infiltration by acute myeloid leukemia, which does not form a tumor mass.

A number of synonyms exist in the literature for myeloid sarcoma including *chloroma, myeloblastoma, granulocytic sarcoma, monocytic sarcoma,* and *extramedullary myeloid cell tumor.* One drawback of using the designation "sarcoma" is that there is a potential risk of the patient being referred to clinicians who specialize in soft tissue sarcomas and the possibility of inappropriate therapy.

Myeloid sarcoma most often occurs in a patient who has acute myeloid leukemia (AML) of any type involving the bone marrow (3,11,13). Myeloid sarcoma (isolated or with bone marrow involvement) can occur following conventional chemotherapy or stem cell transplantation (23) or concurrently with AML involving the bone marrow. These two scenarios represent 75 to 80 percent of all cases of myeloid sarcoma (3,11,13). Less often, myeloid sarcoma represents a blast phase in a patient with a myelodysplastic syndrome (MDS), myeloproliferative neoplasm (MPN), or MDS/MPN. Approximately 5 percent of patients with MPN develop an extramedullary blast phase of disease.

Rarely, myeloid sarcoma occurs as an isolated mass, in other words, without a history of a myeloid neoplasm or evidence of concurrent involvement by AML (3,13,16). Most patients with isolated myeloid sarcoma develop bone marrow involvement by AML, usually within 1 year, but rare patients do not, especially if treated appropriately (4,16,18).

The diagnostic workup for myeloid sarcoma is usually performed on coexistent AML in the bone marrow. The complete workup includes cytochemistry (myeloperoxidase and nonspecific esterase), flow cytometry immunophenotyping, conventional cytogenetic and fluorescence in situ hybridization (FISH) analyses, and molecular studies including next-generation sequencing methods to assess for clinically actionable gene mutations. In patients with isolated myeloid sarcoma in whom AML involving bone marrow is not available, every attempt must be made to obtain fresh tissue and perform a complete workup on the myeloid sarcoma specimen (21).

CLINICAL FEATURES

The epidemiologic features of patients with myeloid sarcoma are similar to those of patients with AML. The male to female ratio is 1.2 to 1.0, with a median age at presentation of 56 years and a wide age range (13,15,17). Myeloid sarcoma is estimated to occur in about 4 percent of children and 10 percent of adults with AML, but may be under-reported as systematic use of current imaging techniques in patients with AML often detects occult extramedullary sites of disease (13).

Any anatomic site can be involved by myeloid sarcoma but the most common are the skin, lymph nodes, gastrointestinal tract, bones, soft tissue, and gingiva (fig. 51-1). In children, skin, the orbital region, and mucosal sites are most commonly involved. Most patients present with a single mass, but at least 10 percent have multiple sites of involvement (3,13,15). Acute myelomonocytic and monocytic leukemias seem to have a preference for involving the skin and gingiva (16).

The symptoms of patients with myeloid sarcoma depend greatly on the anatomic site involved; many patients have more than one site of extramedullary disease at the time of initial diagnosis. Symptoms related to local compression by myeloid sarcoma are common

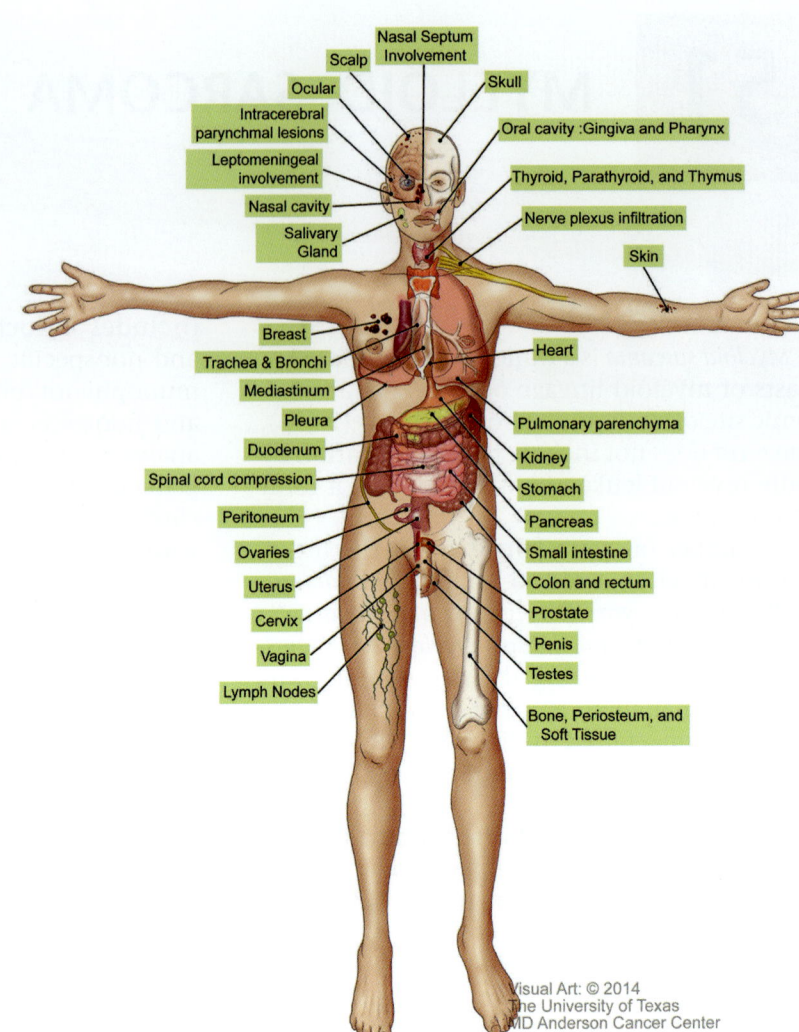

Figure 51-1

ANATOMIC SITES OF MYELOID SARCOMA

Schematic representation of the many anatomic sites that can be involved by myeloid sarcoma.

(16). Myeloid sarcoma uncommonly involves the central nervous system, where it is associated with neurologic deficits related to the mass. Lesions that involve the pituitary gland can impinge on the optic chiasm, leading to visual disturbances. Orbital lesions are more common in children and may be associated with proptosis, eyelid edema, or visual changes (1); the conjunctiva and choroid (rarely) also may be involved. Bleeding is associated with myeloid sarcoma involving mucosal surfaces such as the gingiva, respiratory or gastrointestinal tract, bladder, uterus, and cervix (10,15,24).

Breast involvement is more common in premenopausal women. Patients with breast myeloid sarcoma also seem to have a higher frequency of myeloid sarcoma involving the central nervous system or gynecologic organs (5). Rarely, myeloid sarcoma involves the mediastinum as a large mass and causes superior vena cava syndrome, mimicking lymphomas.

Myeloid sarcoma can involve the pleural, pericardial, or abdominal serous membranes and cause effusions. Involvement of the appendix by AML or myeloid sarcoma can induce symptoms that mimic acute appendicitis (14). Involvement of abdominal organs is commonly associated with abdominal pain (3,13). Massive splenic involvement by myeloid sarcoma can lead to rupture.

Involvement of the prostate gland by myeloid sarcoma is associated with urinary retention. Patients with testicular lesions may undergo orchiectomy for a presumed primary tumor (19).

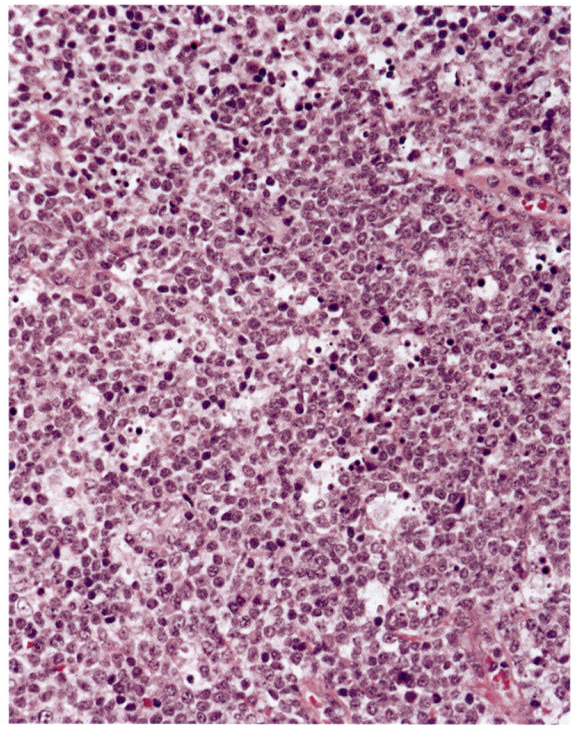

Figure 51-2

MYELOID SARCOMA INVOLVING TONSIL

Abundant single cell apoptosis is seen (hematoxylin and eosin [H&E] stain).

Patients can present with simultaneous involvement of paired organs: about 40 percent of patients with myeloid sarcoma involving the ovaries have bilateral disease (6). Patients with myeloid sarcoma involving lymph nodes can have prominent lymphadenopathy mimicking lymphoma.

HISTOLOGIC FINDINGS

Myeloid sarcoma partially or completely replaces normal tissue architecture in a diffuse pattern (2,15–17). Coagulative necrosis, hemorrhage, or both may be prominent. Mitotic figures are usually common and single cell apoptosis can be abundant (fig. 51-2). Some cases exhibit a prominent starry sky pattern (fig. 51-3). Myeloid sarcoma can infiltrate tissues in a prominent single file pattern reminiscent of a carcinoma (fig. 51-4); this pattern is more common in tumors with monocytic differentiation. Some cases of myeloid sarcoma are associated with fibrosis.

In routine histologic sections, the cells of myeloid sarcoma (and AML) have a high nucleus

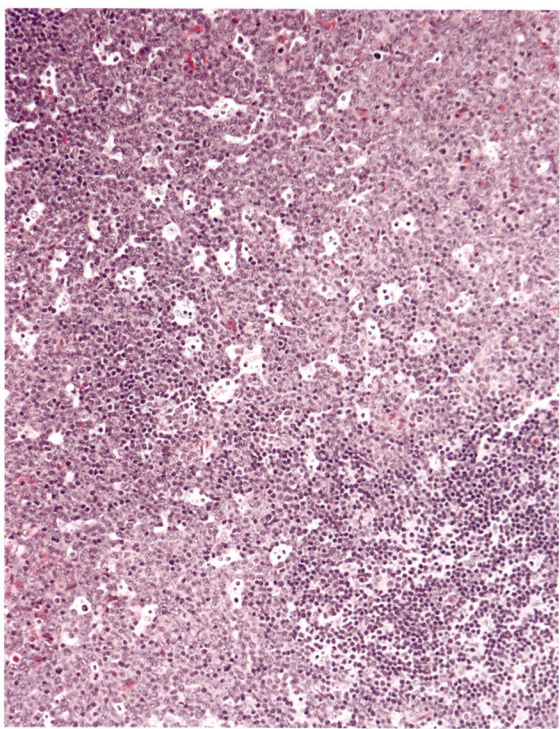

Figure 51-3

MYELOID SARCOMA INVOLVING LYMPH NODE

There is a prominent starry sky pattern. This lymph node was biopsied for suspected lymphoma. Subsequent bone marrow examination showed concurrent acute myeloid leukemia (H&E stain).

to cytoplasm ratio, thin nuclear membranes, often pinpoint nucleoli, and fine nuclear chromatin. The blasts may show maturation or be undifferentiated, but in most cases at least some cells show evidence of maturation, a clue to the diagnosis. Tumors with granulocytic differentiation are characterized by cells with granular cytoplasm resembling promyelocytes, myelocytes, or metamyelocytes (fig. 51-5). Immature eosinophilic precursors are observed in up to half of myeloid sarcomas (fig. 51-6). In rare cases, eosinophilic precursors predominate, and these tumors may be associated with Charcot-Leyden crystals (myeloperoxidase negative). It is unusual to identify Auer rods in granulocytic tumors in routinely processed tissue sections.

In contrast, tumors with monocytic differentiation often exhibit some cells with nuclear folds and less prominent nucleoli that resemble promonocytes (fig. 51-7). Plasmacytoid dendritic cell maturation is identified in some

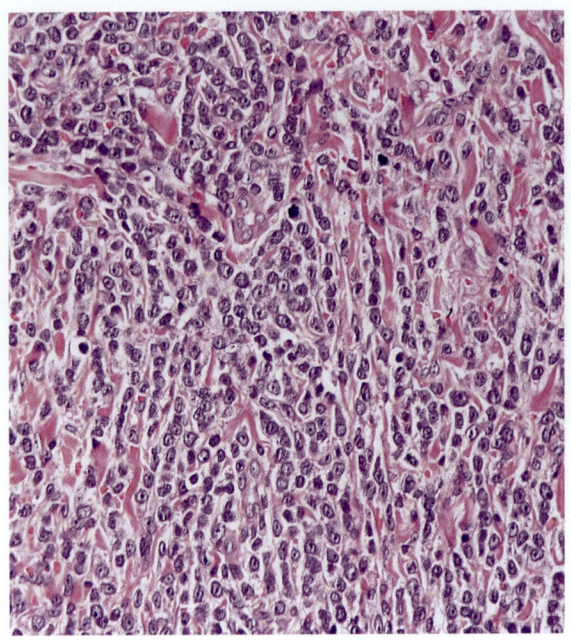

Figure 51-4

MYELOID SARCOMA INVOLVING SKIN

There is a prominent single cell pattern of infiltration. This patient had a history of acute monocytic leukemia and skin was a site of disease relapse (H&E stain).

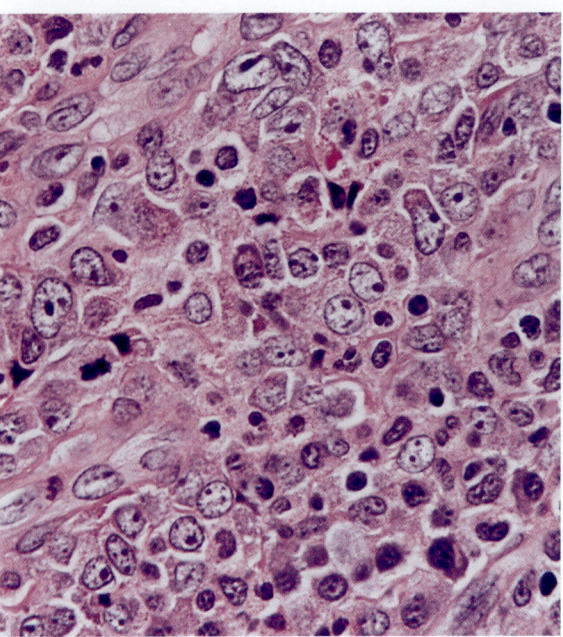

Figure 51-5

MYELOID SARCOMA WITH GRANULOCYTIC DIFFERENTIATION

Some neoplastic cells show maturation with eosinophilic, granular cytoplasm (H&E stain).

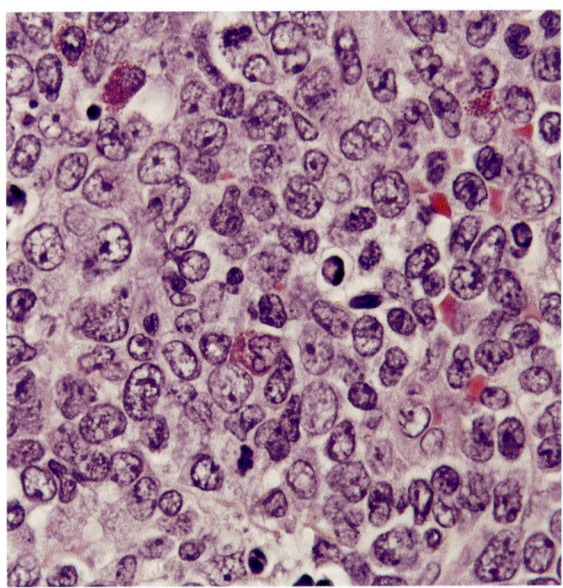

Figure 51-6

MYELOID SARCOMA WITH GRANULOCYTIC DIFFERENTIATION

Eosinophilic metamyelocytes are shown in this field (H&E stain).

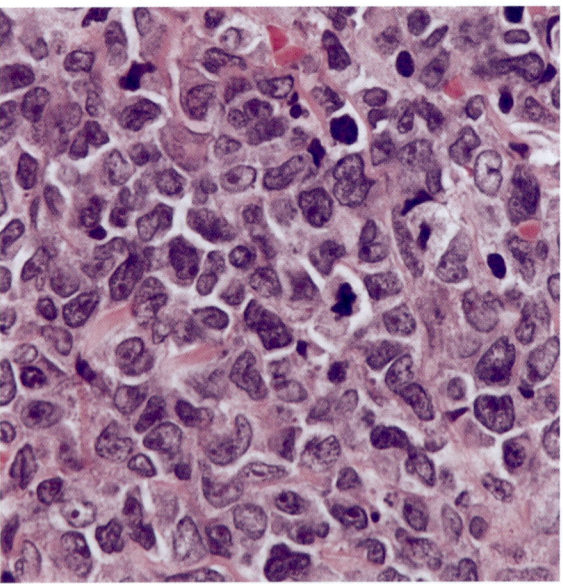

Figure 51-7

MYELOID SARCOMA WITH MONOCYTIC MATURATION (MONOCYTIC SARCOMA)

The neoplastic cells are devoid of granules and some cells have folded nuclei consistent with promonocytes (H&E stain).

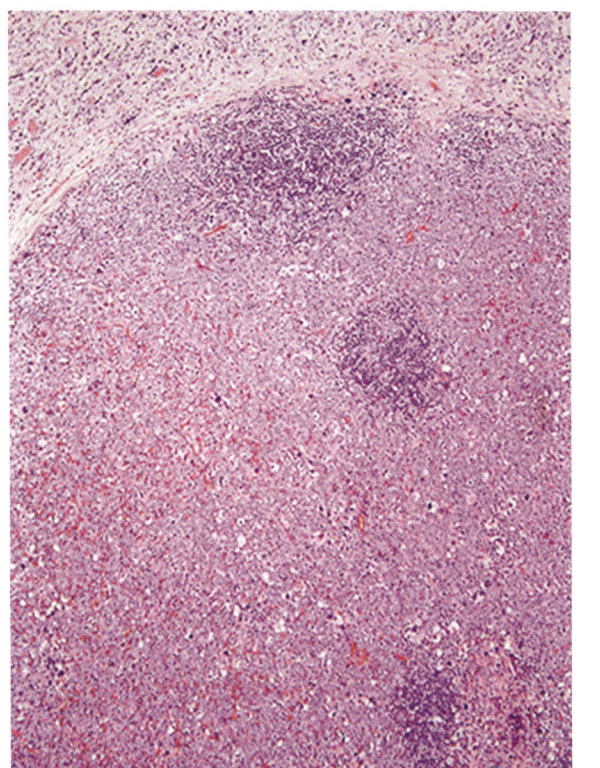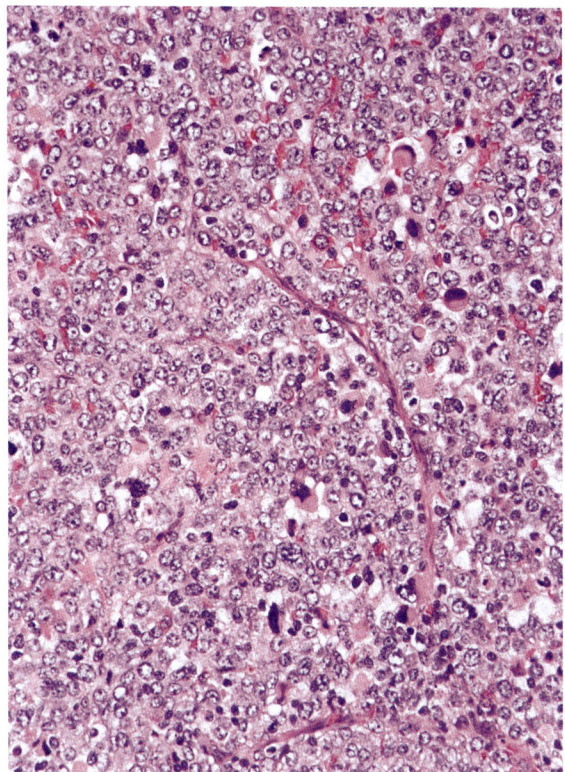

Figure 51-8

MYELOID SARCOMA (BLAST PHASE) IN A PATIENT WITH CHRONIC MYELOID LEUKEMIA

Left: The lymph node architecture is subtotally replaced by tumor.

Right: The neoplastic cells include many blasts but also granulocytes showing a spectrum of maturation and atypical megakaryocytes (H&E stain).

monocytic tumors. Some cases of myeloid sarcoma exhibit both granulocytic and monocytic maturation (and are usually associated with acute myelomonocytic leukemia).

It is rare for cases of myeloid sarcoma to show evidence of megakaryocytic differentiation, except in patients with an underlying MPN or MDS/MPN. In this clinical context, the myeloid sarcoma (i.e., blast phase) is composed of cells with large multilobated nuclei and dense chromatin, consistent with atypical megakaryocytes or smaller, monolobated forms consistent with micromegakaryocytes (fig. 51-8). Pure erythroid differentiation is a rare presentation of myeloid sarcoma that is more likely to occur in the context of the blast phase of MPN or MDS/MPN. Nevertheless, clusters of erythroid blasts are observed in some cases of myeloid sarcoma, although these cells can be difficult to appreciate without immunophenotypic studies.

In earlier studies, cases of myeloid sarcoma were classified into three groups depending on the degree of cell maturation: undifferentiated/blastic, immature, and differentiated. This classification has no prognostic value and is scientifically flawed since the neoplastic cells are blasts or blast equivalents. Nevertheless, this approach is helpful for recognizing the spectrum of cytologic maturation that can be observed in some cases of myeloid sarcoma.

Lymph Node

Lymph node involvement by myeloid sarcoma can show variable patterns of architectural effacement (fig. 51-9). There may be partial involvement, with expansion of the paracortical regions of the lymph node. The neoplasm can surround follicles, mimicking a marginal zone pattern, and a partial sinusoidal pattern is also common. The architecture of other lymph

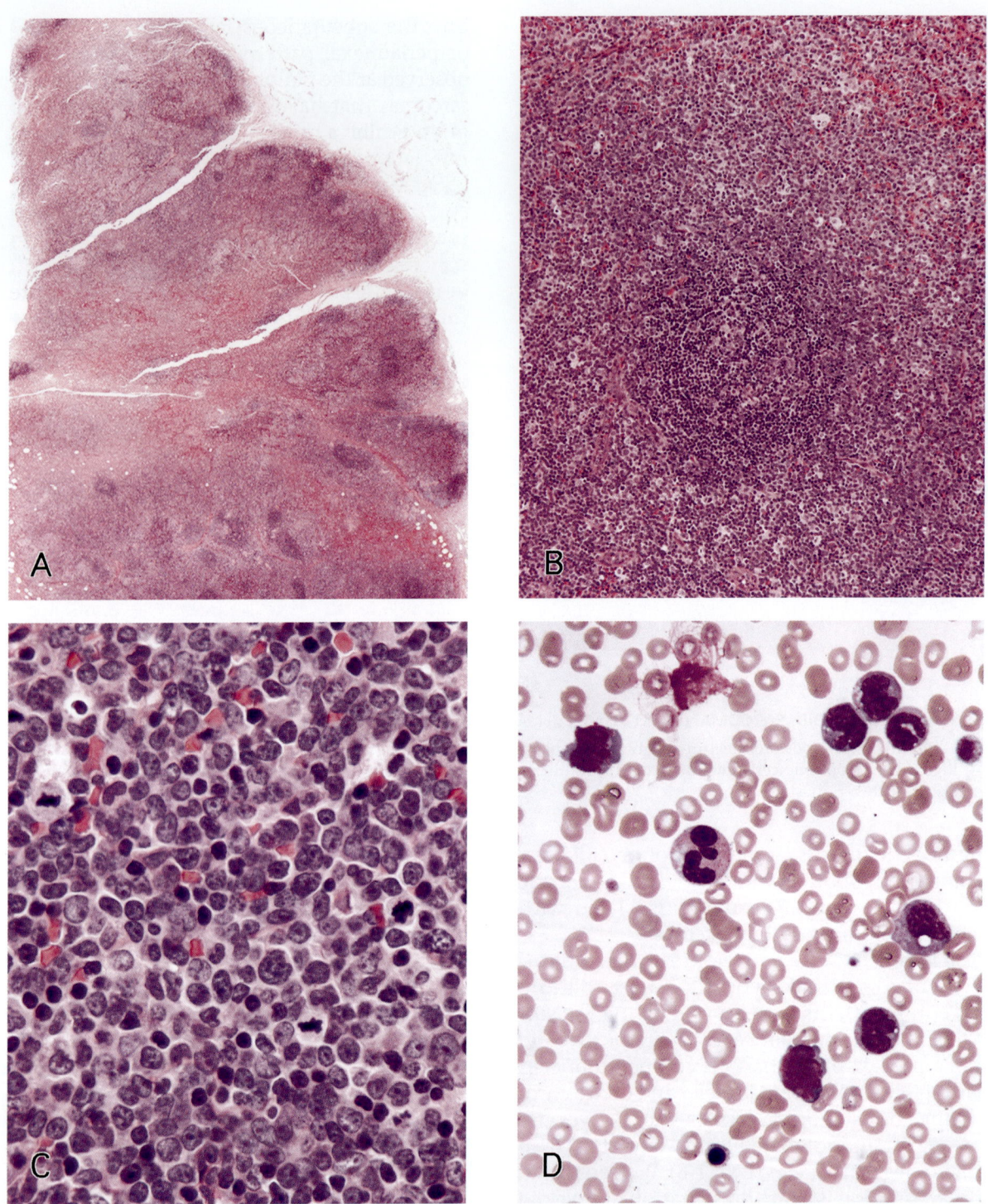

Figure 51-9

MYELOID SARCOMA INVOLVING LYMPH NODE WITH CONCURRENT ACUTE MYELOMONOCYTIC LEUKEMIA

A: The lymph node architecture is subtotally replaced by tumor (A–C: H&E stain).
B: In this field, the myeloid sarcoma surrounds a central lymphoid follicle and has a marginal zone-like pattern.
C: The neoplastic cells are highly immature blasts.
D: The peripheral blood smear shows blasts and immature granulocytes and monocytes (Wright-Giemsa stain).

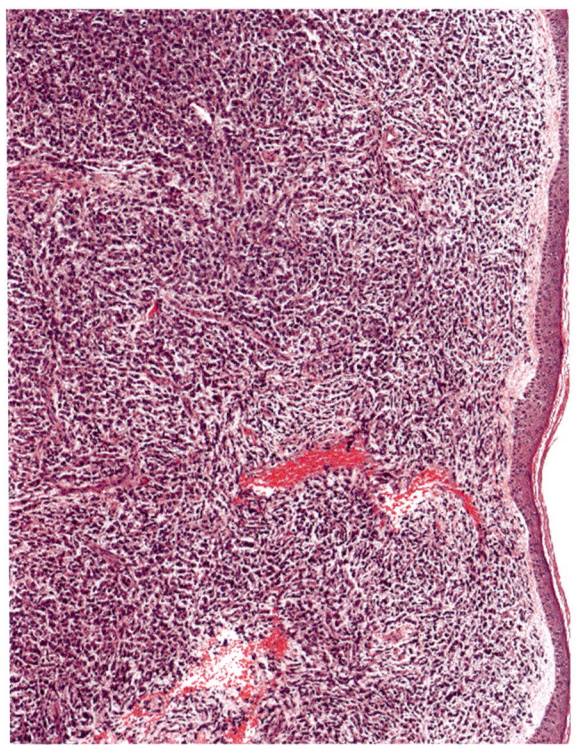

Figure 51-10

MYELOID SARCOMA INVOLVING SKIN

The specimen is characterized by a dense dermal infiltrate of immature cells with fine blastic chromatin associated with prominent blood vessels. There is preservation of the dermal-epidermal junction with attenuation of the overlying epithelium (H&E stain).

nodes is totally effaced without any recognizable nodal structures and the neoplasm can infiltrate through the capsule into perinodal adipose tissue (2,15,17).

As excised lymph nodes are often assessed for tissue adequacy in the frozen section room, this provides an opportunity to triage fresh tissue to various laboratories, thereby facilitating a complete diagnostic workup. Air-dried touch imprints of lymph node can be assessed by cytochemistry for myeloperoxidase, allowing for rapid diagnosis (2).

Skin

Skin is the most common site involved by myeloid sarcoma, and patients may present with papules, plaques, or nodules (2,15–17). Histologically, myeloid sarcoma diffusely replaces the dermis (fig. 51-10). The lesion can extend into the subcutaneous fat and a perivascular or periadnexal pattern of infiltration may be observed at the periphery of the mass. Myeloid sarcomas that have monocytic differentiation often exhibit a prominent single cell pattern of infiltration (fig. 51-4). Chronic myelomonocytic leukemia (CMML) also commonly involves skin and this often occurs as a preterminal phase in the patient's clinical course. The lesion in skin may resemble CMML (with a low blast count) or meet the criteria for myeloid sarcoma (more than 20 percent blasts).

Other Sites

The features described in lymph nodes and skin also apply to other anatomic sites involved by myeloid sarcoma. The neoplasm infiltrates tissues in a diffuse pattern (figs. 51-11, 51-12). In the mouth, myeloid sarcoma can be associated with ulcer, acute and chronic inflammation, or prominent plasmacytosis that can obscure the neoplastic cells (fig. 51-13) (24). At anatomic sites where different organs are in close apposition, myeloid sarcoma commonly infiltrates more than one organ as a part of the formation of a tumor mass (10). In the appendix, myeloid sarcoma can fully infiltrate the wall, resulting in perforation (14). Involvement of the testis is more common as a part of relapsed disease (11).

CYTOLOGIC FINDINGS

In cytologic preparations, the blast cells are often associated with cells showing some evidence of either granulocytic or monocytic maturation (figs. 51-14, 51-15). Tumors of granulocytic lineage may show promyelocytes, myelocytes, and metamyelocytes, and monocytic tumors may show promonocytes and monocytes. In part related to differentiation, cases of myeloid sarcoma are either monomorphic (fig. 51-14) or polymorphic (fig. 51-15). Diff-Quik and Wright-Giemsa stains are particularly helpful because they stain the cytoplasm and granules of myeloid cells. Either azurophilic or secondary granules are observed, and rarely, Auer rods are identified. Basophils and mast cells are also highlighted and rare cases of myeloid sarcoma have a component of mast cell differentiation. Papanicolaou stains are more useful in highlighting the thin nuclear membranes and pinpoint nucleoli common in the blasts of myeloid sarcoma.

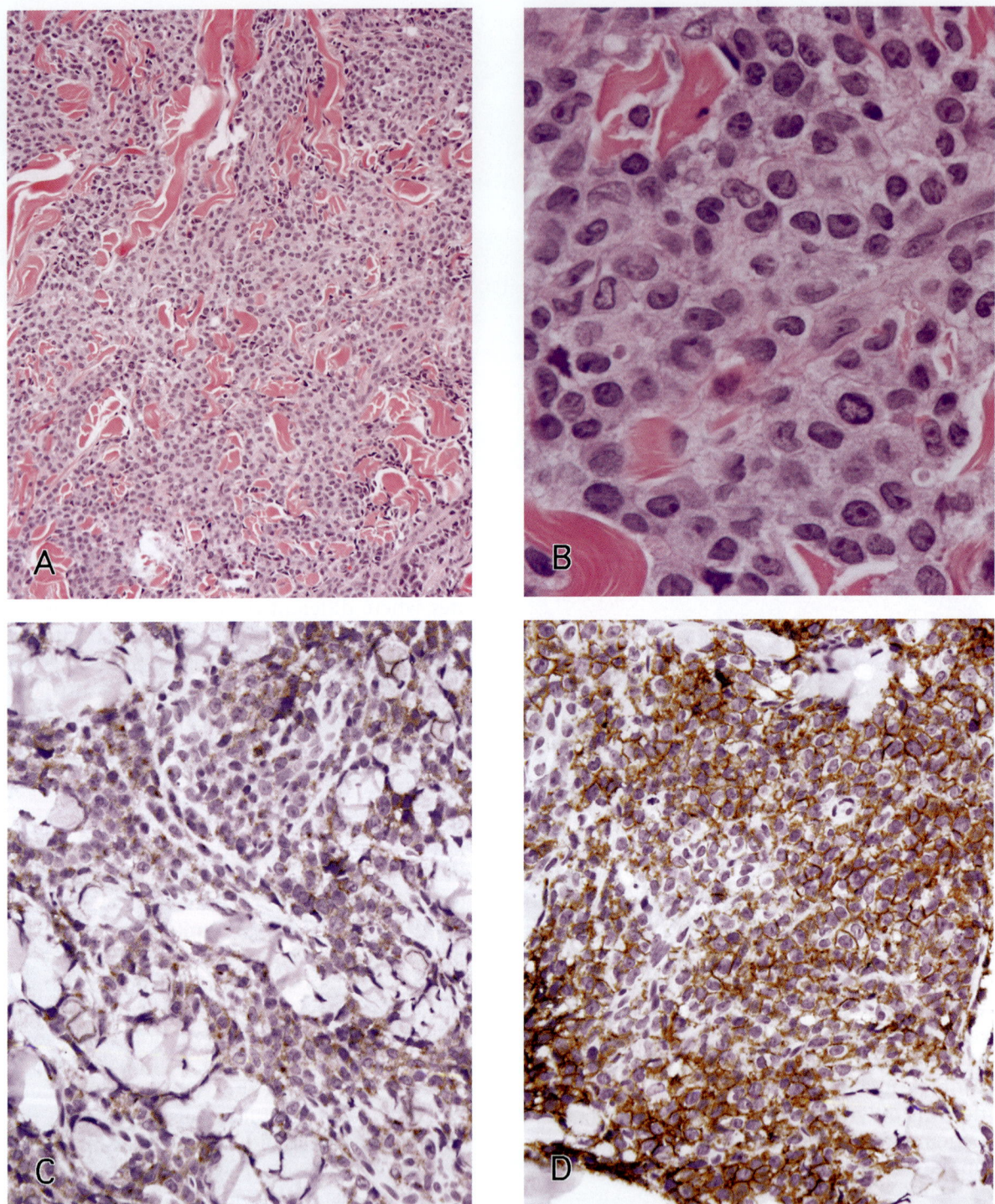

Figure 51-11

MYELOID SARCOMA WITH EXTENSIVE MONOCYTIC DIFFERENTIATION INVOLVING SOFT TISSUE

A: The neoplastic cells diffusely infiltrate fibrous tissue (A,B: H&E stain).

B: Many monoblasts and promonocytes are seen in this field.

C,D: The neoplastic cells are positive for CD4 (C) and CD56 (D) (Immunohistochemistry with hematoxylin counterstain).

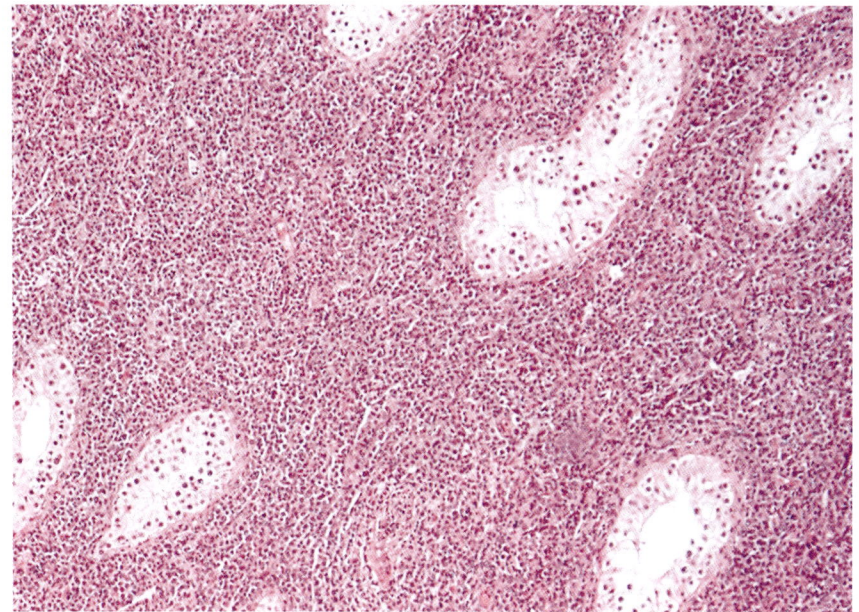

Figure 51-12

MYELOID SARCOMA INVOLVING TESTIS

The myeloblasts infiltrate between seminiferous tubules at the periphery of the tumor mass (H&E stain).

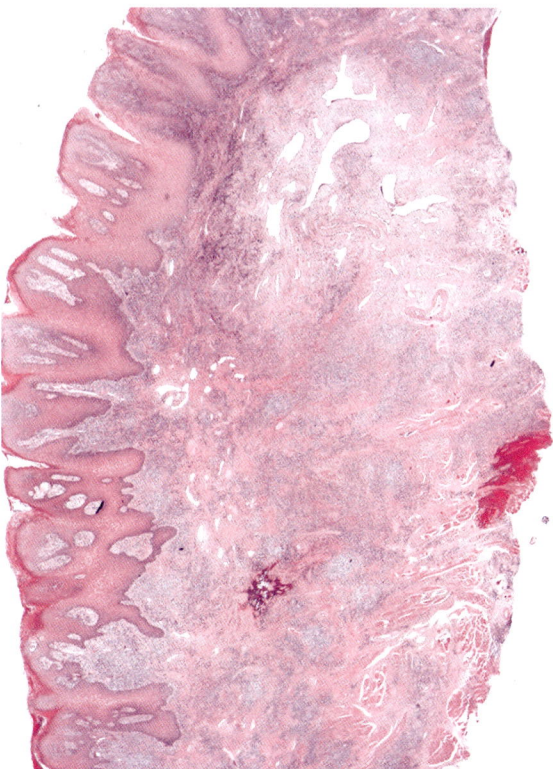
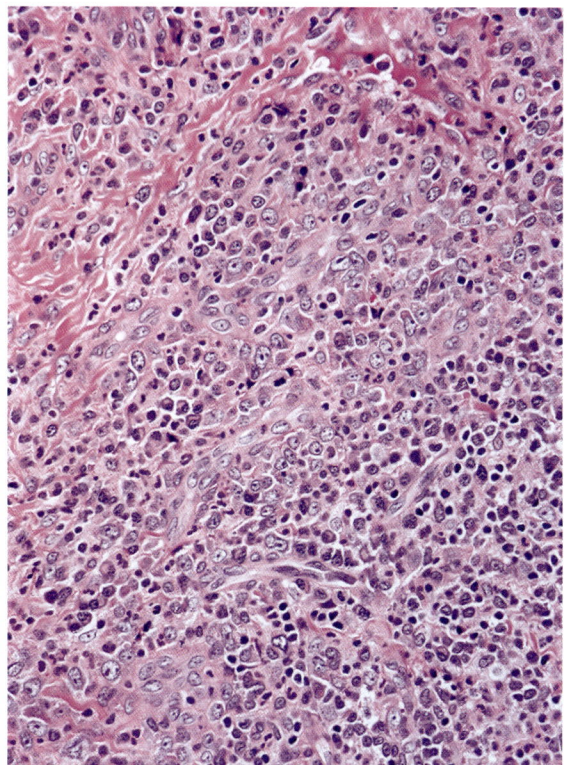

Figure 51-13

MYELOID SARCOMA INVOLVING THE BUCCAL MUCOSA

Left: At low power, the neoplasm is associated with hyperplastic epidermis (H&E stain).

Right: High magnification shows myeloblasts admixed with mature plasma cells that might be mistaken for chronic inflammation.

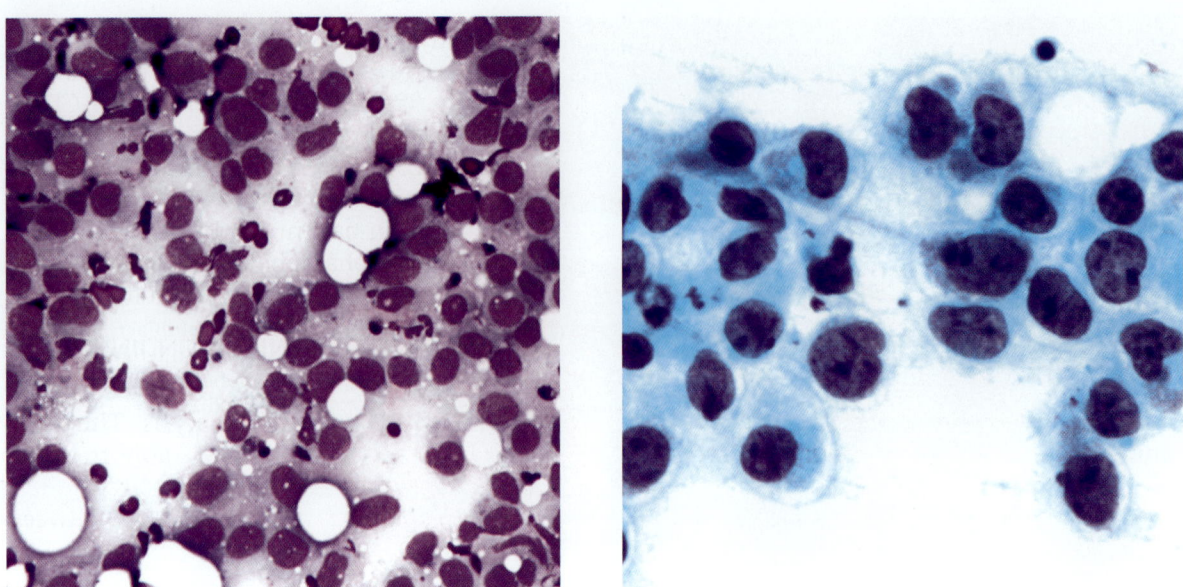

Figure 51-14

MONOMORPHIC MYELOID SARCOMA: CYTOLOGIC FEATURES

A fine-needle aspirate smear shows a monomorphic population of medium-sized neoplastic myeloid cells (left: Diff-Quik stain; right: Papanicolaou stain).

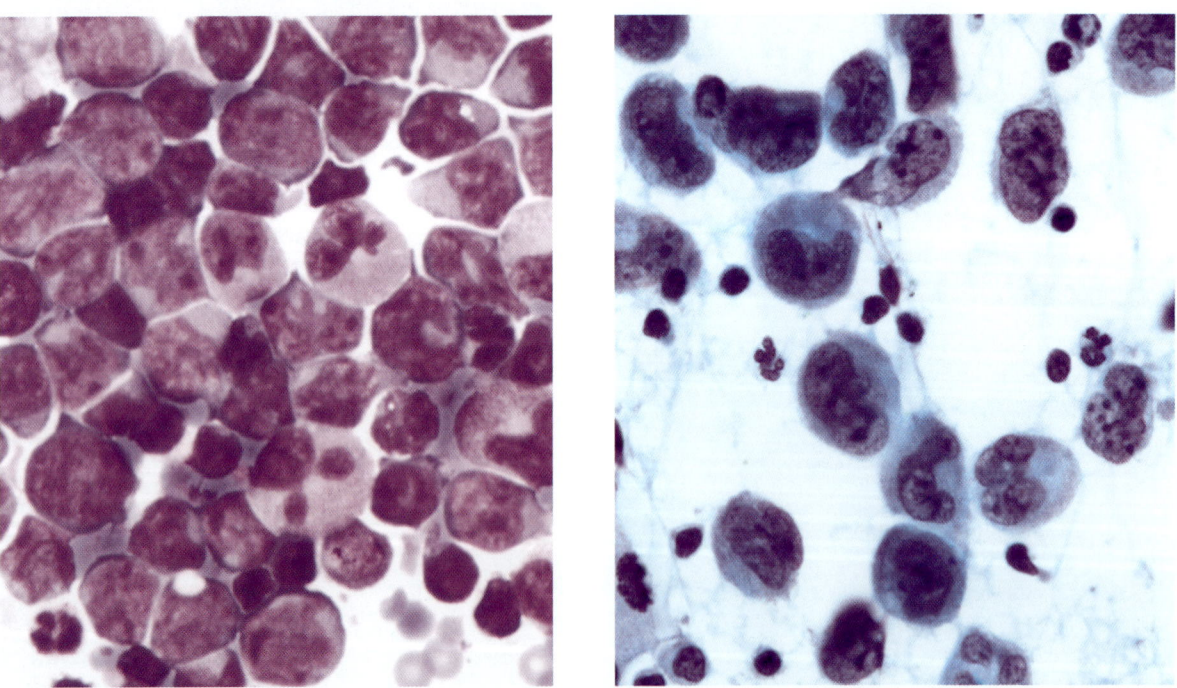

Figure 51-15

POLYMORPHIC MYELOID SARCOMA: CYTOLOGIC FEATURES

Some cases of myeloid sarcoma are more polymorphic, as shown in this fine-needle aspirate smear in which the neoplastic cells have convoluted to lobated nuclear contours, fine chromatin, and variable amounts of cytoplasm. Granules are best seen on the air-dried preparations (left: Diff-Quik stain; right: Papanicolaou stain).

CYTOCHEMICAL FINDINGS

Cytochemical stains for myeloperoxidase (MPO), naphthol-ASD-chloroacetate esterase (CAE), and nonspecific esterase (NSE) can be performed on air-dried touch imprints or smears supporting granulocytic (MPO and CAE) or monocytic (NSE) differentiation. CAE also can be performed on routinely fixed and processed tissue and is positive in about half of myeloid sarcoma cases (16,17).

IMMUNOPHENOTYPIC FINDINGS

Flow cytometry immunophenotyping and immunohistochemistry methods are very helpful for establishing the diagnosis of myeloid sarcoma. Using flow cytometry, antibodies specific for CD4, CD11b, CD11c, CD13, CD14, CD33, CD34, CD36, CD41, CD61, CD64, CD71, CD117, CD123, and other markers establish a granulocytic, monocytic, erythroid, or megakaryocytic lineage.

Immunohistochemistry is useful, but less sensitive than flow cytometry. A number of markers are available to assess routinely processed tissue sections and the following antibodies are the most sensitive: CD43 (fig. 51-16A), CD68/ KP1 (fig. 51-16B), CD117, CD11c (fig. 51-16C), CD33 (fig. 51-16D), lysozyme (fig. 51-16E), and myeloperoxidase (fig. 51-16F) (2,11,15-17). None of these antibodies is entirely specific for myeloid sarcoma. Other antibodies are available that react with half or more cases of myeloid sarcoma: CD34, CD45/LCA, CD56 (fig. 47-11D), CD68/PGM1, CD99, CD163, TdT (usually dim), and Kruppel-like factor 4 (16,17). CD56 and CD68/PGM1 are expressed most often in tumors with monocytic differentiation. Antibodies reactive with factor VIII, CD31, CD42b, CD61, CD71, E-cadherin, glycophorin (A or C), and blood group antigens are positive in some tumors that show evidence of megakaryocytic or erythroid differentiation (2,16). CD15 highlights myeloid sarcomas with maturation, but is negative in immature or blastic tumors. CD30 is rarely positive in myeloid sarcoma (less than 5 percent of cases).

B-cell antigens are usually not expressed by myeloid sarcomas, with the exception of cases associated with t(8;21)(q22;q22)/*RUNX1-RUNX1T1* that commonly express the B-cell antigens CD19 and PAX5 (20). Pan-T-cell antigens are usually negative in myeloid sarcoma, but CD2, CD3, and CD7 can be expressed in a subset of cases, usually infrequently. CD4 positivity (fig. 51-11C) is more common since CD4 is expressed by tumors with monocytic differentiation. CD11c, CD43, CD68, CD163, and Kruppel-like factor 4 are particularly helpful in recognizing monocytic tumors. Rarely, keratin has been reported in cases of myeloid sarcoma (15). In patients with MPN, the extramedullary blast phase may exhibit evidence of two or all three hematopoietic cell lineages.

MOLECULAR GENETIC FINDINGS

Myeloid sarcoma is infrequently assessed by conventional cytogenetic analysis. The cases analyzed have had cytogenetic abnormalities in a frequency similar to that of AML and there are no obvious differences in karyotype between myeloid sarcoma and AML. FISH analysis is used more often to assess cases of myeloid sarcoma.

Approximately half of myeloid sarcomas are associated with cytogenetic abnormalities (13,16). In infants, abnormalities of the chromosome locus 11q23 involve *MLL* (16). Myeloid sarcoma appears to be more common in patients with core-binding factor abnormalities including t(8;21)/*RUNX1-RUNX1T1* or inv(16)(p13.1q22)/t(16;16)(p13.1;q22)/*CBFB-MYH11*. Myeloid sarcoma associated with t(8;21) is more common in children.

Other recurrent cytogenetic abnormalities associated with myeloid sarcoma include t(15;17)(q24.1;q21.2)/*PML-RARA*, t(6;9)(p23;q34)/ *DEK-NUP214*, and inv(3)(q21q26.2) or t(3;3) (q21;q26.2)/*RPN1-EVI1*. Congenital leukemia with t(8;16)(p11;q13) commonly is associated with skin lesions, and presents either as myeloid sarcoma or leukemia cutis (AML infiltrates); spontaneous remission may occur (22).

Array comparative genomic hybridization (aCGH) has been used to assess cases of AML. The results have confirmed known cytogenetic data and identified additional abnormalities; these changes are likely also present in myeloid sarcomas although these tumors have been assessed infrequently. One small study used aCGH to assess seven cases of myeloid sarcoma, all of which showed gains and losses of multiple chromosomal regions; chromosome 8q21.2-q24.3 was one of the more common sites (7).

Little gene mutation data are currently available for myeloid sarcomas. In one study, Falini et al. (8) used cytoplasmic expression of NPM1,

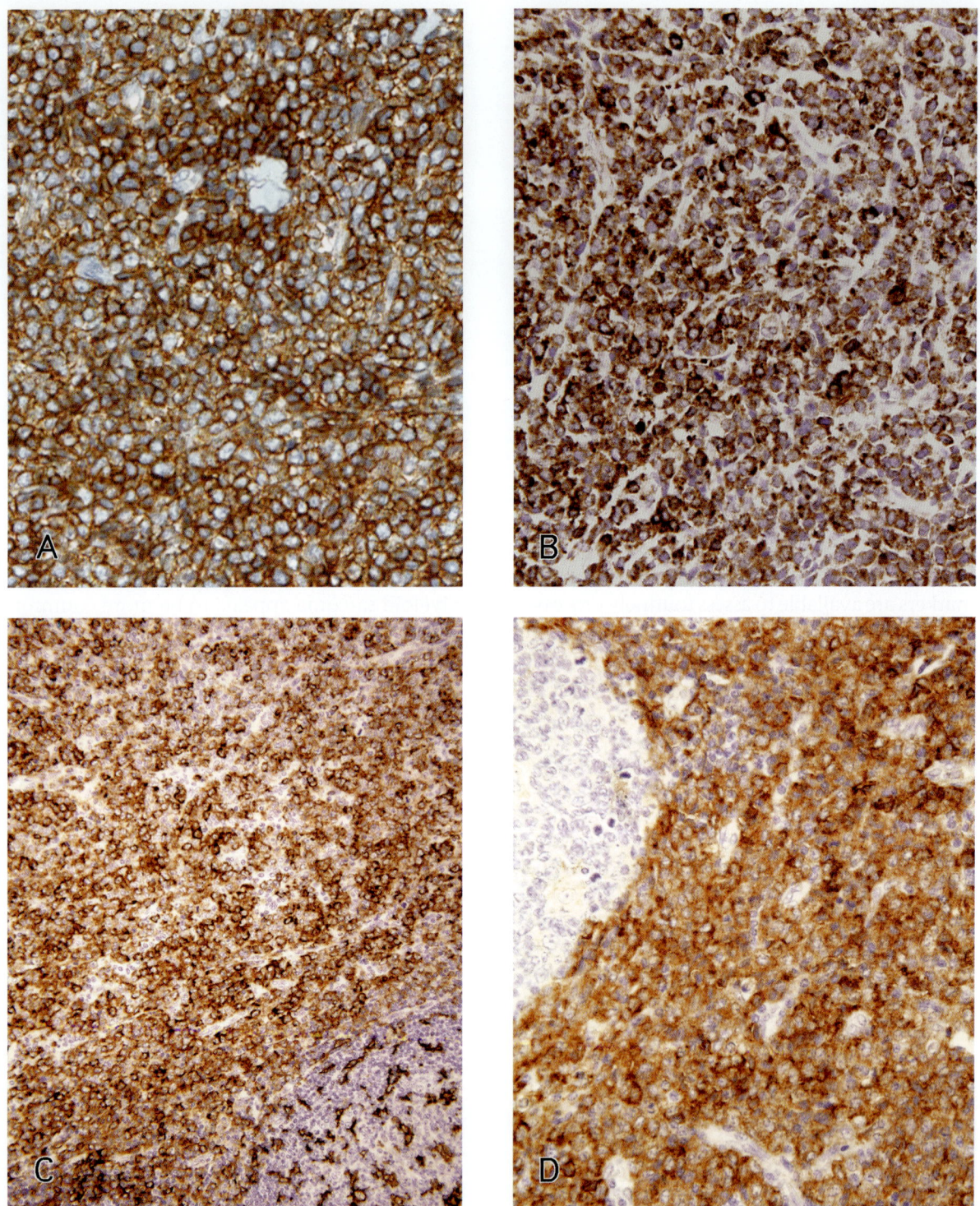

Figure 51-16

IMMUNOHISTOCHEMICAL MARKERS OF MYELOID SARCOMA

A number of antibodies are helpful for establishing the diagnosis of myeloid sarcoma. Examples of positive immunostaining results using many of the more sensitive antibodies are shown (A: CD43; B: CD68; C: CD11c; D: CD33; E: lysozyme; F: myeloperoxidase (immunohistochemistry with hematoxylin counterstain).

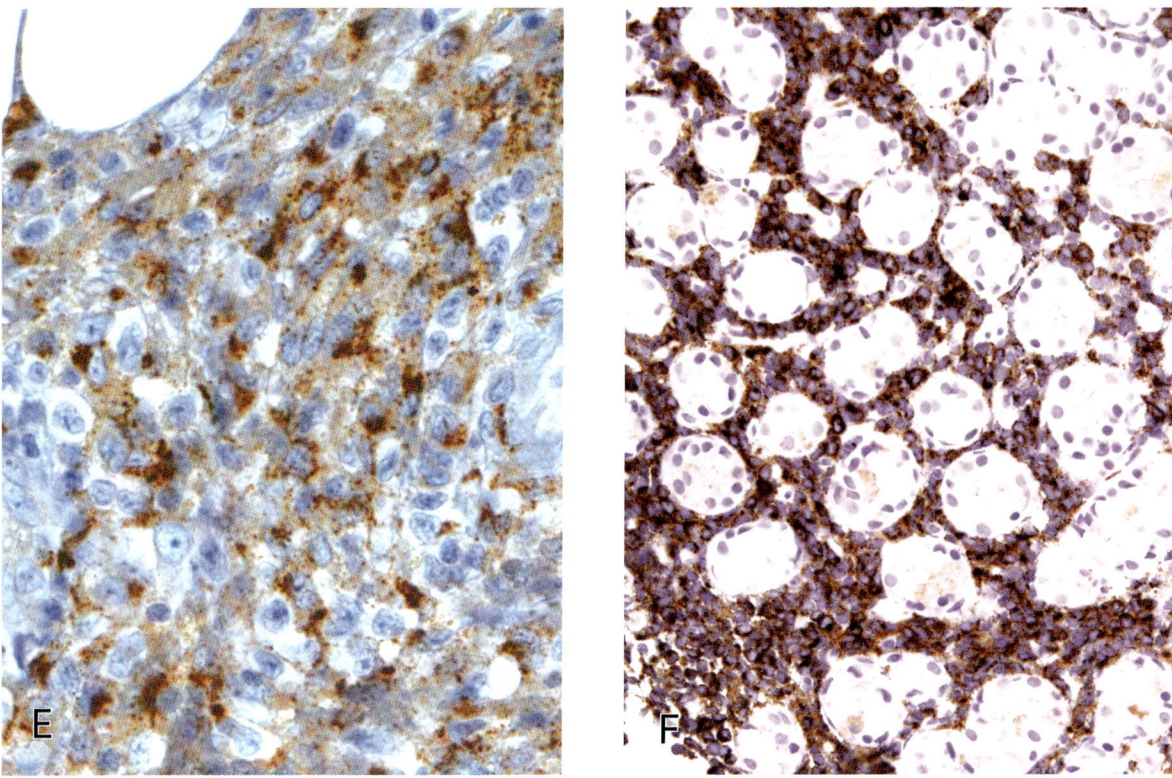

Figure 51-16, continued

assessed by immunohistochemistry, to infer the presence of *NPM1* mutations in approximately 15 percent of myeloid sarcomas. Cases with cytoplasmic NPM1 expression commonly exhibit monocytic differentiation and a normal karyotype, and often have *FLT3* mutations as has been reported in AML (8,9). Next-generation sequencing results in cases of myeloid sarcoma have been reported in a small number of cases. The mutations are similar to those reported in AML, however, the gene profiles can differ between myeloid sarcoma and simultaneous bone marrow involvement by AML (14a). In addition, morphologically negative bone marrow in myeloid sarcoma patients may carry driver gene mutations (14a).

DIFFERENTIAL DIAGNOSIS

Diffuse Large B-Cell Lymphoma (DLBCL). DLBCL is the most common entity in the differential diagnosis of myeloid sarcoma. DLBCL and myeloid sarcoma diffusely replace tissue architecture and can involve extranodal sites or lymph nodes. Unlike myeloid sarcoma, the neoplastic cells of DLBCL have thicker nuclear membranes and more prominent nucleoli, including cells with centroblastic or immunoblastic features. Immunophenotypic or molecular analysis showing B-cell lineage and monoclonal immunoglobulin gene rearrangements supports DLBCL.

Burkitt Lymphoma. Myeloid sarcoma and Burkitt lymphoma have cells of similar size and can exhibit a starry sky pattern, abundant apoptosis, and a high mitotic rate. The cells of Burkitt lymphoma have thick nuclear membranes, hyperchromasia, and 2 to 4 nucleoli, unlike myeloid sarcoma. Immunophenotypic or molecular analysis showing B-cell lineage or *MYC* rearrangements supports Burkitt lymphoma.

Lymphoblastic Lymphoma of B or T Lineage. The cells of lymphoblastic lymphoma and myeloid sarcoma can be of similar size, and both tumors have abundant apoptosis, a high mitotic rate, immature (or blastic) chromatin, and expression of CD43, TdT, and CD99. Lymphoblastic lymphoma cells, however, tend to have less cytoplasm than myeloid sarcoma cells and immunophenotypic analysis shows expression of a number of B- or T-lineage markers. TdT expression is usually much brighter in lymphoblastic lymphoma than myeloid sarcoma.

Anaplastic Large Cell Lymphoma (ALCL). Myeloid sarcoma of monocytic lineage may be composed of cells with folded, almost horseshoe-like nuclei and abundant agranular cytoplasm, and can resemble ALCL. CD43, a T-cell–associated antigen that usually is expressed by myeloid sarcoma, and CD13, a myeloid-associated antigen that is expressed by a subset of cases of ALCL, can be misleading. Expression of CD30 (bright and uniform), ALK, other markers of T-cell lineage, and cytotoxic markers supports the diagnosis of ALCL.

Blastic Plasmacytoid Dendritic Cell Neoplasm (BPDCN). There is substantial morphologic and immunophenotypic overlap between myeloid sarcoma and BPDCN. Further complicating the issue, patients with BPDCN can go on to develop acute or chronic myelomonocytic or acute monocytic leukemia. Usually, BPDCN occurs in older patients with involvement of skin, bone marrow, and lymph nodes whereas myeloid sarcoma can present in a greater variety of anatomic sites. BPDCNs express a number of markers that, in combination, are helpful for diagnosis including CD4, CD56, CD123, BDCA2/CD303, TCL1, and SPIB1, and are negative for myeloperoxidase and lysozyme (21).

In some cases of CMML, extramedullary sites can show prominent clusters of cells with plasmacytoid dendritic cell maturation suggesting a diagnosis of BPDCN. The nodular architecture and clear association with CMML cells preclude the diagnosis of BPDCN.

Extramedullary Sites Involved by MDS, MPN, or MDS/MPN. MDS, MPN, and MDS/MPN can involve extramedullary sites. In many patients, extramedullary disease is associated with numerous blasts (blast phase) and a poor prognosis. Some patients, however, do not have evidence of AML in blood or bone marrow and their extramedullary lesion does not have an adequate percentage of blasts (CD34-positive cells well below 20 percent) to meet the criteria for AML. In this scenario, the extramedullary site of disease should not be designated as blast phase or AML, but instead described as evidence of the primary disease (whether MDS, MPN, or MDS/MPN) involving an extramedullary site (see chapter 62 for additional discussion). Clin-

ical follow-up for these patients can be benign, without progression to AML, although in some patients the disease will progress to blast phase/AML. Extramedullary involvement by CMML commonly heralds the onset of a more aggressive disease course and skin involvement is often a pre-terminal event.

Histiocytic Sarcoma. Distinguishing myeloid sarcoma with monocytic differentiation (i.e., monocytic sarcoma) from histiocytic sarcoma can be difficult using traditional pathologic criteria. Careful attention to the history and laboratory findings is needed. Patients with a biopsy specimen thought to represent histiocytic sarcoma should undergo blood and bone marrow examination to exclude concurrent acute monocytic leukemia. Some histiocytic sarcomas have relapsed as AML after clinical follow-up of a few years, highlighting the difficulty in distinguishing these two entities using current World Health Organization (WHO) criteria.

TREATMENT AND PROGNOSIS

Patients with myeloid sarcoma require systemic chemotherapy similar to that required for AML patients (3,4,13). In the case of isolated myeloid sarcoma, it is clear in the literature that patients treated with local therapies, such as excision or radiation therapy, have a poor prognosis. Radiation therapy, however, may be valuable following chemotherapy as a part of consolidation (4). Hematopoietic (most often allogeneic) stem cell transplantation is likely associated with a higher probability of prolonged survival and possible cure (11a,13,15,23).

In patients with bone marrow–based AML, associated myeloid sarcoma does not portend a worse prognosis and the 5-year overall survival rate ranges between 20 and 30 percent, similar to that of patients with AML overall (3,13). Some authors have suggested, however, that some anatomic sites involved by myeloid sarcoma may be sanctuary sites or sites where the disease is more resistant to standard AML therapies. Central nervous system involvement by myeloid sarcoma is one example in which patients may have a worse prognosis. The prognosis of patients with isolated myeloid sarcoma is not well established; some authors have suggested that patients with isolated myeloid sarcoma have a better prognosis than patients with AML (12,18).

With the development of highly successful therapy for some types of myeloid neoplasms, for example, chronic myeloid leukemia and acute promyelocytic leukemia, some patients have prolonged survival. Nevertheless, late relapse as myeloid sarcoma can occur involving unusual anatomic sites (4,21). For example, long-term survivors following treatment of acute promyelocytic leukemia have an increased frequency of relapse in the central nervous system (4). Therefore, vigilant, long-term clinical follow-up is needed for all patients with myeloid leukemia.

REFERENCES

1. Aggarwal E, Mulay K, Honavar SG. Orbital extra-medullary granulocytic sarcoma: clinicopathologic correlation with immunohistochemical features. Surv Opthalmol 2014;59:232-235.

2. Audouin J, Comperat E, Le Tourneau A, et al. Myeloid sarcoma: clinical and morphologic criteria useful for diagnosis. Int J Surg Pathol 2003;11:271-282.

2a. Arber DA, Orazi A, Hasserjian R, et al. The 2016 revision to the World Health Organization classification of myeloid neoplasms and acute leukemia. Blood 2016;127:2391-2405.

3. Avni B, Koren-Michowitz M. Myeloid sarcoma: current approach and therapeutic options. Ther Adv Hematol 2011;2:309-316.

4. Bakst RL, Tallman MS, Douer D, Yahalom J. How I treat extramedullary acute myeloid leukemia. Blood 2011;118:3785-3793.

5. Cunningham I. A clinical review of breast involvement in acute lekemia. Leuk Lymphoma 2006;47:2517-2526.

6. Cunningham I. The clinical behavior of 124 leukemia ovarian tumors: clues to improving the poor prognosis. Leuk Lymphoma 2013;54:1430-1436.

7. Deeb G, Baer MR, Gaile DP, et al. Genomic profiling of myeloid sarcoma by array comparative genomic hybridization. Genes Chromosomes Cancer 2005;44:373-383.

8. Falini B, Lenze D, Hasserjian R, et al. Cytoplasmic mutated nucleophosmin (NPM) defines the molecular status of a significant fraction of myeloid sarcomas. Leukemia 2007;21:1566-1570.

9. Falini B, Mecucci C, Tiacci E, et al. Cytoplasmic nucleophosmin in acute myelogenous leukemia with a normal karyotype. N Engl J Med 2005;352:254-66.

10. Garcia MG, Deavers MT, Knoblock RJ, et al. Myeloid sarcoma involving the gynecologic tract: a report of 11 cases and review of the literature. Am J Clin Pathol 2006;125:783-790.

11. Kawamoto K, Miyoshi H, Yoshida N, Takizawa J, Sone H, Ohshima K. Clinicopathological, cytogenetic, and prognostic analysis of 131 myeloid sarcoma patients. Am J Surg Pathol 2016;40:1473-1483.

11a. Lazzarotto D, Candoni A, Filì C, et al. Clinical outcome of myeloid sarcoma in adult patients and effect of allogeneic stem cell transplantation. Results from a multicenter survey. Leuk Res 2017;53:74-81.

12. Movassaghian M, Brunner AM, Blonquist TM, et al. Presentation and outcomes among patients with isolated myeloid sarcoma: a Surveillance, Epidemiology, and End Results database analysis. Leuk Lymphoma 2015;56:1698-1703.

13. Ohanian M, Faderl S, Ravandi F, et al. Is acute myeloid leukemia a liquid tumor? Int J Cancer 2013;133:534-543.

14. Palomino-Portilla EA, Valbuena JR, Quinones-Avila MP, Medeiros LJ. Myeloid sarcoma of appendix mimicking acute appendicitis. Arch Pathol Lab Med 2005;129:1027-1031.

14a. Pastoret C, Houot R, Llamas-Gutierrez F, et al. Detection of clonal heterogeneity and targetable mutations in myeloid sarcoma by high-throughput sequencing. Leuk Lymphoma 2017;58:1008-1012.

15. Pileri SA, Ascani S, Cox MC, et al. Myeloid sarcoma: clinico-pathologic, phenotypic and cytogenetic analysis of 92 adult patients. Leukemia 2007;21:340-350.

16. Pileri SA, Orazi A, Falini B. Myeloid sarcoma. In: Swerdlow SH, Campo E, Harris NL, et al., eds. WHO classification of tumours of hematopoietic and lymphoid tissues. Lyon: IARC Press, 2008;140-141.

17. Roth MJ, Medeiros LJ, Elenitoba-Johnson K, Kuchnio M, Jaffe ES, Stetler-Stevenson M. Extramedullary myeloid cell tumors. An immunohistochemical study of 29 cases using routinely fixed and processed paraffin-embedded tissue sections. Arch Pathol Lab Med 1995;119:790-798.

18. Tsimberidou AM, Kantarjian HM, Wen S, et al. Myeloid sarcoma is associated with superior event-free survival and overall survival compared with acute myeloid leukemia. Cancer 2008;113:1370-1378.

19. Valbuena JR, Admirand JH, Lin P, Medeiros LJ. Myeloid sarcoma involving the testis. Am J Clin Pathol 2005;124:445-452.

20. Valbuena JR, Medeiros LJ, Rassidakis GZ, et al. Expression of B cell-specific activator protein/PAX5 in acute myeloid leukemia with t(8;21)(q22;q22). Am J Clin Pathol 2006;126:235-240.

21. Wilson CS, Medeiros LJ. Extramedullary manifestations of myeloid neoplasms. Am J Clin Pathol 2015;144:219-239.

22. Wu X, Sulavik D, Roulston D, Lim MS. Spontaneous remission of congenital acute myeloid leukemia with t(8;16)(p11;13). Pediatr Blood Cancer 2011;56:331-332.

23. Yoshihara S, Ando T, Ogawa H. Extramedullary relapse of acute myeloid leukemia after allogeneic hematopoietic stem cell transplantation: an easily overlooked but significant pattern of relapse. Biol Blood Marrow Transplant 2012;18:1800-1807.

24. Zhou J, Bell D, Medeiros LJ. Myeloid sarcoma of the head and neck region. Arch Pathol Lab Med 2013;137:1560-1568.

52 HISTIOCYTIC SARCOMA

GENERAL FEATURES

Histiocytic sarcoma is a malignant neoplasm with histopathologic, immunophenotypic, and genetic features most consistent with an origin from histiocytes. Acute myeloid leukemia with monocytic differentiation involving an extramedullary site (monoblastic sarcoma) is excluded from this category (11).

Histiocytes are tissue-based cells with phagocytic activity and they also secrete cytokines involved in the inflammatory response. Histiocytes are of myeloid lineage and are derived from bone marrow precursors that mature and enter the bloodstream as monocytes. Monocytes become histiocytes when they exit the blood and reside in tissues. Histiocytes can proliferate in tissues in response to various stimuli.

Our understanding of histiocytic sarcoma has substantially improved over the past 50 years. A number of terms were used for neoplasms thought to be histiocytic tumors in the past that, in retrospect, were not histiocytic sarcoma. For example, the term histiocytic medullary reticulocytosis proposed in 1939 by Scott and Robb-Smith (23) most likely included various tumors, including lymphomas as well as hemophagocytic lymphohistiocytosis (HLH). The term malignant histiocytosis is another older term that included histiocytic tumors, lymphomas, and HLH (2). The designation diffuse histiocytic lymphoma as used by Henry Rappaport in his classification was also incorrectly applied to various types of lymphoma, most often diffuse large B-cell lymphoma (21). This realization lead to the term *true histiocytic lymphoma* being used to distinguish tumors actually thought to be of histiocytic lineage from the much more common lymphomas once designated inappropriately. With the discovery of dendritic cells by Steinman and Cohn (24) and subsequent decades of research by Ralph Steinman and many others (reviewed by Merad et al. in reference 17),

histiocytes were further specified into phagocytic cells and different types of dendritic cells from which malignant neoplasms may arise.

In the World Health Organization (WHO) classification, the term histiocytic sarcoma is used for tumors thought to be derived from histiocytes/macrophages (11,25a). This term was first proposed by Mathe in 1970, but at that time also included a heterogeneous group of tumors (16). This term was reinvigorated in the third edition of the WHO classification, and in the fourth edition and recent revision, histiocytic sarcoma is defined as above. Histiocytic sarcoma is a rare tumor that represents less than 1 percent of all nodal hematolymphoid neoplasms (11).

For the purpose of this chapter, histiocytic sarcoma is divided into three subtypes. The first group is sporadic or de novo histiocytic sarcoma. There is a second, rare subset of cases of histiocytic sarcoma that arise in patients with a history of mediastinal germ cell tumors, often containing teratoma and more specifically yolk sac tumor (6,13). The histiocytic sarcoma and germ cell tumor often share a common chromosomal abnormality, isochromosome 12p, and these tumors may arise from a pluripotential stem cell (6). The third group of histiocytic sarcomas is thought to arise by transdifferentiation from a B-cell lymphoma. As reviewed by Stoecker and Wang (25), the term transdifferentiation implies that a mature neoplastic B cell can become a neoplastic histiocyte (or dendritic cell) as a result of genetic or epigenetic changes. This differs from de-differentiation or origin from a shared progenitor cell (although these possibilities are not completely excluded). Most of this chapter is focused on sporadic histiocytic sarcoma, and the other two subtypes are mentioned where appropriate.

CLINICAL FEATURES

Histiocytic sarcoma most often affects adults in the sixth decade of life, but there is a wide age range from early childhood to the elderly

813

(5,12,14,19,26). There is no evidence of a marked sex preference for this disease. About 40 to 50 percent of patients present with stage I/II disease (10,26). Histiocytic sarcoma has been reported in association with Langerhans cell sarcoma; lineage plasticity may be involved in explaining this occurrence. Histicytic sarcoma also has been reported in association with acute myeloid leukemia or myelodysplasia; in these patients monocytic sarcoma needs to be rigorously excluded and designation as monocytic sarcoma may have been more appropriate (30).

Patients may present with a nodal or extranodal mass and systemic symptoms, in particular, fever and weight loss (5,12,14,19,26). The cervical and axillary lymph nodes are the common nodal regions involved; the most common extranodal sites include the gastrointestinal tract, skin, and soft tissue (14,19,26). Disease involving the intestines may present initially as obstruction. Cutaneous manifestations are highly varied and include innocuous-appearing rashes, isolated nodular cutaneous lesions, or multiple skin nodules.

Staging studies often show advanced stage disease involving liver, spleen, and lymph nodes. Lytic bone lesions can occur. Infrequently, patients present with disseminated disease at diagnosis, imparting a "malignant histiocytosis" type clinical picture (2,19). Rare cases of histiocytic sarcoma apparently can arise in the central nervous system (4,11,29). Rare cases have developed following radiation therapy (29).

HISTOLOGIC FINDINGS

The morphologic features of histiocytic sarcoma, either sporadic or the uncommon tumors associated with germ cell tumors or transdifferentiation from B-cell lymphomas, are similar. Histiocytic sarcoma is characterized by a diffuse growth pattern that usually effaces the architecture of the lymph node or extranodal site (figs. 52-1, 52-2) (5,12,14,19,26). In the lymph nodes as well as the liver and spleen, the neoplasm can preferentially involve sinuses or have a perisinusoidal distribution.

The tumor cells are monomorphic or pleomorphic. They are often large and round or polygonal, with abundant eosinophilic cytoplasm (figs. 52-1B, 52-2B). Tumor cell nuclei may be eccentrically or centrally located, with vesicular chromatin, thin nuclear membranes that may be folded, and a prominent single nucleolus (figs. 52-3, 52-4). A subset of cases exhibits marked nuclear atypia with hyperchromasia (19,26). In these cases the mitotic rate is variable and often high and foci of necrosis may be present (fig. 52-5). Hemophagocytosis is present in some neoplastic cells, but is rarely prominent (19,26). The tumor cell cytoplasm may contain fine vacuoles.

Multinucleated tumor cells, and in some cases, osteoclast-like giant cells (fig. 52-2B), may be observed scattered throughout the neoplasm. Uncommonly, the neoplastic cells have a spindle shape, but these spindled areas usually represent only a minor portion of the entire tumor (5,14,19). A reactive cell infiltrate is common within histiocytic sarcoma, most often composed of small lymphocytes and benign histiocytes, and less often, plasma cells, eosinophils (fig. 52-4), or neutrophils. Histiocytic sarcoma rich in background neutrophils has been observed in the central nervous system (4).

CYTOLOGIC FINDINGS

Fine-needle aspiration smears typically show a dispersed population of large neoplastic cells, but a few loosely cohesive clusters may be present (fig. 52-6). The tumor cells can be admixed with variable numbers of small lymphocytes, benign histiocytes, or other inflammatory cells (18). Otherwise, the features in smears resemble those in tissue sections as described above.

ULTRASTRUCTURAL AND IMMUNOPHENOTYPIC FINDINGS

Electron microscopy shows cells with abundant cytoplasm and numerous lysosomes (11,26). The cells lack Birbeck granules, desmosomes, or other types of cell junctions.

Immunohistochemistry is the primary method for establishing histiocytic lineage. Using fixed, paraffin-embedded tissue sections, the antibodies most often positive in cases of histiocytic sarcoma are CD68 (granular cytoplasmic pattern) (fig. 52-7A), CD163 (membranous and cytoplasmic) (fig. 52-5C), and lysozyme (granular and characteristically accentuated in the Golgi region) (fig. 52-7B) (11,19,26). Other antigens commonly expressed include CD4 (fig. 52-7C), CD11c, CD45/LCA (fig. 52-7D), CD45RO, and alpha-1 antitrypsin. CD123 may be positive.

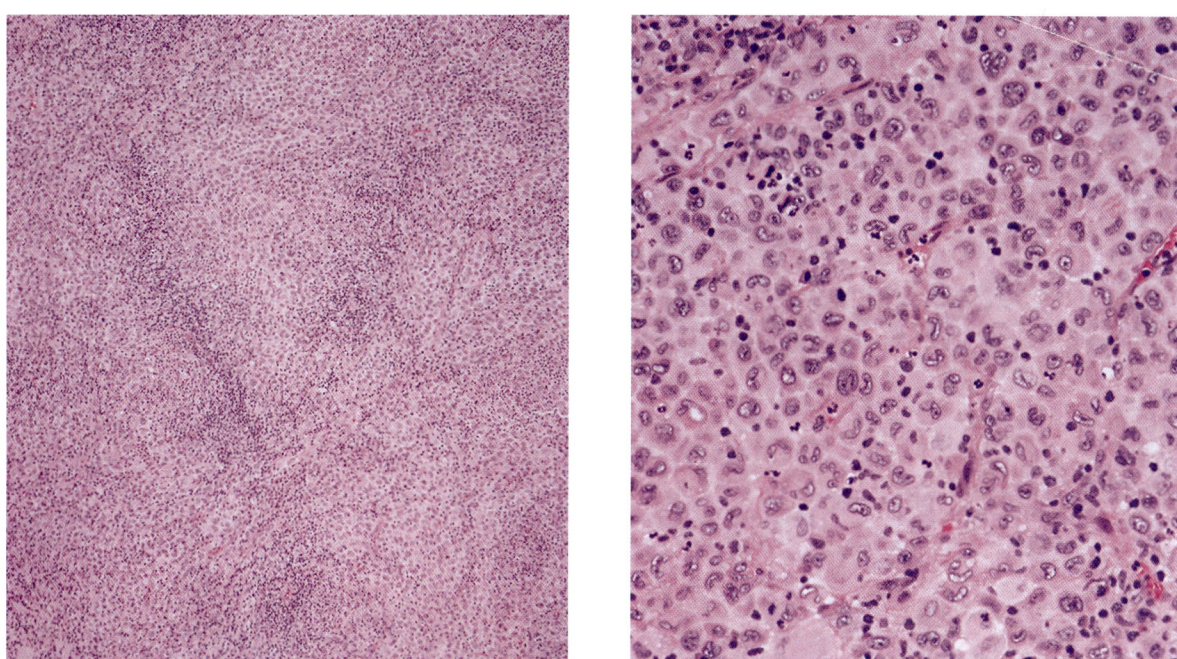

Figure 52-1

HISTIOCYTIC SARCOMA INVOLVING CERVICAL LYMPH NODE

Left: The architecture is almost completely replaced by tumor with a vaguely nodular and diffuse pattern. Small lymphocytes are present in the background (hematoxylin and eosin [H&E] stain).

Right: High magnification shows cells with abundant eosinophilic cytoplasm and folded nuclei, and thin nuclear membranes.

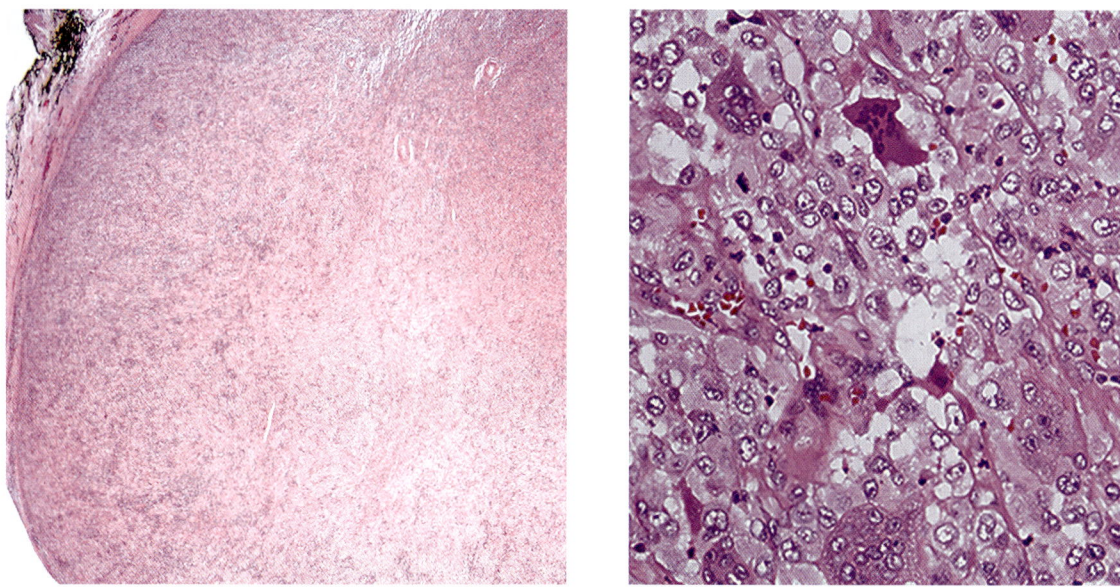

Figure 52-2

HISTIOCYTIC SARCOMA INVOLVING INTRAPAROTID LYMPH NODE

Left: The neoplasm diffusely replaces the lymph node.
Right: Osteoclast-like giant cells are present (left, right: H&E stain).

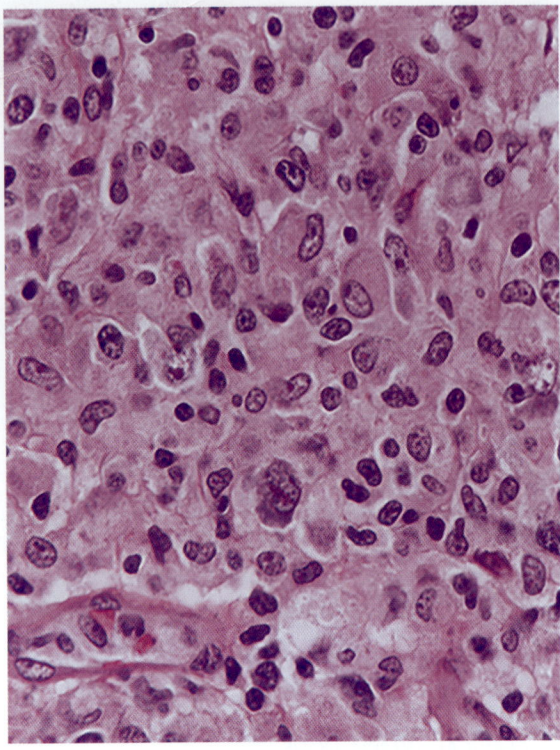

Figure 52-3

**HISTIOCYTIC SARCOMA INVOLVING
INGUINAL LYMPH NODE**

Magnification using oil immersion shows neoplastic cells
with eccentrically located nuclei and abundant eosinophilic
cytoplasm (H&E stain).

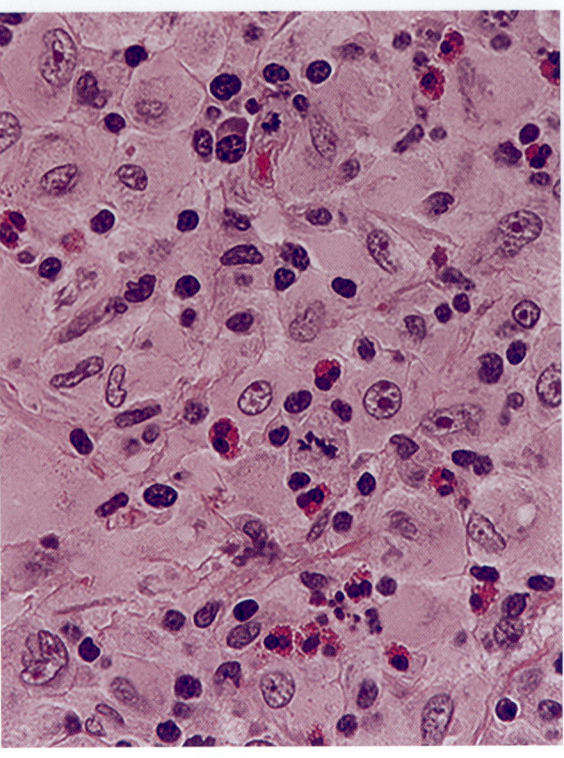

Figure 52-4

**HISTIOCYTIC SARCOMA INVOLVING
CERVICAL LYMPH NODE**

Magnification using oil immersion shows large cells
with abundant plate-like cytoplasm, central nuclei, and
distinct nucleoli. Two mitotic figures are present in this
field. Many eosinophils and one plasma cell are shown in
the background (H&E stain).

Although not widely used, antibodies reactive with T-cell immunoglobulin mucin (TIM)
proteins appear to be helpful for diagnosis
since all cases of histiocytic sarcoma assessed
in one study were strongly positive for TIM-3
and TIM-4 (7). These TIM proteins are normally
expressed on the surface of T cells and are involved in regulating T-cell activation, tolerance,
and phagocytosis of apoptotic cells.

In one small study, 75 percent of cases of
histiocytic sarcoma were positive for platelet-de-
rived growth factor receptor-beta and vascular
endothelial growth factor, and half were positive for epidermal growth factor receptor, suggesting potential targets for therapy (22). The
proliferation (Ki-67) index in cases of histiocytic
sarcoma is highly variable, ranging from 10 to
90 percent (11,19,26).

Other antigens positive in some histiocytic
sarcomas include CD31, CD56 (rare cases), p53

(small subset of cells), CNA.42 (very rare), and
S-100 protein (usually variable) (fig. 52-5D)
(19,26). CD1a and langerin have been reported
in a small subset of cases. Staining is usually
weak and focal, and if both markers are positive, Langerhans cell lineage must be excluded.
Some cases are reported to be positive for B-cell
transcription factors, most often OCT2 or BCL6
but rarely PAX5 (3).

Histiocytic sarcomas are negative for pan-
B-cell (CD19, CD20, CD22, CD79a) and pan-
T-cell (CD2, CD3, CD5, CD7, T-cell receptors)
antigens. In addition, tumor cells are negative
for the follicular dendritic cell-associated markers (CD21, CD23, CD35), CD13, CD30, CD33,
CD34, myeloperoxidase, TCL1, and cyclin D1
(14,19,26). There is no evidence of Epstein-Barr
virus (EBV) infection.

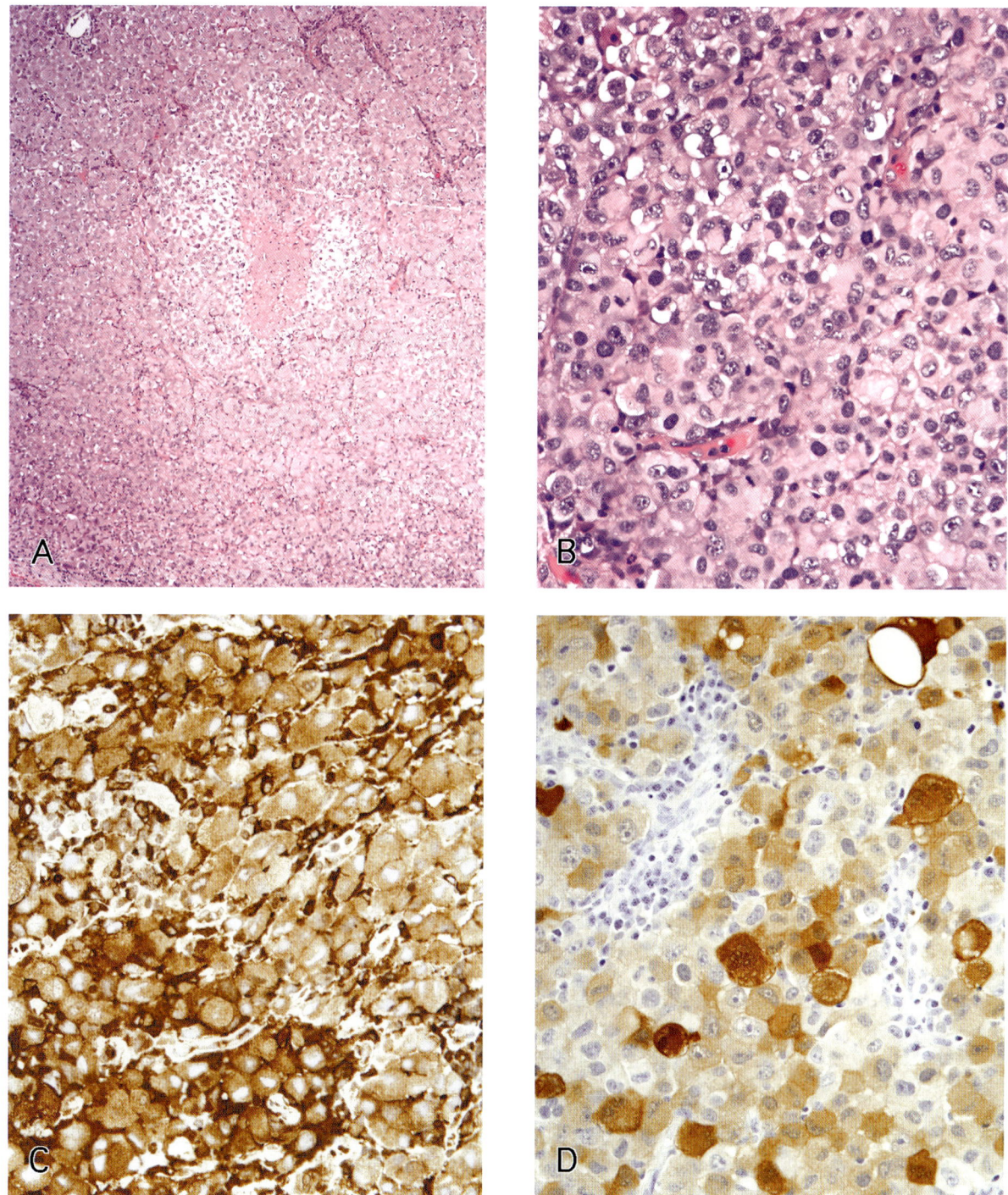

Figure 52-5

HISTIOCYTIC SARCOMA INVOLVING CERVICAL LYMPH NODE

A: In this low-power image, an area of coagulative necrosis is shown (A,B: H&E stain).

B: At high-power (400x) magnification, the cells show nuclear atypia and mitotic figures are identified.

C,D: The cells are strongly positive for CD163 (C) and CD68 (not shown) and variably positive for S-100 protein (D). Based on the S-100 protein reactivity, the possibility of interdigitating dendritic cell sarcoma was entertained but the overall immunophenotype was thought to be more akin to histiocytes (C,D: immunohistochemistry with hematoxylin counterstain).

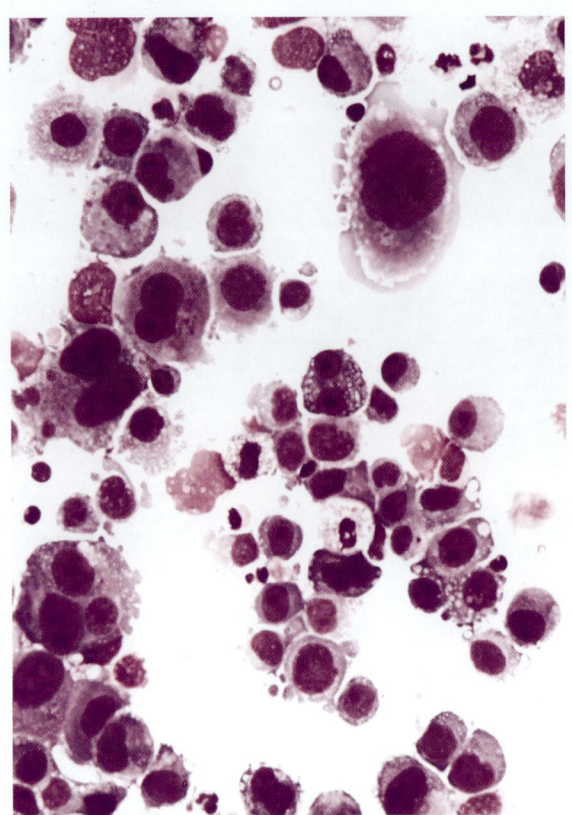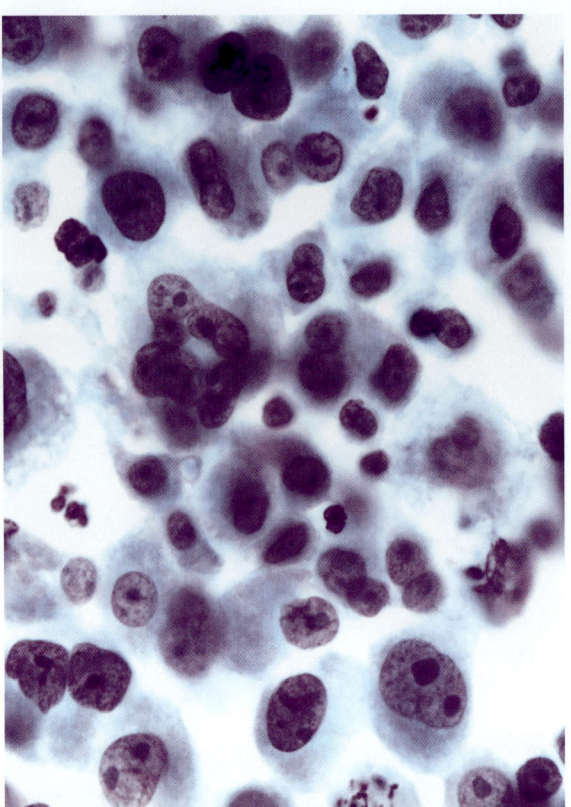

Figure 52-6

HISTIOCYTIC SARCOMA: CYTOLOGIC FINDINGS

A fine-needle aspirate smear shows large and pleomorphic neoplastic cells with prominent nucleoli (left: Diff-Quik stain; right: Papanicolaou stain).

Histiocytic sarcoma can be assessed by flow cytometry immunophenotypic analysis although there are few cases reported. Flow cytometry allows for the use of a larger number of myeloid and histiocyte antibodies. Wang et al. (28) reported a case of histiocytic sarcoma assessed by flow cytometry in which the neoplastic cells were positive for CD11c, CD14, CD45, CD68, CD123, and HLA-DR.

MOLECULAR GENETIC FINDINGS

Little conventional cytogenetic data are available for cases of sporadic histiocytic sarcoma and no characteristic cytogenetic alterations have been identified. Alonso-Dominguez et al. (1) reported a case with a complex karyotype characterized by trisomy 8 and other abnormalities. As this neoplasm involved blood and bone marrow, it may have been an example of acute monoblastic leukemia. The *IGH-BCL2* fusion

has been shown by polymerase chain reaction (PCR) and fluorescence in situ hybridization (FISH) in rare sporadic cases (3).

Using Southern blot analysis, most cases of sporadic histiocytic sarcoma do not carry monoclonal *IGH* or T-cell receptor gene rearrangements. Using more sensitive PCR-based methods, however, monoclonal *IGH* and less often *TRB* or *TRG* rearrangements have been shown in a subset of cases (3,26). *BRAF* mutation was reported in 5 of 8 (62.5 percent) cases of histiocytic sarcoma by Go et al. (9).

Transdifferentiation. Some patients with B-cell lymphoma subsequently (or simultaneously) develop histiocytic sarcoma, and less often, interdigitating dendritic cell sarcoma or Langerhans cell sarcoma (25,26). Follicular lymphoma (fig. 52-8) is the most common B-cell neoplasm, but chronic lymphocytic leukemia/small lymphocytic lymphoma, diffuse large

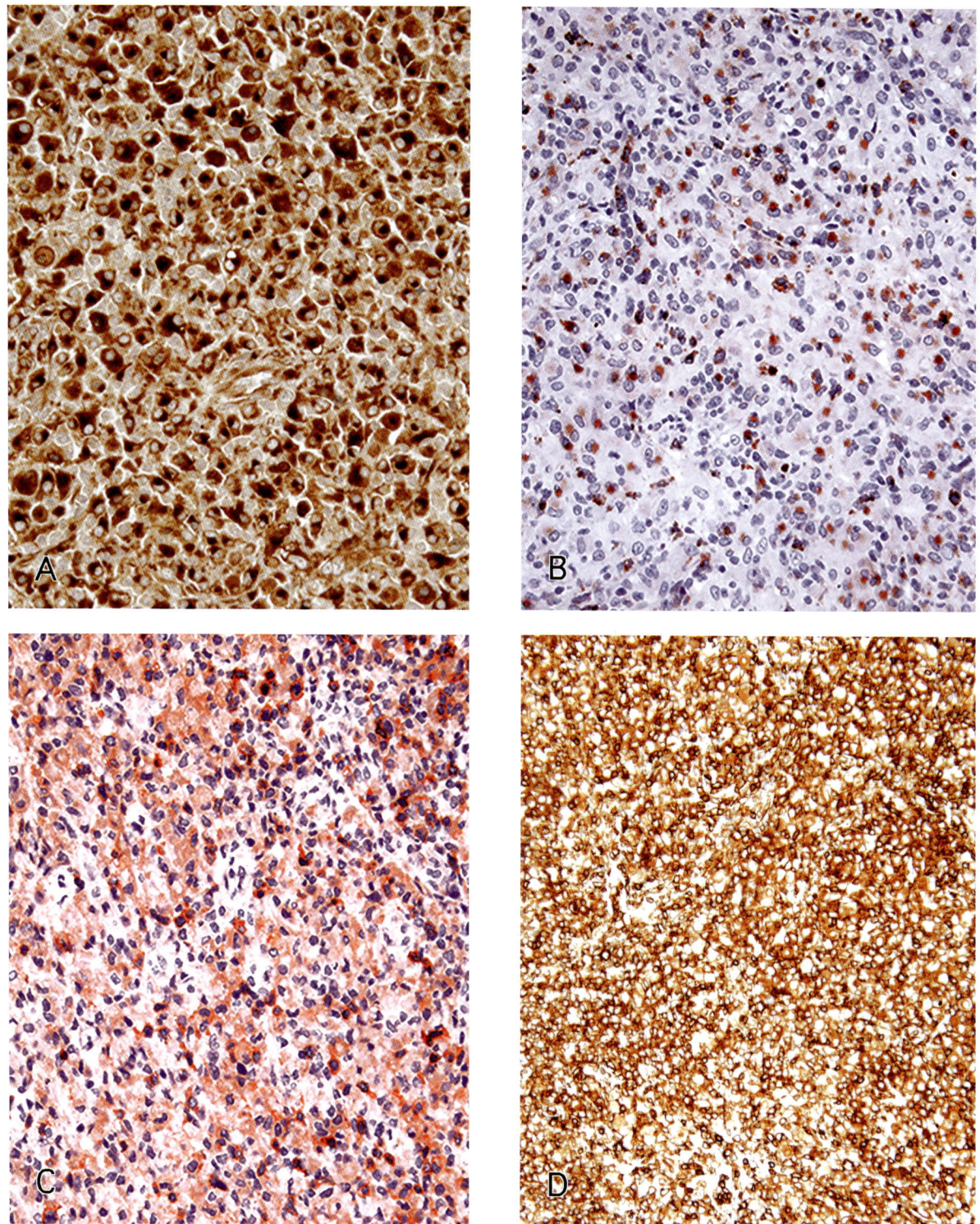

Figure 52-7

HISTIOCYTIC SARCOMA: IMMUNOHISTOCHEMISTRY

These immunohistochemical results correspond to the case of histiocytic sarcoma shown in figure 52-3. A, CD68; B, lysozyme; C, CD4; D. CD45/LCA (immunohistochemistry with hematoxylin counterstain)

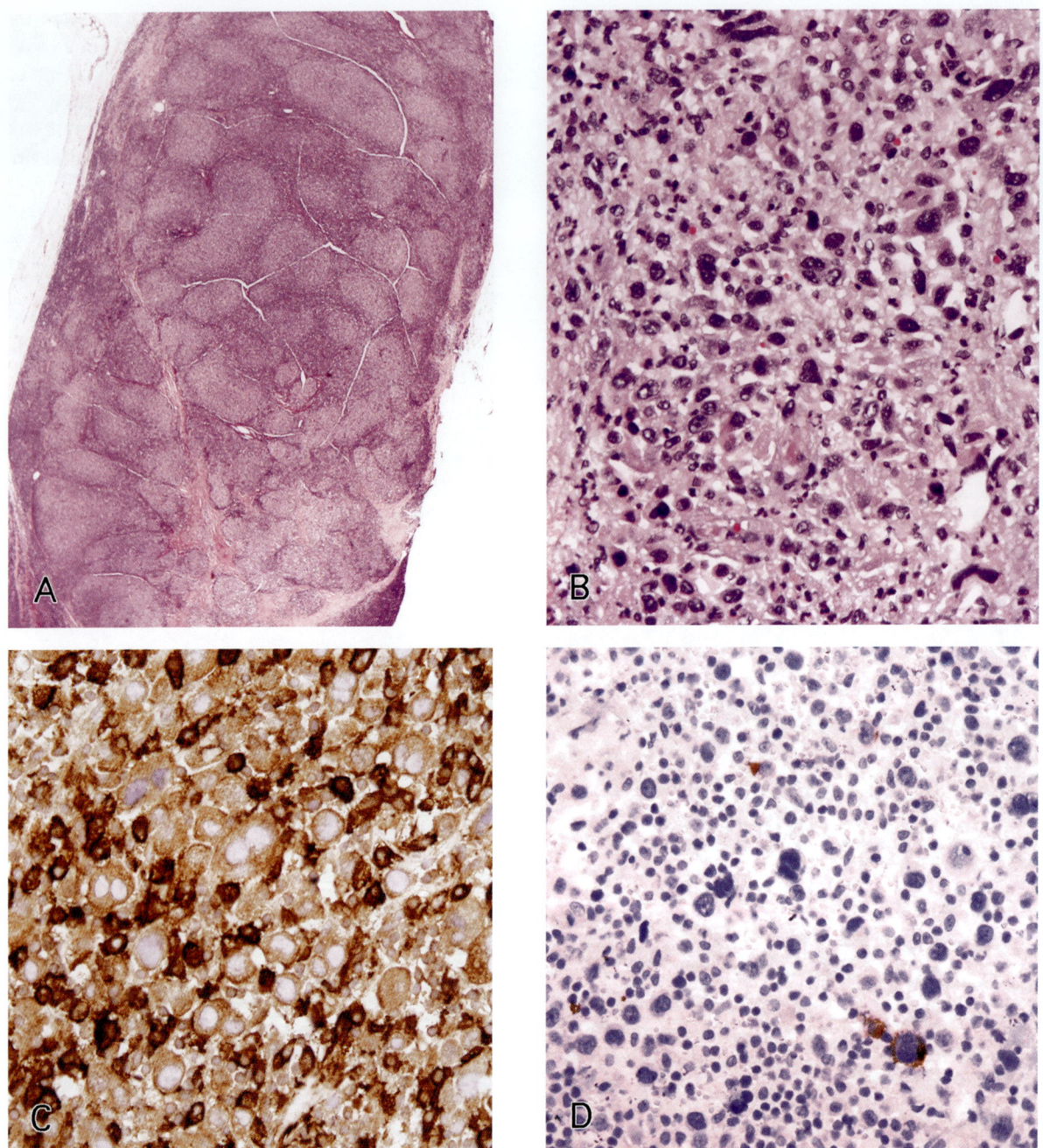

Figure 52-8

TRANSDIFFERENTIATION

A 49-year-old man presented initially with follicular lymphoma in an inguinal lymph node and subsequently developed a pelvic mass involved by histiocytic sarcoma 5 months later.

A: Follicular lymphoma (A,B: H&E stain).

B: Histiocytic sarcoma.

C: The cells of the histiocytic sarcoma are strongly positive for CD163 (C) and other histiocyte-associated antigens (not shown).

D: Some cells in the histiocytic sarcoma are weakly positive for CD20 (D) and PAX5 (not shown). Fluorescence in situ hybridization for *IGH-BCL2* was positive in both the follicular lymphoma and histiocytic sarcoma (not shown) (C,D: immunohistochemistry with hematoxylin counterstain).

B-cell lymphoma, marginal zone lymphomas, and acute lymphoblastic leukemia are also reported. Histiocytic sarcoma and lymphoma may occur simultaneously or histiocytic sarcoma can follow lymphoma with a time interval ranging from 2 months to 17 years (25,26).

Histologically, histiocytic sarcoma arising in the context of a B-cell lymphoma/leukemia (transdifferentiation) closely resembles de novo tumors. At the immunophenotypic and genetic level, however, these tumors are distinctive (25,26). Cases of histiocytic sarcoma that arise via transdifferentiation more often express the B-cell transcription factor OCT2 (less often PAX5) and they have a higher frequency of monoclonal immunoglobulin gene rearrangements or *IGH-BCL2* fusion consistent with t(14;18). In addition, in cases of transdifferentiation, the B-cell lymphoma and histiocytic sarcoma share clonal identity (8,26). Analysis of the *IGH* variable regions in cases of histiocytic sarcoma has shown somatic hypermutation, supporting the idea that the histiocytic sarcoma arose from a follicle center or post-follicle center B cell. This finding argues against a common precursor cell of origin for the B-cell lymphoma and histiocytic sarcoma and supports the concept of transdifferentiation.

From the point of view of the diagnostic workup, it may be beneficial to assess all cases of histiocytic sarcoma for *IGH* rearrangements. The presence of a monoclonal B-cell population does not alter the diagnosis, but its presence raises the possibility of a transdifferentiation event. Likewise, the presence of *IGH/BCL2* is highly unusual in histiocytic sarcoma and may suggest a diagnosis of prior or concurrent follicular lymphoma (8,25,26). Knowledge of transdifferentiation has prognostic importance because the prognosis of patients with histiocytic sarcomas that arise as a result of transdifferentiation is poor, with a median survival period of less than 1 year.

DIFFERENTIAL DIAGNOSIS

Acute Monocytic Leukemia/Monoblastic Sarcoma. In a tissue biopsy specimen, it can be extremely challenging to distinguish histiocytic sarcoma from an extramedullary presentation of acute monocytic leukemia. Blood and bone marrow involvement by blasts supports the diag-

nosis of acute monocytic leukemia. A history of myelodysplastic syndrome or myeloproliferative neoplasm also favors acute monocytic leukemia. Strong immunoreactivity for myeloperoxidase or other immunohistochemical evidence of granulocytic maturation, CD34 expression, and molecular evidence of translocations or mutations associated with acute monocytic leukemia are helpful in this distinction. Nonetheless, we have observed rare patients with an extramedullary mass thought to be histiocytic sarcoma who developed acute monocytic leukemia subsequently within a few months to a year.

Dendritic Cell Sarcomas. Distinguishing histiocytic sarcoma from other dendritic cell sarcomas is based on the immunohistochemical profile and ultrastructural findings (when needed). These differential diagnoses are discussed in more detail in the chapters on follicular dendritic cell and interdigitating dendritic cell sarcomas.

Various Types of Lymphoma. Anaplastic large cell lymphoma (ALCL) is usually composed of large cells with abundant cytoplasm and may resemble histiocytic sarcoma. Like histiocytic sarcoma, ALCL may exhibit a sinusoidal pattern of growth. In ALCL, however, the sinusoidal pattern can be predominant or very prominent and the cells are more anaplastic, with hallmark cells, unlike histiocytic sarcoma. This differential diagnosis is resolved by immunohistochemical analysis. Cases of ALCL are uniformly and brightly positive for CD30 in a membranous and paranuclear (target-like) pattern and many cases of ALCL express ALK and carry translocations involving the *ALK*/2p23 locus.

Hepatosplenic T-cell lymphoma is a rare type of lymphoma, more common in younger men, in which the neoplastic cells fill the sinuses of the liver, spleen, and bone marrow. Most likely, these neoplasms were included in the older category of diseases designated as malignant histiocytosis along with other entities. The cells of hepatosplenic T-cell lymphoma are of T-cell lineage, often positive for TCRγ/δ and characteristically negative for CD4, CD5, and CD8. These cells lack histiocyte-specific markers.

Histiocytic sarcoma often has a diffuse pattern that replaces the normal architecture; this, along with the large cell size, puts diffuse large B-cell lymphoma in the differential diagnosis. Immunohistochemical analysis resolves this issue since most cases of diffuse large B-cell lymphoma express pan-B-cell markers and are negative for lysozyme and CD163.

Metastatic Melanoma. Melanomas diffusely replace normal tissues and are composed of large polygonal cells with abundant cytoplasm that can resemble, at least in part, histiocytic sarcoma. This is particularly true for apigmented melanoma or cases in which melanoma cells show hemophagocytosis. Immunohistochemistry is valuable for sorting out these two neoplasms. Unlike histiocytic sarcoma, malignant melanoma is positive for a variety of melanoma-associated antigens and is negative for CD4, CD11c, CD45/LCA, and CD163. Nevertheless, melanoma can be positive for CD68, attributable to the high lysosomal content of the melanoma cells, and cases of histiocytic sarcoma can express S-100 protein, although usually focal.

Hemophagocytic Lymphohistiocytosis. This term is used for a spectrum of benign diseases in which there is hyperactivation of tissue macrophages as a result of defects in granule-mediated cytotoxicity of T and NK cells (15,20). Although hemophagocytosis is a characteristic morphologic finding of HLH, hemophagocytosis per se is neither sensitive nor specific for the diagnosis of HLH.

HLH can be divided into two forms, primary (hereditary) and secondary (15,20). Primary cases are caused by mutations in *perforin, FAS*, or other genes involved in granule-mediated cytotoxicity of T and NK cells. Primary HLH usually manifests in childhood; secondary HLH is triggered by a malignant neoplasm or an infectious agent in a patient iatrogenically immunosuppressed from chemotherapy. These latter scenarios are designated as malignancy-triggered HLH or HLH during chemotherapy. Patients with secondary HLH are usually adults. The most common tumors associated with HLH are lymphomas; T/NK-cell lymphomas are most frequent followed by diffuse large B-cell lymphoma (fig. 52-9). Other tumors less often associated with HLH include Hodgkin lymphoma, acute leukemias, and uncommonly, solid tumors (less than 5 percent). The most common infectious agent associated with secondary HLH is Epstein-Barr virus; other agents include cytomegalovirus, bacterial infections, and fungal or parasite infections. The net result of HLH, whether primary or secondary, is uncontrolled activation of tissue macrophages with hypersecretion of many proinflammatory cytokines (cytokine storm).

Unlike histiocytic sarcoma, patients with HLH often present with acute disease characterized by fever, splenomegaly, cytopenias, decreased fibrinogen, and elevated serum levels of ferritin (usually pronounced), triglycerides, and serum CD25/IL-2α (20,28a). The pace of the disease can be very fast and therapy needs to be introduced quickly, usually a combination of steroids and etoposide (20). Even if therapy is rapid and appropriate the prognosis is poor with a high mortality rate (20,28a).

Morphologically, the histiocytes in lymph nodes, liver, spleen, and bone marrow of patients with HLH do not form a mass nor do they show cytologic atypia, unlike histiocytic sarcoma. Hemophagocytosis, characterized by the presence of erythrocytes or other blood cells within a histiocyte cytoplasm, may be minimal, even in patients with florid HLH (13). Furthermore, the presence of hemophagocytosis is not specific for HLH and can occur in other benign and malignant conditions, including histiocytic sarcoma.

Rosai-Dorfman Disease. Rosai-Dorfman disease is characterized by large histiocytes with round nuclei, pinpoint nucleoli, and abundant plate-like cytoplasm that usually show abundant emperipolesis in lymph nodes, but much less so at extranodal sites. In lymph nodes, the sinuses are expanded by the characteristic histiocytes and are associated with plasmacytosis. Reactive follicular hyperplasia is often prominent between dilated sinuses. Importantly, the overall lymph node architecture is usually preserved in Rosai-Dorfman disease, unlike histiocytic sarcoma in which the architecture is partially to completely effaced.

TREATMENT AND PROGNOSIS:

Patients who develop histiocytic sarcoma usually have an aggressive clinical course. Low-stage disease has been correlated with better prognosis in some studies. However, Gounder et al. (10) reported that stage did not correlate with overall survival. Therefore, the role of complete surgical excision for histiocytic sarcoma is not well established (unlike for dendritic

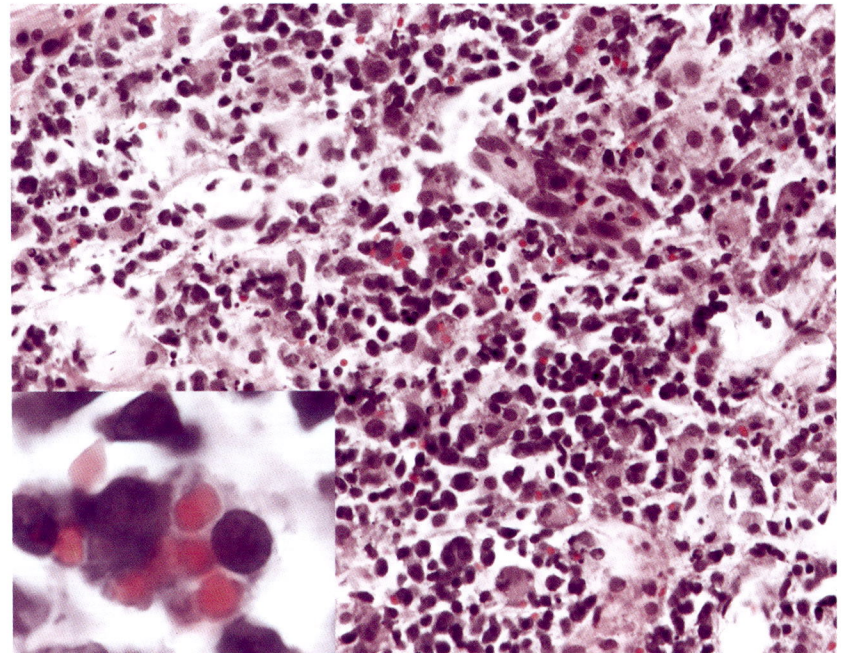

Figure 52-9

LYMPHOMA AND SECONDARY HEMOPHAGOCYTIC LYMPHOHISTIOCYTOSIS (HLH)

This man presented with full-blown HLH and a rapidly growing skin lesion that was biopsied and shown to be primary cutaneous γ/δ T-cell lymphoma. Morphologic evidence of hemophagocytosis is present intermixed with lymphoma cells (H&E stain). The inset shows histiocytes ingesting erythrocytes.

cell sarcomas). Patients have been treated with various regimens, mostly those designed for aggressive lymphomas (e.g., CHOP), but patients often die of disease within a year of diagnosis (11,26). There may be a role for high-dose chemotherapy and autologous stem cell transplantation (27). Patients with histiocytic sarcoma involving the brain appear to have an especially poor prognosis (4,29).

REFERENCES

1. Alonso-Dominguez JM, Calbacho M, Talavera M, et al. Cytogenetics findings in a histiocytic sarcoma case. Case Rep Hematol 2012;2012:428279.
2. Cattoretti G, Villa A, Vezzoni P, Giardini R, Lombardi L, Rilke F. Malignant histiocytosis. A phenotypic and genotypic investigation. Am J Pathol 1990;136:1009-1019.
3. Chen W, Lau SK, Fong D, et al. High frequency of clonal immunoglobulin receptor gene rearrangements in sporadic histiocytic/dendritic cell sarcomas. Am J Surg Pathol 2009;33:863-873.
4. Cheuk W, Walford N, Lou J, et al. Primary histiocytic lymphoma of the central nervous system: a neoplasm frequently overshadowed by a prominent inflammatory component. Am J Surg Pathol 2001;25:1372-1379.
5. Copie-Bergman C, Wotherspoon AC, Norton AJ, Diss TC, Isaacson PG. True histiocytic lymphoma: a morphologic, immunohistochemical, and molecular genetic study of 13 cases. Am J Surg Pathol 1998;22:1386-1392.
6. deMent SH. Association between mediastinal germ cell tumors and hematologic malignancies: an update. Hum Pathol 1990;21:699-703.
7. Dorfman DM, Hornick JL, Shahsafaei A, Freeman GJ. The phosphatidylserine receptors, T cell immunoglobulin mucin proteins 3 and 4, are markers of histiocytic sarcoma and other histiocytic and dendrtic cell neoplasms. Hum Pathol 2010;41:1486-1494.
8. Feldman AL, Minniti C, Santi M, Downing JR, Raffeld M, Jaffe ES. Histiocytic sarcoma after acute lymphoblastic leukaemia: a common clonal origin. Lancet Oncol 2004;5:248-250.
9. Go H, Jeon YK, Huh J, et al. Frequent detection of BRAF (V600E) mutations in histiocytic and dendritic cell neoplasms. Histopathology 2014;65:261-272.

10. Gounder M, Desai V, Kuk D, et al. Impact of surgery, radiation and systemic therapy on the outcomes of patients with dendritic cell and histiocytic sarcomas. Eur J Cancer 2015;51:2413-2422.

11. Grogan TM, Pileri SA, Chan JK, Weiss LM, Fletcher CD. Histiocytic sarcoma. In: Swerdlow SH, Campo E, Harris NL, et al., eds. WHO classification of tumours of haematopoietic and lymphoid tissues. Lyon: IARC Press; 2008:356-357.

12. Hanson CA, Jaszcz W, Kersey JH, et al. True histiocytic lymphoma: histopathologic, immunophenotypic and genotypic analysis. Br J Haematol 1989;73:187-198.

13. Hartmann JT, Nichols CR, Droz JP, et al. Hematologic disorders associated with primary mediastinal nonseminomatous germ cell tumors. J Natl Cancer Inst 2000;92:54-61.

14. Hornick JL, Jaffe ES, Fletcher CD. Extranodal histiocytic sarcoma: clinicopathologic analysis of 14 cases of a rare epithelioid malignancy. Am J Surg Pathol 2004;28:1133-1144.

15. Lehmberg K, Nichols KE, Henter JI, et al. Consensus recommendations for the diagnosis and management of hemophagocytic lymphohistiocytosis associated with malignancies. Haematologica 2015;100:997-1004.

16. Mathé G, Gerard-Marchant R, Texier JL, Schlumberger JR, Berumen L, Paintrand M. The two varieties of lymphoid tissue "reticulosarcomas" histiocytic and histioblastic types. Br J Cancer 1970;24:687–695.

17. Merad M, Sathe P, Helft J, Miller J, Mortha A. The dendritic cell lineage: ontogeny and function of dendritic cells and their subsets in the steady state and the inflamed setting. Annu Rev Immunol 2013;31:563-604.

18. Miliaukas JR. Fine-needle aspiration cytology: true histiocytic lymphoma/histiocytic sarcoma. Diagn Cytopathol 2003;29:233-235.

19. Pileri SA, Grogan TM, Harris NL, et al. Tumours of histiocytes and accessory dendritic cells: an immunohistochemical approach to classification from the International Lymphoma Study Group based on 61 cases. Histopathology 2002;41:1-29

20. Ramos-Casals M, Brito-Zeron P, Lopez-Guillermo A, Khamashta MA, Bosch X. Adult haemophagocytic syndrome. Lancet 2014;383:1503-1516.

21. Rappaport H. Tumors of the hematopoietic system. Atlas of Tumor Pathology, First Series, Fascicle 8. Armed Forces Institute of Pathology; 1966.

22. Schlick K, Aigelsreiter A, Pichler M, et al. Histiocytic sarcoma-targeted therapy: novel therapeutic options? A series of 4 cases. Onkologie 2012; 35:447-450.

23. Scott RB, Robb-Smith AH. Histiocytic medullary reticulocytosis. Lancet 1939;234:194-198.

24. Steinman RM, Cohn ZA. Identification of a novel cell type in peripheral lymphoid organs of mice. I. Morphology, quantitation, tissue distribution. J Exp Med 1973;137:1142-1162.

25. Stoecker MM, Wang E. Histiocytic/dendritic cell transformation of B-cell neoplasms: pathologic evidence of lineage conversion in differentiated hematolymphoid malignancies. Arch Pathol Lab Med 2013;137:865-870.

25a. Swerdlow SH, Campo E, Pileri SA, et al. The 2016 revision of the World Health Organization classification of lymphoid neoplasms. Blood 2016;127:2375-2390.

26. Takahashi E, Nakamura S. Histiocytic sarcoma: an updated literature review based on the 2008 WHO classification. J Clin Exp Hematop 2013;53:1-8.

27. Tsujimura H, Miyaki T, Yamada S, et al. Successful treatment of histiocytic sarcoma with induction chemotherapy consisting of dose-escalate CHOP plus etoposide and upfront consolidation auto-transplantation. Int J Hematol 2014;100:507-510.

28. Wang H, Zhang J, Tao Q, et al. Flow cytometry used to identify histiocytic sarcoma: a case report. Cytometry B Clin Cytom 2016;90:546-550.

28a. Wang YR, Qiu YN, Bai Y, Wang XF. A retrospective analysis of 56 children with hemophagocytic lymphohistiocytosis. J Blood Med 2016;7:227-231.

29. Wu W, Tanrivermis Sayit A, Vinters HV, Pope W, Mirsadraei L, Said J. Primary central nervous system histiocytic sarcoma presenting as a postradiation sarcoma: case report and literature review. Hum Pathol 2013;44:1177-1183.

30. Zhao J, Niu X, Wang Z, Lu H, Lin X, Lu Q. Histiocytic sarcoma combined with acute monocytic leukemia: a case report. Diagn Pathol 2015;10:110.

53 FOLLICULAR DENDRITIC CELL SARCOMA

GENERAL FEATURES

Follicular dendritic cell (FDC) sarcoma is a spindle-shaped (or less often, epithelioid) tumor with immunophenotypic features suggestive of origin from follicular dendritic cells (FDCs) (3). FDCs normally reside in primary and secondary B-cell follicles within lymph nodes and extranodal sites. Their major function is to trap antigens, in the form of immune complexes on their cell surface, to be presented to B lymphocytes. FDCs are thought to be of mesenchymal origin and, unlike other dendritic cells, do not migrate once situated in follicles.

In lymph node follicles, FDCs are recognized in routinely stained tissue sections as spindle-shaped cells that have abutting, rectangular-shaped nuclei. Immunohistochemical analysis using FDC-associated markers (e.g., CD21) highlights concentric rings of FDCs in follicles, both in germinal centers and mantle zones. Electron microscopic examination shows that FDCs have elongated nuclei, long slender cytoplasmic processes, and well-formed desmosomes with few lysosomes and no Birbeck granules.

Although FDC sarcoma is the most common tumor in the category of histiocytic or dendritic cell tumors, it is nonetheless a rare neoplasm that represents less than 1 percent of all tumors that arise primarily in lymph nodes and less than 0.5 percent of all sarcomas (4,12,17). The diagnosis of FDC sarcoma is often challenging and requires a high index of suspicion. An extensive immunohistochemical workup is often needed to arrive at the correct diagnosis, and tumors metastatic to lymph nodes must be rigorously excluded.

A variant of FDC sarcoma, the *inflammatory pseudotumor-like variant*, is distinctive. These lesions usually occur in the spleen or liver and do not arise in lymph nodes (3). Inflammatory pseudotumor-like FDC sarcoma is often positive for Epstein-Barr virus (EBV), likely has a different pathogenesis from nodal FDC sarcoma, and should be viewed as a separate entity. These lesions are covered in chapter 64 and are not further discussed here.

CLINICAL FEATURES

Most patients who develop FDC sarcoma are adults with a median age in the fifth decade, but there is a wide age range, from childhood to the elderly (2,12,13,17,18). The male to female ratio is approximately equal (3). In a small subset of patients, FDC sarcoma arises within the context of preexisting Castleman disease (14).

Up to two thirds of patients present with painless, slowly enlarging lymph nodes often involving the cervical, axillary, or mediastinal region (2,3,14,17). Patients with disease involving abdominal lymph nodes or other intra-abdominal sites may present with abdominal pain. The tumors also arise at extranodal sites including the nasopharynx, tonsil, mouth, lungs, gastrointestinal tract, pancreas, liver, spleen, skin, and soft tissue (3,17). Most patients have localized disease, but FDC sarcoma may metastasize, most often to lymph nodes, lungs, and liver. Paraneoplastic phenomena occur in a small subset of patients, including pemphigus and myasthenia gravis (9,11,19).

HISTOLOGIC FINDINGS

FDC sarcoma may evolve into a large mass, greater than 5 cm, as a result of its slow and painless growth. Histologic examination of lymph nodes shows replacement of the architecture by a tumor that most often exhibits a spindle cell appearance and a whorl-like, fascicular, or storiform growth pattern (figs. 53-1, 53-2) (2,3,5,14). Some cases have a more sheet-like pattern (fig. 53-3).

The neoplastic cells of FDC sarcoma usually have a spindle shape, with moderate to abundant eosinophilic cytoplasm, and indistinct cell

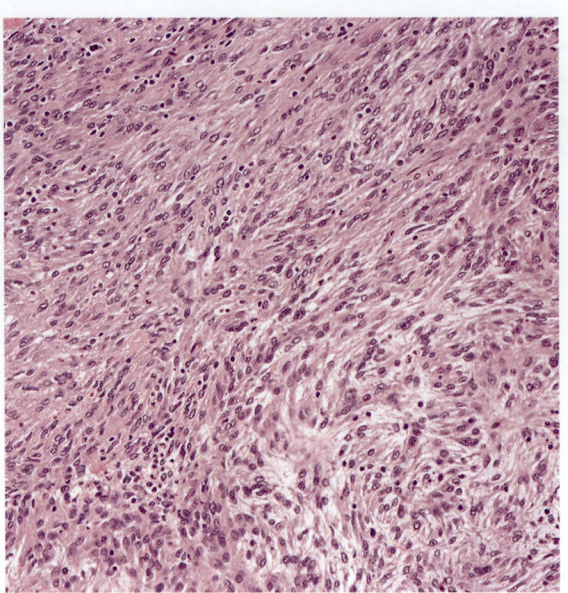
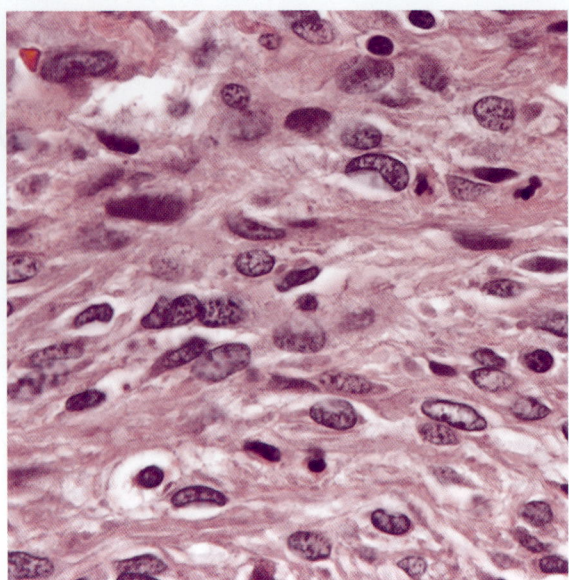

Figure 53-1

FOLLICULAR DENDRITIC CELL SARCOMA REPLACING LYMPH NODE

Left: The neoplastic cells have a spindle shape and are arranged in a storiform pattern.

Right: The neoplastic cells have spindled nuclei with vesicular chromatin and abundant eosinophilic cytoplasm with indistinct cell borders (hematoxylin and eosin [H&E] stain).

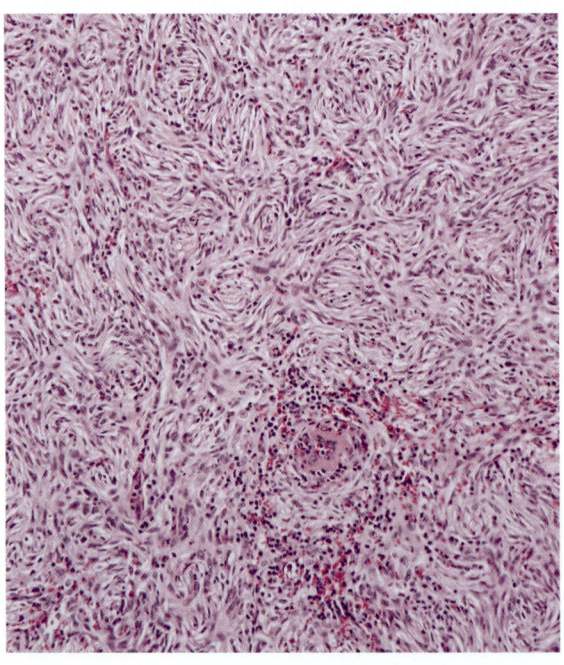
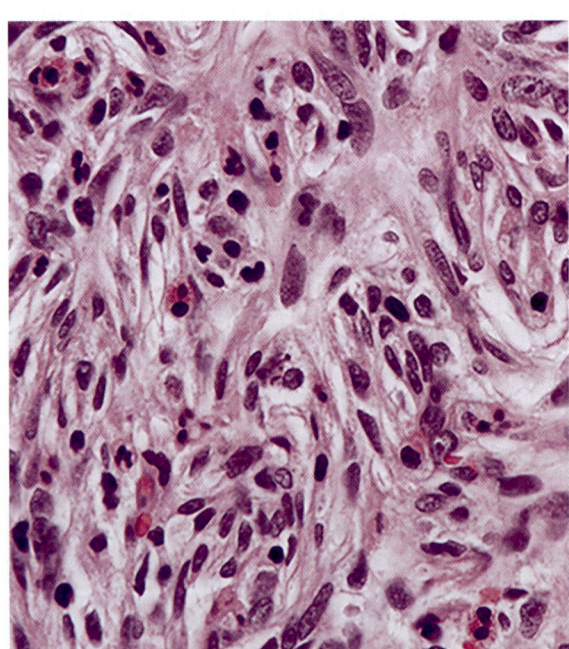

Figure 53-2

FOLLICULAR DENDRITIC CELL SARCOMA INVOLVING CERVICAL LYMPH NODE

Left: The neoplastic spindled cells are arranged in a prominent whorled pattern. One medium-sized blood vessel with a perivascular rim of reactive lymphocytes is present in the field.

Right: High-power magnification shows the spindled cells and an intermixed infiltrate of eosinophils, neutrophils, and small lymphocytes (H&E stain).

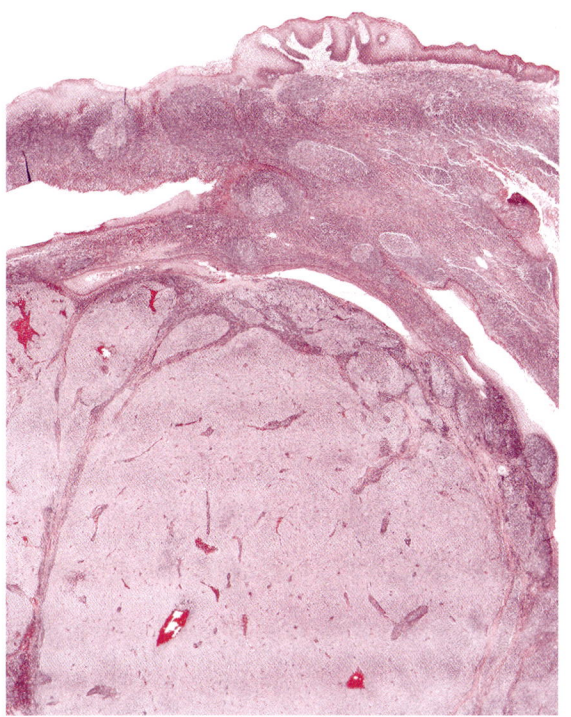 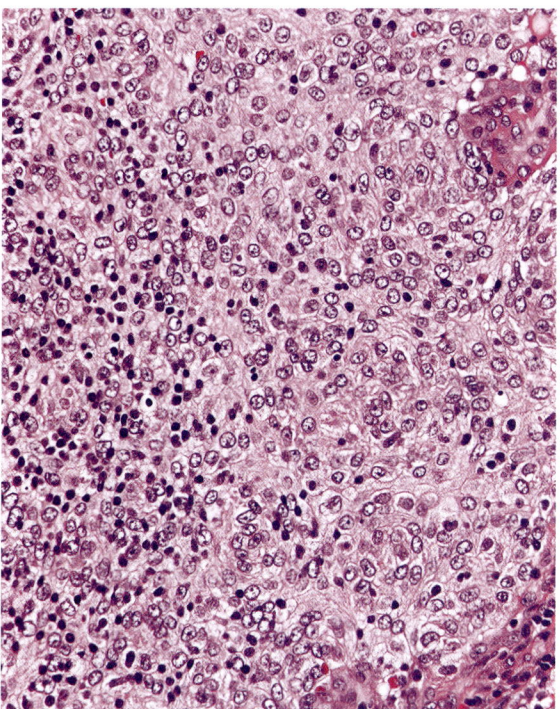

Figure 53-3

FOLLICULAR DENDRITIC CELL SARCOMA PARTIALLY REPLACING TONSIL

Left: The neoplastic cells are arranged in a diffuse, sheet-like pattern. Benign tonsil (top) is also present in this field.
Right: The sarcoma cells are epithelioid with round nuclei, vesicular chromatin, and abundant cytoplasm with defined cell borders. Intermixed reactive lymphocytes (left) are also appreciated in this field (H&E stain).

borders. There is a range of nuclear atypia. In somewhat bland tumors, the tumor cell nuclei are often vesicular, with small nucleoli and thin nuclear membranes (fig. 53-1, right). Other tumors are highly atypical, with hyperchromatic nuclei. Mitotic figures are infrequent in bland tumors, 0 to 1 per 10 high-power fields but are more numerous in atypical tumors, 10 to 30 per 10 high-power fields (fig. 53-4). Foci of coagulative necrosis occur, more common in highly atypical tumors. Binucleated or multinucleated tumor cells are common and nuclear pseudoinclusions (fig. 53-5) are observed occasionally (2,5,14).

The cells of FDC sarcoma can exhibit a broad cytologic spectrum. The tumor cells may have prominent central nucleoli (immunoblast-like) (fig. 53-6), the cells can be epithelioid with eosinophilic or fairly clear cytoplasm with glass-like nuclei, or the cytoplasm can be highly eosinophilic and granular (oncocyte-like). Osteoclast-like giant cells can be interspersed within some tumors (2,3,14).

FDC sarcomas commonly have an inflammatory cell background that is usually composed of small lymphocytes that may form prominent perivascular cuffs (figs. 53-7, 53-8) (2,14). Granulocytes are commonly intermixed and in some cases are prominent (fig. 53-2). These neoplasms may be highly vascular (fig. 53-9). Fibrinoid deposits may be seen within the walls of the blood vessels and foci of hemorrhage may be observed within the tumor. Infrequently, and particularly in a small needle biopsy specimen, FDC sarcoma cells can be outnumbered by the reactive cell infiltrate.

Some cases of FDC sarcoma arise from Castleman disease (1,9a,14). Most often, the hyaline vascular variant has been described, but rare cases of the plasma cell variant are also reported. Usually, histologic evidence of Castleman disease is also present in the pathology specimen. The areas of FDC sarcoma are recognized by their increased cellularity and the fascicular or storiform pattern.

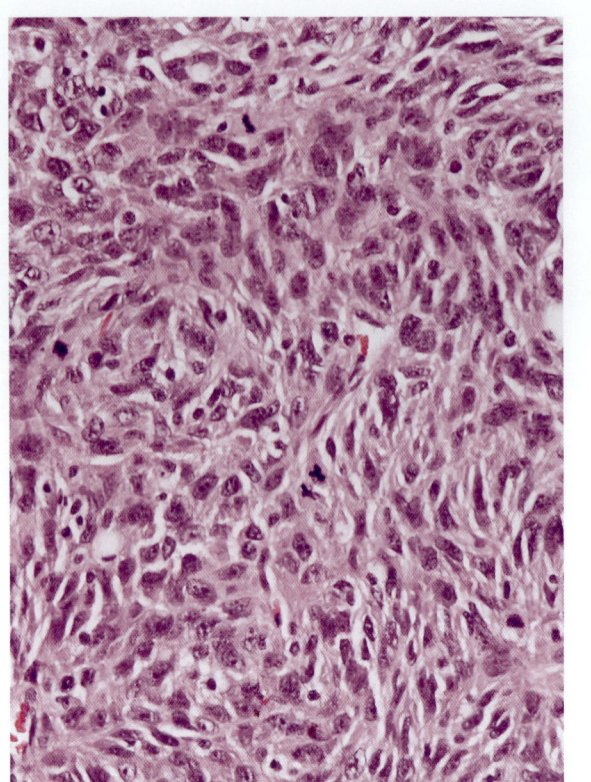
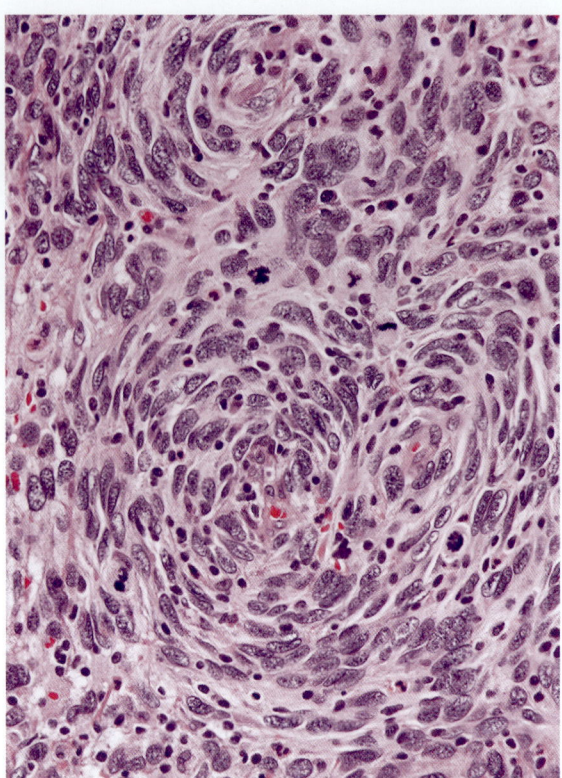

Figure 53-4

FOLLICULAR DENDRITIC CELL SARCOMA WITH CYTOLOGIC ATYPIA

Left: In this case, the spindled cells have a higher nucleus to cytoplasm ratio than the tumors shown in figures 53-1 and 53-2. Mitotic figures are present.

Right: In another case, the neoplastic cells also have a high nucleus to cytoplasm ratio and brisk mitotic rate, including one atypical mitotic figure in this field (H&E stain).

Figure 53-5

FOLLICULAR DENDRITIC CELL SARCOMA WITH MODERATE NUCLEAR ATYPIA AND NUCLEAR PSEUDOINCLUSIONS

Two pseudoinclusions are present in the center of the field along with a number of other pseudoinclusions (H&E stain).

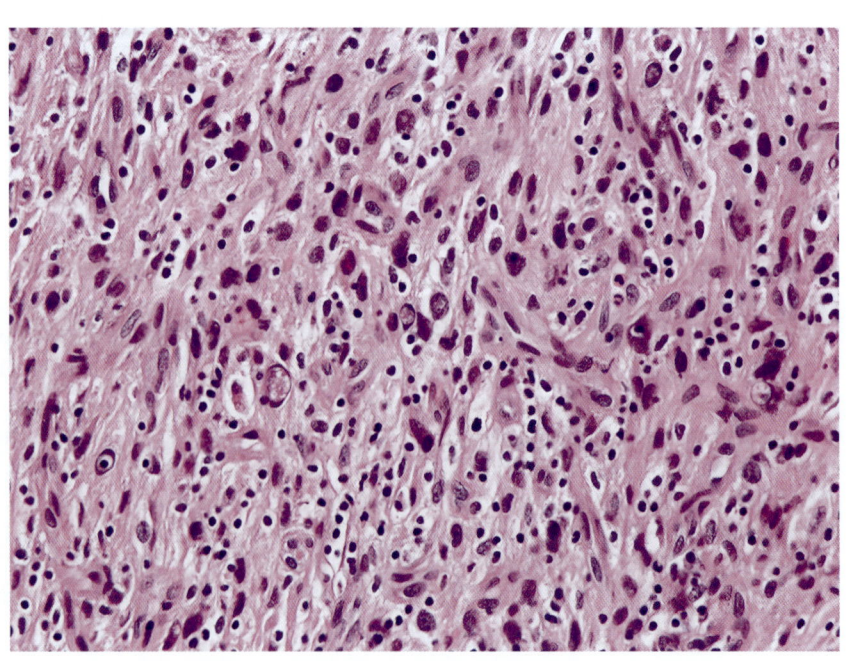

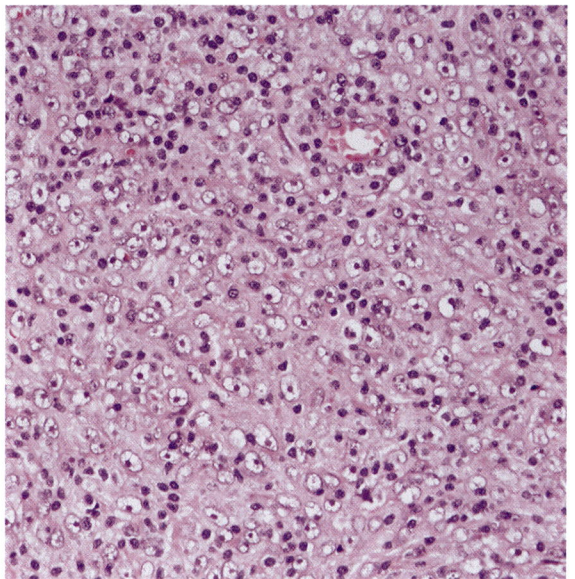

Figure 53-6

FOLLICULAR DENDRITIC CELL SARCOMA WITH PROMINENT NUCLEOLI

In this case of FDC sarcoma, the neoplastic cells are arranged in a sheet-like pattern and the cells are epithelioid. The tumor cells also have vesicular nuclei and prominent nucleoli imparting an immunoblast-like appearance (H&E stain).

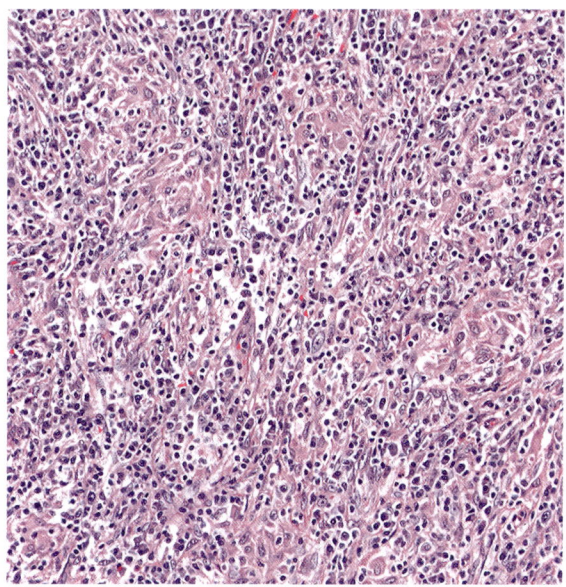

Figure 53-7

FOLLICULAR DENDRITIC CELL SARCOMA WITH MANY REACTIVE LYMPHOCYTES

There is conspicuous vascularity, with many intermixed reactive lymphocytes (H&E stain).

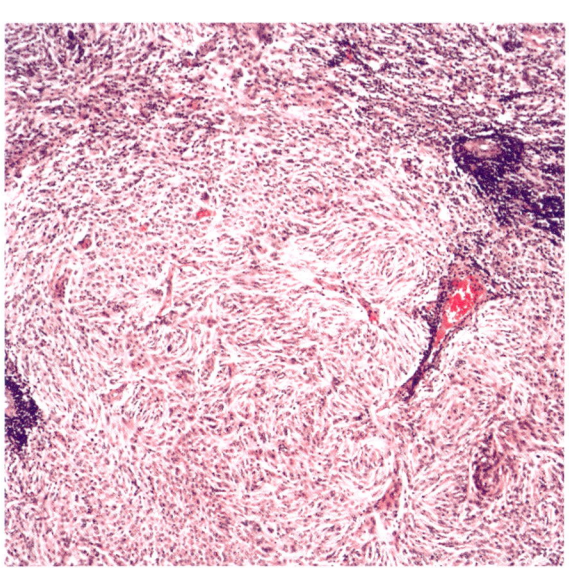

Figure 53-8

FOLLICULAR DENDRITIC CELL SARCOMA WITH REACTIVE PERIVASCULAR CUFFS OF LYMPHOCYTES

In this neoplasm there is a prominent reactive infiltrate of small lymphocytes that formed perivascular cuffs around blood vessels (left and right of field) (H&E stain).

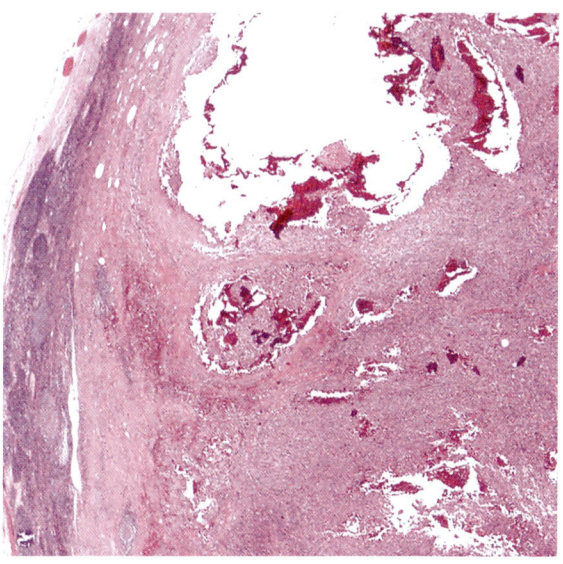

Figure 53-9

FOLLICULAR DENDRITIC CELL SARCOMA ASSOCIATED WITH PROMINENT BLOOD VESSELS

There are prominent, dilated blood vessels and areas of recent hemorrhage within this case of FDC sarcoma. The high-magnification view of this tumor is shown in figure 53-4, left (H&E stain).

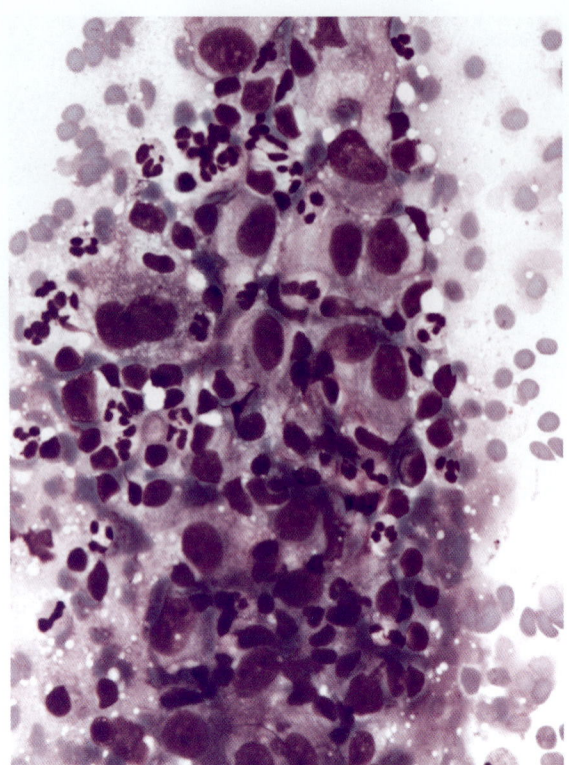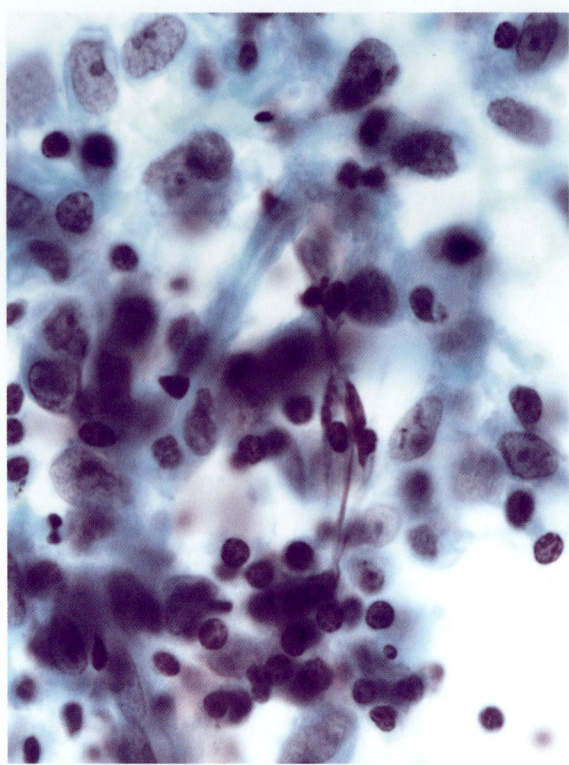

Figure 53-10

FOLLICULAR DENDRITIC CELL SARCOMA: CYTOLOGIC FEATURES

Left: In aspirate smears, the neoplastic cells are present as syncytial groups.

Right: At higher magnification, the neoplastic cells have elongated nuclei, nucleoli, and moderately abundant cytoplasm and are admixed with small lymphocytes and neutrophils (left: Diff-Quik stain; right: Papanicolaou stain). (Courtesy of Dr. U. Kundu, Houston, TX.)

CYTOLOGIC FINDINGS

In fine-needle aspirate smears, the cells of FDC sarcoma are large and often arranged singly and in syncytial groups that are admixed with small lymphocytes (fig. 53-10) (5,10,16). The most common cytologic appearance is that of neoplastic cells that have oval or fusiform nuclei with finely granular chromatin and variably sized nucleoli (figs. 53-10, 53-11). Nuclear pseudoinclusions and grooves may be present.

The variations in the morphology of FDC sarcoma described above are also appreciated in cytologic preparations. The cells can be both spindled and epithelioid, or only epithelioid with moderate to abundant cytoplasm, sometimes with clear cell changes or an oncocytoid appearance (fig. 53-12). Multinucleated and binucleated tumor cells may be present and the nuclei can be pleomorphic and contain promi-

nent nucleoli. In one case reported, the neoplastic cells had long circumferential cytoplasmic extensions resembling hair blown by the wind or starfish (4). The mitotic rate is variable, ranging from low to high and correlates fairly well with the degree of atypia observed within the tumor cells. The background shows many small lymphocytes; plasma cells and necrotic debris also may be present.

ULTRASTRUCTURAL AND IMMUNOPHENOTYPIC FINDINGS

Electron microscopy, although performed rarely, has value in the diagnosis of FDC sarcoma. The neoplastic cells have features similar to those of benign FDCs, including spindle-shaped nuclei and long cytoplasmic processes with mature desmosomes. Birbeck granules are absent (2,5,14).

Immunohistochemistry is the mainstay for the diagnosis of FDC sarcoma. The neoplastic

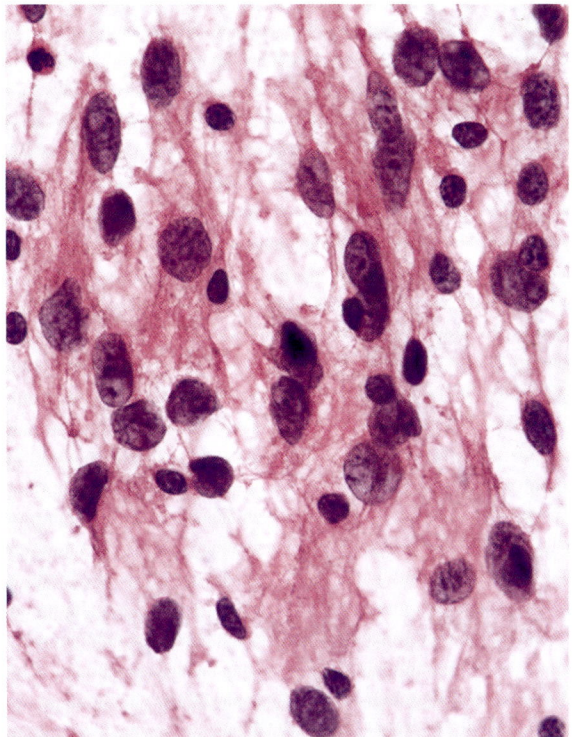

Figure 53-11

**FOLLICULAR DENDRITIC CELL
SARCOMA: SPINDLED CELLS**

A scrape preparation from a case of FDC sarcoma shows spindle-shaped neoplastic cells with abundant, eosinophilic cytoplasm and bland nuclei (H&E stain).

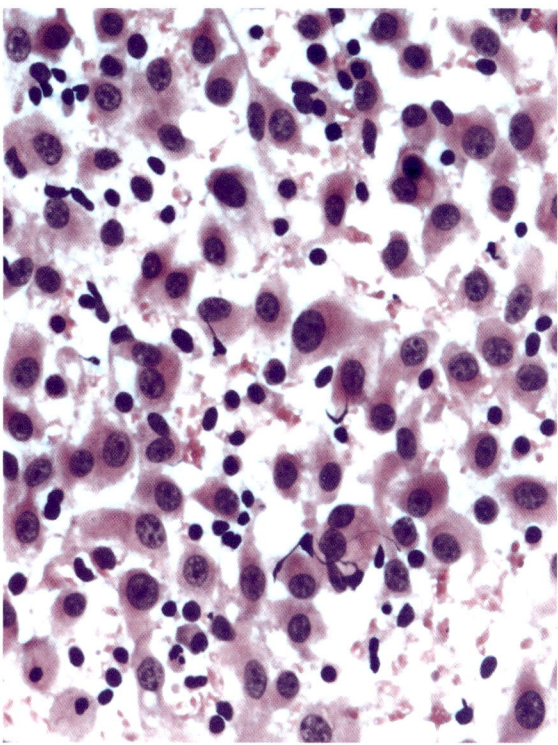

Figure 53-12

**FOLLICULAR DENDRITIC CELL
SARCOMA: EPITHELIOID CELLS**

An aspirate smear shows neoplastic cells that have an epithelioid appearance with abundant, eosinophilic or oncocytoid cytoplasm (Papanicolaou stain).

cells are positive for one or more FDC-associated markers including CD21, CD23, CD35, KiM4p, CNA.42, and clusterin (figs. 53-13–53-15) (2,5,8,14). Two recently reported novel markers that appear to be useful are FDC secreted protein and serglycin (11a). Other markers frequently positive in FDC sarcoma are CD4 (often weakly), desmoplakin, fascin, vimentin, epidermal growth factor receptor (EGFR), CXCL13, PD-L1 (about 50 percent), D2-40/podoplanin, somatostatin receptor 2A (about 40 percent), MDM2 (about 40 percent), and HLA-DR (1,2,3,14). Some cases are variably positive for epithelial membrane antigen (EMA), S-100 protein (usually focal), CD68 (weak, cytoplasmic), and p53; rare cases are positive for CD20 and CD45/LCA. FDC sarcomas are negative for CD1a, CD10, CD19, CD30, CD31, CD34, CD79a, CD163, BCL-6, cyclin D1, langerin/CD207, lysozyme, myeloperoxidase, pan-T-cell antigens, HMB45 and other melanoma-associated antigens, and keratins. The proliferation index,

as measured by Ki-67 expression, is highly variable, ranging from very low to up to about 40 percent in the highly mitotic and atypical cases (2,3,14). There is no evidence of EBV infection. The background lymphocytes in FDC sarcomas may be of B- or T-cell lineage or a mixture of the two. In cases of mediastinal FDC sarcoma, there can be an increased number of immature (TdT-positive) small lymphocytes (9).

MOLECULAR GENETIC FINDINGS

Conventional cytogenetic analysis has been reported for a small number of cases of FDC sarcoma. In 2013, Perry et al. (15) described two cases and noted five others in the literature. Six of the seven cases had complex karyotypes with losses and gains of a number of chromosomal loci. Using molecular inversion probe array, approximately 80 percent of cases of FDC sarcoma have extensive genomic complexity including hemizygous losses of many chromosomes.

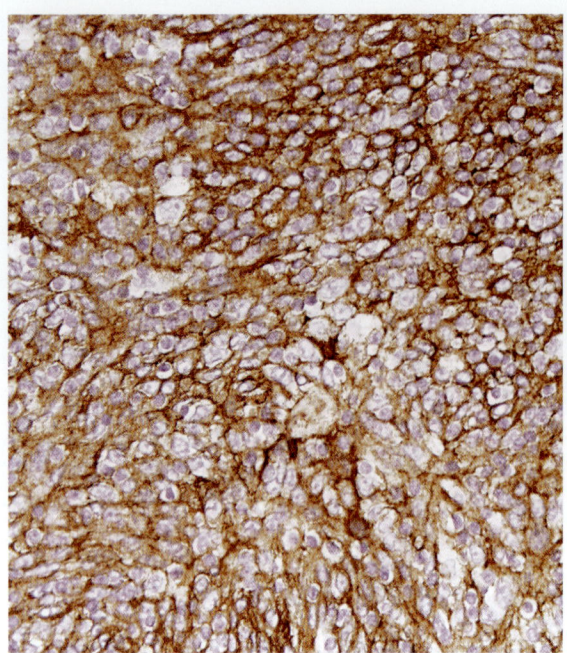
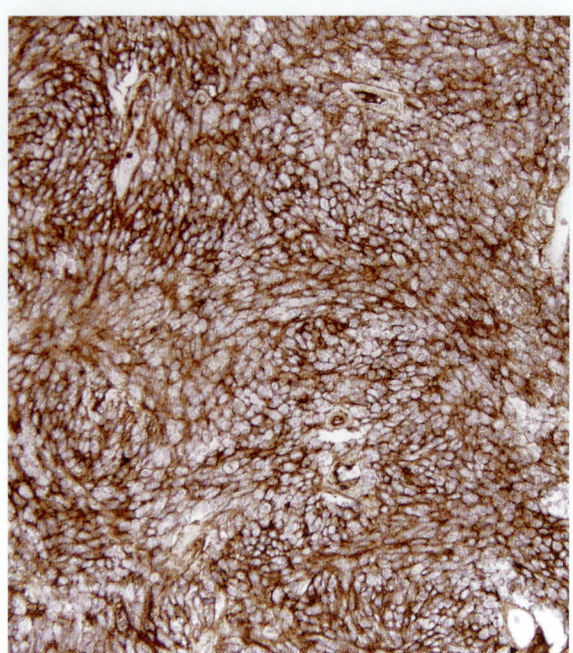

Figure 53-13

FOLLICULAR DENDRITIC CELL SARCOMA: IMMUNOHISTOCHEMISTRY

This case of FDC sarcoma is positive for CD21 (left), and clusterin (right), and was positive for other FDC-associated markers (not shown). This is the same case shown in figures 53-4, left (immunohistochemistry with hematoxylin counterstain).

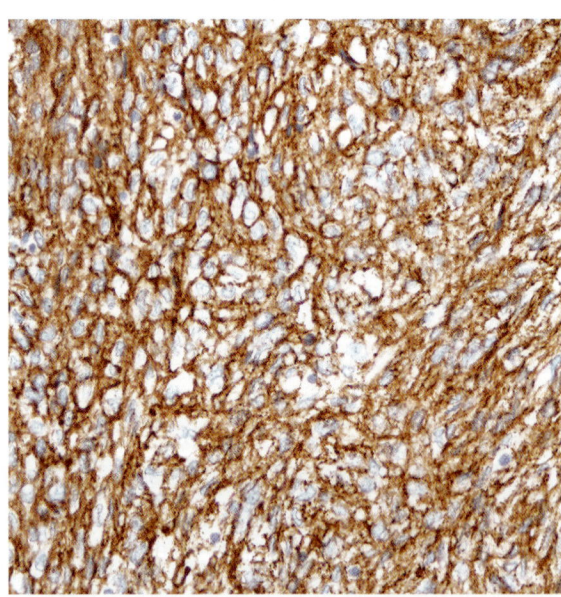

Figure 53-14

FOLLICULAR DENDRITIC CELL SARCOMA: CD23

This FDC sarcoma is positive for CD23 and was also positive for other FDC-associated markers (not shown). This is the same case shown in figure 53-1 (immuno-histochemistry with hematoxylin counterstain).

These results suggest that many tumor suppressor genes are involved in pathogenesis (1a).

Griffin et al. (7a) used next generation sequencing to assess 13 cases of FDC sarcoma and showed loss-of-function mutations in the NK-κB pathway (38 percent) and mutations in cell cycle genes (31 percent) including *CCND1*, *CDKN2A*, and *RB1*. These authors also showed 9p24PD-L1/L2 copy gains in 3 of 13 (23 percent) cases. *BRAF* V600E mutations have been reported in 20 percent of cases (6). The antigen receptor genes are usually in the germline configuration in FDC sarcoma (3).

DIFFERENTIAL DIAGNOSIS

Interdigitating Dendritic Cell Sarcoma. Interdigitating dendritic cell sarcoma cells are commonly spindle-shaped and other histologic findings overlap with those of FDC sarcoma. Unlike FDC sarcoma, the cells of interdigitating dendritic cell sarcoma are strongly positive for S-100 protein and are negative for FDC-associated markers. If ultrastructural examination is performed, interdigitating dendritic cell sarcomas lack desmosomes.

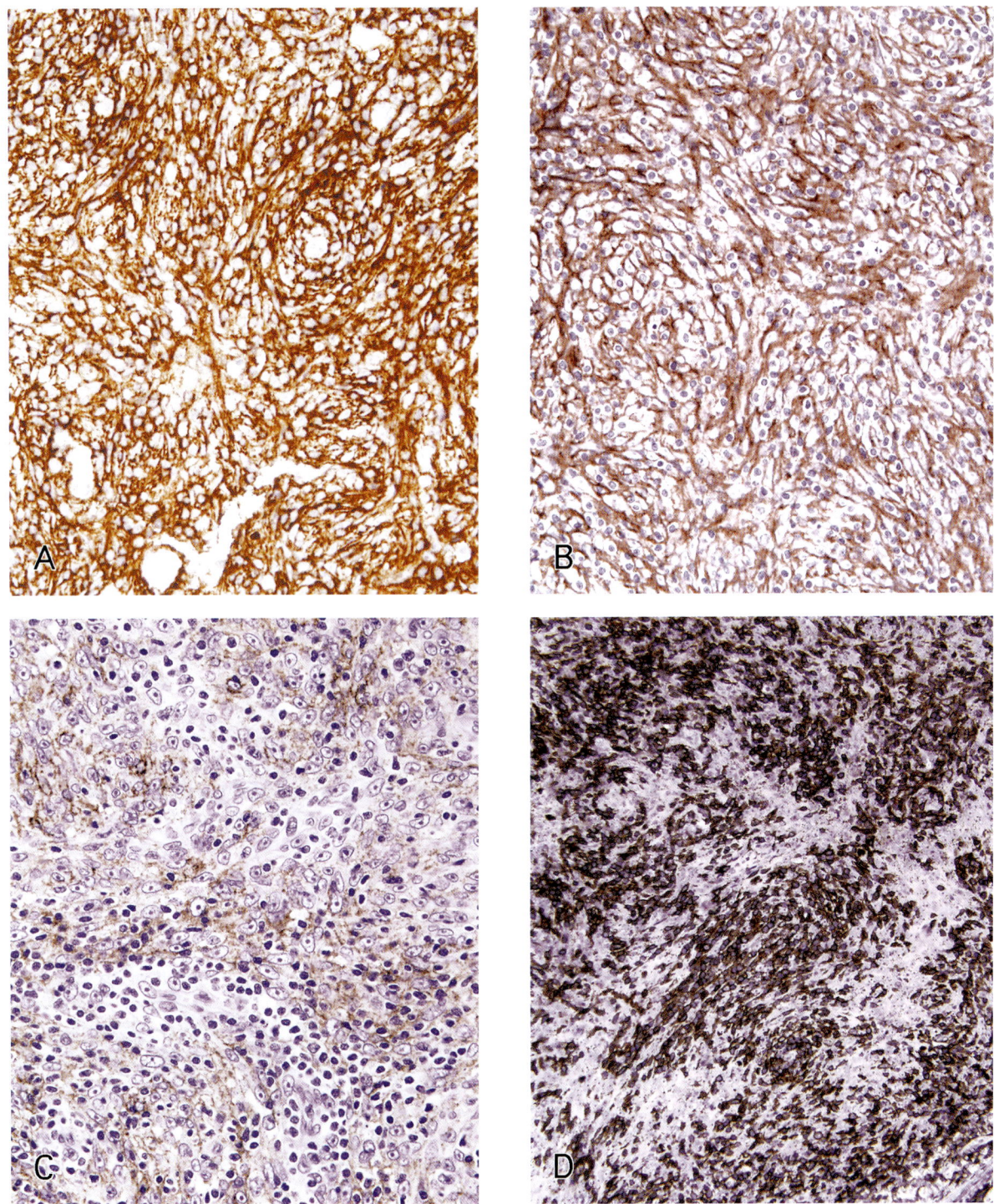

Figure 53-15

FOLLICULAR DENDRITIC CELL SARCOMA: IMMUNOHISTOCHEMISTRY

This FDC sarcoma is positive for CD35 (A), epidermal growth factor receptor (EGFR) (B), and epithelial membrane antigen (C) and is negative for CD20 (D). The anti-CD20 antibody highlights many reactive B lymphocytes intermixed in this neoplasm. This is the same case as is shown in figure 53-3 (immunohistochemistry with hematoxylin counterstain).

Langerhans Cell Sarcoma. The morphologic findings of Langerhans cell sarcoma can overlap with FDC sarcoma. The cells of Langerhans cell sarcoma, however, are positive for CD1a, CD207/langerin, and S-100 protein (usually strongly expressed) and are negative for FDC-associated markers. If ultrastructural examination is performed, Birbeck granules are present in Langerhans cell sarcoma, unlike FDC sarcoma.

Histiocytic Sarcoma. In most cases of histiocytic sarcoma, the tumor cells have an epithelioid appearance which is uncommon in FDC sarcoma. The neoplastic cells of histiocytic sarcoma may express S-100 protein, but usually only weakly and variably. Unlike FDC sarcoma, histiocytic sarcoma cells have a more clearly phagocytic immunophenotype (positive for CD68, CD163, and lysozyme) and are negative for FDC-associated antigens.

Fibroblastic Reticular Cell Sarcoma. Normal fibroblastic reticular cells are of mesenchymal origin and are involved in maintaining the supporting framework of lymph nodes, forming sheaths around postcapillary venules; they also are involved in cytokine transport. Fibroblastic reticular cell sarcoma is the least frequent tumor in the histiocytic and dendritic cell category and, as a result, is the least well characterized. In 2013, Saygin et al. (17) reviewed the literature and identified 19 cases. The prognosis for patients is poor since local recurrence and metastases appear to be common (17).

Fibroblastic reticular cell sarcoma most often occurs in neck or mediastinal lymph nodes and is often composed of highly spindled cells arranged in fascicles or whorls that may resemble FDC sarcoma. Unlike other histiocytic and dendritic cell neoplasms, the tumor cells of fibroblastic reticular cell sarcoma are often positive for smooth muscle actin, desmin, and vimentin and may be positive for the keratins that occur in normal fibroblastic reticular cells. The neoplastic cells are negative for FDC-associated markers, CD1a, CD207/langerin, S-100 protein, and CD68.

Metastatic Carcinoma. Metastatic carcinomas may be spindled and morphologically resemble, at least in part, FDC sarcoma. Based on the common location of FDC sarcoma in neck lymph nodes and the patient age, metastatic squamous cell carcinoma of the head and neck is often part of the differential diagnosis. Any evidence of keratin pearls or intercellular bridges is helpful. Metastatic poorly differentiated adenocarcinoma also can be highly spindled and resemble FDC sarcoma, for example, metastatic breast carcinoma to an axillary lymph node. Immunohistochemical analysis usually resolves this differential diagnosis as carcinomas express keratins and other epithelial-associated markers and are negative for CD21, CD23, and most other FDC-associated antigens.

Sarcoma. The spindled shape of the cells in FDC sarcoma can resemble other spindled tumors such as various types of sarcoma. Location at an extranodal site may particularly raise the suspicion of sarcoma. Immunohistochemical or molecular analysis helps exclude many sarcomas, such as alveolar rhabdomyosarcoma and angiosarcoma. Immunohistochemistry for anaplastic lymphoma kinase (ALK) identifies cases of inflammatory myofibroblastic tumor.

Melanoma. Strong expression of S-100 protein should always lead to consideration of the possibility of metastatic melanoma. The neoplastic cells of melanoma often show foci of melanin pigment, unlike FDC sarcoma. Melanomas express one or more melanoma-associated markers and are negative for FDC-associated markers. Electron microscopic examination of melanoma cases often shows melanosomes.

Diffuse Large B-Cell Lymphoma. When the neoplastic cells of FDC sarcomas have epithelioid features, they may resemble diffuse large B-cell lymphoma (DLBCL). In addition, rare cases of FDC sarcoma express CD20 or CD45. Usually, however, FDC sarcomas have some spindled areas, unusual in DLBCL, and DLBCL cells express a battery of B-cell antigens and are negative for most FDC-associated antigens.

Nodular Sclerosis Hodgkin Lymphoma. Nodular sclerosis Hodgkin lymphoma may have numerous neoplastic cells (so-called syncytial variant) or may be highly spindled (so-called fibroblastic or sarcomatoid variant) and may resemble, in part, FDC sarcoma. The commonly used FDC-associated markers CD21 and CD23 are not specific and may be expressed by Reed-Sternberg and Hodgkin (RS+H) cells. Unlike FDC sarcoma, RS+H cells are usually positive for CD15 (about 70 percent of cases), CD30, PAX5 (dim), and MUM1/IRF4; are negative for CD45/LCA; and are usually negative for other

FDC-associated markers as well as desmoplakin, podoplanin, and EGFR.

Benign Solid Spindle Cell Tumors/Lesions. In the head and neck region, extracranial meningioma may mimic, in part, FDC sarcoma. These tumors are usually close to the skull or follow the pathways of cranial nerves. Histologically, they commonly form whorls and may be associated with psammoma bodies. Most meningiomas are positive for EMA and about one quarter express keratins or S-100 protein. Meningiomas are negative for FDC-associated markers.

In the neck and mediastinum, ectopic thymoma of spindle cell type may mimic FDC sarcoma. Rare FDC sarcomas have a lobulated appearance, with perivascular spaces resembling a thymoma. Thymomas are positive for keratins and p63 and are negative for FDC-associated antigens.

Inflammatory pseudotumor in lymph nodes shows a highly heterogeneous range of morphologic features. Some have a highly spindled appearance and may be confused with FDC sarcoma. Unlike FDC sarcoma, the lymph node architecture is often partially preserved and there is a prominent inflammatory cell background in inflammatory pseudotumor of lymph nodes.

TREATMENT AND PROGNOSIS

FDC sarcoma is a slow-growing lesion and therefore commonly has an indolent clinical course similar to that of low-grade sarcomas (2,14,17). Patients with localized disease have a good chance of cure if the tumor is completely excised (7,9a,13). Adjuvant radiation therapy may reduce the rate of local recurrence as has been suggested by Pang et al. (13). Adjuvant chemotherapy also has been used although the scientific basis for such treatment is not well established. For patients with advanced-stage disease at diagnosis, there is no consensus therapeutic approach at this time. Combination chemotherapy regimens of different types have been used; response is incomplete in most patients.

Various pathologic features correlate with a more aggressive clinical course and therefore deserve specific mention in the surgical pathology report (2,14). Large tumor size, over 6 cm, and intra-abdominal location predict a poorer prognosis, with either local recurrence or metastasis. Other findings that correlate with tumor behavior include the presence of coagulative necrosis, substantial cytologic atypia, and a high mitotic or high proliferation (Ki-67) rate (2,3).

Approximately half of patients with FDC sarcoma develop local recurrences for which repeat surgical excision may be an option. Distant metastases occur in about 25 percent of patients (2,13,14,17,18). Patients with advanced-stage disease or metastases not amenable to excision have a poor prognosis and an appreciable rate of deaths attributable to disease (3,7,9a,17).

REFERENCES

1. Agaimy A, Michal M, Hadravsky L, Michal M. Follicular dendritic cell sarcoma: clinicopathologic study of 15 cases with emphasis on novel expression of MDM2, somatostatin receptor 2A, and PD-L1. Ann Diagn Pathol 2016;23:21-28.
1a. Andersen EF, Paxton CN, O'Malley DP, et al. Genomic analysis of follicular dendritic cell sarcoma by molecular inversion probe array reveals tumor suppressor-driven biology. Mod Pathol 2017. [Epub ahead of print]
2. Chan JK, Fletcher CD, Nayler SJ, Cooper K. Follicular dendritic cell sarcoma. Clinicopathologic analysis of 17 cases suggesting a malignant potential higher than currently recognized. Cancer 1997;79:294-313.
3. Chan JK, Pileri SA, Delsol G, Fletcher CD, Weiss L, Grogg K. Follicular dendritic cell sarcoma. In: Swerdlow SH, Campo E, Harris NL, et al., eds. WHO Classification of tumours of haematopoietic and lymphoid tissues, 4th ed. Lyon: IARC Press; 2008:363-364.
4. Czapla A, Omman RA, Nam MW, Mehrotra S, Pambuccian SE. "Medusa-Head" cells, "Starfish" cells, and interconnecting long cytoplasmic processes as diagnostic cytologic clues for follicular dendritic cell sarcoma in fine needle aspiration samples. Diagn Cytopathol 2017;45:322-326.

5. Dominguez-Malagon H, Cano-Valdez AM, Mosqueda-Taylor A, Hes O. Follicular dendritic cell sarcoma of the pharyngeal region: histologic, cytologic, immunohistochemical, and ultrastructural study of three cases. Ann Diagn Pathol 2004;8:325-332.

6. Go H, Jeon YK, Huh J, et al. Frequent detection of BRAF (V600E) mutations in histiocytic and dendritic cell neoplasms. Histopathology 2014;65:261-272.

7. Gounder M, Desai V, Kuk D, et al. Impact of surgery, radiation and systemic therapy on the outcomes of patients with dendritic cell and histiocytic sarcomas. Eur J Cancer 2015;51:2413-2422.

7a. Griffin GK, Sholl LM, Lindeman NI, Fletcher CD, Hornick JL. Targeted genomic sequencing of follicular dendritic cell sarcoma reveals recurrent alterations in NF-κB regulatory genes. Mod Pathol 2016;29:67-74.

8. Grogg KL, Macon WR, Kurtin PJ, Nascimento AG. A survey of clusterin and fascin expression in sarcomas and spindle cell neoplasms: strong clusterin immunostaining is highly specific for follicular dendritic cell tumor. Mod Pathol 2005;18:260-266.

9. Hartert M, Strobel P, Dahm M, Nix W, Marx A, Vahl CF. A follicular dendritic cell sarcoma of the mediastinum with immature T cells and association with myasthenia gravis. Am J Surg Pathol 2010;34:742-745.

9a. Jain P, Milgrom SA, Patel KP, et al. Characteristics, management, and outcomes of patients with follicular dendritic cell sarcoma. Br J Haematol 2017. [Epub ahead of print]

10. Kure K, Khader SN, Suhrland MJ, Ratech H, Grossberg R, Oktay MH. Fine needle aspiration of follicular dendritic cell sarcoma in an HIV-positive man: a case report. Acta Cytol 2010;54:707-711.

11. Lee IJ, Kim SC, Kim HS, et al. Paraneoplastic pemphigus associated with follicular dendritic cell sarcoma arising from Castleman's tumor. J Am Acad Dermatol 1999;40:294-297.

11a. Lorenzi L, Döring C, Rausch T, et al. Identification of novel follicular dendritic cell sarcoma markers, FDCSP and SRGN, by whole transcriptome sequencing. Oncotarget 2017;8:16463-16472.

12. Nguyen DT, Diamond LW, Hansmann ML, Fischer R. Follicular dendritic cell sarcoma. Identification by monoclonal antibodies in paraffin sections. Appl Immunohistochem 1994;2: 60-64.

13. Pang J, Mydlarz WK, Gooi Z, et al. Follicular dendritic cell sarcoma of the head and neck: case report, literature review, and pooled analysis of 97 cases. Head Neck 2016;38(Suppl 1):E2241-2249.

14. Perez-Ordonez B, Erlandson RA, Rosai J. Follicular dendritic cell tumor: report of 13 additional cases of a distinctive entity. Am J Surg Pathol 1996;20:944-955.

15. Perry AM, Nelson M, Sanger WG, Bridge JA, Greiner TC. Cytogenetic abnormalities in follicular dendritic cell sarcoma: report of two cases and literature review. In Vivo 2013;27:211-214.

16. Ren R, Sun X, Staerkel G, Sneige N, Gong Y. Fine-needle cytology of a liver metastasis of follicular dendritic cell sarcoma. Diagn Cytopathool 2005; 32:38-43.

17. Saygin C, Uzunaslan D, Ozguroglu M, Senocak M, Tuzuner N. Dendritic cell sarcoma: a pooled analysis including 462 cases with presentation of our case series, Crit Rev Hematol Oncol 2013;88:253-271.

18. Vargas H, Mouzakes J, Purdy SS, Cohn AS, Parnes SM. Follicular dendritic cell tumor: an aggressive head and neck tumor. Am J Otolaryngol 2002;23:93-98.

19. Wang J, Bu DF, Li T, et al. Autoantibody production from a thymoma and a follicular dendritic cell sarcoma associated with paraneoplastic pemphigus. Br J Dermatol 2005;153:558-564.

INTERDIGITATING DENDRITIC CELL SARCOMA

GENERAL FEATURES

Interdigitating dendritic cell (IDC) *sarcoma* is a tumor composed of spindle- or oval-shaped neoplastic cells that have an immunophenotype similar to that of interdigitating dendritic cells, thought to be the likely cell of origin (18). Normal IDCs are located in the paracortex of lymph nodes and the periarteriolar lymphoid sheaths of the spleen. Physiologically, IDCs present antigens to T cells and are involved in regulating T-cell immunity (1). They are thought to be of hematopoietic origin, originating from the bone marrow, before migrating to peripheral organs.

IDC sarcoma is a rare neoplasm. In 2013, Saygin et al. (16) reviewed the English literature and identified 100 cases. Description of pathologic findings is available for about two thirds of these cases and ancillary studies (other than immunohistochemistry) have been applied sparingly to the characterization of these tumors.

CLINICAL FEATURES

IDC sarcoma occurs predominantly in adults with a median age in the sixth decade, but the age range is wide, from 2 to 88 years (7,10,14,16). There is a slight male predominance, with a male to female ratio of 1.2 to 1.0. All races have been affected by IDC sarcoma, but too few cases are available to comment on racial preferences (16). These tumors occur mainly in lymph nodes, with the cervical and axillary regions most commonly involved, but any lymph node group may be involved. About half of the patients have extranodal disease, and about 25 percent present with localized extranodal sites of disease (10,16). The most common extranodal sites are skin, soft tissue, gastrointestinal tract, liver, and spleen.

Approximately 50 percent of patients with IDC sarcoma present with asymptomatic lymphadenopathy (10,16). The disease is in an advanced stage in one third of patients, and this subset may have B-type symptoms. The bone marrow is involved infrequently, in less than 10 percent of patients. Feltkamp et al. (5) reported a patient who presented with mediastinal lymphadenopathy and superior vena cava syndrome.

IDC sarcoma can occur in patients with a history of lymphoma or solid tumors; about 10 percent of patients have had lymphoma previously (10,16). These lymphomas include chronic lymphocytic leukemia/small lymphocytic lymphoma (CLL/SLL), follicular lymphoma, diffuse large B-cell lymphoma (DLBCL), mycosis fungoides, and T-cell acute lymphoblastic leukemia (16). In some patients, the IDC sarcoma and lymphoma are coincidental; however, particularly in patients with IDC sarcoma and low-grade B-cell lymphoma, transdifferentiation is thought to have occurred (4,6). The concept of transdifferentiation is discussed in chapter 52 in more detail.

HISTOLOGIC FINDINGS

Lymph nodes are subtotally or completely replaced by neoplasm in a diffuse pattern (10,15–18). In lymph nodes not completely effaced, the neoplasm preferentially involves the paracortical regions. Sinusoidal involvement has been reported. In most cases of IDC sarcoma, the neoplastic cells are spindle-shaped and arranged in a whorled or storiform pattern (fig. 54-1). Some epithelioid neoplastic cells may be present and epithelioid cells can predominate in about one quarter (or less) of cases (fig. 54-2).

The neoplastic cells have abundant eosinophilic cytoplasm and indistinct cell borders. The nuclei have vesicular or hyperchromatic chromatin and nucleoli that are small or prominent. In some cases, the neoplastic cells show emperipolesis, although usually not prominently (10). Multinucleated tumor cells or Reed-Sternberg-like cells have been described in small subsets of cases. Mitotic figures are present, but are usually few, less than 1 per high-power

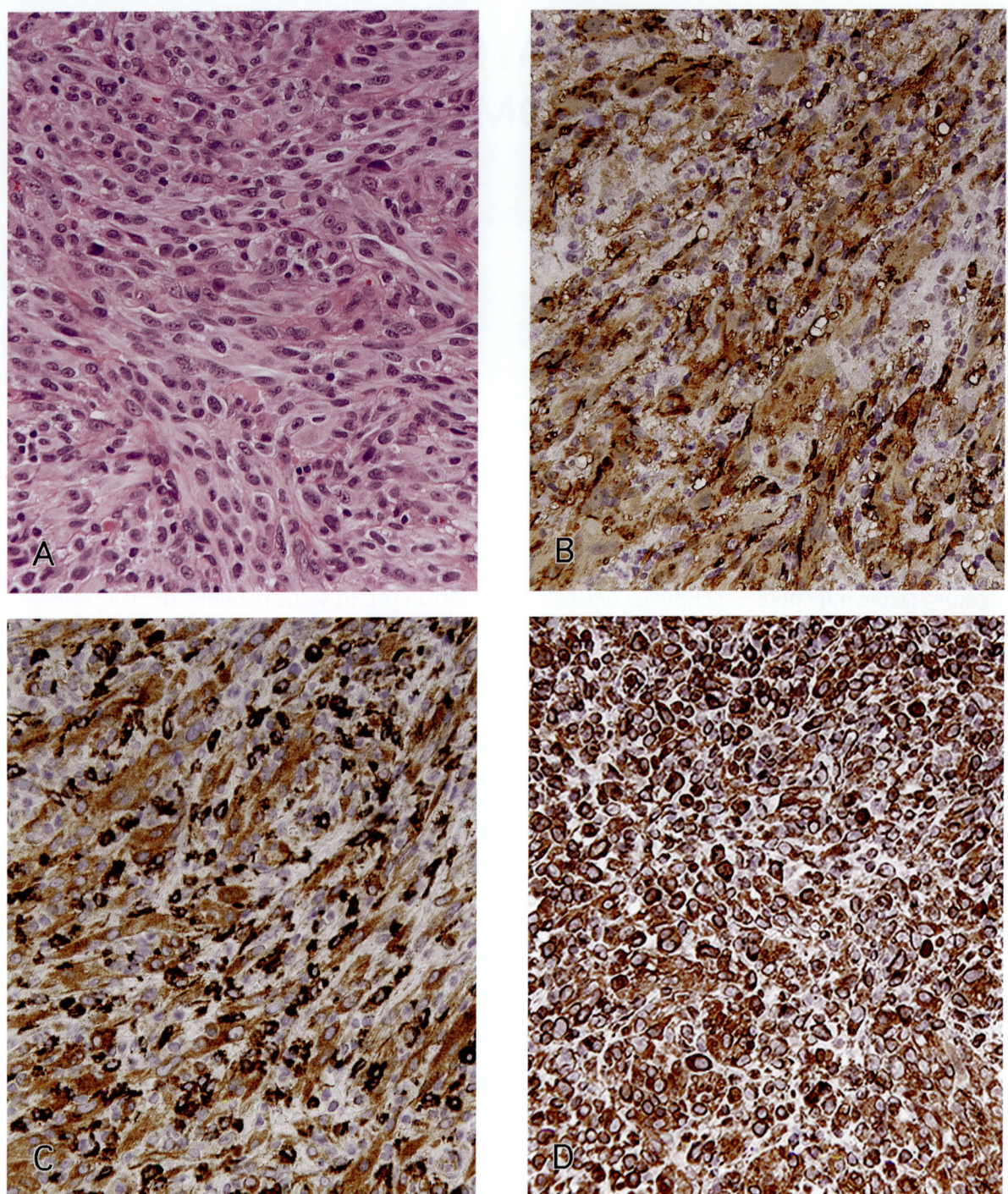

Figure 54-1

INTERDIGITATING DENDRITIC CELL SARCOMA INVOLVING CERVICAL LYMPH NODE

A: The neoplasm is composed of spindle-shaped cells arranged in a storiform pattern (hematoxylin and eosin [H&E] stain).
B–D: The neoplastic cells are positive for S-100 protein (B); weakly positive for CD68 (C), and strongly positive for vimentin (D). Fascin (not shown) and CD45/LCA (not shown) were also positive. All other markers tested were negative including follicular dendritic cell markers, keratins, and melanoma- and muscle-associated antigens (not shown) (B–D: immunohistochemistry with hematoxylin counterstain).

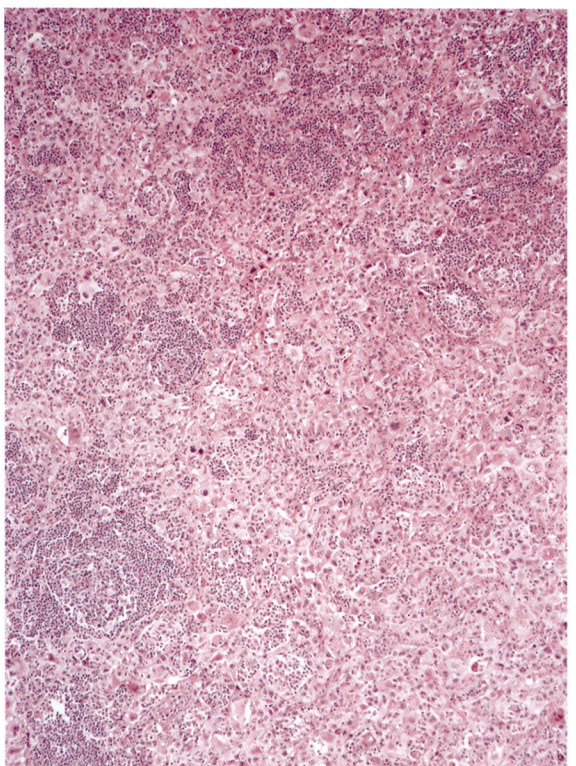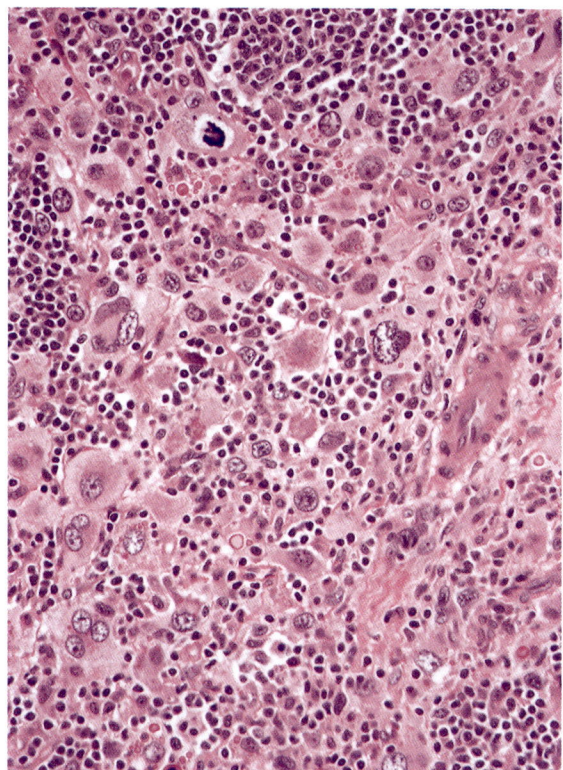

Figure 54-2

INTERDIGITATING DENDRITIC CELL SARCOMA INVOLVING AXILLARY LYMPH NODE

Left: The neoplasm extensively replaces the lymph node but residual islands of lymphoid tissue are appreciated at low-power magnification.

Right: The neoplastic cells have a large and predominantly epithelioid appearance with abundant eosinophilic cytoplasm. Immunohistochemical studies (not shown) showed that the neoplastic cells were strongly positive for S-100 protein and vimentin, weakly positive for CD68, and negative for all other markers tested.

microscopic field (10,18). Areas of coagulative necrosis may be present. The neoplastic cells are often intermixed with reactive cells, most often small lymphocytes, but also plasma cells in many cases and eosinophils in a subset of tumors.

CYTOLOGIC FINDINGS

In fine-needle aspirate smears, the spindle cells of IDC sarcoma are arranged in tight groups or loosely cohesive clusters. The neoplastic cells may have a spindled or ovoid shape and the nuclei may have vesicular or hyperchromatic chromatin with inconspicuous or prominent nucleoli. The tumor cell cytoplasm is abundant and eosinophilic. Mitotic activity is often low. Multinucleated giant cells with bizarre nuclei and admixed reactive lymphocytes, plasma cells, and less often, eosinophils, can be present.

IMMUNOPHENOTYPIC FINDINGS

Immunohistochemical analysis has been the primary ancillary method used to study IDC sarcoma. The neoplastic cells are positive for S-100 protein (moderate to strong), fascin, and vimentin, and are variably positive for CD45/LCA and CD68 (fig. 54-1B-D) (9,13,16,18). Some cases are positive for CD4, CD11c, CD14, CD163, lysozyme, and HLA-DR. In one study, IDC sarcomas were often positive for SOX10, p75, and beta-catenin (17). The anti-Ki-67 antibody usually shows a low proliferation index, in the range of 10 to 20 percent, although some reported cases have a much higher proliferation index (16,18). IDC sarcoma is negative for CD1a, CD207/langerin, follicular dendritic cell-associated antigens (e.g., CD21, CD23), pan-B-cell antigens, T-cell-specific antigens, CD30, CD34, clusterin, D2-40/podoplanin, myeloperoxidase, factor XIIIa, muscle-associated markers, HMB-45, p63, EMA/MUC1, keratins, human herpesvirus 8, and Epstein-Barr virus (EBV) LMP1 (9,13,16). In situ hybridization for EBV small encoded RNA1 (EBER1) is negative.

ULTRASTRUCTURAL FINDINGS

Electron microscopy helps establish the diagnosis of IDC sarcoma. The neoplastic cells usually have a spindle shape, with irregular cytoplasmic borders and complex interdigitating dendritic processes (7,9,18). The cytoplasm also contains abundant rough endoplasmic reticulum and the nuclei have irregular membranes. Birbeck granules and melanosomes are absent in these tumor cells.

MOLECULAR GENETIC FINDINGS

Little genetic data are available for cases of IDC sarcoma. In one small study, array comparative genomic hybridization showed genetic abnormalities in three of four cases assessed (11). The abnormalities included gains of chromosome loci 3q and 13q in one case, trisomy 12 in a second case, and losses of 7p, 12p, 16p, 18q, 19q, and 22q in a third case.

A limited number of cases of IDC sarcoma have been assessed for the *BRAF* V600E mutation, either by molecular methods or mutation-specific immunohistochemistry, and a small percentage of cases has been reported to be positive (2,3). Clonality analysis of IDC sarcoma has shown that the immunoglobulin and T-cell receptor genes are usually in the germline configuration (16,18). However, in IDC sarcoma patients who have a history of coexistent low-grade B-cell lymphoma, either follicular lymphoma or CLL/SLL, monoclonal immunoglobulin gene rearrangements have been identified in the IDC sarcoma that were identical to those present in the low-grade B-cell lymphomas (4,6). Evidence of *IGH-BCL2*/t(14;18)(q32;q21) also has been shown in a patient with both IDC sarcoma and follicular lymphoma, and in one case trisomy 12 was shared between IDC sarcoma and CLL/SLL (4,6,11). These data support the concept of transdifferentiation in these cases.

DIFFERENTIAL DIAGNOSIS

Langerhans Cell Sarcoma. These rare tumors can extensively overlap morphologically with IDC sarcoma and both neoplasms are positive for S-100 protein. Unlike IDC sarcoma, Langerhans cell sarcoma is positive for CD1a and CD207/langerin and electron microscopy shows the presence of Birbeck granules.

Follicular Dendritic Cell Sarcoma. These tumors are often composed of spindle-shaped cells that may morphologically overlap with IDC sarcoma. Unlike IDC sarcoma, the cells of follicular dendritic cell sarcoma are positive for one or more follicular dendritic cell-associated markers, such as CD21, CD23, CD35, and clusterin, among other markers. Ultrastructural examination of follicular dendritic cell sarcoma often shows desmosomes, which are rare in IDC sarcoma.

Histiocytic Sarcoma. In most cases of histiocytic sarcoma the neoplastic cells have an epithelioid appearance which is less common in IDC sarcoma. The neoplastic cells may express S-100 protein, but usually only variably. Unlike IDC sarcoma, the cells of histiocytic sarcoma have a more clearly phagocytic immunophenotype, with strong positivity for CD68, CD163, and lysozyme.

Lymphomas. Cases of IDC sarcoma with an epithelioid appearance may be confused with lymphoma. Two such lymphomas are DLBCL and anaplastic large cell lymphoma. Immunohistochemical studies easily resolve this differential diagnosis.

Sarcomas. The spindled shape of the cells in IDC sarcoma suggests the possibility of other spindled tumors such as various types of sarcoma. Location at an extranodal site may particularly suggest sarcoma. Immunohistochemical analysis helps exclude leiomyosarcoma or rhabdomyosarcoma. IDC sarcoma also may resemble inflammatory myofibroblastic tumors but anaplastic lymphoma kinase (ALK) expression does not occur in IDC sarcoma.

Melanoma. Strong expression of S-100 protein should always lead to the exclusion of metastatic melanoma. However, this differential diagnosis is highly challenging because the immunophenotype of IDC sarcoma and melanoma overlap. In fact, Stowman et al. (17) have made the provocative suggestion that these neoplasms are one and the same. Electron microscopy may be helpful because melanosomes support melanoma.

TREATMENT AND PROGNOSIS

The stage of patients with IDC sarcoma is an important prognostic factor. Patients with localized disease have the best prognosis, with some patients having prolonged survival (12,16). Patients with advanced stage disease have a poor prognosis, with a median survival period of less than 1 year (15,16).

The optimal therapy for patients with localized IDC sarcoma is surgical excision. Some patients with localized disease are treated with radiation therapy alone or after surgical excision. Patients with advanced stage disease are treated with various chemotherapy regimens. Although a few patients respond well to combination chemotherapy as used for aggressive lymphomas (8), most do not respond completely. BRAF inhibitors may have value in the small subset of patients whose tumors carry *BRAF* mutations (1), but new therapeutic regimens are needed for patients with IDC sarcoma.

REFERENCES

1. Chung NP, Chen Y, Chan VS, Tam PK, Lin CL. Dendritic cells: sentinels against pathogens. Histol Histopathol 2004;19:317-324.
2. Di Liso E, Pennelli N, Lodovichetti G, et al. Braf mutation in interdigitating dendritic cell sarcoma: a case report and review of the literature. Cancer Biol Ther 2015;16:1128-1135.
3. Fedoriw Y, Kim YS, Vergilio J, Chen ZW, Weiss LM, O'Malley DP. BRAF V600E mutation-specific immunohistochemistry is a rare finding in dendritic cell- and histiocyte-derived tumors. Leuk Lymphoma 2015;56:1132-1133.
4. Feldman AL, Arber DA, Pittaluga S, et al. Clonally related follicular lymphomas and histiocytic/dendritic cell sarcomas: evidence for transdifferentiation of the follicular lymphoma clone. Blood 2008;111:5433-5439.
5. Feltkamp CA, van Heerde P, Feltkamp-Vroom TM, Koudstaal J. A malignant tumor arising from interdigitating cells; light microscopical, ultrastructural, immuno- and enzyme-histochemical characteristics. Virchows Arch A Pathol Anat Histol 1981;393:183-192.
6. Fraser CR, Wang W, Gomez M, et al. Transformation of chronic lymphocytic leukemia/small lymphocytic lymphoma to interdigitating dendritic cell sarcoma: evidence for transdifferentiation of the lymphoma clone. Am J Clin Pathol 2009;132:928-939.
7. Gaertner EM, Tsokos M, Derringer GA, Neuhauser TS, Arciero C, Andriko JA. Interdigitating dendritic cell sarcoma. A report of 4 cases and review of the literature. Am J Clin Pathol 2001;115:589-597.
8. Lee SY, Lee SR, WJ Chang, Kim HS, Kim BS, Kim IS. Successful treatment of disseminated interdigitating dendritic cell sarcoma with adriamycin, bleomycin, vinblastine, and dacarbazine chemotherapy. Korean J Hematol 2012;47:150-153.
9. Lupato V, Romeo S, Franchi A, et al. Head and neck extranodal interdigitating dendritic cell sarcoma: case report and review of the literature. Head Neck Pathol 2016;10:145-151.
10. Ohtake H, Yamakawa M. Interdigitating dendritic cell sarcoma and follicular dendritic cell sarcoma: histopathological findings for differential diagnosis. J Clin Exp Hematop 2013;53:179-184.
11. O'Malley DP, Zuckerberg L, Smith LB, et al. The genetics of interdigitating dendritic cell sarcoma share some changes with Langerhans cell histiocytosis in select cases. Ann Diagn Pathol 2014;18:18-20.
12. Perkins SM, Shinohara ET. Interdigitating and follicular dendritic cell sarcomas: a SEER analysis. Am J Clin Oncol 2013;36:395-398.
13. Pileri SA, Grogan TM, Harris NL, et al. Tumours of histiocytes and accessory dendritic cells: an immunohistochemical approach to classification from the International Lymphoma Study Group based on 61 cases. Histopathology 2002,41:1-29.
14. Pillay K, Solomon R, Daubenton JD, Sinclair-Smith CC. Interdigitating dendritic cell sarcoma: a report of four paediatric cases and review of the literature. Histopathology 2004;44:283-291.
15. Pokuri VK, Merzianu M, Gandhi S, Baqai J, Loree TR, Bhat S. Interdigitating dendritic cell sarcoma. J Natl Compr Canc Netw 2015;13:128-132.

16. Saygin C, Uzunaslan D, Ozguroglu M, Senocak M, Tuzuner N. Dendritic cell sarcoma: a pooled analysis including 462 cases with presentation of our case series. Crit Rev Oncol Hematol 2013;88:253-271.

17. Stowman AM, Mills SE, Wick MR. Spindle cell melanoma and interdigitating dendritic cell sarcoma: Do they represent the same process? Am J Surg Pathol 2016;40:1270-1279.

18. Weiss LM, Grogan TM, Chan JK. Interdigitating dendritic cell sarcoma. In: Swerdlow SH, Campo E. Harris NL, et al. WHO classification of tumours of haematopoietic and lymphoid tissues. Lyon: IARC Press; 2008:361-362.

55 LANGERHANS CELL TUMORS

LANGERHANS CELL HISTIOCYTOSIS

Langerhans cell histiocytosis (LCH) is a proliferation of Langerhans cells that is monoclonal and thought to be neoplastic in most cases. Langerhans cells have a distinctive immunophenotype, positive for CD1a, langerin/CD207, and S-100 protein, and electron microscopy shows Birbeck granules in their cytoplasm (23,43a).

General Features

Langerhans cells are specialized cells with dendritic cell processes that normally reside in the skin and mucosal surfaces (5,7). In the epidermis, Langerhans cells represent 1 to 2 percent of all cells and function in immune surveillance. After epidermal Langerhans cells encounter antigen, they migrate to lymph nodes and present antigen to T cells in the context of MHC class I and II antigens (7).

In the embryo, Langerhans cells arise mostly from the fetal liver monocytes that populate the epidermis and mucosal surfaces prior to birth. Subsequently, Langerhans cells are maintained in a steady state by maturation from a subset of blood monocytes derived from a common dendritic precursor cell that originates in the bone marrow (5–7). Mature Langerhans cells do not reside in the bone marrow.

In the past, the cytologic and immunophenotypic similarities between normal epidermal Langerhans cells and the cells of LCH led to the suggestion that LCH is derived from epidermal Langerhans cells. This concept, however, seems unlikely in light of studies showing that langerin-positive dendritic cells are not unique to the skin, but are found in virtually all lymphoid and nonlymphoid tissues at low levels (14). In addition, gene expression profiling studies have shown that the cells of LCH have a profile similar to that of immature myeloid dendritic cell precursors, and different from epidermal Langerhans cells (2). Lastly, genetic studies assessing for *BRAF* mutations in LCH patients have shown

that the mutation is present in blood monocytes and bone marrow, in addition to involved tissue sites, in some patients (6).

Because of these results, Berres et al. (6) suggested that the stage of cell differentiation at the time of mutation may explain the highly varied clinical presentations of LCH. If a mutation occurs in a dendritic-myeloid precursor cell, patients will likely have mutated cells in the blood and present with multisystem, high clinical risk disease. In contrast, if the mutation occurs in a more differentiated, tissue-based cell with a Langerhans cell immunophenotype, patients may present with localized LCH (6).

LCH is an uncommon disease that affects 4 to 5 persons per million per year (23). In the United States, LCH most often affects Caucasians, particularly those of northern European descent, and is rare in African Americans. It also occurs in European and Asian countries (24,43). Both children and adults are affected by LCH.

The etiology of LCH may be multifactorial. An infectious origin has been suggested over the years, based on the common presence of inflammatory cells and the fact that LCH has been reported to be more common in the fall and winter seasons (43), but there otherwise is no strong support for this hypothesis. The lesions of LCH are negative for microorganisms including most known viruses. Murakimi et al. (30,31) identified evidence of Merkel cell polyoma virus by quantitative polymerase chain reaction (PCR)-based methods in a small subset of patients with high-risk LCH and Langerhans cell sarcoma; however, these observations need to be confirmed. A genetic predisposition is suggested because rarely LCH clusters in families and there is a high concordance rate in identical twins. An association with HLA-B7 also has been reported (48). The strongest evidence, however, supports the concept that LCH is neoplastic. Many cases of LCH are monoclonal and genetic abnormalities in the RAS pathway are common, leading to activation

Table 55-1

CLINICAL VARIANTS OF LANGERHANS CELL HISTIOCYTOSIS

Variant	Disease Extent	Age	Site Involved	Clinical Features
Solitary eosinophilic granuloma	Unifocal	Older children or adults	Solitary lytic bone lesions involving skull, femur, pelvis, or ribs; skin, lymph node	Erosion of adjacent bone
Hand-Schuller-Christian disease	Multifocal; unisystem	Young children	Multiple bone lesions	Skull involvement with exophthalmos, diabetes insipidus, tooth loss, fever, skin manifestations, hepatosplenomegaly
Letterer-Siwe disease	Multifocal; multisystem	Infants	Bone, liver, skin, spleen, lymph nodes	Bone lesions, pancytopenia

of extracellular signal-related kinase (ERK) which is likely involved in pathogenesis (4,9,46,50).

Clinical Features

The clinical presentation of patients with LCH is highly variable. As a result, a number of eponyms have been used to describe this disease over the years including eosinophilic granuloma, Hand-Schuller-Christian disease, and Letterer-Siwe disease (Table 55-1). These terms are mostly of historical value, although they are still used to describe the varied presentations of LCH. The term histiocytosis X was proposed by Lichtenstein in 1953 as an umbrella term to link together all forms of LCH; since the cell of origin was unclear at that time, the "X" was used (26). For a number of years this term was considered obsolete, but a recent review has suggested that the term may still have value (7).

Children most often develop LCH. Congenital cases occur rarely, usually involving the skin, and can progress or spontaneously regress. More commonly, LCH develops within the first decade of life, with the youngest patients more often having multisystem disease. Males are more often affected in a ratio ranging from 1.2 to 1 to over 3 to 1 in different studies. Localized disease (also known as solitary eosinophilic granuloma) commonly involves a bone, particularly the skull, femur, pelvic bones, or ribs, but can arise in skin, lymph nodes, or other sites. Patients with solitary eosinophilic granuloma tend to be older children or young adults. Skin is the second most common site of localized disease. Skin lesions in patients with LCH are highly variable and can present as nodules, papules, macules, blisters, or vascular tumor-like lesions, and uncommonly can spontaneously resolve (28). Skin lesions also may be part of multisystem disease.

Multifocal, unisystem disease most commonly involves bones, although other organ systems (e.g., lymph nodes) may be involved (23,37). A distinctive triad of features consists of punched-out lesions of the skull, shown by radiologic imaging, exophthalmos, and diabetes insipidus as a result of Langerhans cell infiltration (also known as Hand-Schuller-Christian disease). Multifocal, multisystem disease (Letterer-Siwe disease) involves bones, skin, liver, spleen, lymph nodes, and bone marrow (23,37). Lung involvement by LCH is most common in adults, is highly associated with smoking, and can resolve if smoking is discontinued in some patients.

The stage of disease is the most powerful prognostic factor for patients with LCH. Patients with unifocal disease (stage I) usually survive long-term. In contrast, patients with widespread disease (stage III or IV) require chemotherapy and have an appreciable mortality rate (3,24). Patient age of less than 2 years and involvement of bone marrow, spleen, or liver, are also adverse prognostic factors, but are less important and partially overlap with disease stage.

Histologic Findings

Lymph nodes may be the only site of disease or a part of multisystem involvement by LCH. Histologically, LCH can involve lymph nodes focally or extensively (18,23,37). When involvement is focal, LCH lesions tend to be located in the sinuses (fig. 55-1). With more extensive involvement, LCH involves and expands most of the sinuses (fig. 55-2), spreads into the paracortex (fig. 55-3), or uncommonly completely replaces the lymph node parenchyma. The Langerhans cells are often associated with a background inflammatory infiltrate of eosinophils, neutrophils, phagocytic histiocytes, and small lymphocytes (fig. 55-2, right). Eosinophils can be numerous and form microabscesses, with Charcot-Leyden crystals present in a some cases. Histiocytes may form foreign body-type or osteoclast-type multinucleated giant cells (fig. 55-4). In some cases, the histiocytes are numerous and exhibit lipid-laden (foamy) cytoplasm, in part obscuring the LCH cells. Uncommonly, these phagocytic histiocytes show emperipolesis, although this change is usually minimal. Necrosis can be focal or prominent in LCH lesions (fig. 55-3, right). In some cases, likely those more chronic or advanced, lipid-laden (foamy) histiocytes are numerous and associated with fibrosis. Plasma cells are usually not numerous in LCH lesions, but can be present in more chronic lesions.

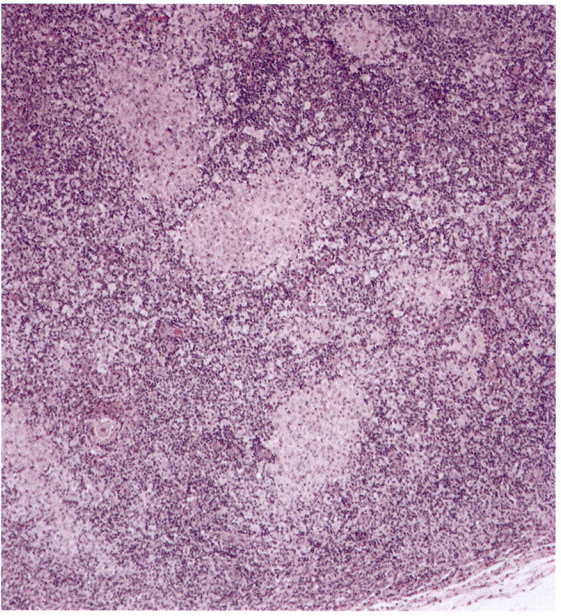

Figure 55-1

LANGERHANS CELL HISTIOCYTOSIS INVOLVING LYMPH NODE

There is a focal and sinusoidal pattern of involvement (hematoxylin and eosin [H&E] stain).

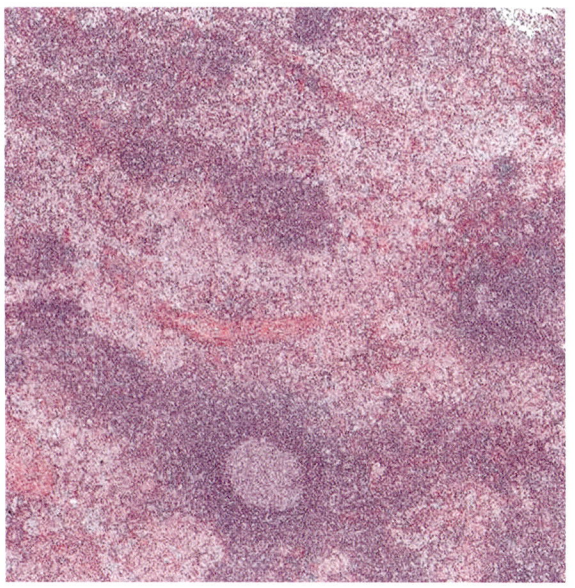

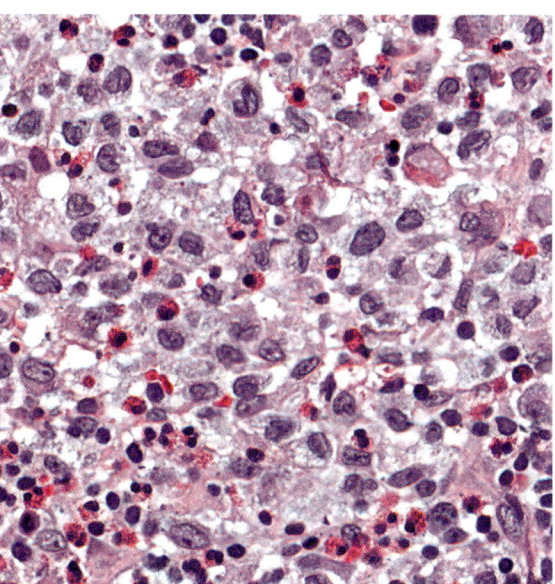

Figure 55-2

LANGERHANS CELL HISTIOCYTOSIS INVOLVING LYMPH NODE

Left: The sinuses are greatly expanded by Langerhans cell histiocytosis (LCH). Residual lymph node parenchyma, including a reactive follicle, is also seen.

Right: High magnification shows Langerhans cells in a background of eosinophils, small lymphocytes, and scattered macrophages. The Langerhans cells have nuclear grooves, thin and folded nuclear membranes, small nucleoli, and abundant pale cytoplasm (H&E stain).

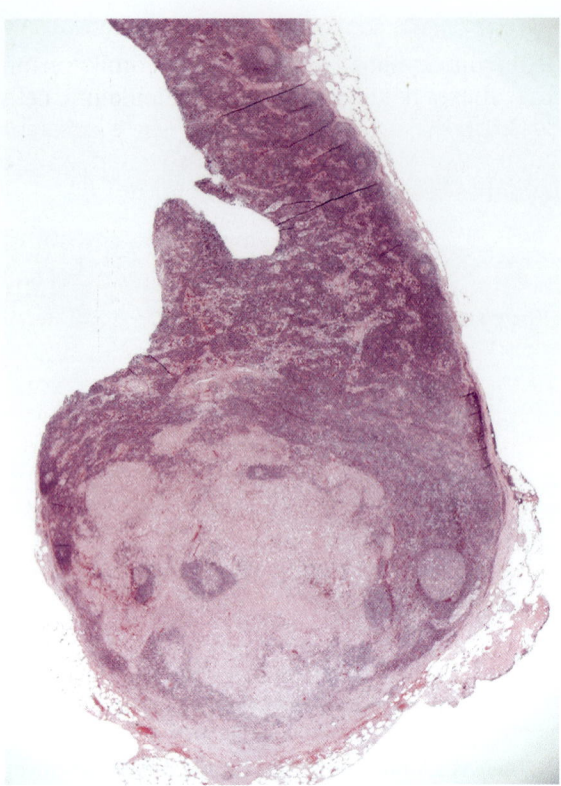
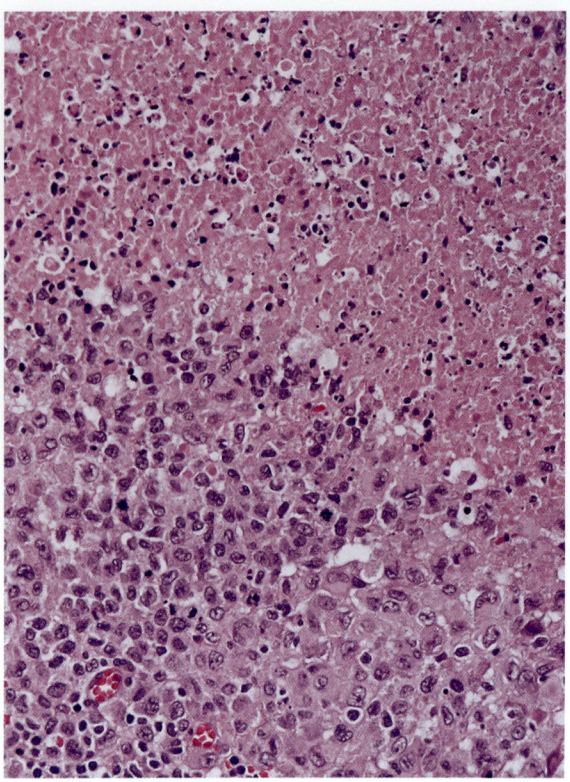

Figure 55-3

LANGERHANS CELL HISTIOCYTOSIS INVOLVING LYMPH NODE

Left: The lesion involves sinusoids but also extends into the paracortex, diffusely replacing the lymph node parenchyma.
Right: At high magnification, sheets of Langerhans cells are present (bottom of field) associated with coagulative necrosis (top of field). Mitotic figures also are seen in this field (H&E stain).

Figure 55-4

LANGERHANS CELL HISTIOCYTOSIS EXPANDING LYMPH NODE SINUS

The Langerhans cells are associated with clusters of eosinophils and histiocytic giant cells (H&E stain).

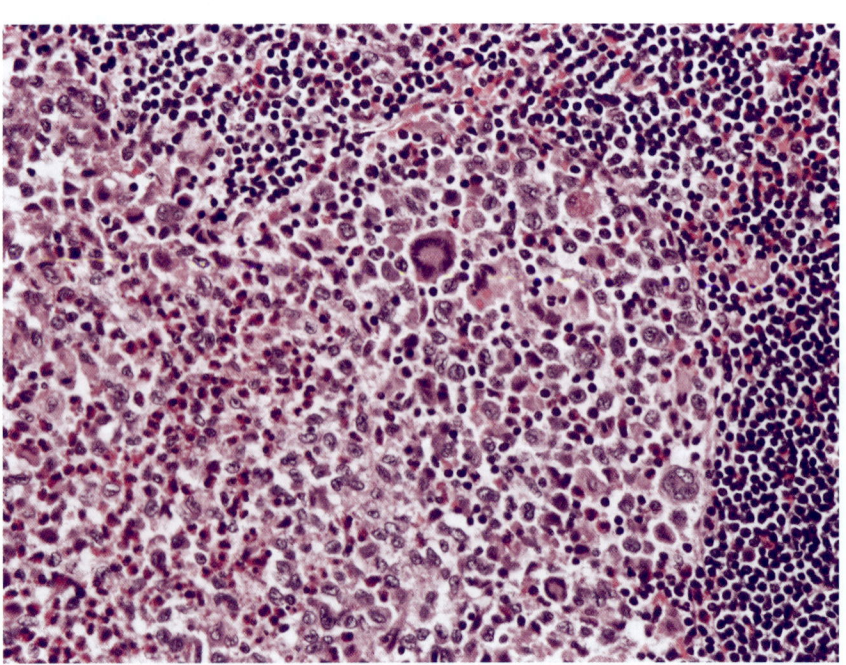

In hematoxylin and eosin (H&E)-stained tissue sections, Langerhans cells are 15 to 25 μm in size. They have abundant, eosinophilic cytoplasm and oval to folded nuclei with linear grooves ("twisted towel" appearance), delicate nuclear membranes, and inconspicuous nucleoli (fig. 55-2, right). Unlike normal epidermal Langerhans cells that have a dendritic morphology, the Langerhans cells in LCH lack dendritic cell processes and are oval or reniform. In rare cases, Langerhans cells may have a spindled shape. Mitotic figures are present in variable number, often few but numerous in some cases (fig. 55-3, right). Atypical mitotic figures are absent and cytologic atypia is absent or minimal.

Tumor-Associated Langerhans Cell Histiocytosis

LCH may be associated with other lymphoproliferative neoplasms. In lymph nodes, tumor-associated LCH is most often associated with classic Hodgkin lymphoma (fig. 55-5), but also with mantle cell lymphoma, diffuse large B-cell lymphoma, peripheral T-cell lymphoma not otherwise specified, and angioimmunoblastic T-cell lymphoma (16,35,38a).

Tumor-associated LCH is usually present as small foci confined to lymph node sinuses; these foci typically represent less than 5 percent of the lesion (fig. 55-5A,C). The lesion is composed of cytologically typical Langerhans cells, often associated with histiocytes, eosinophils, and small lymphocytes. The mixture of reactive cells and histiocytic giant cells common in fully developed LCH is less often present in tumor-associated LCH; necrosis can occur, but less often.

In most patients with lymph nodes involved by lymphoma and tumor-associated LCH, there is no evidence of LCH at other sites. Over 30 years ago, Neumann and Frizzera (35) suggested that these lesions were likely a form of Langerhans cell hyperplasia, and subsequent studies of tumor-associated LCH have not shown evidence of clonality supporting this hypothesis (16). In one study of seven cases of tumor-associated LCH there was no evidence of *BRAF* or *MAP2K1* mutations (38a).

Tumor-associated LCH needs to be distinguished from LCH associated with acute myeloid leukemia or other myeloid neoplasms (48). In these patients, the Langerhans cells are often clonally related to the leukemia. Following therapy, some patients with T- or B-cell acute lymphoblastic leukemia develop a Langerhans cell proliferation that shares the same clone as the leukemic cells (41). These forms of LCH are clearly different from the usually focal tumor-associated LCH in lymph nodes associated with lymphoma.

Cytologic Findings

Fine-needle aspirate specimens typically show Langerhans cells (fig. 55-6) admixed with a background of inflammatory cells (25). Similar to the features in H&E-stained tissue sections, Langerhans cells have oval to reniform nuclei with thin nuclear membranes and characteristic linear grooves, small nucleoli, and moderate to abundant eosinophilic cytoplasm (25). These nuclear features, and in particular, the nuclear grooves, are most readily identified on alcohol-fixed slides (fig. 55-6, right). The background inflammatory cells include small lymphocytes, histiocytes, multinucleated giant cells, eosinophils, and neutrophils in variable numbers (25). In some cases, eosinophils are numerous and Charcot-Leyden crystals are observed. In other cases, background histiocytes with lipid-laden (foamy) cytoplasm may be abundant. Rarely, phagocytic histiocytes may show emperipolesis in aspirate smears; the cells located within the histiocyte cytoplasm are usually small lymphocytes, but neutrophils or eosinophils may be numerous (15).

Immunophenotypic Findings

Neoplastic Langerhans cells are positive for S-100 protein (fig. 55-7, left), CD1a (fig. 55-7, right), langerin/CD207 (fig. 55-5), vimentin, HLA-DR, and CD68 (23,38). About half of cases express (often weakly) lysozyme and CD45/LCA. The cells of LCH also may be positive for CD4, CD11c, and CD14. Unlike normal or hyperplastic Langerhans cells, in LCH the Langerhans cells are commonly positive for cyclin D1 and phosphorylated ERK, consistent with MAPK pathway activation (42a). p53 and CD31 are also restricted to the cells of LCH (22). Langerhans cells are negative for pan-T-cell markers (e.g., CD2, CD3, CD5, and CD7), pan-B-cell markers (e.g., CD19, CD20, and CD79a), and markers of follicular dendritic cells (e.g., CD21, CD23, and CD35). The proliferation index, as assessed by immunohistochemical analysis for Ki-67, is typically low. The VE-1 (*BRAF* V600E specific) antibody highlights Langerhans

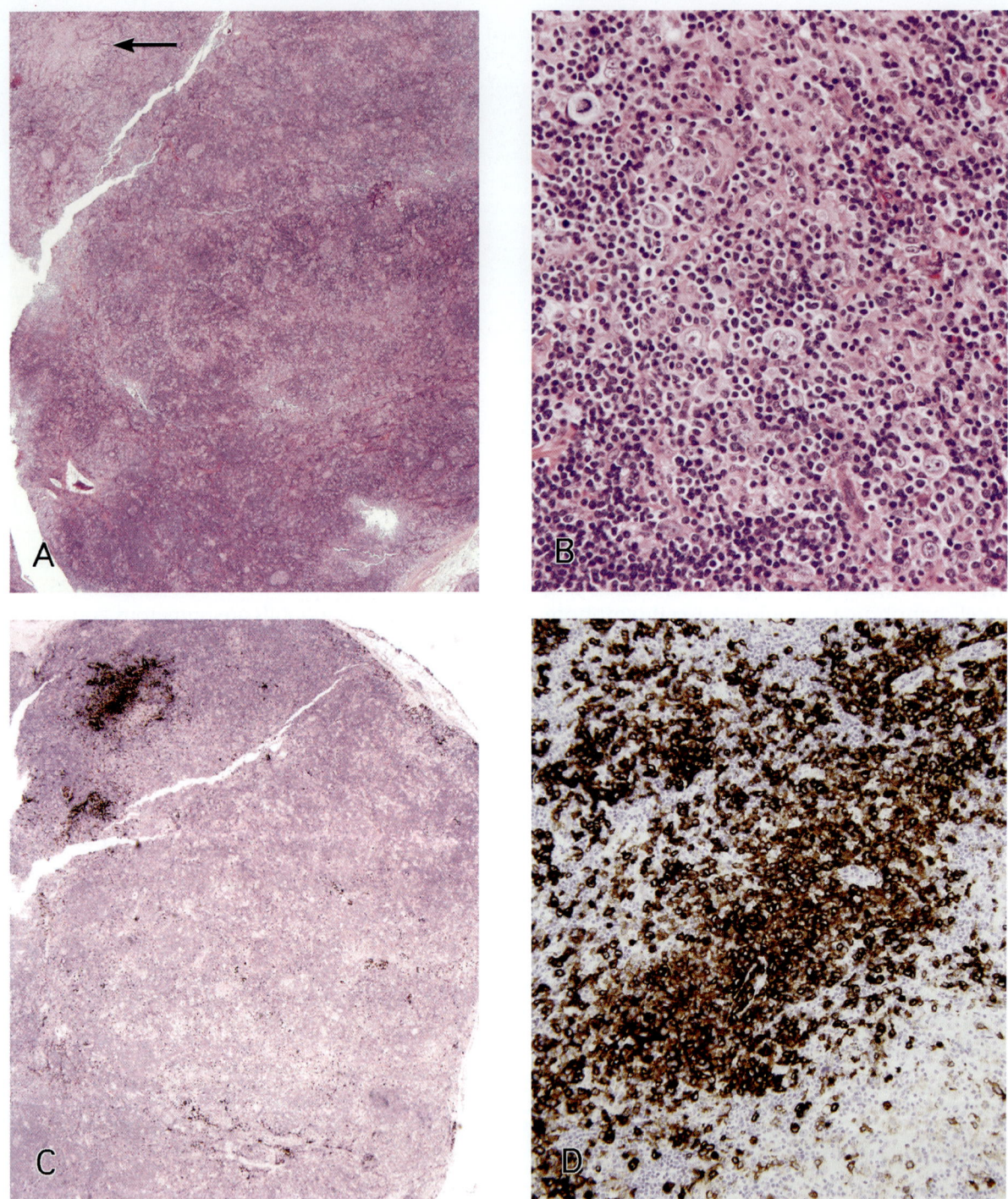

Figure 55-5

MIXED CELLULARITY HODGKIN LYMPHOMA ASSOCIATED WITH LANGERHANS CELL HISTIOCYTOSIS

A: A small (<5%) focus of tumor-associated LCH (arrow at upper left) involves a lymph node that is also involved by Hodgkin lymphoma (A,B: H&E stain).

B: High magnification of Hodgkin lymphoma; a Reed-Sternberg cell (center) and Hodgkin cells are present in the field.

C,D: Immunohistochemical analysis for langerin/CD207 highlights the small focus of LCH at low (C) and higher (D) magnification (C,D: immunohistochemistry with hematoxylin counterstain).

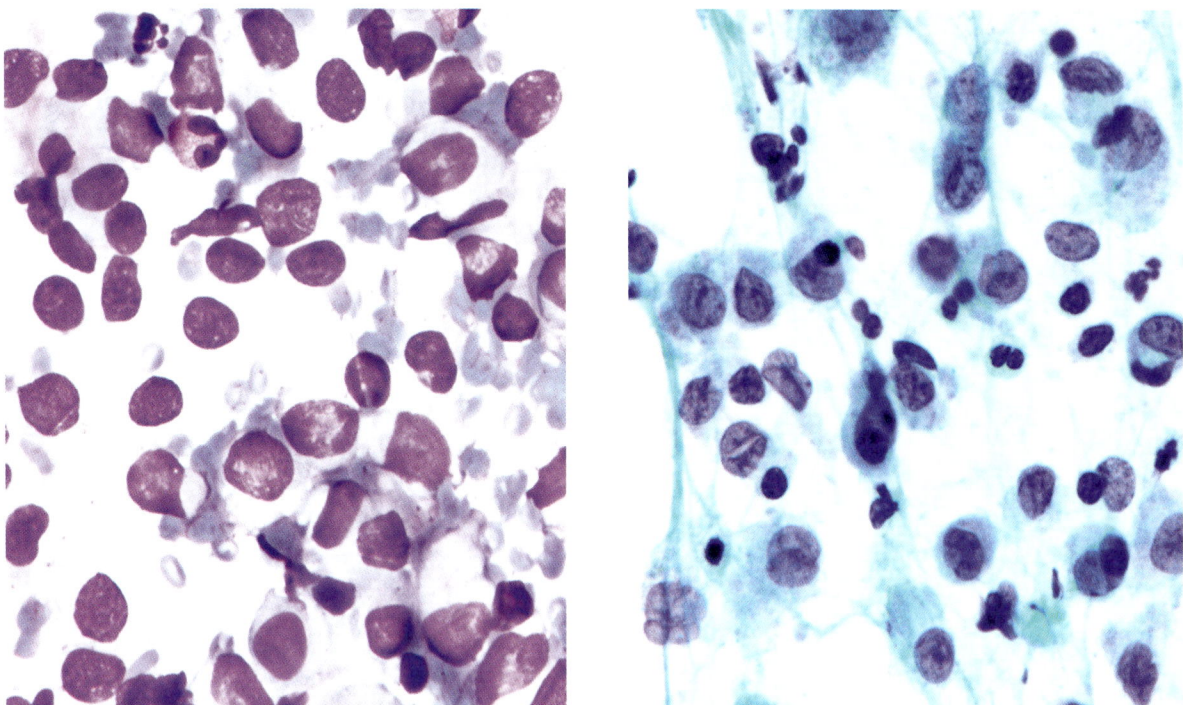

Figure 55-6

LANGERHANS CELL HISTIOCYTOSIS: CYTOLOGIC FINDINGS

Left, Right: Fine-needle aspirate smear shows Langerhans cells with nuclear grooves in a background of lymphocytes, neutrophils, and eosinophils (left: Diff-Quik stain; right: Papanicolaou stain).

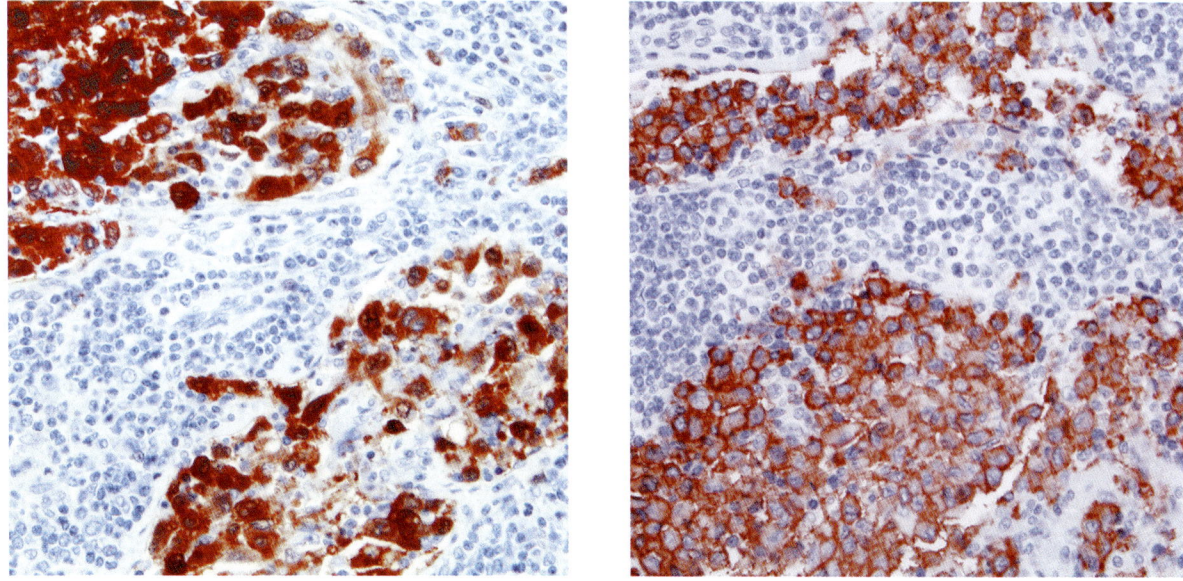

Figure 55-7

LANGERHANS CELL HISTIOCYTOSIS: IMMUNOHISTOCHEMISTRY

The Langerhans cells are positive for S-100 protein (left) and CD1a (right) (immunohistochemistry with hematoxylin counterstain).

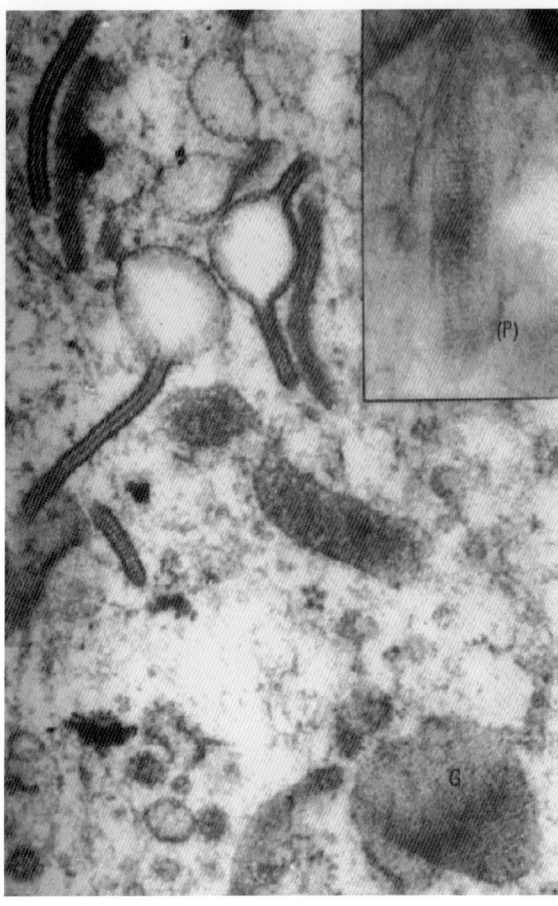

Figure 55-8

BIRBECK GRANULES IN THE CYTOPLASM OF A LANGERHANS CELL

Birbeck granules, seen in an electron micrograph, have a "tennis racket" shape and the linear portion also resembles a "zipper." The inset is a premelanin granule from a melanocyte for comparison (G = granule; P = premelanin granule). (Fig. 9 from Birbeck MS, Breathnach, AS, Everall JD. An electron microscope study of basal melanocytes and high-level clear cells (langerhans cells) in vitiligo. J Invest Dermatol 1961;37:51-64.)

cells in cases with the mutation (1,40,42). Enzyme cytochemical analysis has shown that Langerhans cells express α-naphthyl acetate esterase, α-naphthyl butyrate esterase, and acid phosphatase, and are negative for myeloperoxidase, tartrate-resistant acid phosphatase, and chloroacetate esterase. Osteoclast-type giant cells in LCH express tartrate-resistant acid phosphatase, CD68, and CD1a in some cases (17). The reactive cells associated with Langerhans cells in LCH have an immunophenotype appropriate for their lineage.

Ultrastructural Findings

Electron microscopy has value in the diagnosis of LCH although the role has been diminished because immunohistochemical analysis is more convenient. Langerhans cells contain distinctive cytoplasmic structures known as Birbeck granules. Each Birbeck granule has a "tennis racket" shape, with one bulbous end attached to a pentilaminar rod that is zipper-like (fig. 55-8). In three dimensions, Birbeck granules are composed of two tablet-like structures that meet at a 90 degree angle. The presence of Birbeck granules correlates highly with langerin expression. There is no evidence of junctional complexes, desmosomes, or interdigitating processes in LCH.

Molecular Genetic Findings

Conventional cytogenetic analysis of LCH lesions usually yields a diploid karyotype. In one study of seven bone lesions, comparative genomic hybridization showed recurrent gains at 2q, 4q, and 12 and recurrent losses at 1p, 5, 6, 7, 9, 16, 17, and 22q in about half of cases (29). However, other studies using comparative genomic hybridization or other high-throughput methods have not shown consistent abnormalities or were negative.

An important breakthrough in understanding LCH occurred in the 1994 when Yu et al. (50) and months later Willman et al. (46) used the human androgen receptor assay (HUMARA) to show that a large percentage of LCH cases are monoclonal. Most cases of LCH do not have rearrangements of the antigen receptor genes, especially if Southern blot analysis is used, as expected in histiocytic lesions that theoretically would not rearrange these genes (46). However, Chen et al. (13) reported monoclonal antigen receptor gene rearrangements detected by PCR-based methods in about one third of cases of LCH.

Recently, abnormalities of the RAS pathway, resulting in ERK activation, have been shown to be central to the pathogenesis of LCH. *BRAF* V600E mutations have been identified in various studies, with a frequency ranging from 25 to 70 percent (1,4,9,10,21). Subsequently, about half of LCH cases with wild type *BRAF* were shown to carry *MAP2K1* (encoding MEK) mutations (9,11). *BRAF* and *MAP2K1* mutations combined account for 70 to 80 percent of all LCH cases and these mutations are mutually exclusive (9,11). In 10 to 20 percent of LCH cases, other mutations in this pathway have been identified including *MAP3K1* (encoding MEKK1), *ARAF,* and *ERBB3* (11,33,34). In LCH cases negative for all known mutations, evidence of ERK activation also has been shown, suggesting that there may be other genes in the pathway that are mutated or that other, possibly post-transcriptional mechanisms may result in ERK activation (fig. 55-9). In most studies to date, the presence of gene mutations (present versus absent or *BRAF* V600E versus *MAP2K1*) has not correlated with any clinical features or anatomic sites of disease (1,4,9-11,21). Gene mutations seem to be less common in adults with LCH (1).

A clonal relationship between LCH and concurrent or preexistent follicular lymphoma or acute lymphoblastic leukemia has been documented in rare cases (41,45). West et al. (45) reported a patient with simultaneous follicular lymphoma and LCH involving the lymph nodes. Both components shared *IGH* rearrangements and an *IGH-BCL2* fusion. Transdifferentiation of the lymphoid neoplasm into LCH was thought most likely although other possible explanations, such as two independent neoplasms, could not be excluded entirely (45). Transdifferentiation is discussed in detail in chapter 52.

Differential Diagnosis

Langerhans Cell Sarcoma. Unlike LCH, Langerhans cell sarcoma is overtly malignant with cytologic atypia, many mitotic figures including atypical forms, and often necrosis. This entity is discussed in detail below.

Interdigitating Dendritic Cell Sarcoma (IDCS). These are very rare tumors that can diffusely involve lymph nodes (see chapter 54). They are cytologically malignant, with a high mitotic rate and common association with necrosis. The cells of IDCS express S-100 protein, similar to LCH, but are negative for CD1a and langerin. The neoplastic cells lack Birbeck granules.

Indeterminate Cell Tumor. Indeterminate cell tumors have been described most often in the skin. They may closely resemble LCH, but less often are associated with necrosis or eosinophilia. Indeterminate cell tumors are positive for S-100 protein and CD1a, but lack langerin/CD207, and Birbeck granules are not

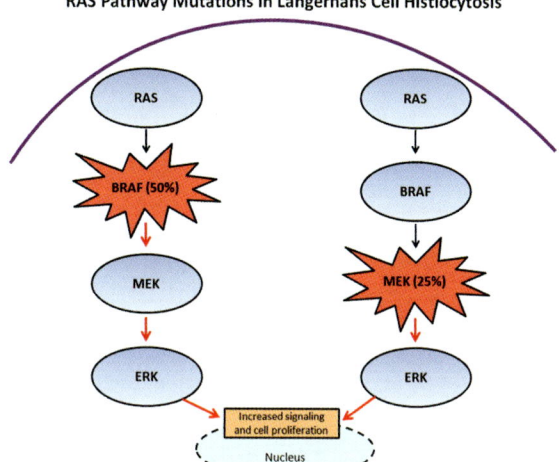

Figure 55-9

TWO MOST COMMON GENES MUTATED IN LANGERHANS CELL HISTIOCYTOSIS

In a schematic of the RAS pathway, *BRAF* is mutated in about 50 percent of cases and *MAP2K1* encoding MEK is mutated in about 25 percent. These mutations are mutually exclusive and result in activation of extracellular signal-related kinase (ERK). The purple line represents the cell membrane.

demonstrable by electron microscopy. Brown et al. (9a) identified *ETV3-NCOA2* gene fusions in 3 cases of indeterminate cell tumor, but not in 11 cases of LCH.

Dermatopathic Lymphadenopathy. Unlike LCH, lymph nodes with dermatopathic changes show expansion of the paracortex by numerous interdigitating dendritic cells, Langerhans cells, small lymphocytes, occasional eosinophils, and macrophages, including a few that contain pigment (fig. 55-10). Giant cells and necrosis are not features of dermatopathic lymphadenopathy. Interdigitating dendritic cells are positive for S-100 protein, but negative for CD1a and langerin whereas the Langerhans cells are positive for all three markers. Patients with LCH of skin may have regional lymph nodes that show dermatopathic lymphadenopathy. In this context, the presence of Langerhans cells in dermatopathic lymphadenopathy should not be over interpreted as LCH involving lymph node.

Rosai-Dorfman Disease (RDD). Like LCH, RDD begins in and expands lymph node sinuses. The RDD histiocytes, however, have distinctive cytologic features: plate-like cytoplasm

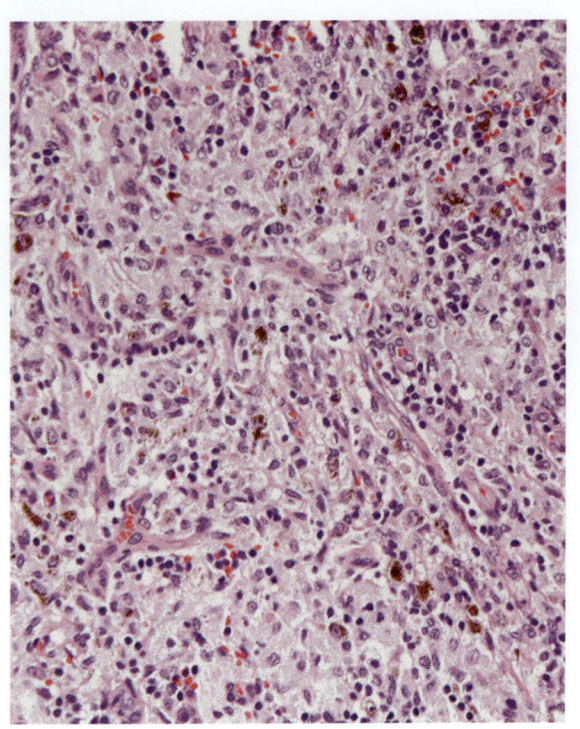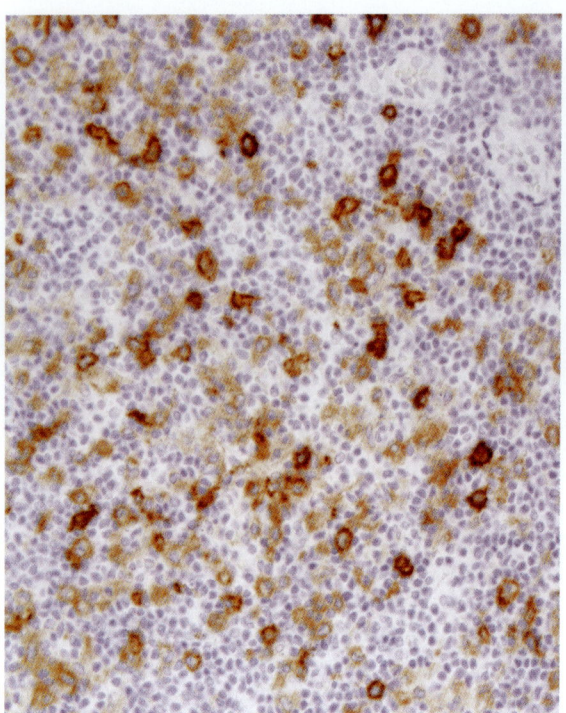

Figure 55-10

DERMATOPATHIC LYMPHADENOPATHY

Left: The lymph node parenchyma is replaced by many interdigitating dendritic cells, fewer Langerhans cells (indistinguishable from interdigitating dendritic cells in H&E sections), macrophages, and small T cells. Pigment is seen within macrophages (H&E stain).

Right: Scattered CD1a-positive Langerhans cells are highlighted (immunohistochemistry with hematoxylin counterstain).

with centrally located round nuclei and small, central nucleoli (fig. 55-11). The histiocytes also can show emperipolesis. In RDD, plasma cells are often numerous and eosinophils are infrequent; the converse is true in LCH. Rarely, LCH and RDD coexist in the same lymph node biopsy specimen (36). RDD, both in clinical and histologic images, is beautifully illustrated in the third series Fascicle on tumors of lymph node and spleen by Warnke et al. (44).

Cat Scratch Disease. Lymph nodes involved by cat scratch disease have stellate microabscesses located mostly in the paracortex; sinuses are not involved preferentially, unlike LCH. The microabscesses are composed of central areas of necrosis containing neutrophils surrounded by small lymphocytes, palisading histiocytes, and sometimes eosinophils (fig. 55-12). More chronic lesions may show abundant chronic granulomatous inflammation. Genetic analysis, cultures, or histochemical stains for the causative

organism, *Bartonella henselae*, support the diagnosis. The histiocytes in cat scratch disease do not resemble Langerhans cells and are negative for CD1a and langerin.

Kikuchi-Fujimoto Disease (KFD). Lymph nodes involved by the proliferative phase of KFD show a paracortical proliferation of histiocytes (many C shaped and CD68 positive), plasmacytoid dendritic cells (CD123 positive), immunoblasts, and small lymphocytes (fig. 55-13). The presence of apoptotic cells is a helpful diagnostic clue. More advanced cases of KFD show necrosis, which is often extensive without neutrophils. Unlike LCH, KFD is a paracortical-based rather than a sinusoidal-based process and the histiocytes neither resemble Langerhans cells nor express CD1a or langerin.

Treatment and Prognosis

The clinical course of LCH patients is related to the number of organs involved (stage

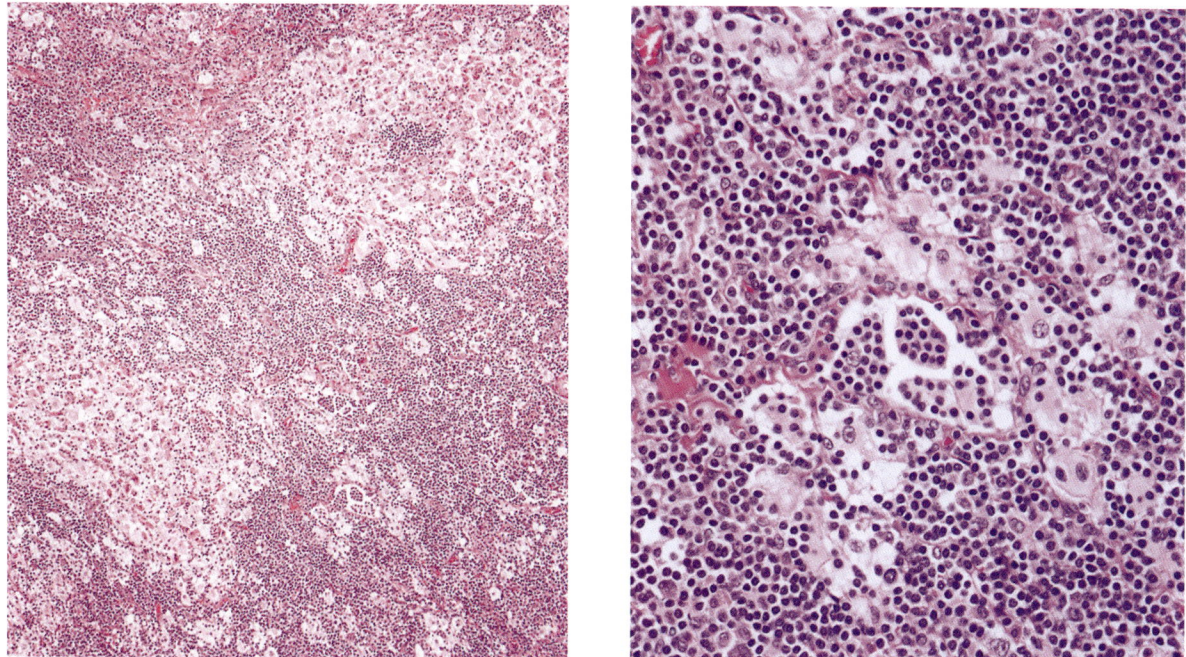

Figure 55-11

ROSAI-DORFMAN DISEASE

Left: In this lymph node Rosai-Dorfman disease (RDD) partially replaces the parenchyma and is mostly located in sinuses. The RDD histiocytes have abundant pale cytoplasm that is appreciated at low power magnification (A–C: H&E stain).

Right: The RDD histiocytes have abundant, pale, plate-like cytoplasm and central nuclei with nucleoli. Numerous small lymphocytes are present within the cytoplasm of some histiocytes, known as emperipolesis (center).

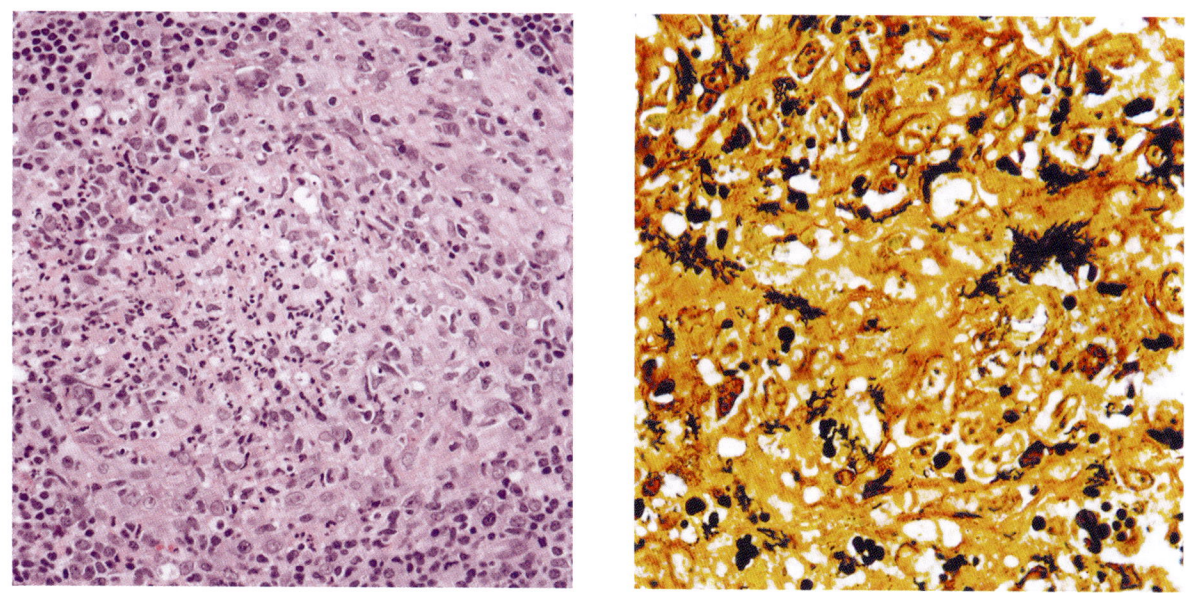

Figure 55-12

CAT SCRATCH DISEASE

Left: An area of the lymph node shows a granuloma with acute inflammatory cells (H&E stain).
Right: A Warthin-Starry stain highlights the *Bartonella henselae* organisms in this case.

Figure 55-13

KIKUCHI-FUJIMOTO DISEASE

A: Low-power magnification image of Kikuchi-Fujimoto lymphadenitis shows a paracortical-based process with extensive necrosis (H&E stain).

B: At the edge of the lesion the disease is proliferative and is characterized by many phagocytic histiocytes (many C shaped), plasmacytoid dendritic cells, immunoblasts, and apoptotic cells.

C: Fully necrotic areas show eosinophilic necrosis and a few apoptotic cells. Granulocytes are absent (A–C: H&E stain).

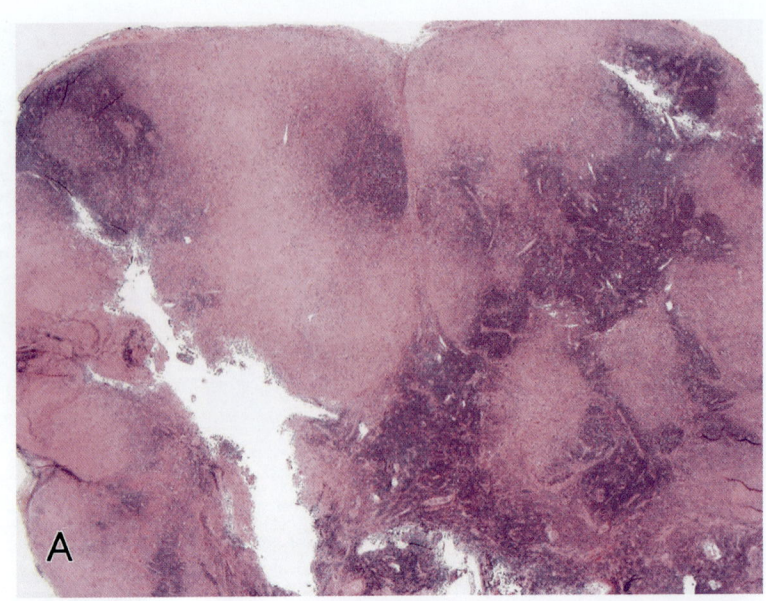

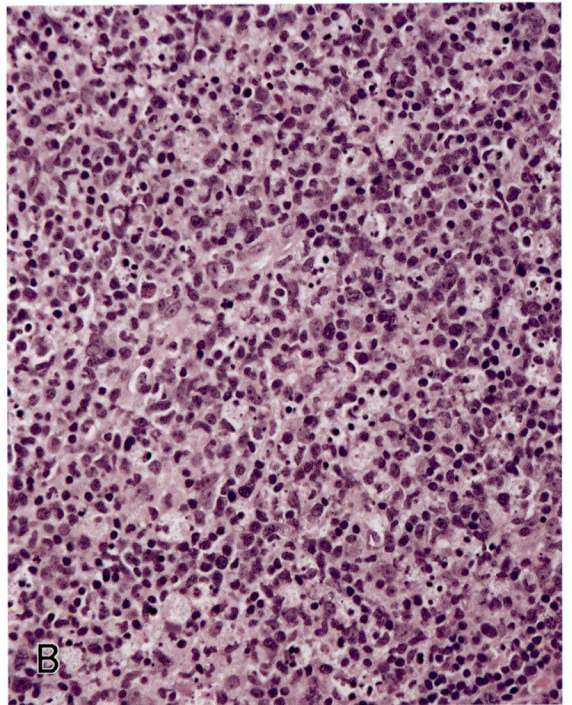

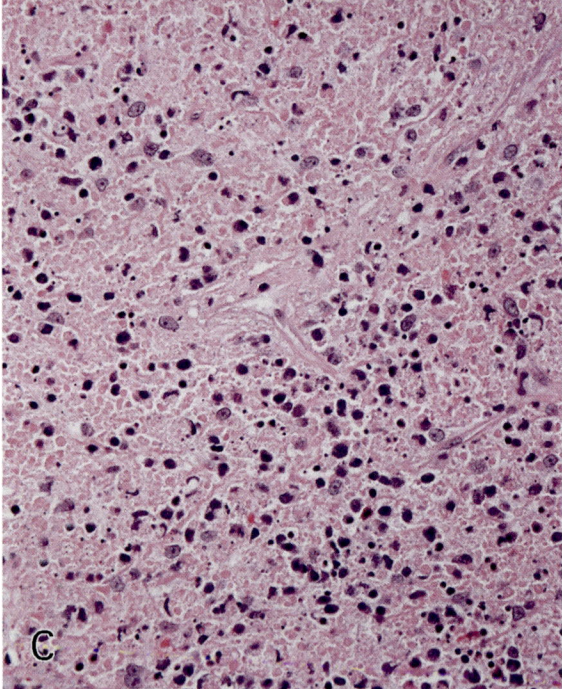

of disease) at time of diagnosis (3,23,24). The overall survival rate of patients with localized (unifocal) disease is high, over 95 percent, but drops to about 75 percent in patients with two or more organs affected. In a study from Korea, the 5-year overall survival rate was 99.8 percent for patients with single site disease, 98.4 percent for multisystem disease without involvement of high-risk organs (liver, spleen, bone marrow), and 77 percent for patients with multisystem disease with involvement of high-risk organs (24). For patients with multisystem disease, failure to respond to initial chemotherapy is a poor prognostic finding. Patients with unifocal disease may undergo regression, but uncommonly progress to multisystem disease.

Therapy is usually conservative for patients with localized LCH. Patients with advanced stage disease and symptoms require chemotherapy. Vinblastine and prednisone, with or without methotrexate, etoposide, and mercaptopurine for patients with involvement of high-risk organs, has been a common approach (3,24). Cladribine also has been used with some success and a subset of patients has been treated by hematopoietic stem cell transplantation. The identification of gene mutations in the RAS pathway, particularly *BRAF* V600E and *MAP2K1* mutations, suggest a potential role for BRAF and MEK inhibitors, and small numbers of LCH patients have shown promising responses (3).

LANGERHANS CELL SARCOMA

Langerhans cell sarcoma is an overtly malignant neoplasm composed of cells that retain the immunophenotypic and ultrastructural features of Langerhans cells (23).

General Features

Langerhans cell sarcoma is a truly rare disease that is far less common than LCH. In a review of the literature, Zwerding et al. (51) identified 53 cases. The epidemiologic features of Langerhans cell sarcoma seem to differ from LCH. The etiology is unknown.

Clinical Features

The median age of patients with Langerhans cell sarcoma is 39 years, but the age range is broad, from 10 to 72 years (8,38). Few children with Langerhans cell sarcoma have been reported (23,51). Women appear to be affected more often than in LCH. The male to female ratio is about 1 to 2.

Patients with Langerhans cell sarcoma may present with localized disease involving the skin or soft tissue, or may have widely disseminated disease with involvement of lymph nodes and visceral organs (8,19,23,51). Advanced stage disease (stage III to IV) is present in approximately half of patients and 10 percent present with pancytopenia.

Histologic Findings

Langerhans cell sarcoma may resemble LCH or an undifferentiated sarcoma, recognized as being of Langerhans cell lineage only following immunohistochemical analysis (23,51). All cases are characterized by overt nuclear atypia and increased mitotic activity (fig. 55-14). Mitotic figures can be numerous, more than 50 per 10 high-power fields. Necrosis is common and can be extensive. Eosinophils are infrequent or absent.

Cytologic Findings

Rare cases of Langerhans cell sarcoma assessed by fine-needle aspiration show large neoplastic cells with scant to moderate amounts of basophilic cytoplasm (fig. 55-15) (27). The nuclei have irregular contours and indentations. Scattered binucleated and multinucleated cells may be seen. Mitotic figures are common. Small lymphocytes, neutrophils, and sparse eosinophils may be observed in the background (27).

Immunophenotypic Findings

The neoplastic cells of Langerhans cell sarcoma express langerin, at least focally. S-100 protein or CD1a reactivity is also present but is less specific (23,51). The neoplastic cells also may express histiocyte-associated markers, such as lysozyme and CD68, although often weakly. Aberrant expression of CD3 has been reported (47) and the proliferation rate, as assessed by Ki-67, is characteristically high (fig. 55-14D).

Molecular Genetic Findings

Few cases of Langerhans cell sarcoma have been assessed by conventional cytogenetics or molecular methods. The *BRAF* V600E mutation has been identified in these tumors, but the frequency is uncertain as few cases have been assessed (51).

A clonal relationship between Langerhans cell sarcoma and concurrent or preexistent lymphoid malignancies has been documented and is considered evidence of transdifferentiation (12,20,45). The evidence for clonality includes shared monoclonal *IGH* rearrangements or a *BRAF* V600E mutation. The lymphoid tumors involved include follicular lymphoma, chronic lymphocytic leukemia/small lymphocytic lymphoma, hairy cell leukemia, and acute lymphoblastic leukemia (12,32,39,45).

Treatment and Prognosis

Langerhans cell sarcoma is an aggressive neoplasm with a poor prognosis and an appreciable mortality rate (51). There is no consensus regarding optimal therapy for these patients.

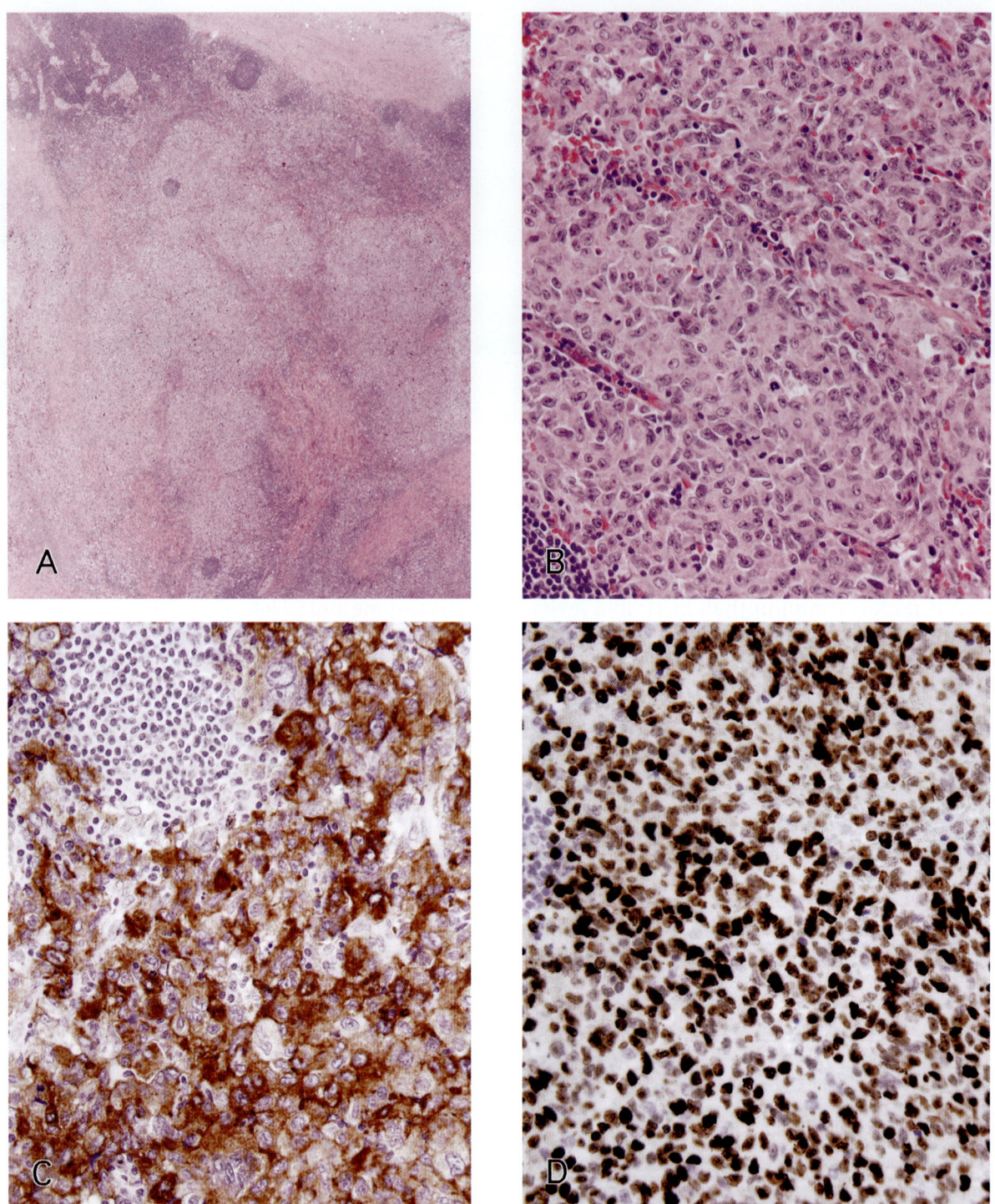

Figure 55-14

LANGERHANS CELL SARCOMA INVOLVING LYMPH NODE

A: The neoplasm extensively replaces the lymph node parenchyma with epithelioid and spindled areas (A,B: H&E stain).
B: The cells have an oval or spindle shape and exhibit nuclear atypia and mitotic figures.
C,D: The neoplastic cells are positive for CD1a (C) and langerin (not shown) and have a high proliferation rate as shown by Ki-67 (D) (C,D: immunohistochemistry with hematoxylin counterstain).

Figure 55-15

CYTOSPIN PREPARATION OF LANGERHANS CELL SARCOMA

Pleomorphic cells with large irregular or indented nuclei, often containing nucleoli, and scant to moderately abundant cytoplasm, are seen in this case. A large binucleated cell is also present (Diff-Quik stain). (Courtesy of Dr. J. Stewart, Houston, Texas.)

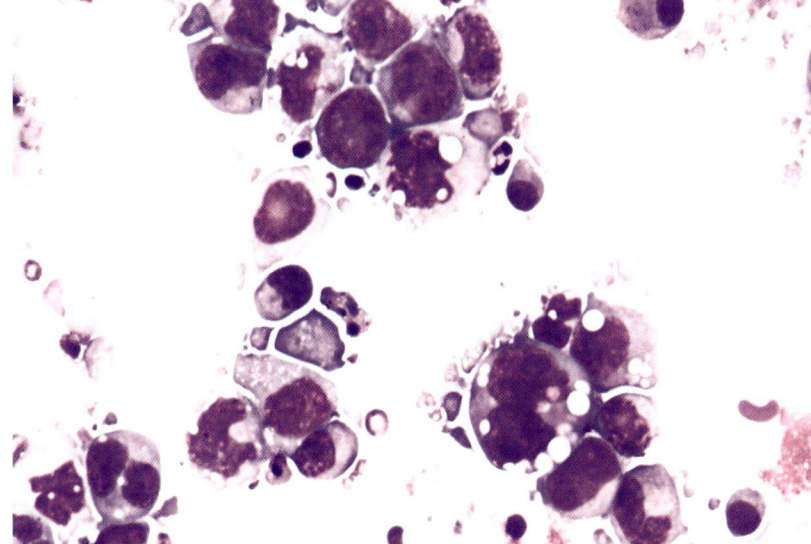

REFERENCES

1. Alayed K, Medeiros LJ, Patel KP, et al. BRAF and MAP2K1 mutations in Langerhans cell histiocytosis: a study of 50 cases. Hum Pathol 2016;52:61-67.
2. Allen CE, Li L, Peters TL, et al. Cell-specific gene expression in Langerhans cell histiocytosis lesions reveals a distinct profile compared with epidermal Langerhans cells. J Immunol 2010;184:4557-4567.
3. Aricò M. Langerhans cell histiocytosis in children: from the bench to bedside for an updated therapy. Br J Haematol 2016;173:663-670.
4. Badalian-Very G, Vergilio JA, Degar BA, et al. Recurrent BRAF mutations in Langerhans cell histiocytosis. Blood 2010;116:1919-1923.
5. Bechan GI, Egeler RM, Arceci RJ. Biology of Langerhans cells and Langerhans cell histiocytosis. Int Rev Cytol 2006;254:1-43.
6. Berres ML, Lim KP, Peters T, et al. BRAF-V600E expression in precursor versus differentiated dendritic cells defines clinically distinct LCH risk groups. J Exp Med 2014;211:669-683.
7. Berres ML, Merad M, Allen CE. Progress in understanding the pathogenesis of Langerhans cell histiocytosis: back to histiocytosis X? Br J Haematol 2015;169:3-13.
8. Bohn OL, Ruiz-Arguelles G, Navarro L, Saldivar J, Sanchez-Sosa S. Cutaneous Langerhans cell sarcoma: a case report and review of the literature. Int J Hematol 2007;85:116-120.
9. Brown NA, Furtado LV, Betz BL, et al. High prevalence of somatic MAP2K1 mutations in BRAF V600E-negative Langerhans cell histiocytosis. Blood 2014;124:1655-1658.
9a. Brown RA, Kwong BY, McCalmont TH, et al. ETV3-NCOA2 in indeterminate cell histiocytosis: clonal translocation supports sui generis. Blood 2015;126:2344-2345.
10. Bubolz AM, Weissinger SE, Stenzinger A, et al. Potential clinical implications of BRAF mutations in histiocytic proliferations. Oncotarget 2014;5:4060-4070.
11. Chakraborty R, Hampton OA, Shen X, et al. Mutually exclusive recurrent somatic mutations in MAP2K1 and BRAF support a central role for ERK activation in LCH pathogenesis. Blood 2014;124:3007-3015.
12. Chen W, Jaffe R, Zhang L, et al. Langerhans cell sarcoma arising from chronic lymphocytic lymphoma/small lymphocytic leukemia: lineage analysis and BRAF V600E mutation study. N Am J Med Sci 2013;5:386-391.
13. Chen W, Wang J, Wang E, et al. Detection of clonal lymphoid receptor gene rearrangements in Langerhans cell histiocytosis. Am J Surg Pathol 2010;34:1049-1057.

14. Chikwava K, Jaffe R. Langerin (CD207) staining in normal pediatric tissues, reactive lymph nodes, and childhood histiocytic disorders. Pediatr Dev Pathol 2004;7:607-614.

15. Chougule A, Srivastava S, Totadri S, Srinivasan R, Trehan A. Nodal Langerhans cell histiocytosis with prominent eosinophilic emperipolesis. Diagn Cytopathol 2015;43:1000-1002.

16. Christie LJ, Evans AT, Bray SE, et al. Lesions resmbling Langerhans cell histiocytosis in association with other lymphoproliferative disorders: a reactive or neoplastic phenomenon? Hum Pathol 2006;37:32-39.

17. da Costa CE, Annels NE, Faaij CM, Forsyth RG, Hogendoorn PC, Egeler RM. Presence of osteoclast-like multinuclear giants cells in the bone and monostotic lesions of Langerhans cell histiocytosis. J Exp Med 2005;201:687-693.

18. Edelweiss M, Medeiros LJ, Suster S, Moran CA. Lymph node involvement by Langerhans cell histiocytosis: a clinicopathologic and immunohistochemical study of 20 cases. Hum Pathol 2007;38:1463-1469.

19. Ferringer T, Banks PM, Metcalf JS. Langerhans cell sarcoma. Am J Dermatopathol 2006;28:36-39.

20. Furmanczyk PS, Lisle AE, Caldwell RB, et al. Langerhans cell sarcoma in a patient with hairy cell leukemia: common clonal origin indicated by identical immunoglobulin gene rearrangements. J Cutan Pathol 2012;39:644-650.

21. Go H, Jeon YK, Huh J, et al. Frequent detection of BRAF(V) (600E) mutations in histiocytic and dendritic cell neoplasms. Histopathology 2014;65:261-272.

22. Grace SA, Sutton AM, Armbrecht ES, Vidal CI, Rosman IS, Hurley MY. p53 Is a helpful marker in distinguishing Langerhans cell histiocytosis from Langerhans cell hyperplasia. Am J Dermatopathol 2016. [Epub ahead of print]

23. Jaffe R, Weiss LM, Facchetti F. Tumours derived from Langerhans cells. In: Swerdlow SH, Campo E, Harris NL, et al., eds. WHO classification of tumours of hematopoietic and lymphoid tissues. Lyon: IARC Press; 2008;358-360.

24. Kim BE, Koh KN, Suh JK, et al. Clinical features and treatment outcomes of Langerhans cell histiocytosis: a nationwide survey from Korea histiocytosis working party. J Pedriatr Hematol Oncol 2014;36:125-133.

25. Kumar PV, Mousavi A, Karimi M, Bedayat GR. Fine needle aspiration of Langerhans cell histiocytosis of the lymph nodes. A report of six cases. Acta Cytol 2002;46:753-756.

26. Lichtenstein L. Histiocytosis X; integration of eosinophilic granuloma of bone, Letterer-Siwe disease, and Schüller-Christian disease as related manifestations of a single nosologic entity. Arch Pathol 1953;56: 84-102

27. Lopez-Ferrer P, Jimenez-Heffernan JA, Alves-Ferreira J, Vicandi B, Viguer JM. Fine needle aspiration cytology of Langerhans cell sarcoma. Cytopathology 2008;19:59-61.

28. Morren MA, Vanden Broecke K, Vangeebergen L, et al. Diverse cutaneous presentations of Langerhans cell histiocytosis in children: a retrospective cohort study. Pediatr Blood Cancer 2016;63:486-492.

29. Murakami I, Gogusev J, Fournet JC, Glorion C, Jaubert F. Detection of molecular cytogenetic aberrations in Langerhans cell histiocytosis of bone. Hum Pathol 2002;33:555-560.

30. Murakami I, Matsushita M, Iwasaki T, et al. High viral load of Merkel cell polyomavirus DNA sequences in Langerhans cell sarcoma tissues. Infect Agent Cancer 2014;9:15

31. Murakami I, Matsushita M, Iwasaki T, et al. Merkel cell polyomavirus DNA sequences in peripheral blood and tissues from patients with Langerhans cell histiocytosis. Human Pathol 2014;45:119-126.

32. Muslimani A, Chisti MM, Blenc AM, Boxwala I, Micale MA, Jaiyesimi I. Langerhans/dendritic cell sarcoma arising from hairy cell leukemia: a rare phenomenon. Ann Hematol 2012;91:1485-1487.

33. Nelson DS, Quispel W, Badalian-Very G, et al. Somatic activating ARAF mutations in Langerhans cell histiocytosis. Blood 2014;123:3152-3155.

34. Nelson DS, Van Halteren A, Quispel WT, et al. MAP2K1 and MAP3K1 mutations in Langerhans cell histiocytosis. Genes Chromosomes Cancer 2015;54:361-368.

35. Neumann MP, Frizzera G. The coexistence of Langerhans' cell granulomatosis and malignant lymphoma may take different forms: report of seven cases with a review of the literature. Hum Pathol 1986;17:1060-1065.

36 O'Malley DP, Duong A, Barry TS, et al. Co-occurrence of Langerhans cell histiocytosis and Rosai-Dorfman disease: possible relationship of two histiocytic disorders in rare cases. Mod Pathol 2010;23:1616-1623.

37. Picarsic J, Jaffe R. Nosology and pathology of Langerhans cell histiocytosis. Hematol Oncol Clin North Am 2015;29:799-823.

38. Pileri SA, Grogan TM, Harris NL, et al. Tumours of histiocytes and accessory dendritic cells: an immunohistochemical approach to classification from the International Lymphoma Study Group based on 61 cases. Histopathology 2002;41:1-29.

38a. Pina-Oviedo S, Medeiros LJ, Li S, et al. Langerhans cell histiocytosis associated with lymphoma: an incidental finding that is not associated with BRAF or MAP2K1 mutations. Mod Pathol 2017;30:734-744.

39. Ratei R, Hummel M, Anagnostopoulos I, et al. Common clonal origin of an acute B-lymphoblastic leukemia and a Langerhans' cell sarcoma: evidence for hematopoietic plasticity. Haematologica 2010; 95:1461-1466.

40. Roden AC, Hu X, Kip S, et al. BRAF V600E expression in Langerhans cell histiocytosis. Clinical and immunohistochemical study on 25 pulmonary and 54 extrapulmonary cases. Am J Surg Pathol 2014;38:548-551.

41. Rodig SJ, Payne EG, Degar BA, et al. Aggressive Langerhans cell histiocytosis following T-ALL: clonally related neoplasms with persistent expression of constitutively active NOTCH1. Am J Hematol 2008;83:116-121.

42. Sahm F, Capper D, Preuser M, et al. BRAFV600E mutant protein is expressed in cells of variable maturation in Langerhans cell histiocytosis. Blood 2012;120:e28-e34.

42a. Shanmugam V, Craig JW, Hornick JL, Morgan EA, Pinkus GS, Pozdnyakova O. Cyclin D1 is expressed in neoplastic cells of langerhans cell histiocytosis but not reactive Langerhans cell proliferations. Am J Surg Pathol 2017. [Epub ahead of print]

43. Stalemark H, Laurencikas E, Karis J, Gavhed D, Fadeel B, Henter JI. Incidence of Langerhans cell histiocytosis in children: a population-based study. Pediatr Blood Cancer 2008;51:76-81.

43a. Swerdlow SH, Campo E, Pileri SA, et al. The 2016 revision of the World Health Organization classification of lymphoid neoplasms. Blood 2016;127:2375-2390.

44. Warnke RA, Weiss LM, Chan JK, Cleary ML, Dorfman RF. Tumors of the lymph nodes and spleen. AFIP Atlas of Tumor Pathology, 3rd Series, Fasicle 14. Washington, DC: American Registry of Pathology; 1994;349-360.

45. West DS, Dogan A, Quint PS, et al. Clonally related follicular lymphomas and Langerhans cell neoplasms: expanding the spectrum of transdifferentiation. Am J Surg Pathol 2013;37:978-986.

46. Willman CL, Busque L, Griffith BB, et al. Langerhans'-cell histiocytosis (histiocytosis X) – a clonal proliferative disease. N Engl J Med 1994;331:154-160.

47. Xu Z, Padmore R, Faught CD, Duffet L, Burns BF. Langerhans cell sarcoma with an aberrant cytoplasmic CD3 expression. Diagn Pathol 2012;7:128.

48. Yohe SL, Chenault CB, Torlakovic EE, Asplund SL, McKenna RW. Langerhans cell histiocytosis in acute leukemias of ambiguous or myeloid lineage in adult patients: support for a possible clonal relationship. Mod Pathol 2014;27:651-656.

49. Yu RC, Chu AC. Langerhans cell histiocytosis—clinicopathological reappraisal and human leukocyte antigen association. Br J Dermatol 1996;135:36-41.

50. Yu RC, Chu C, Buluwela L, Chu AC. Clonal proliferation of Langerhans cells in Langerhans cell histiocytosis. Lancet 1994;343:767-768.

51. Zwerding T, Won E, Shane L, Javahara R, Jaffe R. Langerhans cell sarcoma: case report and review of world literature. J Pediatr Hematol Oncol 2014;36:419-425.

56 HAIRY CELL LEUKEMIA

GENERAL FEATURES

Hairy cell leukemia (HCL) is a clinically indolent, small B-cell lymphoproliferative disorder that usually involves the peripheral blood, bone marrow, and spleen (13,38a). In smears, the neoplastic lymphocytes usually have hair-like cytoplasmic projections; this feature accounts for the distinctive name of this neoplasm.

As reviewed by Andritsos and Grever (1), HCL has a long history of almost 100 years. The disease was initially designated as *leukemic reticuloendotheliosis* in the German literature by Ewald in 1923. In retrospect, however, it seems clear that the initial description included more than one entity, for example, acute monocytic leukemia. Bertha Bouroncle et al. (1) at Ohio State University more fully described leukemic reticuloendotheliosis in 1958 and she deserves much of the credit for our current understanding of the clinical and pathologic features of this neoplasm. The designation *hairy cell* was proposed initially by Schrek and Donnelly in 1966 (32). The term hairy cell leukemia became popular following an important publication by Catovsky et al. in the United Kingdom (6).

Among leukemias, HCL is uncommon, representing only 2 percent of all cases. The incidence of HCL in the United States is 0.33 cases per 100,000 person-years or approximately 600 new cases per year (13,27). HCL occurs most often in Caucasians, who develop the disease three times more frequently than other races; the geographic distribution of HCL reflects this racial preference (39). HCL is rare in Asia. A disease in Japan known as the Japanese variant of HCL is more closely related to the hairy cell leukemia variant (see chapter 57).

The etiology of HCL is unknown. There are some reports of HCL running in families, suggesting a possible genetic predisposition for this disorder (7,8,46). Farmers have an increased risk of HCL, suggesting an etiologic role for occupational exposure (27,39). Exposure to pesticides, petroleum products, and ionizing radiation has been linked to an increased risk of HCL (39). Adult height also has been positively associated with HCL, the importance of which is unclear (27). Cigarette smoking does not appear to be a risk factor (39). Patients with HCL also may have autoimmune disorders, pointing to a possible role for autoimmunity. As reviewed by Tadmor and Polliak (40), associated autoimmune diseases include sarcoidosis, Sjögren syndrome, erythema nodosum, vasculitis, immune cytopenias, Guillain-Barre syndrome, and Behçet disease (40). HCL patients also have a higher risk of second malignancies, most commonly non-Hodgkin lymphoma, Hodgkin lymphoma, and thyroid and lung carcinomas (24,40).

CLINICAL FEATURES

Patients with HCL tend to be middle-aged or older with a median age of 55 years. The disease most often affects men in a ratio of 3.5-4 to 1 (13,19,39). Patients with well-developed disease commonly present with weakness, fatigue, and left upper quadrant fullness, and are predisposed to infections (15,19). Physical examination commonly shows palpable and often massive splenomegaly and hepatomegaly (Table 56-1). Lymphadenopathy is present in about 20 percent of patients at time of initial diagnosis and is often located below the diaphragm (and detected by radiologic studies). Laboratory studies often show anemia, leukopenia, and especially pronounced monocytopenia (13,19,40). Leukocytosis of greater than 10×10^9/L is observed in approximately 10 percent of HCL patients. A monoclonal paraprotein is present uncommonly. Rare cases of HCL present as localized bone disease (21,37).

Although these clinical findings still occur in a subset of HCL patients, with the advent of sensitive methods of diagnosis the presentation of HCL patients has evolved. The disease is often detected earlier in its course, when the

Table 56-1
CLINICAL FINDINGS AND LABORATORY FEATURES IN PATIENTS WITH HAIRY CELL LEUKEMIA

Clinical findings	Frequency
Splenomegaly	60-70%
Hepatomegaly	40-50%
Abdominal lymph node enlargement[a]	15-20%
Laboratory features	
Hairy cells in peripheral blood smear	95%
Monocytopenia: < 0-1 x 10^9/L	90%
Thrombocytopenia	80%
Neutropenia: <1 x 10^9/L	75%
Anemia: Hb < 100 g/L	70%
White blood cell count: < 5 x 10^9/L	65%

[a]By computerized tomography scan investigation.

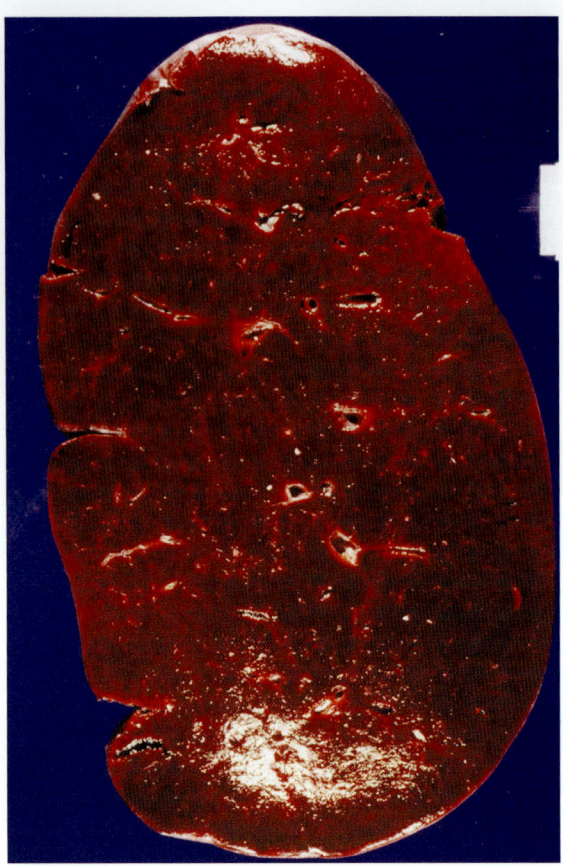

Figure 56-1

HAIRY CELL LEUKEMIA INVOLVING SPLEEN

In this extensively involved spleen, a beefy red appearance is seen, which is typical for processes that diffusely expand the red pulp.

disease burden is lower. HCL can be diagnosed incidentally by hematologic examination as part of a routine checkup or during the workup of other potential diseases.

GROSS FINDINGS

The spleen is enlarged, ranging from 250 to 4,600 g (normal weight, about 170 g or less) (13,15). HCL preferentially involves the red pulp, imparting a red, beefy appearance (fig. 56-1). Blood lakes (described below) may be appreciated grossly as small, cystic, blood-filled spaces in the parenchyma.

HISTOLOGIC FINDINGS

Spleen

The red pulp is diffusely involved by HCL (fig. 56-2) (15,33,48). The neoplastic cells are small to intermediate in size, with oval nuclei (fig. 56-3). They have slightly open chromatin and moderate amounts of pale cytoplasm. The nuclei are commonly centrally placed and nucleoli are absent or inconspicuous. Mitotic figures are typically rare. Due to red pulp expansion, red pulp structures tend to be adjacent to most of the blood vessels and the periarteriolar lymphoid sheath regions are indistinct (fig. 56-4). Blood lakes, or "pseudosinuses," are small areas in the red pulp where erythrocytes accumulate (fig. 56-5). These areas appear to have a lining, but in fact, blood lakes are lined by neoplastic lymphocytes. The white pulp is compressed and indistinct or is replaced completely.

Blood and Bone Marrow

In the blood, HCL cells are usually small to intermediate-sized lymphocytes with round nuclei, spongy chromatin, and moderate amounts of pale cytoplasm (fig. 56-6) (13,33). The cytoplasm has a frayed membrane with delicate hair-like projections that are usually circumferential around the entire cell (33). Rarely, the cytoplasmic projections are larger and more irregular. The HCL cells look similar in bone marrow aspirate smears, but often the smears are hypocellular ("dry tap") due to reticulin fibrosis. Hairy projections are commonly less obvious in aspirate smears.

HCL cells are present in an interstitial distribution in many bone marrow biopsy specimens (22,33,48). Bone marrow specimens diffusely replaced by HCL fit the classic first description

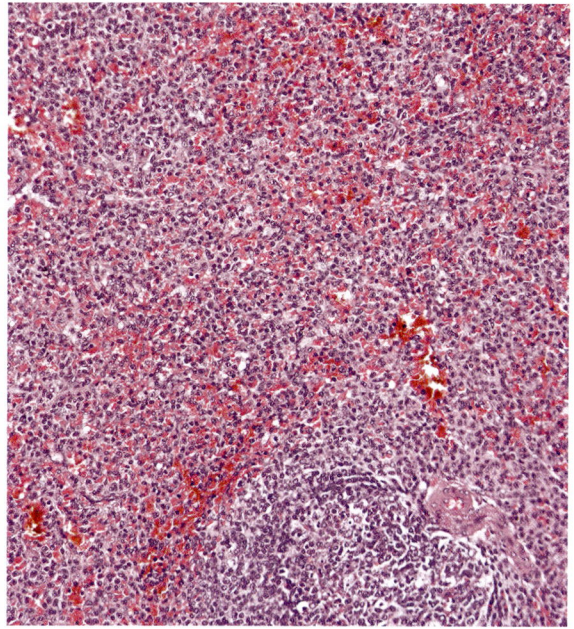

Figure 56-2

HAIRY CELL LEUKEMIA EXPANDING SPLENIC RED PULP

Low magnification image of diffuse red pulp involvement by hairy cell leukemia. The abnormal lymphocytes are located in cords and sinuses. The white pulp (germinal center) is spared in this field (hematoxylin and eosin [H&E] stain.)

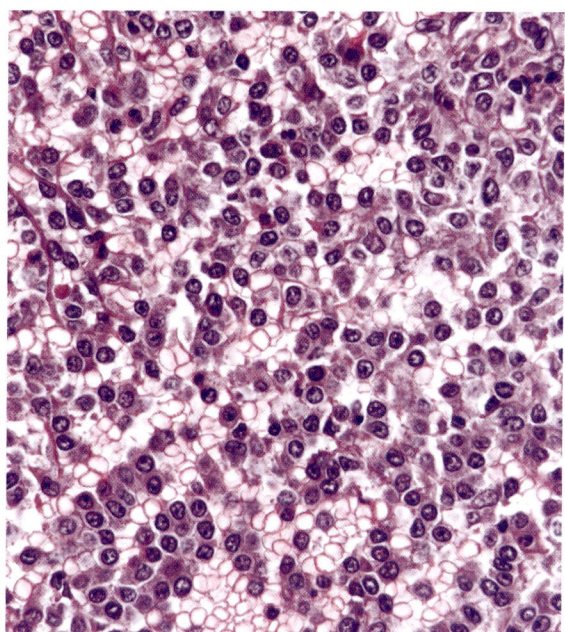

Figure 56-3

HAIRY CELL LEUKEMIA INVOLVING SPLEEN

The nuclei in the red pulp are mostly round with somewhat open chromatin. Each cell has a moderate amount of cytoplasm. The cytoplasmic projections ("hairs") are not usually detectable in tissue sections but can be appreciated in touch imprints of the spleen (H&E stain).

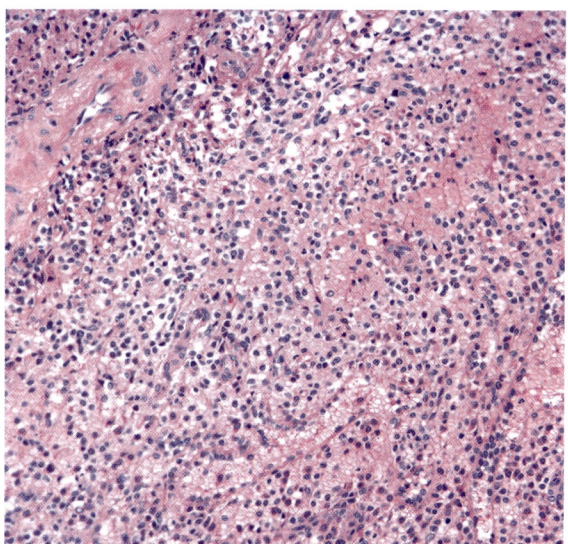

Figure 56-4

HAIRY CELL LEUKEMIA INVOLVING SPLEEN

The number of cells seen in the periarteriolar lymphoid sheath region is reduced leaving bare large-caliber blood vessels. Abnormal cells can be seen in both sinuses and cords (H&E stain).

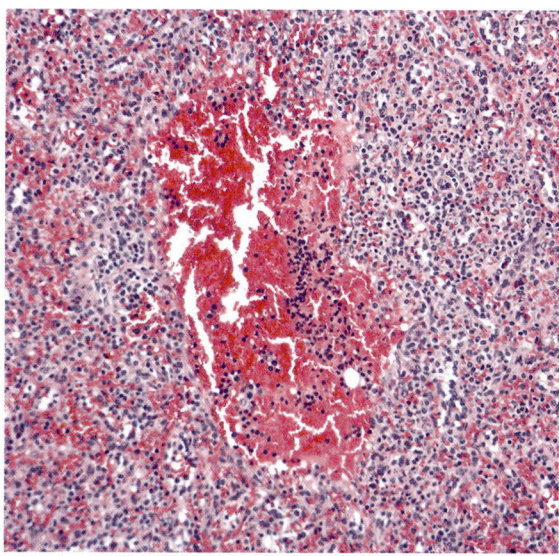

Figure 56-5

HAIRY CELL LEUKEMIA: BLOOD LAKE

A "blood lake" in the spleen is shown. Blood lakes are small cystic areas filled with red blood cells and occasional circulating lymphocytes. These spaces are lined by hairy cells (H&E stain).

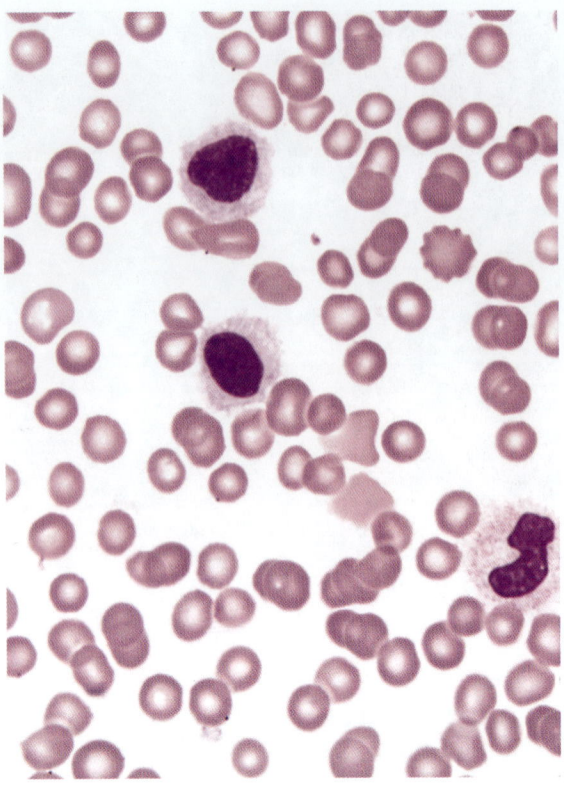

Figure 56-6

HAIRY CELL LEUKEMIA INVOLVING PERIPHERAL BLOOD

The cells are small to intermediate in size, with round nuclei, spongy chromatin, and small to moderate amounts of pale cytoplasm. The characteristic feature is the presence of hair-like projections of cytoplasm (hence the name hairy cells). These projections sometimes indent adjacent red blood cells (Wright-Giemsa stain).

of the disease (15,22). Extensive replacement by hairy cells imparts a pale low-power microscopic appearance and each neoplastic cell resembles a "fried egg," referring to a central round nucleus ("yolk") symmetrically surrounded by pale or clear cytoplasm ("egg white") (fig. 56-7). Severe and diffuse reticulin fibrosis typically is present, likely attributable to substances secreted by the hairy cells (see below).

In patients detected early in the disease course, the bone marrow may be involved only in a patchy, interstitial pattern and the HCL cells can blend in with erythroid precursors and be potentially missed (33,48). Reticulin fibrosis is present to a lesser degree, in association with the areas of HCL infiltration. When evaluating these specimens, immunohistochemical studies are very helpful (almost essential) for recognizing the full extent of disease.

Rare morphologic variants of HCL have been reported. Some HCL cases have cells with spindle-shaped nuclei and pale cytoplasm, and can mimic mast cell disease or nonhematopoietic neoplasms (fig. 56-8). Blastic or large cell variants of HCL have been described (20). Also, cases of HCL with highly irregular or cleaved neoplastic cells have been reported (13).

In areas not involved by HCL, the bone marrow is often hypocellular. This finding has been attributed to possible bone marrow suppression related to HCL. Not all patients with HCL have suppression of myelopoiesis, however, and some have a normocellular bone marrow.

Lymph Node and Extranodal Sites

Although in earlier publications lymphadenopathy was common in patients with HCL, currently lymph node biopsies are performed uncommonly, presumably because lymph nodes are less severely involved at time of diagnosis. Although lymph node involvement is more common in patients with advanced stage, bulky disease (13,33), rare HCL patients present initially with a nodal or soft tissue-based mass, which has been referred to as a lymphomatous presentation (25).

Histologically, HCL diffusely replaces the lymph node architecture, often subtotally with sparing of reactive follicles or sinuses (33,48). The neoplastic cells often have a "fried egg" appearance (described above) (figs. 56-9, 56-10). The liver is also commonly involved and the neoplastic cells are usually distributed within the sinuses (40,48). Rare sites of involvement by advanced HCL include bones, mediastinum, central nervous system, and mucosa-associated lymphoid tissue sites, such as salivary gland (fig. 56-11), skin, breast, and the gastrointestinal tract (40).

CYTOLOGIC FINDINGS

Aspirate smears show small to medium-sized cells with round or oval nuclei that may exhibit irregular nuclear contours (fig. 56-12) (30). On Papanicolaou-stained smears, the cytoplasmic borders are ill-defined. On Romanowsky stained slides, intact cells often show a broad rim of pale cytoplasm. Cytoplasmic projections are usually not identified in smears or touch imprints.

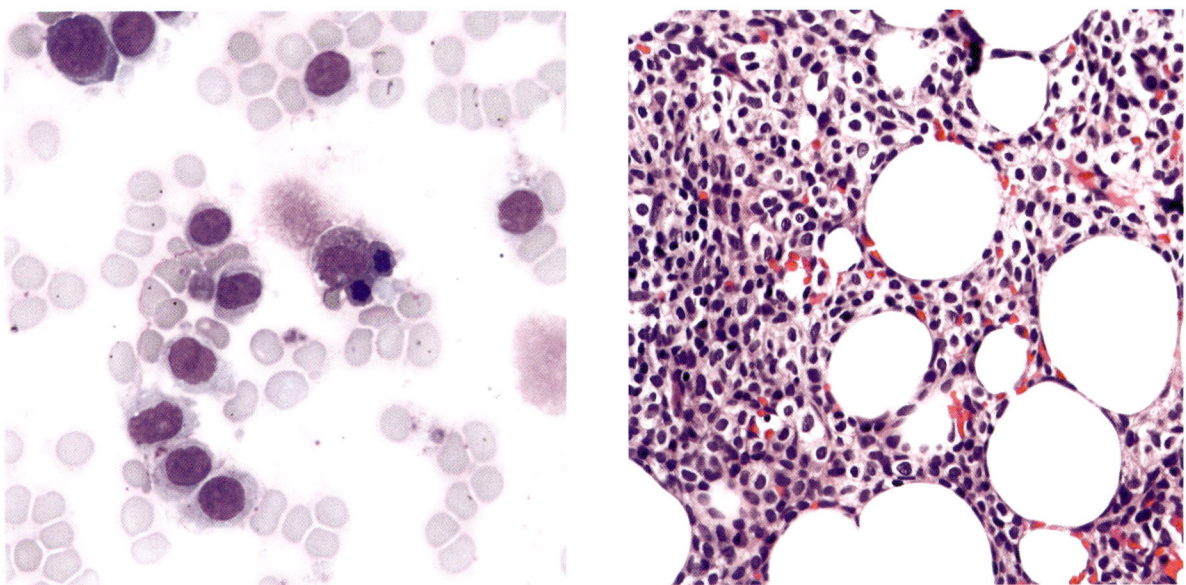

Figure 56-7

HAIRY CELL LEUKEMIA INVOLVING BONE MARROW

Left: An aspirate smear shows hairy cells with shaggy cytoplasm and occasional cytoplasmic "hairs" (Wright-Giemsa stain).

Right: A bone marrow biopsy specimen shows HCL representing most of the bone marrow cells (H&E stain).

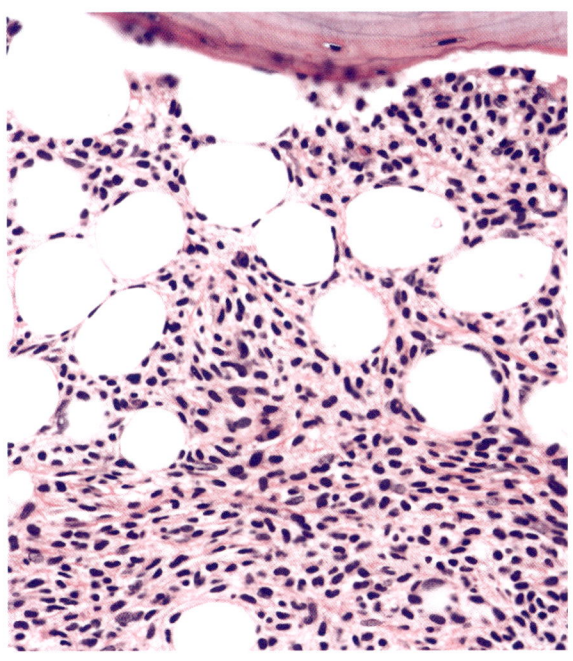

Figure 56-8

HAIRY CELL LEUKEMIA INVOLVING BONE MARROW

In some cases of bone marrow involvement by HCL the neoplastic cells assume a spindled shape. This feature may mimic other diseases in the bone marrow such as systemic mastocytosis (H&E stain).

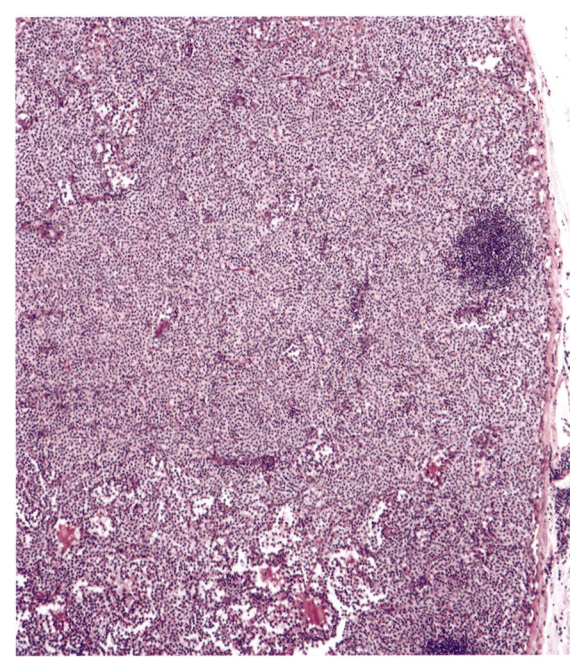

Figure 56-9

HAIRY CELL LEUKEMIA INVOLVING LYMPH NODE

HCL can involve lymph nodes. In this case, there is diffuse involvement of the interfollicular areas by neoplastic cells (periodic acid–Schiff [PAS] stain).

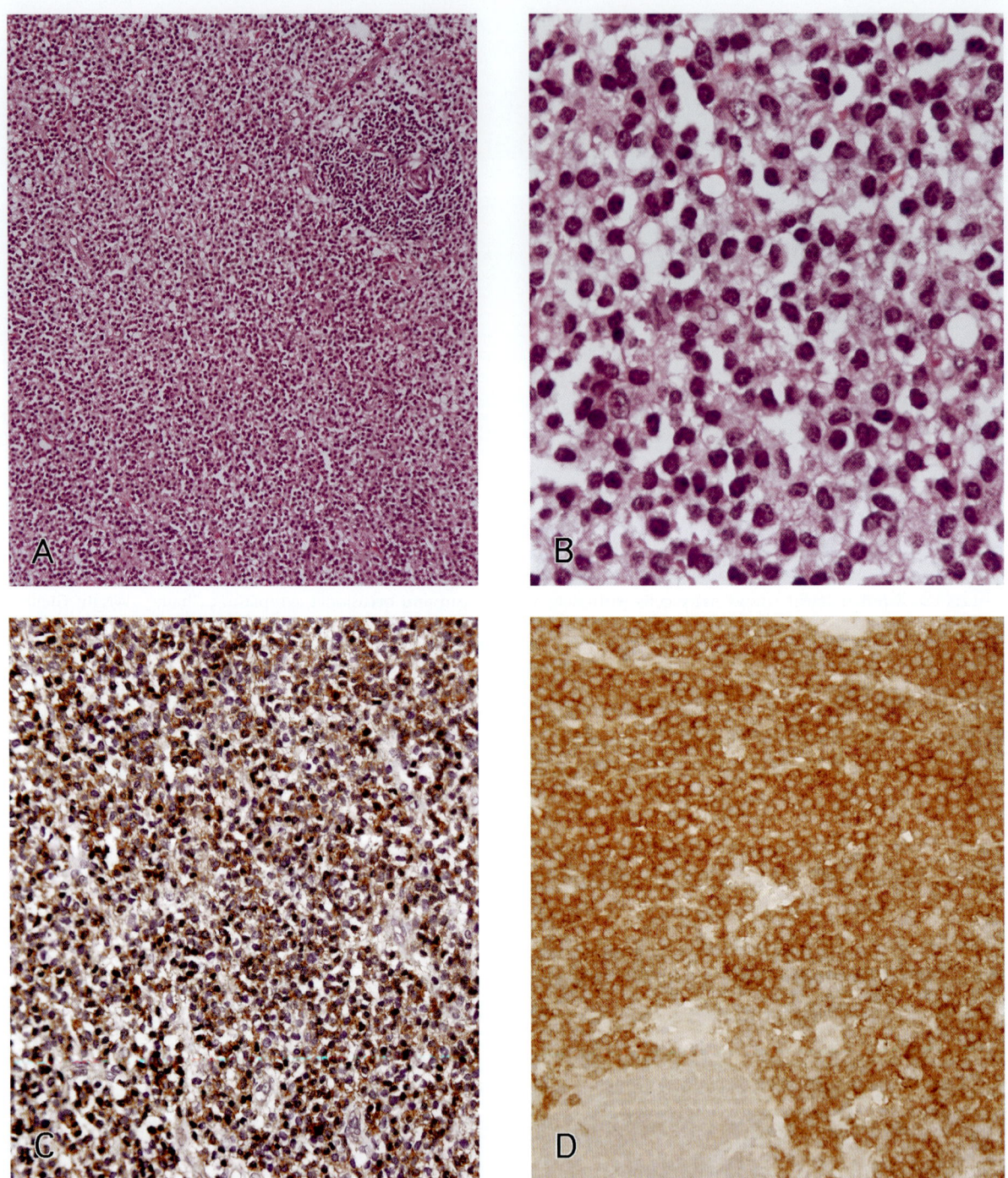

Figure 56-10

HAIRY CELL LEUKEMIA INVOLVING SOFT TISSUE

This case of HCL presented as a mass in the right submandibular region. The patient did not have blood or bone marrow involvement (so-called lymphomatous variant).

A: The biopsy specimen showed diffuse effacement by HCL (A,B: H&E stain).

B: An oil magnification image shows small lymphoid cells with abundant cytoplasm.

C,D: Immunohistochemical analysis showed that the neoplastic cells are positive for annexin A1 (C) and VE-1/*BRAF* V600E (D) (C,D: immunohistochemistry with hematoxylin counterstain).

IMMUNOPHENOTYPIC FINDINGS

Immunophenotypic studies are essential for the diagnosis of HCL and flow cytometry is well suited to the analysis of blood and bone marrow. In side scatter/CD45 gating, HCL cells do not typically fall within the usual lymphocyte gate and have properties that place them within or near the monocyte gate (fig. 56-13). HCL is of B-cell lineage and the cells express CD19, CD20, CD22, and monotypic surface light chain (12,38). Both CD20 and surface light chain are usually brightly expressed by HCL cells (Table 56-2) and HCL is one of the few lymphoid neoplasms that express lambda more commonly than kappa. Other markers characteristically expressed in HCL include CD11c, CD25, CD103, CD123, CD200, and FMC-7. CD11c and FMC7 are typically very brightly expressed and this combination yields a population highly characteristic of HCL. CD5, CD10, CD23, and CD27 are usually negative in HCL (12,38), although CD10 and less frequently CD5 have been reported in some cases.

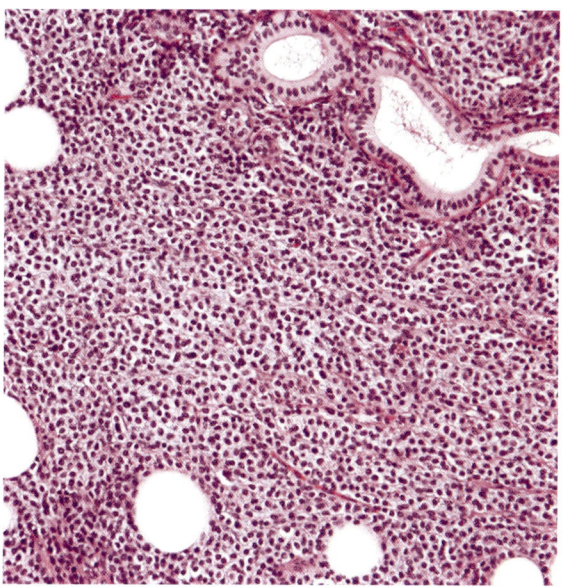

Figure 56-11

HAIRY CELL LEUKEMIA INVOLVING SALIVARY GLAND

This patient also had blood and bone marrow involvement (H&E stain).

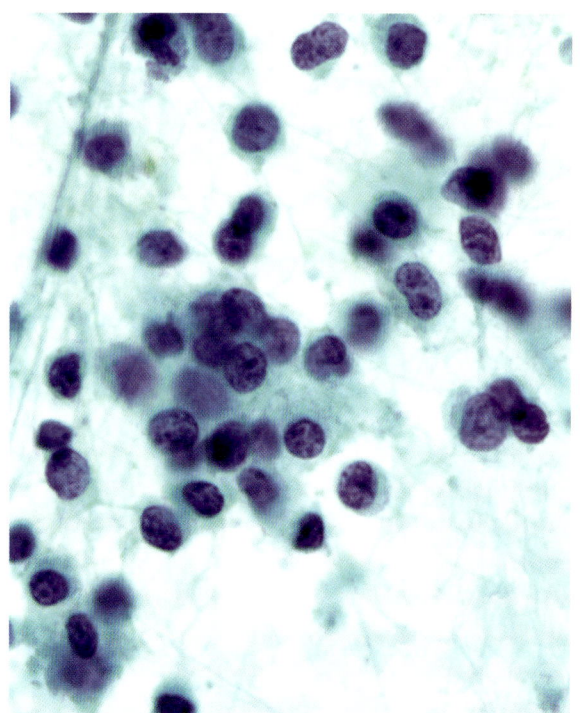
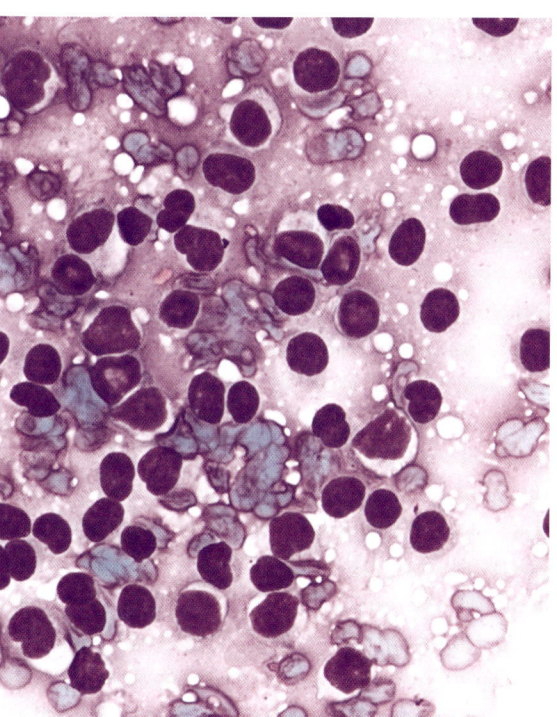

Figure 56-12

CYTOLOGIC FINDINGS IN HAIRY CELL LEUKEMIA

Fine-needle aspirate smears showing many hairy cells (left, Papanicolaou stain; right, Diff-Quik stain). The cytoplasmic processes of hairy cells are rarely seen in aspirate smears.

Table 56-2

FLOW CYTOMETRIC IMMUNOPHENOTYPIC FINDINGS IN HCL AND
OTHER SMALL B-CELL LYMPHOMAS IN THE DIFFERENTIAL DIAGNOSIS

Marker	HCL[a]	SMZL	HCL-V	SDRPL
CD22	+[b]	+	+	+
CD11c	+	+/− (~50%)	−/+ (15-25%)	+
CD25	+	−/+ (up to 33%)	−	−
CD103	+	−/+ (15-25%)	+/− (60-70%)	−/+ (~40%)
CD5	−	−/+ (~20%)	−	−/+ (~15%)
CD123	+	−	−	−/+ (~15%)
FMC7	+	+	+	+
CD23	−	−/+ (~30%)	−	−
CD10	−	infrequent	−	−

[a]HCL= hairy cell leukemia; SMZL = splenic marginal zone lymphoma; HCL-V = hairy cell leukemia variant; SDRPL = splenic diffuse red pulp B-cell lymphoma.
[b]+ in this table indicates that more than 95 percent of cases are positive; – indicates <10%/– of cases are positive.

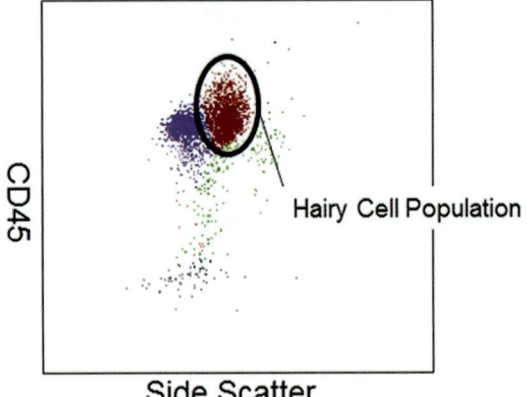

Figure 56-13

FLOW CYTOMETRY HISTOGRAM
OF HAIRY CELL LEUKEMIA

In this histogram of CD45 versus side scatter, lymphocytes are blue (high CD45, low side scatter), and hairy cells are red (CD45 high, intermediate side scatter). In cases of HCL, the neoplastic cells often are found in or near the monocyte gate.

Following therapy, multicolor flow cytometry immunophenotyping is a convenient approach for assessing for minimal residual disease, with a sensitivity of up to 1 hairy cell in 10,000 benign cells (14). Patients with minimal residual disease can otherwise be in complete remission, and therefore the detection of minimal residual disease is not necessarily an indication for therapy. Higher levels of minimal residual disease, however, correlate with a higher rate of relapse (14,38).

Immunohistochemical analysis, although less sensitive than flow cytometry, is also helpful for establishing or supporting a diagnosis of HCL. Pan-B-cell antibodies such as CD20, CD22, and PAX5 help highlight the disease, although these antibodies are not specific. Annexin A1 (fig. 56-10C) is a highly specific marker for HCL, but difficult to interpret in partially involved bone marrow specimens because granulocytes are also positive (10). Other markers reactive with HCL, in decreasing order of specificity, include CD25, phospho-ERK, CD103, HBME-1, CD11c, CD68, cyclin D1, CD200, T-bet/TBX21, DBA.44, and tartrate-resistant acid phosphatase (TRAP) (fig. 56-14) (35,45). The pattern of cyclin D1 expression is nuclear, but HCL cells usually lack the intensity and fairly uniform expression of cyclin D1 observed in mantle cell lymphoma (26).

HCL usually has a very low proliferation rate as shown by Ki-67. *BRAF* is mutated in virtually all cases and the VE-1 antibody specific for the *BRAF* V600E mutation is available (figs. 56-10D, 56-15) (2,5). The correlation between antibody reactivity and the V600E mutation is very good, but as has been shown in solid tumors, can be equivocal in occasional truly mutated cases. The converse is also true uncommonly: patients with minimal disease burden may be negative for mutation by molecular testing but the VE-1 antibody highlights HCL cells (5). The VE-1 antibody does not react in rare cases of HCL with non-*BRAF* V600E mutations (18).

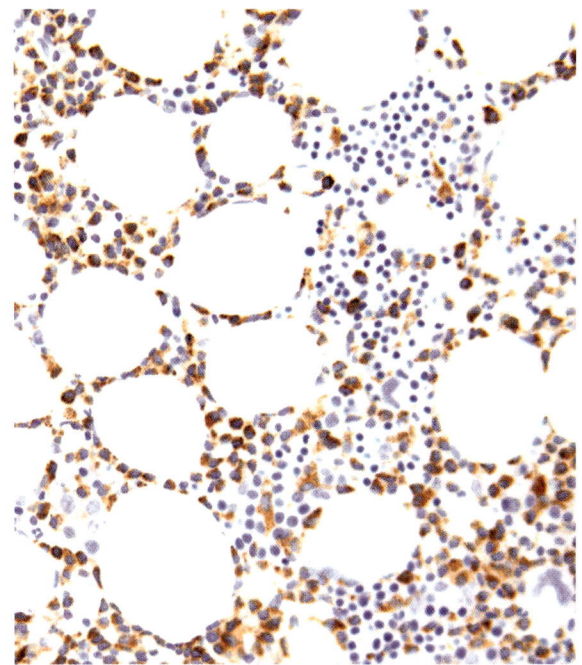

Figure 56-14

HAIRY CELL LEUKEMIA: TRAP

Tartrate-resistant acid phosphatase (TRAP) immuno-histochemical study performed on a bone marrow biopsy specimen involved by HCL shows TRAP positivity in a granular and cytoplasmic distribution. (immunohistochemistry with hematoxylin counterstain.)

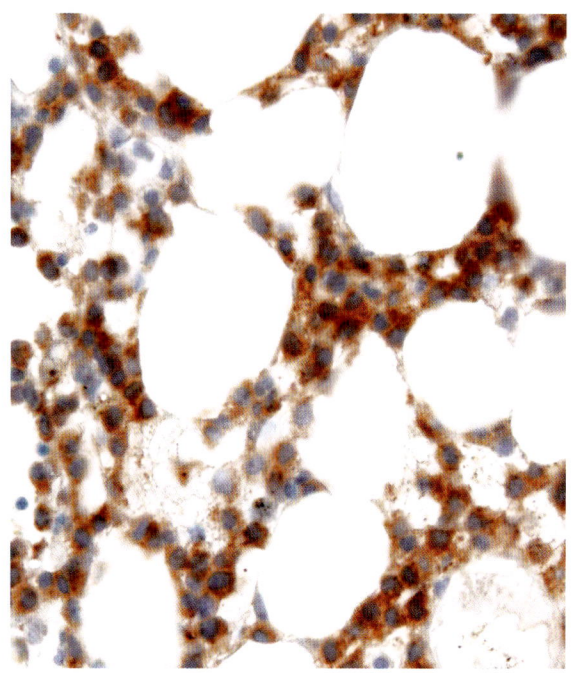

Figure 56-15

HAIRY CELL LEUKEMIA: *BRAF* V600E

Immunohistochemical study for *BRAF* V600E using the VE-1 antibody and performed on a bone marrow biopsy specimen involved by HCL. The neoplastic cells exhibit cytoplasmic reactivity. (immunohistochemistry with hematoxylin counterstain.)

Although cytochemical assessment for TRAP is an older test, perhaps considered "old fashioned" by some pathologists, this test still has value in the assessment of touch imprints or smears. The cells of HCL contain the isoenzyme 5 of acid phosphatase which is resistant to treatment with tartaric acid. Therefore, HCL cells are strongly positive for TRAP with a cytoplasmic granular staining pattern (fig. 56-16). It is recommended that examination of an acid phosphatase reaction prior to the treatment with tartaric acid, in parallel with the TRAP stain, be performed. Usually, HCL cells appear equally bright or brighter in the TRAP slide. In contrast, less intense TRAP positivity is observed in other types of B-cell lymphoma and the reactivity is not specific.

ULTRASTRUCTURAL FINDINGS

In general, the diagnosis of HCL can be established reliably with immunophenotypic and molecular studies; electron microscopy is rarely performed in daily practice. Hairy cells have numerous cytoplasmic projections that interdigitate with those from other cells (23). In addition, ribosome-lamellar complexes are commonly identified in the cells of HCL. Ribosome-lamellar complexes appear to be specific for hematologic malignancies, but they are not entirely specific for HCL (23). The origin and cellular importance of ribosome-lamellar complexes are obscure.

MOLECULAR GENETIC FINDINGS

No characteristic cytogenetic abnormalities have been identified in HCL. Array comparative genomic hybridization and other high-resolution cytogenetic methods have shown that approximately 25 percent of cases have recurrent copy number changes (11,28). Deletions in chromosome 17p or *TP53* have been reported in a small subset of cases and this abnormality correlates with blastic morphology. The t(11;14)(q13;q32)/*CCND1-IGH* does not occur in HCL.

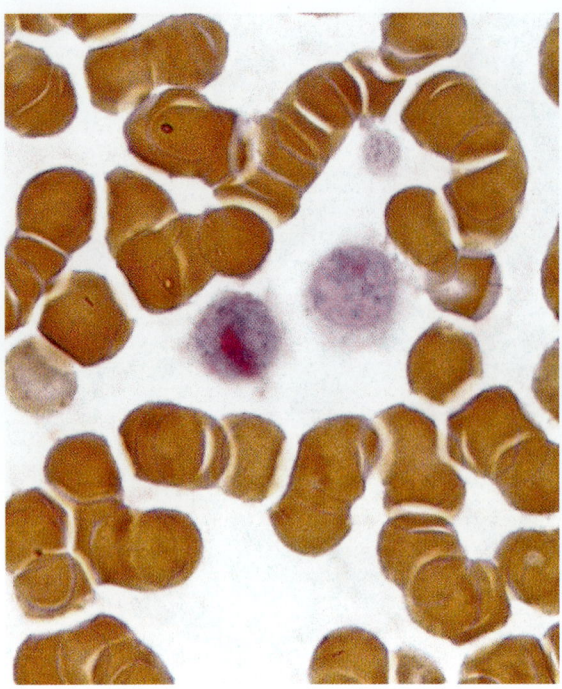

Figure 56-16

HAIRY CELL LEUKEMIA: TRAP CYTOLOTY

This technique is "old fashioned," but is still helpful and can be performed quickly on an unstained air dried smear. Flow cytometry immunophenotyping and immunohistochemistry are more sensitive and more specific, and have superceded the role once held by TRAP cytochemistry (cytochemistry for TRAP performed on a peripheral blood smear).

In keeping with the mature B-cell lineage of HCL, these tumors carry monoclonal immuno-globulin gene rearrangements (13). The *IGH* variable regions are usually mutated in HCL, suggesting that the neoplastic cells traverse the germinal center (31). The *VH-34* gene is used in about 10 percent of cases of HCL (47). The T-cell receptor genes are usually in the germline configuration.

Compared with other B-cell lymphoprolifera-tive disorders, HCL is unusual in that multiple immunoglobulin (Ig) heavy chain isotypes (IgM, IgG, and IgA) are expressed by the neoplastic cells. This finding is thought to be attributable to ongoing class switching, and may be due to the influence of fibroblast growth factors (3).

The explanation for the extensive reticulin and collagenous fibrosis in bone marrow involved by HCL is an area of active research. The cells of HCL secrete substances that can induce fibrosis, such as fibronectin. Genetic dysregulation of fibroblast growth factors or their receptors, as well as the presence of TGF-β1 also may explain the fibrosis (3,34,41).

Gene expression profiling studies of HCL show a profile similar to that of memory B cells (4,41). These studies also show overexpression of genes involved in the RAS and PI3K-AKT pathways and genes involved in cell adhesion. Phospho-ERK and cyclin D1 are downstream targets of the RAS and PI3K-AKT pathway and likely explain their expression in HCL (44). The many adhesion genes overexpressed in HCL may explain the characteristic distribution of the disease in affected patients (41).

The RAS-BRAF-MEK-ERK pathway is frequent-ly constitutively activated in HCL (fig. 56-17). In particular, activating mutations of *BRAF* occur in almost all cases, specifically the *BRAF* V600E mutation in over 95 percent of cases (10,43). In this mutation, glutamate (E) replaces valine (V) at codon 600. *BRAF* is a part of the RAS signaling pathway and encodes B-RAF protein, a 766 amino acid serine/threonine kinase that is involved in signal transduction (43). Mutations in *BRAF* result in constitutive activation and have been described in many types of solid tumors (e.g., melanoma). Mutations in *MAP2K1* (which encodes MEK), also in the RAS pathway, have been reported in a few cases, particularly those that utilize the VH4-34 family (47). Other genes in the RAS-BRAF-MEK-ERK pathway are rarely mutated in HCL. *CDKN1B*, which encodes p27, and *KLF2* are mutated in 10 to 15 percent of HCL cases and may cooperate with *BRAF* V600E in pathogenesis (9,10,44).

DIFFERENTIAL DIAGNOSIS

Primary considerations in the differential diagnosis of HCL are shown in Table 56-2 and include hairy cell leukemia variant (HCL-V), splenic marginal zone lymphoma, and splenic diffuse red pulp B-cell lymphoma. In patients in whom HCL involves lymph nodes or rarely extranodal sites, nodal or extranodal marginal zone lymphoma is also a part of the differential diagnosis. Of these entities, HCL-V is probably the most challenging to distinguish from HCL.

Despite the close similarity in terminology, HCL-V is no longer thought to be biological-ly related to HCL (13). Patients with HCL-V often present with leukocytosis and rarely have monocytopenia. The neoplastic cells of HCL-V

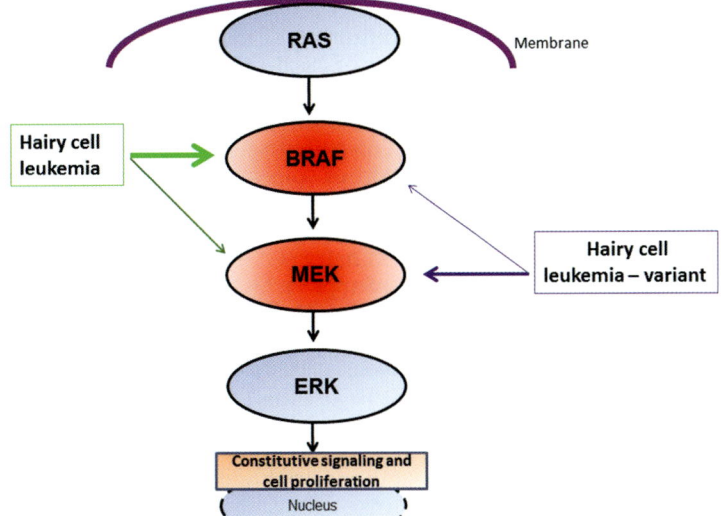

Figure 56-17

RAS PATHWAY MUTATIONS IN HAIRY CELL LEUKEMIA (HCL) AND HCL-VARIANT

Almost all cases of hairy cell leukemia (HCL) have mutations involving BRAF, usually BRAF V600E, encoding mutant BRAF protein (indicated by thick green arrow). A small subset of HCL cases carries MAP2K1 mutations that encode MEK (thinner green arrow). In contrast, in HCL-variant 20-40 percent of cases have MAP2K1 mutations (blue arrow) and very rare cases have been reported to carry BRAF mutations (very thin blue arrow).

in smears differ from hairy cells by having more prominent nucleoli. The immunophenotype of HCL-V is also distinct from HCL; HCL-V cells are usually negative for CD25, CD123, cyclin D1, and annexin A1. *BRAF* mutations are uncommon in HCL-V although *MAP2K1* mutations occur in a subset of cases (47). In some cases, the morphologic and immunophenotypic overlap between HCL and HCL-V can make their distinction challenging even in the most expert hands. However, with genetic analysis even these challenging cases often can be distinguished.

TREATMENT AND PROGNOSIS

After HCL was initially described, for about 20 years the only therapy that provided any relief was splenectomy, and the median survival period was 4 to 6 years (1,17). Splenectomy may still have value in reducing tumor bulk and correcting cytopenias in some patients.

The first effective chemotherapy for HCL patients was interferon alpha, first discovered in 1984 (1,17). Subsequently, it was recognized that HCL is highly responsive to purine analog therapy. Specifically, cladribine and pentostatin have been shown to have great efficacy in most patients with HCL (1,19). However, although most patients go into complete clinical remis-

sion, immunohistochemical and molecular studies have shown that many patients have evidence of minimal residual disease and many HCL patients relapse eventually (16). Patients with de novo or relapsed HCL also respond to rituximab and some recommend combining a purine analog with rituximab as frontline therapy (1). Preliminary studies using this combination have shown good results. Moxetumomab pasudotox is a CD22 antibody drug conjugate that has shown responses in relapsed HCL patients (40a). Preclinical data and early patient trials suggest that ibrutinib may be effective in the treatment of HCL patients (36,40a).

There is a role for BRAF inhibitors in the treatment of HCL. In vitro studies have shown that BRAF and MEK inhibitors can reverse many of the manifestations of HCL, including smoothing of cytoplasmic hairs, downregulation of HCL markers (e.g., CD25), and silencing or loss of BRAF-MEK-ERK pathway effects (29). In early clinical trials of HCL patients treated with standard therapy who subsequently relapsed, treatment with the BRAF inhibitor vemurafenib resulted in an overall response rate of over 90 percent, with complete response rates of 35 to 42 percent (9a,10,42).

REFERENCES

1. Andritsos LA, Grever MR. Historical overview of hairy cell leukemia. Best Pract Res Clin Haematol 2015;28:166-174.
2. Andrulis M, Penzel R, Weichert W, von Deimling A, Capper D. Application of a BRAF V600E mutation-specific antibody for the diagnosis of hairy cell leukemia. Am J Surg Pathol 2012;36:1796-1800.
3. Aziz KA, Till KJ, Chen H, et al. The role of autocrine FGF-2 in the distinctive bone marrow fibrosis of hairy-cell leukemia (HCL). Blood 2003;102:1051-1056.
4. Basso K, Liso A, Tiacci E, et al. Gene expression profiling of hairy cell leukemia reveals a phenotype related to memory B cells with altered expression of chemokine and adhesion receptors. J Exp Med 2004;199:59-68.
5. Brown NA, Betz BL, Weigelin HC, Elenitoba-Johnson KS, Lim MS, Bailey NG. Evaluation of allele-specific PCR and immunohistochemistry for the detection of BRAF V600E mutations in hairy cell leukemia. Am J Clin Pathol 2015;143:89-99.
6. Catovsky D, Pettit JE, Galton DA, Spiers AS, Harrison CV. Leukaemic reticuloendotheliosis ('hairy' cell leukaemia): a distinct clinico-pathological entity. Br J Haematol 1974;26:9-27.
7. Cetiner M, Adigüzel C, Argon D, et al. Hairy cell leukemia in father and son. Med Oncol 2003;20:375-378.
8. Colovic MD, Jankovic GM, Wiernik PH. Hairy cell leukemia in first cousins and review of the literature. Eur J Haematol 2001;67:185-188.
9. Dietrich S, Hullein J, Lee SC, et al. Recurrent CDKN1B (p27) mutations in hairy cell leukemia. Blood 2015;126:1005-1008.
9a. Dietrich S, Pircher A, Endris V, et al. BRAF inhibition in hairy cell leukemia with low-dose vemurafenib. Blood 2016;127:2847-2855.
10. Falini B, Martelli MP, Tiacci E. BRAF V600E mutation in hairy cell leukemia: from bench to bedside. Blood 2016;128:1918-1927.
11. Forconi F, Poretti G, Kwee I, et al. High density genome-wide DNA profiling reveals a remarkably stable profile in hairy cell leukaemia. Br J Haematol 2008;141:622-630.
12. Forconi F, Raspadori D, Lenoci M, Lauria F. Absence of surface CD27 distinguishes hairy cell leukemia from other leukemic B-cell malignancies. Haematologica 2005;90:266-268.
13. Foucar K, Falini B, Catovsky D, Stein H. Hairy cell leukaemia. In: Swerdlow SH, Campo E, Harris NL, et al., eds. WHO classification of tumours of haematopoietic and lymphoid tissues. Lyon: IARC Press; 2008:188-190.
14. Garnache Ottou F, Chandesris MO, Lhermitte L, et al. Peripheral blood 8 colour flow cytometry monitoring of hairy cell leukaemia allows detection of high-risk patients. Br J Haematol 2014;166:50-59.
15. Golomb HM, Vardiman JW. Response to splenectomy in 65 patients with hairy cell leukemia: an evaluation of spleen weight and bone marrow involvement. Blood 1983;61:349-352.
16. Grever MR, Zinzani PL. Long-term follow-up studies in hairy cell leukemia. Leuk Lymphoma 2009;50(Suppl 1):23-26.
17. Habermann TM. Splenectomy, interferon, and treatments of historical interest in hairy cell leukemia. Hematol Oncol Clin North Am 2006;20:1075-1086.
18. Jabbar KJ, Luthra R, Patel K, et al. Comparison of next generation sequencing mutation profiling with BRAF and IDH1 mutation specific immunohistochemistry. Am J Surg Pathol 2015;39:454-461.
19. Jain P, Pemmaraju N, Ravandi F. Update on the biology and treatment options for hairy cell leukemia. Curr Treat Options Oncol 2014;15:187-209.
20. Kanellis G, Garcia-Alonso L, Camacho FI, et al. Hairy cell leukemia, blastic type: description of spleen morphology and immunophenotype of a distinctive case. Leuk Lymphoma 2011;52:1589-1592.
21. Karmali R, Farhat M, Leslie W, McIntire MG, Gregory S. Localized bone disease as a presentation of hairy cell leukemia. Clin Adv Hematol Oncol 2008;6:290-294.
22. Katayama I. Bone marrow in hairy cell leukemia. Hematol Oncol Clin North Am 1988;2:585-602.
23. Katayama I, Schneider GB. Further ultrastructural characterization of hairy cells of leukemic reticuloendotheliosis. Am J Pathol 1977;86:163-182.
24. Kurzrock R, Strom SS, Estey E, et al. Second cancer risk in hairy cell leukemia: analysis of 350 patients. J Clin Oncol 1997;15:1803-1810.
25. Liu H, Wang W, Tang G, et al. Lymphomatous variant of hairy cell leukaemia : a distinctive presentation mimicking low-grade B-cell lymphoma. Histopathology 2015;67:740-745.
26. Miranda RN, Briggs RC, Kinney MC, Veno PA, Hammer RD, Cousar JB. Immunohistochemical detection of cyclin D1 using optimized conditions is highly specific for mantle cell lymphoma and hairy cell leukemia. Mod Pathol 2000;13:1308-1314.
27. Monnereau A, Slager SL, Hughes AM, et al. Medical history, lifestyle, and occupational risk factors for hairy cell leukemia: the InterLymph Non-Hodgkin Lymphoma Subtypes Project. J Natl Cancer Inst Monogr 2014;2014(48):115-124.

28. Nordgren A, Corcoran M, Sääf A, et al. Characterisation of hairy cell leukaemia by tiling resolution array-based comparative genome hybridisation: a series of 13 cases and review of the literature. Eur J Haematol 2010;84:17-25.

29. Pettirossi V, Santi A, Imperi E, et al. BRAF inhibitors reverse the unique molecular signature and phenotype of hairy cell leukemia and exert potent antileukemic activity. Blood 2015;125:1207-1216.

30. Pinto RG, Rocha PD, Vernekar JA. Fine needle aspiration of the spleen in hairy cell leukemia. A case report. Acta Cytol 1995;39:777-780.

31. Rumi E, Passamonti F, Zibellini S, et al. HLA typing and VH gene rearrangement analysis in a family with hairy cell leukaemia. Leuk Lymphoma 2007;48:805-807.

32. Schrek R, Donnelly WJ. "Hairy" cells in blood in lymphoreticular neoplastic disease and 'flagellated' cells or normal lymph nodes. Blood 1966;27:199-211.

33. Sharpe RW, Bethel KJ. Hairy cell leukemia: diagnostic pathology. Hematol Oncol Clin North Am 2006;20:1023-1049.

34. Shehata M, Schwarzmeier JD, Hilgarth M, Hubmann R, Duechler M, Gisslinger H. TGF-beta1 induces bone marrow reticulin fibrosis in hairy cell leukemia. J Clin Invest 2004;113:676-685.

35. Sherman MJ, Hanson CA, Hoyer JD. An assessment of the usefulness of immunohistochemical stains in the diagnosis of hairy cell leukemia. Am J Clin Pathol 2011;136:390-399.

36. Sivina M, Kreitman RJ, Arons E, Ravandi F, Burger JA. The bruton tyrosine kinase inhibitor ibrutinib (PCI-32765) blocks hairy cell leukaemia survival, proliferation and B cell receptor signalling: a new therapeutic approach. Br J Haematol 2014;166:177-188.

37. Spedini P, Tajana M, Bergonzi C. Unusual presentation of hairy cell leukemia. Haematologica 2000;85:548.

38. Stetler-Stevenson M, Tembhare PR. Diagnosis of hairy cell leukemia by flow cytometry. Leuk Lymphoma 2011;52(Suppl 2):11-13.

38a.Swerdlow SH, Campo E, Pileri SA, et al. The 2016 revision of the World Health Organization classification of lymphoid neoplasms. Blood 2016;127:2375-2390.

39. Tadmor T, Polliack A. Epidemiology and environmental risk in hairy cell leukemia. Best Pract Res Clin Haematol 2015; 28:175-179.

40. Tadmor T, Polliack A. Hairy cell leukemia: uncommon clinical features, unusual sites of involvement and some rare associations. Best Pract Res Clin Haematol 2015;28:193-199.

40a.Thompson PA, Ravandi F. How I manage patients with hairy cell leukaemia. Br J Haematol 2017;177:543-556.

41. Tiacci E, Liso A, Piris M, Falini B. Evolving concepts in the pathogenesis of hairy-cell leukaemia. Nat Rev Cancer 2006;6:437-448.

42. Tiacci E, Park JH, DeCarolis L, et al. Targeting mutant BRAF in relapses or refractory hairy-cell leukemia. N Engl J Med 2015;373:1733-1747.

43. Tiacci E, Trifonov V, Schiavoni G, et al. BRAF mutations in hairy-cell leukemia. N Engl J Med 2011;364:2305-2315.

44. Tiacci E, Pettirossi V, Schiavoni G, Falini B. Genomics of hairy cell leukemia. J Clin Oncol 2017;35:1002-1010.

45. Tóth-Lipták J, Piukovics K, Borbényi Z, Demeter J, Bagdi E, Krenács L. A comprehensive immunophenotypic marker analysis of hairy cell leukemia in paraffin-embedded bone marrow trephine biopsies—a tissue microarray study. Pathol Oncol Res 2015;21:203-211.

46. Villemagne B, Bay JO, Tournilhac O, Chaleteix C, Travade P. Two new cases of familial hairy cell leukemia associated with HLA haplotypes A2, B7, Bw4, Bw6. Leuk Lymphoma 2005;46:243-245.

47. Waterfall JJ, Arons E, Walker RL, et al. High prevalence of MAP2K1 mutations in variant and IGHV4-34-expressing hairy-cell leukemias. Nat Genetics 2014;46:8-10.

48. Wotherspoon A, Attygalle A, Sena Texeira Mendes L. Bone marrow and splenic histology in hairy cell leukaemia. Best Pract Res Clin Haematol 2015;28:200-207.

57 HAIRY CELL LEUKEMIA-VARIANT

GENERAL FEATURES

Hairy cell leukemia-variant (HCL-V) is an indolent B-cell lymphoma/leukemia that resembles classic hairy cell leukemia (HCL) but has variant clinical, morphologic, and immunophenotypic features. HCL-V is considered a provisional entity in the World Health Organization (WHO) classification under the umbrella category of splenic B-cell lymphoma/leukemia, unclassifiable (12,15). Patients with HCL-V commonly present with involvement of peripheral blood, bone marrow, and spleen.

HCL-V was initially described by Cawley et al. in 1980 (2). Traditionally, HCL-V has been considered to be closely related to, or a subset of, classic HCL. More recently, however, it has become clear that there is less overlap biologically between the two (10). Based on differences in clinical presentation, immunophenotype, genetic findings, and response to therapy, HCL-V is separated from classic HCL in the WHO classification (12). In retrospect, the name HCL-V seems an unfortunate choice as it is easily confused with classic HCL.

HCL-V is much less common than classic HCL. The incidence is 0.03 per 100,000 persons per year, which translates into 60 to 70 new cases of HCL-V per year in the United Sates (10,13). In Asia, a Japanese variant of HCL has been reported (8). These tumors, characterized by an elevated leukocyte count and poor response to therapies that are effective in classic HCL patients, are most likely examples of HCL-V using current definitions. HCL-V appears to be more common in Asia than in Western nations (8).

It seems likely that cases included in the category of HCL-V are a heterogeneous group. Further refinement of this category of disease seems likely in the future and its relationship to splenic diffuse red pulp small B-cell lymphoma, also a provisional category in the current WHO classification, needs to be clarified (12,15).

CLINICAL FEATURES

Patients with HCL-V tend to be elderly, with a median age in the eighth decade (5,10,13). Men are more frequently affected than women, in a ratio of 1.6-2.0 to 1.0 (5,8,10).

The clinical course of HCL-V is indolent, although more aggressive than classic HCL. Patients commonly present with abdominal discomfort or other symptoms attributable to massive splenomegaly (5,10). B-type symptoms are uncommon. Symptoms may be related to thrombocytopenia and anemia that occur in 40 to 50 percent and about 30 percent of patients, respectively (5,10,12).

The complete blood count in patients with HCL-V usually shows a moderately elevated leukocyte count, often in the range of 20 to 40 x 10^9/L, with an absolute lymphocytosis, although some patients have a very high leukocyte count (3,5,10). Neutropenia is uncommon and monocytopenia is not present in HCL-V patients. Serum lactate dehydrogenase or beta-2 microglobulin levels are elevated in a small subset of patients.

The physical examination and imaging studies show splenomegaly, often massive, in over 90 percent of patients (5,10,13). Hepatomegaly is present in about 20 percent of patients. In 5 to 15 percent of patients, imaging studies show abdominal lymphadenopathy, including enlargement of splenic hilar lymph nodes, but peripheral lymphadenopathy is uncommon (5,10,12).

During the clinical course, patients with HCL-V can develop a more aggressive disease. The leukocyte count can rise to very high levels, over 300 x 10^9/L, and hepatomegaly and lymphadenopathy are more frequent and can be more prominent. Skin lesions have been reported in some patients (10).

Figure 57-1

HAIRY CELL LEUKEMIA-VARIANT INVOLVING SPLEEN

A: The red pulp is prominent and expanded by abnormal lymphocytes whereas the white pulp is almost completely absent.

B: At this magnification, small blood lakes are appreciated.

C: The abnormal lymphocytes are mostly round, with condensed chromatin and small to moderate amounts of pink cytoplasm. Nucleoli are difficult to appreciate in routinely stained tissue sections (A–C: hematoxylin and eosin [H&E] stain).

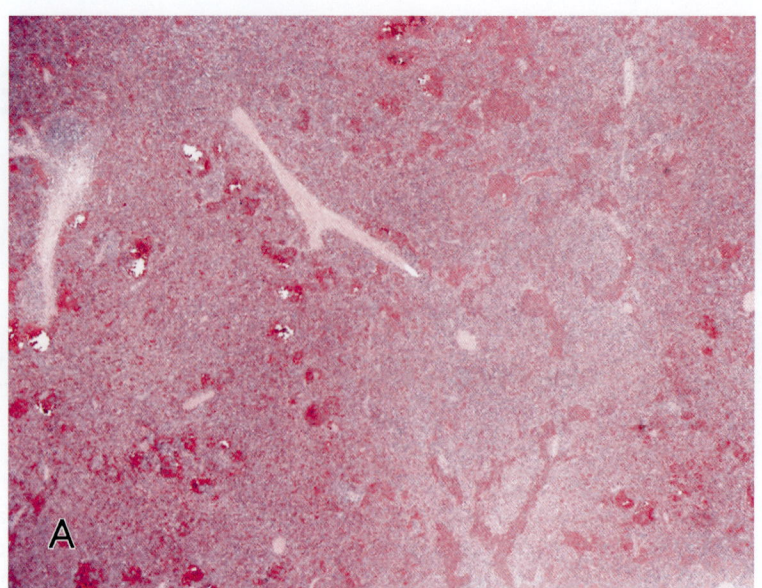

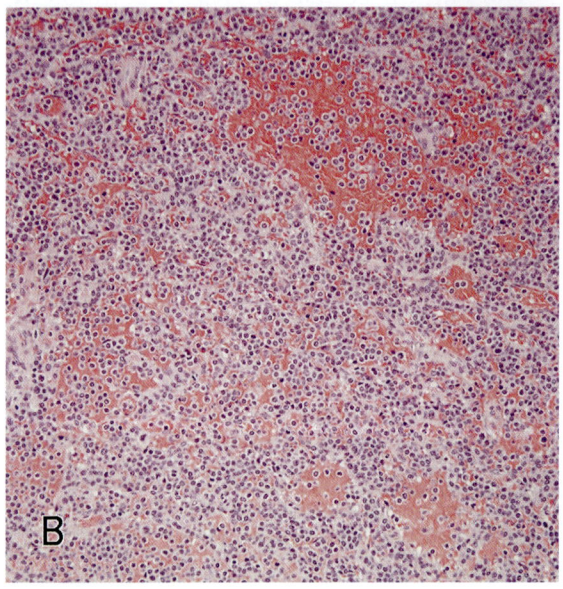

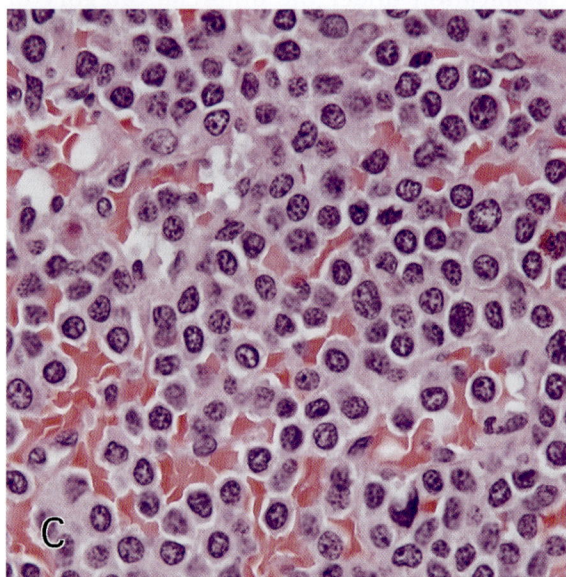

GROSS AND HISTOLOGIC FINDINGS

Spleen

Grossly, the spleen can be very large, with a red, "beefy" cut surface. Small cyst-like structures, consistent with blood lakes, may be appreciated grossly.

Histologic examination shows prominent red pulp and absent or atrophic white pulp (fig. 57-1). Blood lakes can be present (10,12). In the red pulp the splenic sinuses and cords are expanded by small lymphocytes with round nuclei and moderate amounts of pale or clear cytoplasm (fig. 57-2) (10,12). The nucleoli of HCL-V cells are often difficult to appreciate in hematoxylin and eosin (H&E)-stained tissue sections, even when observed by using oil immersion magnification. In some cases, HCL-V cells have more irregular nuclei (fig. 57-3)

Peripheral Blood

The cells of HCL-V in blood smears are typically small to intermediate in size, with abundant cytoplasm, round nuclei, and a single

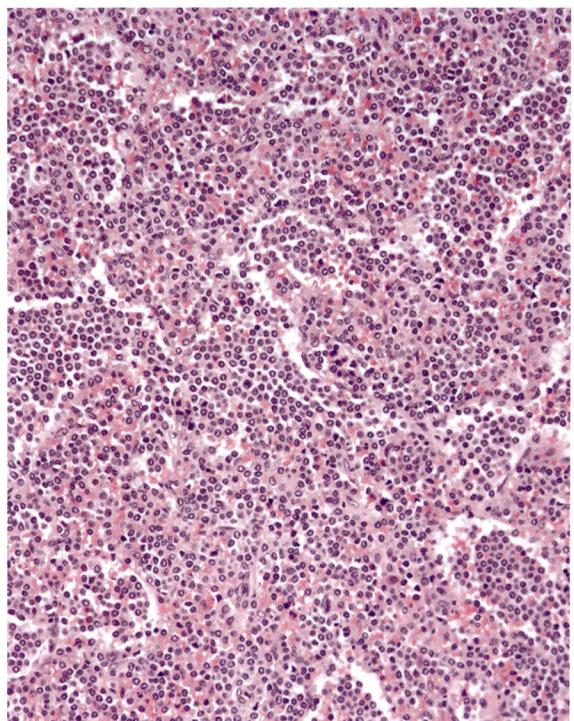

Figure 57-2

HAIRY CELL LEUKEMIA-VARIANT: EXPANDED SPLENIC RED PULP

The red pulp sinuses and cords are expanded by abnormal lymphocytes (H&E stain).

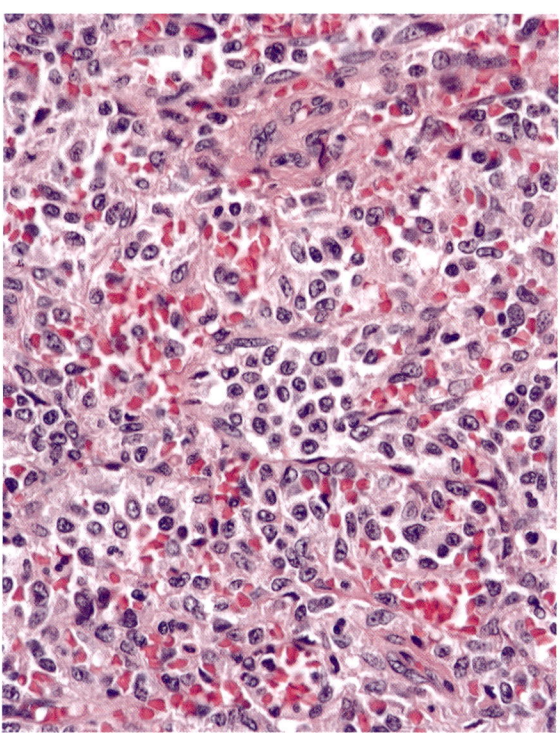

Figure 57-3

HAIRY CELL LEUKEMIA-VARIANT INVOLVING SPLEEN

The neoplastic cells in hairy cell leukemia-variant (HCL-V) can have slightly irregular nuclear contours (H&E stain).

central nucleolus (figs. 57-4, 57-5). Usually the nucleolus is less prominent than is observed in prolymphocytes and a perinucleolar rim is not well-developed. Some cells have two distinct nucleoli. A nucleolus is also not a constant trait since it is usually absent in some HCL-V cells or rarely, most of the neoplastic cells of some patients. The HCL-V cells often have abundant blue or blue-gray cytoplasm and commonly (but not always) have cytoplasmic villous projections (10,13,19). Rare cases of HCL-V are composed of cells with highly convoluted nuclear contours or immature chromatin (so-called convoluted or blastic variants). In some patients, occasional (5 to 10 percent) larger cells are present that may have prominent nucleoli resembling prolymphocytes.

Bone Marrow

The bone marrow is almost always involved in patients with HCL-V. The neoplasm commonly involves the bone marrow in a sinusoidal or interstitial pattern (fig. 57-6, left), but mixed patterns are common and infrequently a diffuse pattern of involvement is present (3,10,17,19). The HCL-V cells may be difficult to appreciate in H&E-stained sections of the bone marrow clot or biopsy specimen. Reticulin fibrosis can occur, but usually is mild or moderate (fig. 57-6, right) and therefore the bone marrow is easily aspirable (10,13). HCL-V cells in bone marrow aspirate smears resemble those in peripheral blood smears except that the villous cytoplasmic projections are more difficult to appreciate (fig. 57-7).

Other Tissues

Splenic hilar lymph nodes are subtotally or completely replaced by HCL-V cells in a diffuse pattern. Small nucleoli are best appreciated using oil immersion. The liver is frequently involved by HCL-V and the neoplastic cells can be distributed throughout the hepatic sinusoids as well as involve the portal tracts (10). Rare skin lesions in patients with HCL-V are dermal infiltrates without evidence of epidermotropism (10).

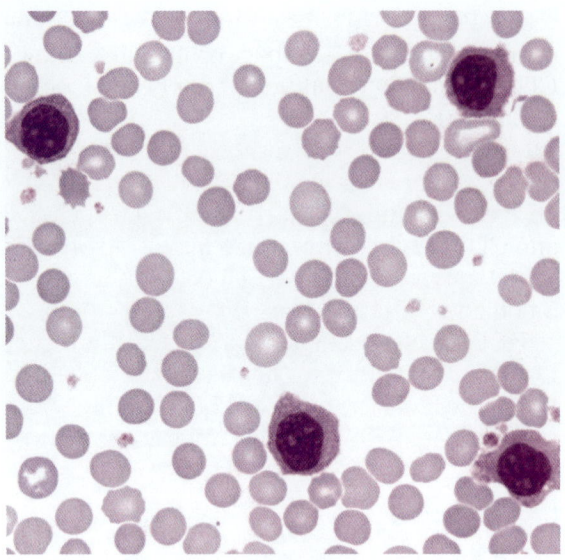

Figure 57-4

**HAIRY CELL LEUKEMIA-VARIANT
INVOLVING PERIPHERAL BLOOD**

The abnormal lymphocytes have distinct nucleoli and shaggy cytoplasmic borders; well-developed villi, however, are not common (Wright-Giemsa stain).

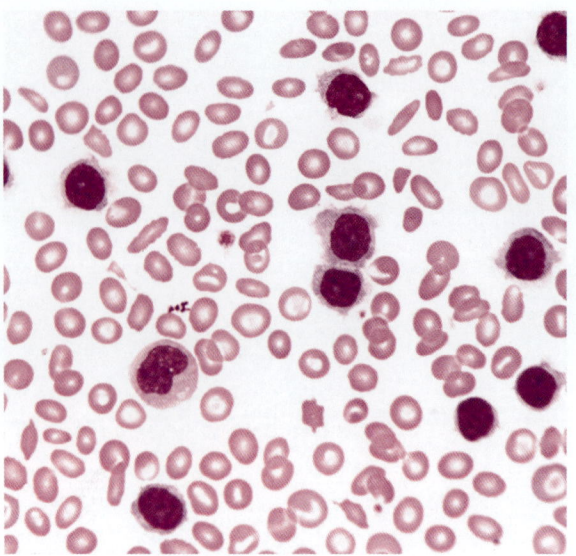

Figure 57-5

**HAIRY CELL LEUKEMIA-VARIANT
INVOLVING PERIPHERAL BLOOD**

The HCL-V cells have coarsely condensed chromatin, distinct nucleoli, pale blue or blue-gray cytoplasm, and irregular (or villous) cytoplasmic borders. The erythrocyte abnormalities also shown are attributable to bone marrow disease (Wright-Giemsa stain).

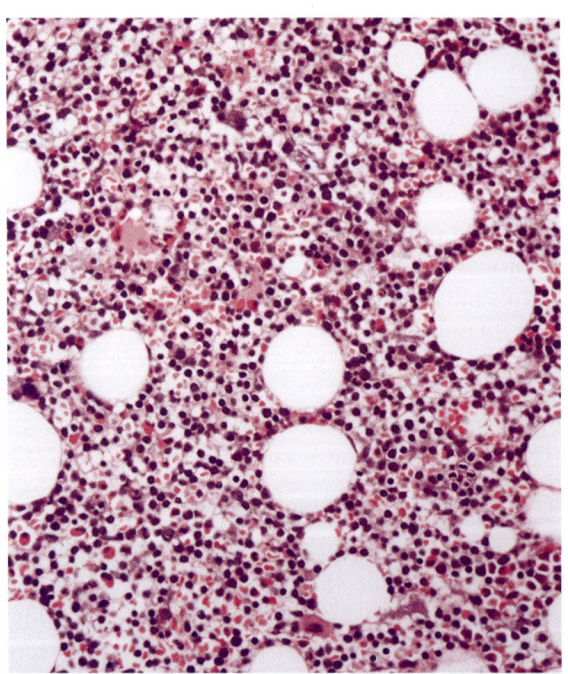

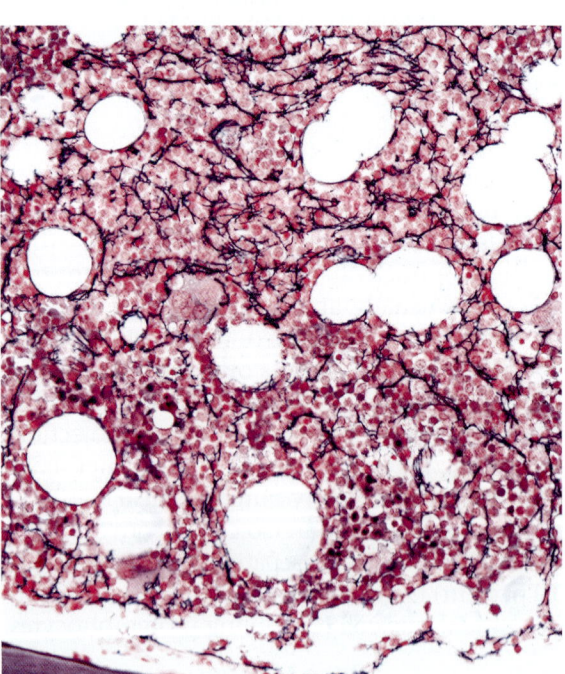

Figure 57-6

HAIRY CELL LEUKEMIA-VARIANT INVOLVING BONE MARROW

Left: A predominantly interstitial pattern is seen (H&E stain).
Right: A reticulin stain shows mild-moderate fibrosis.

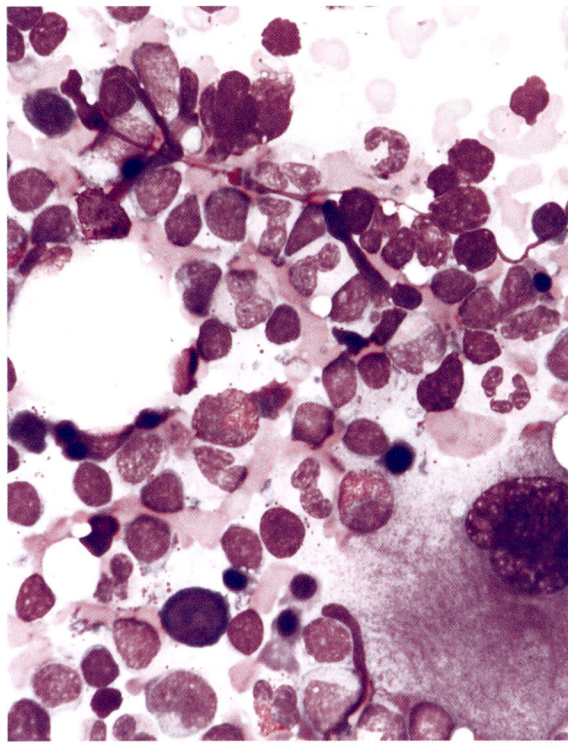

Figure 57-7

**HAIRY CELL LEUKEMIA-VARIANT
INVOLVING BONE MARROW**

This bone marrow aspirate smear shows many HCL-V cells intermixed with normal hematopoietic cells. The villous cytoplasmic projections are difficult to appreciate in this smear (Wright-Giemsa stain).

CYTOLOGIC FINDINGS

In Romanowsky-stained aspirate smears, the lymphocytes are characterized by round, oval, or indented nuclei; single and variably prominent nucleoli; and basophilic cytoplasm. The HCL-V cells may or may not have short blunt cytoplasmic projections.

IMMUNOPHENOTYPIC FINDINGS

Flow cytometry immunophenotypic analysis of HCL-V shows that the neoplastic cells are positive for surface Ig light chain (bright) (3,10,14). IgG is commonly expressed by HCL-V cells, either alone or in combination with IgM or IgD (3,10). The cells are positive for pan-B-cell antigens such as CD19, CD20 (bright), CD22 (bright), and CD79a, as well as for CD11c, CD103, FMC7, and HLA-DR. CD24 or CD79b are positive in about one third of

cases (10). CD123 is often negative, but can be dimly positive in a subset of cases (4,10,14). CD23 is usually negative but has been reported in about 10 percent of HCL-V cases. CD200 is often negative or only dimly expressed (10). Most cases of HCL-V are negative for pan-T-cell antigens (including CD5), CD10, CD23, CD25, and CD27 (3,4,14). Aberrant expression of CD5, CD10, or CD13 has been reported in less than 5 percent of cases (14).

HCL-V cells contain acid phosphatase that is sensitive to tartaric acid and therefore cytochemical analysis for tartrate-resistant acid phosphatase (TRAP) is negative or may show minimal residual acid phosphatase (12,13). Immunohistochemical analysis is very helpful for the analysis of bone marrow and tissue biopsy specimens (11,12). The cells of HCL-V are positive for pan-B-cell markers (fig. 57-8, left) and CD11c. Pan-B-cell antibodies may be critical for distinguishing the extent and distribution of the abnormal B-cell infiltrate in the bone marrow because HCL-V can blend in with erythroid precursors in H&E-stained slides. HCL-V is usually positive for DBA.44/CD76 (fig. 57-8, right) and is negative for CD25, cyclin D1, TRAP, and annexin A1 (fig. 57-9) (11).

MOLECULAR GENETIC FINDINGS

Conventional cytogenetic analysis shows HCL-V to be usually diploid, but about 15 percent of cases have a complex karyotype (10). Using fluorescence in situ hybridization (FISH) analysis or high-resolution genomic profiling with single nucleotide polymorphism arrays, gains of chromosome 5 have been reported in one third of cases and del(7q) in about 20 percent (7). Chromosome 17p deletions or *TP53* mutations also have been reported in up to 30 percent of HCL-V cases (and correlate with a poorer prognosis) (7,10).

HCL-V carries monoclonal immunoglobulin gene rearrangements and is usually negative for T-cell receptor gene rearrangements (12). The *IGH* variable (V) regions show somatic mutations in approximately 75 percent of cases (6). There is also restricted use of *IGHV* in HCL-V; VH4-34 is preferentially used, suggesting a possible role for antigen selection (1,6). Up to 50 percent of HCL-V cases have been reported to use VH4-34, and this finding is associated with

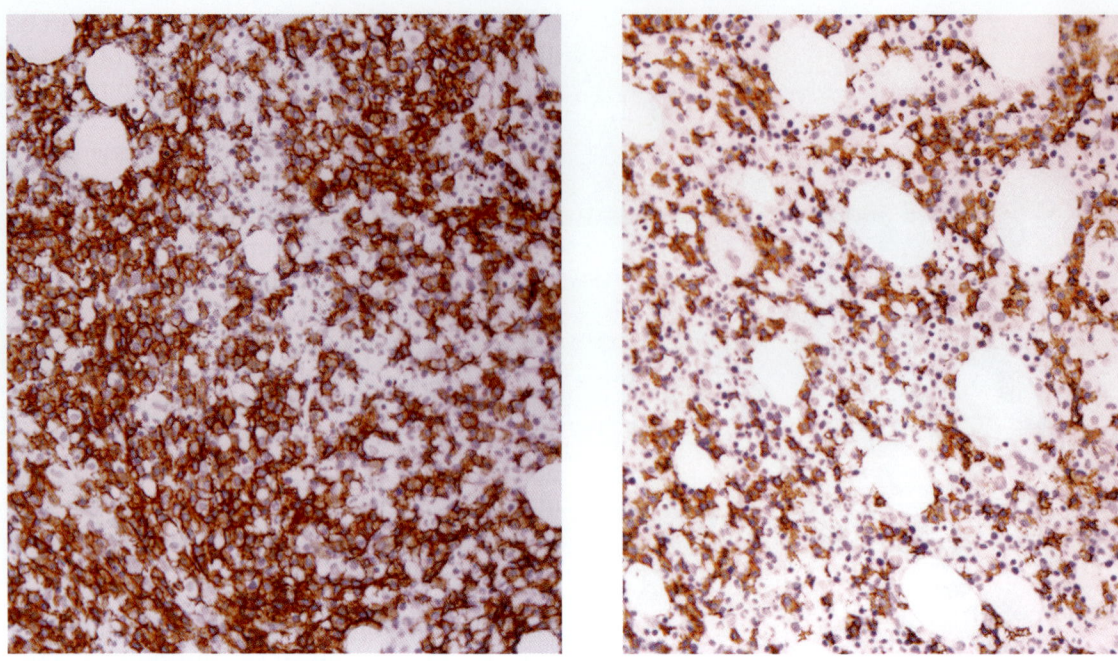

Figure 57-8

HAIRY CELL LEUKEMIA-VARIANT INVOLVING BONE MARROW: IMMUNOHISTOCHEMISTRY

The neoplastic cells are brightly positive for CD20 (left) and DBA.44 (right). This case is the same as is shown in figure 57-6 (immunohistochemistry with hematoxylin counterstain).

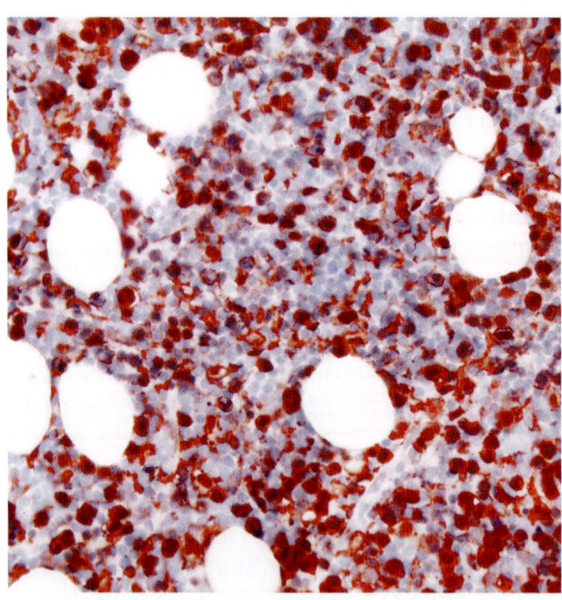

Figure 57-9

HAIRY CELL LEUKEMIA-VARIANT INVOLVING BONE MARROW: ANNEXIN A1

The neoplastic cells are negative for annexin A1 intermixed with many positive granulocytes. This case is the same as is shown in figure 57-6 (immunohistochemistry with hematoxylin counterstain).

an unmutated *IGHV* status (16). Utilization of VH4-34 has been associated with higher disease burden, poorer response to single agent cladribine, and shorter overall survival (16). In one study, shorter telomere length (compared with classic HCL) was shown in cases of HCL-V and was associated with unmutated *IGHV* regions and VH4-34 (1). *IGHV1-2* is not preferentially used in HCL-V, unlike in splenic marginal zone lymphoma (6).

BRAF mutations are rare in HCL-V. Mutations of *MAP2K1*, which encodes MEK in the RAS-BRAF-MEK-ERK pathway, have been reported in 20 to 40 percent of cases of HCL-V (9b,16). *MAP2K1* mutations may be more common in HCL-V cases that utilize VH4-34. Other gene mutations reported in small subsets of cases of HCL-V include *TP53*, *U2AF1* (involved in RNA splicing), and *ARID1A* (involved in chromatin remodeling) (16)

DIFFERENTIAL DIAGNOSIS

Classic Hairy Cell Leukemia. A number of features are helpful for distinguishing HCL-V from classic HCL, summarized here and in

Table 57-1

CLINICOPATHOLOGIC AND LABORATORY FEATURES OF HAIRY CELL LEUKEMIA-VARIANT (HCL-V) AND CLASSIC HAIRY CELL LEUKEMIA (HCL)

Parameter	HCL-V	HCL
White blood cell count	Elevated	Normal or low
Monocyte count	Usually normal	Low to very low
Pancytopenia	Uncommon	Common
Distinct nucleoli in lymphocytes	Usually present	Absent
Bone marrow fibrosis	Mild/moderate or absent	Moderate to severe
TRAP[a] cytochemistry	Rarely positive (variable)	Positive (bright)
CD25, CD123 expression	Uncommon	Usually positive
BRAF V600E	Rare	Usually present
Response to cladribine	Partial or absent	Usually excellent

[a]TRAP = tartrate-resistant acid phosphatase.

Table 57-1. Unlike HCL-V, patients with classic HCL often present with cytopenias, particularly monocytopenia. Classic HCL cells in blood smears have centrally located nuclei without nucleoli. Bone marrow fibrosis is usually prominent in classic HCL, unlike HCL-V in which fibrosis is absent or mild-moderate. Immunophenotypic features helpful for supporting classic HCL include: CD25 (usually bright), annexin A1, and cytochemical and immunohistochemical expression of TRAP. The *BRAF* V600E mutation is very common in classic HCL and rare in HCL-V. Patients with HCL usually respond well to standard therapies such as cladribine or pentostatin unlike HCL-V patients who do not or who may partially respond.

In some cases of HCL, there are minimal immunophenotypic variations from the "usual" that may lead an observer to consider HCL-V. For example, 10 to 20 percent of HCL cases are positive for CD10 and rare cases are CD25 negative. These cases could be diagnosed as HCL-V, but are more appropriately considered as an atypical phenotypic variation of classic HCL if all other data support the diagnosis. The designation of HCL-V should be reserved for cases with significant differences in hematologic and morphologic parameters, immunophenotype, and molecular findings.

Splenic Diffuse Red Pulp Small B-Cell Lymphoma (SDRPBL). There are many similarities between SDRPBL and HCL-V. Some have suggested that these two entities are related since these tumors occur in elderly patients, more

often men, and patients present with lymphocytosis without cytopenias. One morphologic difference between these neoplasms in blood smears is the size of the nucleoli, more prominent in HCL-V. The recent discovery of *MAP2K1* mutations in a subset of HCL-V cases also may be a helpful finding although *MAP2K1* mutation has been reported in rare cases of SDRPBL (9a).

TREATMENT AND PROGNOSIS

Splenectomy is often a first line "therapy" for patients with HCL-V and can result in reduction of symptoms and bulk of disease, as well as providing a specimen for diagnosis (10,13). Sustained responses from splenectomy alone cannot be expected, however. Splenic irradiation has been used with some modest effect, especially in patients who cannot tolerate other therapies. In contrast to classic HCL, patients with HCL-V do not respond well to therapy with interferon alpha or nucleoside analogs, such as cladribine or pentostatin (13). The combination of a nucleoside analog and rituximab, however, has been used with some benefit (9). Other treatments include moxetumomab pasudotox (anti-CD22 combined with pseudomonas exotoxin), anti-CD52 antibody (alemtuzumab), fludarabine, or ibrutinib.

Patients with HCL-V usually have an indolent lymphoproliferative disorder with a median survival period of approximately 9 years (13). Nevertheless, patients with HCL-V often have a more aggressive clinical course and a poorer long-term prognosis than patients with classic HCL. The

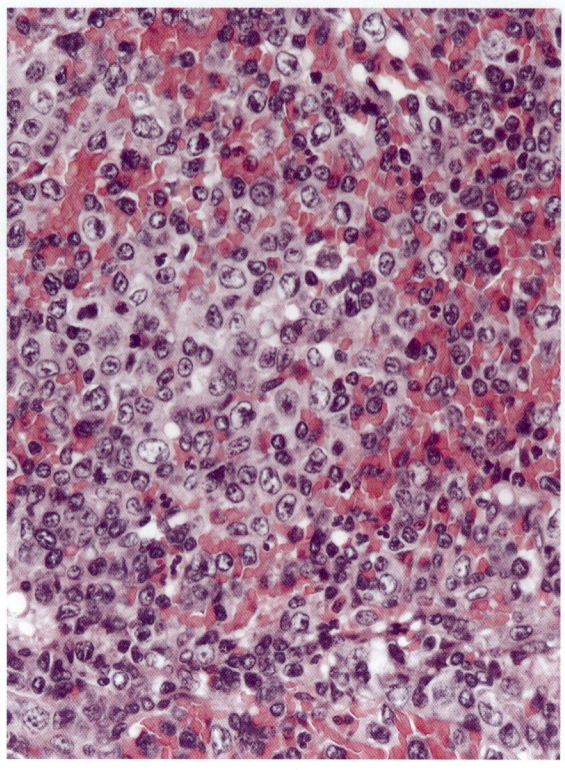

Figure 57-10

HAIRY CELL LEUKEMIA-VARIANT WITH ATYPICAL FEATURES INVOLVING SPLEEN

The cells are intermediate to large in size with occasional mitotic figures, raising the differential diagnosis with diffuse large B-cell lymphoma (H&E stain).

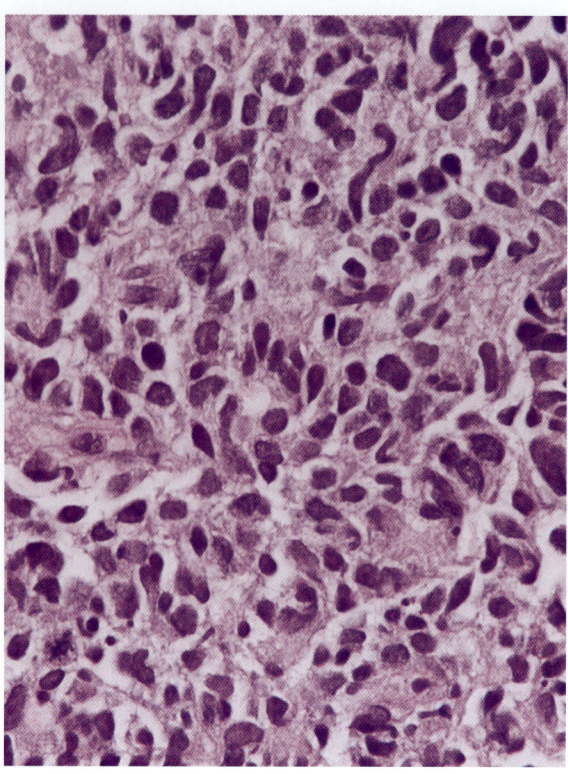

Figure 57-11

HAIRY CELL LEUKEMIA-VARIANT WITH HIGHLY ATYPICAL FEATURES INVOLVING LYMPH NODE

The neoplastic cells have highly irregular nuclei, immature chromatin, and mitotic figures. The patient had a long history of disease and recent clinical findings indicated progression with a change in the pace of disease (H&E stain).

adverse prognostic factors reported by Matutes et al. (10) include older age (over 70 years), anemia (less than 10g/dL), and *TP53* mutations.

Some patients with HCL-V develop a much more aggressive disease, with a very high leukocyte count, extensive bone marrow involvement, and more prominent organomegaly and lymphadenopathy (10,13). In these patients, the neoplastic cells are larger or have blastoid chromatin (figs. 57-10, 57-11) and may be difficult to recognize as HCL-V cells without a history. One case of HCL-V that transformed to a high-grade lymphoma was associated with the use of VH4-34 and the *U2AF1* mutation (18).

REFERENCES

1. Arons E, Zhou H, Edelman DC, et al. Impact of telomere length on survival in classic and variant hairy cell leukemia. Leuk Res 2015;39:1360-1366.
2. Cawley JC, Burns GF, Hayhoe FG. A chronic lymphoproliferative disorder with distinctive features: a distinct variant of hairy-cell leukemia. Leuk Res 1980;4:547-559.
3. Cessna MH, Hartung L, Tripp S, Perkins SL, Bahler DW. Hairy cell leukemia variant: fact or fiction. Am J Clin Pathol 2005;123:132-138.
4. Del Giudice I, Matutes E, Morilla R, et al. The diagnostic value of CD123 in B-cell disorders with hairy or villous lymphocytes. Haematologica 2004;89:303-308.
5. Hockley SL, Else M, Morilla A, et al. The prognostic impact of clinical and molecular features in hairy cell leukaemia variant and splenic marginal zone lymphoma. Br J Haematol 2012;158:347-354.
6. Hockley SL, Giannouli S, Morilla A, et al. Insight into the molecular pathogenesis of hairy cell leukaemia, hairy cell leukaemia variant and splenic marginal zone lymphoma, provided by the analysis of their IGH rearrangements and somatic hypermutation patterns. Br J Haematol 2009;148:666-669.
7. Hockley SL, Morgan GJ, Leone PE, et al. High-resolution genomic profiling in hairy cell leukemia-variant compared with typical hairy cell leukemia. Leukemia 2011;25:1189-1192.
8. Katayama I, Mochino T, Honma T, Fukuda M. Hairy cell leukemia: a comparative study of Japanese and non-Japanese patients. Semin Oncol 1984;11(4 Suppl 2):486-492.
9. Kreitman RJ, Wilson W, Calvo KR, et al. Cladribine with immediate rituximab for the treatment of patients with variant hairy cell leukemia. Clin Cancer Res 2013;19:6873-6881.
9a. Martinez D, Navarro A, Martinez-Trillos A, et al. NOTCH1, TP53, and MAP2K1 mutations in splenic diffuse red pulp small B-cell lymphoma are associated with progressive disease. Am J Surg Pathol 2016;40:192-201.
9b. Mason EF, Brown RD, Szeto DP, et al. Detection of activating MAP2K1 mutations in atypical hairy cell leukemia and hairy cell leukemia variant. Leuk Lymphoma 2017;58:233-236.
10. Matutes E, Martinez-Trillos A, Campo E. Hairy cell leukemia-variant: Disease features and treatment. Best Pract Res Clin Haematol 2015;28:253-263.
11. Petit B, Parrens M, Soubeyran I, et al. Among 157 marginal zone lymphomas, DBA.44 (CD76) expression is restricted to tumour cells infiltrating the red pulp of the spleen with a diffuse architectural pattern. Histopathology 2009;54:626-631.
12. Piris M, Foucar K, Mollejo M, Campo E, Falini B. Splenic B-cell lymphoma/leukemia unclassifiable. In: Swerdlow S, Campo E, Harris NL, et al., eds. WHO classification of tumours of haematopoietic and lymphoid tissues. Lyon: IARC Press; 2008:191-193.
13. Robak T. Hairy-cell leukemia variant: recent view on diagnosis, biology and treatment. Cancer Treat Rev 2011;37:3-10.
14. Shao H, Calvo KR, Gronborg M, et al. Distinguishing hairy cell leukemia variant from hairy cell leukemia: development and validation of diagnostic criteria. Leuk Res 2013;37:401-409.
15. Swerdlow SH, Campo E, Pileri SA, et al. The 2016 revision of the World Health Organization classification of lymphoid neoplasms. Blood 2016;127:2375-2390.
16. Waterfall JJ, Arons E, Walker RL, et al. High prevalence of MAP2K1 mutations in variant and IGHV4-34-expressing hairy-cell leukemias. Nat Genet 2014;46:8-10.
17. Ya-In C, Brandwein J, Pantalony D, Chang H. Hairy cell leukemia variant with features of intrasinusoidal bone marrow involvement. Arch Pathol Lab Med 2005;129:395-398.
18. Zanelli M, Ragazzi M, Valli R, et al. Transformation of IGHV4-34+ hairy cell leukemia-variant with U2AF1 mutation into a clonally-related high grade B-cell lymphoma responding to immunochemotherapy. Br J Haematol 2016;173:491-495.
19. Zhang QY, Chabot-Richards D, Evans M, et al. A retrospective study to assess the relative value of peripheral blood, bone marrow aspirate and biopsy morphology, immunohistochemical stains, and flow cytometric analysis in the diagnosis of chronic B cell lymphoproliferative neoplasms. Int J Lab Hematol 2015;37:390-402.

58 SPLENIC MARGINAL ZONE LYMPHOMA

GENERAL FEATURES

Splenic marginal zone lymphoma (SMZL) is a clinically indolent small B-cell lymphoma associated with prominent splenic involvement, almost invariable bone marrow involvement, and involvement of peripheral blood, liver, and abdominal lymph nodes in decreasing order of frequency. At the molecular level, SMZL is heterogeneous.

These neoplasms have been described in blood smears and the spleen using descriptive names, with the term *splenic lymphoma with villous lymphocytes* the best known (25). In 1992, Schmid et al. (35) described a series of cases using the term splenic marginal zone lymphoma, which is also used in the current World Health Organization (WHO) classification (35a). In retrospect, the term SMZL is somewhat misleading because this neoplasm is distinct from extranodal or nodal marginal zone lymphoma. SMZL represents 1 to 2 percent of all non-Hodgkin lymphomas (16).

The etiology and pathogenesis of SMZL are unknown. There are clues that suggest an infectious etiology. About 5 to 10 percent of patients with SMZL have serologic evidence of hepatitis C infection (23,36). SMZL is more common in geographic regions with a higher prevalence of hepatitis C infection, such as southern Europe (23,36). Evidence of hepatitis B infection is seen in 5 to 10 percent of patients (36). The histologic findings in spleens involved by SMZL show similarities to the spleens of patients with other types of infection.

Molecular analysis of the *IGH* genes in SMZL has shown biased use of *IGH* variable region genes (stereotypy). This suggests a role for antigen drive (selection) in pathogenesis (5,7,11), consistent with either an infectious or autoimmune process. In keeping with a role for autoimmunity, about 10 percent of patients with SMZL have a variety of autoimmune phenomena including autoimmune hemolytic anemia, immune thrombocytopenic purpura, cold agglutinin disease, circulating anticoagulants, or other rare autoimmune manifestations (11,19,37).

CLINICAL FEATURES

SMZL is a disease of adults and the median age in most studies is in the seventh decade (16,24,40). The age range is broad, from about 30 to 90 years. There is no clear sex preference. Some studies have reported a predominance of men, but more recent studies have shown a female predominance (36,40).

Patients most often present with a left upper quadrant mass that may cause pain and early satiety, or is asymptomatic. About 30 to 60 percent of patients also present with B-type symptoms including fever, weight loss, and drenching night sweats (16,24,36). The most common physical finding is splenomegaly, in at least three quarters of all patients, and in some studies over 90 percent (40). Almost all patients have enlarged splenic hilar lymph nodes and about 25 percent have prominent intra-abdominal lymphadenopathy. Peripheral lymphadenopathy is uncommon (10 to 15 percent of patients). Hepatomegaly is present in 10 to 20 percent of SMZL patients. Most patients have stage IV disease at the time of diagnosis.

Laboratory studies show absolute lymphocytosis (although often not marked) in about 50 percent of patients, and anemia, thrombocytopenia, or both in 25 percent (24,36). The anemia may be related to autoimmune hemolytic anemia or is associated with extensive bone marrow replacement by SMZL. A serum paraprotein is detected in up to 25 percent of patients, usually of IgM type, but IgG also has been reported. The paraprotein level is usually low (16,36), but rare patients with SMZL have a high serum IgM paraprotein level associated with serum hyperviscosity. The serum lactate dehydrogenase (LDH) level can be elevated, related to tumor

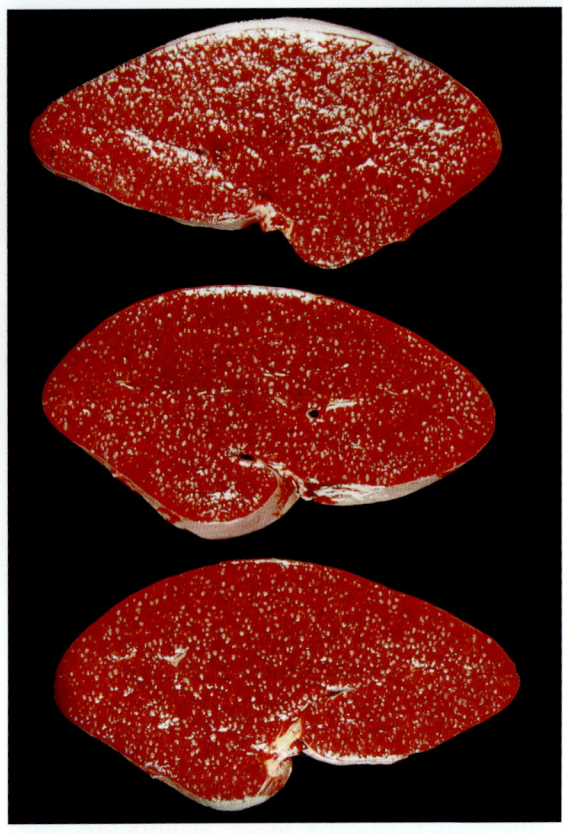

Figure 58-1

SPLENIC MARGINAL ZONE LYMPHOMA

The cut surface shows a massively enlarged spleen with a "miliary" pattern resulting from an increase in the number and size of the splenic white pulp nodules. (Courtesy of Dr. A. Sohani, Boston, MA.)

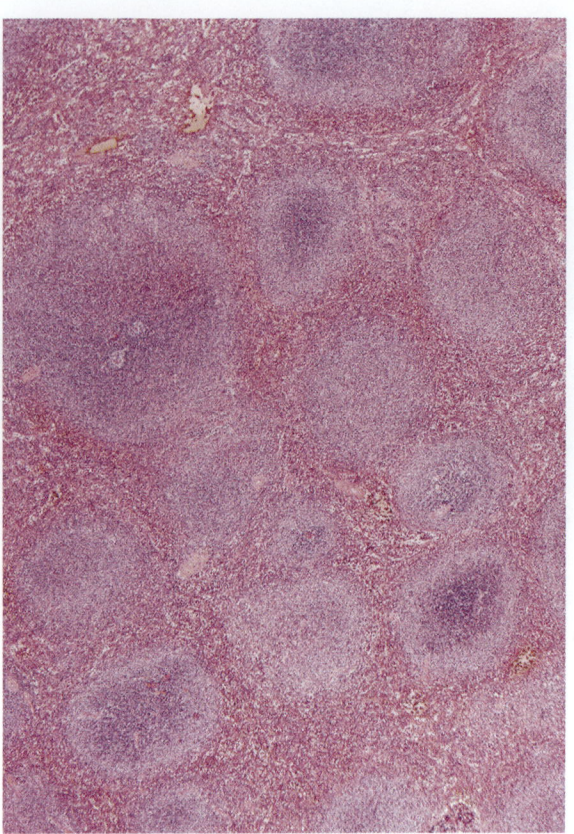

Figure 58-2

SPLENIC MARGINAL ZONE LYMPHOMA

The white pulp nodules are large, with a central darker area and a rim of pale (marginal zone) cells. This is an exaggeration of the normal marginal zone pattern observed in splenic white pulp (hematoxylin and eosin [H&E] stain).

or hemolysis in patients with autoimmune hemolytic anemia. Serum beta-2-microglobulin also may be elevated. A lupus anticoagulant or acquired von Willebrand disease is observed in a small subset of SMZL patients (37).

GROSS AND HISTOLOGIC FINDINGS

Spleen

The spleen is usually markedly enlarged, with a mean weight of 1,300 to 1,800 g (16,24,39). Spleens over 4,000 g have been described. Rarely, the spleen is of normal size, usually excised in patients who initially present with autoimmune-induced anemia or thrombocytopenia (36).

The cut surface of the spleen has a characteristic appearance manifested by expanded white pulp structures and red pulp nodules (with extensive disease), imparting a micro-nodular or miliary pattern (fig. 58-1). In spleens with extensive involvement, large white pulp nodules fuse and diffusely replace the splenic architecture, although some nodular areas are invariably present.

At low magnification, the spleen shows an overall increase in the size and number of white pulp nodules (figs. 58-2, 58-3) (16,17,30,39). In classic SMZL, the white pulp nodules have a biphasic appearance, with slightly larger lymphocytes with abundant pale cytoplasm (monocytoid differentiation) that impart a lighter appearance at the periphery of the white pulp nodules and smaller lymphocytes with minimal cytoplasm (darker appearance) more centrally (fig. 58-2) (16,17,30). In other cases of SMZL, the white pulp nodules are expanded by

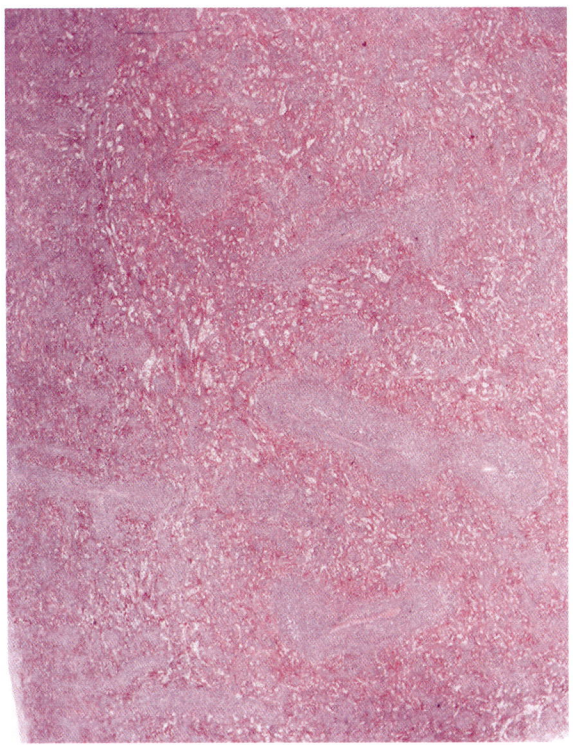

Figure 58-3

SPLENIC MARGINAL ZONE LYMPHOMA

The white pulp nodules are expanded by a more monomorphic population of lymphoma cells. The biphasic pattern observed in figure 58-2 is not present in this case and there is more prominent red pulp involvement (H&E stain).

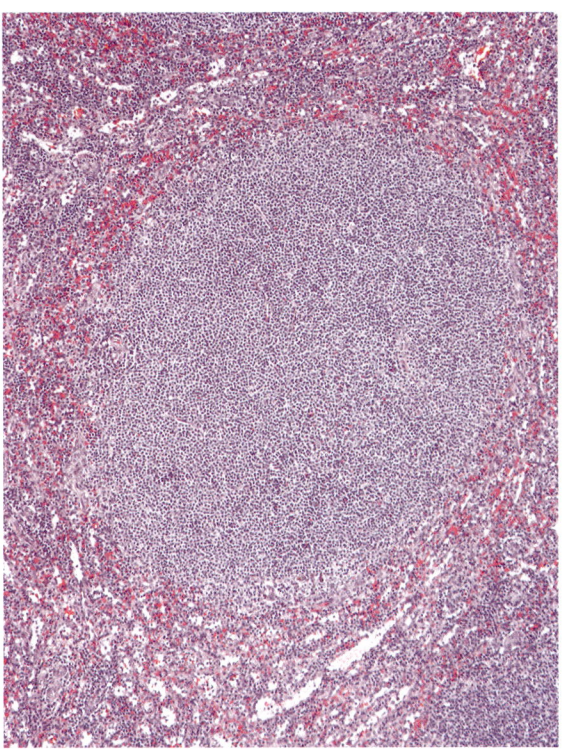

Figure 58-4

SPLENIC MARGINAL ZONE LYMPHOMA

The normal composition of the splenic white pulp nodules is replaced by a uniform population of small lymphoid cells (H&E stain).

a more monotonous infiltrate of cells without the biphasic low-power microscopic pattern (figs. 58-3, 58-4). Residual germinal centers can be appreciated in a subset of white pulp nodules (fig. 58-5). In other cases the periarteriolar lymphoid sheath is surrounded by lymphoma. Lymphoma cells also may colonize germinal centers, imparting a follicle-like appearance. Rarely, SMZL is associated with amyloid deposition.

In almost all cases of SMZL the red pulp is also involved by lymphoma (16,23). Lymphoma cells may be seen singly or in small clusters and small nodules (fig. 58-3). Clusters of epithelioid histiocytes are seen in about one third of SMZL cases, usually in the red pulp (16). Well-formed epithelioid granulomas may be seen and can be florid in occasional cases (21).

At high magnification, the cells of SMZL exhibit a broad spectrum of findings. The cells most commonly are monocytoid with abun-

dant pale cytoplasm (fig. 58-6). Some cells are predominantly small lymphocytes without prominent marginal zone differentiation (fig. 58-4). In 10 to 20 percent of cases, plasmacytoid lymphocytes or plasma cells are common; rarely, they are present in sheets (similar to a plasmacytoma) and Dutcher bodies may be numerous (fig. 58-7) (16,17,30).

Lymph Nodes

Lymph node findings are best described in the splenic hilar lymph nodes (27). The lymph nodes are usually partially involved by SMZL, which forms multiple nodules that are centered on the lymphoid follicles (figs. 58-8, 58-9). These nodules are composed predominantly of small cells, with few (less than 5 percent) admixed large lymphoid cells (monophasic appearance). A biphasic appearance, as observed in the spleen, is less common in lymph nodes. Sinuses are almost always patent, either partially or totally (16,27).

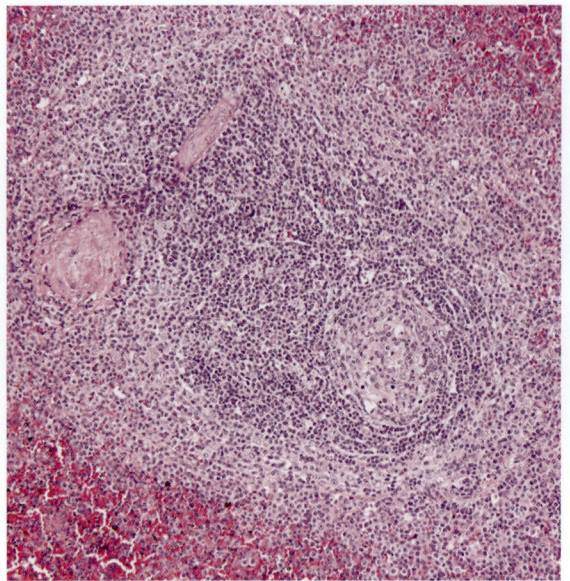

Figure 58-5

SPLENIC MARGINAL ZONE LYMPHOMA

A reactive germinal center is seen surrounded by lymphoma. The periarteriolar sheath region also is seen (H&E stain).

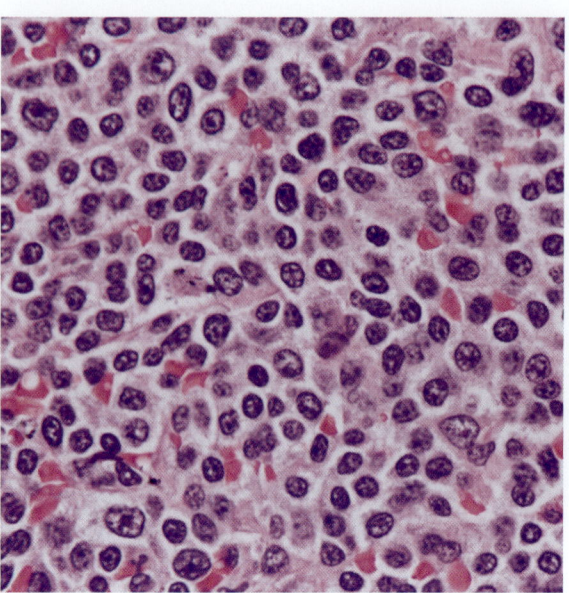

Figure 58-6

SPLENIC MARGINAL ZONE LYMPHOMA

High magnification of this neoplasm shows predominantly small lymphoid cells with round nuclei, dense chromatin, and abundant pale cytoplasm. Scattered large lymphoid cells are also present (H&E stain).

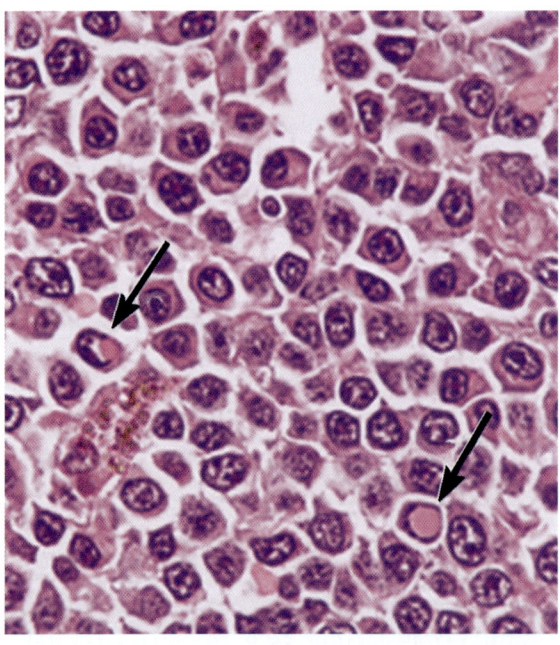

Figure 58-7

SPLENIC MARGINAL ZONE LYMPHOMA

High magnification of this tumor shows lymphoma cells with abundant plasmacytic differentiation. Occasional cells also show nuclear pseudoinclusions or Dutcher bodies (arrows) (H&E stain).

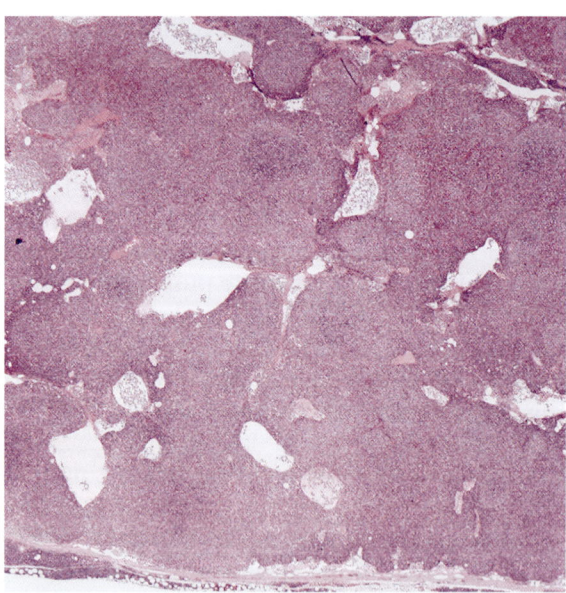

Figure 58-8

SPLENIC MARGINAL ZONE LYMPHOMA EXTENSIVELY INVOLVING SPLENIC HILAR LYMPH NODE

The lymph node is enlarged and most of the parenchyma is replaced by lymphoma, which is pale at this power. A hint of residual follicles is present within the vague nodular areas (H&E stain).

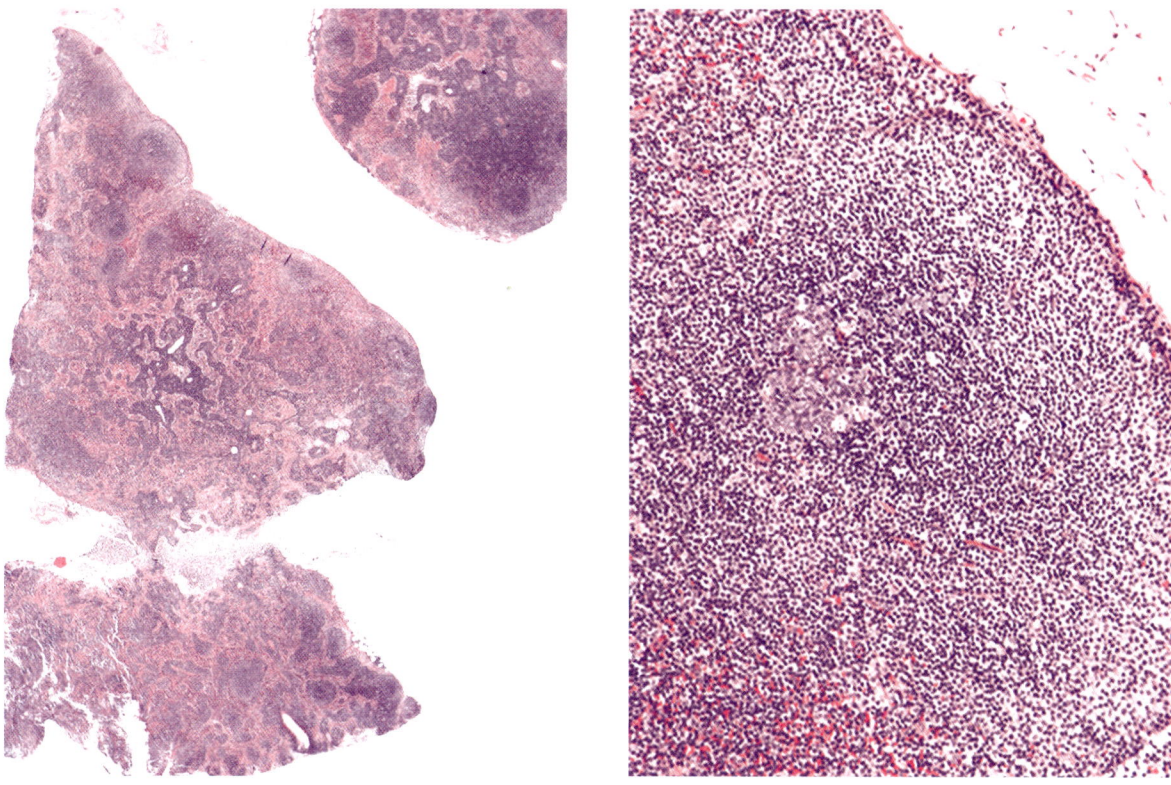

Figure 58-9

SPLENIC MARGINAL ZONE LYMPHOMA PARTIALLY INVOLVING SPLENIC HILAR LYMPH NODE

Left: In areas, the lymphoma cells expand marginal zones around reactive follicles. Most of the lymph node, however, is not involved and sinuses are patent.

Right: Higher magnification shows lymphoma cells with pale (monocytoid) cytoplasm expanding the marginal zone around a reactive germinal center (H&E stain).

Bone Marrow

Bone marrow involvement can be confined to an intrasinusoidal distribution, often difficult to appreciate by standard histologic stains but highlighted by immunohistochemistry (fig. 58-10) (10,15). Nonparatrabecular nodules are also common (fig. 58-11). In about 25 percent of cases, reactive germinal centers with a rim of neoplastic cells with monocytoid differentiation are observed (15). In advanced cases, diffuse bone marrow involvement may be seen.

In contrast with the spleen, SMZL in the bone marrow is more often monomorphic, with fewer apparent large transformed lymphocytes. At high magnification, the lymphoma cells are small lymphocytes with round to slightly irregular nuclei and variable amounts of pale (monocytoid) cytoplasm; a plasmacytoid appearance can be prominent in some cases (10,15).

Peripheral Blood

A low-level absolute lymphocytosis is present in about half of all SMZL patients and a small number of patients present with marked leukocytosis and lymphocytosis (fig. 58-12). The SMZL lymphocytes are most often small, although occasional intermediate-sized lymphocytes may be seen. Most SMZL lymphocytes have round nuclei with dense or dispersed chromatin and moderate to abundant pale cytoplasm. Some of the cells have irregular cytoplasmic projections, often at one or both cell poles (unlike in hairy cell leukemia where the villi are more circumferential), although this feature is not universally present (6,14,25). Lymphocytic villi are more easily appreciable in the peripheral blood than in bone marrow aspirate smears. In some patients with SMZL, prolymphocytes are increased in blood smears and, rarely, prolymphocytes are numerous,

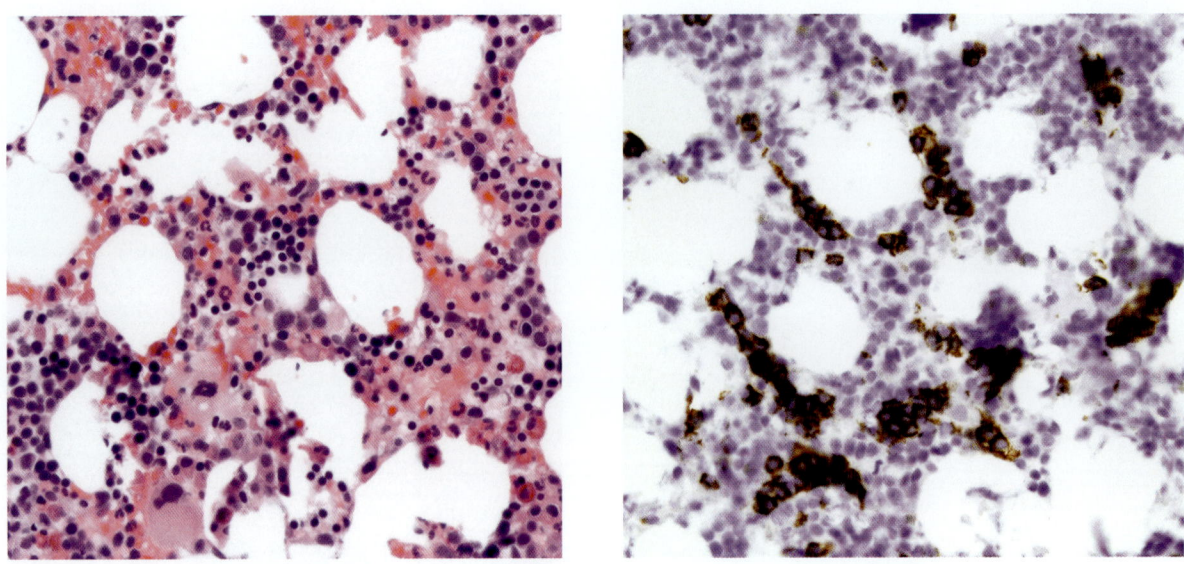

Figure 58-10

SPLENIC MARGINAL ZONE LYMPHOMA INVOLVING BONE MARROW

Left: At this magnification, the bone marrow core biopsy specimen is normocellular and the involvement by lymphoma is subtle (H&E stain).

Right: Immunohistochemistry for CD20 highlights the lymphoma cells in a sinusoidal pattern (immunohistochemistry with hematoxylin counterstain).

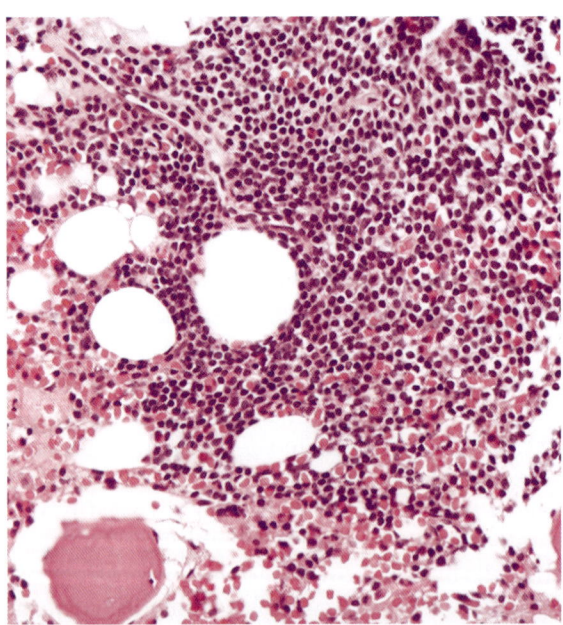

Figure 58-11

SPLENIC MARGINAL ZONE LYMPHOMA INVOLVING BONE MARROW

The core biopsy specimen shows a nonparatrabecular nodule composed of mostly small lymphoid cells. A lipogranuloma is also present (H&E stain).

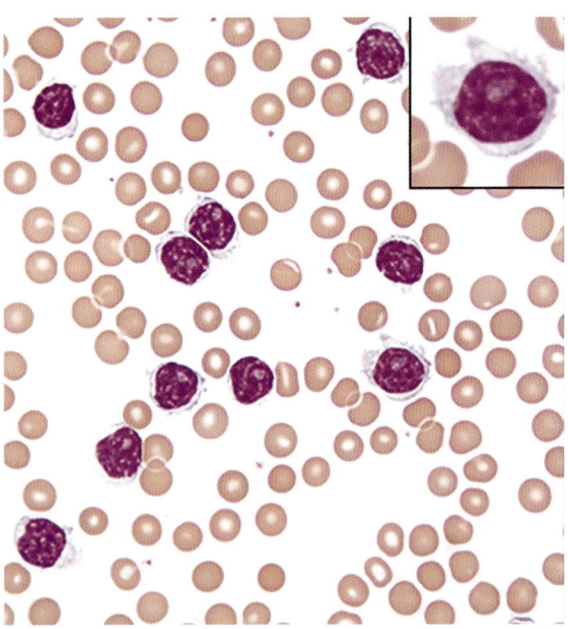

Figure 58-12

SPLENIC MARGINAL ZONE LYMPHOMA IN LEUKEMIC PHASE IN PERIPHERAL BLOOD

The patient had a leukocyte count of 66 x 10⁹/L (normal range, 4-11 x 10⁹/L). The lymphoma cells are small with round nuclei, small nucleoli, and irregular or "villous" cytoplasmic borders (inset) (Wright-Giemsa stain).

resulting in a morphologic picture resembling B-cell prolymphocytic leukemia (fig. 58-13) (14).

Liver

Liver involvement is seen in about one third of SMZL patients who undergo biopsy. The lymphoma cells may be intrasinusoidal or form clusters and aggregates in the portal triads (fig. 58-14) (16,23).

CYTOLOGIC FINDINGS

Although not commonly performed, fine-needle aspiration of the spleen shows small lymphoid cells, many of which have increased pale cytoplasm (fig. 58-15). In all cases, variable numbers of larger lymphocytes are present; plasmacytic differentiation is present in a subset of cases.

IMMUNOPHENOTYPIC FINDINGS

The lymphoma cells are positive for pan-B-cell antigens, such as CD19, CD20, CD22, and CD79a, and are negative for CD3, CD10, CD25, and CD43 (10,16,36). Surface IgM is expressed as well as surface IgD in most cases. The lymphoma

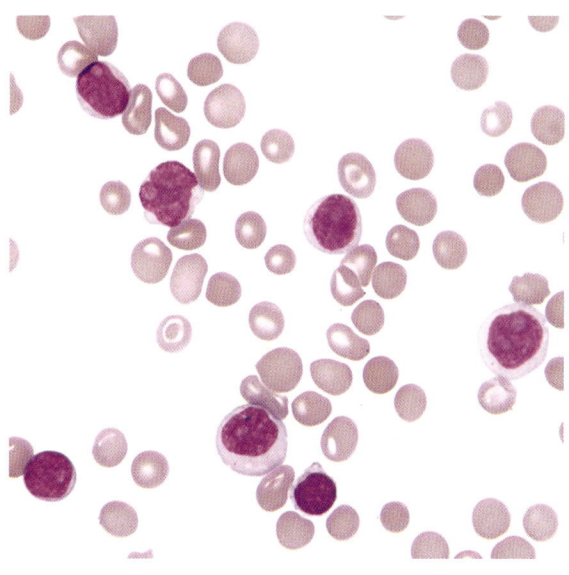

Figure 58-13

SPLENIC MARGINAL ZONE LYMPHOMA WITH INCREASED PROLYMPHOCYTOID CELLS INVOLVING PERIPHERAL BLOOD

This blood smear shows medium-sized and large cells with prominent nucleoli resembling B-prolymphocytic leukemia (Wright-Giemsa stain).

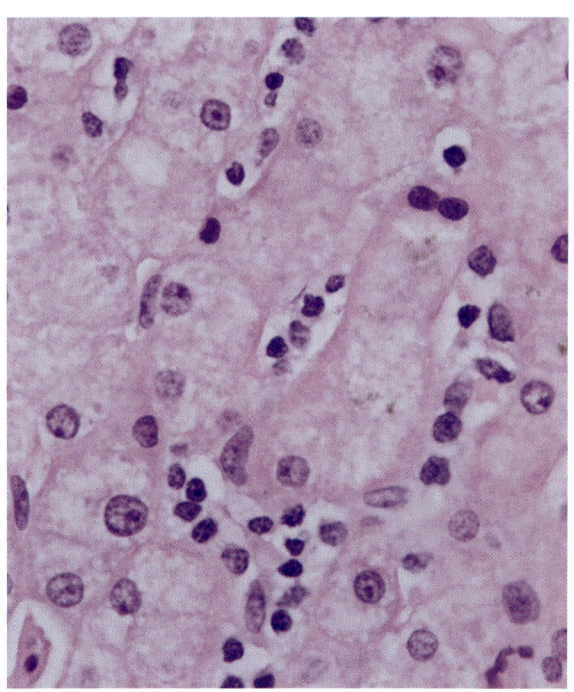
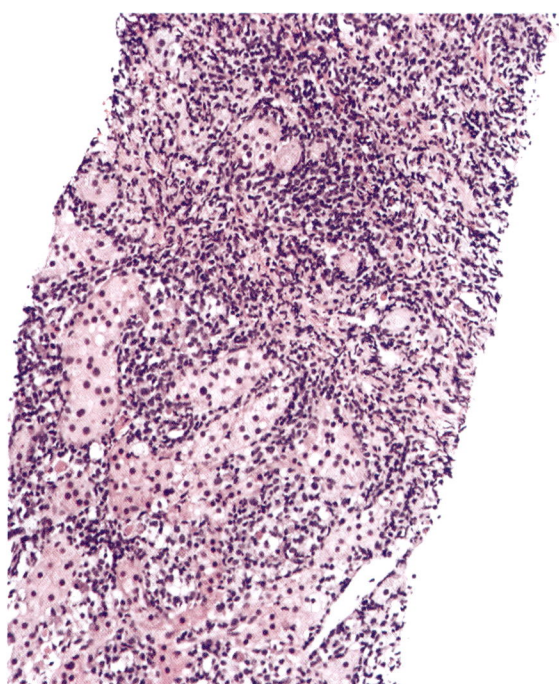

Figure 58-14

SPLENIC MARGINAL ZONE LYMPHOMA INVOLVING LIVER

Left: In this liver biopsy specimen, there is sinusoidal involvement by lymphoma cells.
Right: Another liver biopsy specimen shows extensive involvement of portal tracts and parenchyma (H&E stain).

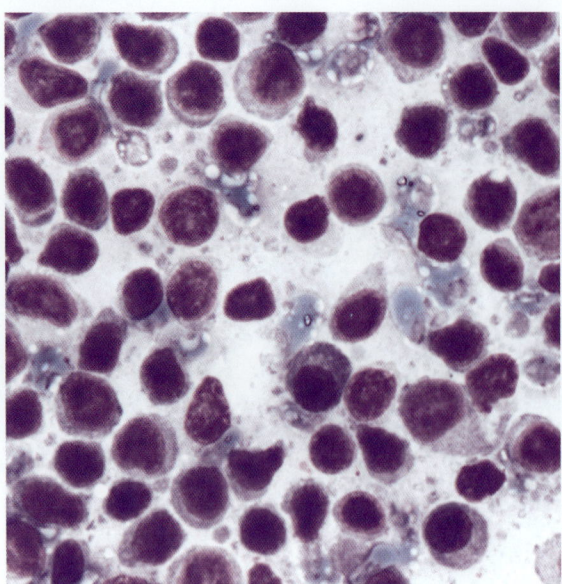
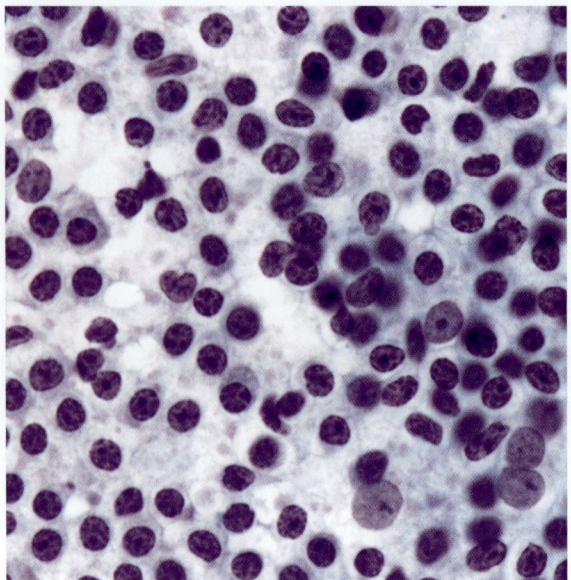

Figure 58-15

SPLENIC MARGINAL ZONE LYMPHOMA: CYTOLOGIC FINDINGS

These fine-needle aspirate smears show monocytoid lymphoma cells with pale blue cytoplasm and occasional plasmacytoid cells (left: Diff-Quik stain; right: Papanicolaou stain).

cells also commonly express CD11c and FMC7, CD200 is often dim, and dim CD123 is seen in some cases (10,12,23). CD5 is usually negative but can be expressed, usually dimly, in about 20 percent of cases. CD5 expression correlates with an increased frequency of marked leukemic involvement (6). CD103 is negative in most cases.

The immunohistochemical findings are comparable with the results of flow cytometric immunophenotyping. SMZL is positive for pan-B-cell antigens including CD20 (fig. 58-16), CD79a, and PAX5. Surface/cytoplasmic IgM is expressed in many cases, whereas IgD is variably expressed. BCL2 is positive (fig. 58-16) and CD11c and DBA.44 are positive in 75 percent of cases (10,24). CD25 and SOX11 reactivity also have been reported (28). The cells of SMZL are negative for pan-T-cell antigens, CD1a, CD10, CD21, CD23, CD43, BCL6, cyclin D1, TRAP, MUM1/IRF4, and annexin A1. Dim CD5 expression detected by flow cytometry is often negative by immunohistochemistry due to the lower sensitivity of the method (6). In cases with plasma cell differentiation, monotypic cytoplasmic immunoglobulin light chain, CD38, and CD138 are often positive. Ki-67 usually shows a low proliferation rate (less than 15 percent). If the overall proliferation rate is high (over 30 percent)

the possibility of transformation to diffuse large B-cell lymphoma (DLBCL) should be considered. In cases of transformation to DLBCL, the lymphoma cells may express BCL6 or MUM1/IRF4 (16).

As mentioned above, intrasinusoidal involvement of the bone marrow may be difficult to appreciate in routinely stained sections but is well highlighted by immunohistochemistry with B-cell antibodies (fig. 58-10, right) (10,15). The presence of lymphoma cells within sinusoids also is accentuated by staining with markers of bone marrow endothelial/sinus cells, such as CD34.

MOLECULAR GENETIC STUDIES

Conventional cytogenetic and fluorescence in situ hybridization (FISH) analysis shows chromosomal aberrations in up to 80 percent of cases of SMZL (16,34). A complex karyotype is common (34). These genetic changes, however, are not specific for SMZL and can be seen in other small B-cell lymphomas, including other lymphomas that involve the spleen.

The most frequent cytogenetic abnormalities are: del 7q, 30 to 40 percent; gains of 3q or +3, 20 to 30 percent; 14q translocations, 10 to 15 percent; and del(6q), about 10 percent (34). Losses of 7q are the most frequent isolated abnormality (1,34).

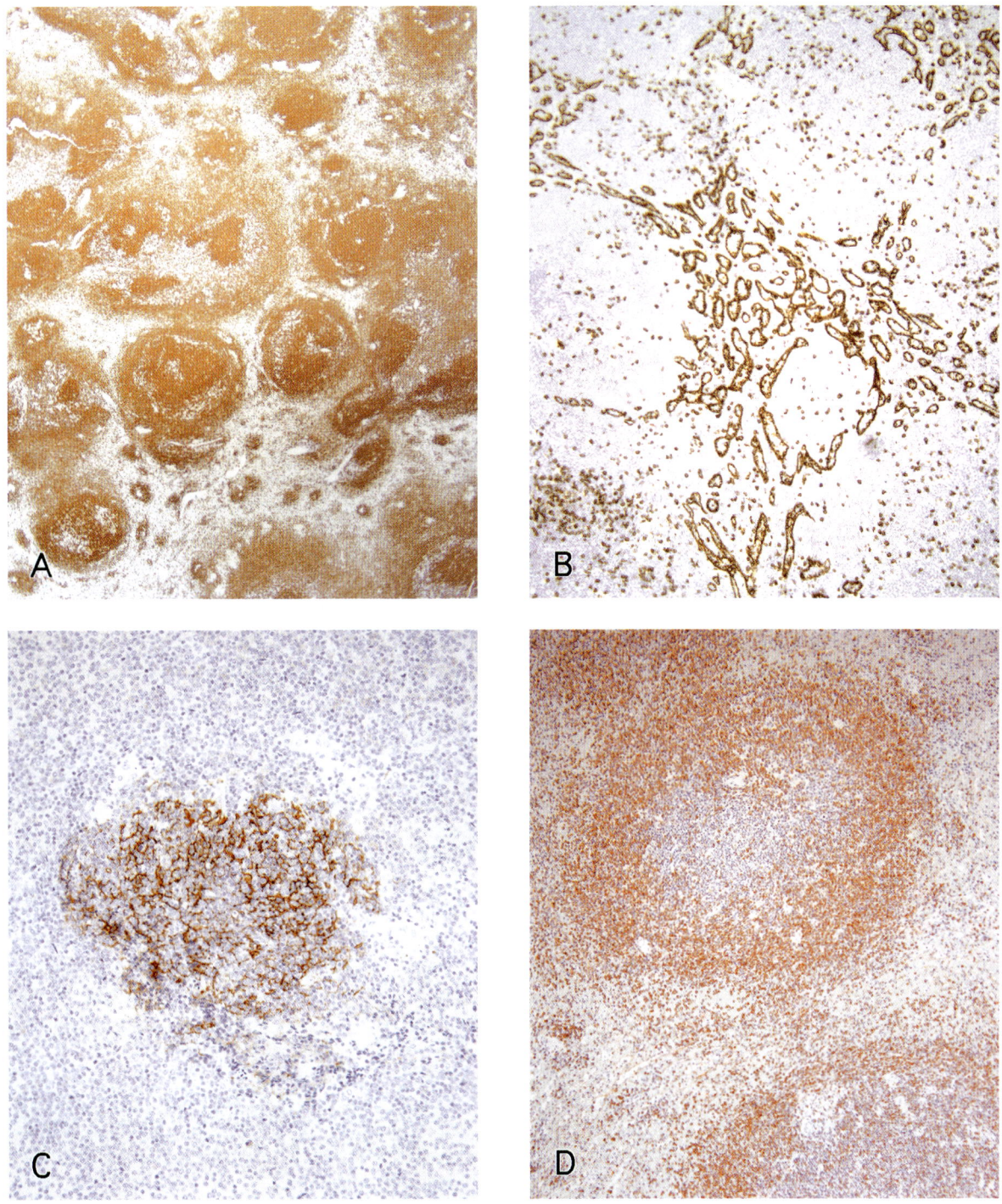

Figure 58-16

SPLENIC MARGINAL ZONE LYMPHOMA: IMMUNOHISTOCHEMISTRY

A: CD20 highlights SMZL in white pulp nodules and also, to a lesser degree, in the red pulp.

B: CD8 highlights the overall decrease of the red pulp components and expansion of white pulp nodules.

C: CD21 highlights the follicular dendritic cell network in a residual germinal center; the lymphoma cells are negative.

D: BCL2 highlights the lymphoma cells. Central residual germinal centers are negative for BCL2 (A–D: Immunohistochemistry with hematoxylin counterstain.)

Abnormalities of *TP53*, as evidenced by del (17p), are detected in about 20 percent of cases by FISH (16,23). Translocations that occur in mucosa-associated lymphoid tissue (MALT) lymphomas do not occur in SMZL. CD5-positive cases of SMZL have a higher frequency +3/3q, del(6q), and trisomy 18 and a lower frequency of del(7q) than CD5-negative SMZL (6). Watkins et al. (38) reported that deletion of 7(q32.1-32.2) is rare in other splenic B-cell lymphomas, and they suggested that this deletion is a fairly specific marker for SMZL.

Array comparative genomic hybridization (CGH) studies of SMZL have shown gains of 3q13.13-q29, about 20 percent; 6q27, about 20 percent, 8p23, about 15 percent; 9q31.1, 13 percent; 12q21.31, 13 percent; 13q11-q12.11, 28 percent; 18q23, 15 percent; and 21p, 17 percent. Losses in SMZL occur in 1p36.21-p36.13, 13 percent; 4p12-11, 13 percent; 7q31.31-q32.3, 25 percent; 8p, 13 percent; and 17p13.3-p13.1, 17 percent (29,32). Other high-resolution array CGH studies have detected abnormalities in 5p, 12p, 20q and 9p (29). Micro (mi) RNA studies have shown overexpression of miR155, miR451, and miR486, and underexpression of miR127, miR139, miR335, and miR411 (3,9). Overexpression of miR21 is reported to be more common in clinically aggressive cases of SMZL.

Evaluation of *IGHV* mutational status in SMZL has shown that about 50 percent of cases have mutated and the other 50 percent has unmutated *IGHV* genes (1,5,24,36). SMZL also has a restricted gene repertoire with the most common being *IGHVH1-2* (about 33 percent), followed by *IGHV4-34* (about 10 percent), and *IGHV3-23* (about 10 percent) (5). These data suggest a role for antigen drive in disease pathogenesis.

Gene expression profiling studies have shown upregulation of genes involved in NF-κB activation, B-cell receptor signaling, tumor necrosis factor signaling, and other genes (3,22). Epigenetic modification of genes also occurs in SMZL. In one study, SMZL was subdivided into two groups based on high versus low promoter methylation (4). The methylation phenotype was associated with *NOTCH2* mutations, del(7q31-32), preferential *IGHV1-02* usage, and a higher frequency of histologic transformation to DLBCL. Cell line experiments using demethylating agents showed that the high methylation phenotype may be reversed, suggesting a potential therapeutic approach (4).

Single gene and next-generation sequencing methods have shown that SMZL is heterogeneous (22,31). In a study by Martinez et al. (22), a variety of genes were mutated in four essential cell processes: marginal zone differentiation, NF-κB activation, chromatin remodeling, and the cytoskeleton. Other studies have shown a high frequency of mutations involving Kruppel-like factor 2 (*KLF2*) and *NOTCH2*, in about 10 to 40 percent and 10 to 30 percent of cases, respectively (13,18,31,33). *KLF2* negatively regulates the NF-κB pathway and inactivation by mutation therefore enhances NF-κB activity (13). *NOTCH2* has many functions including being a master controller of marginal zone differentiation. *TP53* mutations occur in about 15 percent of cases of SMZL and correlate, in part, with shorter overall survival time or histologic transformation to DLBCL (31). Mutations in *TNFAIP3*, *KMT2D/MLL2*, and *ARID1A* occur in 5 to 10 percent of cases (31). The *MYD88* mutation is uncommon (less than 5 percent), but seems to occur in bona fide cases of SMZL (rather than misdiagnosed Waldenstrom macroglobulinemia) (13,31). *BRAF* V600E mutations are rare in SMZL (8).

DIFFERENTIAL DIAGNOSIS

Splenic Marginal Zone Hyperplasia. Marginal zone hyperplasia in the spleen is defined as expansion of the marginal zone to a thickness of greater than 12 cells (fig. 58-17). Cytologically, the cells in expanded, hyperplastic marginal zones are similar to the cells of SMZL. The presence of numerous hyperplastic germinal centers in the white pulp is one clue supporting the diagnosis of hyperplasia, however, previous steroid therapy may suppress germinal center formation without affecting the marginal zone. Clinical findings such as massive splenomegaly or peripheral cytopenias cannot be explained by hyperplasia. Ancillary studies are also helpful as monoclonality or an aberrant B-cell immunophenotype detected in spleen, bone marrow, or blood supports SMZL.

Transformation of SMZL to Diffuse Large B-Cell Lymphoma. DLBCL of the spleen can develop de novo, be a result of transformation of SMZL, or represent secondary involvement by systemic lymphoma. Here the focus is on transformation of SMZL to DLBCL, which occurs in approximately 10 percent of patients with SMZL (16).

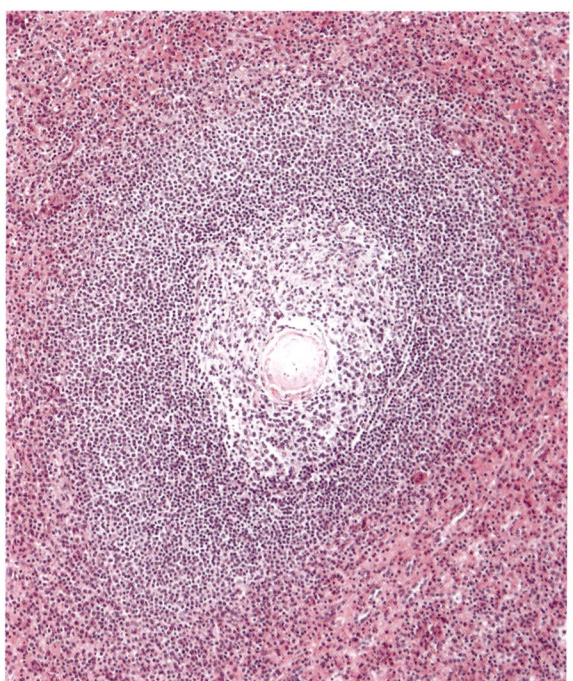

Figure 58-17

SPLENIC MARGINAL ZONE HYPERPLASIA

In this field the marginal zone of a white pulp nodule is expanded. Hyperplasia can overlap with early or subtle involvement by SMZL. In these cases, flow cytometry immunophenotyping or polymerase chain reaction (PCR) studies to assess B-cell clonality may be helpful.

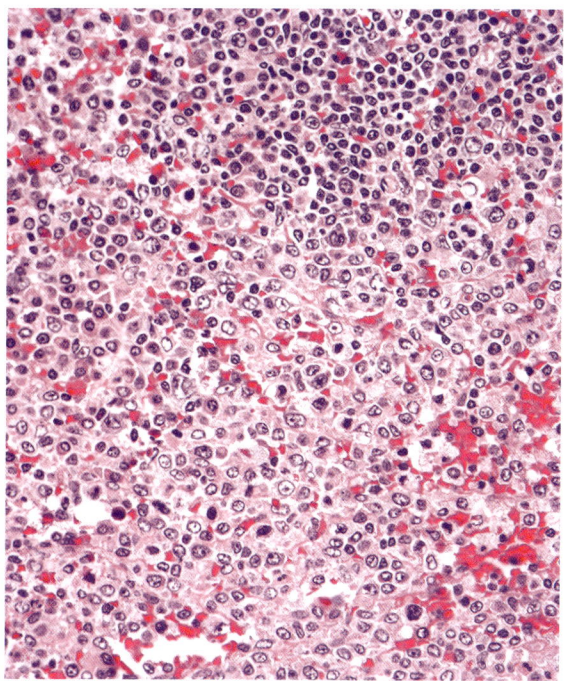

Figure 58-18

SPLENIC MARGINAL ZONE LYMPHOMA WITH TRANSFORMATION TO DIFFUSE LARGE B-CELL LYMPHOMA

The presence of sheets of large B-cells is the only reliable criterion for transformation to diffuse large B-cell lymphoma.

The presence of sheets of large cells replacing the splenic architecture is the best criterion for the diagnosis of transformation of SMZL to DLBCL (fig. 58-18). There are no other consensus criteria that can be applied in non-obvious cases. Others have suggested that the presence of more than 30 percent large cells correlates with more aggressive behavior. Other findings that suggest the possibility of transformation include a high mitotic or proliferation (Ki-67) rate, bright and uniform p53 expression, or *TP53* mutation. Correlation with clinical findings (e.g., B symptoms, high serum LDH level) or radiologic findings (e.g. rapid increase in spleen size or necrosis) can be helpful.

Small B-Cell Lymphomas that Preferentially Involve Splenic White Pulp. These lymphomas include chronic lymphocytic leukemia/small lymphocytic lymphoma (CLL/SLL), mantle cell lymphoma, and follicular lymphoma. If the spleen is examined, the gross appearance can closely resemble SMZL (as described above). Histologically, all three types

of lymphoma can show prominent white pulp involvement, partial or complete replacement of the nodules by lymphoma, and "spillover" of lymphoma cells into the red pulp. Marginal zone differentiation is unusual in these lymphoma types and the cytologic features of lymphoma cells show subtle differences compared with SMZL in well-fixed tissue sections.

Chronic Lymphocytic Leukemia/Small Lymphocytic Lymphoma. Patients with CLL/SLL may have prominent splenomegaly. Clues to support CLL/SLL include small lymphocytes with block-like chromatin (resembling a soccer ball) in blood or bone marrow aspirate smears, proliferation centers in tissue biopsy specimens, and a typical immunophenotype including expression of surface monotypic immunoglobulin (dim), CD5, CD20 (dim), CD23, and CD200 and dim expression or absence of CD11c, CD22, CD79b, and FMC7. Prominent marginal zone differentiation in the spleen, villous lymphocytes in blood and bone marrow aspirate smears, and intrasinusoidal involvement and reactive germinal centers in the bone marrow biopsy specimen support SMZL. Although CD5 and CD23 expression are typical of CLL/SLL, a subset of SMZL can express CD5 and/or CD23, usually dimly.

Mantle Cell Lymphoma. The cell population in mantle cell lymphoma is usually highly monomorphic and composed of small lymphoid cells with slightly to more marked irregular nuclear contours and an absence of centroblasts. Mantle cell lymphoma usually expresses surface immunoglobulin, CD5, SOX11, and CD20, and is usually negative for CD23 and CD200. Mantle cell lymphoma is positive for cyclin D1 and carries t(11;14)(q13;q32)/*CCND1-IGH*, unlike SMZL.

Follicular Lymphoma. Although follicular lymphoma usually has a follicular pattern, in the spleen the neoplastic follicles may not be apparent in white pulp nodules. Follicular lymphoma is composed of centrocytes and centroblasts. Follicular lymphoma cells express bright surface immunoglobulin and CD20; are commonly positive for CD10, BCL6, and other germinal center B-cell markers; and are negative for CD5. The t(14;18)(q32;q21)/*IGH-BCL2* is common in follicular lymphoma and not present in SMZL.

Waldenstrom Macroglobulinemia. Rarely, patients with SMZL can present with a serum IgM paraprotein level and bone marrow involvement by CD5-negative low-grade B-cell lymphoma, adding lymphoplasmacytic lymphoma/ Waldenstrom macroglobulinemia (LPL/WM) to the differential diagnosis. If splenomegaly is prominent, the diagnosis of SMZL is usually suspected. The pattern of bone marrow involvement can be helpful in differential diagnosis. In our experience, a paratrabecular pattern favors SMZL and a sinusoidal pattern is highly unusual in LPL/WM.

Other Splenic B-Cell Lymphomas. Other B-cell lymphomas that arise in the spleen include hairy cell leukemia, hairy cell leukemia-variant, and splenic diffuse red pulp B-cell lymphoma. If the spleen is available for pathologic examination, the pattern of involvement is distinctive as these tumors predominantly involve the red pulp, and the white pulp is often atrophic or effaced. When the spleen is not available, distinguishing these neoplasms from SMZL is more challenging and immunophenotypic and molecular studies are important.

Hairy Cell Leukemia. These tumors have a distinctive cytologic appearance. In blood smears, the cells have central nuclei without nucleoli and abundant cytoplasm with circumferential villi. In tissue sections, the cells are arranged in a diffuse pattern and are widely spaced with a "fried egg" appearance. Hairy cell leukemia also has a distinctive immunophenotype characterized by monotypic surface immunoglobulin (bright), CD11c (bright), CD20 (bright), CD25, CD103, FMC7, and annexin A1. The *BRAF* V600E mutation is almost universally present in hairy cell leukemia (see chapter 56).

Hairy Cell Leukemia-Variant. In blood smears the neoplastic cells may resemble hairy cell leukemia cells except that they usually have distinctive (although usually not prominent) nucleoli. In tissue sections, hairy cell leukemia-variant has a diffuse pattern. Hairy cell leukemia-variant cells express bright monotypic surface immunoglobulin and CD20, often express CD11c and FMC7, and more variably express CD25 or CD103, and are negative for annexin A1. Mutations in *MAP2K1* have been identified in a subset of cases (see chapter 57).

Splenic Diffuse Red Pulp Small B-Cell Lymphoma. This neoplasm is a provisional entity in the WHO classification (35a) and the criteria for these neoplasms are poorly defined. Distinguishing SMZL and splenic diffuse red pulp small B-cell lymphoma is challenging because there is substantial morphologic and immunophenotypic overlap. Examination of the resected spleen specimen may be required to resolve this differential diagnosis (see chapter 59).

Extranodal Marginal Zone Lymphoma. Rarely, MALT lymphomas disseminate to the spleen. The history of MALT lymphoma and the fact that the spleen is not markedly enlarged when involved by MALT lymphoma are helpful. MALT lymphoma, however, has overlapping features with SMZL, including involvement of splenic marginal zones, monocytoid or plasma cell differentiation, follicular colonization, a similar immunophenotype, and some similar genetic features, such as gains of chromosomes 3 and 18.

TREATMENT AND PROGNOSIS

Patients with SMZL have an indolent clinical course with a median survival period of about 10 years (16,23,24). Most patients have stage IV disease at the time of initial diagnosis. As has been reviewed by Arcaini et al. (2), a number of factors correlate with prognosis including low hemoglobin level, low platelet count, high serum LDH level, and extrahilar lymph-adenopathy. These factors can be used to create a score: low risk (0 points), intermediate risk (1-2 points), and high risk (3-4 points). There are a few tumor-associated markers that correlate with prognosis. High proliferation rate, as assessed by Ki-67, is associated with a worse prognosis in some studies. Increased numbers of cytogenetic abnormalities (greater than two abnormalities) is associated with shorter survival time (34). Cytogenetic abnormalities of 14q are also associated with decreased survival (34). The prognostic significance of *IGVH* mutation status in SMZL is presently unclear.

Therapy is usually reserved for SMZL patients with symptoms, substantial cytopenias, or other signs of extensive disease (23,31a). Splenectomy is a reasonable frontline therapeutic approach, providing both diagnostic and therapeutic benefit (20,26,31a,40). Some SMZL patients do not require further therapy, or at least not for a few years. Rituximab, as a single agent or in combination with other therapeutic agents, has benefit (23). Purine analogs, such as fludarabine, are also active. Alkylating agents administered alone provide only marginal benefit. In patients with evidence of hepatitis C virus infection, interferon-based therapies may be helpful, and rare patients have shown regression of disease.

REFERENCES

1. Algara P, Mateo MS, Sanchez-Beato M, et al. Analysis of the IgV(H) somatic mutations in splenic marginal zone lymphoma defines a group of unmutated cases with frequent 7q deletion and adverse clinical course. Blood 2002;99:1299-1304.
2. Arcaini L, Rossi D, Paulli M. Splenic marginal zone lymphoma: from genetics to management. Blood 2016;127:2072-2081.
3. Arribas AJ, Gómez-Abad C, Sánchez-Beato M, et al. Splenic marginal zone lymphoma: comprehensive analysis of gene expression and miRNA profiling. Mod Pathol 2013;26:889-901.
4. Arribas AJ, Rinaldi A, Mensah AA, et al. DNA methylation-profiling identifies two splenic marginal zone lymphoma subgroups with different clinical and genetic features. Blood 2015;125: 1922-1931.
5. Baliakas P, Strefford JC, Bikos V, Parry M, Stamatopoulos K, Oscier D. Splenic marginal-zone lymphoma: ontogeny and genetics. Leuk Lymphoma 2015;56:301-310.
6. Baseggio L, Traverse-Glehen A, Petinataud F, et al. CD5 expression identifies a subset of splenic marginal zone lymphomas with higher lymphocytosis: a clinico-pathological, cytogenetic and molecular study of 24 cases. Haematologica 2010;95:604-612.
7. Bikos V, Stalika E, Baliakas P, et al. Selection of antigen receptors in splenic marginal-zone lymphoma: further support from the analysis of the immunoglobulin light-chain gene repertoire. Leukemia 2012;26:2567-2569.
8. Blombery P, Wong SQ, Hewitt CA, et al. Detection of BRAF mutations in patients with hairy cell leukemia and related lymphoproliferative disorders. Haematologica 2012;97:780-783.
9. Bouteloup M, Verney A, Rachinel N, et al. MicroRNA expression profile in splenic marginal zone lymphoma. Br J Haematol 2012;156:279-281.
10. Boveri E, Arcaini L, Merli M, et al. Bone marrow histology in marginal zone B-cell lymphomas: correlation with clinical parameters and flow cytometry in 120 patients. Ann Oncol 2009;20:129-136.
11. Brisou G, Verney A, Wenner T, et al. A restricted IGHV gene repertoire in splenic marginal zone lymphoma is associated with autoimmune disorders. Haematologica 2014;99:e197-198.
12. Challagundla P, Medeiros LJ, Kanagal-Shamanna R, Miranda RN, Jorgensen JL. Differential expression of CD200 in B-cell neoplasms by flow cytometry can assist in diagnosis, subclassification, and bone marrow staging. Am J Clin Pathol 2014;142:837-844.
13. Clipson A, Wang M, de Leval L, et al. KLF2 mutation is the most frequent somatic change in splenic marginal zone lymphoma and identifies a subset with distinct genotype. Leukemia 2015;29:1177-1185.
14. Hoehn D, Miranda RN, Kanagal-Shamanna R, Lin P, Medeiros LJ. Splenic B-cell lymphomas with more than 55% prolymphocytes in blood: evidence for prolymphocytoid transformation. Hum Pathol 2012;43:1828-1838.
15. Inamdar KV, Medeiros LJ, Jorgensen JL, Amin HM, Schlette EJ. Bone marrow involvement by marginal zone B-cell lymphomas of different types. Am J Clin Pathol 2008;129:714-722.

16. Isaacson PG, Piris MA, Berger F, et al. Splenic marginal zone lymphoma. In: Swerdlow SH, Campo E, Harris NL, Jaffe ES, Pileri SA, Stein H, Thiele J, Vardiman JW, eds. WHO classification of tumours of haematopoietic and lymphoid tissues. Lyon: IARC Press; 2008:185-187.

17. Kansal R, Ross CW, Singleton TP, Finn WG, Schnitzer B. Histopathologic features of splenic small B-cell lymphomas. A study of 42 cases with a definitive diagnosis by the World Health Organization classification. Am J Clin Pathol 2003;120:335-347.

18. Kiel MJ, Velusamy T, Betz BL, et al. Whole-genome sequencing identifies recurrent somatic NOTCH2 mutations in splenic marginal zone lymphoma. J Exp Med 2012;209:1553-1565.

19. Lechner K, Simonitsch I, Haselböck J, Jäger U, Pabinger I. Acquired immune-mediated thrombophilia in lymphoproliferative disorders. Leuk Lymphoma 2011;52:1836-1843.

20. Lenglet J, Traullé C, Mounier N, et al. Long-term follow-up analysis of 100 patients with splenic marginal zone lymphoma treated with splenectomy as first-line treatment. Leuk Lymphoma 2014;55:1854-1860.

21. Manipadam MT, Viswabandya A, Srivastava A. Primary splenic marginal zone lymphoma with florid granulomatous reaction—a case report and review of literature. Pathol Res Pract 2007;203:239-243.

22. Martinez N, Almaraz C. Vaque JP, et al. Whole-exome sequencing in splenic marginal zone lymphoma reveals mutations in genes involved in marginal zone differentiation. Leukemia 2014;28:1334-1340.

23. Matutes E. Splenic marginal zone lymphoma: disease features and management. Expert Rev Hematol 2013;6:735-745.

24. Matutes E, Oscier D, Montalban C, et al. Splenic marginal zone lymphoma proposals for a revision of diagnostic, staging and therapeutic criteria. Leukemia 2008;22:487-495.

25. Melo JV, Robinson DS, Gregory C, Catovsky D. Splenic B-cell lymphoma with "villous" lymphocytes in the peripheral blood: a disorder distinct from hairy cell leukemia. Leukemia 1987;1:294-298.

26. Milosevic R, Todorovic M, Balint B, et al. Splenectomy with chemotherapy vs surgery alone as initial treatment for splenic marginal zone lymphoma. World J Gastroenterol 2009;15:4009-4015.

27. Mollejo M, Lloret E, Menárguez J, Piris MA, Isaacson PG. Lymph node involvement by splenic marginal zone lymphoma: morphological and immunohistochemical features. Am J Surg Pathol 1997;21:772-780.

28. Nakashima MO, Durkin L, Bodo J, et al. Utility and diagnostic pitfalls of SOX11 monoclonal antibodies in mantle cell lymphoma and other lymphoproliferative disorders. Appl Immunohistochem Mol Morphol 2014;22:720-727.

29. Novara F, Arcaini L, Merli M, et al. High-resolution genome-wide array comparative genomic hybridization in splenic marginal zone B-cell lymphoma. Hum Pathol 2009;40:1628-1637.

30. Papadaki T, Stamatopoulos K, Belessi C, et al. Splenic marginal-zone lymphoma: one or more entities? A histologic, immunohistochemical, and molecular study of 42 cases. Am J Surg Pathol 2007;31:438-446.

31. Parry M, Rose-Zerilli MJ, Ljungstrom V, et al. Genetics and prognostication in splenic marginal zone lymphoma: Revelations from deep sequencing. Clin Cancer Res 2015;21:4174-4183.

31a. Perrone S, D'Elia GM, Annechini G, et al. Splenic marginal zone lymphoma: prognostic factors, role of watch and wait policy, and other therapeutic approaches in the rituximab era. Leuk Res 2016;44:53-60.

32. Rinaldi A, Mian M, Chigrinova E, et al. Genome-wide DNA profiling of marginal zone lymphomas identifies subtype-specific lesions with an impact on the clinical outcome. Blood 2011;117:1595-1604.

33. Rossi D, Trifonov V, Fangazio M, et al. The coding genome of splenic marginal zone lymphoma: activation of NOTCH2 and other pathways regulating marginal zone development. J Exp Med 2012;209:1537-1551.

34. Salido M, Baró C, Oscier D, et al. Cytogenetic aberrations and their prognostic value in a series of 330 splenic marginal zone B-cell lymphomas: a multicenter study of the Splenic B-Cell Lymphoma Group. Blood 2010;116:1479-1488.

35. Schmid C, Kirkham N, Diss T, Isaacson PG. Splenic marginal zone lymphoma. Am J Surg Pathol 1992;16:455-466.

35a. Swerdlow SH, Campo E, Pileri SA, et al. The 2016 revision of the World Health Organization classification of lymphoid neoplasms. Blood 2016;127:2375-2390.

36. Traverse-Glehen A, Bachy E, Baseggio L, et al. Immunoarchitectural patterns in splenic marginal zone lymphoma: correlations with chromosomal aberrations, IGHV mutations, and survival. A study of 76 cases. Histopathology 2013;62:876-893.

37. Vinholt PJ, Nybo M. Interference from lupus anticoagulant on von Willebrand factor measurement in splenic marginal zone lymphoma: a case report. Blood Coagul Fibrinolysis 2015;26:454-457.

38. Watkins AJ, Huang Y, Ye H, et al. Splenic marginal zone lymphoma: characterization of 7q deletion and its value in diagnosis. J Pathol 2010; 220:461-474.

39. Wu CD, Jackson CL, Medeiros LJ. Splenic marginal zone cell lymphoma. An immunophenotypic and molecular study of five cases. Am J Clin Pathol 1996;105:277-285.

40. Xing KH, Kahlon A, Skinnider BF, et al. Outcomes in splenic marginal zone lymphoma: analysis of 107 patients treated in British Columbia. Br J Haematol 2015;169:520-527.

59 SPLENIC DIFFUSE RED PULP SMALL B-CELL LYMPHOMA

GENERAL FEATURES

Splenic diffuse red pulp small B-cell lymphoma (SDRPBL) is a clinically indolent B-cell neoplasm that diffusely involves the red pulp of the spleen and commonly involves the peripheral blood and bone marrow (7). More specific criteria for the diagnosis of SDRPBL, however, are not sharply defined and likely in evolution. Before establishing the diagnosis of SDRPBL, other more well-defined B-cell lymphomas that involve the spleen, such as splenic marginal zone lymphoma (SMZL) and hairy cell leukemia (HCL), must be excluded. SDRPBL is a provisional entity in the World Health Organization (WHO) classification and is included with hairy cell leukemia variant (HCL-V) under the umbrella term *splenic B-cell lymphoma/leukemia, unclassifiable* (7,9a).

SDRPBL is a rare entity that has been recently teased out of the larger category of B-cell lymphomas of the spleen. Historically, SDRPBL was included in the heterogeneous category of splenic B-cell lymphoma with villous lymphocytes and also has been referred to as SMZL, diffuse variant, or SMZL with diffuse red pulp involvement (5). The diagnosis of SDRPBL is greatly facilitated by having a splenectomy specimen for evaluation, because recognition of this neoplasm by evaluation of blood or bone marrow specimens is highly challenging (7,8).

SDRPBL is a rare disease that represents less than 10 percent of all lymphomas diagnosed in the spleen and 0.5 to 1.0 percent of all non-Hodgkin lymphomas (10,11). The etiology of SDRPBL is unknown. In contrast with SMZL, there is no association with hepatitis C infection (10).

CLINICAL FEATURES

Patients with SDRPBL are adults, typically elderly with a median age in the eighth decade, and an age range from 40 to 91 years in two of the largest studies to date (2,10). Men develop SDRPBL more often than women, in a ratio reported to range from 1.6–2.4 to 1.0 (2,10).

Patients commonly present with symptoms related to prominent splenomegaly, including abdominal pain. Symptoms also are related to peripheral cytopenias due to hypersplenism (2,5,10). Systemic (B-type) symptoms were infrequent in one study, but were reported in up to one third of patients in another study (2,10).

Abdominal lymphadenopathy may occur and splenic hilar lymph nodes are commonly involved, but peripheral lymphadenopathy is rare. Hepatomegaly is uncommon. Some patients have pruritic skin lesions. Most patients with SDRPBL have clinical stage IV disease (spleen and bone marrow) (2,10).

Hematologic parameters are abnormal in most patients with SDRPBL. Low-level leukocytosis and absolute lymphocytosis are present in most patients (7,11). An extremely high white blood cell count is unusual. Thrombocytopenia occurs in about half of SDRPBL patients. Neutropenia or anemia occurs less often. Importantly, the absolute monocyte count is normal in patients with SDRPBL (unlike patients with HCL). The serum lactate dehydrogenase (LDH) level may be elevated in patients with a large disease burden. Serum protein electrophoresis is usually negative for paraprotein, but a few patients with a paraprotein and rouleaux formation in the blood smear have been described (11).

GROSS AND HISTOLOGIC FINDINGS

Spleen

In most cases of SDRPBL, the spleen is massively enlarged with marked expansion of the red pulp, imparting a typical "beefy" homogeneous appearance (fig. 59-1). Small cystic structures (consistent with blood lakes) may be appreciated. White pulp structures are usually not apparent.

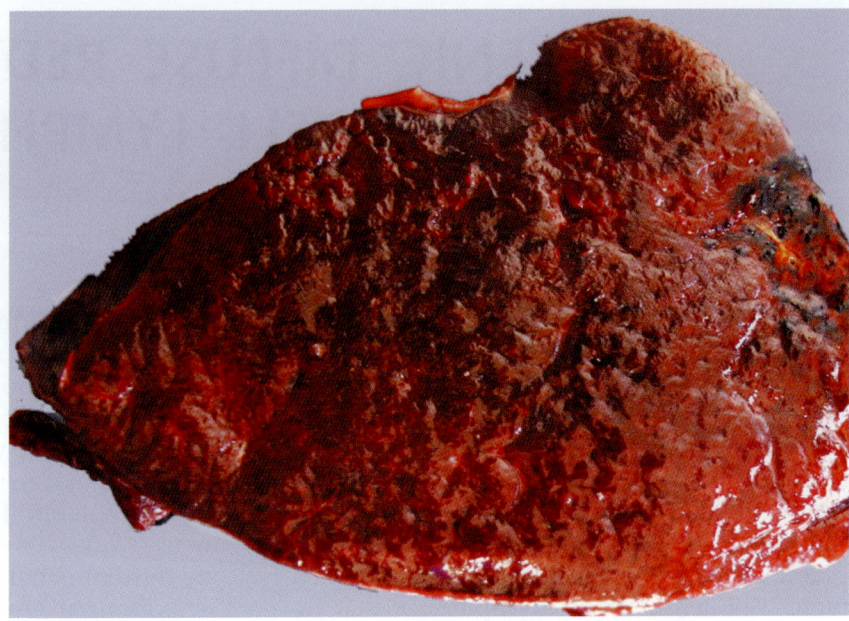

Figure 59-1

SPLENIC DIFFUSE RED PULP SMALL B-CELL LYMPHOMA INVOLVING SPLEEN

The spleen shows a predominantly red pulp pattern, imparting a red "beefy" appearance. (Courtesy of Dr. A. Sohani, Boston, MA).

Histologic evaluation shows diffuse infiltration of the splenic red pulp (2,10). Both cords and sinuses are expanded by abnormal lymphocytes (fig. 59-2). Blood lakes (pseudosinuses lined by lymphoma cells) may be observed. In a small subset of cases, residual white pulp structures may be present but usually these are absent.

Cytologically, the neoplastic lymphocytes are predominantly small, with round nuclei. The chromatin can be dense or vesicular, with small nucleoli. The tumor cell cytoplasm is moderate in amount, with pale to eosinophilic cytoplasm. Scattered large lymphoid cells are also present. Importantly, the white pulp is not involved in SDRPBL. In rare cases of SDRPBL, the large cells are increased or have irregular nuclei with immature chromatin; this presentation likely corresponds to a more aggressive variant of the disease with a higher likelihood of transforming to diffuse large B-cell lymphoma (2,11).

Bone Marrow

In bone marrow, SDRPBL presents in a sinusoidal or interstitial pattern (fig. 59-3) (8,10). In some cases, a partial nodular pattern of lymphoma cells is observed, but reactive follicles are not present (unlike some cases of SMZL). There is usually only mild fibrosis in the bone marrow and aspiration is typically successful (10). The lymphocytes in bone marrow aspirate smears resemble those in blood smears (see below), except that hair-like cytoplasmic projections are uncommon.

Blood

Neoplastic lymphocytes are observed in peripheral blood smears of essentially all patients. The lymphocytes are small to medium in size, with condensed chromatin and round nuclei (2,7,11). Usually, the lymphocytes have indistinct or small nucleoli (2,11). The neoplastic lymphocytes have a variable amount of basophilic cytoplasm (10). Most of the cells in the smear have unevenly distributed, easily seen villous cytoplasmic projections (2). Lymphoplasmacytoid lymphocytes can be observed, and rarely some cells have prominent nucleoli, resembling prolymphocytes.

Other Sites

Mollejo et al. (5) have described skin involvement in rare patients with SDRPBL. These lesions are erythematous papules and histologically show epidermotropism. Other sites of disease are not reported in patients with SDRPBL.

IMMUNOPHENOTYPIC FINDINGS

The immunophenotype of SDRPBL as assessed by flow cytometry is not entirely specific (see Table 56-1). The lymphocytes express monotypic surface light chain (moderate or bright), with kappa and lambda expressed in

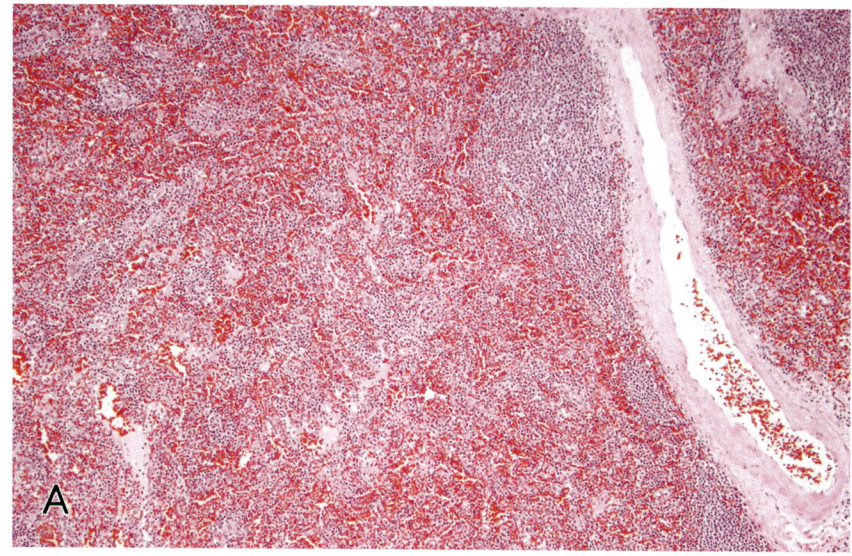

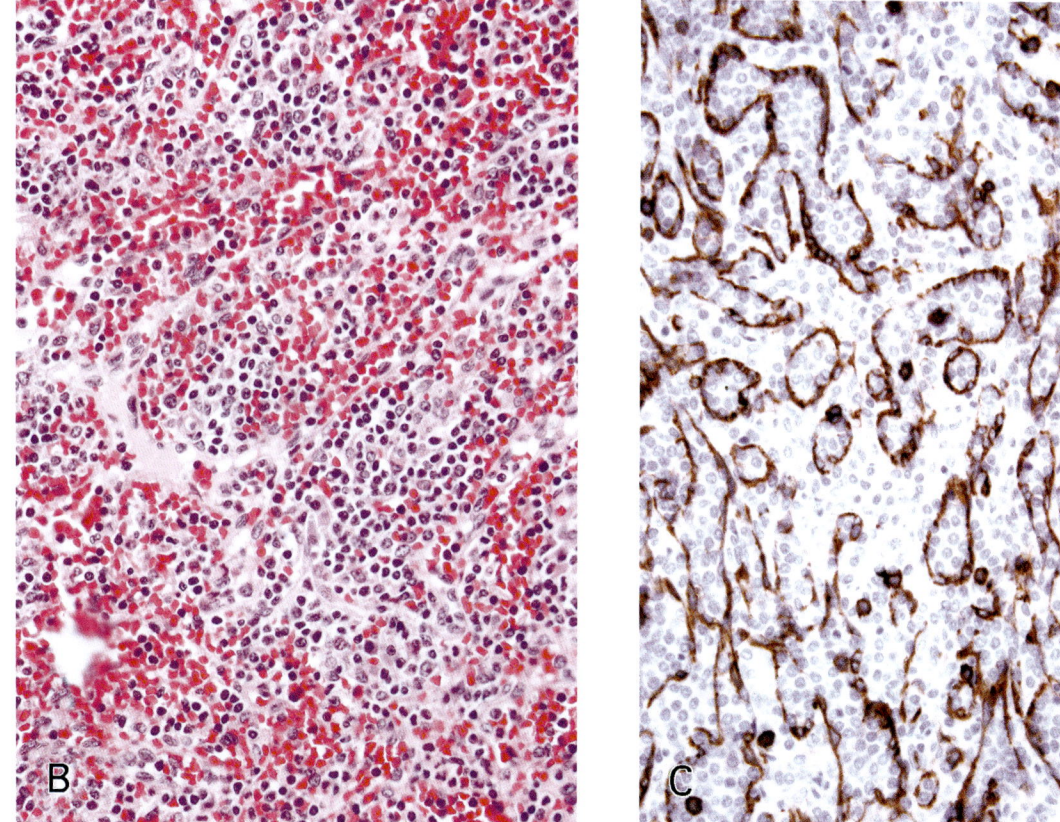

Figure 59-2

SPLENIC DIFFUSE RED PULP SMALL B-CELL LYMPHOMA INVOLVING SPLEEN

A: At low magnification, the red pulp is expanded by lymphoma, with some sparing and compression of the periarteriolar lymphoid sheath regions (A,B: hematoxylin and eosin [H&E] stain).

B: Higher magnification shows small lymphocytes within cords and sinuses of the red pulp.

C: CD8 highlights the splenic sinuses. The cords and sinuses are filled with CD8-negative small lymphoma cells (immunohistochemistry with hematoxylin counterstain).

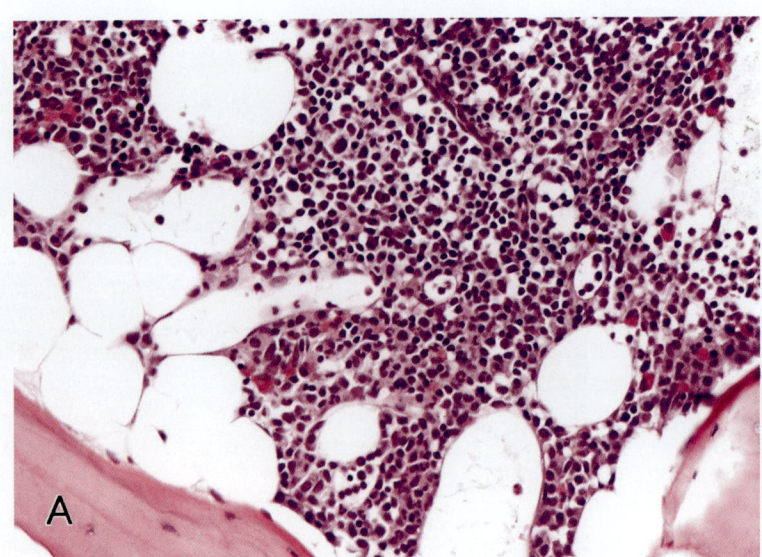

Figure 59-3

SPLENIC DIFFUSE RED PULP SMALL B-CELL LYMPHOMA INVOLVING BONE MARROW

A: The cellularity of the bone marrow appears to be increased but it is difficult to appreciate the lymphoma cells (H&E stain).

B,C: CD20 highlights the lymphoma cells. Most of the cells are sinusoidal (B) but some small nodules (C) are also identified (B,C: immunohistochemistry with hematoxylin counterstain).

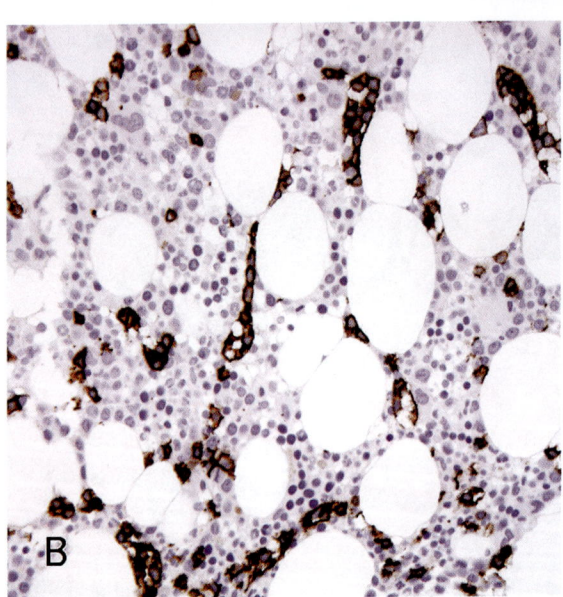

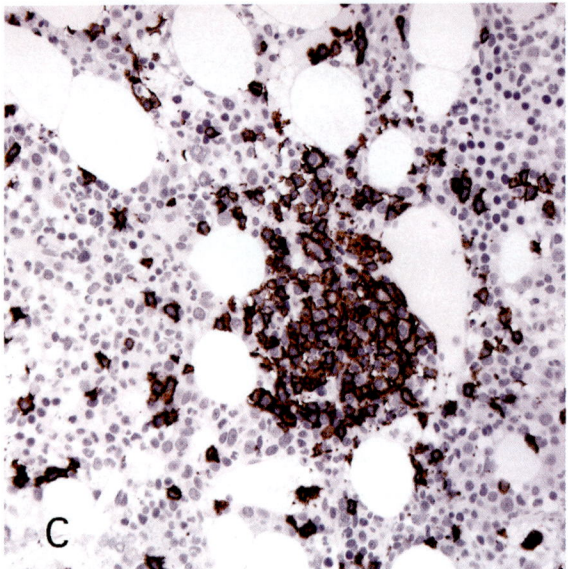

an equal number of cases. The neoplastic cells also express pan-B-cell antigens including CD19, CD20 (bright), CD22 (bright), and CD79a (6,11). Most cases are positive for CD11c. CD180 is positive in most cases (12). In the initial descriptions of SDRPBL a characteristic immunophenotype was reported: positive for IgG and negative for IgD, CD3, CD5, CD10, CD23, CD25, CD27, CD103, and CD123 (6,7,10). Subsequent cases of SDRPBL, however, have been reported that were positive for IgM, IgD, IgG, or a combination of more than one heavy chain. In addition, some cases of SDRPBL express CD103 (about 33 percent), or CD123 (about 10 percent)

(11). Whether these differences are the result of disease heterogeneity or differences in disease definition is unclear.

Using immunohistochemical analysis, the cells of SDRPBL are positive for pan-B-cell antigens (CD19, CD20, CD79a, PAX5) and positive for CD76/DBA.44 in about 90 percent of cases (5,10). Curiel-Olmo et al. (1) have reported that 24 of 33 (73 percent) cases of SDRPBL were positive for cyclin D3. About two thirds of cases are positive for IgG, with about one quarter positive for IgD. BCL2 is usually positive. SDRPBL is usually negative for CD10, CD23, CD43, BCL6, TRAP, annexin A1, and cyclin D1; TRAP, however, can be positive in some cases and one case of SDRPBL reported was positive for annexin A1 (4). The proliferation rate, as assessed by Ki-67, is usually low, less than 10 percent. In rare aggressive variants of SDRPBL, the proliferation rate is higher and P53 may be expressed.

MOLECULAR GENETIC FINDINGS

Conventional cytogenetic analysis has shown abnormalities in about one third of cases of SDRPBL, but no recurrent specific abnormalities have been reported (10,11). Trisomy 18 is seen in a small subset of cases, as is partial trisomy of 3q (10). Del(7q) is observed uncommonly in SDRPL, in 10 percent of cases overall. In cases with an abnormal karyotype, however, del(7q) is one of the more common abnormalities (2,10). A del(8p11) was reported in one case (5). A complex karyotype is present in about 10 percent of cases (3). The t(9;14)(p13;q32)/*PAX5-IGH* has been reported in a splenic lymphoma that may fit in the SDRPBL category (7). There is no evidence of t(11;14)(q13;q32)/*CCND1-IGH*, t(14;18) (q21;q32)/*IGH-BCL2*, or *CCND3* translocations.

Few cases of SDRPBL have been studied using molecular methods. Copy number arrays have shown aberrations in approximately two thirds of cases, including losses of 9p21, 10q23, 14q31-32 and 17p13 in some tumors (3). TP53 deletions detected by fluorescence in situ hybridization (FISH) have been reported in a subset of cases. *CCND3* is mutated in about 40 percent of SDRPBL cases (1). Mutations in *TP53, NOTCH1, MAP2K1, BRAF*, and SF3B1 have been reported, each in 5 to 10 percent of cases (3,12). One case of SDRPBL carried a *BRAF* V600E mutation (9).

SDRPBL is a B-cell neoplasm that carries monoclonal *IGH* rearrangements and usually the T-cell receptor genes are in the germline configuration. The IGH variable (*VH*) genes *VH3-23* and *VH4-34* appear to be preferentially utilized, each in up to 15 percent of cases (10–12). The *IGV* region genes commonly show evidence of somatic mutation (3,10).

DIFFERENTIAL DIAGNOSIS

The recent report of cyclin D3 expression and CCND3 mutations in SDRPBL, once confirmed, will be a very useful tool in differential diagnosis. SDRPBL shares morphologic and immunophenotypic features with HCL, HCL-V, and SMZL (11) (see chapters 56 to 58).

Hairy Cell Leukemia. Patients with HCL often present with monocytopenia, unlike patients with SDRPBL. Immunophenotypic analysis is very helpful for distinguishing HCL from SDRPBL. HCL cells are positive for CD11c, CD22, CD25, CD103, and CD123 and fall within a characteristic gate in CD45/side scatter analysis using flow cytometry. In histologic sections, HCL cells are positive for annexin A1 and commonly positive for cyclin D1. *BRAF* V600E mutation is nearly universal in HCL, but has been reported rarely in SDRPBL (9).

Hairy Cell Leukemia-Variant. Distinguishing HCL-V from SDRPBL may be challenging and some authors suggest that these two entities are part of a spectrum of disorders. The placing of HCL-V with SDRPBL within the same category of splenic B-cell lymphoma/leukemia unclassifiable in the WHO classification also implies a close relationship (7). One helpful morphologic feature is the presence of a distinct nucleolus in the cells of HCL-V, which is typically not present in the cells of SDRPBL. This is best appreciated in peripheral blood smears. A subset of cases of HCL-V carry *MAP2K1* mutations.

Splenic Marginal Zone Lymphoma. If the spleen is available for examination, SMZL involves the white pulp with a common biphasic appearance. In contrast, SDRPBL involves the red pulp and is composed of a monomorphous population of small lymphocytes. Most cases of SMZL express IgD and up to 50 percent have del(7q). These findings are uncommon in SDRPBL.

TREATMENT AND PROGNOSIS

There is no consensus regarding the optimal therapeutic approach for patients with SDRPBL. Splenectomy is a primary therapy in many patients and often results in a good clinical response (11). There appears to be a role for rituximab either upfront or at time of relapse. Cytotoxic chemotherapy has been used for some patients, particularly those who have relapsed.

Patients with SDRPBL have an indolent but incurable disease. The 5-year overall survival rate in a case series by Kanellis et al. (2) was 93 percent. Some patients progress to diffuse large B-cell lymphoma (10,11).

REFERENCES

1. Curiel-Olmo S, Mondéjar R, Almaraz C, et al. Splenic diffuse red pulp small B-cell lymphoma displays increased expression of cyclin D3 and recurrent CCND3 mutations. Blood 2017;129:1042-1045.

2. Kanellis G, Mollejo M, Montes-Moreno S, et al. Splenic diffuse red pulp small B-cell lymphoma: revision of a series of cases reveals characteristic clinico-pathologic features. Haematologica 2010;95:1122-1129.

3. Martinez D, Navarro A, Martinez-Trillos A, et al. NOTCH1, TP53, and MAP2K1 mutations in splenic diffuse red pulp small B-cell lymphoma are associated with progressive disease. Am J Surg Pathol 2016;40:192-201.

4. Mendes LS, Attygalle A, Matutes E, Wotherspoon A. Annexin A1 expression in a splenic diffuse red pulp small B-cell lymphoma: report of the first case. Histopathology 2013;63:590-600.

5. Mollejo M, Algara P, Mateo MS, et al. Splenic small B-cell lymphoma with predominant red pulp involvement: a diffuse variant of splenic marginal zone lymphoma? Histopathology 2002;40:22-30.

6. Petit B, Parrens M, Soubeyran I, et al. Among 157 marginal zone lymphomas, DBA.44 (CD76) expression is restricted to tumour cells infiltrating the red pulp of the spleen with a diffuse architectural pattern. Histopathology 2009;54:626-631.

7. Piris M, Foucar K, Mollejo M, et al. Splenic B-cell lymphoma/leukaemia, unclassifiable. In: Swerdlow SH, Campo E, Harris NL, Jaffe ES, Pileri SA, Stein H, Thiele J, Vardiman JW, eds. WHO classification of tumours of haematopoietic and lymphoid tissues. Lyon: IARC Press; 2008:191-192.

8. Ponzoni M, Kanellis G, Pouliou E, et al. Bone marrow histopathology in the diagnostic evaluation of splenic marginal-zone and splenic diffuse red pulp small B-cell lymphoma: a reliable substitute for spleen histopathology? Am J Surg Pathol 2012;36:1609-1618.

9. Raess PW, Mintzer D, Husson M, et al. BRAF V600E is also seen in unclassifiable splenic B-cell lymphoma/leukemia, a potential mimic of hairy cell leukemia. Blood 2013;122:3084-3085.

9a. Swerdlow SH, Campo E, Pileri SA, et al. The 2016 revision of the World Health Organization classification of lymphoid neoplasms. Blood 2016;127:2375-2390

10. Traverse-Glehen A, Baseggio L, Bauchu EC, et al. Splenic red pulp lymphoma with numerous basophilic villous lymphocytes: a distinct clinicopathologic and molecular entity? Blood 2008;111:2253-2260.

11. Traverse-Glehen A, Baseggio L, Salles G, Coiffier B, Felman P, Berger F. Splenic diffuse red pulp small-B cell lymphoma: toward the emergence of a new lymphoma entity. Discov Med 2012;13:253-265.

12. Traverse-Glehen A, Verney A, Gazzo S, et al. Splenic diffuse red pulp lymphoma has a distinct pattern of somatic mutations amongst B-cell malignancies. Leuk Lymphoma 2017;58:666-675.

60 PRIMARY SPLENIC LARGE B-CELL LYMPHOMA

GENERAL FEATURES

Primary splenic large B-cell lymphoma is a neoplasm with a diffuse growth pattern that is composed of large B cells. It involves the spleen with no (or little) evidence of disease at other anatomic sites.

Diffuse large B-cell lymphomas (DLBCLs) involving the spleen are a heterogeneous group that includes primary neoplasms that arise in the spleen and systemic neoplasms that secondarily involve the spleen. For tumors thought likely to arise in the spleen de novo, the term primary splenic large B-cell lymphoma is used. DLBCLs also arise via histologic transformation from two types of low-grade B-cell lymphoma involving the spleen: primary low-grade splenic lymphoma (most often splenic marginal zone lymphoma) and low-grade B-cell lymphoma that has disseminated to the spleen (3,16). Histologic transformation of low-grade B-cell lymphoma is excluded from the category of primary splenic large B-cell lymphoma in this chapter.

There are differences of opinion regarding the definition of primary splenic large B-cell lymphoma. Some authors believe that following the diagnosis of large B-cell lymphoma, an interval of 6 months without involvement of other sites is required to establish the diagnosis of primary splenic large B-cell lymphoma with certainty (2). Other authors have a broader definition that allows for predominant involvement of the spleen with only minimal involvement of regional lymph nodes, bone marrow, or both (9). When defined strictly, primary splenic large B-cell lymphoma is rare (less than 1 percent of all lymphomas).

Primary splenic large B-cell lymphoma and systemic DLBCL involving the spleen may present in a similar fashion and may be indistinguishable morphologically (6,15). A clinical history and staging studies help exclude systemic disease disseminated to the spleen. Patients with systemic DLBCL involving the spleen commonly have a high International Prognostic Index (IPI) score or undergo imaging studies that show evidence of widespread lymphoma at non-splenic sites. Other patients have a history of low-grade B-cell lymphoma or current low-grade B-cell lymphoma coexistent with DLBCL.

No specific etiology is known for primary splenic large B-cell lymphoma. Cases associated with hepatitis C infection have been reported, most often in Italy, Japan, and Taiwan where there is a high seroprevalance (10,21). In one study from Taiwan, 44 percent of patients with early stage primary splenic large B-cell lymphoma had serologic evidence of hepatitis C infection (21)

CLINICAL FEATURES

Primary splenic large B-cell lymphoma is the most common type of lymphoma to arise in the spleen, accounting for 40 to 50 percent of all primary splenic lymphomas in some studies (15). Patients are usually older (over 50 years). The sex ratio has varied in different, albeit small, clinicopathologic studies, ranging from about equal (13) to an almost 2 to 1 male predominance (15).

Patients may have symptoms associated with prominent splenic disease including a splenic mass, splenomegaly, abdominal fullness, left upper quadrant pain, and cytopenias (1,7,13,18). Approximately half of patients have B-type symptoms including fever, weight loss, and night sweats (1). Fever is reported more often in primary splenic large B-cell lymphoma with predominant red pulp involvement. Rarely, patients present with an acute abdomen secondary to splenic rupture. The lymphoma also can be associated with a hemophagocytic syndrome (20).

A staging system for patients with primary splenic large B-cell lymphoma and other splenic lymphomas has been proposed by Kehoe and Straus (11) as follows: stage I–only splenic

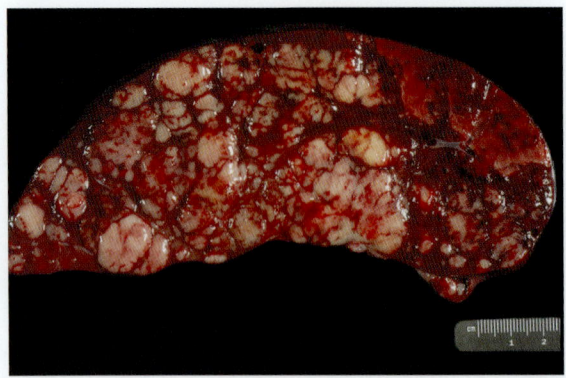

Figure 60-1

PRIMARY SPLENIC LARGE B-CELL LYMPHOMA: MACRONODULAR PATTERN

Large, fleshy macronodules of tumor involve otherwise normal splenic parenchyma. (Courtesy of Dr. S. Konoplev, Houston, TX.)

disease; stage II–disease involving the spleen and hilar lymph nodes; and stage III–involvement of the spleen, liver, and lymph nodes beyond the splenic hilum or involvement of bone marrow. It is debatable whether patients with systemic sites of disease have true primary lymphoma arising in the spleen. This is especially true for patients with primary splenic large B-cell lymphoma with predominant red pulp involvement since these patients commonly have low-level disease in the bone marrow, liver, blood, or various combinations of these sites (9). These patients do not have systemic lymphadenopathy, although they can have minimally enlarged splenic hilar or regional abdominal lymph nodes. Primary splenic large B-cell lymphoma with predominant red pulp involvement also overlaps with intravascular large B-cell lymphoma.

GROSS FINDINGS

Spleens involved by primary splenic large B-cell lymphoma are almost always enlarged and can be massive, greater than 1 kg (7,13). In most cases, the spleen contains one or multiple distinct, large tumor nodules or masses (fig. 60-1). These masses may contain areas of hemorrhage and necrosis, or occasionally, fibrosis. The tumor masses are associated with varying degrees of adjacent, uninvolved splenic parenchyma. Less often, primary splenic large B-cell lymphoma is more subtle grossly, involving the white pulp as small nodules in a miliary pattern or primar-

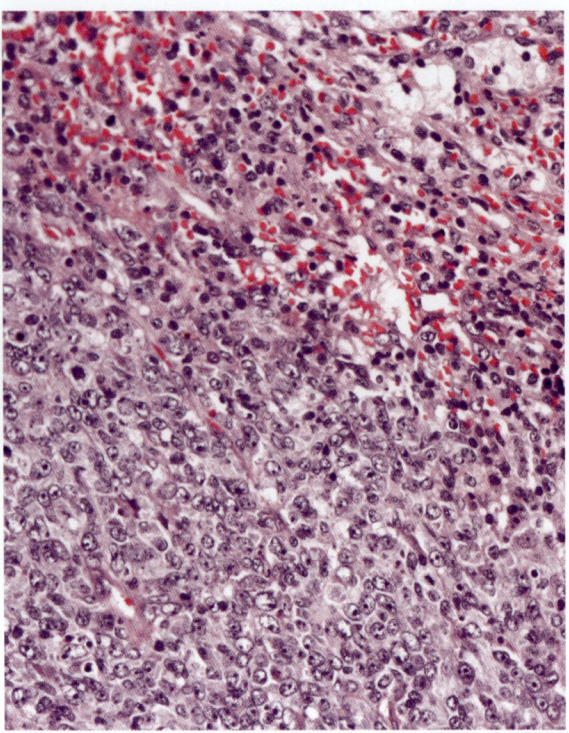

Figure 60-2

PRIMARY SPLENIC LARGE B-CELL LYMPHOMA

There is an abrupt transition between normal splenic parenchyma (upper right) and lymphoma (hematoxylin and eosin [H&E] stain).

ily involving the red pulp. Splenic hilar lymph nodes are often involved, although these lymph nodes are usually not large.

HISTOLOGIC FINDINGS

The histologic patterns described in primary splenic large B-cell lymphoma relate to the gross distribution of disease. They are subdivided into macronodular, micronodular, or predominantly red pulp involvement. One or more patterns may occur in a patient.

In *macronodular disease*, the large lymphoma cells form a mass that diffusely replaces the splenic architecture. The transition between lymphoma and adjacent splenic parenchyma is usually abrupt (fig. 60-2) (6,7,13,18). In most cases, the lymphoma has moderate to numerous apoptotic cells and mitotic figures (fig. 60-3). Coagulative necrosis may be prominent. In the uninvolved spleen, extramedullary hematopoiesis may be present; cells of the erythroid lineage are most common.

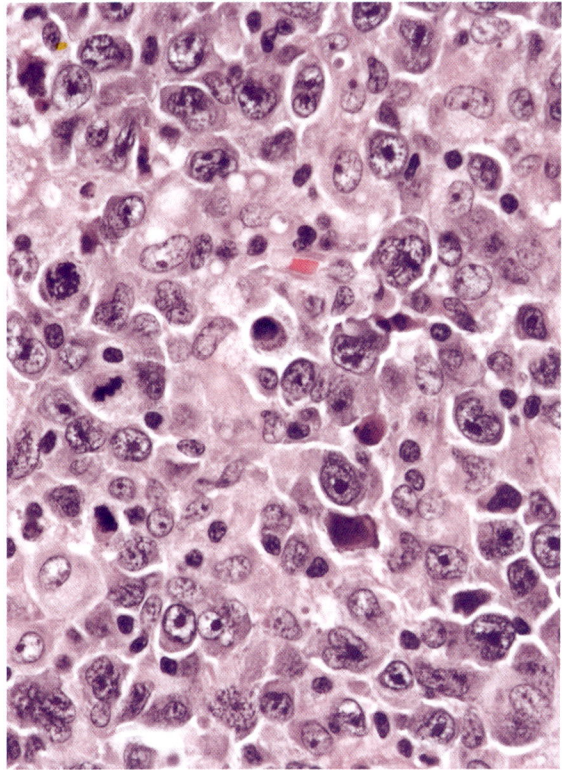

Figure 60-3

PRIMARY SPLENIC LARGE B- CELL LYMPHOMA

The lymphoma cells are large and show a mixture of multilobated centroblasts and occasional immunoblasts. Mitotic figures and apoptotic cells are present in this field (H&E stain).

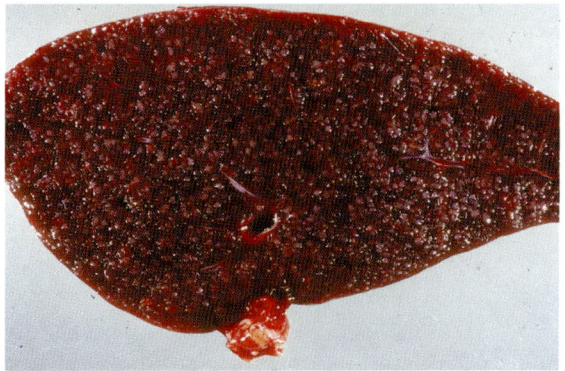

Figure 60-4

PRIMARY SPLENIC LARGE B-CELL LYMPHOMA: MICRONODULAR PATTERN

Extensive involvement and expansion of white pulp nodules are seen.

The *micronodular pattern* is multifocal, predominantly involves the white pulp (fig. 60-4), and may be inapparent by gross examination (5,8,12). A distinctive form of micronodular disease is T-cell/histiocyte-rich large B-cell lymphoma. By definition, the large B cells represent 10 percent or less of the cellularity and these neoplasms are rich in reactive small T cells and histiocytes (fig. 60-5) (5). Uncommonly, the histiocytes are epithelioid and may be numerous, imparting a Lennert-like pattern (12).

The *predominant red pulp pattern* is uncommon, representing 5 to 10 percent of all cases (9,13). The red pulp is expanded and diffusely involved by large B-lymphoma cells that infiltrate the cords and sinuses, often in a noncohesive pattern (fig. 60-6). Extramedullary hematopoiesis and hemophagocytosis may be present. Overall, the white pulp is preferentially spared.

In all patterns of involvement, the cells of primary splenic large B-cell lymphoma exhibit variable cytologic features. In most cases, the large lymphoid cells resemble centroblasts (fig. 60-3); in other cases, however, the large cells have prominent nucleoli more in keeping with immunoblasts. The cells may also have plasmablastic, pleomorphic, or anaplastic features (fig. 60-7).

CYTOLOGIC FINDINGS

Fine-needle aspirate smears most often show a monomorphic population of large lymphoid cells with round to oval nuclei, coarse and clumped chromatin, and conspicuous nucleoli. Lymphoglandular bodies are often present in the background. In some cases, aspirate smears show primarily necrotic debris with only scattered, large, atypical lymphoid cells. These cases may be difficult to recognize as large B-cell lymphoma (14).

IMMUNOPHENOTYPIC FINDINGS

The neoplastic cells of primary splenic large B-cell lymphoma have a mature B-cell immunophenotype. The lymphoma cells are positive for pan-B-cell antigens such as CD19, CD20 (figs. 60-5, right; 60-7, right), CD22, CD79a, OCT2, and PAX5 (fig. 60-6C), and are negative for pan-T-cell antigens (5,15). CD5 is usually negative. If assessed by flow cytometry, many cases express monotypic surface immunoglobulin light chain, but in paraffin sections, immunoglobulins are usually negative unless

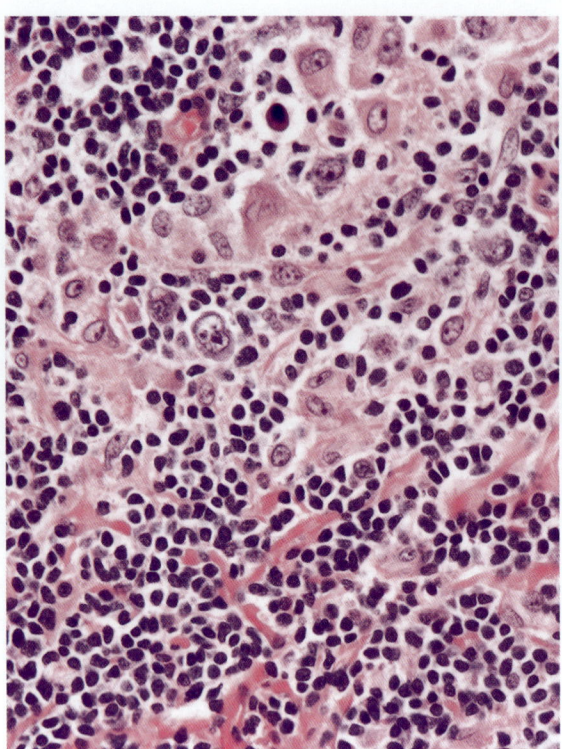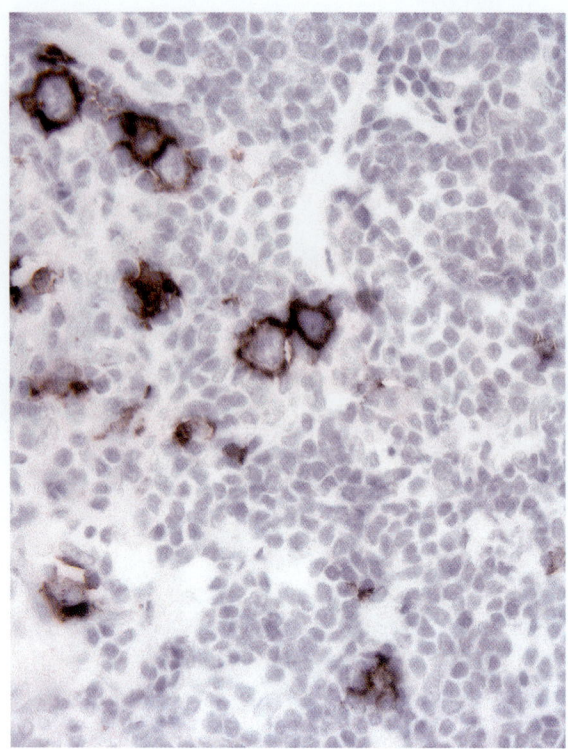

Figure 60-5

MICRONODULAR T-CELL/HISTIOCYTE-RICH LARGE B-CELL LYMPHOMA INVOLVING SPLEEN

Left: Scattered large lymphoma cells are present in a background of numerous lymphocytes and histiocytes (H&E stain).
Right: The lymphoma cells are positive for CD20 (immunohistochemistry with hematoxylin counterstain).

plasmacytoid differentiation is present. Cases of primary splenic large B-cell lymphoma are often positive for MUM1 (fig. 60-6D) and BCL6 (dim or moderate), and are usually negative for CD10, supporting a nongerminal center B-cell immunophenotype (13). A subset of cases is positive for BCL2 (often bright). MYC can be expressed, usually with dim or moderate intensity. CD30 is often negative, but it can be expressed variably, as can epithelial membrane antigen (EMA) or CD23. Primary splenic large B-cell lymphoma is negative for CD21, CD35, CD68, CD138, and lysozyme. P53 is usually negative, but can be positive in a small subset of cases.

Since these tumors have a diffuse pattern, no follicular dendritic cell networks are identified, including cases of micronodular T-cell/histiocyte-rich large B-cell lymphoma (5). Primary splenic large B-cell lymphomas usually have a high proliferation rate as assessed by Ki-67. There is no evidence of infection by Epstein-Barr virus or human herpesvirus 8.

MOLECULAR GENETIC FINDINGS

Few cases of primary splenic large B-cell lymphoma have been assessed by conventional cytogenetic analysis and cases with red pulp involvement seem to be over-represented. The most common loci involved include 14q32, 9p24, del(3q21), add(7p22), t(3;6), del(8p22), add(19p13), and trisomy 18. About half of patients have a complex karyotype (9,20).

Molecular analysis has shown monoclonal *IGH* rearrangements. There are currently no known distinctive gene mutations in primary splenic large B-cell lymphoma.

DIFFERENTIAL DIAGNOSIS

Systemic DLBCL Involving the Spleen. Systemic DLBCL involving the spleen is far more common than primary splenic large B-cell lymphoma. Patients with systemic DLBCL may have de novo disease or low-grade B-cell lymphoma with histologic transformation to DLBCL that is first detected in the spleen (fig. 60-8).

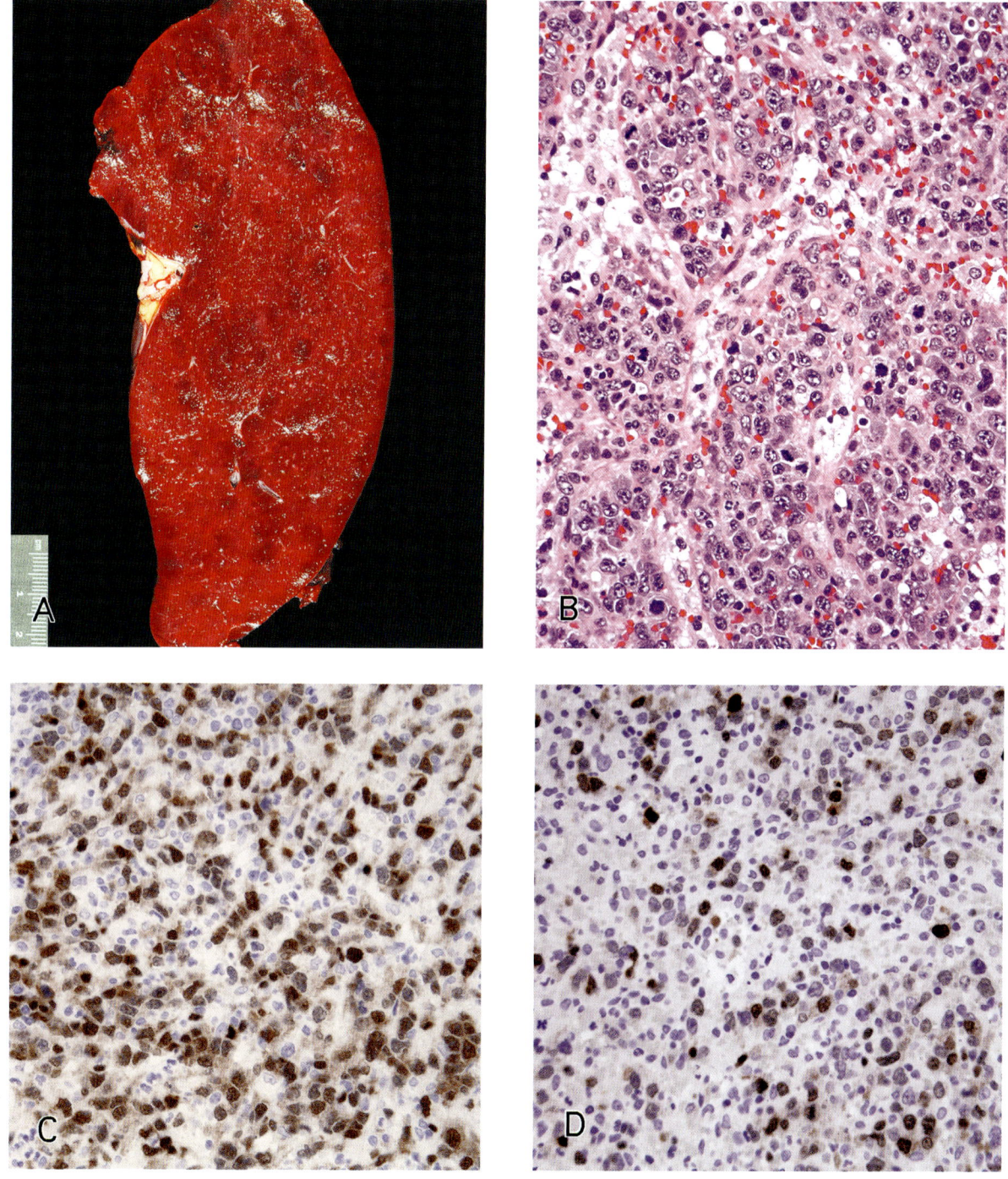

Figure 60-6

PRIMARY SPLENIC LARGE B-CELL LYMPHOMA WITH PREDOMINANT RED PULP INVOLVEMENT

A: This gross image shows a large spleen (1,410 g) with expanded red pulp, but no nodules.

B: The red pulp is expanded by lymphoma cells located predominantly in the cords of Billroth whereas sinusoids are relatively spared. The lymphoma cells are large with vesicular chromatin and mitotic figures are numerous (A,B: H&E stain).

C,D: Immunohistochemical analysis shows that the lymphoma cells are positive for PAX5 (C) and MUM1 (D). The lymphoma cells were also positive for BCL2 and Ki-67 was high (not shown) (C,D: immunohistochemistry with hematoxylin counterstain). (Courtesy of Drs. W. Wang and S. Li, Houston, TX.)

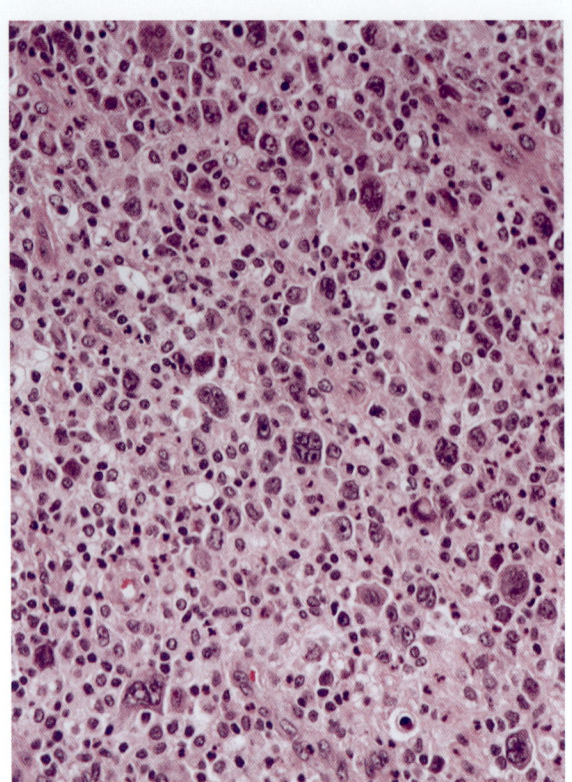 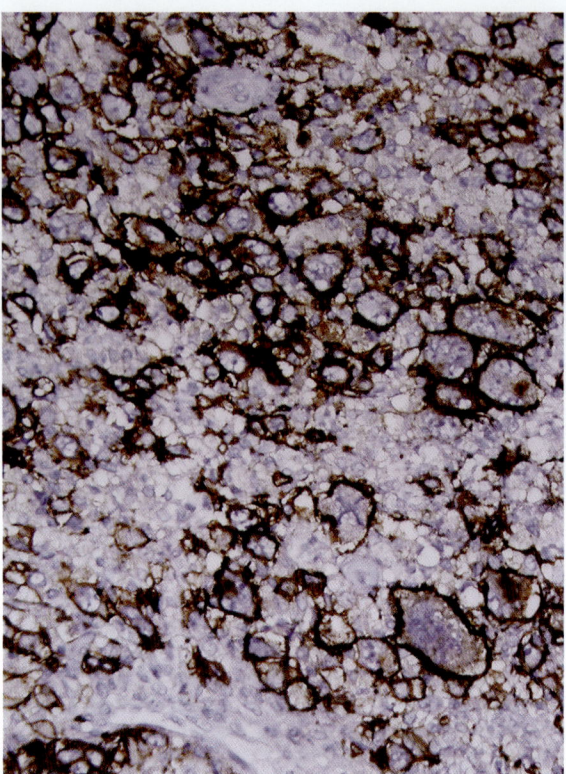

Figure 60-7

PRIMARY SPLENIC LARGE B-CELL LYMPHOMA

Left: Many of the lymphoma cells are large and multinucleated, and some have anaplastic features (H&E stain).
Right: The lymphoma cells are brightly positive for CD20 (immunohistochemistry with hematoxylin counterstain).

In patients with systemic DLBCL, evidence of disease elsewhere is usually known, either as a result of the history or staging studies. Morphologically, disseminated disease in the spleen presents as multiple smaller nodules, but also may form a large tumor mass and can closely resemble primary splenic large B-cell lymphoma. Expression of CD10 or bright BCL6 suggests a germinal center B-cell origin or transformation from an underlying follicular lymphoma. Expression of CD5 and CD23 raises the possibility of transformation of chronic lymphocytic leukemia/small lymphocytic lymphoma, so-called Richter syndrome (fig. 60-8).

T-Cell/Histiocyte-Rich Large B-Cell Lymphoma. In the spleen, systemic T-cell/histiocyte-rich large B-cell lymphoma usually forms macronodules composed of numerous T cells and histiocytes with less than 10 percent large B cells. Rare cases, however, involve the spleen in a micronodular pattern and are difficult to distin-guish from primary splenic large B-cell lymphoma with a micronodular T-cell/histiocyte-rich pattern. The clinical history and the presence of disease elsewhere help distinguish the two.

Intravascular Large B-Cell Lymphoma. Most patients with intravascular large B-cell lymphoma have systemic disease. In the spleen, intravascular large B-cell lymphoma is nearly always confined to the red pulp, almost exclusively in the sinuses (fig. 60-9). The large cells are present in clusters, but may be focally distributed. There is one case of splenic DLBCL with a micronodular pattern that transformed to intravascular large B-cell lymphoma (6a).

Nodular Lymphocyte-Predominant Hodgkin Lymphoma (NLPHL). About 10 to 20 percent of patients with NLPHL present with advanced-stage disease, usually stage III, and the spleen is a common site of involvement. Unlike primary splenic large B-cell lymphoma, NLPHL usually forms nodules that are composed of

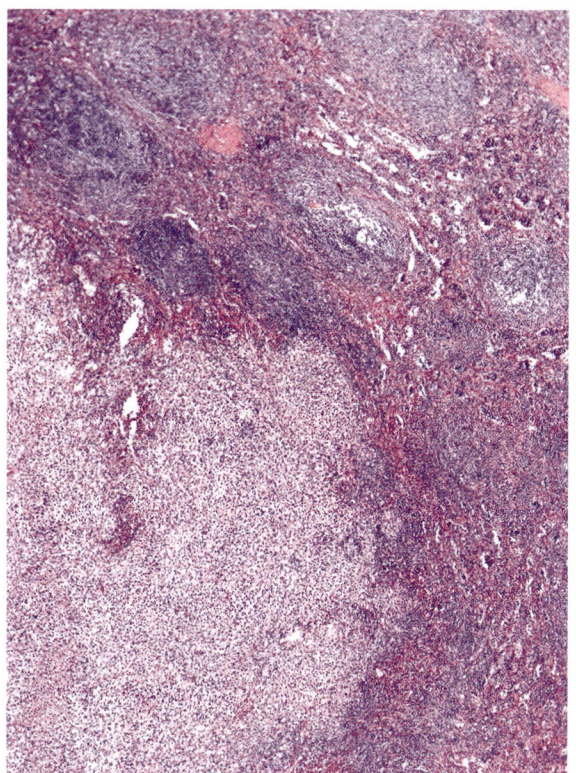 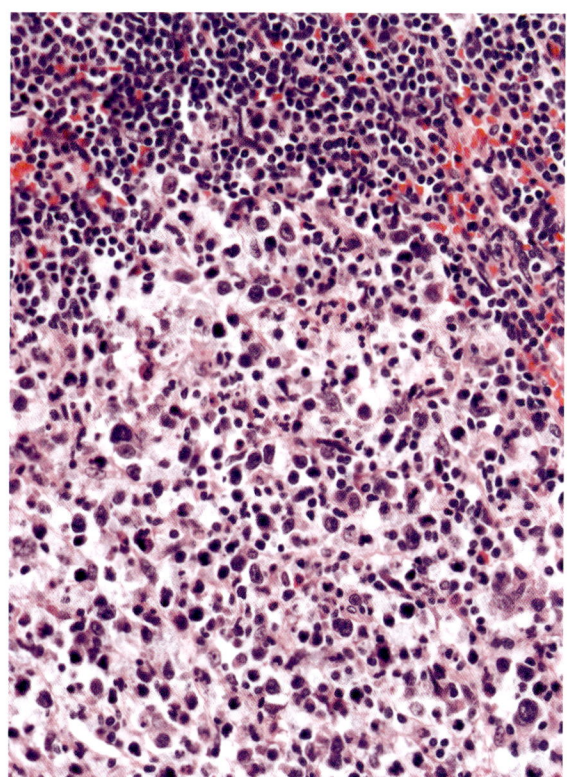

Figure 60-8

**CHRONIC LYMPHOCYTIC LEUKEMIA/SMALL LYMPHOCYTIC LYMPHOMA (CLL/SLL)
AND DIFFUSE LARGE B-CELL LYMPHOMA (DLBCL) INVOLVING SPLEEN**

Left: At this magnification, the CLL/SLL involves and expands white pulp nodules (upper part of field) and the DLBCL forms a large nodule replacing splenic parenchyma (lower left).

Right: High magnification shows the small CLL/SLL cells (top) and large DLBCL cells (bottom) (left, right: H&E stain).

scattered lymphocyte-predominant cells in a background of small and reactive B and T lymphocytes and histiocytes. Tumor nodularity and small B lymphocytes in the background are clues that point to the diagnosis of NLPHL.

Classic Hodgkin Lymphoma (HL). All types of HL may involve the spleen, usually as one or multiple macronodules. Classic HL is characterized by the presence of Reed-Sternberg and Hodgkin (RS+H) cells in a mixed inflammatory background. Some cases of primary splenic large B-cell lymphoma have large pleomorphic or anaplastic cells that can superficially resemble RS+H cells of classic HL (fig. 60-7). Immunohistochemical analysis is helpful because RS+H cells in classic HL have a CD15(+), CD30(+), CD20(-) immunophenotype as opposed to CD20(+), CD15(-), CD30(-) of large cells in primary splenic large B-cell lymphoma.

Splenic Marginal Zone Lymphoma (SMZL). Most cases of SMZL involve the white pulp as nodules with a target-like appearance composed of a central reactive germinal center (if present), surrounded by a zone of small lymphocytes (dark area), and further surrounded at the periphery by cells with abundant monocytoid cytoplasm (pale rim). Small lymphoid cells predominate in SMZL; large cells usually represent no more than 15 percent of the neoplastic cell population. These tumors are usually easy to distinguish from primary splenic large B-cell lymphoma.

About 10 percent of SMZL cases undergo transformation to DLBCL. The most reliable criterion for transformation to DLBCL is the presence of sheets of large B cells. A high proliferation (Ki-67) rate and p53 expression are also findings that support transformation. The DLBCL is often macronodular. Rarely, SMZL transforms to a

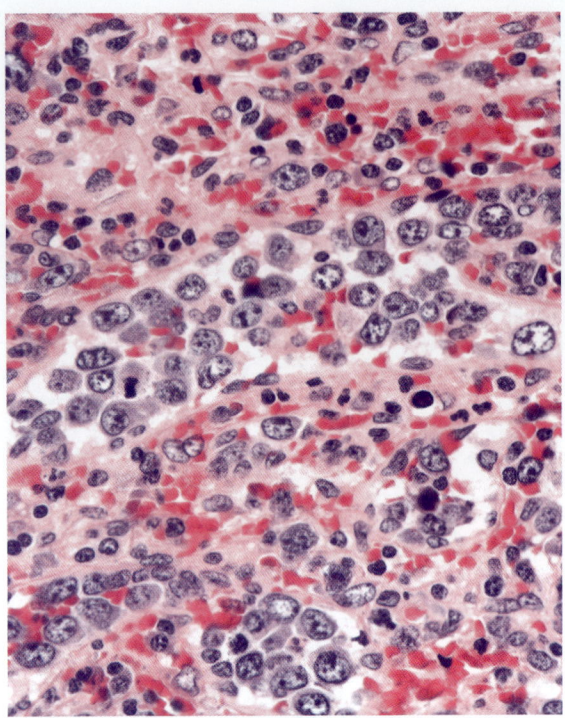

Figure 60-9

INTRAVASCULAR LARGE B-CELL LYMPHOMA INVOLVING SPLEEN

The lymphoma cells are located within the splenic sinuses (H&E stain)

T-cell/histiocyte-rich large B-cell lymphoma that can involve the red pulp (17). In cases in which SMZL has transformed to DLBCL, there is usually some evidence of coexistent low-grade SMZL in the spleen or bone marrow, allowing distinction from primary splenic large B-cell lymphoma.

Inflammatory Pseudotumor of the Spleen. These benign lesions involve the spleen, often as a single, macronodular mass that grossly mimics primary splenic large B-cell lymphoma. Inflammatory pseudotumor of the spleen is rare. It is most often detected in adults who present with left upper quadrant pain or fever; the splenic lesion may be detected incidentally. Histologic examination shows a mixed, inflammatory infiltrate, often associated with sclerosis. Foci of necrosis can be present. There is no histologic or immunohistochemical evidence of large B-cell lymphoma (see chapter 64).

Localized Lymphoid Hyperplasia of the Spleen. Rarely, a splenectomy specimen shows

one or a few macronodules that resemble primary splenic large B-cell lymphoma grossly. Histologic examination, however, shows a conglomeration of reactive follicles into a larger nodule(s) or prominent immunoblastic hyperplasia with fewer follicles. There are no other sites of disease and there is no evidence of a monotypic B-cell population. These cases usually are incidental findings in splenectomy specimens removed for other reasons (e.g., staging laparotomy, trauma) or in patients who have autoimmune hemolytic anemia or immune thrombocytopenia.

Postchemotherapy Histiocyte-Rich Pseudotumor. This is a rare lesion that occurs in patients with lymphoma involving the spleen, usually systemic DLBCL, who have been treated with chemotherapy (4). Postchemotherapy histiocyte-rich pseudotumor most often is detected within the first year following treatment, as a mass in the spleen observed by radiologic studies. Gross examination of the splenectomy specimen shows one or more macronodular lesions that can resemble, in part, primary splenic large B-cell lymphoma. Histologic examination shows abundant ghosts of cells, amorphous areas of necrosis, and numerous lipid-laden histiocytes without viable lymphoma. Immunohistochemical analysis shows that the necrotic cell ghosts are of B-cell lineage and likely represent necrotic B-cell lymphoma that responded to chemotherapy.

TREATMENT AND PROGNOSIS

Usually splenectomy is performed in patients with primary splenic large B-cell lymphoma for diagnostic purposes, but debulking also has the potential of modifying the disease course (19). In one study, Bairey et al. (1) showed improved overall survival for patients who underwent splenectomy. Patients with primary splenic large B-cell lymphoma are usually treated as are other patients with DLBCL, with R-CHOP being the frontline therapy.

The prognosis of patients with primary splenic large B-cell lymphoma is strongly associated with stage and response to chemotherapy (6,17). Patients with disease confined to the spleen have the best response to therapy and often experience complete remission and cure (13).

REFERENCES

1. Bairey O, Shvidel L, Perry C, et al. Characteristics of primary splenic diffuse large B-cell lymphoma and role of splenectomy in improving survival. Cancer 2015;121:2909-2916.

2. Brox A, Bishinsky JI, Berry G. Primary non-Hodgkin lymphoma of the spleen. Am J Hematol 1991;38:95-100.

3. Canelhas A, Compérat E, Le Tourneau A, et al. Marginal zone lymphoma of both spleen and kidney displaying transformation into large B-cell lymphoma. Int Urol Nephrol 2006;38:431-437.

4. Chandra P, Wen YH, Tuli S, et al. Postchemotherapy histiocyte-rich pseudotumor involving the spleen. Am J Clin Pathol 2009;132:342-348.

5. Dogan A, Burke JS, Goteri G, Stitson RN, Wotherspoon AC, Isaacson PG. Micronodular T-cell/histiocyte-rich large B-cell lymphoma of the spleen: histology, immunophenotype, and differential diagnosis. Am J Surg Pathol 2003;27:903-911.

6. Falk S, Stutte HJ. Primary malignant lymphomas of the spleen. A morphologic and immunohistochemical analysis of 17 cases. Cancer 1990;66:2612-2619.

6a. Hall JM, Meyers N, Andrews J. Hemophagocytosis-related (Asian variant) intravascular large B-cell lymphoma in a Hispanic patient: a case report highlighting a micronodular pattern in the spleen. Am J Clin Pathol 2016;145:727-735.

7. Harris NL, Aisenberg AC, Meyer JE, Ellman L, Elman A. Diffuse large cell (histiocytic) lymphoma of the spleen. Clinical and pathologic characteristics of ten cases. Cancer 1984;54:2460-2467.

8. Kan E, Levy I, Benharroch D. Splenic micronodular T-cell/histiocyte-rich large B-cell lymphoma. Ann Diagn Pathol 2008;12:290-292.

9. Kashimura M, Noro M, Akikusa B, et al. Primary splenic diffuse large B-cell lymphoma manifesting in red pulp. Virchows Arch 2008;453:501-509.

10. Kedmi M, Fridlander T, Ilan Y, Shibolet O. Large solitary splenic diffuse large B cell lymphoma in a hepatitis C virus-infected patient. Isr Med Assoc J 2005;7:346-347.

11. Kehoe J, Straus DJ. Primary lymphoma of the spleen. Clinical features and outcome after splenectomy. Cancer 1988;62:1433-1438.

12. Li S, Mann KP, Holden JT. T-cell-rich B-cell lymphoma presenting in the spleen: a clinicopathologic analysis of 3 cases. Int J Surg Pathol 2004;12:31-37.

13. Mollejo M, Algara P, Mateo MS, et al. Large B-cell lymphoma presenting in the spleen: identification of different clinicopathologic conditions. Am J Surg Pathol 2003;27:895-902.

14. Ramdall RB, Cai G, Alaiso TM, Levine P. Fine-needle aspiration biopsy for the primary diagnosis of lymphoproliferative disorders involving the spleen: one institution's experience and review of the literature. Diagn Cytopathol 2006;34:812-817.

15. Shimizu-Kohno K, Kimura Y, Kiyasu J, et al. Malignant lymphoma of the spleen in Japan: a clinicopathologic analysis of 115 cases. Pathol Int 2012;62:577-582.

16. Türköz HK, Polat N, Akin I, Ozcan D. Micronodular T-cell/histiocyte-rich B-cell lymphoma of the spleen in a case of small lymphocytic lymphoma: a Richter's transformation. Ups J Med Sci 2010;115:217-219.

17. Wang SA, Olson N, Zukerberg L, Harris NL. Splenic marginal zone lymphoma with micronodular T-cell rich B-cell lymphoma. Am J Surg Pathol 2006;30:128-132.

18. Wani NA, Parray FQ. Primary lymphoma of the spleen: an experience with seven patients. Int Surg 2005;90:279-283.

19. Xiros N, Economopoulos T, Christodoulidis C, et al. Splenectomy in patients with malignant non-Hodgkin's lymphoma. Eur J Haematol 2000;64:145-150.

20. Yeh YM, Chang KC, Chen YP, et al. Large B cell lymphoma presenting initially in bone marrow, liver and spleen: an aggressive entity associated frequently with haemophagocytic syndrome. Histopathology 2010;57:785-795.

21. Yu SC, Lin CW. Early-stage splenic diffuse large B-cell lymphoma is highly associated with hepatitis C virus infection. Kaohsiung J Med Sci 2013;29:150-156.

61 HEPATOSPLENIC T-CELL LYMPHOMA

GENERAL FEATURES

Hepatosplenic T-cell lymphoma (HSTCL) is defined in the World Health Organization (WHO) classification as a systemic, extranodal T-cell neoplasm derived from cytotoxic T cells; the tumor characteristically involves the spleen, liver, and bone marrow (7,24). In most cases, the lymphoma cells express the γ/δ T-cell receptor (TCR); isochromosome 7q is a characteristic, but not specific, cytogenetic abnormality. A subset of cases currently considered a variant of HSTCL expresses the α/β TCR (7,24).

Normal γ/δ T cells are a part of the innate immune system and normally populate a variety of body sites. γ/δ T cells represent approximately 15 percent of T cells in the spleen and are located mostly within the red pulp. γ/δ T cells also represent 2 to 4 percent of T cells in lymph nodes, 1 percent in the thymic cortex, 3 to 5 percent in the thymic medulla, and 5 percent in the peripheral blood (27). γ/δ T cells also populate mucosal sites and the skin. HSTCL is thought to be derived from normal γ/δ T cells in the spleen that preferentially utilize the *Vδ1* gene and express Vδ1 protein (21).

HSTCL is rare, representing far less than 1 percent of all non-Hodgkin lymphomas and less than 5 percent of peripheral T-cell lymphomas (7). Little data are available regarding the pathogenesis of HSTCL. Two factors likely to be involved are immunodeficiency or immuno-dysregulation and chronic antigen stimulation (29). The incidence of HSTCL is increased in patients with immunosuppression, particularly iatrogenic immune suppression, as a result of solid organ transplantation (22,24). There is a history of organ transplantation in 10 to 20 percent of patients. Other examples of immunosuppression associated with HSTCL include pregnancy and the post-therapy setting for patients treated for acute myeloid leukemia or classic Hodgkin lymphoma (3,7). Chronic antigen stimulation and increased risk of HSTCL

have been reported in patients with malaria infection and inflammatory bowel disease, usually in patients treated with azathioprine, 6-mercaptopurine, or monoclonal antibodies directed against tumor necrosis factor alpha (TNFα), such as infliximab (3,9,11,13,23).

There is no strong evidence linking HSTCL with viral infection, including hepatitis C, human T-cell leukemia lymphoma virus-1, human herpesvirus 8, or human immunodeficiency virus. Epstein-Barr virus (EBV) infection is present in a small subset of HSTCL patients, most often in the post-transplant setting. Rare cases of HSTCL are associated with hepatitis B infection (4,18,20).

CLINICAL FEATURES

HSTCL usually arises in young patients, including adolescents and younger adults (3,7,32). Patients with classic γ/δ HSTCL often first develop disease in the third decade. The male to female ratio is approximately 5 to 1. Patients with the α/β TCR variant of HSTCL are older, with a median age of 36 years and women are more often affected (14,32). These differences in age and sex preference suggest differences in etiology between the γ/δ and α/β variants of HSTCL.

Patients frequently have B symptoms including fever, weight loss, night sweats, and fatigue (Table 61-1) (7,32). Most patients present with marked splenomegaly and 60 to 70 percent also have hepatomegaly (3,31,32). Jaundice, secondary to liver involvement, occurs in about 30 to 40 percent of patients and left upper quadrant pain, associated with splenomegaly occurs in about 25 percent. Peripheral lymphadenopathy is uncommon (15 to 20 percent of patients) (32). All patients with HSTCL have Ann Arbor stage IV disease and most patients have a high International Prognostic Index (IPI) score (3). Rarely, patients develop manifestations of a full-blown hemophagocytic syndrome, either at the time of diagnosis or during the clinical course of disease (1).

Table 61-1

CLINICAL AND LABORATORY FINDINGS IN PATIENTS WITH HEPATOSPLENIC T-CELL LYMPHOMA

Finding	Frequency
Splenomegaly	80-90%
B symptoms	~80%
Hepatomegaly	60-70%
Elevated serum lactate dehydrogenase	60-70%
Thrombocytopenia	60-70%
Anemia	50-60%
Neutropenia	~50%
Jaundice	30-40%
Abnormal liver function tests (mild)	30-40%
Abdominal pain	~25%
Monocytosis	~20%
Lymphadenopathy	15-20%
History of solid organ transplant	15-20%
Skin lesions	~5%

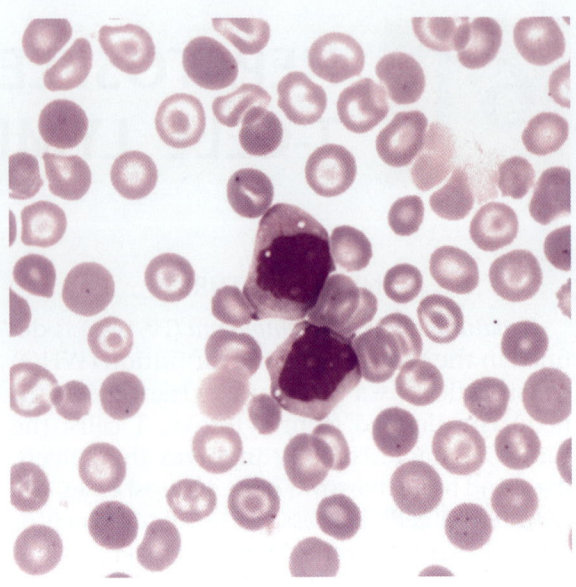

Figure 61-1

γ/δ HEPATOSPLENIC T-CELL LYMPHOMA

A peripheral blood smear shows intermediate-sized cells, with irregular nuclear contours, nucleoli, and slightly blue cytoplasm (Wright-Giemsa stain).

Laboratory abnormalities are common in patients with HSTCL. The serum lactate dehydrogenase (LDH) level is elevated in over half of all patients (7,32). Rare patients with cold agglutinin disease have been reported (15). Serum liver function tests are mildly elevated in 30 to 40 percent of patients. Hematologic abnormalities are common (3,7,31): thrombocytopenia is the most common, in 60 to 70 percent of patients, but anemia and leukopenia also occur (3,7,31). The mechanisms that explain cytopenias in HSTCL are poorly understood. Cytokine secretion by γ/δ T cells has been suggested as a possible explanation. In occasional patients, there are immune hematologic complications, including immune thrombocytopenic purpura and hemolytic anemia. Monocytosis has been reported in about 20 percent of patients (3).

An overt leukemic presentation is rare in HSTCL patients, but some lymphoma cells can be observed in the peripheral blood smears of up to half of patients. Compared with normal small lymphocytes, HSTCL cells have enlarged nuclei, folded or irregular nuclear contours, coarser or more blastic nuclear chromatin, and increased amounts of cytoplasm that often has a blue tinge (fig. 61-1). In advanced stages of disease, a leukemic phase with marked lymphocytosis is observed (3).

GROSS AND HISTOLOGIC FINDINGS

Spleen

The spleen is often massively enlarged, ranging from 1,000 to 3,000 g (7,31,32). In one study, Belhadj et al. (3) reported an upper weight range of 6,000 g. The cut surface of the spleen is homogeneous red-purple and without focal lesions. Necrosis is unusual but can occur after therapy (fig. 61-2). Splenic hilar lymph nodes are not prominent.

The red pulp is diffusely involved and the white pulp is attenuated or absent (fig. 61-3) (4,7,31). HSTCL cells are present in sinuses and cords. Frequently, there is massive expansion of the splenic sinuses, giving an appearance of islands of abnormal cells, surrounded by a thin delimiting cell lining (splenic littoral cells). In addition, the cords are often expanded by HSTCL cells (fig. 61-4). Areas of coagulative necrosis are uncommon.

The cytologic appearance of HSTCL cells is variable (7,28,29). Most often, they are small, mature-appearing lymphocytes with dense, mature chromatin and scant cytoplasm. The cells often have folded or irregular nuclear contours,

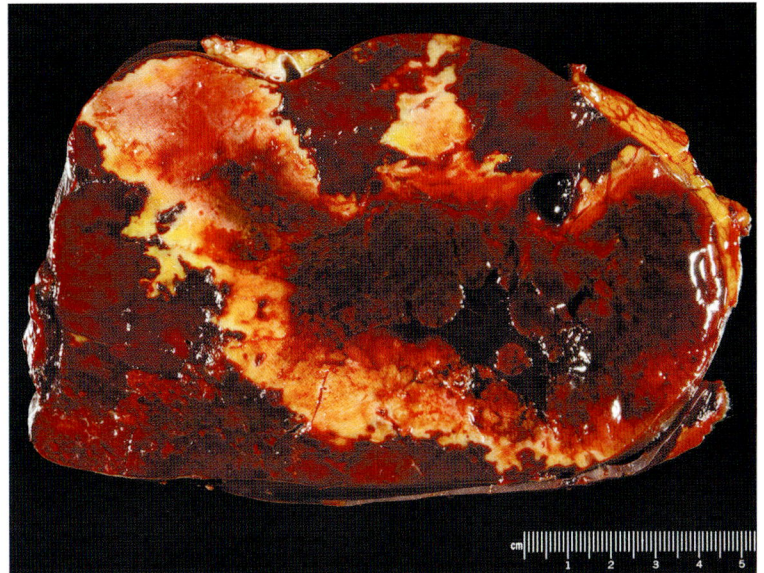

Figure 61-2

γ/δ HEPATOSPLENIC T-CELL LYMPHOMA

This man with γ/δ hepatosplenic T-cell lymphoma (HSTCL) who was being treated with combination chemotherapy when he developed left upper quadrant pain and splenomegaly, which prompted splenectomy. The spleen was 3,090 g. The cut surface shows large yellow zones representing necrosis, presumably in response to therapy. The uniform, congested and red appearance of the non-necrotic splenic parenchyma is typical of HSTCL.

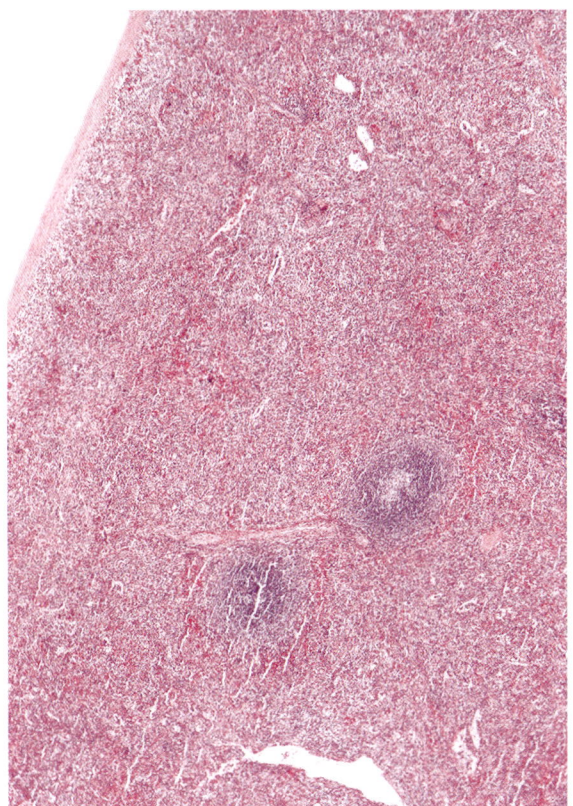

Figure 61-3

γ/δ HEPATOSPLENIC T-CELL LYMPHOMA INVOLVING SPLEEN

The red pulp is expanded by abnormal lymphocytes present in cords and sinuses. The white pulp is relatively spared (hematoxylin and eosin [H&E] stain).

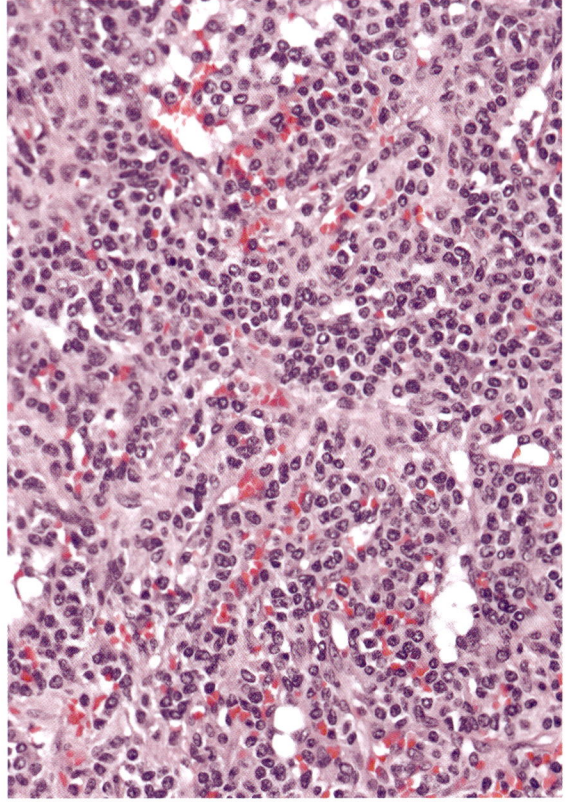

Figure 61-4

γ/δ HEPATOSPLENIC T-CELL LYMPHOMA INVOLVING SPLEEN

The splenic red pulp is extensively involved by small tumor cells with dense chromatin and only small amounts of cytoplasm. These cells expand the cords and sinuses (H&E stain).

917

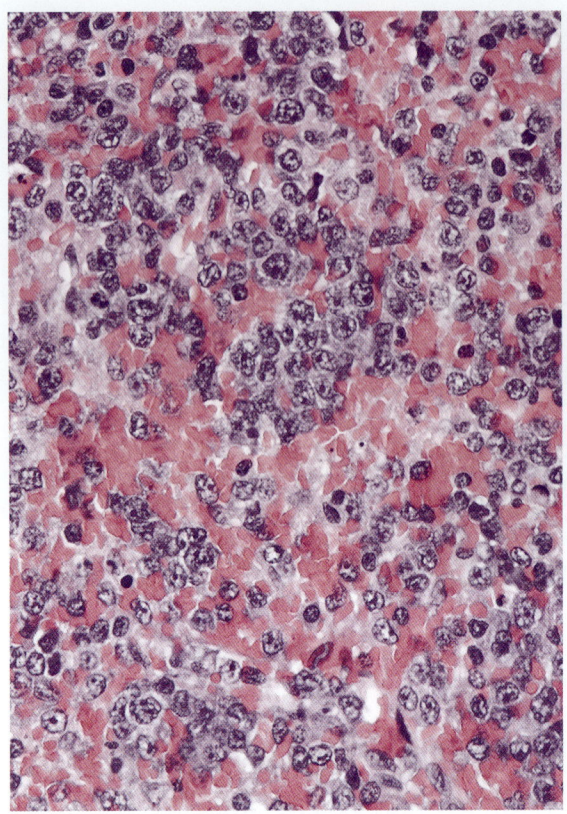

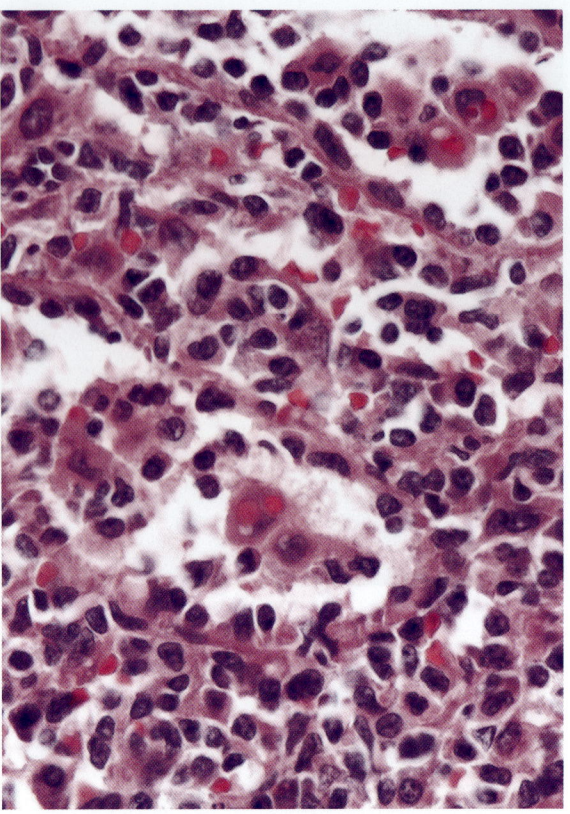

Figure 61-5

γ/δ HEPATOSPLENIC T-CELL LYMPHOMA: LARGE CELL VARIANT

The tumor cells in the spleen are large, with vesicular chromatin and exhibit more nuclear pleomorphism than observed in typical HSTCL cases (H&E stain).

Figure 61-6

γ/δ HEPATOSPLENIC T-CELL LYMPHOMA INVOLVING SPLEEN WITH HEMOPHAGOCYTOSIS

Extensive replacement by lymphoma and hemophago-cytosis are evident. In this field erythrocytes are prominent within the cytoplasm of histiocytes (H&E stain).

although in some cases the cell nuclei are round-er. Rarely, cytoplasmic granules are seen. Some cases of HSTCL have intermediate-sized cells with a more blastoid appearance. These cells have more open and delicate chromatin and minimal cytoplasm. In other cases, the neo-plastic cells are large with vesicular chromatin and more cytoplasm (fig. 61-5). The increasing size of HSTCL cells may correlate with disease progression (29).

Evidence of hemophagocytosis is identified in the spleen (and other sites) in HSTCL (fig. 61-6). The cytoplasm of the histiocytes con-tains neoplastic lymphocytes as well as benign hematopoietic elements. Only a small subset of patients with histologic evidence of hemo-phagocytosis has overt clinical evidence of a hemophagocytic syndrome (1,3).

Other Sites

Splenic hilar lymph nodes, although not grossly abnormal, may be involved. These lymph nodes often have a predominantly si-nusoidal pattern of involvement, but they can be diffusely replaced by tumor (27). Periph-eral lymph nodes are involved infrequently (7,31).

Liver biopsy specimens show HSTCL cells in a sinusoidal distribution (fig. 61-7). Involve-ment of the portal tracts also occurs but is less prominent (3,4). In patients with advanced stage or recurrent disease, other extranodal sites that may be involved include skin, mucosal surfaces, and kidney (fig. 61-8). The cytologic features of HSTCL at these sites are similar to those described in the spleen.

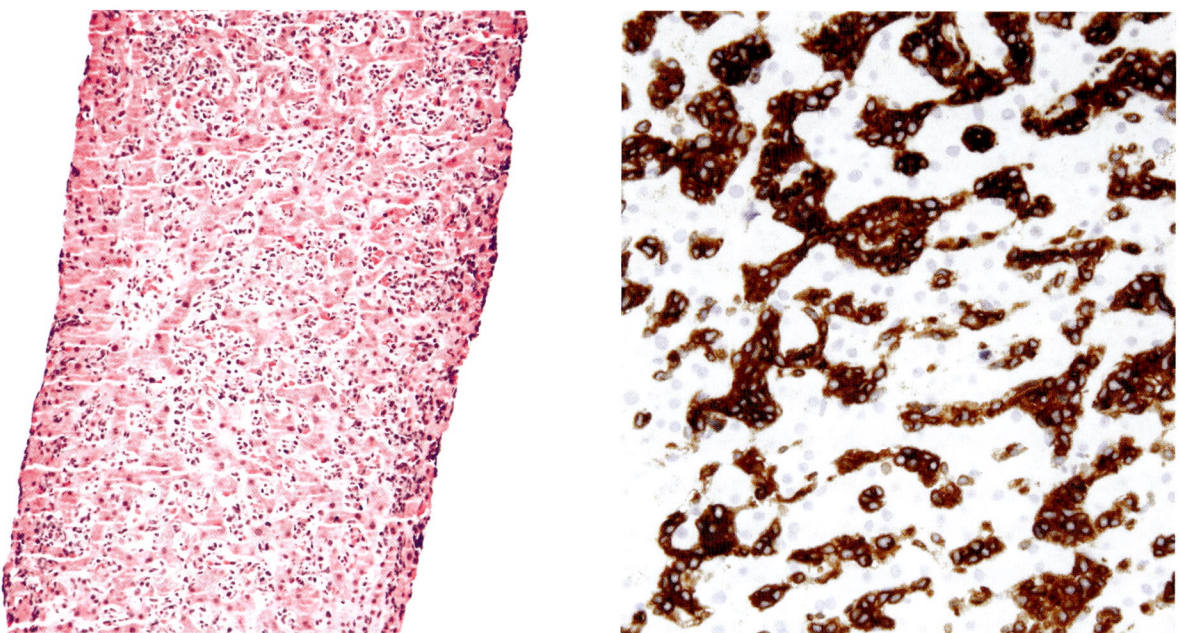

Figure 61-7

γ/δ HEPATOSPLENIC T-CELL LYMPHOMA INVOLVING LIVER

Left: The lymphoma cells are distributed within and expand the sinusoids (H&E stain).
Right: The lymphoma cells are positive for CD3 (immunohistochemistry with hematoxylin counterstain).

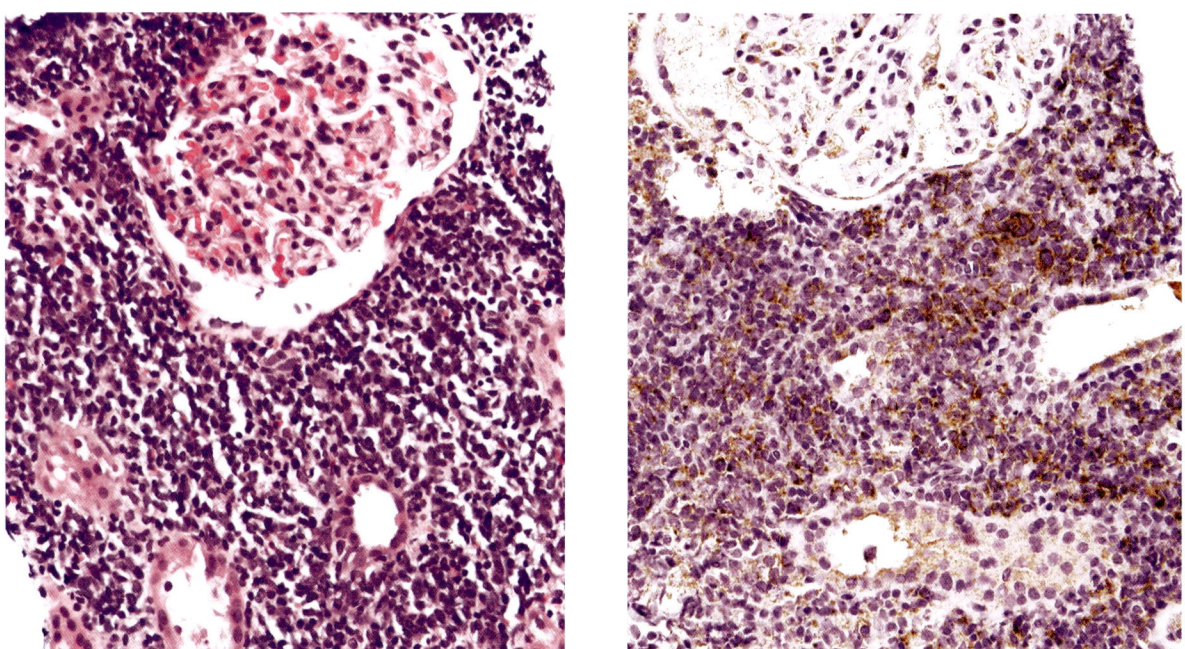

Figure 61-8

γ/δ HEPATOSPLENIC T-CELL LYMPHOMA INVOLVING KIDNEY

Left: The lymphoma cells extensively replace the parenchyma, but a few tubules and one glomerulus are spared (H&E stain).
Right: The lymphoma cells are positive for T-cell receptor (TCR) gamma (immunohistochemistry with hematoxylin counterstain).

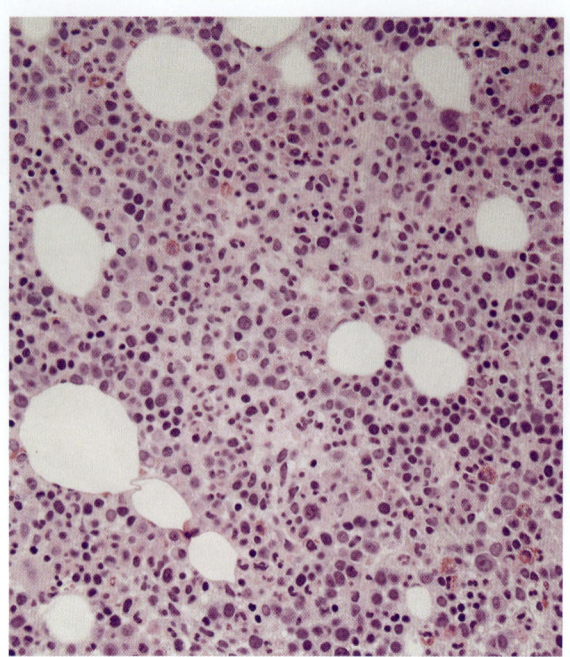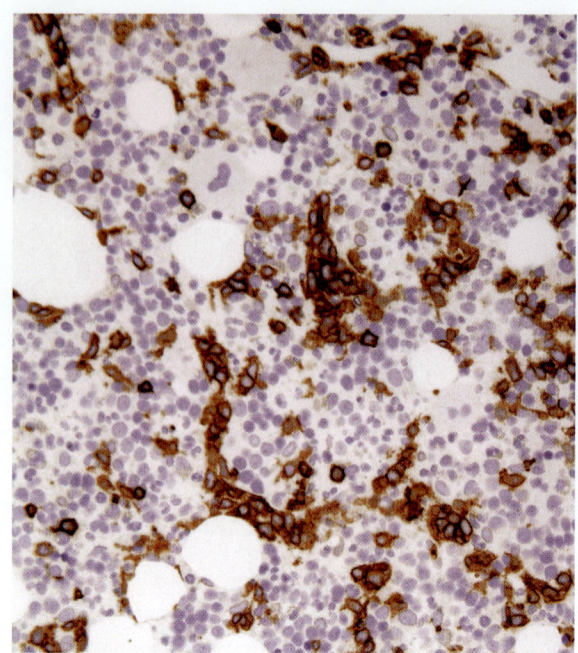

Figure 61-9

γ/δ HEPATOSPLENIC T-CELL LYMPHOMA INVOLVING BONE MARROW

This patient had Crohn disease and was being treated with immunomodulating agents including an inhibitor of tumor necrosis factor alpha (infliximab).

Left: The biopsy specimen shows a hypercellular bone marrow. The HSTCL cells blend in with hematopoietic cells and are difficult to discern in this field (H&E stain).

Right: Immunohistochemistry for CD3 highlights the lymphoma cells which are distributed in a sinusoidal pattern (immunohistochemistry with hematoxylin counterstain).

Bone Marrow

Bone marrow aspirate smears from patients with HSTCL show trilineage hematopoiesis. The lymphoma cells, particularly when small, may be difficult to appreciate (7,28), although some cases have larger and easier to recognize lymphoma cells (fig. 61-10A). Slight to moderate plasmacytosis is common and monocytosis also occurs (3). In some cases, the cells appear cohesive on smears and resemble, in part, nonhematopoietic neoplasms. Hemophagocytosis, most often erythrophagocytosis, is observed (1).

In aspirate smears, evidence of dyspoiesis is common but usually mild (fig. 61-11) (28,33). The changes include hypolobated or small megakaryocytes, nuclear budding or megaloblastoid changes in erythroid precursors, and hypogranular or abnormally segmented granulocytes. As a result, the possibility of a myelodysplastic syndrome may be considered. If the HSTCL cells are larger and contain nucleoli, they may be misconstrued as myeloblasts, further complicating analysis (28). The dyspoietic changes in HSTCL do not correlate with peripheral cytopenias, however, and true myeloblasts are not increased. Therefore, these changes are not thought to be evidence of myelodysplastic syndrome (33). The pathogenesis of these changes is unknown.

Bone marrow biopsy specimens are typically hypercellular (figs. 61-9, 61-10, 61-12). Increased trilineage hematopoietic elements may make it difficult to identify the lymphoma cells. (28). The lymphoma cells are usually present in an intrasinusoidal and interstitial pattern (figs. 61-9, right; 61-12, right). In more advanced cases, a diffuse pattern of involvement becomes apparent, which is easier to recognize in routinely stained tissue sections (fig. 61-10). The lymphoma cells are usually small, but intermediate-sized cells or more blastoid or large and pleomorphic cells may be observed. The abnormal lymphocytes tend to have moderate amounts of basophilic

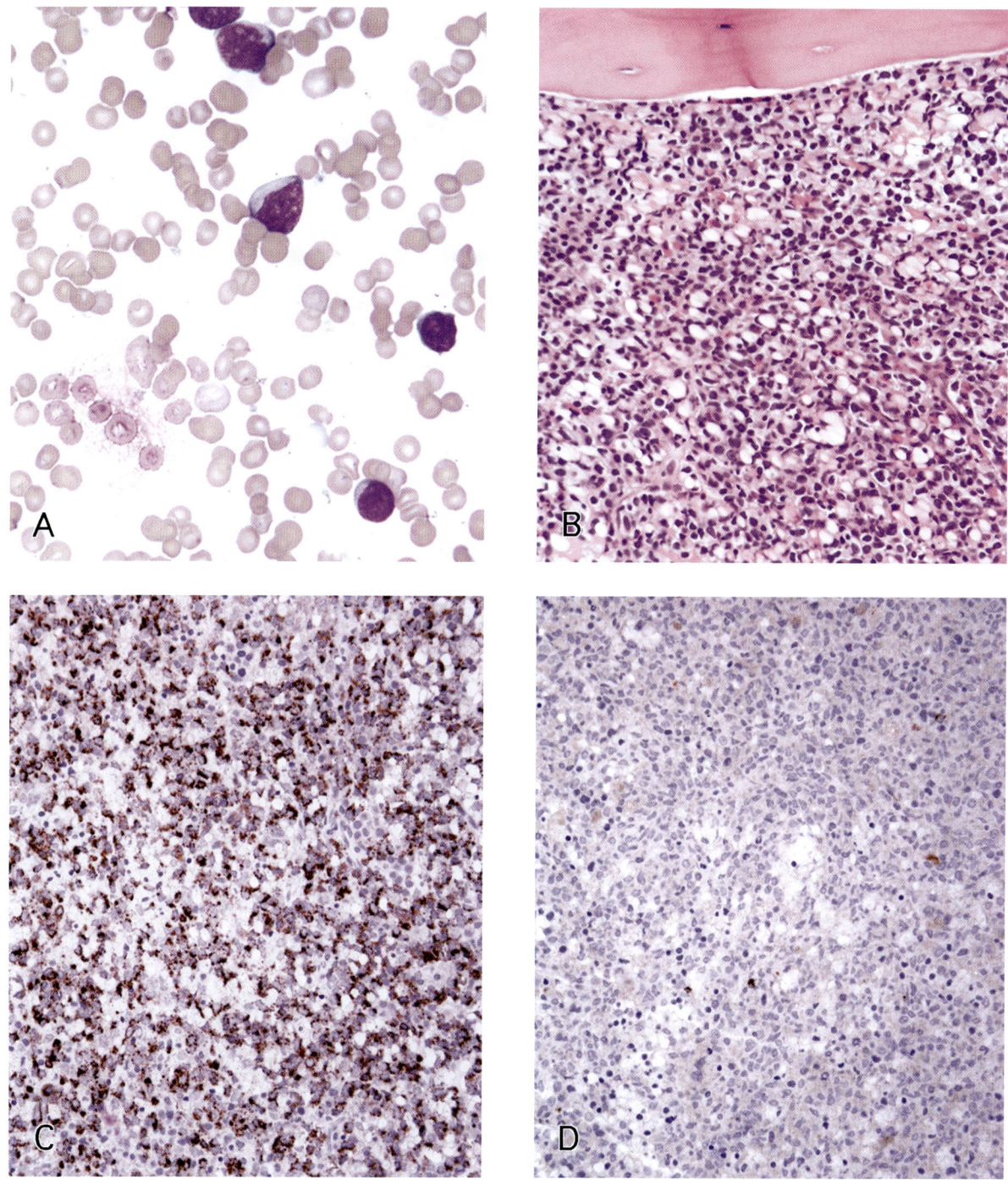

Figure 61-10

α/β HEPATOSPLENIC T-CELL LYMPHOMA INVOLVING BONE MARROW

A: The aspirate smear shows multiple small and larger lymphoma cells (Wright-Giemsa stain).

B: The biopsy specimen shows a markedly hypercellular bone marrow in which many lymphoma cells are appreciated (H&E stain).

C,D: Immunohistochemical analysis shows an immature cytotoxic T-cell immunophenotype: positive for TIA-1 (C) and negative for granzyme B (D). These cells were also positive for TCR α/β and CD3 and negative for CD4, CD5, and CD8 (not shown) (C,D: immunohistochemistry with hematoxylin counterstain).

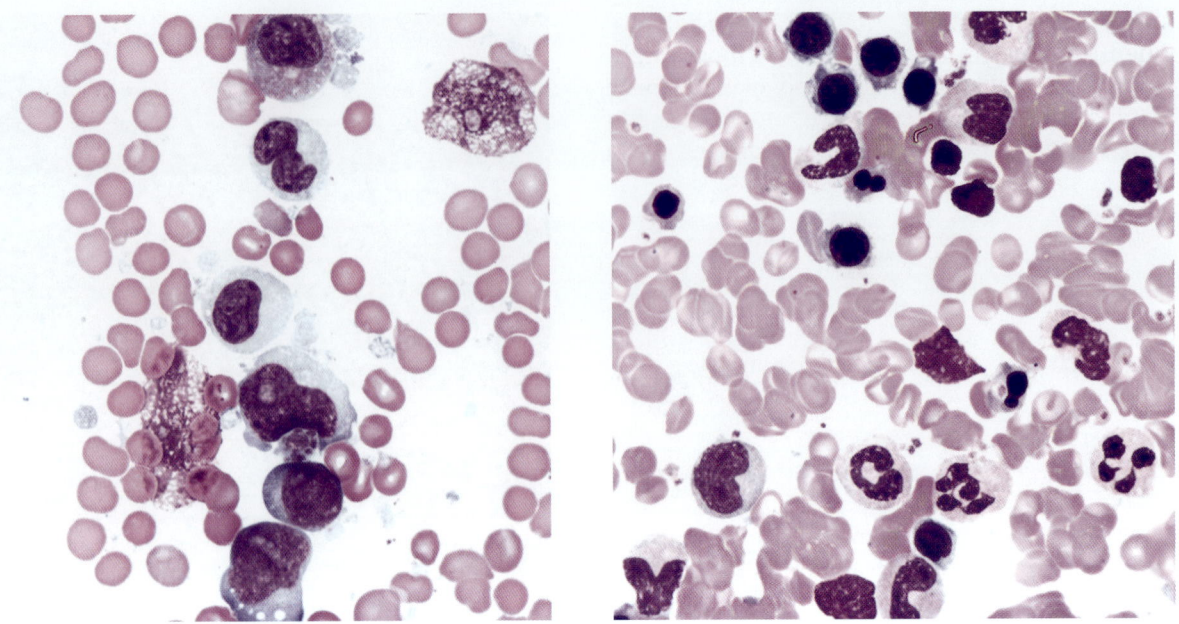

Figure 61-11

γ/δ HEPATOSPLENIC T-CELL LYMPHOMA: DYSPOIETIC CHANGES IN BONE MARROW

Left: In this aspirate smear, two granulocytes have markedly hypogranular cytoplasm. Three lymphoma cells are also present in this field, which could possibly be misinterpreted as blasts.

Right: In this aspirate smear from a different patient there are hypogranular granulocytes and asymmetrically budded erythroid precursors (Wright-Giemsa stain).

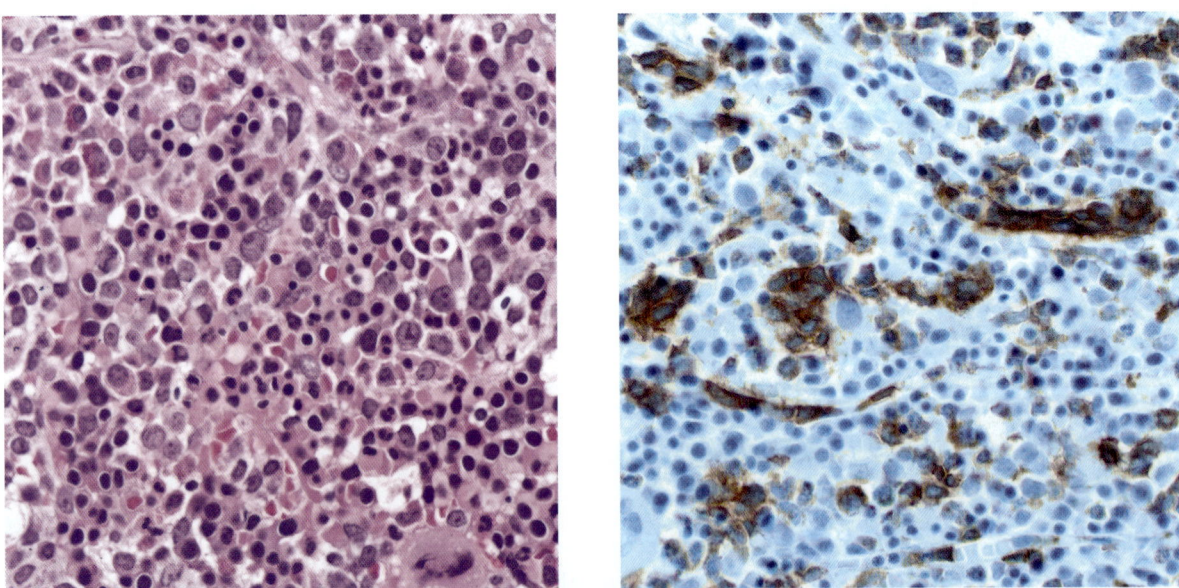

Figure 61-12

γ/δ HEPATOSPLENIC T-CELL LYMPHOMA INVOLVING BONE MARROW

Left: The bone marrow is markedly hypercellular but lymphoma cells also are appreciated in a sinusoid (especially in retrospect after reviewing immunohistochemistry results) (H&E stain).

Right: Immunohistochemistry for CD3 highlights the lymphoma cells which expand sinusoids (immunohistochemistry with hematoxylin counterstain).

cytoplasm. In almost all cases, immunohisto-chemical analysis using a T-cell antibody high-lights a sinusoidal pattern and usually more extensive disease than is originally appreciated by examination of the hematoxylin and eosin (H&E) stained slides (figs. 61-9, 61-10, 61-12) (7,28,29).

CYTOLOGIC FINDINGS

Cytologic preparations commonly show a dispersed population of small to intermediate-sized lymphoid cells characterized by irregular, convoluted, or ovoid nuclei; mature chromatin; inconspicuous nucleoli; and pale cytoplasm (fig. 61-13). On air-dried preparations, the tumor cell cytoplasm is often blue (12). Nuclear features vary from case to case and include intermedi-ate-sized nuclei with blastoid chromatin and large cells with vesicular chromatin.

IMMUNOPHENOTYPIC FINDINGS

Flow cytometry and immunohistochemistry are equally helpful as well as complementary for determining the immunophenotype of HSTCL. The cells of HSTCL are positive for surface CD2, CD3, and CD7, and lack CD5 (3,7,31,32). CD43 is usually positive and CD56 is expressed in 70 to 80 percent of cases (3). CD16 is often expressed. About 75 percent of cases express surface γ/δ TCR, but some cases express α/β TCR (7,32). About 10 percent of cases are neg-ative for both γ/δ and α/β TCR (so-called TCR silent). The cells of HSTCL usually express killer immunoglobulin-like receptors (KIR) and some express CD94/NKG2 (17). In contrast to normal γ/δ TCR cells, HSTCL cells show a lower (dim) expression of surface CD3 as well as surface TCR (10). ZAP70 is often positive. CD8 is usually negative but can be expressed, often partially, in about 20 percent of cases (3). CD1a, CD4, CD10, CD25, CD30, CD57 (less than 5 percent positive), myeloid-associated and B-cell anti-gens, and TdT are negative (3,7,32).

Using immunohistochemistry, the immuno-phenotype of HSTCL cells closely matches the flow cytometry findings (fig. 61-14). In addition, HSTCL cells are invariably positive for TIA-1 and granzyme M, but granzyme B and perforin are often negative. This combination of cytotoxic markers implies that the tumor cells have an immature cytotoxic T-cell immunophenotype.

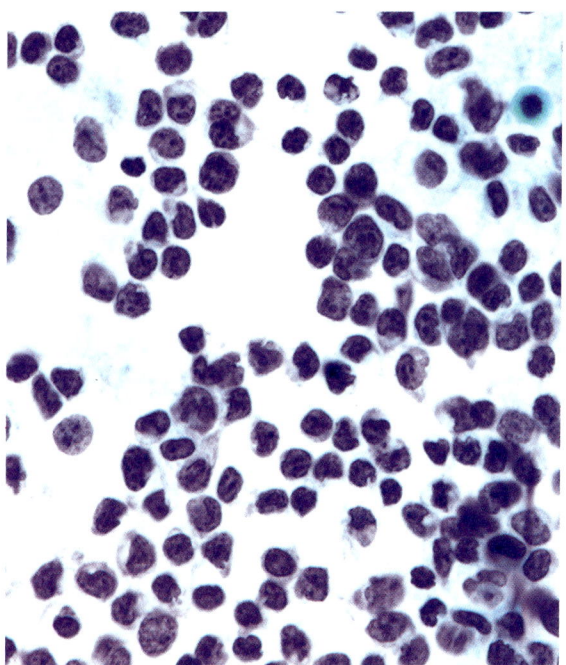

Figure 61-13

γ/δ HEPATOSPLENIC T-CELL: LYMPHOMA CYTOLOGIC FEATURES

This pleural fluid specimen was obtained from a patient with γ/δ HSTCL who after therapy developed infections and a leukemic phase of disease. The lymphoma cells are medium-sized, with irregular convoluted nuclear contours and pale cytoplasm (Papanicolaou stain).

Nevertheless, up to one third of HSTCL cases are positive for granzyme B (32) and perforin also can be positive, although less frequently (fig. 61-14).

Assessment of Ki-67 shows a variable prolif-eration rate in HSTCL, which can be brisk. TCR γ and β expression can be assessed by immuno-histochemistry using fixed, paraffin-embedded tissue sections. TCRδ assessment has been per-formed using fixed, paraffin-embedded tissue sections but in our experience is more reliably done using fresh or frozen tissue. BCL2 is dim-ly positive or negative in HSTCL, p53 is rarely positive, and cyclin D1 is negative.

Rare cases of HSTCL are reported to express S-100 protein (5). While thought to be unusual, the frequency of S-100 expression by HSTCL is unknown since S-100 staining is not routinely performed. EBV latent membrane protein type 1 (LMP1) is negative, but about 10 percent of cases of HSTCL are positive for EBV encoded

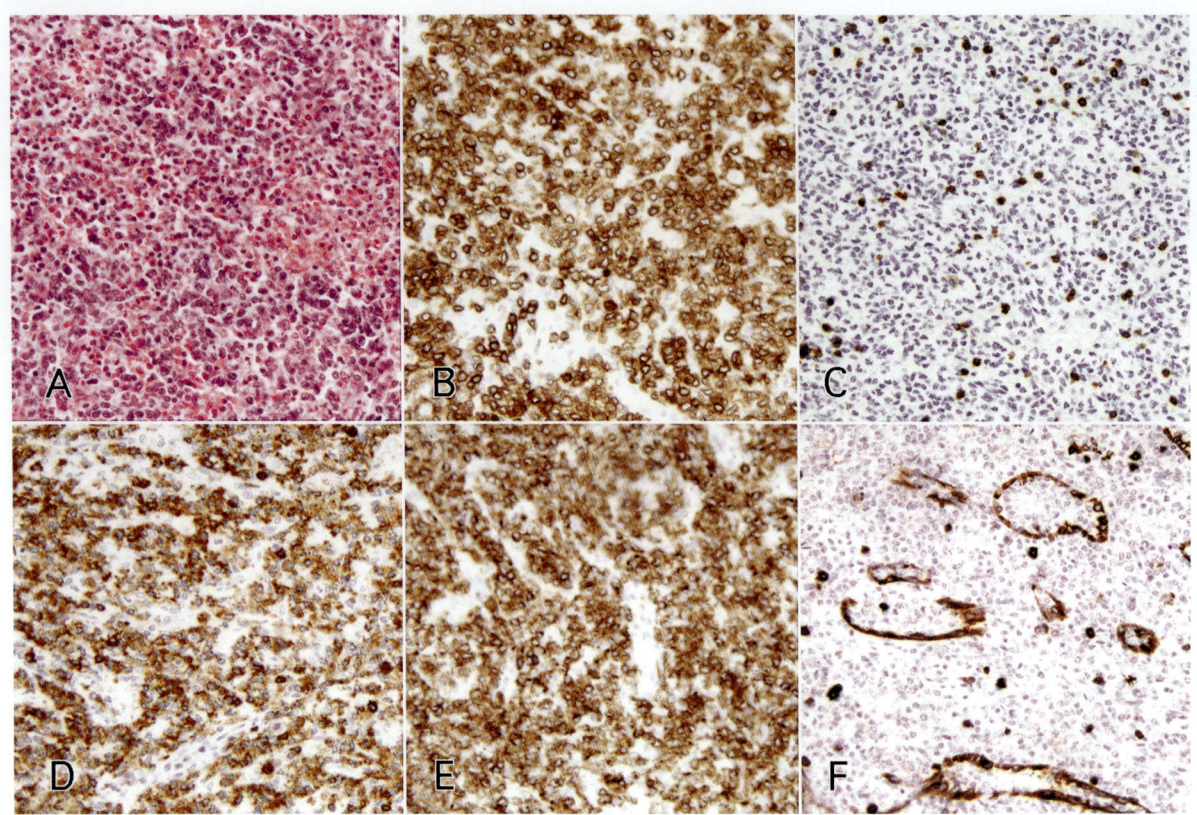

Figure 61-14

γ/δ HEPATOSPLENIC T-CELL LYMPHOMA INVOLVING SPLEEN: IMMUNOHISTOCHEMISTRY

A: High magnification shows the splenic red pulp packed with lymphoma cells (H&E stain).

B–F: Immunohistochemical analysis of the spleen showed that the lymphoma cells are positive for CD3 (B), negative for CD5 (C), positive for CD7 (D), positive for perforin (E), and negative for CD8 (F). The anti-CD8 antibody highlights splenic sinuses. Expression of perforin is not typical, but it occurs in a small subset of HSTCL cases (B–F: immunohistochemistry with hematoxylin counterstain).

RNA1 (EBER1) by in situ hybridization (3). EBER positivity occurs most often in cases with pleomorphic cytologic features or in the post-transplant setting (3).

MOLECULAR GENETIC FINDINGS

Isochromosome (7q10) is present in about 50 percent of cases of HSTCL (2,3,28,30). Rarely, ring chromosome 7 or other structural rearrangements and numerical abnormalities of chromosome 7q are observed. Isochromosome (7q) may be the sole abnormality in HSTCL and is therefore thought to be an early (driver) event in pathogenesis. The common deleted region in cases of HSTCL has been localized to 7p22.1p14.1 and the common gained region to 7q22.11q31.1 (6). These changes are associated with increased expression of *CHN2,* which encodes for β-chimerin (loss of 7p22.1-7p14.1) and overexpression of a number of genes including *ABCB1*, a multidrug resistance gene (gain of 7q22.11-7q31.1) (6). Overexpression of *CHN2*/β-chimerin may result in NFAT pathway downregulation and cell proliferation (6). The TCRγ (7p14.1) and TCRβ (7q32) loci are involved in the ring (7) abnormality (6).

Isochromosome (7q) is commonly associated with additional cytogenetic abnormalities, and trisomy 8 and loss of either an X or Y chromosome are common in HSTCL. In one study, trisomy 8 was localized within the lymphoma cells in most of the cases assessed (33). Importantly, isochromosome (7q) is not specific for HSTCL and has been reported in other tumors, including acute myeloid and lymphoblastic leukemias, myelodysplastic syndromes, Wilms tumor, and rarely, NK/T cell lymphomas.

Gene expression profiling studies have shown, for the most part, that the expression profiles of HSTCL are similar regardless of TCR expression and that HSTCL can be distinguished from other types of T-cell lymphoma (6,16,26). Finalet-Ferreiro et al. (6) proposed a 24-gene panel that distinguishes HSTCL from other T-cell lymphomas. Travert et al. (26) reported that HSTCL cases have a gene expression profile similar to that of NK/T-cell lymphomas, with overexpression of genes involved in the JAK-STAT pathway, *SYK*, cell trafficking genes (e.g., sphingosine-1-phosphate receptor [*S1PR5*]), and multidrug resistance (e.g., *MDR1*) (26).

McKinney et al. (14a) performed whole exome sequencing on 68 cases of HSTCL. The most common gene mutated was *SETD2* in about 25 percent of cases. *SETD2* encodes a methyltransferase that methylates lysine 36 on histone H3. Other mutations identified likely important in pathogenesis included *STAT5B* (31 percent), *STAT3* (9 percent), *PIK3CD* (9 percent), and less frequently *INOSO*, *E2H2*, *KRAS*, and *TP53* (14a). *ARIDIB* mutations also were identified but their functional significance is unclear. *STAT5B* mutations occur most often in a hotspot, resulting in a p.N642H mutation thought to result in JAK-STAT pathway activation (19). *STAT5B* and *STAT3* mutations are mutually exclusive (14a,19).

Analysis for T-cell receptor gene rearrangements shows monoclonal *TRG* rearrangements in almost all cases of HSTCL (7,32). About one third of cases carry *TRB* gene rearrangements. The immunoglobulin genes are usually in the germline configuration. Cases of γ/δ HSTCL preferentially utilize the *Vδ1* gene in about 75 percent of cases (3,21).

DIFFERENTIAL DIAGNOSIS

Hairy Cell Leukemia. Grossly and histologically, hairy cell leukemia in the spleen may resemble HSTCL. In both diseases, the red pulp is expanded by small lymphoid cells. Immunophenotypic analysis resolves the issue: hairy cell leukemia is composed of B cells that express immunoglobulin, B-cell antigens, CD11c, CD25, and CD103. In addition, bone marrow involvement by hairy cell leukemia is diffuse rather than sinusoidal, and patients with HSTCL are usually more ill than patients with hairy cell leukemia.

Splenic Marginal Zone Lymphoma (SMZL). The sinusoidal infiltration of the bone marrow by SMZL resembles that of HSTCL morphologically. SMZL, however, preferentially involves the splenic white pulp and is a B-cell neoplasm, positive for immunoglobulin and B-cell antigens, unlike HSTCL. Deletion (7q31) occurs in about half of patients with SMZL, and these patients often have an indolent clinical course and are not as ill as patients with HSTCL.

Extranodal Lymphomas that Express γ/δ TCR. A number of other extranodal lymphoid neoplasms can express γ/δ TCR. These include primary cutaneous γ/δ T-cell lymphoma and rare extranodal lymphomas arising at other mucosal sites. These tumors, like HSTCL, likely arise from γ/δ T cells of the innate immune system, but otherwise are not thought to be closely related to HSTCL. The diagnosis of HSTCL is based on the characteristic clinical presentation of hepatosplenomegaly and cytopenias, bone marrow disease, a characteristic immunophenotype, and cytogenetic findings.

T-Cell Large Granular Lymphocytic (T-LGL) Leukemia. Although most cases of T-LGL leukemia express the α/β TCR, some cases express γ/δ TCR. Patients with T-LGL leukemia are typically older adults who have clinically indolent disease (34). Patients may be asymptomatic or have a history of autoimmune diseases or cytopenias. Mild to moderate lymphocytosis is usually present. In the bone marrow, T-LGL leukemia exhibits an interstitial pattern of infiltration and the tumor cells have cytoplasmic azurophilic granules and are positive for CD8 and CD57. Features that support HSTCL include massive splenomegaly, bone marrow sinuses expanded by lymphoma cells, and lymphoma cells devoid of cytoplasmic granules (35).

Aggressive Natural Killer-Cell (NK-Cell) Leukemia. Patients with aggressive NK-cell leukemia present with B symptoms, cytopenias, and splenomegaly, mimicking the presentation of patients with HSTCL. Unlike HSTCL, the neoplastic cells of aggressive NK-cell leukemia have a NK cell immunophenotype; usually express the cytotoxic molecules TIA-1, granzyme B, and perforin (a mature cytotoxic immunophenotype); and can be positive for EBV infection (7).

Reactive γ/δ T-cell Proliferations. There are rare reports of florid γ/δ T-cell proliferations that can mimic HSTCL. In one report, a patient with HSTCL had persistently increased non-neoplastic γ/δ T cells in the cerebrospinal fluid (10). In another report, Zhang and Bayer (36) described two patients who underwent splenectomy for reactive γ/δ T-cell proliferations that expanded the splenic red pulp. Flow cytometry immunophenotyping and molecular studies were essential to exclude HSTCL in these cases (10,36).

TREATMENT AND PROGNOSIS

There is no consensus regarding the best therapy for patients with HSTCL. A number of different combination chemotherapy regimens have been used with limited success (7,31). There appears to be a role for hematopoietic stem cell transplantation and, particularly, al-logeneic transplantation; some patients treated in this manner have had a prolonged survival period (25,32). There are some reports in the literature that suggest that early splenectomy may lead to improvement of thrombocytopenia, thereby contributing to improved patient management and potentially survival (8). Recurrence of thrombocytopenia usually heralds relapse of disease.

HSTCL is a highly aggressive type of lymphoma and the overall survival period is typically less than 2 years (3,31,32). The median survival rate of patients with α/β HSTCL appears to be worse than that of patients with γ/δ HSTCL (14,32).

REFERENCES

1. Allory Y, Challine D, Haioun C, et al. Bone marrow involvement in lymphomas with hemaphagocytic syndrome at presentation: a clinicopathologic study of 11 patients in a Western institution. Am J Surg Pathol 2001;25:865-874.
2. Alonsozana EL, Stamberg J, Kumar D, et al. Isochromosome 7q: the primary cytogenetic abnormality in hepatosplenic gammadelta T cell lymphoma. Leukemia 1997;11:1367-1372.
3. Belhadj K, Reyes F, Farcet JP, et al. Hepatosplenic gammadelta T-cell lymphoma is a rare clinicopathologic entity with poor outcome: report on a series of 21 patients. Blood 2003;102:4261-4269.
4. Chan JK. Splenic involvement by peripheral T-cell and NK-cell neoplasms. Semin Diagn Pathol 2003;20:105-120.
5. Dong J, Chong YY, Meyerson HJ. Hepatosplenic alpha beta T-cell lymphoma: a report of an S100-positive case. Arch Pathol Lab Med 2003;127:e119-122.
6. Finalet Ferreiro J, Rouhgharabaei L, Urbankova H, et al. Integrative genomic and transcriptomic analysis identified candidate genes implicated in the pathogenesis of hepatosplenic T-cell lymphoma. PLoS One 2014;9:e102977.
7. Gaulard P, Jaffe ES, Krenacs L, Macon WR. Hepatosplenic T-cell lymphoma. In: Swerdlow SH, Campo E, Harris NL, et al., eds. WHO classification of tumours of haematopoietic and lymphoid tissues. Lyon: IARC Press; 2008:292-293.
8. Gumbs AA, Zain J, Neylon E, MacGregor-Cortelli B, Patterson M, O'Connor OA. Importance of early splenectomy in patients with hepatosplenic T-cell lymphoma and severe thrombocytopenia. Ann Surg Oncol 2009;16:2014-2017.
9. Hassan R, Franco SA, Stefanoff CG, et al. Hepatosplenic gammadelta T-cell lymphoma following seven malaria infections. Pathol Int 2006;56:668-673.
10. Jiang L, Abati AD, Wilson W, Stetler-Stevenson M, Yuan C. Persistent non-neoplastic gammadelta-T cells in cerebrospinal fluid of a patient with hepatosplenic (gammadelta) T cell lymphoma: a case report with 6 years of flow cytometry follow-up. Int J Clin Exp Pathol 2009;3:110-116.
11. Kotlyar DS, Osterman MT, Diamond RH, et al. A systematic review of factors that contribute to hepatosplenic T-cell lymphoma in patients with inflammatory bowel disease. Clin Gastroenterol Hepatol 2011;9:36-41.
12. Kumar R, Dey P, Das A, Sachdeva MS, Varma S. Hepatosplenic T-cell lymphoma is a distinct rare entity: diagnosis by fine-needle aspiration cytology. Diagn Cytopathol 2011;39:677-680.
13. Mackey AC, Green L, Leptak C, Avigan M. Hepatosplenic T cell lymphoma associated with infliximab use in young patients treated for inflammatory bowel disease: update. J Pediatr Gastroenterol Nutr 2009;48:386-388.
14. Macon WR, Levy NB, Kurtin PJ, et al. Hepatosplenic alphabeta T-cell lymphomas: a report of 14 cases and comparison with hepatosplenic gammadelta T-cell lymphomas. Am J Surg Pathol 2001;25:285-296.

14a. McKinney M, Moffitt AB, Gaulard P, et al. The genetic basis of hepatosplenic T-cell lymphoma. Cancer Discov 2017;7:369-379.

15. Minauchi K, Nishio M, Itoh T, et al. Hepatosplenic alpha/beta T cell lymphoma presenting with cold agglutinin disease. Ann Hematol 2007;86:155-157.

16. Miyazaki K, Yamaguchi M, Imai H, et al. Gene expression profiling of peripheral T-cell lymphoma including gammadelta T-cell lymphoma. Blood 2009;113:1071-1074.

17. Morice WG, Macon WR, Dogan A, Hanson CA, Kurtin PJ. NK-cell-associated receptor expression in hepatosplenic T-cell lymphoma, insights into pathogenesis. Leukemia 2006;20:883-886.

18. Nagai Y, Ikegame K, Mori M, et al. Hepatosplenic alphabeta T cell lymphoma. Int J Clin Oncol 2010;15:215-219.

19. Nicolae A, Xi L, Pittaluga S, et al. Frequent STAT5B mutations in gammadelta hepatosplenic T-cell lymphomas. Leukemia 2014;28:2244-2248.

20. Ozaki S, Ogasahara K, Kosaka M, et al. Hepatosplenic gamma delta T-cell lymphoma associated with hepatitis B virus infection. J Med Invest 1998;44:215-217.

21. Przybylski GK, Wu H, Macon WR, et al. Hepatosplenic and subcutaneous panniculitis-like gamma/delta T cell lymphomas are derived from different Vdelta subsets of gamma/delta T lymphocytes. J Mol Diagn 2000;2:11-19.

22. Roelandt PR, Maertens J, Vandenberghe P, et al. Hepatosplenic gammadelta T-cell lymphoma after liver transplantation: report of the first 2 cases and review of the literature. Liver Transpl 2009;15:686-692.

23. Rosh JR, Gross T, Mamula P, Griffiths A, Hyams J. Hepatosplenic T-cell lymphoma in adolescents and young adults with Crohn's disease: a cautionary tale? Inflamm Bowel Dis 2007;13:1024-1030.

24. Swerdlow SH, Campo E, Pileri SA, et al. The 2016 revision of the World Health Organization classification of lymphoid neoplasms. Blood 2016;127:2375-2390.

25. Tanase A, Schmitz N, Stein H, et al. Allogeneic and autologous stem cell transplantation for hepatosplenic T-cell lymphoma: a retrospective study of the EBMT Lymphoma Working Party. Leukemia 2015;29:686-688.

26. Travert M, Huang Y, de Leval L, et al. Molecular features of hepatosplenic T-cell lymphoma unravels potential novel therapeutic targets. Blood 2012;119:5795-5806.

27. Tripodo C, Iannitto E, Florena AM, et al. Gammadelta T-cell lymphomas. Nat Rev Clin Oncol 2009;6:707-717.

28. Vega F, Medeiros LJ, Bueso-Ramos C, et al. Hepatosplenic gamma/delta T-cell lymphoma in bone marrow. A sinusoidal neoplasm with blastic cytologic features. Am J Clin Pathol 2001;116:410-419.

29. Vega F, Medeiros LJ, Gaulard P. Hepatosplenic and other gammadelta T-cell lymphomas. Am J Clin Pathol 2007;127:869-880.

30. Wang CC, Tien HF, Lin MT, et al. Consistent presence of isochromosome 7q in hepatosplenic T gamma/delta lymphoma: a new cytogenetic-clinicopathologic entity. Genes Chromosomes Cancer 1995;12:161-164.

31. Weidmann E. Hepatosplenic T cell lymphoma. A review on 45 cases since the first report describing the disease as a distinct lymphoma entity in 1990. Leukemia 2000;14:991-997.

32. Yabe M, Medeiros LJ, Tang G, et al. Prognostic factors of hepatosplenic T-cell lymphoma: Clinicopathologic study of 28 cases. Am J Surg Pathol 2016;50:109-117.

33. Yabe M, Medeiros LJ, Tang G, et al. Dyspoietic changes associated with hepatosplenic T-cell lymphoma are not a manifestation of a myelodysplastic syndrome. Hum Pathol 2016;40:676-688

34. Yabe M, Medeiros LJ, Wang SA, et al. Clinicopathologic, immunophenotypic, cytogenetic and molecular features of γδ T-cell large granular lymphocytic leukemia: an analysis of 14 patients suggests biologic differences with αβ T-cell large granular lymphocytic leukemia. Am J Clin Pathol 2015;144:607-619.

35. Yabe M, Medeiros LJ, Wang SA, et al. Distinguishing between hepatosplenic T-cell lymphoma and γ/δ T-cell large granular lymphocytic leukemia: a clinicopathologic, immunophenotypic, and molecular analysis. Am J Surg Pathol 2017;41:82-93.

36. Zhang S, Bayerl MG. Florid splenic gamma/delta T-cell proliferation in patients with splenomegaly and cytopenias: a "high stakes" diagnostic challenge. Hum Pathol 2017. [Epub ahead of print]

62 MYELOID NEOPLASMS INVOLVING THE SPLEEN

Myeloid neoplasms manifest predominantly in the bone marrow and peripheral blood, and their diagnosis is usually established by a complete blood count assessment, morphologic review of the peripheral blood smear, and bone marrow examination integrating the results of ancillary studies. Myeloid neoplasms also may involve extramedullary sites, but these sites are uncommonly assessed by morphologic examination unless a mass is formed or the extramedullary disease causes symptoms or prominent laboratory abnormalities. Virtually any extramedullary site can be involved, but the most common are the spleen, lymph nodes, and skin (34). In the spleen, myeloid neoplasms preferentially involve the red pulp.

In the literature, the presence of hematopoietic cells in the spleen (or other extramedullary sites) has been referred to traditionally as *extramedullary hematopoiesis* (EMH) or *myeloid metaplasia*. This terminology, however, has limitations because the cells of EMH may be benign or neoplastic. Examples of benign diseases that cause EMH include thalassemia, autoimmune hemolytic anemia, and hemolytic uremic syndrome/thrombotic thrombocytopenic purpura, as well as following stem cell transplantation (10). EMH also occurs in spleens extensively involved by nonmyeloid malignant neoplasms. In these circumstances, the EMH is thought to be a compensatory event in which benign bone marrow elements recapitulate "normal" hematopoiesis.

Myeloid neoplasms involving the blood and bone marrow are commonly associated with hematopoietic cells in the spleen. The hematopoietic cells in the spleen are often malignant and share clonal molecular abnormalities with the myeloid neoplasm in the bone marrow (4,6,13). Presumably, neoplastic myeloid elements have been released from the bone marrow prematurely, as a result of an altered bone marrow microenvironment, and then filtered out of the bloodstream by the spleen. For this reason, others have suggested the term *neoplastic myeloid proliferation* for the presence of neoplastic myeloid cells involving the spleen (11).

In this chapter, neoplastic myeloid proliferations are distinguished from EMH; the latter term is used for benign hematopoietic cells in the spleen. Neoplastic myeloid proliferations involving the spleen are more extensive and cause a greater degree of splenomegaly than benign EMH (11). The myeloid neoplasms specified in the World Health Organization (WHO) classification include myeloproliferative neoplasms, myelodysplastic/myeloproliferative neoplasms, myelodysplastic syndromes, and myeloid sarcoma.

MYELOPROLIFERATIVE NEOPLASMS

General Features. *Myeloproliferative neoplasms* (MPNs) are a heterogeneous group of diseases that are characterized by the overproduction of immature and mature cells of myeloid lineage. In the WHO classification, there are seven types of MPNs: chronic myeloid leukemia (CML), chronic neutrophilic leukemia, polycythemia vera, primary myelofibrosis, essential thrombocythemia, chronic eosinophilic leukemia, and an unclassifiable group (1). The MPNs are uncommon to rare diseases, with an overall annual incidence rate that ranges from 1.15 to 4.99 per 100,000 per year (29,30). CML is most frequent, occurring two to three times more often than polycythemia vera, essential thrombocytopenia, or primary myelofibrosis. Chronic neutrophilic leukemia is rare, with less than 200 cases reported in the literature (8).

Each of these diseases has unique clinical and laboratory findings, and each commonly exhibits distinct phases of disease. For example, CML patients usually present in chronic phase and after a variable time interval undergo transformation, initially to accelerated phase and then

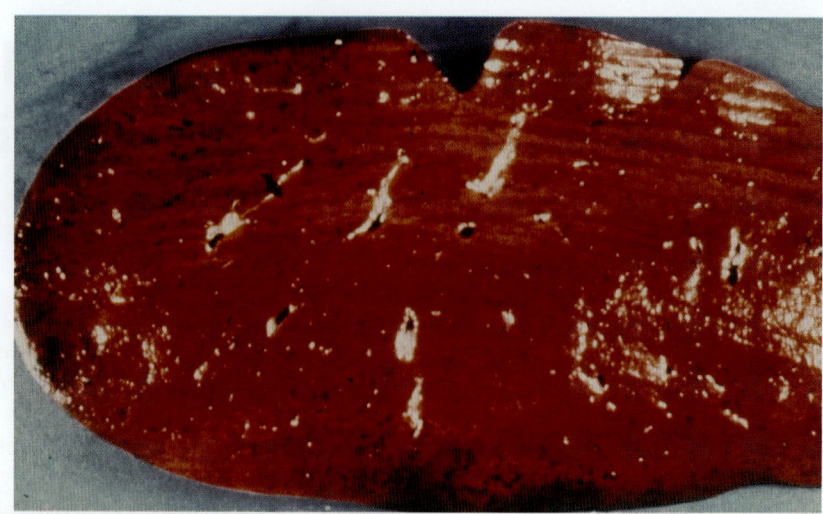

Figure 62-1

CHRONIC MYELOID LEUKEMIA INVOLVING SPLEEN

The red pulp of this massive spleen is diffusely expanded, imparting a uniform "beefy" red appearance to the cut surface. White pulp nodules cannot be appreciated.

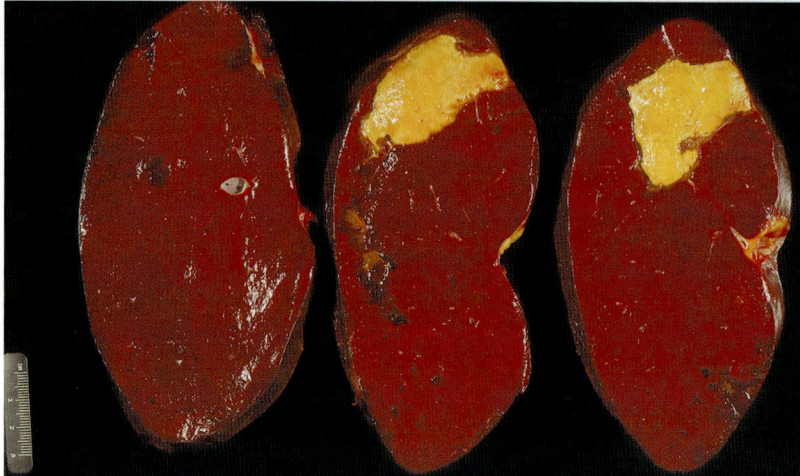

Figure 62-2

PRIMARY MYELOFIBROSIS INVOLVING SPLEEN

The red pulp of this enlarged spleen is diffusely expanded, appearing red with small infarcts (dense yellow areas). Infarcts in the spleen may occur secondary to vascular compromise. (Courtesy of Dr. W. Greaves, Trinidad.)

to blast phase or acute myeloid leukemia (AML) (24). Similarly, patients with polycythemia vera can exhibit prepolycythemic, polycythemic, and postpolycythemic (spent) phases and patients with primary myelofibrosis can show prefibrotic (cellular) and fibrotic phases.

Splenomegaly is observed in virtually all patients with CML, polycythemia vera, and primary myelofibrosis (9,17,29). Splenomegaly is also common in patients with chronic neutrophilic leukemia. In other patients with MPN, splenomegaly is variably present. Splenomegaly is present in 30 to 50 percent of patients with chronic eosinophilic leukemia, and tends to be modest in a minority subset of patients with essential thrombocytopenia (24).

Gross Findings. Grossly, the spleen in patients with CML, primary myelofibrosis, and polycythemia vera is large, with expanded red pulp imparting a beefy red appearance (figs. 62-1, 62-2). There may be focal purple nodules, known as "megakaryocytic plums," so named because these nodules have an expansile cut surface and histologically are rich in megakaryocytes. Infarcts may be seen in association with myeloid disorders of the spleen, likely due to massive enlargement and vascular compromise by the presence of tumor (fig. 62-2) (9).

Histologic Findings. The spleen is involved by a mixture of bone marrow hematopoietic cells in the splenic red pulp, with the percentage of cells dependent on MPN type (11,17). In CML, the red pulp is often markedly expanded, predominantly by sheets of mature granulocytes as well as band forms, myelocytes, and fewer promyelocytes; myeloblasts are rare (fig. 62-3).

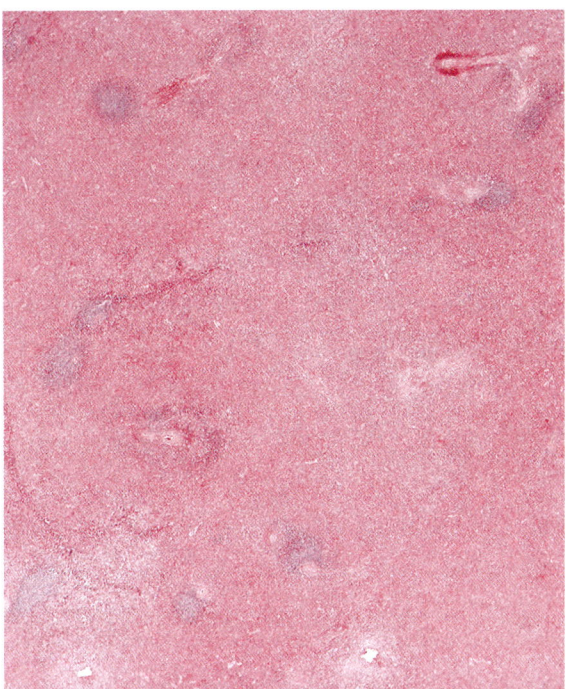 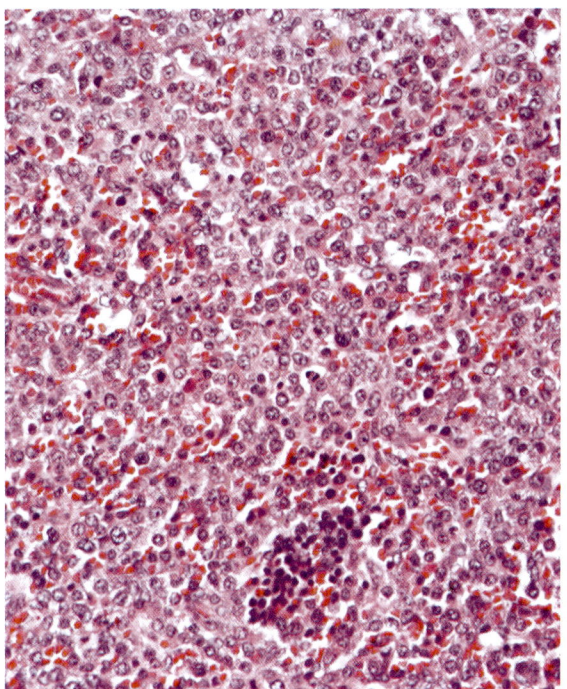

Figure 62-3

CHRONIC MYELOID LEUKEMIA INVOLVING SPLEEN

Left: In this histologic section the red pulp the spleen is markedly and diffusely expanded.

Right: Numerous mature and immature granulocytic elements in sheets replace the red pulp. A cluster of erythroid precursors is also present (lower center) in this field (hematoxylin and eosin [H&E] stain).

Eosinophils are also common as are a lesser number of erythroid elements and megakaryocytes (11,24). The megakaryocytes in CML are often small and the histiocytes may show sea blue or pseudo-Gaucher features attributable to high cell turnover (24).

In primary myelofibrosis (fig. 62-4) and polycythemia vera, a mixed population of hematopoietic cells is present. Three patterns of involvement are recognized: diffuse, nodular, and mixed (17). In the diffuse pattern, granulocytic elements predominate and are located mostly in the splenic cords. In the nodular pattern, all three hematopoietic cell lineages are often present. Erythroid precursors tend to be intravascularly located whereas megakaryocytes are present in the cords and intravascular compartment (17). In primary myelofibrosis, the megakaryocytes are atypical and bizarre, with enlarged and hyperchromatic ("cloud-like") nuclei, and are often present in clusters (figs. 62-4, 62-5) (9,29). In polycythemia vera, the findings are more variable, but erythroid precursors are usually

plentiful (24). Little information is available regarding the morphologic findings of the spleen in patients with chronic neutrophilic leukemia.

Cytologic Findings. Air-dried touch imprints of the spleen help in the assessment of myeloid cells. Imprints stained with Wright-Giemsa stain allow for delineation of cytologic features and blast cell percentage. Unstained air-dried imprints also facilitate cytochemical analysis and fluorescence in situ hybridization (FISH) testing.

Immunophenotypic Findings. Since the neoplastic cells in the spleen are usually readily recognizable by routine morphologic examination, there is a limited role for immunophenotyping in their identification. As expected, the immature cells express granulocytic, monocytic, erythroid, or megakaryocytic antigens. A more important role for immunophenotyping is excluding the presence of increased blasts or immature cells that signal transformation to AML. Antibodies specific for CD34 and CD117 are helpful for identifying immature myeloid elements. Sheets or large aggregates of immature

931

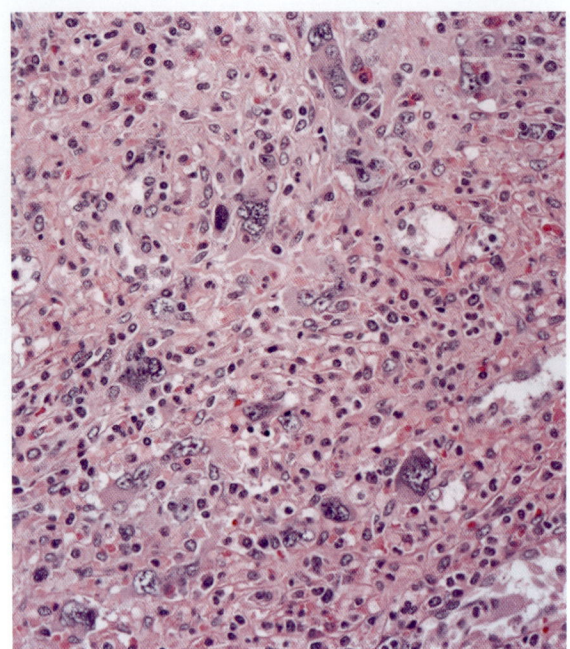
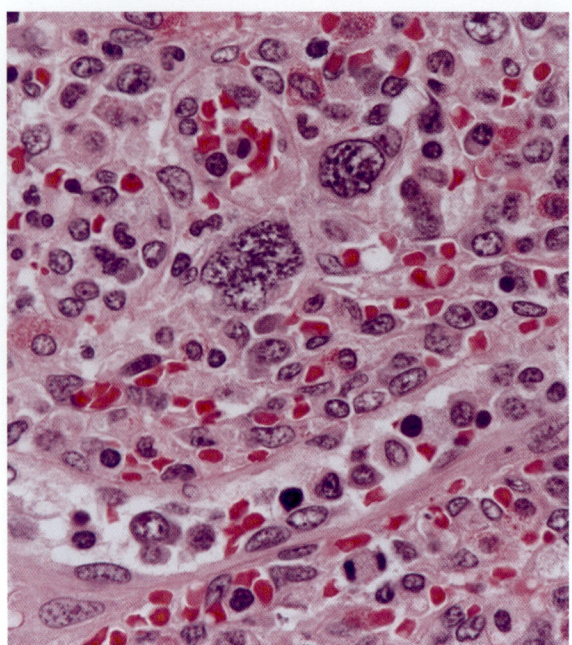

Figure 62-4

PRIMARY MYELOFIBROSIS INVOLVING SPLEEN

Left: Numerous large and atypical megakaryocytes and immature granulocytes, including eosinophils, are present.
Right: Oil magnification image shows megakaryocytes with cloud-like nuclei, granulocytic precursors, and immature erythroid precursors within vascular spaces (H&E stain).

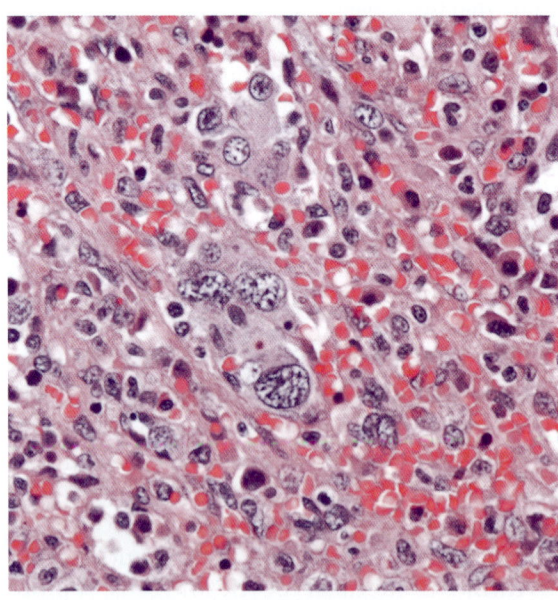

Figure 62-5

PRIMARY MYELOFIBROSIS INVOLVING SPLEEN

This intermediate-magnification view shows splenic red pulp with atypical megakaryocytes, many erythroid cells in the vascular compartment, and few granulocytic precursors (H&E stain).

cells that express CD34 suggest that blastic transformation of the underlying myeloid disorder has occurred (11,24). Blast transformation can begin in the spleen.

Molecular Genetic Findings. CML is defined by t(9;22)(q34;q11.2) and more specifically *BCR-ABL1*, which is usually tested in blood or bone marrow rather than the spleen (24). *JAK2* is mutated in over 95 percent of polycythemia vera, about 50 percent of primary myelofibrosis, and about 60 percent of essential thrombocythemia cases. *CALR* (25 to 40 percent) and *MPL* (5 to 10 percent) are also mutated in essential thrombocythemia and primary myelofibrosis and mutations in these three genes are largely mutually exclusive (24,30). Activating *CSF3R* mutations are characteristic of chronic neutrophilic leukemia (8).

A variety of abnormalities have been identified by conventional cytogenetic analysis and loss of heterozygosity (LOH) studies, including abnormalities of chromosomal loci 7q, 8q, 9p, 13q, and 20q as well as 17p/*TP53* (12,13). In a small number of patients, molecular abnormalities have been compared in spleen and bone marrow. Splenic samples can have a greater number of genetic abnormalities than the bone marrow, supporting the spleen as an initial site of blastic transformation.

Differential Diagnosis. *Distinguishing between MPNs.* Based on morphologic findings in the spleen, it may be highly challenging to distinguish between different types of MPN. The splenic findings need to be correlated with the clinical history and the results of the morphologic examination of blood and bone marrow. Molecular testing is also required for the definitive diagnosis of MPNs.

Benign Extramedullary Hematopoiesis. Benign hematopoietic cells (EMH) in the spleen can show some morphologic overlap with neoplastic proliferations as occur in MPN (10,11). In patients with benign EMH there is often a physiologic explanation, such as an underlying benign hematologic disorder, compromise of the bone marrow medullary space, or a physiologic stimulus to overproduce bone marrow elements at extramedullary sites. In EMH, unilineage proliferations can occur, most often erythroid elements due to benign conditions resulting in abnormal red blood cell or hemoglobin production.

Trilineage proliferations also can occur in EMH when there is underproduction of all bone marrow elements (figs. 62-6, 62-7). In these cases, there is typically evidence of orderly maturation of hematopoietic cells. Uncommonly, megakaryocytes in EMH appear mildly or moderately enlarged and atypical, likely a result of these cells being in the "foreign" microenvironment of the spleen.

The morphologic features that support a neoplastic myeloid proliferation over benign EMH include: an extensive myeloid proliferation, erythroid immaturity, and prominent megakaryocytic atypia including clustering of megakaryocytes, dwarf forms, and megakaryoblasts (11). Immunophenotypic assessment for CD34 is also very helpful as CD34-positive cells may be numerous in neoplastic myeloid tumors and are not increased in benign EMH.

MASTOCYTOSIS

General Features. *Mastocytosis* or *mast cell disease* is a monoclonal hematopoietic stem cell disorder that was included in the group of MPNs

in the 2008 WHO classification (24). However, in the 2016 revision of the WHO classification mast cell disease is now distinguished from the MPN group (1). Approximately 70 percent of patients with generalized mast cell disease have splenomegaly (3). Mastocytosis is discussed in detail in chapter 49. The findings in the spleen are the focus of this section.

Gross Findings. Splenomegaly in patients with mastocytosis can be prominent. In a study by Horny et al. (3), the spleen weight ranged from 160 to 2,300 g, with 80 percent over 500 g. Most patients with splenomegaly have involvement by mastocytosis. Some patients, however, also have associated myeloid diseases that are often clonally related including chronic myelomonocytic leukemia, myelodysplastic syndrome (MDS), MPN, or rarely AML (32). These myeloid neoplasms may also involve the spleen and cause splenomegaly, with, or less often, without associated involvement by mastocytosis (1,32).

Histologic Findings. Mastocytosis tends to surround small and larger blood vessels in the red and white pulp of the spleen (figs. 62-8, 62-9). In the red pulp, mast cells appear to begin as small nodules that can become large and replace the red pulp. Mast cells also track along blood vessels that surround the white pulp and along radial arterioles that penetrate into germinal centers. The periarteriolar lymphoid sheath region is often involved. In some cases, germinal centers are lymphocyte depleted and the overall appearance can superficially resemble a hyaline-vascular lesion as seen in Castleman disease (fig. 62-8D).

Mast cell aggregates are frequently associated with fibrosis that can form dense, collagenous layers around blood vessels (fig. 62-9). They are also commonly associated with a polymorphous mixture of cells including eosinophils, histiocytes, small lymphocytes, and less often, plasma cells. In some cases, histiocytes are numerous and the lesions resemble, in part, granulomas.

Mast cell nodules, especially if prominent, may be associated with hemorrhage and organization. Small foci of EMH can be present, associated with the mast cells or in the uninvolved areas of the spleen.

Cytologic Findings. Mast cells may be round or spindle-shaped, and their cytoplasm may be agranular or vaguely granular (fig. 62-10). Mast cells show minimal atypia or mitotic figures, with

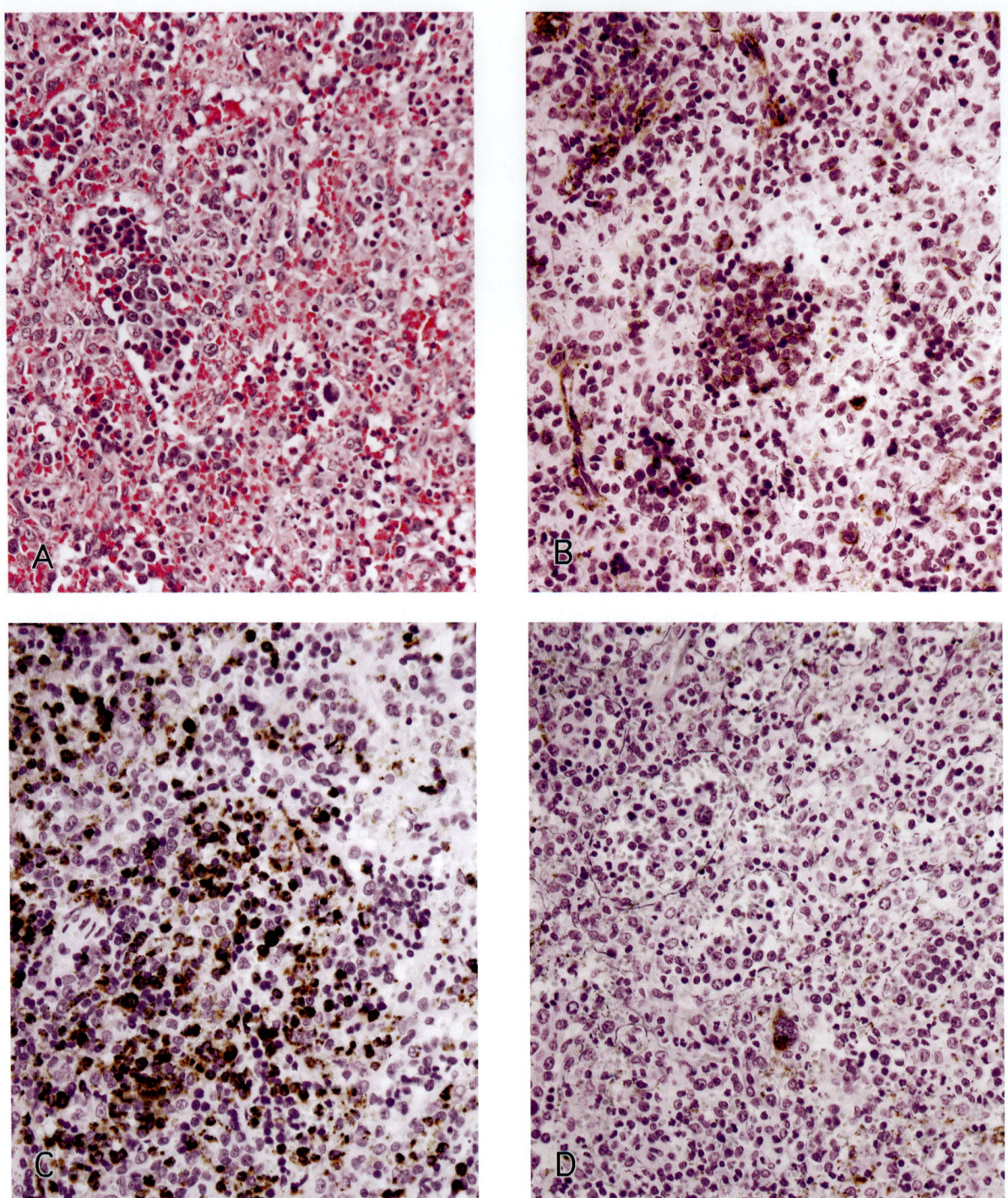

Figure 62-6

EXTRAMEDULLARY HEMATOPOIESIS INVOLVING SPLEEN

A: Numerous clusters of immature hematopoietic cells are present in a patient with Evan syndrome (autoimmune anemia and thrombocytopenia) (H&E stain).

B: Erythroid precursors are positive for E-cadherin (B–D: immunohistochemistry with hematoxylin counterstain).

C: Granulocytic precursors are positive for myeloperoxidase.

D: CD61 highlights occasional megakaryocytes.

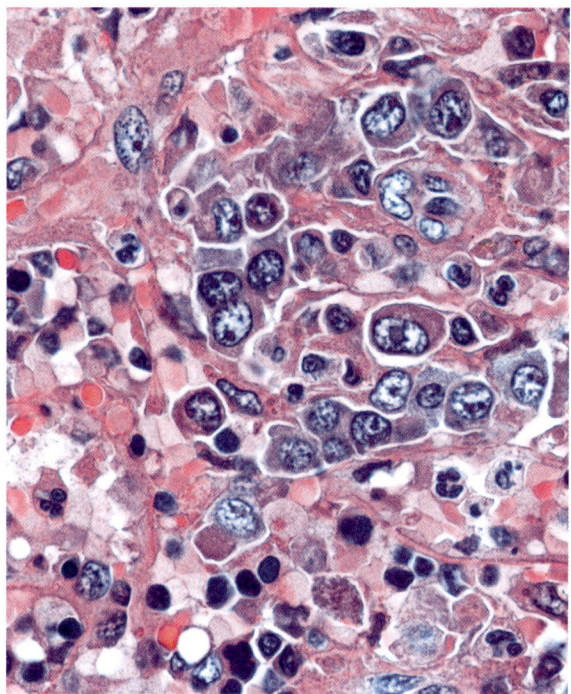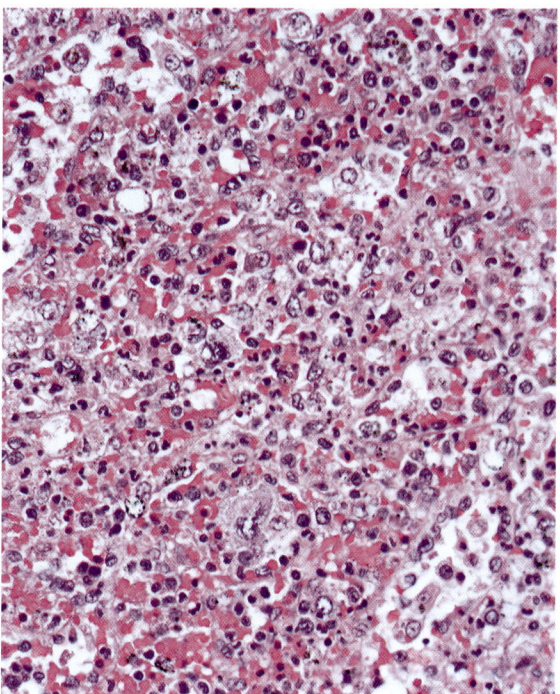

Figure 62-7

EXTRAMEDULLARY HEMATOPOIESIS INVOLVING SPLEEN

Left: Oil magnification of spleen section from a patient with autoimmune hemolytic anemia shows immature hematopoietic cells including many erythroid precursors.

Right: In this spleen from a patient who underwent stem cell transplantation, immature myeloid cells and atypical megakaryocytes are seen and mimic, in part, the findings associated with neoplastic myeloid disorders (H&E stain).

the exception of rare cases of mast cell sarcoma in which pleomorphism, mitotic figures, and often necrosis are present. In hematoxylin and eosin (H&E)-stained sections, mast cells may be difficult to recognize as they can resemble, in part, monocytoid B cells or fibroblasts. Giemsa or toluidine blue metachromatic stains highlight purple mast cell granules. Mast cells are also positive for chloroacetate esterase.

Immunophenotypic Findings. Mast cells can be identified by flow cytometry immuno-phenotypic analysis. They are positive for CD33, CD43, CD45, CD68, and CD117 (bright) and are negative for T- and B-cell antigens, CD34, and CD123 (5,31). Compared with normal mast cells, neoplastic mast cells are commonly posi-tive for CD2 and CD25, with the latter marker more sensitive (5,31). Some cases, particularly cases with high-grade morphologic features, express CD30 (31).

Immunohistochemical analysis is well suited for assessing mast cell disease in tissue sections

and is the most common method employed for detecting mastocytosis in the spleen. Mast cells are positive for CD43, CD68, CD117/KIT (bright), and mast cell tryptase (fig. 62-11), and are commonly aberrantly positive for CD2 and CD25.

Molecular Genetic Findings. Molecular analysis is an important tool for diagnosis. Mastocytosis is associated with *KIT* mutations, usually D816V, but other uncommon mutations are also described (1).

MYELODYSPLASTIC/ MYELOPROLIFERATIVE NEOPLASMS

General Features. There are five categories of *myelodysplastic/myeloproliferative neoplasms* (MDS/MPN) recognized in the WHO classifica-tion: *chronic myelomonocytic leukemia* (CMML), *atypical CMML, juvenile CMML, MDS/MPN with ring sideroblasts and thrombocytosis,* and *MDS/ MPN unclassified* (1,25). These diseases are hy-brid neoplasms that have myelodysplastic and myeloproliferative features. Splenic involvement

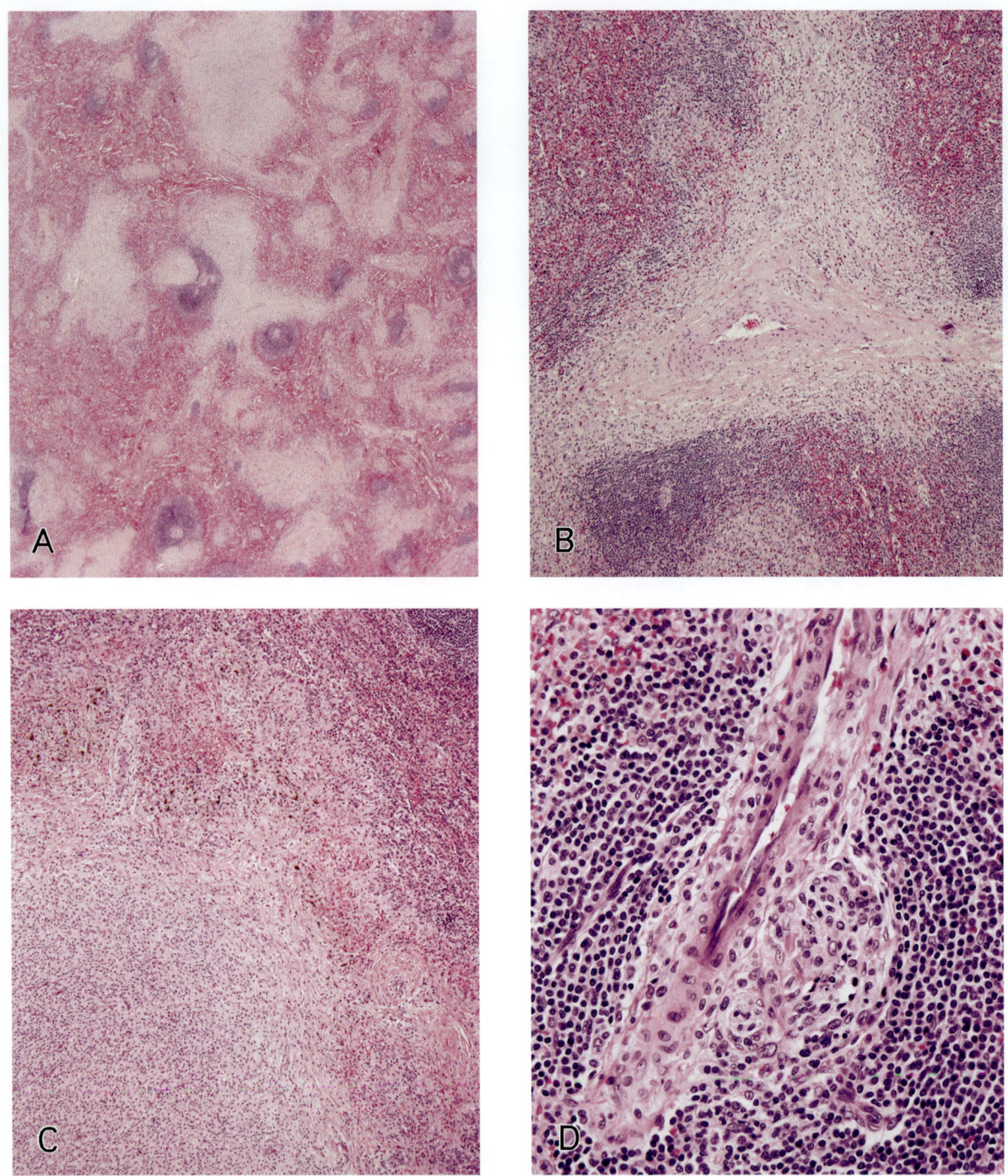

Figure 62-8

MASTOCYTOSIS INVOLVING SPLEEN

A: Low-magnification view shows mast cells (pale at low power) surrounding blood vessels in the red and white pulp.

B: Higher magnification shows mast cells surrounding a large blood vessel and extending into the splenic parenchyma. The mast cells are associated with eosinophils and fibrosis.

C: A large nodule of mast cells replaces the red pulp parenchyma.

D: Mast cells track along an arteriole, penetrating into a germinal center in the white pulp. At low power, this finding imparts a hyaline-vascular lesion-like or Castleman-like appearance (A–D: H&E stain).

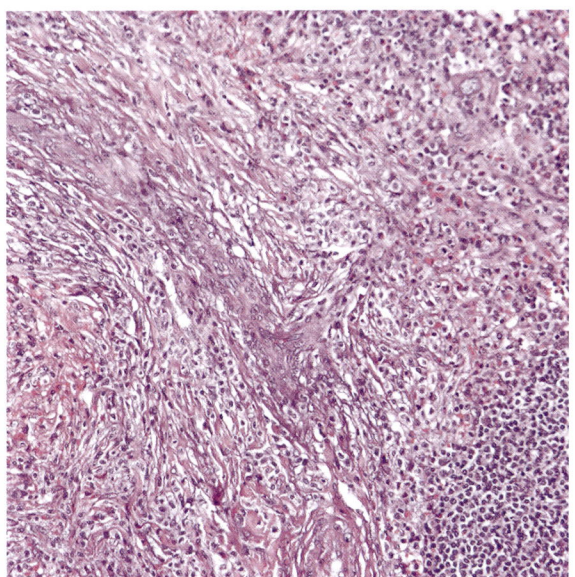

Figure 62-9

MASTOCYTOSIS INVOLVING SPLEEN

A central blood vessel is surrounded by mast cells associated with extensive fibrosis and scattered eosinophils. White pulp is at the lower right of this image (H&E stain).

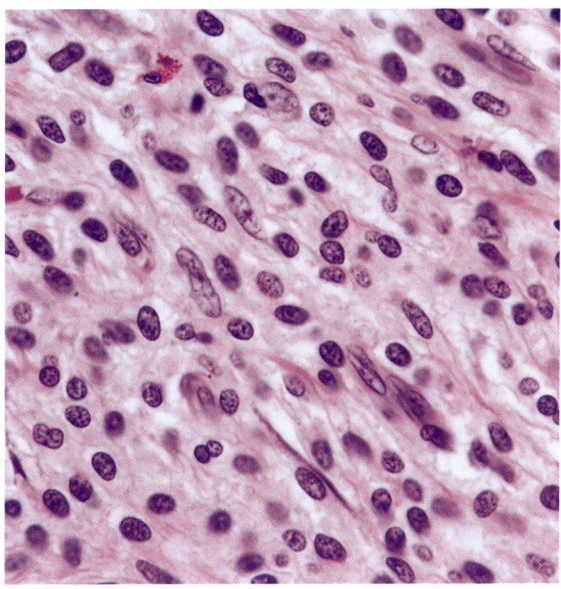

Figure 62-10

MASTOCYTOSIS INVOLVING SPLEEN

Oil magnification of mast cells from a large mast cell nodule in the red pulp of the spleen. An associated eosinophil (upper center), fibroblasts, and endothelial cells are also present (H&E stain). (Same case as shown in fig. 62-8).

occurs in a subset of patients with all types of MDS/MPN. Here the focus is on the most common type, CMML.

CMML is defined as involvement of blood and bone marrow by a myeloid neoplasm that is characterized by an absolute monocytosis of greater than 1 x 10^9/L (often with more than 10 percent monocytes), dysplasia in at least one hematopoietic cell lineage, myeloblasts less than 20 percent, and the absence of disease-defining genetic abnormalities, such as *BCR-ABL1* (1,15). In the WHO classification, CMML is subdivided into three subtypes: CMML-0, with less than 2 percent blasts in blood and less than 5 percent blasts in bone marrow; CMML-1, with less than 5 percent blasts in blood and less than 10 percent blasts in bone marrow; and CMML-2, with 5 to 19 percent blasts in blood and 10 to 19 percent blasts in bone marrow, or if Auer rods are present regardless of the blast counts (1,15).

CMML is an uncommon disease, occurring in about 1,000 patients per year in the United States (15,16). The median age of patients is 65 to 75 years and men outnumber women in a ratio of about 2 to 1 (16). Patients typically present with blood and bone marrow involvement,

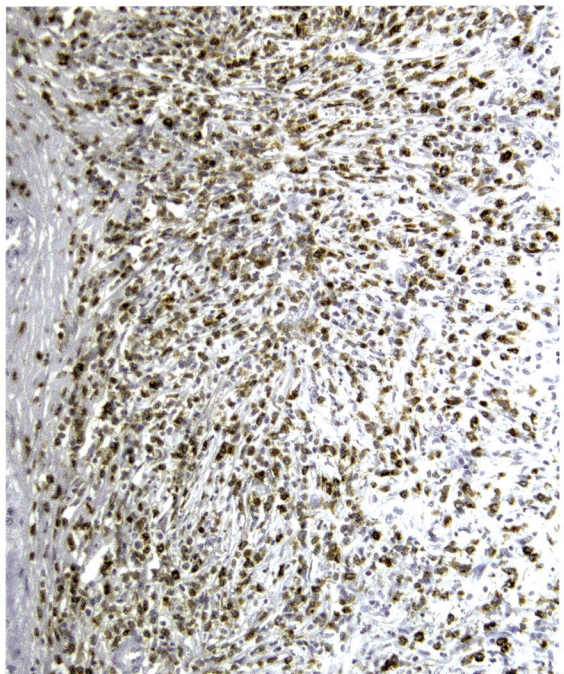

Figure 62-11

MASTOCYTOSIS INVOLVING SPLEEN

Mast cells are positive for tryptase (immunohistochemistry with hematoxylin counterstain).

but splenomegaly occurs in 30 to 50 percent of patients. Patients with CMML can present with cytopenias and transfusion dependence and closely resemble patients with MDS, or they can present with leukocytosis and hepatosplenomegaly and more closely resemble those with MPN (16,23). Splenomegaly is more common in the myeloproliferative subset of CMML patients.

Histologic Findings. In patients with CMML, the splenic red pulp is commonly involved by mature and immature granulocytes and monocytes that tend to diffusely expand the red pulp (fig. 62-12). Erythroid precursors and megakaryocytes are also commonly present. Foamy histiocytes can be numerous in the marginal zones, consistent with platelet consumption (analogous to histiocytes in immune thrombocytopenic purpura) (23). Proliferation or nodules of plasmacytoid dendritic cells may be seen in the spleen and rarely, are prominent (15,18). In touch imprints, dysplasia can be observed in one or more hematopoietic cell lineages.

About 15 to 30 percent of patients with CMML go on to develop AML (15,16). An increased number of immature cells in the splenic red pulp (fig. 62-12D) or increased CD34-positive cells in the spleen suggest progression/transformation to AML.

Cytologic Findings. The cells of CMML include granulocytes, monocytes, and often hybrid cells that exhibit evidence of granulocytic and monocytic differentiation (15). These cells may be difficult to appreciate by routine morphologic examination of the spleen, but cytochemical analysis on touch imprints shows cells with granulocytic differentiation (myeloperoxidase or chloroacetate esterase positive) and monocytic differentiation (nonspecific or butyrate esterase positive). So-called hybrid cells are reactive for both chloroacetate esterase and nonspecific/butyrate esterase.

Immunophenotypic Findings. Using flow cytometry immunophenotypic analysis, the neoplastic cells are positive for granulocyte- and monocyte-associated antigens including CD13, CD14, CD33, CD64, and CD68 (16,22). Aberrant expression of antigens (e.g., CD2 or CD56) and either loss or aberrant intensity of other myeloid antigens is common.

Using immunohistochemistry, myeloperoxidase, CD68, CD163, and lysozyme are helpful markers. Several markers highlight plasmacytoid dendritic cells in the spleen including CD4, CD43, CD68, CD56, CD123, CD303, and TCL1 (18,34).

Molecular Genetic Findings. About 20 to 40 percent of patients with CMML carry abnormalities that are detectable by conventional cytogenetics, although there are no characteristic, recurrent translocations (27,33). Frequent chromosomal abnormalities include trisomy 8, monosomy or deletion of chromosome 7, del(20q), trisomy 21, and chromosomal 12p abnormalities. Loss of the Y chromosome is common in men, but may be age-related rather than disease-associated. Cytogenetic abnormalities are more common in patients with CMML-2. Patients with a complex karyotype, trisomy 8, or abnormalities of chromosome 7 have a poorer prognosis (27,33).

As has been reviewed by others (8,16), gene mutations have been identified in up to 90 percent of patients with CMML and can be subdivided into four subgroups: 1) epigenetic regulator genes (e.g., *ASXL1*, *EZH2*, *TET*, *IDH1*, and IDH2); 2) genes involved in the spliceosome pathway (e.g., *SF3B1*, *SRSF2*, *U2AF1*); 3) DNA damage response genes (e.g., *TP53*); and 4) genes encoding cellular/receptor tyrosine kinases (e.g., *RAS*, *JAK2*, *FLT3*, and *RUNX1*). *TET2* (ten eleven translocation 2) and *ASXL1* (additional sex combs like transcriptional regulator 1) are mutated in about half of CMML cases. Mutations in RNA-splicing genes occur in 50 to 60 percent of CMML cases, with the most common being *SRSF2* (serine/arginine-rich splicing factor 2). *RUNX1* is mutated in 15 to 40 percent of cases.

The patterns of gene mutations in CMML differ between MDS-like versus MPN-like tumors. *KRAS* and *NRAS* mutations occur most often in MPN-like CMML, in up to 40 percent of cases, and *BRAF* mutations have been identified in a subset of cases with wild-type *RAS* (15,35). *ASXL1* and *SF3B1* mutations are more common in patients with an abnormal karyotype (16,33).

MYELODYSPLASTIC SYNDROMES

General Features. The *myelodysplastic syndromes* (MDS) are a group of diseases characterized by insufficient hematopoiesis of at least one hematopoietic cell lineage. In the 2016 revision of the WHO classification there are six types of MDS (1,26). Patients with MDS have one or

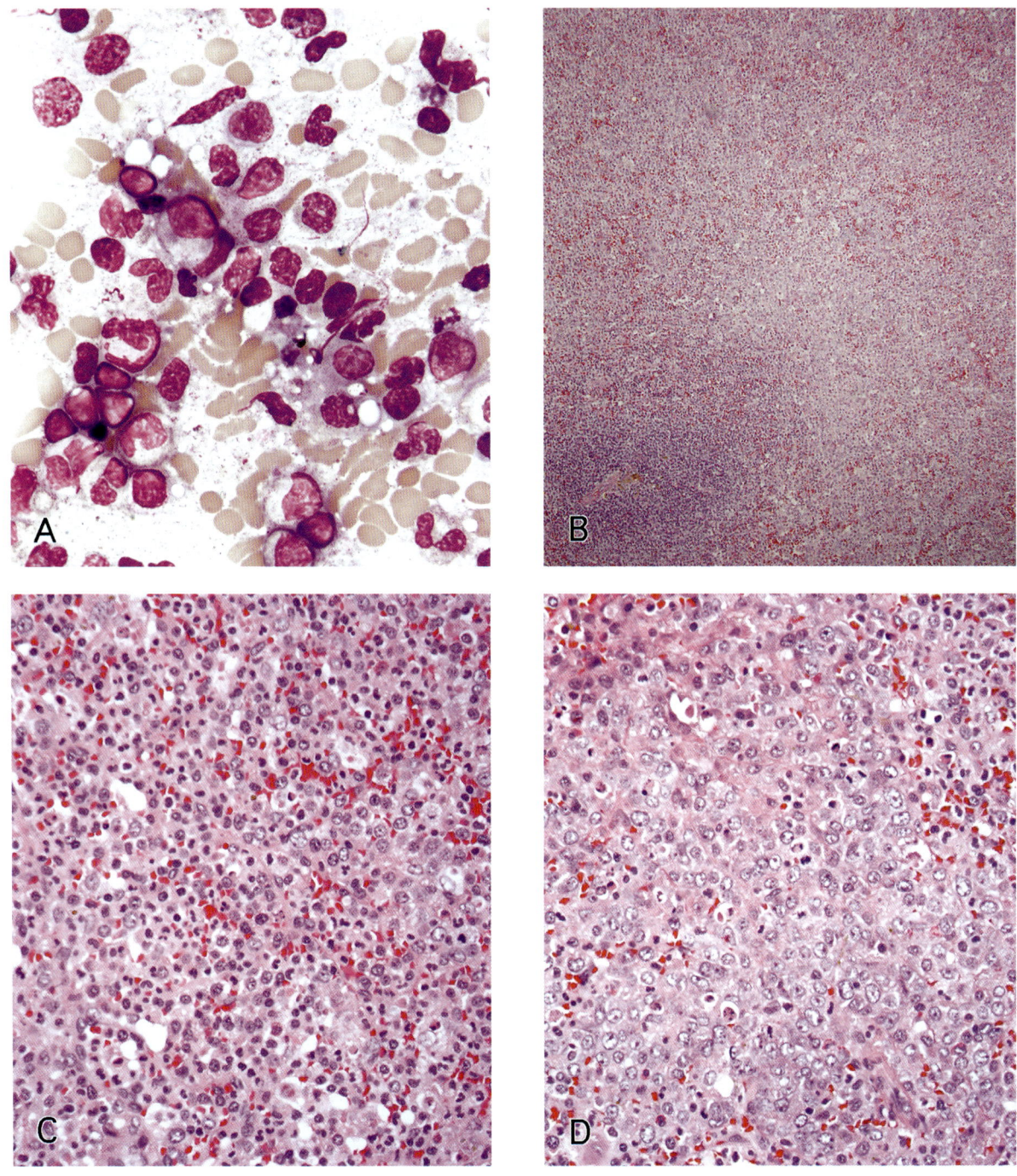

Figure 62-12

CHRONIC MYELOMONOCYTIC LEUKEMIA INVOLVING SPLEEN

A: A touch imprint shows mature and immature granulocytes and monocytes from an enlarged spleen. The monocytes were positive for butyrate esterase by cytochemistry (not shown) (Wright-Giemsa stain).

B: The red pulp is diffusely expanded by granulocytic and monocytic cells. Residual compressed white pulp is at lower left of image.

C: High magnification of the splenic red pulp shows granulocytes and monocytes with a spectrum of maturation.

D: In areas of the red pulp, nodules of immature cells are present which correlate with an increased risk of transformation to acute myeloid leukemia (B–D: H&E stain).

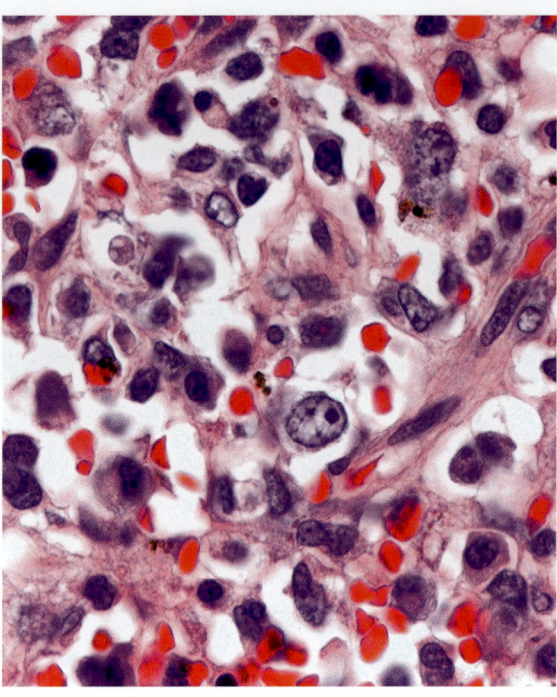

Figure 62-13

HIGH-GRADE MYELODYSPLASTIC SYNDROME CLASSIFIED AS REFRACTORY ANEMIA WITH EXCESS BLASTS

Oil magnification image shows immature and mature myeloid elements within the red pulp of the spleen (H&E stain).

more peripheral cytopenias and may have a hypercellular bone marrow. MDS can be divided into low- versus high-grade myeloid neoplasms, based in large part on the myeloblast count in the bone marrow (less than 5 percent versus 5 percent or more). Splenomegaly occurs in less than 10 percent of patients with low-grade MDS, but in up to 25 percent of patients with high-grade MDS.

The spleen is uncommonly removed in patients with MDS (7,26). One reason for splenectomy is refractory cytopenia(s), most often thrombocytopenia, but less often another cell lineage or pancytopenia. Cytopenia(s) may improve following splenectomy. Another indication for splenectomy is clinical or laboratory evidence suggesting that transformation to AML in the spleen has occurred.

Histologic Findings. A number of findings have been described in the spleen of MDS patients. Kraus et al. (7) described 11 cases of MDS in spleens removed surgically or examined at autopsy. In some cases, dyspoiesis is minimal and the spleen may show erythrophagocytosis or red pulp plasmacytosis. In other cases, the hematopoietic cells of MDS are identified in the red pulp. Myeloid cells often predominate with varying stages of maturation (fig. 62-13). Erythroid precursors and megakaryocytes also occur. The megakaryocytes may be dysplastic, with monolobated or hypolobated nuclei. The presence of a monomorphic population of immature myeloid elements supports progression/transformation of MDS to AML/myeloid sarcoma.

In air-dried touch imprints of spleen stained with Wright-Giemsa, dysplasia involving one or more cell lineages may be observed. An iron stain may show abnormal iron incorporation, or rarely, ring sideroblasts. Cytochemical analysis for myeloperoxidase, Sudan black B, and nonspecific esterase can be performed to assess for cell differentiation and dysplastic features.

Immunophenotypic Findings. Flow cytometry immunophenotypic and immunohistochemical analyses are useful to assess for the presence of myeloid, erythroid, or megakaryocytic elements of MDS in the spleen (26). In the blood and bone marrow, flow cytometry shows decreased side scatter, a decreased number of immature B-cell precursors (hematogones), aberrant patterns of antigen expression, and an increased percentage of CD34-positive blasts in many MDS cases (21,28). As far as we are aware, these methods have been rarely used on MDS cases involving the spleen and presumably this workup would rarely be necessary at this point.

Immunohistochemical analysis, using a small antibody panel (CD34, CD68, CD71, E-cadherin, and CD61) can assess for dysplastic hematopoietic cells in the spleen. Other antibody panels are also suitable for this purpose. The presence of a uniform population of immature cells or CD34-positive cells present in sheets or large aggregates (20 to 50 cells) suggests AML or transformation to myeloid sarcoma.

Molecular Genetic Findings. Conventional cytogenetic analysis and FISH are valuable for the diagnosis and prognostic stratification of patients with MDS and these findings are well covered in the WHO classification (1,26). As reviewed by Cazzola et al. (2), about 90 percent of MDS cases carry gene mutations and there is much overlap in the genes involved in CMML (discussed above) and other MDS cases. Depending on the study, only four to six genes are mutated with a frequency of over 10 percent in MDS cases, but there are about 50 other genes that are mutated at a lower frequency. Although conventional cytogenetics, FISH, and gene mutation analysis can be assessed on spleen specimens in patients with MDS, usually this testing already has been performed on blood and/or bone marrow, and analysis of a spleen specimen is unnecessary.

MYELOID SARCOMA

General Features. *Myeloid sarcoma* is defined in the WHO classification as an extramedullary tumor mass composed of myeloblasts that effaces normal architecture (1,20). Approximately 5 percent of patients with AML develop myeloid sarcoma during the course of their disease. Myeloid sarcoma also occurs in patients with MPN, MDS/MPN, and MDS and, rarely, occurs de novo before the onset of AML. Myeloid sarcoma can occur at virtually any extramedullary site including the spleen, and rarely can present initially in the spleen. Myeloid sarcoma is discussed in detail in chapter 51. The pathologic findings in the spleen are the focus of the discussion here.

Histologic Findings. Myeloid sarcoma usually diffusely involves the red pulp of the spleen. The abnormal cells are commonly distributed within red pulp cords and sinuses, although when there is extensive involvement, the normal splenic architecture is completely effaced.

Cytologically, myeloid sarcoma cells may be primitive blasts or they can show evidence of maturation (34). Undifferentiated blasts are intermediate-sized cells, usually with scant cytoplasm, round nuclei, open and finely reticulated (blastic) chromatin (fig. 62-14), and thin nuclear membranes. Nucleoli, if present, are often pinpoint. In cases with maturation, the maturing cells have irregular or folded nuclei and increased amounts of cytoplasm, sometimes with recognizable granules.

Promyelocytes or promonocytes can be numerous, resulting in tumors that can be further specified as granulocytic or monocytic sarcoma. A useful finding in granulocytic sarcoma is the presence of immature eosinophilic precursors (eosinophilic myelocytes and metamyelocytes)

admixed with myeloblasts. These cells occur in about 50 percent of all cases of myeloid sarcoma. Knowledge of differentiation is helpful for the diagnosis of myeloid sarcoma, but is not associated with prognosis. In cases of myeloid sarcoma arising from MPN, MDS/MPN, or MDS, evidence of the underlying disorder (e.g., dysplastic megakaryocytes) often accompanies myeloid sarcoma in the spleen.

Rare cases of myeloid sarcoma in the spleen can exhibit megakaryoblastic or erythroid (fig. 62-15) differentiation. In most cases, in routinely stained tissue sections the blasts cannot be identified as megakaryoblasts or erythroblasts without immunophenotypic studies. In touch imprints, in some cases the blasts are large, with increased amounts of deep blue cytoplasm and cytoplasmic blebs (suggesting abortive platelet production). Features suggestive of erythroid differentiation in touch imprints include perfectly round nuclei, peripheral condensation of chromatin, and a concentric rim of deep blue cytoplasm.

Touch imprints of splenic myeloid sarcoma are useful for cytochemical analysis as well as FISH. In tissue sections, the chloroacetate esterase (Leder) stain is useful, positive in about 50 to 60 percent of all cases of myeloid sarcoma, about one third of immature and blastic tumors, and much more frequent in differentiated cases.

Immunophenotypic Findings. Flow cytometry immunophenotyping and immunohistochemical analysis are both well suited to the diagnosis of myeloid sarcoma (34). Myeloid markers useful to establish lineage include CD11c, CD13, CD33, CD43, CD68, CD163, myeloperoxidase, and lysozyme. Using immunohistochemistry, antibodies specific for CD43, CD68, and lysozyme are very sensitive, but not specific, since they can be expressed by both granulocytic and monocytic sarcomas as well as other nonmyeloid tumors. Myeloperoxidase and CD117/KIT highlight most cases of granulocytic myeloid sarcoma, but purely monoblastic tumors are often negative. CD4, CD123, and CD163 are expressed by monocytic sarcoma, and CD163 is specific. Of these, only CD123 will react with a subset of the most immature cases. CD15 and Mac387 are markers of granulocytic/monocytic differentiation, but do not react with immature tumors and are not lineage specific.

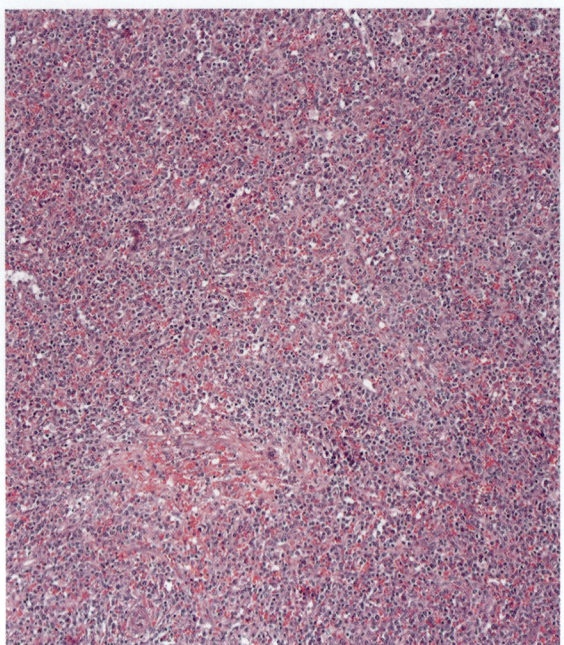
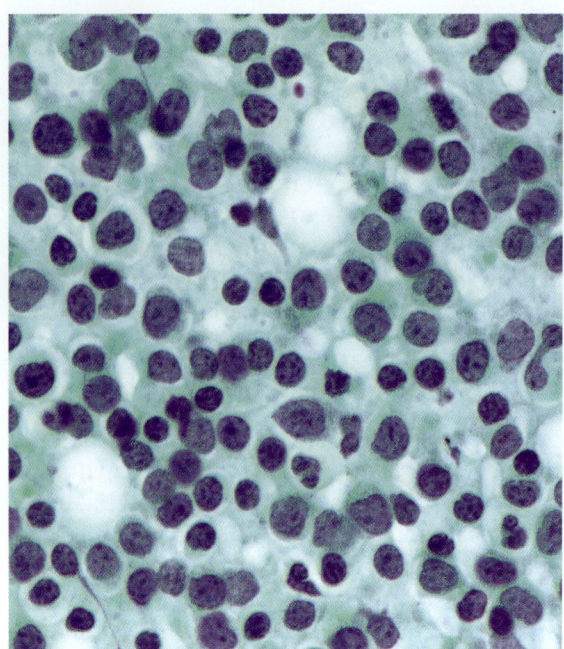

Figure 62-14

MYELOID SARCOMA INVOLVING SPLEEN

Left: The red pulp is diffusely expanded by sheets of immature cells, many of which were CD34-positive myeloblasts (CD34 results not shown) (H&E stain).

Right: Fine-needle aspirate smear of myeloid sarcoma of spleen shows intermediate-sized blasts admixed with small lymphocytes (Papanicolaou stain).

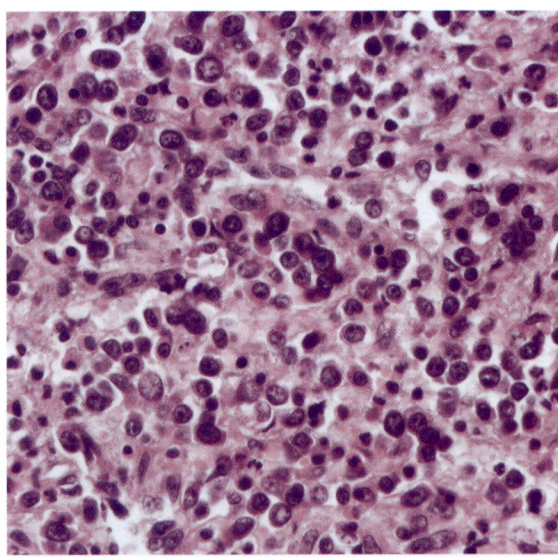

Figure 62-15

ERYTHROLEUKEMIA INVOLVING SPLEEN

Many immature cells, which were proven to be erythroblasts by immunohistochemistry, are seen in the red pulp. Cytologic clues of erythroid lineage include the round nuclei and delicate margination of the chromatin in some cells (H&E stain).

About 75 percent of cases of myeloid sarcoma are positive for CD45/LCA. CD34 highlights immature myeloid sarcomas with many blasts. Monoblastic sarcomas are often negative for CD34. CD99 and TdT are positive in some cases, but neither marker is sensitive or specific and both markers can be expressed by acute lymphoblastic leukemia.

Myeloid sarcomas usually have a high proliferation rate as shown by Ki-67 and are negative for T-cell- and B-cell-specific antigens and CD30. Megakaryoblastic differentiation is highlighted by CD41, CD42b, CD61, factor VIII antigen, and anti-linker of activated T cells (anti-LAT). Immunohistochemical markers for erythroid cells include CD71, E-cadherin, hemoglobin A, and glycophorin A.

Molecular Genetic Findings. Genetic changes that are specific for various types of AML are detected in myeloid sarcoma of the spleen, thereby supporting the diagnosis. Additional discussion of molecular findings in myeloid sarcoma is found in chapter 51.

Differential Diagnosis. *Other Neoplasms.* The diagnosis of myeloid sarcoma is particularly challenging in patients without antecedent myeloid disease. The differential diagnosis includes various types of non-Hodgkin lymphoma, histiocytic tumors, and undifferentiated carcinomas (34). Immunohistochemical analysis easily resolves this issue. A complete discussion of the differential diagnosis of myeloid sarcoma is provided in chapter 51.

Extramedullary Proliferations Associated with Cytokines. Cytokines, which affect the proliferation of bone marrow elements, specifically granulocyte-colony stimulating factor (G-CSF) and granulocyte macrophage-colony stimulating factor (GM-CSF), may cause extramedullary proliferation (fig. 62-16) (10,19). These cytokines are administered most commonly for cytopenias or for stem cell proliferation/mobilization. Usually, the extramedullary myeloid cells are a mixture of a few blasts and more numerous immature myeloid cells such as promyelocytes, myelocytes, and promonocytes, but in H&E-stained slides it may be difficult to distinguish between blasts and immature, nonblastic cells. A history of cytokine administration is very helpful in preventing overdiagnosis as myeloid sarcoma. Rare patients have developed splenic rupture as a result of prominent splenomegaly following cytokine therapy (10).

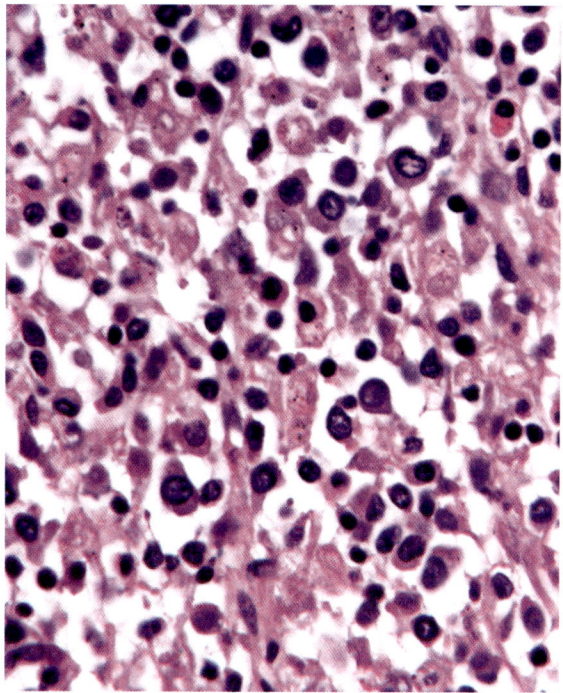

Figure 62-16

GRANULOCYTE-COLONY STIMULATING FACTOR AFFECTING SPLEEN

A splenectomy specimen in a patient who had received G-CSF therapy. There is massive expansion of the red pulp by myeloid cells, mostly promyelocytes or myelocytes. These cells were positive for myeloperoxidase (not shown) by immunohistochemistry (H&E stain).

REFERENCES

1. Arber DA, Orazi A, Hasserjian R, et al. The 2016 revision to the World Health Organization classification of myeloid neoplasms and acute leukemia. Blood 2016;127:2391-2405.
2. Cazzola M, Della Porta MG, Malcovati L. The genetic basis of myelodysplasia and its clinical relevance. Blood 2013;122:4021-4034.
3. Horny HP, Ruck MT, Kaiserling E. Spleen findings in generalized mastocytosis. A clinicopathologic study. Cancer 1992;70:459-468.
4. Hsieh PP, Olsen RJ, O'Malley DP, et al. The role of Janus Kinase 2 V617F mutation in extramedullary hematopoiesis of the spleen in neoplastic myeloid disorders. Mod Pathol 2007;20:929-935.
5. Jabbar KJ, Medeiros LJ, Wang SA, et al. Flow cytometric immunophenotypic analysis of systemic mastocytosis involving bone marrow. Arch Pathol Lab Med 2014;138:1210-1214.
6. Konoplev S, Hsieh PP, Chang CC, Medeiros LJ, Lin P. Janus kinase 2 V617F mutation is detectable in spleen of patients with chronic myeloproliferative diseases suggesting a malignant nature of splenic extramedullary hematopoiesis. Hum Pathol 2007;38:1760-1763.
7. Kraus MD, Bartlett NL, Fleming MD, Dorfman DM. Splenic pathology in myelodysplasia: a report of 13 cases with clinical correlation. Am J Surg Pathol 1998;22:1255-1266.
8. Li B, Gale RP, Xiao Z. Molecular genetics of chronic neutrophilic leukemia, chronic myelomonocytic leukemia and atypical chronic myeloid leukemia. J Hematol Oncol 2014;7:93.
9. Mesa RA, Li CY, Schroeder G, Tefferi A. Clinical correlates of splenic histopathology and splenic karyotype in myelofibrosis with myeloid metaplasia. Blood 2001;97:3665-3667.

10. O'Malley DP. Benign extramedullary myeloid proliferations. Mod Pathol 2007;20:405-415.

11. O'Malley DP, Kim YS, Perkins SL, Baldridge L, Juliar BE, Orazi A. Morphologic and immunohistochemical evaluation of splenic hematopoietic proliferations in neoplastic and benign disorders. Mod Pathol 2005;18:1550-1561.

12. O'Malley DP, Orazi A, Dunphy CH, et al. Loss of heterozygosity identifies genetic changes in chronic myeloid disorders, including myeloproliferative disorders, myelodysplastic syndromes and chronic myelomonocytic leukemia. Mod Pathol 2007;20:1166-1171.

13. O'Malley DP, Orazi A, Wang M, et al. Analysis of loss of heterozygosity and X chromosome inactivation in spleens with myeloproliferative disorders and acute myeloid leukemia. Mod Pathol 2005;18:1562-1568.

14. O'Malley DP, Whalen M, Banks PM. Spontaneous splenic rupture with fatal outcome following G-CSF administration for myelodysplastic syndrome. Am J Hematol 2003;73:294-295.

15. Orazi A, Bennett JM, Germing U, Brunning RD, Bain BJ, Thiele J. Chronic myelomonocytic leukemia. In: Swerdlow SH, Campo E, Harris NL, et al., eds. WHO classification of tumours of haematopoietic and lymphoid tissues. Lyon: IARC Press; 2008:76-79.

16. Patnaik MM, Tefferi A. Chronic myelomonocytic leukemia: 2016 update on diagnosis, risk stratification, and management. Am J Hematol 2016;91:631-642.

17. Prakash S, Hoffman R, Barouk S, et al. Splenic extramedullary hematopoietic proliferation in Philadelphia chromosome-negative myeloproliferative neoplasms: heterogeneous morphology and cytological composition. Mod Pathol 2012;25:815-827.

18. Petrella T, Facchetti F. Tumoral aspects of plasmacytoid dendritic cells: what do we know in 2009? Autoimmunity 2010;43:210-214.

19. Picardi M, De Rosa G, Selleri C, et al. Spleen enlargement following recombinant human granulocyte colony-stimulating factor administration for peripheral blood stem cell mobilization. Haematologica 2003;88:794-800.

20. Pileri SA, Orazi A, Falini B. Myeloid sarcoma. In: Swerdlow SH, Campo E, Harris NL, et al. eds. WHO classification of tumours of haematopoietic and lymphoid tissues. Lyon: IARC Press; 2008:140-141.

21. Porwit A, Rajab A. Flow cytometry immunophenotyping in integrated diagnostics of patients with newly diagnosed cytopenia: one tube 10 color 14-antibody screening panel and 3-tube extensive panel for detection of MDS-related features. Int J Lab Hematol 2015;37(Suppl 1):133-143.

22. Shen Q, Ouyang J, Tang G, et al. Flow cytometry immunophenotypic findings in chronic myelomonocytic leukemia and its utility in monitoring treatment response. Eur J Haematol 2015;95:168-176.

23. Steensma DP, Tefferi A, Li CY. Splenic histopathological patterns in chronic myelomonocytic leukemia with clinical correlations: reinforcement of the heterogeneity of the syndrome. Leuk Res 2003;27:775-782.

24. Swerdlow SH, Campo E, Harris NL, et al., eds. Myeloproliferative neoplasms. In: Swerdlow SH, Campo E, Harris NL, et al., eds. WHO classification of tumours of haematopoietic and lymphoid tissues. Lyon: IARC Press; 2008:32-65.

25. Swerdlow SH, Campo E, Harris NL, et al., eds. Myelodysplastic/myeloproliferative neoplasms. In: Swerdlow SH, Campo E, Harris NL, et al., eds. WHO classification of tumours of haematopoietic and lymphoid tissues. Lyon: IARC Press; 2008:76-86.

26. Swerdlow SH, Campo E, Harris NL, et al., eds. Myelodysplastic syndromes. In: Swerdlow SH, Campo E, Harris NL, et al., eds. WHO classification of tumours of haematopoietic and lymphoid tissues. Lyon: IARC Press; 2008:88-107.

27. Tang G, Fu B, Hu S, et al. Prognostic impact of acquisition of cytogenetic abnormalities during the course of chronic myelomonocytic leukemia. Am J Hematol 2015;90:882-887.

28. Tang G, Jorgensen JL, Zhou Y, et al. Multi-color CD34+ progenitor-focused flow cytometric assay in evaluation of myelodysplastic syndromes in patients with post cancer therapy cytopenia. Leuk Res 2012;36:974-981.

29. Tefferi A. Myeloproliferative neoplasms: a decade of discoveries and treatment advances. Am J Hematol 2016;91:50-58.

30. Titmarsh GJ, Duncombe AS, McMullin MF, et al. How common are myeloproliferative neoplasms? A systematic review and meta-analysis. Am J Hematol 2014;89:581-587.

31. Valent P, Cerny-Reiterer S, Herrmann H, et al. Phenotypic heterogeneity, novel diagnostic markers, and target expression profiles in normal and neoplastic human mast cells. Best Pract Res Clin Haematol 2010;23:369-378.

32. Wang SA, Hutchinson L, Tang GL, et al. Systemic mastocytosis with associated clonal hematological non-mast cell lineage disease: clinical significance and comparison of chromosomal abnormalities in SM and AHNMD components. Am J Hematol 2013;88:219-224.

33. Wassie EA, Itzykson R, Lasho TL, et al. Molecular and prognostic correlates of cytogenetic abnormalities in chronic myelomonocytic leukemia: a Mayo Clinic-French Consortium Study. Am J Hematol 2014;89:1111-1115.

34. Wilson CS, Medeiros LJ. Extramedullary manifestations of myeloid neoplasms. Am J Clin Pathol 2015;144:219-239.

35. Zhang L, Singh RR, Patel KP, et al. BRAF kinase domain mutations are present in a subset of chronic myelomonocytic leukemia with wild type RAS. Am J Hematol 2014;89:499-504.

VASCULAR TUMORS OF THE SPLEEN

HAMARTOMA

General Features. *Splenic hamartoma* is a benign tumor that is composed of unorganized vascular channels and intervening disorganized red pulp stroma. The incidence of splenic hamartoma is low, far less than 1 percent, in reviews of the pathology of splenectomy and autopsy spleen specimens reported in the literature (35). In most patients, splenic hamartoma is asymptomatic and detected incidentally. Other names used previously for splenic hamartoma include splenoma, splenoadenoma, spleen-in-spleen, and splenic splenunculus (2,35,48).

The pathogenesis of splenic hamartoma is uncertain. The possibilities include a congenital malformation of the red pulp, a true neoplasm of red pulp vascular origin, and a reactive proliferation that may be related to prior trauma (32,35).

Clinical Features. Splenic hamartoma can occur at any age (range, 11 months to 86 years), but the average age range at diagnosis is 40 to 50 years (2,35). There is no gender preference. About 15 percent of patients have symptoms, and in this subset, women outnumber men. This is because women tend to have larger, symptomatic lesions, perhaps suggesting a role for sex hormones in hamartoma growth (32,35).

The most common manifestations of splenic hamartoma are hematologic abnormalities including anemia, thrombocytopenia, and pancytopenia (2,35,48). Following abdominal trauma a splenic hamartoma may sequester platelets, producing a Henoch-Schonlein purpura-like clinical picture. Fever, malaise, and weight loss are seen in some patients (26,35).

Splenic hamartoma is associated with a variety of benign and malignant diseases (Table 63-1). Some of these associations may point to a shared predisposition or etiology, but in others, the splenic hamartoma is detected when the associated disease prompts a splenectomy or autopsy.

Gross Findings. Splenic hamartoma is usually a single lesion, but patients may have multiple lesions. The median lesion size is 4 to 5 cm, but the size ranges from small (less than 1 cm) to very large (20 cm that distorts the normal splenic architecture). Viewing the splenic cut surface, the hamartoma often bulges outward from the surrounding parenchyma and is typically well-circumscribed but not encapsulated (figs. 63-1–63-3).

Histologic Findings. Splenic hamartoma is composed predominantly of disorganized red pulp components that otherwise resemble normal red pulp. Splenic hamartoma contains tortuous, slit-like vascular spaces lined by plump endothelial cells of littoral cell derivation that are of similar size to endothelial cells in normal red pulp (fig. 63-4). These vascular spaces are separated by disorganized stroma (Table 63-2).

Table 63-1

DISEASES REPORTED TO BE ASSOCIATED WITH SPLENIC HAMARTOMA

Benign hematologic disorders
Aplastic anemia
Hereditary spherocytosis
Sickle cell anemia
Hemolytic anemia
Congenital dyserythroblastic anemia

Other benign diseases
Tuberous sclerosis
Congestive heart failure
Cerebral vascular accident
Hypertension
Myocardial infarct
Myocarditis
Cirrhosis and portal hypertension

Neoplasms
Hairy cell leukemia
Hodgkin lymphoma
Non-Hodgkin lymphoma
Chronic lymphocytic leukemia
Chronic myeloid leukemia (CML)
Myeloproliferative disorders (not CML)
Different types of carcinoma (breast, lung, stomach, and bladder)
Different types of sarcoma
Thymoma

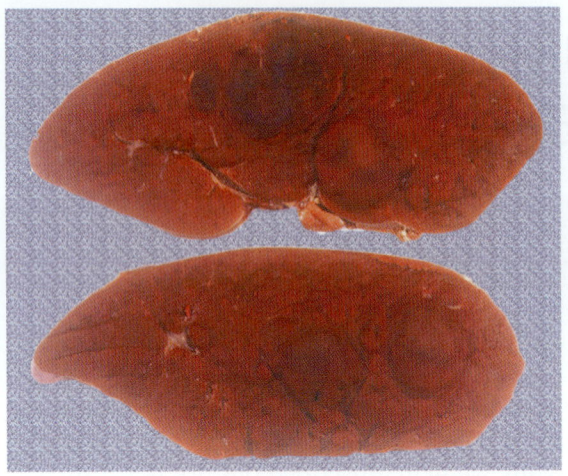

Figure 63-1

SPLENIC HAMARTOMA

Two fairly well-circumscribed masses are seen. (Courtesy of Dr. R. Neiman, Harpswell, ME).

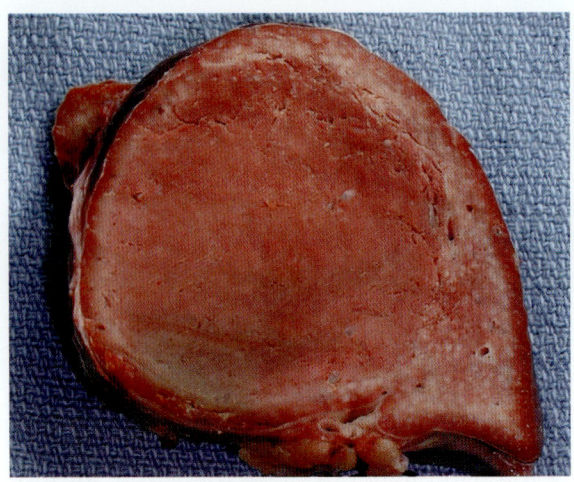

Figure 63-2

SPLENIC HAMARTOMA

The rim of normal tissue surrounding the hamartoma shows multiple small nodules of white pulp, but otherwise is similar to the composition of the hamartoma.

Figure 63-3

SPLENIC HAMARTOMA

The tumor appears hemorrhagic and bulges above the cut surface of the splenic parenchyma.

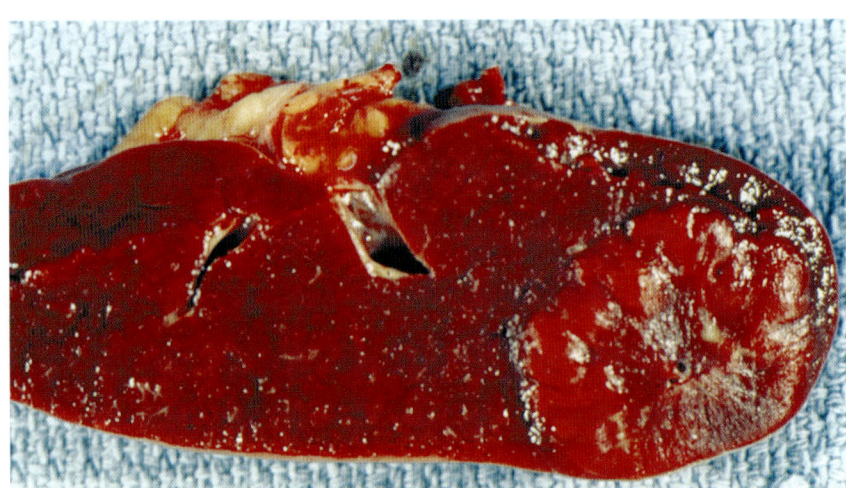

Capillaries also are observed within the cordal areas. White pulp structures are usually atrophic and haphazardly arranged or completely absent (18,32).

Variable numbers of inflammatory cells are present including macrophages, lymphocytes, and plasma cells. Eosinophils and neutrophils may be seen rarely. Foci of macrophages with granular or lipid-filled cytoplasm may be seen. Fibrosis, hemorrhage, and calcifications are present in varying degrees. Extramedullary hematopoiesis is detected frequently. A complex network of reticulin fibers is present in virtually all cases of splenic hamartoma.

Krishnan and Frizzera (32) proposed that there are three subtypes of splenic hamartoma: *classic*, which is the most common, and two rare subtypes known as *myoid angioendothelioma* and *histiocyte-rich hamartoma*. Each subtype has a dominant expression of one or more components of the red pulp. Myoid angioendothelioma, originally described as a benign vascular neoplasm of the spleen with myoid and angioendotheliomatous features, is a vascular lesion lined by CD34-positive cells, with prominent stromal cells positive for smooth muscle actin and muscle-specific actin (31). The histiocyte-rich type of hamartoma has a predominance of histiocytes,

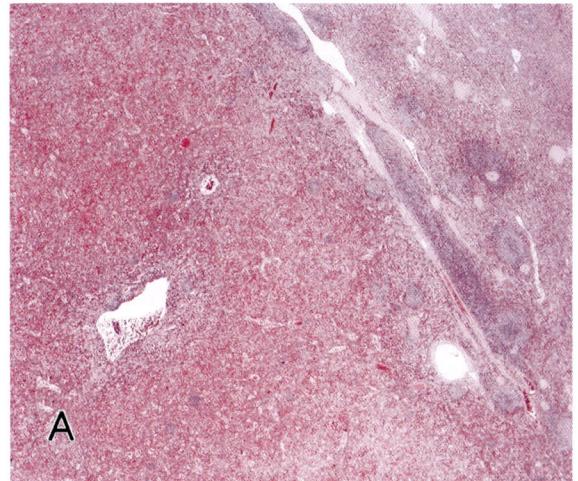

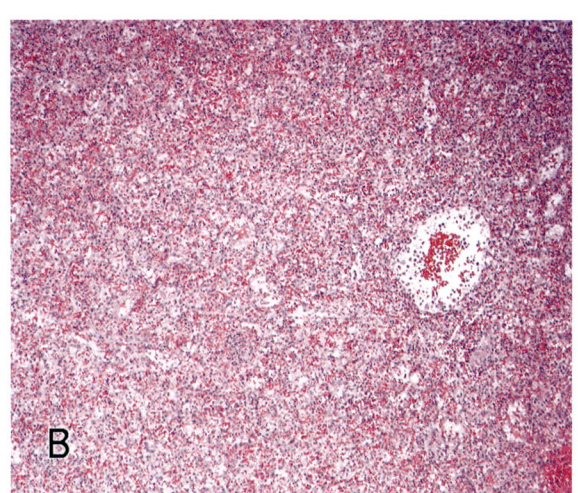

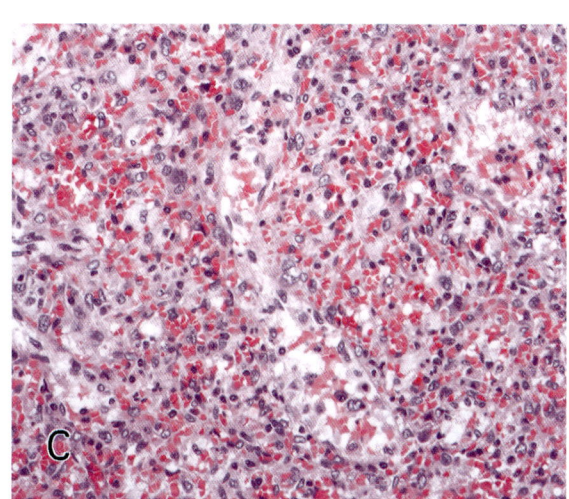

Figure 63-4

SPLENIC HAMARTOMA

A: Normal spleen with white pulp is seen at the upper right. The border between uninvolved spleen and hamartoma is not well defined.

B: At intermediate magnification, disorganized red pulp sinuses and cords within the hamartoma are appreciated.

C: High magnification shows bland splenic red pulp sinuses and cords within the hamartoma (A–C: hematoxylin and eosin [H&E] stain).

Table 63-2

KEY FEATURES OF SPLENIC VASCULAR TUMORS

Tumor	Histologic Findings	Immunoprofile	Outcome
Hamartoma	Disorganized vascular channels intermixed with red pulp stroma	CD8+, ERG+, CD21-, CD34 variably+, CD68-	Benign
Hemangioma	Vascular channels lined by flat endothelial cells	CD31+, CD34+, ERG+, Factor VIII+, CD8-	Benign
Littoral cell angioma	Vascular channels lined by plump cuboidal cells (tombstone-like)	CD21+, CD68+, ERG+, CD8-, CD34-	Benign
Hemangioendothelioma	Anastomosing vascular channels lined by mild-moderately atypical endothelial cells	CD31+, Factor VIII+, ERG+, CD34 variably+, CD21-	Indeterminate; some behave as low-grade malignant
Kaposi sarcoma	Slit-like vascular spaces with extravasation of erythrocytes and cytoplasmic hyaline globules	CD31+, CD34+, ERG+, HHV-8+, CD8-, CD21-	Malignant; aggressive in untreated AIDS[a] patients
Angiosarcoma	Anastomosing vascular channels lined by markedly atypical endothelial cells with mitotic figures	CD31+, CD34+, CD68+, Factor VIII+, ERG+	Malignant, usually highly aggressive

[a]AIDS = acquired immunodeficiency syndrome.

including pseudosinuses lined by CD68-positive histiocytes as opposed to endothelial cells (fig. 63-5). The three subtypes of splenic hamartoma are not thought to have any clinical importance.

Rarely, splenic hamartoma contains large and bizarre stromal cells (10). These cells appear to represent altered stromal cells, have a low mitotic rate, and lack the immunohistochemical features of megakaryocytes, lymphocytes, histiocytes, endothelial cells, or epithelial cells. These stromal cells may be analogous to the "ancient changes" described in ancient schwannoma (fig. 63-6).

Immunophenotypic Findings. A broad array of vascular markers is available to assess splenic hamartomas. A summary of the diagnostic value of these markers and potential pitfalls is presented in Table 63-3.

The lining cells of splenic hamartoma are positive for CD8 and CD68 (35,56). Small capillaries in cordal areas are positive for CD34. The red pulp vascular components are strongly positive for ERG, WT1, CD31, factor VIII, and vimentin, similar to normal red pulp. The proliferation (Ki-67) rate within hamartomas is low (less than 5 percent), although proliferation may be observed in foci of extramedullary hematopoiesis within the lesion (2).

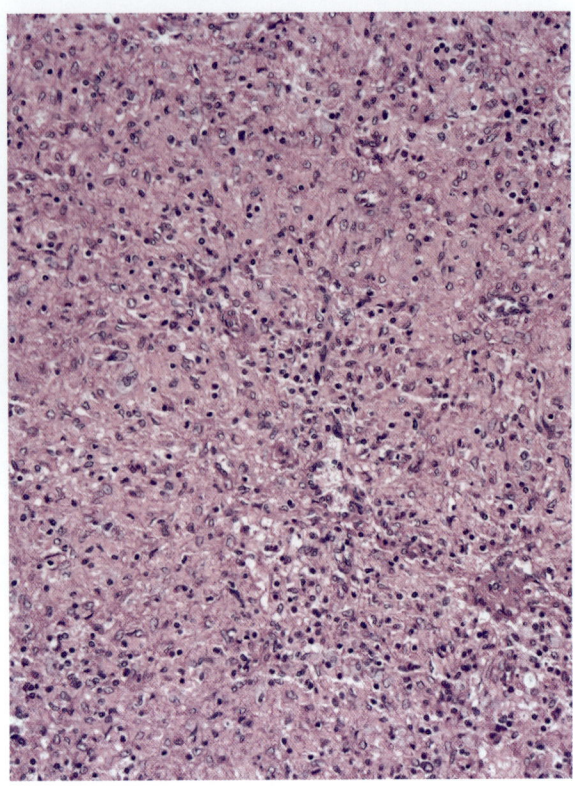

Figure 63-5

HISTIOCYTE-RICH VARIANT OF SPLENIC HAMARTOMA

In this case of splenic hamartoma vascular spaces are inconspicuous and numerous histiocytes are present (H&E stain).

Table 63-3

VASCULAR MARKERS AND POSSIBLE INTERPRETIVE PITFALLS

Marker	Specificity	Possible Pitfalls, Comments
Ulex europaeus	Positive in most vascular elements	Lacks sensitivity
Factor VIII antigen	Broad specificity	Positive in platelets and megakaryocytes
CD34	Reacts with arteries and arterioles in spleen; positive in subset of vascular tumors	Negative in most littoral cell-derived splenic neoplasms
CD31	Sensitive marker; positive in arterial, venular, and lymphatic vessels	Highlights histiocytes
FLI1	Positive in nearly all vessels; nuclear pattern	Positive in some small blue cell tumors
WT1	Positive in nearly all vessels; nuclear and cytoplasmic pattern	Positive in some small blue cell tumors and T cells
ERG	Highly sensitive; nuclear pattern	Positive in bone marrow precursors, some myeloid tumors, Ewing sarcoma with *EWSR1-ERG*, and prostate carcinoma
D2-40/podoplanin	Lymphatic	Many tumor types are reactive for D2-40
LYVE1	Lymphatic	Reactivity not restricted to lymphatics
VEGFR3 (FLT4)	Lymphatic	Reactivity not restricted to lymphatics

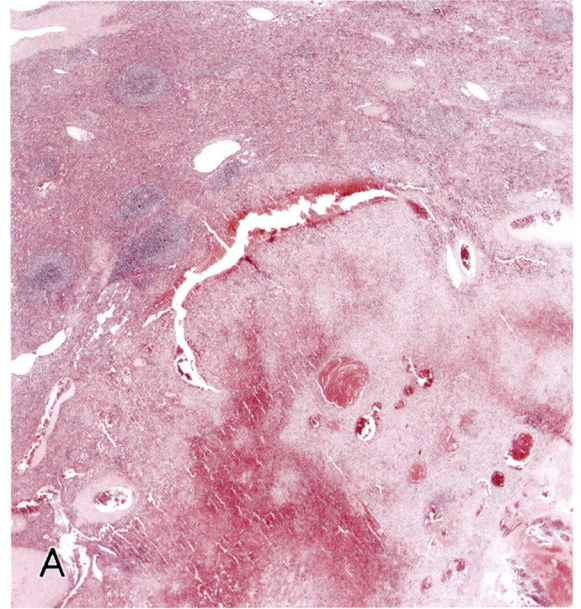

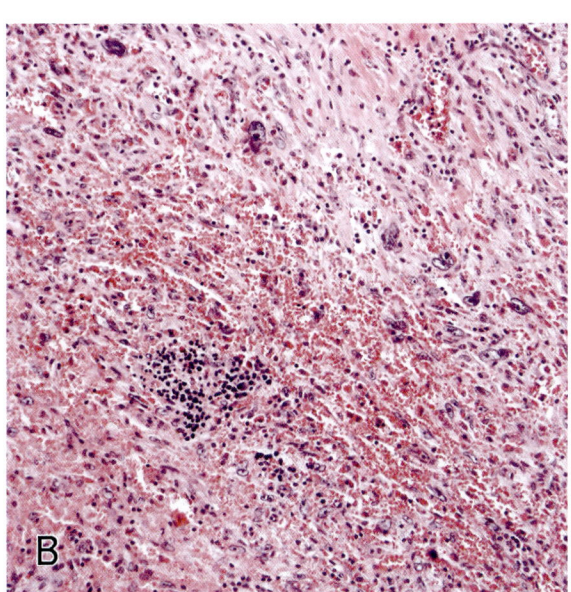

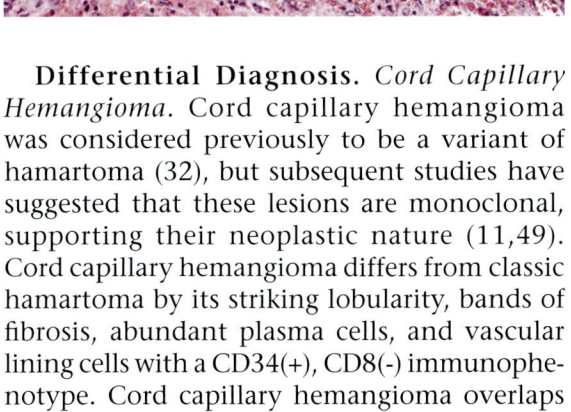

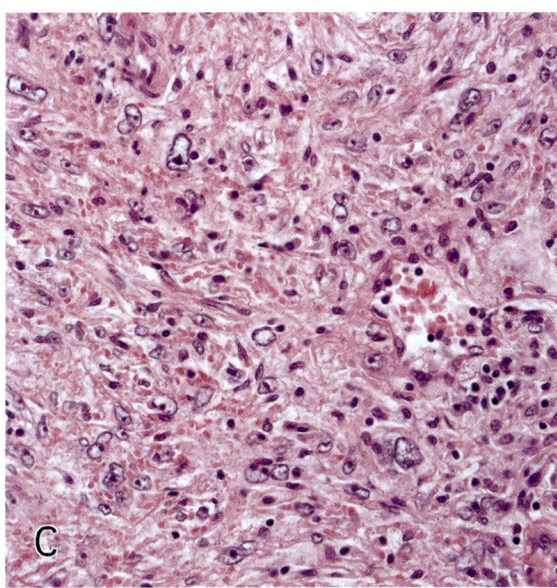

Figure 63-6

**SPLENIC HAMARTOMA WITH
BIZARRE STROMAL CELLS**

A: At low magnification, the hamartoma (bottom of field) is vascular and circumscribed from the normal spleen (top of field).

B: Bizarre stromal cells and a focus of extramedullary hematopoiesis are seen.

C: High magnification image shows large, bizarrely shaped stromal cells, some of which have prominent nucleoli. In spite of these atypical cells, splenic hamartoma with bizarre stromal cells is a benign lesion (A–C: H&E stain).

Differential Diagnosis. *Cord Capillary Hemangioma.* Cord capillary hemangioma was considered previously to be a variant of hamartoma (32), but subsequent studies have suggested that these lesions are monoclonal, supporting their neoplastic nature (11,49). Cord capillary hemangioma differs from classic hamartoma by its striking lobularity, bands of fibrosis, abundant plasma cells, and vascular lining cells with a CD34(+), CD8(-) immunophenotype. Cord capillary hemangioma overlaps morphologically with splenic capillary heman-gioma with sclerosis and sclerosing angiomatoid nodular transformation of the spleen.

Littoral Cell Angioma. Littoral cell angioma (see below) is a benign vascular neoplasm unique to the spleen that is likely derived from cells lining red pulp sinuses (littoral cells). Splenic hamartoma lacks the distinctive cytologic features of littoral cell angioma and is negative for CD21 and WT1.

Sclerosing Angiomatoid Nodular Transformation (SANT) of the Spleen. SANT of the spleen may resemble splenic hamartoma either clinically or radiologically. The designation of SANT was coined by Martel et al. (36). In a 2016 review, Wang et al. (53a) identified 132 cases of SANT reported in the literature.

Patients with SANT are almost always adults, between 20 and 75 years (36,42,53a). This lesion is more common in women and the male to female ratio is about 1 to 2 (36). In about half of patients, SANT is an incidental finding; a subset of patients presents with abdominal pain or splenomegaly. Excision is curative.

Unlike splenic hamartoma, the cut surface of the spleen involved by SANT shows red-brown nodules embedded within fibrous stroma. Histologically, SANT is composed of splenic red pulp entrapped by a non-neoplastic proliferation of stromal cells with fibroblastic and often myofibroblastic features (36,42,53a). In the center of the nodules, blood vessels are lined by plump endothelial cells (fig. 63-7). There is no or only minimal nuclear atypia, mitotic figures are absent or rare, and there is no necrosis.

Immunohistochemical analysis of SANT shows three types of blood vessels in which the lining cells have different immunophenotypes: CD31(+), CD8(+), and CD34(-) sinusoids; CD31(+), CD34(+), and CD8(-) capillaries; and CD31+, CD34- and CD8- venules. The lining cells are negative for CD68 and podoplanin/D2-40 (36,42). Stromal cells with myofibroblastic differentiation are positive for S-100 protein. Assessment of human androgen receptor gene (HUMARA) in cases of SANT has shown that these lesions are polyclonal (9a).

Treatment and Prognosis. Splenic hamartoma is a benign lesion. No specific therapy is required although these lesions are usually resected completely for diagnostic purposes (35). In patients who have associated hematologic abnormalities, resection of hamartoma may lead to resolution of these issues (13). Rarely, a hamartoma ruptures and the patient presents with hemoperitoneum; this is a medical emergency with risk of death.

HEMANGIOMA

General Features. *Hemangioma* is a benign, neoplastic proliferation of vascular elements that occurs in spleen (more commonly) and lymph nodes. It can be sporadic or associated with congenital syndromes. *Diffuse hemangi-*

omatosis is a congenital condition in which multiple organs are involved by hemangiomas (14,38), including the liver, bone marrow, and less commonly, skin.

Congenital syndromes may be associated with large hemangiomas. Kasabach-Merritt syndrome is a coagulopathy attributable to the consumption of platelets and coagulation factors within hemangiomas (38). Klippel-Trenaunay syndrome is a rare disorder characterized by an abnormal vascular proliferation and rare visceral involvement that has been described in the spleen (14). These syndromes suggest that a genetic basis underlies the pathogenesis of at least some hemangiomas, but the etiology and pathogenesis of splenic hemangiomas are unknown.

Clinical Features. Splenic hemangioma occurs most often in older adults. In a study from the Mayo Clinic, the mean age was 63 years, with a range from 23 to 94 years (56). There is no sex preference. In about 20 percent of patients, the symptoms related to splenic hemangioma are usually related to a large tumor causing pain or displacing contiguous structures. Rarely, in about 10 percent of patients, the spleen is enlarged and palpable. In most patients, splenic hemangioma is identified incidentally, either by radiologic imaging or splenectomy performed for another purpose (33,56). Splenic hemangiomas rupture on rare occasion (56).

Gross Findings. Hemangioma of the spleen is usually solitary, but can be multiple. In one study, the size ranged from 0.3 to 7 cm (56). It is commonly an unencapsulated, red-purple mass with irregular borders that is hemorrhagic and has a sponge-like surface. Prominent cystic changes, thrombosis, and infarction may occur.

Histologic Findings. Histologically, hemangioma of the spleen is characterized by variably sized vascular spaces lined by bland, flat endothelial cells (fig. 63-8) (33,56). The spaces are commonly cavernous and distended by blood cells and proteinaceous fluid (cavernous hemangioma) or the vascular spaces are small (capillary hemangioma). The vascular spaces in hemangioma are often anastomosing, but the lumens are generally patent. Some cases of hemangioma are associated with abundant sclerosis (fig. 63-9). In these cases many of the lumens may be obliterated by sclerosis.

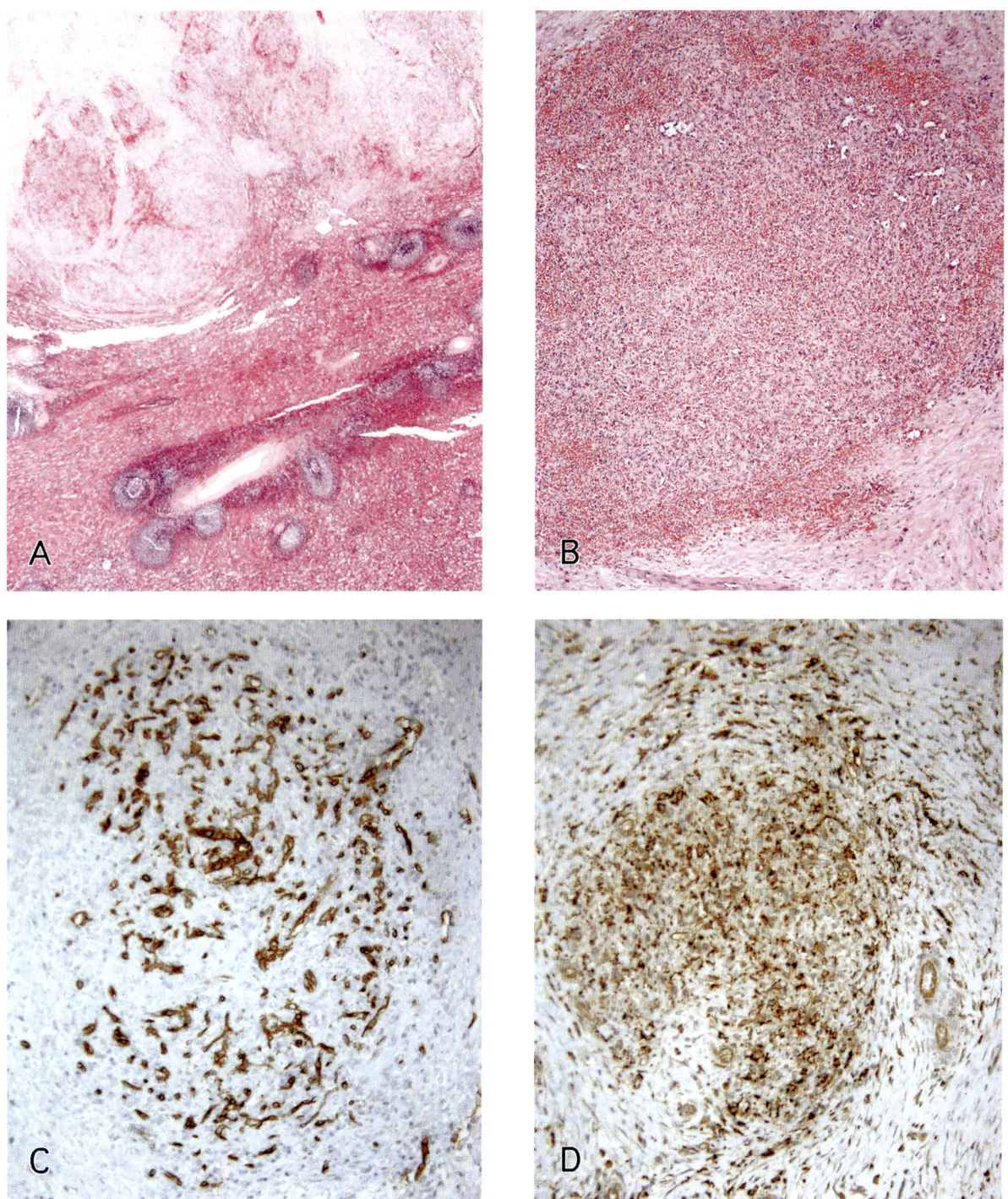

Figure 63-7

SCLEROSING ANGIOMATOID NODULAR TRANSFORMATION (SANT) INVOLVING SPLEEN

A: Low-power image of SANT (top), with normal spleen (bottom). SANT has a multinodular appearance, with the nodules surrounded by bands of stroma (A,B: H&E stain).

B: A nodule within SANT composed of blood vessels and surrounded by stroma (at the periphery of the field).

C,D: Immunohistochemistry for CD34 (C) and CD68 (D) highlights blood vessels and histiocytes within a nodule of SANT (C,D: immunohistochemistry with hematoxylin counterstain).

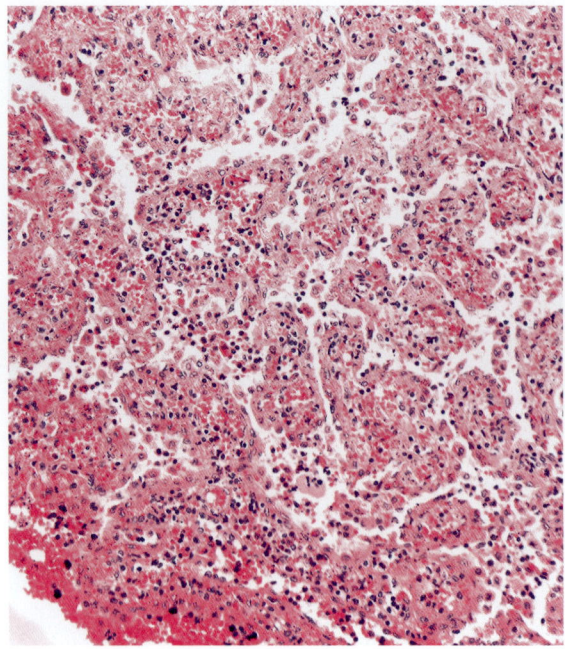

Figure 63-8

SPLENIC HEMANGIOMA

The tumor is composed of many blood vessels lined by bland endothelial cells (H&E stain).

Immunophenotypic Findings. Hemangiomas are lined by cells positive for vascular-associated markers including CD31, CD34, WT1, ERG, FLI1, and factor VIII, and negative for CD8 (33,58). In one report, cavernous hemangioma lining cells were positive for vascular endothelial growth factor (VEGF), but not capillary hemangioma (29). BCL2 is often positive and Ki-67 is low in hemangiomas (29).

Differential Diagnosis. *Splenic Hamartoma.* Unlike splenic hemangioma, the lining cells of hamartoma are positive for CD8, and CD34 is expressed variably.

Malignant Vascular Neoplasms. Diffuse hemangiomatosis associated with congenital syndromes may suggest a malignant vascular tumor such as angiosarcoma of the spleen. Unlike angiosarcoma, the lining cells of the lesions in diffuse hemangiomatosis are cytologically bland and lack tufting, cytologic atypia, or mitotic figures.

Treatment and Prognosis. Splenic hemangioma is a benign lesion. Small asymptomatic neoplasms may be managed by watch-and-wait. The treatment for larger tumors is simple resection. For patients with associated congenital

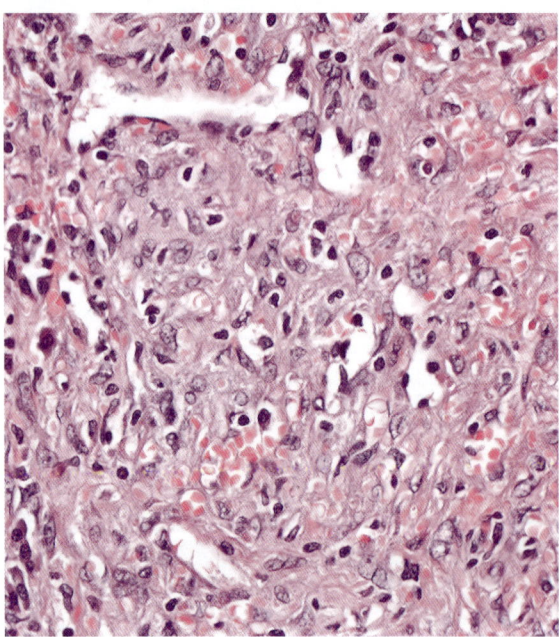 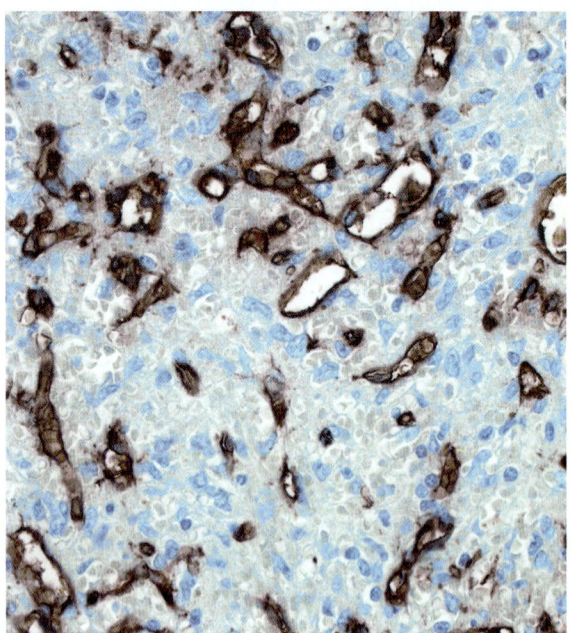

Figure 63-9

SCLEROSING HEMANGIOMA INVOLVING SPLEEN

Left: The neoplasm is composed of numerous blood vessels, unlike splenic hamartoma. Some patent blood vessel lumens are appreciated in this field (H&E stain).

Right: The lining cells of blood vessels are positive for CD34 (immunohistochemistry with hematoxylin counterstain)

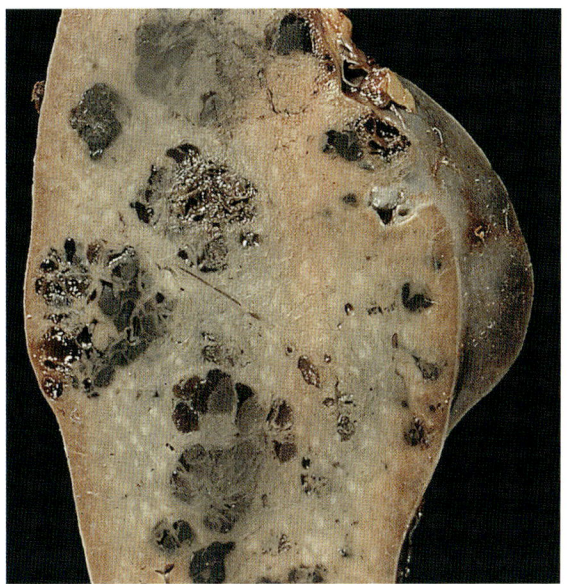

Figure 63-10

LITTORAL CELL ANGIOMA INVOLVING SPLEEN

At this magnification, multiple blood-filled nodules are seen scattered throughout the spleen.

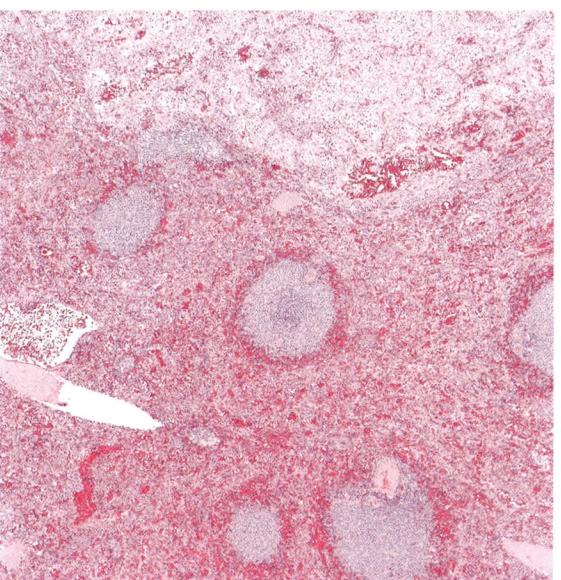

Figure 63-11

LITTORAL CELL ANGIOMA INVOLVING SPLEEN

The littoral cell angioma is at the top of the field. The border between the angioma and normal splenic parenchyma is somewhat ill-defined and no capsule is present (H&E stain).

syndromes, the prognosis is dependent on impingement and dysfunction of involved organs.

LITTORAL CELL ANGIOMA

General Features. Littoral cell angioma is a benign vascular neoplasm that likely arises from the littoral cells that line red pulp sinuses. The cause of littoral cell angioma is unknown, but immune dysregulation may play a role in pathogenesis (25). In a subset of patients, littoral cell angioma is associated with primary immunodeficiency syndromes, autoimmune disorders, therapy with immunosuppressive and immunomodulatory medications, and malignant neoplasms or other causes of immune suppression (4,8,25). In one interesting patient, littoral cell angioma was identified in the spleen and in an intrapancreatic accessory spleen, suggesting an underlying genetic defect that affected all splenic tissues (40). Littoral cell angioma occurs uniquely in the spleen and there is no known lymph node or soft tissue counterpart (19,33).

Clinical Features. Littoral cell angioma usually occurs in adults and there is no sex preference (19). Most patients are asymptomatic and the tumor is usually detected as an incidental finding during radiologic evaluation. Some patients have splenomegaly or hematologic abnormalities (6,33).

Gross and Histologic Findings. Grossly, littoral cell angioma appears as multiple spongy and cystic nodules (fig. 63-10). Histologically, littoral cell angioma is composed of plump and cuboidal endothelial cells (figs. 63-11–63-13) (19,33). Papillary projections of endothelial cells may protrude into the vascular spaces. Vascular lumens also contain abundant desquamated littoral cells and macrophages; the latter may exhibit erythrophagocytosis. Mild cytologic atypia may be present. A distinctive feature in littoral cell angioma is the presence of intracytoplasmic eosinophilic globules, often in aggregates (33).

Immunophenotypic Findings. CD21, CD31, CD68 (focal), and CD163 are positive in most cases of littoral cell angioma and CD34 is consistently negative (fig. 63-14) (33). Unlike normal splenic littoral cells, the cells in littoral cell angioma are negative for CD8.

Differential Diagnosis. *Angiosarcoma.* Although littoral cell angioma and low-grade angiosarcoma can resemble each other, at least in part, unequivocal malignant features such as

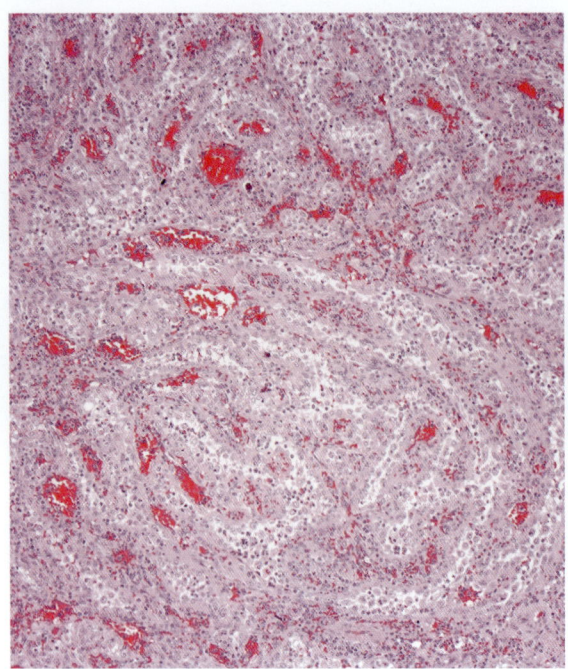

Figure 63-12

LITTORAL CELL ANGIOMA INVOLVING SPLEEN

In this example of littoral cell angioma, many channel-like vascular spaces are lined by littoral type cells. Littoral cells are plump and surround fibrovascular cores. A mixture of cell types is present within the vascular spaces (H&E stain).

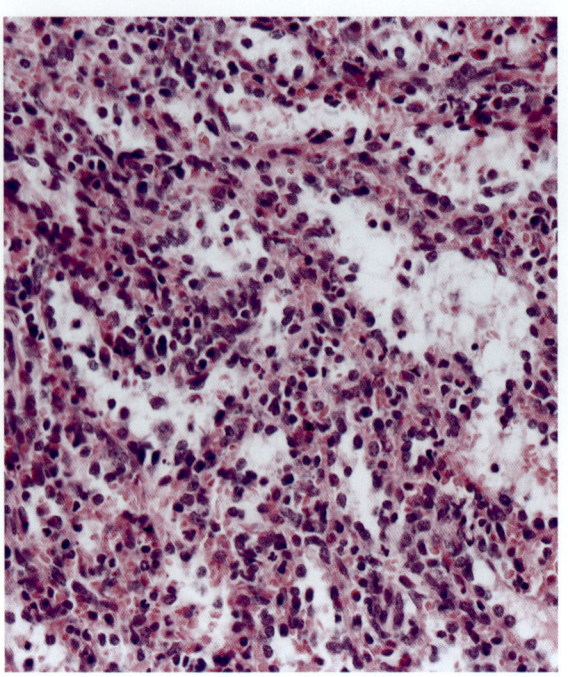

Figure 63-13

LITTORAL CELL ANGIOMA INVOLVING SPLEEN

The neoplastic cells are plump, with a "tombstone" appearance. Although the cells are large, there is no cytologic atypia. The cells in the vascular lumens consist of desquamated littoral cells and macrophages (H&E stain).

atypia and mitotic figures are absent in littoral cell angioma (17,19).

Recent studies suggest that littoral cell lesions show a spectrum of clinical behavior and morphologic features. Littoral cell angioma is, by far, the most common. A tumor with features intermediate between littoral cell angioma and angiosarcoma has been designated as *littoral cell hemangioendothelioma* (3). This tumor has more aggressive clinical behavior than littoral cell angioma and is characterized by solid areas with clear cell morphology, atypia, and a low frequency of mitotic figures. Rare cases of overtly malignant littoral cell tumors, designated as *littoral cell angiosarcoma*, also have been reported (34,45,46). These tumors are characterized by distinctly malignant features including an arborizing, highly anastomotic or solid pattern of growth, necrosis, marked cytologic atypia, and high mitotic activity.

Treatment and Prognosis. Littoral cell angioma is a benign lesion that is best treated by surgical resection and does not recur. The

prognosis of patients with littoral cell hemangioendothelioma and particularly, littoral cell angiosarcoma, is guarded and metastases occur.

HEMANGIOENDOTHELIOMA

General Features. *Hemangioendothelioma* is a vascular tumor of the spleen that has morphologic features intermediate between hemangioma and angiosarcoma. These tumors are thought to have borderline or intermediate malignant potential (33,54).

Hemangioendothelioma arising in the spleen is an exceedingly rare neoplasm. These tumors are most often observed in young or middle-aged adults (1).

Gross and Histologic Findings. Splenic hemangioendothelioma usually involves the red pulp. It is often a well-circumscribed, unencapsulated mass (1,33,54).

Histologically, hemangioendothelioma shows a range of features, with poorly formed vascular spaces, epithelioid cells, and spindle cells in varying proportions in an individual

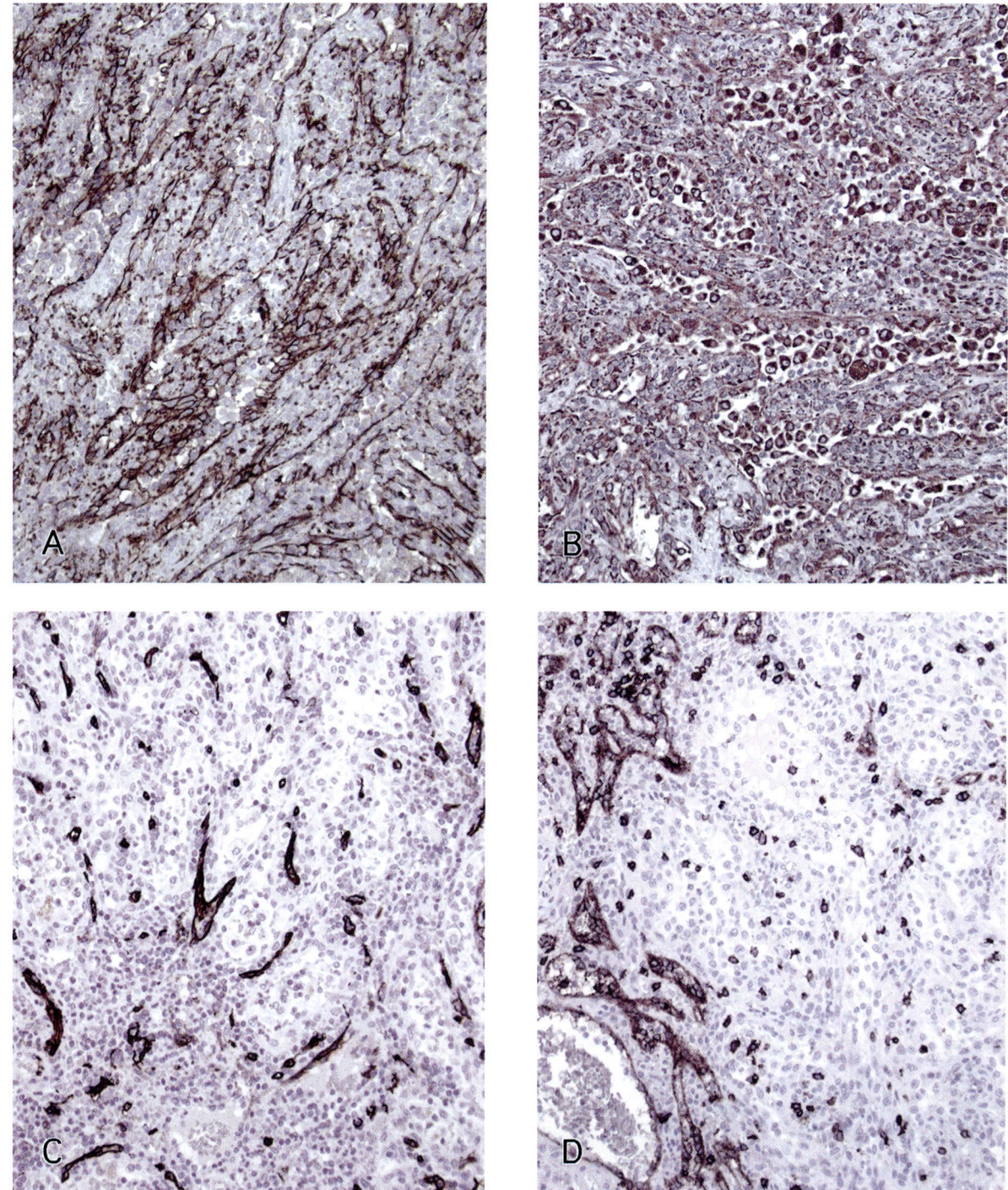

Figure 63-14

IMMUNOHISTOCHEMISTRY OF LITTORAL CELL ANGIOMA INVOLVING SPLEEN

A,B: CD31 (A) and CD68 (B) are positive in the littoral cell angioma, highlighting the shared vascular and macrophage characteristics.

C: CD34 is negative in littoral cell angioma, although small feeder vessels are positive.

D: CD8 is negative in littoral cell angioma (right), but normal splenic sinuses (left) are positive (Immunohistochemistry with hematoxylin counterstain).

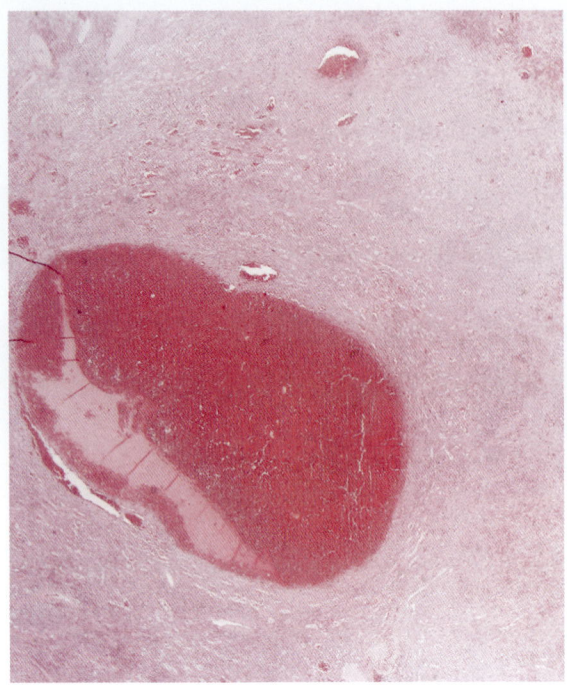

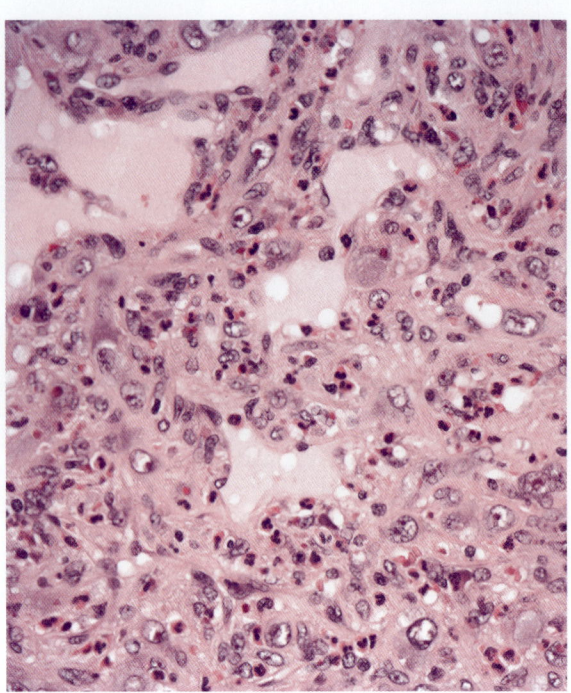

Figure 63-15

HEMANGIOENDOTHELIOMA INVOLVING SPLEEN

The tumor has a vaguely nodular pattern, and typically has a margin that is poorly demarcated from uninvolved spleen (H&E stain). (Courtesy of Dr. C. Fisher, London, England.)

Figure 63-16

HEMANGIOENDOTHELIOMA INVOLVING SPLEEN

The abnormal cells exhibit some epithelioid differentiation and have enlarged and atypical nuclei with dispersed nuclear chromatin. There is considerable variation in cell size and shape. No necrosis or mitotic figures are seen (H&E stain).

tumor (figs. 63-15–63-17). In many cases, the features of the underlying blood vessels are maintained, with some formation of cavernous and honeycombed vascular spaces. Abnormal tumor cells line the vascular spaces and may radiate outward from a central lumen of abnormal structures, imparting a nodular appearance.

Individual tumor cells, in contrast with other vasoformative tumors, usually do not have an intracellular lumen or intracellular or intraluminal red blood cells and most often resemble endothelial cells. Epithelioid variants can mimic epithelial malignancies, but have characteristic central vascular spaces and an immunophenotype of vascular elements.

Mitotic activity is usually low, less than 1 mitosis per 10 high-power microscopic fields. Tumor necrosis is absent and cellular atypia is usually absent or only focal.

Cytologic Findings. Aspirates of hemangioendothelioma are often hypocellular, with mostly single neoplastic cells, and occasionally contain small cell clusters with scalloped borders. The cells are polymorphic and can be ovoid, polygonal, or spindle in shape (51). The cells have ovoid or reniform nuclei with variable numbers of intranuclear inclusions (fig. 63-18). Typically, the cytoplasm is abundant and dense, but cytoplasmic vacuoles may occur. Blister cells with clear cytoplasm may be observed (51). These tumors can be mistaken for metastatic carcinoma on cytology preparations.

Immunophenotypic Findings. Almost all cases of hemangioendothelioma are positive for WT1, FLI1, CD31, and CD34 (22). Ulex europaeus lectin and factor VIII are also usually positive as is vimentin (33). In tumors with epithelioid differentiation there may be aberrant expression of epithelial-associated markers such as pankeratin and epithelial membrane antigen (EMA). Smooth muscle actin and CD10 may be positive in epithelioid variants of hemangioendothelioma (55). Doyle et al. (16) reported that calmodulin-binding transcription activator 1 (CAMTA1) expression in a nuclear

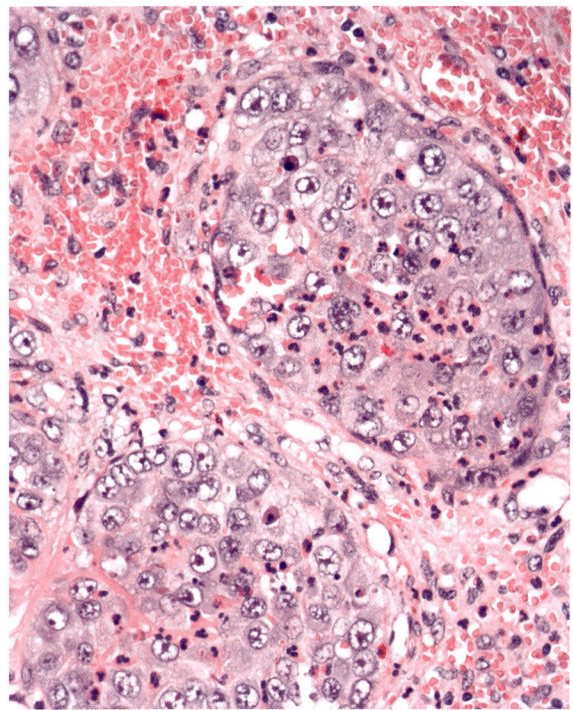

Figure 63-17

HEMANGIOENDOTHELIOMA INVOLVING SPLEEN

Vascular spaces are lined by layers of enlarged atypical epithelioid cells (H&E stain).

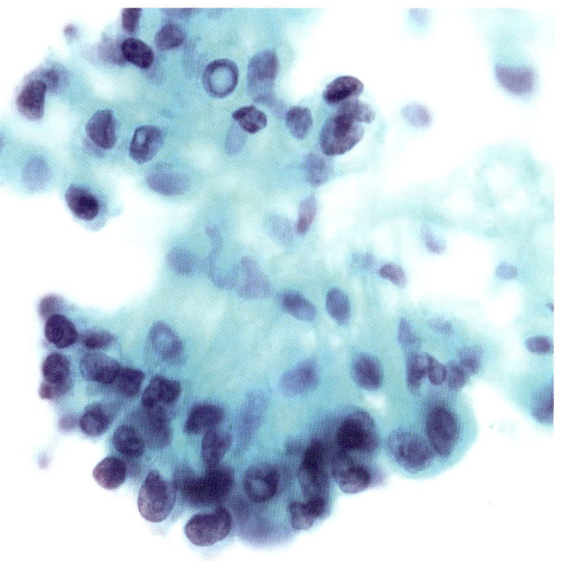

Figure 63-18

HEMANGIOENDOTHELIOMA INVOLVING SPLEEN

The aspirate smear shows a cluster of atypical cells with scalloped borders, abundant cytoplasm, and intranuclear inclusions (Papanicolaou stain). (Courtesy of Dr. G. Staerkel, Houston, TX.)

pattern is common in epithelioid hemangioendothelioma and rare in other epithelioid vascular tumors. Tumors negative for nuclear CAMTA1 are often positive for transcription factor binding to IGHM enhancer 3 (TFE3) (16).

Molecular Genetic Findings. Little is known about the genetic abnormalities specific to splenic hemangioendothelioma. General findings in hemangioendotheliomas are: loss of chromosome Y, complex translocations involving chromosomes 7 and 22, and abnormalities of chromosomal loci 11q and 12q (7,52).

Epithelioid hemangioendothelioma is better understood at the molecular level. t(1;3) (p36;q25) resulting in the *WWTR1-CAMTA1* fusion gene is present in about 90 percent of tumors (16,39). The *YAP1-TFE3* fusion gene is detected in about 5 percent of epithelioid hemangioendotheliomas that are negative for *WWTR1-CAMTA1* (16,39). In one case, altered expression of *TP53, MDM2, CAV1,* and *VEGF* was reported (50).

Differential Diagnosis. *Kaposi Sarcoma.* Spindle cell hemangioendothelioma may be confused with Kaposi sarcoma (see below). Unlike hemangioendothelioma, Kaposi sarcoma as a rule does not show epithelioid differentiation or cavernous vascular formations. However, rare cases of kaposiform hemangioendothelioma, including a case that involved the spleen, have been reported (57). Hemangioendothelioma is negative for human herpes virus 8 (HHV-8), unlike Kaposi sarcoma.

Angiosarcoma. Extensive tumor necrosis, marked cellular atypia, a high mitotic rate, and sheets of neoplastic cells support the diagnosis of angiosarcoma over hemangioendothelioma.

Treatment and Prognosis. The prognosis of patients with splenic hemangioendothelioma is variable. A minority develop metastases, most often to the liver or regional lymph nodes, but patients with distant metastases, including the brain, have been reported (54).

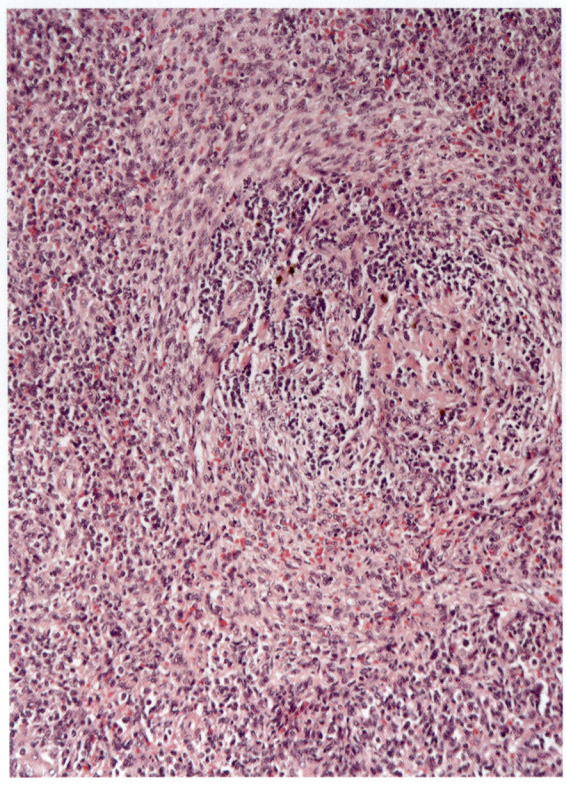

Figure 63-19

KAPOSI SARCOMA INVOLVING SPLEEN

There is a proliferation of spindle-shaped cells surrounding white pulp structures. These cells form small irregular vascular channels (H&E stain).

KAPOSI SARCOMA

General Features. *Kaposi sarcoma* is a malignant vascular neoplasm that is associated with infection by HHV-8, also known as Kaposi sarcoma-associated virus. There are four general forms of Kaposi sarcoma (5). Moritz Kaposi in 1872 initially described the sporadic form. These patients tend to be elderly persons who live in areas endemic for infection, for example, the Mediterranean basin.

The most common form of Kaposi sarcoma is the so-called epidemic form, associated with human immunodeficiency virus (HIV) infection and acquired immunodeficiency syndrome (AIDS). Other forms of Kaposi sarcoma include the endemic form, which affects patients (often children) in equatorial Africa and cases associated with immunosuppression resulting from iatrogenic causes or inherited immunodeficien-

cy diseases (5). The pathogenesis of all forms of Kaposi sarcoma is related to infection by HHV-8 and its viral-associated effects. The virus encodes for a number of proteins that can mimic human cellular genes or bind to the promoter regions of cellular genes, thereby hijacking normal cellular pathways.

Clinical Features. The skin is the most common site of Kaposi sarcoma, but any site with vasculature can be involved. The spleen is involved uncommonly. In the United States and other nonendemic regions, most cases of Kaposi sarcoma occur in patients with AIDS.

Gross and Histologic Findings. Grossly, Kaposi sarcoma often involves the splenic red pulp or trabeculae in a multifocal fashion. The lesions vary from hemorrhagic and necrotic to solid masses.

Histologically, Kaposi sarcoma is characterized by poorly formed or slit-like vascular spaces formed by spindle-shaped endothelial cells (figs. 63-19, 63-20) (5). These small vessels may be associated with larger, normal blood vessels and appear to radiate outward. The blood vessels may have a sieve-like arrangement. Deposition of red blood cells and hemosiderin may occur, presumably from interstitial hemorrhage and breakdown of red blood cells. Individual tumor cells commonly have periodic acid–Schiff (PAS)-positive cytoplasmic globules that may represent fragments of partially digested erythrocytes.

Typical cases of Kaposi sarcoma show mild to moderate atypia; highly pleomorphic cells are seen in a small subset of cases. Mitotic figures are present, but are not numerous.

Cytologic Findings. Aspirates of Kaposi sarcoma are typically hypocellular, containing loosely cohesive clusters of bland spindle cells, sometimes with a radial arrangement (fig. 63-21). The cells have bland oval nuclei and scant to moderately abundant cytoplasm; eosinophilic cytoplasmic globules may be observed (21). Kaposi sarcoma can be challenging to diagnose in cytology specimens.

Immunophenotypic Findings. The neoplastic cells of Kaposi sarcoma are positive for most pan-vascular markers, such as CD31, CD34, ERG, FLI1, and WT1 (44). Most cases express the lymphatic-associated markers D2-40/podoplanin and VEGFR-3 (20,44) and virtually all cases are positive for HHV-8 with a nuclear pattern of

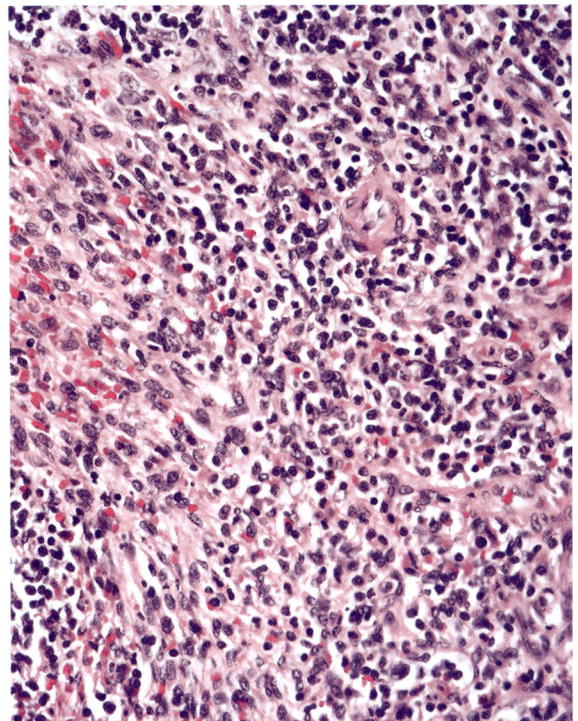

Figure 63-20

KAPOSI SARCOMA INVOLVING SPLEEN

At high magnification, the spindle-shaped cells form irregular and sometimes slit-like vascular spaces. Red blood cell fragments with associated splenic lymphocytes are seen (H&E stain).

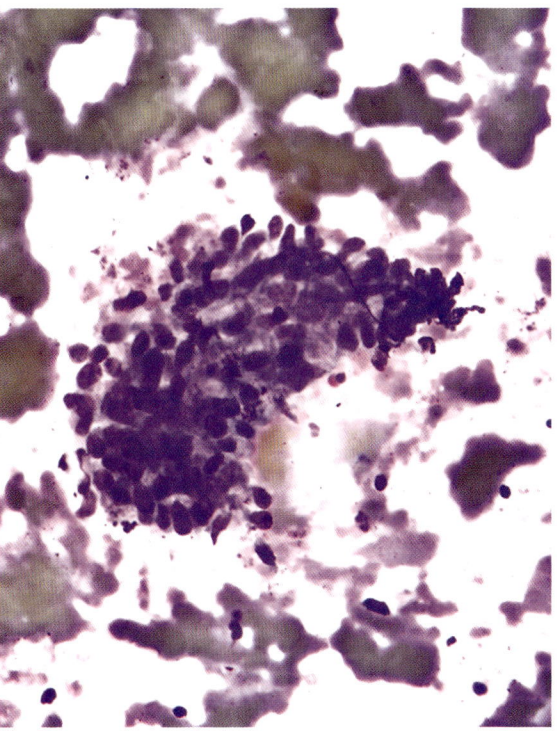

Figure 63-21

KAPOSI SARCOMA INVOLVING SPLEEN

Aspirate smears are typically hypocellular and contain aggregates of ovoid to spindle cells (Diff-Quik stain).

expression as observed using the LANA-1 antibody (5).

Molecular Genetic Findings. Kaposi sarcoma shows structural and numerical chromosomal abnormalities. Comparative genomic hybridization has shown loss of chromosome Y in a large percentage of cases in men (43). Loss of chromosome Y may therefore be an early event in pathogenesis. Other abnormalities, likely later events in pathogenesis, include loss of chromosomes 14 and 21; nonrandom translocations and deletions involving the 3p14 locus; recurrent gains of 1q, 8q, and 11q13; and rearrangements of 1p, 7q, 8p, 13p, 13q, 16, 17, and 19q (9,43).

Treatment and Prognosis. Kaposi sarcoma can exhibit locally aggressive behavior and also can recur and metastasize (33). The clinical course depends greatly on the clinical context. In patients with AIDS and disseminated Kaposi sarcoma, the prognosis is poor.

ANGIOSARCOMA

General Features. *Angiosarcoma* involving the spleen is a clinically aggressive and high-grade neoplasm derived from endothelial cells. The spleen is an uncommon site of angiosarcoma, representing less than 5 percent of all cases. In 2005, Valbuena reviewed the literature and identified about 200 reported cases (53).

The etiology of splenic angiosarcoma is unknown. A case report of two siblings with coincidental littoral cell angioma and angiosarcoma of spleen suggests the possibility of a genetic predisposition (30). Splenic angiosarcoma is associated with radiation therapy; genetic syndromes; foreign materials including shrapnel, steel, plastic and synthetic vascular graft material, surgical sponges, and bone wax; and toxic exposure to agents such as thorium dioxide (Thorotrast), arsenic containing materials, vinyl chloride, insecticides, and anabolic steroids (37,53).

Clinical Features. Most affected patients are adults with a mean age of about 60 years, but

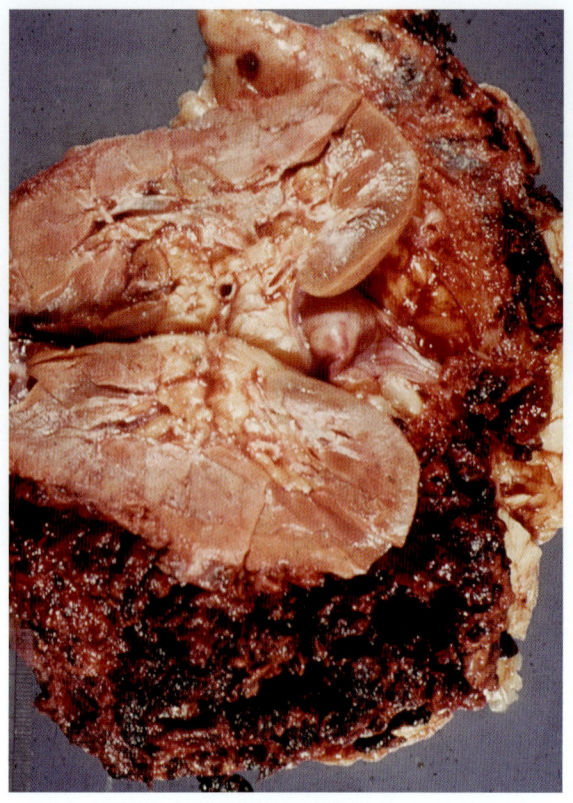

Figure 63-22

ANGIOSARCOMA INVOLVING SPLEEN

This large friable, dark red tumor encased the left kidney (center of the image). (Courtesy of Dr. D. Farhi, Marietta, GA.)

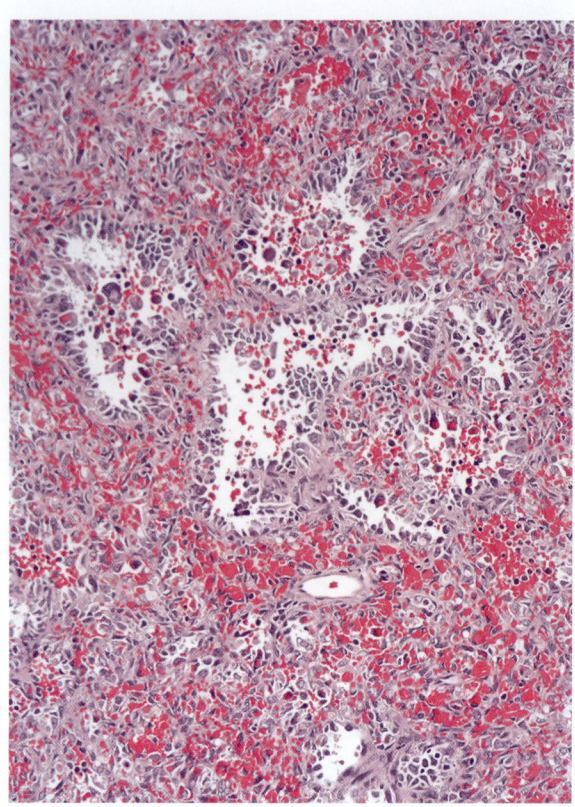

Figure 63-23

ANGIOSARCOMA INVOLVING SPLEEN

Patent vascular spaces in a case of angiosarcoma (H&E stain).

splenic angiosarcoma also occurs in children (17,27,37). There is no clear sex preference (17,37). Patients are often symptomatic, with fever, malaise, and abdominal pain (17,37,47). Splenomegaly is common and rarely patients present initially with splenic rupture (17,23,37). Accessory spleens also may be involved by angiosarcoma (17). Common laboratory findings in patients include anemia, thrombocytopenia, or pancytopenia (17). Microangiopathic hemolytic anemia also has been reported (47).

Gross Findings. Splenectomy specimens involved by angiosarcoma are often massive, with a mean size of approximately 1,000 g (17) and maximum size of over 3,000 g. The cut surface of the spleen can be hemorrhagic, necrotic, spongy, or solid (figs. 63-22). Cystic spaces, corresponding to areas of blood deposition, are frequent. The tumor can be confined to the red pulp as a single mass, or may be multifocal;

diffuse splenic involvement is uncommon. Extension beyond the splenic capsule and entrapment of other abdominal tissues can occur in patients with advanced tumors.

Histologic Findings. Low-grade and well-differentiated angiosarcomas may resemble, in part, littoral cell angioma, but always contain areas of cellular atypia, mitotic activity, and an arborizing, highly anastomotic or solid pattern of growth (figs. 63-23–63-25). The pattern of abnormal vasoformative elements can be cavernous, honeycomb, or slit-like. Individual cells may be spindle-shaped, polygonal, round, or epithelioid.

High-grade angiosarcoma of the spleen usually contains solid areas with a spindle-cell morphology, high mitotic activity, and little evidence of vascular differentiation. These tumors may resemble other types of sarcoma (figs. 63-26, 63-27) (17,37). Hemophagocytosis, intracytoplasmic hyaline globules, hemorrhage, hemosiderin

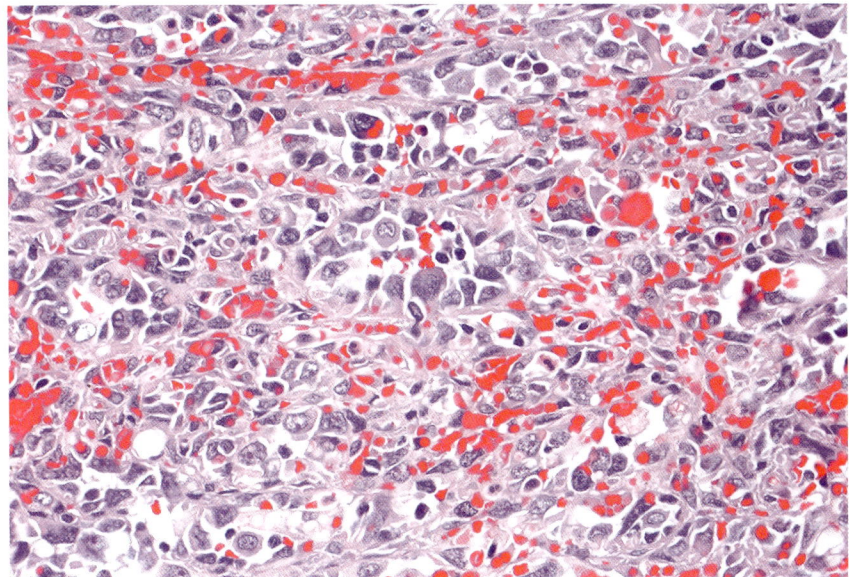

Figure 63-24

ANGIOSARCOMA INVOLVING SPLEEN

In addition to abnormally anastomosing vascular spaces, individual cells have intracellular lumens, some with red blood cells, supporting their nature as endothelial-derived cells. Atypia is also present (H&E stain).

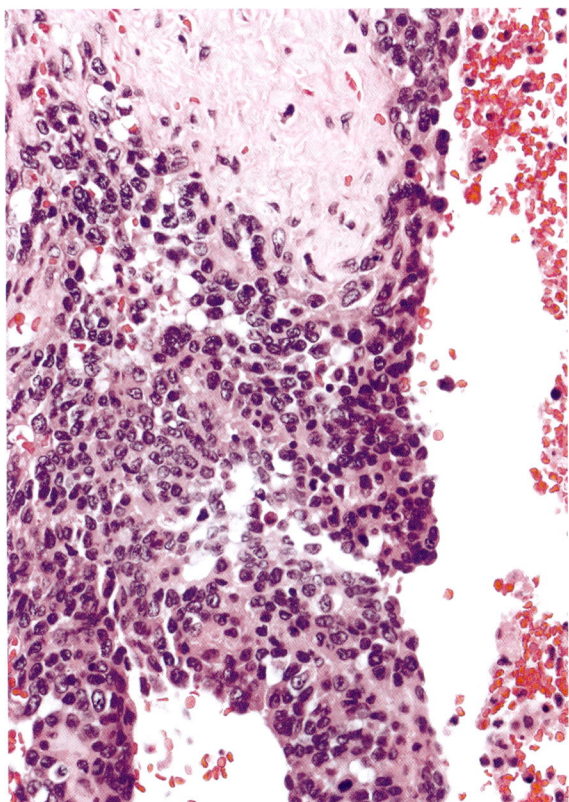

Figure 63-25

ANGIOSARCOMA INVOLVING SPLEEN

In this well-differentiated angiosarcoma of spleen, the cells have a uniform appearance. However, they are proliferative and line abnormal vascular spaces (H&E stain). (Courtesy of Dr. J. Goldblum, Cleveland, OH).

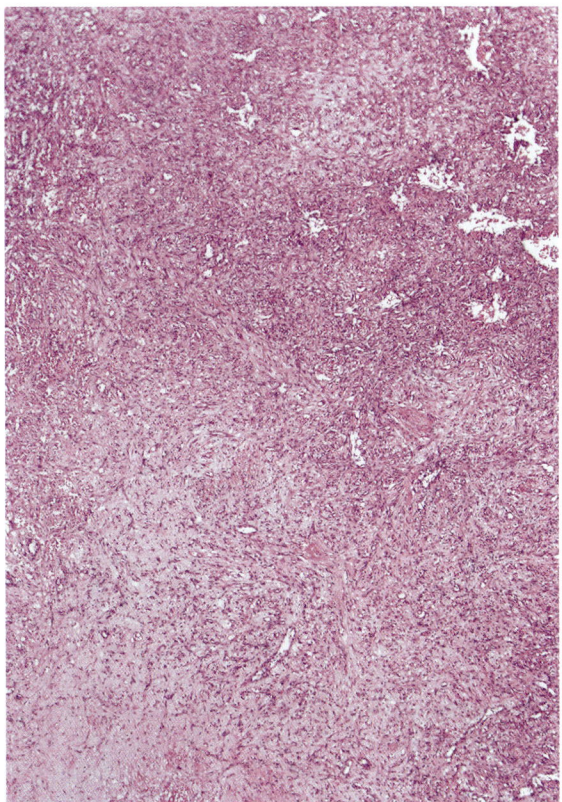

Figure 63-26

ANGIOSARCOMA INVOLVING SPLEEN

At low magnification, a more solid appearance of angiosarcoma is seen. Some vascular spaces are present. No normal splenic architecture is appreciated (H&E stain).

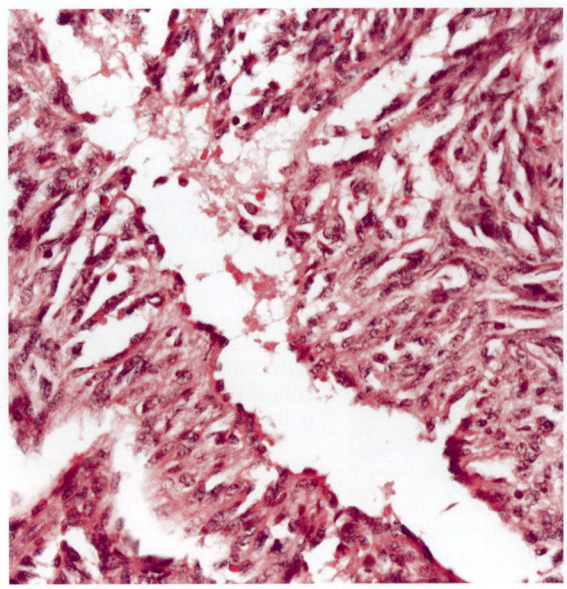

Figure 63-27

ANGIOSARCOMA INVOLVING SPLEEN

High magnification of the spindle cell variant of angiosarcoma shows narrow vascular spaces that are more slit-like, similar to those seen in Kaposi sarcoma (H&E stain).

deposition, extramedullary hematopoiesis, and calcification may be present.

Cytologic Findings. Aspirates of angiosarcoma are usually cellular, and the neoplastic cells are often dissociated, but also occur in small tissue fragments with eosinophilic stroma. The tumor cells have a spectrum of cytomorphologic features ranging from predominantly epithelioid to predominantly spindle-shaped or a mixture of both cell types (15).

The epithelioid cells are pleomorphic or carcinoma-like. In the pleomorphic type, the tumor cells often have a plasmacytoid appearance and contain large hyperchromatic nuclei with coarse chromatin and nucleoli. Binucleated and multinucleated cells range from few to numerous.

In the spindle cell type, the cells are arranged in dense cell groups with marked variation in nuclear size (fig. 63-28). The nuclei are hyperchromatic with multiple nucleoli. Branching papillary-like clusters and pseudoacini or rosette-like groups also are described.

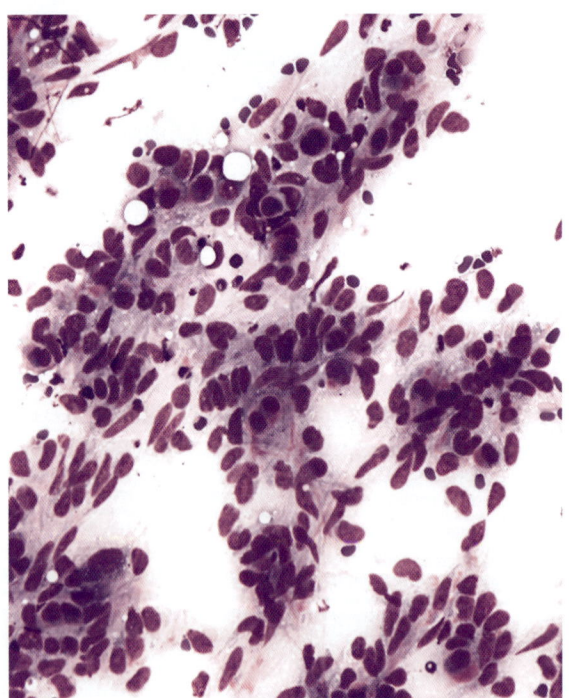
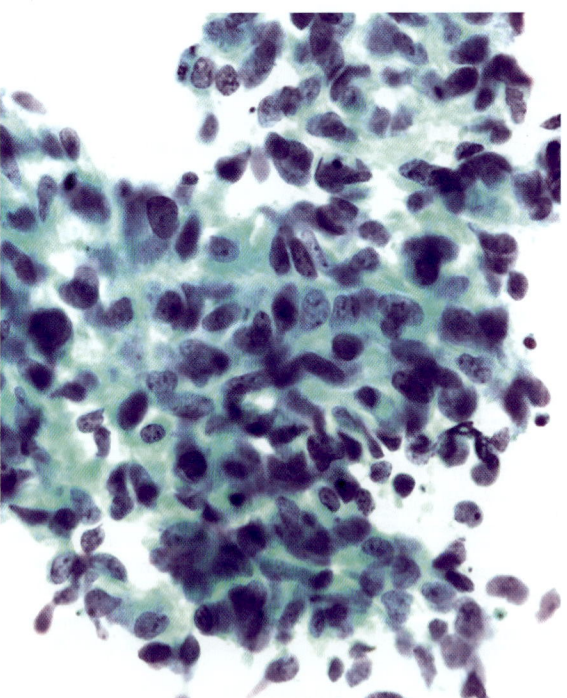

Figure 63-28

ANGIOSARCOMA INVOLVING SPLEEN

Aspirate smears of angiosarcoma show loosely cohesive clusters of spindled to epithelioid tumor cells (left: Diff-Quik stain; right: Papanicolaou stain).

Immunophenotypic Findings. Vascular-associated markers are present in most cases of splenic angiosarcoma and include CD31, CD34, factor VIII, ERG, FLI1, and Ulex europaeus (17,37). Vimentin is positive in virtually all cases (17). S-100 protein is positive in a subset of cases (37). Some cases are positive for CD68 (37) and, less commonly, CD8, suggesting derivation from splenic sinusoidal endothelium (i.e., littoral cell origin) (45,46). Angiosarcomas with epithelioid differentiation may be positive for epithelial-associated markers, such as various keratins.

Many angiosarcomas are partially or strongly positive for lymphatic-related antigens including D2-40/podoplanin, VEGFR3, and LYVE1 (20,37). These results suggest possible lymphatic derivation for some of these neoplasms, although a lack of differentiation also may account for aberrant expression. At present, distinguishing lymphatic from endothelial-derived vascular neoplasms is not associated with prognosis or therapeutic decisions.

Molecular Genetic Findings. Little is known about the underlying genetics of angiosarcoma arising at any anatomic site (24). In the small number of cases that have been assessed, complex karyotypes are common. The most common chromosomal imbalances are gains of 5p, 8p, and 20p; losses of 4p and 7p; and aberrations involving 20q (24).

Differential Diagnosis. *Low-Grade Vascular Lesions.* In benign or low-grade vascular tumors, areas of cytologic atypia can mimic angiosarcoma. Individual areas of an angiosarcoma also may deceptively resemble a benign vascular neoplasm and therefore incomplete sampling, for example needle biopsy, can lead to misdiagnosis (12,17,37). In an adequate tissue biopsy sample, angiosarcoma is characterized by cytologic atypia, mitotic figures, and tufting of endothelial cells, unlike benign or low-grade vascular neoplasms.

Diffuse hemangiomatosis and diffuse lymphangiomatosis are congenital conditions with multiple organ involvement by hemangiomas. The extent of involvement may raise the possibility of angiosarcoma. However, cytologic atypia and mitotic activity are absent in these congenital lesions, unlike angiosarcoma.

Other Types of Sarcoma. High-grade variants of angiosarcoma may be confused with other types of sarcoma. In older publications, some angiosarcomas were regarded as examples of malignant fibrous histiocytoma. Metastatic poorly differentiated carcinoma or melanoma also may be considered. The presence of unequivocal vascular channel formation by neoplastic cells is a helpful histologic finding in angiosarcoma. Lacking morphologic evidence, confirmation of the endothelial nature of the neoplasm, usually by immunohistochemistry, is required to support the diagnosis of angiosarcoma.

Treatment and Prognosis. If the neoplasm is localized, surgical resection is indicated. Nevertheless, patients with splenic angiosarcoma have a poor prognosis with a median survival of only months (37,47,53). The features associated with a poorer outcome include older patient age, large tumor size, and high proliferation (Ki-67) rate. A retroperitoneal location (presumably including splenic tumors) is associated with a poorer prognosis. Splenic rupture, often associated with early metastases, is also associated with a worse prognosis (1,17,37).

Metastases are frequent in patients with splenic angiosarcoma, occurring in over 85 percent and often occurring early in the course of disease (1,17,37,47). Metastases (in order of frequency) occur to the liver, lungs, bones or bone marrow, lymph nodes, gastrointestinal tract, brain, and adrenal glands (17,37). Metastases to bone marrow are usually associated with fibrosis and we have observed a case of splenic angiosarcoma metastatic to bone marrow that mimicked a myeloproliferative neoplasm (primary myelofibrosis) (28).

REFERENCES

1. Abbott RM, Levy AD, Aguilera NS, Gorospe L, Thompson WM. From the archives of the AFIP: primary vascular neoplasms of the spleen: radiologic-pathologic correlation. Radiographics 2004;24:1137-1163.

2. Abramowsky C, Alvarado C, Wyly JB, Ricketts R. "Hamartoma" of the spleen (splenoma) in children. Pediatr Dev Pathol 2004;7:231-236.

3. Ben-Izhak O, Bejar J, Ben-Eliezer S, Vlodavsky E. Splenic littoral cell haemangioendothelioma: a new low-grade variant of malignant littoral cell tumour. Histopathology 2001;39:469-475.

4. Berman E, Ikpatt F, Wang D, Dembner A, Zauber NP. Rapid progression of littoral cell angioma of the spleen in a man with multiple infections. Rare Tumors 2010;2:e17.

5. Bhutani M, Polizzotto MN, Uldrick TS, Yarchoan R. Kaposi sarcoma-associated herpesvirus-associated malignancies: epidemiology, pathogenesis, and advances in treatment. Semin Oncol 2015;42:223-246.

6. Bierenbaum J, Alapat DV, Godinez C, Park AE, Zhao XF, Baer MR. Littoral cell angioma: a correctable cause of progressive pancytopenia in a patient with myelodysplastic syndrome. Leuk Res 2010;34:e117-119.

7. Boudousquie AC, Lawce HJ, Sherman R, Olson S, Magenis RE, Corless CL. Complex translocation [7;22] identified in an epithelioid hemangioendothelioma. Cancer Genet Cytogenet 1996;92:116-121.

8. Cappello M, Bravatà I, Cocorullo G, Cacciatore M, Florena AM. Splenic littoral cell hemangioendothelioma in a patient with Crohn's disease previously treated with immunomodulators and anti-TNF agents: a rare tumor linked to deep immunosuppression. Am J Gastroenterol 2011;106:1863-1865.

9. Casalone R, Albini A, Righi R, Granata P, Toniolo A. Nonrandom chromosome changes in Kaposi sarcoma: cytogenetic and FISH results in a new cell line (KS-IMM) and literature review. Cancer Genet Cytogenet 2001;124:16-19.

9a. Chang KC, Lee JC, Wang YC, et al. Polyclonality in sclerosing angiomatoid nodular transformation of the spleen. Am J Surg Pathol 2016;40:1343-1351.

10. Cheuk W, Lee AK, Arora N, Ben-Arie Y, Chan JK. Splenic hamartoma with bizarre stromal cells. Am J Surg Pathol 2005;29:109-114.

11. Chiu A, Czader M, Cheng L, et al. Clonal X-chromosome inactivation suggests that splenic cord capillary hemangioma is a true neoplasm and not a subtype of splenic hamartoma. Mod Pathol 2011;24:108-116.

12. Chun YS, Robu VG. Spectrum of primary vascular neoplasms of the spleen. J Clin Oncol 2011;29:e116-117.

13. Compton CN, McHenry CR, Aijazi M, Chung-Park M. Thrombocytopenia caused by splenic hamartoma: resolution after splenectomy. South Med J 2001;94:542-544.

14. Dekeyzer S, Houthoofd B, De Potter A, Van Bockstal M, Smeets P, Vogelaers D. Hemangiomatosis of the spleen in a patient with Klippel-trénaunay syndrome. JBR-BTR 2013;96:357-359.

15. Delacruz V, Jorda M, Gomez-Fernandez C, Benedetto P, Ganjei P. Fine-needle aspiration diagnosis of angiosarcoma of the spleen: a case report and review of the literature. Arch Pathol Lab Med 2005;129:1054-1056.

16. Doyle LA, Fletcher CD, Hornick JL. Nuclear expression of CAMTA1 distinguishes epithelioid hemangioendothelioma from histologic mimics. Am J Surg Pathol 2016;40:94-102.

17. Falk S, Krishnan J, Meis JM. Primary angiosarcoma of the spleen. A clinicopathologic study of 40 cases. Am J Surg Pathol 1993;17:959-970.

18. Falk S, Stutte HJ. Hamartomas of the spleen: a study of 20 biopsy cases. Histopathology 1989;14:603-612.

19. Falk S, Stutte HJ, Frizzera G. Littoral cell angioma. A novel splenic vascular lesion demonstrating histiocytic differentiation. Am J Surg Pathol 1991;15:1023-1033.

20. Folpe AL, Veikkola T, Valtola R, Weiss SW. Vascular endothelial growth factor receptor-3 (VEGFR-3): a marker of vascular tumors with presumed lymphatic differentiation, including Kaposi's sarcoma, kaposiform and Dabska-type hemangioendotheliomas, and a subset of angiosarcomas. Mod Pathol 2000;13:180-185.

21. Gamborino E, Carrilho C, Ferro J, et al. Fine-needle aspiration diagnosis of Kaposi's sarcoma in a developing country. Diagn Cytopathol 2000;23:322-325.

22. Gill R, O'Donnell RJ, Horvai A. Utility of immunohistochemistry for endothelial markers in distinguishing epithelioid hemangioendothelioma from carcinoma metastatic to bone. Arch Pathol Lab Med 2009;133:967-972.

23. Giordano G, Gnetti L. Spontaneous rupture of spleen: histological, immunohistochemical and ultrastructural study. Adv Clin Path 2003;7:39-45.

24. Guillou L, Aurias A. Soft tissue sarcomas with complex genomic profiles. Virchows Arch 2010;456:201-217.

25. Harmon RL, Cerruto CA, Scheckner A. Littoral cell angioma: a case report and review. Curr Surg 2006;63:345-350.

26. Hayes TC, Britton HA, Mewborne EB, Troyer DA, Saldivar VA, Ratner IA. Symptomatic splenic hamartoma: case report and literature review. Pediatrics 1998;101:E10.

27. Hsu JT, Ueng SH, Hwang TL, Chen HM, Jan YY, Chen MF. Primary angiosarcoma of the spleen in a child with long-term survival. Pediatr Surg Int 2007;23:807-810.

28. Hu S, Bueso-Ramos CE, Verstovsek S, et al. Metastatic splenic angiosarcoma presenting with thrombocytopenia and bone marrow fibrosis mimicking idiopathic thrombocytopenic purpura and primary myelofibrosis: a diagnostic challenge. Clin Lymphoma Myeloma Leuk 2013;13:629-633.

29. Huang Y, Mu G, Qin X, Lin J, Li S, Zeng Y. 21 case reports on haemangioma of spleen. J Cancer Res Ther 2016;12:1323.

30. Kranzfelder M, Bauer M, Richter T, et al. Littoral cell angioma and angiosarcoma of the spleen: report of two cases in siblings and review of the literature. J Gastrointest Surg 2012;16:863-867.

31. Kraus MD, Dehner LP. Benign vascular neoplasms of the spleen with myoid and angioendotheliomatous features. Histopathology 1999;35:328-336.

32. Krishnan J, Frizzera G. Two splenic lesions in need of clarification: hamartoma and inflammatory pseudotumor. Semin Diagn Pathol 2003;20:94-104.

33. Kutok JL, Fletcher CD. Splenic vascular tumors. Semin Diagn Pathol 2003;20:128-139.

34. Larsen BT, Bishop MC, Hunter GC, Renner SW. Low-grade, metastasizing splenic littoral cell angiosarcoma presenting with hepatic cirrhosis and splenic artery aneurysm. Int J Surg Pathol 2013;21:618-626.

35. Lee H, Maeda K. Hamartoma of the spleen. Arch Pathol Lab Med 2009;133:147-151.

36. Martel M, Cheuk W, Lombardi L, Lifschitz-Mercer B, Chan JK, Rosai J. Sclerosing angiomatoid nodular transformation (SANT): report of 25 cases of a distinctive benign splenic lesion. Am J Surg Pathol 2004;28:1268-1279.

37. Neuhauser TS, Derringer GA, Thompson LD, et al. Splenic angiosarcoma: a clinicopathologic and immunophenotypic study of 28 cases. Mod Pathol 2000;13:978-987.

38. Pampin C, Devillers A, Treguier C, et al. Intratumoral consumption of indium-111-labeled platelets in a child with splenic hemangioma and thrombocytopenia. J Pediatr Hematol Oncol 2000;22:256-258.

39. Patel NR, Salim AA, Sayeed H, et al. Molecular characterization of epithelioid haemangioendotheliomas identifies novel WWTR1–CAMTA1 fusion variants. Histopathology 2015;67:699-708.

40. Pilz JB, Sperschneider T, Lutz T, Loosli B, Maurer CA. Littoral cell angioma in main and accessory intrapancreatic spleen presenting as splenic rupture. Am J Surg 2011;201:e15-17.

41. Pohar-Marinsek Z, Lamovec J. Angiosarcoma in FNA smears: diagnostic accuracy, morphology, immunocytochemistry and differential diagnoses. Cytopathology 2010;21:311-319.

42. Pradhan D, Mohanty SK. Sclerosing angiomatoid nodular transformation of the spleen. Arch Pathol Lab Med 2013;137:1309-1312.

43. Pyakurel P, Montag U, Castaños-Vélez E, et al. CGH of microdissected Kaposi's sarcoma lesions reveals recurrent loss of chromosome Y in early and additional chromosomal changes in late tumour stages. AIDS 2006;20:1805-1812.

44. Rosado FG, Itani DM, Coffin CM, Cates JM. Utility of immunohistochemical staining with FLI1, D2-40, CD31, and CD34 in the diagnosis of acquired immunodeficiency syndrome-related and non-acquired immunodeficiency syndrome-related Kaposi sarcoma. Arch Pathol Lab Med 2012;136:301-304.

45. Rosso R, Paulli M. Littoral cell angiosarcoma: a truly malignant tumor. Am J Surg Pathol 2004;28:1255.

46. Rosso R, Paulli M, Gianelli U, Boveri E, Stella G, Magrini U. Littoral cell angiosarcoma of the spleen. Case report with immunohistochemical and ultrastructural analysis. Am J Surg Pathol 1995;19:1203-1208.

47. Sordillo EM, Sordillo PP, Hajdu SI. Primary hemangiosarcoma of the spleen: report of four cases. Med Pediatr Oncol 1981;9:319-324.

48. Steinberg JJ, Suhrland M, Valensi Q. The spleen in the spleen syndrome: the association of splenoma with hematopoietic and neoplastic disease--compendium of cases since 1864. J Surg Oncol 1991;47:193-202.

49. Tajima S, Koda K. A case of cord capillary hemangioma of the spleen: a recently proven true neoplasm. Pathol Int 2015;65:254-258.

50. Theurillat JP, Vavricka SR, Went P, et al. Morphologic changes and altered gene expression in an epithelioid hemangioendothelioma during a ten-year course of disease. Pathol Res Pract 2003;199:165-170.

51. Tong GX, Hamele-Gena D, Borczuk A, Monaco S, Khosh MM, Greenebaum E. Fine needle aspiration biopsy of epithelioid hemangioendothelioma of the oral cavity: report of one case and review of the literature. Diagn Cytopathol 2006;34:218-223.

52. Tsarouha H, Kyriazoglou AI, Ribeiro FR, Teixeira MR, Agnantis N, Pandis N. Chromosome analysis and molecular cytogenetic investigations of an epithelioid hemangioendothelioma. Cancer Genet Cytogenet 2006;169:164-168.

53. Valbuena JR, Levenback C, Mansfield P, Liu J. Angiosarcoma of the spleen clinically presenting as metastatic ovarian cancer. A case report and review of the literature. Ann Diagn Pathol 2005;9:289-292.

53a. Wang TB, Hu BG, Liu DW, Gao ZH, Shi HP, Dong WG. Sclerosing angiomatoid nodular transformation of the spleen: A case report and literature review. Oncol Lett 2016;12:928-932.

54. Wang Z, Zhang L, Zhang B, Mu D, Cui K, Li S. Hemangioendothelioma arising from the spleen: a case report and literature review. Oncol Lett 2015;9:209-212.

55. Weinreb I, Cunningham KS, Perez-Ordoñez B, Hwang DM. CD10 is expressed in most epithelioid hemangioendotheliomas: a potential diagnostic pitfall. Arch Pathol Lab Med 2009;133:1965-1968.

56. Willcox TM, Speer RW, Schlinkert RT, Sarr MG. Hemangioma of the spleen: presentation, diagnosis, and management. J Gastrointest Surg 2000;4:611-613.

57. Yu L, Yang SJ. Kaposiform hemangioendothelioma of the spleen in an adult: an initial case report. Pathol Oncol Res 2011;17:969-972.

58. Zukerberg LR, Kaynor BL, Silverman ML, Harris NL. Splenic hamartoma and capillary hemangioma are distinct entities: immunohistochemical analysis of CD8 expression by endothelial cells. Hum Pathol 1991;22:1258-1261.

64 STROMAL TUMORS AND TUMOR-LIKE LESIONS OF THE SPLEEN

GENERAL FEATURES

Stromal tumors and tumor-like lesions of the spleen are a heterogeneous and rare group of diseases that usually present as a mass lesion and are characterized histologically by a proliferation of spindled cells associated with a mixed inflammatory infiltrate. This group of diseases includes: *inflammatory pseudotumor of the spleen, inflammatory pseudotumor-like follicular dendritic cell tumor,* and *inflammatory myofibroblastic tumor.* In the literature, these three terms have been used somewhat interchangeably and the diagnostic criteria used to distinguish between these entities are not entirely defined.

Historically, inflammatory pseudotumor of the spleen has been used as a catchall designation for rare mass lesions that occur in the spleen. As the name implies, most patients have a benign clinical course. In a review published in 2013, Ma et al. (20) identified 114 cases of inflammatory pseudotumor of the spleen in the literature. However, as our understanding of these lesions has increased, the heterogeneous nature of these tumors has been recognized. It now seems clear that cases once designated as inflammatory pseudotumor of the spleen include cases of unknown etiology as well as true monoclonal neoplasms. For cases of unknown etiology still designated as inflammatory pseudotumor of the spleen, an infectious etiology seems likely, at least in many cases, and an unusual tissue response to infection (or other type of injury) also has been postulated. The neoplastic group of lesions includes tumors highly associated with Epstein-Barr virus (EBV) infection, which is a suspected etiologic agent (1,14,17) and cases associated with characteristic genetic alterations (e.g., anaplastic lymphoma kinase [*ALK*] rearrangements) known to be involved in oncogenesis (2,19).

CLINICAL FEATURES

Although the different stromal tumors and tumor-like lesions of the spleen are biologically distinct, their clinical and pathologic findings overlap, likely explaining the historical use of the term inflammatory pseudotumor. The age range of patients with splenic stromal tumors and tumor-like lesions is broad, ranging from 6 to 81 years, with a median age of 47 years (20). There is a slight dominance of women with a male to female ratio of 1.0 to 1.3 (14,20,28).

About one third of patients are symptomatic and present with left upper quadrant abdominal pain or a sense of fullness (20,28). Fever occurs in 5 to 10 percent of patients (20). The remaining two thirds are asymptomatic and a spleen mass is detected incidentally during the workup of other presenting symptoms or physical findings.

Imaging studies highlight a distinct mass in the spleen that may be small or large, with cases over 20 cm reported (14,20,25). A splenic mass is detected by a variety of imaging techniques including ultrasound, computerized tomography (CT) (fig. 64-1), magnetic resonance imaging (MRI), and 18F-fluorodeoxyglucose positron emission tomography (18F-FDG-PET). The splenic mass is often heterogeneous and of low density; calcifications are present in some lesions and these masses may be 18F-FDG-PET avid (25).

Although the diagnosis of a splenic stromal tumor or tumor-like lesion may be suspected by the clinical history and radiologic findings, in most patients definitive diagnosis depends on splenectomy. In a few patients, however, the diagnosis of inflammatory pseudotumor of spleen has been successfully established by fine-needle aspiration analysis (11,22).

GROSS AND HISTOLOGIC FINDINGS

Stromal tumors and tumor-like lesions of the spleen have similar gross features. Usually, there is a solitary, circumscribed, white or tan mass; foci of necrosis are common (fig. 64-2) (14,20,28). The size can be variable. The borders of the mass may be well-circumscribed or vague and indefinite. Rarely, multiple nodules are seen.

Histologically, the lesions have pushing peripheral borders and are not encapsulated (20). Adjacent splenic parenchyma may be compressed but is otherwise not affected. It seems likely that stromal tumors and tumor-like lesions of the spleen are evolving and dynamic disease processes, and that their gross and histologic features depend on the stage of evolution.

Inflammatory Pseudotumor

Inflammatory pseudotumor of the spleen, a tumor-like process, is the most common of these rare lesions. Although over 100 cases have been reported in the literature (20), the true number is likely less (as discussed above). In most patients with inflammatory pseudotumor of the spleen, an etiology cannot be determined; in others, a review of their history may suggest an associated infectious etiology, but cultures of blood or splenic tissue are usually negative for organisms.

Inflammatory pseudotumor of spleen is composed of a proliferation of bland-appearing spindle cells arranged in a more or less storiform pattern that is associated with marked vascularity, a mixed inflammatory cell infiltrate, and often a collagenous background (figs. 64-3–64-5) (15,16,28). The spindled cells are few or numerous. The mixed inflammatory cell infiltrate is composed of lymphocytes, histiocytes, and plasma cells in most cases, but also neutrophils and eosinophils in some lesions. Areas of recent or older hemorrhage may be present with hemosiderin-laden histiocytes. There may be multinucleated and giant histiocytes. Plasma cells may be numerous and may show binucleation, intracytoplasmic globules (Russell bodies), or intranuclear pseudoinclusions (Dutcher bodies). The plasma cells also may show enlarged nuclei, although nucleoli are minimal or absent. Areas of necrosis can be seen, especially within the central portion of the mass. Extensive sclerosis may be present in a subset of cases. In rare cases, a prominent non-necrotizing chronic granulomatous reaction is present (29).

Postchemotherapy Histiocyte-Rich Pseudotumor of the Spleen. This lesion is a distinctive form of inflammatory pseudotumor. It occurs in patients with a history of lymphoma, most often diffuse large B-cell lymphoma, who have been treated with multiagent chemotherapy (3). These lesions are tumor-like masses that are composed of necrotic ghosts of cells, numerous histiocytes (that are often lipid-laden), a variable degree of hemorrhage and coagulative necrosis, and often spindled fibroblasts and lymphocytes (fig. 64-6).

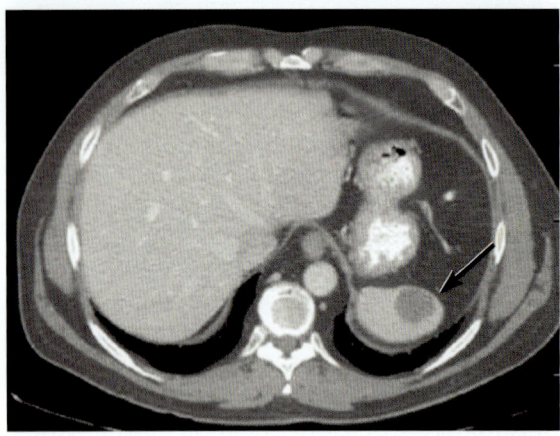

Figure 64-1

SMALL INFLAMMATORY PSEUDOTUMOR OF SPLEEN

In this computerized tomography (CT) scan, the arrow points to a hypodense mass within the spleen.

Figure 64-2

INFLAMMATORY PSEUDOTUMOR OF SPLEEN

Gross image of the same patient as in figure 64-1 shows no apparent capsule. The central portion shows a variegated yellow-white-tan appearance with some focal hemorrhage. Most cases of inflammatory pseudotumor of the spleen have a similar gross appearance. (Courtesy of Dr. C. Bueso-Ramos, Houston, TX.)

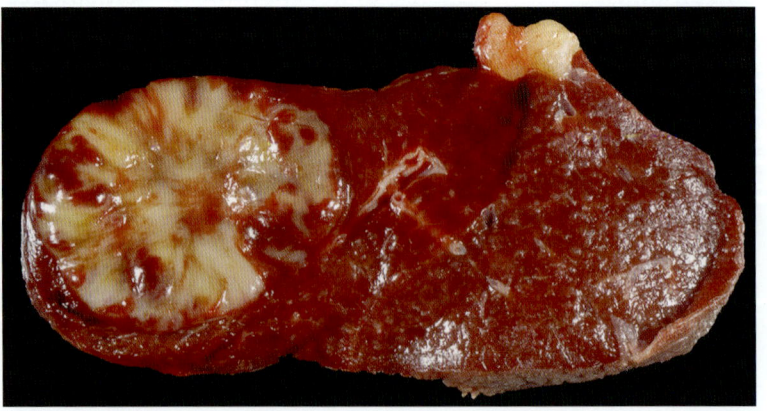

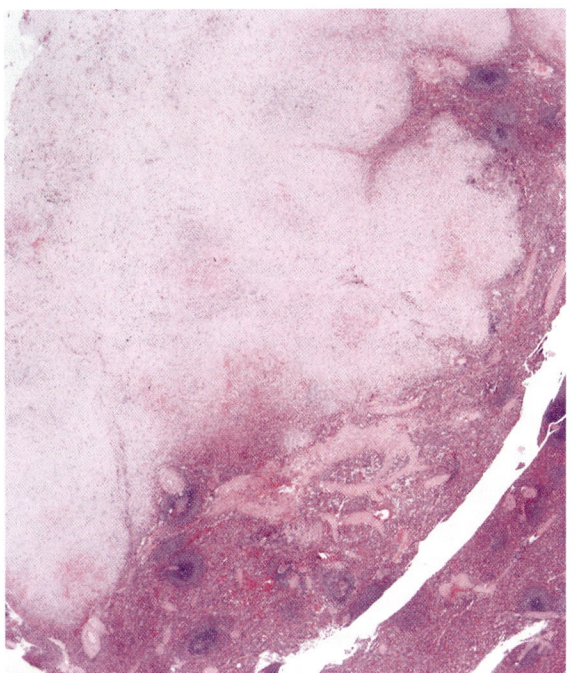 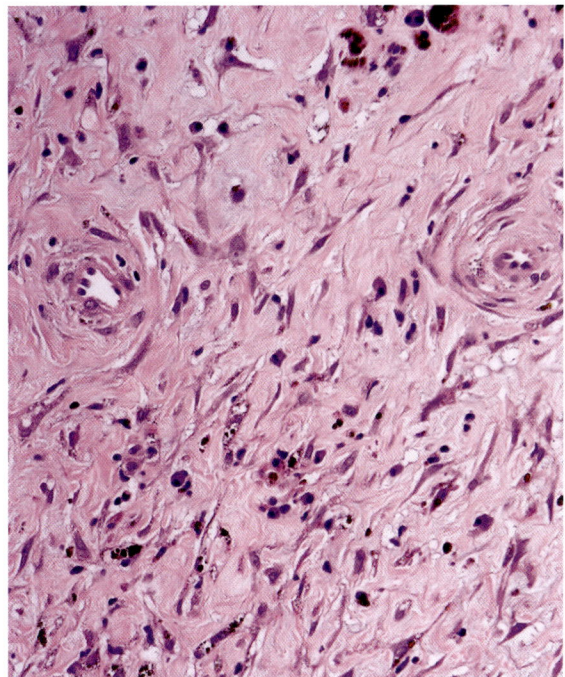

Figure 64-3

INFLAMMATORY PSEUDOTUMOR OF SPLEEN

Left: A capsule cannot be appreciated at this low magnification of the same tumor as shown in figures 64-1 and 64-2.

Right: The mass is hypocellular and composed of spindled cells, hemosiderin-laden macrophages, plasma cells, and lymphocytes with a collagenous background. An infectious etiology was suspected but unproven in this patient (hematoxylin and eosin [H&E] stain).

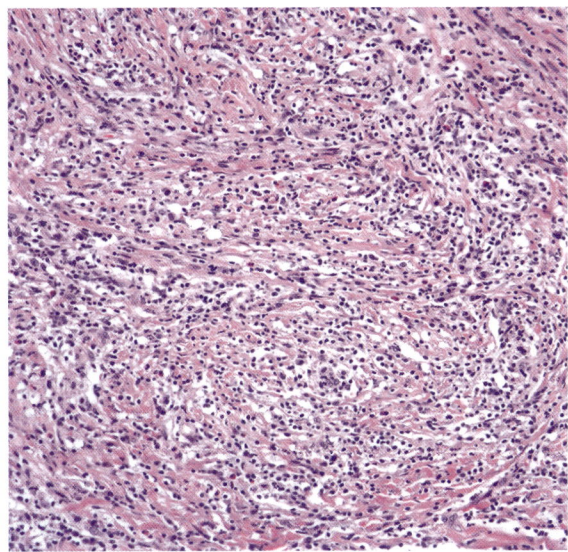 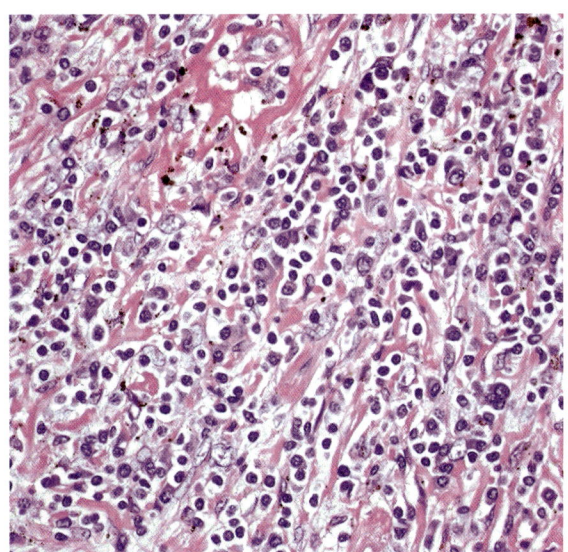

Figure 64-4	**Figure 64-5**
INFLAMMATORY PSEUDOTUMOR OF SPLEEN	**INFLAMMATORY PSEUDOTUMOR OF SPLEEN**
This lesion is more cellular, and scattered streaming bands of spindle-shaped cells with a polymorphous cellular infiltrate are seen (H&E stain).	Numerous plasma cells and small lymphocytes are present in a background of sclerosis in this case (H&E stain).

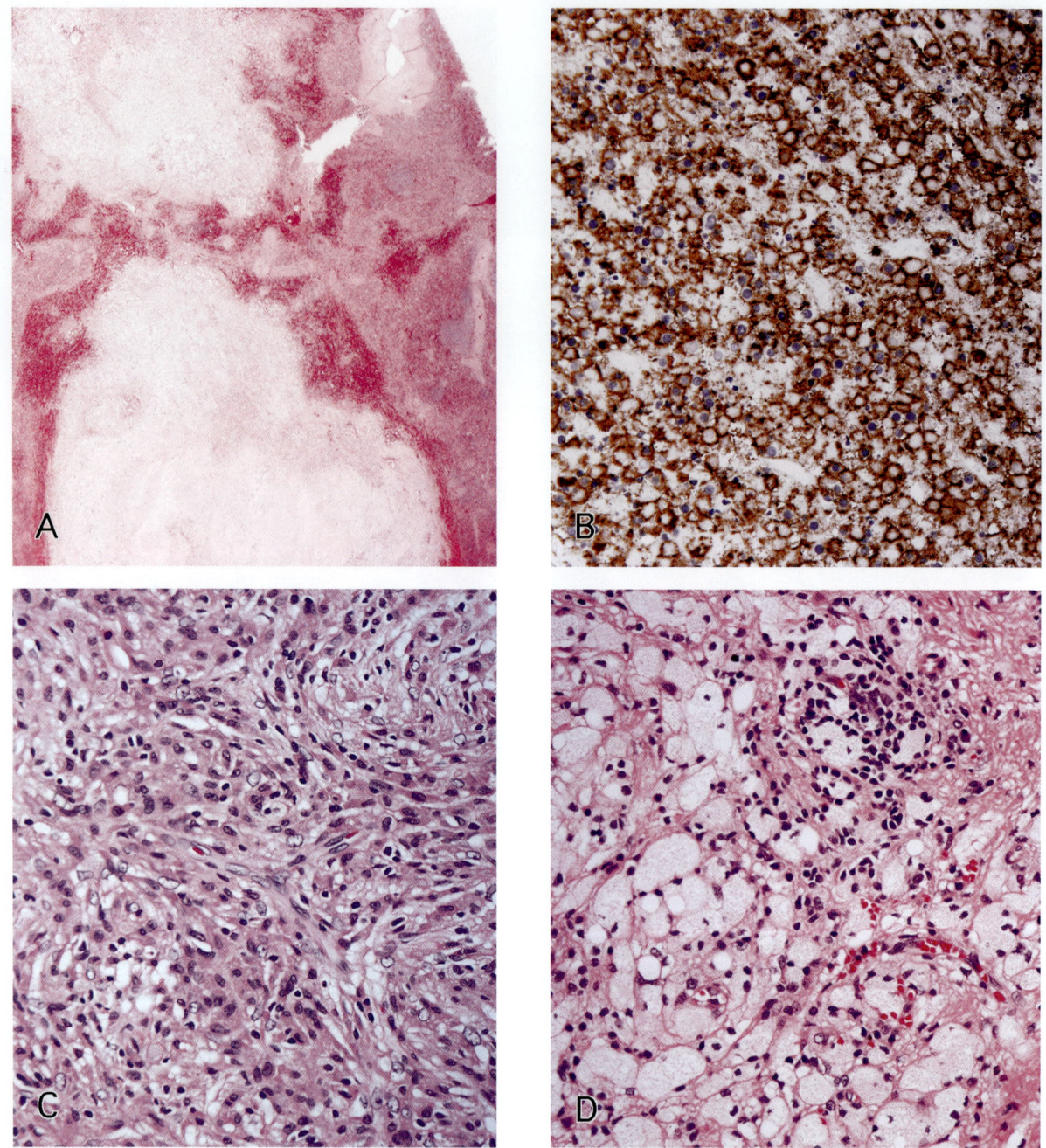

Figure 64-6

POSTCHEMOTHERAPY HISTIOCYTE-RICH PSEUDOTUMOR INVOLVING SPLEEN

These rare lesions occur in patients with lymphoma following chemotherapy and appear to be an exuberant reaction to tumor necrosis. This patient had a history of diffuse large B-cell lymphoma.

A: At low magnification, large nodules with central necrosis associated with an inflammatory reaction replace the splenic parenchyma.

B: Immunohistochemistry for CD20 highlights ghosts of necrotic lymphoma cells.

C: Some areas of these lesions are composed of spindled cells and histiocytes, and resemble inflammatory pseudotumor of the spleen.

D: Other areas show abundant lipid-laden histiocytes. (A,C,D: H&E stain; B: immunohistochemistry with hematoxylin counterstain).

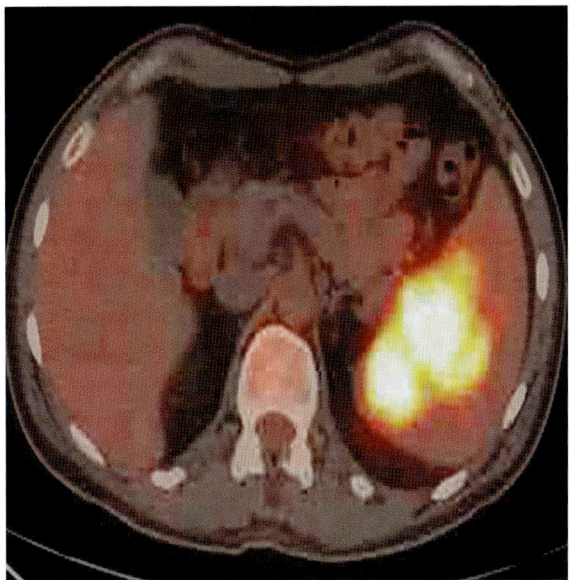

Figure 64-7

INFLAMMATORY PSEUDOTUMOR-LIKE FOLLICULAR DENDRITIC CELL TUMOR OF SPLEEN

CT/positron emission tomography (PET) scan shows a large lesion that is metabolically active.

Inflammatory Pseudotumor-Like Follicular Dendritic Cell Tumor

Inflammatory pseudotumor-like follicular dendritic cell tumor of the spleen is a monoclonal and neoplastic proliferation of follicular dendritic cells (4-6,18). These lesions are rare: about 35 well-characterized cases have been reported in the literature (10). Patients are most often women. In the older literature, cases were designated as EBV-positive inflammatory pseudotumor of the spleen (1,27). It seems likely that some of these cases, if the lesions had been assessed more rigorously by immunohistochemical methods for follicular dendritic cell (FDC) markers, would be currently designated as inflammatory pseudotumor-like follicular dendritic cell tumor.

Radiologically and grossly, inflammatory pseudotumor-like follicular dendritic cell tumor of the spleen can resemble inflammatory pseudotumor of the spleen (figs. 64-7, 64-8). Histologically, these tumors are composed of spindled FDCs associated with a variable mixed inflammatory infiltrate (fig. 64-9) (4–6). The spindled cells are usually bland, but can be larger with nucleoli resembling Hodgkin cells in some

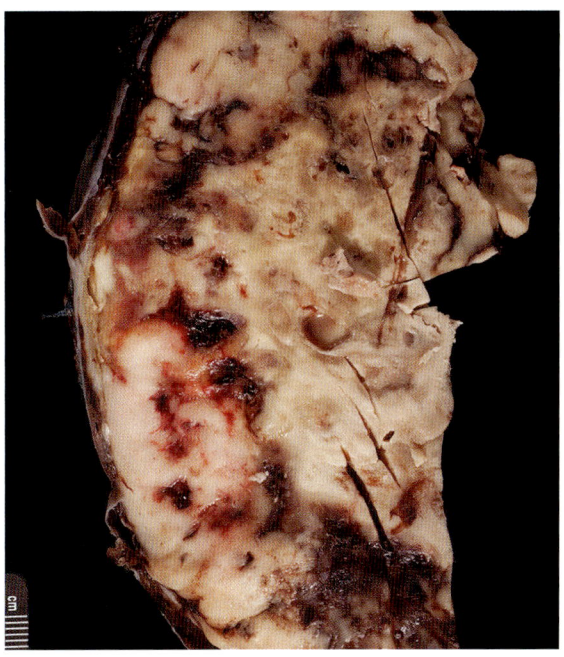

Figure 64-8

INFLAMMATORY PSEUDOTUMOR-LIKE FOLLICULAR DENDRITIC CELL TUMOR OF SPLEEN

The lesion is firm, tan-white, with areas of hemorrhage and compresses uninvolved spleen. No capsule is identified.

cases (11a). The inflammatory cells include numerous small lymphocytes, histiocytes, plasma cells, and granulocytes. In some cases, marked chronic granulomatous inflammation or numerous granulocytes (eosinophils or neutrophils) are present (18). Immunohistochemical and in situ hybridization studies for EBV are essential for establishing the diagnosis (see below) (fig. 64-9).

Inflammatory Myofibroblastic Tumor

Inflammatory myofibroblastic tumor is a monoclonal neoplasm of myofibroblastic cells (7). These neoplasms have been reported at many anatomic sites throughout the body, most often in the abdomen or pelvis and the lungs (7). Rare cases involve the spleen (13,23).

The symptoms are usually local and related to the anatomic site of involvement, but 10 to 20 percent of patients present with fever, weight loss, and various laboratory abnormalities such as anemia, elevated erythrocyte sedimentation rate, and thrombocytosis (7). Inflammatory myofibroblastic tumors exhibit features of low-grade malignant neoplasms. Local recurrences,

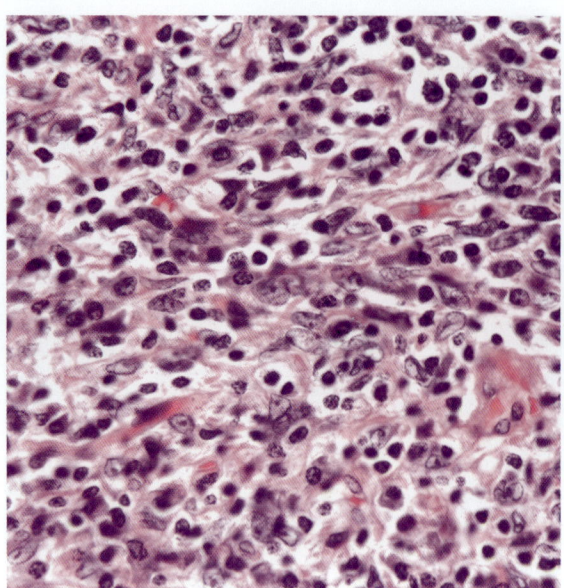 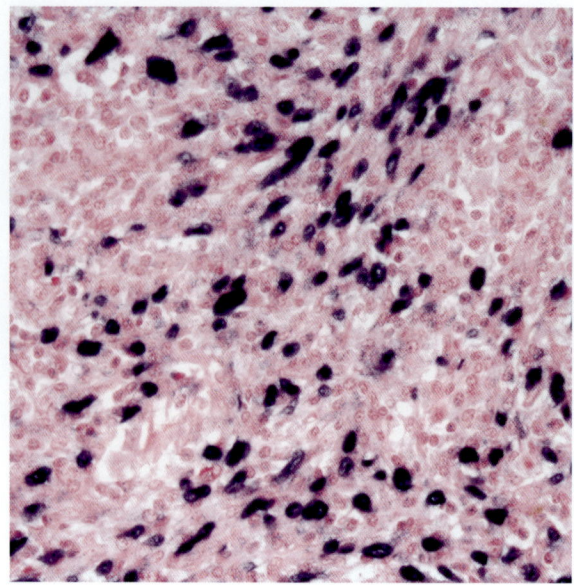

Figure 64-9

INFLAMMATORY PSEUDOTUMOR-LIKE FOLLICULAR DENDRITIC CELL TUMOR OF SPLEEN

Left: In this field, many spindled cells are associated with a prominent lymphoplasmacytic infiltrate.
Right: The spindled cells are positive for Epstein-Barr virus (EBV) and were also positive for follicular dendritic cell markers (not shown) (right: H&E stain; left: in situ hybridization for EBER1 with eosin counterstain).

including multiple recurrences occur, particularly when tumors involve the abdomen and pelvis, but distant metastases are uncommon (7).

Inflammatory myofibroblastic tumors consist of a proliferation of spindled cells associated with a background of lymphocytes, histiocytes, and plasma cells, with a variable number of eosinophils (fig. 64-10) (7,19). Neutrophils are uncommon. Sclerosis is variable. The histologic features associated with more aggressive behavior include hypercellularity, a prominent storiform pattern, necrosis, epithelioid cells, and cytologic atypia (7).

IMMUNOPHENOTYPIC FINDINGS

Inflammatory Pseudotumor of Spleen

Histochemical stains for microorganisms are warranted in some of cases, particularly when large areas of necrosis or a granulomatous infiltrate is present. Usually these stains are negative (28).

Immunohistochemical analysis of inflammatory pseudotumor of the spleen is essential to exclude mimics. The spindled cells are often positive for vimentin and may express (usually focally) smooth muscle actin, but are negative for FDC-associated markers. The inflammatory cells present are composed of a mixture of predominantly T cells with fewer B cells, the latter often in small follicles. Histiocytes are present (CD68 and CD163 positive) and scattered immunoblasts may be present that express CD30 and are negative for CD15. Plasma cells are polytypic (28).

EBV has been described in a subset of cases designated as inflammatory pseudotumor in the literature (1,14,17,24,26). Many of these EBV-positive cases are incompletely described and robust immunohistochemical analysis to exclude a follicular dendritic cell tumor was not performed. It seems likely that some of these cases are truly inflammatory pseudotumor-like follicular dendritic cell tumors; it is also seems likely that a few cases of inflammatory pseudotumor of the spleen have a small subset of EBV-positive cells.

In cases of postchemotherapy histiocyte-rich pseudotumor of the spleen, the cell ghosts often express CD20 or other B-cell antigens consistent with necrotic B-cell lymphoma, but in some cases relatively few cells are reactive with B-cell antibodies (3). The small lymphocytes are T cells and histiocytes express CD68 and CD163.

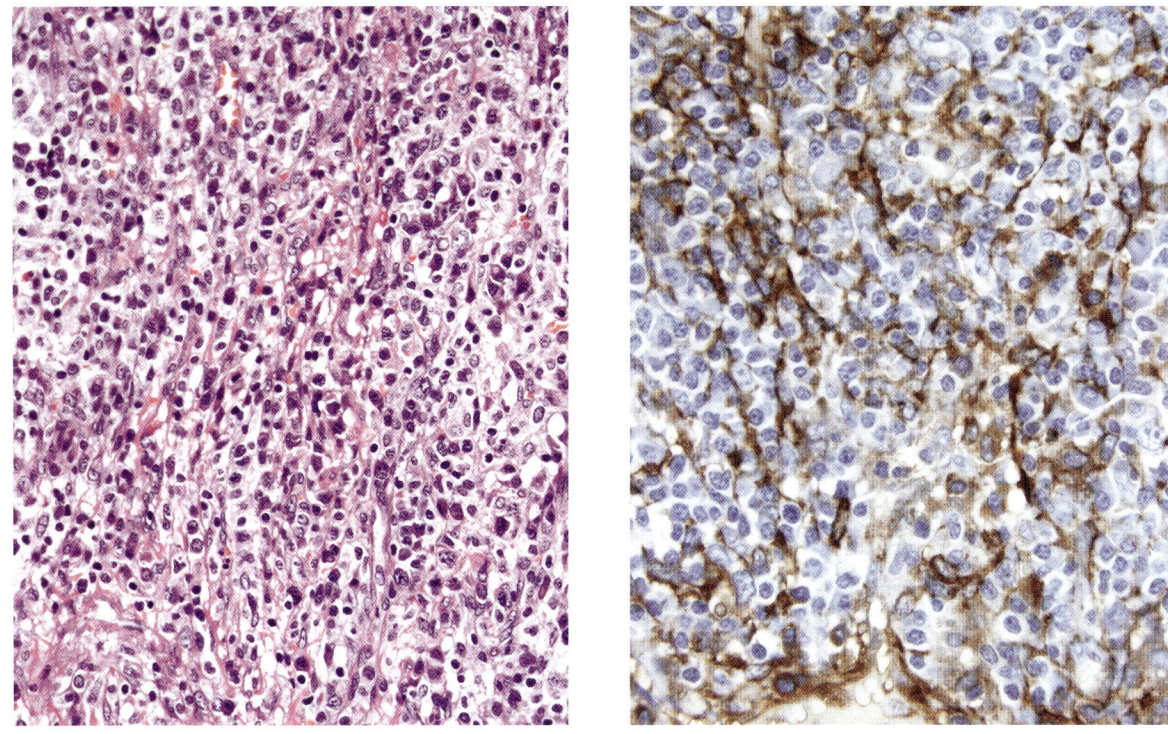

Figure 64-10

INFLAMMATORY MYOFIBROBLASTIC TUMOR OF SPLEEN

Left: The cellular infiltrate is very similar to true inflammatory pseudotumor of spleen (H&E stain).

Right: The spindled cells are positive for smooth muscle actin and had an immunophenotype supporting a myofibroblastic origin (immunohistochemistry with hematoxylin counterstain).

Inflammatory Pseudotumor-Like Follicular Dendritic Cell Tumor

In these tumors, the spindled cells express FDC-associated markers including CD21, CD23, CD35, clusterin, epidermal growth factor receptor (EGFR) as well as others (4,6,18). As expression of one or more of these antigens may be focal or absent, use of a panel of FDC-associated markers is suggested. The spindled cells are almost invariably positive for EBV, best evaluated by in situ hybridization for EBV-encoded RNA1 (EBER1). Many cases are also positive for EBV latent membrane protein type 1 (18). The Inflammatory cells in these lesions are similar to those described above for inflammatory pseudotumor of spleen.

Inflammatory Myofibroblastic Tumor

The spindled cells of these tumors are often reactive with smooth muscle actin (fig. 64-10, right), desmin, and vimentin; variably reactive for CD68; and negative for FDC-associated markers and EBV, supporting a fibroblastic/myofibroblastic origin (7). The spindled cells in most cases also express cyclin D1, MYC, MCL1, MDM2, and p53 and are negative for CD56 and BCL2 (7). ALK is expressed in 40 to 60 percent of cases, usually in a cytoplasmic pattern (2,7,19). ALK expression does not occur in inflammatory pseudotumor or inflammatory pseudotumor-like follicular dendritic cell tumor (5,18). The inflammatory cells in these lesions are similar to those described above in inflammatory pseudotumor of spleen.

MOLECULAR GENETIC FINDINGS

There is no evidence of monoclonal *IGH* or T-cell receptor gene rearrangements in splenic tumors and tumor-like lesions. For inflammatory pseudotumor of the spleen, no recurrent cytogenetic abnormalities have been identified and there are currently no genetic clues pointing to

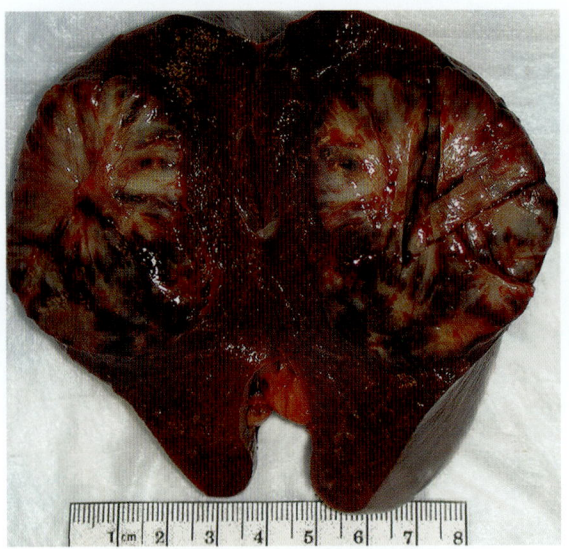

Figure 64-11

**SCLEROSING NODULAR
TRANSFORMATION (SANT) OF SPLEEN**

The gross appearance of this vascular-based lesion is similar to that of inflammatory pseudotumor. (Courtesy of Dr. R. Dewar, Ann Arbor, MI.)

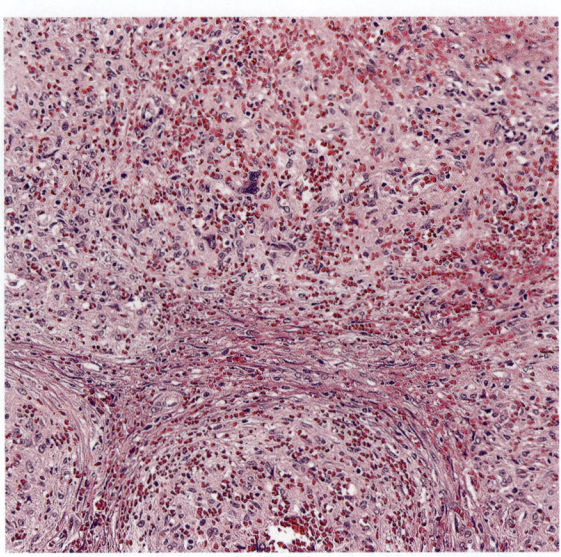

Figure 64-12

SCLEROSING NODULAR TRANSFORMATION OF SPLEEN

The lesion is composed of a proliferation of spindled cells and a lymphoplasmacytic infiltrate. In contrast with inflammatory pseudotumor of spleen, SANT tends to have a nodular pattern and is centered around small to intermediate-sized vascular elements (H&E stain).

a possible etiology or pathogenesis. In cases of inflammatory pseudotumor-like follicular dendritic cell tumor, Southern blot analysis using EBV terminal repeat probes has shown that the virus is present in monoclonal form (17). As this finding indicates that the virus is present at the onset of disease, EBV may be involved in pathogenesis.

Using targeted next-generation sequencing analysis, Lovly et al. (19) showed that up to 85 percent of inflammatory myofibroblastic tumors carry translocations that result in fusion genes. These fusions most often involve *ALK*, but *ROS1*, *PDGRFβ*, and rarely, *RET,* also have been identified (2,19). For fusion genes involving *ALK*, at least 10 different partner genes have been identified. Using conventional cytogenetic analysis or fluorescence in situ hybridization (FISH), translocations/rearrangements involving the 2p23/*ALK* locus can be identified in 40 to 50 percent of inflammatory myofibroblastic tumors (2,7).

Most cases with *ALK* abnormalities also express ALK by immunohistochemistry, but rarely, *ALK* fusion genes have been identified in ALK-negative tumors (19). Fusions involving *ROS1*, *PDGRFβ*, or *RET* have been reported only in the ALK-negative group of tumors (19). Gene fusions are more common in inflammatory

myofibroblastic tumors of children than adults and about 90 percent of fusion-negative cases occur in adults (2).

DIFFERENTIAL DIAGNOSIS

Splenic Hamartoma. These lesions are typically surrounded by a rim of compressed red pulp, usually without associated fibrosis (9,15). Splenic hamartomas are composed predominantly of red pulp structures such as splenic sinuses and cord-like spaces with minimal white pulp. In some cases, histiocytes are prominent. Unlike splenic hamartoma, no splenic sinuses or cord-like spaces are observed in inflammatory pseudotumor of the spleen. Splenic hamartomas lack expression of FDC-associated markers or ALK.

Sclerosing Angiomatoid Nodular Transformation (SANT). These lesions occasionally resemble inflammatory pseudotumor of spleen (figs. 64-11–64-13) (8,21). However, SANT tends to have a predominant component of small blood vessels with increased numbers of histiocytes, and their low-power microscopic pattern often appears to be lobular. Some authors have suggested that all cases of splenic inflammatory pseudotumor are, in fact, SANT (8), but many

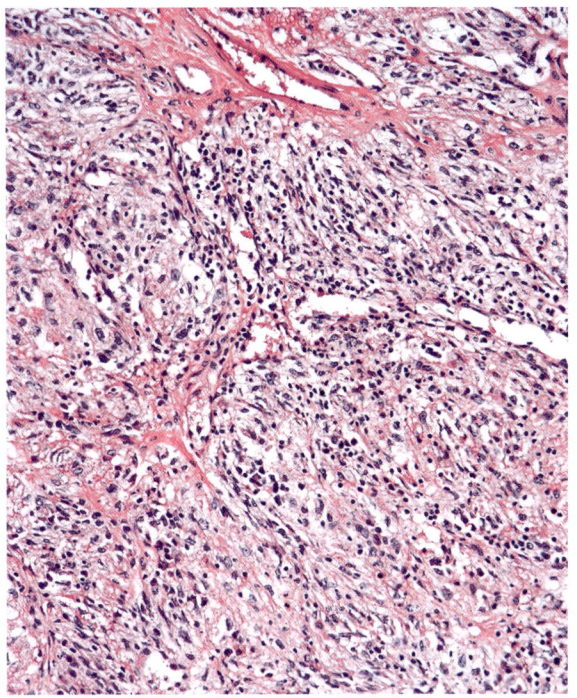

Figure 64-13

SCLEROSING NODULAR TRANSFORMATION OF SPLEEN

Higher-magnification image shows prominent vascular spaces in SANT (H&E stain).

cases of inflammatory pseudotumor of the spleen lack the characteristic lobular angiomatoid pattern that defines SANT. Furthermore, unlike inflammatory pseudotumor of spleen, SANT is a vascular lesion and immunohistochemical analysis highlights its vascular nature.

IgG4-Related Disease. Patients with IgG4-related disease develop fibrotic lesions with an inflammatory infiltrate, often with numerous plasma cells. Many of these features overlap with those described in inflammatory pseudotumor of the spleen. Some have suggested a relationship between IgG4-related disease and inflammatory pseudotumor-like follicular dendritic cell tumor (6,12). In lesions with a substantial number of IgG4-positive plasma cells, or if the IgG4/IgG ratio is high, a workup to exclude IgG4-related disease is warranted.

Diffuse Large B-Cell Lymphoma (DLBCL) of Spleen. Rare cases of DLBCL exhibit prominent sclerosis or the lymphoma cells exhibit spindled lymphocyte morphology that mimics inflammatory pseudotumor of spleen or other stromal tumors. In DLBCL, however, the lymphoid cells are large and atypical. These tumors express pan-B-cell markers and carry monoclonal immunoglobulin gene rearrangements.

TREATMENT AND PROGNOSIS

The first line therapy for patients with stromal tumors and tumor-like lesions of the spleen is surgical excision. Inflammatory pseudotumor of the spleen is a benign disease and surgical excision is curative (28). For patients with inflammatory pseudotumor-like follicular dendritic cell tumor of the spleen, local recurrences and relapses occur rarely (5,18,23). Similarly, patients with inflammatory myofibroblastic tumor of the spleen develop recurrences, and rarely, develop metastases (7,14a).

REFERENCES

1. Akatsu T, Kameyama K, Tanabe M, Endo T, Kitajima M. Epstein-Barr virus-positive inflammatory pseudotumor of the spleen with concomitant rectal cancer: a case report and review of the literature. Dig Dis Sci 2007;52:2806-2812.
2. Antonescu CR, Suurmeijer AJ, Zhang L, et al. Molecular characterization of inflammatory myofibroblastic tumors with frequent ALK and ROS1 gene fusions and rare novel RET rearrangement. Am J Surg Pathol 2015;39:957-967.
3. Chandra P, Wen YH, Tuli S, et al. Postchemotherapy histiocyte-rich pseudotumor involving the spleen. Am J Clin Pathol 2009;132:342-348.
4. Chen Y, Shi H, Li H, Zhen T, Han A. Clinicopathological features of inflammatory pseufotumor-like follicular dendritic cell tumor of the abdomen. Histopathology 2016;68:858-865.
5. Cheuk W, Chan JK, Shek TW, et al. Inflammatory pseudotumor-like follicular dendritic cell tumor: distinctive low-grade malignant intra-abdominal neoplasm with consistent Epstein-Barr virus association. Am J Surg Pathol 2001;25:721-731.

6. Choe JY, Go H, Jeon YK, et al. Inflammatory pseudotumor-like follicular dendritic cell sarcoma of the spleen: a report of six cases with increased IgG4-positive plasma cells. Pathol Int 2013;63:245-251.

7. Coffin CM, Hornick JL, Fletcher CD. Inflammatory myofibroblastic tumor. Comparison of clinicopathologic, histologic, and immunohistochemical features including ALK expression in atypical and aggressive cases. Am J Surg Pathol 2007;31:509-520.

8. Diebold J, Le Tourneau A, Marmey B, et al. Is sclerosing angiomatoid nodular transformation (SANT) of the splenic red pulp identical to inflammatory pseudotumour? Report of 16 cases. Histopathology 2008;53:299-310.

9. Falk S, Stutte HJ. Hamartomas of the spleen: a study of 20 biopsy cases. Histopathology 1989;14:603-612.

10. Ge R, Liu C, Yin X, et al. Clinicopathologic characteristics of inflammatory pseudotumor-like follicular dendritic cell sarcoma. Int J Clin Exp Pathol 2014;7:2421-2429.

11. Handa U, Tiwari A, Singhal N, Mohan H, Kaur R. Utility of ultrasound-guided fine-needle aspiration in splenic lesions. Diagn Cytopathol 2013;41:1038-1042.

11a. Hang JF, Wang LC, Lai CR. Cytological features of inflammatory pseudotumor-like follicular dendritic cell sarcoma of spleen: A case report. Diagn Cytopathol 2017;45:230-234.

12. Kashiwagi S, Kumasaka T, Bunsei N, et al. Detection of Epstein-Barr virus-encoded small RNA-expressed myofibroblasts and IgG4-producing plasma cells in sclerosing angiomatoid nodular transformation of the spleen. Virchows Arch 2008;453:275-282.

13. Kirli EA, Orhan D, Haliloglu M, et al. Invasive inflammatory myofibroblastic tumor of the spleen treated with partial splenectomy in a child. J Pediatr Hematol Oncol 2012;34:e131-133.

14. Kiryu S, Takeuchi K, Shibahara J, et al. Epstein-Barr virus-positive inflammatory pseudotumour and inflammatory pseudotumour-like follicular dendritic cell tumour. Br J Radiol 2009;82:e67-71.

14a. Koechlin L, Zettl A, Koeberle D, von Flüe M, Bolli M. Metastatic inflammatory myofibroblastic tumor of the spleen: a case report and review of the literature. Case Rep Surg 2016;2016:8593242.

15. Krishnan J, Frizzera G. Two splenic lesions in need of clarification: hamartoma and inflammatory pseudotumor. Semin Diagn Pathol 2003;20:94-104.

16. Kutok JL, Pinkus GS, Dorfman DM, Fletcher CD. Inflammatory pseudotumor of lymph node and spleen: an entity biologically distinct from inflammatory myofibroblastic tumor. Hum Pathol 2001;32:1382-1387.

17. Lewis JT, Gaffney RL, Casey MB, Farrell MA, Morice WG, Macon WR. Inflammatory pseudotumor of the spleen associated with a clonal Epstein-Barr virus genome. Case report and review of the literature. Am J Clin Pathol 2003;120:56-61.

18. Li XQ, Cheuk W, Lam PW, et al. Inflammatory pseudotumor-like follicular dendritic cell tumor of liver and spleen. Granulomatous and eosinophil-rich variants mimicking inflammatory or infective lesions. Am J Surg Pathol 2014;38:646-653.

19. Lovly CM, Gupta A, Lipson D, et al. Inflammatory myofibroblastic tumors harbor multiple potentially actionable kinase fusions. Cancer Discov 2014;4:889-895.

20. Ma ZH, Tian XF, Ma J, Zhao YF. Inflammatory pseudotumor of the spleen: a case report and review of published cases. Oncol Lett 2013;5:1955-1957.

21. Martel M, Cheuk W, Lombardi L, Lifschitz-Mercer B, Chan JK, Rosai J. Sclerosing angiomatoid nodular transformation (SANT): report of 25 cases of a distinctive benign splenic lesion. Am J Surg Pathol 2004;28:1268-1279.

22. Mundi I, Singhal N, Punia RP, Dalal U, Mohan H. Inflammatory pseudotumor of the spleen: A rare case diagnosed on FNAC. Diagn Cytopathol 2012;40:1104-1106.

23. Neuhauser TS, Derringer GA, Thompson LD, et al. Splenic inflammatory myofibroblastic tumor (inflammatory pseudotumor): a clinicopathologic and immunophenotypic study of 12 cases. Arch Pathol Lab Med 2001;125:379-385.

24. Oz Puyan F, Bilgi S, Unlu E, et al. Inflammatory pseudotumor of the spleen with EBV positivity: report of a case. Eur J Haematol 2004;72:285-291.

25. Rao L, Yang Z, Wang X, et al. Imaging findings of inflammatory pseudotumor-like follicular dendritic cell tumor of spleen. Clin Nucl Med 2014;39:e286-289.

26. Rosenbaum L, Fekrazad MH, Rabinowitz I, Vasef MA. Epstein-Barr virus-associated inflammatory pseudotumor of the spleen: report of two cases and review of the literature. J Hematop 2009;2:127-131.

27. Sarker A, An C, Davis M, Praprotnik D, McCarthy LJ, Orazi A. Inflammatory pseudotumor of the spleen in a 6-year-old child: A clinicopathologic study. Arch Pathol Lab Med 2003;127:e127-130.

28. Thomas RM, Jaffe ES, Zarate-Osorno A, Medeiros LJ. Inflammatory pseudotumor of the spleen. A clinicopathologic and immunophenotypic study of eight cases. Arch Pathol Lab Med 1993;117:921-926.

29. Zhang MQ, Lennerz JK, Dehner LP, Brunt LM, Wang HL. Granulomatous inflammatory pseudotumor of the spleen: association with Epstein-Barr virus. Appl Immunohistochem Mol Morphol 2009;17:259-263.

65 CYSTS OF SPLEEN

GENERAL FEATURES

Splenic cysts are composed of completely or partly encapsulated spaces within the spleen that are usually fluid filled. Cysts have a variety of etiologies, including infectious, congenital, and neoplastic.

Cysts of the spleen can be divided dichotomously in several relevant ways: benign versus malignant, infectious versus noninfectious, and "true" cysts versus pseudocysts. This approach underlies the fact that cyst formation is a common pathway for a variety of insults to the splenic parenchyma (13). When evaluating cysts, it is important to evaluate the lining and the contents to determine the most appropriate diagnosis. Splenic cysts and hematomas occur with a higher frequency in patients with chronic pancreatitis (14).

Masses in the spleen also undergo cystic change and are included here as part of the overall spectrum of splenic cysts. Cystic masses may be due to congenital, inflammatory, vascular, post-traumatic, and neoplastic causes (21).

CLINICAL FEATURES

Many patients with splenic cysts are asymptomatic and a cyst is found incidentally during radiologic examination or splenectomy performed for other reasons. Abdominal pain may be present. With infectious causes, fever and neutrophilic leukocytosis may be observed. In some patients, serum markers associated with carcinoma, such as CA19-9, CA125, and carcinoembryonic antigen (CEA), may be elevated in association with benign cysts of the spleen (8,18). Splenomegaly is present in many patients.

Hemorrhage, rupture, and secondary bacterial infections are potential serious complications associated with splenic cysts of any type. When splenic cysts rupture patients often present with an acute abdomen and possibly massive intraperitoneal hemorrhage. A rare complication is the unmooring of the spleen from its fibrous connections and its displacement to the pelvis (20).

GROSS AND HISTOLOGIC FINDINGS

The gross features of splenic cysts are highly variable depending on the etiology, age of the cyst, and other findings. Features that should be noted in the gross evaluation are: size of the intact cyst (if evaluable), whether there is a capsule lining the cyst that separates the cyst from normal parenchyma, whether the cyst lining is smooth or rough, and the quality of the material filling the cyst. Mesothelial cysts commonly have a smooth and shiny cyst lining. Clear fluid is likely serous, and is most typically seen in mesothelial cysts. Epidermoid cysts have a smooth and shiny lining or the lining can be trabecular or rough (figs. 65-1, 65-2). Bloody fluid may be seen in a variety of cysts. The cyst fluid of echinococcal cysts is typically described as hydatid sand, with small gritty matter composed of fragments of the organisms.

Mesothelial Cyst

Mesothelial cysts, also known as *congenital* or *true cysts*, account for approximately 20 percent of the cysts found in the spleen (13). These lesions are thought to arise as a result of developmental entrapment of mesothelial cells within the splenic parenchyma. Mesothelial cysts are unilocular (most common) or multilocular. Multiple mesothelial cysts that are not connected also may be present.

Mesothelial cysts have a true lining of mesothelial cells, which are often attenuated. There may be focal destruction or absence of the mesothelial lining, so adequate sampling is important to identify lining cells. The cytologic features of the lining cells are bland and the fluid is most often clear serous fluid, although brown, yellow, or red fluid may be seen. Rarely, small tufts of mesothelial cells are present.

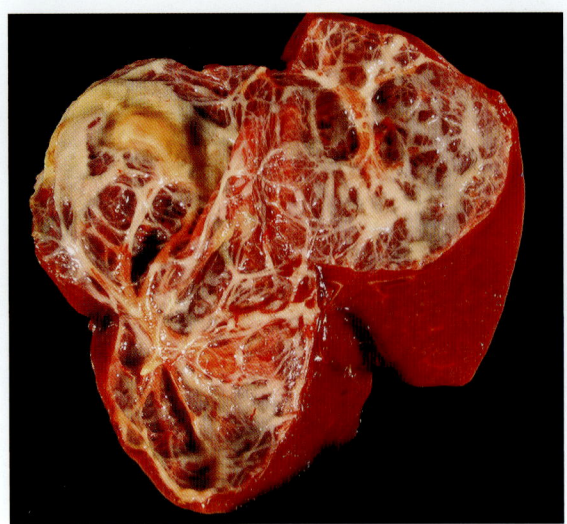

Figure 65-1

EPIDERMOID CYST OF SPLEEN

The cyst has a trabecular inner lining. (Courtesy of Dr. A. Sohani, Boston, MA.)

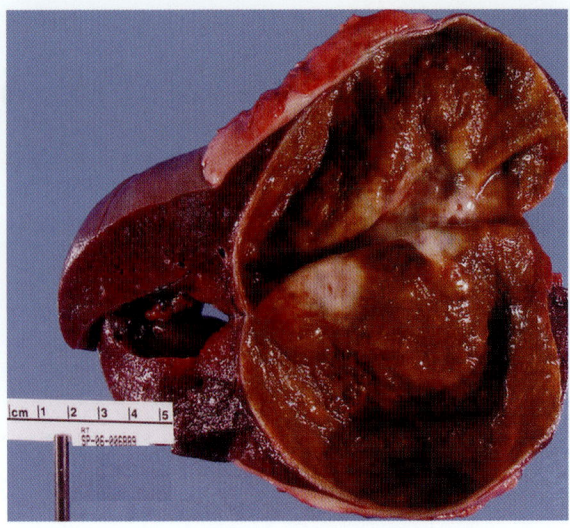

Figure 65-2

EPIDERMOID CYST OF SPLEEN

The cyst has a rough inner surface. Adjacent normal splenic parenchyma is also present. (Courtesy of Dr. M. Drachenberg, Long Beach, CA.)

Epidermoid/Epithelial Cyst

Epidermoid cysts are lined by true epithelium, rather than mesothelium (fig. 65-3). The epithelial lining is most often flattened and bland in appearance, but occasionally is composed of more polygonal cells (7,9,16). The cyst contents vary from clear or colored fluid to a more grumous material, such as is seen in epidermoid cysts of the skin. The presence of significant proliferations of epithelial cells (greater than 2 to 3 cells thick) or significant cytologic atypia should raise the possibility of a cystic neoplasm. *True dermoid cysts*, similar to benign cystic teratomas of the ovary, rarely have been reported in the spleen (13). Skin appendage structures are present in dermoid cysts.

Rarely, cysts arise within the distal pancreas in intrapancreatic accessory spleens (6,9). These are typically identified by the presence of residual splenic parenchyma, often highlighted by CD8 staining of splenic sinus-lining cells. Epidermoid cysts can recur if not completely excised (2a). An exceedingly rare complication of epidermoid/epithelial cysts is malignant transformation of the cyst lining. Rare reports of squamous cell carcinoma, cystadenocarcinoma, and malignant teratoma are reported; these are presumed to be derived from intrasplenic cystic structures.

Pseudocyst

Pseudocysts ("false cysts") represent up to 80 percent of all splenic cysts (13,17). Infarction or remote hemorrhage (hematoma) may lead to the formation of a cystic cavity in the spleen. A pseudocyst may arise as a result of ischemia (arterial effects) or hemorrhage (venous effects), or may represent cystic degeneration of an angioma or hamartoma. Although most patients with splenic pseudocyst do not report a history of trauma, a pseudocyst can occur in up to 7.5 percent of patients following blunt splenic injury (12).

Pseudocysts are small or large (4,17,19). The pseudocyst wall is fibrotic and may be calcified, imparting an "egg shell" radiographic appearance (19). The wall lacks an epithelial, mesothelial, or endothelial lining (fig. 65-4). The luminal wall may be shaggy and hemorrhagic, although some older cysts have a smooth fibrous wall. The contents may be fluid or contain debris (13,17).

Echinococcal Cyst

The most common parasitic cyst of the spleen is caused by larvae of the tapeworm of the genus *Echinococcus*. Infection by *E. granulosus*, also referred to as hydatid disease, is the most common form, although other *Echinococcus* species also rarely cause human infections. The lungs and

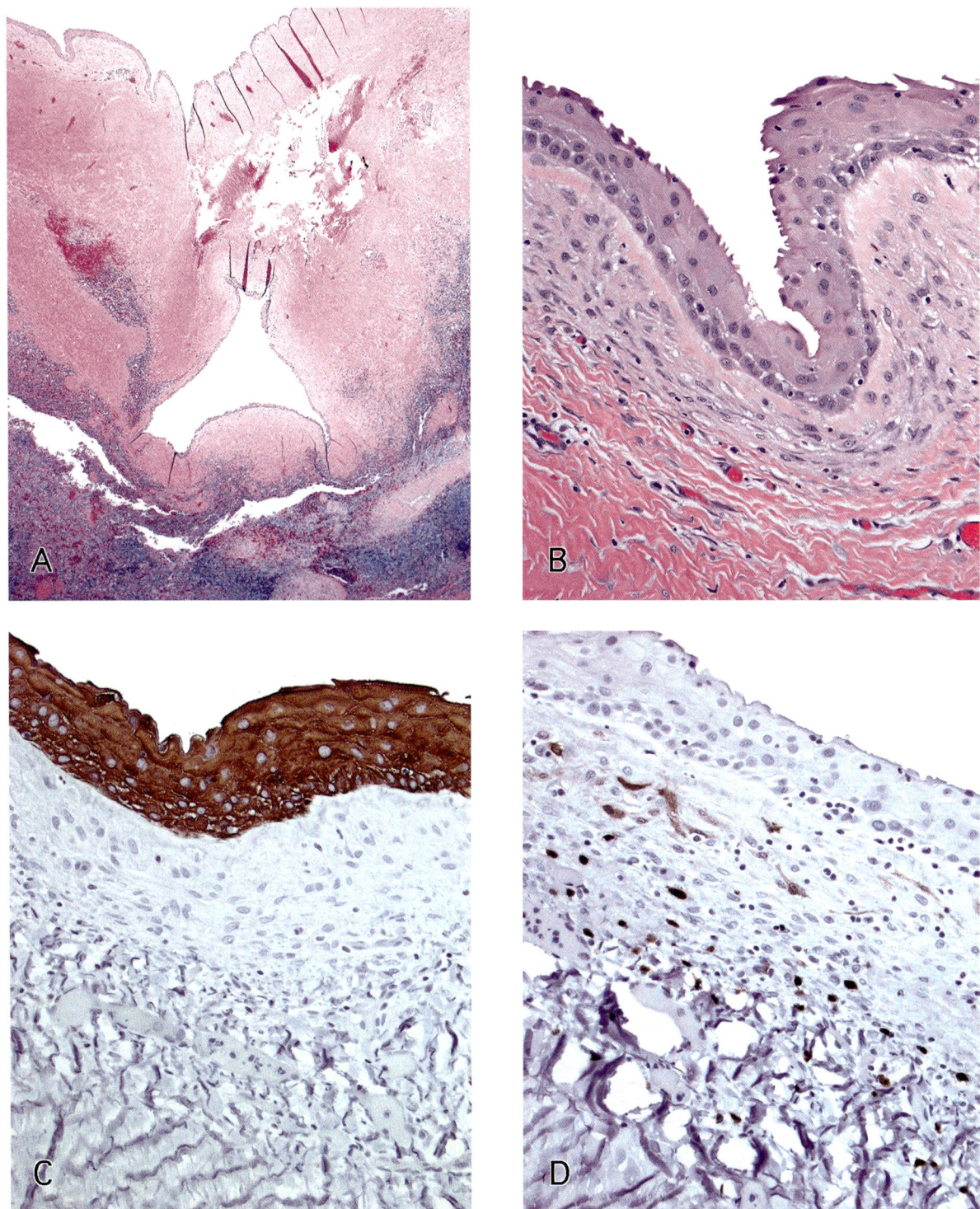

Figure 65-3

EPIDERMOID CYST OF SPLEEN

A,B: Low- (A) and high- (B) power magnification (hematoxylin and eosin [H&E] stain).

C,D: Epithelial cysts are positive for pankeratin (C) and negative for calretinin (D) (C,D: immunohistochemistry with hematoxylin stain).

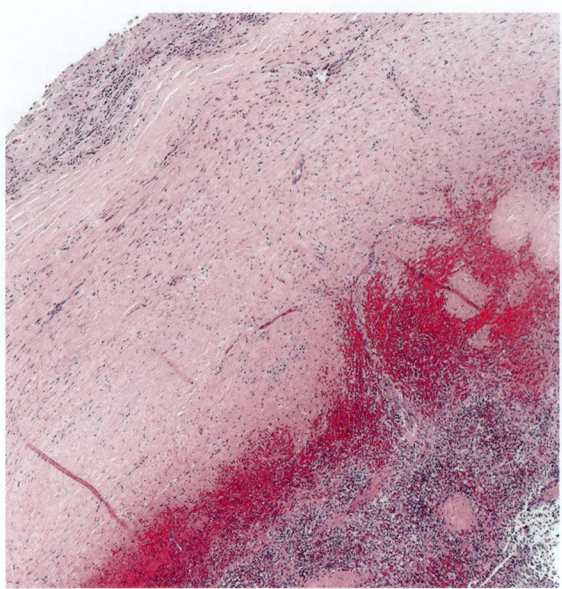

Figure 65-4

PSEUDOCYST OF SPLEEN

The wall of the pseudocyst is composed of macrophages and fibrous tissue. A distinct epithelial lining is not present (H&E stain).

liver are most frequently involved, but splenic cysts also occur (3,15,17). Up to 60 percent of *echinococcal cysts* are asymptomatic. Serum antibody testing is available for confirmation of the diagnosis, although false-negative results occur

The size of the cyst is variable and ranges usually between 1 and 15 cm, but much larger cysts have been noted (3,5,15,17a). The outer surface of the cyst is composed of dense fibrous tissue, often with calcification. There is an inner germinative layer which has many daughter cysts, termed "brood capsules." The cysts may have an associated inflammatory response, often with prominent eosinophilia. Calcification and fibrosis of the cyst wall are common in long-lasting cysts. The mouth portions of the echinococcal larvae, or scolices, are a characteristic finding (fig. 65-5). They are small and appear hook or sickle shaped. These parts in the fluid account for the gross appearance of "hydatid sand."

Other Types of Cysts

Abscesses may appear as cystic spaces in the spleen. These may be caused by a variety of infectious organisms, and are filled with neutrophils and necrotic debris. An organism may be identifiable by histologic evaluation or special stains (5,10,13). Infectious causes of cystic splenic lesions are more common in underdeveloped countries and include tuberculosis and kala-azar (1,4). Neoplasms in the spleen may become secondarily infected with an associated abscess. Histologic examination reveals abnormal, neoplastic cells in addition to the usual features of an abscess.

A variety of malignant neoplasms can metastasize to the spleen, most often carcinomas but also melanoma and other tumors (2,10). In some patients, splenic metastases undergo necrosis and cystic degeneration. Similarly, Hodgkin lymphomas and non-Hodgkin lymphomas often disseminate to the spleen and can undergo necrosis with cystic degeneration (2,10).

An exceedingly rare phenomenon is the development fibrin-associated Epstein-Barr virus (EBV)-positive large B-cell lymphoma within a splenic cyst (11). In these microscopic tumors the large lymphoma cells are confined to the cyst. Surgical excision may be adequate for these rare tumors.

A number of primary splenic neoplasms may become cystic, including benign vascular neoplasms such as hemangioma and lymphangioma as well as malignant vascular neoplasms (see chapter 63). Peliosis is a lesion composed of cystic blood-filled spaces and sinuses, without an endothelial lining, of unknown etiology, and may be seen in the spleen or liver (discussed in chapter 66).

CYTOLOGIC FINDINGS

A number of studies have shown that cystic splenic lesions can be aspirated safely. The cytologic findings depend on the etiology of the splenic cyst. Mesothelial cysts are often paucicellular or acellular. Epidermoid cysts have anucleated and pyknotic squamous cells, macrophages, and amorphous debris (10). The squamous cells lack nuclear atypia and pleomorphism. In some cases, aspirates contain primarily macrophages (fig. 65-6), with few or no epithelial cells. Fine needle aspiration of infectious cysts can show the causative organism. Aspirates of malignant splenic cystic lesions often show neoplastic cells (2,5,10).

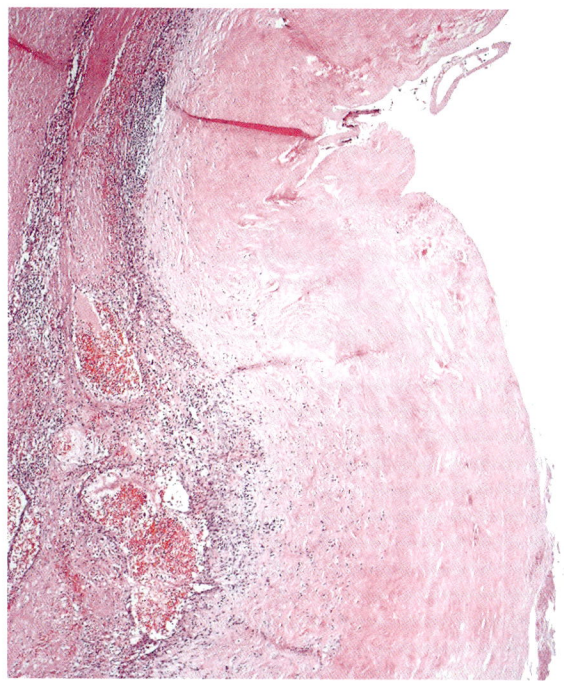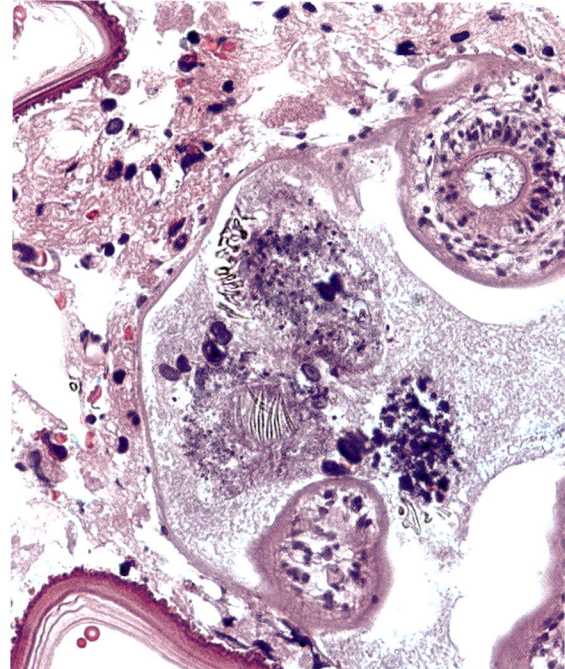

Figure 65-5

ECHINOCOCCAL CYST OF SPLEEN

The wall (left) and contents (right) of an echinococcal cyst are shown. The refractile structures (right) are the hooklets or mouthparts of the tapeworm larvae (H&E stain).

IMMUNOPHENOTYPIC FINDINGS

Immunohistochemical studies help distinguish various types of splenic cyst. The lining of an epidermoid cyst is positive for pankeratin (such as AE1/AE3) and keratin 7; however, an epidermoid cyst is negative for calretinin, D2-40, and WT1 (fig. 65-3C,D). In contrast, the lining of a mesothelial cyst is positive for pankeratin, keratin 7, calretinin, D2-40, WT1, and keratin 5/6 (13).

The lining of a pseudocyst does not express keratins or mesothelial markers. The cells are mostly histiocyte derived and may express markers such as CD68 and CD163. Specific metastatic tumors or lymphomas that are cystic should be evaluated by more extensive antibody panels tailored toward the suspected diagnosis.

TREATMENT AND PROGNOSIS

Echinococcal cysts require specialized therapy which includes: surgery, PAIR (puncture, aspiration, injection, reaspiration), and antimicrobial agents. If the cyst is small, partial splenectomy may be performed (3). Long-term antimicrobial

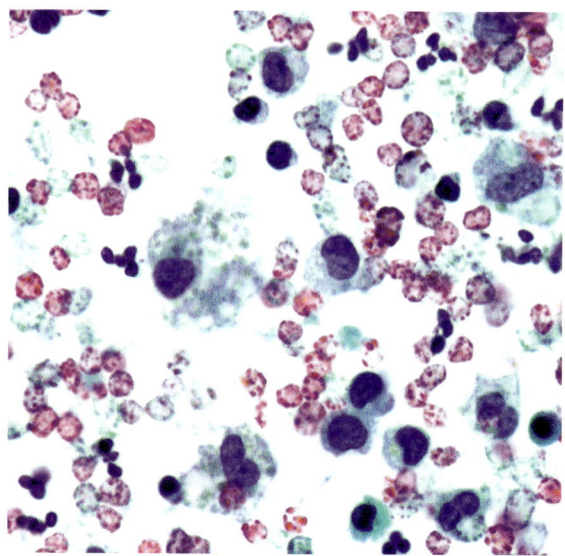

Figure 65-6

EPIDERMOID CYST OF SPLEEN

Cytospin preparation of an aspirate specimen from a splenic cyst shows numerous foamy histiocytes and degenerated blood elements, but lacks the characteristic epithelial cells that were identified in the resection specimen (Papanicolaou stain).

treatment is mandatory for patients with inoperable lesions or after incomplete resection of lesions (15).

Other benign cysts are managed conservatively, undergo surgical removal, or are drained percutaneously. If a splenic cystic lesion is symptomatic and large (over 10 cm), surgical excision is often recommended. Spleen sparing surgeries such as partial splenectomy and "marsupialization" have been advocated (17,20).

REFERENCES

1. Acharya PR, Anand R, Acharya VK, Sahoo RC. PUO-a rare (and forgotten) cause! J Assoc Physicians India 2014;62:66-68

2. Caraway NP, Fanning CV. Use of fine-needle aspiration biopsy in the evaluation of splenic lesions in a cancer center. Diagn Cytopathol 1997;16:312-316.

2a. Cianci P, Tartaglia N, Altamura A, et al. A recurrent epidermoid cyst of the spleen: report of a case and literature review. World J Surg Oncol 2016;14:98.

3. Costi R, Castro Ruiz C, Zarzavadjian le Bian A, Scerrati D, Santi C, Violi V. Spleen hydatidosis treated by hemi-splenctomy: A low-morbidity, cost-effective management by a recently imporved surgical technique. Int J Surg 2015;20:41-45.

4. Galyfos G, Touloumis Z, Palogos K, et al. Oversized pseudocysts of the spleen: Report of two cases: Optimal magement of oversized pseudocysts of the spleen. Int J Surg Case Rep 2014;5:104-107.

5. Handa U, Tiwari A, Singhal N, Mohan H, Kaur R. Utility of ultrasound-guided fine-needle aspiration in splenic lesions. Diagn Cytopathol 2013;41:1038-1042.

6. Hwang HS, Lee SS, Kim SC, Seo DW, Kim J. Intrapancreatic accessory spleen: clinicopathologic analysis of 12 cases. Pancreas 2011;40:956-965.

7. Ingle SB, Hinge Ingle CR, Patrike S. Epithelial cysts of the spleen: a minireview. World J Gastroenterol 2014;20:13899-13903.

8. Inokuma T, Minami S, Suga K, Kusano Y, Chiba K, Furukawa M. Spontaneously ruptured giant splenic cyst with elevated serum levels of CA 19-9, CA 125 and carcinoembryonic antigen. Case Rep Gastroenterol 2010;4:191-197.

9. Iwasaki Y, Tagaya N, Nakagawa A, et al. Laparoscopic resection of epidermoid cyst arising from an intrapancreatic accessory spleen: a case report with a review of the literature. Surg Laparosc Endosc Percutan Tech 2011;21:e275-279.

10. Kumar PV, Monabati A, Raseki AR, et al. Splenic lesions: FNA findings in 48 cases. Cytopathology 2007;18:151-156.

11. Loong F, Chan AC, Ho BC, et al. Diffuse large B-cell lymphoma associated with chronic inflammation as an incidental finding and new clinical scenarios. Mod Pathol 2010;23:493-501.

12. Moore HB, Vane DW. Long-term follow-up of children with nonoperative management of blunt splenic trauma. J Trauma 2010;68:522-525.

13. O'Malley DP, George TI, Orazi A, Abbondanzo SL. Splenic cysts. In: Benign and reactive conditions of lymph node and spleen. AFIP Atlas of Nontumor Pathology, Fascicle 7. Washington, DC: American Registry of Pathology; 2009;553-560.

14. Patil PV, Khalil A, Thaha MA. Splenic parenchymal complications in pancreatitis. JOP 2011; 12:287-291.

15. Pawlowski ZS, Eckert J, Vuitton DA, et al. Chapter 2: Echinococcosis in humans: clinical aspects, diagnosis and treatment. In: WHO/OIE Manual on Echinococcosis in Humans and Animals: a Public Health Problem of Global Concern. Eckert J, Gemmell MA, Meslin FX, Pawlowski ZS, eds. World Organisation for Animal Health 2001:20-72.

16. Shanthi V, Reddy VC, Rao NM, Grandhi B, Kona S. Epithelial cyst of the spleen with squamous metaplasia: a rare entity. J Clin Diagn Res 2014;8: FD05-6.

17. Sucandy I, Klar A, Pezzi CM. Large pseudocyst of the spleen: etiology, diagnosis, and treatment for general surgeons. Am Surg 2015;81:E234-235.

17a. Taxy JB, Gibson WE, Kaufman MW. Echinococcosis: unexpected occurrence and the diagnostic contribution of routine histopathology. Am J Surg Pathol 2017;41:94-100.

18. Uludag M, Yetkin G, Citgez B, Karakoc S, Polat N, Yener S. Giant true cyst of the spleen with elevated serum markers, carbohydrate antigen 19-9 and cancer antigen 125. BMJ Case Rep 2009;2009:1691.

19. Urrutia M, Mergo PJ, Ros LH, Torres GM, Ros PR. Cystic masses of the spleen: radiologic-pathologic correlation. Radiographics 1996;16:107-129.

20. Ward EV, O'Brien J, Conlon K, Torreggiani WC. Unusual long-term complications of a splenic cyst. JBR-BTR 2010;93:7-9.

21. Williams RJ, Glazer G. Splenic cysts: changes in diagnosis, treatment and aetiological concepts. Ann R Coll Surg Engl 1993;75:87-89.

66 NONHEMATOLYMPHOID TUMORS AND TUMOR-LIKE LESIONS

Many of the more common benign tumors or tumor-like lesions that occur in lymph nodes and spleen (if not covered elsewhere in this book) are reviewed in this chapter. The reader is referred to the Fascicle on benign lymph node diseases for a more detailed discussion of many of these entities (45).

INFLAMMATORY PSEUDOTUMOR

General Features. *Inflammatory pseudotumor* (IPT) *of lymph node* is a rare benign lesion that likely has a number of etiologies. These lesions show a broad range of morphologic and immunophenotypic findings, but most cases are characterized by a proliferation of spindle cells with a variable, mixed inflammatory infiltrate.

Strictly defined, IPT of lymph node is a rare lesion that was first characterized in detail by Perrone et al. in 1988 (46). The etiology and pathogenesis of IPT of lymph node are poorly understood. Unknown infectious agents have been suggested as etiologic factors. An unusual tissue response to injury or infection also has been postulated. Lesions similar to IPT of lymph node occur at other anatomic sites including the orbital region, lungs, spleen, retroperitoneum, and urinary bladder, and have been designated in the literature as plasma cell granuloma or idiopathic retroperitoneal fibrosis. As a result, others have included IPT of lymph node within the spectrum of idiopathic fibrosclerotic disorders (15) or IgG4-related disorders (17).

Clinical Features. IPT of lymph node occurs at any age. There is a male predominance of approximately 1.5 to 1.0 (32,33). About two thirds of patients present with symptoms that include fever of unknown origin, night sweats, weight loss, nausea, fatigue, and abdominal pain (32,33,44). One third of patients are asymptomatic. Some patients report a history of infection. Laboratory abnormalities occur in about half of the patients (32).

Usually, a single lymph node is involved and any lymph node site may be affected. Ten to 20 percent of patients present with two separate lymph nodes involved simultaneously and rarely, patients have widespread lymphadenopathy or concurrent involvement of liver or spleen (32,33,42,44).

Gross and Histologic Findings. Lymph nodes may be enlarged up to 3 cm. The gross findings depend on the extent of nodal involvement. Smaller lesions are often firm and pale, with variably circumscribed borders. Larger lesions may entirely replace the lymph node with firm, fibrous tissue.

Histologically, the spectrum of findings observed suggests that IPT of lymph node is an evolving, dynamic process with histologic features that depend on the stage of evolution of disease (14,20,32,33). Moran et al. (44) suggested that IPT of lymph node be divided into three stages based on the degree of cellularity and fibrosis, the overall architectural pattern, and the extent of the lesion (Table 66-1). Common features of IPT of lymph node are: 1) a proliferation of spindle cells with a storiform pattern involving primarily the connective tissue framework

Table 66-1

HISTOPATHOLOGIC GRADING SYSTEM FOR INFLAMMATORY PSEUDOTUMOR OF LYMPH NODE[a]

Stage	Histologic Findings
Stage I	Small, localized nodules; preservation of normal lymph node architecture
Stage II	Disruption/distortion of lymph node archichitecture; replacement of lymph node by a mixed inflammatory infiltrate and myofibroblastic spindle cell proliferation
Stage III	Total or near-total replacement of lymph node; dense sclerosis with minimal inflammatory infiltrate; only small islands of residual lymphoid tissue

[a]Modified from a table in reference 44.

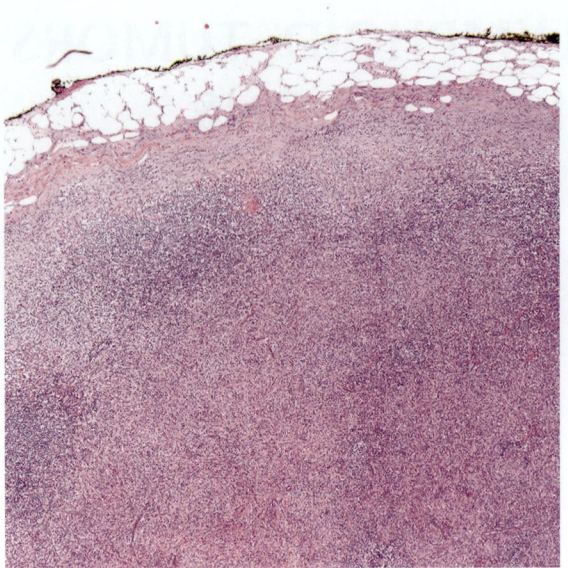
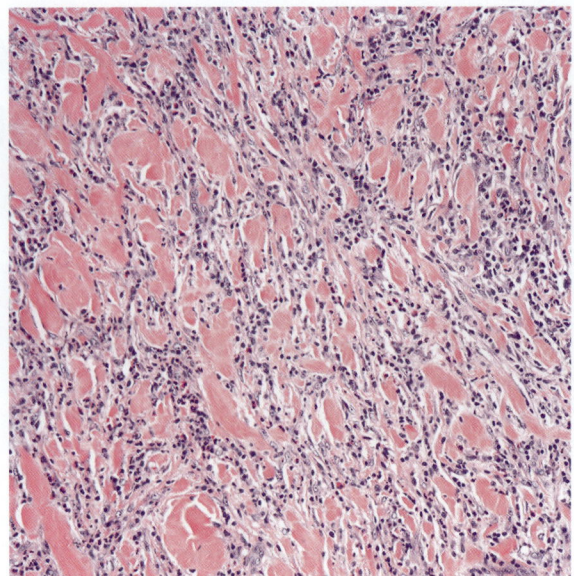

Figure 66-1

INFLAMMATORY PSEUDOTUMOR INVOLVING LYMPH NODE

Left: At low magnification, the lymph node has a thickened capsule and normal parenchyma is almost completely replaced by spindle cells with a mixed inflammatory infiltrate.

Right: High magnification shows a mixture of fibrosis/sclerosis with admixed small lymphocytes, plasma cells, and rare granulocytes (hematoxylin and eosin [H&E] stain).

of the lymph node; 2) prominent vascularity with obliteration of vessel lumens; and 3) a mixed inflammatory cell infiltrate composed of variable numbers of plasma cells, lymphocytes, and histiocytes, and less commonly, neutrophils and eosinophils (fig. 66-1) (14,32,33,44). In early lesions, the spindle cells have features of myofibroblasts, but in later lesions these features may be less prominent and there is often collagenous sclerosis (20,33,44,46). Necrosis and infarction also may be observed (44). Inflammatory pseudotumor of lymph node can extend into perinodal tissues.

Immunophenotypic Findings. The spindle cells of IPT of lymph node are reactive for vimentin, with variable reactivity for CD68 and smooth-muscle actin, supporting a fibroblastic/myofibroblastic origin (20,32,33,44). Immunohistochemical markers for vimentin or smooth-muscle actin highlight the storiform pattern. The spindle cells are negative for anaplastic lymphoma kinase (ALK) (33).

The lymphocytes in IPT of lymph node are a mixture of B and T cells, in a variable ratio, with T cells usually predominant (14,20,32,44). Scat-tered CD30-positive immunoblasts are present. Plasma cells express polytypic light chains. In situ hybridization is positive for Epstein-Barr virus (EBV) encoded RNA1 (EBER1) in approximately 10 percent of cases (2,33). There is no evidence of human herpesvirus (HHV)-8 infection (33).

Molecular Genetic Findings. Although few cases of IPT of lymph node have been assessed by conventional cytogenetic or molecular methods, no evidence of cytogenetic abnormalities has been reported to date. Fluorescence in situ hybridization (FISH) is negative for *ALK* translocations (33). There is no evidence of monoclonal antigen receptor gene rearrangements.

Differential Diagnosis. In large part, the diagnosis of IPT of lymph node is a diagnosis of exclusion. The differential diagnosis is broad and includes both benign and malignant lesions.

Infections. The inflammatory morphologic appearance of IPT of lymph node is suggestive of infection, and stains to exclude microorganisms are indicated as a part of the diagnostic workup. Evidence of active infection excludes the diagnosis of IPT of lymph node. Although any infection of lymph node can theoretically

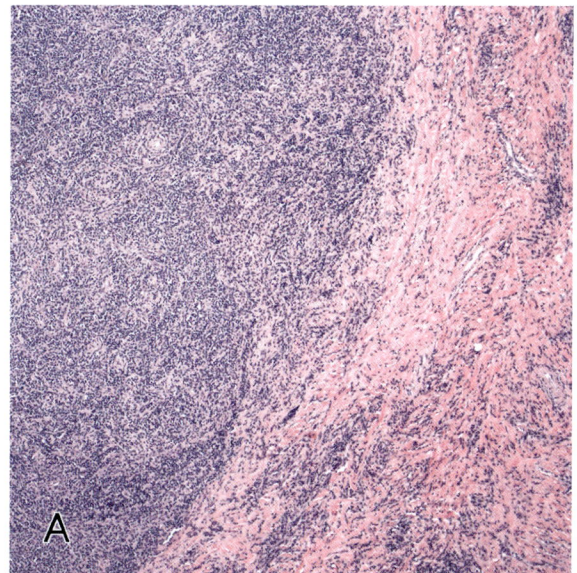

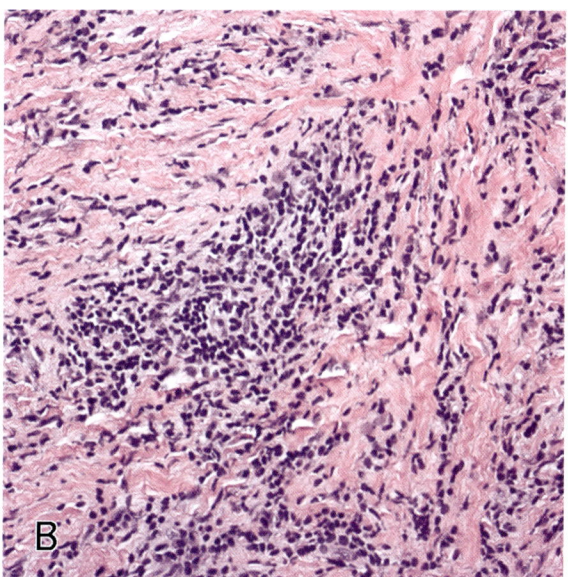

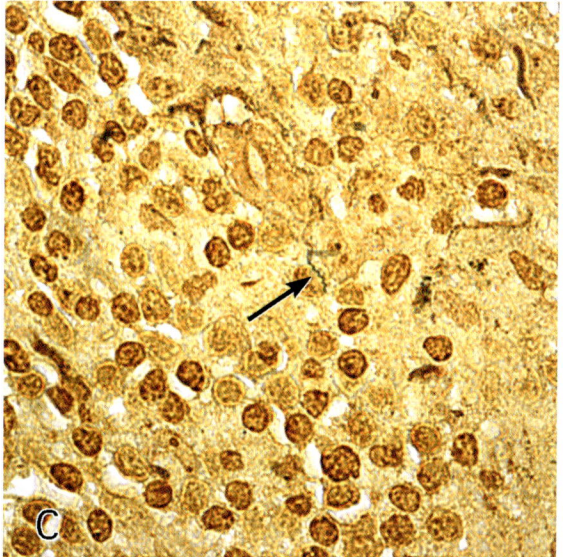

Figure 66-2

SYPHILITIC (LUETIC) LYMPHADENOPATHY

A: There is extensive capsular fibrosis (A,B: H&E stain).

B: A spindle cell proliferation has admixed inflammatory elements including lymphocytes, plasma cells, and histiocytes.

C: Steiner stain for syphilis shows a dark, corkscrew-shaped *Treponema pallidum* organism in the center of the field.

mimic the features of IPT, two infectious agents are mentioned here in more detail.

Syphilis. Syphilitic infection of lymph node (luetic lymphadenopathy) has a number of histologic features similar to IPT including fibrosis, vascular proliferation and often vasculitis, plasmacytosis, and a mixed chronic inflammatory infiltrate (fig. 66-2). Small granulomas and follicular hyperplasia also are observed (21,26,43). In rare cases of luetic lymphadenopathy, a prominent spindle cell proliferation with occasional mitotic figures is present, leading to consideration of a possible diagnosis of sarcoma (43).

The diagnosis of luetic lymphadenopathy is highly challenging in developed nations, because of the low prevalence of the disease and because a high index of suspicion is required to consider the possibility. The clinical history of a high-risk sexual lifestyle is a helpful clue, if available. Most cases of syphilis infection of lymph nodes involve the inguinal region and therefore location is also a clue. Once the possibility of syphilis is considered, a workup to identify *Treponema pallidum* can be performed (fig. 66-2C) (21,43).

Mycobacterial Pseudotumor. This rare manifestation of mycobacterial infection occurs in

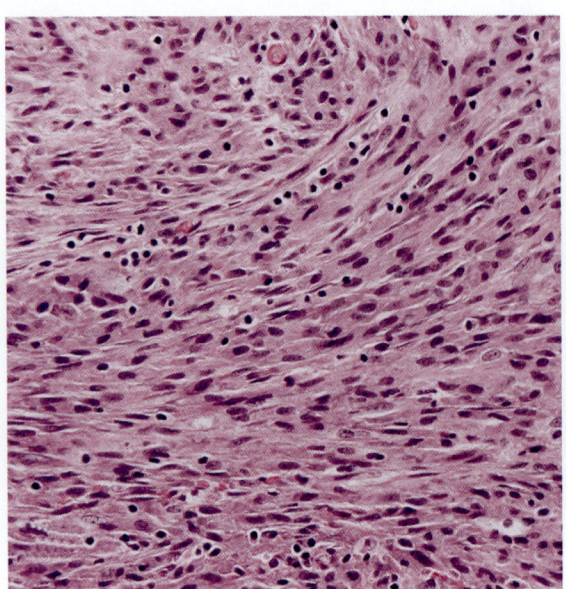 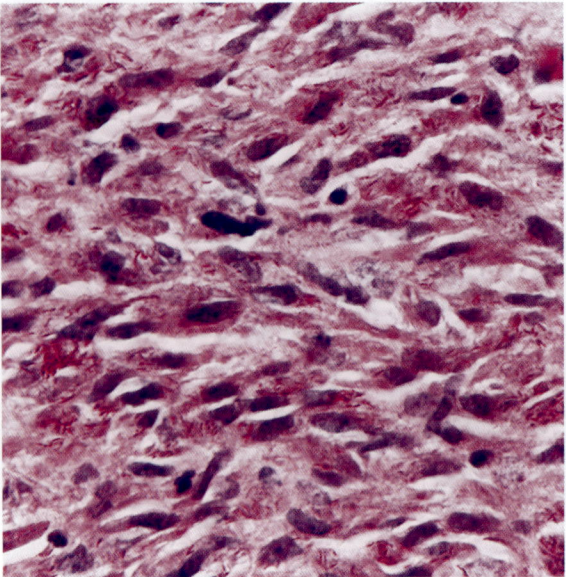

Figure 66-3

MYCOBACTERIAL SPINDLE CELL PSEUDOTUMOR REPLACING LYMPH NODE

Left: The lymph node parenchyma is replaced by intersecting spindle cells with eosinophilic cytoplasm in a patient with acquired immunodeficiency syndrome (AIDS) (H&E stain).

Right: An acid fast stain highlights numerous mycobacterial species shown by culture to be *Mycobacterium avium-intracellulare* (acid fast stain).

patients with human immunodeficiency virus (HIV) infection and acquired immunodeficiency syndrome (AIDS). The normal lymph node parenchyma is replaced by an exuberant proliferation of spindle-shaped histiocytes, with a lesser number of epithelioid histiocytes (fig. 66-3). Inflammatory cells are often present and these lesions can resemble IPT of lymph node (37). Unlike IPT of lymph node, the histiocytes contain numerous acid-fast bacilli, usually *Mycobacterium avium intracellulare* (37,59).

Inflammatory Myofibroblastic Tumor. IPT of lymph node and inflammatory myofibroblastic tumor (IMT) are both composed of spindle cells of myofibroblastic lineage and can resemble each other. In the literature, cases of IMT have been classified as IPT of lymph node and vice versa. However, unlike IPT of lymph node, IMT is usually located in soft tissues or the spleen and rarely primarily involves lymph nodes (10,33). IMT, at least in most cases, is a neoplastic lesion that can recur locally and less often metastasizes (10). The spindle cells are uniformly positive for smooth muscle actin whereas the spindle cells of IPT of lymph node are more variably positive. In addi-

tion, about 50 percent of IMTs are positive for ALK or carry translocations involving *ALK/2p23*; less often other gene fusions involving *ROS1* or *PDGFRB* are identified (33,38).

Spindle Cell Neoplasms of Lymph Node. A number of spindle cell neoplasms mimic IPT of lymph node. These include palisaded myofibroblastoma, tumors of histiocyte/accessory cells including follicular or interdigitating dendritic cell sarcoma, Langerhans cell histiocytosis/sarcoma, and metastatic tumors. Immunohistochemical analysis is helpful for distinguishing these tumors from IPT of lymph node. Unlike palisaded myofibroblastoma, the spindle cells of IPT do not express nuclear β-catenin or cyclin D1. The spindle cells of follicular dendritic cell sarcoma are positive for CD21, CD23, or other follicular dendritic cell markers. S-100 protein positivity supports interdigitating dendritic cell sarcoma and immunoreactivity for CD1a or CD207/langerin supports Langerhans cell lineage. Immunoreactivity for CD31, CD34, other vascular-associated markers, and HHV-8 supports Kaposi sarcoma over IPT of lymph node. Antibodies specific for keratins/epithelial markers and melanoma-associated antigens are helpful to exclude metastatic spindle cell carcinoma and melanoma, respectively.

Lymphomas with a Prominent Fibroblastic/ Fibrohistiocytic Response. Rarely, lymphomas are associated with a prominent fibroblastic or fibrohistiocytic reaction and can mimic IPT of lymph node. Examples include the fibroblastic variant of nodular sclerosis Hodgkin lymphoma and some types of peripheral T-cell lymphoma. The differential diagnosis is usually resolved by immunohistochemical analysis. The cells of classic Hodgkin lymphoma are CD15(+/-), CD30(+), MUM1/IRF4(+), and PAX5 (weak+) and are negative for CD45/LCA. The cells of peripheral T-cell lymphoma express a variety of T-cell antigens and often have an aberrant immunophenotype. Molecular studies of peripheral T-cell lymphoma show monoclonal T-cell receptor gene rearrangements, unlike IPT of lymph node.

Treatment and Prognosis. IPT of lymph node is a benign lesion that is usually localized, and resection is curative in virtually all patients. Local recurrence can occur, but only rarely, and therefore recurrence should prompt consideration of histologic mimics that are associated with aggressive clinical behavior (12).

PALISADED MYOFIBROBLASTOMA

General Features. *Palisaded myofibroblastoma* is a rare, benign neoplasm of lymph nodes with myofibroblastic features. It is likely derived from cells of the lymph node capsule or stroma.

Although these tumors were described in the past using a variety of names, in 1989 three groups described these tumors in detail, at which time the terms *palisaded myofibroblastoma*, *intranodal hemorrhagic spindle cell tumor with amianthoid fibers*, and *solitary spindle cell tumor with myoid differentiation of lymph node* were suggested (35,53,57). Although palisaded myofibroblastoma is the most commonly used term for this neoplasm, the other terms also have value as they convey different aspects of the clinical and pathologic features of this entity (35,53).

Clinical Features. Patients with palisaded myofibroblastoma are adults with a wide age range. There is a slight male predominance (3). Patients present with localized lymphadenopathy that is often asymptomatic, but the affected lymph node may be tender. Over 90 percent of

cases involve the inguinal lymph nodes, but rarely, these tumors are reported in other lymph node areas including the cervical region and mediastinum (3,53,57).

Gross and Histologic Findings. Grossly, these tumors are firm and gray-white, and have foci of hemorrhage. The tumor size ranges from less than 1 cm to 5 cm. Residual lymph node may be grossly visible at one side of the tumor (53,57).

The most salient histologic feature is a storiform pattern of palisaded, intersecting spindle cells surrounding eosinophilic collagenous areas (fig. 66-4) (34,35,53,57). The distinctive, so-called amianthoid fibers consist of stellate areas of collagen deposits that may be calcified. Extracellular and intracellular perinuclear hyaline globules are common in these tumors. The spindle cell nuclei often show palisading and are bland without atypia. Mitotic figures are uncommon. Variable amounts of fibrosis or granulation tissue may be present. Residual normal lymph node, if present, is compressed and often is associated with recent or old areas of hemorrhage.

Cytologic Findings. Few cases of palisaded myofibroblastoma assessed by fine-needle aspiration biopsy have been reported, likely attributable to the rarity of these tumors. Skagias et al. (51) reported the cytologic findings in lymph node touch imprints. Bland spindle cells, areas of vague palisading, extravasation of red blood cells into interstitial areas, and crystalline fibers consistent with amianthoid fibers may be appreciated (51).

Ultrastructural and Immunophenotypic Findings. Electron microsopy has shown that the spindle cells have features of myofibroblasts with discontinuous basal laminae, abundant microfilaments with focal densities, rough endoplasmic reticulum, and pinocytotic vesicles (41). The amianthoid fibers are composed of collagen.

Immunohistochemical analysis shows that the spindle cells are reactive with vimentin, D2-40/podoplanin, smooth muscle actin, muscle-specific actin, factor XIIIa (variable), and cyclin D1 and are negative for desmin, S-100 protein, factor VIII-related antigen, synaptophysin, keratin, epithelial membrane antigen (EMA), and CD45/LCA and other lymphoid markers (3,31,34,53,57). The amianthoid-like fibers are positive for collagen types I and III and actin (53,57). The cytoplasmic globules are commonly positive for actin. There is no evidence of EBV infection.

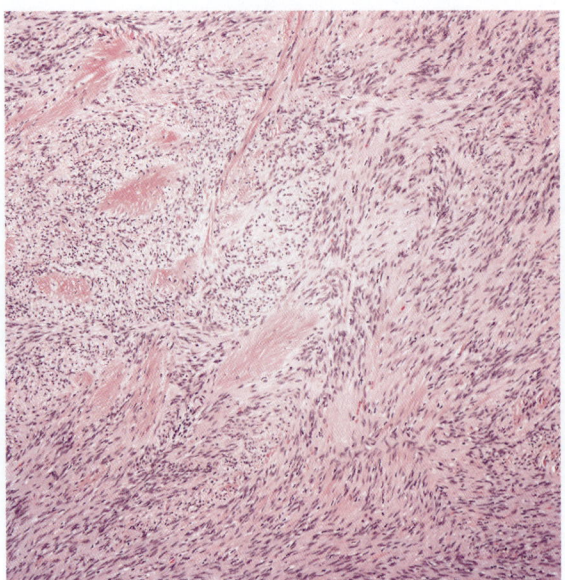 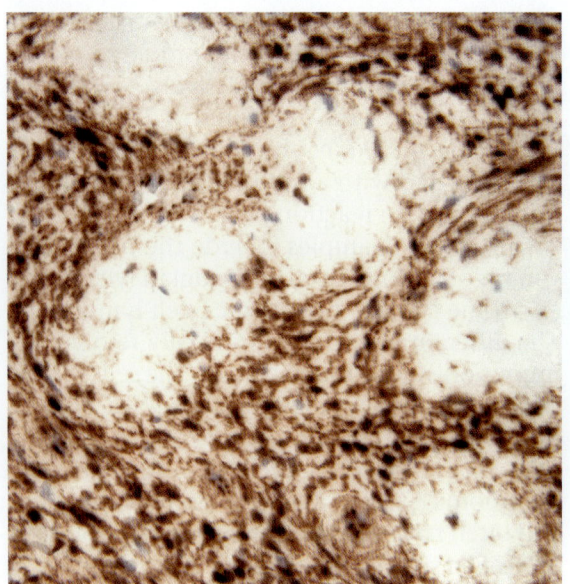

Figure 66-4

PALISADED MYOFIBROBLASTOMA INVOLVING LYMPH NODE

Left: The neoplasm is composed of a proliferation of spindle cells with nuclear palisading and nodules of collagen (amianthoid fibers) (H&E stain).

Right: These tumors are positive for β-catenin with a nuclear pattern. Nuclear expression of β-catenin is abnormal and supports the presence of a *CTNNB1* mutation (immunohistochemistry with hematoxylin counterstain).

Molecular Genetic Findings. Laskin et al. (34) used Sanger sequencing to show mutations in exon 3 of the β-catenin gene glycogen synthase kinase-3β (*CTNNB1*) in 7 of 8 (88 percent) cases of palisaded myofibroblastoma. This pathway is therefore thought to be important in pathogenesis. Immunohistochemical analysis also can be used to screen for these mutations. The spindle cells of palisaded myofibroblastoma express β-catenin in an abnormal nuclear and cytoplasmic pattern, unlike normal cells that exhibit cytoplasmic reactivity (fig. 66-4, right) (34). Cyclin D1 is positive in palisaded myofibroblastoma because it is downstream of activated β-catenin (31,34).

Differential Diagnosis. *Inflammatory Pseudotumor of Lymph Node.* As discussed above, IPT of lymph node is centered on the lymph node framework and is more heterogeneous in terms of the spindle cell population and the degree of inflammation. Amianthoid fibers do not occur in IPT of lymph node.

Benign Spindle Cell Tumors of Lymph Node. Schwannoma may be suggested by the palisading pattern of the spindle cells in palisaded myofi-broblastoma. Unlike schwannoma, palisaded myofibroblastoma does not have Antoni type A or B areas and is negative for S-100 protein. Schwannoma also occurs rarely in lymph nodes.

Primary nodal or benign metastasizing leiomyoma may be considered. Unlike palisaded myofibroblastoma, the spindle cells of leiomyoma have cigar-shaped nuclei and no amianthoid fibers. In addition, leiomyoma is usually positive for desmin.

Follicular Dendritic Cell Sarcoma. Although follicular dendritic cell (FDC) sarcoma can be composed of highly spindled cells, similar to palisaded myofibroblastoma, the spindle cells of FDC sarcoma are often more plump, may be arranged in whorls or nests (as well as a storiform pattern), and are positive for CD21, CD23, or other FDC-associated markers.

Kaposi Sarcoma. The presence of spindle cells and hemorrhage in palisaded myofibroblastoma may resemble Kaposi sarcoma. In palisaded myofibroblastoma, however, there is no evidence of blood vessel formation. Unlike palisaded myofibroblastoma, in Kaposi sarcoma there may be a history of immunodeficiency, the spindle cells often show nuclear atypia and a higher mitotic rate, and the spindle cells are positive for HHV-8, CD34, and other vascular-associated markers.

Metastatic Spindle Cell Tumors to Lymph Node. In general, metastatic tumors show more pleomorphism and nuclear atypia, and a higher mitotic rate than palisaded myofibroblastoma. Immunohistochemical analysis is helpful for distinguishing palisaded myofibroblastoma from metastatic carcinoma (keratin and EMA positive) and melanoma (S-100 protein and HMB-45 positive).

Treatment and Prognosis. Palisaded myofibroblastoma is a benign neoplasm and resection is typically curative, even with incomplete resection. Rare cases have recurred (3,13).

ANGIOMYOLIPOMA

General Features. *Angiomyolipoma* is a benign tumor characterized by a proliferation of smooth muscle cells, thick-walled blood vessels, and adipose tissue. It is thought to be derived from perivascular epithelioid cells (39).

Angiomyolipoma can arise sporadically or as a manifestation of tuberous sclerosis complex. In general, sporadic angiomyolipoma is approximately four times more common than cases associated with tuberous sclerosis (39). The kidney is most commonly affected, but other organs such as the liver and spleen may be involved, usually as a part of multifocal disease (1,54). Regional lymph nodes also may be involved. In the literature, the frequency of perirenal lymph node involvement has been reported to be low, but this apparent low frequency may be related to suboptimal sampling.

Tuberous sclerosis is an inherited neurocutaneous disorder characterized by multiple benign neoplasms that primarily involve the kidneys, skin, and brain, but are not limited to these organs. Patients have loss-of-function mutations in the tumor suppressor gene *TSC1* on chromosome 9q34 or *TSC2* on chromosome 16p13. These genes normally encode for hamartin or tuberin, respectively (30,39). Hamartin and tuberin form a complex that is involved in regulation of the mTOR and AKT cellular pathways.

Clinical Features. The median patient age at the time of diagnosis of sporadic angiomyolipoma is 45 to 55 years. There is a 4 to 1 female predominance (39). In patients with angiomy-

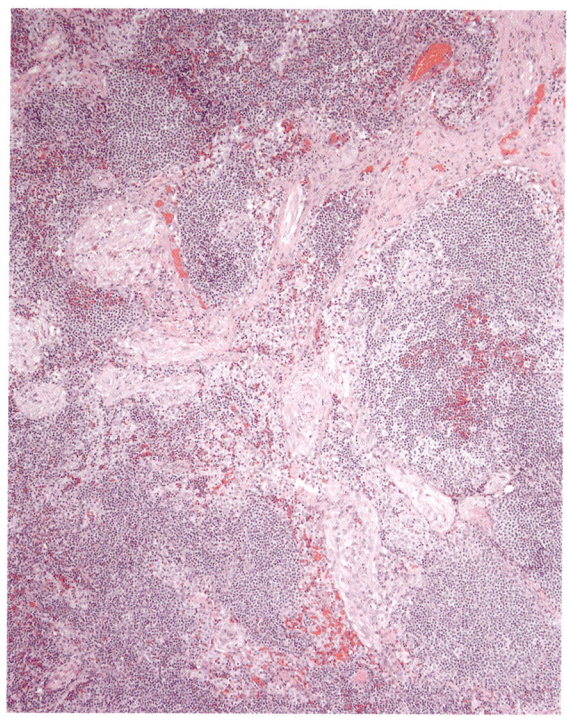

Figure 66-5

ANGIOMYOLIPOMA PARTIALLY INVOLVING LYMPH NODE

The tumor is mostly located in sinusoids and there is a predominance of spindle cells (H&E stain).

olipoma associated with tuberous sclerosis, the median patient age at diagnosis is 25 to 35 years and there is no apparent sex predilection (39).

Histologic Findings. Angiomyolipomas contain variable mixtures of blood vessels, smooth muscle, and adipose tissue (figs. 66-5, 66-6) (39). In most cases all three components are present, but sometimes two or rarely only one component may predominate. The components are arranged in a haphazard fashion. The blood vessels are thick-walled and abnormal in appearance. Smooth muscle cells often appear to be arranged radially around blood vessels.

Cytologic Findings. In most cases, the cells appear bland, although some cases exhibit mild to moderate atypia, which is of little clinical consequence. In some cases, however, the cells are large and polygonal, with abundant cytoplasm, marked nuclear atypia, mitotic figures, and necrosis and these features correlate with malignant behavior (5).

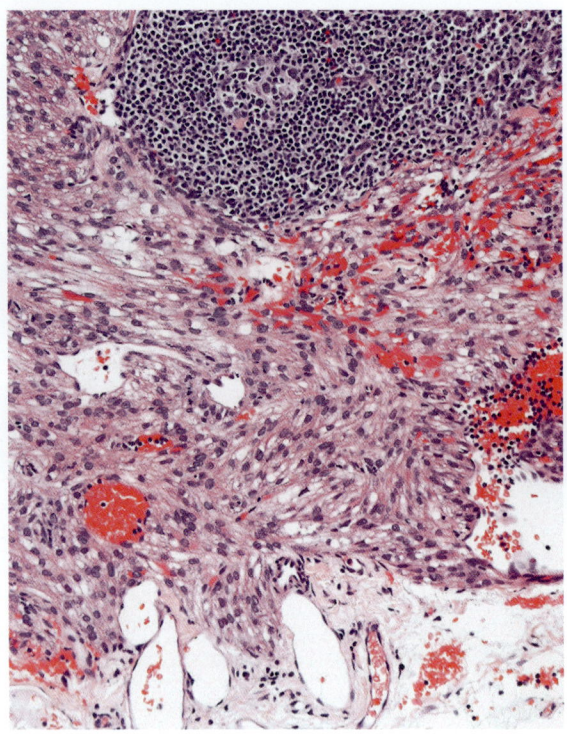

Figure 66-6

ANGIOMYOLIPOMA PARTIALLY INVOLVING LYMPH NODE

Both spindle cells and blood vessels are present (H&E stain).

Immunophenotypic Findings. Immunohistochemical analysis of angiomyolipomas shows that the muscle component is positive for smooth muscle actin and HMB-45 (1,30,39). The cells of angiomyolipoma also express other melanoma-associated markers including SOX10, MART1/melan A, tyrosinase, and micro-ophthalmia transcription factor (MITF). Epithelioid angiomyolipomas are more commonly positive for p53 and often have a higher proliferation (Ki-67) rate (36).

Molecular Genetic Findings. DNA content analysis, as assessed by flow cytometry in angiomyolipomas, is usually diploid (1,54). Conventional cytogenetic analysis has shown clonal karyotypes, but no consistent cytogenetic abnormalities (61). By assessing the human androgen receptor gene on chromosome Xq11-12, about 40 to 50 percent of cases are of monoclonal origin (9,48). *TP53* mutations were identified in 6 of 11 (55 percent) cases of epithelioid angiomyolipoma in one study (36).

Differential Diagnosis. *Kaposi Sarcoma.* The spindled nature of the cellular component of angiomyolipoma may be confused with a primary vascular neoplasm, most notably Kaposi sarcoma. Correlation with clinical findings is important. In addition, the spindle cells are negative for vascular markers and HHV-8 in angiomyolipoma, unlike the spindle cells of Kaposi sarcoma.

Lymphangioleiomyomatosis. Lymphangioleiomyomatosis (see below) may be considered in the differential diagnosis of angiomyolipoma involving lymph nodes. Some patients with lymphangioleiomyomatosis also have renal angiomyolipoma, and both neoplasms are composed of spindle cells that are positive for HMB-45 and associated with *TSC* mutations. The common development of progressive lung disease is unique to patients with lymphangioleiomyomatosis. Histologically, the haphazard mixture of the muscle, fat, and blood vessel components in most cases of angiomyolipoma is not present in lymphangioleiomyomatosis.

Treatment and Prognosis. Most cases of angiomyolipoma are benign including neoplasms that involve the inferior vena cava or regional lymph nodes, and resection alone is sufficient therapy (39). However, a small subset of cases may locally recur or metastasize, particularly cases of epithelioid angiomyolipoma (5).

LYMPHANGIOLEIOMYOMATOSIS

General Features. *Lymphangioleiomyomatosis* (also known as *lymphangiomyomatosis*) is a neoplastic proliferation of lymphatic channels and abnormal smooth muscle-like cells (11,50). This disease involves the lungs, thoracic duct, and axial lymph nodes (11,50). Localized lesions are designated as *lymphangioleiomyoma*.

Most cases of lymphangioleiomyomatosis are sporadic, but a subset of patients has tuberous sclerosis (50). Sporadic cases usually have biallelic mutations of *TSC2* whereas patients with tuberous sclerosis have mutations of either *TSC1* or *TSC2* (50). These mutations result in a loss-of-function of these genes and result in abnormal mTOR signaling (reviewed in reference 31a). About half of patients with lymphangioleiomyomatosis also have renal angiomyolipoma.

Lymphangioleiomyomatosis begins as small proliferations of spindle cells that protrude into the lumens of lymphatic vessels. Fragmentation of the protruding cells is thought to be the mechanism of spread from site to site (50). Growth factors, such as vascular endothelial growth factor (VEGF) types C and D, are also involved in the proliferation of the spindle cells. Serum VEGF-D levels correlate with disease activity as assessed by radiologic methods. Patients who have undergone lung transplantation for lymphangioleiomyomatosis have developed recurrent disease in the allografts, presumably by spread from axial lymph nodes and lymphatic vessels (50).

Clinical Features. Lymphangioleiomyomatosis occurs almost exclusively in women, usually during the child-bearing years, but rarely men are affected (11,50,53a,56). Patients most often present with respiratory symptoms including exertional dyspnea, cough, hemosputum, and spontaneous pneumothorax. These manifestations are a result of the proliferation of spindle cells and lymphatic vessels, which form numerous pleural cysts and destroy alveolar lung parenchyma (11,50,53a).

Rarely, as a result of involvement of lymphatics or lymph nodes, chyle leaks into body cavities, airways, or urine (50). Some patients present with lymphedema of the lower extremities. Lymphangioleiomyomatosis may progress during pregnancy because the spindle cells proliferate in response to stimulation by female hormones (50).

Lymphangioleiomyomatosis may be detected incidentally in lymph node dissection specimens of women who have undergone gynecologic surgery for cancer. Schoolmeester and Park (49) reported 19 patients, all adults (age range, 35 to 71 years) who did not have a history of either tuberous sclerosis or renal angiomyolipoma. Typically, only one or a few lymph nodes were involved by lesions less than 1 cm (mean, 0.43 cm). None of these women went on to develop lymphangioleiomyomatosis of the lungs.

Lymphangioleiomyoma can arise theoretically in any axial lymph node, but most often arises in retroperitoneal and pelvic lymph nodes. These lesions are usually asymptomatic and are detected as incidental findings during surgery performed for another reason.

Histologic Findings. In lymph nodes, lymphangioleiomyomatosis is characterized by sinusoidal involvement by a proliferation of spindled, smooth muscle-like cells associated with an anastomosing network of endothelium-lined spaces (7,11,49,50,60). In fully developed lesions, the gross cut surface of a lymph node has been described as having a shredded appearance (50). The spindle cell proliferation is bland, without mitotic figures, and in early lesions can be subtle and difficult to recognize.

Immunophenotypic Findings. The spindle cells of lymphangioleiomyomatosis are reactive with smooth muscle actin, desmin, and HMB-45. The pattern of HMB-45 expression is cytoplasmic and granular (7,49,50). The spindle cells are also positive for estrogen and progesterone receptors, and β-catenin is often positive in a cytoplasmic pattern (49). D2-40/podoplanin and E-cadherin are positive in some cases, which correlates with advanced stage (23). Epidermal growth factor receptor (EGFR) is also positive in some cases, but is not associated with gene amplification (23). Intermixed endothelial cells are often positive for vascular-associated antigens.

Differential Diagnosis. Smooth muscle proliferations of lymph node can resemble lymphangioleiomyomatosis or lymphangioleiomyoma. In contrast to lymphangioleiomyomatosis, the smooth muscle cells are plump, with clear or pale cytoplasm. Immunohistochemical analysis is helpful as smooth muscle tumors express a variety of muscle-associated antigens and are negative for HMB-45.

Treatment and Prognosis. The treatment of patients with lymphangioleiomyomatosis is highly challenging. Over time and usually after a prolonged interval of 10 or more years, patients may die of lung failure (11,50). Lung transplantation has been employed for some patients. Inhibitors of the mTOR pathway (e.g., sirolimus) have been used for patients with progressive disease (4,53a).

LEIOMYOMATOSIS

General Features. *Leiomyomatosis* is a smooth muscle proliferation that replaces lymph node. *Leiomyoma* is a benign tumor of smooth muscle that is usually confined to one lymph node or the spleen.

Leiomyomatosis most often involves intra-abdominal or pelvic lymph nodes. Possible etiologies have been suggested and include: 1) metastasis of a uterine leiomyoma; 2) organization

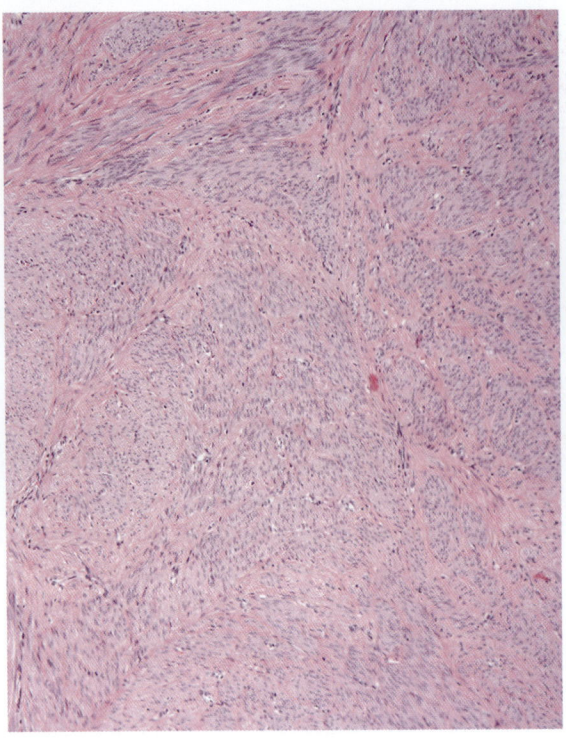

Figure 66-7

LEIOMYOMA INVOLVING LYMPH NODE

The lymph node parenchyma is replaced by intersecting fascicles of smooth muscle (H&E stain).

of decidua or endometriosis in lymph node; and 3) direct derivation from subcoelomic mesenchyme (27). Leiomyoma of lymph node or spleen is thought to arise from the smooth muscle walls of blood vessels.

Clinical Features. Leiomyomatosis is usually detected incidentally during gynecologic surgery performed for another purpose (40). Intranodal leiomyoma may cause lymphadenopathy or be an incidental finding (22). Other than palpable lymphadenopathy, patients have no other symptoms. Leiomyoma of the spleen may be associated with leiomyomas involving other sites, bilateral testicular microlithiasis, and an empty sella turcica (16).

Histologic Findings. Leiomyomatosis (and leiomyoma) of lymph node is characterized by a proliferation of smooth muscle cells that partially or totally replace the lymph node architecture (fig. 66-7) (22,40,52). The smooth muscle cells have spindle-shaped nuclei with blunt ends and do not exhibit atypia or mitotic figures. Leiomy-

oma resembles benign smooth muscle tumors at other anatomic sites.

Differential Diagnosis. Lymphangioleiomyomatosis is an important entity in the differential diagnosis, as discussed above.

ANGIOMYOMATOUS HAMARTOMA

Clinical Features. *Angiomyomatous hamartoma* is a smooth muscle proliferation that occurs predominantly in the lymph node hilum, with extension into the medulla and cortex. Patients are usually adults but there is a wide age range. Men are more frequently affected. Patients present with enlarged, often matted lymph nodes almost exclusively in the inguinal region (6,18).

Gross and Histologic Findings. Grossly, the lymph nodes in angiomyomatous hamartoma are firm and white, and also may be fibrotic. Histologically, the proliferation is based in the lymph node hilum and extends into the nodal parenchyma. The proliferation is composed of smooth muscle bundles irregularly arranged in fibrotic stroma and is associated with medium-sized, thick-walled blood vessels (fig. 66-8) (6,18). Congestion and thrombosis of blood vessels may be present.

In our experience, dermatopathic changes commonly coexist in lymph nodes involved by angiomyomatous hamartoma and some patients have concurrent skin disease. Whether this combination of findings is related or simply coincidental is unknown. The smooth muscle cells of angiomyomatous hamartoma show reactivity for desmin, actin, and other muscle-associated antigens (6,18).

Treatment and Prognosis. Angiomyomatous hamartoma is a benign lesion. No specific therapy is required.

LYMPHANGIOMA AND LYMPHANGIOMATOSIS

General and Clinical Features. *Lymphangioma* is a proliferation of lymphatic-derived, thin-walled cystic structures often filled with fluid. *Lymphangiomatosis* is a rare disease with diffuse or multifocal involvement of tissues by lymphangioma. Lymph nodes and spleen may be involved.

Lymphangioma is usually an isolated finding in lymph node. Lymphangiomatosis is rare and is usually observed in infants.

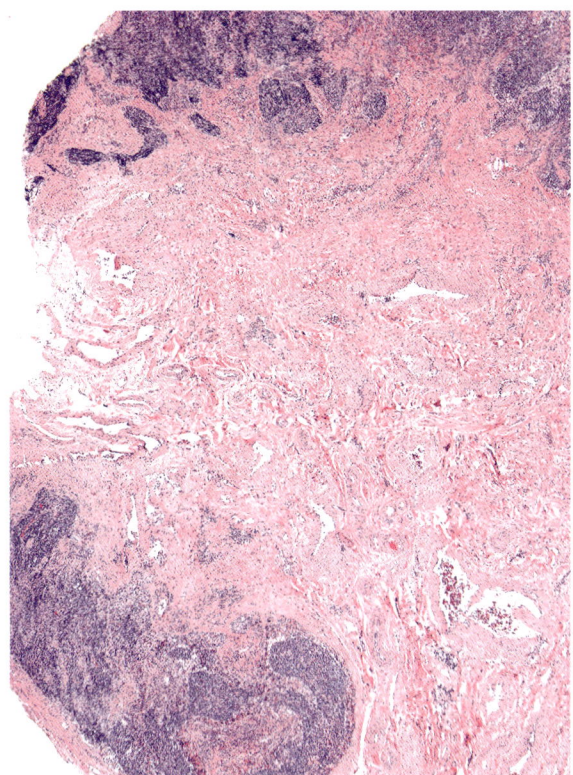

Figure 66-8

**ANGIOMYOMATOUS HAMARTOMA
INVOLVING INGUINAL LYMPH NODE**

The hilum of the lymph node is replaced by large-caliber blood vessels, smooth muscle bundles, and fibrous tissue.

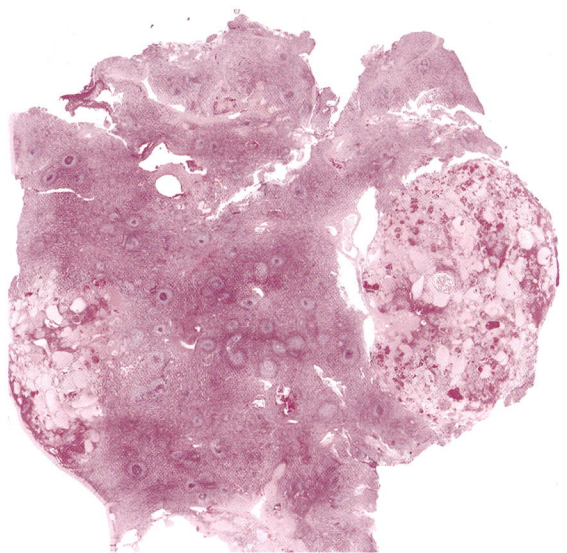

Figure 66-9

LARGE LYMPHANGIOMA INVOLVING SPLEEN

The smooth walled cystic spaces are filled with clear or eosinophilic lymph fluid (H&E stain).

Gross and Histologic Findings. Gross examination of lymphangioma reveals a variably sized multicystic appearance or, less commonly, a solid appearance (29,58,60). In the spleen, lymphangioma, especially if small, may be located in a subcapsular location. Histologically, the cystic spaces are lined by flat, bland endothelial cells (fig. 66-9). Papillary tufts of lining cells are present in most cases. The cystic spaces are separated by collagenous stroma, sometimes with bundles of smooth muscle (29,45). The cysts are filled with watery, eosinophilic proteinaceous fluid. Foamy macrophages or cholesterol clefts may be seen within the cysts.

Immunophenotypic Findings. Immunohistochemical staining confirms the lymphatic derivation of the lining cells. Podoplanin/D2-40 is positive and the vascular-associated antigens CD31, CD34, ERG, and FLI1 are variably positive in lymphatic vessels and can highlight the cells of lymphangioma.

Differential Diagnosis. Isolated lymphangioma of spleen may be mistaken for a mesothelial cyst. Both lesions are lined by bland, flattened cells. Immunohistochemical analysis is helpful. If the lining cells are positive for keratin, the diagnosis of mesothelial cyst is supported over lymphangioma.

Treatment and Prognosis. If incompletely excised, a lymphangioma may recur.

LIPOMATOSIS AND LIPOMA

General and Clinical Features. *Lipomatosis* refers to the non-neoplastic infiltration or replacement of lymph node by mature adipose tissue. *Lipoma* is a benign tumor of fat cells that occurs within lymph node or spleen.

Lipomatosis or fatty infiltration of the lymph node is a common cause of lymphadenopathy, especially in axillary lymph nodes. It is usually an incidental finding that is not clinically important (45). Lipoma of lymph node can involve any lymph node group. Adipose tissue is not a normal finding in spleen, and is always associated with a pathologic process.

Gross and Histologic Findings. Grossly, lymph nodes are soft, greasy, and often bright

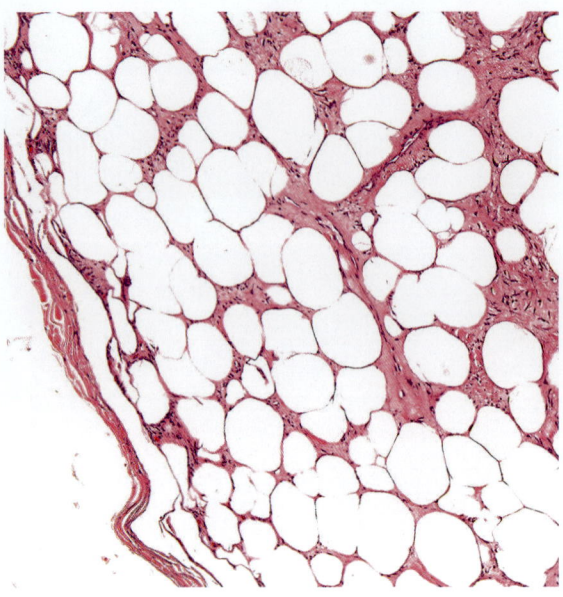

Figure 66-10

LIPOMATOSIS OR LIPOMA INVOLVING LYMPH

The lymph node is replaced by mature adipose tissue consistent with lipomatosis or lipoma. The lymph node sinus is maintained (H&E stain).

yellow. The lymph node size depends on the site and duration of the lesion. In some cases, the distinct borders of the lymph node are difficult to distinguish from perinodal fat. Occasionally, a thin rim of residual lymph node is seen at the periphery and near a thinned capsule.

Lipomatosis is characterized by a nodular/lobular infiltrate of mature adipocytes (fig. 66-10). There is subtotal or total effacement of the normal lymph node architecture (especially the hilum) by mature adipose cells (45). Distinguishing lipoma from lipomatosis can be challenging by histologic analysis, but this distinction is of no clinical consequence.

Ancillary studies are rarely employed in the evaluation of lipomatosis and lipoma. The cytoplasm of adipose tissue cells is reactive for S-100 protein. Conventional cytogenetic analysis performed on cases of lipoma has shown chromosomal abnormalities of *HMGA2*/12q15 in many cases (62).

Differential Diagnosis. In lymph node, it is important to distinguish lipoma from angiomyolipoma with a predominance of mature adipose tissue.

Treatment and Prognosis. Lipomatosis and lipomas are benign lesions and no treatment beyond excision is required.

VASCULAR TRANSFORMATION OF LYMPH NODE SINUSES

General and Clinical Features. *Vascular transformation of lymph node sinuses* (VTS), also known as *nodal angiomatosis*, is a proliferation of small vascular channels that form an anastomosing network within the subcapsular and medullary sinuses of lymph nodes. It is uncommon and has no gender or age predilection (8,28). It appears to occur most commonly in abdominal lymph nodes, but VTS can involve all lymph node groups. In many patients, VTS is an incidental finding, usually associated with lymph node excision for other causes, such as tumor staging. Less frequently, VTS presents as isolated lymphadenopathy. Although VTS most often involves a single lymph node, in some patients involvement of groups of lymph nodes, multiple individual lymph nodes, or bilateral lymph nodes can be observed (8,28).

About 70 percent of cases of VTS are associated with vascular obstruction (8) due to adjacent tumor, thrombosis, congestive heart failure, constrictive pericarditis, or previous surgery/radiation to the area of the involved lymph node. Unspecified angiogenic factors also have been postulated in the pathogenesis of VTS.

Gross and Histologic Findings. Lymph nodes involved by VTS typically appear normal on gross examination. Histologic examination shows small, endothelial-lined channels in the lymph node sinuses (fig. 66-11). Several microscopic patterns, alone or in combination, have been described and include: cleft-like spaces, about 70 percent of cases; rounded vascular spaces, 60 percent; solid areas, 40 percent; and a plexiform pattern (rare) (8,47). In some cases, VTS can form a nodule within a lymph node (47). Fibrosis may be present. Extravasation of erythrocytes and, rarely, hyaline globules, similar to those of Kaposi sarcoma, can be observed (8,28). Hemosiderin deposits may be prominent.

Immunophenotypic Findings. Immunohistochemical stains are useful for highlighting the vascular nature of VTS, especially in areas that are solid. Antibodies specific for CD31, CD34, ERG, and FLI1 confirm the vascular nature of

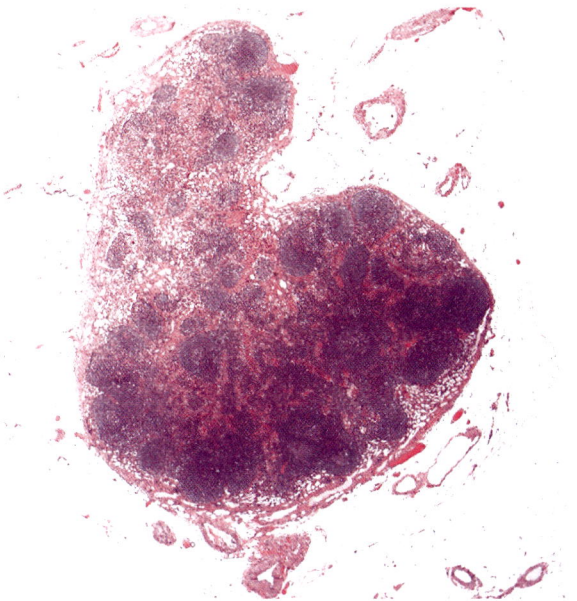 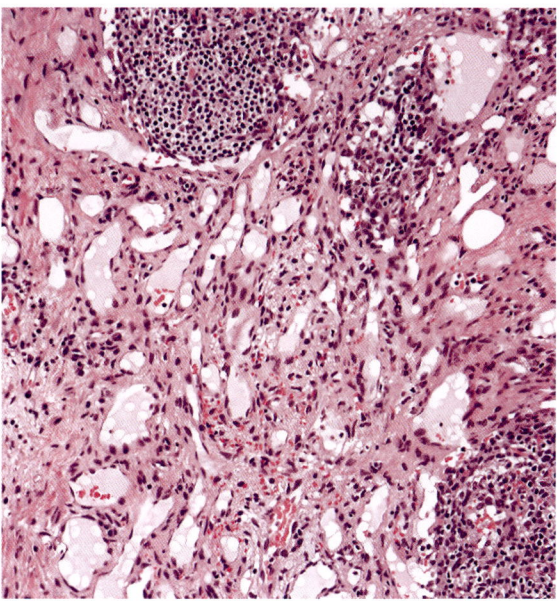

Figure 66-11

VASCULAR TRANSFORMATION OF LYMPH NODE SINUSES

Left: At low magnification the subcapsular and some medullary sinuses are expanded by a proliferation of vascular channels.
Right: The vascular channels are lined by bland endothelial cells (H&E stain).

the process. Some reports have shown that VTS is positive for D2-40/podoplanin, a marker of lymphatic differentiation. Human herpesvirus 8 (HHV-8) is negative.

Differential Diagnosis. *Kaposi Sarcoma.* The most important entity in the differential diagnosis of VTS is Kaposi sarcoma (Table 66-2). Both VTS and Kaposi sarcoma are vascular processes, and cytoplasmic hyaline globules can occur in either entity. Unlike VTS, Kaposi sarcoma involves the lymph node capsule. Other features that support the diagnosis of Kaposi sarcoma over VTS include nuclear atypia, numerous hyaline globules, and predominance of short slit-like vascular spaces. In addition, Kaposi sarcoma is positive for HHV-8, unlike VTS.

Other Vascular Tumors. As discussed elsewhere, other malignant vascular neoplasms occur in lymph node or spleen. Unlike malignant tumors, the cells in VTS are cytologically bland, without atypia or mitotic figures (8,47).

Treatment and Prognosis. No specific treatment is required for VTS since this lesion is unlikely to cause specific problems. Removing the underlying cause of lymphatic blockage may improve the condition.

LYMPHANGIECTASIA

Lymphangiectasis of lymph node is characterized by an abnormal dilatation of pre-existing sinuses and lymphatic channels. It is a reactive process that is usually associated with proximal soft tissue obstruction and involves preexisting structures, unlike nodal lymphangioma, which is of hamartomatous or neoplastic origin (58).

The dilated lymphatic vessels in lymphangiectasis are filled with eosinophilic, protein-

Table 66-2		
DISTINGUISHING VASCULAR TRANSFORMATION OF LYMPH NODE SINUSES (VTS) FROM KAPOSI SARCOMA		
Features	**VTS**	**Kaposi Sarcoma**
Slit-like vascular spaces	Some	Predominant
Spindle-shaped cells	Present	Present
Extravasated RBC	Occasional	Frequent
Capsular involvement	Absent	Frequent
Cytologic atypia	Absent	Subset of cases
Hyaline globules	Rare	Common
HHV-8[a]	Absent	Present

[a]HHV-8 = human herpesvirus 8.

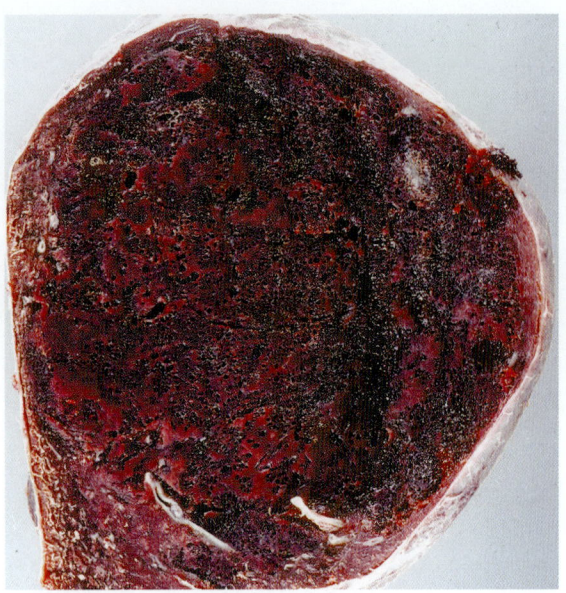
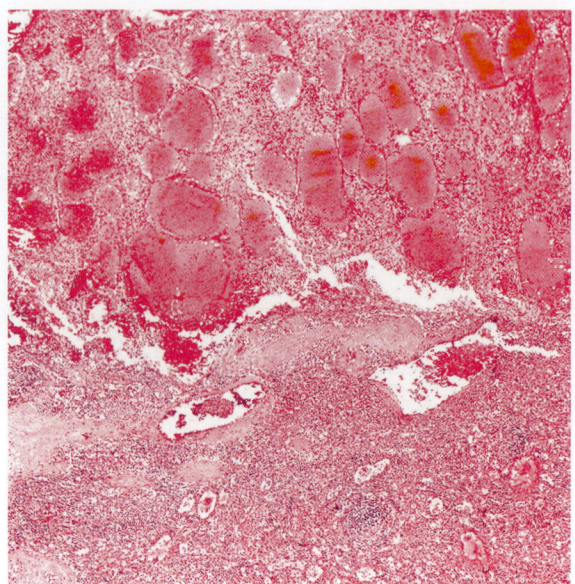

Figure 66-12

PELIOSIS INVOLVING SPLEEN

Left: Gross image illustrates the spongy appearance and blood-filled spaces of peliosis. (Courtesy of Dr. Diane Farhi, Atlanta, GA.)

Right: Histologic section shows the numerous blood-filled spaces of peliosis (top) and normal spleen (bottom) (H&E stain).

aceous fluid. Occasional lymphocytes and red blood cells may be present. The lining cells are flattened, with benign cytologic features. Antibodies specific for lymphatic endothelium, such as D2-40/podoplanin, allow distinction of lymphatics from other vascular-derived processes.

Lymphangiectasia shows morphologic overlap with VTS (see previous section), isolated lymphangioma, and systemic lymphangiomatosis, and these entities may share an underlying etiology, such as stasis. With the exception of systemic lymphangiomatosis, which is extensive, distinguishing between these other entities has little clinical importance.

Lymphangiectasia is typically detected as an incidental finding. It has little clinical consequence.

PELIOSIS

General Features. *Peliosis* is a rare, non-neoplastic proliferation of blood-filled cavities that most commonly occurs in the liver, but spleen, lymph nodes, and other organs can be involved. Peliosis can be localized to spleen or lymph node (55). Other rare anatomic sites that may be involved by peliosis include the lungs, kidneys, bone marrow, and parathyroid glands.

A number of diseases and lifestyle choices are associated with peliosis including tuberculosis, hematologic neoplasms, chemotherapy and steroid treatment, chronic alcoholism and cirrhosis, and intravenous drug abuse (55). The exact etiology of peliosis is unknown. The pathogenesis may be related to underlying vascular malformations that are made apparent by local alterations of vascular pressure.

Gross and Histologic Findings. Cross sections of the spleen involved by peliosis show multiple round to oval cavities filled with blood (fig. 66-12) (55). These cavities are clustered, often abutting the white pulp, but can be widely distributed throughout the splenic parenchyma. The blood may be liquid, clotted, or associated with thrombus. Histologic sections show widely dilated spaces, many of which appear to be sinusoids lined by cytologically bland, flattened cells without atypia or mitotic figures (55).

Differential Diagnosis. *Infections.* Peliosis may be associated with a variety of infectious agents. Special stains should be performed to exclude microorganisms.

Vascular Neoplasms. Vascular neoplasms show a proliferation of vascular elements, rather than

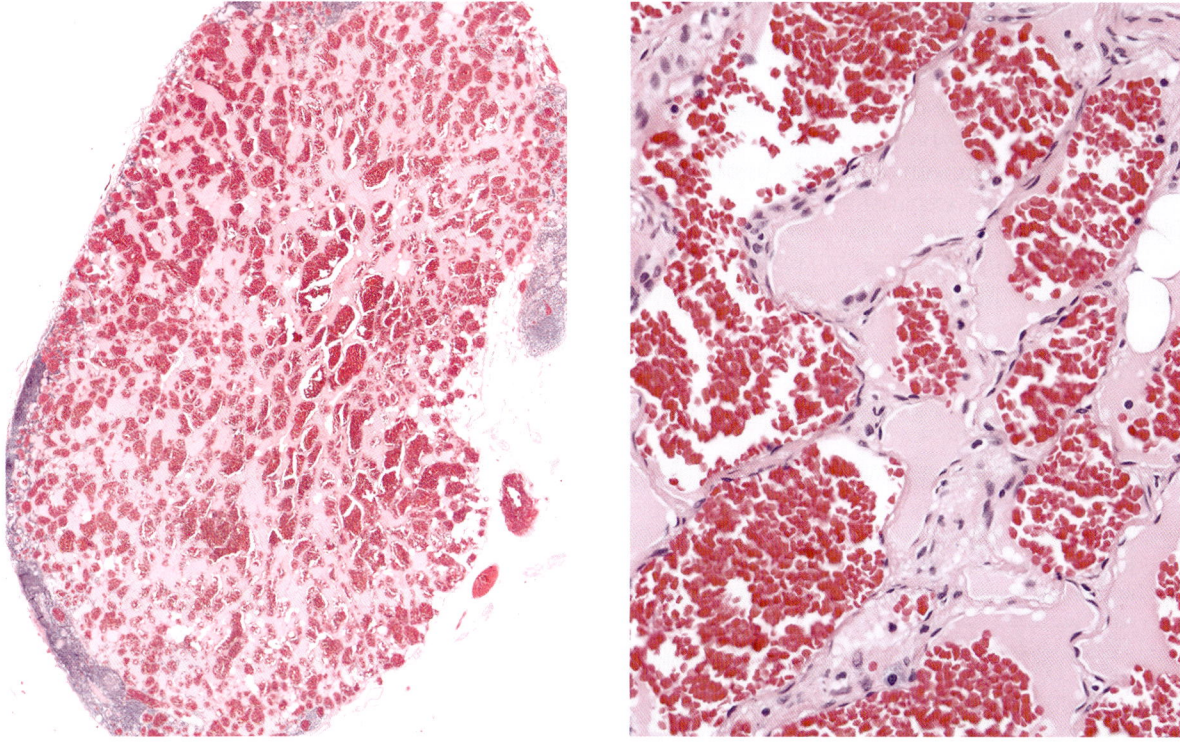

Figure 66-13

CAVERNOUS HEMANGIOMA INVOLVING LYMPH NODE

Left: Vascular spaces distended with blood replace over 90 percent of the parenchyma. A rim of lymph node tissue is present at the edge of the tumor.

Right: The vascular spaces are lined by bland endothelial cells (H&E stain).

dilatation and cyst formation of preformed elements. Cytologic atypia is associated with many vascular neoplasms, unlike peliosis.

Treatment and Prognosis. The clinical importance of peliosis lies in its association with spontaneous splenic rupture, due to a combination of splenomegaly and the fragility of the dilated, cystic sinusoids. Splenic rupture can result in hemoperitoneum and, rarely, death (55).

HEMANGIOMA

General Features. *Hemangioma* is a benign, neoplastic proliferation of vascular elements that can occur in lymph nodes or spleen. Hemangioma of lymph node is usually detected incidentally, but rarely is a cause of lymphadenopathy (19,25). Hemangioma occurs more commonly in spleen and is discussed in more detail in chapter 63.

Histologic Findings. Hemangioma of lymph node is characterized by variably sized vascular spaces lined by bland, flat endothelial cells (figs.

66-13) (19,25). These spaces are large and distended by blood cells and proteinaceous fluid (cavernous hemangioma), or are small (capillary hemangioma). The vascular spaces in hemangioma are often anastomosing, but the lumens are generally patent.

Hemangiomas are lined by endothelial cells positive for CD31, CD34, WT1, ERG, FLI1, and factor VIII and are negative for CD8.

Differential Diagnosis. *Lymphangioma.* Lymphangioma and hemangioma of lymph node overlap histologically and immunophenotypically. Lymphangioma is composed of cystic spaces lined by bland lining cells separated by collagenous stroma, sometimes associated with smooth muscle. Immunohistochemical analysis shows that the lining cells are positive for D2-40/podoplanin and variably positive for vascular-associated antigens. Distinguishing lymphangioma from hemangioma of lymph node does not have clinical importance.

Angiomyomatous Hamartoma. Unlike hemangioma, angiomyomatous hamartoma is based primarily in the lymph node hilum and extends into the lymph node cortex and medulla. This lesion usually involves inguinal or femoral lymph nodes. Angiomyomatous hamartoma does not have an expansile appearance as is seen in hemangioma.

Vascular Transformation of Lymph Node Sinuses. Unlike hemangioma, VTS is located within lymph node sinuses and does not form an expansile mass. As stated above, VTS may be associated with solid areas and a plexiform pattern, which do not occur in hemangioma.

Treatment and Prognosis

Hemangiomas are benign lesions and when isolated they can be treated by simple resection.

REFERENCES

1. Abdulla M, Bui HX, del Rosario AD, Wolf BC, Ross JS. Renal angiomyolipoma. DNA content and immunohistochemical study of classic and multicentric variants. Arch Pathol Lab Med 1994;118:735-739.
2. Arber DA, Kamel OW, van de Rijn M, et al. Frequent presence of the Epstein-Barr virus in inflammatory pseudotumor. Hum Pathol 1995;26:1093-1098.
3. Bhullar JS, Varshney N, Dubay L. Intranodal palisaded myofibroblastoma: a review of the literature. Int J Surg Pathol 2013;21:337-341.
4. Bissler JJ, McCormack FX, Young LR, et al. Sirolimus for angiomyolipoma in tuberous sclerosis complex or lymphangioleiomyomatosis. N Engl J Med 2008;358:140-151.
5. Brimo F, Robinson B, Guo C, Zhou M, Latour M, Epstein JI. Renal epithelioid angiomyolipoma with atypia: a series of 40 cases with emphasis on clinicopathologic prognostic indicators of malignancy. Am J Surg Pathol 2010;34:715-722.
6. Chan JK, Frizzera G, Fletcher CD, Rosai J. Primary vascular tumors of lymph nodes other than Kaposi's sarcoma. Analysis of 39 cases and delineation of two new entities. Am J Surg Pathol 1992;16:335-350.
7. Chan JK, Tsang WY, Pau MY, Tang MC, Pang SW, Fletcher CD. Lymphangiomyomatosis and angiomyolipoma: closely related entities characterized by hamartomatous proliferation of HMB-45-positive smooth muscle. Histopathology 1993;22:445-455.
8. Chan JK, Warnke RA, Dorfman R. Vascular transformation of sinuses in lymph nodes. A study of its morphological spectrum and distinction from Kaposi's sarcoma. Am J Surg Pathol 1991;15:732-743.
9. Cheng L, Gu J, Eble JN, et al. Molecular genetic evidence for different clonal origin of components of human renal angiomyolipomas. Am J Surg Pathol 2001;25:1231-1236.
10. Coffin CM, Dehner LP, Meis-Kindblom JM. Inflammatory myofibroblastic tumor, inflammatory fibrosarcoma, and related lesions: an historical review with differential diagnostic considerations. Semin Diagn Pathol 1998;15:161-173.
11. Corrin B, Liebow AA, Friedman PJ. Pulmonary lymphangiomyomatosis: a review. Am J Pathol 1975;79:348-382.
12. Cossu A, Lissia A, Dedola MF, et al. Classic follicular dendritic reticulum cell tumor of the lymph node developing in a patient with a previous inflammatory pseudotumor-like proliferation. Hum Pathol 2005;36:207-211.
13. Creager AJ, Garwacki CP. Recurrent intranodal palisaded myofibroblastoma with metaplastic bone formation. Arch Pathol Lab Med 1999;123:433-436.
14. Davis RE, Warnke RA, Dorfman RF. Inflammatory pseudotumor of lymph nodes. Additional observations and evidence for an inflammatory etiology. Am J Surg Pathol 1991;15:744-756.
15. Dehner LP, Coffin CM. Idiopathic fibrosclerotic disorders and other inflammatory pseudotumors. Semin Diagn Pathol 1998;15:161-173.
16. Demirel S, Erk O, Akkaya V, et al. Multiple vascular leiomyomas involving bilateral adrenal glands, spleen, and epicardium, associated with bilateral testicular microlithiasis and empty sella turcica. J Pediatr Surg 1997;32:1365-1367.
17. Deshpande V. The pathology of IgG4-related disease: critical issues and challenges. Semin Diagn Pathol 2012;29:191-196.
18. Dzombeta T, Francina M, Matkovi K, et al. Angiomyolipomatous hamartoma of the inguinal lymph node—report of two cases and literature review. In Vivo 2012;26:459-462.
19. Elgoweini M, Chetty R. Primary nodal hemangioma. Arch Pathol Lab Med 2012;136:110-112.
20. Facchetti F, De Wolf Peeters C, De Wever I, Frizzera G. Inflammatory pseudotumor of lymph nodes. Immunohistochemical evidence for its fibrohistiocytic nature. Am J Pathol 1990;137:281-289.

21. Facchetti F, Incardona P, Lonardi S, et al. Nodal inflammatory pseudotumor caused by luetic infection. Am J Surg Pathol 2009;33:447-453.
22. Girhotra M, Virk SS, Verma S, Bansal K, Gupta R. Intranodal leiomyoma in a young child: report of a rare spindle cell lesion. Pediatr Dev Pathol 2014;17:118-121.
23. Grzegorek I, Lenze D, Chabowski M, et al. Immunohistochemical evaluation of pulmonary lymphangioleiomyomatosis. Anticancer Res 2015;35:3353-3360.
24. Gulwani H, Chopra P. Inflammatory pseudotumor of lymph nodes presenting as pyrexia of unknown origin. Indian J Pathol Microbiol 2008;51:67-69.
25. Har-El G, Heffner DK, Ruffy M. Haemangioma in a cervical lymph node. J Laryngol Otol 1990;104:513-515.
26. Hartsock RJ, Halling LW, King FM. Luetic lymphadenitis: a clinical and histologic study of 20 cases. Am J Clin Pathol 1970;53:304-314.
27. Hsu YK, Rosenshein NB, Parmley TH, Woodruff JD, Elberfeld HT. Leiomyomatosis in pelvic lymph nodes. Obstet Gynecol 1981;57:91s-93s.
28. Ide F, Shimoyama T, Horie N. Vascular transformation of sinuses in bilateral cervical lymph nodes. Head Neck 1999;21:366-369.
29. Ioannidis I, Kahn AG. Splenic lymphangioma. Arch Pathol Lab Med 2015;139:278-282.
30. Kimura N, Watanabe M, Date F, et al. HMB-45 and tuberin in hamartomas associated with tuberous sclerosis. Mod Pathol 1997;10:952-959.
31. Kleist B, Poetsch M, Schmoll J. Intranodal palisaded myofibroblastoma with overexpression of cyclin D1. Arch Pathol Lab Med 2003;127:1040-1043.
31a. Krymskaya VP, McCormack FX. Lymphangioleiomyomatosis: a monogenic model of malignancy. Annu Rev Med 2017;68:69-83.
32. Kojima M, Nakamura S, Shimizu K, et al. Inflammatory pseudotumor of lymph nodes: clinicopathologic and immunohistological study of 11 Japanese cases. Int J Surg Pathol 2001;9:207-14.
33. Kutok JL, Pinkus GS, Dorfman DM, Fletcher CD. Inflammatory pseudotumor of lymph node and spleen: an entity biologically distinct from inflammatory myofibroblastic tumor. Hum Pathol 2001;32:1382-1387.
34. Laskin WB, Lasota JP, Fetsch JF, Felisiak-Golabek A, Wang ZF, Miettinen M. Intranodal palisaded myofibroblastoma: another mesenchymal neoplasm with CTNNB1 (β-catenin gene) mutations: clinicopathologic, immunohistochemical, and molecular genetic study of 18 cases. Am J Surg Pathol 2015;39:197-205.
35. Lee JY, Abell E, Shevechik GJ. Solitary spindle cell tumor with myoid differentiation of the lymph node. Arch Pathol Lab Med 1989;113:547-550.
36. Li W, Guo L, Ma J, Zheng S. Immunohistochemistry of p53 and Ki-67 and p53 mutation analysis in renal epithelioid angiomyolipoma. Int J Clin Exp Pathol 2015;8:9446-9451.
37. Logani S, Lucas DR, Cheng JD, Ioachim HL, Adsay NV. Spindle cell tumors associated with mycobacteria in lymph nodes of HIV-positive patients: 'Kaposi sarcoma with mycobacteria' and 'mycobacterial pseudotumor'. Am J Surg Pathol 1999;23:656-661.
38. Lovly CM, Gupta A, Lipson D, et al. Inflammatory myofibroblastic tumors harbor multiple potentially actionable kinase fusions. Cancer Discov 2014;4:889-895.
39. Martignoni G, Reuter VF, Cheville J, et al. Mesenchymal tumours occurring mainly in adults. In: Moch H, Humphrey PA, Ulbright TM, Reuter VE, eds. Tumours of the urinary system and male genital organs. IARC Press; 2016:62-66.
40. Mazzoleni G, Salerno A, Santini D, Marabini A, Martinelli G. Leiomyomatosis in pelvic lymph nodes. Histopathology 1992;21:588-589.
41. Michal M, Chlumská A, Skálová A, Fakan F. Palisaded intranodal myofibroblastoma. Electron microscopic study. Zentralbl Pathol 1993;139:81-88.
42. Miras-Parra FJ, Parra-Ruiz J, Gomez-Morales M, Gómez-Jiménez FJ, de la Higuera-Torres-Puchol J. Inflammatory pseudotumor of lymph nodes with focal infiltration in liver and spleen. Dig Dis Sci 2003;48:2003-2004.
43. Montes-Moreno S, García OA, Santiago-Ruiz G, Ferreira JA, García JF, Pinilla MA. Primary luetic lymphadenopathy simulating sarcoma-like inflammatory pseudotumour of the lymph node. Histopathology 2010;56:656-658.
44. Moran CA, Suster S, Abbondanzo SL. Inflammatory pseudotumor of lymph nodes: a study of 25 cases with emphasis on morphological heterogeneity. Hum Pathol 1997;28:332-338.
45. O'Malley DP, George TI, Orazi A, Abbondanzo SL. Benign and reactive conditions of lymph node and spleen. AFIP Atlas of Non-Tumor Pathology, First Series, Fascicle 7. Washington, DC;: American Registry of Pathology; 2009.
46. Perrone T, De Wolf-Peeters C, Frizzera G. Inflammatory pseudotumor of lymph nodes. A distinctive pattern of nodal reaction. Am J Surg Pathol 1988;15:351-361.
47. Pirola S, Shenjere P, Nonaka D. Combined usual and nodular types of vascular transformation of sinuses in the same lymph node. Int J Surg Pathol 2012;20:175-177.
48. Saxena A, Alport EC, Custead S, Skinnider LF. Molecular analysis of clonality of sporadic angiomyolipoma. J Pathol 1999;189:79-84.
49. Schoolmeester JK, Park KJ. Incidental nodal lymphangioleiomyomatosis is not a harbinger of pulmonary lymphangioleiomyomatosis. A study of 19 cases with evaluation of diagnostic immunohistochemistry. Am J Surg Pathol 2015;39: 1404-1410.
50. Seyama K, Kumasaka T, Kurihara M, Mitani K, Sato T. Lymphangioleiomyomatosis: a disease involving the lymphatic system. Lymphat Res Biol 2010;8:21-31.

999

51. Skagias L, Vasou O, Kondi-Pafiti A, Politi E. Imprint cytology of intranodal palisaded myofibroblastoma. Diagn Cytopathol 2010;38:272-273.

52. Starasoler L, Vuitch F, Albores-Saavedra J. Intranodal leiomyoma: another distinctive primary spindle cell neoplasm of lymph node. Am J Clin Pathol 1991;95:858-862.

53. Suster S, Rosai J. Intranodal hemorrhagic spindle-cell tumor with "amianthoid" fibers. Report of six cases of a distinctive mesenchymal neoplasm of the inguinal region that simulates Kaposi's sarcoma. Am J Surg Pathol 1989;13:347-357.

53a. Taveira-DaSilva AM, Moss J. Epidemiology, pathogenesis and diagnosis of lymphangioleiomyomatosis. Expert Opin Orphan Drugs 2016;4:369-378.

54. Terris B, Fléjou JF, Picot R, Belghiti J, Hénin D. Hepatic angiomyolipoma. A report of four cases with immunohistochemical and DNA-flow cytometric studies. Arch Pathol Lab Med 1996;120:68-72.

55. Tsokos M, Erbersdobler A. Pathology of peliosis. Forensic Sci Int 2005;149:25-33.

56. Wakida K, Watanabe Y, Kumasaka T, et al. Lymphangioleiomyomatosis in a male. Ann Thor Surg 2015;100:1105-1107.

57. Weiss SW, Gnepp DR, Bratthauer GL. Palisaded myofibroblastoma. A benign mesenchymal tumor of lymph node. Am J Surg Pathol 1989;13:341-346.

58. Williams HB. Hemangiomas and lymphangiomas. Adv Surg 1981;15:317-349.

59. Wolf DA, Wu CD, Medeiros LJ. Mycobacterial pseudotumors of lymph node. A report of two cases diagnosed at the time of intraoperative consultation using touch imprint preparations. Arch Pathol Lab Med 1995;119:811-814.

60. Wolff M. Lymphangiomyoma: clinicopathologic study and ultrastructural confirmation of its histogenesis. Cancer 1973; 31:988-1007.

61. Wullich B, Henn W, Siemer S, Seitz G, Freiler A, Zang KD. Clonal chromosome aberrations in three of five sporadic angiomyolipomas of the kidney. Cancer Genet Cytogenet 1997;96:42-45.

62. Zhang H, Erickson-Johnson M, Wang X, et al. Molecular testing for lipomatous tumors: critical analysis and test recommendations based on the analysis of 405 extremity-based tumors. Am J Surg Pathol 2010;34:1304-1311.

67 METASTATIC TUMORS

GENERAL FEATURES

Metastasis, or the spread of neoplastic cells from a primary site of tumor to another, distant anatomic site, is a fundamental feature and defining characteristic of malignant tumors.

Lymph Node Versus Spleen

Metastases may occur via blood vessels (hematogenous spread), but most often travel from the primary neoplasm via the lymphatic system to regional lymph nodes which are rich in afferent lymphatic vessels. In autopsy studies of patients with solid tumors who develop metastases, about the 30 percent have metastases to regional lymph nodes (29,46). Regional lymph nodes are often the first site of metastases, preceding widespread metastatic disease by a variable time interval. Lymph node metastases may occur at a great distance from the primary site and the primary neoplasm may be unknown at the time the metastases are detected.

In contrast, the spleen is an uncommon site of metastases. In different autopsy studies the spleen is involved by metastases in less than 10 percent of patients, and in most studies, less than 5 percent (8,46). In living patients, refined radiologic imaging studies have improved the detection of splenic metastases, but in general, splenic metastases are uncommon and occur most often in patients with widespread metastatic disease (34,37). One potential explanation for the apparent "resistance" of the spleen to metastases is that the spleen lacks afferent lymphatics, restricting metastases to those that occur only via the bloodstream. This anatomic difference likely explains the higher frequency of metastases to lymph nodes versus spleen. In patients with hematogenous metastases, however, the spleen is still involved less frequently than other organs (e.g., liver, lung). Other theories that have been proposed to explain splenic "resistance" to metastases include: 1) the spleen is innately hostile to metastases; 2) the reticuloendothelial system of the spleen may inhibit seeding of the spleen by metastatic cells; and 3) splenic contraction may expunge small groups of malignant cells before clinically evident metastases develop. There is little scientific data to support or refute these theories.

As splenic metastases are rare, most of this chapter is focused on metastases to lymph nodes. The spleen is discussed briefly at the end of the chapter.

Biology of Metastases

The underlying mechanisms of metastases are complex and our understanding is incomplete. The efficiency of the metastatic process is minimal and mathematical models predict that only a truly minute percentage (about 1 in 60 million) circulating tumor cells are able to successfully metastasize (17). Tumor metastases arise from a series of nonrandom, sequential events that involve cell adhesion, chemotaxis, cell invasion, and interactions with the extracellular matrix (ECM) (14). Tumor cells must change from differentiated, specialized phenotypes to a migratory and invasive phenotype. Other processes in the development of metastases include: development of new blood vessels, disruption and invasion of the basement membrane and ECM, intravasation into blood or lymphatic vessels, adhesion to capillaries in target organs, invasion into endothelium, and extravasation into target organs (9,47).

Most epithelial tumor cells have cellular adhesion molecules that must be downregulated and their processes remodeled; this process makes epithelial tumor cells biologically more akin to mesenchymal cells, also known as epithelial to mesenchymal transition (EMT) (49). A number of coordinated genetic events occur that underlie this process. In addition, metastatic tumor cells are thought to have stem cell-like characteristics, including mobility, self-renewal, and resistance to stress. The stresses that determine "success" (or spread) of metastatic cells include hypoxia, reactive oxygen and nitrogen species, inflammation, and high or low pH, among others. Hypoxia induces c-Met activation which induces angiogenesis and tumor cell migration and invasion (14,49). Stromal cells likely contribute to the process of support and development of tumor cell metastases (15).

Transforming growth factor-beta (TGFβ) promotes EMT, immune suppression, tumor invasion, and dissemination of tumor cells (14). Other factors that play key roles in the development of metastases include hepatocyte growth factor, epidermal growth factor, insulin-like growth factors, fibroblast growth factors, and matrix metalloproteinases. The adhesion of cells to other cells and to matrix is also a factor in the development of metastases. In many epithelial tumors, loss of E-cadherin is associated with tumor progression, by disrupting interactions between neighboring cells (14,47). The development of new lymphatic channels, enabling metastatic cells to gain access and be transported to regional lymph nodes, is also important in promoting metastases to lymph nodes. Vascular endothelial growth factors (VEGF) play an important role in lymphangiogenesis (14).

Role of Metastases in Staging

The presence or absence of metastases makes up a fundamental portion of the staging evaluation of most tumors (5). The American Joint Committee on Cancer (AJCC) (5) uses a tumor (T), lymph node (N), metastasis (M) system. The T component is tailored for the unique features of different malignant neoplasms. In contrast, the N and M components of the system are more universal. M is based on the presence or absence of distant metastases. N is defined as follows: "the N (node) component is defined by the absence, or presence and extent of cancer in the regional draining lymph nodes. Nodal involvement is categorized by the number of positive nodes and for certain cancer sites by the involvement of specific regional nodal groups" (5).

When there is a known primary site and a temporal and often physical association with metastatic tumor (e.g., axillary lymph node metastasis associated with breast carcinoma), then the identification of the tumor type is presumed to be from the known primary. However, when there is no known primary site, or less frequently, when there is more than one possible primary site, a more thorough evaluation of the lymph node metastasis may be necessary. A patient with lymph node metastasis from an unknown primary site is staged as T0 N1 M0 (AJCC).

The extent of metastatic tumor in the lymph nodes has prognostic value. As a result, metastases to regional lymph nodes are often classified based on their size: single tumor cells, micrometastases, and macrometastases. Micrometastases (fig. 67-1) are defined as aggregates of tumor cells greater than 0.2 mm but not greater than 2.0 mm. Macrometastases are characterized by somewhat arbitrary cutoffs, for example, below or above 5 cm in diameter. Systems to semi-quantify metastatic tumor in lymph nodes correlate (imperfectly) with the size of the primary tumor as well as the overall extent of metastatic disease, and are therefore indicators of overall tumor burden. The clinical and prognostic impact of single tumor cells versus micrometastases versus macrometastases is often different, and therefore leads to changes in the treatment approach.

CLINICAL FEATURES

In this section the focus is on patients with lymph node metastases in whom the primary site is unknown. Three to 5 percent of patients with cancer present with positive lymph nodes without a known primary tumor (21). Unknown primary tumors most often are metastatic carcinomas, but 1 to 2 percent of patients with melanoma and a lower frequency of patients with germ cell tumors or sarcomas also present initially with lymphadenopathy as a result of metastases (31).

The evaluation of an unknown primary tumor in lymph nodes is an important diagnostic challenge about which much is written in the literature. The challenge is amplified when using fine-needle aspiration cytology or small needle core biopsy specimens for diagnosis (27,43). The basic principles and approach to these tumors, as well as some potential diagnostic pitfalls, are addressed briefly.

Patient age, medical history, and location of the involved lymph nodes are helpful factors in guiding diagnosis. The patient age narrows down the myriad of possibilities, as certain

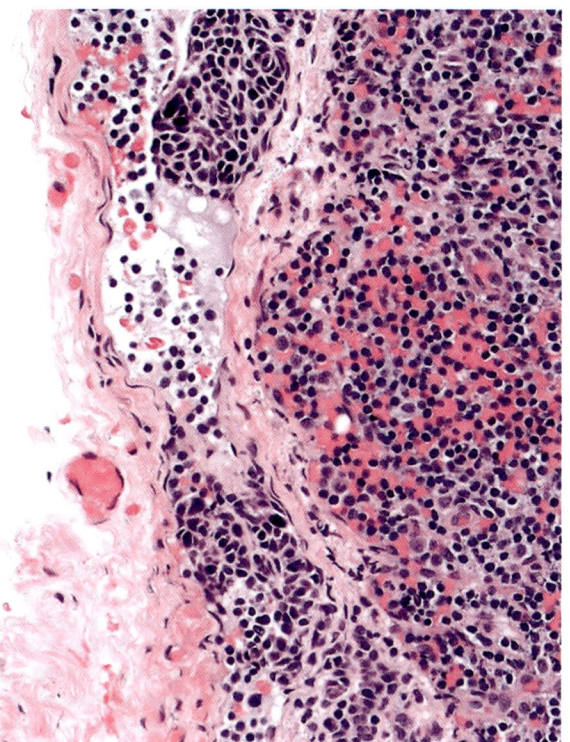 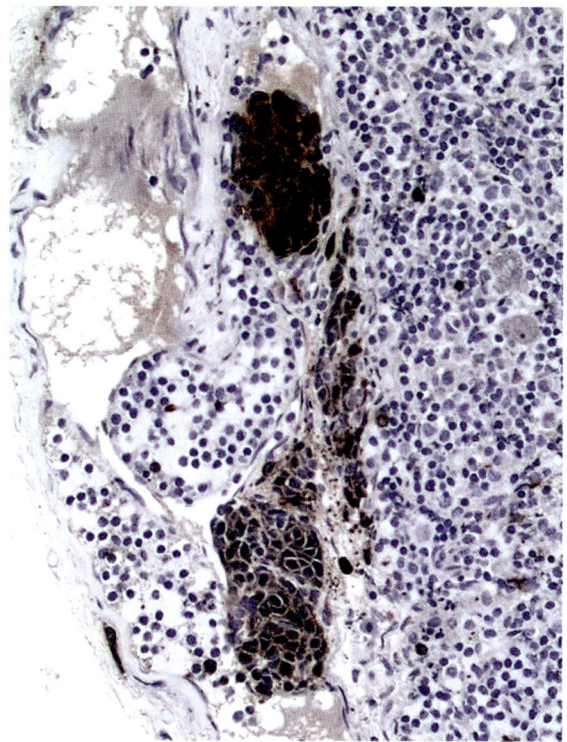

Figure 67-1

MICROMETASTASIS OF MELANOMA TO LYMPH NODE

Left: Small aggregates of melanoma cells are present in an afferent lymphatic vessel and subcapsular sinus (hematoxylin and eosin [H&E] stain).

Right: The cells are positive for S-100 protein (immunohistochemistry with hematoxylin counterstain).

tumors occur almost exclusively in generally restricted age groups (31). For example, metastatic carcinoma affects adults and is highly unusual in children. In contrast, neuroblastoma is most often a disease of young children. The medical history, if available, is another helpful clue. Perhaps the best example is a history of cigarette smoking, which raises the suspicion for a primary lung cancer. Smoking is also risk factor for head and neck carcinomas as well as tumors at other sites.

The location of the lymph nodes involved by metastatic tumor is an important guiding factor. Occult metastases to cervical lymph nodes are commonly metastatic squamous cell carcinoma from a head and neck site (43). Posterior cervical lymph nodes are a site of metastasis from nasopharyngeal carcinoma (42). The left supraclavicular lymph node, known as Virchow node, named after the German pathologist Rudolf Virchow, is a common site of metastasis from

intra-abdominal and pelvic tumors. A patient who presents with an enlarged, hard left supraclavicular lymph node is known to have Troisier sign, named after the French pathologist Charles E. Troisier (38). The association between the left supraclavicular lymph node and intra-abdominal and pelvic tumors is explained by drainage of the thoracic duct into the left subclavian vein. Both supraclavicular lymph nodes are also sites of metastases from primary neoplasms arising in the lung, head and neck, breast, and esophagus as well as lymphomas (11,23,43).

Lymph nodes in the axilla are most often involved by metastatic breast carcinoma in women, and less commonly, melanoma, cutaneous squamous cell carcinoma, and lung carcinoma in both genders (31,44). Mediastinal and pulmonary hilar lymph nodes are a common site of metastatic lung carcinoma of all types. The inguinal lymph nodes are a common site for metastases from prostate carcinoma in men or gynecologic tumors in women (25). Melanoma also metastasizes to inguinal lymph nodes. Retroperitoneal lymph nodes are a common site for the spread of germ cell tumors. All of these lymph nodes are also sites for the dissemination of lymphoid neoplasms, but since these tumors are addressed in detail elsewhere in this text, they are not emphasized here.

Although not a lymph node, the Sister Mary Joseph nodule is another example of a specific site of metastasis suggesting primary tumor location. This term refers to metastatic tumor presenting as a palpable nodule of the umbilicus. The most common primary tumors that metastasize to this site arise in intra-abdominal (e.g., gastric carcinoma) or gynecologic organs. The mechanism of metastasis is uncertain but may occur by travel along embryologic remnants of the umbilicus, spread via lymphatic or blood vessels, direct spread, or possibly more than one of these proposed mechanisms perhaps correlating with the type of primary neoplasm. This association was described in 1928 by William J. Mayo who attributed the observation to Sister Mary Joseph, a surgical nurse (18).

GROSS FINDINGS

Metastases within lymph nodes are often identified by their differences in consistency and appearance compared with normal lymphoid tissue. Normal lymph nodes have a soft, tan, and fleshy appearance. By contrast, metastatic tumor is often firm and has a different color and consistency (figs. 67-2, 67-3). Furthermore, products of the neoplastic cells, such as melanin or mucin, may be seen in association with melanoma or adenocarcinomas, respectively. Recent hemorrhage or hemosiderin deposition is also associated with metastatic tumors.

HISTOLOGIC FINDINGS

Metastatic tumors, when they initially involve lymph nodes, most commonly are distributed in the lymph node sinuses, especially the subcapsular sinus. Invasion of tumor-associated or nearby lymphatic channels then leads to spread of tumor cells into other compartments of the lymph node (fig. 67-4). When involvement by metastases is extensive, only a few residual nodal structures may be present or the lymph node architecture may be completely effaced (fig. 67-5).

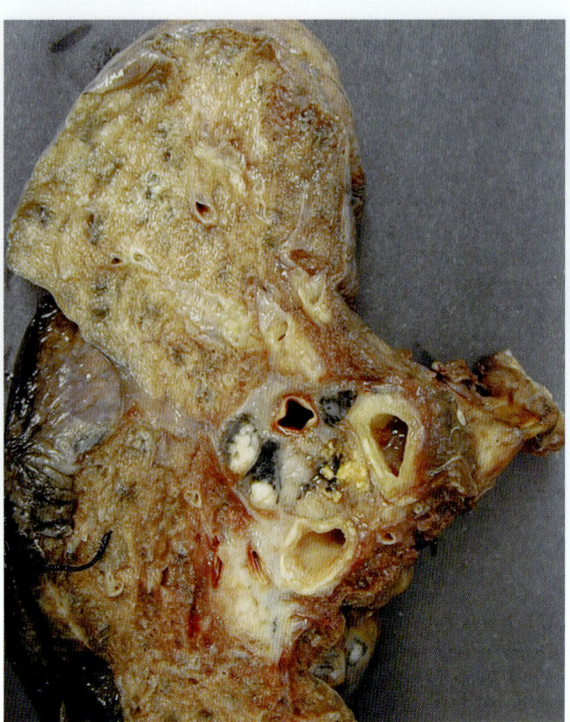

Figure 67-2

HILAR LYMPH NODES REPLACED BY METASTATIC LUNG CARCINOMA

In this gross lung resection specimen, the large white nodules in the hilum represent lymph nodes replaced by metastases. (Courtesy of Dr. R. N. Miranda, Houston, TX.)

The histologic appearance of metastatic tumors in lymph node provides clues to the primary site. Cellular differentiation is indicated by keratinization in squamous cell carcinoma, gland formation and mucin in adenocarcinoma (fig. 67-6), rosette formation in neuroendocrine tumors, melanin pigment in melanoma (fig. 67-7) (27), and extracellular matrix in sarcomas (31). Papillary adenocarcinoma (arising in a number of anatomic sites) metastatic to lymph nodes may show papillae, nuclear pseudoinclusions, and psammoma bodies (fig. 67-8). Small intracellular lumens are a feature of metastatic hemangioendothelioma and angiosarcoma.

Necrosis is a feature that is particularly common in certain types of metastases and therefore is a "soft" finding that has some value in the differential diagnosis. Colonic adenocarcinoma metastatic to lymph nodes commonly shows central necrosis within neoplastic glands (fig. 67-9) (32). Germ cell tumors, in general, often

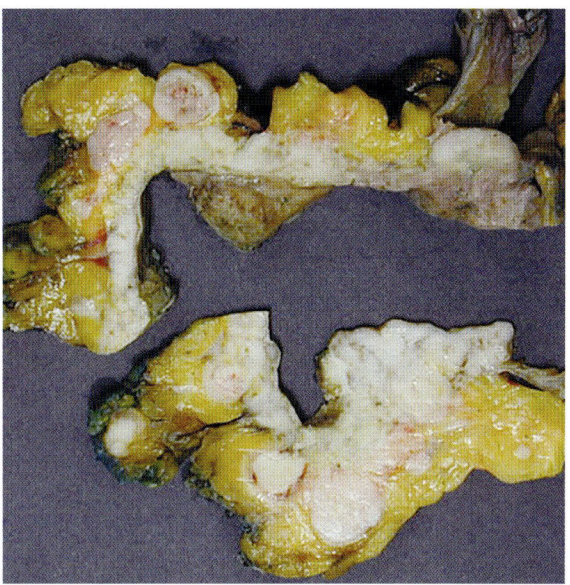

Figure 67-3

**PERICOLONIC LYMPH NODES INVOLVED
BY METASTATIC COLON CARCINOMA**

This image of a segmental colectomy specimen shows a thickened colonic wall and large white nodules in pericolonic adipose tissue that represent lymph nodes replaced by metastatic carcinoma. (Courtesy of Dr. R. Miranda, Houston, TX.)

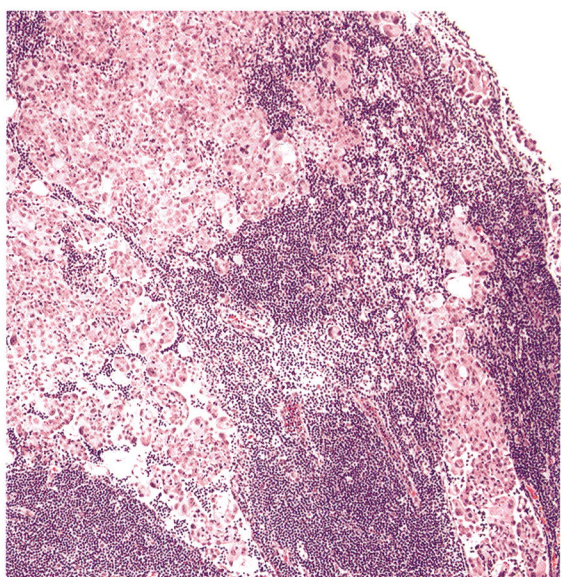

Figure 67-4

**METASTATIC ADENOCARCINOMA
WITHIN LYMPH NODE SINUSES**

Metastatic tumor expands the lymph node sinuses (H&E stain.)

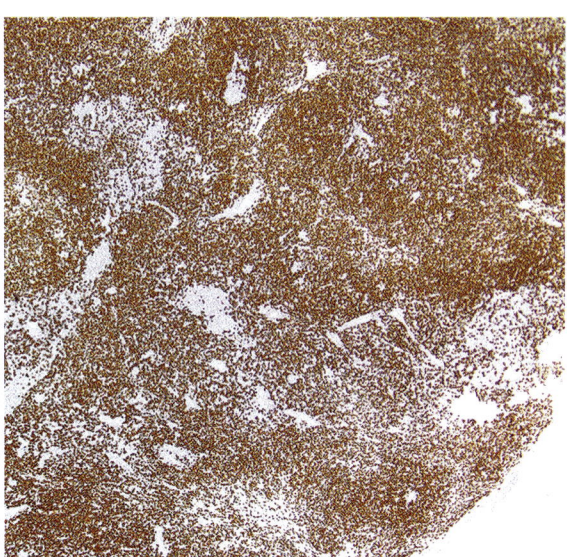

Figure 67-5

**LYMPH NODE ALMOST COMPLETELY
REPLACED BY METASTATIC CARCINOMA**

A pancytokeratin antibody, AE1/AE3, highlights numerous metastatic carcinoma cells. Little residual lymph node parenchyma remains in this field (immunohistochemistry with hematoxylin counterstain).

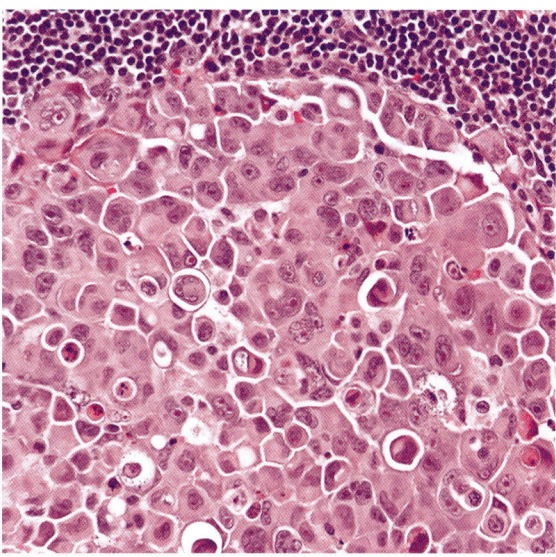

Figure 67-6

**METASTATIC LUNG ADENOCARCINOMA
IN A PULMONARY HILAR LYMPH NODE**

The neoplastic cells are cohesive, with apoptosis, and show small vacuoles within the cytoplasm. The vacuoles were positive for mucin (not shown) (H&E stain).

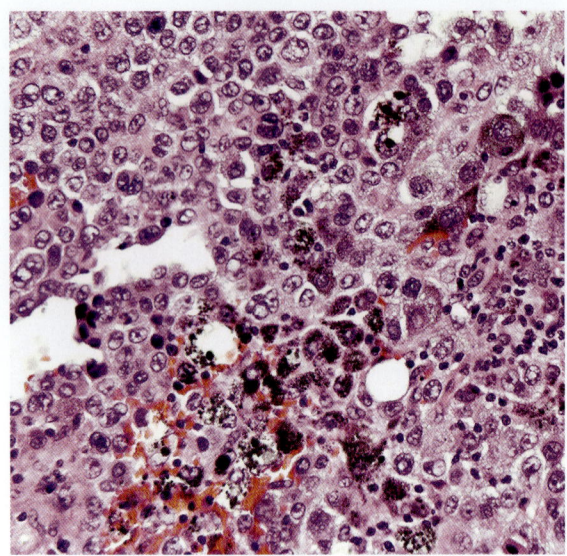

Figure 67-7

METASTATIC MELANOMA IN AXILLARY LYMPH NODE

This image shows many neoplastic cells, some of which contain melanin, supporting the diagnosis of metastatic melanoma (H&E stain).

show extensive necrosis at sites of metastases. Small cell carcinoma of the lung is extensively necrotic and, as a result, basophilic, cell-free DNA may be observed within the tumor (fig. 67-10). The DNA also can be deposited on blood vessels, known as nuclear encrustation, or the Azzopardi phenomenon, since it was described by John G. Azzopardi in 1959.

MORPHOLOGIC DIFFERENTIATION OF METASTASES

The morphologic evaluation of metastases is an essential first step in the assessment of lymph node metastases. In many cases, however, ancillary methods of analysis are essential to establish the diagnosis or the likely primary site of origin. Ancillary methods are especially needed to identify the primary site of metastatic tumors that lack histologic evidence of differentiation. The most commonly used ancillary method, by far, is immunohistochemical analysis and therefore immunohistochemistry is emphasized in this chapter and summarized in many tables

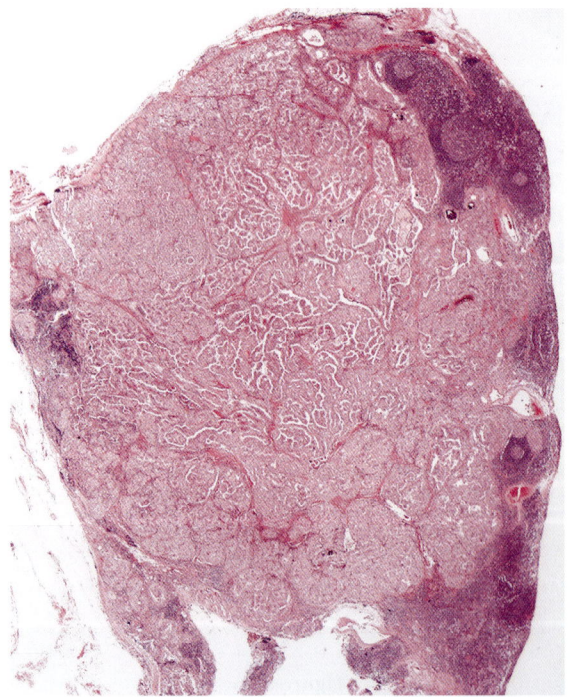
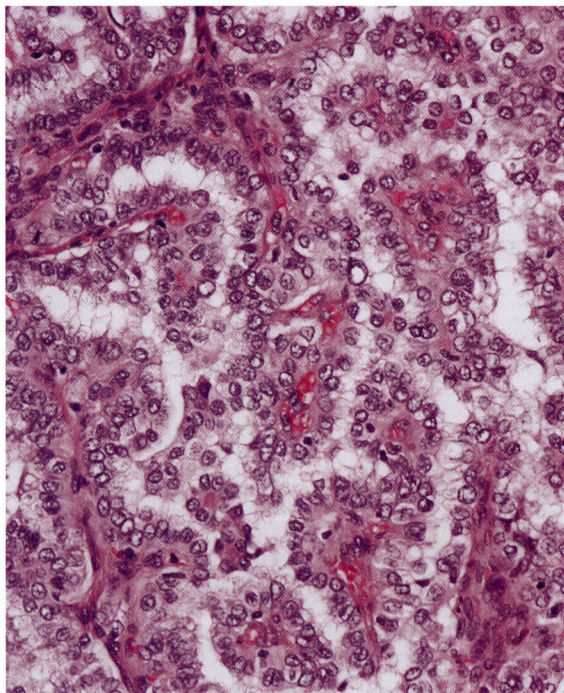

Figure 67-8

METASTATIC PAPILLARY CARCINOMA OF THYROID GLAND IN CERVICAL LYMPH NODE

Left: At low magnification, the metastasis replaces most of the lymph node parenchyma.

Right: High magnification shows papillae lined by cells with squared nuclear contours and clear ("orphan Annie") nuclei (H&E stain).

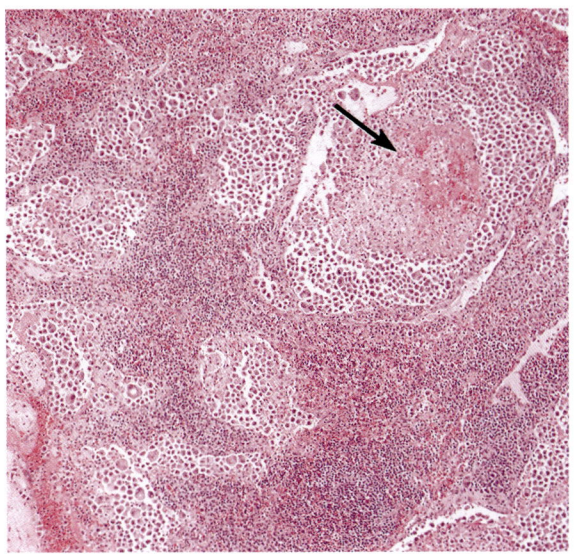

Figure 67-9

**METASTATIC COLON CARCINOMA
IN A PERICOLONIC LYMPH NODE**

In this field, the neoplastic cells are filling lymph node sinuses. Coagulative necrosis is associated with this tumor (arrow) (H&E stain).

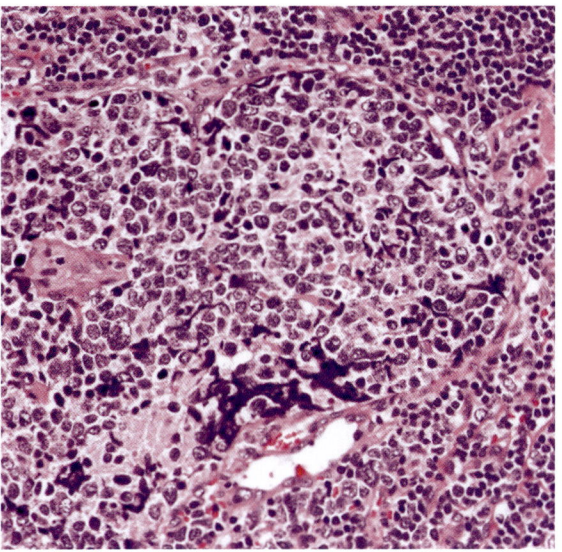

Figure 67-10

**METASTATIC SMALL CELL CARCINOMA
OF THE LUNG IN CERVICAL LYMPH NODE**

Basophilic, cell-free DNA is present within the neoplasm and is near a blood vessel in this field. These findings do not strictly meet criteria for the Azzopardi phenomenon because the blood vessel is not encrusted by the DNA (H&E stain).

(Tables 67-1–67-6). Other methods that have a role in the workup of metastases in lymph nodes include electron microscopy, conventional cytogenetic analysis, fluorescence in situ hybridization (FISH) analysis, and molecular testing.

A helpful general approach to the examination of poorly differentiated metastases in lymph nodes from an unknown primary site is to subdivide these tumors into four morphologic categories: small cell, epithelioid, anaplastic, and spindle cell (16,32,51). This approach has the advantage of narrowing down the possibilities somewhat, although the differential diagnosis for each category remains broad and an inclusive approach to cover all possibilities is required.

Small Cell Tumors

The use of the term *small cell* in this context refers to metastatic tumor cells that are small relative to normal epithelial cells (31). Metastatic small cells, however, are often appreciably larger than benign small lymphocytes. In most circumstances, metastatic small cells have round to slightly irregular nuclei with scant cytoplasm (figs. 67-11–67-14). The tumor cell chromatin

varies from dense to delicate or fine, with a "dusty" or "salt and pepper" appearance (31).

The differential diagnosis of small cell metastasis includes a subset of carcinomas, a number of neuroendocrine tumors (including carcinoid and small cell carcinoma), neuroblastoma, "small blue cell tumors" including some mesenchymal sarcomas, lymphomas, and myeloid sarcoma (Table 67-2; figs. 67-11, 67-12). Although any poorly differentiated carcinoma can exhibit a small cell appearance, small cell morphologic features are most commonly observed in lobular breast carcinoma, prostate carcinoma, and undifferentiated carcinomas. Most neuroendocrine tumors also exhibit a small cell appearance; the "salt and pepper" nuclear appearance is classically seen in neuroendocrine carcinomas. Neuroblastoma occurs in a variety of sites and has features that overlap with those of neuroendocrine carcinoma.

Primitive sarcomas are often lumped into the category of "small blue cell tumors." Included in this group are Ewing sarcoma/primitive neuroectodermal tumor (fig. 67-13), neuroblastoma, small cell rhabdomyosarcoma (fig. 67-14),

Table 67-1

EVALUATION OF METASTATIC TUMOR BY IMMUNOHISTOCHEMICAL ANALYSIS TO DETERMINE PRIMARY SITE[a]

Cytokeratin (CK)	Initial Antibody Panel	Additional Antibodies[b]	Likely Primary Tumor
CK7+/CK20-	OCT4, pankeratin (OSCAR), CD117, SALL4, PLAP[c]	CD30 (embryonal), AFP and glypican-3 (yolk sac), EMA (negative)	Germ cell tumor
	WT1, ER, PAX8		Ovarian carcinoma, nonmucinous
	TTF1, thyroglobulin	Calcitonin (medullary), chromogranin A (medullary)	Thyroid carcinoma
	ER, PAX8, p53 (serous)	p63 (adenosquamous), CK5/6 (adenosquamous), p16 (classic – patchy, weak; serous – diffuse, strong)	Endometrial carcinoma
	P16 (strong, diffuse), HR-HPV (in situ), m-CEA, vimentin (usually negative)		Endocervical carcinoma
	ER, PR, GATA3	Mammaglobin, GCDFP-1	Breast carcinoma
	SMAD4/DPC4 (negative), p63, CK17	CDX2, mesothelin and MUC5, PAX8 (pan-neuroendocrine)	Pancreaticobiliary carcinoma (most cases)
	CDX2	HepPar (hepatoid-), arginase-1 (hepatoid)	Upper GI carcinoma/ pancreaticobiliary carcinoma (minority)
	TTF1, napsin	MOC31, BerEp4	Lung adenocarcinoma
CK7-/CK20+	Synaptophysin, chromogranin A, CK20 (dot-like)	CD56, NSE, CM2B4 (anti-Merkel cell polyoma virus T antigen)	Merkel cell carcinoma
	CDX2	Villin, SATB2	Colorectal carcinoma
	CDX2	HepPar (hepatoid), arginase-1 (hepatoid)	Gastric carcinoma (minority)
CK7+/CK20+	CK5/6, p63, p40	Uroplakin III, GATA3, PAX8, thrombomodulin	Urothelial carcinoma
	PAX8, villin		Ovarian/appendiceal mucinous carcinoma
	DPC4/SMAD4 (negative), p63, CK17	CDX2, mesothelin and MUC5	Pancreaticobiliary carcinoma (minority)
	CDX2	HepPar (hepatoid), arginase-1 (hepatoid)	Gastric carcinoma (minority)
CK7-/CK20-	HepPar, arginase 1, glypican-3	CEA-poly, CD10, TTF1 (cytoplasmic)	Hepatocellular carcinoma
	PSA, p501s	PSAP, NKX3.1, androgen receptor, AMACR	Prostate carcinoma
	PAX8, CD10, vimentin	CK18, PAX2	Renal cell carcinoma
	Synaptophysin, chromogranin	CD56, NSE	Neuroendocrine carcinoma
	P63, p40	CK5/6, CK14	Squamous cell carcinoma
	calretinin, melan-A, inhibin, SF-1		Adrenocortical carcinoma

[a]This Table summarizes the common immunophenotypic findings in metastatic tumor sites beginning by using anticytokeratin (CK) 7 and 20 antibodies. The Table is not intended to be comprehensive, and individual tumors may vary from the patterns described.

[b]The initial antibody panel is composed of antibodies the authors believe are most helpful in the first round of immunohistochemical studies. The additional antibodies listed are also helpful, but may be better used at a later stage, based on the initial antibody results. This order of antibody use is only a suggestion and other sequences and combinations of the antibodies listed, as well as other antibodies not included in the Table, are equally valid.

[c]PLAP = placental alkaline phosphatase; AFP = alpha-fetoprotein; EMA = epithelial membrane antigen; HR-HPV = high-risk human papillomavirus; CEA = carcinoembryonic antigen; ER = estrogen receptor; PR = progesterone receptor; GCDFP = gross cystic disease fluid protein; NSE = neuron-specific esterase; GI = gastrointestinal; PSA = prostate-specific antigen; PSAP = prostate-specific acid phosphatase; SF-1 = steroidogenic factor (adrenal 4-binding protein); TTF = thyroid transcription factor.

Table 67-2

SMALL CELL TUMORS: DIFFERENTIAL DIAGNOSIS AND IMMUNOHISTOCHEMISTRY

Tumor	Initial Antibodies	Additional Antibodies/Studies
Poorly differentiated carcinoma	Pancytokeratin (CK)	(See Table 67-1)
Neuroendocrine carcinoma	CK, synaptophysin, chromogranin	CD56, CK20 (dot-like positivity)
Neuroblastoma	Neurofilament protein (NF), NB84, ALK1	
Ewing sarcoma/PNET[a]	CD99, FLI1	Genetic analysis
Rhabdomyosarcoma, small cell	Desmin, myogenin, MyoD	Genetic analysis
Wilms tumor	CK, CD56, WT1	Desmin (blastema), genetic analysis
Desmoplastic small round cell tumor	WT1, CK	Genetic analysis
Liposarcoma, small round cell	S-100 protein	
Small cell lymphoma	CD3, CD20, cyclin D1, BCL6	BCL2, CD5, CD23; Genetic analysis, flow cytometry
Lymphoblastic lymphoma	TdT, CD3 (T cell), PAX5 (B cell)	CD34, CD19; flow cytometry, genetic analysis
Myeloid sarcoma	Myeloperoxidase, CD68, CD117, lysozyme	CD11c, CD34, CD43, flow cytometry, genetic analysis

[a]PNET = peripheral neuroectodermal tumor.

Table 67-3

EPITHELIOID TUMORS: DIFFERENTIAL DIAGNOSIS AND IMMUNOHISTOCHEMISTRY

Tumor	Initial Antibodies	Additional Antibodies
Carcinoma	Pancytokeratin	(See Table 67-1)
Melanoma	S-100, SOX10, HMB-45, melan A	Tyrosinase, MITF
Seminoma	OCT4, SALL4	CK, CD117, PLAP
Myeloid sarcoma	Myeloperoxidase, CD68, CD117, lysozyme	CD11c, CD34, CD43, flow cytometry, genetic analysis
Large cell lymphoma	CD3 (T cell), CD20 (B cell)	CD2 and CD5 (T cell), CD22 and CD79a (B cell), CD30, CD45/LCA
Plasmacytoma	CD138, kappa/lambda, MUM1/IRF4	CD38, VS38, BLIMP1
Epithelioid sarcoma	CK, INI1 (loss)	CD34, genetic analysis
Epithelioid angiosarcoma	CD31, CD34, ERG, FLI1	Thrombomodulin, CK, factor VIII antigen
Epithelioid fibrosarcoma	MUC4, CK (focal, weak)	
Epithelioid leiomyosarcoma	SMA[a], desmin	
Perivascular epithelioid cell tumor (PEComa)	Desmin, HMB-45	

[a]SMA = smooth muscle actin; MITF = microphthalmia-associated transcription factor; PLAP = placental alkaline phosphatase.

liposarcoma, Wilms tumor, lymphomas, and myeloid sarcoma (31,33,51). While most of these occur in pediatric patients, some are seen in adults and may present as lymph node metastases.

In general, the identification of a carcinoma is accomplished by the presence of cytokeratin (CK) within the neoplastic cells. Highly sensitive pan-CK antibodies are useful. Neuroendocrine differentiation is determined by the presence of synaptophysin, chromogranin A, or neuron-specific enolase (NSE). CD56 expression is a secondary, supportive finding of neuroendocrine differentiation. Squamous differentiation is highlighted by expression of CK5/6, p63, and

Table 67-4

ANAPLASTIC TUMORS: DIFFERENTIAL DIAGNOSIS AND IMMUNOHISTOCHEMISTRY

Tumor	Initial Antibodies	Additional Antibodies
Anaplastic carcinoma	Pancytokeratin (CK)	(See Table 67-1)
Nasopharyngeal carcinoma	CK, EBV[a] (in situ)	
Melanoma	S-100, SOX10, HMB-45, melan A	
Angiosarcoma	CD34, ERG, WT1, FLI1	CD31, factor VIII antigen
Leiomyosarcoma	Desmin, SMA	
Malignant fibrous histiocytoma		
Embryonal rhabdomyosarcoma	Desmin, MyoD1, myogenin	
Osteosarcoma	SATB2	
Malignant epithelioid hemangioendothelioma	CD34, factor VIII antigen, ERG	
Seminoma	OCT4, SALL4	CK, CD117, PLAP
Anaplastic large cell lymphoma	CD30	ALK, CD2, CD4, CD43, cytotoxic antigens
Classic Hodgkin lymphoma	CD15, CD30, CD45 (negative), PAX5 (weak)	EBV (in situ; subset of cases)
Follicular dendritic cell sarcoma	CD21, CD23, CD35, clusterin	Fascin, D2-40/podoplanin, EGFR
Interdigitating dendritic cell sarcoma	S100, CD68, CD163	
Histiocytic sarcoma	CD68, CD163, CD11c	CD4, lysozyme

[a]EBV = Epstein-Barr virus; SMA = smooth muscle actin; SATB2 = special AT-rich sequence binding protein 2; ALK = anaplastic lymphoma kinase; EGFR = epidermal growth factor receptor.

Table 67-5

SPINDLE CELL TUMORS: DIFFERENTIAL DIAGNOSIS AND IMMUNOHISTOCHEMISTRY

Tumor	Initial Antibodies	Additional Antibodies
Sarcomatoid carcinoma	Pancytokeratin (CK)	(See Table 67-1)
Melanoma	SOX10, HMB-45, melan A, S-100 (often negative)	MITF[a]
Kaposi sarcoma	CD34, ERG, HHV-8	CD31, factor VIII-related antigen
Follicular dendritic cell sarcoma	CD21, CD23, CD35, clusterin	Fascin, D2-40/podoplanin, EGFR
Sarcoma	S-100, CD34, CD117, desmin, SMA	
Non-Hodgkin lymphomas with fibrosis	CD3 (T cell), CD20 (B cell), CD45/LCA	CD2 and CD5 (T-cell), CD22 and CD79a (B cell), CD30
Nodular sclerosis Hodgkin lymphoma	CD15, CD30, CD45 (negative), PAX5 (weak)	EBV (in situ; subset of cases)

[a]MITF = microphthalmia-associated transcription factor; HHV = human herpesvirus; SMA = smooth muscle actin; EGFR = epidermal growth factor receptor; EBV = Epstein-Barr virus.

p40, although these antibodies are not entirely specific. In cases of metastatic poorly differentiated carcinoma of the head and neck region, identification of human papilloma virus (HPV), usually by in situ hybridization, supports a primary carcinoma of the head and neck region (43). Similar metastatic tumors in inguinal lymph nodes positive for HPV support metastasis from the uterine cervix, vulva, or penis.

Epithelioid Tumors

The term *epithelioid* is used for tumors with cells that resemble epithelial-derived tumor cells. An epithelioid appearance refers to cells of large size, often with moderate to large amounts of cytoplasm, arranged in diffuse, often cohesive sheets. The differential diagnosis of metastatic cells with an epithelioid appearance is broad and

Table 67-6

HEMATOPOIETIC-ASSOCIATED MARKERS THAT MAY BE EXPRESSED
IN NONHEMATOPOIETIC TUMORS AND NORMAL TISSUES[a]

Hematopoietic Marker	Other Tissues and Tumors	Notes
CD5	Thymoma, thymic epithelium	Expressed in about 10% of non-hematopoietic tumors.
CD7	Subset of carcinomas and melanoma	Expressed in about 20% of non-hematopoietic tumors
CD10	Large variety of tumors and tissue types	
CD15	Broad range of carcinomas	
CD20	Thymoma	B cells intermixed with epithelial cells that often have asteroid/dendritic features; also can focally highlight epithelial cells
CD30	Embryonal carcinoma, other carcinomas, some yolk sac tumors, rare mesotheliomas, rare sarcomas	
CD43	Mesothelioma, adrenocortical carcinoma, lung carcinoma	
CD56 (NCAM)	Neuroendocrine tumors, CNS[b] tumors, neural crest-derived cells, adrenocortical tumors, thyroid tumors, variety of sarcomas	
CD138	Large variety of tumor and tissue types	~60% of carcinomas are positive
ALK	Inflammatory myofibroblastic tumors, rhabdomyosarcoma, lipogenic tumors, Ewing/PNET, leiomyosarcoma, lung adenocarcinoma (small subset)	
BCL2	Large variety of tumors and tissue types	
BCL6	Bronchial epithelium, some lung tumors, squamous cell carcinoma, urothelial carcinoma	
Cyclin D1	Wide variety of proliferating epithelial and mesenchymal tissues	Endothelial cells in lymph nodes are positive and serve as internal control
MUM1/IRF4	Melanoma	
PAX5	Merkel cell carcinoma, alveolar rhabdomyosarcoma	Small cell carcinoma of lung usually negative
TdT	Merkel cell carcinoma, small cell carcinoma	Reactivity can be bright and uniform (similar to lymphoblastic lymphoma)

[a]This Table is a general summary of antigens commonly used in the diagnosis of hematopoietic tumors that also may be positive in nonhematopoietic tumors and normal tissues. The Table is not intended to be comprehensive.
[b]CNS = central nervous system; PNET = peripheral neuroectodermal tumor.

includes carcinomas of various types, melanoma, seminoma and other germ cell tumors, a small number of sarcomas, and a limited number of hematopoietic neoplasms, such as diffuse large B-cell lymphoma, anaplastic large cell lymphoma, and myeloid sarcoma (Table 67-3).

The most common types of metastatic carcinoma are those derived from the kidney, prostate gland, and breast. The presence of any gland formation is suggestive of adenocarcinoma (fig. 67-15), with only the most poorly differentiated adenocarcinomas lacking this feature. Melanoma may have an epithelioid appearance, either focally or throughout, and must always be considered (figs. 67-16, 67-17). Germ cell tumors, such as embryonal carcinoma and seminoma, may present initially as metastatic disease in lymph nodes (fig. 67-18); the primary site may be occult and rarely can regress (6,7).

The immunohistochemical approach to this group of tumors is somewhat distinctive, and is guided by the morphologic findings. In the initial evaluation, a small battery of antibodies may be useful including those specific for pan-CK, S-100 protein, and CD45/LCA. This is simply a "scout" approach to gain a preliminary

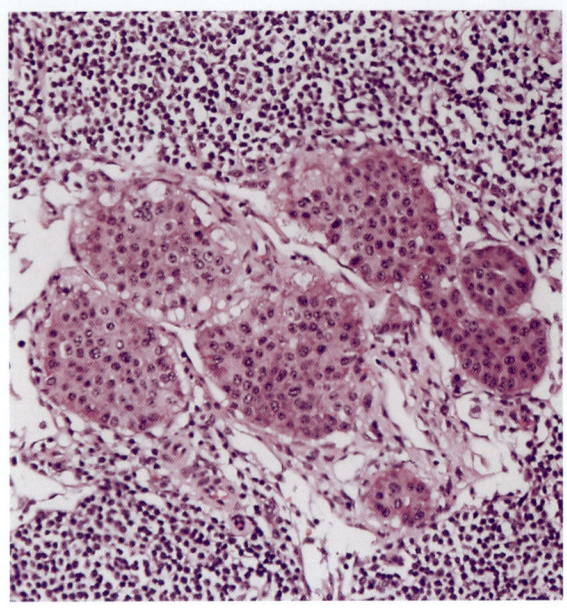

Figure 67-11

**METASTATIC CARCINOID
IN ABDOMINAL LYMPH NODE**

The neoplastic cells are present as small aggregates in the lymph node sinus. The cells have abundant eosinophilic cytoplasm (H&E stain).

impression and is almost never adequate. Additional analysis for specific cytokeratins, such as CK7 and CK20, provides better information to more appropriately identify a primary site (Table 67-1).

Some melanomas are negative for S-100 protein and therefore, if clinically indicated, other melanoma markers (e.g., HMB-45 or Melan A) should be included in the antibody panel and while many germ cell tumors are positive for pan-CKs and CK7, more specific markers, including SALL-4 and OCT4 should be used. Seminoma is commonly positive for KIT/CD117. CD45/LCA highlights most tumors of lymphoid and myeloid lineage, but can be negative. If a hematolymphoid neoplasm is a primary consideration, then more specific antibodies reactive with T cells, B cells, and myeloid cells (e.g., CD3, CD20, CD68, myeloperoxidase) should be employed.

Anaplastic large cell lymphomas do not always have anaplastic cytologic features; these tumors are notorious for being negative for some T-cell antigens (e.g., CD3) and CD45/LCA and expressing epithelial membrane antigen

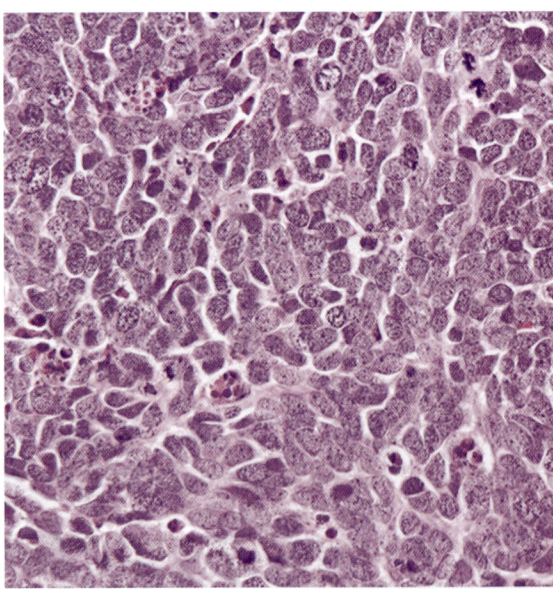 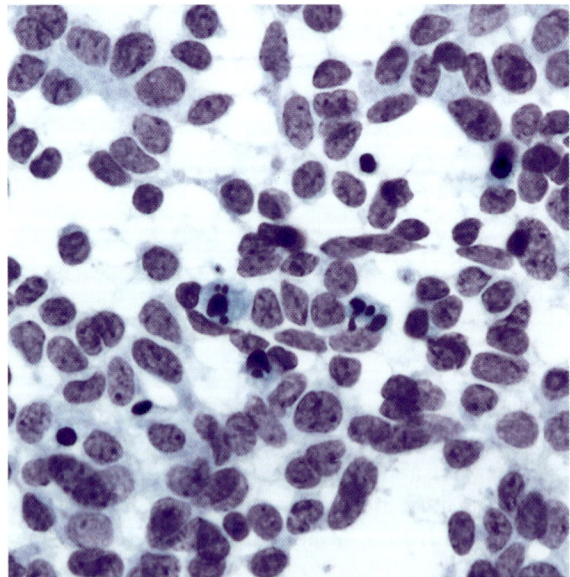

Figure 67-12

METASTATIC SMALL CELL CARCINOMA IN LYMPH NODE

Left: In a biopsy specimen the chromatin has a delicately distributed pattern, referred to as "dusty" or "salt and pepper" (H&E stain).

Right: These nuclear features also are appreciated on aspirate smears. Metastatic small cell carcinoma may mimic lymphoma; however, the presence of cohesive clusters of small tumor cells with nuclear molding and fine chromatin help avoid this pitfall (Papanicolaou stain).

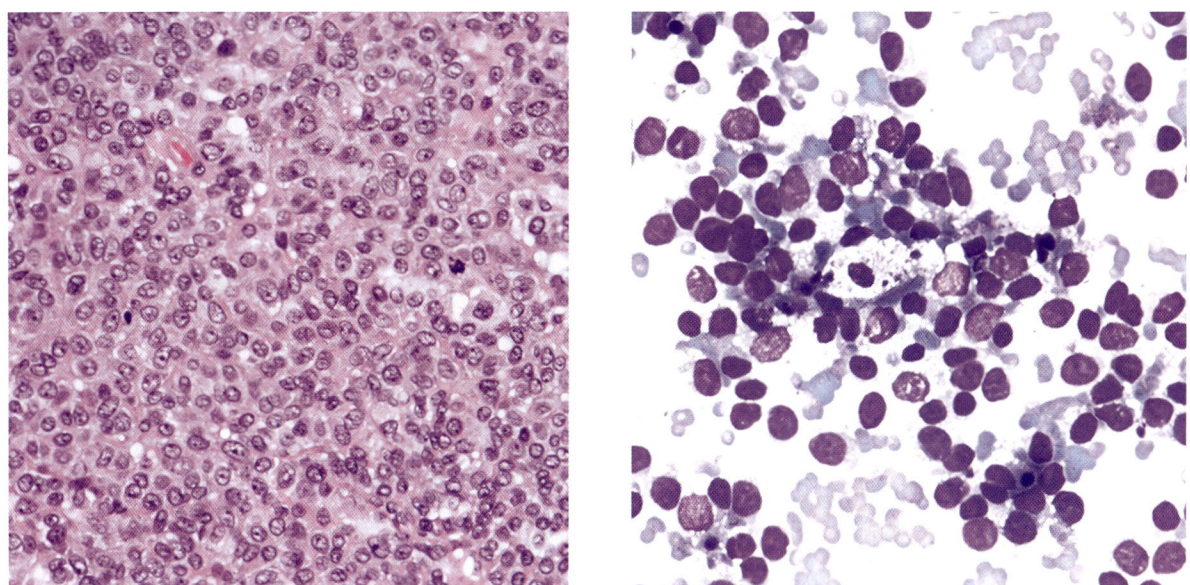

Figure 67-13

METASTATIC EWING SARCOMA IN LYMPH NODE

Left: The neoplastic cells completely and diffusely replace the lymph node parenchyma in this field.
Right: Fine-needle aspirate smear shows a dispersed population of small round tumor cells (Diff-Quik stain).

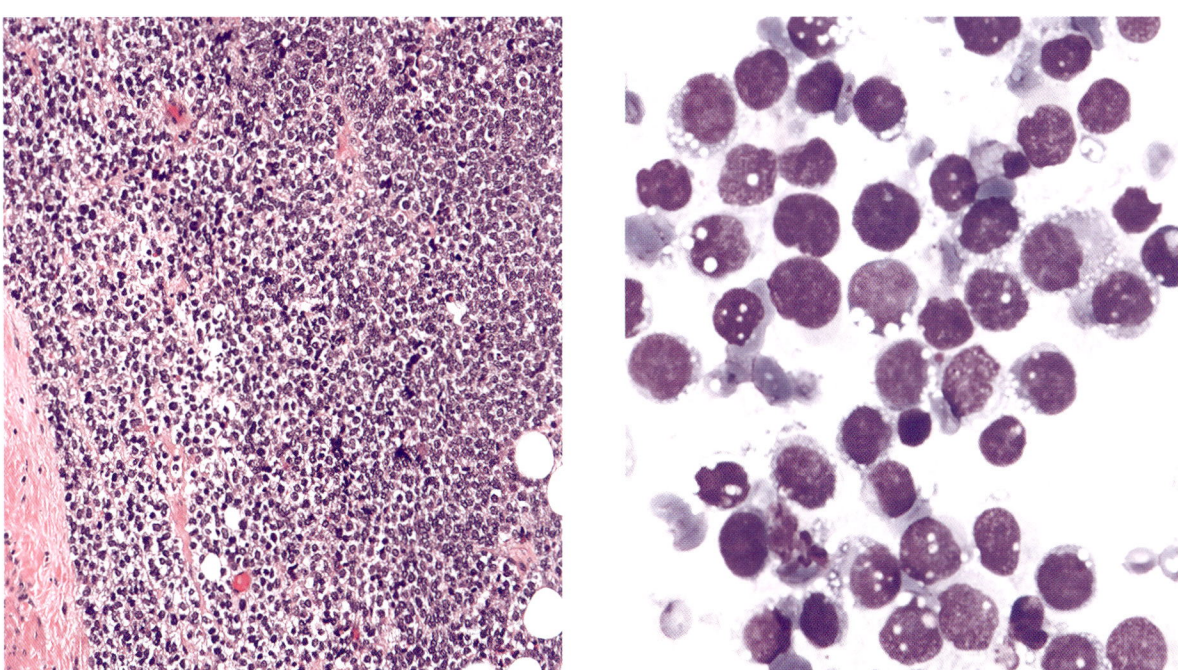

Figure 67-14

METASTATIC RHABDOMYOSARCOMA IN LYMPH NODE

Left: The biopsy specimen shows diffuse replacement of nodal parenchyma by metastatic "small" (medium-sized) cells (H&E stain).

Right: The fine-needle aspirate smear shows medium-sized cells with variable amounts of cytoplasm that may have vacuoles (Diff-Quik stain).

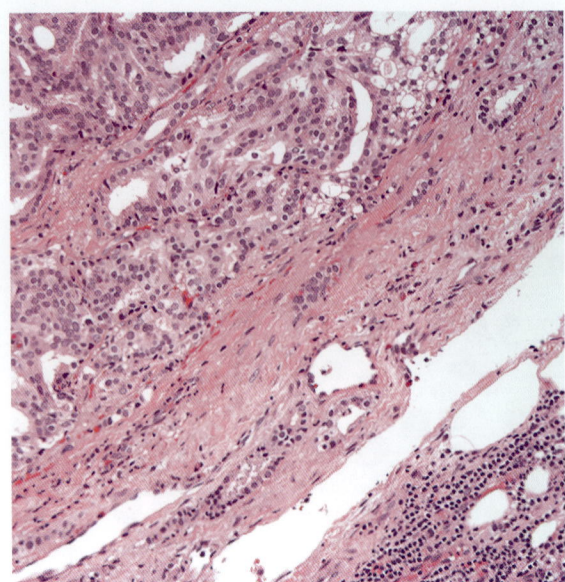

Figure 67-15

METASTATIC ADENOCARCINOMA FROM PROSTATE GLAND IN LYMPH NODE

There is prominent gland formation in this tumor that was positive for prostate-specific antigen (not shown) (H&E stain).

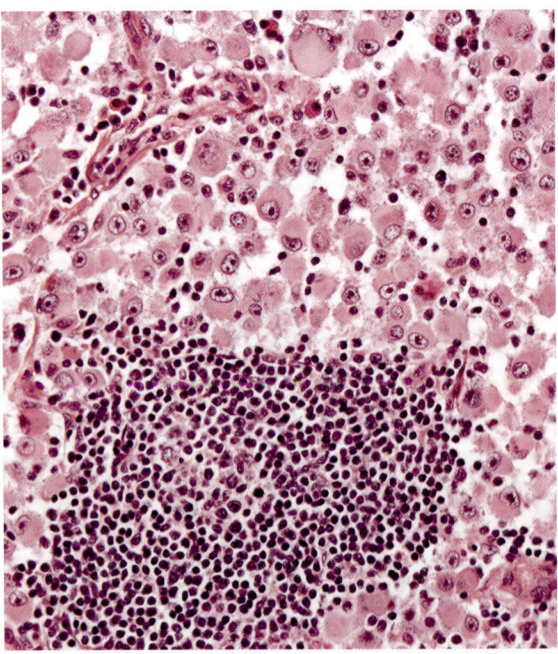

Figure 67-16

METASTATIC MELANOMA WITH A PROMINENT EPITHELIOID APPEARANCE IN LYMPH NODE

The tumor cells are epithelioid and large as compared to the size of small lymphocytes (bottom, middle) (H&E stain).

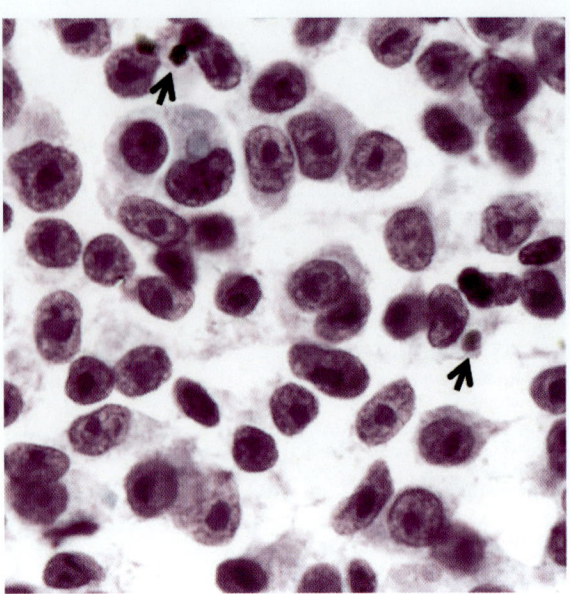

Figure 67-17

METASTATIC MELANOMA IN LYMPH NODE

In this fine-needle aspirate smear, the tumor mimics large cell lymphoma, however, the presence of intracellular pigment (arrows) is a clue to the diagnosis. Other features suggestive of melanoma in this field are mirror image nuclei and eccentrically located nuclei (Papanicolaou stain).

(EMA) suggesting an epithelial tumor. It is important to use anti-CD30 and anti-ALK to exclude cases of anaplastic large cell lymphoma with an epithelioid appearance.

Anaplastic Tumors

The term *anaplastic* refers to tumors that bear little or no resemblance to normal cells and that have a high proliferation rate. The differential diagnosis for anaplastic metastatic tumors is extensive (Table 67-4) and includes a number of carcinomas, especially those derived from the nasopharynx (fig. 67-19), thyroid gland, lung, breast, and bladder. Other metastatic solid tumors in the differential diagnosis include melanoma, germ cell tumors (figs. 67-20, 67-21), and sarcomas, particularly angiosarcoma, embryonal rhabdomyosarcoma, and leiomyosarcoma. Dendritic cell neoplasms, either metastatic to or arising in the lymph node being examined, are part of this differential as are anaplastic large cell lymphoma, anaplastic variants of diffuse large B-cell lymphoma (fig. 67-22), and Hodgkin lymphoma, either the syncytial variant of

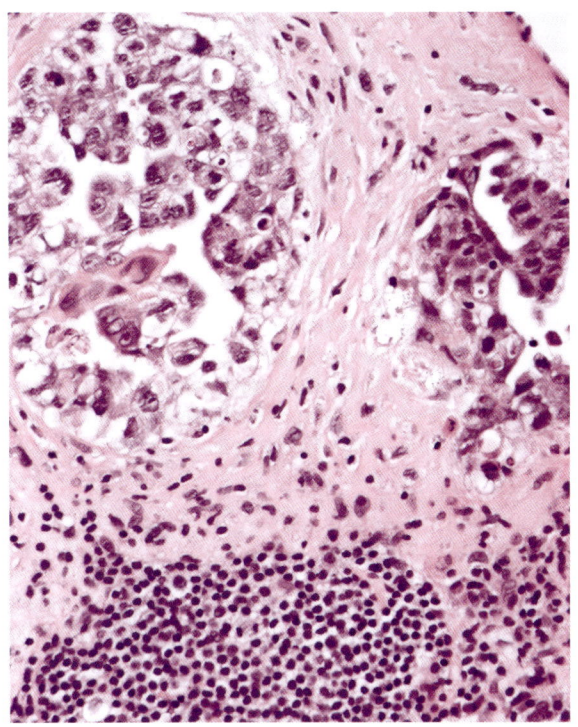

Figure 67-18

METASTATIC EMBRYONAL CARCINOMA OF TESTIS IN LYMPH NODE

The neoplastic cells are arranged in nodules and have an epithelioid appearance (H&E stain).

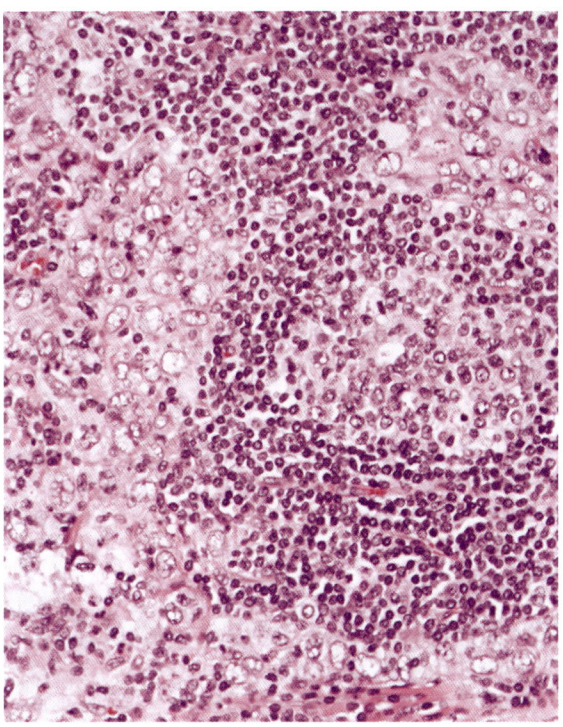

Figure 67-19

METASTATIC NASOPHARYNGEAL CARCINOMA IN LYMPH NODE

The anaplastic carcinoma cells are located within the lymph node sinuses (H&E stain).

nodular sclerosis or the lymphocyte-depleted type (discussed elsewhere in the text).

Immunohistochemical analysis is essential to the workup of metastatic anaplastic tumors (16,51). Metastatic carcinoma and melanoma should be excluded using anti-CK and melanoma-associated antibodies before more esoteric diagnoses are considered. The possibility of metastatic angiosarcoma is addressed by using several markers associated with vascular differentiation, including antibodies reactive with CD31, CD34, ERG, FLI1, WT1, factor VIII antigen, and the lymphatic-associated marker D2-40/podoplanin. These antigens are variably expressed in cases of metastatic angiosarcoma, particularly in poorly differentiated tumors. Metastatic leiomyosarcoma is identified by the expression of smooth muscle actin or desmin (22,32).

Many antibodies used diagnostically have overlapping reactivity with other tumor types. For example, some leiomyosarcomas express keratin, typically low-molecular weight forms (22). There-

fore, a panel of antibodies is highly recommended and often required to establish a diagnosis.

Spindle Cell Tumors

The term *spindle cell* is used for cells that have an elongated or spindled shape and therefore may have a sarcoma-like appearance. Primary spindle cell tumors in lymph nodes are uncommon and thus most spindle cell tumors in lymph nodes are metastases. The more common metastatic tumors with a spindle cell morphology include sarcomatoid carcinoma (fig. 67-23), melanoma (particularly desmoplastic melanoma), various types of sarcoma, and nerve sheath tumors (Table 67-5) (16,50,51).

Soft tissue tumors that metastasize to lymph nodes most often include angiosarcoma, Kaposi sarcoma, leiomyosarcoma (fig. 67-24), and nerve sheath tumors. Dendritic cell sarcomas (discussed in chapters 53 and 54) are also in the differential diagnosis. Although spindle cell morphologic features are unusual

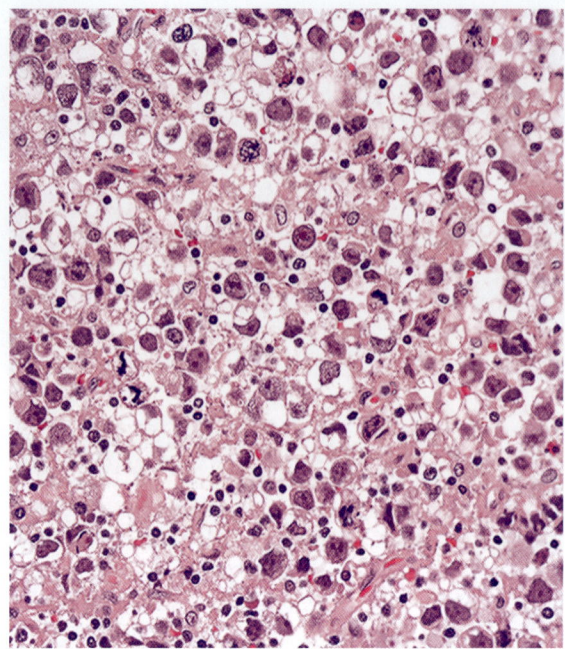

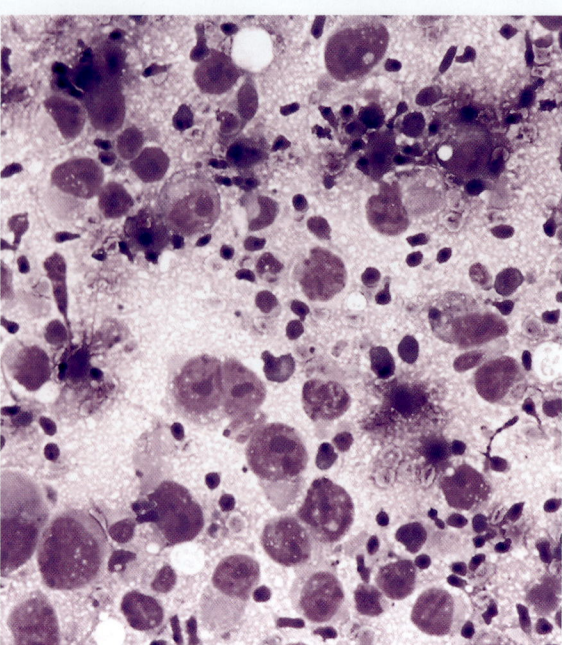

Figure 67-20

METASTATIC SEMINOMA IN LYMPH NODE

In this case the neoplastic cells are large and anaplastic with poorly defined cell borders and prominent nucleoli. The cells were positive for OCT4 (not shown) (H&E stain).

Figure 67-21

METASTATIC SEMINOMA IN LYMPH NODE

A dispersed population of large tumor cells with round nuclei, nucleoli, and pale delicate cytoplasm are admixed with small lymphocytes. A tigroid background is seen which is a clue to the diagnosis (Diff-Quik stain).

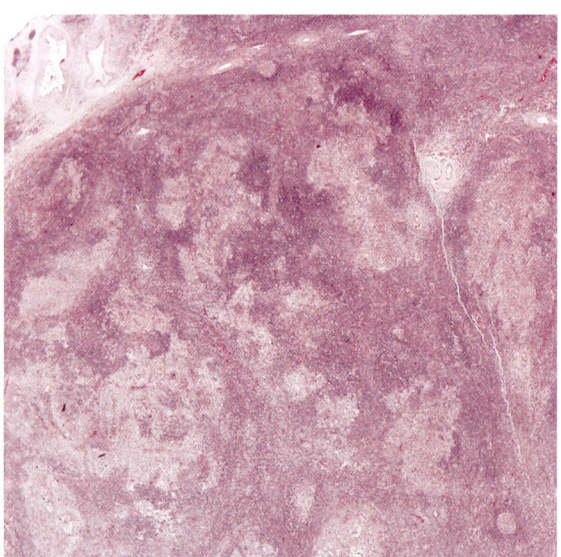

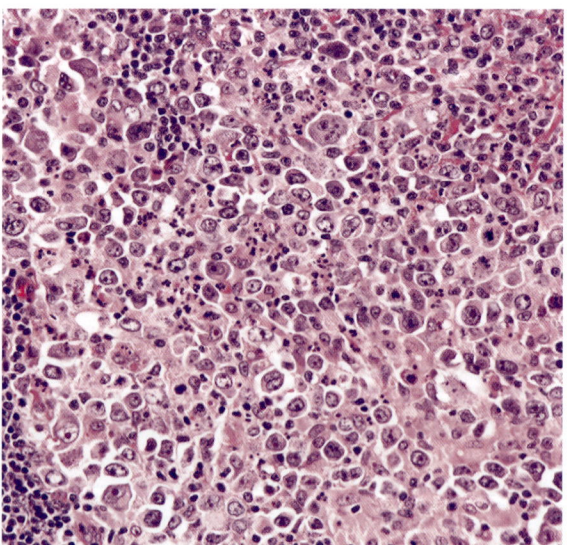

Figure 67-22

DIFFUSE LARGE B-CELL LYMPHOMA WITH ANAPLASTIC FEATURES INVOLVING LYMPH NODE

Left: At low magnification, the lymphoma partially replaces the lymph node with a pattern similar to that of a metastatic solid tumor (left, right: H&E stain).

Right: At high magnification, the neoplastic cells are large and anaplastic. The neoplastic cells were positive for CD20 and other lymphoid antigens (not shown), supporting a diagnosis of diffuse large B-cell lymphoma.

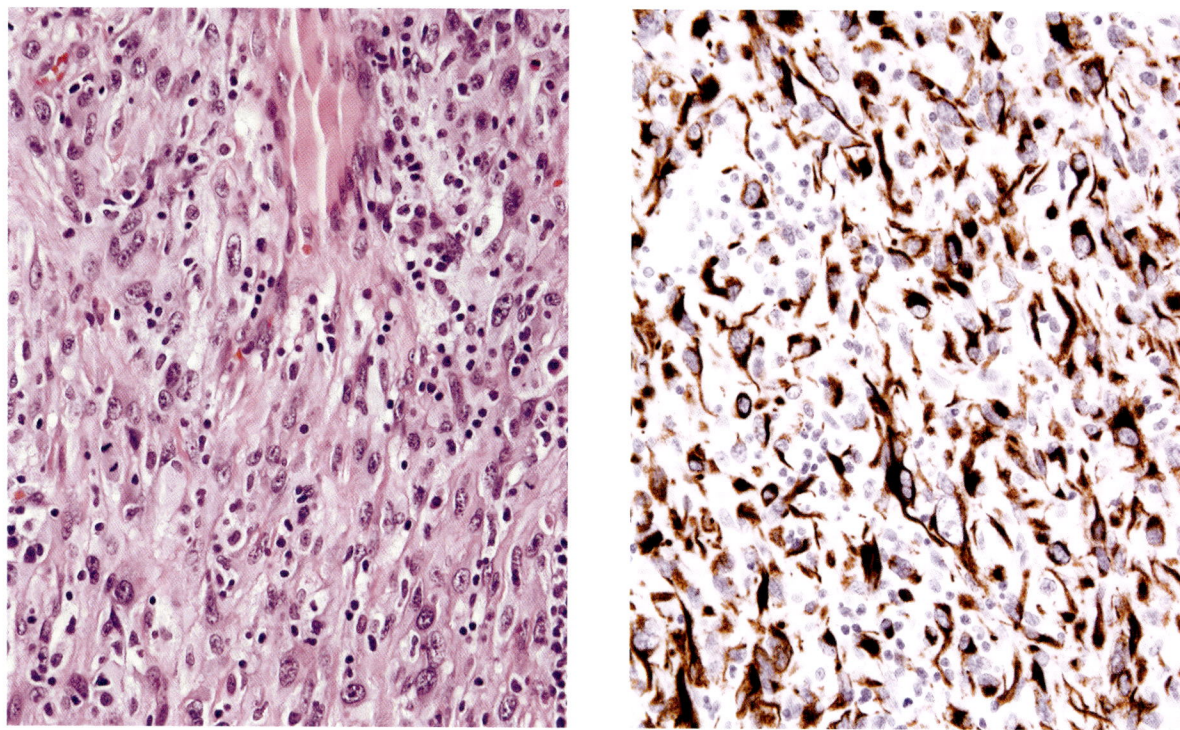

Figure 67-23

METASTATIC SPINDLE CELL CARCINOMA IN LYMPH NODE

Left: The carcinoma cells have a prominent spindle shape and exhibit cytologic atypia (H&E stain).
Right: The neoplastic cells are positive for keratin (immunohistochemistry with hematoxylin counterstain).

in lymphomas, some cases of nodular sclerosis Hodgkin lymphoma and diffuse large B-cell lymphoma also are composed of spindle cells.

Kaposi Sarcoma. Kaposi sarcoma is discussed in chapter 63, but lymph node involvement is the focus here. Patients with Kaposi sarcoma present with generalized lymphadenopathy or localized disease draining a skin site of Kaposi sarcoma. This tumor is driven by HHV-8 infection and is most common in patients with immunodeficiency, particularly those with human immunodeficiency virus (HIV)/acquired immunodeficiency syndrome (AIDS). In a study of patients with HIV and lymphadenopathy, 6.5 percent had Kaposi sarcoma (10).

Grossly, Kaposi sarcoma involving the lymph node is hemorrhagic or has tan, solid areas. The tumor may be adjacent to the lymph node capsule or replace the entire lymph node.

Histologically, Kaposi sarcoma is characterized by a spindle cell proliferation that forms fascicles and abnormal slit-like vascular spaces (fig. 67-25). The spindle cells exhibit mild-

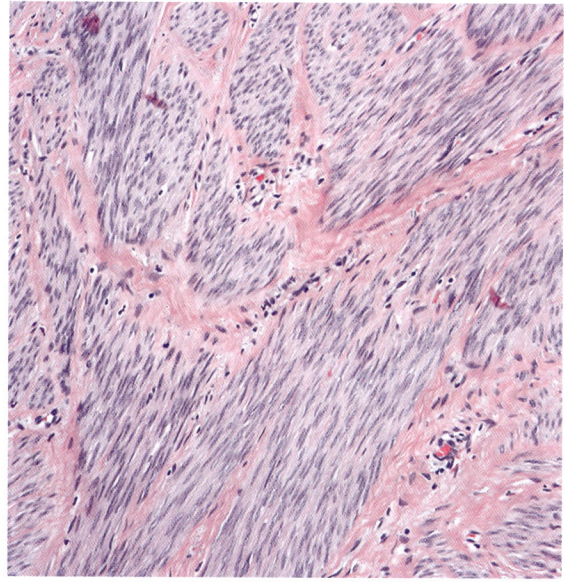

Figure 67-24

METASTATIC LEIOMYOSARCOMA IN LYMPH NODE

The neoplastic cells are highly spindled and were positive for muscle-associated antigens (not shown) (H&E stain).

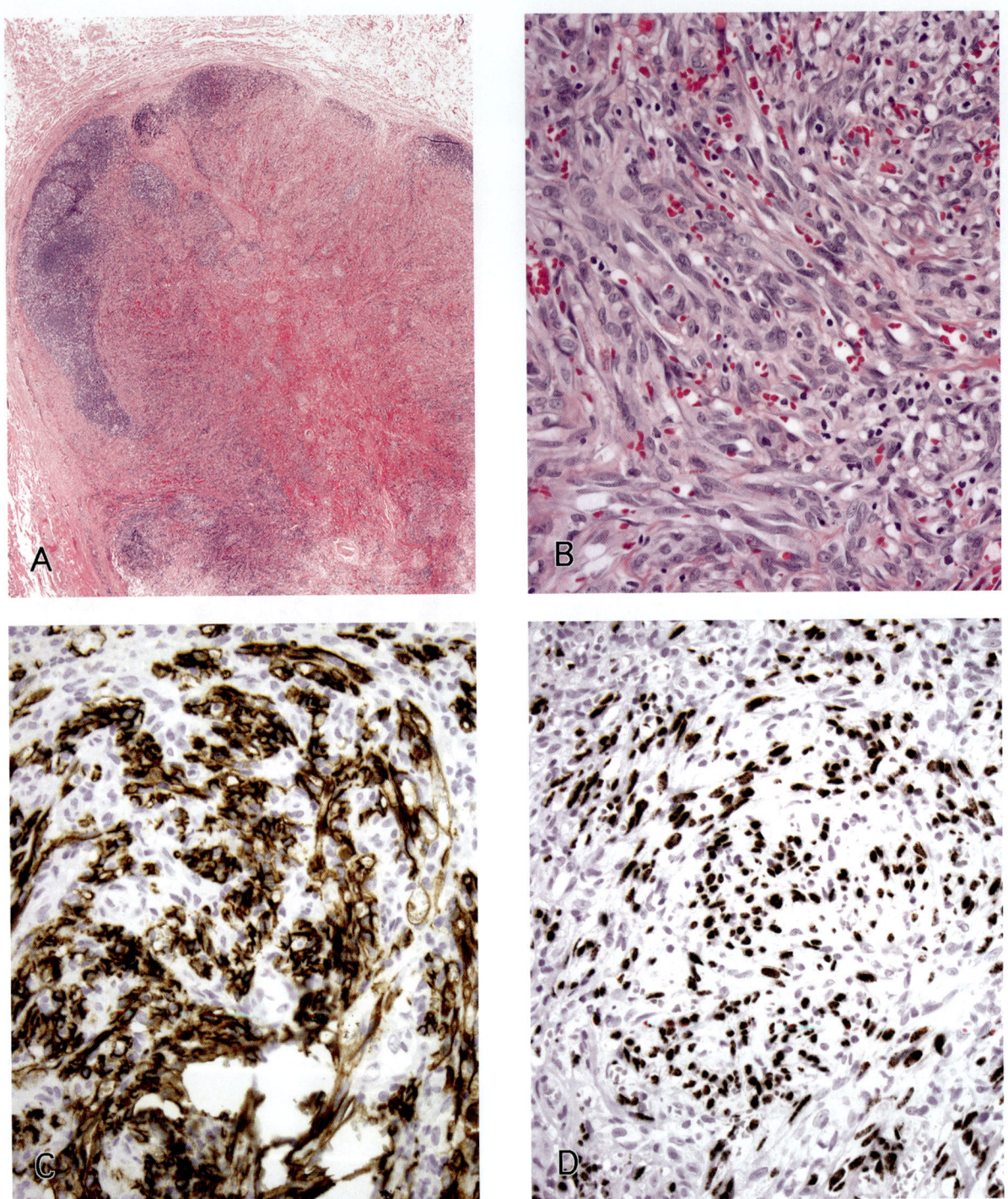

Figure 67-25

METASTATIC KAPOSI SARCOMA IN LYMPH NODE

A: The lymph node has a hemorrhagic appearance, radiating from the more central portions of the lymph node (where there are more vascular elements) (A,B: H&E stain).

B: Higher magnification shows slit-like vascular spaces, with intracellular lumens and moderate cytologic atypia.

C,D: The tumor is positive for D2-40/podoplanin (C) and human herpesvirus (HHV)-8 (D) (C,D: immunohistochemistry with hematoxylin counterstain).

moderate cellular pleomorphism and nuclear atypia. The tumor often begins in or near the lymph node capsule and extends through fibrous trabeculae before replacing the lymph node parenchyma. The tumor may surround hilar blood vessels. Individual tumor cells may contain cytoplasmic globules (periodic acid–Schiff [PAS] positive). Extravasated erythrocytes, hemosiderin deposits, and plasma cells are commonly present. Multicentric Castleman disease associated with HHV-8 infection (see chapter 22) is associated with Kaposi sarcoma in lymph nodes.

Immunohistochemical analysis helps establish the diagnosis of Kaposi sarcoma in lymph nodes. The neoplastic cells are positive for panvascular markers (e.g., CD31, CD34, ERG) and for HHV-8 in a nuclear, granular pattern when assessed with an antibody specific for latency-associated nuclear antigen 1 (LANA-1). Among metastatic spindle cell tumors, HHV-8 reactivity is unique to Kaposi sarcoma.

Metastatic Solid Tumors Associated with a Prominent Infiltrate of Benign Hematopoietic Cells

Some nonhematopoietic malignant tumors are commonly associated with a prominent infiltrate of reactive, hematopoietic cells. Most often, the reactive cells are lymphocytes and histiocytes, but plasma cells or granulocytes also may be numerous. When these tumors metastasize to lymph nodes, the reactive cells are commonly associated with the metastatic cells, and in some cases, may be so numerous that they obscure the neoplastic cells. This event is problematic diagnostically, especially in small needle biopsy specimens. In this scenario, the metastatic tumor may resemble non-Hodgkin or Hodgkin lymphoma.

The metastatic tumors that most often are associated with a prominent reactive infiltrate are nasopharyngeal carcinoma, seminoma, melanoma, and lymphoepithelioma-like carcinomas, and less often, medullary carcinoma. Rare cases of metastatic thymoma and thymic carcinoma also involve regional lymph nodes or other local structures and are associated with a prominent infiltrate of reactive thymocytes. In addition to the location of the lymph node metastasis (discussed above), a high index of suspicion and immunohistochemical analysis will confirm the diagnosis is most instances.

Nasopharyngeal Carcinoma. Approximately half of all patients with nasopharyngeal carcinoma present with metastases to cervical lymph nodes with an occult primary neoplasm (42). Nasopharyngeal carcinoma commonly exhibits squamous cell differentiation that can be keratinizing or nonkeratinizing (fig. 67-19). These tumors uncommonly present a diagnostic challenge when they metastasize to lymph nodes, even when reactive lymphocytes, histiocytes, or eosinophils are plentiful (42). In contrast, metastatic undifferentiated nasopharyngeal carcinoma, also known as lymphoepithelioma, or Schmincke type, is notorious for being confused with lymphoma and some cases closely mimic classic Hodgkin lymphoma (fig. 67-26) (52). The histologic clues to the correct diagnosis include the cohesive tendency of the metastatic cells and the opaque or "hard" quality of their cytoplasm.

POTENTIAL PITFALLS USING IMMUNOHISTOCHEMISTRY

It is not possible in one chapter to cover the numerous pitfalls that are associated with using immunohistochemical analysis to assess metastases. Here many of the more common pitfalls are summarized. Potential pitfalls can be avoided by using a panel of antibodies that yields expected positive and negative results.

CKs, which are intermediate filament proteins that are usually abundant in epithelial tissues and their tumors, are not restricted to epithelial tumors. There are a wide variety of CKs with 54 functional keratin genes in the human genome (16). Different CKs are of low or high molecular weight, and different normal tissues or tumors may be rich in either low or high molecular weight CKs (16,51). For example, hepatocellular carcinoma expresses abundant low molecular weight CKs such as CK8. In contrast, squamous cell carcinomas express high molecular weight CKs. Accordingly, certain anti-CK antibodies are more reactive with low molecular weight CKs (e.g., CAM5.2) whereas other antibodies are reactive with high molecular weight CKs (e.g., AE1/AE3). The antibody must be matched with the suspected site of metastasis. For this reason, a cocktail of anti-CK

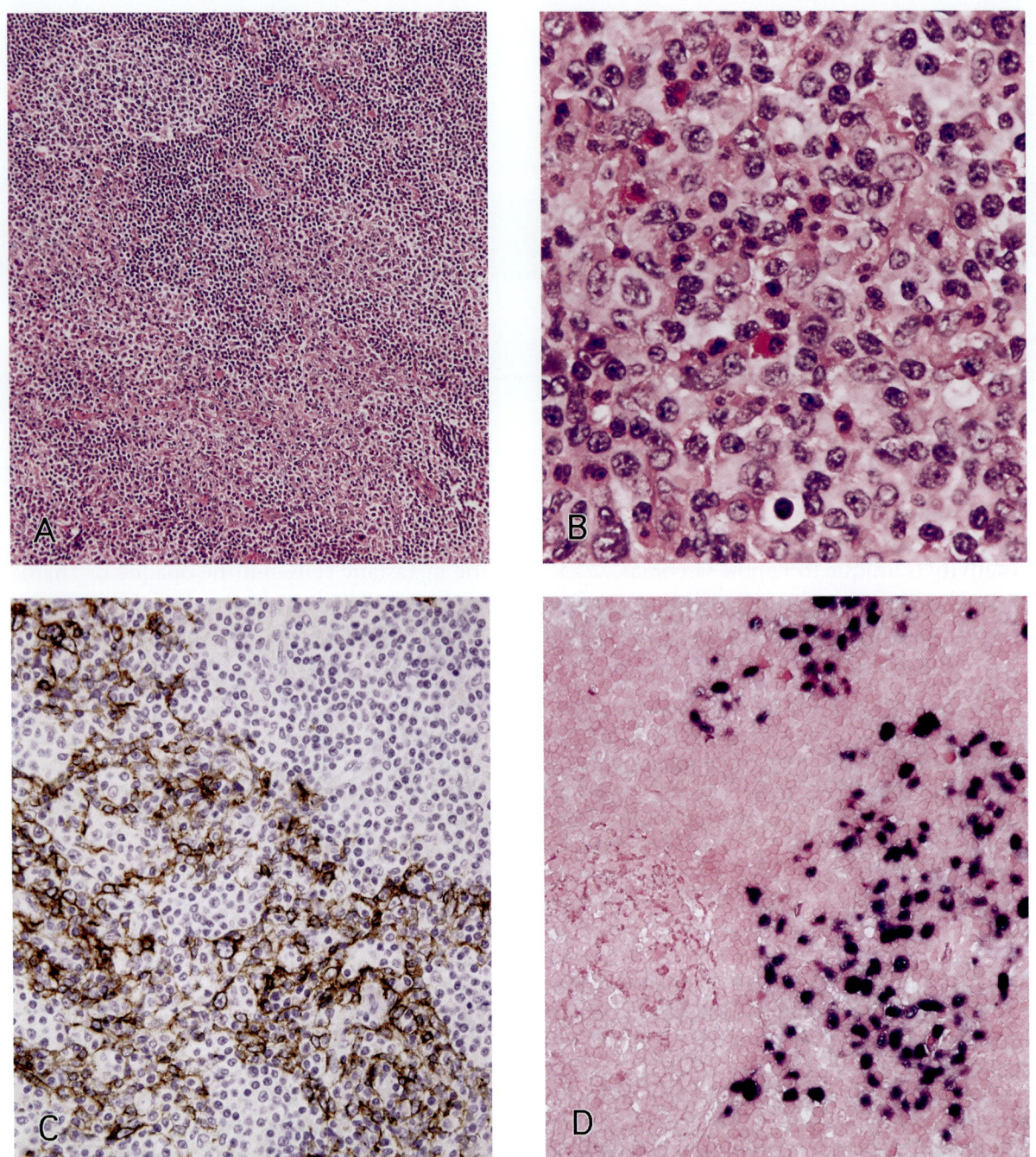

Figure 67-26

**METASTATIC NASOPHARYNGEAL CARCINOMA, ALSO KNOWN AS
SCHMINKE TYPE OR LYMPHOEPITHELIOMA, IN CERVICAL LYMPH NODE**

A: The neoplasm partially replaces the lymph node parenchyma. Residual lymphoid tissue, including a reactive germinal center, is present in this field (top left) (A,B: H&E stain).

B: Oil magnification shows scattered large neoplastic cells with prominent nucleoli associated with reactive lymphocytes, histiocytes, and eosinophils.

C: The neoplastic cells are positive for pancytokeratin (immunohistochemistry with hematoxylin counterstain).

D: The neoplastic cells are positive for Epstein-Barr virus encoded RNA1 (EBER1) (in situ hybridization with eosin counterstain).

antibodies that includes reactivity for all CKs is popular and helpful.

There are many lineage-specific antibodies that are available for different types of carcinoma. For example, antibodies specific for gross cystic disease fluid protein-15 (GCDP-15) or thyroglobulin are highly specific for breast carcinoma or thyroid carcinoma, respectively. The challenge, however, is that these antibodies are not very sensitive for poorly differentiated breast and thyroid carcinomas. As summarized by Conner and Hornick (16), the lack of sensitivity in the analysis of poorly differentiated tumors is a major issue for most of the currently available lineage-specific antibodies. This problem is further magnified in the analysis of metastatic carcinomas as many studies have shown that the sensitivity of these antibodies is lower in metastatic versus primary tumors, in part because metastatic tumors are more commonly poorly differentiated (16,32,51). In some metastatic tumors this issue is worsened by the loss of many characteristic antigens as the tumor devolves into a more and more undifferentiated state.

A small subset of metastatic poorly differentiated carcinomas lacks one or multiple keratins (16,32,51). Metastatic melanoma may not express one or more melanoma-associated antigens and rarely, multiple melanoma-associated antigens are missing (2). Some lymphomas, 5 to 10 percent, are negative for CD45/LCA. In anaplastic large cell lymphoma, the absence of CD45/LCA combined with the presence of EMA may lead to an erroneous diagnosis of metastatic carcinoma.

Another potential issue is cross reactivity of antibodies. Unexpected patterns of antibody reactivity may be attributable to the true expression of antigen by another tumor type. In other cases, however, the unusual reaction pattern may be a form of nonspecific cross reactivity. An example of cross reactivity involves PAX8. Anti-PAX8 antibodies are commonly used as a marker of kidney and thyroid carcinomas and tumors of mullerian origin, particularly from the ovary (16). Anti-PAX8 antibodies are reactive with a subset of B-cell lymphomas, but this phenomenon is not true expression of PAX8, but instead cross reactivity between PAX8 and PAX5, the latter a well-established pan-B-cell antigen (fig. 67-27) (41).

Epithelial- and Mesenchymal-Related Antigens in Hematopoietic Tumors

Epithelial- or mesenchymal-related antigens are detected in a small subset of hematopoietic tumors. In a large survey, Adams et al. (1) showed CKs in 1.5 percent of lymphomas. In most cases, CK immunoreactivity was finely granular and present in less than 10 percent of tumor cells (1); rarely, however, keratin expression is prominent. A variety of CK types have been reported and in some cases prominently expressed in plasma-cell derived neoplasms, including plasmablastic lymphoma, plasmacytoma, and plasma cell myeloma.

CD31, also known as platelet endothelial cell adhesion molecule 1 (PECAM-1), is an excellent marker of endothelial cells and vascular tumors, but is also expressed by monocytes and macrophages, and therefore, histiocytic tumors. CD31 is also expressed in a subset of cases of chronic lymphocytic leukemia and lymphoblastic lymphoma (39).

p63, often positive in epithelial tumors, is expressed in a variety of B-cell lymphomas, including primary mediastinal large B-cell lymphoma. S-100 protein, a hallmark of melanoma, also is expressed in a small subset of T-cell lymphomas, including T-cell prolymphocytic leukemia, peripheral T-cell lymphoma, anaplastic large cell lymphoma, and hepatosplenic T-cell lymphoma (3,45).

Common Hematopoietic Antigens in Epithelial and Mesenchymal Tumors

Many antibodies used routinely in the assessment of hematopoietic tumors are also reactive in epithelial and mesenchymal tumors (Table 67-6). CD5, a T-cell antigen that is also expressed by chronic lymphocytic leukemia and mantle cell lymphoma, may be expressed by thymic epithelial tumors, particularly thymic carcinoma (36). CD10 expression, seen commonly in many follicular lymphomas, large cell lymphomas, and a subset of T-cell lymphomas, is also expressed in a number of carcinomas. CD15, expressed by Reed-Sternberg and Hodgkin cells in about 70 percent of cases of classic Hodgkin lymphoma, is expressed in a number of types of adenocarcinoma. CD20, a pan-B-cell antigen, is expressed by cells with stellate shapes, so-called asteroid cells,

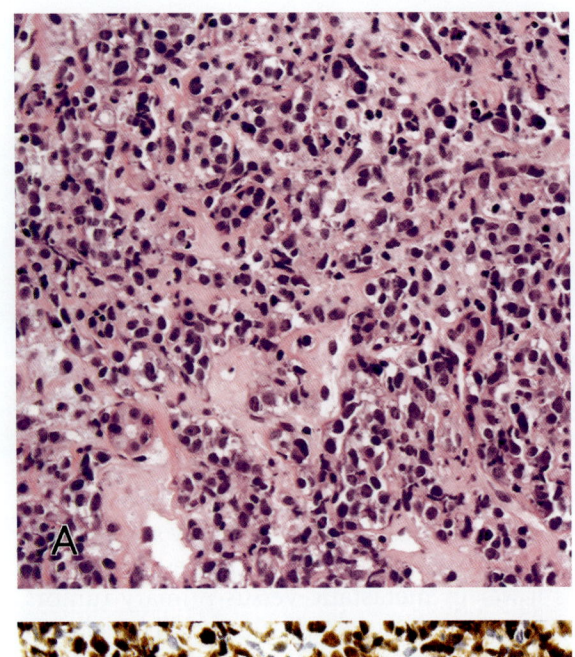

Figure 67-27

**DIFFUSE LARGE B-CELL LYMPHOMA
POSITIVE FOR PAX5 AND PAX8**

A: The neoplastic cells are arranged in a diffuse pattern and are large (H&E stain).

B: The lymphoma cells are strongly and uniformly positive for PAX5, a pan-B-cell antigen (B,C: immunohistochemistry with hematoxylin counterstain).

C: The lymphoma cells are also positive for PAX8. The PAX8 positivity is likely attributable to cross-reactivity with PAX5.

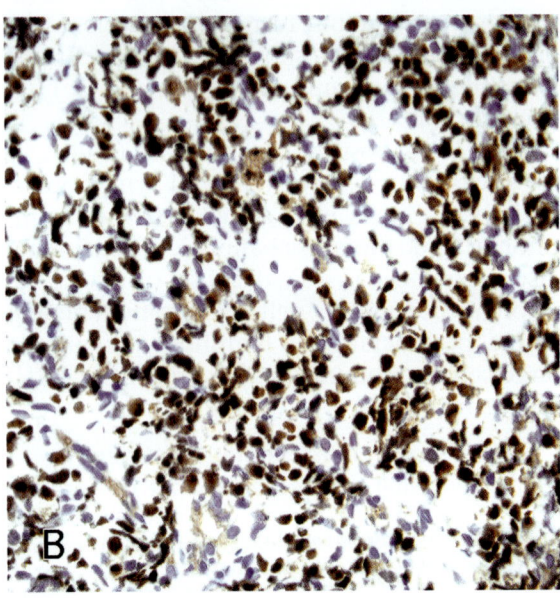

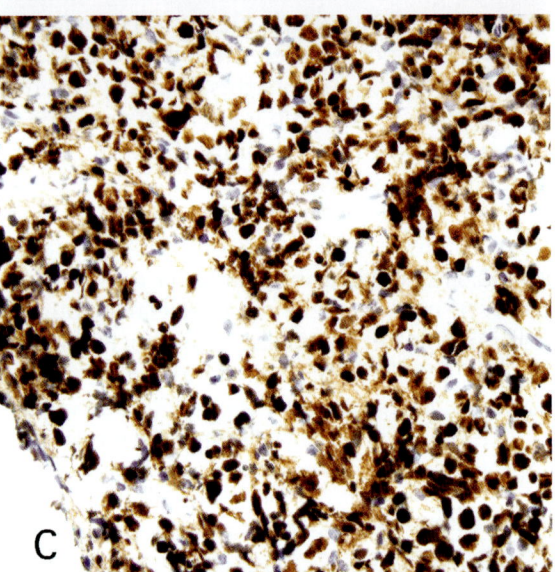

in a subset of thymomas (13,48). Many of these CD20-positive cells correspond to B cells also located in the medulla of the normal thymus (48). However, Chilosi et al. (13) showed that thymoma cells also can express CD20. CD30, characteristically expressed in classic Hodgkin lymphoma and anaplastic large cell lymphoma, also is expressed by a variety of epithelial and mesenchymal tumors, including embryonal carcinoma of the testis and mesothelioma.

CD45/LCA is commonly positive in the cytoplasm (but not the membrane) of metastatic breast carcinoma cells. CD56, also known as neural cell adhesion molecule (NCAM), although used as a natural killer cell-associated marker in lymphoma diagnosis, is expressed in neuroendocrine carcinomas and a wide variety of central nervous system and neural crest-derived cells and associated tumors (fig. 67-28). CD138, strongly expressed by plasma cells, is also present in a wide variety of carcinomas.

BCL2, a protein originally identified in follicular lymphoma where it is over-expressed as a result of t(14;18)(q32;q21)/*IGH-BCL2*, is expressed in many normal tissue types and malignant neoplasms. Cyclin D1, which is

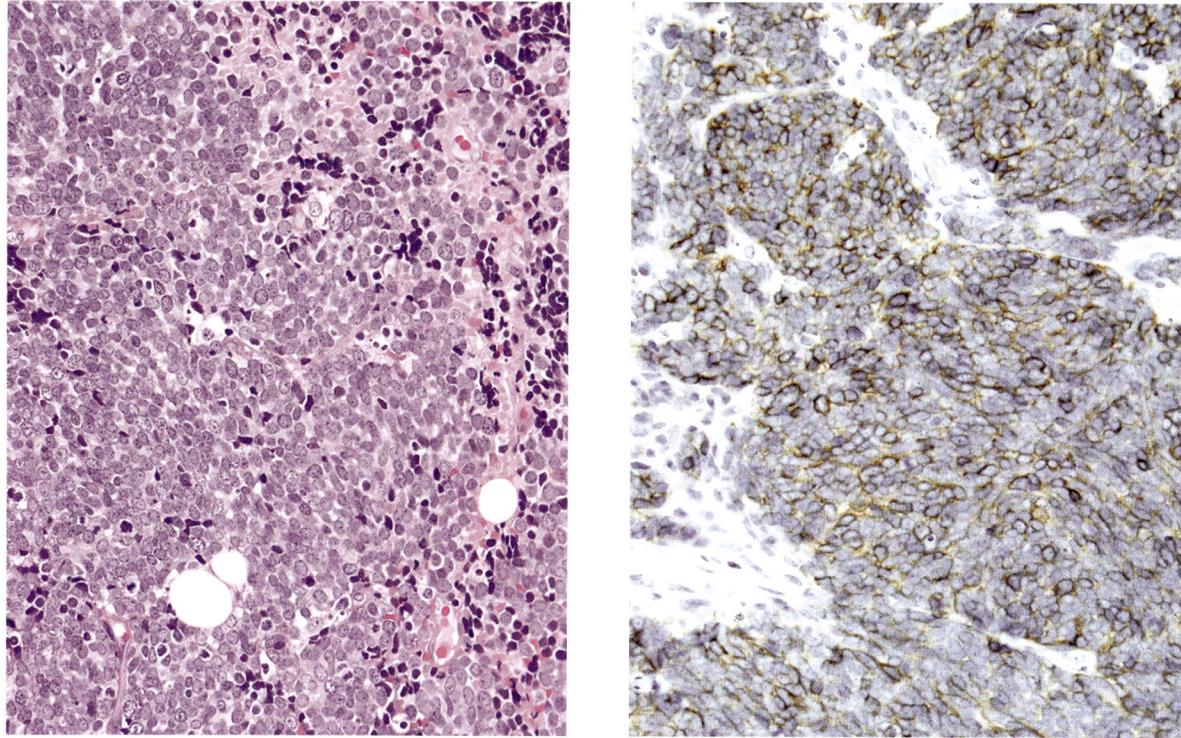

Figure 67-28

METASTATIC NEUROENDOCRINE CARCINOMA WITH EXPRESSION OF CD56

Left: A routinely stained section of the tumor shows that the neoplastic cells are cohesive and have neuroendocrine features (H&E stain).

Right: The tumor is positive for CD56. Although CD56 is used as a marker of natural killer cells in lymphoma diagnosis, expression of CD56 is seen in a variety of hematopoietic and nonhematopoietic tumors (immunohistochemistry with hematoxylin counterstain).

overexpressed in mantle cell lymphoma as a result of t(11;14)(q13;q32)/*CCND1-IGH*, is constitutively expressed in a variety of epithelial cells, epithelial tumors (fig. 67-29), and proliferating stromal elements, especially endothelial cells. ALK, originally detected in anaplastic large cell lymphoma by its fusion with nucleophosmin in t(2;5)(p23;q35), is also expressed in inflammatory myofibroblastic tumors, a subset of rhabdomyosarcomas, lung adenocarcinomas, and Wilms tumors, and uncommonly other neoplasms (12,24,33). PAX5, which is useful as a pan-B-cell marker, is also positive in most cases of Merkel cell carcinoma, but not small cell carcinoma of the lung (35,53). Merkel cell carcinoma and small cell carcinoma of the lung are also positive for terminal deoxynucleotidyl transferase (TdT), an antigen of immature lymphocytes considered to be characteristic of B- and T-cell lymphoblastic lymphoma/leukemia (fig. 67-30) (35,53).

Normal Cells Usually Not Appreciated in Routinely Stained Tissue Sections

Highly sensitive monoclonal antibodies may result in the recognition of normal or benign cells that could potentially be confused with a metastatic tumor. For example, sensitive pan-CK antibodies such as OSCAR, highlight normal fibroblastic reticular cells within lymph nodes and these cells should not be confused with metastatic carcinoma (fig. 67-31). This may be an issue in the analysis of sentinel lymph node biopsy specimens from patients with breast carcinoma. Similarly, anti-S-100 antibody and other melanocytic markers may highlight single or small groups of nevus cells, usually located in the capsule or fibrous trabeculae of lymph nodes. These nevus cells must not be confused with metastatic melanoma in sentinel lymph node biopsy specimens.

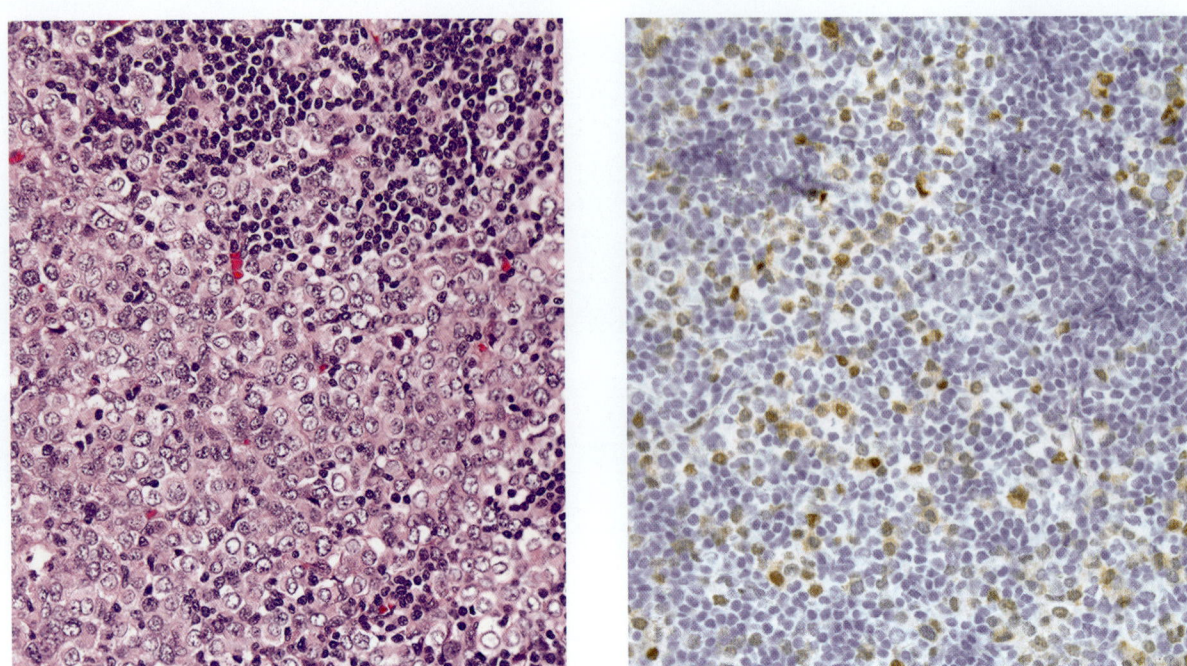

Figure 67-29

METASTATIC CARCINOMA POSITIVE FOR CYCLIN D1

Left: A routinely stained section of a poorly differentiated carcinoma that subtotally replaces lymph node (H&E stain).

Right: The nuclei of some carcinoma cells are positive for cyclin D1 (immunohistochemistry with hematoxylin counterstain).

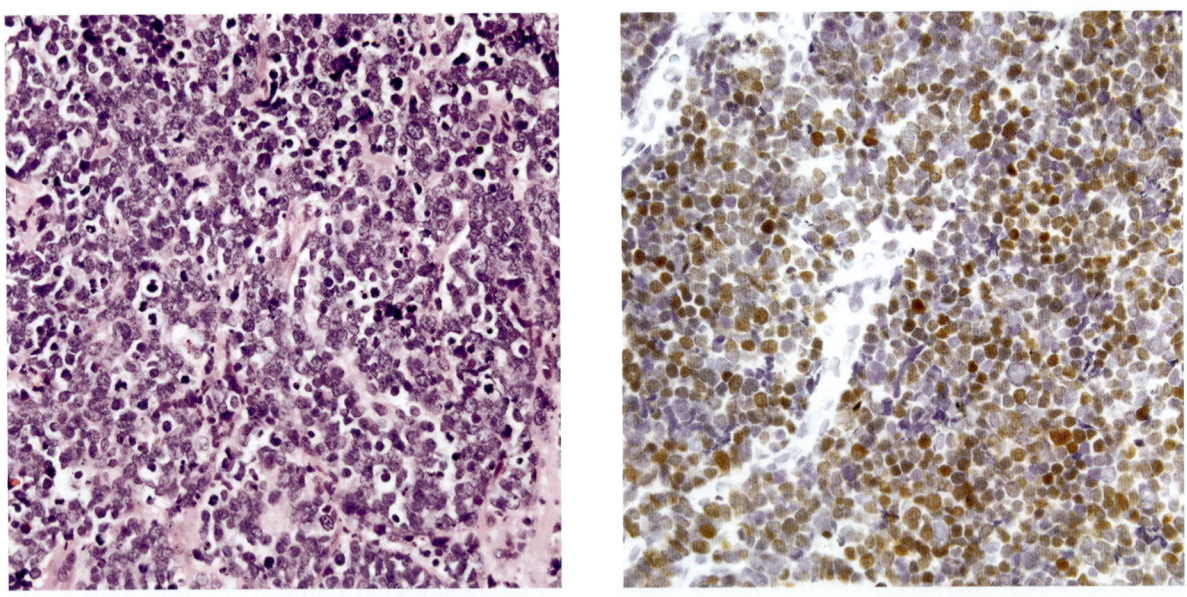

Figure 67-30

METASTATIC SMALL CELL CARCINOMA WITH EXPRESSION OF TDT

Left: A routinely stained section of the tumor shows that the neoplastic cells are cohesive and have neuroendocrine features.

Right: The nuclei of some carcinoma cells are positive for TdT (left: H&E stain; right: immunohistochemistry with hematoxylin counterstain).

OTHER ANCILLARY METHODS FOR DIAGNOSIS OF METASTASES

Although immunohistochemical analysis has a very prominent role in the diagnosis of lymph node metastases, other methods are also helpful. Electron microscopy has much value in the workup of poorly differentiated tumors. Electron microscopy may identify cell junctions that are a feature of carcinomas or melanosomes that are characteristic of melanoma, as well as cytoplasmic granules in some neuroendocrine tumors and muscle filaments in rhabdomyosarcomas.

Conventional cytogenetic analysis and fluorescence in situ hybridization (FISH) help evaluate childhood small blue cell tumors as well as blastoid tumors and sarcomas in adults. Some chromosomal translocations are highly characteristic of specific tumor types. For example, alveolar rhabdomyosarcoma is usually associated with either t(2;13)(p35;q14)/ *PAX3-FKHR* or t(1;13)(p36;q14)/*PAX7-FKHR*. Ewing sarcoma is associated with translocations involving *EWS*, most often t(11;22)(q24;q12)/ *EWS-FLI1*. Conventional cytogenetic analysis requires fresh tissue, a potential drawback that can be overcome by using FISH and fixed, paraffin-embedded tissue sections.

High-throughput molecular methods help in the analysis of metastatic tumors. As has been reviewed by Economopoulou et al. (20), gene expression profiling, microRNA arrays, and next-generation sequencing methods are used for this purpose. Due to the cost and complexity of these techniques, it seems unlikely that high-throughput methods will replace immunohistochemistry. However, immunohistochemical analysis has some limitations and does not identify the primary tumor in up to one third of metastatic tumors of unknown primary site (19). In a study in which immunohistochemistry was directly compared with gene expression profiling, the latter was more sensitive and accurate than immunohistochemistry, particularly for extremely poorly differentiated tumors (28).

It seems likely that in the future high throughput methods will have their greatest value in the workup of poorly differentiated tumors as well as metastatic tumors of unknown primary origin. High-throughput analysis also will have the simultaneous advantage of identifying potential therapeutic targets.

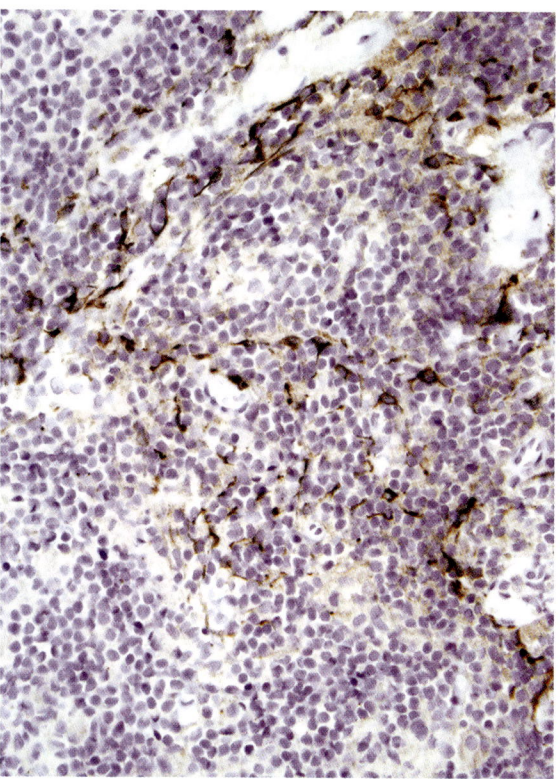

Figure 67-31

NORMAL KERATIN-POSITIVE DENDRITIC CELLS IN LYMPH NODE

Pancytokeratin antibodies with broad reactivity, such as OSCAR, often highlight small, spindled cells with dendritic cell processes in lymph nodes. These cells are "keratin-positive dendritic cells," a subset of dendritic/ accessory cells normally observed in lymph nodes, and must not be confused with metastatic carcinoma (immunohistochemistry with hematoxylin counterstain).

SPLEEN

As mentioned, the spleen is an uncommon site of metastases of solid tumors. Most studies that have assessed metastases to spleen have been autopsy studies. The frequency of splenic metastases in these studies is usually less than 5 percent (8,46). Splenic metastases are more common in patients with widespread metastatic disease (e.g., liver, lungs, bones), suggesting that splenic metastases are a late event in the disease course, and likely occur via hematogenous spread.

The spleen is usually not enlarged as a result of metastasis. In an autopsy study by Schon et al. (46), about 80 percent of patients had a normal spleen size. The 20 percent of patients with enlarged spleens usually had only modest

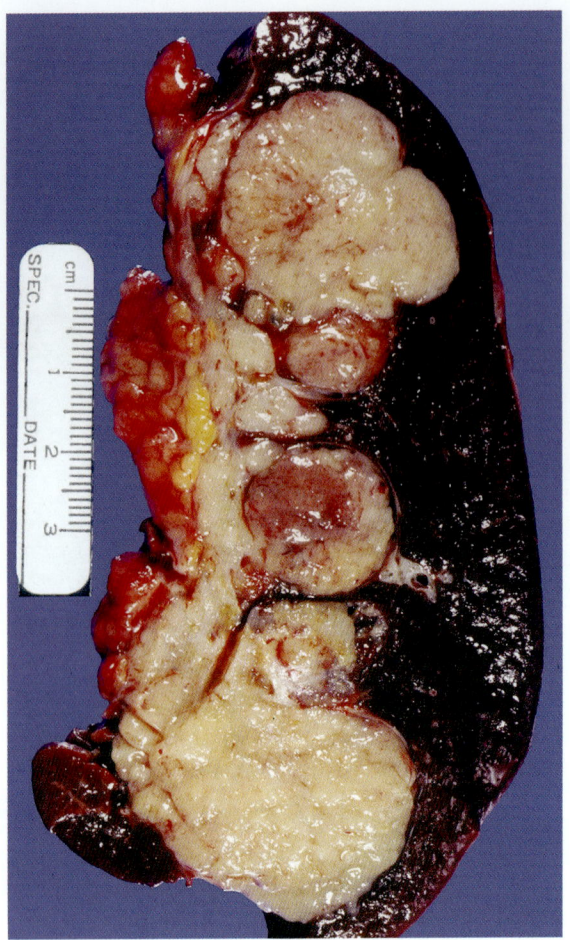
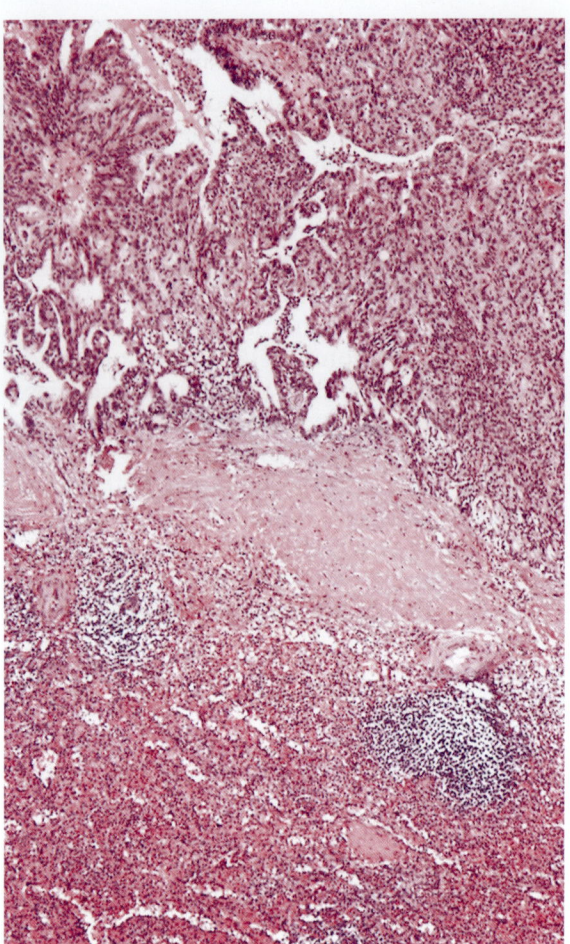

Figure 67-32

METASTATIC OVARIAN ADENOCARCINOMA IN SPLEEN

Left: The tumor involved the spleen as a large mass.
Right: A histologic section shows metastatic adenocarcinoma (top) and uninvolved spleen (bottom) (H&E stain).

splenomegaly, with only rare patients with a spleen up to 1,000 g. Splenic metastases are usually large enough to be detected grossly; about 15 percent of patients have metastases that are only detected by microscopic examination. Extramedullary hematopoiesis is commonly present in spleen specimens with metastases and may explain splenomegaly in some patients (46).

Few studies have assessed splenic metastases in living patients, but the availability of imaging studies has resulted in more frequent detection of such metastases in patients with solid tumors (4,34). Usually, metastases are a manifestation of widespread disease, but some patients have single metastases (fig. 67-32). Patients with single

or isolated splenic metastases most often have a metastatic carcinoma of some type. Melanoma rarely spreads to the spleen in the absence of widespread metastatic disease (4).

Virtually any primary tumor may metastasize to the spleen, but the most common metastatic tumors in order of frequency are: gynecologic (most often from the ovary); colorectal, lung, and breast carcinomas; and melanoma (8,46). This frequency is, in part, attributable to the overall frequency of these diseases. The tendency for a certain type of tumor to metastasize to the spleen is higher for ovarian carcinoma and melanoma than it is for colorectal, lung, and breast carcinomas (4,46). Among lung carcinomas, small cell carcinoma has the greatest tendency to metastasize to the spleen. It is uncommon for patients with splenic metastases to have an unknown primary tumor.

Patients with single or isolated splenic metastases may present with left upper quadrant pain or weight loss (4). Rarely, large splenic metastases cause spontaneous rupture of the spleen, resulting in hemoperitoneum and a high mortality rate (26,40). Splenectomy is often recommended for patients with metastases localized to the spleen, to alleviate symptoms and to avoid the risk of splenic rupture (4,37).

REFERENCES

1. Adams H, Schmid P, Dirnhofer S, Tzankov A. Cytokeratin expression in hematological neoplasms: a tissue microarray study on 866 lymphoma and leukemia cases. Pathol Res Pract 2008;204:569-573.
2. Agaimy A, Specht K, Stoehr R, et al. Metastatic malignant melanoma with complete loss of differentiation markers (undifferentiated/dedifferentiated melanoma): analysis of 14 patients emphasizing phenotypic plasticity and the value of molecular testing as surrogate diagnostic marker. Am J Surg Pathol 2016;40:181-191.
3. Aggarwal N, Pongpruttipan T, Patel S, et al. Expression of S100 protein in CD4-positive T-cell lymphomas is often associated with T-cell prolymphocytic leukemia. Am J Surg Pathol 2015;39:1679-1687.
4. Agha-Mohammadi S, Calne RY. Solitary splenic metastasis: case report and review of the literature. Am J Clin Oncol 2001;24:306-310.
5. Edge S, Byrd DK, Compton CC, Fritz AG, Greene FL, Trotti A, eds. AJCC Cancer Staging Manual New York: Springer-Verlag; 2010.
6. Angulo JC, González J, Rodríguez N, et al. Clinicopathological study of regressed testicular tumors (apparent extragonadal germ cell neoplasms). J Urol 2009;182:2303-2310.
7. Balzer BL, Ulbright TM. Spontaneous regression of testicular germ cell tumors: an analysis of 42 cases. Am J Surg Pathol 2006;30:858-865.
8. Berghe T. Splenic metasteses. Frequencies and patterns. Acta Pathol Microbiol Scand 1974; 82A:499-506.
9. Bidard FC, Pierga JY, Vincent-Salomon A, Poupon MF. A "class action" against the microenvironment: do cancer cells cooperate in metastasis? Cancer Metastasis Rev 2008;27:5-10.
10. Bogoch II, Andrews JR, Nagami EH, Rivera AM, Gandhi RT, Stone D. Clinical predictors for the aetiology of peripheral lymphadenopathy in HIV-infected patients. HIV Med 2013;14:82-86.
11. Cervin JR, Silverman JF, Loggie BW, Geisinger KR. Virchow's node revisited. Analysis with clinicopathologic correlation of 152 fine-needle aspiration biopsies of supraclavicular lymph nodes. Arch Pathol Lab Med 1995;119:727-730.
12. Cessna MH, Zhou H, Sanger WG, et al. Expression of ALK1 and p80 in inflammatory myofibroblastic tumor and its mesenchymal mimics: a study of 135 cases. Mod Pathol 2002;15:931-938.
13. Chilosi M, Castelli P, Martignoni G, et al. Neoplastic epithelial cells in a subset of human thymomas express the B cell-associated CD20 antigen. Am J Surg Pathol 1992;16:988-997.
14. Christofori G. New signals from the invasive front. Nature 2006;441:444-450.
15. Chung LW, Baseman A, Assikis V, Zhau HE. Molecular insights into prostate cancer progression: the missing link of tumor microenvironment. J Urol 2005;173:10-20.
16. Conner JR, Hornick JL. Metastatic carcinoma of unknown primary: diagnostic approach using immunohistochemistry. Adv Anat Pathol 2015;22:149-167.
17. Coumans FA, Siesling S, Terstappen LW. Detection of cancer before distant metastasis. BMC Cancer 2013;13:283.
18. Dar IH, Kamili MA, Dar SH, Kuchaai FA. Sister Mary Joseph nodule-A case report with review of the literature. J Res Med Sci 2009;14:385-387.
19. DeYoung B, Wick MR. Immunohistologic evaluation of metastatic carcinomas of unknown origin: an algorithmic approach. Semin Diagn Pathol 2000;17:184-193.
20. Economopoulou P, Mountzios G, Pavlidis N, Pentheroudakis G. Cancer of unknown primary origin in the genomic era: elucidating the dark box of cancer. Cancer Treat Rev 2015;41:598-604.
21. Fizazi K, Greco FA, Pavlidis N, et al. Cancers of unknown primary site: ESMO Clinical Practice Guidelines for diagnosis, treatment and follow-up. Ann Oncol 2015;26(Suppl 5):v133-v138.
22. Folpe AL, Cooper K. Best practices in diagnostic immunohistochemistry: pleomorphic cutaneous spindle cell tumors. Arch Pathol Lab Med 2007;131:1517-1524.
23. Giridharan W, Hughes J, Fenton JE, Jones AS. Lymph node metastases in the lower neck. Clin Otolaryngol Allied Sci 2003;28:221-226.

24. Gruber K, Kohlhäufl M, Friedel G, Ott G, Kalla C. A novel, highly sensitive ALK antibody 1A4 facilitates effective screening for ALK rearrangements in lung adenocarcinomas by standard immunohistochemistry. J Thorac Oncol 2015;10:713-716.

25. Guarischi A, Keane TJ, Elhakim T. Metastatic inguinal nodes from an unknown primary neoplasm. A review of 56 cases. Cancer 1987;59:572-577.

26. Gupta PB, Harvey L. Spontaneous rupture of the spleen secondary to metastatic carcinoma. Br J Surg 1993;80:613.

27. Hall BJ, Schmidt RL, Sharma RR, Layfield LJ. Fine-needle aspiration cytology for the diagnosis of metastatic melanoma: systematic review and meta-analysis. Am J Clin Pathol 2013;140:635-642.

28. Handorf CR, Kulkarni A, Grenert JP, et al. A multicenter study directly comparing the diagnostic accuracy of gene expression profiling and immunohistochemistry for primary site identification in metastatic tumors. Am J Surg Pathol 2013;37:1067-1075.

29. Hess KR, Varadhachary GR, Taylor SH, et al. Metastatic patterns in adenocarcinoma. Cancer 2006;106:1624-1633.

30. Iezzoni JC, Mills SE. "Undifferentiated" small round cell tumors of the sinonasal tract: differential diagnosis update. Am J Clin Pathol 2005;124(Suppl):S110-121.

31. Jones D, Medeiros LJ. Nonlymphoid lesions of the lymph nodes. In: Jaffe ES, Harris NL, Vardiman JW, Campo E, Arber DA, eds. Hematopathology. Philadelphia: Elsevier; 2011:951-964.

32. Kandalaft PL, Gown AM. Practical applications in immunohistochemistry: carcinomas of unknown primary site. Arch Pathol Lab Med 2016;140:508-523.

33. Karakus E, Emir S, Kaçar A, Karakus R, Demir HA, Özyörük D. Anaplastic lymphoma kinase gene expression in small round cell tumors of childhood—a comparative immunohistochemical study. Ann Diagn Pathol 2015;19:239-42.

34. Klein B, Stein M, Kuten A, et al. Splenomegaly and solitary spleen metastasis in solid tumors. Cancer 1987;60:100-102.

35. Kolhe R, Reid MD, Lee JR, Cohen C, Ramalingam P. Immunohistochemical expression of PAX5 and TdT by Merkel cell carcinoma and pulmonary small cell carcinoma: a potential diagnostic pitfall but useful discriminatory marker. Int J Clin Exp Pathol 2013;6:142-147.

36. Kornstein MJ, Rosai J. CD5 labeling of thymic carcinomas and other nonlymphoid neoplasms. Am J Clin Pathol 1998;109:722-726.

37. Lee S, Morgenstern L, Phillips E, Hiatt JR, Margulies DR. Splenectomy for splenic metastasis: a changing spectrum. Am J Surg 2000;66:837-840.

38. Loh KY, Yushak AW. Images in clinical medicine. Virchow's node (Troisier's sign). N Engl J Med 2007;357:282.

39. Mainou-Fowler T, Porteous A, Nicolle A, Proctor SJ, Anderson JJ, Summerfield G. CD31 density is a novel risk factor for patients with B-cell chronic lymphocytic leukemia. Int J Oncol 2008;33:169-174.

40. Massarweh S, Dhingra H. Unusual sites of malignancy: case 3. Solitary splenic metastasis in lung cancer with solitary rupture. J Clin Oncol 2001;19:1574-1575.

41. Moretti L, Medeiros LJ, Kunkalla K, Williams MD, Singh RR, Vega F. N-terminal PAX8 polyclonal antibody shows cross-reactivity with N-terminal region of PAX5 and is responsible for reports of PAX8 positivity in malignant lymphomas. Mod Pathol 2012;25:231-236.

42. Petersson F. Nasopharyngeal carcinoma: a review. Semin Diagn Pathol 2015;32:54-73.

43. Pusztaszeri MP, Faquin WC. Cytologic evaluation of cervical lymph node metastases from cancers of unknown primary origin. Semin Diagn Pathol 2015;32:32-41.

44. Rosen PP, Kimmel M. Occult breast carcinoma presenting with axillary lymph node metastases: a follow-up study of 48 patients. Hum Pathol 1990;21:518-523.

45. Rust R, Visser L, van der Leij J, et al. High expression of calcium-binding proteins, S100A10, S100A11 and CALM2 in anaplastic large cell lymphoma. Br J Haematol 2005;131:596-608.

46. Schon CA, Gorg C, Ramaswamy A, Barth PJ. Splenic metastases in a large unselected autopsy series. Pathol Res Pract 2006;202:351-356.

47. Spano D, Heck C, De Antonellis P, Christofori G, Zollo M. Molecular networks that regulate cancer metastasis. Semin Cancer Biol 2012;22:234-249.

48. Taubenberger JK, Jaffe ES, Medeiros LJ. Thymoma with abundant L26-positive "asteroid" cells. A case report with an analysis of normal thymus and thymoma specimens. Arch Pathol Lab Med 1991;115:1254-1257.

49. Tiwari N, Gheldof A, Tatari M, Christofori G. EMT as the ultimate survival mechanism of cancer cells. Semin Cancer Biol 2012;22:194-207.

50. Turner MS, Goldsmith JD. Best practices in diagnostic immunohistochemistry: spindle cell neoplasms of the gastrointestinal tract. Arch Pathol Lab Med 2009;133:1370-1374.

51. Wick MR. Immunohistochemical approaches to the diagnosis of undifferentiated malignant tumors. Ann Diagn Pathol 2008;12:72-84.

52. Zarate-Osorno A, Jaffe ES, Medeiros LJ. Metastatic nasopharyngeal carcinoma initially presenting as cervical lymphadenopathy. A report of two cases that resembled Hodgkin's disease. Arch Pathol Lab Med 1992;116:862-865.

53. Zur Hausen A, Rennspiess D, Winnepenninckx V, Speel EJ, Kurz AK. Early B-cell differentiation in Merkel cell carcinomas: clues to cellular ancestry. Cancer Res 2013;73:4982-4987.

Index*

A

Acquired immunodeficiency syndrome-related polymorphic lymphoproliferative disorder, 684

Acute monocytic leukemia/monoblastic sarcoma, differentiation from histiocytic sarcoma, 821

Acute myeloid leukemia, 163, 461
    differentiation from B-lymphoblastic leukemia/lymphoma, 163; from T-lymphoblastic leukemia/lymphoma, 461

Adult T-cell leukemia/lymphoma, 140, **501**, 589
    clinical features, 503
    cytologic findings, 509
    differential diagnosis, 513: differentiation from T-cell prolymphocytic leukemia, 513; from anaplastic large cell lymphoma, 513; from angioimmunoblastic T-cell lymphoma, 513; from mycosis fungoides, 589
    general features, 501
    histologic findings, 505
    human T-cell lymphotropic virus type 1 (HTLV-1) association, 140, **501**
    immunophenotypic findings, 510
    molecular genetic findings, 511
    treatment and prognosis, 513
    variants, 504
        acute, 504
        chronic, 505
        lymphomatous, 504
        smoldering, 505

Aggressive NK-cell leukemia/lymphoma, 556

Aggressive systemic mastocytosis, 767

Agranular CD4-positive natural killer cell leukemia, *see* Blastic plasmacytoid dendritic cell neoplasm

Amyloidosis, 399

Anaplastic large cell lymphoma, 810, 821
    differentiation from myeloid sarcoma, 810; from histiocytic sarcoma, 821

Anaplastic large cell lymphoma, Hodgkin related, 441

Anaplastic large cell lymphoma, primary cutaneous, see Primary cutaneous anaplastic large cell lymphoma

Anaplastic lymphoma kinase (ALK), 355, 359

Anaplastic lymphoma kinase (ALK)-negative anaplastic large cell lymphoma (ALCL), **539**, 623
    clinical features, 539
    cytologic findings, 540
    differential diagnosis, 548: differentiation from ALK-positive ALCL, 534, 548; from primary cutaneous ALCL, 548; from lymphomatoid papulosis, 549; from peripheral T-cell lymphoma, 549; from Hodgkin lymphoma, 549, 623; from breast implant-associated ALCL, 540
    general features, 539
    histologic findings, 539
    immunophenotypic findings, 540
    molecular genetic findings, 543
    treatment and prognosis, 552

Anaplastic lymphoma kinase (ALK)-positive anaplastic large cell lymphoma (ALCL), **517**, 548, 623
    clinical features, 518
    cytologic findings, 526
    differential diagnosis, 534: differentiation from ALK-negative ALCL, 534, 548; from primary cutaneous ALCL, 534; from peripheral T-cell lymphoma, 534; from Hodgkin lymphoma, 534, 623; from CD30-positive DLBCL, 534; from metastatic tumors, 535
    general features, 517
    histologic findings, 518
    immunohistochemical findings, 528
    molecular genetic findings, 532
    treatment and prognosis, 536
    variants, 520
        common (classic), 520
        Hodgkin-like, 522
        lymphohistiocytic, 520
        small cell, 522

Anaplastic lymphoma kinase (ALK)-negative large B-cell lymphoma, 479, 513
    differentiation from peripheral T-cell lymphoma, 479; from adult T-cell leukemia/lymphoma, 513

Anaplastic lymphoma kinase (ALK)-positive large B-cell lymphoma, 355, 385
    clinical features, 355
    cytologic findings, 355
    differential diagnosis, 360; differentiation from lymphoblastic lymphoma, 385
    general features, 355
    histologic findings, 355

*In a series of numbers, those in boldface indicate the main discussion of the entity.

immunophenotypic findings, 358

molecular genetic findings, 358

treatment and prognosis, 361

Anatomy, normal, 1

  lymph node, 1

    B cells, 4

    cortex, 2

    fibroblastic reticular cells, 8

    follicles, 2

    follicular dendritic cells, 5

    germinal centers, 3

    gross, 1

    high endothelial venule, 10

    marginal zone, 4

    medulla, 11

    microscopic, 1

    paracortex, 8

    plasmacytoid dendritic cells, 9

    primary follicles, 2

    secondary follicles, 2

    sinuses, 11

    T cells, 7

    tingible body macrophages, 7

  spleen, 12

    gross, 12

    microscopic, 12

    red pulp, 14

    white pulp, 12

Angioimmunoblastic lymphadenopathy with
  dysproteinemia, 483

Angioimmunoblastic T-cell lymphoma (AITL), 136,
  248, 263, 340, 479, 483, 513, 590, 700

  clinical features, 484

  cytologic findings, 490

  differential diagnosis, 496: differentiation from
    nodal marginal zone lymphoma, 248; from
    extranodal marginal zone lymphoma, 263;
    from EBV-positive DLBCL, 340, 497; from
    peripheral T-cell lymphoma, 479, 497; from
    reactive paracortical hyperplasia, 496; from
    Castleman disease, 496; from angiolymphoid
    hyperplasia with eosinophilia, 497; from T-cell/
    histiocyte-rich large B-cell lymphoma, 497;
    from Hodgkin lymphoma, 497; from adult
    T-cell lymphoma, 513; from mycosis fun-
    goides, 590

  Epstein-Barr virus association, 136

  general features, 483

  histologic findings, 484

  iatrogenic, 799

immunohistochemical findings, 490

molecular genetic findings, 495

relationship to T(FH) lymphomas, 496

risk of other lymphomas, 496

treatment and prognosis, 498

variants, 486

  AITL with Reed-Sternberg and Hodgkin cells, 488

  Lennert-like AITL, 486

  plasma cell-rich AITL, 486

Angiolymphoid hyperplasia with eosinophilia,
  differentiation from angioimmunoblastic T-cell
  lymphoma, 497

Angiomyolipoma, 989

Angiomyomatous hamartoma, 992

Angiosarcoma, spleen, 953, 957, **959**

  differential diagnosis, 963: differentiation from
    littoral cell angioma, 953; from hemangioen-
    dothelioma, 957; from other sarcomas, 963

Ann Arbor lymphoma staging system, 110

Ataxia-telangiectasia, 720

Autoimmune lymphoproliferative syndrome, 723

B

B-acute lymphoblastic leukemia (B-ALL), 149

  BCR-ABL1-like/Philadelphia chromosome-like
    B-ALL, 161

  genetic abnormalities, 162

  with functional pre-B-cell receptor signaling, 162

B cells, normal, 4

B-cell lymphoma, not otherwise specified, high-
    grade, see High-grade B-cell lymphoma, not
    otherwise specified

B-cell lymphoma, unclassifiable, with features in-
    termediate between DLBCL and Hodgkin lym-
    phoma (gray zone lymphoma), 441, 623

  clinical features, 441

  cytologic findings, 443

  differential diagnosis, 446: differentiation from
    nodular sclerosis Hodgkin lymphoma, 446,
    623; from primary mediastinal large B-cell
    lymphoma, 446

  general features, 441

  histologic findings, 442

  immunophenotypic findings, 444

  mediastinal gray zone lymphoma, 441

  molecular genetic findings, 445

B-cell prolymphocytic leukemia, differentiation
    from CLL/SLL, 178

B-lymphoblastic leukemia/lymphoma, **149**, 461,
    759, 809

B-acute lymphoblastic leukemia (B-ALL), 149
BCR-ABL1-like/Philadelphia chromosome-like
    B-ALL, 161
  genetic abnormalities, 162
  with functional pre-B-cell receptor signaling, 162
 clinical features, 151
 cytologic findings, 153
 differential diagnosis, 162: differentiation from
    T-lymphoblastic leukemia/lymphoma, 162,
    461; from Burkitt lymphoma, 163; from
    DLBCL, 163; from mantle cell lymphoma, 163;
    from acute myeloid leukemia, 163; from blas-
    tic plasmacytoid dendritic cell neoplasm, 163;
    from Ewing sarcoma, 163; from blastic plasma-
    cytic dendritic cell lymphoma, 759; from
    myeloid sarcoma, 809
 general features, 149
 genetic abnormalities, 150
 histologic findings, 151
 immunophenotypic findings, 153
 lymphoblastic lymphoma (LBL), 149
 molecular genetic findings, 159
 treatment and prognosis, 163
Bing-Neel syndrome, 268
Blastic hematopoietic neoplasms associated with
    t(8;13)(p11;q12)/*ZMYM2-FGFR1*, 787
 clinical features, 788
 cytologic findings, 790
 differential diagnosis, 794
 general features, 787
 histologic findings, 788
 immunophenotypic findings, 790
 molecular genetic findings, 791
 treatment and prognosis, 795
Blastic plasmacytoid dendritic cell neoplasm, 163,
    461, **751**, 810
 clinical features, 751
 cytochemical findings, 755
 cytologic findings, 754
 differential diagnosis, 758: differentiation from
    B-lymphoblastic leukemia/lymphoma, 163,
    759; from T-lymphoblastic leukemia/lym-
    phoma, 461, 759; from benign proliferations
    of plasmacytoid dendritic cells, 758; from
    myeloid sarcoma/leukemia, 758, 810; from
    extramedullary chronic myelomonocytic
    leukemia, 759; mycosis fungoides, 760;
    extranodal NK/T-cell lymphoma, 760; mantle
    cell lymphoma, 760
 general features, 751
 histologic findings, 751

 immunophenotypic findings, 755
 molecular genetic findings, 758
 treatment and prognosis, 761
BRC-ABL1-like/Philadelphia chromosome-like
    B-acute lymphoblastic leukemia, 161
Breast implant-associated ALCL, differentiation
    from ALK-negative ALCL, 549
Brill-Symmers disease, see Follicular lymphoma
Burkitt lymphoma, 132, 163, 403, 426, 438, 461,
    685, 700, 738, 809
 arbovirus association, 404
 clinical features, 405
 cytologic findings, 410
 differential diagnosis, 417: differentiation from
    B-lymphocytic leukemia/lymphoma, 163; from
    DLCBL, 417 from high-grade B-cell lymphoma,
    NOS, 417, 426; from mantle cell lymphoma,
    418; from peripheral T-cell lymphoma, 418;
    from double-hit lymphomas, 417, 438; from
    T-lymphoblastic leukemia/lymphoma, 418,
    461; from myeloid sarcoma, 809
 Epstein-Barr virus association, 132, 404
 general features, 403
 histologic findings, 406
 human immunodeficiency virus association, 685
 iatrogenic, 700
 immunophenotypic findings, 412
 leukemic presentation, 409
 molecular genetic findings, 412
 pathogenesis, 404
 Plasmodium falciparum association, 404
 post-transplant, 738
 staging, 406
 treatment and prognosis, 418
 variants, 403
  endemic, 403, 405
  immunodeficiency-associated, 403, 406
  sporadic, 403, 405

C

Cancer therapy-associated lymphoproliferative
    disorders, see Lymphoproliferative disorders,
    cancer therapy associated
Cartilage hair hypoplasia syndrome, 722
Castleman disease, 234, 396, 496
 differentiation from follicular lymphoma, 234;
    from plasmacytoma, 396; from angioimmuno-
    blastic T-cell lymphoma, 496
 HHV-8 association, see HHV-8-positive multi-
    centric Castleman disease

Cat scratch disease, differentiation from Langerhans cell histiocytosis, 852
CD4/CD56-positive hematodermic neoplasm, *see* Blastic plasmacytoid dendritic cell neoplasm
CD5-positive follicular lymphoma, 218
CD8-positive aggressive epidermotropic cytotoxic T-cell lymphoma, differentiation from mycosis fungoides, 589
CD30-positive diffuse large B-cell lymphoma, differentiation from ALK-positive ALCL, 534
Centroblastic/centrocytic lymphoma, *see* Follicular lymphoma
Chloroma, see Myeloid sarcoma
Chronic lymphocytic leukemia/small lymphocytic lymphoma (CLL/SLL), 85, 167, 200, 263, 700, 895
    clinical features, 167
    cytologic findings, 172
    differential diagnosis, 178: differentiation from monoclonal B-cell lymphocytosis, 178; from B-cell prolymphocytic leukemia, 178; from mantle cell lymphoma, 178, 200; from extranodal marginal zone lymphoma, 263; from splenic marginal zone lymphoma, 895
    general features, 167
    histologic findings, 168
    histologic transformation, 85, 177
    iatrogenic, 700
    immunophenotypic findings, 172
    molecular genetic findings, 174
    staging, 180
    treatment and prognosis, 179
Chronic lymphocytic leukemia/small lymphocytic lymphoma-like mantle cell lymphoma, 187
Chronic myelomonocytic leukemia, spleen, 937
Classification of lymphomas, 65, 283
    current lymphoma classification, 71, 283
        2016 World Health Organization classification update, 76
        World Health Organization classification of B-cell neoplasms, 74
        World Health Organization classification of DLBCL, 283
        World Health Organization classification of T- and NK-cell neoplasms, 75
        World Health Organization classification of Hodgkin lymphomas, 75
    historical background, 65
        international working formulation of non-Hodgkin lymphomas, 71
        revised European American Classification of lymphoid neoplasms, 72
        updated Kiel classification of non-Hodgkin lymphomas, 70
        updated Lukes and Collins classification of non-Hodgkin lymphomas, 69
        updated Rappaport classification of non-Hodgkin lymphomas, 68
Clear cell lymphoma, *see* Primary mediastinal large B-cell lymphoma
Common variable immunodeficiency syndrome, 718
Composite lymphomas, 75
Crystal-storing histiocytosis, 399
Cutaneous anaplastic large cell lymphoma, iatrogenic, 700
Cutaneous mastocytosis, *see* Mastocytosis
Cysts, spleen, 977
    clinical features, 977
    cytologic findings, 980
    echinococcal cyst, 978
    epidermoid/epithelial cyst, 978
    general features, 977
    histologic findings, 977
    immunophenotypic findings, 981
    mesothelial cyst, 977
    pseudocyst, 978
    treatment and prognosis, 981
Cytotoxic peripheral T-cell lymphoma, differentiation from extranodal NK/T-cell lymphoma, nasal type, 568

D

Dendritic cell sarcomas, 821, 832
    differentiation from histiocytic sarcoma, 821
    follicular dendritic cell sarcoma, *see* Follicular dendritic cell sarcoma
    interdigitating dendritic cell sarcoma, 832
Dermatopathic lymphadenopathy, differentiation from Langerhans cell histiocytosis, 851
Diffuse large B-cell lymphoma (DLBCL), 79, 92, 133, 163, **283**, 333, 335, 340, 351, 385, 426, 438, 461, 534, 568, 695, 738, 809, 834, 894, 908, 975
    anaplastic variant, 289
    association with chronic inflammation, 298
    association with nodular lymphocyte-predominant Hodgkin lymphoma, 668
    CD30 positive, 534
    centroblastic variant, 286
    classification, World Health Organization, 283
    clinical features, 285
    cytologic findings, 303
    differential diagnosis, 314: differentiation from B-lymphoblastic leukemia/lymphoma, 163;

from reactive conditions, 314; from metastatic tumors, 315; from hematolymphoid neoplasms, 315; from T-cell/histiocyte-rich large B-cell lymphoma, 333; from EBV-positive DLBCL, 340; from primary mediastinal large B-cell lymphoma, 351; from plasmablastic lymphoma, 385; from Burkitt lymphoma, 418; from high-grade B-cell lymphoma, NOS, 426; from double-hit lymphomas, 438; from T-lymphoblastic leukemia/lymphoma, 461; from extranodal NK/T-cell lymphoma, nasal type, 568; from myeloid sarcoma, 809; from follicular dendritic cell sarcoma, 834; from primary splenic large B-cell lymphoma, 908; from splenic stromal tumors, 975
  Epstein-Barr virus association, 133, 335
  Epstein-Barr virus-positive DLBCL, 335, *see also* Epstein-Barr virus-positive DLBCL
  general features, 283
  histologic downgrading, 92
  histologic findings, 285
  histologic transformation, 79, 293, 314
  human immunodeficiency virus association, 686
  human herpesvirus 8 association, 370
  iatrogenic, 695
  immunoblastic variant, 286
  immunophenotypic findings, 303
  intravascular large B-cell lymphoma, 296
  lymphomatoid granulomatosis, 298
  molecular genetic findings, 311
  post-transplantation, 738
  primary cutaneous DLBCL, leg type, 298
  primary DLBCL of central nervous system, 295
  primary splenic, *see* Primary splenic large B-cell lymphoma
  prognosis, 316
    clinical features, 316
    gene expression profile, 317
    gene mutations, 319
    immunophenotypic findings, 317
    morphologic features, 317
    prognostic markers, 310
  testicular DLBCL, 302
  transformation from splenic marginal zone lymphoma, 894
  treatment, 315
Diffuse lymphocyte-predominant Hodgkin lymphoma, 670
Discordant lymphoma histology, 76
Double-hit lymphomas, 417, 426, **429**
  atypical *MYC/BCL2* double-hit lymphoma, 437

  BCL2 and *BCL6* translocation, 438
  clinical features, 429
  cytologic findings, 435
  differential diagnosis, 438: differentiation from DLBCL, 438; from Burkitt lymphoma, 417, 438
  double-positive lymphoma, 423, 437
  general features, 429
  histologic findings, 430
    MYC/BCL2 double-hit lymphoma, 430
    MYC/BCL6 double-hit lymphoma, 433
  immunophenotypic findings, 435
  molecular genetic findings, 437
  treatment and prognosis, 438
Double-positive (double-expressor) lymphoma, 423, 437

E

8p11 myeloproliferative syndrome, *see* Blastic hematopoietic neoplasms associated with t(8;13)(p11;q12)/*ZMYM2-FGFR1*
Early T-cell acute precursor leukemia, 458
Echinococcal cyst, spleen, 978
Epidemiology of lymphomas, 119
  geographic variation, 123
  patient age, 120
  patient sex and race, 123
  relative frequency, 119
  risk factors, 125
  statistics, 119
Epidermoid/epithelial cyst, spleen, 978
Epstein-Barr virus (EBV), 130, 225, 335, 337, 375, 555, 595, 694
  associated lymphomas, 132
    angioimmunoblastic T-cell lymphoma, 136
    Burkitt lymphoma, 132
    DLBCL, 133, 134, 335
    extranodal NK/T-cell lymphoma, nasal type, 555
    follicular lymphoma, 225
    Hodgkin lymphoma, 132, 595
    hydroa vacciniforme-like T-cell lymphoproliferative disorder, 137
    iatrogenic lymphoproliferative disorders, 694
    lymphomatoid granulomatosis, 133
    NK/T-cell lymphoma, 136
    plasmablastic lymphoma, 133, 375
    post-transplant lymphoproliferative disorders, 134
    T-cell lymphoma of childhood, 136
  immunophenotypic findings, 337
  lymphomagenesis, 130
Epstein-Barr virus (EBV)-positive diffuse large B-cell

lymphoma (DLBCL), **335**, 497
clinical features, 336
cytologic findings, 337
differential diagnosis, 339: differentiation from other EBV-positive lymphoproliferative disorders, 339; from DLBCL, 340; from T-cell/histiocyte-rich large B-cell lymphoma, 340; classic Hodgkin lymphoma, 340; from angio-immunoblastic-like T-cell lymphoma, 340, 497
general features, 335
histologic findings, 336
immunophenotypic findings, 337
molecular genetic findings, 339
oncogenic effects, 335
treatment and prognosis, 340
Epstein-Barr virus-positive follicular lymphoma, 225
Epstein-Barr virus-positive mucocutaneous ulcer, 699
Ewing sarcoma, differentiation from B-lympho-blastic leukemia/lymphoma, 163
Extramedullary chronic myelomonocytic leukemia, differentiation from blastic plasmacytoid dendritic cell neoplasm, 759
Extramedullary hematopoiesis, 929
Extramedullary myeloid cell tumor, *see* Myeloid sarcoma
Extramedullary plasmacytoma, 385, 389, *see also* Plasmacytoma
  differentiation from plasmablastic lymphoma, 385
Extranodal marginal zone lymphoma of mucosa-associated lymphoid tissue, see Marginal zone lymphoma, extranodal, of mucosa-associated lymphoid tissue
Extranodal NK/T-cell lymphoma, nasal type, 555, 700, 760
  aggressive NK-cell leukemia/lymphoma, 556
  clinical features, 555
  cytologic findings, 563
  differential diagnosis, 568: differentiation from cytotoxic peripheral T-cell lymphoma, 568; DLBCL, 568; lymphomatoid granulomatosis, 568; from cutaneous and gastrointestinal NK/T-cell lymphomas, 568; from Wegener granulomatosis, 569; from blastic plasmacy-toid dendritic cell lymphoma, 760
  Epstein-Barr virus association, 555
  general features, 555
  histologic findings, 556
  iatrogenic, 700
  immunophenotypic findings, 563
  molecular genetic findings, 566
  treatment and prognosis, 569

F

Fine-needle aspiration biopsy, 17, 43, **47**
Follicular center lymphoma, *see* Follicular lymphoma
Follicular dendritic cells, normal, 5
Follicular dendritic cell sarcoma, **825**, 840
  clinical features, 825
  cytologic findings, 830
  differential diagnosis, 832: differentiation from interdigitating dendritic cell sarcoma, 832, 840; from Langerhans cell sarcoma, 832; from histiocytic sarcoma, 834; from fibroblastic reticular cell sarcoma, 834; from DLBCL, 834; from nodular sclerosis Hodgkin lymphoma, 834
  general features, 825
  histologic findings, 825
  immunophenotypic findings, 830
  molecular genetic findings, 831
  treatment and prognosis, 834
Follicular hyperplasia, 233, 733
  differentiation from follicular lymphoma, 233
  post-transplantation, 733
Follicular lymphoma, 79, 98, 113, 200, **205**, 262, 480, 671, 700, 733, 896
  CD5-positive follicular lymphoma, 218
  clinical features, 206
  cytologic findings, 227
  del1p36/TNFRSF14 abnormalities, 225
  differential diagnosis, 233: differentiation from mantle cell lymphoma, 200, 234; from reactive follicular hyperplasia, 233; from progressive transformation of germinal centers, 234; from Castleman disease, 234; from nodular lymphocyte-predominant Hodgkin lymphoma, 234, 671; from nodal marginal zone lymphoma, 234, 247; from extranodal marginal zone lymphoma, 262; from peripheral T-cell lymphoma, 480; from splenic marginal zone lymphoma, 896
  DLBCL coexistence, 214
  duodenal-type follicular lymphoma, 218
  Epstein-Barr virus-positive follicular lymphoma, 225
  general features, 205
  genetic abnormalities, 232
  grading, 210
  histologic findings, 206
  histologic transformation, 79
  iatrogenic, 700
  immunophenotypic findings, 227
  in situ neoplasia, 98
  international prognostic index, 113

IRF4 rearrangement, 222
microenvironment, 232
molecular genetic findings, 230
pediatric-type follicular lymphoma, 221
post-transplantation, 733
primary cutaneous follicular lymphoma, 225
t(14;18)(q32;q21)/*IGH-BCL2* in pathogenesis,
205, 230
testicular follicular lymphoma, 225
treatment and prognosis, 234
variants, 214
abundant extracellular PAS-positive material, 215
floral follicular lymphoma, 214
in situ follicular neoplasia, 214
monocytoid B-cell differentiation, 215
partial follicular lymphoma involvement, 214
signet ring cell follicular lymphoma, 214
Follicular lymphoma in situ, 98
Follicular lymphoma-like B cells of uncertain
significance, 98
Follicular T-cell lymphoma, 469
Follicular T-helper cell lymphoma, differentiation
from lymphocyte-rich Hodgkin lymphoma, 634

G

Germinotropic lymphoproliferative disorder,
human herpesvirus 8 association, 140, 370
Granulocytic sarcoma, *see* Myeloid sarcoma
Gray zone lymphoma, *see* B-cell lymphoma,
unclassifiable, with features intermediate
between DLBCL and Hodgkin lymphoma

H

Hairy cell leukemia, 782, **861**, 896, 903, 925
clinical features, 861
cytologic findings, 864
differential diagnosis, 870: differentiation from
mastocytosis, 782; from hairy cell leukemia
variant, 870; from splenic marginal zone lymphoma, 896; from splenic diffuse red pulp
small B-cell lymphoma, 903; from hepatosplenic T-cell lymphoma, 925
general features, 861
gross findings, 862
histologic findings, 862
immunophenotypic findings, 867
molecular genetic findings, 869
treatment and prognosis, 871
ultrastructural findings, 869
Hairy cell leukemia variant, 870, **875**, 896
clinical features, 875

cytologic findings, 879
differential diagnosis, 880: differentiation from
hairy cell leukemia, 870, 880; from splenic
diffuse red pulp small B-cell lymphoma, 881;
from splenic marginal zone lymphoma, 896
general features, 875
histologic findings, 876
immunophenotypic findings, 879
molecular genetic findings, 879
treatment and prognosis, 881
Hamartoma, spleen, 945, 952, 974
associated diseases, 945
differentiation from cord capillary hemangioma,
949; littoral cell angioma, 949; sclerosing angiomatoid nodular transformation, 950; from
splenic hemangioma, 952; from stomal tumors
of spleen, 974
subtypes, 946
Hemangioendothelioma, spleen, 954
differentiation from Kaposi sarcoma, 957; from
angiosarcoma, 957
Hemangioma, **950**, **997**
lymph nodes, 997
differentiation from lymphangioma, 997; from
angiomyomatous hamartoma, 998; from
vascular transformation of lymph node
sinuses, 998
spleen, 950
differentiation from splenic hamartoma, 952;
from malignant vascular neoplasms, 952
Hemophagocytic lymphohistiocytosis, differentiation from histiocytic sarcoma, 822
Hepatitis C virus, associated lymphomas, 143
Hepatosplenic T-cell lymphoma, 700, 741, 821, **915**
alpha/beta variant, 915
clinical features, 915
cytologic findings, 923
differential diagnosis, 925: differentiation from
histiocytic sarcoma, 821; from hairy cell
leukemia, 925; from splenic marginal zone
lymphoma, 925; from extranodal gamma/delta
TCR lymphomas, 925; T-cell large granular
lymphocytic leukemia, 925; from aggressive
NK-cell leukemia, 925
gamma/delta variant, 915
general features, 915
histologic findings, 916
iatrogenic, 700
immunophenotypic findings, 923
molecular genetic findings, 924
post-transplant, 744

treatment and prognosis, 926
High-grade B-cell lymphoma, not otherwise
    specified, 417, **421**
  clinical features, 421
  cytologic findings, 423
  differential diagnosis, 426: differentiation from
      DLBCL, 426; from Burkitt lymphoma, 417, 426
  double-hit lymphomas, 426, **429**
  double-positive (double-expressor) lymphoma, 423
  general features, 421
  histologic findings, 421
  immunophenotypic findings, 423
  molecular genetic findings, 423
  single-hit lymphoma, 426
  treatment and prognosis, 427
Histiocytic sarcoma, 810, **813**, 834, 840
  clinical features, 813
  cytologic findings, 814
  differential diagnosis, 821: differentiation from
      myeloid sarcoma, 810; from acute monocytic
      leukemia, 821; from dendritic cell sarcomas,
      821, 834, 840; from anaplastic large cell lym-
      phoma, 821; from hepatosplenic lympho-
      ma, 821; from metastatic melanoma, 822;
      from hemophagocytic lymphohistiocytosis,
      822; from Rosai-Dorfman disease, 822
  general features, 813
  histologic findings, 814
  immunophenotypic findings, 814
  molecular genetic findings, 818
  transdifferentiation, 818
  treatment and prognosis, 822
Histologic transformation of lymphoma, 79
  follicular lymphoma, 79
    variants, 83
  chronic lymphocytic leukemia/small lympho-
      cytic lymphoma, 85
  marginal zone lymphoma, 89
  mycosis fungoides, 91
  nodular lymphocyte-predominant Hodgkin
      lymphoma, 91
  Waldenstrom macroglobulinemia, 89
Hodgkin lymphomas, 65, 110, 132, 333, 340, 480,
    497, 534, 549, **593**, 695, 741, 911, *see also
    under individual Hodgkin lymphoma types*
  classification, 65, 593
  clinical features, 596
  differential diagnosis, 604; differentiation from
      T-cell/histiocyte-rich large B-cell lymphoma,
      333; from EBV-positive DLBCL, 340; from
      peripheral T-cell lymphoma, 480; from angio-

immunoblastic T-cell lymphoma, 497; from
    ALK-positive ALCL, 534; from ALK-negative
    ALCL, 549; from mycosis fungoides, 589; from
    primary splenic large B-cell lymphoma, 911
  epidemiology, 119, *see also* Epidemiology of
    lymphomas
  Epstein-Barr virus association, 132, 595
  general features, 593
  histologic downgrading, 92
  histologic findings, *see under individual
    Hodgkin lymphoma types*
  histologic transformation, 79
  human immunodeficiency virus association, 688
  iatrogenic, 695
  immunophenotypic findings, 597
  incidence, 595
  lymphocyte-depleted Hodgkin lymphoma, *see*
    Lymphocyte-depleted Hodgkin lymphoma
  lymphocyte-rich Hodgkin lymphoma, *see*
    Lymphocyte-rich Hodgkin lymphoma
  mixed cellularity Hodgkin lymphoma, *see*
    Mixed cellularity Hodgkin lymphoma
  molecular genetic findings, 601
  nodular lymphocyte-predominant Hodgkin
    lymphoma, *see* Nodular lymphocyte-
    predominant Hodgkin lymphoma
  nodular sclerosis Hodgkin lymphoma, *see*
    Nodular sclerosis Hodgkin lymphoma
  post-transplant, 741
  Reed-Sternberg and Hodgkin cells, 593
  risk factors, 596
  staging system, 110
  treatment and prognosis, 112, 603
Human herpesvirus 4, *see* Epstein-Barr virus
Human herpesvirus 8, 137, 363
  associated lymphomas, 138, 363
    DLBCL, 370
    germinotropic lymphoproliferative disorder,
      140, 370
    multicentric Castleman disease and large B-cell
      lymphoma, 139, 363, *see also* Human her-
      pesvirus 8-positive multicentric Castleman
      disease *and* Human herpesvirus 8-positive
      large B-cell lymphoma
    plasmablastic/large B-cell proliferations in
      multicentric Castleman disease, 368
    primary effusion lymphoma, 138, 363
  lymphomagenesis, 137
Human herpesvirus-positive diffuse large B-cell
    lymphoma, 370

Human herpesvirus-positive germinotropic
 lymphoproliferative disorder, 370
Human herpersvirus 8-positive large B-cell
 lymphomas, 363
 germinotropic lymphoproliferative disorder, 370
 multicentric Castleman disease, 363
 plasmablastic/large B-cell proliferations arising in
 HHV-8-positive Castleman disease, 368
Human herpesvirus 8-positive multicentric
 Castleman disease, 363
 clinical features, 364
 general features, 363
 histologic findings, 364
 immunophenotypic findings, 366
 Kaposi sarcoma-associated herpesvirus inflammatory cytokine syndrome, 364
 molecular genetic findings, 368
 plasmablastic/large B-cell proliferations, 368
 treatment and prognosis, 368
Human immunodeficiency virus (HIV), 145, 375
 associated lymphomas, 145
 plasmablastic lymphoma, 375
Human immunodeficiency virus (HIV)-associated
 lymphoproliferative disorders, 675
 AIDS-related polymorphic lymphoproliferative
 disorder, 684
 associated benign lymphadenopathy, 677
 Burkitt lymphoma, 685
 clinical features, 679
 DLBCL, 686
 extranodal marginal zone lymphoma, 689
 general features, 675
 HIV-positive multicentric Castleman disease, 680
 Hodgkin lymphoma, 688
 peripheral T-cell lymphoma, 689
 plasma cell myeloma, 688
 plasmablastic lymphoma, 688
 primary DLBCL of central nervous system, 687
 primary effusion lymphoma, 680
 risk of lymphoma, 675
 treatment and prognosis, 689
 viral structure and replication, 675
Human immunodeficiency virus-positive multicentric Castleman disease, 680
Human T-cell lymphotropic virus type 1 (HTLV-1),
 140, **501**
 adult T-cell leukemia/lymphoma association,
 140, 501
 associated diseases, 503
 epidemiology, 501
 lymphomagenesis, 140

Hydroa vacciniforme-like T-cell lymphoproliferative
 disorder, Epstein-Barr virus association, 137
Hyper-IgM syndrome, 721

I

Iatrogenic lymphoproliferative disorders, see
 Lymphoproliferative disorders, iatrogenic
IgM monoclonal gammopathy, differentiation
 from lymphoplasmacytic lymphoma, 278
Immunohistochemical antigens, 19
 BCL2, 21
 CD3, 19
 CD5, 20
 CD10, 21
 CD20, 19
 CD30, 21
 cyclin D1, 20
 Ki-67, 22
 PAX5, 19
Incipient follicular lymphoma, 98
Indolent systemic mastocytosis, 767
Infectious agents and lymphomas, 129
 direct oncogenic effects, 130
 Epstein-Barr virus, 130, *see also* Epstein-Barr
 virus
 human herpesvirus 8, 137, *see also* Human
 herpesvirus 8
 human T-cell lymphotropic virus type 1, 140,
 see also Human T-cell lymphotropic virus
 type 1
 indirect oncogenic effects, 141
 Helicobacter pylori and marginal zone
 lymphoma association, 140
 hepatitis C virus, 143
 human immunodeficiency virus, 145
Inflammatory myofibroblastic tumor of spleen, 971
Inflammatory pseudotumor, 968, 983
 lymph nodes, 983
 grading, 983
 spleen, 968
Inflammatory pseudotumor-like follicular dendritic
 cell tumor of spleen, 971
In situ neoplasia, 97
 in situ follicular neoplasia, 98
 in situ mantle cell neoplasia, 101
 in situ nodular lymphocyte-predominant
 Hodgkin lymphoma, 102
Interdigitating dendritic cell sarcoma, 832, **837**
 association with lymphoma, 836
 clinical features, 837
 cytologic findings, 839

differential diagnosis, 840: differentiation from follicular dendritic cell sarcoma, 832,840; from Langerhans cell sarcoma, 840; histiocytic sarcoma, 840; melanoma, 840; from Langerhans cell histiocytosis, 851
general features, 837
histologic findings, 837
immunophenotypic findings, 839
molecular genetic findings, 840
treatment and prognosis, 841
ultrastructural findings, 840
Interleukin-2-inducible T-kinase deficiency, 725
International pediatric non-Hodgkin lymphoma staging system, 112
International prognostic index, 113
Intrafollicular neoplasia, 98
Intranodal hemorrhagic spindle cell tumor with amianthoid fibers, 987
Intravascular large B-cell lymphoma, **296**, 910
differentiation from primary splenic large B-cell lymphoma, 910

K

Kaposi sarcoma, lymph nodes, 1017
Kaposi sarcoma, spleen, 957, **958**, 995
differentiation from splenic hemangioendothelioma, 957; from vascular transformation of lymph node sinuses, 995
Kaposi sarcoma-associated herpesvirus, *see* Human herpesvirus 8
Kaposi sarcoma-associated herpesvirus inflammatory cytokine syndrome, 364

L

Langerhans cell histiocytosis, 782, 832, 840, **843**
clinical features, 844
cytologic findings, 847
differential diagnosis, 851: differentiation from mastocytosis, 782; from follicular dendritic cell sarcoma, 832; from interdigitating dendritic cell sarcoma, 840, 851; from Langerhans cell sarcoma, 851; from dermatopathic lymphadenopathy, 851; from Rosai-Dorfman disease, 851; from cat scratch disease, 852; from Kikuchi-Fujimoto disease, 852
general features, 843
histologic findings, 844
immunophenotypic findings, 847
molecular genetic findings, 850
treatment and prognosis, 852
tumor-associated disease, 847

ultrastructural findings, 850
Langerhans cell sarcoma, 851, **855**
differentiation from Langerhans cell histiocytosis, 851
Large B-cell lymphoma with Hodgkin features, 441
Leiomyomatosis, 991
Lennert lymphoma, 468
Lipoma/lipomatosis, 993
Littoral cell angioma, spleen, 949, **953**
differentiation from splenic hamartoma, 949; from angiosarcoma, 953
Lymph node anatomy, 1
Lymph node cortex, 2
germinal centers, 3
marginal zone, 4
primary follicles, 2
secondary follicles, 2
Lymph node medulla, 11
Lymph node paracortex, 8
fibroblastic reticular cell, 8
high endothelial venules, 10
plasmacytoid dendritic cell, 9
Lymph node sinuses, 11
Lymphangiectasia, 995
Lymphangioleiomyomatosis, 990
Lymphangioma/lymphangiomatosis, 992
Lymphoblastic lymphoma, 149, 418, 759, 809, *see also* B-lymphoblastic leukemia/lymphoma differentiation from Burkitt lymphoma, 418; from blastic plasmacytoid dendritic cell lymphoma, 759; from myeloid sarcoma, 809
Lymphocyte-depleted Hodgkin lymphoma, 645
clinical features, 645
cytologic findings, 648
differential diagnosis, 648
general features, 645
histologic findings, 645
immunophenotypic findings, 648
molecular genetic findings, 648
treatment and prognosis, 649
Lymphocyte-rich classic Hodgkin lymphoma, **627**, 643, 671
clinical features, 627
cytologic findings, 631
differential diagnosis, 633: differentiation from nodular lymphocyte-predominant Hodgkin lymphoma, 633, 671; from nodular sclerosis Hodgkin lymphoma, 633; from mixed cellularity Hodgkin lymphoma, 634, 643; from T-cell/histiocyte-rich large B-cell lymphoma, 634; from follicular T-helper cell lymphoma,

634; from B-cell non-Hodgkin lymphomas, 634
diffuse variant, 627
general features, 627
histologic findings, 627
immunohistochemical findings, 631
molecular genetic findings, 633
nodular variant, 627
relationship to nodular sclerosis Hodgkin
lymphoma, 630
treatment and prognosis, 634
Lymphocyte-rich thymoma, differentiation from
T-lymphoblastic leukemia/lymphoma, 461
Lymphoepithelial T-cell lymphoma, 468
Lymphoma, overview, 65, 109, 119, 129
classification, 65, *see also* Classification of
lymphomas
clinical workup, 109
epidemiology, 119, *see also* Epidemiology of
lymphomas
grading, 116
infectious agents, 129, *see also* Infectious agents
and lymphomas
prognostic factors, 112
biomarkers, 114
follicular lymphoma international prognostic
index, 113
Hodgkin lymphoma, 112
international prognostic index, 113
non-Hodgkin lymphoma, 113, 115
staging, 110
Ann Arbor staging system, 110
Hodgkin lymphoma, 110
international pediatric non-Hodgkin lymphoma staging system, 112
non-Hodgkin lymphoma, 111
Lymphomatoid granulomatosis, 133, **298**, 568
differentiation from extranodal NK/T-cell lymphoma, nasal type, 568
Epstein-Barr association, 133
Lymphomatoid papulosis, differentiation from
ALK-negative ALCL, 549
Lymphoplasmacytic lymphoma, 248, **262**, 267,
700, *see also* Waldenstrom macroglobulinemia
association with Waldenstrom macroglobulinemia, 267
clinical features, 267
cytologic findings, 273
differential diagnosis, 278: differentiation from
nodal marginal zone lymphoma, 248, 278;
from extranodal marginal zone lymphoma,
262, 278; from macroglobulinemia, 267; from

IgM monoclonal gammopathy, 278; from
splenic marginal zone lymphoma, 278; from
plasma cell myeloma, 278; from gamma heavy
chain disease, 278
general features, 267
histologic findings, 268
iatrogenic, 700
immunophenotypic findings, 273
molecular genetic findings, 274
treatment and prognosis, 279
Lymphoproliferative disorders, cancer therapy
associated, 707
hematologic malignancies, 707
pathogenesis, 708
Lymphoproliferative disorders, iatrogenic, 693
cancer therapy associated, 707, *see also* Lymphoproliferative disorders, cancer therapy
associated
clinical features, 694
cytologic findings, 703
differential diagnosis, 704
EBV association, 694
frequency, 695
general features, 693
histologic findings, 695
Burkitt lymphoma, 700
DLBCL, 695
EBV-positive mucocutaneous ulcer, 699
hepatosplenic T-cell lymphoma, 700
Hodgkin lymphoma, 695
low-grade B-cell lymphomas, 700
polymorphic lymphoproliferative disorders, 697
T-cell lymphomas, 700
methotrexate association, 693
molecular genetic findings, 703
treatment and prognosis, 704
Lymphoproliferative disorders, post-transplant,
see Post-transplant lymphoproliferative disorder
Lymphoproliferative disorders, primary immunodeficiency associated, 715
associated primary immunodeficiency diseases, 717
clinical features, 718
cytologic findings, 727
differential diagnosis, 727
general features, 715
histologic findings, 725
immunophenotypic findings, 727
IUIS grouping, 716
molecular genetic findings, 727
treatment and prognosis, 727
types, 718

activated phosphoinositide 3-kinase delta syndrome, 724
ataxia-telangiectasia, 720
autoimmune lymphoproliferative syndrome, 723
cartilage hair hypoplasia syndrome, 722
common variable immunodeficiency syndrome, 718
hyper-IgM syndrome, 721
interleukin-2-inducible T-cell kinase deficiency, 725
Nijmegen breakage syndrome, 721
severe combined immunodeficiency, 721
Wiskott-Aldrich syndrome, 721
X-linked agammaglobulinemia, 722
X-linked lymphoproliferative syndrome, 722

M

MALT lymphoma, *see* Marginal zone lymphoma, extranodal, of mucosa-associated lymphoid tissue
Mantle cell lymphoma (MCL), 101, 163, 178, **183**, 247, 263, 761, 896
  aggressive variants, 188
    blastoid MCL, 188
    pleomorphic MCL, 188
    prolymphocytoid MCL, 189
  clinical features, 183
  composite MCL, 189
  cyclin D1-negative MCL, 200
  cytologic findings, 191
  differential diagnosis, 200: differentiation from B-lymphoblastic leukemia/lymphoma, 163; from CLL/SLL, 178, 200; from follicular lymphoma, 200, 234; from marginal zone B-cell lymphoma, 200, 247; from other cyclin D1-positive neoplasms, 201; from extranodal marginal zone lymphoma, 263; from T-lymphoblastic leukemia/lymphoma, 461; from blastic plasmacytoid dendritic cell lymphoma, 761; from splenic marginal zone lymphoma, 896
  general features, 183
  histologic findings, 184
  immunophenotypic findings, 195
  indolent variants, 187
    CLL/SLL-like MCL, 187
    in situ mantle cell neoplasia, 187
    marginal zone-like MCL, 187
  in situ, 101
  molecular genetic findings, 197
  treatment and prognosis, 201
Mantle cell lymphoma in situ, 101
Mantle cell lymphoma-like cells of uncertain

significance, 101
Mantle cell neoplasia, 187
Marginal zone hyperplasia, differentiation from marginal zone lymphoma, 246
Marginal zone-like mantle cell lymphoma, 187
Marginal zone lymphoma, extranodal, of mucosa-associated lymphoid tissue, **251**, 689, 700, 896
  associated infections, 251
  clinical features, 251
  cytologic findings, 256
  differential diagnosis, 261: differentiation from reactive lesions, 251; from nodal marginal zone lymphoma, 261; from lymphoplasmacytic lymphoma, 262, 278; from follicular lymphoma, 262; from mantle zone lymphoma, 263; from CLL/SLL, 263; from angioimmunoblastic T-cell lymphoma, 263; from splenic marginal zone lymphoma, 896
  general features, 251
  genetic abnormalities, 261
  histologic findings, 252
  human immunodeficiency virus association, 689
  iatrogenic, 700
  immunophenotypic findings, 256
  molecular genetic findings, 257
  transformation to DLBCL, 263
  treatment and prognosis, 263
Marginal zone lymphoma, nodal, 89, 141, 200, 234, **239**, 261, 480, 781
  clinical features, 239
  cytologic findings, 244
  differential diagnosis, 246: differentiation from mantle cell lymphoma, 200, 247; from follicular lymphoma, 234, 247; from marginal zone hyperplasia, 246; from progressive transformation of germinal centers, 247; from lymphoplasmacytic lymphoma, 248, 278; from angioimmunoblastic T-cell lymphoma, 248; from extranodal marginal zone lymphoma, 261; from peripheral T-cell lymphoma, 480; from mastocytosis, 781
  general features, 239
  Helicobacter pylori association, 141, 239
  histologic findings, 239
  histologic transformation, 89
  immunophenotypic findings, 244
  molecular genetic findings, 246
  treatment and prognosis, 248
Mast cell disease, *see* Mastocytosis
Mast cell hyperplasia, differentiation from mastocytosis, 781

Mast cell leukemia, 767
Mast cell sarcoma, 767
Mast cell syndrome, differentiation from masto-
    cytosis, 781
Mastocytosis, lymph nodes, 763
    classification, 764, 765
    clinical features, 764
    cytologic and cytochemical findings, 779
    cutaneous mastocytosis, 763
        urticaria pigmentosa, 763
    differential diagnosis, 781: differentiation from
        mast cell syndromes, 781; from mast cell hy-
        perplasia, 781; from nodal marginal zone
        lymphoma, 781; from peripheral T-cell lym-
        phoma, 782; from hairy cell leukemia, 782;
        from Langerhans cell histiocytosis, 782; from
        acute myeloid leukemia, 782; from acute baso-
        philic leukemia, 782
    general features, 763
    histologic findings, 767
    immunophenotypic findings, 779
    molecular genetic findings, 780
    systemic mastocytosis, 763
        aggressive systemic mastocytosis, 767
        indolent systemic mastocytosis, 767
        mast cell leukemia, 767
        mast cell sarcoma, 767
        smoldering systemic mastocytosis, 767
        well-differentiated systemic mastocytosis, 767
        with an associated hematologic neoplasm, 767
    treatment and prognosis, 782
Mastocytosis, spleen, 933
Mediastinal germ cell tumors, differentiation from
    nodular sclerosis Hodgkin lymphoma, 624
Melanoma, differentiation from interdigitating
    dendritic cell sarcoma, 840
Mesothelial cyst, spleen, 977
Metastatic melanoma, differentiation from
    histiocytic sarcoma, 822
Metastatic tumors, 1001
    biology of metastases, 1001
    clinical features, 1002
    epithelial- and mesenchymal-related antigens, 1021
    gross findings, 1004
    hematopoietic markers for nonhematopoietic
        tumors, 1011
    histologic findings, 1004
    immunohistochemical analysis, 1008
        pitfalls, 1019
    lymph node versus spleen, 1001
    morphologic differentiation, 1006

anaplastic tumors, 1014
    epithelioid tumors, 1010
    Kaposi sarcoma, 1017
    nasopharyngeal carcinoma, 1019
    small cell tumors, 1007
    spindle cell tumors, 1015
    splenic metastases, 1025
    staging, 1002
Methotrexate and iatrogenic lymphoproliferative
    disorders, 693
Mixed cellularity Hodgkin lymphoma, 634, **637**
    Castleman-like changes, 640
    clinical features, 637
    cytologic findings, 641
    differential diagnosis, 643: differentiation from
        lymphocyte-rich Hodgkin lymphoma, 634,
        643; from chronic granulomatous inflamma-
        tion, 643; from nodular sclerosis Hodgkin lym-
        phoma, 643; from T-cell/histiocyte-rich large
        B-cell lymphoma, 643; from peripheral T-cell
        lymphoma, 643
    general features, 637
    histiocyte-rich variant, 639
    histologic findings, 637
    immunophenotypic findings, 641
    interfollicular variant, 639
    molecular genetic findings, 641
    sinusoidal involvement associated with marginal
        zone B-cell clusters, 640
    treatment and prognosis, 644
Monoclonal asymptomatic lymphocytosis, cyclin
    D1 positive, 106
Monoclonal B-cell lymphocytosis, 103
    CLL-like, 104
    differentiation from CLL/SLL, 178
    with atypical CLL-like immunophenotype, 106
    with mantle cell lymphoma-like immunopheno-
        type, 106
    with non-CLL immunophenotype, 107
Monoclonal immunoglobulin deposition diseases,
    399
    amyloidosis, 399
    crystal-storing histiocytosis, 399
Monoclonal plasma cells of uncertain significance
    in lymph node, differentiation from plasma-
    cytoma, 396
Monocytic sarcoma, *see* Myeloid sarcoma
Multicentric Castleman disease, 680
    human herpesvirus 8 association, *see* Human
        herpesvirus-8-positive multicentric Castleman
        disease

human immunodeficiency virus-positive, 680

Mycosis fungoides, 91, 573, 760

clinical features, 573

cytologic findings, 581

differential diagnosis, 588: differentiation from benign skin diseases, 588; from spongiotic dermatitis, 588; from interface dermatitis, 589; from primary cutaneous gamma/delta T-cell lymphoma, 589; from CD8-positive epidermotropic cytotoxic T-cell lymphoma, 589; from primary cutaneous ALCL, 589; from adult T-cell leukemia/lymphoma, 589; from Hodgkin lymphoma, 589; from angioimmunoblastic T-cell lymphoma, 590; from T-cell prolymphocytic leukemia, 590; from blastic plasmacytoid dendritic cell lymphoma, 760

general features, 573

histologic findings, 575

histologic transformation, 91

immunophenotypic findings, 582

molecular genetic findings, 586

Sezary syndrome, 586

staging systems, 574

treatment and prognosis, 590

Myeloblastoma, *see* Myeloid sarcoma

Myelodysplastic/myeloproliferative neoplasms, spleen, 935

chronic myelomonocytic leukemia (CMML), 937

Myelodysplastic syndromes, spleen, 938

Myeloid/lymphoid neoplasms with *FGFR1* rearrangements, *see* Blastic hematopoietic neoplasms associated with t(8;13)(p11;q12)/*ZMYM2-FGFR1*

Myeloid metaplasia, 929

Myeloid neoplasms involving spleen, 929

Myeloid sarcoma, lymph nodes, 758, 782, **797**

clinical features, 797

cytochemical findings, 807

cytologic findings, 803

differential diagnosis, 809: differentiation from blastic plasmacytoid dendritic cell neoplasm, 758, 810; from mastocytosis, 782; differentiation from DLBCL, 809; from Burkitt sarcoma, 809; from lymphoblastic lymphoma, 809; from anaplastic large cell lymphoma, 810; from histiocytic sarcoma, 810

general features, 797

histologic findings, 799

immunophenotypic findings, 807

molecular genetic findings, 807

treatment and prognosis, 810

Myeloid sarcoma, spleen, 941

Myeloproliferative neoplasms, 929

N

Needle core biopsy, 43

Neoplastic myeloid proliferation, 929

Nijmegen breakage syndrome, 721

NK/T-cell lymphomas, Epstein-Barr virus association, 136

Nodal angiomatosis, 994

Nodal marginal zone lymphoma, *see* Marginal zone lymphoma, nodal

Nodular lymphocyte-predominant Hodgkin lymphoma, 91, 102, 234, 332, 633, 651, 910

clinical features, 652

cytologic findings, 659

differential diagnosis, 670: differentiation from progressive transformation of germinal centers, 670; from follicular lymphoma, 234, 671; from T-cell/histiocyte-rich large B-cell lymphoma, 332, 671; from lymphocyte-rich Hodgkin lymphoma, 633, 671; from primary splenic large B-cell lymphoma, 910

diffuse lymphocyte-predominant Hodgkin lymphoma, 670

DLBCL association, 668

general features, 651

histologic findings, 653

histologic transformation, 91

immunophenotypic findings, 659

in situ, 102

molecular genetic findings, 667

Rosai-Dorfman disease association, 659

treatment and prognosis, 671

variant patterns, 654

Nodular lymphoma, *see* Follicular lymphoma

Nodular paragranuloma, *see* Nodular lymphocyte-predominant Hodgkin lymphoma, 651

Nodular sclerosis Hodgkin lymphoma, 351, 446, **611**, 633, 643, 834

clinical features, 611

cytologic findings, 617

differential diagnosis, 623: differentiation from other types of Hodgkin lymphoma, 623, 633, 643; from primary mediastinal large B-cell lymphoma, 351, 623; from B-cell lymphoma, unclassifiable, 446, 623; from follicular dendritic cell sarcoma, 834; from T-cell/histiocyte-rich large B-cell lymphoma, 623; ALK-positive and -negative anaplastic large cell lymphoma, 623; from peripheral T-cell lymphoma,

623; from mediastinal germ cell tumors, 624
general features, 611
grading, 615
histologic findings, 611
immunohistochemical findings, 620
molecular genetic findings, 621
morphologic variants, 615
relationship to lymphocyte-rich Hodgkin
 lymphoma, 630
treatment and prognosis, 624
Non-Hodgkin lymphomas, 67, 111, 119, *see also
 under individual lymphoma*s
classification, 67, *see also* Classification of
 lymphomas
epidemiology, 119, *see also* Epidemiology of
 lymphomas
histologic downgrading, 92
histologic transformation, 79
prognostic factors, 113, 115
staging, 111

P

Palisaded myofibroblastoma, 987
Peliosis, 996
Peripheral T-cell lymphoma, not otherwise specified, 418, 465, 534, 549, 624, 643, 689, 700, 782
classification, 465
clinical features, 466
cytologic findings, 472
differential diagnosis, 479: differentiation from
 Burkitt lymphoma, 418; from angioimmunoblastic T-cell lymphoma, 479, 497; from
 ALK-negative ALCL, 479, 549; from small
 T-cell lymphomas, 479; from Hodgkin lymphoma, 480, 624, 643; from nodal marginal
 zone lymphoma, 480; from follicular lymphoma, 480; from ALK-positive ALCL, 534;
 from mastocytosis, 782
general features, 465
histologic findings, 466
human immunodeficiency virus association, 689
iatrogenic, 700
immunophenotypic findings, 472
molecular genetic findings, 477
treatment and prognosis, 480
variants, 468
 follicular variant, 469
 lymphoepithelioid variant, 468
 T-zone variant, 468
Plasma cell myeloma, 278, 385, 688
 differentiation from Waldenstrom macroglobu-

linemia, 278; from plasmablastic lymphoma, 385
 human immunodeficiency virus association, 688
Plasma cell myeloma, post-transplantation, 738
Plasma cell neoplasms, 389
Plasmablastic lymphoma, 133, **375**, 398, 688, 741
 autoimmune disease association, 377
 clinical features, 375
 cytologic findings, 378
 differential diagnosis, 385: differentiation from
 plasma cell myeloma, 385; from extramedullary plasmacytoma, 385, 398; from DLBCL,
 385; from ALK-positive large B-cell lymphoma,
 385; from primary effusion lymphoma, 386
 Epstein-Barr virus association, 133, 375
 general features, 375
 histologic findings, 377
 human immunodeficiency virus (HIV) association, 375, 688
 immunophenotypic findings, 378
 molecular genetic findings, 384
 transplantation associated, 377, 741
 treatment and prognosis, 386
Plasmacytic lymphoma, 398, 741
 differentiation from plasmacytoma, 398
 post-transplant, 741
Plasmacytoma, 385, **389**
 clinical features, 390
 cytologic findings, 391
 differential diagnosis, 396: differentiation from
 plasma cell Castleman disease, 396; from
 monoclonal plasma cells of uncertain significance in lymph node, 396; from extranodal
 marginal zone lymphoma, 397; from lymphoplasmacytic lymphoma, 398; from plasmablastic lymphoma, 398
 extramedullary plasmacytoma, 385, 389
 general features, 389
 histologic findings, 391
 immunophenotypic findings, 391
 molecular genetic findings, 394
 nodal plasmacytoma, 390
 solid plasmacytoma of bone, 389
 treatment and prognosis, 398
Polymorphic lymphoproliferative disorders, 684, 697
 acquired immunodeficiency syndrome associated, 684
 iatrogenic, 697
Postchemotherapy histiocyte-rich pseudotumor of
 spleen, 968
Post-transplant lymphoproliferative disorders, 134,
 731

clinical features, 732
cytologic findings, 744
differential diagnosis, 746
Epstein-Barr virus association, 134, 731
general features, 731
histologic findings, 733
  Hodgkin lymphoma, 741
  monomorphic B-cell lesions, 738
  monomorphic T-cell lesions, 743
  nondestructive lesions, 733
  polymorphic lesions, 735
molecular genetic findings, 744
treatment and prognosis, 746
Primary cutaneous follicular lymphoma, 225
Primary cutaneous ALCL, differentiation from
    ALK-positive ALCL, 534; from ALK-negative
    ALCL, 548; from mycosis fungoides, 589
Primary cutaneous DLBCL, leg type, 298
Primary DLBCL of nervous system, 295, 687
Primary effusion lymphoma, 138, 386, 680
  differentiation from plasmablastic lymphoma, 386
  human herpesvirus 8 association, 138
  human immunodeficiency virus association, 680
Primary immunodeficiency disorders, 718
  activated phosphoinositide 3-kinase delta
      syndrome, 724
  ataxia-telangiectasia, 720
  autoimmune lymphoproliferative syndrome, 723
  cartilage hair hypoplasia syndrome, 722
  CD27 deficiency, 725
  common variable immunodeficiency syndrome, 718
  coronin-1A deficiency, 725
  hyper-IgM syndrome, 721
  interleukin-2-inducible T-cell kinase deficiency, 725
  Nijmegen breakage syndrome, 721
  severe combined immunodeficiency, 721
  Wiscott-Aldrich syndrome, 721
  X-linked agammaglobulinemia, 722
  X-linked lymphoproliferative syndrome, 722
Primary mediastinal (thymic) large B-cell lympho-
    ma, 343, 446, 623
  clinical features, 343
  cytologic findings, 344
  differential diagnosis, 351: differentiation from
      DLCBL, 351; from nodular sclerosis Hodgkin
      lymphoma, 351, 623; from thymic tumors,
      351; from mediastinal germ cell tumors, 351;
      from B-cell lymphoma, unclassifiable, 446
  genetic abnormalities, 350
  general features, 343
  histologic findings, 343

immunophenotypic findings, 348
molecular genetic findings, 348
treatment and prognosis, 351
Primary splenic large B-cell lymphoma, 905
  clinical features, 905
  cytologic findings, 907
  differential diagnosis, 908: differentiation from
      systemic DLBCL involving spleen, 908; from
      T-cell/histiocyte-rich large B-cell lymphoma,
      910; from intravascular large B-cell lymphoma,
      910; from nodular lymphocyte predominant
      Hodgkin lymphoma, 910; from classic Hodgkin
      lymphoma, 911; from splenic marginal zone
      lymphoma, 911; from inflammatory pseudo-
      tumor of spleen, 912; from lymphoid hyperplasia
      of spleen, 912; from post-chemotherapy
      histiocyte-rich pseudotumor, 912
  general features, 905
  gross findings, 906
  histologic findings, 906
    macronodular pattern, 906
    micronodular pattern, 907
    predominant red pulp pattern, 907
  immunophenotypic findings, 907
  molecular genetic findings, 908
  treatment and prognosis, 912
Progressive transformation of germinal centers,
    234, 247, 670
  differentiation from follicular lymphoma, 234;
      from marginal zone lymphoma, 247; from
      nodular lymphocyte-predominant Hodgkin
      lymphoma, 670
Pseudocyst, spleen, 978

R

Reed-Sternberg and Hodgkin cells, 593
Richter syndrome, 85
Richter transformation, 85
Rosai-Dorfman disease, 659, 822, 851
  association with nodular lymphocyte-predom-
      inant Hodgkin lymphoma, 659
  differentiation from histiocytic sarcoma, 822;
      from Langerhans cell histiocytosis, 851

S

Sclerosing angiomatoid nodular transformation,
    spleen, 949, 974
  differentiation from splenic hamartoma, 949;
      from splenic stromal tumors, 974
Severe combined immunodeficiency, 721
Sezary syndrome, 586

Single-hit lymphomas, 426
Small noncleaved cell lymphoma, non-Burkitt type, *see* High-grade B-cell lymphoma, not otherwise specified
Smoldering systemic mastocytosis, 767
Solitary spindle cell tumor with myoid differentiation, 987
Specimen processing, 17
  cytogenetic abnormalities, 28
    API2-MALT1, 31
    BCL2 translocations, 29
    BCL6 translocations, 29
    CCND1 translocation, 30
    MYC translocations, 28
    NPM-ALK, 30
  cytogenetic/molecular analysis, **25**, 60
    clonality detection, 33
    conventional karyotyping, 26
    fluorescence in situ hybridization, 26
    high-throughput genetic techniques, 35
      Comparative genomic hybridization, 35
      Gene expression profiling, 36
      MicroRNA analysis, 36
      Mutational anaysis, 38
      Proteomics, 36
    in situ hybridization, 32
    lineage infidelity, 34
    polymerase chain reaction, 31
    southern blot hybridization, 31
  excisional biopsy, 17
  fine-needle aspiration biopsy, 17, 43, **47**
  flow cytometry, 22
  gross evaluation, 17
  histologic stains, 18
  immunophenotypic analysis, **18**, 58
    BCL2, 21
    CD3, 19
    CD5, 20
    CD10, 21
    CD20, 19
    CD30, 21
    cyclin D1, 20
    Ki-67, 22
    PAX5, 19
  needle core biopsy, 43
  pathology report, 38
Spleen, anatomy, 12
Splenic B-cell lymphoma/leukemia, unclassifiable, 899
Splenic cysts, *see* Cysts, spleen
Splenic diffuse red pulp small B-cell lymphoma, 881, 896, 899

  clinical features, 899
  differential diagnosis, 903: differentiation from hairy cell lymphoma variant, 881, 903; from splenic marginal zone lymphoma, 896, 903; from hairy cell leukemia, 903
  general features, 899
  histologic findings, 899
  immunophenotypic findings, 900
  molecular genetic findings, 903
  treatment and prognosis, 903
Splenic hamartoma, *see* Hamartoma, spleen
Splenic hemangioendothelioma, *see* Hemangioendothelioma, spleen
Splenic hemangioma, *see* Hemangioma, spleen
Splenic marginal zone hyperplasia, differentiation from splenic marginal zone lymphoma, 894
Splenic marginal zone lymphoma, 278, 885, 911, 925
  clinical features, 885
  cytologic findings, 891
  differential diagnosis, 894: differentiation from lymphoplasmacytic lymphoma, 278; from splenic marginal zone hyperplasia, 894; from chronic lymphocytic leukemia/small lymphocytic lymphoma, 895; from mantle cell lymphoma, 896; from follicular lymphoma, 896; from Waldenstrom macroglobulinemia, 896; from hairy cell leukemia, 896; from hairy cell leukemia variant, 896; from splenic diffuse red pulp small B-cell lymphoma, 896; from extranodal marginal zone lymphoma, 896; from primary splenic large B-cell lymphoma, 911; from hepatosplenic T-cell lymphoma, 925
  general features, 885
  histologic findings, 886
  immunophenotypic findings, 891
  molecular genetic findings, 892
  transformation to DLBCL, 894
  treatment and prognosis, 896
Stromal tumors and tumor-like lesions, spleen, 967
  clinical features, 967
  differential diagnosis, 974: differentiation from splenic hamartoma, 974; from sclerosing angiomatoid nodular transformation, 974; from IgG4-related disease, 975; from DLBCL, 975
  general features, 967
  histologic findings, 967
  immunophenotypic findings, 972
  inflammatory myofibroblastic tumor, 971
  inflammatory pseudotumor, 968
    postchemotherapy histiocyte-rich pseudotumor of spleen, 968

inflammatory pseudotumor-like follicular dendritic cell tumor, 971

molecular genetic findings, 973

treatment and prognosis, 975

Systemic mastocytosis, 765, *see also* Mastocytosis

aggressive systemic mastocytosis, 767

extracutaneous mastocytosis, 767

indolent systemic mastocytosis, 767

involving bone marrow, 773

involving gastrointestinal tract, 770

involving lymph nodes, 768

mast cell leukemia, 767

mast cell sarcoma, 767

smoldering systemic mastocytosis, 767

well-differentiated systemic mastocytosis, 767

with associated hematologic neoplasm, 767

T

T-acute lymphoblastic leukemia, 449

T cells, normal, 7

T-cell/histiocyte-rich large B-cell lymphoma, **325**, 340, 497, 623, 634, 643, 671, 910

clinical features, 325

cytologic findings, 328

differential diagnosis, 332: differentiation from nodular lymphocyte-predominant Hodgkin lymphoma, 332, 671; from classic Hodgkin lymphoma, 333; from DLBCL, 333; from peripheral T-cell lymphoma, 333; from histiocytic sarcoma, 333; from EBV-positive DLBCL, 340; from angioimmunoblastic T-cell lymphoma, 497; from nodular sclerosis Hodgkin lymphoma, 623; from lymphocyte-rich Hodgkin lymphoma, 634; from mixed cellularity Hodgkin lymphoma, 643; from primary splenic large B-cell lymphoma, 910

general features, 325

histologic findings, 325

immunophenotypic findings, 330

molecular genetic findings, 332

treatment and prognosis, 333

T-cell lymphoblastic lymphoma, differentiation from myeloid sarcoma, 809

T-cell lymphoma of childhood, Epstein-Barr virus association, 136

T-cell prolymphocytic leukemia, 513, 590

differentiation from adult T-cell leukemia/lymphoma, 513; from mycosis fungoides, 590

T-lymphoblastic leukemia/lymphoma, 162, **449**

clinical features, 449

cytologic findings, 453

differential diagnosis, 460: differentiation from B-lymphoblastic leukemia/lymphoma, 162, 460; indolent T-lymphoblastic proliferation, 460; Burkitt lymphoma, 460; DLBCL, 460; mantle zone lymphoma, 461; acute myeloid leukemia, 461; blastic plasmacytoid dendritic cell neoplasm, 461; lymphocyte-rich thymoma, 461

early T-cell acute precursor leukemia, 458

general features, 449

histologic findings, 449

immunophenotypic findings, 453

molecular genetic findings, 455

T-acute lymphoblastic leukemia, 449

T-lymphoblastic lymphoma, 449

treatment and prognosis, 461

T-lymphoblastic lymphoma, 449

T-zone lymphoma, 468

Thymic B-cell lymphoma, *see* Primary mediastinal large B-cell lymphoma

Tingible body macrophages, 7

Transformation of lymphoma, *see* Histologic transformation of lymphoma

Triple-hit lymphomas, 429, 433

U

Undifferentiated lymphoma, non-Burkitt type, *see* High-grade B-cell lymphoma, not otherwise specified

V

Vascular transformation of lymph node sinuses, 994

differentiation from Kaposi sarcoma, 995

Vascular tumors, spleen, 945

angiosarcoma, 959

hamartoma, 945

hemangioendothelioma, 954

hemangioma, 950

Kaposi sarcoma, 958

littoral cell angioma, 953

W

Waldenstrom macroglobulinemia, 89, 248, 262, **267**, 896

association with lymphoplasmacytic lymphoma, 267

Bing-Neel syndrome, 268

clinical features, 267

cytologic findings, 273

differential diagnosis, 278: differentiation from nodal marginal zone lymphoma, 248, 278; from IgM monoclonal gammopathy, 278;

from splenic marginal zone lymphoma, 278, 896; from extranodal marginal zone lymphoma, 262, 278; from plasma cell myeloma, 278; from gamma heavy chain disease, 278; from primary cold agglutinin-associated lymphoproliferative disease, 279
general features, 267
histologic findings, 268
histologic transformation, 89
immunophenotypic findings, 273
molecular genetic findings, 274
Schnitzler syndrome, 267 add

treatment and prognosis, 279
Wegener granulomatosis, differentiation from extranodal NK/T-cell lymphoma, nasal type, 569
Well-differentiated systemic mastocytosis, 767
Wiskott-Aldrich syndrome, 721
World Health Organization classification, lymphomas, *see* classification of lymphomas

X

X-linked agammaglobulinemia, 722
X-linked lymphoproliferative syndrome, 722